# LOWINSON AND RUIZ'S
Substance Abuse

A Comprehensive Textbook

FIFTH EDITION

LOWINSON AND RUIZ'S

Substance Abuse

A Comprehensive Textbook

FIFTH EDITION

EDITORS

Pedro Ruiz, M.D.

Professor and Executive Vice Chair
Department of Psychiatry and Behavioral Sciences
University of Miami Miller School of Medicine
Miami, Florida
President Elect (2008–2011)
World Psychiatric Association
Past President (2006–2007)
American Psychiatric Association

Eric C. Strain, M.D.

Professor
Director, Johns Hopkins Center for Substance Abuse Treatment and Research
Medical Director, Behavioral Pharmacology Research Unit
Johns Hopkins University School of Medicine
Baltimore, Maryland

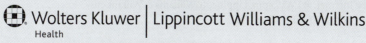

Philadelphia • Baltimore • New York • London
Buenos Aires • Hong Kong • Sydney • Tokyo

Acquisitions Editor: Charles Mitchell
Product Manager: Tom Gibbons
Vendor Manager: Bridgett Dougherty
Senior Manufacturing Manager: Benjamin Rivera
Marketing Manager: Brian Freiland
Design Coordinator: Steve Druding
Production Service: MPS Limited, a Macmillan Company

© 2011 by LIPPINCOTT WILLIAMS & WILKINS, a WOLTERS KLUWER business
Two Commerce Square
2001 Market Street
Philadelphia, PA 19103 USA
LWW.com

All rights reserved. This book is protected by copyright. No part of this book may be reproduced in any form by any means, including photocopying, or utilized by any information storage and retrieval system without written permission from the copyright owner, except for brief quotations embodied in critical articles and reviews. Materials appearing in this book prepared by individuals as part of their official duties as U.S. government employees are not covered by the above-mentioned copyright.

Printed in China

Library of Congress Cataloging-in-Publication Data

Lowinson and Ruiz's substance abuse: a comprehensive textbook.—5th ed./editors, Pedro Ruiz, Eric C. Strain.
   p. ; cm.
Substance abuse
Rev. ed. of: Substance abuse/editors, Joyce H. Lowinson... [et al.]. 4th ed. c2005.
Includes bibliographical references and index.
ISBN-13: 978-1-60547-277-5
ISBN-10: 1-60547-277-8
1. Substance abuse. 2. Substance abuse—Treatment. 3. Substance abuse—Social aspects. I. Ruiz, Pedro, 1936– II. Strain, Eric C. III. Lowinson, Joyce H. IV. Substance abuse. V. Title: Substance abuse.
  [DNLM: 1. Substance-Related Disorders. WM 270]
RC564.S826 2011
362.29—dc22

2010040016

Care has been taken to confirm the accuracy of the information presented and to describe generally accepted practices. However, the authors, editors, and publisher are not responsible for errors or omissions or for any consequences from application of the information in this book and make no warranty, expressed or implied, with respect to the currency, completeness, or accuracy of the contents of the publication. Application of the information in a particular situation remains the professional responsibility of the practitioner.

   The authors, editors, and publisher have exerted every effort to ensure that drug selection and dosage set forth in this text are in accordance with current recommendations and practice at the time of publication. However, in view of ongoing research, changes in government regulations, and the constant flow of information relating to drug therapy and drug reactions, the reader is urged to check the package insert for each drug for any change in indications and dosage and for added warnings and precautions. This is particularly important when the recommended agent is a new or infrequently employed drug.

   Some drugs and medical devices presented in the publication have Food and Drug Administration (FDA) clearance for limited use in restricted research settings. It is the responsibility of the health care provider to ascertain the FDA status of each drug or device planned for use in their clinical practice.

To purchase additional copies of this book, call our customer service department at (800) 638-3030 or fax orders to (301) 223-2320. International customers should call (301) 223-2300.

Visit Lippincott Williams & Wilkins on the Internet: at LWW.com. Lippincott Williams & Wilkins customer service representatives are available from 8:30 am to 6 pm, EST.

10 9 8 7 6 5 4 3 2 1

I wish to dedicate this textbook to Pablo Antonio Holgin, who at two years of age taught me what love, courage and resilience were all about.
—Pedro Ruiz, M.D.

I wish to dedicate this textbook to my family—Grace, Andrew, Kate and Cori—who have provided me with love and support through the years and have helped me to keep perspective on those things that matter most at the end of my day.
—Eric C. Strain, M.D.

We wish to dedicate this textbook to those who suffer from alcohol and drug use, abuse and dependence; they deserve the best possible care that our field can offer them.
—Pedro Ruiz, M.D.
—Eric C. Strain, M.D.

Preface

This fifth edition of *Lowinson and Ruiz's Substance Abuse: A Comprehensive Textbook* symbolizes a major effort by the profession to address the devastating effects of alcohol and drug use, abuse, and dependence. Addictive disorders and the conditions associated with drug use clearly have a direct deleterious impact on a person's physical and mental health, but this impact is also felt in numerous other aspects of life—including relationships with family and friends, spiritual life, work and education, the legal system, and the broader communities in which we all live. One goal of this book is to bring together current, state-of-the-art knowledge of what we know about addictions, so that the interested reader has a single resource that can provide answers to questions about all aspects of addictive disorders.

The target audience for this textbook includes medical students, psychiatric residents and residents from other specialties, addiction fellows, physicians in practice, nurses, social workers, and counselors, and other health and mental health practitioners at large. The goal is to provide all health care professionals with a comprehensive textbook on addictive disorders. The content of this book represent the most up-to-date information related to every possible aspect of addiction, that is, the epidemiology, diagnosis, and treatment of all addictive disorders and conditions. All major drug classes are addressed in this textbook, and chapters include information about both our understanding of how a particular drug affects the brain and body and what is known about the most effective approaches to treat the consequences of the abuse of that drug. In addition, this book addresses public policy–related issues, special populations, and other related addictive conditions. Overall, all aspects of addiction are addressed in this edition, including health, mental health, forensic, legal and correctional, judicial, socioeconomic, ethical, and governmental aspects of drug misuse and abuse.

As was the goal and objective of the previous editions, we wanted to provide practitioners and the public at large with the most authoritative and comprehensive resource on the subject of alcohol and drug use and abuse. We believe this textbook continues to be the definitive text for students at large, as well as for mental health professionals, clinicians, and scientists. The previous editions of this book have also served as an important source of information for primary care professionals and professionals at large in the fields of medicine and law, and we hope this objective continues with this edition.

In preparing this edition, we sought authors with the best current and comprehensive expertise in the topic areas covered by this textbook. A large majority of the senior authors of this edition are new additions. In addition to new authors, we also added new relevant and important topics in this edition. The field of addiction has expanded considerably, and we therefore included these new and relevant topics that needed to be addressed in this edition (e.g., a current perspective on the international epidemiology of drug use; the behavioral aspects of addiction; the use of vaccines as possible treatment agents; contingency management procedures as treatment interventions; new knowledge on medication interactions; and other relevant topics as well). In addition, in recognition that a variety of health care workers currently provide treatment to persons with substance use disorders, new chapters were added for the purpose of specifically addressing professions such as psychology, nursing, social work, and counseling as they participate in the training and treatment of persons with substance use disorders. We hope that these new chapters are useful to the wide variety of health care workers, who devote their professional careers to help persons suffering from addictive disorders and conditions.

Addictive disorders have no geographical boundaries, and thus we hope that this book is of use to persons from all countries of the world. A substantial body of addiction-related research has occurred in the United States, and many large epidemiological studies focusing on addictions have been also conducted in the United States over the last several decades; however, research in addictions is certainly not limited to the United States. In fact, new and effective treatments of addictive disorders occur throughout the world, and there are also a growing number of excellent national and regional epidemiological studies on addictive disorders that are conducted in different regions of the world. We have tried to be mindful of this—while previous editions have tended to focus on the United States, the goal of this new edition (and hopefully in subsequent ones) is to be a valuable resource that reflects the world community—both in authors of chapters and in the content of work presented.

Without question, the addiction field has expanded a great deal since the last edition of this textbook, which was published in 2005. In the United States, the recently approved health care reform might positively affect the delivery of health and mental health care vis-à-vis the population suffering from alcohol and drug abuse in this country. At the same time, the availability of substance abuse treatments in other countries can be hampered by health care financing that fails, at times, to recognize addictions as medical illnesses (or treatments as being effective)—even in systems that provide universal health coverage. The financing of health care—in the United States and in other parts of the world—is an area that continues to evolve, and it will be of great interest to see the balance achieved in the use of health care resources for medical disorders such as substance abuse and dependence.

We are, of course, indebted to the team of distinguished contributors who made this new edition possible; certainly, they have all fully satisfied our expectations. We should also thank Charles Mitchell and Tom Gibbons from Lippincott Williams & Wilkins for their outstanding assistance and support in this new edition. Finally, we deeply thank the readers of this new edition. We hope to meet all of their expectations.

Pedro Ruiz, MD
Eric C. Strain, MD

Foreword

Since its first printing in 1981, *Lowinson and Ruiz's Substance Abuse: A Comprehensive Textbook* has served as a primary source of knowledge and practice advice for clinicians treating substance use disorders. The three updates in 1992, 1997, and 2004 chronicle the extraordinary progress in medical understanding about substance abuse and about better means of treating and managing the addiction-related changes in cognition, emotion, desire, and behavior that remain so troubling to affected individuals, their families, and society as a whole. This fifth edition reflects more advances in basic, clinical, epidemiological, and behavioral research, and the volume is being released at a particularly historic and important time. At this writing, there is a historic confluence of scientific discoveries and policy changes that may lead to much greater progress in preventing, treating, and managing substance use problems.

Continuing Substance Use Problems – As was true when each of the four prior editions of this volume were published, our country continues to experience significant and broadly destructive substance use problems. Many of the traditional drug problems continue but with new features. For example, at this writing, a large contingent of U.S. soldiers is again returning from a foreign war and is suffering from dependence upon opioids. But it is pharmaceutical opioids from diverted pain prescriptions, rather than heroin that is the source of this current, lethal epidemic. In fact, opioid overdose deaths are currently the number two cause of accidental death in the United States—second only to automobile accidents.

Other traditional drugs of abuse continue to plague our national health and safety. Specifically, alcohol use remains the major factor contributing to automobile accidents, and binge drinking is largely responsible for most injuries and accidents, especially among adolescents and young adults. Although rates of cigarette and all other forms of nicotine dependence continue to fall among most adolescents, college-attending girls have shown disturbing increases in cigarette use.

Still another indication of our nation's continuing problems with substance use comes from the 2009 report of the National Highway and Traffic Safety Administration. That report indicated that approximately 16% of drivers who were randomly stopped at various locations throughout our nation and voluntarily drug tested (oral swab) were found to be positive for illicit and/or prescribed drugs (11% was marijuana). That this was a voluntary test, and that the oral testing method was only sensitive for drug ingestion within the past 3 to 4 hours, suggests that these already alarming findings may well be a significant under representation of the true prevalence of "drugged driving."

Changes in U.S. Approach to Substance Use Problems – There have been significant changes in U.S. substance abuse policies expressed within the 2010 National Drug Control Strategy and particularly within the recently enacted healthcare reform legislation. These two new policies bring unprecedented emphasis upon public health–oriented, "demand reduction" efforts including prevention, early intervention, and treatment. The text that follows describes how these new policies set the stage for, and will rely heavily upon the basic information and clinical practice suggestions from this fifth edition of *Lowinson and Ruiz's Substance Abuse: A Comprehensive Textbook*.

The 2010 National Drug Control Strategy – For a long while, it was possible to believe that the U.S. drug problem had been created by a few drug-producing and drug-transit countries, and that significant efforts to disrupt the production, prevent the export, and punish the domestic users of those substances would destroy the market and eliminate U.S. drug problems. This thinking contributed to the decades-long U.S. strategy of waging a "war on drugs." That strategy did have some positive results on the production and export of several drugs such as cocaine and heroin, but that approach ignored a fundamental part of any market economy—the United States has long been the world's largest market for substances of abuse and that market has continued to expand and differentiate; there is a new or re-emergent drug problem almost every year. As would be expected in any market where foreign suppliers are seen to be meeting, and profiting from internal demand, domestic suppliers within the United States have risen to meet that demand. Indeed, five of the major drug problems now affecting the United States are "Made in the USA" (e.g., tobacco, alcohol, marijuana, methamphetamine, and prescription medications). Moreover, because of several foreign countries' efforts to meet U.S. demand for drugs, the resulting increase in local availability of these drugs appears to have promoted unprecedented levels of local addiction in those countries. Ironically, it is likely that U.S. demand for drugs may be in part responsible for both increased development and export of drugs from foreign countries, as well as significant drug-related health and social problems within those countries. For these reasons, there has been increased interest among countries (particularly in this hemisphere) for technical assistance in developing local drug demand reduction efforts (prevention, intervention, treatment, drug courts, community organization) to deal with the social consequences of illegal drugs. Thus, it will be increasingly important to implement national and international demand reduction efforts—as well as ongoing supply reduction efforts—if we are to reduce the scope and devastation of drug problems in our country and the rest of the world.

Importantly, and abundantly documented in the present volume, scientific research has now produced potent, practical interventions, therapies, and medications that can play an important role in reducing demand for substances. The United States thus has a unique opportunity to promote demand reduction initiatives at home and to assist key partners in addressing their domestic drug problems. Promoting effective internal and international demand reduction programs will help all partnering countries to control their internal demand for drugs and should thereby help reduce drug production and trafficking around the world.

Healthcare Reform: The American Care Accountability Act – The second change in national policy that will significantly increase emphasis upon substance use demand reduction efforts is the recent passing of healthcare reform through the American Care Accountability Act. This historic legislation will expand and integrate treatments for substance use disorders into mainstream healthcare as never before, as part of an overall effort to improve general healthcare quality, efficiency, and effectiveness. Specialty care providers will of course continue to be necessary—likely more necessary than ever—to treat severe and complicated forms of addiction. But this legislation creates a national requirement for primary care providers to learn and practice screening and brief interventions with emerging cases of "harmful" or "hazardous" substance use, and also to become facile with office-based monitoring, managing, and medicating mild-to-moderate cases of substance "abuse" and "dependence."

Historical Significance – Like many other illnesses, substance use disorders can be arrayed on a continuum of severity and prevalence. This continuum ranges from "harmful or hazardous use," which affects more than 50 million adults, through the most serious forms of "abuse or dependence" (i.e., addiction), which affect about 24 million adults. But only "addiction" has been eligible for treatment and then almost exclusively in specialty "addiction treatment programs." Importantly, very few of these specialty care programs are affiliated with any other part of healthcare. Currently, fewer than 20% of the approximately 13,000 addiction treatment programs are affiliated with a larger healthcare system; less than half of the programs have a part-time physician; only a third have a nurse; even fewer have access to an electronic healthcare record.

Because care for substance use disorders has been divorced from care for all other illnesses, few physicians, nurses, pharmacists, or psychologists have received training or clinical experience in the treatment of substance use disorders. If they do, that experience is typically in an emergency room with the most severely and chronically affected patients in a clinical crisis. It is safe to say that this clinical presentation rarely evokes a strong desire to pursue a career in addiction medicine among young physicians, nurses, pharmacists, or other healthcare professionals.

A second effect of this segregation has been to reduce willingness to enter treatment among affected patients—especially those with less severe or emerging forms of the illness. In fact, only about one tenth of those who meet diagnostic criteria for "addiction" enter treatment each year, and the great majority of these cases are stipulated to attend treatment by an employer, spouse, or particularly some part of the criminal justice system. Because of the severe, multiple, and complex nature of the problems presented in this subgroup of patients, 6- to 12-month outcomes from treatment in these specialty care settings typically show at least 50% have experienced serious relapses.

For these reasons public perception—but also medical perception—of the potential benefit from medical treatments of "substance use disorders" is unnecessarily negative. This type of perception would be—and has been—true for any illness where treatment was available only to the most severely, chronically affected cases, was offered exclusively by provider organizations outside the rest of mainstream healthcare and relied upon methods (e.g., group counseling, therapeutic communities, and court-ordered care) that have rarely been trained or practiced by the rest of healthcare.

Consider, for example, that diseases such as tuberculosis, AIDS, depression, and cancer were also treated almost exclusively in specialty care settings. Because the available treatments were often intrusive, invasive, and had a poor reputation for effectiveness, few patients were interested in early detection. Consequently, these specialty care facilities generally treated the most severely and chronically affected, and these areas of healthcare had trouble in attracting young professionals. In all these cases an important part of improving the quality of care for the full spectrum of those disorders was the creation of care options—"first-line treatments"— for the less severely affected cases that could be practically and effectively applied by primary care providers.

Again, as documented in this volume, scientific research has now produced potent, practical first-line interventions, therapies, and medications that can be used by primary care providers to treat many substance use disorders. These first-line treatments are likely to be important in three ways. First, the availability of these treatments should increase physicians' willingness to screen and identify emerging cases. Few physicians want to identify conditions they are not able to address. Second, the privacy and convenience of primary care, coupled with the availability of many choices in treatment options, should increase those willing to seek treatment earlier, before the illness and its complications become chronic. Third, first-line treatments that may not work well for the most severely and chronically affected may show effectiveness with those whose condition is identified early. Even those who are not adequately treated with first-line treatments often come to accept the need for a more intensive specialty care while there is still time for the condition to be arrested and managed. In turn, experiences like these should increase the perceived effectiveness of available treatments in the eyes of care providers, insurers, pharmaceutical firms, and the public at large—and could bring new patients, new care providers, more research, teaching and training in schools, and more investment into treatment quality.

Implications for the Treatment of Substance Use Disorders – As illustrated in this brief discussion there is a clear need for primary care involvement and, in turn, first-line treatments that can be attractive to patients, practically applied by physicians and reimbursed by insurers. Research over the past 10 years has provided effective screening and brief interventions for emerging substance use problems, and a number of FDA-approved medications for the first-line treatment of mild-to-moderate addictions within an office-based setting. Because of these scientific developments and because healthcare reform legislation now demands it, primary care providers will soon begin to learn to recognize and provide appropriate treatments for the full range of "substance use disorders."

Of course, there are important hurdles that remain. Most practicing primary care physicians, nurses, and pharmacists will have to become educated and trained, as most did not receive adequate education in their schools or residency programs. Existing providers will require support and technical assistance from the relatively small number of primary care providers who are experienced in substance abuse treatment.

Traditional specialty treatment programs will also have to change their practices. Many will find new lines of business from medical referrals. Medically referred patients are likely to have a different constellation of health and social problems than those now referred from the legal system. Those patients and their referring physicians will likely demand new types of services and different types of information exchange; most primary care physicians will expect regular reports of progress and the assurance of referral back to them for continuing care and management. Thus, traditional specialty care treatment programs will likely have to learn a new language and a new working format and culture—but those who develop these new skills are likely to see a new line of clinical business.

Pharmaceutical firms may have to assist primary and specialty care providers in using addiction treatment medications. Early successful experiences may prompt a market for more and even better medications to assist these providers in managing previously undiagnosed substance use disorders—often in their existing patients. Electronic health record providers will have to work out the complicated issues surrounding the collection and exchange of information on patient alcohol and other drug use in a way that maintains patient privacy but enhances patient safety.

Conclusion – These broad and important implications from the suggested integration of care for "substance use disorders" into primary care set a historic context for the publication of the fifth edition of *Lowinson and Ruiz's Substance Abuse: A Comprehensive Textbook*. The work presented in this edition is likely to be particularly relevant to the training and basic knowledge needs of both primary and specialty care providers as they face the challenges of integrating treatment for "substance use disorders" into mainstream healthcare in the coming years.

A. Thomas McLellan, PhD
The White House Office of National Drug Control Policy
Washington, DC

Contributors

Evaristo Akerele, M.D., M.P.H., D.F.A.P.A.
Co-Director, Addiction Psychiatry Fellowship Program
Associate Professor of Psychiatry
Mount Sinai School of Medicine
New York, New York
Associate Clinical Professor of Psychiatry
New York State Psychiatric Institute
Columbia University
Vice President, Medical Director
Phoenix House
New York, New York

Britta L. Anderson, M.A.
Ph.D. Candidate in Psychology
American University
Washington, D.C.

Robert M. Anthenelli, M.D.
Professor of Psychiatry, Psychology, and Neuroscience
Substance Dependence Program
University of Cincinnati College of Medicine
Cincinnati Veterans Affairs Medical Center
Cincinnati, Ohio

Francisco (Sebastian) P. Bacatan, Jr., Ph.D.
Special Assistant to the President
Daytop Village, Inc.
New York, New York
Associate Pastor
Church of Saint Pius X
Scarsdale, New York

Sudie E. Back, Ph.D.
Associate Professor of Psychiatry
Medical University of South Carolina
Charleston, South Carolina

David A. Baron, M.S.Ed., D.O.
Professor of Psychiatry
Keck School of Medicine, University of Southern California
Los Angeles, California

Mark J. Biscone

Gilbert J. Botvin, Ph.D.
Professor of Public Health and Professor of Psychiatry
Weill Cornell Medical College
Cornell University
New York, New York

J. Wesley Boyd, M.D., Ph.D.
Assistant Clinical Professor of Psychiatry
Harvard Medical School
Staff Psychiatrist
Cambridge Health Alliance
Boston, Massachusetts

Kathleen T. Brady, M.D., Ph.D.
Professor of Psychiatry
Medical University of South Carolina
Ralph H. Johnson VA Medical Center
Charleston, South Carolina

Harry A. Brandt, M.D.
Clinical Associate Professor of Psychiatry
University of Maryland School of Medicine
Baltimore, Maryland
Director, Center for Eating Disorders
Sheppard Pratt Health System
Towson, Maryland

Robert M. Bray, Ph.D.
Senior Program Director
Behavioral Health Criminal Justice Division
RTI International
Research Triangle Park, North Carolina

Gregory S. Brigham, Ph.D.
Research Scientist in Psychiatry
University of Cincinnati
Cincinnati, Ohio
Chief Research Officer
Research Institute, Maryhaven
Columbus, Ohio

Adriaan W. Bruijnzeel, Ph.D.
Assistant Professor of Psychiatry
University of Florida College of Medicine
McKnight Brain Institute
Gainesville, Florida

Alan J. Budney, Ph.D.
Professor of Psychiatry and Behavioral Sciences
University of Arkansas for Medical Sciences
Little Rock, Arkansas

Robert Paul Cabaj, M.D.
Associate Clinical Professor of Psychiatry
University of California, San Francisco
San Francisco, California

John S. Cacciola, M.D.
Senior Scientist
Treatment Research Institute (TRI)
Adjunct Associate Professor of Psychiatry
University of Pennsylvania School of Medicine
Philadelphia, Pennsylvania

L. Brett Caram

Kathleen M. Carroll, Ph.D.
Professor of Psychiatry
Yale University School of Medicine
New Haven, Connecticut
MIRECC, Department of Psychiatry
VA Connecticut Healthcare System
West Haven, Connecticut

Joseph Cerimele, M.D.
Resident Physician
Department of Psychiatry
Mount Sinai School of Medicine
New York, New York

Domenic A. Ciraulo, M.D.
Professor and Chairman of Psychiatry
Boston University School of Medicine
Psychiatrist-in-Chief
Boston Medical Center
Boston, Massachusetts

Christopher J. Combs, Ph.D.
Assistant Professor of Psychiatry
Temple University School of Medicine
Psychologist
Temple University Hospital
Philadelphia, Pennsylvania

Wilson M. Compton, M.D., M.P.E.
Director, Division of Epidemiology, Services and Prevention Research
National Institute on Drug Abuse, National Institutes of Health
Bethesda, Maryland

Steven F. Crawford, M.D.
Clinical Associate Professor of Psychiatry
University of Maryland School of Medicine
Baltimore, Maryland
Associate Director, Center
 for Eating Disorders
Sheppard Pratt Health Systems
Towson, Maryland

Cai-Lian Cui, M.D.
Professor of Neurobiology
Neuroscience Research Institute
Peking University
Beijing, China

Kathryn Ann Cunningham, Ph.D.
Chauncey Leake Distinguished Professor
 of Pharmacology
Interim Chair of Pharmacology and
 Toxicology
Director, UTMB Center for Addiction
 Research
University of Texas Medical Branch
Galveston, Texas

Dennis C. Daley, Ph.D.
Professor of Psychiatry
Chief, Addiction Medicine Services
Western Psychiatric Institute and Clinic
Pittsburgh, Pennsylvania

Anthony DeFulio, Ph.D.
Instructor in Psychiatry and Behavioral
 Sciences
Johns Hopkins University School of
 Medicine
Baltimore, Maryland

Michael L. Dennis, Ph.D.
Senior Research Psychologist
Director, GAIN Coordinating Center
Chestnut Health Systems
Normal, Illinois

Sylvia J. Dennison, M.D.
Consulting Psychiatrist
Department of Medicine
Aspirus Hospital
Wausau, Wisconsin

Helen Dermatis, Ph.D.
Research Associate Professor of Psychiatry
New York University School of Medicine
New York, New York

Elise Eva DeVito, B.A.
Postgraduate Associate in Psychiatry
Yale University
New Haven, Connecticut

Stephen L. Dewey, Ph.D.
Senior Scientist
Brookhaven National Laboratory
Upton, New York

Daniel Lee Dickerson, D.O., M.P.H.
Assistant Research Psychiatrist
Integrated Substance Abuse Programs
University of California, Los Angeles
Addiction Psychiatrist, Seven Generations
United American Indian Involvement, Inc.
Los Angeles, California

Carlo C. DiClemente, Ph.D.
Professor of Psychology
University of Maryland, Baltimore County
Baltimore, Maryland

Antoine Douaihy, M.D.
Associate Professor of Psychiatry
University of Pittsburgh Medical Center
Medical Director, Addiction Medicine
 Services
Western Psychiatric Institute and Clinic
Pittsburgh, Pennsylvania

Karen Drexler, M.D.
Associate Professor of Psychiatry and
 Behavioral Sciences
Emory University School of Medicine
Atlanta, Georgia
Director, Substance Abuse Treatment
 Program
Atlanta Veterans Affairs Medical Center
Decatur, Georgia

Ernest Drucker, Ph.D.
Professor Emeritus of Family and Social
 Medicine
Montefiore Medical Center/Albert Einstein
 College of Medicine
Adjunct Professor of Epidemiology
Mailman School of Public Health
Columbia University
Scholar in Residence and Senior Research
 Associate
John Jay College of Criminal Justice
City University of New York.
New York, New York

Thomas M. Dunn, Ph.D.
Associate Professor of Psychological
 Sciences
University of Northern Colorado
Greeley, Colorado
Psychologist, Behavioral Health Service
Denver Health Medical Center
Denver, Colorado

Robert L. DuPont, M.D.
Clinical Professor of Psychiatry
Georgetown University
Washington, D.C.

Nady el-Guabaly, M.D.
Professor of Psychiatry and Head,
 Addiction Division
University of Calgary
Consultant, Foothills Addiction Centre
Calgary, Canada

Paul F. Engelhart, M.S., M.A.
Chief Operating Officer
Catholic Charities---Diocese of Rockville
 Centre
Hicksville, New York

David H. Epstein, Ph.D.
Associate Scientist, Treatment Section
National Institute on Drug Abuse
Baltimore, Maryland

Anita S. Everett, M.D.
Assistant Professor of Psychiatry
Johns Hopkins University
Division Director, Community Psychiatry
Johns Hopkins Bayview
Baltimore, Maryland

Jeffrey J. Everly, Ph.D.
Psychiatry and Behavioral Sciences
Johns Hopkins University School of
 Medicine
Baltimore, Maryland

**William Fals-Stewart, Ph.D.
(deceased)**
University of Rochester
School of Nursing
Rochester, New York

Stephanie A. Fearer, Ph.D.
Research Associate III in Psychiatry
College of Medicine
University of Arkansas for Medical
 Sciences
Little Rock, Arkansas

Jacqueline Maus Feldman, M.D.
Patrick H. Linton Professor of Psychiatry
Director, Division of Public Psychiatry
University of Alabama at Birmingham
Birmingham, Alabama

Francisco Fernandez, M.D.
Professor and Chairperson, Department
 of Psychiatry and Neurosciences
University of South Florida College of
 Medicine
Tampa, Florida

Bennet W. Fletcher, Ph.D.
Senior Research Psychologist, Services
 Research Branch
National Institute on Drug Abuse
Bethesda, Maryland

Paul J. Fudala, Ph.D.
Affiliate Associate Professor of
 Epidemiology and Community Health
Virginia Commonwealth University
Director, Clinical and Scientific Affairs
Reckitt Benckiser Pharmaceuticals Inc.
Richmond, Virginia

Marc Galanter, M.D.
Professor of Psychiatry
New York University School of Medicine
Director, Division of Alcoholism and
 Drug Abuse
New York University Medical Center
New York, New York

Stuart Gitlow, M.D., M.P.H., M.B.A.
Associate Clinical Professor of Psychiatry
Executive Director, Annenberg Physician
 Training Program in Addictive Disease
Mount Sinai School of Medicine
New York, New York

Harold W. Goforth, M.D.
Assistant Professor of Medicine and
 Psychiatry
Duke University Medical Center
Attending Physician
Duke University Medical Center and
 Durham VA Medical Center
Durham, North Carolina

Mark S. Gold, M.D.
Donald R. Dizney Eminent Scholar,
 Distinguished Professor and Psychiatry
 Chairman
University of Florida College of Medicine
McKnight Brain Institute
Gainesville, Florida

Michael S. Gordon, D.P.A.
Research Scientist
Friends Research Institute
Baltimore, Maryland

Marc N. Gourevitch, M.D., Ph.D.
Director, Division of General Internal
 Medicine
Dr. Adolph and Margaret Berger Professor
 of Medicine
New York University School of Medicine
New York, New York

Shelley F. Greenfield, M.D., M.P.H.
Associate Professor of Psychiatry
Harvard Medical School
Boston, Massachusetts
Chief Academic Officer
Associate Clinical Director, Division of
 Alcohol and Drug Abuse
McLean Hospital
Belmont, Massachusetts

Kenneth W. Griffin, Ph.D., M.P.H.
Professor of Public Health
Weill Cornell Medical College
Cornell University
New York, New York

Roland R. Griffiths, Ph.D.
Professor of Psychiatry and Behavioral
 Sciences
Johns Hopkins University School of
 Medicine
Baltimore, Maryland

Carolina L. Haass-Koffler, Pharm.D.
Transitional Research Medications
 Development
Ernest Gallo Clinic and Research Center
University of California, San Francisco
San Francisco, California

Katherine A. Halmi, M.D.
Professor of Psychiatry
DeWitt Wallace Senior Scholar
Weill Cornell Medical College
New York, New York

Ji-Sheng Han, M.D.
Professor
Neuroscience Research Institute
Peking University Health Science Center
Beijing, China

Emily L.R. Harrison, Ph.D.
Postdoctoral Fellow in Psychiatry
Yale University School of Medicine
New Haven, Connecticut

Jaimee L. Heffner, Ph.D.
Research Assistant Professor of Psychiatry
 and Behavioral Neuroscience
University of Cincinnati College of
 Medicine
Cincinnati, Ohio

Sarah H. Heil, Ph.D.
Research Assistant Professor of Psychiatry
 and Psychology
University of Vermont
Burlington, Vermont

Carlos A. Hernandez-Avila, M.D., Ph.D.
Assistant Professor of Psychiatry
University of Connecticut School of
 Medicine
Farmington, Connecticut

Jessica Herrera, M.D.
Post-graduate in Psychiatry
Howard University Hospital
Washington, D.C.

Stephen T. Higgins, Ph.D.
Professor of Psychiatry and Psychology
Vice Chair of Research
University of Vermont
Burlington, Vermont

Kevin P. Hill, M.D., M.H.S.
Instructor in Psychiatry
Harvard Medical School
Psychiatrist-in-Charge, Division of Alcohol
 and Drug Abuse
McLean Hospital
Boston, Massachusetts

A. Tom Horvath, Ph.D.
Instructor in Psychology
Alliant International University
San Diego, California
President, Practical Recovery
La Jolla, California
President, SMART Recovery
Mentor, Ohio

Matthew O. Howard, Ph.D.
Frank A. Daniels Distinguished Professor
School of Social Work
University of North Carolina at Chapel Hill
Chapel Hill, North Carolina

Yujiang Jia, M.D., Dr.PH.
Chief Epidemiologist
HIV/AIDS, Hepatitis, STD, and TB
 Administration
Department of Health
Washington, D.C.

Per Johansson

Christopher W. Johnson, B.A.
Research Associate in Psychiatry
University of Massachusetts Medical
 School
Worcester, Massachusetts

Rolley E. Johnson, Pharm.D.
Adjunct Professor of Psychiatry and
 Behavioral Sciences
Johns Hopkins University School of
 Medicine
Baltimore, Maryland

Hendrée E. Jones, Ph.D.
Professor of Psychiatry
Johns Hopkins University
Baltimore, Maryland

Laura M. Juliano, Ph.D.
Associate Professor of Psychology
American University
Washington, D.C.

David Kalman, Ph.D.
Associate Professor of Psychiatry
University of Massachusetts
Worcester, Massachusetts
Health Research Scientist, Research Service
Edith Nourse Rogers Memorial VA Medical Center
Bedford, Massachusetts

Karol Kaltenbach, Ph.D.
Clinical Associate Professor of Pediatrics
Jefferson Medical College
Director, Maternal Addiction Treatment, Education and Research
Thomas Jefferson University
Philadelphia, Pennsylvania

Timothy W. Kinlock, Ph.D.
Senior Research Scientist
Friends Research Institute
Adjunct Professor of Criminology, Criminal Justice, and Forensic Studies
University of Baltimore
Baltimore, Maryland

Berma M. Kinsey, Ph.D.
Assistant Professor of Medicine
Baylor College of Medicine
Houston, Texas

Herbert D. Kleber, M.D.
Professor of Psychiatry
Columbia University College of Physicians and Surgeons
Director, Division on Substance Abuse
New York State Psychiatric Institute
Attending
New York Presbyterian Hospital
New York, New York

Clifford M. Knapp, Ph.D.
Associate Professor of Psychiatry
Boston University School of Medicine
Boston, Massachusetts

John R. Knight, M.D.
Associate Professor of Pediatrics
Harvard Medical School
Senior Associate
Children's Hospital Boston
Boston, Massachusetts

Thomas Kosten, M.D.
J.H. Waggoner Professor of Psychiatry
Baylor College of Medicine
Director, SUD-QUERI (Quality Evaluation Research Initiative)
Michael DeBakey VA Medical Center
Houston, Texas

Henry R. Kranzler, M.D.
Professor of Psychiatry
University of Connecticut Health Center
Farmington, Connecticut

Colleen T. LaBelle, R.N., C.A.R.N.
Program Director
Office-Based Opioid Treatment Program
Clinical Addiction Research and Education Unit (CARE)
Boston University Medical Center
Boston, Massachusetts

Wendy K. K. Lam

Katie M. Lawson, M.A.
Program Coordinator of Psychiatry and Behavioral Sciences
Medical University of South Carolina
Charleston, South Carolina

Robert G. Lawson

William B. Lawson, M.D., Ph.D., D.F.A.P.A.
Professor and Chairman of Psychiatry and Behavioral Sciences
Howard University Hospital
Washington, D.C.

Joshua D. Lee, M.D., M.Sc.
Assistant Professor of Medicine
New York University School of Medicine
Bellevue Hospital Center
New York, New York

Jack Levinson, Ph.D.
Assistant Professor of Sociology
City College of New York
New York, New York

Show W. Lin, M.D.
Associate Clinical Professor of Psychiatry
University of Cincinnati College of Medicine
Cincinnati, Ohio

Mercedes Lovrecic
Institute of Public Health of the Republic of Slovenia
Ljubjiana, Slovenia

(The Honorable) Bertha K. Madras, B.Sc., Ph.D.
Professor, NEPRC
Harvard Medical School
Southborough, Massachusetts
Research Associate
Massachusetts General Hospital
Boston, Massachusetts

Jorge L. Maldonado, M.D.
Clinical Assistant Professor of Psychiatry
University of Texas Health Science Center at San Antonio
St. Luke's Baptist Hospital
Christus Santa Rosa Hospital
San Antonio, Texas

Kasia Malinowska-Sempruch
Director, Global Drugs Policy Program
Open Society Institute
Warsaw, Poland

Icro Maremmani, M.D.
Professor of Addiction Medicine
University of Pisa
Chief, Vincent P. Dole Dual Diagnosis Unit
Santa Chiara University Hospital
Pisa, Italy

G. Alan Marlatt, Ph.D.
Professor of Psychology
University of Washington
Seattle, Washington

David C. Marsh, M.D., C.C.S.A.M.
Associate Dean, Community Engagement and Clinical Professor
Northern Ontario School of Medicine
Sudbury, Canada

Elinore McCance-Katz, M.D., Ph.D.
Professor of Psychiatry
University of California, San Francisco
Director, Addiction Medicine Research
San Francisco General Hospital
San Francisco, California

Una D. McCann, M.D.
Professor of Psychiatry and Behavioral Sciences
Director, Anxiety Disorders Program
Johns Hopkins School of Medicine
Baltimore, Maryland

Jennifer McNeely, M.D., M.S.
Assistant Professor
NYU School of Medicine
Department of Medicine, Division of General Internal Medicine
New York, New York

Gerard M. Meenan, M.S.
Laboratory Manager, Clinical and Forensic Toxicology
Ammon Analytical Laboratory
Linden, New Jersey

Contributors **xvii**

Robert Milin, M.D., F.R.C.P.C.
Associate Professor of Psychiatry
University of Ottawa
Director, Adolescent Day Treatment Unit,
  Youth Psychiatry Program
Royal Ottawa Mental Health Centre
Ottawa, Ontario, Canada

Karen A. Miotto, M.D.
Clinical Professor of Psychiatry and
  Behavioral Sciences
David Geffen School of Medicine at UCLA
Director, Addiction Medicine Service
Semel Institute of Neuroscience and
  Human Behavior
Los Angeles, California

Lisa A. Mistler, M.D., M.S.
Assistant Professor of Psychiatry
University of Massachusetts Medical
  School
Worcester, Massachusetts

Rudolf H. Moos, Ph.D.
Professor of Psychiatry and Behavioral
  Sciences
Stanford University
Senior Research Career Scientist
Department of Veterans Affairs Health
  Care System
Palo Alto, California

**Betty D. Morgan, Ph.D.,
  P.M.H.C.N.S., B.C.**
Associate Professor of Nursing
University of Massachusetts, Lowell
Lowell, Massachusetts

David F. Musto, M.A., M.D. (deceased)
Professor of Child Psychiatry
  and History of Medicine
Yale University
New Haven, Connecticut

Ethan Nadelmann, J.D., Ph.D.
Executive Director
Drug Policy Alliance
New York, New York

Niru S. Nahar, M.D., M.P.H.
Assistant Clinical Professor of Psychiatry
Columbia University
Attending Outpatient Psychiatrist
Harlem Hospital Center
New York, New York

Robert G. Newman, M.D., M.P.H.
Director, Baron Edmond de Rothschild
  Chemical Dependency Institute
Beth Israel Medical Center
Professor, Departments of Epidemiology
  and Population Health, and Psychiatry
  and Behavioral Sciences
Albert Einstein College of Medicine
New York, New York

Thomas Anh Nguyen, M.D.
Assistant Professor of Clinical Psychiatry
University of Cincinnati College of
  Medicine
Cincinnati, Ohio

Benjamin R. Nordstrom, M.A., M.D.
Ph.D. Candidate in Criminology
University of Pennsylvania
Medical Director, Addiction Treatment
  Services
Penn Presbyterian Medical Center
Philadelphia, Pennsylvania

William B. O'Brien
President
Daytop Village, Inc.
New York, New York

Frank M. Orson, M.D.
Associate Professor of Medicine
Baylor College of Medicine
Chief, Allergy/Immunology
Veterans Affairs Medical Center
Houston, Texas

Eugene Oscapella, B.A., L.L.B., L.L.M.
Barrister and Solicitor
Department of Criminology
University of Ottawa
Canadian Foundation for Drug Policy
Ottawa, Canada

Matteo Pacini
G. De Lisio Institute of Behavioral Sciences
Pisa, Italy

Richard Paczynski, M.D.
Fellow in Psychiatry
University of Florida College of Medicine
McKnight Brain Institute
Gainesville, Florida

Pier Paolo Pani, M.D.
Chief, Social-Health Direction
Health District 8 (ASL 8), Cagliari
Cagliari, Italy

Robert N. Pechnick, Ph.D.
Professor of Psychiatry
David Geffen School of Medicine at University of California, Los Angeles
Associate Director of Research in Psychiatry and Behavioral Neurosciences
Cedars-Sinai Medical Center
Los Angeles, California

Michael R. Pemberton, Ph.D.
Research Psychologist
Behavioral Health and Criminal Justice
RTI International
Research Triangle Park, North Carolina

Ismene L. Petrakis, M.D.
Professor of Psychiatry
Yale University School of Medicine
New Haven, Connecticutt

Karran A. Phillips, M.D., M. Sc.
Staff Clinician
National Institute on Drug Abuse,
  Intramural Research Program
National Institutes of Health
Baltimore, Maryland

Edmond H. Pi, M.D.
Professor of Clinical Psychiatry
University of Southern California Keck
  School of Medicine
Associate Chair for Clinical Affairs
Director of Psychiatric Consultation-
  Liaison Service
Los Angeles County and University of
  Southern California Medical Center
Los Angeles, California

J. Gabriel Piedrahita, M.A., M.S.W.
Consultant
Daytop Village, Inc.
New York, New York

R. Christopher Pierce, Ph.D.
Associate Professor of Psychiatry
University of Pennsylvania School of
  Medicine
Philadelphia, Pennsylvania

Russell K. Portenoy, M.D.
Professor of Neurology and Anesthesiology
Albert Einstein College of Medicine
Chairman and Gerald J. Friedman Chair in
  Pain Medicine and Palliative Care
Beth Israel Medical Center
New York, New York

Marc N. Potenza, M.D., Ph.D.
Associate Professor of Psychiatry and
  Child Study
Yale University School of Medicine
New Haven, Connecticut

Kenzie L. Preston, Ph.D.
Chief, Clinical Pharmacology and
 Therapeutics Research Branch
National Institute on Drug Abuse
 Intramural Research Program
Baltimore, Maryland

Richard N. Rosenthal, M.D.
Professor of Clinical Psychiatry
Columbia University
Chairman, Department of Psychiatry and
 Behavioral Health
St. Luke's Roosevelt Hospital Center
New York, New York

Pedro Ruiz, M.D.
Professor and Executive Vice Chair
Department of Psychiatry and Behavioral
 Sciences
University of Miami Miller School of
 Medicine
Miami, Florida
President Elect (2008-2011)
World Psychiatric Association
Past President (2006-2007)
American Psychiatric Association

Virginia A. Sadock, M.D.
Clinical Professor of Psychiatry
New York University School of Medicine
Director, Program in Human Sexuality
New York University-Langione Medical
 Center
New York, New York

Ihsan M. Salloun, M.D., M.P.H.
Professor of Psychiatry
Chief, Division of Alcohol and Drug
 Abuse: Treatment and Research
University of Miami Miller School of
 Medicine
Miami, Florida

Andrew J. Saxon, M.D.
Professor of Psychiatry and Behavioral
 Sciences
University of Washington
Seattle, Washington

Wynne K. Schiffer, Ph.D.
Associate Scientist, Medical Department
Brookhaven National Laboratory
Upton, New York

Heath D. Schmidt

Joy M. Schmitz, Ph.D.
Professor of Psychiatry
University of Texas Medical School
Houston, Texas

Grant Schroeder

Robert P. Schwartz, M.D.
Medical Director, Social Research Center
Friends Research Institute
Senior Fellow, Drug Addiction Treatment
 Program
Open Society Institute
Baltimore, Maryland

Charles W. Sharp, M.D. (Retired)
Division of Basic Neuroscience and Behavioral Research
National Institute on Drug Abuse
National Institutes of Health
Rockville, Maryland

Steven Shoptaw, Ph.D.
Professor and Vice Chair for Academic
 Afffairs
Department of Family Medicine
David Geffen School of Medicine at UCLA
Los Angeles, California

Stacey C. Sigmon, Ph.D.
Associate Professor of Psychiatry
University of Vermont
Burlington, Vermont

Kenneth Silverman, Ph.D.
Professor of Psychiatry and Behavioral
 Sciences
Johns Hopkins University School of
 Medicine
Baltimore, Maryland

Natasha Slesnick, Ph.D.
Associate Professor of Human
 Development and Family Science
Ohio State University
Columbus, Ohio

LaVerne Hanes Stevens, Ph.D.
GAIN Clinical Training and Product
 Developer
GAIN Coordinating Center
Chestnut Health Systems
Normal, Illinois

Angela L. Stotts, Ph.D.
Associate Professor and Director of
 Research of Family and Community
 Medicine
University of Texas Medical School at
 Houston
Houston, Texas

Eric C. Strain, M.D.
Professor
Director, Johns Hopkins Center for Substance Abuse Treatment and Research
Medical Director, Behavioral Pharmacology Research Unit
Johns Hopkins University School of Medicine
Baltimore, Maryland

Zebulon Taintor, M.D.
Clinical Dean
Touro College of Osteopathic Medicine
Adjunct Professor of Psychiatry
New York University School of Medicine
New York, New York

Cindy Taormina, M.S., C.R.C., L.M.H.C.
Vocational Rehabilitation Counselor
EAC, Inc.
Hempstead, New York

Christine Timko, Ph.D.
Consulting Professor of Psychiatry and
 Behavioral Sciences
Stanford University
Stanford, California
Research Career Scientist, Health Services
 Research and Development Service
VA Health Care System
Menlo Park, California

D. Andrew Tompkins, M.D.
Assistant Professor of Psychiatry and
 Behavioral Sciences
Johns Hopkins University
Staff Psychiatrist
Johns Hopkins Bayview Medical Center
Baltimore, Maryland

John W. Tsuang, M.D.
Clinical Professor of Psychiatry
David Geffen School of Medicine at UCLA
Los Angeles, California
Director of Dual Diagnosis Treatment
 Program
Harbor/UCLA Medical Center
Torrance, California

Michelle Tuten, M.S.W.
Assistant Professor of Psychiatry
Johns Hopkins University School of
 Medicine
Baltimore, Maryland

Ryan L. Vandrey, Ph.D.
Assistant Professor of Psychiatry and
 Behavioral Science
Johns Hopkins University School of
 Medicine
Baltimore, Maryland

Onna R. Van Orden, M.A.
Graduate Assistant, Psychology Department
University of Maryland, Baltimore County
Baltimore, Maryland

Fair M. Vassoler

Karl Verebey, Ph.D., D.A.B.F.T., H.C.L.D.
Associate Professor Emeritus of Psychiatry
State University of New York
Brooklyn, New York
Director, Clinical and Forensic Toxicology
Ammon Analytical Laboratory
Linden, New Jersey

Richard C. Oude Voshaar, M.D., Ph.D.
Associate Professor
University Center of Psychiatry
University Medical Center Groningen
Groningen, The Netherlands

Selena Walker, M.A.
Program Evaluation Coordinator
Youth Psychiatry Program
Royal Ottawa Mental Health Centre
Ottawa, Ontario, Canada

Arnold M. Washton, Ph.D.
Executive Director
Recovery Options
New York, New York/Princeton, New Jersey

Philippe Weintraub, M.D.
Associate Professor of Psychiatry
University of Colorado Denver School of Medicine
Aurora, Colorado

Roger D. Weiss, M.D.
Professor of Psychiatry
Harvard Medical School
Boston, Massachusetts
Chief, Division of Alcohol and Drug Abuse
McLean Hospital
Belmont, Massachusetts

A. P. Wells

Joseph Westermeyer, M.D., Ph.D.
Professor of Psychiatry
University of Minnesota
Psychiatrist, Mental Health Service
Minneapolis VA Medical Center
Minneapolis, Minnesota

Laurence M. Westreich, M.D.
Clinical Associate Professor of Psychiatry
Division of Alcoholism and Drug Abuse
New York University School of Medicine
New York, New York

Donna M. White, R.N., Ph.D., C.S., C.A.D.A.C.
Addiction Specialist
Addiction Services
Lemuel Shattuck Hospital
Boston, Massachusetts

Charles Winick, Ph.D.
Professor Emeritus of Sociology
City University of New York Graduate School
New York, New York

Eric D. Wish, Ph.D.
Director, Center for Substance Abuse Research (CESAR)
University of Maryland
College Park, Maryland

Alex Wodak, A.M., F.R.A.C.P., F.A.Ch.A.M.
Director, Alcohol and Drug Service
St. Vincent's Hospital
President, Australian Drug Law Reform Foundation
Darlinghurst, New South Wales, Australia

Daniel Wolfe, M.P.H.
Director, International Harm Reduction Development Program
Open Society Foundations
New York, New York

George E. Woody, M.D.
Professor of Psychiatry
University of Pennsylvania
Philadelphia, Pennsylvania

Katherine S. Wright, B.A.
Graduate Assistant, Psychology Department
University of Maryland, Baltimore County
Baltimore, Maryland

Joel Yager, M.D.
Professor of Psychiatry
University of Colorado School of Medicine
Attending Psychiatrist
University of Colorado Medical Center
Aurora, Colorado

Douglas M. Ziedonis, M.D., M.P.H.
Professor of Psychiatry
University of Massachusetts Medical School
Chairman, Psychiatry Department
University of Massachusetts Memorial Healthcare
Worcester, Massachusetts

Joan E. Zweben, M.D.
Clinical Professor of Psychiatry
University of California, San Francisco
San Francisco, California
Executive Director, East Bay Community Recovery Project
Oakland, California

Preface   vii
Foreword   ix

SECTION 1:
Foundations

1. Historical Perspectives 1
   David F. Musto and Eric D. Wish

2. Epidemiology—The United States 17
   Charles Winick and Jack Levinson

3. Epidemiology—A European Perspective 26
   Icro Maremmani, Matteo Pacini, Mercedes Lovrecic, and Pier Paolo Pani

SECTION 2:
Determinants of Abuse and Dependence

4. Genetic Factors in the Risk for Substance Use Disorders 36
   Thomas A. Nguyen, Jaimee L. Heffner, Show W. Lin, and Robert M. Anthenelli

5. Neurobiological Factors of Drug Dependence and Addiction 55
   Heath D. Schmidt, Fair M. Vassoler, and R. Christopher Pierce

6. Psychological Factors (In Determinants of Abuse and Dependence) 79
   Steven Shoptaw

7. Behavioral Aspects 88
   Kenneth Silverman, Anthony DeFulio, and Jeffery J. Everly

8. Sociocultural Factors and Their Implications 99
   Nady el-Guebaly and Pedro Ruiz

SECTION 3:
Evaluation

9. Clinical Assessment 107
   LaVerne Hanes Stevens and Michael L. Dennis

10. Diagnosis and Classification: *DSM-IV-TR* and *ICD-10* 117
    George E. Woody and John Cacciola

11. Diagnostic Laboratory: Screening for Drug Abuse 123
    Karl G. Verebey and Gerard Meenan

SECTION 4:
Substances of Abuse

12. Alcohol Use Disorders 138
    Carlos A. Hernandez-Avila and Henry R. Kranzler

13. Opioids 161
    David H. Epstein, Karran A. Phillips, and Kenzie L. Preston

14. Cocaine and Crack 191
    Richard P. Paczynski and Mark S. Gold

15. Cannabis 214
    Alan J. Budney, Ryan L. Vandrey, and Stephanie Fearer

16. Amphetamines and Other Stimulants 238
    Kevin P. Hill and Roger D. Weiss

17. Sedative–Hypnotics 255
    Domenic A. Ciraulo and Clifford Knapp

18. Hallucinogens 267
    Robert N. Pechnick and Kathryn A. Cunningham

19. PCP/Designer Drugs/MDMA 277
    Una D. McCann

20. Inhalants 284
    Charles W. Sharp, Matthew O. Howard, and Wynne K. Schiffer

21. Nicotine 319
    Joy M. Schmitz and Angela L. Stotts

22. Caffeine 335
    Laura M. Juliano, Britta L. Anderson, and Roland R. Griffiths

23. Anabolic–Androgenic Steroids 354
    Laurence M. Westreich

SECTION 5:
Compulsive and Addictive Behaviors

24. Eating Disorders and Substance Use Disorders 373
    Harry A. Brandt, Steven F. Crawford, and Katherine A. Halmi

25. Pathologic Gambling 384
    Elise E. DeVito and Marc Potenza

26. Sexual Addiction 393
    Virginia A. Sadock

27. Internet Addiction 284
    Philippe Weintraub, Thomas M. Dunn, Joel Yager, and Zebulon Taintor

xxi

SECTION 6:
Treatment Approaches

Part 1: Neurobiologic Treatments

28 Methadone Maintenance 419
    Andrew J. Saxon and Karen Miotto

29 Buprenorphine in the Treatment of Opioid
    Dependence 437
    D. Andrew Tompkins and Eric C. Strain

30 Naltrexone Pharmacotherapy 447
    Emily Harrison and Ismene Petrakis

31 Vaccines for Substance Abuse 457
    Frank M. Orson, Mark J. Biscone, Berma M. Kinsey, and
    Thomas R. Kosten

32 Acupuncture 466
    Ji-Sheng Han and Cai-Lian Cui

33 Alcohol Abstinence Management 477
    Richard N. Rosenthal

34 Alternative Pharmacotherapies for Opioid
    Addiction 494
    Paul J. Fudala and Rolley E. Johnson

35 Sedative-Hypnotics Abstinence 501
    R.C. Oude Voshaar

36 Nicotine Dependence Management 510
    Douglas Ziedonis, David Kalman, Chris W. Johnson,
    and Lisa A. Mistler

Part 2: Psychosocial and Other Treatments

37 Self-Help Programs Focused on Substance Use:
    Active Ingredients and Outcomes 523
    Rudolf H. Moos and Christine Timko

38 Alternative Support Groups 533
    Arthur T. Horvath

39 The Therapeutic Community 543
    William B. O'Brien, J. Gabriel Piedrahita, and Francisco
    (Sebastian) P. Bacatan, Jr.

40 Network Therapy 551
    Marc Galanter and Helen Dermatis

41 Individual Psychotherapy 562
    Joan E. Zweben

42 Group Therapy 575
    Arnold M. Washton

43 Family/Couples Approaches to Treatment
    Engagement and Therapy 584
    William Fals-Stewart and Wendy K. K. Lam

44 Cognitive Behavioral Therapy 593
    Kathleen M. Carroll

45 Contingency Management in the Treatment
    of Substance Use Disorders: Trends in
    the Literature 603
    Stephen T. Higgins, Stacey C. Sigmon, and Sarah H. Heil

46 Motivational Interviewing and Enhancement 622
    Carlo C. DiClemente, Onna R. Van Orden, and
    Katherine S. Wright

47 Relapse Prevention 633
    Dennis C. Daley, G. Alan Marlatt, and Antoine Douaihy

SECTION 7:
Management of Associated Medical Conditions

48 Maternal and Neonatal Complications of
    Alcohol and Other Drugs 648
    Karol Kaltenbach and Hendrée Jones

49 Medical Complications of Drug Use/Dependence . . 663
    Joshua D. Lee, Jennifer McNeely, and Marc N. Gourevitch

50 Psychiatric Complications of HIV-1 Infection
    and Drug Abuse 682
    Harold W. Goforth, L. Brett Caram, Jorge Maldonado,
    Pedro Ruiz, and Francisco Fernandez

51 Acute and Chronic Pain 695
    Russell K. Portenoy

52 Substance Use Disorders in Individuals with
    Co-occurring Psychiatric Disorders 721
    Sylvia J. Dennison

53 Medication Interactions 730
    Carolina L. Haass-Koffler and Elinore F. McCance-Katz

SECTION 8:
Models of Prevention

54 School-Based Programs 742
    Gilbert J. Botvin and Kenneth W. Griffin

55 Harm Reduction: New Drug Policies and Practices . . 754
    Ernest Drucker, Robert G. Newman, Ethan Nadelmann, Alex Wodak,
    Daniel Wolfe, David Marsh, Eugene Oscapella, Jennifer Mcneely,
    Yujiang Jia, and Kasia Malinowska-Sempruch

56 Work Setting 777
    Paul F. Engelhart and Cindy Taormina

SECTION 9:
Life Cycle

57 Adolescent Substance Abuse 786
    Robert Milin and Selena Walker

58 The Older Drug Abuser 802
    Bennett W. Fletcher and Wilson M. Compton

SECTION 10:
Special Populations

59 African Americans: Alcohol and Substance
    Abuse 813
    William B. Lawson, Jessica Herrera, and Robert G. Lawson

60 Hispanic Americans 819
   Pedro Ruiz

61 Asian Americans and Pacific Islanders 829
   John W. Tsuang and Edmond H. Pi

62 American Indians and Alaska Natives 837
   Daniel Dickerson

63 Women and Addiction 847
   Shelly F. Greenfield, Sudie E. Back, Katie Lawson, and
   Kathleen T. Brady

64 Gays, Lesbians, and Bisexuals 871
   Robert Paul Cabaj

65 Incarcerated Populations 881
   Timothy W. Kinlock, Michael S. Gordon, and
   Robert P. Schwartz

66 Substance Use Disorders among Health Care
   Professionals 892
   J. Wesley Boyd and John R. Knight

67 The Homeless 901
   Jacqueline Maus Feldman

68 Disability, Impairment, and Addiction 908
   Stuart Gitlow

69 New Immigrants and Refugees 918
   Joseph Westermeyer

70 Substance Use in the Armed Forces 926
   Robert M. Bray and Michael R. Pemberton

SECTION 11:

Training and Education

71 Medical Education on Addiction 937
   Karen Drexler

72 Psychologists: Training and Education 949
   D. Baron, C.J. Combs, and A.P. Wells

73 Nursing Education in Addictions and
   Substance Abuse 957
   Betty D. Morgan and Donna M. White, and Colleen T. LaBelle

74 Social Worker Education and Training in the Care of
   Persons with Substance Use Disorders 965
   Michelle Tuten

75 Counselor Training and Education 971
   Gregory S. Brigham, Natasha Slesnick, and Grant Schroeder

76 Other Mental Health Professionals 979
   E. Akerele, N. Nahar, and J. Cerimele

SECTION 12:

Policy Issues

77 Drug Policy: A Biological Science Perspective 988
   Robert L. DuPont, Bertha K. Madras, and Per Johansson

78 Substance Abuse Policy and Payment 1011
   Anita Everett

79 Forensics 1019
   Ihsan M. Salloum

80 Clinical and Societal Implications of Drug
   Legalization 1034
   Benjamin R. Nordstrom and Herbert D. Kleber

81 Future Directions 1046
   Pedro Ruiz and Eric C. Strain

Index   1051

LOWINSON AND RUIZ'S
Substance Abuse

| A Comprehensive Textbook | FIFTH EDITION |

SECTION 1 — FOUNDATIONS

CHAPTER 1 — Historical Perspectives

David F. Musto ■ Eric D. Wish

The last three decades of the 19th century saw far-reaching transformations in American life. With immigration from all parts of Europe and from Asia, the population expanded greatly and became heterogeneous in speech, religion, and way of life. Many of the immigrants, unprepared to join the agricultural sector of the economy, crowded into the growing cities, which soon began to exhibit today's familiar urban problems. With the industrial revolution, large enterprises grew and attained a new level of economic power; with the construction of the railroads, vast areas of the West were opened for settlement and exploitation of the timber and mineral resources. In social terms, the geographic dispersal of the population that occurred as many moved west spelled the end of the once close-knit family. In political terms, these changes terminated the hegemony of the Protestant, North European group that had controlled the affairs of the nation through the Civil War.

The variety of social ills that inevitably attended these rapid changes in all aspects of life gave rise to a spirit of reform that ran through American culture from the mid-19th century to 1920. This reformist or "progressive" impulse stemmed largely from the fear of social disorder among the same middle- and upper-class citizens whose political and economic power was increasingly insecure. Rapid transformation seemed to threaten the heart of American life. While most reforms of the Progressive Era (1890 to 1917) were aimed at curing the disorder itself, some movements naturally responded to specific evils that seemed to result from the upheaval (1). Increasingly, crime and immorality were blamed on easily obtained narcotics and alcohol. This goal of moral uplift of the underprivileged was shared by Progressive Era temperance activists, political reformers, and crusaders against the indiscriminate use of psychoactive substances such as opium and cocaine.

THE BACKGROUND OF PROGRESSIVE ERA REFORMS

Alcohol and the Prohibition Movement

Alcohol had been the object of recurrent prohibition crusades in the 19th century, and as the Progressive Era developed, some sociologists began to speculate that alcohol abuse was actually the result, rather than the cause, of poverty. However, alcohol seemed to exacerbate almost all the evils of a disorderly society. Even if it could not be wholly blamed for economic failure, it certainly did not help. Alcohol lowered efficiency and productivity and, in the eyes of the reformers, increased all the evils of the urban scene: prostitutes worked in and around saloons; alcohol apparently made men more susceptible to the influence of corrupt city bosses; and it broke up families and invited violence. It reduced the chances for freedom, prosperity, and happiness and did not contribute to the virtue and enlightened character of an electorate needed by a democracy.

Furthermore, alcohol worsened the situation of Protestant Christianity. Not only was the saloon associated with Catholic immigrants, but it also seemed to make people incapable of responding to evangelical Protestantism (2). If it made a person unconcerned about something as urgent as salvation, then surely it would make that person oblivious to public concerns. Democratization, therefore, made it even more important that the saloon be abolished. Extending the powers of the landless class, in itself, posed quite a threat to stability; drunken masses would constitute an intolerable danger (3).

With the final temperance movement that led to the adoption in 1919 of the Eighteenth Amendment, the nation moved toward implementation of a prohibition justified on moral, religious, and scientific grounds (4). It is quite likely that by 1919 a majority of Americans believed that liquor prohibition would be a great benefit in reducing poverty, crime, broken families, lost work time, and immorality. Eventually, every state except Rhode Island and Connecticut ratified the amendment.

Narcotics, Cocaine, and Cannabis

By the end of the 19th century, the narcotics problem was also worrying reform-minded legislators, health professionals, and the laity. Opium in its crude form had been imported into North America from the time of the earliest European settlements. Various medicines were made from it. Alcohol extracts of crude opium included laudanum and paregoric, and opium was mixed with other drugs in patent medicines, among the most popular of which was Dover's powder, originating in England in the 18th century. American statistics on opium imports were not kept until the 1840s, but from that time on, domestic consumption rose rapidly until the mid-1890s, when the annual importation of crude opium leveled off at about a half million pounds (5). After passage of federal laws in 1914 strictly limiting importation of opium, the import statistics became less helpful in estimating national consumption, and smuggling became a greater problem. Yet, statistics for the pre–World War I period provide good evidence that a steady increase of opium use in the United States occurred in the 19th century and that when the 20th century began, there was already a substantial consumption of the drug for medicinal and nonmedicinal purposes. State laws regulating the availability of narcotics were first enacted around the time of the Civil War, and many states attempted to control the drugs by the 1890s.

Several major technologic and chemical advances made the most powerful ingredients in opium available in pure, cheap form. In the first decade of the 19th century, morphine was isolated from opium, and by 1832, American pharmaceutical manufacturers were preparing morphine from imported crude opium. Codeine was isolated in 1832, and this less-addicting substance became a common form of manufactured derivative, particularly after morphine and heroin were severely restricted in the United States after World War I (6,7). Heroin, a trade name of the Bayer Company for diacetylmorphine, was introduced commercially in 1898, with the hope that acetylation of the morphine molecule would reduce its side effects while maintaining its effectiveness in suppressing the cough reflex. A similar hope was entertained the next year for acetylation of salicylic acid, a mild analgesic with undesirable side effects, which was then marketed as Aspirin, the Bayer trademark for sodium acetylsalicylic acid. Heroin, of course, proved to be at least as addictive as morphine and eventually ousted morphine as the drug of choice among American drug habitués (8). The increasing use of heroin in this period is an example of the effectiveness of three innovations adopted by 19th-century industrial enterprises: manufacturing, rapid distribution, and effective marketing techniques.

Coca leaves, in their indigenous growth areas in South America, were known to have stimulant properties and had been used for centuries by natives. Coca's unusual properties were popularized in Europe and America in the mid-19th century, and an alcohol extract of the leaves, which contained some of the active stimulant cocaine, often appeared under the name "wine of coca." In the 1880s, pure cocaine became more easily available because of advances in manufacturing technology, and it was immediately praised, especially in the United States. Its stimulating and euphoric properties were touted for athletes, workers, and students, and bottlers of popular soda drinks, and easily obtained "tonics" added cocaine to obtain a stimulant effect. Medical uses were soon discovered, and worldwide experimentation established cocaine as an anesthetic for the surface of the eye and as a block to pain stimuli when injected near a nerve. The stimulant properties were bothersome side effects of cocaine when used as an anesthetic, but within a few decades, satisfactory substitutes were developed that were considered less habituating, such as procaine in 1905. Cocaine was also convenient for shrinking nasal and sinus membranes, and it became one of the early effective remedies for "hay fever," allergies, and sinusitis. As an over-the-counter remedy for hay fever or "nasal catarrh," in powder form to be sniffed or as a spray, cocaine began to be criticized as misused or carelessly dispensed for mere pleasure or dissipation.

In the period from about 1895 to 1915, cocaine became associated in the popular and medical press with southern blacks' hostility toward whites. Vicious crimes said to have been perpetrated by blacks were commonly attributed to the effects of cocaine. In efforts to pass antinarcotic legislation, this association was repeated by federal officials and spokesmen for the health professions, although direct evidence for such a close and specifically racial association was wanting or even contradictory (9). Eighty years ago, cocaine was considered a typically "Negro" drug, whereas opiates, and specifically heroin, were described as characteristically "white," illustrating the influence of social tensions and racial stereotypes on interpretation of the narcotics problem.

Cannabis, or marihuana, in the form of "reefers" or "joints," seems to have been unfamiliar in the United States until the 20th century, yet there has been a long-standing fear of hashish, a concentrated and powerful form of cannabis. Hashish was known from its use as an esoteric and perilous drug popular in the Middle East and from the description of its bizarre effects by literary figures who experimented with it in the mid-19th century (10).

PROGRESSIVE ERA FOOD AND DRUG REFORMS (1898 TO 1906)

Faced with what they perceived as social breakdown associated with the pernicious effects of drugs and alcohol, reformers turned to the federal government. In the period leading to the Progressive Era, state and local laws were losing credibility as effective measures to control distribution and consumption of both alcohol and psychoactive drugs. The failure was usually ascribed to the patchwork-quilt character of laws below the federal level of government (11). But federal action was limited by the few constitutional bases for laws that would affect abuses. Other than the tariff, the federal government was restricted mostly to regulating interstate commerce and levying taxes. Police and health powers, obviously the most appropriate for combating addiction and illicit drugs, were the province of the states. For example, the United States Public Health Service and its antecedent agencies were limited to dealing with communicable diseases and gathering and disseminating such medical information as vital statistics and public health advice; they could not provide direct delivery of health services except to their legal wards, chiefly the Merchant Marine and American Indians (12). The armed services excepted, federal police agencies included alcohol tax agents, members of the Coast Guard, and customs and immigration officers. Therefore, there was little precedent for federal regulation of dangerous drugs, and no federal policing agency could easily add this burden to its current duties. As a result, the range of activities that were left to an individual's or company's sense of fair play was remarkably large. In the 19th century, federal law did not require the labeling of drugs on over-the-counter proprietaries. Thus, these patent medicines could contain any amount of, say, morphine without acknowledgment, and could even aver that the potion contained no morphine. The percentage of alcohol in some popular remedies was higher than that in many cocktails today. Claims that a proprietary could cure cancer, tuberculosis, or any other ailment were legally unchallengeable; no tests of efficacy, purity, or standardization were required. In addition, newspapers, the primary source of information for most Americans, were chary of offending their advertisers, and many papers had contracts with proprietary manufacturers that would become invalid with the enactment of any state law requiring disclosure of contents or any modification of advertising claims (13).

Hence, it is not surprising that no federal law requiring content information and some accuracy of claims was enacted until 1906, when public concern reached a pitch sufficient to propel the government to resort to its power over interstate commerce to enact such a measure. The law, the Pure Food and Drug Act, contained some of the earliest federal provisions affecting narcotics; if any over-the-counter remedy in interstate commerce contained an opiate, cannabis, cocaine, or chloral hydrate, the label was required to state its contents and percentage. The effect of this simple measure apparently was to reduce the amount of such drugs in popular remedies and also to hurt their sales, although other proprietaries flourished. The Proprietary Association of America, dismayed at the accusation of being "dopers," favored strict limitation of dangerous drugs in their products and ostracized manufacturers who continued to put such drugs as cocaine in "asthma cures."

Although a step had been taken to warn proprietary users of the amount of dangerous drugs in the remedies, still nothing had been done to bring under control another target of reform: "dope doctors" and pharmacists who purveyed opiates and cocaine to anyone who asked for them. The percentage of such deviants in each profession was not large, but they took advantage of the broad authority given to all licensed pharmacists and physicians to use their professional judgment in the delivery of medicines and services, and the dominance of the state in the licensing of the health professions seemed unassailable by the federal government. In addition to purchasing drugs from professional miscreants, one could order them from mail-order houses. How to rectify this promiscuous distribution of narcotics presented another difficult constitutional problem for federal action.

TOWARD PROHIBITION OF NARCOTIC DRUGS (1909–1919)

The Shanghai Commission and the Smoking Opium Act (1909)

Several bills directed at the traffic in narcotics had been introduced into Congress before 1908, but federal legislation was accomplished only after President Theodore Roosevelt convened the Shanghai Opium Commission in 1909 to aid the Chinese Empire in its desire to stamp out opium addiction, particularly opium smoking (14). The measure, intended more as evidence of America's good faith in convening the commission than as an adequate weapon against American narcotic abuse, was modest and limited. Called The Smoking Opium Exclusion Act, it outlawed importation of opium prepared for smoking (15). Its passage while the Shanghai Commission was in session under the chairmanship of an American, the Right Reverend Charles H. Brent, Episcopal bishop of the Philippine Islands, was designed to show the delegates of other nations that the United States was willing to take steps to aid control of world opium traffic. American delegates reported back to the State Department that the announcement of the act's passage was met with an impressive response from the other 12 nations represented.

The American delegates, however, and indeed the departments most closely associated with narcotic policy planning—State, Treasury, and Agriculture—were aware that the legislation against smoking opium was but the first step in controlling a national problem described as serious and threatening to progress. The nation needed a law that more closely controlled sales of over-the-counter remedies, excessive or careless prescribing of narcotics, and other avenues of easy access to narcotics. The question, of course, was how the federal government could accomplish this by constitutional means. Both the power to regulate interstate commerce and to levy taxes provided some basis for federal narcotics control. The State Department, which coordinated domestic legislation and planning until 1914, eventually opted for the latter, reasoning that by using tax administration, all narcotics could be traced, not just drugs shipped from one state to another.

The first of the administration's proposed bills, drafted in 1909, provided for extremely harsh penalties and was intricately detailed but without exemption for proprietaries that contained very small amounts of the narcotics (16). The effect of such bills would have been to make the handling of narcotic preparations so risky and complicated for retail outlets that the whole narcotic traffic would fall into the hands of physicians. The physicians would be limited only by their good judgment and by restrictions that state legislatures might enact (e.g., record keeping, prohibiting the refilling of narcotic prescriptions, or maintaining addicts) (17).

Such tough proposals met with opposition from the rank and file of the drug trades, proprietary manufacturers, and some members of Congress who feared, among other things, that such a precedent might be extended to alcohol. Before the Webb–Kenyon Act was passed over President Taft's veto in 1913 and upheld by the Supreme Court, it was legal to live in a dry state, purchase liquor from a wet state, and have it delivered via interstate commerce.

The Hague Treaty (1912)

While domestic debate continued among the specific interests affected by the proposed narcotic legislation, the United States continued its campaign to regulate the international traffic in narcotics. Because the Shanghai Commission was not empowered to draft a treaty (the delegates could only make recommendations), American diplomats sought a second meeting for the preparation of an international treaty. After much persuasion and repeated setbacks, the Netherlands, at America's request, convened the International Opium Conference at The Hague in December 1911. Again, Bishop Brent, head of the American delegation, was chosen to preside, and after weeks of debate and compromise, the delegates signed The Hague Opium Convention in January 1912 (5). The title is somewhat misleading; the treaty also sought to control cocaine. An American and Italian suggestion that cannabis be included was not accepted.

The Hague Treaty emphasized enactment of legislation in each nation to control the production of crude substances, their manufacture into pharmaceutical products, and their distribution within the nation and abroad (18). The United States government believed that its people were extravagant consumers of opiates; federal publications reported that the country was, by far, the largest consumer of opium per capita among Western nations. In the words of the State Department's opium commissioner, Dr. Hamilton Wright, "Uncle Sam is the worst drug fiend in the world," consuming, he claimed, more opium per capita than the fabled opium-using Chinese (19). The thought within the State Department was that if the nations that grew opium and coca enacted strict legislation in the spirit of the treaty, the American problem would be greatly reduced, perhaps would even vanish. The challenge was to persuade other nations to have a "correct" view of narcotic use and to enforce legislation in accord with this view.

Yet the stern international measures envisaged by such reformers as Dr. Wright were not adopted before World War I. The Hague Treaty was not airtight; its vague phrases did not compel the ratifying nations to enact strict laws to reduce narcotic distribution to solely medical purposes. Moreover, American domestic legislation, now promoted as the American implementation of The Hague Treaty, was still hampered by doctrines of states' rights and constitutional interpretation, to say nothing of the competing interests of physicians, pharmacists, and manufacturers of proprietary medicines.

The Harrison Act (1914)

In 1913, the administration of President Woodrow Wilson drafted legislation grounded in its constitutional taxation power. It was hoped that the new measure would, at the very least, bring into the open the vast narcotic traffic so that the states could take appropriate health and police measures or step up enforcement of existing laws. At the most, Wright hoped the Harrison Act, as the legislation was called, would be recognized as the fulfillment of an international obligation in accord with Article VI of the Constitution and thus take precedence over the rights of states. If this were the case, the general phraseology of the Harrison Bill, such as requiring the prescription of narcotics "in good faith," could be interpreted broadly and would allow prosecution of "dope doctors," other malpracticing professionals, and peddlers.

The measure passed the House of Representatives relatively easily but slowed down in the Senate and did not finally pass into law until December 1914. It was to come into effect on March 1, 1915 (20). In its final form, the act allowed proprietary medicines to include small amounts of narcotics, and physicians were not required to keep records of medicines dispensed while they personally attended a patient. Legitimate purveyors of opiate and cocaine preparations were required to register with the Bureau of Internal Revenue and obtain a tax stamp, for which they paid one dollar per year. Detailed record keeping was required for most transactions, and legal possession by a consumer was made dependent on a physician's or dentist's prescription. Individual consumers were forbidden to register (21). But when federal personnel sought to arrest the dope doctors for prescribing, they discovered that many federal district court judges thought the action was an infringement of state police powers. In 1916, a crucial Supreme Court interpretation, known as the first *Jin Fuey Moy* decision, held that it was beyond federal powers to prohibit narcotics possession by anyone to whom the Treasury Department had refused registration, such as a peddler or addict (22).

Not until the height of the war effort—and in the midst of a zealous drive to rid the nation of perceived threats to its integrity and security—was a successful campaign mounted to strengthen the Harrison Act to prevent health professionals from dispensing narcotics to persons whose only problem was addiction itself.

DRUG CONTROL IN A PERIOD OF DIMINISHING USE (1919–1962)

Size and Symbolism of the Addiction Problem

The true size of the drug abuse problem in the early decades of the 20th century (Dr. Wright's hyperbole not withstanding) was a matter of public debate, much as it is today. Whereas the Public Health Service in rather sober studies published in 1915 and 1924 argued that there were probably never more than a quarter million habitual users of opiates and cocaine in the nation, the Treasury Department assessed the number at slightly more than one million, who were described as moral wretches for the most part (23,24). New York City officials claimed that heroin addicts were responsible for huge numbers of crimes and estimated that in 1924, the remarkable figure of 75% of all crimes were committed by addicts (25). In 1919, the mayor of New York City linked heroin with anarchism and political bombings (26)—and his was not an isolated opinion. There was fear in the nation about several groups that were considered extreme domestic threats: socialists, members of the Industrial Workers of the World, Bolsheviks, and addicts (27). The image of the addict as immoral and criminal, a belief dating back among respectable writers and observers well into the 19th century, made them an obvious target for serious social reformers, as well as for ambitious politicians and bureaucrats. If one accepted that they numbered more than 1 million in a nation of 100 million, stern action and uncompromising control seemed entirely justified. Nevertheless, this sentiment coexisted with experiments in public-health-based addiction management and medical theories of addiction as a treatable disease. When the results of attempts at treatment proved disappointing, faith in treatment waned, and the punitive model of drug abuse control won, as it were, by default.

Maintenance Clinics (1912 to 1925)

Beginning in 1912 in Jacksonville, Florida, 40 odd clinics were established in various parts of the country to supply addicts with maintenance doses of narcotics in what were designed to be controlled conditions. The clients were usually those too poor or socially marginal to have access to private physicians. A relatively small percentage of the nation's addicts were enrolled in these clinics, particularly if one accepted the extravagant estimate of more than a million addicts for the whole nation. It is likely that the number of addicts registered at any one time in maintenance clinics did not exceed 5,000 (28). The average age of patrons was about 30 years, and they had usually been addicts for at least several years before joining the clinic. Some clinics were operated by police departments (e.g., New Haven) and others by health departments (e.g., Atlanta), and attitudes toward the clinics varied from one city to another. Some were clearly operated under political patronage and for a profit. In a few instances, as in Albany, New York, both cocaine and morphine were dispensed.

An exception to the policy of almost all these clinics, which was to maintain addicts indefinitely on morphine, was the clinic operated in 1919 and 1920 by the New York City Department of Health. Here heroin was used to entice addicts into a detoxification and rehabilitation program. After almost a year of operation, the city ended its experiment. It found that almost all addicts, even if detoxified, returned to heroin after release from 6 weeks of hospital treatment. The Health Department concluded that restriction of availability by the police and federal agents was necessary if addiction was to be effectively diminished. About 7,500 persons registered at the clinic, and almost all received gradually decreasing doses of heroin; 10% were younger than age 19 years (29).

Adoption of a Federal Antimaintenance Policy

Given the inadequacy and variety of state laws, there seemed no way to control physicians and pharmacists—even though the unethical percentage was small—other than by imposition of federal authority. If a physician could exercise judgment as to when and whom to maintain in an opiate habit, it was certain that some physicians would be unscrupulous, thus spreading the habit and reaping a profit. Therefore, in addition to reforms in the medical and pharmaceutical professions, the goal of the federal government was to restrict that breadth of medical judgment by law. The undertaking was hazardous, for such federal encroachment on medicine was unprecedented; the physician would be allowed to maintain an opiate addict only if approved by a local narcotics agent. These exceptions would be chiefly iatrogenically addicted and middle-class patients. (One should keep in mind that some observers believed that physicians created about half of American opiate addiction.)

In 1918, partly to counteract the *Jin Fuey Moy* decision, the Treasury Department established a Special Committee on Narcotics Traffic. The committee helped persuade Congress to pass strengthening legislation in February 1919 (30). Then, aiding the government effort, the Supreme Court, in two fundamental interpretations of the act, rejected by a vote of five to four the argument that it was legal to maintain an addict by prescription if the addict had no problem except addiction (31). To carry out the strict Supreme Court ruling that addiction maintenance be severely limited in the United States, a Narcotics Division was established in the Treasury Department in December 1919. It was part of the newly formed Prohibition Unit of the Internal Revenue Bureau, which had been created to enforce liquor prohibition. Its first head was Levi G. Nutt, a pharmacist from Ohio who had risen in the ranks of the tax unit. He now oversaw about 150 narcotic agents scattered across the nation.

Addiction Disease and Law Enforcement

One result of antimaintenance law enforcement, which was backed by leading physicians and such reformers as Dr. Alexander Lambert, president of the American Medical Association (AMA) in 1919, was a curious decline in the respectability of a certain medical theory that would have admitted maintenance as a rational therapy response: the immunochemical theory of opiate addiction. This happened because both reformers and government agents feared maintenance and were disgusted by the subterfuges some health professionals used to justify a profitable trade. Their fear and disgust extended to suspicion of any justification for maintenance. Supplying drugs to an addict came to be considered a form of medical malpractice that endangered society by perpetuating criminal and immoral persons in their esoteric pleasures.

In the immunologic reasoning that was popular among some addiction experts prior to 1919, the argument ran that ingestion of, say, morphine stimulated the formation of antibodies, like those produced against smallpox virus, or of antitoxins, like those produced against the toxins of the diphtheria bacterium. Such theories were popular explanations for illnesses in the late 19th and early 20th centuries, and in many cases, saved lives. With regard to addiction, and according to several competent and respected clinicians, the theory held that maintenance doses of an opiate would be required to bring an addict's physiology into balance with the level of antibodies or antitoxins present. If too little opiate were administered, the body would begin to experience withdrawal symptoms as a result of the action of unneutralized antibodies or antitoxins; if too much opiate were administered, the body would experience the physiologic effects of opiates. According to Dr. Ernest Bishop of New York, the amount of opiate required to balance an individual's physiology could be determined with great precision, and the addict would remain a fully normal person only so long as this exact dose was maintained. However, Dr. Bishop did not rule out cure in some instances by various popular medical regimens (32).

The intimate link between this scientific theory and its implications for public policy made its adherents suspect. Those who practiced medicine in accordance with the theory could be indicted and convicted of violating the laws defining what was legitimate medical practice as interpreted by 1919 Supreme Court decisions. When Dr. A.G. DuMez of the Hygienic Laboratory (now the National Institutes of Health), one of the leading addiction experts of the United States Public Health Service, published his endorsement of some of the immunologic experiments in 1919, he was asked by the AMA's Committee on Addiction to retract his statement, which he did, in part, by qualifying his previous endorsement (33,34). Within 2 years, the question of the cause of addiction was so controversial that the Surgeon General of the Public Health Service wrote to the president of the Louisiana State Board of Health to advise that the phrase "physiological balance" was too controversial to be included in a description of narcotic treatment and the enforcement problem (14).

It was soon demonstrated that immunologic substances could not be found in the blood; the adherents of "addiction disease" caused by a simple and easily detectable immunologic process were evidently in error. Yet the intense political nature of the addiction question and the fear of addicts, whose numbers were very likely overestimated, had an impact on the exchange of scientific information and medical practice. At the level of social planning, maintenance was judged poor public policy, and it was to be eliminated if at all possible. This decision might, indeed, have been the correct one, but the suddenness of implementation and the emotionally charged attitude toward addicts and their maintainers caused policy to collide dramatically with research and medical opinion.

The events of 1919 spelled the eventual end of the clinic experiment and of the concept of addiction as a health problem. Maintenance of nonmedical addicts had become illegal, even if records were carefully kept and a physician examined every patient and tried to keep the drug down to a minimum. By 1925, all the clinics known to the Narcotics Division had been closed.

The rapidity with which opinion on controversial questions like addiction and narcotics can be crystallized is one of the most interesting features of narcotic control in the United States. To resist the closure of maintenance was difficult; the new policy ensued from the anger, scapegoating, fatigue, and frustration of the lawmakers because a simple answer to addiction was still not available. The burden for the next several decades would rest on law enforcement to prevent illegal access to narcotic supplies. The hope for a simple medical cure had been dashed.

Fear of Federal Control on the Part of Health Professions

Court decisions continued to restrict what remained of a physician's right to maintain an addict. Procedures used by agents to get information led to hostility and suspicion, but the reason that enforcement personnel used such methods as informers was that they had repeatedly encountered determined profit-making physicians whose concern for the welfare of their patients and the community was nil. A further disagreement between the federal government and the medical profession arose from a question even more fundamental than maintenance: Did the federal government have the right to interfere with medical practice and exempt certain classes of patients from a doctor's judgment? The medical profession came out of the social agitation associated with World War I with a fear that the federal government would enter into "state medicine" or compulsory health insurance. After 1920, the AMA greatly resisted the various federal measures concerning health, such as the Sheppard-Towner Act for Maternal and Child Care, which was to be financed by matching grants to the states. The medical profession fought such federal intervention with great vigor and generally with success (35).

Yet the Harrison Act remained a thorn in the side of professional medicine. If it was constitutional for government to say who could be maintained or not, a precedent was set for further incursions into medical practice. A similar problem for the AMA was the Willis-Campbell Act of 1921, which limited a physician's prescriptions for alcohol to a fairly modest number and placed other restrictions on the kind and amount of alcohol that could be prescribed. Hence, physicians were disturbed at the Harrison and Willis-Campbell Acts in part not because they wanted to maintain addicts or become saloon-keepers (although at times a few seemed quite willing to do just that), but because they were fearful of where this unprecedented use of federal power in the health fields might lead.

Narcotic Drugs Import and Export Act (1922)

After the outlawing of addiction maintenance, a series of federal statutes in the 1920s sought to fill gaps in the federal control of narcotics. The first, the Narcotic Drugs Import and Export Act of 1922, permitted only crude narcotics to enter the United States; American drug companies would manufacture them into pure substances (36). Any subsequently manufactured foreign narcotic product in the United States, like Swiss morphine or German cocaine, was illegal. Intricate restrictions were placed on American export and transshipment of narcotics because it was feared that a great deal of morphine was arriving in China, via Japan, in this manner or that it was being smuggled back into the United States after export to Canada or Mexico. Finally, the Federal Narcotic Control Board, composed of the secretaries of Treasury, Commerce, and State, was established to authorize legitimate imports and exports.

Restrictions on Heroin (1924)

In the mid-1920s, the United States attempted to obtain international sanctions against the manufacture of heroin, which by then was considered the most dangerous narcotic, particularly for adolescents. Most of the crime in New York City was blamed on heroin, including daring bank robberies, senseless violence, and murders. The danger of heroin was exaggerated by respectable antinarcotic reformers in order to inform the American people of its peril. One excellent example is the educational campaign of Captain Richmond Pearson Hobson, a hero of the Spanish-American War, former congressman, and ardent prohibitionist, who directed his speaking and organizational talents against narcotics shortly after the Eighteenth Amendment's ratification. Captain Hobson was wont to warn women who habitually used any particular face powder to have it checked for heroin, lest they become addicted. He claimed that one dose of heroin was addictive, and that an ounce of heroin could addict 2,000 persons. He blamed a national crime wave on heroin, claiming that it was a stimulant to senseless violence. He desired that a compilation of such warnings be sent into every American home and requested Congress to print 50 million copies of his eight-page brochure, "The Peril of Narcotics" (37). The pamphlet was not printed, but a revised version of his message was printed in the Congressional Record and distributed by sympathetic congressmen (38). Hobson represents a popularizer of heroin dangers who disseminated grossly erroneous information on addiction that tended to alarm the public while providing a convenient explanation for unrelated, serious social problems.

In 1924, partly to encourage other nations to regulate narcotics and partly to assist in the American fight against addiction, Congress prohibited importation of crude opium into the United States for the manufacture of heroin (39). The author of this legislation, Representative Stephen Porter of Pittsburgh, chairman of the House Foreign Affairs Committee, took the leading congressional role in the international negotiations and planning for domestic control of narcotics in the 1920s.

Federal Narcotic Farms (1929)

Porter's second major effort was to provide for two "narcotic farms" where addicts could be treated as sick individuals and detoxified, and where they could perhaps assist investigators in the search for a cure (40). A factor in this legislation was that federal prisons were becoming jammed with Harrison Act violators, most of whom were also addicts. Congress had to build either two new prisons or two treatment centers. Thus came into being the Lexington, Kentucky, and Fort Worth, Texas, narcotic hospitals operated by the United States Public Health Service. This legislation also provided for the Public Health Service Narcotics Division, which evolved into the present National Institute of Mental Health (NIMH) and National Institute on Drug Abuse (NIDA).

The Federal Bureau of Narcotics (1930)

Finally, Representative Porter sought to establish in the Treasury Department an independent narcotics agency. The Narcotics Division had accompanied the Prohibition Unit when the latter was raised to the rank of bureau in 1927, and although still subordinate and headed by an assistant commissioner, it was gradually expanding. In 1930, shortly before his death, Porter shepherded through Congress the act creating the Federal Bureau of Narcotics (FBN) (41). When the Prohibition Bureau moved from the Treasury Department to the Justice Department in the mid-1920s, the Narcotics Division remained behind, but its head, Levi G. Nutt, was not to become the first commissioner of narcotics. Nutt's son and son-in-law were implicated by a federal grand jury in "indiscreet" dealings with the recently slain New York narcotics underworld figure, Arnold Rothstein (42). Nutt was transferred from his post a week after the filing of the grand jury's report, which also touched on his own activities and those of the New York district office. Assistant Prohibition Commissioner Harry J. Anslinger was picked from the international control section of the Prohibition Bureau to take temporary charge of the Narcotics Division.

Anslinger had not been deeply involved with narcotics; his training was in the foreign service and in international negotiations to cut off rum running. To Representative Porter, however, he seemed the ideal candidate. Accustomed to what Porter likely regarded as foreign wiles and ulterior motives in areas of American moral concern, he could ably represent the United States in its struggle, dating back to 1906, to achieve international control of narcotics traffic. The medical aspect of the question seemed secondary, for if smuggling could be ended, the narcotics problem would take care of itself.

Thus began the 32-year tenure of Commissioner Anslinger. Most of the enforcement questions had been settled: maintenance was illegal; the image of the heroin addict was well-publicized by such spokesmen as Captain Hobson; and a national system of agents was established with fairly well-defined styles of enforcement, although there was the eternal integrity problem in the agents' dealings with smugglers. The most profound effect on narcotics enforcement in the immediate future was not new policies but the Depression, which drastically reduced the FBN's budget, led to detailed scrutiny of even its telephone bills by Congress, and probably helped explain the parsimony characteristic of the Anslinger tenure. Even in the 1960s, the Bureau made a fetish of a low budget.

The Marihuana Problem (1930 to 1937)

Commissioner Anslinger's first major issue appeared even as he took office—a quickly burgeoning fear centered in the Southwest about a plant grown and used by Mexicans who had poured into the region as farm laborers in the prosperous 1920s. This drug or plant was known as locoweed, marihuana, or, more scientifically, cannabis. As the fear of marihuana grew, so did the belief that it stimulated violence and was being slyly sold to American schoolchildren. In the early 1930s, the FBN tried to minimize these fears and suggested that state laws were the appropriate response. The Uniform State Narcotic Drug Act proposed in 1932 included marihuana regulations as an option for state legislation; the Bureau thought it had found the solution. The plant grew in the United States, so the best response would be from local government, not from an agency that had its eyes on the smuggling of drugs from Turkey, France, Bolivia, China, and Siam.

Yet, recalled Anslinger, the Treasury Department decided to make marihuana use a federal offense, more as a gesture to the fearful Southwest than as a comprehensive and probably effective plan for marihuana control. The Department's bill was modeled on the National Firearms Act, which was declared constitutional by the Supreme Court in March 1937. In April, Treasury representatives went before Congress to ask for a similar "transfer tax" and licensing system for marihuana. Congress passed the Marihuana Tax Act of 1937 without dissent, and by October it was in effect (43). Opposition to the act in committee came from an AMA representative, Dr. William C. Woodward, who stated that this was an area of state concern, and that it should not become one more example of federal encroachment on the medical profession.

In the enforcement of the act, the Bureau described marihuana as a fearsome substance, but played down any suggestion that it was a problem out of control. The apparent goal was to make the drug unattractive, but not to create a panic over claims that it was widely disseminated to schoolchildren (10).

Adoption of Mandatory Minimum Sentences (1951 to 1956)

World War II brought narcotic use, particularly opiates, to a low point. Control over the growth of opium poppies had been sought in 1942 by the Opium Poppy Control Act (44). There was other legislation at this time to resolve technical problems, strengthen penalties, and include synthetic narcotics, such as meperidine, under federal regulations (45). At the close of hostilities, however, the FBN anticipated a resumption of illicit world narcotic trade. The Bureau looked back to World War I when, it was claimed, there had been a postwar upsurge. Consequently, when there was a rise in addiction among ghetto youth in Chicago and New York City in the late 1940s, and authorities noted a lower age among those sent to prisons or narcotic hospitals, the Bureau asked Congress for stronger penalties. The variability in judges' sentences and disposition of cases—a short sentence or probation for a trafficker the Bureau might have spent years trying to convict—led to the proposal to take sentencing of certain offenders out of the hands of judges. Also, a mandatory sentence might deter the potential trafficker or even the drug user.

Such legislation was introduced by Representative Hale Boggs and enacted in 1951 (46). In 1956, after Senate hearings chaired by Senator Price Daniel, the death penalty was allowed at the jury's discretion in some instances of heroin sales (47). This was the peak of punitive legislation against drug addiction in the United States. In a half century, the federal response to dangerous drugs had advanced from requiring accurate labeling of narcotics in over-the-counter remedies (but with no limit on how much could be present) to the possibility of the death penalty or, at least, a mandatory sentence for conveying heroin to a minor (regardless of the quantity of heroin).

Voices were raised against such harsh measures, but they were not very effective in modifying the course of events up to 1956. The American Bar Association (ABA) questioned the wisdom of mandatory minimum sentences, and a joint ABA–AMA committee began to examine the narcotics question with a philosophy far different from that embodied in the Boggs-Daniel acts. Staff of the committee looked at the British experience, in which legal heroin maintenance was available to the several hundred known addicts, and wondered whether some similar system would be suitable for the United States (48). Presidential and congressional confidence in various forms of psychological and chemical treatment flourished and was expressed in such national projects as the Community Mental Health Center program of 1963. Narcotic maintenance programs reappeared, using the synthetic narcotic methadone. The police effort to make narcotic supplies scarce—which seemed so reasonable to progressive medical leadership in 1919—began to seem crude, ineffective, and conducive to gross malfeasance. A turning point in the national approach to narcotics was again at hand.

DRUG CONTROL IN A PERIOD OF RISING USE (1962 TO 1980)

Medical and Psychological Response to Addiction (1962 to 1970)

After Anslinger announced his retirement in 1962—a sign of hope to those wanting to see some form of maintenance or at least less reliance on mandatory prison sentences—President John F. Kennedy called the White House Conference on Narcotics and Drug Abuse (49). Its participants represented the various conflicting points of view; after the conference was over, the President's Advisory Commission on Narcotics and Drug Abuse considered how to carry out the spirit of reexamination and make specific recommendations. The Commission's *Final Report*, published in 1963, marks a definite, if small, shift from the trend to see all "narcotics" as equal in the sight of the law. There was a suggestion that psychological treatment might be useful and that some variations in prison sentencing, such as civil commitment, might prove effective against addiction (50).

In the 1960s, the appearance of psychedelic substances, such as lysergic acid diethylamide (LSD), and the quick rise in marihuana use drew attention to the varieties of drugs available and abusable. Further studies of marihuana suggested that it was less dangerous than had been assumed in the early 1930s, and the fact that millions of individuals were estimated to have used it in the 1960s also suggested that marihuana was not so very dangerous in moderate use. Other drugs, like amphetamines and barbiturates, became as popular in the streets as they had previously been common in middle-class homes. The number of heroin addicts began to rise, and the nation perceived itself under attack by a "drug culture" linked by many observers to a youth "counterculture."

Both the legislative and executive branches of the government began to respond to the drug problem in ways that reflected, at the same time, concern about increasing drug use and changing opinions on the nature of drugs and the best ways to prevent abuse. The Drug Abuse Amendments of 1965 created the Bureau of Drug Abuse Control in the Department of Health, Education, and Welfare to address diversion and misuse of barbiturates and amphetamines; and the Narcotic Addict Rehabilitation Act of 1966 approved civil commitment as an alternative to prison for addicted drug offenders (51,52).

The high hopes held for civil commitment of drug addicts were not to be realized. At first such commitment seemed in keeping with advanced notions of psychological and milieu treatment, but it was modified to guarantee that the addict would remain for treatment. Yet the cost and length of treatment, as well as the dismal success rate, brought this apparently more sophisticated form of confinement into question. Civil commitment may also have conflicted with the legal rights of the individual: An addict could be confined for several years, not for a crime but because he or she had a disease. These many difficulties with civil commitment caused a shift from optimism in the Advisory Commission's report of 1963 to a close questioning of the concept in the report of the President's Commission on Law Enforcement and the Administration of Justice in 1967 (53).

Reorganization of the Federal Drug Control Bureaucracy

In response to political and social pressures similar to those that had prompted the transfer of the Prohibition Unit from the Treasury Department to the Justice Department in the late 1920s, the FBN was joined with the Bureau of Drug Abuse and Control in 1968 and moved to Justice under the name, Bureau of Narcotics and Dangerous Drugs (BNDD).

When Richard Nixon took office as president in 1969, his advisors saw almost immediately that narcotics control offered an opportunity to make good on Nixon's campaign promise to reduce crime (54). The first major legislative initiative of the Nixon administration was the Comprehensive Drug Abuse Prevention and Control Act of 1970, which brought together and rationalized all previous drug legislation under the interstate commerce powers of the federal government. The new law also established schedules that differentiated among the various drugs of abuse and formed the basis for a new penalty structure that abandoned mandatory minimum sentences (55).

In the spring of 1971, President Nixon issued an executive order that established the Special Action Office for Drug Abuse Prevention (SAODAP), a White House office that was meant to oversee the prevention and treatment programs of a host of cabinet departments and agencies. SAODAP was given statutory existence through the Drug Abuse Office and Treatment Act of 1972 (56). That same year a special unit in aid of local law enforcement called the Office of Drug Abuse Law Enforcement (ODALE) was also established through executive order, as was the Office of National Narcotics Intelligence (ONNI). The expenditure of the BNDD in fiscal year 1972 was more than $60 million, a remarkable amount when compared with the FBN expenditures in 1962 of about $4 million.

In 1973, ODALE and ONNI were combined with BNDD to form the Drug Enforcement Administration. Also in 1973, the NIDA evolved from SAODAP and the Division of Narcotics and Drug Abuse to the NIMH. To date, the Drug Enforcement Agency (DEA) and the NIDA have pursued the law enforcement and drug research components of national drug policy (16).

Methadone Maintenance

Perhaps the most fundamental change in narcotics control of this period was the widespread use of methadone maintenance in control and treatment of narcotic addiction. The technique, begun in the 1960s, was given enthusiastic support by the Nixon administration, in no small measure because of its apparent effectiveness in reducing addict crime. Methadone is a long-acting synthetic narcotic that was developed in Germany during World War II. It is given orally to lessen or even eliminate the desire for heroin. Some of the similarities between the use of and theoretical justification for methadone maintenance now and morphine maintenance in the World War I period are obvious, and both have encountered some of the same practical problems.

Some experts say that methadone may be required by a hard-core addict indefinitely; that is, it does not end narcotic addiction but makes it more socially acceptable or feasible. This policy runs counter to an old theme in American attitudes, namely, that addiction should be stopped, not catered to. As realized a half century ago, however, a maintenance system, if deployed across the nation, is difficult to regulate, and diversion of supplies to nonaddicts can be a problem. One objection to the old maintenance clinics was the enormous profits garnered by some individuals who operated them; the implication was that profits stimulated the distribution of narcotics and the temptation to recruit new customers. Another problem was the failure of neat scientific explanations, such as Dr. Bishop's theory that a patient in precise opiate maintenance balance is quite normal. This did not work out so conveniently in practice. Maintenance, which was legal, for example, in New York State in 1918 and 1919, eventually led to abuses among health professionals and, in times of national fear, made the thousands of addicts scapegoats for social problems. Legal maintenance systems can thus become unpalatable or abhorred. They are sensitive to public pressure and political influences, and their existence is precarious, especially when the public believes that addiction itself is the cause of immorality, criminal behavior, and loss of productivity.

Changing Mores, Changing Laws

Gerald R. Ford brought a markedly different political style to the White House in August 1974. The new president wanted to distance himself from Nixon's heated antidrug rhetoric and from his management style that had concentrated power in the White House at the expense of the cabinet departments. To these ends, Ford adamantly resisted congressional attempts to institute an Office of Drug Control Policy in the White House to continue SAODAP-style oversight functions. He did sign amendments to the Drug Abuse Office and Treatment Act of 1972 that mandated establishment of such a body in the Executive Office of the President, but did not seek appropriations to fund it.

In March 1975, in the face of what appeared to be a worsening drug situation, the administration ordered a comprehensive study of the nature and extent of drug use and directions for future remedial policy. The study, known as the *White Paper on Drug Abuse*, was published in September 1975, and set a new tone for drug abuse policy in the years to come. It recognized that the "total elimination of drug abuse is unlikely, but government actions can contain the problem and limit its adverse effects," a view that presaged the "harm reduction" argument of today. It also established antidrug priorities: "All drugs are not equally dangerous, and all drug use is not equally destructive …. Priority in both supply and demand reduction should be directed toward those drugs which inherently pose a greater risk—heroin, amphetamines (particularly when used intravenously), and mixed barbiturates" (57).

In the end, Ford turned away from the spirit of the *White Paper* and, in an attempt to bolster his chances in the 1976 presidential elections, resorted to the law-and-order approach to narcotics control that still paralleled the sentiments of an ever-narrowing majority of voters. In April 1976, he introduced the Narcotic Sentencing and Seizure Act of 1976, which tried to revive the concept of mandatory minimum sentences for drug-trafficking offenses, and established cabinet committees for drug policy oversight and coordination. Whatever the merits of the bill, Ford was defeated, and the trend toward greater toleration of drug use and less emphasis on control of abuse through law enforcement accelerated.

The election of Jimmy Carter was most welcome to those who supported profound revision of the laws governing possession and use of recreational drugs, particularly marihuana. Carter appointed Dr. Peter Bourne as his special assistant for health issues and decided after some delay to implement the legislation establishing the Office of Drug Abuse Policy with Dr. Bourne as its head. Dr. Bourne set a tone of accommodation to the view that possession of marihuana in small amounts for personal use ought to be decriminalized as a step toward wiser and more just use of law-enforcement resources. Dr. Bourne was also of the opinion, as he wrote in August 1974, that "Cocaine … is probably the most benign of illicit drugs currently in widespread use. At least as strong a case could be made for legalizing it as for legalizing marihuana. Short-acting—about 15 minutes—not physically addicting, and acutely pleasurable, cocaine has found increasing favor at all socioeconomic levels in the last year" (58). But the career of Dr. Bourne dramatically illustrates that toleration of recreational drug use would not become characteristic of more than a vocal minority of Americans.

Bourne served the Carter administration from January 1977 until July 1978. During this time, drug policy continued to focus on the international aspects of the heroin problem and on domestic control of barbiturates and amphetamines. The Drug Strategy Council was revitalized and published national strategies for the duration of the administration. Bourne was able to report an apparent reversal of the 1974 and 1975 trends that had indicated a worsening heroin situation: Overdose death rates were declining, as were heroin prices and purity. In early 1977, President Carter decided to advocate decriminalization of marihuana in accordance with a trend that was being acted on by state legislatures throughout the nation. This was startling evidence of the profound change in attitudes toward drug consumption that had taken place since the 1960s. But in July 1978, Dr. Bourne resigned because of allegations that he had written a fraudulent prescription for methaqualone for a member of his staff and that he himself had used cocaine—an accusation that Bourne denied; the Carter administration was suddenly in no position to appear soft on the drug issue. Although not obvious to most observers at the time, the wave of toleration that had been rising since the 1960s had crested, and both public opinion and public policy were about to change course.

THE NEW WAR ON DRUGS (1980 TO THE PRESENT)

Cocaine and Drug Intolerance

As the 1980s opened, cocaine use became more common but seemed to be characteristic of an economic elite who preferred to sniff or inject it. But by the middle of the decade, the method of consuming cocaine was shifting to smoking. Cocaine hydrochloride had to be converted to a base form for successful volatilizing. At first, smokers would use a "free-base kit," a dangerous method involving open flames and ether, often purchased at a drug paraphernalia store or "head shop." Then, about 1985, drug dealers began distributing "crack" to the streets of America's large urban centers. "Crack" was a rocklike base form of cocaine that could be volatilized easily without requiring any preliminary ether treatment. The extraordinary blood levels of cocaine one could achieve by inhaling cocaine fumes from "crack," and its availability in units costing only a few dollars, greatly expanded the cocaine market among poor and minority populations. Accompanying the "crack epidemic" were turf wars in urban areas as sellers competed for territory. Through the latter part of the decade, the street price drifted lower until eventually, in terms of equivalent value, crack sold for less than cocaine had on New York City streets prior to the Harrison Act of 1914 (59).

The arrival of crack, coupled with the overdose deaths of well-known youthful sports stars, combined with growing political pressure from anxious and angry parents, contributed to a new sense of national crisis over the cocaine problem. From the historian's perspective, the shift in attitude was rapid, widespread, and profound. The perception of cocaine for many moved from that of a safe, nonaddictive tonic to that of a feared substance linked to ruined careers and families. The stereotypic "coke head"—anxious, fearful, paranoid, hyperactive, and out of touch with others—may be the most fear-producing drug image to the American public. Perhaps the change in attitude is so striking because the initial image of cocaine was so optimistic (60). The fear of cocaine as well as popular and, at times, expert opinion that cocaine use would continue unabated unless legislators took drastic action spurred Congress and President Reagan into dramatic attacks on the drug problem.

In the fall of 1986, shortly before congressional elections, the executive and legislative branches of the federal government competed to enact the most severe laws against drug use. Billions were authorized by the Anti-Drug Abuse Act of 1986, although much less was later appropriated by Congress (61). Many observers, especially those within the treatment community, believed that the actual impact and funding of the law was a discouraging anticlimax to the promises and expectations that had accompanied its passage.

In 1988, as the presidential election approached, the fear of cocaine was reflected in enormous media coverage. Democrats and Republicans were each expressing outrage over drugs and drug use, neither side wanting to appear less determined than its opponent. An emphasis on law enforcement, so characteristic of the decline phase of the earlier wave of drug use, was most clearly demonstrated by the competition between the two major presidential contenders in which the Democratic candidate proposed greatly expanding the number of DEA agents, a stance in favor of law enforcement that eloquently illustrated the great change that had taken place in American attitudes since the Carter–Ford campaign. In 1976, the candidates had vied with one another as to which would be more understanding of casual or recreational use of what were considered to be "soft" drugs.

The 1988 Anti-Drug Abuse Act, like the one passed 2 years earlier, authorized substantial sums for treatment, but about two thirds of funding went to law enforcement (62). Also, the 1988 act targeted the casual user much more prominently, with provisions such as fines for possession of personal amounts of drugs. An indication that the concern over drugs was expanding to include alcohol was the 1988 act's provision that a year after enactment, every bottle of beverage alcohol manufactured in the United States would have to carry a warning label.

One of the most significant provisions of the 1988 law was its Title I, known as the National Narcotics Leadership Act. Reaching back to the 1972 Drug Abuse Office and Treatment Act and the 1974 amendments to it, this title again established an Office of National Drug Control Policy (ONDCP) in the Executive Office of the President and with it the position of Director of National Drug Control Policy—the so-called "drug czar" (Table 1.1). The legislation also included a requirement that the executive branch provide a comprehensive national strategy with guidelines to measure its success. A series of federal strategies have been published since September 1989, including the latest one, put out by the George W. Bush White House in February 2002.

CONCLUSION

We can now look back on nearly four decades of continuous and widespread exposure to illicit drugs. Those who have lived through this most recent "drug epidemic" can testify to the remarkable change in attitude toward drugs since the 1970s. When we recall Jerry Rubin's claim in 1970 that "marijuana makes each person God," Timothy Leary's recommendation to youth to "turn on, tune in, and drop out," and a *Time* magazine cover in 1981 attractively exhibiting cocaine in a martini glass, we know that a shift in social norms has taken place. Legislatively, we have moved from softening of antidrug laws in the 1970s to renewing their severity since the late 1980s.

Our society has been through two "experiments in nature" regarding cocaine in the United States: twice (once beginning in the 1880s and again around 1970) a young population with no deeply held antagonism to the drug or even information about it has been exposed to the euphoric effects of cocaine. In each instance, 15 to 20 years passed before the nation started to change its mind on the value and risks of cocaine.

An important difference between the earlier cocaine problem and the present one is that the first anticocaine laws came as public attitudes turned against the drug, while in the current episode, severe anticocaine laws were on the statute books at the very beginning of the new infatuation. The result has been a much longer controversy over control of cocaine and the efficacy of legal restrictions than was the case early in the 20th century.

Debate over legalization of drugs received public prominence during the current wave of drug use, both as drug toleration was quickly rising—in the mid-1970s—and as drug toleration was rapidly falling—in the late 1980s. The dominant argument for legalizing or "decriminalizing" cocaine, marihuana, and opiates in each case reflects the shift in the public's assumptions about drugs. In the 1970s, the argument was commonly made that the drugs were relatively safe, especially when compared with alcohol or tobacco; in the recent controversy, the argument has seldom been made that a drug like cocaine is safe, but rather that availability of a cheaper product would end turf wars and allow the dollars spent on interdiction to be spent improving conditions in the inner city. Comparison with alcohol and tobacco seems

TABLE 1.1	Drug Czars[a]				
Name	Birth year	Appointed by	Term	Title	Field/prior experience	Summary
Dr. Jerome Jaffe	1933	Nixon	(1971–1973)	Director of SAODAP, Special Action Office for Drug Abuse Prevention	Pharmacology/psychiatry	Public health policy model; focus on treating heroin with methadone
Dr. Robert DuPont	1936	Nixon, continued under Ford	(1973–1977)	Director of NIDA, and head of Narcotics Treatment Administration	Psychiatry	Originally treatment/Methadone oriented
Dr. Peter Bourne	1939	Carter	(1977–1978)	Head of Office on Drug Abuse Policy	Physician/psychiatrist /treatment provider	Wanted to decriminalize marijuana possession. Focus on harm reduction. First to have control over both supply and demand
Lee Dogoloff	1939	Carter	(1978–1981)	Head of Office on Drug Abuse Police	Social work	Supported treatment. Came to focus on prevention of teenage marijuana use
Carlton Turner	1940	Reagan	(1981–1986)	Head of Office on Drug Abuse Police	Pharmacology. Director of the University of Mississippi Marijuana Research Program	Strongly supported parents' campaign to prevent adolescent use of marijuana. Less concerned about hard drugs or treatment for them
Dr. D. Ian MacDonald	1931	Carter	(1986–1988)	Deputy Director of Office on Drug Abuse Police	Pediatrician	Supported parents' antimarijuana activities
William Bennett	1943	George H.W. Bush	(1989–1990)	Director of ONDCP, Office of National Drug Control Policy	Secretary of Education	First Cabinet-level drug czar. Bennett, called for an "all-out war on drugs—with more resources for police, more prosecutors, more convictions." Resigned after 19 months

Robert Martinez	1934	(1991–1993)	George H.W. Bush	Director of ONDCP, Office of National Drug Control Policy	Governor of Florida	Continued Bennett's policies
Lee P. Brown	1937	(1993–1995)	Clinton	Director of ONDCP, Office of National Drug Control Policy	Law enforcement	Initially supported treatment as opposed to war on drugs, but had to change focus to marijuana use, in accordance with White House political stances
General Barry McCaffrey	1942	(1996–2001)	Clinton	Director of ONDCP, Office of National Drug Control Policy	Military	Supported treatment and stopping drug smuggling
John Walters	1952	(2001–1909)	George W. Bush	Director of ONDCP, Office of National Drug Control Policy	Career civil servant	Focused on marijuana, drug war, and stopping drug smuggling
Gil Kerlikowske	1942	(2009–)	Obama	Director of ONDCP, Office of National Drug Control Policy	Law enforcement	Renewed emphasis on treatment and public health as opposed to the war on drugs and incarceration. Drug czar is no longer a cabinet level post

[a]The title "drug czar" does not appear in a statute; it is an informal honorific that has been resisted by some of those listed in the table. President Nixon started the fashion by declaring that Dr. Jaffe was his drug czar.

Sources: Baum, D. *Smoke and Mirrors*. Boston, MA: Little, Brown, 1996; Massing, M. *The Fix*. New York, NY: Simon & Schuster, 1998; Frontline (PBS). *Thirty Years of America's Drug War*, 2000 (http://www.pbs.org/wgbh/pages/frontline/shows/drugs/).

to have diminished as the public has become increasingly alarmed at these two legal substances.

Crime reduction was a core goal of the Nixon administration's broad campaign against drugs. Interestingly, property crime has fallen since 1980 by about 63%. Violent crime has fallen by 48% in the past 10 years. Curiously, neither side in the drug debate makes much mention of these astounding statistics, which imply that much progress has been made toward the goal of the original impetus for national drug strategies.

The rise of acquired immune deficiency syndrome (AIDS) adds another dimension to drug abuse control; the epidemic is now spreading most rapidly among intravenous drug users, many of whom engage in both needle sharing and unprotected sex. Here the debate about relaxing legal restrictions has centered on the wisdom of distributing sterile syringes and needles, condoms, and methadone without many of the elaborate regulations now controlling this opioid. The full social and medical impact of AIDS lies in the future, but it would not be surprising if the stress of these concerns—as happened in the history of other chronic, often fatal diseases, such as tuberculosis—tended toward restrictive public policies (63).

Change in the perception of alcohol over the past 10 years is another marker of evolving attitudes toward psychoactive substances of all kinds. More people now regard alcohol as a dangerous substance, rather than as a beverage to be used in moderation with meals and on festive occasions. In 1984, the federal government required states to raise the drinking age to 21 years or lose a part of highway taxes; in 1989, as noted, all beverage alcohol had to carry warning labels; the federal government has pressured states to lower the driving under the influence level to 0.08% for those older than age 21 years, and to 0.02% for those younger than age 21 years. In the past, antagonism to alcohol has led, over three or four decades, to extreme restrictions, which, in turn, were followed by a backlash against alcohol's tarnished image. For almost 50 years following repeal of national prohibition in 1933, it was difficult to discuss the problems associated with alcohol consumption without being accused of sympathy with discredited prohibitionists. Now the mood has changed, and the task will be to see whether this time the nation can establish a sustainable alcohol policy that will not be swept aside in frustration and resentment.

Recent legislation bearing on drug abuse control attempts once again to make the consequences of violating drug laws more dire. The Violent Crime Control and Law Enforcement Act of 1994 enhanced penalties for drug trafficking in prisons and drug-free zones, allowed the president to declare a violent crime or drug emergency in a specific area on request of the state or local executive, and amended the National Narcotics Leadership Act of 1988 to strengthen ONDCP (64).

The question for public policy is the degree to which a growing reliance on law enforcement will be balanced by availability of treatment and sustained support for research.

As this chapter goes to press, there are a number of current trends that we would like to mention. First of all, the crack cocaine epidemic in the United States that began in the 1980s appears to be over, as evidenced by the statistics from national surveys and the D.C. Pretrial Services Administration's arrestee drug testing program. The percentage of arrestees in Washington, D.C. testing positive for cocaine metabolite peaked in 1988 at 64% and in the first 10 months of 2009 is averaging 29%, a level not seen since the mid-1980s at the beginning of the epidemic (65). This is an impressive trend, given that criminals would be expected to be among those least likely to desist from use of the drug. The national household survey statistics also reflect this decline but peaked earlier, with a peak of 17% of 18 to 25 years old reporting use of cocaine in the past year in the 1979 survey, compared with 5.5% in 2008 (66). The reasons behind the end of this Nation's second love affair with cocaine will be debated by historians and politicians for years.

As cocaine use recedes, the misuse of prescription drugs has expanded. In 2008, U.S. youths in grades 7 to 12 indicated that after marijuana, the misuse of inhalants and prescription drugs were tied as the second most prevalent drugs ever tried (67). In 2007, about one fourth of youths ages 12 to 17 who first started using drugs in the past year started with the nonmedical use of prescription-type drugs (68). The most commonly misused prescription drugs at all age levels are pain relievers (69). Furthermore, with the growing recognition of and treatment of attention deficit hyperactivity disorder, the misuse of prescription stimulants is being increasingly found among college students (70). The recent approval and expansion of the prescribing of buprenorphine for opiate addiction in the United States is another trend worthy of monitoring over the next decade, given other countries' experience with the abuse of this drug (71).

Finally, we must note the growing approval by states of the use of medical marijuana. As of this writing, 13 states have approved the prescribing of this drug (72). With the steep decline in cigarette use among high school seniors since 1997, the percentage of 12th grade students reporting use of marijuana in the past month in 2009 is virtually identical to the percentage who reported cigarette use (73). It remains to be seen how much marijuana use will grow as the medical use of marijuana becomes more prevalent and visible across the United States.

REFERENCES

1. Clark N. *Deliver us from Evil: An Interpretation of American Prohibition*. New York: WW Norton; 1976:29.
2. Beecher L. Six sermons on the nature, occasions, signs, evils and remedy of intemperance. 4th ed. 1828. In: Musto DF, ed. *Drugs in America: A Documentary History*. New York: New York University Press; 2002:44–86.
3. Timberlake JH. *Prohibition and the Progressive Movement*. Cambridge, MA: Harvard University Press; 1963.
4. Sinclair A. *Era of Excess: A social history of the Prohibition Movement*. New York: Harper & Row; 1962:36–49.
5. Terry CE, Pellens M. *The Opium Problem*. New York: Bureau of Social Hygiene; 1928:50–51, 929–937.
6. Sonnedecker G. Emergence of the concept of opiate addiction. *J Mon Pharm*. 1962;6:275.

7. Sonnedecker G. Emergence of the concept of opiate addiction. *J Mon Pharm.* 1963;7:27.
8. Musto DF, ed. *One Hundred Years of Heroin*. Westport, CT: Auburn House; 2002.
9. Wright H. Report on the international opium commission and on the opium problem as seen within the United States and its possession. In: 61st Congress, 2nd Session. *Opium Problem: Message from the President of the United States, February 21, 1910*. Senate document no. 377. Washington, DC: Government Printing Office; 1910:49.
10. Musto DF. The Marihuana Tax Act of 1937. *Arch Gen Psychiatry.* 1972;26:101–108.
11. Wilbert MI, Motter MG. *Digest of Laws and Regulations in Force in the United States Relating to the Possession, Use, Sale, and Manufacture of Poisons and Habit-forming Drugs*. Public Health Bulletin no. 56. Washington, DC: US Government Printing Office; 1912.
12. Dupree AH. *Science in the Federal Government: A History of Policies and Activities to 1940*. Cambridge, MA: Harvard University Press; 1957:267–270.
13. Young JH. *The Toadstool Millionaires: A Social History of Patent Medicines in America before Federal Regulation*. Princeton, NJ: Princeton University Press; 1961.
14. Taylor AH. *American Diplomacy and the Narcotics Traffic, 1900–1939: A Study in International Humanitarian Reform*. Durham, NC: Duke University Press; 1969:48–81.
15. United States 60th Congress. Public law no. 221. An act to prohibit the importation and use of opium for other than medicinal purposes. Approved February 9, 1909.
16. Musto DF. *The American Disease: Origins of Narcotic Control*. 3rd ed. New York: Oxford University Press; 1999:41–42.
17. State of Massachusetts, Acts of 1914, Chapter 694. An act to regulate the sale of opium, morphine and other narcotic drugs. Approved June 22, 1914.
18. Renborg BA. *International Drug Control: A Study of International Administration By and Through the League of Nations*. Washington, DC: Carnegie Endowment for International Peace; 1947:15–17.
19. Wright H. Uncle Sam is the worst drug fiend in the world. *New York Times.* 1911; March 12:(sect 5):12.
20. United States 63rd Congress. Public law no. 233. To provide for the registration of, with collectors of internal revenue, and to impose a special tax upon all persons who produce, import, manufacture, compound, deal in, dispense, sell, distribute, or give away opium or coca leaves, their salts, derivatives or preparations. Approved December 17, 1914.
21. United States Treasury Department. Treasury decision no. 2172. March 9, 1915.
22. *United States v. Jin Fuey Moy,* 241 U.S. 394 (1916).
23. Kolb L, DuMez AG. The prevalence and trend of drug addiction in the United States and factors influencing it. *Public Health Rep.* 1924;39:1179.
24. United States Treasury Department. *Traffic in Narcotic Drugs*. Washington, DC: US Government Printing Office; 1919.
25. Kuhne G. Statement of Gerhard Kuhne, head of Identification Bureau, New York City Department of Correction. In: *Conference on Narcotic Education: Hearings Before the Committee on Education of the House of Representatives, December 16, 1925*. Washington, DC: US Government Printing Office; 1926:175.
26. Mayor appoints drug committee. *New York Times.* 1919; May 27:9.
27. Murray RK. *Red Scare: A Study of National Hysteria, 1919–1920*. Minneapolis: University of Minnesota; 1955.
28. Federal Bureau of Narcotics. *Narcotic Clinics in the United States*. Washington, DC: US Government Printing Office; 1955.
29. Hubbard SD. New York City narcotic clinic and differing points of view on narcotic addiction. *New York City Department of Health Monthly Bulletin.* 1920; Jan:45–47.
30. United States 65th Congress. Public law no. 254, sections 1006 to 1009. An act to provide revenue, by paying special taxes for every person who imports, manufactures, produces, compounds, sells, deals in, dispenses or gives away opium. Approved February 24, 1919.
31. *Webb et al. v. United States,* 249 U.S. 96 (1919); *United States v. Doremus* 249 U.S. 86 (1919).
32. Bishop ES. *The Narcotic Drug Problem*. New York: Macmillan; 1920. Partially reprinted in David F. Musto, ed. *Drugs in America: A Documentary History*. New York: New York University Press; 2002:265–270.
33. American Medical Association, House of Delegates. Report of the committee on the narcotic drug situation in the United States. *JAMA.* 1920;74:1326.
34. DuMez AG. Increased tolerance and withdrawal phenomena in chronic morphinism. *JAMA.* 1919;72:1069.
35. Burrow JG. *AMA, Voice of American Medicine*. Baltimore: Johns Hopkins University Press; 1963.
36. United States 67th Congress. Public law no. 227. To amend the act of February 9, 1909, as amended, to prohibit the importation and use of opium for other than medicinal purposes. Approved May 26, 1922.
37. United States Senate, Committee on Printing. *Use of Narcotics in the United States, June 3, 1924*. Washington, DC: US Government Printing Office; 1924.
38. Hobson RP. The peril of narcotic drugs. *Congressional Record.* 1925; Feb 18:4088–4091.
39. United States 68th Congress. Public law no. 274. Prohibiting the importation of crude opium for the purpose of manufacturing heroin. Approved June 7, 1924.
40. United States 70th Congress. Public law no. 672. To establish two United States narcotic farms for the confinement and treatment of persons addicted to the use of habit-forming narcotic drugs who have been convicted of offenses against the United States. Approved January 19, 1929.
41. United States 71st Congress. Public law no. 357. To create in the Treasury Department a Bureau of Narcotics. Approved June 14, 1930.
42. United States House of Representatives, Committee on Ways and Means. *Bureau of Narcotics: Presentment and Report by the Grand Jury on the Subject of the Narcotic Traffic*. Filed February 19, 1930. Washington, DC: US Government Printing Office. 1930;Feb 19:73–77.
43. United States 75th Congress. Public law no. 238. To impose an occupational excise tax upon certain dealers in marihuana, to impose a transfer tax upon certain dealings in marihuana. Approved August 2, 1937.
44. United States 77th Congress. Public law no. 797. Opium poppy control act of 1942. Approved December 12, 1942.
45. Udell GG, compiler. *Opium and Narcotic Laws*. Washington, DC: US Government Printing Office; 1968.
46. United States 82nd Congress. Public law no. 255. To amend the penalty provision applicable to persons convicted of violating certain narcotic laws. Approved November 2, 1951.
47. United States 84th Congress. Public law no. 728. Narcotic control act of 1956. Approved July 18, 1956.
48. Joint Committee of the American Bar Association and the American Medical Association on Narcotic Drugs. *Interim and Final*

Reports. Drug Addiction: Crime or Disease? Bloomington, IN: Indiana University Press; 1961.
49. *Proceedings of the White House Conference on Narcotic and Drug Abuse.* Washington, DC: US Government Printing Office; 1962.
50. President's Advisory Commission on Narcotics and Drug Abuse. *Final Report.* Washington, DC: US Government Printing Office; 1963.
51. United States 89th Congress. Public law no. 89–74. Drug abuse control amendment act of 1965. Approved February 1965.
52. United States 89th Congress. Public law no. 793. Narcotic addict rehabilitation act of 1966. Approved November 8, 1966.
53. President's Commission on Law Enforcement and the Administration of Justice. *The Challenge of Crime in a Free Society.* Washington, DC: US Government Printing Office; 1967:228–229.
54. Musto DF, Korsmeyer P. *The Quest for Drug Control: Politics and Federal Policy in a Period of Increasing Substance Abuse, 1963–1981.* New Haven, CT: Yale University Press; 2002.
55. United States 91st Congress. Public law no. 513. Comprehensive drug abuse prevention and control act of 1970. Approved October 27, 1970.
56. United States 92nd Congress. Public law no. 92–255. Drug abuse office and treatment act of 1972. Approved March 21, 1972.
57. Domestic Council on Drug Abuse Task Force. *White Paper on Drug Abuse.* Washington, DC: US Government Printing Office. 1975:97–98.
58. Bourne PG. The great cocaine myth. *Drugs and Drug Abuse Education Newsletter.* 1974;5:5.
59. Musto DF. Illicit price of cocaine in two eras: 1908–1914 and 1982–1989. *Conn Med.* 1990;54:321–326.
60. Musto DF. America's first cocaine epidemic. *Wilson Q.* 1989;13:59–64.
61. United States 99th Congress. Public law no. 570. Anti-drug abuse act of 1986. Approved October 27, 1986. For summary, see *Congressional Quarterly Wkly Rep.* 1986;44(Oct 25):2699–2707.
62. United States 100th Congress. Public law no. 690. Anti-drug abuse act of 1988. Approved November 18, 1988. For summary, see *Congressional Quarterly Wkly Rep.* 1988;46(Nov 19):3145–3151.
63. Musto DF. Quarantine and the problem of AIDS. *Milbank Q.* 1986;64(suppl 1):97–117.
64. United States 103rd Congress. Public law no. 103–322. Violent crime control and law enforcement act of 1994. Approved September 13, 1994.
65. D.C. Pretrial Services Agency, Adult Drug Test Statistics. Available at: http://www.dcpsa.gov/foia/foiaERRpsa.htm. Accessed January 12, 2009.
66. Substance Abuse and Mental Health Services Administration. Cocaine use in the past year, by age group: percentages,1971–2008. *2008 NSDUH Detailed Tables, Table 8.40B;* 2009. Available at: http://www.oas.samhsa.gov/NSDUH/2K8NSDUH/tabs/Sect8peTabs39to40.pdf.
67. Center for Substance Abuse Research (CESAR). Marijuana, inhalants, and prescription drugs are top three substances abused by teens. *CESAR FAX* 18(9), March 9, 2009, Available at:http://www.cesar.umd.edu/cesar/cesarfax/vol18/18-09.pdf.
68. Center for Substance Abuse Research (CESAR). 56% of youths who first started using drugs in the past year began with marijuana; around one-fourth started with nonmedical use of prescription-yype drugs. *CESAR FAX* 18(15), April 20, 2009. Available at: http://www.cesar.umd.edu/cesar/cesarfax/vol18/18-20.pdf.
69. Substance Abuse and Mental Health Services Administration. *Results from the 2008 National Survey on Drug Use and Health: National Findings;* 2009.
70. Center for Substance Abuse Research (CESAR). Prescription stimulants: the "New Caffeine" for enhancing college students' academic performance? *CESAR FAX* 14(34), August 22, 2005. Available at: http://www.cesar.umd.edu/cesar/cesarfax/vol18/18-09.pdf.
71. Agar M, Bourgois P, French J, et al. Buprenorphine: "field trials" of a new drug. *Qual Health Res.* 2001;11(1):69–84.
72. Marijuana Policy Project. *State-by-State Medical Marijuana Laws;* 2008. Available at: http://www.mpp.org/assets/pdfs/download-materials/SBSR_NOV2008_1.pdf.
73. Center for Substance Abuse Research (CESAR). U.S. high school seniors now as likely to be smoking cigarettes as marijuana. *CESAR FAX* 18(2), January 29, 2009. Available at: http://www.cesar.umd.edu/cesar/cesarfax/vol18/18-02.pdf.

CHAPTER 2: Epidemiology—The United States

Charles Winick ■ Jack Levinson

Epidemiology—the population distribution and determinants of the use and problems related to alcohol, tobacco, and other drugs (ATOD)—plays a central role in drug control and health policies in the United States. It permits us to track changes in substance use and abuse through time, and across groups and regions. Epidemiology contributes to the social ecology of substance use, as in its clarification of how the visibility of drug problems—though traditionally associated with neighborhood disadvantage, concentration of minorities, and population density—is not related to levels of drug use (1).

MAJOR SOURCES OF EPIDEMIOLOGICAL DATA

Since 1971, the National Survey on Drug Use and Health (NSDUH) (formerly the National Household Survey on Drug Abuse), sponsored by the Substance Abuse and Mental Health Services Administration (SAMHSA), has been the leading source on incidence and prevalence of ATOD. Since 1999, NSDUH uses an interactive, bilingual, computer-assisted home interview with an annual sample of roughly 67,500 persons 12 and older (2). Between 2002 and 2007, the overall rate of illicit drug use has remained stable.

Beginning in 1975, the University of Michigan has annually conducted Monitoring the Future (MTF), sponsored by the National Institute on Drug Abuse (NIDA). MTF, using self-report questionnaires in schools, is the primary source for survey data on ATOD use by secondary school students. The 2008 MTF sample was about 46,000 students from 386 schools. From 2002 to 2008, annual rates of illicit drug use by 8th, 10th, and 12th graders remained stable or showed modest declines (3).

The National Institute on Alcohol Abuse and Alcoholism (NIAAA) sponsors the National Alcohol Survey (NAS), conducted by the Alcohol Research Group, University of California at Berkeley. NIAAA has also sponsored the longitudinal National Epidemiologic Survey on Alcohol and Related Conditions (NESARC), the largest comorbidity study of alcohol use disorder and treatment utilization among the civilian population, with a sample of roughly 43,000; the first wave of computer-assisted home interviews was conducted in 2001 to 2002 and the second in 2004 to 2005 (4). Among findings from the second wave was that 5.6% of American adults used both alcohol and drugs in the past year and 1.1% had comorbid alcohol and drug use disorders. Past week use of an illicit drug, other drug use, and drug use disorders increased among those with increasing levels of alcohol use and alcohol use disorders (5).

Data on alcohol consumption, along with tobacco and other drug use, are collected by the NSDUH and MTF. The Centers for Disease Control and Prevention (CDC) also provide national data on alcohol and tobacco, via two surveys. First, the Behavioral Risk Factor Surveillance System (BRFSS) is an annual state-based telephone survey of the adult civilian population that began in 1984 and by 1994 had incorporated all 50 states and additional U.S. territories. Second, the Youth Risk Behavior Survey (YRBS), started in 1990, is conducted every 2 years with a sample size of 12,000 to 16,000.

The Drug Abuse Warning Network (DAWN) reports drug-related emergency visits from hospitals in major metropolitan areas and since 1992, has been administered by SAMHSA's Office of Applied Studies (OAS). DAWN tracks all drugs, including over the counter medications and dietary supplements. Fatalities directly or indirectly related to drug use are reported by a sample of coroners and medical examiners. For alcohol alone, drug-related emergency department visits are recorded only for patients under 21. DAWN drug-related visits may result from chronic or unexpected reactions; accidental ingestion or reactions that do not suggest abuse are excluded. The 2006 DAWN national estimates were derived from a sample of 205 hospitals, with 28% of DAWN visits involving pharmaceutical drugs only and 31% illicit drugs only (6). For the most often reported major illicit drugs—cocaine, marihuana, heroin, and stimulants—there were no significant changes from 2004 through 2006.

A key source of regional data is the Community Epidemiology Work Group (CEWG), established in 1976 by NIDA to conduct surveillance in 21 major metropolitan areas, where working groups use survey and qualitative methods to gather data. CEWG epidemiologists meet biannually to assess patterns of use, substance purity, prices, and distribution (7).

SOCIODEMOGRAPHIC FACTORS AND SPECIAL POPULATIONS

Gender Differences

Males' higher use rate than females of most illicit substances increases with age (2). In 2007, among those aged 12 to 17, 10% of males and 9.1% of females were current users of illicit drugs (defined as use in the past month). Among 18 to 25 year olds, 24.1% of males but 15.3% of females reported past month use and for those 26 and older, only 8% of men and 3.8% of women did so. Some 27.1% of men smoked cigarettes in the past month compared to 21.5% of women, while 56% of men and 46% of women reported binge or heavy alcohol use.

Race and Ethnicity

Rates of illicit drug use in the past month in 2007 for persons aged 12 and older were 4.2% for Asians, 6.6% for Hispanics, 8.2% for whites, 9.5% for blacks, and 12.6% for American and Alaskan Natives (2). Though current use of illicit drugs by black adults roughly equals that of whites, black adolescents have always had substantially lower rates of illicit drug use and cigarette smoking than whites (3). Hispanic adolescents also have lower rates than whites except for some drugs in both the 8th and 12th grades.

The race/ethnicity age crossover effect refers to the consistent finding that despite varying rates of use across racial groups during adolescence and young adulthood, by the mid-thirties such rates are roughly equivalent. Analysis of NSDUH data from 1999 to 2002 suggests that this difference between black and white substance use can be explained by sociodemographic factors, such as patterns of availability and exposure in adulthood (8). When sociodemographic factors are controlled, the crossover effect between whites and blacks disappears and the rates of illegal drug use among black men and heavy drinking among black women are lower than among whites. ATOD use has different meanings and functions for specific subgroups, and risk and protective factors relevant to such use may operate differently across ethnic/racial subgroups (9).

National civilian use rates are inconsistent with those of different racial/ethnic groups in treatment and prison settings. Treatment admissions for marihuana, the most commonly used illicit drug, were 13.5% white and 21.9% black in 2007 (10).

Drug Users and Drug-Related Offenders in the Criminal Justice System

Substance abuse or dependence among individuals involved in the criminal justice system, incarcerated or otherwise, is more than four times that of the general population (11). A large proportion of the incarcerated are presumed to have a substance abuse disorder, with a range from half to more than two-thirds (12, 13). In 2004, 53% of state and 45% of federal inmates met DSM-IV criteria for abuse or dependence (14). Some 32% of state and 26% of federal prisoners in 2004 had used a psychoactive drug at the time they committed their crimes (15).

Some 2.3 million Americans are behind bars; the United States has 5% of the world's population but nearly 25% of its prisoners (16). From 2000 to 2006, persons incarcerated in federal prisons increased by 5% and by another 1.7% from 2006 to 2007 (17). The sharp increase in U.S. prison inmates since the 1980s has resulted from changes in law enforcement and sentencing procedures. Drug offenders accounted for 24.9% of federal prisoners in 1980, 52.2% in 1990, increased to 60.7% in 1994 and 1995, and declined to 54.1% in 2004 (18). The proportion of drug offenders in federal prisons increased by 4% from 2000 to 2006 and by another 1.7% from 2006 to 2007 (17). In state prisons in 2007, drug offenders represented 19.5% of the total population and 15.4% of white prisoners, compared to 22.5% of black and 21.3% of Hispanic prisoners.

Most correctional facilities offering substance abuse programs are less likely to involve clinical treatment than education and awareness activities, offered in 74% of prisons and 61% of jails, or low-intensity group counseling (for less than 4 hours per week), offered in 55% of prisons and 60% of jails (19). However, less than a quarter of those incarcerated actually have access to these services and few correctional agencies have the means to identify the offender pool needing treatment.

The Life Cycle and Substance Use

The concept of "maturing out" of narcotic addiction directed attention to the relationship between substance use and the life cycle (20). Different subgroups appear to have different rates of loosening and/or maintaining their ties to a substance. Such rates are associated with a range of social and individual variables (21). Current drug use has consistently reached a peak in late adolescence and young adulthood and then declined dramatically. In 2007, current use of any illicit drug was 3.3% for ages 12 or 13, 8.9% for those 14 or 15, 16% for those 16 or 17, and 21.6% for those 18 to 20 (2). For persons aged 21 to 25, rates decline to 18.5% and for those 26 to 34 to 10.9%. Current drug use continues to decline further with age to 4.1% for those 55 to 59, 1.9% for those 60 to 64, and 0.7% for those 65 and older.

Across age groups, the highest rates of past month illicit drug use are associated with heavy alcohol use (defined as 5 or more drinks on the same occasion on each of 5 days in the past 30 days); rates decline for binge alcohol users (defined as 5 or more drinks on the same occasion) who are not heavy users and also for alcohol users who do not binge (2). Concurrent alcohol and illicit drug use declines consistently with age: in 2007, for persons aged 12 to 17, 60.1% of heavy drinkers used illicit drugs, 48.4% of those aged 18 to 25 did so, along with 22.8% of the 26+ age group.

Epidemiological research has recently examined the association between population-based factors and the life cycle of drug use, showing how some common sociodemographic factors have a different impact on the transitions in drug use careers (22). Birth cohort was strongly associated with access and opportunity to try drugs for the first time, as well as to remission from drug use disorders. However, birth cohort was not associated with transition to abuse or dependence. The specific type of drug and individual history of drug use were strongly associated with transition from use to abuse and to dependence. Women abusers were more likely than men to transition to dependence but also more likely to transition to remission.

Employment status is a significant predictor of past month illicit drug use and is related to age. In 2007, for unemployed persons aged 18 or older, the rate of past month use was 18.3% but 8.4% for those employed full time and 10.1% for those employed part time (2). However, studies since the early 1970s have shown that some occupational environments involve factors that increase the risk of substance misuse (23). Notably, physicians and other medical workers have had historically higher rates and/or different patterns of substance abuse because of the combination of access to and knowledge about drugs, including a sense of invulnerability to potential drug problems, and the unique pressures and role strain related to medical work conditions (24). Research has shown higher rates of nonprescription use of certain drugs among physicians (25), anesthesiology residents (26), nurses (27), pharmacists (28), and hospital employees with access to drugs (29).

Geographic Factors

Local and regional variation can be best explained by factors such as different populations, social class and subcultural differences, proportion of age groups, and climate. In 2007, 8.3% of those aged 12 or older reported past month illicit drug use in large metropolitan areas but only 4.1% did so in rural areas (2). Rates of current cigarette use for those 12 and above in 2007 are lower in large urbanized metropolitan areas (22.7%) than in small metropolitan areas (24.8%), urbanized nonmetropolitan areas (28%), and in less urbanized nonmetropolitan areas (29.5%).

In 2007, illicit drug use was 9.3% in the West, 7.9% in the Midwest, 7.8% in the Northeast, and 7.4% in the South (2). Methamphetamine's history of high prevalence in the West stretches back to the 1960s. Between 2002 and 2005, 1.2% in the West reported using it in the past year as opposed to 0.5% in the Midwest and South and 0.1% in the Northeast (30). Not only are there strong regional preferences for types of alcoholic beverages but rates of use also vary: in 2007, for those aged 12 and above, past month alcohol use was lower in the South (46.8%) and West (50.8%) than in the Northeast (56%) and Midwest (54.6%) (2).

COMORBIDITY

Mental Health

Since the 1990s, there has been growing interest in the comorbidity of drug use disorders with each other and with psychiatric syndromes, such as depression, antisocial personality disorder, generalized anxiety disorder, and mood disorders (31). In 2007, among people with drug abuse or dependence aged 18 or older, past month use of alcohol or illicit drugs was 8.8% among those who had a major depressive episode in the past year compared to 2.1% who had not (2). For alcohol alone, past month use was reported by 17% of those who had a major depressive episode in the past year compared with 7% who had not.

Comorbidity research was facilitated in part by the DSM-IV because it categorized co-occurring disorders as primary (31). Most people with substance abuse disorders do not receive treatment, and treatment disparities exist among those at high risk even though they have disability and co-occurring disorders (31,33). In the preparation of DSM-V, some researchers argue that further refinement of primary co-occurring disorders would improve clinical reliability and encourage longitudinal research (32,33).

HIV and HCV

Since the advent of human immunodeficiency virus (HIV) in the early 1980s, men who have unprotected sex with men (MSM) have accounted for the vast majority of cases; the next largest group consists of injection drug users (IDUs) and their mostly female sexual partners. HIV incidence has declined dramatically from the late 1980s. Although HIV increased slightly among MSM since the 1990s, it continued to decline among IDUs. For the estimated annual incidence of HIV between 2003 and 2006, approximately 56% are MSM, 11% are IDUs, and 3% are both MSM and IDUs (34).

In 2008, all 50 states began reporting new HIV diagnoses to the CDC and relatively new assay technology makes it possible to determine the recency of infection. Since the late 1990s, HIV incidence among IDUs has dropped 80% because of the growth of syringe exchange programs (SEPs), decriminalization and availability of syringes, and education/awareness programs of needle sharing and cleaning (34).

Since the 1990s, there has been concern about the association between noninjection illicit drug and alcohol use and sexual transmission of HIV and other infections among MSM. In particular, the increasing popularity of methamphetamine among certain segments of gay men has been associated with increasing rates of sexually transmitted infection (35). The connection between substance abuse and behaviors that facilitate transmission among those who are already HIV infected remains a growing concern (36).

The vast majority of hepatitis C virus (HCV) cases in the United States are from IDUs. HCV incidence peaked in the mid to late 1990s and then declined substantially from 5.2 cases per 100,000 population in 1995 to 0.5 in 2007 among the age group that historically had the highest rates of infection (25–39 years) (37). The drop in HCV incidence could be attributable to the growth of services, however limited, that provide or enable access to clean syringes and information about cleaning and sharing needles. Still, the prevalence of chronic HCV in 2007 was substantial, with approximately 3.2 million persons infected, largely among those aged 40 to 49, most of whom were likely infected through needle use in the 1970s and 1980s.

SUBSTANCES

Alcohol

Alcohol is the most commonly used psychoactive substance in the United States. NSDUH reported that 60.8% of Americans 26 and older were current alcohol users in 2007 (2).

For those 18 and older in that year, BRFSS reported that 54.8% were current users (38). In the 2007 NSDUH, 31.4% of those over 26 reported binge drinking and 10.1% reported heavy drinking (as defined above) (2). BRFSS, which defines binge drinking by gender (five drinks at a time for men, four for women), in 2007 found that 15.8% of respondents reported an episode of binge drinking in the last month (21.2% of men and 10.1% of women) (38). Even though the BRFSS threshold of heavy drinking (two drinks per day for men and one for women) is lower than the NSDUH, only 6.1% of men and 4% of women reported that they are heavy drinkers.

In the 2007 NSDUH, of the 56.1% of whites who reported past month use, 16.8% reported binge use and 7.8% reported heavy use; of the 39.3% of blacks who were past month users, 15% reported binge drinking and 4.1% heavy drinking (2). American and Alaskan Natives had the highest proportion of binge and heavy use: of the 44.7% who are past month users, 16.6% are binge users and 11.6% are heavy users. Hispanics also have a higher proportion of binge and heavy alcohol use than whites and blacks: of the 42.1% who are past month users, 17.9% reported binging and 5.5% heavy use. Asians have the lowest proportion of all groups: of the 35.2% past month users, only 10% reported an episode of binging and 2.6% heavy use.

According to the BRFSS, between 2001 and 2007, current alcohol use among adults (at least one drink in the past month) appears relatively stable for whites at roughly 59% and for blacks at roughly 43% (38). For both these groups, there was an increase: for whites, from 58.6% (2001) to 60.4% (2002) and 62.1% (2003); and for blacks, from 41.5% (2001) to 45.4% (2002) and 45% (2003). For Hispanics, however, past month use has declined consistently from 52.2% in 2001 to 44.8% in 2007 without increasing in 2002 and 2003. NAS researchers have shown that social disadvantage is associated with psychological distress and problem drinking across racial/ethnic groups (39).

Underage drinking is a continuing concern. Past month alcohol use among those aged 12 to 17 has dropped slightly but significantly from 17.6% in 2002 to 15.9% in 2007 and, consistent with the life cycle, rates of past month use in this group increased with age (2). MTF shows steady but significant declines over the past 10 years in past month alcohol use (28% of 8th, 10th, and 12th graders combined in 2008) and having been drunk in the past month (14.9%) (3). However, trend analysis data from six NASs between 1979 and 2005 suggest that although mean values of drinking measures have declined for those over 26, there has been an increase both in alcohol volume and drinking days among those 18 to 25, indicating the possibility of a sustained increase in future U.S. alcohol consumption (40).

Driving under the influence of alcohol became a major concern in the 1980s, when states increased the legal drinking age to 21. In the past 30 years, there has been a substantial decline in the number of social drinkers arrested for driving under the influence (DUI) (41). DUI rates in the past year reflect, in part, the relationship between drinking behavior and age: 7.8% for the 16- to 17-year-old group, 18.3% for the 18 to 20 group, and 25.8% of 21 to 25 year olds. For the 26- to 29-year-old group, the rate declined to 20.1%. Overall, for Americans 12 and older, past year DUI declined modestly but significantly from 2002 (14.2%) to 2008 (12.7%). Up to 70% of drivers arrested have previous alcohol- or drug-related offenses, and binge/heavy drinkers accounted for most episodes of alcohol-impaired driving (51.3%).

NSDUH annual estimates of Americans with substance abuse or dependence have remained stable between 2002 and 2007 at just above 22 million (2). The vast majority—roughly 15.5 million—abuse or are dependent on alcohol alone; 3.2 million abuse or are dependent on both alcohol and illicit drugs. In an analysis of 2006 and 2007 data, 5.6% of past month alcohol users also used an illicit drug within 2 hours of drinking. Binge drinkers were far more likely to use an illicit drug (13.9%) than nonbinge past month alcohol users (3.8%). Adolescents and young adults who were past month alcohol users were far more likely than older age groups also to have used illicit drugs: 14.2% for the 12 to 17 group and 13.5% for 18 to 25, 7.7% for 26 to 34, 4.3% for 35 to 49, and 1.1% for 50 and over (42). The illicit drug used most frequently in concurrence with alcohol was marihuana (4.8%) followed by cocaine (0.06%) and pain relievers (0.04%). There is no evidence, over time, of a displacement effect between teen alcohol and marihuana use, which have run in parallel (3).

Marihuana

Since the 1970s, marihuana has been by far the most commonly used illicit drug. In 2007, of Americans 12 or older, 40.6% had tried marihuana at least once, 10.1% had used in the past year, and 5.8% or 14.4 million in the past month (2). Some 31 states and the District of Columbia currently have laws that recognize marihuana's medical value. Since 1996, 13 of these states have enacted laws, 9 of which were established by popular ballot, that permit patients to use marihuana despite the conflict with the federal zero-tolerance policy.

The declining stigma of marihuana may have contributed to slight increases in its use during the 1990s. Along with more marihuana-related emergency room visits, there were substantial increases in arrests and treatment admissions. There has been a slight but significant decline in past month use from 11% in 2002 to 10.1% in 2007 (2). Even youths aged 12 to 17, whose rates of past month marihuana use had increased through the 1990s, declined from 8.2% in 2002 to 6.8% in 2005 and had remained stable (43). Despite these declines, analysis of substantial national increases in annual marihuana arrests suggests that low-level marihuana offenders have become a focus of drug enforcement strategy. National arrests for marihuana, which had declined to about 325,000 in 1991, increased to more than 725,000 in 2000 (44) and even as use declined further, the number of arrests continued to increase to about 873,000 in 2007 (45). Few of these arrests were for serious offenses and in 2000 only 6% resulted in a felony conviction. By 2002, marihuana arrests represented 45% of the 1.5 million drug arrests annually (44). Between 1990 and

2000, U.S. marihuana arrests increased two and a half times but in New York City, marihuana possession arrests increased tenfold (46). From 1997 to 2006, in New York City, 335,000 people were arrested and jailed for possessing small amounts of marihuana, 11 times the number in the previous decade. These arrests disproportionately involve young racial/ethnic minority men: between 1997 and 2006, 52% of arrestees were black, 31% Hispanic, and 15% white.

Marihuana was considered the primary drug in the gateway theory of substance abuse, which suggested that teenagers using marihuana were likely to begin using substances such as heroin or cocaine. Some researchers now treat alcohol and tobacco as the initial substances in a normative sequence of drug initiation (47) with marihuana viewed as a terminus rather than a gateway (48).

However, in 2007 only 1.6% of Americans were estimated to have marihuana dependence or abuse, representing a slight but significant decline from 1.8% in 2002 (2). SAMHSA's Treatment Episode Data Set (TEDS) reports that primary treatment admissions for marihuana increased from 11.7% of all admissions in 1996 to 15.8% in 2007 (10,49). Nationally, between 1996 and 2006, the rate of marihuana user admissions increased by 32% from 91 to 120 per 100,000 population aged 12 and over (49). Fifty-seven percent of marihuana admissions resulted from criminal justice referrals (10). Considering the relatively low rate of marihuana dependence/abuse overall and that 63.1% of its treatment admissions are aged 24 and under (49), a sizable number of these referrals could have come to the attention of law enforcement for reasons unrelated to marihuana but attributed to problem use.

Tobacco

Of all substance use, cigarette smoking has the most substantial long-term negative health effects. Rates of current cigarette use have been declining, especially since the late 1990s, with the continued expansion of legal prohibitions, higher taxes, and increasingly negative attitudes toward smokers and smoking (3,50,51). Between 2002 and 2007, past month American cigarette smokers declined from 26% to 24.2% (60.1 million) (2).

Most smokers begin in adolescence and, after a decline through most of the 1980s, current cigarette use among teenagers and young adults began to increase and peaked in the mid-1990s (3,50). Still, the declines in this age group are greater than the overall decline: among 12 to 17 year olds, 9.8% were past month users in 2007, down from 13% in 2002 (2). Between 1996 and 2008, current smoking has declined substantially among 8th graders (67%) and 10th graders (60%) and a cohort effect seems to explain the more modest 44% decline among 12th graders (3).

Heroin and Other Opiates

During the 1990s, heroin of relatively high purity and lower cost became widely available and was accompanied by a rise in intranasal sniffing and smoking in some areas (52). By the end of the decade, increased "cutting" of heroin began to decrease purity (53) and through the 2000s, fluctuating and generally lower purity has usually been accompanied by increased prices (7). Only 0.1% of Americans 12 and older have reported past month heroin use between 2002 and 2007 (2). Among 12th graders, the annual prevalence of heroin use between 1975 and 1979 fell from 1% to 0.5% and then remained steady until the early 1990s, peaking at 1.5% in 2000 (3). Since then, annual prevalence among 12th graders has declined, fluctuating slightly, to 0.9% in 2007 and 0.7% in 2008.

Since the early 2000s, most parts of the country have reported growing nonprescription use of pharmaceutical opiates such as oxycodone (OxyContin) and hydrocodone (Vicodin). Between 2002 and 2007, previous year illicit use of pharmaceutical pain relievers rose slightly but significantly, from 4.7% to 5% among Americans 12 and older (2). OxyContin has remained steady at 0.5% since 2004. Similarly, past month use of pain relievers in Americans 12 and older has increased slightly from 1.6% in 2002 to 2.1% in 2007 and 2008. In 2007, oxycodone and hydrocodone appeared in the top 10 ranked drugs identified in forensic laboratories in CEWG areas and were the two most frequently identified narcotic analgesics/opiates (7). However, they represented about 1% or less of drugs reported. Among 12th graders, after trending down, the early 1990s saw a rise in annual use of narcotics other than heroin from 3.3% in 1992, peaking at 9.5% in 2004 (3). In contrast to the overall declines in drug use by adolescents since 2004, their prevalence rates of narcotics other than heroin have remained steady at about 9%.

Cocaine

Between 2002 and 2007, the prevalence of past month use of cocaine hydrochloride by Americans 12 and older has remained stable, hovering at 0.9% in 2002, 0.8% in 2004, 1% in 2006, and 0.8% in 2007 (2). Relatively few Americans used crack in the past month: 0.2% in 2002, 0.3% in 2005, and 0.3% in 2007. In 2008, 1.9% of 12th graders reported use of cocaine in the past 30 days, a rate which has been stable since 1991 (3). For crack, 0.9% of 12th graders used in the last 30 days, a rate which has also remained stable since 1991.

Despite low overall rates of use, the majority of drug-related emergency room visits involved cocaine, with blacks and whites accounting for roughly equal numbers (6). Among cocaine abusers, crack remains predominant across 11 CEWG areas in 2008, when between 56% and 95% of cocaine treatment admissions were crack smokers (7).

Club Drugs

Since the 1980s, drugs such as MDMA, GHB, and ketamine have been referred to as club drugs because they have been associated with dance parties and nightclubbing. However, these drugs, especially MDMA or ecstasy, the most commonly used club drug, are also used in different settings for other reasons (54,55). Past month ecstasy use among Americans 12 and older dropped slightly but significantly from 0.3% in 2002 to 0.2% in 2003 through 2007 (2). In 2008, 2.9% of 8th, 10th, and 12th graders had used ecstasy at least once and 0.9% and 1.2% had used GHB and ketamine, respectively (3). Ecstasy use dropped in this group from a peak of 2.4% in 2002 to 1.2% in 2008.

Amphetamine-Like Stimulants

Methamphetamine

In the early 1990s, concern grew about the expectation that methamphetamine would move eastward. By 1996, methamphetamine became a focus of legislation and drug-abuse agencies. Through the late 1990s, both methamphetamine-related emergency room visits and treatment admissions increased, although these numbers began to decline overall. The number of Americans 12 and older who used methamphetamine nonmedically in the past year changed little from 1999 (0.5%) to 2004 (0.6%) (56).

There were relatively low rates of methamphetamine use between 2002 and 2005 by Americans 12 and older, both for annual use (0.7% in 2002 and 0.5% in 2005) and past month use (0.3% in 2002 and 0.2% in 2005) (57). The 18 to 25 group in 2002 used 0.5% in the past month and 0.6% in 2005. Previous month use has remained stable, with 0.2% of those 12 and older using in the past month in 2007 (2).

Concerns about the eastward movement of methamphetamine have not been confirmed. Its regional appeal is confirmed in rates of use (30), treatment admissions, and laboratory forensics (7). In high-use areas, the major routes of administration are smoking or injecting; in contrast, in New York City the primary route of administration is inhalation.

Pharmaceutical Stimulants

The nonmedical use of pharmaceutical stimulant drugs such as amphetamine (Adderall) and methylphenidate (Ritalin) has been a growing concern since the 1990s, especially among youth and college students. As with other teenage drug use, pharmaceutical stimulant use peaked in 1996, when 4.8% of 8th, 10th, and 12th graders combined used in the past 30 days, but their use declined to 3.9% in 2003 and 2.6% in 2008 (3). In contrast to these rates of use, more high schoolers perceive these drugs as easily available. In 2008, 12.8% of 8th graders said the drug was "fairly" or "very" easy to obtain, along with 32% of 10th graders and 47.9% of 12th graders. The higher rate among 12th graders is curious in light of their high rates of disapproval: 87.2% disapprove of using amphetamine once or twice and 94.2% disapprove of its regular use.

Among college students and their age peers, amphetamine use also increased through the 1990s, with college students having lower rates. Even so, in the 1990s and 2000s, rates for college students, their noncollege age peers, and 12th graders were substantially lower than in the 1980s. In the 2000s, use among 12th graders and the noncollege group declined, while annual use among college students increased to 7.2% in 2001 and remained stable at 6.9% in 2007 (58). Monthly prevalence rates among college students reflect a similar pattern, with 3.3% in 2001 and 3.1% in 2007. College students vastly overestimate the levels of nonmedical use of pharmaceutical drug among their peers, as they also do with alcohol and other substances (59).

NSDUH indicates that college students nonmedically using Adderall were more likely to use other drugs (60). Among Adderall users, 8.6% were white, 2.2% were Hispanic, 2.1% were Asian, and 1% were black. There is also difference in rates of use by family income, with the highest use (8.9%) among college students from families earning under $20,000 per year, followed by students from families with incomes of $75,000 or more (6%). Only 3% of students from families with incomes between $20,000 and $49,000 and 2% from those earning $50,000 and $75,000 are users.

DRUG ABUSE AND TREATMENT

In 2007, 22.3 million Americans aged 12 and older were classified with substance dependence or abuse in the past year (based on DSM-IV), a number that has remained stable since 2002 (2). Roughly 15.5 million were dependent on or abusing alcohol only, 3.7 million illicit drugs only, and 3.2 million were dependent on or abused both alcohol and illicit drugs. In 2007, men were twice as likely (3.8%) as women (2.1%) to report past year abuse or dependence. Past year dependence or abuse changes dramatically with age: in 2007, 4.3% of the 12 to 17 group had problems with illicit drugs and 5.4% with alcohol; 7.9% of those 18 to 25 had problems with illicit drugs and 16.8% with alcohol. For those 26 or older, 1.7% had problems with illicit drugs and 6.2% with alcohol. There are racial/ethnic differences among those classified as having substance abuse or dependence: white 9.4%, black 8.5%, Hispanic 8.3%, and Native Americans/Alaskans 13.4% in 2007. The disproportion is greater for those who received treatment: 18.2% of blacks who needed treatment received it in contrast with 9.9% of whites, possibly because relatively more African Americans are involved with public agencies.

In 2007, 7.5 million Americans aged 12 or older needed treatment for an illicit drug problem but only 1.3 million (17.8%) received it at a specialty facility, leaving 6.2 million in need of treatment (2). Of the 19.3 million people who needed treatment for alcohol, only 1.6 million (8.1%) received it, so that 17.7 million people remained without treatment. In 2007, 2.7 million people received treatment for a problem with alcohol or an illicit drug in the past year at a rehabilitation facility. Just less than 2.2 million of the people who received treatment in 2007 did so in self-help groups. These figures changed little between 2002 and 2007. Based on combined 2004 to 2007 NSDUH data, 35.9% of those who tried to get treatment failed because of lack of funds or health coverage.

The proportion of dependence on or abuse of specific drugs has remained stable since 2002, with the exception of a slight but significant decline for marihuana and hashish (1.8% in 2002, 1.9% in 2004, and 1.6% in 2007). Of those persons classified as having substance abuse or dependence, the largest proportion is for marihuana, with approximately 3.9 million in 2007. Approximately 1.7 million used pain relievers and 1.5 million used cocaine.

From 1996 to 2006, roughly 40% of TEDS treatment admissions were not in the labor force and 30% were unemployed (49). Well over half the admissions during this period were between the ages of 25 and 44, roughly 70% were men, and about 60% of all admissions were white, while blacks comprised 25.7% in 1996 and 21.3% in 2006.

Five substances represented 96% of TEDS admissions in 2007: alcohol (40%); opiates, primarily heroin (19%); marihuana/hashish (16%); cocaine (13%); and stimulants, primarily methamphetamine (8%) (10). Between 1996 and 2006, 40% of admissions were for problems with both alcohol and an illicit drug. Primary admission for treatment of alcohol alone dropped to 40% from 51% in 1996 (49). Although 58.1% of primary heroin admissions were self-referrals, 14.2% came through the criminal justice system; in contrast, for primary marihuana admissions, 56.9% came through the criminal justice system and 14.8% were self-referrals (10).

In 2007, 213,000 Americans were dependent on or abusing heroin (2). From 1996 to 2006, heroin treatment admissions increased 10%, however, the number receiving medication-assisted therapy decreased by 22% (49) and in 2007 only 29.1% received methadone or buprenorphine (10). This is noteworthy, considering not only the growing emphasis on pharmacological treatment for addiction but also, by the mid-2000s, the easing of regulations governing methadone, buprenorphine, and naloxone meant to encourage greater use of these treatments for heroin addiction, especially in physicians' offices.

Since the 1990s there has been a growing body of research on those individuals who change their addictive behaviors without treatment or self-help programs (61,62). Natural recovery (also referred to sometimes as self-change) is the most common form of managing addictive behaviors. Studies suggest the important role of personal and social resources, as well as cultural variation, both in the meaning of drug and alcohol problems and in what constitutes recovery (62,63). Recruiting subjects for studies of natural recovery poses a challenge to epidemiologists who cannot rely on convenience samples (64) but there is a need for more systematic research in this area given that the majority of people with drinking and drug use problems change their behavior without treatment or mutual support programs.

ROLE OF EPIDEMIOLOGICAL INDICATORS

Epidemiology's importance for understanding substance abuse was recognized in the 1970s, with the first systematic national studies on rates of prevalence and incidence of ATOD. By the early 1980s, studies of substances and their users documented the decline in use which began at that time. Since then, new epidemiological approaches and studies have been undertaken. When there are differences between measures, for example, between NSDUH and NESARC, detailed analysis of methodologies illuminates the reasons for the lack of agreement (65). Such triangulation of multiple approaches is an essential dimension of epidemiology and the role it plays in defining and evaluating goals for programs and policy at all levels of government and in the private sector.

REFERENCES

1. Ford JM, Beveridge AA. Varieties of substance use and visible drug problems: individual and neighborhood factors. *J Drug Issues*. 2006;36:377–391.
2. Office of Applied Studies. *Results from the 2007 National Survey on Drug Use and Health: National Findings*. Rockville, MD: Department of Health and Human Services; 2008.
3. Johnston LD, O'Malley PM, Bachman JG, et al. *Monitoring the Future National Results on Adolescent Drug Use: Overview of Key Findings, 2008*. Bethesda, MD: National Institute on Drug Abuse; 2009.
4. Grant B, Dawson D. Introduction to the National Epidemiological Survey on Alcohol and Related Conditions. *Alcohol Res Health*. 2006;29:74–78.
5. Falk D, Yi H, Hiller-Sturmhöfel S. An epidemiological analysis of co-occurring alcohol and drug use and disorders: findings from the National Epidemiological Survey of Alcohol and Related Conditions (NESARC). *Alcohol Res Health*. 2008;31:100–110.
6. Office of Applied Statistics. *Drug Abuse Warning Network, 2006: National Estimates of Drug-Related Emergency Department Visits*. Rockville, MD: Department of Health and Human Services; 2008.
7. Community Epidemiology Work Group. *Proceedings of the Community Epidemiology Work Group, January 2008*. Bethesda, MD: National Institute on Drug Abuse; 2008.
8. Watt T. The race/ethnic age crossover effect in drug use and heavy drinking. *J Ethn Sub Abuse*. 2008;7:93–114.
9. Resnicow K, Soler R, Braithwaite RL. Cultural sensitivity in substance use prevention. *Am J Community Psychol*. 2000;28:270–290.
10. Office of Applied Studies. *Treatment Episode Data Set (TEDS) Highlights-2007 National Admissions to Substance Abuse Treatment Services*. Rockville, MD: Department of Health and Human Services; 2009.
11. Office of National Drug Control Policy. *National Drug Control Strategy*. Washington, DC: Government Printing Office; 2009.
12. Whitten L. Research addresses needs of criminal justice staff and offenders. *NIDA Notes*. 2009;22(3):4–5.
13. Bureau of Justice Statistics. *Substance Dependence, Abuse, and Treatment of Jail Inmates, 2002*. Washington, DC: Department of Justice; 2005.
14. Bureau of Justice Statistics. *Drug Use and Dependence, State and Federal Prisoners, 2004*. Washington, DC: Department of Justice; 2006.
15. Office of National Drug Control Policy. *National Drug Control Strategy*. Washington, DC: Government Printing Office; 2008.
16. Senator Webb's call for prison reform. *The New York Times*. Jan 1, 2009:A24.
17. Bureau of Justice Statistics. *Prisoners in 2007*. Washington, DC: Department of Justice; 2008.
18. Bureau of Justice Statistics. *Sourcebook of Criminal Justice Statistics 2003*. Washington, DC: Department of Justice; 2005.
19. Taxman F, Perdoni M, Harrison L. Drug treatment services for adult offenders: the state of the state. *J Subst Abuse Treat*. 2007;32:239–254.
20. Winick C. Maturing out of narcotic addiction. *Bull Narc*. 1962;14:1–7.

21. Prins EH. *Maturing Out: An Empirical Study of Personal Histories and Processes in Hard-drug Addiction*. Rotterdam, Holland: Van Gorcum; 1995.
22. Swendsen J, Anthony J, Conway K, et al. Improving targets for the prevention of drug use disorders: sociodemographic predictors of transitions across drug use stages in the national co-morbidity survey replication. *Prev Med*. 2008;47:629–634.
23. Trice H, Roman P. *Spirits and Demons at Work: Alcohol and Other Drugs on the Job*. Ithaca, NY: Cornell University Press; 1972.
24. Winick C. Physician narcotic addicts. *Soc Probl*. 1961;9:174–186.
25. Hughes PH, Brandenburg N, Baldwin DC, et al. Prevalence of substance abuse among US physicians. *JAMA*. 1992;267:2333–2340.
26. Wischmeyer PE, Johnson BR, Wilson JE, et al. A survey of propofol abuse in academic anesthesia programs. *Anesth Analg*. 2007;105:1066–1071.
27. Trinkoff A, Zhou Q, Storr C, et al. Workplace access, negative proscriptions, job strain, and substance use in registered nurses. *Nurs Res*. 2000;49:83–90.
28. Hollinger RC, Dabney DA. Social factors associated with pharmacists' unauthorized use of mind-altering medications. *J Drug Issues*. 2002;32:231–264.
29. Inciardi JA, Suratt HL, Kurts S, et al. The diversion of prescription drugs by health care workers in Cincinnati, Ohio. *Subst Use Misuse*. 2006;41:255–264.
30. Office of Applied Statistics. *Methamphetamine Use: the NSDUH Report*. Rockville, MD: Department of Health and Human Services; 2007.
31. Compton WM, Thomas YF, Stinson FS, et al. Prevalence, correlates, disability, and co-morbidity of *DSM-IV* drug abuse and dependence in the United States: results from the national epidemiological survey on alcohol and related conditions. *Arch Gen Psychiatry*. 2007;64:566–576.
32. Nunes EV, Rounsaville BJ. Co-morbidity of substance use with depression and other mental disorders: from Diagnostic and Statistical Manual of Mental Disorders, fourth edition (DSM-IV) to DSM-V. *Addiction*. 2006;101(suppl 1):89–96.
33. Hasin DS, Stinson FS, Ogburn E, et al. Prevalence, correlates, disability, and co-morbidity of *DSM-IV* alcohol abuse and dependence in the United States: results from the National Epidemiological Survey on Alcohol and Related Conditions. *Arch Gen Psychiatry*. 2007;64:830–842.
34. Hall HI, Song R, Rhodes P, et al. Estimation of HIV incidence in the United States. *JAMA*. 2008;300:520–529.
35. Shoptaw S, Reback CJ. Methamphetamine use and infectious disease-related behaviors in men who have sex with men: implications for interventions. *Addiction*. 2007;102(suppl 1):130–135.
36. Samet JH, Walley AY, Bridden C. Illicit drugs, alcohol, and addiction in human immunodeficiency virus. *Panminerva Med*. 2007;49:67–77.
37. Centers for Disease Control and Prevention. Surveillance for acute viral hepatitis—United States, 2007. *MMWR Morb Mortal Wkly Rep*. 2009;58(SS-3):1–27.
38. Centers for Disease Control and Prevention. *Behavioral Risk Factor Surveillance System Survey Data*. Atlanta, GA: Centers for Disease Control and Prevention; 2001–2007.
39. Mulia N, Ye Y, Zemore SE, et al. Social disadvantage, stress, and alcohol use among black, Hispanic, and white Americans: findings from the 2005 U.S. National Alcohol Survey. *J Stud Alcohol Drugs*. 2008;69:824–833.
40. Kerr WC, Greenfield TK, Bond J, et al. Age-period-cohort modeling of alcohol volume and heavy drinking days in the US National Alcohol Surveys: divergence in younger and older adult trends. *Addiction*. 2009;104:27–37.
41. Flowers N, Naimi T, Brewer R, et al. Patterns of alcohol consumption and alcohol-impaired driving in the United States. *Alcohol Clin Exp Res*. 2008;32:639–644.
42. Office of Applied Statistics. *Concurrent Illicit Drug and Alcohol Use: the NSDUH Report*. Rockville, MD: Department of Health and Human Services; 2009.
43. Office of Applied Statistics. *Marihuana Use and Perceived Risk of Use Among Adolescents, 2002 to 2007: the NSDUH Report*. Rockville, MD: Department of Health and Human Services; 2009.
44. King R, Mauer M. The war on marihuana: the transformation of the war on drugs in the 1990s. *Harm Reduct J*. 2006;3:6.
45. National Organization for the Reform of Marijuana Laws. Annual marijuana arrests in the US. Available at: http://www.norml.org/index.cfm?Group_ID=7042. Accessed July 3, 2009.
46. Levine H, Small D. *Marihuana Arrest Crusade: Racial Bias and Police Policy in New York City, 1997–2006*. New York: New York Civil Liberties Union; 2008.
47. Degenhardt L, Chiu WT, Conway K, et al. Does the 'gateway' matter? Associations between the order of drug use initiation and the development of drug dependence in the National Co-morbidity Study Replication. *Psychol Med*. 2009;39:157–167.
48. Zimmer L, Morgan JP. *Marihuana Myths, Marihuana Facts*. New York: The Lindesmith Center; 1997.
49. Office of Applied Studies. *Treatment Episode Data Set (TEDS): 1996–2006. National Admissions to Substance Abuse Treatment Services*. Rockville, MD: Department of Health and Human Services; 2008.
50. Nelson DE, Mowery P, Asman K, et al. Long-term patterns in adolescent and young adult smoking in the United States: meta-patterns and implications. *Am J Pub Health*. 2008;98:905–914.
51. Sweanor D, Alcabes P, Drucker, E, et al. Tobacco harm reduction: how rational public policy could transform a pandemic. *Int J Drug Pol*. 2007;18:70–74.
52. Andrade X, Sifaneck SJ, Neaigus A. Dope sniffers in New York City: an ethnography of heroin markets and patterns of use. *J Drug Issues*. 1999;29:271–298.
53. Furst RT. The re-engineering of heroin: an emerging heroin "cutting" trend in New York City. *Addict Res*. 2000;8:357–379.
54. Beck J, Rosenbaum M. *Pursuit of Ecstasy: the MDMA Experience*. Albany, NY: SUNY Press; 1994.
55. Sales P, Murphy S. San Francisco's freelancing ecstasy dealers: towards a sociological understanding of drug markets. *J Drug Issues*. 2007;37:919–950.
56. Colliver JD, Kroutil LA, Dai L, et al. *Misuse of Prescription Drugs: Data from the 2002, 2003, and 2004 National Surveys on Drug Use and Health*. Rockville, MD: Office of Applied Studies, Department of Health and Human Services; 2006.
57. Office of Applied Statistics. Tables of methamphetamine data. Available at: http://www.oas.samhsa.gov/methTabs.htm. Accessed July 6, 2009.
58. Johnston LD, O'Malley PM, Bachman JG, et al. *Monitoring the Future National Survey Results on Drug Use, 1975–2007: Volume II, College Students and Adults Ages 19–45*. Bethesda, MD: National Institute on Drug Abuse; 2008.
59. McCabe SE. Misperceptions of non-medical prescription drug use: a web survey of college students. *Addict Behav*. 2008;33:713–724.
60. Office of Applied Statistics. *Nonmedical Use of Adderall among Full-time College Students: the NSDUH Report*. Rockville, MD: US Department of Health and Human Services; 2009.

61. Dawson DA, Grant BF, Stinson FS, et al. Recovery from DSM-IV alcohol dependence: United States, 2001–2002. *Addiction*. 2005;100:281–292.
62. Klingemann H, Carter-Sobell L. *Promoting Self-change from Addictive Behaviors: Practical Implications for Policy, Prevention, and Treatment*. New York: Springer; 2007.
63. Mohatt G, Rasmus SM, Thomas L. Risk, resilience, and natural recovery: a model of recovery from alcohol abuse for Alaska Natives. *Addiction*. 2007;103:205–215.
64. Caraballo JL, Fernández-Hermida JR, Secades-Villa R, et al. Effectiveness and efficiency of methodology for recruiting participants in natural recovery from alcohol and drug addiction. *Addiction Res Theory*. 2009;17:80–90.
65. Grucza RA, Abbacchi AM, Przybeck TR, et al. Discrepancies in estimates of substance use and disorders between two national surveys. *Addiction*. 2007;102:623–629.

CHAPTER 3

Epidemiology—A European Perspective

Icro Maremmani ■ Matteo Pacini ■ Mercedes Lovrecic ■ Pier Paolo Pani

INTRODUCTION

The principal font of information regarding trends of European drug problems is the European Monitoring Centre for Drugs and Drug Addiction (EMCDDA). It provides decision makers and professionals, institutions, and other organizations involved in drug-related interventions with evidence-based information to support the drugs debate and decisions at both political and technical levels. The EMCDDA produces annual reports on the drug situation in Europe, including data about drug trafficking, estimation of consumption, and information about treatment requests and availability (1).

To develop a European overview of drug prevalence, the EMCDDA coordinates a network of National Focal Points (NFPs) set up in the 27 EU Member States, Norway, the European Commission, and the candidate countries. Together, these information collection and exchange points form Reitox, the European Information Network on Drugs and Drug Addiction. Under the responsibility of their respective governments, the NFPs are the national authorities providing drug information to the EMCDDA.

Given the national or regional level of the system of data collection, combining and comparing reported drug prevalence is problematic. Epidemiologic reasoning is conditioned by the heterogeneity of the data regarding the time frame considered, the context of the collection of data, the age range considered, the data collection procedure, the sampling frame and sampling procedure, and the weighting procedure.

In this chapter, we have selected information about treatment demand, which is the best filter to make meaningful comparisons between different use-groups, and describe longitudinal trends. Nevertheless, treatment demand may correspond to a different rate of actual problematic drug use, depending on the availability and accessibility of treatment, the level of information about treatment options in the general population, and not least to the legal consequences of enrolling into treatment. As a result, opiates may be the only substance class for which treatment demand might parallel incidence and prevalence of abuse/addiction cases. On the other hand, the presumption that treatment demands equate to addiction, or indeed any disease at all, is problematic: for example, treatment demand due to drug law offences as an alternative to jail have created an abnormal channel toward therapeutic settings, especially if substance based and not diagnosis based. In fact, although therapeutic parole is reserved to those who display features of pathologic drug use, some laws draw a direct link between the illicit status of a substance and the possibility of treatment, mistaking therapy for some kind of (re)education or legally oriented behavioral conditioning.

One important restriction applied in EMCDDA reports, to be considered in our reasoning on treatment demand, refers to the case definition, which includes only people entering treatment for drug use. Therefore EMCDDA data do not necessarily include clients in continued treatment from previous years. Moreover, it should be considered that treatment demand data come from each country with varying degrees of national coverage (from 24% to 100% of treatment units covered).

Finally, the EMCDDA definition of "problem drug use" as a key indicator of drug use epidemics is "injecting drug use or long duration/regular use of opioids, cocaine and/or amphetamines." Such a definition omits noninjectable drug use, at any stage, but does include prescribed opioid use, provided that the opioids are prescribed on a regular basis. Thereby, overall data corresponding to such a definition cannot be easily interpreted.

In our presentation we will refer principally to EMCDDA reports. Other data reported from surveys, prevalence studies, national reports, and observational and experimental studies will be considered for specific subjects.

PATTERN OF SUBSTANCE TREATMENT DEMAND

All Drugs

In Europe, primary heroin use rose from 108,000 in 2002 (63% of all treatment episodes) to 129,000 in 2007 (52%); primary cocaine use rose from 22,000 (13%) to 47,000 (19%); and primary cannabis use from 27,000 (16%) to 50,000 (20%). Stimulants other than cocaine accounted for 15,000 cases of primary problem drug use in 2002 (9%) and 20,000 (8%) in 2007. Among new clients entering treatment, heroin use rose slightly from 36,000 (48%) in 2002 to 38,000 (34%) in 2007, while cocaine increased sharply from 13,000 (17%) to 28,000 (25%) and cannabis from 18,829 (25%) to 34,312 (31%). There was a smaller increase for stimulants other than cocaine, from 8,000 (10%) to 10,000 (9%).

Primary heroin treatment demand increased in number but decreased as a rate of all treatment demand (+20% from 2002 to 2007), due to the absolute and relative rise of treatment demand for cocaine (+135%), cannabis (+85%), and other stimulants (+33%). The trend is more evident among new clients (+5% for heroin, +115% for cocaine, +82% for cannabis, and +25% for other stimulants). The rise in emerging use, as calculated by the ratio between new client numbers in 2002 and 2007, was twice as much for cocaine than for heroin.

The fact that standardized treatments are available and known for heroin addiction but not generally for cocaine abuse, increases the significance of the rise in problem cocaine use: cocaine abusers may be less likely to enter treatment if no specific treatment perspective is available and may be less likely to make further attempts after the first treatment failure (2).

Alcohol

The EMCDDA report features alcohol as a secondary substance; however, no European data about alcohol treatment episodes are presented. For licit substances such as alcohol, estimates of abuse and addiction epidemiology are problematic. In fact, alcohol use may be regular and heavy but this pattern of use does not necessarily equate with addiction, whereas such a relationship is often presumed with illicit drugs such as heroin.

Increasing alcohol abuse, such as recurrent episodes of heavy drinking, was reported in most countries across the late 1990s, among both men and women. More recently, no uniform course can be observed. By 2006, approximately 5% of male and 2% of female drinkers report negative consequences of habitual drinking on their job or study performance. A significant rate of premature deaths, and disability, are related to alcohol, at least as a contributing risk factor for the cause of death or accident (12% in men and 2% in women). The role of alcohol as a cause of death among young people is relevant: 25% of young men and 10% of young women die of alcohol-related causes. Specifically, 1 out of 3 lethal car accidents, 4 out of 10 killings, and 1 out of 6 suicides are directly related to alcohol use. Further, as many as 17,000 deaths due to neuropsychiatric problems are related to alcohol. Beyond such data, the specific weight and trends of alcoholism remain unclear (3).

Opiates

In most European countries supplying data, between 50% and 80% of all treatment demand (about 387,000 for 24 countries in 2006) is related to opioids as the primary drugs, in the remaining countries the proportion varies between 1% and 40%. Opioids are infrequently reported as a secondary drug (11% to 13%), and are generally less frequent among clients entering their first treatment episode (40%). As a rule, treatment demand related to opioid use has been increasing in recent years. Data from nine countries show that opioids are the most frequent primary drug of abuse among clients who are already in treatment (59%) but account for only 40% of clients entering treatment for the first time in their lives.

Injecting drug use is not as frequent as one may presume: 63% of all opioid users applying for, or currently receiving, treatment reported injecting opioids at the time of treatment entry. Percentages vary between 25% and over 80% across different countries. While some countries, such as Ukraine, report higher percentages such as 97% (4). Among those entering treatment for the first time, the percentage of opioid injectors is generally lower and decreased from 43% to 35% between 2003 and 2006, although there has been a more recent reprise up to 42%.

Generally, the rates of reported injecting opioid use show a decreasing trend over time. In some countries, smoked or snorted opiates are the prominent mode of administration. However, another plausible explanation may be that the availability of opiate addiction treatment has favored a trend toward earlier involvement into treatment, assuming that the transition to injecting drug use is a sign of increasing severity of use. Further, the availability and marketing of newer opioid formulations that are not automatically linked with the risk of addiction, such as smoked opium, may be becoming more popular.

The mean age of patients entering outpatient treatment for primary opiate use is 33 years and has been increasing since 2003. Men outnumber women by 3.5 to one. Among those who develop opioid-related problems and apply for treatment later in life, opioid use is likely to start before the age of 25, and unlikely to start after 25 years. An average time interval of 7 to 9 years stands between first use of opioids and first contact with drug treatment. Men spend a longer time using opioids before entering treatment. However, the mean age of first opioid use is decreasing (one year lower among new clients). A possible reason for this is higher rates of treatment re-entry among previously treated addicts who have been prematurely discharged or dropped out of treatment: thus, the whole population is aging while the average age of new clients is decreasing.

To summarize, mean age at treatment entrance is 32 years, which is usually 7 to 9 years from the very first episode of drug use. Men spend a longer time using opioids before entering treatment. On the whole, new clients tend to be younger, use more frequently, and they may have spent longer snorting or smoking the drugs before starting injecting drug use.

For details consult http://www.emcdda.europa.eu/situation/analysis (5).

Cannabis

The rate of treatment requests for a primary cannabis-related drug problem rose to 12% of all clients, and 30% of all new clients, in 2002. Although rates vary across different countries, cannabis appears to be an increasing problem in all European countries for the 1996 to 2002 period. In 2007 primary cannabis-related demands are 20% of all cases and 28% of new cases.

The peculiarity of cannabis-related treatment demand is the high prevalence of compulsory treatment or nonspontaneous treatment requests, such as in the case of treatment requests to avoid jail or other legal consequences. According to EMCDDA in several countries, cannabis users, regardless of a thorough assessment of their possible addictive state, are referred to hypothetical treatment programs for implicitly supposed problematic cannabis use, thus confusing a legal option with a medical condition of cannabis abuse/dependence. In fact, the majority of presumed abusers, about two thirds, do not use cannabis on a regular basis (less than daily), and in half of those cases consumption is actually infrequent (once a week or less often) (6). In 2007, 24% of clients were classified as occasional users, or had not been using the substance during the last month. As such, the reason for cannabis-related treatment seeking does not always appear related to intensive cannabis use. It may be either that cannabis-related treatment seeking is mostly due to legal problems related to cannabis possession and consumption, or that occasional intoxication or cannabis-related adverse events, rather than addiction, may be the primary reason. Cannabis use generally commenced before the age of 20, while the mean age at treatment request is 24.

Stimulants

In Europe (5), cocaine was the primary drug in 17% of treatment-seeking drug users in 2007, and the secondary drug in 18% of cases. The rate among new clients is higher (22%) and has been increasing in recent years (on the whole, 19% of cases were cocaine related at some level). Spain, in particular, has experienced an increasing rate of primary and secondary cocaine-related treatment demand (over 40% and over 60%, respectively). Most countries report a higher prevalence of primary cocaine problem use among new clients than among all clients, indicating a generally increasing trend in problematic cocaine use. Treatment demand is linked to recent regular consumption in 60% of cases, whereas in other cases clients apply for treatment while not using on a regular basis or during periods of abstinence. Intravenous use is rare (6%) and does not seem to be increasing (being lower among new clients and with respect to previous years, despite the increase in treatment demand).

The rate of cocaine and amphetamine-related problems appear to be inversely related, which may suggest that these two stimulants are seen as equivalent to each other, alternatively dominating each territory's market. Crack cocaine use is limited to some urban areas, and rather uncommon (at any level in 2% of all treatment requests).

Treatment for primary amphetamine use is usually below 5%, although some countries have rates of 25% to 35%, notably Sweden (34%), Finland (Helsinky) 23%. Methamphetamine has become a trend in exceptional cases, up to 59% of treatment demands as a primary drug in 2006. In treatment settings, problematic methamphetamine use is predominantly via injecting. MDMA treatment requests are relatively rare (0.5% down to irrelevant numbers for most countries, a few countries reporting up to 4%). As a rule, MDMA problem users applying for treatment are polydrug abusers, mostly of alcohol, cannabis, or other stimulants. Fifty-two percent of primary noncocaine stimulant clients are occasional users.

Polydrug Abuse

As many as 57% of clients reported at least one secondary drug (33% one drug, 20% two, 4% three or more) (7). Clients entering treatment for the first time are more likely to be polyabusers, except for first-time heroin treatment clients. The lowest rate of polyabuse is among cannabis clients (43%), while crack-cocaine abusers report the highest (69%). This latter category, however, corresponds to a very small proportion of all clients receiving treatment in most European countries.

The list of secondary drugs reported by polydrug users includes cocaine (32%), alcohol (40%), cannabis (27%), and other stimulants (11%). The involvement of cocaine in polyabuse patterns plausibly increases the weight of this drug in the course and outcome of treatment for primary drug abuse pictures such as heroin (8).

Cannabis polyabuse accounts for most cannabis-related treatment demands (85%), with cannabis predominantly being the secondary substance of abuse. Most featured combinations are with alcohol, cocaine, or both. Primary cocaine users in treatment report 63% of polyabuse, mainly alcohol (42%), cannabis (28%), and heroin (17%).

Opiate clients often engage in polyabuse during the relapsing course of their disease: as such, the likelihood of polyabuse is higher among re-entering clients or those who have been in treatment for some time. A Swedish study reported a history of hospitalization due to alcohol-related problems in 1 out of 3 heroin addicts entering methadone treatment (9). An Irish study reported a 56% rate of alcohol polyabuse among methadone patients (10).

Benzodiazepine use is also frequent, although to a variable extent (11% to 70%). Cocaine polyabuse in methadone maintenance is also common, and seems to mirror the estimated trend of use in the general population. Cocaine polyabusers during methadone treatment are also likely to report alcohol abuse.

POPULATION SUBGROUPS

Gender Differences

Male to female sex ratios show male predominance in all age groups and across all countries (ranging from 1.6 to 9:1). A relatively higher rate of females is found among very young and elderly clients (<15 and >45), which suggests a lowering trend for sex ratios in the future, at least for clients who will stay in long-term treatment or display the usual addictive pattern of recurrent relapse and subsequent re-entering into treatment. The relatively higher proportion of females within the over-45 age group may suggest a gender-specific feature, either the concentration of late-onset drug abuse among women or the higher rate of long-term treatment adherence for females, especially within standard maintenance treatments (i.e., opiate addiction) (11).

TABLE 3.1	Pattern of substance abuse				
	Mean age (years)	Started using at (years)	Sex ratio (M/F)	IDUs	Regular use (daily or several times a week)
Cocaine	33	15–24	5:1	6%	60%
Amphetamine	29	<20	2:1	14% (all)	42%
MDMA	24	<20	n.d.	n.d.	n.d.
Methamphetamines	24–25	<20	(less than 2:1)	41%–82%	n.d.
Cannabis	24	<20	5.5:1	n.d.	76%
Opiates	31–33	<25	3.5:1	63%	60%–70%
Sedatives-hypnotics	n.d.	n.d.	1.4:1	n.d.	n.d.

Data from http://www.emcdda.europa.eu/

Table 3.1 presents the sex ratios for the primary reported drug categories. Females may outnumber men just in the case of sedatives-hypnotics, but the number of male sedative-abusers has been increasing as a whole. Some countries report ratios below 1; on average it was 0.9 in 2003 but it rose to 1.4 recently (up to date). Some countries still report ratios below 1, so it may be that in some samples men are fewer (to be noted, the body of data about primary sedative clients is quite small with respect to other drug categories). The mean age of new clients for any drug is similar (about 27) between sexes. Injecting drug use is rather typical of males. Age of onset of drug use is higher for females just in the case of sedatives. The rate of female clients is lower in subgroups of "at-least-daily" users for all substances, except for cannabis and sedatives. Female clients are more likely to have been referred by the health system (36% vs. 27%) and less likely to be referred by the criminal justice system (10.6% vs. 22%). It was estimated that the latency period from drug use to treatment is about 2 years shorter for women.

Drug-related deaths have been a predominantly male phenomenon. However, recent data show that the incidence of drug-related deaths have not been decreasing by the same rate in the two sexes (half as much among women). Thereby, factors affecting drug-related deaths do not seem to have the same impact among women as among men. Despite similar rates of infection, the seroconversion of female clients is higher when controlling for the prevalence of intravenous drug use. Given the similar rates of Hepatitis C Virus (HCV) infection, it is plausible that sexual transmission is the basis for such increased risk (5,12).

Younger People, Under 15 Years

In most European countries, fewer than 2% of drug clients are under 15 years of age, although that subpopulation increased between 1999 and 2005, while in 2006 as many as 80% of reported cases came from the United Kingdom. Their primary drug is almost always cannabis or inhalants, to a lesser extent opiates with other substances being very rare. The male/female sex ratio in younger clients is 2.5:1 versus 4.1:1 among clients over 19 years. Among the younger clients, 78% of under-15 year olds and 67% of 15- to 19-year-old clients are in treatment for primary cannabis use (13). In 2005, 18 drug-related deaths among children under the age of 15 were reported, which represents 0.2% of the total number of drug-related deaths in Europe.

Immigration and Problem Drug Use

Studies about addiction and problem drug use among immigrants are lacking, and no European network aiming at the characterization of immigration-related drug risks has thus far been established. This is surprising, considering migrants are becoming an increasing part of European society. Nevertheless, in the field of drug use and addiction, little attention has been paid to this subject.

Among foreigners immigrating to Italy, mostly in a clandestine way at least when crossing the border, addictive drug use is closely related to immigration. Three out of four of foreigner heroin addicted clients in Rome report starting heroin use after moving to Italy. Successfully settling in Italy is not always protective against the development of addiction: immigrants who have been in Italy for a short time (less than 4 years) report lower rates of injecting and noninjecting drug problems than those who immigrated earlier (4 or more years before). Such a difference is particularly evident for heroin, but has been documented for cocaine too. (14,15).

Data from studies across Europe suggest that the prevalence of migrants with addictive disorders corresponds to, or even exceeds, the general population, yet there are still substantial barriers to accessing facilities that provide help to addicts (16). The literature reports a number of barriers to treatment access, including language difficulties, diffidence, condition of clandestinely, fear of losing residency rights, culturally different understanding of the causes and treatment of addictive behavior, and a lack of intercultural competence of people working in health and psychosocial care institutions (17). For example, in Hamburg, where migrants represent 33% to 35% of the drug addict population and 16% of the city's total population, only 8% to 10% of people attending drug addiction facilities were migrants (18).

Infectious Disease and Drug Use: The European Experience and the Russian Paradigm

In the epidemiologic study of addictive diseases, infectious needle-borne diseases, especially Human Immunodeficiency Virus (HIV), HCV, and Hepatitis B Virus (HBV) can be regarded as behavioral indicators of drug abuse and treatment outcome. Likewise, prevention strategies and responses to drug-related infectious disease should be founded on a synergy between core addiction treatment and harm reduction, particularly for those initially resistant to treatment.

In several countries, both in and out of the European Community (Middle East, Asia), the increase in the rate of HIV incidence raised the first political concern about the need to limit the impact of injecting drug use upon public health. The control of infectious disease epidemics, together with effective crime control strategies, highlights the relationship between addiction treatment and the more general issue of health and safety for the wider population. The history of opiate addiction treatment in Europe clearly shows the relationship between delivering effective addiction treatment and reducing the rates of infections among injecting drug users. The resistance to the spread of opioid agonist replacement therapy has caused, and is still causing, a paradox of prevention: HIV infection should be considered an exceptional condition for agonist maintenance treatment to be allowed, and not just a priority condition for the access to it. In Germany and Scotland, when methadone was limited exclusively to HIV-positive addicts, cases of drug users who would infect themselves voluntarily in order to access treatment were reported. This paradoxical fact was reported by J. Mordaunt during the "Fourth International Conference on the Reduction of Drug Related Harm" that was held in Rotterdam (March 14 to 18, 1993).

The above situation corresponds to a paradigm where agonist maintenance treatment is not spread evenly throughout Europe. At the beginning of the 1990s, over 90% of AIDS cases among drug users were registered in 3 out of the 12 current European community countries: France, Italy, and Spain, which accounted for less than 50% of the current European community population. Apparently, in 9 out of 11 countries a relationship stood between AIDS prevalence and/or incidence rates among Injecting Drug Users (UDUs) and the percentage of IDUs enrolled in methadone treatment. Countries with a low prevalence and relatively stable incidence were those for which the introduction of methadone treatment dates back to the 1980s or late 1970s. Thus, despite territorial contiguity and membership to a common economic system, the differential impact of HIV infection among high-risk categories such as IDU was directly related to the availability of treatment in different territories (19,20).

Among countries with a more recent history of opioid addiction epidemics, the Russian Federation shows a higher prevalence and incidence rate of HIV infection among injecting drug users. These data may illustrate the situation of a country facing an epidemic of opioid addiction with no or few specific resources to respond to it, despite nonspecific efforts aiming at detoxification, re-education, or drug-free rehabilitation. The prevalence rate of officially registered cases of drug addiction in Russia leaped from about 60/100,000 in 1997 to 154.8/10,000 in 1999, and 241/100,000 by the end of 2003 (343,000 individuals). The vast majority of cases correspond to opioid addiction (133.1/10,000 in 1999 and 211.6 in 2003, standing at 210.9/10,000 in 2004). The highest prevalence is among young people, with 1025/100,000 in the 18 to 19 age range and a 976.5/100,000 in the 20 to 39 range.

Approximately 87% of drug addicts are primarily engaged with heroin use. The incidence of female cases of drug abuse has risen to 14 times its value across a 15 years period. Injecting drug use accounted for 75% of registered cases of HIV infection registered by June 2004. HIV prevalence demonstrated a 310-fold increase from 1995 to 2003; HIV incidence has risen by a factor of 276. The prevalence of HIV infection among injecting drug users reached 2081/100,000 in 2005.

In one subregion, the seroconversion rate was as high as 41% in a 1-year period in a sample of 426 IDUs, and prevalence of HIV positivity reached 64.5% in another sample. In 2005, this value reached 80% for injecting opiate addicts (21,22).

The majority of HIV infected people in Russia is aged between 20 and 29, and one third are women, mostly within the 15 to 25 age range (25% in the 15 to 20 age group and 50% in the 20 to 30 age group). The incidence of HIV among women has risen 450 times its initial value, and current prevalence among pregnant women is 114.7/100,000. Moreover, 48% of commercial sex workers who are IDUs are also HIV infected. Up to 80% of people with HIV infection are IDUs with variable patterns of use and have had at least occasional experience of sex trading for money. As much as 60% of viral hepatitis B and 90% of hepatitis C are due to injecting drug use.

The role of addictive drug use in the spread of HIV infection becomes "overwhelming" to any nonspecific public health strategy when the availability of evidence-based treatment for opioid addiction is either none or low. The Russian experience demonstrates how the relative neutralization of protective factors (i.e., gender-related protective factors in the case of injecting drug use) may lead to an amplifying effect, as females become more vulnerable to seroconversion. In this background it is difficult to understand why some Russian psychiatrists could openly take sides against the introduction of methadone in Russia (23).

TREATMENT POLICY AND PROCEDURE

In the case of heroin addiction, there are reliable predictors of treatment effectiveness, including the dose of the replacement pharmacotherapy, retention in treatment, and integration with facilities for concurrent health and social issues. Surprisingly, data about these important predictors of dose and duration of treatment are not reported by EMCDDA. To be more precise, data about duration are incidentally reported in a way that reveals an alarming misconception about gold standards of agonist maintenance. In fact, the distinction between short- and long-term treatment is usually fixed at some months of treatment duration, regardless of dosage regimens. Such a view results in the misclassification as "agonist treatments" of those interventions that do not effectively manage opioid addiction (i.e., detoxification or medium-term tapering). Furthermore, methadone treatment programs that are delivered for a short period of time (e.g., a few months) are grouped together with recognizable methadone maintenance programs, leading to an overestimation of methadone maintenance availability. Moreover, no detail of dosage or regimen is provided, apart from those reported in single subnational studies. Nor is detail provided about the rate of re-entries, dropouts, or accomplishment of therapeutic goals, since no uniform encoding is utilized. In our opinion, it is not appropriate to dilute the results of high-performing services with those of centers where tapering opioid medication dosages is accepted as a therapeutic procedure or 1-month's program rated as a success. Finally, the EMCDDA makes no discrimination between opioid use, abuse, and addiction, so that it is not possible to determine the adequacy of treatment programs in relation to the actual diagnosis.

Treatment Provision

In general, treatment provision is provided mostly from outpatient settings. Some countries continue to offer no specific treatment approaches for opioid addiction (Hungary, Poland, and Sweden), although agonist treatment is available. It appears that broad-spectrum treatments are increasing in those countries. Further, the provision of agonist treatment does not appear to depend on the duration of the opioid use epidemic: countries with decades of experience such as England and Germany show similar coverage rates with newcomers such as Croatia, Italy, and the Czech Republic. However, the availability of agonist treatment is quite dissimilar among countries with shorter experiences of opioid addiction treatment (e.g., 5% in Slovakia compared with approximately 40% in the Czech Republic).

Surprisingly, in some territories, profiles of drug users entering treatment are changing in a way that suggests improvement in the outreach to problem drug users. In Ukraine, for example, the rate of young people aged up to 20 years enrolled in treatment programs has increased from 16.4% to 21%, with a decrease in the percentage of those between 30 and 40 years of age from 19.3% to 16.4%. Also, the mean duration of opioid use at first-time treatment entry has reduced, from 3.9 to 3.0 years. Thus, the availability of treatment is expected to favor earlier treatment of younger people, with clear improvement in rehabilitation (4).

The involvement of General Practitioners (GPs) in the treatment of heroin addiction is somewhat surprising in some countries. On one hand, in some countries GPs are the primary treatment provider, representing about 80% in France and 90% in Germany. Such a status should correspond to the capillary spread of specific knowledge about heroin addiction and mental disorders. In the absence of such a situation, the provision of treatment would rather correspond to detoxification or longer-term prescription without specific therapeutic goals (i.e., rehabilitation and relapse prevention at average effective dosages). On the other hand, some countries that are theoretically enabled to provide GP-based methadone treatment fail to do so, or do it exceptionally, as in the case of Italy. Although the feasibility of GP-based methadone maintenance has been documented both in Germany and in Italy, other factors seem to influence such diverging national situations (24,25).

As for harm-reduction campaigns, to date they have been primarily focussed upon the personal and social needs of heroin addicts, with an aim to prevent the consequences of addictive behaviors. An incorrect distinction appears to be employed when comparing harm-reduction interventions to specific treatments for heroin addiction. Nevertheless, some of the specific targets in the treatment of heroin addiction, as well as features of mentally ill subpopulations, may be reasonable targets for harm reduction. Although a tacit dichotomy stands between the two approaches, they may be viewed as different stages in the process of rehabilitation of socially impaired drug addicts, or shared components of large treatment campaigns when waiting lists cannot be avoided.

Convergence upon overlapping targets may be considered when harm-reduction and specific treatment interventions share the same therapeutic components and goals. Opioid agonists, the primary option for the specific treatment of heroin addiction, may also serve as a harm-reduction approach, as long as harm reduction is conceived as a means to act upon the same disease, although at a low-threshold level. From a treatment point of view, what is specifically targeted at treating addiction is also likely to function as an effective form of harm reduction.

The personal and social impact of agonist-mediated harm reduction is particularly important for higher-risk populations, such as mentally ill heroin users, who may demonstrate poorer retention and outcome in standard opioid agonist replacement pharmacotherapies. Harm reduction should be regarded as a lower intensity of treatment delivery for more severely disabled subjects, bridging the gap between the street and the clinical settings by offering less demanding treatment requirements and services but retaining the essence of evidence-based pharmacotherapy. Such low threshold–low intervention methadone programs have been shown to be effective in retaining clients within the treatment system (26). Graduating from a lower threshold harm reduction program to a higher level of intervention should represent the ultimate goal of harm reduction itself. Transition to specific treatment is of particular importance for dually diagnosed addicts who are expected to experience greater relative benefit and who otherwise may be excluded from the opportunity of a positive outcome (27).

The Epidemiologic Black Hole of Heroin Addiction: A Possible Sign of Inadequacy of Treatment Standards or Blindness to Changes in Drug Use Behavior

Opiate addiction is a curable disease, with a standard approach consisting of long-term treatment aimed at the maintenance of rehabilitation through relapse prevention. Agonist treatment is an effective technical instrument for such a purpose. Some information is available about the availability and spread of agonist treatment, but no clear data exist to permit an evaluation that evidence-based treatment standards and principles have been applied.

In 2002, 72,000 "old" clients are recorded in Europe, plus 36,000 new clients. On theoretical grounds, ideally in 2003 some 100,000 clients are expected to be in treatment, and the number of agonist-maintenance clients should increase by the cumulative effect of each year's new and old clients re-entering treatment. In fact, a stabilizing effect would be expected if older patients who have failed previous treatment attempts were maintained on the gold standard treatment (i.e., agonist maintenance), also providing with the highest retention rates.

Assuming that some 30,000 new clients have applied for primary problem heroin use from 2002 to 2007, and that some 70,000 have been "trying treatment again," the resulting number of recorded methadone maintenance clients would be presumably higher than the 650,000 reported in 2007 (+150,000 in 6 years). Therefore, out of some cumulative 700,000 theoretical new clients throughout a 6-year period, approximately 550,000 were not recorded after 6 years. Omitting clients lost to treatment due to reasons such as death, emigration, incarceration, or possible switching to other primary substances, the number of "disappeared" clients still remains significant. It can be hypothesized that these clients either dropped out of treatment or were prematurely discharged with no subsequent re-entry in a 6-year period, or were definitely abstinent after a short-/medium-term intervention with no known relapses in a 6-year period. Also, it may be that part of those clients are the same ones re-entering treatment programs each year, or being addressed toward short-term treatment programs every time, regardless of their treatment failure history. Given that no brief intervention is known or reported to be effective in opiate-addiction, the only plausible conclusion is that the majority of opiate addicts, even if treated by agonist drugs, are prematurely discharged or leave treatment in a way that does not favor subsequent re-entry into the same treatment, at least in the following years. The fact that in several countries a 6-month term is referred to as the threshold between short- and long-term treatment is consistent with such a hypothesis.

It is obvious that no increase as such has taken place, which means that longer-term maintenance treatments are not being offered according to best practice principles. Thus, the availability of agonist treatment programs does not necessarily guarantee the effective, evidence-based delivery of treatment. In Italy, for instance, it was documented that 8 treatment programs out of 10 are characterized by methadone dosages below the minimum effective dose of 60 mg/day, and methadone dose increases did not take place in response to the lack of response in the months following treatment entry (28).

Another study conducted in a university center for the treatment of dual-diagnosis patients investigated new clients' characteristics across a 10-year period. In this retrospective study, more recent treatment demands came from older patients (33 years on average) with a history of earlier treatment but a lower rate of previous methadone maintenance (regardless of outcome). Thus, earlier intervention had not led those patients to potentially effective treatment options (27%), and patients had continued to be addicted to heroin. The reasons for treatment requests by a University Center demonstrated the relative resistance to treatment re-entry for clients who had previously attempted programs at local addiction treatment units. This phenomenon of missed re-entry after the failure of nonspecific short-term treatments may be a major issue behind the poor outcomes among heroin addicts (29).

Finally, moving from one primary drug of abuse to another remains poorly characterized. An Italian survey in a specialized hospital center for alcohol dependence in a major urban area (Rome) investigated the history of past drug use among new clients. Approximately 15% of clients entering treatment for alcohol abuse or dependence reported a past or present history of heroin use, although heroin was currently a secondary substance. Alcohol consumption started usually before heroin consumption, but reached higher mean and maximum levels with respect to other categories of alcoholics. In those subjects, a history of long-term opioid agonist treatment was quite unlikely, while current mean methadone dosages were lower than the effective average dose of 60 mg/day (30).

Methadone and Buprenorphine Misuse: An Epidemiologic Pitfall Due to Abnormal Treatment Profiles

Some countries report significant rates of primary abuse of opioids other than heroin. Therapeutic opiates are featured, with notably high rates of reported primary abuse in Finland for buprenorphine (51%) and in Denmark for methadone (20.6%). However, it can be difficult to distinguish between addictive use, abuse, and simple generic misuse of prescribed opioids, as indicated in the Danish report.

"Misuse" is an ambiguous term, which does not permit a clear distinction between treatment demands corresponding to addictive use or infrequent supply and handling use of potentially harmful substances. "Street methadone" use is a known phenomenon, but the presence of nontherapeutic methadone use at treatment entry does not necessarily equate to methadone abuse or addiction. The use of illicit long-acting opioids may either correspond to self-medication, with the purpose of withdrawal prevention or sedation, or else to actual misuse and addiction-like behavior (which usually means a change in the route of administration to injection, since a change in the administration route is required to elicit intoxication by oral formulations of methadone and buprenorphine). It is not clear how many clients have entered treatment due to nontherapeutic use and loss of control upon methadone or buprenorphine, with no history of heroin abuse. Further, the fact that problem drug users may apply for treatment with a goal to leave and detoxify from methadone or buprenorphine does not usually reflect addiction to those compounds, but the request to manage withdrawal discomfort and reverse acquired tolerance.

Curiously, the Danish data show a significant rate of methadone misusers among older clients (<25 years old) rather than younger clients. It is possible that older clients have a greater tendency to self-medicate withdrawal discomfort or have re-entered treatment as they became tolerant to street methadone, and were classified as primary methadone misusers for such a reason. In that case, the improper classification of "street use" as addiction would create the false impression of a rising methadone epidemic. If the following therapeutic response was to detoxify those subjects from methadone instead of offering methadone maintenance at higher dosages, this vicious circle would perpetuate. In fact, the misconception that therapeutic opioids are merely a substitute for heroin has caused many treatment policies to shift from the prevention of relapse to heroin addiction to the short-term tapering of any opiate. In fact, in most countries (Denmark included) national authorities classify maintenance over some months as "long-term" treatment (instead of short-term as it actually is), which mirrors the negative attitudes toward the application of agonist treatment and feeds this misconception. Indeed, the Danish data also show, consistent with other countries, that despite the increasing rate of clients in "long-term" treatment, such a solution is more likely to be adopted for older clients (over 30), which suggests that drug-free approaches or detoxification are still very common, especially among clients in treatment for the first time and younger addicts.

As a consequence, the public (patient and physicians included) often believe that therapeutic opiates create a new dependence. Patients who succeed in reducing their illicit drug use by lower dose methadone, with occassional heroin use, may indeed report methadone as their "primary" drug problem. Paradoxically, their condition at treatment entry (heroin addicted with harm reduction through methadone) would be still rated by many as better than at treatment exit (heroin addicted and methadone-free).

It is important to diagnose addiction to methadone (i.e., psychological and physical dependence) based upon standard objective criteria for addiction (as in Diagnostic and Statistical Manual, Fourth Edition, Text Revision - DSM-IV-TR criteria) rather than relying upon patient self-report or physical dependence criteria alone.

There have been documented cases of the illicit, nontherapeutic use and abuse of Buprenorphine. Buprenorphine misusers are concentrated in France and Finland, countries where buprenorphine treatment was launched earlier than in the rest of Europe, and for many years was the primary agonist treatment option (31).

In Finland, the 2008 National Report reported that 56% of agonist treatment episodes are buprenorphine based (32).

As many as 33% of clients reported buprenorphine as their primary drug of abuse, with a clear trend indicating a decrease in primary heroin use and an increase in primary buprenorphine use (from 7% to 33% and from 20% to 2%, respectively, in the 2000 to 2007 period). Buprenorphine misusers tend to be younger, enter treatment earlier, start injecting sooner and inject more often. In a French survey (32) among low-threshold facilities, 54% of attendees reported using nonprescribed buprenorphine as self-medication, 13% to get "high," and 34% for both reasons. Older clients tended to use buprenorphine for self-medication of withdrawal discomfort rather than for intoxication.

Given its pharmacological profile as a partial opioid agonist, injecting buprenorphine will produce a "high" (euophoria and intoxication). However, habitual use is somewhat surprising, due to its long half-life and the rapid experience of the ceiling effect on the opioid effects. In a context where long-term maintenance agonist treatment is uncommon, older clients may re-enter treatment reporting injecting buprenorphine use, which may represent an attempt to maintain some direct opioid effects with a reduced reliance upon the use of heroin. Further, it is likely that patients will report polydrug abuse, as pharmacodynamic interactions between buprenorphine and other central nervous system (CNS) depressants (such as benzodiazepines) may increase the likelihood of experiencing sedation, intoxication, and euphoria. Conversely some primary stimulant abusers may use opioids to manage the negative consequences or withdrawal symptoms of the psychostimulants (33).

The introduction of the buprenorphine–naloxone combination product may help to discriminate different patterns of buprenorphine abuse and reduce its nontherapeutic use.

Drug-Related Crime

Data are available regarding drug law offences (EMCCDA). However, the interrelationship of drug use, pathologic drug use (i.e., addictive), and involvement in criminal behavior provides complexity. Specific indicators of drug addiction (as opposed to drug use) are missing from the EMCCDA reports, which makes it difficult to identify addiction-related criminal records from drug law offences and general crime committed by nonaddicted individuals. Further, drug use data from prison populations also fails to discriminate between addicts and recreational users.

The rate of drug users who are in treatment at the time of arrest may provide a marker of treatment effectiveness within a region. According to various reports to Italian Parliament (years 1986 to 2002), the number of addicts in jail increased from about 6,000 in 1986 to about 15,000 in 2002. The rate of addicts in treatment at the time of arrest rose from below 5% in 1986 to over 20% in 1989, congruent with the greater availability of methadone programs throughout the territory. The 2002 trend continues. Thus, the spread of methadone treatment in the wider community has not directly translated into a reduction in criminal behavior, although the increased numbers of clients receiving methadone, and the classification criteria used, may explain the apparent rise in the number of addicts being incarcerated. The initiation of methadone maintenance in jail is quite unlikely in Italy; however, the rate of continued maintenance among existing clients in jail has been growing to a small extent up to date.

Drug-Related Deaths

The EMCCDA data permit the monitoring of the incidence of drug-related deaths, poisonings, or overdoses in several European countries. Overall, drug-related deaths have been stable since the early 1990s, although a wide variability of incidence exists between different countries. As a general rule, the age of drug-related deaths has been increasing over the years. While in some countries drug-related deaths have remained relatively stable, in others there have been changes over time. In Poland, the mean age of drug-related deaths has increased from around 40 years in the middle of 1990s to over 45 years by 2006. In Bulgaria, the mean age of death was approximately 45 years in the early 1990s and has fallen to 30 by 2007.

Data are difficult to interpret, since different drugs are considered together as one cause of death, and polydrug abuse precludes specific causal linkage. It is commonly thought that drug-related deaths take place after the onset of intensive and heavier use (than usual), during relapses (where tolerance may be lower) or in the period between treatment episodes. The greater availability of treatment programs should theoretically lead to a decrease in death rate and the average age of death.

Data suggest that there has been a decrease in deaths due to acute drug intoxication throughout the 1990s up to 2005. Nevertheless, studies on the profile of either lethal or nonlethal heroin overdoses show unexpected features. In Italy, for instance, almost 70% of overdoses reported in 1997 occurred among people who had gone through some nonspecific form of addiction approach, had been discharged from jail in a drug-free state or had stopped taking naltrexone (i.e., had no tolerance) (34). Such practices endure despite another Italian study (35) clearly showing the protective effect of methadone maintenance treatment against the likelihood of lethal overdose. However, effective daily dosage of methadone is still rare in many treatment services, which may explain the findings that the average age of drug-related deaths rose from about 30 to about 35 in the period from 1996 to 2005, while the rate of drug-related deaths in the over-35 age range rose from about 25% to about 55% in the same period.

Limited case numbers in many countries does not permit firm conclusions to be drawn. Other consequences of drug use, such as infectious diseases and drug-related deaths, seem to be very rare in the youngest drug users, partly because of their short drug career.

FINAL REMARKS AND FUTURE PROSPECTS

We believe that epidemiology should be built upon foundations of clinical medicine. The bedside clinical observation, which includes the classic stages of diagnosis and therapy, is not inconsistent with the epidemiological medical science that studies the disease: in fact, it just implies a different perspective on the distribution and evolution over time of its determinants in the population.

Epidemiological tradition is not uniform across Europe. There seem to be areas where the epidemiological tradition appears more entrenched than others. A "leopard skin" map (spotted pattern) covers up most of Europe's territory. In England there is a strong home-grown tradition and at the same time close ties with North America. We could say that metaphorically "The Atlantic Ocean is shorter than the Channel!" In the map of continental Europe, Scandinavian countries and the Netherlands are countries whose academic structures have evolved more quickly, while France's, Germany's, and Italy's academic structures have been growing more slowly. Eastern Europe countries have recently displayed considerable attention and commitment to public health. However, in the long term, this commitment has suffered from a lack of original research and associated infrastructure.

Across Europe, many clinicians remain unfamiliar about the methodology of evaluation of diagnostic interventions; their degree of reliability, efficacy; the safety of therapeutic interventions; and other features of clinical epidemiology. The culture of evaluation is, however, essential to interpret the large body of available research data and to provide evidence-based treatment and best practice. Therefore, we need to promote the transition from clinical epidemiology to etiologic epidemiology and workforce development.

The questions we ask are: (1) "What will be the future of epidemiology." (2) "Will there be a conflict between the clinician and the epidemiologist?"

We believe that there are positive signs for the continued integration of clinical epidemiology as a key component of public health. The second question really should not exist. Clinicians should be supported to integrate epidemiological research within their clinical practice.

REFERENCES

1. About EMCDDA, 1993. Available at: *http://www.emcdda.europa.eu/about*. Accessed October 28, 2008.
2. Gowing L, Proudfoot H, Henry-Edwards S, et al. *Evidence Supporting Treatment: The Effectiveness of Interventions for Illicit Drug Use. ANCD Research Paper No 3*. Canberra ACT: Australian National Council on Drugs; 2001.
3. Anderson P, Baumberg B. *Alcohol in Europe—A Public Health Perspective. A Report for the European Commission*. UK: Institute of Alcohol Studies; 2006. Available at: http://ec.europa.eu/health-eu/news_alcoholineurope_en.htm. Accessed October 10, 2009.
4. Dvoryak S. Evaluation of effectiveness of drug treatment programmes in Ukraine. *Heroin Addict Relat Clin Probl*. 2004;6(3):33–36.
5. EMCDDA. *Annual Report 2009—The State of Drugs Problem in Europe*; 2009. Available at: http://www.emcdda.europa.eu/attachments.cfm/att_93236_EN_EMCDDA_AR2009_EN.pdf. Accessed October 10, 2009.
6. EMCDDA. Cannabis problems in context—understanding the increase in European treatment demands. EMCDDA 2004 selected

issue. *EMCDDA 2004 Annual Report on the State of the Drugs Problem in the European Union and Norway*; 2004. Available at: http://www.emcdda.europa.eu/attachements.cfm/att_37361_EN_sel2004_2-en.pdf. Accessed October 28, 2009.

7. EMCCDDA. *Polydrug Use: Patterns and Response—Selected Issue 2009*; 2009. Available at: http://www.emcdda.europa.eu/attachements.cfm/att_93217_EN_EMCDDA_SI09_polydrug%20 use.pdf. Accessed November 1, 2009.

8. DeMaria PA Jr., Sterling R, Weinstein SP. The effect of stimulant and sedative use on treatment outcome of patients admitted to methadone maintenance treatment. *Am J Addict*. 2000;9(2): 145–153.

9. Stenbacka M, Leifman A, Romelsjö A. Mortality among opiate abusers in Stockholm: a longitudinal study. *Heroin Addict Relat Clin Probl*. 2007;9(3):41–50.

10. McManus E, Fitzpatrick C. Alcohol dependence and mood state in a population receiving methadone maintenance treatment. *Ir J Psychol Med*. 2007;24:19–22.

11. EMCDDA. *Differences in Patterns of Drug Use Between Women and Men*; 2005. Available at: http://www.emcdda.europa.eu/attachements.cfm/att_34281_EN_TDS_gender.pdf. Accessed November 1, 2009.

12. EMCDDA. *Annual Report 2006—Selected Issues*; 2006. Available at: http://www.emcdda.europa.eu/attachements.cfm/att_37291_EN_sel2006_2-en.pdf. Accessed November 1, 2009.

13. EMCDDA. *Drug Use and Related Problems among Very Young People (under 15 Years Old)*; 2007. Available at: http://www.emcdda.europa.eu/attachements.cfm/ att_44741_EN_TDSI07001ENC.pdf. Accessed November 1, 2009.

14. Casella PP. *La salute dei migranti*; 2000. Available at: http://www.istitutosanti.org.

15. Salvioni P, Soria A, Feltrin R. Tossicodipendenza e immigrazione: analisi sociodemografica degli utenti di un servizio a bassa soglia a Milano. *Boll Farmacodip e Alcoolis*. 2002;XXV(1–2):101–110.

16. Selten JP, Wierdsma A, Mulder N, et al. Treatment seeking for alcohol and drug use disorders by immigrants to the Netherlands: retrospective, population-based, cohort study. *Soc Psychiatry Psychiatr Epidemiol*. 2007;42(4):301–306.

17. Lindert J, Schouler-Ocak M, Heinz A, et al. Mental health, health care utilisation of migrants in Europe. *Eur Psychiatry*. 2008; 23(suppl 1):14–20.

18. Penka S, Heimann H, Heinz A, et al. Explanatory models of addictive behaviour among native German, Russian-German, and Turkish youth. *Eur Psychiatry*. 2008;23(suppl 1):36–42.

19. Reisinger M. Methadone treatment and the epidemiology of AIDS in the European community. In: Tagliamonte A, Maremmani I, eds. *Drug Addiction and Related Clinical Problems*. Wien/New York: Springer-Verlag; 1995:175–180.

20. Reisinger M. Methadone Treatment and spread of AIDS in Europe in the 1987–1993 years. *Heroin Addict Relat Clin Probl*. 1999;1(2):19–26.

21. Kozlov AA, Perelygin VV, Rohlina ML, et al. Heroin dependence in the Russian Federation: the current situation. *Heroin Addict Relat Clin Probl*. 2006;8(1):11–24.

22. Dolzhanskaya NA, Bouzina TS, Kozlov AA, et al. Knowledge and attitudes of drug treatment professionals towards HIV prevention and care activities in the Russian Federation. *Heroin Addict Relat Clin Probl*. 2006;8(2):23–35.

23. Maremmani I, Pacini M, Pani PP, et al. Say "Yes" to Methadone and Buprenorphine in Russian Federation. *Heroin Addict Relat Clin Probl*. 2006;8(2):5–22.

24. Strang J, Sheridan J, Hunt C, et al. The prescribing of methadone and other opioids to addicts: national survey of GPs in England and Wales. *Br J Gen Pract*. 2005;55(515):444–451.

25. Michelazzi A, Vecchiet F, Leprini R, et al. GPs' office based Metadone Maintenance Treatment in Trieste, Italy. Therapeutic efficacy and predictors of clinical response. *Heroin Addict Relat Clin Probl*. 2008;10(2):27–38.

26. Torrens M, Castillo C, Perez-Sola V. Retention in a low-threshold methadone maintenance program. *Drug Alcohol Depend*. 1996; 41(1):55–59.

27. Maremmani I, Pacini M, Lubrano S, et al. Harm reduction and specific treatments for heroin addiction. Different approaches or levels of intervention?. An illness-centred perspective. *Heroin Addict Relat Clin Probl*. 2002;4(3):5–11.

28. Schifano F, Bargagli AM, Belleudi V, et al. Methadone treatment in clinical practice in Italy: need for improvement. *Eur Addict Res*. 2006;12(3):121–127.

29. Maremmani I, Pacini M. Resistance to treatment. In: Maremmani I, ed. *The Principles and Practice of Methadone Treatment*. Pisa: Pacini Editore Medicina; 2009:135–140.

30. Ceccanti M, Vitali M. Alcoholics With a history of heroin consumption: clinical features and chronology of substance abuse. *Heroin Addict Relat Clin Probl*. 2009;11(3):35–38.

31. EMCDDA. *2008 National Report (2007 Data) to the EMCDDA by the Finnish National Focal Point, STAKES. Finland Drug Situation 2008. New Developments, Trends and In-depth Information on Selected Issues*; 2008. Available at: http://www.emcdda.europa.eu/attachements.cfm/att_86775_EN_NR_2008_FI.pdf. Accessed November 5, 2009.

32. EMCDDA. *Buprenorphine—Treatment, Misuse and Prescription Practices*. Lisbon: EMCDDA; 2005. Accessed November 5, 2009.

33. Cruickshank CC, Dyer KR. A review of the clinical pharmacology of methamphetamine. *Addiction*. 2009;104(7):1085–1099.

34. Ferrari A, Manaresi S, Castellini P, et al. Overdose da oppiacei: analisi dei soccorsi effettuati dal Servizio Emergenze Sanitarie "118", Modena Soccorso, nel 1997 [Opioid overdose: analysis of the aid interventions effected by the Emergency Service "118", Modena Soccorso, in 1997]. *Boll Farmacodip e Alcoolis*. 2001; XXIV(2):31–41.

35. Galli M, Musicco M, for the Comcat Study Group. Mortality of intravenous drug users living in Milan, Italy. Role of HIV-1 infection. *AIDS*. 1994;8:1457–1463.

SECTION 2 ■ DETERMINANTS OF ABUSE AND DEPENDENCE

CHAPTER 4 — Genetic Factors in the Risk for Substance Use Disorders

Thomas A. Nguyen ■ Jaimee L. Heffner ■ Show W. Lin ■ Robert M. Anthenelli

INTRODUCTION

More than a decade ago, the *New York Times* reported that "scientists (had) link (ed) alcoholism to a specific gene, … opening the window of hope for the prevention of a deadly disease." Although the accuracy of the finding on which the headline was based is controversial (1,2), the story remains historically significant.

Sixty years ago there were those who doubted they would ever read such a headline (3). As our understanding of alcoholism (i.e., alcohol dependence) and other substance use disorders has advanced, so, too, have our ideas about their pattern of transmission. The importance of environmental, developmental, and social factors championed by Jellinek and others in the 1940s has had to share the stage with compelling evidence supporting a genetic vulnerability to the disorder. All are important. No one headline tells the whole story, and it is the interaction of genes, environment, and developmental influences that ultimately predict susceptibility to substance use disorders (4,5).

This updated chapter reviews the role of genetic factors in the risk for alcohol, tobacco, cocaine, opioid, and cannabis dependence. Because the preponderance of data is from studies on alcohol and tobacco, these two drugs are emphasized. Reflecting the clinical nature of this text and the authors' area of expertise, this chapter focuses primarily on human genetic aspects of substance use disorders. Comprehensive reviews of the animal and preclinical literature are available elsewhere (6,7).

GENETIC INFLUENCES IN ALCOHOLISM

Traditionally, the search for genetic influences in any complex disorder begins with studies of families, twins, and adoptees affected with the condition. These investigations can provide preliminary evidence on the probable importance of genetic factors and serve as the foundation for subsequent research. The following sections briefly review the results of more than four decades of family, twin, and adoption studies in alcoholism.

Although these investigations are not unanimous in their results, when taken together, they provide compelling evidence for the importance of genetic influences in this disorder and indicate that 40% to 60% of the phenotypic variance in alcoholism can be attributed to genetic factors (8).

Family, Twin, and Adoption Studies of Alcoholism

Family Studies

For centuries, philosophers, writers, and clergy have commented on the familial nature of alcoholism. Plutarch's assertion that "drunks beget drunkards" was based on anecdotal observation alone, and it was not until the last few decades that this contention came under careful scientific scrutiny (9).

The basic design for family studies of any complex illness is to compare the risk for developing the disorder in relatives of probands (individuals manifesting the phenotype or trait) with the rate for relatives of control groups or for the general population (10).

Numerous studies have found that rates of alcoholism are substantially higher in relatives of alcoholics than in relatives of nonalcoholics, with children of alcoholics demonstrating a four- to fivefold increased risk for developing the disorder (7,11). Furthermore, Bierut et al. have reported that, relative to controls without alcohol dependence, the siblings of alcohol-dependent probands have elevated rates of the disorder (up to 50% for men and 25% for women) (12). This increased risk appears to be relatively specific to alcoholism, with most family studies showing an increased prevalence of the disorder among relatives of alcoholic probands, without accompanying higher prevalence of other mental disorders, such as schizophrenia or bipolar disorder (13,14).

Although family studies provide preliminary evidence that alcoholism might be inherited, in themselves, they are inconclusive. Familial aggregation might also reflect the shared social and developmental influences of being raised in the same environment by biologic parents. To disentangle these factors, other approaches are required.

Twin Studies

Research with twins evaluates the relative contributions of genetic and environmental factors by comparing the similarity or concordance rates for the condition in pairs of monozygotic (identical) twins with those of dizygotic (fraternal) twins. The twin study design allows researchers to estimate the contribution of genetic and environmental effects to the individual's liability for alcoholism and other substance use disorders. The liability identified in twin research generally has three components: (a) additive genetic effects; (b) common environmental effects shared by twins (e.g., intrauterine environment, parental upbringing); and (c) specific, nonshared environmental experiences (14). Additive genetic influences are shared 100%, on average, between members of monozygotic twin pairs, while dizygotic twin pairs share 50% of their additive genetic influences (15).

Several major twin studies have directly addressed the concordance rates for alcoholism in identical versus fraternal twins. The first of these was conducted in Sweden where Kaij found that the concordance rate for alcoholism in male monozygotic pairs was greater than that for dizygotic twins (approximately 60% vs. 39%) (16). Interestingly, the discrepancy between concordance rates increased in proportion to the severity of alcoholism in these male twin pairs, favoring a genetic diathesis. A Veterans Administration twin register study in the United States revealed similar higher concordance rates for identical male twin pairs (17) as did two other smaller studies (18,19). These findings were further corroborated in a population-based sample of twins in the United States (20). However, not all studies agree (21).

While results among male–male twin pairs had consistently demonstrated that genetic factors were important in the etiology of alcoholism in men, results in women were initially less consistent. Several smaller twin studies found no (19,21) or relatively little (18) genetic influence in females compared to males. However, in a large sample of female same-sex twin pairs in the United States, the concordance for alcoholism was greater in monozygotic than in dizygotic twin pairs (22).

These results were corroborated in a study of Australian twin pairs that found genetic factors play as important a role in determining alcoholism risk in women as in men (23). Thus, the vast majority of twin studies support the notion that alcoholism is genetically influenced and that heritable factors are important in the vulnerability for the disorder in both men and women.

Adoption Studies

Perhaps the most convincing way to separate genetic from environmental effects is to study individuals who were separated soon after birth from their biologic parents and those who were raised by nonrelative adoptive parents (24). This can be done through classical adoption studies or through a half-sibling approach.

There have been several half-sibling and adoption studies evaluating the possibility that alcoholism, at least in part, has genetic determinants. Regarding the half-sibling approach, Schuckit and colleagues evaluated a group of individuals who had been raised apart from their biologic parents but who had either a biologic or surrogate parent with alcoholism (25). Subjects who had a biologic parent with severe alcohol problems were significantly more likely to have alcoholism themselves than if their surrogate parents were alcoholics.

Comparing the similarities between the offspring behavior and the biologic and adoptive parents' characteristics is the basis of adoption studies. If there are strong associations between the offspring and biologic parents then this is indicative of genetic impact, whereas strong associations between the offspring and the adoptive parents are suggestive of environmental impact (26).

Over the last three decades, several adoption studies in Denmark, Sweden, and the United States have yielded similar results. In Denmark, Goodwin and coworkers found that the sons of alcoholics were about four times more likely to be alcoholic than were sons of nonalcoholics, and that being raised by either nonalcoholic adoptive parents or by biologic parents did not affect this increased risk (27). Furthermore, although the sons of alcoholics were found to be at highest risk for developing alcoholism, they were no more likely to have other psychiatric disorders than were sons of nonalcoholics (24,27). As with some of the twin studies cited above, results for women in the Copenhagen Adoption Study were not significant, but the sample size for women was too small to reach any firm conclusions about potential gender differences in genetic vulnerability. Similar results were found in another large study done in Stockholm, Sweden, where Cloninger and colleagues showed significantly higher rates of alcohol abuse in adopted sons of biologic fathers registered with alcohol problems (28). Data from two smaller-scale adoption studies in Iowa largely confirmed the results of the larger European studies (29,30); however, one of the studies detected genetic influences in female adoptees, as well (31). Only one adoption study has found contrary results (32), and most authors agree that the disparity probably reflects methodologic problems in its design (e.g., small sample size and lack of rigorous diagnostic criteria for alcohol problems in the parents) or differences in the subpopulations studied (9,24,33).

The Search for Genetically Mediated Markers of Alcoholism

The results of family, twin, and adoption studies offer ample support for the heredity of alcohol dependence, thereby justifying a search for what might be inherited to increase the risk for this disorder. However, before such a search can be optimally conducted, it is important to consider several major factors that obscure our ability to identify the genetic factors that predispose individuals to develop alcoholism.

Clinical and Etiologic Heterogeneity

First, when studying complex disorders like alcoholism and other kinds of drug dependence, it is essential to realize that a diagnosis is made at the clinical syndrome level and that it is likely that many different pathways or etiologies can lead to this combination of symptoms and signs (34,35). As a result of this etiologic heterogeneity and the likelihood that multiple genes are involved for each of the various pathways that may lead to the broad clinical phenotype of alcoholism, consideration of the sample in which the genetic analyses are conducted is of paramount importance.

Comorbidity with Other Psychiatric Disorders

A second, related consideration is that problematic use of alcohol or other drugs may co-occur with other disorders in the same individual. In fact, at least 30% of alcoholic men have evidence of preexisting disorders (36), and this figure soars to 60% to 70% among alcoholic women (37). Alcoholism has been found to co-occur with internalizing disorders (e.g., depression, bipolar disorder) as well as externalizing disorders (e.g., antisocial personality disorder [ASPD], conduct disorder [CD], and attention deficit hyperactivity disorder [ADHD]) (38). Approximately 70% of men with ASPD have secondary alcohol problems during the course of their disorder (36), and during the manic phase of bipolar illness, approximately 50% of patients develop severe ethanol-related difficulties (39). The phenotypic differences between these groups of "alcoholics" are obvious, but genetic influences specific to the development of alcohol dependence become much less clear in the context of psychiatric comorbidity.

Subtypes of Alcoholism

Several overlapping approaches have been used to categorize alcoholics into clinical phenotypes or subgroups based on family history of alcohol dependence, age-at-onset of the disorder, clinical symptoms, and personality traits (24,40–42). Although each of these methods has its strengths and limitations, the validity of any one method over the others has not yet been established (43,44). Reviewed in detail elsewhere (45), the underlying philosophy behind their use is an attempt to better define subtypes of alcoholics who vary in genetic risk for the disorder.

Among the many typologies of alcohol dependence that have been identified, one theory proposed by Cloninger and colleagues gained considerable popularity (28,33,41,46,47). Using a discriminant function analysis of their large sample of Swedish adoptees, this group initially proposed two subtypes of alcoholism (types 1 and 2) that could be distinguished on the basis of the biologic parents' history of alcohol abuse and the degree to which postnatal environmental factors affected the inheritance of susceptibility to alcoholism (28,46). Type 1, or "milieu-limited," alcoholism was posited to predominate among female alcoholics and their male relatives, and characterized by loss of control of drinking after the age of 25 years, pronounced environmental reactivity to drinking, minimal associated criminality, and "passive-dependent personality traits" marked by high degrees of harm avoidance, reward dependence, and low levels of novelty seeking as measured by Cloninger's Tridimensional Personality Questionnaire (TPQ) (41). In contrast, the "male-limited," or type 2, subgroup was postulated to have an inheritance pattern less dependent on environmental factors for phenotypic expression and an earlier age of onset, more associated criminal behavior, and a triad of personality traits that run opposite those of the prototypic "milieu-limited" alcoholic (33,41,48). This group later refined their theory to include a *third* class of alcoholism, which they called "antisocial behavior disorder with alcohol abuse" (33,48,49).

Babor and colleagues (42) used an empirical clustering technique and described a subgrouping scheme for alcoholics that included type A and type B alcoholics, named after the Roman gods Apollo and Bacchus. Type A alcoholics are characterized by later age-at-onset, fewer childhood risk factors, less-severe dependence, fewer alcohol-related problems, and less psychopathologic dysfunction. Type B alcoholics typically exhibit an early onset of alcohol-related problems, higher levels of childhood risk factors and familial alcoholism, greater severity of dependence, multiple substance use, a long-term treatment history, greater psychopathologic dysfunction, and greater life stress (42,50). The type A/B dichotomy was replicated in another large sample of alcohol-dependent subjects even after the exclusion of individuals with ASPD and those with an onset of alcohol dependence before age 25 years, further supporting this subtyping method's potential usefulness (51).

In summary, the search for what is inherited in the predisposition toward alcoholism is challenging because alcoholism is a clinically and etiologically heterogeneous disorder. Moreover, because of the comorbidity between alcoholism and certain other psychiatric disorders, studies that do not adequately control for this increased variability may yield spurious genetic associations. Furthermore, among the broad clinical phenotype of alcoholism, subgroups may exist who differ in the degree of genetic susceptibility.

Intermediate Phenotypes

One way of discovering gene effects in etiologically complex disorders is through restructuring of the complexity into factors that are likely to be less etiologically heterogeneous (52). Prior to the explosion in molecular genetics research (see "Molecular Genetic Studies"), the search for these vulnerability factors for alcoholism focused on identifying endophenotypes or intermediate phenotypes that might be associated with the predisposition toward the disease. These are neurobiologic or neurobehavioral characteristics associated with alcoholism whose manifestation may be more closely linked to gene expression than the broad clinical phenotype of alcoholism itself (53). The focus of many older articles (34,54) and book chapters (55) dedicated to the topic of the genetics of alcoholism, these intermediate phenotypes remain relevant because they may represent some of the end-stage pathophysiologic processes through which genetic factors influence susceptibility to the disease. Because of space limitations, only some of these phenotypic markers are discussed here, and interested readers may seek more detailed reviews of these broad phenotypes elsewhere (53).

Electrophysiologic Markers

Electrophysiologic measurements of brain activity have been demonstrated as potentially promising neurobiologic markers that might be associated with the predisposition toward alcoholism, at least among some subgroups of individuals (56,57). Event-related brain potentials (ERPs) have been used extensively to study information processing in both long-term abstinent alcoholics and unaffected high- and low-risk populations who differ on the presence or absence of a family history of alcoholism, respectively (34). The amplitude of one important component of the ERP, the positive wave observed at 300 to 500 milliseconds after a rare but expected stimulus (P3), has been demonstrated to be significantly decreased in about one third of the sons of alcoholic fathers when compared to controls (56,58). Moreover, this decrease is more dramatic in alcohol-dependent individuals who also have a diagnosis of illicit drug abuse or dependence, especially those with ASPD (59). Although some studies do not agree with these results (60,61), differences probably reflect variations in the studies' designs, including the sample population chosen. Bergleiter and Porjesz have proposed that such ERP anomalies may reflect brain disinhibition and/or hyperexcitability (impulsivity) that is critically involved in the vulnerability toward alcohol dependence (53).

In addition to this elicited brain-wave marker, a second approach has relied on measurements of the power of waveforms on the background cortical electroencephalogram (EEG) (34). Male alcoholics and their sons might demonstrate a decreased amount of slow-wave (e.g., alpha wave) activity at baseline when compared with controls (62,63). Similarly, Ehlers and Schuckit reported that sons of alcoholics differ from lower-risk, matched controls at baseline on the amount of activity in one part of the frequency range of alpha waves (i.e., men with a positive family history of alcoholism had more energy in the fast alpha range than did controls) (64,65).

Low Level of Response to Alcohol

Schuckit et al. and others have documented differences in the response to alcohol between high-risk and control populations. Otherwise healthy groups of 18- to 25-year-old sons of primary alcoholic men were selected as higher risk, or family history positive (FHP), subjects who were then compared with controls comprised of lower-risk, family history negative (FHN) individuals. Each FHP–FHN matched pair was carefully evaluated at baseline and then observed for 3 to 4 hours after consuming placebo or the equivalent of 3 to 5 drinks of beverage alcohol.

After drinking the alcohol, the two family history groups developed similar patterns of blood alcohol concentrations (BACs) over time, making it unlikely that group differences depended on the rate of absorption or metabolism of ethanol (34,66). However, a major consistent difference between FHP and FHN subjects was in the intensity of their subjective feelings of intoxication after imbibing alcohol (66–68). Using an analogue scale and asking subjects to rate the intensity of different aspects of intoxication, FHP men rated themselves as significantly less intoxicated than did their FHN matched controls after drinking ethanol (66–68). This decreased intensity of reaction to alcohol among FHP men was also observed for at least one measure of motor performance; the level of sway in the upper body (69). Furthermore, following the ethanol challenge, FHP men also exhibited less-intense change in the levels of cortisol and prolactin, two hormones shown to be altered after ethanol ingestion (70,71).

Schuckit et al. hypothesized that a decreased intensity of reaction to lower doses of alcohol might make it more difficult for susceptible individuals to discern when they are becoming drunk at low enough blood levels to be able to stop drinking during an evening.

Without this feedback, and especially in the setting of a heavy drinking society, predisposed individuals may be inclined to drink more and thus run an increased risk for subsequent alcohol-related life problems (13). Consequently, viewers blind to the initial family history and the determination of the level of response to alcohol located all 453 subjects an average of 8.2 years after the time of their initial evaluation (72,73). The data revealed that the family groups had been correctly identified, and that the sons of alcoholics had a threefold increased risk for alcohol dependence. The results also demonstrated a strong and significant relationship between a low level of response to alcohol and the future development of alcoholism. A possible explanation for the low response to alcohol is the genetic variation in the serotonin transporter gene and in the gene encoding the subunit alpha-6 of the gamma-aminobutyric acid receptor A, both of which are discussed later in the chapter (74).

Early Onset of Alcohol Use and the Development of Alcohol Dependence

Multiple studies have demonstrated that the early onset of alcohol consumption is associated with increased rates of subsequent alcohol dependence (75,76). Hingson et al. found that the lifetime prevalence of alcohol dependence was 47% among those whose first drink was at 14 years or younger as compared to 9% among those whose first drink was at 21 years or older (75). This finding is comparable between males and females (77). The timing of first alcohol drink is attributable, in part, to both heritable factors and shared environment, although heritable factors appear to exert a greater influence (77).

These studies demonstrate some important attributes regarding genetic influences in alcoholism risk. First, a family history of alcoholism is associated with increased risk for this disorder among people of diverse socioeconomic classes. Second, it is likely that there are multiple roads into the heightened alcohol risk, with, for example, some individuals developing alcoholism in part through very high levels of impulsivity, others having increased risk of alcoholism due to a low level of response to alcohol in the context of a heavy drinking society, and so on (78). Third, it is unlikely that any single gene explains alcoholism risk; but rather, it is multiple genes interacting with the environment.

Molecular Genetic Studies

With the advent of modern molecular genetic techniques blossoming over the past two decades, more recent efforts have attempted to identify genes that influence susceptibility to alcoholism. Although the details of the molecular genetic techniques used to identify such genetic markers are beyond the scope of this chapter, briefly, they involve the meticulous dissection of deoxyribonucleic acid (DNA) into specific nucleotide (i.e., the building blocks of DNA) patterns called markers or microsatellites (for details see references) (57,79,80). Such markers are then analyzed to determine whether there is *linkage* between the marker and the phenotype (i.e., the marker is transmitted along with the disease in families) or whether there is an *association* between the polymorphism and the phenotype (81,82) (i.e., a given marker allele is more common among those individuals with the disease in a population). Indeed, such genetic strategies have been used extensively in the large multicenter effort entitled the Collaborative Study on the Genetics of Alcoholism (COGA) (83).

A number of candidate genes for alcohol dependence have been proposed thus far; interested readers are urged to see other recent reviews of this to appreciate the full breadth of this massive research effort (7,8,84,85). Because genes encoding the alcohol-metabolizing enzymes are the only genes consistently demonstrated to contribute to alcoholism susceptibility, these genes are highlighted.

Alcohol Dehydrogenase and Aldehyde Dehydrogenase

BAC and an individual's subjective response to alcohol represent a complex interaction of pharmacokinetic and pharmacodynamic effects of ethanol in the brain and body. There is a large degree of interindividual variation, as a function of genetic, gender, and ethnic influences, in how one responds to alcohol that involves the drug's absorption, distribution, metabolism, and elimination. Alcohol dehydrogenase (ADH) and aldehyde dehydrogenase (ALDH) are the major enzymes involved in the sequential degradation of ethanol; ADH catabolizes alcohol into acetaldehyde, which ALDH breaks down to acetate and water (86,87). Numerous studies have found that allelic variants of ADH and ALDH genes play an important role in influencing the metabolism of alcohol and that these polymorphisms are associated with the risk for developing alcohol dependence. ALDH is the major enzyme that catabolizes acetaldehyde in the liver and other organs. There are many ALDH gene families distributed on several different chromosomes (88). Family 2 genes (ALDH 2) have been the most well studied genes regarding an association with alcohol dependence. This family of genes encodes mitochondrial enzymes that oxidize acetaldehyde. ALDH 2 has a deficient allelic variant (ALDH 2∗2), when compared with the wild type of ALDH 2 (ALDH 2∗1). The ALDH 2∗2 variant gene is found in approximately 16–35% of Han Chinese, Japanese, Koreans, and Vietnamese (89–93). ALDH 2∗2 rarely occurs in other ethnic groups (94). Individuals with the ALDH 2∗2 variant typically experience aversive responses (e.g., facial flushing, tachycardia, headache, hypotension, and a burning sensation in the stomach) to alcohol consumption as a result of the accumulation of acetaldehyde. Several studies demonstrate the protective effect of ALDH 2∗2 gene carriers from developing alcohol dependence with homozygosity providing full protection whereas heterozygosity (ALD∗1/∗2) can only afford partial protection against alcoholism (93–97).

The association between polymorphisms in ADH genes (located on chromosome 4) and alcohol dependence is not as robust as for ALDH genes. The variant allele ADH 2∗2 (more recently renamed the ADH 1B∗2 allele) encodes a high-activity enzyme involved in the oxidation of ethanol to acetaldehyde exhibiting no appreciable cardiovascular responses and subjective perceptions following the consumption of alcohol (8,94). ADH 1B∗2 homozygosity is associated with an eightfold decrease in the risk of alcohol dependence in East Asians (98). Interestingly, it has been found that having the combination of the ADH 2∗2 and ALDH 2∗2 gene variants is associated with the lowest risk for alcoholism (96,99). Taken together, then, there is compelling evidence that the interaction between a genetically controlled alcohol-metabolizing enzyme system and environmental factors (such as attitudes about drinking and drunkenness) appears to contribute significantly to the lower alcoholism risk among a subgroup of Asians and Ashkenazi Jews (100,101).

Dopaminergic System

The dopaminergic system is involved in the reinforcing effects of drugs of abuse. As alluded to at the beginning of this chapter, the first report of an "alcoholism gene" occurred in 1990, when Blum et al. identified an allele of the gene encoding the D2 dopamine receptor (DRD2) that appeared to be implicated in severe cases of alcoholism (102). The finding had good face validity because the mesolimbic dopamine reward circuit in the brain has been repeatedly demonstrated to play a major role in ethanol's rewarding effects (103,104). The subject of much debate, with studies both finding (1,81,105–111) and not finding (2,112–115) an association with alcoholism, the DRD2 controversy remains relevant because it heralded the advent of modern molecular genetic approaches to this complex genetic disease. Interestingly, there is also some evidence to implicate the DRD2 gene in other substance use disorders, leading some investigators to label it a potential "reward gene" as discussed subsequently in this chapter (107,116).

Ebstein et al. (117) reported an association between a polymorphism of the dopamine D4 receptor (DRD4) and the novelty seeking subscale as measured by Cloninger's TPQ (41). The DRD4 is expressed predominantly in the limbic system. Ebstein and colleagues' finding, along with other confirmatory results (118) published in the same journal issue, provided the first replicated association between a specific genetic polymorphism and a personality trait that has been linked with alcoholism and other substance use disorders (117). Although the subjects in this study were nonalcoholic normal controls, it is intriguing that a personality trait believed to predict an increased risk for alcoholism might have heritable components. Studies examining the associations among the DRD1 gene polymorphism (affecting the D1 receptor) (119,120) and the dopamine D3 gene (affecting dopamine D3 receptors) (121–123) and alcoholism have yielded inconsistent and generally negative results.

GABAergic System

Gamma-aminobutyric acid (GABA) receptor genes, which encode the GABAa and GABAb receptors that bind GABA (the human brain's major inhibitory neurotransmitter), have also been identified as promising candidate genes for alcoholism (8,124,125). *In vitro* studies have found that ethanol potentiates GABAergic neurotransmission (126) and preclinical studies in experimental animals have determined that GABA plays an important role in alcohol's brain depressant behavioral effects (127). Specifically, the cluster of GABAa receptor genes is found on chromosome 4, and this chromosomal region has been implicated in linkage scans for alcoholism. One variation of this gene is GABRA2, which has been strongly associated with alcohol use disorders (128). Studies in Southwest American Indians have identified GABRA2 as a susceptibility factor for alcoholism (129). These findings have been confirmed in some studies in Caucasian populations, and provocative associations have been described between quantitative trait loci of GABAa receptor genes and potential intermediate phenotypes such as electroencephalographic markers (130). Furthermore, a study by Enoch et al. identified the gene adjacent to GABRA2, GABRG1, through linkage disequilibrium studies and found that GABRG1 haplotypes and single nucleotide polymorphisms (SNPs) were significantly associated with alcoholism in both Finnish Caucasian men and Plains Indian men and women (131).

Serotonergic System

The serotonergic system has been studied extensively in clinical populations and has been implicated in alcoholism, aggression, impulsivity, and mood disorders (132). Serotonergic dysfunction has also been repeatedly implicated in both preclinical (133,134) and clinical (74,135,136) studies examining the vulnerability for alcoholism. Two main alleles of the serotonin transporter–linked polymorphic region (5-HTTLPR) of the SLC6A4-1 gene have either 14 (short [S]) or 16 (long [L]) copies of a 22 base-pair imperfect repeat. The L allele increases transcriptional activity of the 5-HTT gene, which results in increased production of 5-HTT and more rapid reuptake of serotonin. Conversely, the S allele decreases transcription of the message, the end result of which is a reduction in transporter number and slower serotonin reuptake. It is thought that more rapid reuptake, associated with the L allele, results in lower level of this neurotransmitter and potentially decreased alcohol effects (74). Reviewed in greater detail elsewhere (8), there is controversial support for an association between alcoholism and the L allele of 5-HTTLPR; (74,137–140) however, not all studies agree with other studies finding that the S allele contributes significantly to risk for alcohol dependence (141–144).

Opioidergic System

The mu-opioid receptor (MOR) OPRM1 plays a central role in the rewarding process of alcohol, opioids, and other substances of abuse such as cocaine and nicotine (145). Ethanol produces some of its rewarding effects through the release of endogenous opioids interacting with the mesocorticolimbic dopaminergic pathways. One of the most widely studied polymorphisms of the OPRM1 gene is the A118G variant in which aspartic acid (Asp40 allele) replaces asparagine (Asn40 allele) at position 40 of the receptor. This single amino acid substitution alters its endogenous ligand's (beta-endorphin's) activity at the receptor, resulting in beta-endorphin binding with threefold greater affinity to variant Asp40 than to the Asn40 MOR (116,146). Some investigators have found an association between the A118G SNP and linkage (147,148); whereas others have not found this association (149–151). Individuals with one copy of the Asp40 allele were found to have a greater response to the effects of alcohol than those who were homozygous for the Asn40 allele (105,152).

Genetic variants in the OPRM1 gene may also influence the response to antirelapse medications used to treat alcohol dependence (153). The therapeutic effects of naltrexone are based on the "endorphin compensation" theory, which suggests that alcohol-dependent subjects have a relative deficiency in endogenous opioids at baseline and possibly following stress, and that alcohol helps restore these levels (116). Naltrexone is a pure opioid receptor antagonist with the greatest affinity for MORs. Among alcohol-dependent patients, naltrexone reduces the occurrence of heavy drinking days (154), increases the time to first relapse (155,156), and reduces the number of drinking days (157) as well as the number of drinks per drinking occasion (158). Using a pharmacogenetic approach, it has been found that alcoholic subjects with the Asp40 allele treated with naltrexone were more likely to have good clinical outcome (87.1%) than those individuals homozygous for the Asn40 allele (54.8%) (159).

In summary, advances in molecular genetics and an explosion of studies in this field within the last decade have added important information to our understanding of the genetic factors associated with the susceptibility to alcoholism. Many potential candidate genes have been identified that might be associated with the risk for the disorder; only a few of these have been highlighted as examples of the findings accumulating from this massive search. What is clear is that many genes likely influence the vulnerability for alcoholism and that different combinations of genes are likely to be more or less salient for each endophenotype associated with the disorder. Certain genes (e.g., the ALDH 2*2 gene) may provide protection against developing serious alcohol-related problems, while others (e.g., the DRD2 gene) might predispose certain individuals to alcoholism and other substance use disorders that are discussed next.

GENETIC INFLUENCES IN TOBACCO AND OTHER DRUG DEPENDENCE

This section focuses on nicotine dependence because of its high prevalence, associated morbidity and mortality, and common co-occurrence with alcohol and other substance use disorders. There is also significant overlap in the genetic vulnerability to alcohol and nicotine dependence, especially in heavy drinkers and smokers (26); about 50% of the genetic liability to nicotine dependence is shared with alcoholism and 15% of the genetic liability to alcoholism is shared with nicotine dependence (128). Genetic influences on other drugs of abuse (cocaine and other stimulants, opioids, and cannabinoids) are discussed subsequently.

Nicotine/Tobacco Dependence

Cigarette smoking is still the leading preventable cause of death each year in the United States, with more than 440,000 deaths being attributed to tobacco smoking (160). The estimated annual smoking attributable costs in the United States were $96 billion for direct medical care for adults and $97 billion for lost productivity (160). Alarmingly, every day nearly 5000 young people under the age of 18 years try their first cigarette (160). Thus, searching for the genetic and environmental factors that contribute to the initiation and persistence of cigarette smoking is of paramount importance in the prevention and treatment of nicotine dependence. This section reviews the role of genetic factors in the initiation and maintenance of tobacco smoking and organizes this literature into population versus molecular genetics studies.

Family, Twin, and Adoption Studies of Tobacco Dependence

Family Studies

In contrast to the large literature on family studies in the genetics of alcoholism, there are fewer studies examining the familial transmission of tobacco smoking. Initiation of cigarette smoking is strongly associated with parental and sibling smoking, thus, the prevalence of smoking among teenagers is two to four times higher in individuals whose parents or siblings smoke (161). For example, Hughes reported that individuals whose parents smoked during the probands' adolescence were more likely to be smokers (52%) than were individuals whose parents did not smoke during the subjects' adolescence (20%) (161). In the Collaborative Study on the Genetics of Alcoholism (COGA), Bierut et al. found that siblings of habitual smoking probands had a roughly twofold (relative risk = 1.77) elevated risk of becoming smokers when compared with siblings of nonsmoking probands (12). However, as stated previously, family studies have difficulty disentangling genetic from environmental factors because the study subjects involved lived together and shared the same environment. For this reason, more recent studies examining the genetic influences on cigarette smoking have focused on twin pairs raised in the same or mixed families, and on combined twin and adoption studies, in order to tease out more precisely the relative contributions of genetic and environmental factors that lead to the initiation and perpetuation of tobacco use (162,163).

Twin Studies

Twin studies are a very powerful tool to explore the relative contribution of genetic factors in the etiology of nicotine dependence. Taken together, results of several twin studies indicate there is a significant genetic influence on the development and continuation of habitual cigarette smoking. Carmelli et al. compared male monozygotic and dizygotic twins in the genetic influence on smoking. They found that the concordance rate for smoking was significantly higher in monozygotic twins than among dizygotic twins across all three categorizations (i.e., among never, former, and current smokers) of smokers they examined (164). Interestingly, the data also suggested that genetic factors appear to influence an individual's ability to quit smoking; monozygotic twins were more likely than dizygotic twins to be concordant for quitting smoking (rate ratio = 1.24).

As alluded to earlier, recent studies on the genetics of cigarette smoking not only focus on nicotine dependence itself, but also investigate the related process of initiating tobacco smoking behavior (165–169). Parsing the relative genetic contributions to the various component behaviors that ultimately contribute to tobacco addiction (i.e., initiation, amount smoked, continuation), it appears that approximately 50% of the initiation of smoking behavior is genetically influenced, while persistence of smoking and amount smoked have approximately a 70% genetic contribution (170). Heath et al. retrospectively analyzed 3810 adult Australian twin pairs on age-at-onset of smoking to determine the role of genetic and environmental factors in the onset of smoking (167). For female twins and younger male twins, the onset of smoking was strongly influenced by genetic factors. Kendler et al., studying female twins on smoking initiation and nicotine dependence, suggested that heritable factors played an important etiologic role in both smoking initiation and nicotine dependence (169). However, while the liabilities to smoking initiation and nicotine dependence were highly correlated, they were not identical, suggesting that both independent and common genetic factors may underlie these behaviors.

Even though the twin study design is an important tool in the study of genetic factors in nicotine dependence, studies have found that monozygotic twins cosocialized more, spent more time together, and shared peer groups more closely than dizygotic twins (171,172). Thus, based on these studies, the higher concordance rate of monozygotic twins could be inflated as a consequence of the cosocialization (shared environment), requiring other population genetic techniques be used.

Adoption Studies

Adoption studies provide another approach to disentangle the environmental and genetic contributions to tobacco smoking. An older adoption study found that parental and child smoking was significantly correlated among biologic pairs, but was not correlated among adoptive parents and adoptees (173). These results were extended in an analysis of the Danish Adoption Register, where it was demonstrated that adoptees' smoking status was strongly associated with their biologic full-siblings' smoking status (174).

Another novel strategy to combine both twin and adoption designs is by examining concordance rates in twins reared together versus those reared apart. Consistent with results from regular twin studies, both male monozygotic twins reared together and reared apart had higher correlations in smoking behavior when compared with their dizygotic twin counterparts. However, the monozygotic twins reared together exhibited greater concordance rates in smoking than monozygotic twins reared apart, providing further evidence that the rearing environment and genetics interact to influence an individual's risk to be a smoker (175).

Gender Differences

An interesting observation from studies of smokers is a potential gender difference in the magnitude of the relative contribution of genetic and environmental effects. Social or cultural constraints might influence the expression of these genetic influences on smoking. This is evident in certain countries such as China and India, as reflected by the lower prevalence of smoking in women as compared to men (176). As far as the ability to stop smoking, there appear to be greater genetic effects on women's ability to quit (68%) than that seen in men (54%) (177).

Molecular Genetic Studies

The evidence to date has been very consistent with respect to the significance of genetic contributions to smoking initiation and tobacco dependence. As was the case for alcoholism, the more daunting task is to determine the genes responsible for nicotine dependence susceptibility. As with other addictive disorders, the inheritance of tobacco smoking is most likely polygenic and multifactorial, involving a complex web of genetic, environmental, and developmental influences. Indeed, the severity of the disorder may reflect on how many different genes are involved.

The search for genetic factors contributing to nicotine dependence susceptibility is focused primarily on genetic variations (polymorphisms) between smokers and nonsmokers. A variety of potential candidate genes are implicated that affect multiple aspects of nicotine metabolism and other components of the mesolimbic brain reward system, including various neurotransmitters, receptors, and transporters, as briefly described in the next four subsections.

Dopaminergic System

Much attention is focused on the mesolimbic dopamine system as playing an important role in mediating the vulnerability for tobacco dependence. There are five categories of dopamine receptor subtypes labeled D1 to D5. Since the first report of an association of the A1 allele of the dopamine D2 receptor (DRD2) gene with alcoholism described previously (178), the DRD2 gene has been intensively studied in other substance use disorders, including nicotine dependence. DRD2 SNPs including the A1 allele have been associated with decreased dopamine binding sites (176). Both past and current cigarette smokers were found to have higher prevalence of the A1 allele of the DRD2 than did nonsmoking controls (179). Moreover, the prevalence of the A1 allele increased progressively from nonsmokers to past smokers to active smokers. Another study found a significantly higher A1 allele frequency (48.7%) of the DRD2 in smokers who made unsuccessful quit attempts, when compared with controls (25.9%) (180). (Interestingly, Spitz et al. suggested that smokers had significantly higher B1 allele frequency of the DRD2 gene than nonsmokers (181).) In addition, subjects with the A1 allele had significant inverse associations between the prevalence of the A1 allele and (a) the age-at-onset of smoking and (b) the number of attempts at quitting smoking. However, other studies have not found any increase in A1 allele frequency when comparing smokers with nonsmokers (182), raising concerns that population stratification in some case control studies might have influenced the results.

How may the A1 allele DRD2 polymorphism influence the risk for developing and maintaining tobacco dependence? As previously mentioned and reported in some studies, the subjects carrying the A1 allele in the DRD2 gene may have significantly reduced D2 receptor density (176,183), as indexed by a lower mean relative glucose metabolic rate on positron emission tomography testing (184). Thus, it has been hypothesized that individuals may use nicotine (and other drugs of abuse) to compensate for a deficiency of their dopaminergic system (185).

As reviewed elsewhere, many other polymorphisms have also been found in genes encoding other dopamine receptors, some of which have been associated with tobacco smoking (186–191).

Lerman et al. compared the dopamine transporter gene (SLC6A3) and the DRD2 genes in a group of smokers and nonsmokers and found that individuals with allele 9 of the SLC6A3 gene (SLC6A3-9) were significantly less likely to be smokers, especially when this polymorphism was found in combination with the A2 allele of the DRD2 genotype (192). Sabol et al. replicated this finding (193). Thus, it has been hypothesized that the presence of the A2 allele of the DRD2 gene may be negatively associated with tobacco smoking or might yield a protective effect against smoking.

Serotonergic System

Several studies have found that nicotine increases central nervous system (CNS) serotonin release and that acute nicotine withdrawal is marked by a relative depletion in central serotonin (194,195). As alluded to previously in the alcoholism section, after serotonin is released into the synaptic cleft from terminals of serotonergic neurons, it is promptly taken back up into the presynaptic neuron via the actions of serotonin transporter (5-HTT). Two functional alleles of the serotonin transporter-linked polymorphic region (5-HTTLPR) have been identified and labeled the long (L) and short (S) types (196,197). The S-type allele decreases the transcriptional activity of the 5-HTT gene, as compared to the L-type allele, and subsequently decreases the function of the 5-HTT. A strong association between tobacco smoking and the S allele of the 5-HTTLPR has been reported by several investigators (198–200). However, another study failed to confirm this finding (201). Another study found that the short (S/S or S/L) genotype interacted with neuroticism such that neurotic traits were associated with the rate of nicotine intake, nicotine dependence, and smoking motivation in S carriers as compared to those individuals carrying the homozygous long (L/L) genotype (202,203).

Although the relationship between the 5-HTTLPR and cigarette smoking has been studied widely, a recent meta-analysis revealed that this association remains equivocal (204). This same group of investigators found that there was not an effect of 5-HTTLPR genotype on smoking cessation or on nicotine replacement therapy (NRT) response compared with placebo (205). Another study by Trummer et al., supported this finding by showing that neither smoking status nor Fagerström Test for Nicotine Dependence (FTND) score, pack years, number of cigarettes smoked daily, or previous attempts to quit smoking were related to 5-HTTLPR genotype (206). However, a more recent study found that the L/L and the S/L genotypes were significantly higher in smokers than in nonsmokers among Chinese males. Furthermore, this study demonstrated that the number of cigarettes per day and FTND score were significantly higher in smokers with the L/L and S/L genotypes than in smokers with S/S genotype (207). Clearly, these mixed results point to the complexity of these issues and the relatively early stages of this line of inquiry.

To our knowledge, there are no published reports of an association between cigarette smoking and the multiple serotonin-receptor-subtype polymorphisms. However, polymorphic variants in the gene encoding the protein involved with serotonin synthesis are also implicated in tobacco smoking behavior. Tryptophan hydroxylase (TPH) is the enzyme that performs the initial and rate-limiting step in the production of serotonin from tryptophan. Individuals with the A/A genotype of the TPH gene were found to have started smoking earlier than other genotypes, but there was no association of TPH alleles with subjects' current smoking status (208). Interestingly, Sullivan et al. also found that TPH markers were significantly associated with the onset of smoking initiation (209).

Cytochrome P450 Enzyme System

The cytochrome P450 enzyme system plays an important role in the metabolism of drugs and other xenobiotic agents. In vivo, the majority of nicotine is metabolized by CYP2A6 into cotinine (210). CYP2A6 genetic polymorphisms may result in decreased nicotine metabolism, and this reduction in nicotine metabolism may produce favorable outcomes in smokers as reflected in lower amounts of daily cigarette consumption, lower smoking intensity, and improved quit rates. Individuals who carry the inactive alleles of the CYP2A6 also have a lower risk of becoming smokers because of decreased nicotine metabolism, resulting in lower levels of cotinine in urine (211). Furthermore, individuals carrying these alleles smoke fewer cigarettes if they do smoke (212,213). In those subjects who are homozygous for the CYP2A6 deletion, the systemic levels of nicotine following smoking are about four times higher (214) and the urinary levels of cotinine are approximately 85% higher (215) than smokers who are heterozygous for this deletion. Having one loss-of-function CYP2A6 allele reduces the CYP2A6 activity by 50% and elevates the plasma levels of nicotine by 44% in smokers who are treated with the transdermal patch (210). Conversely, individuals with the CYP2A6 wild-type genotype (faster metabolizers of nicotine) smoke more cigarettes per day and are less likely to successfully quit smoking (186).

CYP2B6 polymorphisms also appear to influence smoking behaviors; smokers of European ancestry who have the CYP2B6*6 genotype have been found to have higher rates of relapse when trying to quit than those with other cytochrome P450 genotypes (216). Thus, as was the case with genes regulating the metabolism of alcohol, CYP2A6 and CYP2B6 are genetically regulated modulators of nicotine metabolism that appear to influence smoking behaviors.

Nicotinic Acetylcholine Receptors

Nicotine is the major addictive ingredient in tobacco smoke (170). Nicotine activates the nicotinic acetylcholine receptors (nAChRs) and stimulates dopamine release in the mesolimbic brain reward system. nAChRs are widely distributed in the CNS and peripheral nervous system. These receptors are excitatory, ligand-gated channels, and are composed of five subunits. Twelve subunit genes have been identified and labeled alpha2 to alpha10 and beta2 to beta4 (213,217,218). The properties of these receptors depend on the various compositions of these subunit combinations.

Genes encoding nAChR subunits have been found adjacent to those genetic loci that are associated with greater susceptibility to nicotine dependence (219). Candidate gene association studies have yielded evidence that several variants of the alpha4 nAChR subunit (CHRNA4) are protective against smoking-related behaviors (220). Feng et al. reported in a study of Chinese men, two SNPs of the CHRNA4 gene that were associated with reduced risk of nicotine dependence (221). Another study found an association between a different SNP in CHRNA4 and heaviness of smoking index (222). Genome-wide association studies (GWAS) have identified a SNP encoding the alpha3 nAChR subunit (CHRNA3) associated with increased smoking quantity (223,224). Using a candidate gene approach, a strong association with nicotine dependence and early subjective response to nicotine was seen with a SNP in CHRNB3 (224). Zeiger et al. found evidence for an association between a SNP in CHRNA6 and early subjective response to nicotine suggesting that the genomic region containing CHRNB3 and CHRNA6 plays an important role in mediating early subjective response to nicotine (225). While the clinical implications of these findings remain unclear, it is interesting to note that genetic variants of nAChR subunits, especially those involving the alpha7 subunit (226), have been implicated in the cognitive and attentional deficits associated with schizophrenia—one of the serious mental illnesses frequently associated with nicotine dependence.

Other Drugs of Abuse

Before embarking on a brief synopsis of the genetic influences implicated in other categories of drug abuse, some general comments bear mentioning. First, as for nicotine dependence where we focused on genetic factors involved in the initiation of smoking behavior versus those involved in the development of nicotine dependence, a few studies have examined the related process of making the transition from substance use to heavy use to abuse and on to dependence in male–male twin pairs (227,228). In general, these twin studies found that the genetic factors play a significant role in these transitions from drug initiation to dependence. Second, many studies have found that personality variables such as sensation seeking play a salient role in the prediction of both substance abuse and dependence (229–231). Thus, in searching for genes that contribute to the risk of developing substance use disorders, genes affecting personality traits have received consideration.

Cocaine and Other Stimulants

Approximately 5 million Americans have used cocaine and other stimulants within the last 12 months (232,233). Cocaine addiction liability appears to be related to heritable factors (234). Personality traits such as impulsivity and novelty seeking, as well as an individual's response to stress, may contribute to cocaine addiction. Furthermore, vulnerability to cocaine's reinforcing properties is influenced by genetically influenced neurobiologic pathways within the CNS (235).

Kendler et al. estimated that common additive genetic factors account for 50% of the variance in cocaine use. (234). Population genetic studies of cocaine users and addicts found that cocaine use, and especially cocaine abuse and dependence in women, is substantially influenced by genetic factors. One study suggested that twin resemblance for liability to cocaine use was a result of genetic and familial-environmental factors, while twin resemblance for cocaine abuse and dependence was solely a result of genetic factors (236).

Cocaine inhibits the reuptake of dopamine and other monoamines via its blockade effects at monoamine transporters. These mechanisms of action result in an acute accumulation of extracellular dopamine in the synaptic cleft. Although a large preclinical literature exists, there is relatively limited information available about genetic variants affecting dopamine transporter function and cocaine dependence in humans. Regarding dopamine receptor subtypes, Comings et al. reported that the dopamine D3 (DRD3) receptor gene may play a modest role in the susceptibility to cocaine dependence (237), a finding that corroborates results obtained in animals (238). Allelic variants in the DRD2 gene have also been associated with cocaine dependence (239). However, as was the case for the DRD2 gene and alcoholism, other reports have been unable to replicate this finding (240).

Cocaine and other stimulants also affect serotonin reuptake, prompting some interest in genetic variants in the serotonergic system and their relation to stimulant dependence. To date, these studies have yielded mostly negative results (235). Patkar et al. found that polymorphisms in the serotonin transporter gene were not associated with cocaine dependence among African-American subjects (241,242), and another group reported no association between single-nucleotide polymorphisms in the serotonin B1 receptor gene and cocaine abuse or dependence (243).

Opiates

Opiates, including morphine and codeine, are drugs that originate from opium. Regardless whether they are naturally occurring or synthetic, all opioids are composed of substances with morphine-like activity. There are three types of opioid receptors: mu, kappa, and delta. However, opiates that are misused primarily act as MOR agonists. The MOR is a transmembrane G-protein–coupled receptor consisting of seven subunits that regulates pain responsivity, stress behaviors, immune activity, and gastrointestinal function (244). As discussed previously, a polymorphism at position 118 (A118G) of the mu receptor gene has been found that changes the receptor's ability to bind opioid ligands, especially endogenous beta-endorphin. The differences in binding of beta-endorphin and activation of the A118G variant receptors *in vitro* has led some investigators to assume that persons carrying this polymorphism might show altered function in the response to pain and stress (244). Szeto et al. found that the 118G allele was associated with opiate addiction in Han Chinese individuals (245). Like the study of Szeto and colleagues, another study found a substantial attributable risk for heroin dependence contributed by the 118G allele (244). However, not all studies have been able to replicate this association (246,247).

Oral opioid analgesics (e.g., oxycodone, hydrocodone, and codeine) are common medications prescribed for pain. The prevalence of oral opioid abuse has increased in the United States from 2002 to 2004, with oxycodone exhibiting the highest increase (248). Some patients become addicted to these oral opioids to the extent that they fulfill the *Diagnostic and Statistical Manual of Mental Disorders, 4th Edition (DSM-IV)* diagnosis of opioid dependence. These oral opioids are metabolized by CYP2D6 to morphine in order to exert their analgesic effects. Individuals with two nonfunctional alleles of CYP2D6 (2D6*3 and 2D6*4) are poor metabolizers of these drugs. These poor metabolizers are less responsive to codeine analgesia and its side effects than individuals with active CYP2D6 who are known as "extensive metabolizers" (244). Intriguingly, Tyndale et al. found no poor metabolizers in a sample of opioid-dependent cases, suggesting that the CYP2D6 defective genotype may provide pharmacogenetic protection against developing opioid dependence (249).

Cannabinoids

Marijuana is the most commonly used illicit drug in the United States, accounting for 75% of all illicit drug use. Family studies have reported that the use, abuse of, and dependence on cannabis seem to aggregate in families (250). Moreover, another study found that among first-degree relatives of probands who abused cannabis, there is a near sixfold increase in the likelihood of cannabis abuse as compared to the relatives of the control group (251). For cannabis use, estimates of heritability range from 0.17 to 0.67. Lynskey et al., studying Australian twins, found that genetic factors were important determinants for the risk of developing cannabis dependence among men, but results among women were less certain (246). However, Kendler and Prescott found that the heavy use of cannabis, as well as cannabis abuse and dependence, were largely attributable to genetic factors, with heritabilities ranging from 62% to 79% in female twins (252).

There is growing evidence that cannabis use may lead to the development of nicotine dependence (253,254). Furthermore, there is a relationship between the use of cannabis and the subsequent use of hard drugs, and this is seen across various populations, sexes, ethnicities, and socioeconomic strata (255). Other studies have suggested that cannabis is a potential gateway drug for harder substances, such as heroin and cocaine (202,256,257). Karkowski et al. observed that the association between cannabis and other illicit drug use may be a consequence of shared genetic factors and common environmental experiences (258).

Recent research suggests that the endogenous cannabinoid (endocannabinoid) system plays an important role in the brain's reward pathways (259). There are at least two cannabinoid receptor subtypes: CB1, primarily located in the CNS, and CB2, located mainly in immune tissues (260). CB1 receptors are the most numerous G-protein–coupled receptors found in the CNS (261). High concentrations of CB1 receptors are located within the dopaminergic mesolimbic system, an area central to the reward process of abused substances, including cannabis. Activation of these CB1 receptors by a CB1 receptor agonist, such as tetrahydrocannabinol, the psychoactive ingredient in cannabis, produces rewarding effects in humans (259). The result of this process is the enhancement of the rewarding properties of food and certain drugs of abuse, including heroin, nicotine, and alcohol (262). However, other investigators have found no effects (263) or a decrease of the CNS reward activity from CB1 synthetic agonists (264). The CB1 receptor antagonist/inverse agonists (e.g., rimonabant and others) diminish the rewarding effects of some drugs of abuse including nicotine (265), opioids (266), and alcohol (267). These consequences of CB1 receptor antagonism appear to be mediated by blocking dopamine accumulation in the nucleus accumbens (266). With regard to food consumption, CB1 receptor antagonism reduces the intake of food, especially sweet food (268). Thus, CB1 blockers have been found to be efficacious in the treatment of obesity (269).

The most important cannabinoid-related candidate genes for substance use disorders are named CNR1 and CNR2, respectively, corresponding to the receptor proteins (i.e., CB1 and CB2) they encode. The CNR1 gene is located on chromosome 6q14–15, and some studies have found evidence for associations among SNPs in CNR1 and vulnerabilities to substance use disorders (270). Specifically, Agrawal et al. found that SNPs in CNR1 were linked with the development of cannabis dependence (85). Recently, other SNPs in CNR1 were found to be associated with alcohol and illicit drug use disorders in Americans of European descent (271). Another study found a relationship between SNPs in CNR1 and nicotine dependence (272). However, other investigators have reported little or no association between substance use disorders and SNPs in CNR1 (273,274).

The gene encoding the CB2 receptor (CNR2) is found on chromosome 1p35.11. Although most of the CB2 receptors are found among leukocytes in the periphery, there is evidence of CB2 receptors located in the CNS (275). Only a few studies have examined the relationship between CRN2 and substance use disorders. In one study, Ishiguro et al., reported SNPs in CNR2 to be linked with alcoholism (276); however, more studies are necessary to confirm this finding.

In summary, genetic factors play an important role in the initiation (in tobacco studies) and persistence of substance dependence. The search for candidate genes that contribute to the risk of developing and maintaining substance use disorders is still in its early stages. The task of identifying such genes is made more arduous because it is likely that variation in substance dependence susceptibility results not only from genotypic differences and environmental influences, but also from their interactions (5). Thus, genetic factors are background sources of variance that can be minimized or exaggerated by environmental factors before the phenotype (substance dependence) can be expressed.

CONCLUSIONS AND IMPLICATIONS

This chapter organizes more than four decades of diverse findings into a format that is understandable and illustrative of the promise of this line of research, while not minimizing the complexity of the issues at hand. The clinical, societal, and research implications of this body of work have already emerged, with results from family, twin, and adoption studies having already shaped programs aimed at preventing the illness by educating children at high risk for alcoholism, tobacco dependence, and other drug use disorders early on, allowing them to modify their drinking and drug use patterns. Individuals already suffering from the disorders are matched to more appropriate therapies using the information obtained from studies of alcoholic subtypes. Pharmacogenetic approaches are offering a powerful new tool to match specific elements of an individual's complex blueprint (e.g., allelic variants in genes encoding various neurotransmitter receptors or transporters) with targeted pharmacotherapies to which that person may optimally respond.

Studies pointing to the importance of gene–environment interactions have demonstrated the need for cooperation among researchers in different disciplines, and they highlight the fact that unitary hypotheses arguing exclusively for any one approach are inadequate in explaining these heterogeneous disorders.

ACKNOWLEDGMENTS

This work was supported, in part, by the National Institute on Alcohol Abuse and Alcoholism (NIAAA) grant award #s R01AA013307 and R01AA013957, NIDA/VA CSP#1022, and by the Department of Veterans Affairs Research Service. Dr. Heffner also receives support from NIDA Award #K23DA026517.

The authors would like to thank Reene Cantwell for her technical assistance.

REFERENCES

1. Noble EP. The D2 dopamine receptor gene: a review of association studies in alcoholism and phenotypes. *Alcohol.* 1998;16(1):33–45.
2. Gelernter J, Kranzler H. D2 dopamine receptor gene (DRD2) allele and haplotype frequencies in alcohol dependent and control subjects: no association with phenotype or severity of phenotype. *Neuropsychopharmacology.* 1999;20(6):640–649.
3. Goodwin DW. The gene for alcoholism. *J Stud Alcohol.* 1989;50:397–398.
4. Rutter M. The interplay of nature, nurture, and developmental influences: the challenge ahead for mental health. *Arch Gen Psychiatry.* 2002;59:996–1000.
5. Gunzerath L, Goldman D. G × E: a NIAAA workshop on gene-environment interactions. *Alcohol Clin Exp Res.* 2003;27(3):540–562.
6. Schumann G, Spanagel R, Mann K. Candidate genes for alcohol dependence: animal studies. *Alcohol Clin Exp Res.* 2003;27(5):880–888.
7. Enoch MA, Goldman D. Molecular and cellular genetics of alcohol addiction. In: Davis KL, Charney D, Coyle JT, et al., eds. *Neuropsychopharmacology: The Fifth Generation of Progress.* Philadelphia: Lippincott Williams & Wilkins; 2002:1413–1423.
8. Dick DM, Foroud T. Candidate genes for alcohol dependence: a review of genetic evidence from human studies. *Alcohol Clin Exp Res.* 2003;27(5):868–879.
9. Goodwin DW. Alcoholism and genetics: the sins of the fathers. *Arch Gen Psychiatry.* 1985;42:171–174.
10. Pardes H, Kaufmann CA, Pincus HA, et al. Genetics and psychiatry: past discoveries, current dilemmas, and future directions. *Am J Psychiatry.* 1989;164(4):435–443.
11. Cotton NS. The familial incidence of alcoholism. *J Stud Alcohol.* 1979;40(1):89–116.
12. Bierut LJ, Dinwiddie SH, Begleiter H, et al. Familial transmission of substance dependence: alcohol, marijuana, cocaine, and habitual smoking. *Arch Gen Psychiatry.* 1998;55:982–988.
13. Schuckit MA. Biological vulnerability to alcoholism. *J Consult Clin Psychol.* 1987;55:1–9.
14. Schuckit MA. Genetic and clinical implications of alcoholism and affective disorder. *Am J Psychiatry.* 1986;143:140–147.
15. Horwitz AV, Videon TM, Schmitz MF, et al. Rethinking twins and environments: possible social sources for assumed genetic influences in twin research. *J Health Soc Behav.* 2003;44(2):111–129.
16. Kaij L. Studies on the etiology and sequels of abuse of alcohol. Lund: University of Lund Press; 1960.
17. Hrubec Z, Omenn GS. Evidence of genetic predisposition to alcoholic cirrhosis and psychosis: twin concordances for alcoholism and its biological end points by zygosity among male veterans. *Alcohol Clin Exp Res.* 1981;5:207–215.
18. Pickens RW, Svikis DS, McGue M, et al. Heterogeneity in the inheritance of alcoholism. *Arch Gen Psychiatry.* 1991;48:19–28.
19. McGue M, Pickens RW, Svikis DS. Sex and age effects on the inheritance of alcohol problems: a twin study. *J Abnorm Psychol.* 1992;101:3–17.
20. Prescott CA, Kendler KS. Genetic and environmental contributions to alcohol abuse and dependence in a population-based sample of male twins. *Am J Psychiatry.* 1999;156(1):34–40.
21. Gurling HM, Oppenheim BE, Murray RM. Depression, criminality and psychopathology associated with alcoholism: evidence from a twin study. *Acta Genet Med Gemellol.* 1984;33:333–339.
22. Kendler KS, Heath AC, Neale MC, et al. A population-based twin study of alcoholism in women. *JAMA.* 1992;268:1877–1882.
23. Heath AC, Bucholz KK, Madden PA, et al. Genetic and environmental contributions to alcohol dependence risk in a national twin sample: consistency of findings in women and men. *Psychol Med.* 1997;27(6):1381–1396.
24. Goodwin DW. Familial alcoholism: a separate entity? *Subst Alcohol Actions Misuse.* 1983;4:129–136.
25. Schuckit MA, Goodwin DW, Winokur GA. A study of alcoholism in half-siblings. *Am J Psychiatry.* 1972;128:1132–1136.
26. Ducci F, Goldman D. Genetic approaches to addiction: genes and alcohol. *Addiction.* 2008;103(9):1414–1428.
27. Goodwin DW. Alcoholism and heredity. *Arch Gen Psychiatry.* 1979;36:57–61.
28. Cloninger CR, Bohman M, Sigvardsson S. Inheritance of alcohol abuse: cross-fostering analysis of adopted men. *Arch Gen Psychiatry.* 1981;38:861–868.
29. Cadoret RJ, Cain CA, Grove WM. Development of alcoholism in adoptees raised apart from alcoholic biologic relatives. *Arch Gen Psychiatry.* 1980;37:561–563.
30. Cadoret RJ, Troughton E, O'Gorman TW. Genetic and environmental factors in alcohol abuse and antisocial personality. *J Stud Alcohol.* 1987;48:1–8.
31. Cadoret RJ, O'Gorman TW, Troughton E, et al. Alcoholism and antisocial personality: interrelationships, genetic and environmental factors. *Arch Gen Psychiatry.* 1985;42:161–167.
32. Roe A. The adult adjustment of children of alcoholic parents raised in foster homes. *J Stud Alcohol.* 1994;5:378–393.
33. Cloninger CR, Sigvardsson S, Reich T, et al. Inheritance of risk to develop alcoholism. In: Braude MC, Chao HM, eds. *Genetic and Biological Markers in Drug Abuse and Alcoholism.* NIDA Research Monograph 66, Rockville, MD: National Institute on Drug Abuse (NIDA);1986:86–96.
34. Anthenelli RM, Schuckit MA. Genetic studies on alcoholism. *Int J Addict.* 1990;25:81–94.
35. McHugh PR, Slavney PR. *The Perspectives of Psychiatry.* Baltimore: Johns Hopkins University Press; 1983.
36. Helzer JE, Pryzbeck TR. The co-occurence of alcoholism with other psychiatric disorders in the general population and its impact on treatment. *J Stud Alcohol.* 1988;49:219–224.

37. Kessler RC, Crum RM, Warner LA, et al. Lifetime co-occurence of DSM-III-R alcohol abuse and dependence with other psychiatric disorders in the national comorbidity survey. *Arch Gen Psychiatry*. 1997;54:313–321.
38. Grant BF, Stinson FS, Dawson DA, et al. Prevalence and co-occurrence of substance use disorders and independent mood and anxiety disorders: results from the National Epidemiologic Survey on Alcohol and Related Conditions. *Arch Gen Psychiatry*. 2004;61(8):807–816.
39. Strakowski SM, DelBello MP, Fleck DE, et al. The impact of substance abuse on the course of bipolar disorder. *Biol Psychiatry*. 2000;48(6):477–485.
40. Schuckit MA. The clinical implications of primary diagnostic groups among alcoholics. *Arch Gen Psychiatry*. 1985;42:1043–1049.
41. Cloninger CR. Neurogenetic adaptive mechanisms in alcoholism. *Science*. 1987;236:410–416.
42. Babor TF, Hofmann M, DelBoca FK, et al. Types of alcoholics, I: evidence for an empirically derived typology based on indicators of vulnerability and severity. *Arch Gen Psychiatry*. 1992;49:599–608.
43. Penick EC, Powell BJ, Nickel EJ, et al. Examination of Cloninger's type I and type II alcoholism with a sample of men alcoholics in treatment. *Alcohol Clin Exp Res*. 1990;14:623–629.
44. Anthenelli RM, Smith TL, Irwin MR, et al. A comparative study of criteria for subgrouping alcoholics: the primary/secondary diagnostic scheme versus variations of the type 1/type 2 criteria. *Am J Psychiatry*. 1994;151(10):1468–1474.
45. Epstein EE, Labouvie E, McCrady BS, et al. A multi-site study of alcohol subtypes: classification and overlap of unidimensional and multi-dimensional typologies. *Addiction*. 2002;97(8):1041–1053.
46. Bohman M, Sigvardsson S, Cloninger CR. Maternal inheritance of alcohol abuse: cross-fostering analysis of adopted women. *Arch Gen Psychiatry*. 1991;38:965–969.
47. von Knorring L, von Knorring AL, Smigan L, et al. Personality traits in subtypes of alcoholics. *J Stud Alcohol*. 1987;48:523–527.
48. Bohman M, Cloninger R, Sigvardsson S, et al. The genetics of alcoholisms and related disorders. *J Psychiat Res*. 1987;21(4):447–452.
49. Devor EJ, Cloninger CR. Genetics of alcoholism. *Annu Rev Genet*. 1989;23:19–36.
50. Anthenelli RM, Tabakoff B. The search for biochemical markers. *Alcohol Health Res World*. 1995;19:176–181.
51. Schuckit MA, Tipp JE, Smith TL, et al. An evaluation of Type A and B alcoholics. *Addiction*. 1995;90:1189–1203.
52. Gottesman II, Gould TD. The endophenotype concept in psychiatry: etymology and strategic intentions. *Am J Psychiatry*. 2003;160(4):636–645.
53. Begleiter H, Porjesz B. What is inherited in the predisposition toward alcoholism? a proposed model. *Alcohol Clin Exp Res*. 1999;23(7):1125–1135.
54. Schuckit MA. A clinical model of genetic influences in alcohol dependence. *J Stud Alcohol*. 1994;55:5–17.
55. Anthenelli RM, Schuckit MA. Genetics. In: Lowinson JH, Ruiz P, Millman RB, eds. *Substance Abuse: A Comprehensive Textbook*. Baltimore: Williams & Wilkins; 1992:39–50.
56. Begleiter H, Porjesz B, Bihari B, et al. Event-related brain potentials in boys at risk for alcoholism. *Science*. 1984;227:1493–1496.
57. Begleiter H. The collaborative study on the genetics of alcoholism. *Alcohol Health Res World*. 1995;19:228–236.
58. Hesselbrock V, O'Connor S, Tasman A, et al. Cognitive and evoked potential indications of risk for alcoholism in young men. In: Kuriyamam K, Takada A, Ishii H, eds. *Biomedical and Social Aspects of Alcohol and Alcoholism*. Amsterdam: Elsevier Science Publishers; 1988.
59. Malone SM, Iacono WG, McGue M. Event-related potentials and comorbidity in alcohol-dependent adult males. *Psychophysiology*. 2001;38(3):367–376.
60. Polich J, Bloom FE. Event-related brain potentials in individuals at high and low risk for developing alcoholism: failure to replicate. *Alcohol Clin Exp Res*. 1988;12:368–373.
61. Hill SY, Steinhauer SR, Zubin J, et al. Event-related potentials as markers for alcoholism risk in high density families. *Alcohol Clin Exp Res*. 1988;12:368–373.
62. Pollock VE, Volavka J, Goodwin DW. The EEG after alcohol administration in men at risk for alcoholism. *Arch Gen Psychiatry*. 1983;40:857–861.
63. Volavka J, Pollock VE, Gabrielli WF, et al. *The EEG in Persons at Risk for Alcoholism: currents in Alcoholism*. New York: Grune & Stratton; 1982.
64. Ehlers CL, Schuckit MA. Evaluation of EEG alpha activity in sons of alcoholics. *Neuropsychopharmacology*. 1991;4:199–205.
65. Ehlers CL, Phillips E. EEG low-voltage alpha and alpha power in African American young adults: relation to family history of alcoholism. *Alcohol Clin Exp Res*. 2003;27(5):765–772.
66. Schuckit MA. Subjective responses to alcohol in sons of alcoholics and control subjects. *Arch Gen Psychiatry*. 1984;41:879–884.
67. Schuckit MA. Reactions to alcohol in sons of alcoholics and controls. *Alcohol Clin Exp Res*. 1988;12:465–470.
68. Schuckit MA, Gold EO. A simultaneous evaluation of multiple markers of ethanol/placebo challenges in sons of alcoholics. *Arch Gen Psychiatry*. 1988;45:211–216.
69. Schuckit MA. Ethanol-induced changes in body sway in men at high alcoholism risk. *Arch Gen Psychiatry*. 1985;42:375–379.
70. Schuckit MA, Gold E, Risch C. Serum prolactin levels in sons of alcoholics and control subjects. *Am J Psychiatry*. 1987;144:854–859.
71. Schuckit MA. Differences in plasma cortisol after ethanol in relatives of alcoholics and controls. *J Clin Psychiatry*. 1984;45:374–379.
72. Schuckit MA. A long-term study of sons of alcoholics. *Alcohol Health Res World*. 1995;19:172–175.
73. Schuckit MA, Smith TL. An 8-year follow-up of 450 sons of alcoholic and control subjects. *Arch Gen Psychiatry*. 1996;53:202–210.
74. Hu X, Oroszi G, Chun J, et al. An expanded evaluation of the relationship of four alleles to the level of response to alcohol and the alcoholism risk. *Alcohol Clin Exp Res*. 2005;29(1):8–16.
75. Hingson RW, Heeren T, Winter MR. Age at drinking onset and alcohol dependence: age-at-onset, duration, and severity. *Arch Pediatr Adolesc Med*. 2006;160(7):739–746.
76. McGue M, Iacono WG, Legrand LN, et al. Origins and consequences of age at first drink. II. Familial risk and heritability. *Alcohol Clin Exp Res*. 2001;25(8):1166–1173.
77. Sartor CE, Lynskey MT, Bucholz KK, et al. Timing of first alcohol use and alcohol dependence: evidence of common genetic influences. *Addiction*. 2009;104(9):1512–1518.
78. Anthenelli RM, Schuckit MA. Genetics. In: Lowinson JH, Ruiz P, Millman RB, et al., eds. *Substance Abuse: A Comprehensive Textbook*. Baltimore: Williams & Wilkins; 1997:41–51.
79. Mullan M. Alcoholism and the 'new genetics'. *Br J Addict*. 1989;84:1433–1440.
80. Goldman D. Identifying alcoholism vulnerability alleles. *Alcohol Clin Exp Res*. 1995;19:824–831.

81. Cloninger CR. D2 dopamine receptor gene is associated but not linked with alcoholism. *JAMA*. 1991;266:1833–1834.
82. Parsian A, Todd RD, Devor EJ, et al. Alcoholism and alleles of the human D2 dopamine receptor locus. *Arch Gen Psychiatry*. 1991;48:655–666.
83. Begleiter H, Reich T, Nurnberger J Jr, et al. Description of the genetic analysis workshop 11 collaborative study on the genetics of alcoholism. *Genet Epidemiol*. 1999;17(suppl 1):S25–S30.
84. Treutlein J, Cichon S, Ridinger M, et al. Genome-wide association study of alcohol dependence. *Arch Gen Psychiatry*. 2009;66(7):773–784.
85. Agrawal A, Lynskey MT. Are there genetic influences on addiction: evidence from family, adoption and twin studies. *Addiction*. 2008;103(7):1069–1081.
86. Neumark YD, Friedlander Y, Thomasson HR, et al. Association of the ADH2*2 allele with reduced ethanol consumption in Jewish men in Israel: a pilot study. *J Stud Alcohol*. 1998;59(2):133–139.
87. Yoshida A, Rzhetsky A, Hsu LC, et al. Human aldehyde dehydrogenase gene family. *Eur J Biochem*. 1998;251(3):549–557.
88. Vasiliou V, Bairoch A, Tipton KF, et al. Eukaryotic aldehyde dehydrogenase (ALDH) genes: human polymorphisms, and recommended nomenclature based on divergent evolution and chromosomal mapping. *Pharmacogenetics*. 1999;9(4):421–434.
89. Yin SJ, Peng GS. Overview of ALDH polymorphism: relation to cardiovascular effects of alcohol. In: Preedy VR, Watson RR, eds. *Comprehensive Handbook of Alcohol Related Pathology*. London: Elsevier Academic; 2005:409–424.
90. Goedde HW, Agarwal DP, Fritze G, et al. Distribution of ADH2 and ALDH2 genotypes in different populations. *Hum Genet*. 1992;88(3):344–346.
91. Goedde HW, Harada S, Agarwal DP. Racial differences in alcohol sensitivity: a new hypothesis. *Hum Genet*. 1979;51(3):331–334.
92. Agarwal DP. Genetic polymorphisms of alcohol metabolizing enzymes. *Pathol Biol (Paris)*. 2001;49(9):703–709.
93. Barr CS, Newman TK, Becker ML, et al. The utility of the non-human primate; model for studying gene by environment interactions in behavioral research. *Genes Brain Behav*. 2003;2(6):336–340.
94. Peng GS, Yin SJ. Effect of the allelic variants of aldehyde dehydrogenase ALDH2*2 and alcohol dehydrogenase ADH1B*2 on blood acetaldehyde concentrations. *Hum Genomics*. 2009;3(2):121–127.
95. Peng GS, Yin JH, Wang MF, et al. Alcohol sensitivity in Taiwanese men with different alcohol and aldehyde dehydrogenase genotypes. *J Formos Med Assoc*. 2002;101(11):769–774.
96. Chen CC, Lu RB, Chen YC, et al. Interaction between the functional polymorphisms of the alcohol- metabolism genes in protection against alcoholism. *Am J Hum Genet*. 1999;65(3):795–807.
97. Ramchandani VA, Bosron WF, Li TK. Research advances in ethanol metabolism. *Pathol Biol (Paris)*. 2001;49(9):676–682.
98. Chen YC, Peng GS, Wang MF, et al. Polymorphism of ethanol-metabolism genes and alcoholism: correlation of allelic variations with the pharmacokinetic and pharmacodynamic consequences. *Chem Biol Interact*. 2009;178(1–3):2–7.
99. Chen YC, Peng GS, Tsao TP, et al. Pharmacokinetic and pharmacodynamic basis for overcoming acetaldehyde-induced adverse reaction in Asian alcoholics, heterozygous for the variant ALDH2*2 gene allele. *Pharmacogenet Genomics*. 2009;19(8):588–599.
100. Wall TL, Ehlers CL. Genetic influences affecting alcohol use among Asians. *Alcohol Health Res World*. 1995;19:184–189.
101. Mayfield RD, Harris RA, Schuckit MA. Genetic factors influencing alcohol dependence. *Br J Pharmacol*. 2008;154(2):275–287.
102. Blum K, Noble EP, Sheridan PJ, et al. Allelic association of human dopamine D2 receptor gene in alcoholism. *JAMA*. 1990;263:2055–2060.
103. McBride WJ, Murphy JM, Lumeng L, et al. Serotonin, dopamine and GABA involvement in alcohol drinking of selectively bred rats. *Alcohol*. 1990;7:199–205.
104. Koob GF, Rassnick S, Heinrichs S, et al. Alcohol, the reward system and dependence. *EXS*. 1994;71:103–114.
105. Gelernter J, Kranzler HR, Panhuysen C, et al. Dense genome wide linkage scan for alcohol dependence in African Americans: significant linkage on chromosome 10. *Biol Psychiatry*. 2009;65(2):111–115.
106. Yang BZ, Kranzler HR, Zhao H, et al. Association of haplotypic variants in DRD2, ANKK1, TTC12 and NCAM1 to alcohol dependence in independent case control and family samples. *Hum Mol Genet*. 2007;16(23):2844–2853.
107. Noble EP. Polymorphisms of the D2 dopamine receptor gene and alcoholism and other substance use disorders. *Alcohol*. 1994;235–43.
108. Noble EP, Blum K, Ritchie T, et al. Allelic association of the D2 dopamine receptor gene with receptor-binding characteristics in alcoholism. *Arch Gen Psychiatry*. 1991;48:648–654.
109. Limosin F, Gorwood P, Loze JY, et al. Male limited association of the dopamine receptor D2 gene TaqI a polymorphism and alcohol dependence. *Am J Med Genet*. 2002;112(4):343–346.
110. Connor JP, Young RM, Lawford BR, et al. D(2) dopamine receptor (DRD2) polymorphism is associated with severity of alcohol dependence. *Eur Psychiatry*. 2002;17(1):17–23.
111. Noble EP, Zhang X, Ritchie TL, et al. Haplotypes at the DRD2 locus and severe alcoholism. *Am J Med Genet*. 2000;96(5):622–631.
112. Goldman D, Brown GL, Albaugh B, et al. D2 receptor genotype and linkage disequilibrium and function in Finnish, American Indian and U.S. Caucasian patients. In: Gershon ES, Cloninger CR, eds. *Genetic Approaches to Mental Disorders*. Washington D.C.: American Psychiatric Press, Inc.; 1994:327–344.
113. Bolos AM, Dean M, Lucas-Derse S, et al. Population and pedigree studies reveal a lack of association between the dopamine D2 receptor gene and alcoholism. *JAMA*. 1990;264:3156–3160.
114. Edenberg HJ, Foroud T, Koller DL, et al. A Family-based analysis of the association of the Dopamine D2 Receptor (DRD2) with alcoholism. *Alcohol Clin Exp Res*. 1998;22:505–512.
115. Blomqvist O, Gelernter J, Kranzler HR. Family-based study of DRD2 alleles in alcohol and drug dependence. *Am J Med Genet*. 2000;96(5):659–664.
116. Haile CN, Kosten TA, Kosten TR. Pharmacogenetic treatments for drug addiction: alcohol and opiates. *Am J Drug Alcohol Abuse*. 2008;34(4):355–381.
117. Ebstein RP, Novick O, Umansky R, et al. Dopamine D4 receptor (D4DR) rcon III polymorphism associated with the human personality trait of novelty seeking. *Nat Genet*. 1996;12:78–80.
118. Benjamin J, Greenberg B, Murphy DL, et al. Population and familial association between the d4 dopamine receptor gene and measures of Novelty seeking. *Nat Genet*. 1996;12:81–84.
119. Thompson M, Comings DE, Feder L, et al. Mutation screening of the dopamine D1 receptor gene in Tourette's syndrome and alcohol dependent patients. *Am J Med Genet*. 1998;81(3):241–244.
120. Sander T, Harms H, Podschus J, et al. Dopamine D1, D2 and D3 receptor genes in alcohol dependence. *Psychiatr Genet*. 1995;5(4):171–176.

121. Gorwood P, Limosin F, Batel P, et al. The genetics of addiction: alcohol-dependence and D3 dopamine receptor gene. *Pathol Biol (Paris)*. 2001;49(9):710–717.
122. Lee MS, Ryu SH. No association between the dopamine D3 receptor gene and Korean alcohol dependence. *Psychiatr Genet*. 2002;12(3):173–176.
123. Parsian A, Chakraverty S, Fisher L, et al. No association between polymorphisms in the human dopamine D3 and D4 receptors genes and alcoholism. *Am J Med Genet*. 1997;74(3):281–285.
124. Covault J, Gelernter J, Hesselbrock V, et al. Allelic and haplotypic association of GABRA2 with alcohol dependence. *Am J Med Genet B Neuropsychiatr Genet*. 2004;129B(1):104–109.
125. Krystal JH, Staley J, Mason G, et al. Gamma-aminobutyric acid type A receptors and alcoholism: intoxication, dependence, vulnerability, and treatment. *Arch Gen Psychiatry*. 2006;63(9):957–968.
126. Aguayo LG, Peoples RW, Yevenes GE, et al. GABA(A) receptors as molecular sites of ethanol action. Direct or indirect actions. *Curr Top Med Chem*. 2002;2(8):869–885.
127. McBride WJ, Li TK. Animal models of alcoholism: neurobiology of high alcohol-drinking behavior in rodents. *Crit Rev Neurobiol*. 1998;12(4):339–369.
128. Goldman D, Oroszi G, Ducci F. The genetics of addictions: uncovering the genes. *Nat Rev Genet*. 2005;6(7):521–532.
129. Li MD, Burmeister M. New insights into the genetics of addiction. *Nat Rev Genet*. 2009;10(4):225–231.
130. Porjesz B, Begleiter H, Wang K, et al. Linkage and linkage disequilibrium mapping of ERP and EEG phenotypes. *Biol Psychol*. 2002;61:229–248.
131. Enoch MA, Hodgkinson CA, Yuan Q, et al. GABRG1 and GABRA2 as independent predictors for alcoholism in two populations. *Neuropsychopharmacology*. 2009;34(5):1245–1254.
132. Johnson BA. Role of the serotonergic system in the neurobiology of alcoholism: implications for treatment. *CNS Drugs*. 2004;18(15):1105–1118.
133. Yoshimoto K, McBride WJ, Lumeng L, et al. Alcohol stimulates the release of dopamine and serotonin in the nucleus accumbens. *Alcohol*. 1991;9:17–22.
134. Roberts AJ, McArthur RA, Hull EE, et al. Effects of amperozide, 8-OH-DPAT, and FG 5974 on operant responding for ethanol. *Psychopharmacology*. 1998;137(1):25–32.
135. Anthenelli RM, Maxwell RA, Geracioti TD Jr, et al. Stress hormone dysregulation at rest and following serotonergic stimulation among alcohol-dependent men with extended abstinence and controls. *Alcohol Clin Exp Res*. 2001;25(5):692–703.
136. Heinz A, Mann K, Weinberger DR, et al. Serotonergic dysfunction, negative mood states, and response to alcohol. *Alcohol Clin Exp Res*. 2001;25(4):487–495.
137. Covault J, Tennen H, Armeli S, et al. Interactive effects of the serotonin transporter 5-HTTLPR polymorphism and stressful life events on college student drinking and drug use. *Biol Psychiatry*. 2007;61(5):609–616.
138. Kaufman J, Yang BZ, Douglas-Palumberi H, et al. Genetic and environmental predictors of early alcohol use. *Biol Psychiatry*. 2007;61(11):1228–1234.
139. Sander T, Harms H, Dufeu P, et al. Serotonin transporter gene variants in alcohol-dependent subjects with dissocial personality disorder. *Biol Psychiatry*. 1998;43(12):908–912.
140. Hammoumi S, Payen A, Favre JD, et al. Does the short variant of the serotonin transporter linked polymorphic region constitute a marker of alcohol dependence? *Alcohol*. 1999;17(2):107–112.
141. Dick DM, Wang JC, Plunkett J, et al. Family-based association analyses of alcohol dependence phenotypes across DRD2 and neighboring gene ANKK1. *Alcohol Clin Exp Res*. 2007;31(10):1645–1653.
142. Kranzler H, Lappalainen J, Nellissery M, et al. Association study of alcoholism subtypes with a functional promoter polymorphism in the serotonin transporter protein gene. *Alcohol Clin Exp Res*. 2002;26(9):1330–1335.
143. Edenberg HJ, Reynolds J, Koller DL, et al. A family-based analysis of whether the functional promoter alleles of the serotonin transporter gene HTT affect the risk for alcohol dependence. *Alcohol Clin Exp Res*. 1998;22(5):1080–1085.
144. Feinn R, Nellissery M, Kranzler HR. Meta-analysis of the association of a functional serotonin transporter promoter polymorphism with alcohol dependence. *Am J Med Genet B Neuropsychiatr Genet*. 2005;133B(1):79–84.
145. Kreek MJ, Nielsen DA, Butelman ER, et al. Genetic influences on impulsivity, risk taking, stress responsivity and vulnerability to drug abuse and addiction. *Nat Neurosci*. 2005;8(11):1450–1457.
146. Beyer A, Koch T, Schroder H, et al. Effect of the A118G polymorphism on binding affinity, potency and agonist-mediated endocytosis, desensitization, and resensitization of the human mu-opioid receptor. *J Neurochem*. 2004;89(3):553–560.
147. Schinka JA, Town T, Abdullah L, et al. A functional polymorphism within the mu-opioid receptor gene and risk for abuse of alcohol and other substances. *Mol Psychiatry*. 2002;7(2):224–228.
148. Tan EC, Tan CH, Karupathivan U, et al. Mu opioid receptor gene polymorphisms and heroin dependence in Asian populations. *Neuroreport*. 2003;14(4):569–572.
149. Arias A, Feinn R, Kranzler HR. Association of an Asn40Asp (A118G) polymorphism in the mu-opioid receptor gene with substance dependence: a meta-analysis. *Drug Alcohol Depend*. 2006;83(3):262–268.
150. Luo X, Kranzler HR, Zhao H, et al. Haplotypes at the OPRM1 locus are associated with susceptibility to substance dependence in European-Americans. *Am J Med Genet B Neuropsychiatr Genet*. 2003;120B(1):97–108.
151. Loh eW, Fann CS, Chang YT, et al. Endogenous opioid receptor genes and alcohol dependence among Taiwanese Han. *Alcohol Clin Exp Res*. 2004;28(1):15–19.
152. Ray LA, Hutchison KE. A polymorphism of the mu-opioid receptor gene (OPRM1) and sensitivity to the effects of alcohol in humans. *Alcohol Clin Exp Res*. 2004;28(12):1789–1795.
153. Ray LA, Hutchison KE. Effects of naltrexone on alcohol sensitivity and genetic moderators of medication response: a double-blind placebo-controlled study. *Arch Gen Psychiatry*. 2007;64(9):1069–1077.
154. Balldin J, Berglund M, Borg S, et al. A 6-month controlled naltrexone study: combined effect with cognitive behavioral therapy in outpatient treatment of alcohol dependence. *Alcohol Clin Exp Res*. 2003;27(7):1142–1149.
155. Kim SG, Kim CM, Choi SW, et al. A micro opioid receptor gene polymorphism (A118G) and naltrexone treatment response in adherent Korean alcohol-dependent patients. *Psychopharmacology (Berl)*. 2009;201(4):611–618.
156. Guardia J, Caso C, Arias F, et al. A double-blind, placebo-controlled study of naltrexone in the treatment of alcohol-dependence disorder: results from a multicenter clinical trial. *Alcohol Clin Exp Res*. 2002;26(9):1381–1387.

157. O'Malley SS, Jaffe AJ, Chang G, et al. Naltrexone and coping skills therapy for alcohol dependence: a controlled study. *Arch Gen Psychiatry*. 1992;49:881–887.
158. Morris PL, Hopwood M, Whelan G, et al. Naltrexone for alcohol dependence: a randomized controlled trial. *Addiction*. 2001;96(11):1565–1573.
159. Anton RF, Oroszi G, O'Malley S, et al. An evaluation of mu-opioid receptor (OPRM1) as a predictor of naltrexone response in the treatment of alcohol dependence: results from the Combined Pharmacotherapies and Behavioral Interventions for Alcohol Dependence (COMBINE) study. *Arch Gen Psychiatry*. 2008;65(2):135–144.
160. Fiore MC. Treating tobacco use and dependence. Clinical Practice Guideline: 2008 Update. US Department of Health and Human Services Public Health Service 2008.
161. Hughes JR. Genetics of smoking: a brief review. *Behav Ther*. 1986;17:335–345.
162. Flannery BA, Allen JP, Pettinati HM, et al. Using acquired knowledge and new technologies in alcoholism treatment trials. *Alcohol Clin Exp Res*. 2002;26(3):423–429.
163. Boomsma DI, Koopmans JR, Van Doornen LJ, et al. Genetic and social influences on starting to smoke: a study of Dutch adolescent twins and their parents. *Addiction*. 1994;89(2):219–226.
164. Carmelli D, Swan GE, Robinette D, et al. Genetic influence on smoking—a study of male twins. *N Engl J Med*. 1992;327(12):829–833.
165. Heath AC, Madden PA, Martin NG. Statistical methods in genetic research on smoking. *Stat Methods Med Res*. 1998;7(2):165–186.
166. Griesler PC, Kandel DB, Davies M. Ethnic differences in predictors of initiation and persistence of adolescent cigarette smoking in the National Longitudinal Survey of Youth. *Nicotine Tob Res*. 2002;4(1):79–93.
167. Heath AC, Kirk KM, Meyer JM, et al. Genetic and social determinants of initiation and age-at-onset of smoking in Australian twins. *Behav Genet*. 1999;29(6):395–407.
168. Heath AC, Martin NG, Lynskey MT, et al. Estimating two-stage models for genetic influences on alcohol, tobacco or drug use initiation and dependence vulnerability in twin and family data. *Twin Res*. 2002;5(2):113–124.
169. Kendler KS, Neale MC, Sullivan P, et al. A population-based twin study in women of smoking initiation and nicotine dependence. *Psychol Med*. 1999;29(2):299–308.
170. Stolerman IP, Jarvis MJ. The scientific case that nicotine is addictive. *Psychopharmacology (Berl)*. 1995;117(1):2–10.
171. Kendler KS, Heath A, Martin NG, et al. Symptoms of anxiety and depression in a volunteer twin population. The etiologic role of genetic and environmental factors. *Arch Gen Psychiatry*. 1986;43(3):213–221.
172. Kendler KS, Gardner CO Jr. Twin studies of adult psychiatric and substance dependence disorders: are they biased by differences in the environmental experiences of monozygotic and dizygotic twins in childhood and adolescence? *Psychol Med*. 1998;28(3):625–633.
173. Hall W, Madden P, Lynskey M. The genetics of tobacco use: methods, findings and policy implications. *Tob Control*. 2002;11:119–124.
174. Osler M, Holst C, Prescott E, et al. Influence of genes and family environment on adult smoking behavior assessed in an adoption study. *Genet Epidemiol*. 2001;21(3):193–200.
175. Kendler KS, Thornton LM, Pedersen NL. Tobacco consumption in Swedish twins reared apart and reared together. *Arch Gen Psychiatry*. 2000;57(9):886–892.
176. Lessov-Schlaggar CN, Pergadia ML, Khroyan TV, et al. Genetics of nicotine dependence and pharmacotherapy. *Biochem Pharmacol*. 2008;75(1):178–195.
177. Lessov CN, Martin NG, Statham DJ, et al. Defining nicotine dependence for genetic research: evidence from Australian twins. *Psychol Med*. 2004;34(5):865–879.
178. Blum K, Noble EP, Sheridan PJ, et al. Association of the A1 allele of the D2 dopamine receptor gene with severe alcoholism. *Alcohol*. 1991;8(5):409–416.
179. Noble EP, St. Jeor ST, Syndulko K, et al. D2 dopamine receptor gene and cigarette smoking: a reward gene? *Med Hypotheses*. 1994;42:257–260.
180. Comings DE, Ferry L, Bradshaw-Robinson S, et al. The dopamine D2 receptor (DRD2) gene: a genetic risk factor in smoking. *Pharmacogenetics*. 1996;6(1):73–79.
181. Spitz MR, Shi H, Yang F, et al. Case-control study of the D2 dopamine receptor gene and smoking status in lung cancer patients. *J Natl Cancer Inst*. 1998;90(5):358–363.
182. Singleton AB, Thomson JH, Morris CM, et al. Lack of association between the dopamine D2 receptor gene allele DRD2*A1 and cigarette smoking in a United Kingdom population. *Pharmacogenetics*. 1998;8(2):125–128.
183. Pohjalainen T, Rinne JO, Nagren K, et al. The A1 allele of the human D2 dopamine receptor gene predicts low D2 receptor availability in healthy volunteers. *Mol Psychiatry*. 1998;3(3):256–260.
184. Noble EP, Gottschalk LA, Fallon JH, et al. D2 dopamine receptor polymorphism and brain regional glucose metabolism. *Am J Med Genet*. 1997;74(2):162–166.
185. Blum K, Cull JG, Braverman ER, et al. Reward deficiency syndrome. *Am Sci*. 1996;84(132):145.
186. Ray R, Schnoll RA, Lerman C. Nicotine dependence: biology, behavior, and treatment. *Annu Rev Med*. 2009;60:247–260.
187. Davies GE, Soundy TJ. The genetics of smoking and nicotine addiction. *S D Med*. 2009;Spec No:43–49.
188. Uhl GR, Liu QR, Drgon T, et al. Molecular genetics of successful smoking cessation: convergent genome-wide association study results. *Arch Gen Psychiatry*. 2008;65(6):683–693.
189. Lerman C, Caporaso N, Main D, et al. Depression and self-medication with nicotine: the modifying influence of the dopamine D4 receptor gene. *Health Psychol*. 1998;17(1):56–62.
190. Sullivan PF, Neale MC, Silverman MA, et al. An association study of DRD5 with smoking initiation and progression to nicotine dependence. *Am J Med Genet*. 2001;105(3):259–265.
191. Shields PG, Lerman C, Audrain J, et al. Dopamine D4 receptors and the risk of cigarette smoking in African-Americans and Caucasians. *Cancer Epidemiol Biomarkers Prev*. 1998;7(6):453–458.
192. Lerman C, Caporaso NE, Audrain J, et al. Evidence suggesting the role of specific genetic factors in cigarette smoking. *Health Psychol*. 1999;18(1):14–20.
193. Sabol SZ, Nelson ML, Fisher C, et al. A genetic association for cigarette smoking behavior. *Health Psychol*. 1999;18(1):7–13.
194. Mihailescu S, Palomero-Rivero M, Meade-Huerta P, et al. Effects of nicotine and mecamylamine on rat dorsal raphe neurons. *Eur J Pharmacol*. 1998;360(1):31–36.
195. Ribeiro EB, Bettiker RL, Bogdanov M, et al. Effects of systemic nicotine on serotonin release in rat brain. *Brain Res*. 1993;621(2):311–318.
196. Eichhammer P, Langguth B, Wiegand R, et al. Allelic variation in the serotonin transporter promoter affects neuromodulatory effects of a selective serotonin transporter reuptake inhibitor (SSRI). *Psychopharmacology (Berl)*. 2003;166(3):294–297.

197. Mancama D, Kerwin RW. Role of pharmacogenomics in individualising treatment with SSRIs. *CNS Drugs.* 2003;17(3):143–151.
198. Gerra G, Garofano L, Zaimovic A, et al. Association of the serotonin transporter promoter polymorphism with smoking behavior among adolescents. *Am J Med Genet B Neuropsychiatr Genet.* 2005;135B(1):73–78.
199. Kremer I, Bachner-Melman R, Reshef A, et al. Association of the serotonin transporter gene with smoking behavior. *Am J Psychiatry.* 2005;162(5):924–930.
200. Ishikawa H, Ohtsuki T, Ishiguro H, et al. Association between serotonin transporter gene polymorphism and smoking among Japanese males. *Cancer Epidemiol Biomarkers Prev.* 1999;8(9):831–833.
201. Lerman C, Shields PG, Audrain J, et al. The role of the serotonin transporter gene in cigarette smoking. *Cancer Epidemiol Biomarkers Prev.* 1998;7(3):253–255.
202. Lessem JM, Hopfer CJ, Haberstick BC, et al. Relationship between adolescent marijuana use and young adult illicit drug use. *Behav Genet.* 2006;36(4):498–506.
203. Lerman C, Caporaso NE, Audrain J, et al. Interacting effects of the serotonin transporter gene and neuroticism in smoking practices and nicotine dependence. *Mol Psychiatry.* 2000;5(2):189–192.
204. Munafo M, Clark T, Johnstone E, et al. The genetic basis for smoking behavior: a systematic review and meta-analysis. *Nicotine Tob Res.* 2004;6(4):583–597.
205. David SP, Munafo MR, Murphy MF, et al. The serotonin transporter 5-HTTLPR polymorphism and treatment response to nicotine patch: follow-up of a randomized controlled trial. *Nicotine Tob Res.* 2007;9(2):225–231.
206. Trummer O, Koppel H, Wascher TC, et al. The serotonin transporter gene polymorphism is not associated with smoking behavior. *Pharmacogenomics J.* 2006;6(6):397–400.
207. Chu SL, Xiao D, Wang C, et al. Association between 5-hydroxytryptamine transporter gene-linked polymorphic region and smoking behavior in Chinese males. *Chin Med J (Engl).* 2009;122(12):1365–1368.
208. Lerman C, Caporaso NE, Bush A, et al. Tryptophan hydroxylase gene variant and smoking behavior. *Am J Med Genet.* 2001;105(6):518–520.
209. Sullivan PF, Jiang Y, Neale MC, et al. Association of the tryptophan hydroxylase gene with smoking initiation but not progression to nicotine dependence. *Am J Med Genet.* 2001;105(5):479–484.
210. Malaiyandi V, Goodz SD, Sellers EM, et al. CYP2A6 genotype, phenotype, and the use of nicotine metabolites as biomarkers during ad libitum smoking. *Cancer Epidemiol Biomarkers Prev.* 2006;15(10):1812–1819.
211. Wall TL, Schoedel K, Ring HZ, et al. Differences in pharmacogenetics of nicotine and alcohol metabolism: review and recommendations for future research. *Nicotine Tob Res.* 2007;9(suppl 3):S459–S474.
212. Raunio H, Rautio A, Gullsten H, et al. Polymorphisms of CYP2A6 and its practical consequences. *Br J Clin Pharmacol.* 2001;52(4):357–363.
213. Elgoyhen AB, Johnson DS, Boulter J, et al. Alpha 9: an acetylcholine receptor with novel pharmacological properties expressed in rat cochlear hair cells. *Cell.* 1994;79(4):705–715.
214. Xu C, Rao YS, Xu B, et al. An in vivo pilot study characterizing the new CYP2A6*7, *8, and *10 alleles. *Biochem Biophys Res Commun.* 2002;290(1):318–324.
215. Zhang X, Su T, Zhang QY, et al. Genetic polymorphisms of the human CYP2A13 gene: identification of single-nucleotide polymorphisms and functional characterization of an Arg257Cys variant. *J Pharmacol Exp Ther.* 2002;302(2):416–423.
216. Lee AM, Jepson C, Hoffmann E, et al. CYP2B6 genotype alters abstinence rates in a bupropion smoking cessation trial. *Biol Psychiatry.* 2007;62(6):635–641.
217. Lindstrom J. Neuronal nicotinic acetylcholine receptors. *Ion Channels.* 1996;4:377–450.
218. Elgoyhen AB, Vetter DE, Katz E, et al. alpha10: a determinant of nicotinic cholinergic receptor function in mammalian vestibular and cochlear mechanosensory hair cells. *Proc Natl Acad Sci USA.* 2001;98(6):3501–3506.
219. Portugal GS, Gould TJ. Genetic variability in nicotinic acetylcholine receptors and nicotine addiction: converging evidence from human and animal research. *Behav Brain Res.* 2008;193(1):1–16.
220. Hutchison KE, Allen DL, Filbey FM, et al. CHRNA4 and tobacco dependence: from gene regulation to treatment outcome. *Arch Gen Psychiatry.* 2007;64(9):1078–1086.
221. Feng Y, Niu T, Xing H, et al. A common haplotype of the nicotine acetylcholine receptor alpha 4 subunit gene is associated with vulnerability to nicotine addiction in men. *Am J Hum Genet.* 2004;75(1):112–121.
222. Li MD, Beuten J, Ma JZ, et al. Ethnic- and gender-specific association of the nicotinic acetylcholine receptor alpha4 subunit gene (CHRNA4) with nicotine dependence. *Hum Mol Genet.* 2005;14(9):1211–1219.
223. Berrettini W, Yuan X, Tozzi F, et al. Alpha-5/alpha-3 nicotinic receptor subunit alleles increase risk for heavy smoking. *Mol Psychiatry.* 2008;13(4):368–373.
224. Saccone SF, Hinrichs AL, Saccone NL, et al. Cholinergic nicotinic receptor genes implicated in a nicotine dependence association study targeting 348 candidate genes with 3713 SNPs. *Hum Mol Genet.* 2007;16(1):36–49.
225. Zeiger JS, Haberstick BC, Schlaepfer I, et al. The neuronal nicotinic receptor subunit genes (CHRNA6 and CHRNB3) are associated with subjective responses to tobacco. *Hum Mol Genet.* 2008;17(5):724–734.
226. Waldo MC, Adler LE, Leonard S, et al. Familial transmission of risk factors in the first-degree relatives of schizophrenic people. *Biol Psychiatry.* 2000;47(3):231–239.
227. Kendler KS, Karkowski LM, Neale MC, et al. Illicit psychoactive substance use, heavy use, abuse, and dependence in a US population-based sample of male twins. *Arch Gen Psychiatry.* 2000;57(3):261–269.
228. Tsuang MT, Lyons MJ, Harley RM, et al. Genetic and environmental influences on transitions in drug use. *Behav Genet.* 1999;29(6):473–479.
229. Martin CS, Clifford PR, Clapper RL. Patterns and predictors of simultaneous and concurrent use of alcohol, tobacco, marijuana, and hallucinogens in first-year college students. *J Subst Abuse.* 1992;4(3):319–326.
230. Brook JS, Whiteman M, Finch S, et al. Mutual attachment, personality, and drug use: pathways from childhood to young adulthood. *Genet Soc Gen Psychol Monogr.* 1998;124(4):492–510.
231. Kosten TA, Ball SA, Rounsaville BJ. A sibling study of sensation seeking and opiate addiction. *J Nerv Ment Dis.* 1994;182(5):284–289.
232. Substance Abuse and Mental Health Services Administration. The NSDUH Report: Cocaine Use: 2002 and 2003 (August 12,

2005). Rockville, MD: Substance Abuse and Mental Health Services Administration; 2005.
233. Substance Abuse and Mental Health Services Administration. The NSDUH Report: Methamphetamine Use (January 26, 2007). Rockville, MD: Substance Abuse and Mental Health Services Administration; 2007.
234. Kendler KS, Jacobson KC, Prescott CA, et al. Specificity of genetic and environmental risk factors for use and abuse/dependence of cannabis, cocaine, hallucinogens, sedatives, stimulants, and opiates in male twins. *Am J Psychiatry.* 2003;160(4): 687–695.
235. Haile CN, Kosten TR, Kosten TA. Genetics of dopamine and its contribution to cocaine addiction. *Behav Genet.* 2007;37(1): 119–145.
236. Kendler KS, Prescott CA. Cocaine use, abuse and dependence in a population-based sample of female twins. *Br J Psychiatry.* 1998;173:345–350.
237. Comings DE, Gonzalez N, Wu S, et al. Homozygosity at the dopamine DRD3 receptor gene in cocaine dependence. *Mol Psychiatry.* 1999;4(5):484–487.
238. Vorel SR, Ashby CR Jr, Paul M, et al. Dopamine D3 receptor antagonism inhibits cocaine-seeking and cocaine- enhanced brain reward in rats. *J Neurosci.* 2002;22(21):9595–9603.
239. Noble EP, Blum K, Khalsa ME, et al. Allelic association of the D2 dopamine receptor gene with cocaine dependence. *Drug Alcohol Depend.* 1993;33(3):271–285.
240. Gelernter J, Kranzler H, Satel SL. No association between D2 dopamine receptor (DRD2) alleles or haplotypes and cocaine dependence or severity of cocaine dependence in European- and African-Americans. *Biol Psychiatry.* 1999;45(3):340–345.
241. Patkar AA, Berrettini WH, Hoehe M, et al. No association between polymorphisms in the serotonin transporter gene and susceptibility to cocaine dependence among African-American individuals. *Psychiatr Genet.* 2002;12(3):161–164.
242. Patkar AA, Berrettini WH, Hoehe M, et al. Serotonin transporter (5-HTT) gene polymorphisms and susceptibility to cocaine dependence among African-American individuals. *Addict Biol.* 2001;6(4):337–345.
243. Cigler T, LaForge KS, McHugh PF, et al. Novel and previously reported single-nucleotide polymorphisms in the human 5-HT(1B) receptor gene: no association with cocaine or alcohol abuse or dependence. *Am J Med Genet.* 2001;105(6):489–497.
244. Kreek MJ, Bart G, Lilly C, et al. Pharmacogenetics and human molecular genetics of opiate and cocaine addictions and their treatments. *Pharmacol Rev.* 2005;57(1):1–26.
245. Szeto CY, Tang NL, Lee DT, et al. Association between mu opioid receptor gene polymorphisms and Chinese heroin addicts. *Neuroreport.* 2001;12(6):1103–1106.
246. Kranzler HR, Gelernter J, O'Malley S, et al. Association of alcohol or other drug dependence with alleles of the mu opioid receptor gene (OPRM1). *Alcohol Clin Exp Res.* 1998;22(6): 1359–1362.
247. Franke P, Wang T, Nothen MM, et al. Nonreplication of association between mu-opioid-receptor gene (OPRM1) A118G polymorphism and substance dependence. *Am J Med Genet.* 2001;105(1):114–119.
248. Kahan M, Srivastava A, Wilson L, et al. Misuse of and dependence on opioids: study of chronic pain patients. *Can Fam Physician.* 2006;52(9):1081–1087.
249. Tyndale RF, Droll KP, Sellers EM. Genetically deficient CYP2D6 metabolism provides protection against oral opiate dependence. *Pharmacogenetics.* 1997;7:375–379.
250. Agrawal A, Lynskey MT. The genetic epidemiology of cannabis use, abuse and dependence. *Addiction.* 2006; 101(6):801–812.
251. Merikangas KR, Stolar M, Stevens DE, et al. Familial transmission of substance use disorders. *Arch Gen Psychiatry.* 1998; 55(11):973–979.
252. Kendler KS, Prescott CA. Cannabis use, abuse, and dependence in a population-based sample of female twins. *Am J Psychiatry.* 1998;155(8):1016–1022.
253. Timberlake DS, Haberstick BC, Hopfer CJ, et al. Progression from marijuana use to daily smoking and nicotine dependence in a national sample of U.S. adolescents. *Drug Alcohol Depend.* 2007;88(2–3):272–281.
254. Patton GC, Coffey C, Carlin JB, et al. Reverse gateways? Frequent cannabis use as a predictor of tobacco initiation and nicotine dependence. *Addiction.* 2005;100(10):1518–1525.
255. Golub A, Johnson BD. Variation in youthful risks of progression from alcohol and tobacco to marijuana and to hard drugs across generations. *Am J Public Health.* 2001;91(2): 225–232.
256. Lynskey MT, Vink JM, Boomsma DI. Early onset cannabis use and progression to other drug use in a sample of Dutch twins. *Behav Genet.* 2006;36(2):195–200.
257. Kandel DB. Does marijuana use cause the use of other drugs? *JAMA.* 2003;289(4):482–483.
258. Karkowski LM, Prescott CA, Kendler KS. Multivariate assessment of factors influencing illicit substance use in twins from female-female pairs. *Am J Med Genet.* 2000;96(5):665–670.
259. Gardner EL. Endocannabinoid signaling system and brain reward: emphasis on dopamine. *Pharmacol Biochem Behav.* 2005;81(2):263–284.
260. Ameri A. The effects of cannabinoids on the brain. *Prog Neurobiol.* 1999;58(4):315–348.
261. Howlett AC, Barth F, Bonner TI, et al. International Union of Pharmacology. XXVII. Classification of cannabinoid receptors. *Pharmacol Rev.* 2002;54(2):161–202.
262. Solinas M, Goldberg SR, Piomelli D. The endocannabinoid system in brain reward processes. *Br J Pharmacol.* 2008;154(2): 369–383.
263. Antoniou K, Galanopoulos A, Vlachou S, et al. Behavioral pharmacological properties of a novel cannabinoid 1',1'-dithiolane delta8-THC analog, AMG-3. *Behav Pharmacol.* 2005;16(5–6):499–510.
264. Vlachou S, Nomikos GG, Stephens DN, et al. Lack of evidence for appetitive effects of Delta 9-tetrahydrocannabinol in the intracranial self-stimulation and conditioned place preference procedures in rodents. *Behav Pharmacol.* 2007;18(4): 311–319.
265. Forget B, Hamon M, Thiebot MH. Cannabinoid CB1 receptors are involved in motivational effects of nicotine in rats. *Psychopharmacology (Berl).* 2005;181(4):722–734.
266. Caille S, Parsons LH. Cannabinoid modulation of opiate reinforcement through the ventral striatopallidal pathway. *Neuropsychopharmacology.* 2006;31(4):804–813.
267. Lallemand F, De Witte P. SR147778, a CB1 cannabinoid receptor antagonist, suppresses ethanol preference in chronically alcoholized Wistar rats. *Alcohol.* 2006;39(3):125–134.
268. Thornton-Jones ZD, Vickers SP, Clifton PG. The cannabinoid CB1 receptor antagonist SR141716A reduces appetitive and consummatory responses for food. *Psychopharmacology (Berl).* 2005;179(2):452–460.
269. Padwal RS, Majumdar SR. Drug treatments for obesity: orlistat, sibutramine, and rimonabant. *Lancet.* 2007;369(9555):71–77.

270. Hutchison KE, Haughey H, Niculescu M, et al. The incentive salience of alcohol: translating the effects of genetic variant in CNR1. *Arch Gen Psychiatry*. 2008;65(7):841–850.
271. Wegener N, Koch M. Neurobiology and systems physiology of the endocannabinoid system. *Pharmacopsychiatry*. 2009;42(suppl 1):S79–S86.
272. Chen X, Williamson VS, An SS, et al. Cannabinoid receptor 1 gene association with nicotine dependence. *Arch Gen Psychiatry*. 2008;65(7):816–824.
273. Herman AI, Kranzler HR, Cubells JF, et al. Association study of the CNR1 gene exon 3 alternative promoter region polymorphisms and substance dependence. *Am J Med Genet B Neuropsychiatr Genet*. 2006;141B(5):499–503.
274. Heller D, Schneider U, Seifert J, et al. The cannabinoid receptor gene (CNR1) is not affected in German i.v. drug users. *Addict Biol*. 2001;6(2):183–187.
275. Onaivi ES, Ishiguro H, Gong JP, et al. Discovery of the presence and functional expression of cannabinoid CB2 receptors in brain. *Ann N Y Acad Sci*. 2006;1074:514–536.
276. Ishiguro H, Iwasaki S, Teasenfitz L, et al. Involvement of cannabinoid CB2 receptor in alcohol preference in mice and alcoholism in humans. *Pharmacogenomics J*. 2007;7(6):380–385.

CHAPTER 5

Neurobiological Factors of Drug Dependence and Addiction

Heath D. Schmidt ■ Fair M. Vassoler ■ R. Christopher Pierce

INTRODUCTION

Drug addiction is a chronically relapsing disorder characterized by compulsive use of one or more drugs of abuse, the inability to control drug intake, and continued drug use despite its associated negative consequences. The complex neurochemical, biochemical, and structural changes in the brain that underlie addiction are steadily coming into focus, and there are many excellent recent review articles addressing these topics (1–6). In this chapter, we focus on the neurobiological factors that mediate the reinforcing effects of five major classes of abused drugs (psychostimulants, opiates, ethanol, cannabinoids, and nicotine). Particular focus is placed on preclinical studies utilizing the drug self-administration paradigm, which is the most homologous model of human drug taking. In self-administration studies, animals are trained to perform an operant response (e.g., pressing a lever) in order to obtain a drug reinforcer. In some instances, critical hypotheses have been addressed only using paradigms such as conditioned place preference, intracranial self-stimulation, drug discrimination, or behavioral hyperactivity. Where appropriate, important findings using these models also are presented. A discussion of the neurobiological factors underlying withdrawal from chronic drug taking is outside the scope of this chapter; however, there are a number of outstanding recent reviews on these phases of drug addiction (see (7–12)).

Although different classes of abused drugs have different mechanisms of action, there are several striking similarities in terms of the brain circuits modified by repeated exposure to these drugs. Thus, the reinforcing effects of all drugs of abuse are due to actions in the limbic system, a circuit of nuclei that is responsible for the influence of motivational, emotional, contextual, and affective information on behavior. Limbic nuclei including the amygdala, hippocampus, and medial prefrontal cortex (mPFC) send major glutamatergic efferent projections to the nucleus accumbens, which is broadly subdivided into limbic and motor subregions known as the shell and core, respectively (13). The nucleus accumbens sends two main GABAergic efferents to the ventral pallidum and ventral tegmental area (VTA), both of which send GABAergic projections to the medial dorsal thalamus. This limbic circuit is closed via glutamatergic projections from the medial dorsal thalamus to the mPFC (14–18). Dopaminergic axons from the VTA innervate the nucleus accumbens, amygdala, hippocampus, mPFC, and ventral pallidum, and changes in dopaminergic transmission in these nuclei play a critical role in modulating the flow of information through the limbic nuclei comprising this neuronal network (19–22). An overwhelming body of evidence compiled over the last 30 years indicates that increased dopamine neurotransmission contributes significantly to the reinforcing efficacy of psychostimulants, opiates, ethanol, cannabinoids, and nicotine (23,24). The current review is an update of a paper we published in 2006, which focused on the role of dopamine in drug addiction (18). Here, we also have expanded the scope to include information on the role of other neurotransmitter systems in the reinforcing effects of five major classes of abused drugs.

PSYCHOSTIMULANTS

Mechanisms of Action

It is estimated that approximately 3.0 million Americans regularly use a psychostimulant, a class of drugs that includes cocaine and amphetamine-like compounds (25). Psychostimulants produce euphoria, elation, mood elevation, alertness, attention focusing, fatigue reduction, and appetite suppression by interacting with biogenic amine transporters (26). Whereas cocaine inactivates dopamine, norepinephrine, and serotonin transporters, amphetamine and most of its derivatives promote the release of these biogenic amines by reverse transport (26–28). Thus, although the specific mechanisms of action differ, all psychostimulants increase extracellular levels of dopamine, serotonin, and norepinephrine in the nervous system.

Dopamine and Psychostimulant Reinforcement

Although the psychostimulants bind to all of the biogenic amine transporters with high affinity (29), the reinforcing potency of psychostimulants, particularly cocaine, is correlated with their affinity at dopamine but not serotonin or norepinephrine transporters (29,30). Consistent with this finding, selective dopamine reuptake inhibitors are self-administered by rodents and nonhuman primates (30–33). Similarly, in humans there is a positive correlation between dopamine transporter (DAT) occupancy and the desirable subjective effects produced by cocaine (34). Collectively, these data show that increased dopamine transmission plays a critical role in psychostimulant reinforcement.

A substantial body of evidence from animal studies indicates that enhanced dopamine transmission in the nucleus accumbens is important for the initiation and maintenance of psychostimulant self-administration behavior. Thus, whereas removal of dopaminergic inputs to the nucleus accumbens, but not the neostriatum, substantially reduce self-administration of cocaine or D-amphetamine (35,36), destruction of norepinephrinergic neurons has little impact on cocaine self-administration (37). During cocaine or D-amphetamine self-administration, extracellular levels of dopamine in the striatum and nucleus accumbens of rats and monkeys increase markedly, but rapidly decrease when drug access is removed (38–40). Moreover, there is a close correspondence between falling accumbal dopamine levels between psychostimulant infusions and responding for cocaine or amphetamine. That is, operant responding for psychostimulants appears to be initiated in order to maintain extracellular dopamine above a threshold level (39,41).

Dopamine Receptors and Psychostimulant Reinforcement

The five dopamine receptors were classified as D1-like (D1 and D5) or D2-like (D2, D3, and D4) based on pharmacology and sequence homology (42). D1-like agonists are self-administered by rats (43) (but see also (44)) and monkeys (45,46), whereas D1-like antagonists decrease cocaine reinforcement (see (18,47)). Similarly, D2-like agonists are self-administered by rats (48,49) and monkeys (50,51) and D2-like antagonists reduce the reinforcing effects of cocaine (see (18,47)) and D-amphetamine reinforcement (52,53). Collectively, these results clearly show that both D1-like and D2-like dopamine receptors are critically involved in psychostimulant reinforcement (47,54).

Currently, there are no ligands that effectively distinguish between D1 and D5 receptors, a limitation that has severely interfered with the elucidation of specific roles for D1 or D5 dopamine receptors in psychostimulant reinforcement (see Ref. 55). Despite the absence of appropriate pharmacological tools, the roles of D1 and D5 dopamine receptors in various psychostimulant-mediated behaviors has been assessed using transgenic mice. D1 dopamine receptor–deficient mice were developed in the 1990s and were shown to have a decreased hyperactive behavioral response to cocaine relative to controls (56–58) as well as a lack of behavioral sensitization to cocaine (56,59). It was subsequently shown that these transgenic animals have increased thresholds for intracranial self-stimulation (60). However, cocaine-mediated conditioned place preference was observed in D1 dopamine receptor–deficient mice (61). Self-administration experiments showed that D1 dopamine receptor knockout mice were impervious to the reinforcing effects of cocaine or a D1-like dopamine receptor agonist as well as (somewhat surprisingly) a D2-like dopamine receptor agonist (62). These results indicate that D1 dopamine receptors contribute specifically to cocaine reinforcement and also play a permissive role in the reinforcing effects of dopamine receptor agonists. Although D5 dopamine receptor knockout mice have been created, cocaine self-administration has not yet been assessed in these transgenic animals. The available behavioral data with D5 dopamine receptor knockout mice has thus far been inconsistent. Some studies have failed to discern a role for D5 receptors in the behavioral effects of psychostimulants. Thus, D5 dopamine receptor knockout mice showed normal behavioral responses to acute and repeated injections of cocaine (56) and the discriminative stimulus properties of cocaine were intact (63). In contrast, other studies have shown that the behavioral hyperactivity induced by cocaine (63) or D1/D5 agonists (64,65) was blunted in D5 dopamine receptor knockout mice. Moreover, D5 dopamine receptor antisense oligodeoxynucleotides (ODNs) administered into the nucleus accumbens disrupted the ability of rats to discriminate cocaine from saline (66), and injections of D5 ODNs into the ventricles actually enhanced the rotations induced by D1-like dopamine receptor agonists in unilateral dopamine-depleted rats (67).

Although there are more options in terms of the availability of relatively selective D2, D3, and D4 ligands, distinctions among the D2-like dopamine receptors in terms of psychostimulant reinforcement remain somewhat unclear. Mice lacking D3 dopamine receptors display increased locomotor activity when challenged with amphetamine or cocaine (68). Although there are no truly selective D3 receptor agonists, the agonists that are most selective for D3 relative to D2 receptors are self-administered (69,70). Consistent with these findings, selective D3 dopamine receptor antagonists or partial agonists attenuated cocaine reinforcement in rats and monkeys (71,72) (but see also (73)). In contrast, although mice lacking D4 dopamine receptors have an enhanced behavioral response to psychostimulants (74–76), a selective D4 dopamine receptor antagonist had no influence on cocaine self-administration in rodents (73). Genetic deletion of D2 dopamine receptors substantially attenuated the behavioral activating effect of cocaine (77). However, D2 receptor knockout mice not only readily self-administered cocaine, but also their rates of consumption of higher doses of cocaine were actually higher than those of wild-type controls (73), which was likely due to compensatory developmental neuroadaptations. Taken together these results indicate that D2 and perhaps D3 dopamine receptors play critical roles in cocaine reinforcement; however, there is little evidence to date supporting a role for D4 dopamine receptors in the reinforcing effects of psychostimulants.

A number of nuclei receiving dopaminergic projections have been shown to be involved in psychostimulant reinforcement. For example, there is evidence suggesting that increased dopamine transmission in the mPFC (78), olfactory tubercle (79), and the amygdala (80–82) contributes to psychostimulant reinforcement. However, the nucleus that has received the greatest attention in terms of psychostimulant reinforcement is the nucleus accumbens and, in particular, the shell subregion of the accumbens. Thus, cocaine and D-amphetamine are self-administered directly into the rat nucleus accumbens including the limbic system–associated shell subregion (79,83–85). This effect is dopamine dependent in that it can be blocked by coinfusion of D1-like or D2-like dopamine receptor antagonists (83,85). Consistent with these findings, intra-accumbal administration of D1-like or D2-like dopamine receptor antagonists attenuates the reinforcing effects of intravenous cocaine (81,82,86).

Cocaine Self-Administration in DAT Knockout Mice

As reviewed above, an overwhelming body of evidence indicates that the action of psychostimulants at DATs plays a key role in psychostimulant reinforcement (30,31). It was very surprising, therefore, when initial reports indicated that mice lacking the DAT were able to self-administer cocaine in the absence of increases in extracellular dopamine in the striatum (87). It was subsequently shown, however, that cocaine increased extracellular dopamine specifically in the nucleus accumbens of these DAT knockout mice (88,89) via compensatory neuroadaptations involving norepinephrine transporters (NETs) (88) and/or serotonin transporters (SERTs) (89) (for reviews see Refs. 90 and 91). More recently, a different line of DAT knockout mice was developed in which cocaine had no influence on extracellular dopamine in the nucleus accumbens (92). Interestingly, cocaine self-administration was dramatically decreased in these DAT knockout mice (93). In addition, mice expressing a cocaine-insensitive DAT failed to self-administer cocaine (94). Thus, although initial results examining cocaine self-administration in mice with genetic deletion of DAT were interpreted as inconsistent with the dopamine hypothesis of the reinforcing effects of cocaine, subsequent behavioral and neurochemical results confirmed that the DAT plays a fundamental role in cocaine reinforcement. Moreover, results from experiments using DAT mutant mice ultimately supported the prevailing notion that increased dopamine transmission in the limbic system generally, and the nucleus accumbens shell in particular, underlies the reinforcing effects of cocaine.

Norepinephrine, Serotonin, and Cocaine Reinforcement

Even though most research on the mechanisms underlying cocaine reinforcement has focused on dopamine systems, there is also evidence that norepinephrine and serotonin contribute to the behavioral effects of cocaine. Although increased norepinephrine transmission may be involved in the discriminative stimulus effects of cocaine (95) as well as the reinstatement of cocaine seeking (96–98) (but see also (99)), norepinephrine does not appear to play a significant role in cocaine reinforcement (100). Thus, selective NET inhibitors are not self-administered and have no effect on cocaine self-administration (101,102), although NET knockout mice actually self-administered cocaine at higher rates than wild-type controls (90).

Although serotonin contributes to the discriminative stimulus properties of cocaine (103), the role of serotonin in cocaine reinforcement remains unclear. Selective SERT inhibitors do not maintain self-administration (104,105) and genetic deletion of SERT had no effect on cocaine self-administration (93). Moreover, direct and indirect serotonin receptor agonists actually attenuate cocaine reinforcement (106,107). However, there is evidence that specific serotonin receptors modulate the reinforcing effects of cocaine. Thus, cocaine reinforcement and cocaine-induced increases in extracellular dopamine in the nucleus accumbens were enhanced in 5-HT2C knockout mice (108), presumably via effects on dopaminergic neuronal activity in the VTA (109,110). In contrast, administration of 5-HT1B receptor agonists augments cocaine-induced reinforcement (111) as well as cocaine-mediated increases in accumbal dopamine (112). Taken together, the currently available evidence indicates that to the extent that norepinephrine and serotonin influence cocaine reinforcement they do so by modulating mesolimbic dopamine transmission.

Glutamate and Cocaine Reinforcement

Although cocaine does not have a direct effect on glutamatergic neurons, a growing body of evidence indicates that altered glutamate transmission contributes substantially to cocaine-induced neuronal and behavioral plasticity. This is exemplified by the fact that whereas an acute cocaine injection had little or no effect on extracellular accumbal glutamate levels (113,114) (but see also (115)), repeated cocaine administration followed by a cocaine challenge injection increased extracellular glutamate in the core subregion of the nucleus accumbens (114,116,117). Interestingly, repeated exposure to cocaine without subsequent cocaine re-exposure resulted in decreased basal levels of extracellular accumbal glutamate in the nucleus accumbens (114,118). Thus, repeated cocaine administrations reduce basal extracellular glutamate in the nucleus accumbens core but a challenge injection of cocaine increases glutamate release in this structure.

There are several subtypes of glutamate receptors including ionotropic (AMPA [α-amino-3-hydroxyl-5-methyl-4-isoxazole-propionate], kainate, and NMDA [N-methyl-D-aspartic acid]) and metabotropic classes. AMPA/kainate and NMDA receptors allow sodium, potassium, and in some cases calcium to pass through the ion channel, while metabotropic glutamate receptors are G-protein-coupled and therefore increase activation of intracellular effectors. AMPA and NMDA receptors are tetrameric and composed of four different subunits: GluR1–4 (119) and NR1-3 (120), respectively. There are three classes of metabotropic glutamate receptors. The group I metabotropic receptors, which include mGluR1 and mGluR5, stimulate phospholipase C and are predominantly postsynaptic (121). Group II includes mGluR2 and mGluR3, while group III encompasses mGluR4, mGluR6, mGluR7, and mGluR8. Both groups II and III are negatively coupled to adenylyl cyclase (AC) and are mainly located presynaptically (121).

A number of studies indicate that repeated exposure to cocaine influences the expression of AMPA and NMDA receptor subunit protein expression. Repeated cocaine injections or cocaine self-administration result in increased GluR1, GluR2/3 (122–125), and phospho-GluR1 (126,127) expression in the nucleus accumbens and also increased NR1 and NR2B in accumbens (122,126) (but see also Ref. 128). Collectively, these studies indicate that following a period of forced abstinence following repeated exposure to cocaine, there is increased expression of AMPA and NMDA receptor subunits in the nucleus accumbens. Recent evidence suggests that the trafficking of AMPA receptors to and from synapses in the nucleus accumbens plays a critical role in cocaine-induced behavioral and neuronal plasticity. Thus, following repeated administrations of cocaine there is increased surface expression of the GluR1 and GluR2/3 AMPA receptor subunits in the nucleus accumbens (128,129) as well as enhanced accumbal AMPA receptor–mediated synaptic transmission (130). However, these effects were transient and reversed 24 hours following a challenge injection of cocaine (130,131). These results indicate that repeated cocaine exposure produces changes in the expression of AMPA and NMDA subunits as well as bidirectional plasticity of AMPA transmission in the nucleus accumbens (130,131). Although it is not clear to what extent AMPA receptor trafficking contributes to the reinforcing effects of cocaine, emerging evidence indicates that transport of GluR1 and GluR2 subunits in the nucleus accumbens plays an important role in the reinstatement of cocaine seeking (132–134).

Not surprisingly, modulation of AMPA and NMDA receptor–mediated glutamate transmission influences psychostimulant self-administration. Thus, systemic or intra-accumbal administration of an AMPA receptor antagonist decreased cocaine reinforcement (135–137). NMDA receptor antagonists, some of which are reinforcing in their own right (138), disrupt the acquisition of cocaine self-administration (139). Moreover, systemic or intra-accumbal administration of an NMDA receptor antagonist decreases responding for cocaine on an FR schedule (136,140,141) (see also Ref. 142). In terms of metabotropic glutamate receptors, mGluR5 receptor knockout mice do not self-administer cocaine (143). Consistent with this finding, the mGluR5 antagonist, MPEP, decreases self-administration of cocaine and methamphetamine (144–147). A growing literature indicates that stimulation of mGluR2/3 receptors also attenuates cocaine reinforcement (148–150). These findings, collectively, suggest that modulators of ionotropic and metabotropic glutamate receptors may be viable targets for the development of therapeutics for psychostimulant addiction.

OPIATES

Mechanisms of Action

Opiates are analgesic drugs that also have euphorigenic properties that may lead to chronic drug-taking behavior and dependence. Opiates are classified as any natural or synthetic drug with morphine-like actions. Clinical opiate use has escalated over the past 15 years with approximately 9.4 billion dosage units of opiates prescribed annually in the United States of America (151). In terms of illicit drug use, abuse of prescription opiates is second only to marijuana in the United States (25). Moreover, mortality rates related to abuse of prescription opiates continue to rise annually at an alarming rate (152).

Opiates bind to and activate opioid receptors and, thereby, mimic the effects of endogenous opioids (endorphins, enkephalins, dynorphins, and endomorphins) at μ, κ, δ, and/or opioid receptor–like (ORL1) opioid receptors (153,154). Opioid receptors are G-protein–coupled receptors that can form homodimeric as well as heterodimeric protein complexes with other opioid receptors or nonopioid receptors (i.e., α2a-adrenoreceptors, β2-adrenoreceptors, D1-like dopamine receptors, chemokine receptors), respectively (155–157). Heterodimerization of opioid receptors results in altered pharmacology of the individual receptors as well as changes in receptor trafficking and coupling to intracellular signal transduction pathways (153). Stimulation of opioid receptors leads to a variety of physiological and psychological effects, including euphoria, analgesia, sedation, diuresis, miosis, constipation, and/or respiratory depression. Of the opioid receptors, stimulation of μ opioid receptors is mainly responsible for the reinforcing effects of morphine-like opiates, although δ opioid receptors also may contribute to opiate reinforcement (54,154). With regard to localization, μ opioid receptors are widely distributed throughout the central nervous system (CNS), including relatively heavy expression in the VTA and nucleus accumbens (158).

Opiates reduce membrane excitability and subsequently slow cell firing by activating a variety of potassium channels in the plasma membrane of cells in brain regions that send afferents to the VTA (including the nucleus accumbens, ventral pallidum, prefrontal cortex, and amygdala) (159). Furthermore, opiates inhibit voltage-gated calcium channels in presynaptic terminals and thereby modulate neuronal function/networks mainly by inhibiting release of glutamate, gamma aminobutyric acid (GABA), and glycine throughout the CNS (159). Opiates decrease synaptic transmission, in part, by inhibiting AC and, thus, decreasing intracellular levels of cyclic adenosine monophosphate (cAMP) (153). Repeated exposure to opiates results in robust upregulation of AC activity, specifically activity of AC1, AC5, and AC8 isoforms (160). Consistent with these findings, morphine-induced behavioral and physiological changes are modulated in mutant mice lacking AC1, AC5, or AC8 (161).

Dopamine and Opiate Reinforcement

A substantial literature implicates the mesoaccumbens dopamine system in mediating the reinforcing effects of opiates. Opiates exert their effects in the VTA and accumbens through both dopamine-dependent and dopamine-independent mechanisms (36,162,163). Rats will self-administer opioids directly into the VTA (164) or nucleus accumbens (165). Moreover, excitotoxic kainic acid lesions of accumbal cell bodies disrupt opiate self-administration behavior in laboratory animals (166,167). The precise role of the accumbens shell and core subregions in opioid self-administration behavior remains to be determined. However, recent evidence suggests that the core, but not the shell, plays a critical role in the acquisition of heroin self-administration behavior that is under the control of drug-associated stimuli (168). Nucleus accumbens shell dopamine levels are increased in rodents self-administering systemic infusions of opioids (169,170). In contrast, extracellular dopamine levels are not altered within the nucleus accumbens of animals self-administering opioids directly into this nucleus. Thus, pretreatment with the D2/D3 dopamine receptor antagonist, sulpiride, had no effect on intra-accumbal morphine self-administration (171). Rather, the reinforcing effect of opioids self-administered into the nucleus accumbens appears to result from either direct inhibition of GABAergic accumbal projection neurons (172) or inhibition of excitatory neurotransmitter release from glutamatergic terminals within the accumbens (173).

In contrast to the GABAergic- and glutamatergic-dependent mechanisms underlying the reinforcing effects of opiates in the accumbens, a substantial literature suggests that self-administration of opiates directly into the VTA relies on the activation of the mesoaccumbens dopamine system. Only a very small percentage of dopaminergic neurons in the VTA express μ opioid receptors (174). Therefore, μ opioid receptors most likely influence VTA dopaminergic transmission through an indirect mechanism. Stimulation of μ opioid receptors in the VTA inhibits GABA release, which disinhibits dopaminergic neurons, resulting in increased extracellular dopamine levels in the nucleus accumbens. Consistent with this hypothesis, (i) VTA μ opioid receptors are found primarily on the terminals of inhibitory neurons, many of which synapse onto dopaminergic neurons (174); (ii) opioids do not directly influence the excitability of dopaminergic neurons, but do function to hyperpolarize GABAergic interneurons and thereby disinhibit dopamine neurons (175); (iii) intra-VTA microinjection of μ opioid receptor agonists increases the firing rate of dopaminergic neurons (176,177); (iv) local administration of opiates into the VTA increases dopamine release in the nucleus accumbens (178); and (v) pretreating rodents with a GABAergic receptor agonist prior to microinfusing a μ opioid receptor agonist directly into the VTA impairs intra-VTA μ opioid receptor agonist-induced dopamine release in the nucleus accumbens (179).

The role of dopamine in opiate reinforcement is complex and may depend on prior drug history (180). Recent studies demonstrate that in nondependent, drug-naive subjects, the acute rewarding effects of opiates are produced through dopamine-independent mechanisms that are mediated, in part, by cholinergic input from brain stem nuclei, including the pedunculopontine tegmental nucleus, to the VTA (181, 182). However, in subjects that are experiencing a state of withdrawal from repeated opioid administration, the motivational effects of opioids are mediated, in part, by the mesolimbic dopamine system (183), which suggests that dopamine transmission may underlie opiate craving that is independent from the acute rewarding effects of opiates. The VTA is one nucleus wherein opiates produce their rewarding effects through functionally distinct dopamine-independent (opiate-naive) and dopamine-dependent (opiate-dependent or opiate-withdrawn) signaling mechanisms depending upon prior history of drug use (182). Furthermore, $GABA_A$ receptors in the VTA play a critical role in gating bidirectional reward transmission through these two motivation systems (184). The transition from a dopamine-independent to dopamine-dependent opiate reward state is associated with a physiological switch from inhibitory to excitatory signaling in $GABA_A$ receptors that is facilitated by brain-derived neurotrophic factor (BDNF) in the VTA (185).

Dopamine and Opiate Self-Administration

Preclinical studies using the drug self-administration paradigm suggest that activation of the mesolimbic dopamine system plays an important role in opiate reinforcement. Lesions of dopaminergic inputs to the nucleus accumbens impair the acquisition of heroin self-administration (186) and decrease the reinforcing efficacy of morphine (187). Consistent with these findings, self-administration of morphine directly into the VTA was disrupted by administration of the D2/D3 dopamine receptor antagonist, sulpiride (171). In addition, morphine self-administration behavior was not observed in mutant mice lacking the D2 dopamine receptor (188), which suggests that D2-like dopamine receptors play a critical role in the reinforcing effects of opiates. However, it should be noted that several reports indicate that dopamine receptor antagonists do not consistently alter opiate self-administration behavior (189,190).

The hypothesis that the reinforcing effects of opiates are at least partially due to the disinhibition of dopaminergic neurons in the VTA was also confirmed in experiments using the drug self-administration paradigm. Thus, heroin self-administration behavior is associated with an increase in the firing rate of dopaminergic neurons in the VTA (191) and a corresponding increase in extracellular dopamine levels in the nucleus accumbens (170). Moreover, increases in GABA transmission in the VTA attenuate the reinforcing efficacy of heroin as well as heroin-induced increases in accumbal dopamine (192). Also, rodents will self-administer a $GABA_A$ receptor antagonist directly into the VTA (193,194), an effect that is extinguished by pretreatment with a D2 dopamine receptor antagonist (194). Taken together, these findings suggest that the reinforcing effects of opiates are mediated, in part, by altered GABA transmission in the VTA and subsequent effects on neuronal excitability of dopaminergic neurons in the VTA.

Glutamate, Norepinephrine, Cannabinoids, and Opiate Self-Administration

Turnover of a number of neurotransmitters, including biogenic amine and amino acid neurotransmitters, in limbic nuclei is altered in animals self-administering morphine (195). Blocking ionotropic glutamate receptors in the VTA generally (196) or within the anterior VTA specifically (197) reduces heroin self-administration. Furthermore, noncontingent injections of morphine are associated with decreased expression of the AMPA receptor subunit GluR1 in D1-like dopamine receptor expressing neurons in the accumbens shell and non–D1-containing cells in the accumbens core (198). Taken together, these results suggest that chronic opioid exposure induces plasticity in glutamatergic systems within the VTA and nucleus accumbens. The role of norepinephrine in opioid self-administration is less clear (100), although recent evidence suggests that α1b-adrenergic receptors play a role in the reinforcing efficacy of morphine (199).

A growing body of evidence indicates that cannabinoids contribute to opiate reinforcement. For example, CB1 cannabinoid receptor antagonist administration attenuates the self-administration of heroin (200–202). Further evidence that

CB1 receptors mediate the reinforcing effects of opiates comes from studies demonstrating that mutant mice lacking CB1 receptors do not acquire morphine self-administration (203,204). Moreover, intra-accumbens administration of a CB1 receptor antagonist attenuates heroin self-administration behavior (205). In contrast, administration of a CB1 receptor agonist enhances the reinforcing efficacy of heroin through a mechanism that involves interactions with μ opioid receptors (206). Taken together, these findings suggest that cannabinoid receptors exert their influence on opiate reinforcement via interactions with the mesoaccumbens dopamine system. Consistent with this hypothesis, CB1 receptor agonists increase the firing rate of dopaminergic neurons in the VTA and subsequently increase extracellular accumbal dopamine levels (207). However, administration of a CB1 receptor antagonist reduced heroin self-administration but did not influence heroin-induced increases in accumbal dopamine (201), which suggests that cannabinoids can modulate opiate self-administration behavior in a dopamine-independent manner.

Opioid Receptor Knockout Mice and Opiate Self-Administration

Mutant mice lacking one of three opioid receptor genes encoding μ, δ, or κ opioid receptors have been generated using homologous recombination technology and have been used to study the cellular and molecular mechanisms underlying the pharmacological effects and behavioral response of opiates (for review see Ref. 208). Constitutive homozygous and heterozygous μ opioid receptor knockout mice display reduced morphine self-administration behavior compared to wild-type controls (209,210), effects that may depend on κ opioid receptor activation in these mice (210). Furthermore, development of somatic withdrawal signs is absent in μ opioid receptor knockout mice (209,211). In addition to mediating the reinforcing effects of opioids, μ opioid receptors have been demonstrated to mediate the reinforcing effects of other drugs of abuse including cannabinoids, ethanol, and nicotine (212). In contrast, morphine withdrawal was attenuated in mutant mice lacking the κ opioid receptor (213), which suggests that the dysphoric effects of opiates are mediated by κ opioid receptors and that these receptors oppose μ opioid receptors in regulating hedonic tone (214). Behavioral phenotypes of δ and κ opioid receptor knockout mice and mutant mice lacking one of three opioid precursor propeptide genes in self-administration paradigms of opiates and other drugs of abuse remain to be fully characterized.

ETHANOL

Mechanisms of Action

Alcohol use and abuse remains a serious public health issue. In 2007, 18.6 million people in the United States over 12 were classified as dependent on alcohol (25). This represents 7.5% of the population, a number that has remained stable since 2002. Ethanol produces numerous neurochemical and physiological effects on both excitatory and inhibitory neurotransmitter systems in the brain, which result in mood elevation, sedative, anxiolytic, and ataxic effects. Ethanol positively modulates $GABA_A$ receptors, inhibits NMDA and kainate glutamate receptors, inhibits N- and P/Q-type calcium channels, has both inhibitory and excitatory effects at nicotinic acetylcholine receptors, enhances the activity of calcium-activated potassium channels, and modulates inwardly rectifying potassium channels (215).

Effects of Ethanol on Mesolimbic Dopamine Transmission

A number of studies suggest that ethanol increases extracellular dopamine levels in the nucleus accumbens (216,217) by increasing the firing rate of dopaminergic neurons in the VTA (218,219) rather than an effect in the nucleus accumbens itself (220,221). There are several potential mechanisms whereby ethanol might influence the firing rate of dopaminergic neurons including effects on potassium channels and $GABA_A$ receptors in the VTA. In terms of potassium channels, ethanol reduces potassium currents in the VTA leading to the attenuation of after-hyperpolarizations following spontaneous action potentials (222,223). In contrast, stimulation of $GABA_A$ receptors on GABAergic interneurons in the VTA by ethanol or a $GABA_A$ receptor agonist disinhibits dopaminergic neuronal activity (179,224) (but see also (225)). However, since $GABA_A$ receptors also are expressed by dopaminergic cells in the VTA (226), GABAergic interneurons must be more sensitive to $GABA_A$ receptor agonists than dopaminergic cells (227).

Dopamine and Ethanol Self-Administration

Much of the research examining the reinforcing effects of ethanol using the self-administration paradigm has focused on differences between ethanol-preferring lines of rodents in comparison to non–ethanol-preferring lines. The behavioral phenotype of ethanol-preferring rats satisfies criteria for an animal model of alcoholism, including freely consuming large quantities of ethanol sufficient to produce intoxicating blood alcohol concentrations, willingness to work to obtain ethanol, self-administration of ethanol for the pharmacological effects as opposed to gustatory or olfactory reinforcement, and development of tolerance to and dependence on ethanol (228). In contrast, other lines of rats require a sucrose-substitution procedure in which rats are initially allowed to drink freely a rewarding sucrose solution and the concentration of sucrose is slowly decreased while simultaneously increasing the concentration of ethanol in order to obtain ethanol self-administration behavior.

There are numerous findings that support the hypothesis that ethanol-induced increases in firing rates of dopaminergic neurons in the VTA and the subsequent increased release of dopamine in the nucleus accumbens may underlie the reinforcing effects of ethanol. For example, ethanol is self-administered directly into the VTA by rats (229), an effect that is blocked by the stimulation of D2-like dopamine autoreceptors in the VTA (230). In addition, ethanol self-administration behavior is associated with increased extracellular dopamine levels in the nucleus accumbens of rodents (231–233) and rhesus monkeys (234). Moreover, administration of the D2-like dopamine receptor antagonist sulpiride or low doses of the indirect dopamine agonist D-amphetamine increase ethanol self-administration behavior in ethanol-preferring rats (235).

D1-like and D2-like dopamine receptor agonists and antagonists modify ethanol self-administration behavior (236–239) (but see also (238)). Moreover, intra-accumbal microinjection of D1-like (240) or D2-like (240–242) dopamine receptor antagonists reduces ethanol self-administration behavior in rats. Consistent with these findings, genetic deletion of D1 (243) or D2 (244,245) dopamine receptors as well as antisense oligonucleotide-induced decreases in D2 dopamine receptor expression in the nucleus accumbens (246,247) suppressed ethanol self-administration behavior. In contrast, ethanol self-administration behavior was not influenced in constitutive D3 dopamine receptor knockout mice (248,249). Taken together, these results suggest that D1 and D2, but not D3, dopamine receptors in the nucleus accumbens contribute significantly to the reinforcing effects of ethanol. Interestingly, reduced expression of striatal D2 dopamine receptors was observed in alcoholics (250), which may lead to compensatory increases in ethanol intake (250).

GABA, Opiates, Serotonin, Cannabinoids, and Ethanol Self-Administration

The precise role of GABA transmission in the behavioral and physiological effects of ethanol continues to be elucidated. It has been hypothesized that lower doses of ethanol have direct effects on GABA receptor complexes (251). Ethanol appears to be a positive allosteric modulator of the $GABA_A$ receptor in that it potentiates GABA-induced hyperpolarization either through $GABA_A$ receptors or by directly stimulating chloride channel opening (251). GABAergic terminals synapsing on dopaminergic neurons in the VTA have been implicated in the acute rewarding effects of ethanol, and $GABA_B$ receptors appear to play a critical role in this process. Further evidence supporting the role of enhanced GABA transmission in mediating ethanol self-administration behavior comes from animal studies demonstrating that $GABA_A$ receptor antagonists and $GABA_B$ receptor agonists or positive allosteric modulators decrease ethanol self-administration behavior (252–255) (but see also Ref. 256). Moreover, the firing rate of VTA GABAergic neurons increases in animals self-administering intravenous ethanol (257).

The opioid system also mediates ethanol self-administration behavior. The endogenous opioids beta-endorphin and enkephalins, which activate μ and δ opioid receptors, respectively, play a critical role in the reinforcing effects of ethanol (258). In contrast, dynorphin, which activates κ opioid receptors, appears to mediate the dysphoric properties of ethanol (258). Opioid receptor agonists increase ethanol self-administration behavior at low doses and decrease ethanol self-administration at high doses (for review see Ref. 259). These dose-dependent effects may be due to interspecies variability in the behavioral response to ethanol (260). The selective μ opioid receptor antagonists β-funaltrexamine (261) and CTOP (-Pen-Cys-Tyr- -Trp-Orn-Thr-Pen-Thr-NH2) (262) decrease ethanol consumption in rodents. Results examining the effects of selective δ opioid receptor antagonist have been less clear. Thus, ICI (174864), a selective δ opioid receptor antagonist, had no affect on ethanol intake (262), but naltrindole was effective in reducing ethanol self-administration behavior (263). The κ opioid receptor antagonist, norbinaltorphimine, did not impair ethanol self-administration behavior, but it attenuated ethanol-induced increases in extracellular levels of dopamine in the nucleus accumbens (264). Buprenorphine, a partial opioid receptor agonist with high affinity for the μ and κ opioid receptors, reduced ethanol intake for 1.5 hours but increased ethanol intake 4 hours post buprenorphine injection (265). Collectively, these data support a role of endogenous opioid systems in ethanol reinforcement. Indeed, the opiate antagonist naltrexone is used in the treatment of alcoholism (266).

The role of serotonin (5-HT) in the reinforcing effects of ethanol has been extensively studied for over 30 years. Serotonergic efferents from the dorsal raphe nucleus to the nucleus accumbens play a critical role in the reinforcing effects of ethanol. Ethanol-preferring rats have lower 5-HT content in the nucleus accumbens and the prefrontal cortex (235, 267). Moreover, administration of 5-HT reuptake inhibitors, fluoxetine and fluvoxamine, markedly decreased ethanol self-administration behavior in ethanol-preferring rats as well as other lines such as Long Evans (268). In addition, administration of the serotonin depleter p-chlorophenylalanine increases self-administration behavior (269). However, the role of individual 5-HT receptors in ethanol reinforcement is ambiguous. The vast majority of studies examining the role of 5-HT receptors in the reinforcing effects of ethanol have focused on the 5-HT1a, 5-HT1B, 5-HT2, and 5-HT3 receptor subtypes due to a lack of selective pharmacological compounds required to distinguish between other 5-HT receptors (for reviews see (163,228)). Paradoxically, 5-HT receptor agonists and antagonists have both been shown to increase and decrease ethanol self-administration behavior. Thus, direct infusion of a 5-HT receptor agonist into the nucleus accumbens of ethanol-preferring rats enhances ethanol self-administration behavior (270), while systemic and intra-accumbens core injections of the 5-HT1A receptor agonists 8-OH-DPAT and isapirone reduce ethanol intake (271–273). Systemic and intra-accumbens core administration of 5-HT1B receptor agonists also reduces ethanol self-administration behavior (271,273,274). Similarly, administration of a 5-HT2 receptor agonist or risperidone, which preferentially antagonizes the 5-HT2 receptor at low doses, reduced ethanol self-administration behavior (273,275). Systemic administration of the specific 5-HT2A receptor agonist amperozide also reduced ethanol self-administration behavior (276). Furthermore, administration of FG 5974, which has 5HT1A receptor agonist and 5HT2A receptor antagonist actions, also reduced ethanol self-administration behavior (277). 5-HT3 receptor antagonists decrease ethanol self-administration behavior (278–280) and have synergistic effects when combined with opiates (279), which suggests that 5-HT3 receptors and opioid receptors activated overlapping mechanisms to produce the reinforcing effects of ethanol. The effects of 5-HT3 receptor antagonists may be dependent upon temporal-environmental cues associated with the presentation of ethanol (281). However, a different study found that three different 5-HT3 receptor antagonists were not effective in reducing ethanol self-administration (282), indicating that the role of 5-HT3 receptors in the rewarding properties of ethanol need to be further examined. Ethanol preference can be induced in rats by administration of the aldehyde dehydrogenase inhibitor cyanamide. In these pharmacologically ethanol-preferring rats, the 5-HT2 receptor antagonist amperozide significantly reduced ethanol consumption (283,284) but the 5-HT2 antagonists with no effect on reuptake, trazodone or ritanserin, have no effect on ethanol self-administration behavior (283). In animals self-administering ethanol into the posterior VTA, the 5-HT2a and 5-HT3, but not the 5-HT1B, receptors have been shown to mediate the reinforcing effects of ethanol administered into this brain region (285).

Finally, a literature has begun to emerge indicating a role for the cannabinoid system in ethanol reinforcement. Administration of the cannabinoid CB1 receptor agonist CP 55,940 increased breakpoints for the self-administration of beer in rats (286). This effect was reversed with the CB1 receptor antagonist SR 141716 and the opioid receptor antagonist naloxone (286). The CB1 receptor antagonist SR 141716A dose-dependently suppressed responding for intravenous infusions of ethanol as well as intra-VTA and intra-accumbens ethanol self-administration (287,288) (but see also (289)). Moreover, ethanol intake is increased following systemic administration of the CB1 receptor agonist WIN 55,212-2 (288). Blocking the transporter for the endogenous cannabinoid anandamide also reduces ethanol self-administration behavior (290).

Genetically Altered Mice and Ethanol Self-Administration

Constitutive knockout and transgenic mice have been used to further our understanding of the roles of different neurotransmitter systems in the reinforcing effects of ethanol. Mice lacking the alpha1 subunit of the $GABA_A$ receptor display reduced ethanol self-administration behavior when compared to controls and a significant increase in locomotor activity following administration of ethanol, an effect blocked by administration of either a dopamine or benzodiazepine receptor antagonist (291,292). Intracellular mechanisms responsible for interactions between GABA and dopamine signaling during ethanol self-administration may involve specific kinases as it was recently shown using protein kinase C epsilon null mice that $GABA_A$ receptor regulation of ethanol self-administration was absent (293). Furthermore, mice lacking κ opioid receptors display impaired ethanol self-administration behavior when compared to wild-type littermates (294). Interestingly, these same mice showed decreased saccharin preference and higher quinine preference, consonant with previous observations of the involvement of opioids in regulating food intake (294). Moreover, beta-endorphin–deficient mice self-administer ethanol more readily than wild-type controls (295,296). Overexpression of 5-HT3 receptors in the forebrain using a CaMKII-specific promoter decreases ethanol self-administration in mice (297). Genetic deletion of 5-HT1B receptors produces slight preference for ethanol compared to wild-type controls (298). CB1 receptor knockout mice have a significantly lower baseline ethanol consumption compared with wild-type mice (299). Finally, BDNF (+/−) mice, which display abnormal serotonergic neurotransmission and forebrain innervation, have increased ethanol consumption (300). Taken together, these studies examining the phenotype of genetically altered mice support a role of GABA, opioid, serotonergic, and cannabinoid neurotransmitter systems in the reinforcing effects of ethanol.

CANNABINOIDS

Mechanisms of Action

Marijuana remains one of the most widely abused drugs in the United States of America. Forty-one percent of Americans 12 years and older have used marijuana at least once in their lifetime and 10% of the US population has used marijuana within the past year (25). Marijuana smoke contains numerous chemical compounds, including around 60 different cannabinoids (301). However, there is a general consensus that Δ^9-tetrahydrocannabinol (Δ^9-THC) is the primary cannabinoid responsible for the psychoactive effects of marijuana, which include euphoria, enhanced sensory perception, increased appetite, analgesia, disrupted cognitive functioning, anxiety, paranoia and, at higher doses, sedation (301,302). Exogenous cannabinoids appear to mimic the action of endogenous cannabinoids, or endocannabinoids, in the brain by binding to and activating G-protein–coupled cannabinoid receptors. Endocannabinoids constitute a class of compounds that includes anandamide and 2-arachidonoylglyceryl (2-AG), which are the best characterized of the endocannabinoids, and 2-arachidonoylglyceryl ether, N-arachidonoyldopamine, and O-arachidonoylethanolamine (302). Cannabinoids produce their physiological and psychoactive effects by interacting with cannabinoid receptors, which include CB1 and CB2 subtypes. However, since CB2 receptors are only expressed in the immune system, whereas CB1 receptors are expressed extensively in the brain (303), CB1 receptors are responsible for the psychoactive effects of Δ^9-THC.

Cannabinoid–Dopamine Interactions

Unlike classical neurotransmitters, endocannabinoids are not stored in vesicles but, instead, are synthesized and released in an activity-dependent manner (302). In the CNS, endocannabinoids act as retrograde messengers that are released from a postsynaptic neuron and subsequently inhibit the release of classical neurotransmitters from presynaptic terminals via the stimulation of presynaptic CB1 receptors (304).

CB1 receptors are abundantly and widely distributed in the brain (301) including the mesoaccumbal system (305) and the nucleus accumbens shell in particular (306).

Although systemic administration of Δ^9-THC or CB1 receptor agonists increases extracellular accumbal dopamine levels (307,308), particularly in the accumbens shell (308), CB1 receptors are not found on dopaminergic terminals or cell bodies (305,309). It seems likely that, similar to opioids, stimulation of CB1 receptors on GABAergic terminals in the VTA disinhibits dopaminergic neuronal activity, resulting in increased dopamine release in the nucleus accumbens (but see also (310)). Consistent with this hypothesis, administration of a $GABA_A$ receptor antagonist blocked cannabinoid-induced increases in dopaminergic neuronal activity (311–313). Moreover, administration of a cannabinoid receptor agonist decreased $GABA_A$ receptor–mediated inhibitory postsynaptic currents in VTA dopaminergic neurons (314). Taken together, these results suggest that cannabinoids increase dopaminergic neuronal activity by decreasing inhibitory GABAergic tone on these cells.

Dopamine and Cannabinoid Self-Administration

Due to a number of issues, including slow onset of action and a relatively long half-life, reliable self-administration of Δ^9-THC in animal models has proven to be difficult although not insurmountable (315–317). Nonetheless, much of the behavioral pharmacology of cannabinoid self-administration has focused on self-administration of the CB1 receptor agonist WIN 55,212-2 (318,319). WIN 55,212-2 self-administration increases dopamine release in the nucleus accumbens shell and to a lesser extent in the core (320,321). It also has been shown that the nicotinic α7 acetylcholine receptor antagonist, methyllycaconitine, reduced intravenous self-administration of WIN 55,212-2 and Δ^9-THC–induced dopamine elevations in the shell subregion of the nucleus accumbens (322), which suggests that nicotinic receptor antagonists may represent a possible therapeutic modality to treat marijuana addiction.

Opioid–Dopamine Interactions and Cannabinoid Self-Administration

A number of studies indicate that there are functional interactions between cannabinoid and opioid systems (323). For example, Δ^9-THC–induced increases in extracellular dopamine in the nucleus accumbens are attenuated by the systemic or intra-VTA administration of an opiate receptor antagonist (308,324), which suggests that cannabinoids increase dopamine release in the nucleus accumbens by enhancing the firing rate of dopaminergic neurons in the VTA. However, an opioid receptor antagonist had no effects on the increased firing rates of dopaminergic neurons in the VTA produced by Δ^9-THC (207). Although the precise mechanisms underlying cannabinoid–opioid interactions in the mesoaccumbal dopamine system remain unclear, behavioral studies revealed that an opioid receptor antagonist attenuated self-administration of a CB1 receptor agonist (202,325) or Δ^9-THC (308,326).

CRF Cannabinoid Interactions

Due to the difficulties maintaining reliable self-administration of cannabinoids, many studies have sought to examine the neurobiological factors underlying addiction to marijuana through noncontingent administration of Δ^9-THC. Using this experimental design, researchers discovered that Δ^9-THC, along with other cannabinoids, interacts with the hypothalamic pituitary adrenal (HPA) system. It was shown as early as 1978 that plasma corticosterone levels are increased following noncontingent administration of Δ^9-THC (see (327)). Acute Δ^9-THC, anandamide, or HU-210 (a potent CB1 receptor agonist) administration stimulates secretion of adrenocorticotropic hormone (ACTH) and subsequently corticosterone levels in rats in a dose-dependent manner (328,329). Moreover, these effects can be blocked by administration of the selective cannabinoid receptor antagonist, SR 141716A but not the corticotropin-releasing factor (CRF) receptor antagonist D-Phe CRF, suggesting that the stimulation of the HPA axis and consequent increase in plasma corticosterone levels are mediated by activation of cannabinoid receptors (323,330).

NICOTINE

Mechanisms of Action

The World Health Organization estimates that there were approximately 1.3 billion tobacco smokers worldwide in 2003, and this number is expected to increase to 1.7 billion by 2020 (331). If smoking patterns remain the same, approximately 1 billion people will die from smoking-related diseases in the 21st century (332). Although tobacco smoke contains at least 4000 separate chemical compounds, the principal psychoactive chemical is nicotine, which mediates tobacco's reinforcing effects (333). Stimulation of nicotinic acetylcholine receptors in the CNS is responsible for the diverse psychoactive effects of nicotine including mood elevation, decreased anxiety, increased arousal, improved attentiveness, decreased appetite, muscle relaxation, and cognitive enhancement (333). Twelve nicotinic receptor subunits have been identified in the brain ($\alpha 2$–$\alpha 10$, $\beta 2$–$\beta 4$) (334,335). These receptors are heterogenous cation channels that are typically composed of combinations of five α and β subunits; pentameric homomers formed from $\alpha 7$ also have been identified (336).

Nicotine–Dopamine Interactions

In the VTA, nicotinic receptors are found on dopaminergic cell bodies ($\alpha 4\alpha 5\beta 2$, $\alpha 4\alpha 6\alpha 5\beta 2$, $\alpha 7$), glutamatergic terminals ($\alpha 7$) as well as GABAergic cell bodies ($\alpha 4\beta 2\alpha 5$, $\alpha 7$) and terminals ($\alpha 4\beta 2^*$) (333,337,338). In the nucleus accumbens, nicotinic receptors are localized on presynaptic dopamine terminals ($\alpha 4\beta 2$, $\alpha 4\alpha 5\beta 2$, $\alpha 6\beta 2\beta 3$, $\alpha 4\alpha 6\beta 2\beta 3$) as well as presynaptic GABAergic and glutamatergic terminals ($\alpha 4\beta 2^*$) (333,339,340). Systemic administration of nicotine increases extracellular dopamine in the nucleus accumbens (341,342), particularly in the shell subregion (343). Moreover, administration of nicotine into either the VTA (344,345) or the nucleus accumbens (344,346,347) increases extracellular dopamine levels in the nucleus accumbens.

Dopamine release in the nucleus accumbens following the local administration of nicotine into this brain region mainly results from the direct stimulation of β2-containing nicotinic receptors (α4β2* and α6β2*) on presynaptic dopamine terminals (333,348,349), although nicotine-induced glutamate release may also contribute to this process (350). In experiments performed in ex vivo striatal synaptosome preparations, it was demonstrated that there are four major nicotinic receptors on presynaptic dopamine terminals (α4β2, α4α5β2, α6β2β3, α4α6β2β3) that contribute to nicotine-induced dopamine release (338,351,352). In contrast, experiments performed in vivo indicate that nicotine-induced dopamine release is attenuated by intra-accumbal administration of nicotine receptor antagonists that target α7-containing receptors (353).

Nicotine administration also increases phasic burst firing of dopaminergic neurons in the VTA that target the nucleus accumbens shell (354). By increasing the ratio of burst (high-frequency) firing relative to tonic (low-frequency) firing of midbrain dopamine neurons, nicotine effectively increases the signal-to-noise ratio of dopamine afferents in the accumbens shell thereby facilitating dopamine-dependent reinforcement processes that contribute to nicotine addiction. Systemic administration of nicotine increases burst firing of midbrain dopamine neurons (355,356), which results in increased release of dopamine in the nucleus accumbens. This effect is almost completely blocked following administration of a nicotinic receptor antagonist directly into the VTA (345,353). Collectively, these findings indicate that stimulation of nicotinic receptors in the VTA is the primary mechanism underlying nicotine-induced increases in extracellular accumbal dopamine (357), whereas stimulation of nicotinic receptors in the nucleus accumbens appears to modulate the amplitude of this response (353). However, although stimulation of nicotinic receptors on midbrain dopaminergic neurons increases their firing rates, these receptors rapidly desensitize (356). Interestingly, microinjection of a receptor antagonist that targets α7 subunit–containing nicotinic receptors into the VTA decreased dopamine release in the nucleus accumbens induced by nicotine (358). It has been suggested that α7 subunit–containing receptors located on glutamatergic in the VTA desensitize more slowly than other nicotinic receptors, resulting in prolonged glutamate release and stimulation of dopaminergic neuronal activity in the VTA (333,359).

Dopamine and Nicotine Self-Administration

Nicotine is self-administered by a number of species in addition to humans, including primates, dogs, rats, and mice (360). Not surprisingly, nicotinic receptor antagonists attenuate nicotine self-administration (361,362) and blunt nicotine-induced increases in accumbal dopamine levels (363). Interestingly, rodents will self-administer nicotine directly into the posterior VTA and these effects are blocked by coadministration of a nicotinic receptor antagonist, suggesting that the reinforcing effects of nicotine are mediated by these brain regions (364). Activation of the mesoaccumbal dopamine system appears to contribute significantly to nicotine reinforcement. Thus, the acquisition (365) and maintenance (366) of nicotine self-administration was disrupted following the accumbal dopamine depletion. In addition, D1-like or D2-like dopamine receptor antagonists administered systemically attenuated nicotine self-administration (367) and coadministration of a D2-like dopamine receptor antagonist attenuates intra-VTA self-administration of nicotine (364). Administration of a nicotinic receptor antagonist into the VTA attenuated nicotine self-administration (368), which further indicates that the reinforcing effects of nicotine are due to activation of the mesoaccumbal dopamine system (see Refs. 333, 357, 360, and 369).

GABA and Nicotine Self-Administration

Neurochemical studies suggest that the prolonged stimulation of dopaminergic neuronal activity in the VTA following nicotine exposure is due to decreases in GABAergic and increases in glutamatergic transmission (370). Enhancing GABAergic transmission or stimulating $GABA_B$ receptors has been shown to decrease nicotine self-administration behavior (371,372) as well as nicotine-induced increases in extracellular dopamine levels in the nucleus accumbens (373). Moreover, infusion of $GABA_A$ or $GABA_B$ receptor agonists directly into the VTA reduces nicotine self-administration behavior (374) and suggests that GABAergic mechanisms are involved in mediating the reinforcing efficacy of nicotine (375). GABAergic neurons in the VTA express β2-containing nicotinic receptors (342), and nicotine self-administration as well as nicotine-induced increases in burst firing of VTA dopaminergic neurons and striatal dopamine release were attenuated in mice lacking the β2 subunit of the nicotinic receptor (376). Similarly, administration of a high-affinity nicotinic receptor antagonist (including the α4β2 subtype) decreases the reinforcing efficacy of nicotine (377,378). Collectively, these results suggest that nicotine-induced decreases in VTA GABA transmission disinhibit dopaminergic neuronal activity, which in turn promotes the reinforcing effects of nicotine.

Glutamate and Nicotine Self-Administration

Glutamate also has been demonstrated to play a critical role in mediating the reinforcing effects of nicotine (379–381). Systemic administration of NMDA receptor antagonists (382), metabotropic glutamate (mGlu) 5 receptor antagonists (379–381), or presynaptic mGlu(2) and mGlu(3) receptor agonists (383) decreases nicotine self-administration behavior, which suggests that decreasing glutamatergic transmission may reduce the reinforcing effects of nicotine. It has been proposed that the effect of nicotine on glutamate transmission in the VTA is due to interactions with α7 subunit–containing nicotinic receptors (359,384,385). Consistent with this hypothesis, an α7-selective nicotinic receptor antagonist significantly reduced nicotine self-administration (386). However, in another study, the same α7-selective nicotinic receptor antagonist had no effect on nicotine self-administration behavior in rats (377). Taken together, these results suggest that glutamate activation and GABA inhibition act concurrently to activate dopamine cells in the VTA following nicotine self-administration. Thus, although it seems likely that both GABA and glutamate play important roles in nicotine reinforcement, the precise interactions among GABA, glutamate, and dopamine in the VTA that combine to support the reinforcing efficacy of nicotine remain to be determined.

Norepinephrine, Opioids, Cannabinoids, and Nicotine Self-Administration

Although these data clearly indicate that interactions among dopamine, GABA, and glutamate transmitter systems play a critical role in the reinforcing efficacy of nicotine, emerging evidence suggests that other neurotransmitter systems are involved as well. In particular, bupropion influences nicotine self-administration behavior by modulating both dopamine and norepinephrine transmission in the CNS (387,388), which suggests a potential role for norepinephrine in nicotine reinforcement. Extracellular norepinephrine levels are increased in the paraventricular nucleus of the hypothalamus (389) and the amygdala (390) of rodents self-administering nicotine, which suggests that nicotine modulates neuroendocrine function and consolidation of amygdala-dependent memories, respectively. Moreover, inhibiting the norepinephrine transporter, which increases extracellular levels of norepinephrine in the brain, attenuates both nicotine and food self-administration behaviors (362,391,392).

Cannabinoids also have been shown to mediate, in part, the reinforcing effects of nicotine. Although CB1 cannabinoid receptor knockout mice self-administer nicotine to a similar extent as their wild-type littermates (203), pharmacological studies indicate that CB1 receptors may contribute to nicotine reinforcement. For example, administration of a CB1 receptor antagonist attenuates nicotine self-administration behavior (393,394) as well as nicotine-induced dopamine release in the nucleus accumbens (393). These findings provided the rationale for clinical studies designed to assess the efficacy of CB1 receptor antagonists as a smoking cessation therapy (395). Systemic administration of nicotine increases opioid levels in the nucleus accumbens (396). While clinical studies have demonstrated that administration of an opioid receptor antagonist attenuates the reinforcing effects of nicotine in human cigarette smokers (397,398), preclinical studies have demonstrated that systemic (367,399,400) or intra-VTA administration (374) of opioid receptor antagonists has no effect on the reinforcing efficacy of nicotine in rodents. However, opioid receptors outside of the dopamine system may play a role in the reinforcing effects of nicotine (401). Thus, the reinforcing efficacy of nicotine may be mediated by both dopamine-dependent and dopamine-independent mechanisms (402).

Nicotine Receptor Knockout Mice and Nicotine Self-Administration

Nicotinic receptors are pentomeric protein complexes with different pharmacological and electrophysiological properties depending on their subunit composition. The effects of nicotine on nicotinic receptors in the brain are complex and consist of both activation and desensitization of nicotinic receptors (403). Therefore, nicotine-induced neuroadaptations are likely to be mediated by differential activation and desensitization of nicotinic receptors in neural networks underlying the behavioral response(s) to nicotine. However, identification of precise subunit compositions that comprise functional neuronal nicotinic receptors in vivo is limited due to lack of selective pharmacological compounds that target individual subunits (404). The role of nicotine receptor subunits in nicotine-mediated behaviors has recently been examined using genetically modified mice with null mutations in the genes that encode individual nicotinic receptor subunits. While a number of nicotinic receptor mutant mice have been generated to date (404), the reinforcing effects of nicotine have been studied mainly in constitutive β2 knockout mice (376,405). Mutant mice lacking the β2 subunit do not self-administer nicotine when compared to wild-type controls, suggesting the β2 nicotinic receptor subunit plays a critical role in the reinforcing efficacy of nicotine (376,405). Consistent with these results, constitutive β2 knockout mice re-establish nicotine self-administration behavior when the β2 subunit is selectively re-expressed in the VTA using viral-mediated gene transfer techniques (406,407). Furthermore, nicotine self-administration increases extracellular dopamine levels in constitutive β2 knockout mice re-expressing the β2 subunit to similar levels observed in wild-type animals self-administering nicotine (407). Recently, the contribution of different alpha subunit partners of the β2 subunit of nicotinic receptors in the reinforcing effects of nicotine was examined by re-expressing α4, α6, or α7 subunits in the VTA of mutant mice in which the corresponding α subunit was knocked out (406). Constitutive α4 or α7 knockout mice do not self-administer nicotine and re-expressing α4 or α6 subunits in the VTA promotes nicotine self-administration in mice lacking these individual subunits (406). In contrast, mutant mice lacking the α7 nicotinic receptor subunit self-administer nicotine in patterns similar to those of wild-type animals which suggests that α7-containing nicotinic receptors do not mediate the reinforcing efficacy of nicotine (406). Taken together, these results indicate that functional α4β2*- and α6β2*-containing nicotinic receptors, but not α7-containing nicotinic receptors, in the VTA are required for the reinforcing effects of nicotine.

SUMMARY/CONCLUSIONS

As reviewed above, a rapidly expanding literature indicates that changes in the function of diverse neurotransmitter systems independently and in concert underlie the reinforcing

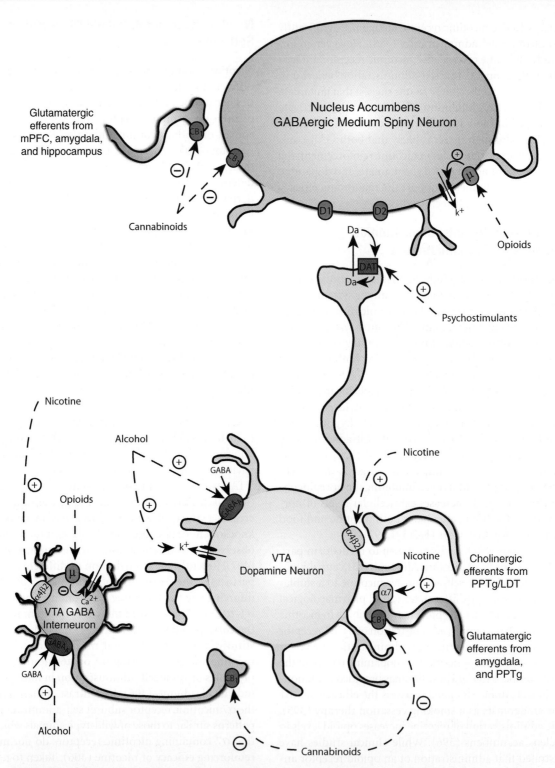

Figure 5.1. Influences of psychostimulants, opioids, cannabinoids, nicotine, and alcohol on the mesoaccumbens dopamine system. See text for details. α4β2, α4β2 nicotinic receptor subtype; α7, α7 nicotinic receptor subtype; CB1, cannabinoid 1 receptor; D1, D1-like dopamine receptor; D2, D2-like dopamine receptor; Da, dopamine; DAT, dopamine transporter; μ, μ opioid receptor; VTA, ventral tegmental area.

effects of abused drugs. Although various drugs of abuse influence glutamate, GABA, acetylcholine, opioid, cannabinoid, and other neurotransmitter systems, the mesolimbic dopamine system is the common denominator in terms of the reinforcing effects of psychostimulants, opiates, ethanol, cannabinoids, and nicotine (see Fig. 5.1). Whereas psychostimulants act directly on dopaminergic neurons by interacting with DATs, the other drugs of abuse increase dopamine release and/or dopaminergic neuronal activity in the mesoaccumbens pathway through interactions with a number of ionotropic receptors, metabotropic receptors, ion channels, and transporters. Drug self-administration experiments indicate that enhanced dopamine transmission in the nucleus accumbens plays at least a partial role in the reinforcing effects of psychostimulants, opiates, ethanol, cannabinoids, and nicotine, which suggest that the mesoaccumbal dopamine system is the final common pathway underlying the reinforcing effects of the major classes of abused drugs.

ACKNOWLEDGMENTS

The authors thank Thomas Hopkins and Michael McMullen for their help in preparing this chapter. This work was supported by grants from the National Institutes of Health (NIH) to RCP (RO1 DA15214, R01 DA22339, and K02 DA18678).

REFERENCES

1. Volkow ND, Fowler JS, Wang GJ, et al. Imaging dopamine's role in drug abuse and addiction. *Neuropharmacology*. 2009;56(suppl 1):3–8.
2. Russo SJ, Mazei-Robison MS, Ables JL, et al. Neurotrophic factors and structural plasticity in addiction. *Neuropharmacology*. 2009;56(suppl 1):73–82.
3. Koob GF. Neurobiological substrates for the dark side of compulsivity in addiction. *Neuropharmacology*. 2009;56(suppl 1):18–31.
4. Thomas MJ, Kalivas PW, Shaham Y. Neuroplasticity in the mesolimbic dopamine system and cocaine addiction. *Br J Pharmacol*. 2008;154:327–342.
5. Renthal W, Nestler EJ. Epigenetic mechanisms in drug addiction. *Trends Mol Med*. 2008;14:341–350.
6. Kalivas PW, O'Brien C. Drug addiction as a pathology of staged neuroplasticity. *Neuropsychopharmacology*. 2008;33:166–180.
7. Koob GF. Dynamics of neuronal circuits in addiction: reward, antireward, and emotional memory. *Pharmacopsychiatry*. 2009;42(suppl 1):S32–S41.
8. Kalivas PW, Lalumiere RT, Knackstedt L, et al. Glutamate transmission in addiction. *Neuropharmacology*. 2009;56(suppl 1):169–173.
9. Aston-Jones G, Harris GC. Brain substrates for increased drug seeking during protracted withdrawal. *Neuropharmacology*. 2004;47(suppl 1):167–179.
10. Shalev U, Grimm JW, Shaham Y. Neurobiology of relapse to heroin and cocaine seeking: a review. *Pharmacol Rev*. 2002;54:1–42.
11. Lu L, Grimm JW, Hope BT, et al. Incubation of cocaine craving after withdrawal: a review of preclinical data. *Neuropharmacology*. 2004;47(suppl 1):214–226.
12. Schmidt HD, Anderson SM, Famous KR, et al. Anatomy and pharmacology of cocaine priming-induced reinstatement of drug seeking. *Eur J Pharmacol*. 2005;526:65–76.
13. Heimer L, Alheid GF, de Olmos JS, et al. The accumbens: beyond the core-shell dichotomy. *J Neuropsychiatry Clin Neurosci*. 1997;9:354–381.
14. Haber S. Parallel and integrative processing through the Basal Ganglia reward circuit: lessons from addiction. *Biol Psychiatry*. 2008;64:173–174.
15. Heimer L. A new anatomical framework for neuropsychiatric disorders and drug abuse. *Am J Psychiatry*. 2003;160:1726–1739.
16. Zahm DS. An integrative neuroanatomical perspective on some subcortical substrates of adaptive responding with emphasis on the nucleus accumbens. *Neurosci Biobehav Rev*. 2000;24:85–105.
17. Groenewegen HJ, Uylings HB. The prefrontal cortex and the integration of sensory, limbic and autonomic information. *Prog Brain Res*. 2000;126:3–28.
18. Pierce RC, Kumaresan V. The mesolimbic dopamine system: the final common pathway for the reinforcing effect of drugs of abuse? *Neurosci Biobehav Rev*. 2006;30:215–238.
19. Wheeler RA, Carelli RM. Dissecting motivational circuitry to understand substance abuse. *Neuropharmacology*. 2009;56(suppl 1):149–159.
20. Sesack SR, Carr DB, Omelchenko N, et al. Anatomical substrates for glutamate–dopamine interactions: evidence for specificity of connections and extrasynaptic actions. *Ann N Y Acad Sci*. 2003;1003:36–52.
21. Wise RA. Brain reward circuitry: insights from unsensed incentives. *Neuron*. 2002;36:229–240.
22. Schultz W. Getting formal with dopamine and reward. *Neuron*. 2002;36:241–263.
23. Wise RA. Catecholamine theories of reward: a critical review. *Brain Res*. 1978;152:215–247.
24. Fibiger HC. Drugs and reinforcement mechanisms: a critical review of the catecholamine theory. *Annu Rev Pharmacol Toxicol*. 1978;18:37–56.
25. Substance Abuse and Mental Health Services Administration S. *Results from the 2007 National Survey on Drug Use and Health: National Findings*. Rockville, MD: Office of Applied Studies; 2008.
26. Ritz MC, Cone EJ, Kuhar MJ. Cocaine inhibition of ligand binding at dopamine, norepinephrine and serotonin transporters: a structure–activity study. *Life Sci*. 1990;46:635–645.
27. Sulzer D, Maidment NT, Rayport S. Amphetamine and other weak bases act to promote reverse transport of dopamine in ventral midbrain neurons. *J Neurochem*. 1993;60:527–535.
28. Seiden LS, Sabol KE, Ricaurte GA. Amphetamine: effects on catecholamine systems and behavior. *Annu Rev Pharmacol Toxicol*. 1993;33:639–677.
29. Ritz MC, Kuhar MJ. Relationship between self-administration of amphetamine and monoamine receptors in brain: comparison with cocaine. *J Pharmacol Exp Ther*. 1989;248:1010–1017.
30. Ritz MC, Lamb RJ, Goldberg SR, et al. Cocaine receptors on dopamine transporters are related to self-administration of cocaine. *Science*. 1987;237:1219–1223.
31. Bergman J, Madras BK, Johnson SE, et al. Effects of cocaine and related drugs in nonhuman primates. III. Self-administration by squirrel monkeys. *J Pharmacol Exp Ther*. 1989;251:150–155.
32. Roberts DC. Self-administration of GBR 12909 on a fixed ratio and progressive ratio schedule in rats. *Psychopharmacology (Berl)*. 1993;111:202–206.
33. Woolverton WL, Hecht GS, Agoston GE, et al. Further studies of the reinforcing effects of benztropine analogs in rhesus monkeys. *Psychopharmacology (Berl)*. 2001;154:375–382.
34. Volkow ND, Wang GJ, Fischman MW, et al. Relationship between subjective effects of cocaine and dopamine transporter occupancy. *Nature*. 1997;386:827–830.
35. Roberts DC, Koob GF, Klonoff P, et al. Extinction and recovery of cocaine self-administration following 6-hydroxydopamine lesions of the nucleus accumbens. *Pharmacol Biochem Behav*. 1980;12:781–787.
36. Pettit HO, Ettenberg A, Bloom FE, et al. Destruction of dopamine in the nucleus accumbens selectively attenuates

cocaine but not heroin self-administration in rats. *Psychopharmacology (Berl)*. 1984;84:167–173.
37. Roberts DC, Corcoran ME, Fibiger HC. On the role of ascending catecholaminergic systems in intravenous self-administration of cocaine. *Pharmacol Biochem Behav*. 1977;6:615–620.
38. Hurd YL, Weiss F, Koob GF, et al. Cocaine reinforcement and extracellular dopamine overflow in rat nucleus accumbens: an in vivo microdialysis study. *Brain Res*. 1989;498:199–203.
39. Wise RA, Newton P, Leeb K, et al. Fluctuations in nucleus accumbens dopamine concentration during intravenous cocaine self-administration in rats. *Psychopharmacology (Berl)*. 1995;120:10–20.
40. Bradberry CW, Barrett-Larimore RL, Jatlow P, et al. Impact of self-administered cocaine and cocaine cues on extracellular dopamine in mesolimbic and sensorimotor striatum in rhesus monkeys. *J Neurosci*. 2000;20:3874–3883.
41. Ranaldi R, Pocock D, Zereik R, et al. Dopamine fluctuations in the nucleus accumbens during maintenance, extinction, and reinstatement of intravenous D-amphetamine self-administration. *J Neurosci*. 1999;19:4102–4109.
42. Civelli O, Bunzow JR, Grandy DK. Molecular diversity of the dopamine receptors. *Annu Rev Pharmacol Toxicol*. 1993;33:281–307.
43. Self DW, Belluzzi JD, Kossuth S, et al. Self-administration of the D1 agonist SKF 82958 is mediated by D1, not D2, receptors. *Psychopharmacology (Berl)*. 1996;123:303–306.
44. Caine SB, Negus SS, Mello NK. Method for training operant responding and evaluating cocaine self-administration behavior in mutant mice. *Psychopharmacology (Berl)*. 1999;147:22–24.
45. Grech DM, Spealman RD, Bergman J. Self-administration of D1 receptor agonists by squirrel monkeys. *Psychopharmacology (Berl)*. 1996;125:97–104.
46. Weed MR, Paul IA, Dwoskin LP, et al. The relationship between reinforcing effects and in vitro effects of D1 agonists in monkeys. *J Pharmacol Exp Ther*. 1997;283:29–38.
47. Platt DM, Rowlett JK, Spealman RD. Behavioral effects of cocaine and dopaminergic strategies for preclinical medication development. *Psychopharmacology (Berl)*. 2002;163:265–282.
48. Wise RA, Murray A, Bozarth MA. Bromocriptine self-administration and bromocriptine-reinstatement of cocaine-trained and heroin-trained lever pressing in rats. *Psychopharmacology (Berl)*. 1990;100:355–360.
49. Caine SB, Negus SS, Mello NK, et al. Effects of dopamine D(1-like) and D(2-like) agonists in rats that self-administer cocaine. *J Pharmacol Exp Ther*. 1999;291:353–360.
50. Woolverton WL, Goldberg LI, Ginos JZ. Intravenous self-administration of dopamine receptor agonists by rhesus monkeys. *J Pharmacol Exp Ther*. 1984;230:678–683.
51. Ranaldi R, Wang Z, Woolverton WL. Reinforcing effects of D2 dopamine receptor agonists and partial agonists in rhesus monkeys. *Drug Alcohol Depend*. 2001;64:209–217.
52. Amit Z, Smith BR. Remoxipride, a specific D2 dopamine antagonist: an examination of its self-administration liability and its effects on D-amphetamine self-administration. *Pharmacol Biochem Behav*. 1992;41:259–261.
53. Fletcher PJ. A comparison of the effects of risperidone, raclopride, and ritanserin on intravenous self-administration of D-amphetamine. *Pharmacol Biochem Behav*. 1998;60:55–60.
54. Mello NK, Negus SS. Preclinical evaluation of pharmacotherapies for treatment of cocaine and opioid abuse using drug self-administration procedures. *Neuropsychopharmacology*. 1996;14:375–424.
55. Waddington JL, Daly SA, Downes RP, et al. Behavioural pharmacology of 'D-1-like' dopamine receptors: further subtyping, new pharmacological probes and interactions with 'D-2-like' receptors. *Prog Neuropsychopharmacol Biol Psychiatry*. 1995;19:811–831.
56. Karlsson RM, Hefner KR, Sibley DR, et al. Comparison of dopamine D1 and D5 receptor knockout mice for cocaine locomotor sensitization. *Psychopharmacology (Berl)*. 2008;200:117–127.
57. Karasinska JM, George SR, Cheng R, et al. Deletion of dopamine D1 and D3 receptors differentially affects spontaneous behaviour and cocaine-induced locomotor activity, reward and CREB phosphorylation. *Eur J Neurosci*. 2005;22:1741–1750.
58. Xu M, Moratalla R, Gold LH, et al. Dopamine D1 receptor mutant mice are deficient in striatal expression of dynorphin and in dopamine-mediated behavioral responses. *Cell*. 1994;79:729–742.
59. Xu M, Guo Y, Vorhees CV, et al. Behavioral responses to cocaine and amphetamine administration in mice lacking the dopamine D1 receptor. *Brain Res*. 2000;852:198–207.
60. Tran AH, Tamura R, Uwano T, et al. Dopamine D1 receptors involved in locomotor activity and accumbens neural responses to prediction of reward associated with place. *Proc Natl Acad Sci U S A*. 2005;102:2117–2122.
61. Miner LL, Drago J, Chamberlain PM, et al. Retained cocaine conditioned place preference in D1 receptor deficient mice. *Neuroreport*. 1995;6:2314–2316.
62. Caine SB, Thomsen M, Gabriel KI, et al. Lack of self-administration of cocaine in dopamine D1 receptor knock-out mice. *J Neurosci*. 2007;27:13140–13150.
63. Elliot EE, Sibley DR, Katz JL. Locomotor and discriminative-stimulus effects of cocaine in dopamine D5 receptor knockout mice. *Psychopharmacology (Berl)*. 2003;169:161–168.
64. O'Sullivan GJ, Kinsella A, Sibley DR, et al. Ethological resolution of behavioural topography and D1-like versus D2-like agonist responses in congenic D5 dopamine receptor mutants: identification of D5:D2-like interactions. *Synapse*. 2005;55:201–211.
65. Holmes A, Hollon TR, Gleason TC, et al. Behavioral characterization of dopamine D5 receptor null mutant mice. *Behav Neurosci*. 2001;115:1129–1144.
66. Filip M, Thomas ML, Cunningham KA. Dopamine D5 receptors in nucleus accumbens contribute to the detection of cocaine in rats. *J Neurosci*. 2000;20:RC98.
67. Dziewczapolski G, Menalled LB, García MC, et al. Opposite roles of D1 and D5 dopamine receptors in locomotion revealed by selective antisense oligonucleotides. *Neuroreport*. 1998;9:1–5.
68. Xu M, Koeltzow TE, Santiago GT, et al. Dopamine D3 receptor mutant mice exhibit increased behavioral sensitivity to concurrent stimulation of D1 and D2 receptors. *Neuron*. 1997;19:837–848.
69. Caine SB, Koob GF. Modulation of cocaine self-administration in the rat through D-3 dopamine receptors. *Science*. 1993;260:1814–1816.
70. Nader MA, Mach RH. Self-administration of the dopamine D3 agonist 7-OH-DPAT in rhesus monkeys is modified by prior cocaine exposure. *Psychopharmacology (Berl)*. 1996;125:13–22.
71. Xi ZX, Gilbert JG, Pak AC, et al. Selective dopamine D3 receptor antagonism by SB-277011A attenuates cocaine reinforcement as assessed by progressive-ratio and variable-cost-variable-payoff fixed-ratio cocaine self-administration in rats. *Eur J Neurosci*. 2005;21:3427–3438.
72. Claytor R, Lile JA, Nader MA. The effects of eticlopride and the selective D3-antagonist PNU 99194-A on food- and cocaine-

maintained responding in rhesus monkeys. *Pharmacol Biochem Behav.* 2006;83:456–464.
73. Caine SB, Negus SS, Mello NK, et al. Role of dopamine D2-like receptors in cocaine self-administration: studies with D2 receptor mutant mice and novel D2 receptor antagonists. *J Neurosci.* 2002;22:2977–2988.
74. Kruzich PJ, Suchland KL, Grandy DK. Dopamine D4 receptor-deficient mice, congenic on the C57BL/6J background, are hypersensitive to amphetamine. *Synapse.* 2004;53:131–139.
75. Katz JL, Chausmer AL, Elmer GI, et al. Cocaine-induced locomotor activity and cocaine discrimination in dopamine D4 receptor mutant mice. *Psychopharmacology (Berl).* 2003;170:108–114.
76. Rubinstein M, Phillips TJ, Bunzow JR, et al. Mice lacking dopamine D4 receptors are supersensitive to ethanol, cocaine, and methamphetamine. *Cell.* 1997;90:991–1001.
77. Welter M, Vallone D, Samad TA, et al. Absence of dopamine D2 receptors unmasks an inhibitory control over the brain circuitries activated by cocaine. *Proc Natl Acad Sci U S A.* 2007;104:6840–6845.
78. Goeders NE, Smith JE. Cortical dopaminergic involvement in cocaine reinforcement. *Science.* 1983;221:773–775.
79. Ikemoto S. Involvement of the olfactory tubercle in cocaine reward: intracranial self-administration studies. *J Neurosci.* 2003;23:9305–9311.
80. Chevrette J, Stellar JR, Hesse GW, et al. Both the shell of the nucleus accumbens and the central nucleus of the amygdala support amphetamine self-administration in rats. *Pharmacol Biochem Behav.* 2002;71:501–507.
81. McGregor A, Roberts DC. Dopaminergic antagonism within the nucleus accumbens or the amygdala produces differential effects on intravenous cocaine self-administration under fixed and progressive ratio schedules of reinforcement. *Brain Res.* 1993;624:245–252.
82. Caine SB, Heinrichs SC, Coffin VL, et al. Effects of the dopamine D-1 antagonist SCH 23390 microinjected into the accumbens, amygdala or striatum on cocaine self-administration in the rat. *Brain Res.* 1995;692:47–56.
83. Rodd-Henricks ZA, McKinzie DL, Li TK, et al. Cocaine is self-administered into the shell but not the core of the nucleus accumbens of Wistar rats. *J Pharmacol Exp Ther.* 2002;303:1216–1226.
84. Hoebel BG, Monaco AP, Hernandez L, et al. Self-injection of amphetamine directly into the brain. *Psychopharmacology (Berl).* 1983;81:158–163.
85. Phillips GD, Robbins TW, Everitt BJ. Bilateral intra-accumbens self-administration of D-amphetamine: antagonism with intra-accumbens SCH-23390 and sulpiride. *Psychopharmacology (Berl).* 1994;114:477–485.
86. Bari AA, Pierce RC. D1-like and D2 dopamine receptor antagonists administered into the shell subregion of the rat nucleus accumbens decrease cocaine, but not food, reinforcement. *Neuroscience.* 2005;135:959–968.
87. Rocha BA, Fumagalli F, Gainetdinov RR, et al. Cocaine self-administration in dopamine-transporter knockout mice. *Nat Neurosci.* 1998;1:132–137.
88. Carboni E, Spielewoy C, Vacca C, et al. Cocaine and amphetamine increase extracellular dopamine in the nucleus accumbens of mice lacking the dopamine transporter gene. *J Neurosci.* 2001;21:RC141:141–144.
89. Mateo Y, Budygin EA, John CE, et al. Role of serotonin in cocaine effects in mice with reduced dopamine transporter function. *Proc Natl Acad Sci U S A.* 2004;101:372–377.
90. Rocha BA. Stimulant and reinforcing effects of cocaine in monoamine transporter knockout mice. *Eur J Pharmacol.* 2003;479:107–115.
91. Gainetdinov RR, Caron MG. Monoamine transporters: from genes to behavior. *Annu Rev Pharmacol Toxicol.* 2003;43:261–284.
92. Shen HW, Hagino Y, Kobayashi H, et al. Regional differences in extracellular dopamine and serotonin assessed by in vivo microdialysis in mice lacking dopamine and/or serotonin transporters. *Neuropsychopharmacology.* 2004;29:1790–1799.
93. Thomsen M, Hall FS, Uhl GR, et al. Dramatically decreased cocaine self-administration in dopamine but not serotonin transporter knock-out mice. *J Neurosci.* 2009;29:1087–1092.
94. Thomsen M, Han DD, Gu HH, et al. Lack of cocaine self-administration in mice expressing a cocaine-insensitive dopamine transporter. *J Pharmacol Exp Ther.* 2009;331:204–211.
95. Spealman RD. Noradrenergic involvement in the discriminative stimulus effects of cocaine in squirrel monkeys. *J Pharmacol Exp Ther.* 1995;275:53–62.
96. Platt DM, Rowlett JK, Spealman RD. Noradrenergic mechanisms in cocaine-induced reinstatement of drug seeking in squirrel monkeys. *J Pharmacol Exp Ther.* 2007;322:894–902.
97. Erb S, Hitchcott PK, Rajabi H, et al. Alpha-2 adrenergic receptor agonists block stress-induced reinstatement of cocaine seeking. *Neuropsychopharmacology.* 2000;23:138–150.
98. Lee B, Tiefenbacher S, Platt DM, et al. Pharmacological blockade of alpha2-adrenoceptors induces reinstatement of cocaine-seeking behavior in squirrel monkeys. *Neuropsychopharmacology.* 2004;29:686–693.
99. Schmidt HD, Pierce RC. Systemic administration of a dopamine, but not a serotonin or norepinephrine, transporter inhibitor reinstates cocaine seeking in the rat. *Behav Brain Res.* 2006;175:189–194.
100. Weinshenker D, Schroeder JP. There and back again: a tale of norepinephrine and drug addiction. *Neuropsychopharmacology.* 2007;32:1433–1451.
101. Mello NK, Lukas SE, Bree MP, et al. Desipramine effects on cocaine self-administration by rhesus monkeys. *Drug Alcohol Depend.* 1990;26:103–116.
102. Woolverton WL. Evaluation of the role of norepinephrine in the reinforcing effects of psychomotor stimulants in rhesus monkeys. *Pharmacol Biochem Behav.* 1987;26:835–839.
103. Filip M, Bubar MJ, Cunningham KA. Contribution of serotonin (5-HT) 5-HT2 receptor subtypes to the discriminative stimulus effects of cocaine in rats. *Psychopharmacology (Berl).* 2006;183:482–489.
104. Vanover KE, Nader MA, Woolverton WL. Evaluation of the discriminative stimulus and reinforcing effects of sertraline in rhesus monkeys. *Pharmacol Biochem Behav.* 1992;41:789–793.
105. Roberts DC, Phelan R, Hodges LM, et al. Self-administration of cocaine analogs by rats. *Psychopharmacology (Berl).* 1999;144:389–397.
106. Grottick AJ, Fletcher PJ, Higgins GA. Studies to investigate the role of 5-HT(2C) receptors on cocaine- and food-maintained behavior. *J Pharmacol Exp Ther.* 2000;295:1183–1191.
107. Czoty PW, Ginsburg BC, Howell LL. Serotonergic attenuation of the reinforcing and neurochemical effects of cocaine in squirrel monkeys. *J Pharmacol Exp Ther.* 2002;300:831–837.
108. Rocha BA, Goulding EH, O'Dell LE, et al. Enhanced locomotor, reinforcing, and neurochemical effects of cocaine in serotonin 5-hydroxytryptamine 2C receptor mutant mice. *J Neurosci.* 2002;22:10039–10045.

109. Gobert A, Rivet JM, Lejeune F, et al. Serotonin(2C) receptors tonically suppress the activity of mesocortical dopaminergic and adrenergic, but not serotonergic, pathways: a combined dialysis and electrophysiological analysis in the rat. *Synapse.* 2000;36:205–221.
110. Di Giovanni G, Di Matteo V, La Grutta V, et al. m-Chlorophenylpiperazine excites non-dopaminergic neurons in the rat substantia nigra and ventral tegmental area by activating serotonin-2C receptors. *Neuroscience.* 2001;103:111–116.
111. Parsons LH, Weiss F, Koob GF. Serotonin1B receptor stimulation enhances cocaine reinforcement. *J Neurosci.* 1998;18:10078–10089.
112. Parsons LH, Koob GF, Weiss F. RU 24969, a 5-HT1B/1A receptor agonist, potentiates cocaine-induced increases in nucleus accumbens dopamine. *Synapse.* 1999;32:132–135.
113. Miguens M, Del Olmo N, Higuera-Matas A, et al. Glutamate and aspartate levels in the nucleus accumbens during cocaine self-administration and extinction: a time course microdialysis study. *Psychopharmacology (Berl).* 2008;196:303–313.
114. Pierce RC, Bell K, Duffy P, et al. Repeated cocaine augments excitatory amino acid transmission in the nucleus accumbens only in rats having developed behavioral sensitization. *J Neurosci.* 1996;16:1550–1560.
115. Smith JA, Mo Q, Guo H, et al. Cocaine increases extraneuronal levels of aspartate and glutamate in the nucleus accumbens. *Brain Res.* 1995;683:264–269.
116. McFarland K, Lapish CC, Kalivas PW. Prefrontal glutamate release into the core of the nucleus accumbens mediates cocaine-induced reinstatement of drug-seeking behavior. *J Neurosci.* 2003;23:3531–3537.
117. Reid MS, Berger SP. Evidence for sensitization of cocaine-induced nucleus accumbens glutamate release. *Neuroreport.* 1996;7:1325–1329.
118. Baker DA, McFarland K, Lake RW, et al. Neuroadaptations in cystine–glutamate exchange underlie cocaine relapse. *Nat Neurosci.* 2003;6:743–749.
119. Derkach VA, Oh MC, Guire ES, et al. Regulatory mechanisms of AMPA receptors in synaptic plasticity. *Nat Rev Neurosci.* 2007;8:101–113.
120. Paoletti P, Neyton J. NMDA receptor subunits: function and pharmacology. *Curr Opin Pharmacol.* 2007;7:39–47.
121. Conn PJ, Pin JP. Pharmacology and functions of metabotropic glutamate receptors. *Annu Rev Pharmacol Toxicol.* 1997;37:205–237.
122. Lu L, Grimm JW, Shaham Y, et al. Molecular neuroadaptations in the accumbens and ventral tegmental area during the first 90 days of forced abstinence from cocaine self-administration in rats. *J Neurochem.* 2003;85:1604–1613.
123. Tang W, Wesley M, Freeman WM, et al. Alterations in ionotropic glutamate receptor subunits during binge cocaine self-administration and withdrawal in rats. *J Neurochem.* 2004;89:1021–1033.
124. Churchill L, Swanson CJ, Urbina M, et al. Repeated cocaine alters glutamate receptor subunit levels in the nucleus accumbens and ventral tegmental area of rats that develop behavioral sensitization. *J Neurochem.* 1999;72:2397–2403.
125. Sutton MA, Schmidt EF, Choi KH, et al. Extinction-induced upregulation in AMPA receptors reduces cocaine-seeking behaviour. *Nature.* 2003;421:70–75.
126. Zhang X, Lee TH, Davidson C, et al. Reversal of cocaine-induced behavioral sensitization and associated phosphorylation of the NR2B and GluR1 subunits of the NMDA and AMPA receptors. *Neuropsychopharmacology.* 2007;32:377–387.
127. Edwards S, Graham DL, Bachtell RK, et al. Region-specific tolerance to cocaine-regulated cAMP-dependent protein phosphorylation following chronic self-administration. *Eur J Neurosci.* 2007;25:2201–2213.
128. Ghasemzadeh MB, Windham LK, Lake RW, et al. Cocaine activates Homer1 immediate early gene transcription in the mesocorticolimbic circuit: differential regulation by dopamine and glutamate signaling. *Synapse.* 2009;63:42–53.
129. Boudreau AC, Wolf ME. Behavioral sensitization to cocaine is associated with increased AMPA receptor surface expression in the nucleus accumbens. *J Neurosci.* 2005;25:9144–9151.
130. Kourrich S, Rothwell PE, Klug JR, et al. Cocaine experience controls bidirectional synaptic plasticity in the nucleus accumbens. *J Neurosci.* 2007;27:7921–7928.
131. Boudreau AC, Reimers JM, Milovanovic M, et al. Cell surface AMPA receptors in the rat nucleus accumbens increase during cocaine withdrawal but internalize after cocaine challenge in association with altered activation of mitogen-activated protein kinases. *J Neurosci.* 2007;27:10621–10635.
132. Conrad KL, Tseng KY, Uejima JL, et al. Formation of accumbens GluR2-lacking AMPA receptors mediates incubation of cocaine craving. *Nature.* 2008;454:118–121.
133. Famous KR, Kumaresan V, Sadri-Vakili G, et al. Phosphorylation-dependent trafficking of GluR2-containing AMPA receptors in the nucleus accumbens plays a critical role in the reinstatement of cocaine seeking. *J Neurosci.* 2008;28:11061–11070.
134. Anderson SM, Famous KR, Sadri-Vakili G, et al. CaMKII: a biochemical bridge linking accumbens dopamine and glutamate systems in cocaine seeking. *Nat Neurosci.* 2008;11:344–353.
135. Suto N, Ecke LE, Wise RA. Control of within-binge cocaine-seeking by dopamine and glutamate in the core of nucleus accumbens. *Psychopharmacology (Berl).* 2009;205:431–439.
136. Pierce RC, Meil WM, Kalivas PW. The NMDA antagonist, dizocilpine, enhances cocaine reinforcement without influencing mesoaccumbens dopamine transmission. *Psychopharmacology (Berl).* 1997;133:188–195.
137. Cornish JL, Duffy P, Kalivas PW. A role for nucleus accumbens glutamate transmission in the relapse to cocaine-seeking behavior. *Neuroscience.* 1999;93:1359–1367.
138. Carlezon WA Jr, Wise RA. Rewarding actions of phencyclidine and related drugs in nucleus accumbens shell and frontal cortex. *J Neurosci.* 1996;16:3112–3122.
139. Schenk S, Valadez A, Worley CM, et al. Blockade of the acquisition of cocaine self-administration by the NMDA antagonist MK-801 (dizocilpine). *Behav Pharmacol.* 1993;4:652–659.
140. Pulvirenti L, Maldonado-Lopez R, Koob GF. NMDA receptors in the nucleus accumbens modulate intravenous cocaine but not heroin self-administration in the rat. *Brain Res.* 1992;594:327–330.
141. Allen RM, Carelli RM, Dykstra LA, et al. Effects of the competitive N-methyl-D-aspartate receptor antagonist, LY235959 [(-)-6-phosphonomethyl-deca-hydroisoquinoline-3-carboxylic acid], on responding for cocaine under both fixed and progressive ratio schedules of reinforcement. *J Pharmacol Exp Ther.* 2005;315:449–457.
142. Ranaldi R, French E, Roberts DC. Systemic pretreatment with MK-801 (dizocilpine) increases breaking points for self-administration of cocaine on a progressive-ratio schedule in rats. *Psychopharmacology (Berl).* 1996;128:83–88.
143. Chiamulera C, Epping-Jordan MP, Zocchi A, et al. Reinforcing and locomotor stimulant effects of cocaine are absent in mGluR5 null mutant mice. *Nat Neurosci.* 2001;4:873–874.

144. Gass JT, Osborne MP, Watson NL, et al. mGluR5 antagonism attenuates methamphetamine reinforcement and prevents reinstatement of methamphetamine-seeking behavior in rats. *Neuropsychopharmacology*. 2009;34:820–833.
145. Platt DM, Rowlett JK, Spealman RD. Attenuation of cocaine self-administration in squirrel monkeys following repeated administration of the mGluR5 antagonist MPEP: comparison with dizocilpine. *Psychopharmacology (Berl)*. 2008;200:167–176.
146. Lee B, Platt DM, Rowlett JK, et al. Attenuation of behavioral effects of cocaine by the metabotropic glutamate receptor 5 antagonist 2-methyl-6-(phenylethynyl)-pyridine in squirrel monkeys: comparison with dizocilpine. *J Pharmacol Exp Ther*. 2005;312:1232–1240.
147. Kenny PJ, Boutrel B, Gasparini F, et al. Metabotropic glutamate 5 receptor blockade may attenuate cocaine self-administration by decreasing brain reward function in rats. *Psychopharmacology (Berl)*. 2005;179:247–254.
148. Adewale AS, Platt DM, Spealman RD. Pharmacological stimulation of group II metabotropic glutamate receptors reduces cocaine self-administration and cocaine-induced reinstatement of drug seeking in squirrel monkeys. *J Pharmacol Exp Ther*. 2006;318:922–931.
149. Xie X, Steketee JD. Effects of repeated exposure to cocaine on group II metabotropic glutamate receptor function in the rat medial prefrontal cortex: behavioral and neurochemical studies. *Psychopharmacology (Berl)*. 2009;203:501–510.
150. Baptista MA, Martin-Fardon R, Weiss F. Preferential effects of the metabotropic glutamate 2/3 receptor agonist LY379268 on conditioned reinstatement versus primary reinforcement: comparison between cocaine and a potent conventional reinforcer. *J Neurosci*. 2004;24:4723–4727.
151. Katz N. Opioids: after thousands of years, still getting to know you. *Clin J Pain*. 2007;23:303–306.
152. Paulozzi LJ, Budnitz DS, Xi Y. Increasing deaths from opioid analgesics in the United States. *Pharmacoepidemiol Drug Saf*. 2006;15:618–627.
153. Corbett AD, Henderson G, McKnight AT, et al. 75 years of opioid research: the exciting but vain quest for the Holy Grail. *Br J Pharmacol*. 2006;147(suppl 1):S153–S162.
154. De Vries TJ, Shippenberg TS. Neural systems underlying opiate addiction. *J Neurosci*. 2002;22:3321–3325.
155. Juhasz JR, Hasbi A, Rashid AJ, et al. Mu-opioid receptor heterooligomer formation with the dopamine D1 receptor as directly visualized in living cells. *Eur J Pharmacol*. 2008;581:235–243.
156. Jordan BA, Trapaidze N, Gomes I, et al. Oligomerization of opioid receptors with beta 2-adrenergic receptors: a role in trafficking and mitogen-activated protein kinase activation. *Proc Natl Acad Sci U S A*. 2001;98:343–348.
157. George SR, Fan T, Xie Z, et al. Oligomerization of mu- and delta-opioid receptors. Generation of novel functional properties. *J Biol Chem*. 2000;275:26128–26135.
158. Mansour A, Fox CA, Akil H, et al. Opioid-receptor mRNA expression in the rat CNS: anatomical and functional implications. *Trends Neurosci*. 1995;18:22–29.
159. Williams JT, Christie MJ, Manzoni O. Cellular and synaptic adaptations mediating opioid dependence. *Physiol Rev*. 2001;81:299–343.
160. Christie MJ. Cellular neuroadaptations to chronic opioids: tolerance, withdrawal and addiction. *Br J Pharmacol*. 2008;154:384–396.
161. Pierre S, Eschenhagen T, Geisslinger G, et al. Capturing adenylyl cyclases as potential drug targets. *Nat Rev Drug Discov*. 2009;8:321–335.
162. Hnasko TS, Sotak BN, Palmiter RD. Morphine reward in dopamine-deficient mice. *Nature*. 2005;438:854–857.
163. Koob GF. Drugs of abuse: anatomy, pharmacology and function of reward pathways. *Trends Pharmacol Sci*. 1992;13:177–184.
164. Devine DP, Wise RA. Self-administration of morphine, DAMGO, and DPDPE into the ventral tegmental area of rats. *J Neurosci*. 1994; 14:1978–1984.
165. Goeders NE, Lane JD, Smith JE. Self-administration of methionine enkephalin into the nucleus accumbens. *Pharmacol Biochem Behav*. 1984;20:451–455.
166. Dworkin SI, Guerin GF, Goeders NE, et al. Kainic acid lesions of the nucleus accumbens selectively attenuate morphine self-administration. *Pharmacol Biochem Behav*. 1988;29:175–181.
167. Zito KA, Vickers G, Roberts DC. Disruption of cocaine and heroin self-administration following kainic acid lesions of the nucleus accumbens. *Pharmacol Biochem Behav*. 1985;23:1029–1036.
168. Hutcheson DM, Parkinson JA, Robbins TW, et al. The effects of nucleus accumbens core and shell lesions on intravenous heroin self-administration and the acquisition of drug-seeking behaviour under a second-order schedule of heroin reinforcement. *Psychopharmacology (Berl)*. 2001;153:464–472.
169. Lecca D, Valentini V, Cacciapaglia F, et al. Reciprocal effects of response contingent and noncontingent intravenous heroin on in vivo nucleus accumbens shell versus core dopamine in the rat: a repeated sampling microdialysis study. *Psychopharmacology (Berl)*. 2007;194:103–116.
170. Wise RA, Leone P, Rivest R, et al. Elevations of nucleus accumbens dopamine and DOPAC levels during intravenous heroin self-administration. *Synapse*. 1995;21:140–148.
171. David V, Durkin TP, Cazala P. Differential effects of the dopamine D2/D3 receptor antagonist sulpiride on self-administration of morphine into the ventral tegmental area or the nucleus accumbens. *Psychopharmacology (Berl)*. 2002;160:307–317.
172. Lee RS, Criado JR, Koob GF, et al. Cellular responses of nucleus accumbens neurons to opiate-seeking behavior: I. Sustained responding during heroin self-administration. *Synapse*. 1999;33:49–58.
173. Jiang ZG, North RA. Pre- and postsynaptic inhibition by opioids in rat striatum. *J Neurosci*. 1992;12:356–361.
174. Garzon M, Pickel VM. Plasmalemmal mu-opioid receptor distribution mainly in nondopaminergic neurons in the rat ventral tegmental area. *Synapse*. 2001;41:311–328.
175. Johnson SW, North RA. Opioids excite dopamine neurons by hyperpolarization of local interneurons. *J Neurosci*. 1992;12:483–488.
176. Matthews RT, German DC. Electrophysiological evidence for excitation of rat ventral tegmental area dopamine neurons by morphine. *Neuroscience*. 1984;11:617–625.
177. Gysling K, Wang RY. Morphine-induced activation of A10 dopamine neurons in the rat. *Brain Res*. 1983;277:119–127.
178. Spanagel R, Herz A, Shippenberg TS. Opposing tonically active endogenous opioid systems modulate the mesolimbic dopaminergic pathway. *Proc Natl Acad Sci U S A*. 1992;89: 2046–2050.
179. Kalivas PW, Duffy P, Eberhardt H. Modulation of A10 dopamine neurons by gamma-aminobutyric acid agonists. *J Pharmacol Exp Ther*. 1990;253:858–866.
180. Bechara A, Nader K, van der Kooy D. A two-separate-motivational-systems hypothesis of opioid addiction. *Pharmacol Biochem Behav*. 1998;59:1–17.

181. Olmstead MC, Munn EM, Franklin KB, et al. Effects of pedunculopontine tegmental nucleus lesions on responding for intravenous heroin under different schedules of reinforcement. *J Neurosci*. 1998;18:5035–5044.
182. Nader K, van der Kooy D. Deprivation state switches the neurobiological substrates mediating opiate reward in the ventral tegmental area. *J Neurosci*. 1997;17:383–390.
183. Laviolette SR, Nader K, van der Kooy D. Motivational state determines the functional role of the mesolimbic dopamine system in the mediation of opiate reward processes. *Behav Brain Res*. 2002;129:17–29.
184. Laviolette SR, Gallegos RA, Henriksen SJ, et al. Opiate state controls bi-directional reward signaling via GABAA receptors in the ventral tegmental area. *Nat Neurosci*. 2004;7:160–169.
185. Vargas-Perez H, Kee RT, Walton CH, et al. Ventral tegmental area BDNF induces an opiate-dependent-like reward state in naive rats. *Science*. 2009;324:1732–1734.
186. Singer G, Wallace M. Effects of 6-OHDA lesions in the nucleus accumbens on the acquisition of self injection of heroin under schedule and non schedule conditions in rats. *Pharmacol Biochem Behav*. 1984;20:807–809.
187. Smith JE, Guerin GF, Co C, et al. Effects of 6-OHDA lesions of the central medial nucleus accumbens on rat intravenous morphine self-administration. *Pharmacol Biochem Behav*. 1985;23:843–849.
188. Elmer GI, Pieper JO, Rubinstein M, et al. Failure of intravenous morphine to serve as an effective instrumental reinforcer in dopamine D2 receptor knock-out mice. *J Neurosci*. 2002;22:RC224.
189. Van Ree JM, Ramsey N. The dopamine hypothesis of opiate reward challenged. *Eur J Pharmacol*. 1987;134:239–243.
190. Ettenberg A, Pettit HO, Bloom FE, et al. Heroin and cocaine intravenous self-administration in rats: mediation by separate neural systems. *Psychopharmacology (Berl)*. 1982;78:204–209.
191. Kiyatkin EA, Rebec GV. Impulse activity of ventral tegmental area neurons during heroin self-administration in rats. *Neuroscience*. 2001;102:565–580.
192. Xi ZX, Stein EA. Increased mesolimbic GABA concentration blocks heroin self-administration in the rat. *J Pharmacol Exp Ther*. 2000;294:613–619.
193. Ikemoto S, Murphy JM, McBride WJ. Self-infusion of GABA(A) antagonists directly into the ventral tegmental area and adjacent regions. *Behav Neurosci*. 1997;111:369–380.
194. David V, Durkin TP, Cazala P. Self-administration of the GABAA antagonist bicuculline into the ventral tegmental area in mice: dependence on D2 dopaminergic mechanisms. *Psychopharmacology (Berl)*. 1997;130:85–90.
195. Smith JE, Co C, Freeman ME, et al. Neurotransmitter turnover in rat striatum is correlated with morphine self-administration. *Nature*. 1980;287:152–154.
196. Xi ZX, Stein EA. Blockade of ionotropic glutamatergic transmission in the ventral tegmental area reduces heroin reinforcement in rat. *Psychopharmacology (Berl)*. 2002;164:144–150.
197. Shabat-Simon M, Levy D, Amir A, et al. Dissociation between rewarding and psychomotor effects of opiates: differential roles for glutamate receptors within anterior and posterior portions of the ventral tegmental area. *J Neurosci*. 2008;28:8406–8416.
198. Glass MJ, Lane DA, Colago EE, et al. Chronic administration of morphine is associated with a decrease in surface AMPA GluR1 receptor subunit in dopamine D1 receptor expressing neurons in the shell and non-D1 receptor expressing neurons in the core of the rat nucleus accumbens. *Exp Neurol*. 2008;210:750–761.
199. Drouin C, Darracq L, Trovero F, et al. Alpha1b-adrenergic receptors control locomotor and rewarding effects of psychostimulants and opiates. *J Neurosci*. 2002;22:2873–2884.
200. De Vries TJ, Homberg JR, Binnekade R, et al. Cannabinoid modulation of the reinforcing and motivational properties of heroin and heroin-associated cues in rats. *Psychopharmacology (Berl)*. 2003;168:164–169.
201. Caille S, Parsons LH. SR141716A reduces the reinforcing properties of heroin but not heroin-induced increases in nucleus accumbens dopamine in rats. *Eur J Neurosci*. 2003;18:3145–3149.
202. Navarro M, Carrera MR, Fratta W, et al. Functional interaction between opioid and cannabinoid receptors in drug self-administration. *J Neurosci*. 2001;21:5344–5350.
203. Cossu G, Ledent C, Fattore L, et al. Cannabinoid CB1 receptor knockout mice fail to self-administer morphine but not other drugs of abuse. *Behav Brain Res*. 2001;118:61–65.
204. Ledent C, Valverde O, Cossu G, et al. Unresponsiveness to cannabinoids and reduced addictive effects of opiates in CB1 receptor knockout mice. *Science*. 1999;283:401–404.
205. Caille S, Parsons LH. Cannabinoid modulation of opiate reinforcement through the ventral striatopallidal pathway. *Neuropsychopharmacology*. 2006;31:804–813.
206. Solinas M, Panlilio LV, Tanda G, et al. Cannabinoid agonists but not inhibitors of endogenous cannabinoid transport or metabolism enhance the reinforcing efficacy of heroin in rats. *Neuropsychopharmacology*. 2005;30:2046–2057.
207. French ED. delta9-Tetrahydrocannabinol excites rat VTA dopamine neurons through activation of cannabinoid CB1 but not opioid receptors. *Neurosci Lett*. 1997;226:159–162.
208. Kieffer BL, Gaveriaux-Ruff C. Exploring the opioid system by gene knockout. *Prog Neurobiol*. 2002;66:285–306.
209. Sora I, Elmer G, Funada M, et al. Mu opiate receptor gene dose effects on different morphine actions: evidence for differential in vivo mu receptor reserve. *Neuropsychopharmacology*. 2001;25:41–54.
210. Becker A, Grecksch G, Brödemann R, et al. Morphine self-administration in mu-opioid receptor-deficient mice. *Naunyn Schmiedebergs Arch Pharmacol*. 2000;361:584–589.
211. Matthes HW, et al. Loss of morphine-induced analgesia, reward effect and withdrawal symptoms in mice lacking the mu-opioid-receptor gene. *Nature*. 1996;383:819–823.
212. Contet C, Kieffer BL, Befort K. Mu opioid receptor: a gateway to drug addiction. *Curr Opin Neurobiol*. 2004;14:370–378.
213. Simonin F, Valverde O, Smadja C, et al. Disruption of the kappa-opioid receptor gene in mice enhances sensitivity to chemical visceral pain, impairs pharmacological actions of the selective kappa-agonist U-50,488H and attenuates morphine withdrawal. *EMBO J*. 1998;17:886–897.
214. Kieffer BL, Evans CJ. Opioid receptors: from binding sites to visible molecules in vivo. *Neuropharmacology*. 2009;56(suppl 1):205–212.
215. Fleming M, Mihic SJ, Harris RA. *Ethanol. Goodman and Gilman's The Pharmacological Basis of Therapeutics*. 10th ed. New York: McGraw-Hill; 2001:429–445.
216. Gonzales RA, Job MO, Doyon WM. The role of mesolimbic dopamine in the development and maintenance of ethanol reinforcement. *Pharmacol Ther*. 2004;103:121–146.
217. Yim HJ, Gonzales RA. Ethanol-induced increases in dopamine extracellular concentration in rat nucleus accumbens are accounted for by increased release and not uptake inhibition. *Alcohol*. 2000;22:107–115.

218. Bunney EB, Appel SB, Brodie MS. Electrophysiological effects of cocaethylene, cocaine, and ethanol on dopaminergic neurons of the ventral tegmental area. *J Pharmacol Exp Ther*. 2001; 297:696–703.
219. Brodie MS, Shefner SA, Dunwiddie TV. Ethanol increases the firing rate of dopamine neurons of the rat ventral tegmental area in vitro. *Brain Res*. 1990;508:65–69.
220. Budygin EA, Phillips PE, Wightman RM, et al. Terminal effects of ethanol on dopamine dynamics in rat nucleus accumbens: an in vitro voltammetric study. *Synapse*. 2001;42:77–79.
221. Yim HJ, Schallert T, Randall PK, et al. Comparison of local and systemic ethanol effects on extracellular dopamine concentration in rat nucleus accumbens by microdialysis. *Alcohol Clin Exp Res*. 1998;22:367–374.
222. Appel SB, Liu Z, McElvain MA, et al. Ethanol excitation of dopaminergic ventral tegmental area neurons is blocked by quinidine. *J Pharmacol Exp Ther*. 2003;306:437–446.
223. Brodie MS, McElvain MA, Bunney EB, et al. Pharmacological reduction of small conductance calcium-activated potassium current (SK) potentiates the excitatory effect of ethanol on ventral tegmental area dopamine neurons. *J Pharmacol Exp Ther*. 1999;290:325–333.
224. Mereu G, Gessa GL. Low doses of ethanol inhibit the firing of neurons in the substantia nigra, pars reticulata: a GABAergic effect? *Brain Res*. 1985;360:325–330.
225. Stobbs SH, Ohran AJ, Lassen MB, et al. Ethanol suppression of ventral tegmental area GABA neuron electrical transmission involves N-methyl-D-aspartate receptors. *J Pharmacol Exp Ther*. 2004;311:282–289.
226. Okada H, Matsushita N, Kobayashi K. Identification of GABAA receptor subunit variants in midbrain dopaminergic neurons. *J Neurochem*. 2004;89:7–14.
227. Grace AA, Bunney BS. Paradoxical GABA excitation of nigral dopaminergic cells: indirect mediation through reticulata inhibitory neurons. *Eur J Pharmacol*. 1979;59:211–218.
228. McBride WJ, Murphy JM, Lumeng L, et al. Serotonin and ethanol preference. *Recent Dev Alcohol*. 1989;7:187–209.
229. Rodd-Henricks ZA, McKinzie DL, Crile RS, et al. Regional heterogeneity for the intracranial self-administration of ethanol within the ventral tegmental area of female Wistar rats. *Psychopharmacology (Berl)*. 2000;149:217–224.
230. Rodd ZA, Melendez RI, Bell RL, et al. Intracranial self-administration of ethanol within the ventral tegmental area of male Wistar rats: evidence for involvement of dopamine neurons. *J Neurosci*. 2004;24:1050–1057.
231. Melendez RI, Rodd-Henricks ZA, Engleman EA, et al. Microdialysis of dopamine in the nucleus accumbens of alcohol-preferring (P) rats during anticipation and operant self-administration of ethanol. *Alcohol Clin Exp Res*. 2002; 26:318–325.
232. Olive MF, Mehmert KK, Messing RO, et al. Reduced operant ethanol self-administration and in vivo mesolimbic dopamine responses to ethanol in PKCepsilon-deficient mice. *Eur J Neurosci*. 2000;12:4131–4140.
233. Weiss F, Lorang MT, Bloom FE, et al. Oral alcohol self-administration stimulates dopamine release in the rat nucleus accumbens: genetic and motivational determinants. *J Pharmacol Exp Ther*. 1993;267:250–258.
234. Bradberry CW. Dose-dependent effect of ethanol on extracellular dopamine in mesolimbic striatum of awake rhesus monkeys: comparison with cocaine across individuals. *Psychopharmacology (Berl)*. 2002;165:67–76.
235. McBride WJ, Murphy JM, Gatto GJ, et al. CNS mechanisms of alcohol self-administration. *Alcohol Alcohol Suppl*. 1993;2:463–467.
236. Boyce JM, Risinger FO. Dopamine D3 receptor antagonist effects on the motivational effects of ethanol. *Alcohol*. 2002; 28:47–55.
237. Cohen C, Perrault G, Sanger DJ. Effects of D1 dopamine receptor agonists on oral ethanol self-administration in rats: comparison with their efficacy to produce grooming and hyperactivity. *Psychopharmacology (Berl)*. 1999;142:102–110.
238. Silvestre JS, O'Neill MF, Fernandez AG, et al. Effects of a range of dopamine receptor agonists and antagonists on ethanol intake in the rat. *Eur J Pharmacol*. 1996;318:257–265.
239. Pfeffer AO, Samson HH. Haloperidol and apomorphine effects on ethanol reinforcement in free feeding rats. *Pharmacol Biochem Behav*. 1988;29:343–350.
240. Hodge CW, Samson HH, Chappelle AM. Alcohol self-administration: further examination of the role of dopamine receptors in the nucleus accumbens. *Alcohol Clin Exp Res*. 1997;21:1083–1091.
241. Samson HH, Chappell A. Dopaminergic involvement in medial prefrontal cortex and core of the nucleus accumbens in the regulation of ethanol self-administration: a dual-site microinjection study in the rat. *Physiol Behav*. 2003;79:581–590.
242. Rassnick S, Pulvirenti L, Koob GF. Oral ethanol self-administration in rats is reduced by the administration of dopamine and glutamate receptor antagonists into the nucleus accumbens. *Psychopharmacology (Berl)*. 1992;109:92–98.
243. El-Ghundi M, George SR, Drago J, et al. Disruption of dopamine D1 receptor gene expression attenuates alcohol-seeking behavior. *Eur J Pharmacol*. 1998;353:149–158.
244. Risinger FO, Freeman PA, Rubinstein M, et al. Lack of operant ethanol self-administration in dopamine D2 receptor knockout mice. *Psychopharmacology (Berl)*. 2000;152:343–350.
245. Phillips TJ, Brown KJ, Burkhart-Kasch S, et al. Alcohol preference and sensitivity are markedly reduced in mice lacking dopamine D2 receptors. *Nat Neurosci*. 1998;1:610–615.
246. Myers RD, Robinson DE. Mmu and D2 receptor antisense oligonucleotides injected in nucleus accumbens suppress high alcohol intake in genetic drinking HEP rats. *Alcohol*. 1999;18: 225–233.
247. Thanos PK, Taintor NB, Rivera SN, et al. DRD2 gene transfer into the nucleus accumbens core of the alcohol preferring and nonpreferring rats attenuates alcohol drinking. *Alcohol Clin Exp Res*. 2004;28:720–728.
248. McQuade JA, Xu M, Woods SC, et al. Ethanol consumption in mice with a targeted disruption of the dopamine-3 receptor gene. *Addict Biol*. 2003;8:295–303.
249. Boyce-Rustay JM, Risinger FO. Dopamine D3 receptor knockout mice and the motivational effects of ethanol. *Pharmacol Biochem Behav*. 2003;75:373–379.
250. Volkow ND, Wang GJ, Fowler JS, et al. Decreases in dopamine receptors but not in dopamine transporters in alcoholics. *Alcohol Clin Exp Res*. 1996;20:1594–1598.
251. Koob GF. A role for GABA mechanisms in the motivational effects of alcohol. *Biochem Pharmacol*. 2004;68:1515–1525.
252. Liang JH, Chen F, Krstew E, et al. The GABA(B) receptor allosteric modulator CGP7930, like baclofen, reduces operant self-administration of ethanol in alcohol-preferring rats. *Neuropharmacology*. 2006;50:632–639.
253. Walker BM, Koob GF. The gamma-aminobutyric acid-B receptor agonist baclofen attenuates responding for ethanol in ethanol-dependent rats. *Alcohol Clin Exp Res*. 2007;31:11–18.

254. Maccioni P, Fantini N, Froestl W, et al. Specific reduction of alcohol's motivational properties by the positive allosteric modulator of the GABAB receptor, GS39783—comparison with the effect of the GABAB receptor direct agonist, baclofen. *Alcohol Clin Exp Res.* 2008;32:1558–1564.
255. Janak PH, Michael Gill T. Comparison of the effects of allopregnanolone with direct GABAergic agonists on ethanol self-administration with and without concurrently available sucrose. *Alcohol.* 2003;30:1–7.
256. Czachowski CL, Legg BH, Stansfield KH. Ethanol and sucrose seeking and consumption following repeated administration of the GABA(B) agonist baclofen in rats. *Alcohol Clin Exp Res.* 2006;30:812–818.
257. Steffensen SC, Walton CH, Hansen DM, et al. Contingent and non-contingent effects of low-dose ethanol on GABA neuron activity in the ventral tegmental area. *Pharmacol Biochem Behav.* 2009;92:68–75.
258. Herz A. Endogenous opioid systems and alcohol addiction. *Psychopharmacology (Berl).* 1997;129:99–111.
259. Ulm RR, Volpicelli JR, Volpicelli LA. Opiates and alcohol self-administration in animals. *J Clin Psychiatry.* 1995;56(suppl 7):5–14.
260. Williams KL, Kane EC, Woods JH. Interaction of morphine and naltrexone on oral ethanol self-administration in rhesus monkeys. *Behav Pharmacol.* 2001;12:325–333.
261. Froehlich JC, Harts J, Lumeng L, et al. Naloxone attenuates voluntary ethanol intake in rats selectively bred for high ethanol preference. *Pharmacol Biochem Behav.* 1990;35:385–390.
262. Hyytia P. Involvement of mu-opioid receptors in alcohol drinking by alcohol-preferring AA rats. *Pharmacol Biochem Behav.* 1993;45:697–701.
263. Le AD, Poulos CX, Quan B, et al. The effects of selective blockade of delta and mu opiate receptors on ethanol consumption by C57BL/6 mice in a restricted access paradigm. *Brain Res.* 1993;630:330–332.
264. Doyon WM, Howard EC, Shippenberg TS, et al. Kappa-opioid receptor modulation of accumbal dopamine concentration during operant ethanol self-administration. *Neuropharmacology.* 2006;51:487–496.
265. June HL, Cason CR, Chen SH, et al. Buprenorphine alters ethanol self-administration in rats: dose–response and time-dependent effects. *Psychopharmacology (Berl).* 1998;140:29–37.
266. Pettinati HM, O'Brien CP, Rabinowitz AR, et al. The status of naltrexone in the treatment of alcohol dependence: specific effects on heavy drinking. *J Clin Psychopharmacol.* 2006; 26:610–625.
267. Zhou FC, Pu CF, Murphy J, et al. Serotonergic neurons in the alcohol preferring rats. *Alcohol.* 1994;11:397–403.
268. Ginsburg BC, Koek W, Javors MA, et al. Effects of fluvoxamine on a multiple schedule of ethanol- and food-maintained behavior in two rat strains. *Psychopharmacology (Berl).* 2005; 180:249–257.
269. Lyness WH, Smith FL. Influence of dopaminergic and serotonergic neurons on intravenous ethanol self-administration in the rat. *Pharmacol Biochem Behav.* 1992;42:187–192.
270. McBride WJ, Murphy JM, Gatto GJ, et al. Serotonin and dopamine systems regulating alcohol intake. *Alcohol Alcohol Suppl.* 1991;1:411–416.
271. Czachowski CL. Manipulations of serotonin function in the nucleus accumbens core produce differential effects on ethanol and sucrose seeking and intake. *Alcohol Clin Exp Res.* 2005; 29:1146–1155.
272. Schreiber R, Manze B, Haussels A, et al. Effects of the 5-HT1A receptor agonist ipsapirone on operant self-administration of ethanol in the rat. *Eur Neuropsychopharmacol.* 1999;10:37–42.
273. Wilson AW, Neill JC, Costall B. An investigation into the effects of 5-HT agonists and receptor antagonists on ethanol self-administration in the rat. *Alcohol.* 1998;16:249–270.
274. Tomkins DM, O'Neill MF. Effect of 5-HT(1B) receptor ligands on self-administration of ethanol in an operant procedure in rats. *Pharmacol Biochem Behav.* 2000;66:129–136.
275. Ingman K, Honkanen A, Hyytia P, et al. Risperidone reduces limited access alcohol drinking in alcohol-preferring rats. *Eur J Pharmacol.* 2003;468:121–127.
276. Maurel S, De Vry J, Schreiber R. 5-HT receptor ligands differentially affect operant oral self-administration of ethanol in the rat. *Eur J Pharmacol.* 1999;370:217–223.
277. Roberts AJ, McArthur RA, Hull EE, et al. Effects of amperozide, 8-OH-DPAT, and FG 5974 on operant responding for ethanol. *Psychopharmacology (Berl).* 1998;137:25–32.
278. Silvestre JS, Palacios JM, Fernandez AG, et al. Comparison of effects of a range of 5-HT receptor modulators on consumption and preference for a sweetened ethanol solution in rats. *J Psychopharmacol.* 1998;12:168–176.
279. Le AD, Sellers EM. Interaction between opiate and 5-HT3 receptor antagonists in the regulation of alcohol intake. *Alcohol Alcohol Suppl.* 1994;2:545–549.
280. Hodge CW, Samson HH, Lewis RS, et al. Specific decreases in ethanol- but not water-reinforced responding produced by the 5-HT3 antagonist ICS 205-930. *Alcohol.* 1993;10:191–196.
281. McKinzie DL, McBride WJ, Murphy JM, et al. Effects of MDL 72222, a serotonin3 antagonist, on operant responding for ethanol by alcohol-preferring P rats. *Alcohol Clin Exp Res.* 2000;24:1500–1504.
282. Beardsley PM, Lopez OT, Gullikson G, et al. Serotonin 5-HT3 antagonists fail to affect ethanol self-administration of rats. *Alcohol.* 1994;11:389–395.
283. McMillen BA, Walter S, Williams HL, et al. Comparison of the action of the 5-HT2 antagonists amperozide and trazodone on preference for alcohol in rats. *Alcohol.* 1994;11:203–206.
284. Myers RD, Lankford M, Bjork A. Irreversible suppression of alcohol drinking in cyanamide-treated rats after sustained delivery of the 5-HT2 antagonist amperozide. *Alcohol.* 1993;10: 117–125.
285. Ding ZM, Toalston JE, Oster SM, et al. Involvement of local serotonin-2A but not serotonin-1B receptors in the reinforcing effects of ethanol within the posterior ventral tegmental area of female Wistar rats. *Psychopharmacology (Berl).* 2009;204: 381–390.
286. Gallate JE, Saharov T, Mallet PE, et al. Increased motivation for beer in rats following administration of a cannabinoid CB1 receptor agonist. *Eur J Pharmacol.* 1999;370:233–240.
287. Economidou D, Mattioli L, Ubaldi M, et al. Role of cannabinoidergic mechanisms in ethanol self-administration and ethanol seeking in rat adult offspring following perinatal exposure to Delta9-tetrahydrocannabinol. *Toxicol Appl Pharmacol.* 2007; 223:73–85.
288. Malinen H, Hyytia P. Ethanol self-administration is regulated by CB1 receptors in the nucleus accumbens and ventral tegmental area in alcohol-preferring AA rats. *Alcohol Clin Exp Res.* 2008;32:1976–1983.
289. Ginsburg BC, Lamb RJ. Cannabinoid effects on behaviors maintained by ethanol or food: a within-subjects comparison. *Behav Pharmacol.* 2006;17:249–257.

290. Cippitelli A, Bilbao A, Gorriti MA, et al. The anandamide transport inhibitor AM404 reduces ethanol self-administration. *Eur J Neurosci.* 2007;26:476–486.
291. Stephens DN, Pistovcakova J, Worthing L, et al. Role of GABAA alpha5-containing receptors in ethanol reward: the effects of targeted gene deletion, and a selective inverse agonist. *Eur J Pharmacol.* 2005;526:240–250.
292. June HL Sr, Foster KL, Eiler WJ II, et al. Dopamine and benzodiazepine-dependent mechanisms regulate the EtOH-enhanced locomotor stimulation in the GABAA alpha1 subunit null mutant mice. *Neuropsychopharmacology.* 2007;32:137–152.
293. Besheer J, Lepoutre V, Mole B, et al. GABAA receptor regulation of voluntary ethanol drinking requires PKCepsilon. *Synapse.* 2006;60:411–419.
294. Kovacs KM, Szakall I, O'Brien D, et al. Decreased oral self-administration of alcohol in kappa-opioid receptor knock-out mice. *Alcohol Clin Exp Res.* 2005;29:730–738.
295. Grisel JE, Mogil JS, Grahame NJ, et al. Ethanol oral self-administration is increased in mutant mice with decreased beta-endorphin expression. *Brain Res.* 1999;835:62–67.
296. Grahame NJ, Low MJ, Cunningham CL. Intravenous self-administration of ethanol in beta-endorphin-deficient mice. *Alcohol Clin Exp Res.* 1998;22:1093–1098.
297. Engel SR, Lyons CR, Allan AM. 5-HT3 receptor over-expression decreases ethanol self administration in transgenic mice. *Psychopharmacology (Berl).* 1998;140:243–248.
298. Risinger FO, Doan AM, Vickrey AC. Oral operant ethanol self-administration in 5-HT1b knockout mice. *Behav Brain Res.* 1999;102:211–215.
299. Thanos PK, Dimitrakakis ES, Rice O, et al. Ethanol self-administration and ethanol conditioned place preference are reduced in mice lacking cannabinoid CB1 receptors. *Behav Brain Res.* 2005;164:206–213.
300. Hensler JG, Ladenheim EE, Lyons WE. Ethanol consumption and serotonin-1A (5-HT1A) receptor function in heterozygous BDNF (+/−) mice. *J Neurochem.* 2003;85:1139–1147.
301. Ameri A. The effects of cannabinoids on the brain. *Prog Neurobiol.* 1999;58:315–348.
302. van der Stelt M, Di Marzo V. The endocannabinoid system in the basal ganglia and in the mesolimbic reward system: implications for neurological and psychiatric disorders. *Eur J Pharmacol.* 2003;480:133–150.
303. Howlett AC, Bidaut-Russell M, Devane WA, et al. The cannabinoid receptor: biochemical, anatomical and behavioral characterization. *Trends Neurosci.* 1990;13:420–423.
304. Ralevic V. Cannabinoid modulation of peripheral autonomic and sensory neurotransmission. *Eur J Pharmacol.* 2003;472:1–21.
305. Julian MD, Martin AB, Cuellar B, et al. Neuroanatomical relationship between type 1 cannabinoid receptors and dopaminergic systems in the rat basal ganglia. *Neuroscience.* 2003;119:309–318.
306. Pickel VM, Chan J, Kash TL, et al. Compartment-specific localization of cannabinoid 1 (CB1) and mu-opioid receptors in rat nucleus accumbens. *Neuroscience.* 2004;127:101–112.
307. Cheer JF, Wassum KM, Heien ML, et al. Cannabinoids enhance subsecond dopamine release in the nucleus accumbens of awake rats. *J Neurosci.* 2004;24:4393–4400.
308. Tanda G, Pontieri FE, Di Chiara G. Cannabinoid and heroin activation of mesolimbic dopamine transmission by a common mu1 opioid receptor mechanism. *Science.* 1997;276:2048–2050.
309. Herkenham M, Lynn AB, de Costa BR, et al. Neuronal localization of cannabinoid receptors in the basal ganglia of the rat. *Brain Res.* 1991;547:267–274.
310. Gardner EL, Vorel SR. Cannabinoid transmission and reward-related events. *Neurobiol Dis.* 1998;5:502–533.
311. Cheer JF, Kendall DA, Mason R, et al. Differential cannabinoid-induced electrophysiological effects in rat ventral tegmentum. *Neuropharmacology.* 2003;44:633–641.
312. Gessa GL, Melis M, Muntoni AL, et al. Cannabinoids activate mesolimbic dopamine neurons by an action on cannabinoid CB1 receptors. *Eur J Pharmacol.* 1998;341:39–44.
313. Wu X, French ED. Effects of chronic delta9-tetrahydrocannabinol on rat midbrain dopamine neurons: an electrophysiological assessment. *Neuropharmacology.* 2000;39:391–398.
314. Szabo B, Siemes S, Wallmichrath I. Inhibition of GABAergic neurotransmission in the ventral tegmental area by cannabinoids. *Eur J Neurosci.* 2002;15:2057–2061.
315. Tanda G, Goldberg SR. Cannabinoids: reward, dependence, and underlying neurochemical mechanisms—a review of recent preclinical data. *Psychopharmacology (Berl).* 2003;169:115–134.
316. Maldonado R, Rodriguez de Fonseca F. Cannabinoid addiction: behavioral models and neural correlates. *J Neurosci.* 2002;22:3326–3331.
317. Justinova Z, Tanda G, Redhi GH, et al. Self-administration of delta9-tetrahydrocannabinol (THC) by drug naive squirrel monkeys. *Psychopharmacology (Berl).* 2003;169:135–140.
318. Mendizabal V, Zimmer A, Maldonado R. Involvement of kappa/dynorphin system in WIN 55,212-2 self-administration in mice. *Neuropsychopharmacology.* 2006;31:1957–1966.
319. Fattore L, Viganò D, Fadda P, et al. Bidirectional regulation of mu-opioid and CB1-cannabinoid receptor in rats self-administering heroin or WIN 55,212-2. *Eur J Neurosci.* 2007;25:2191–2200.
320. Lecca D, Cacciapaglia F, Valentini V, et al. Monitoring extracellular dopamine in the rat nucleus accumbens shell and core during acquisition and maintenance of intravenous WIN 55,212-2 self-administration. *Psychopharmacology (Berl).* 2006;188:63–74.
321. Fadda P, Scherma M, Spano MS, et al. Cannabinoid self-administration increases dopamine release in the nucleus accumbens. *Neuroreport.* 2006;17:1629–1632.
322. Solinas M, Scherma M, Fattore L, et al. Nicotinic alpha 7 receptors as a new target for treatment of cannabis abuse. *J Neurosci.* 2007;27:5615–5620.
323. Manzanares J, Corchero J, Fuentes JA. Opioid and cannabinoid receptor-mediated regulation of the increase in adrenocorticotropin hormone and corticosterone plasma concentrations induced by central administration of delta(9)-tetrahydrocannabinol in rats. *Brain Res.* 1999;839:173–179.
324. Chen JP, Paredes W, Li J, et al. Delta 9-tetrahydrocannabinol produces naloxone-blockable enhancement of presynaptic basal dopamine efflux in nucleus accumbens of conscious, freely-moving rats as measured by intracerebral microdialysis. *Psychopharmacology (Berl).* 1990;102:156–162.
325. Braida D, Pozzi M, Parolaro D, et al. Intracerebral self-administration of the cannabinoid receptor agonist CP 55,940 in the rat: interaction with the opioid system. *Eur J Pharmacol.* 2001;413:227–234.
326. Justinova Z, Tanda G, Munzar P, et al. The opioid antagonist naltrexone reduces the reinforcing effects of Delta 9 tetrahydrocannabinol (THC) in squirrel monkeys. *Psychopharmacology (Berl).* 2004;173:186–194.
327. Sarnyai Z, Shaham Y, Heinrichs SC. The role of corticotropin-releasing factor in drug addiction. *Pharmacol Rev.* 2001;53:209–243.

328. Martin-Calderon JL, Muñoz RM, Villanúa MA, et al. Characterization of the acute endocrine actions of (-)-11-hydroxy-delta8-tetrahydrocannabinol-dimethylheptyl (HU-210), a potent synthetic cannabinoid in rats. *Eur J Pharmacol*. 1998; 344:77–86.
329. Weidenfeld J, Feldman S, Mechoulam R. Effect of the brain constituent anandamide, a cannabinoid receptor agonist, on the hypothalamo-pituitary-adrenal axis in the rat. *Neuroendocrinology*. 1994;59:110–112.
330. Rodriguez de Fonseca F, Rubio P, Menzaghi F, et al. Corticotropin-releasing factor (CRF) antagonist [D-Phe12,Nle21,38,C alpha MeLeu37]CRF attenuates the acute actions of the highly potent cannabinoid receptor agonist HU-210 on defensive-withdrawal behavior in rats. *J Pharmacol Exp Ther*. 1996;276:56–64.
331. Jong-wook L. World Health Organization directors general's speech to the 12th World Congress on Tobacco and Health. Helsinki, Finland, 2003.
332. Mackay J, Eriksen M, Shafey O. *The Tobacco Atlas*. 2nd ed. Atlanta, GA: American Cancer Society; 2006.
333. Picciotto MR. Nicotine as a modulator of behavior: beyond the inverted U. *Trends Pharmacol Sci*. 2003;24:493–499.
334. Greenbaum L, Lerer B. Differential contribution of genetic variation in multiple brain nicotinic cholinergic receptors to nicotine dependence: recent progress and emerging open questions. *Mol Psychiatry*. 2009;14:912–945.
335. Gotti C, Zoli M, Clementi F. Brain nicotinic acetylcholine receptors: native subtypes and their relevance. *Trends Pharmacol Sci*. 2006;27:482–491.
336. Corringer PJ, Le Novere N, Changeux JP. Nicotinic receptors at the amino acid level. *Annu Rev Pharmacol Toxicol*. 2000;40: 431–458.
337. Jones IW, Wonnacott S. Precise localization of alpha7 nicotinic acetylcholine receptors on glutamatergic axon terminals in the rat ventral tegmental area. *J Neurosci*. 2004;24: 11244–11252.
338. Champtiaux N, Gotti C, Cordero-Erausquin M, et al. Subunit composition of functional nicotinic receptors in dopaminergic neurons investigated with knock-out mice. *J Neurosci*. 2003; 23:7820–7829.
339. Wonnacott S, Sidhpura N, Balfour DJ. Nicotine: from molecular mechanisms to behaviour. *Curr Opin Pharmacol*. 2005;5: 53–59.
340. Luetje CW. Getting past the asterisk: the subunit composition of presynaptic nicotinic receptors that modulate striatal dopamine release. *Mol Pharmacol*. 2004;65:1333–1335.
341. Zocchi A, Girlanda E, Varnier G, et al. Dopamine responsiveness to drugs of abuse: a shell-core investigation in the nucleus accumbens of the mouse. *Synapse*. 2003;50:293–302.
342. Livingstone PD, Wonnacott S. Nicotinic acetylcholine receptors and the ascending dopamine pathways. *Biochem Pharmacol*. 2009;78:744–755.
343. Pontieri FE, Tanda G, Orzi F, et al. Effects of nicotine on the nucleus accumbens and similarity to those of addictive drugs. *Nature*. 1996;382:255–257.
344. Ferrari R, Le Novere N, Picciotto MR, et al. Acute and long-term changes in the mesolimbic dopamine pathway after systemic or local single nicotine injections. *Eur J Neurosci*. 2002;15:1810–1818.
345. Nisell M, Nomikos GG, Svensson TH. Infusion of nicotine in the ventral tegmental area or the nucleus accumbens of the rat differentially affects accumbal dopamine release. *Pharmacol Toxicol*. 1994;75:348–352.
346. Mifsud JC, Hernandez L, Hoebel BG. Nicotine infused into the nucleus accumbens increases synaptic dopamine as measured by in vivo microdialysis. *Brain Res*. 1989;478:365–367.
347. Quarta D, Ciruela F, Patkar K, et al. Heteromeric nicotinic acetylcholine–dopamine autoreceptor complexes modulate striatal dopamine release. *Neuropsychopharmacology*. 2007;32: 35–42.
348. Klink R, de Kerchove d'Exaerde A, Zoli M, et al. Molecular and physiological diversity of nicotinic acetylcholine receptors in the midbrain dopaminergic nuclei. *J Neurosci*. 2001;21:1452–1463.
349. Grilli M, Zappettini S, Zoli M, et al. Pre-synaptic nicotinic and D receptors functionally interact on dopaminergic nerve endings of rat and mouse nucleus accumbens. *J Neurochem*. 2009;108:1507–1514.
350. Wonnacott S, Kaiser S, Mogg A, et al. Presynaptic nicotinic receptors modulating dopamine release in the rat striatum. *Eur J Pharmacol*. 2000;393:51–58.
351. Salminen O, Murphy KL, McIntosh JM, et al. Subunit composition and pharmacology of two classes of striatal presynaptic nicotinic acetylcholine receptors mediating dopamine release in mice. *Mol Pharmacol*. 2004;65:1526–1535.
352. Cui C, Booker TK, Allen RS, et al. The beta3 nicotinic receptor subunit: a component of alpha-conotoxin MII-binding nicotinic acetylcholine receptors that modulate dopamine release and related behaviors. *J Neurosci*. 2003;23:11045–11053.
353. Fu Y, Matta SG, Gao W, et al. Local alpha-bungarotoxin-sensitive nicotinic receptors in the nucleus accumbens modulate nicotine-stimulated dopamine secretion in vivo. *Neuroscience*. 2000;101:369–375.
354. Zhang T, Zhang L, Liang Y, et al. Dopamine signaling differences in the nucleus accumbens and dorsal striatum exploited by nicotine. *J Neurosci*. 2009;29:4035–4043.
355. Grillner P, Svensson TH. Nicotine-induced excitation of midbrain dopamine neurons in vitro involves ionotropic glutamate receptor activation. *Synapse*. 2000;38:1–9.
356. Pidoplichko VI, DeBiasi M, Williams JT, et al. Nicotine activates and desensitizes midbrain dopamine neurons. *Nature*. 1997;390: 401–404.
357. Di Chiara G. Role of dopamine in the behavioural actions of nicotine related to addiction. *Eur J Pharmacol*. 2000;393: 295–314.
358. Schilstrom B, Svensson HM, Svensson TH, et al. Nicotine and food induced dopamine release in the nucleus accumbens of the rat: putative role of alpha7 nicotinic receptors in the ventral tegmental area. *Neuroscience*. 1998;85:1005–1009.
359. Wooltorton JR, Pidoplichko VI, Broide RS, et al. Differential desensitization and distribution of nicotinic acetylcholine receptor subtypes in midbrain dopamine areas. *J Neurosci*. 2003;23: 3176–3185.
360. Corrigall WA. Nicotine self-administration in animals as a dependence model. *Nicotine Tob Res*. 1999;1:11–20.
361. Neugebauer NM, Zhang Z, Crooks PA, et al. Effect of a novel nicotinic receptor antagonist, N,N -dodecane-1,12-diyl-bis-3-picolinium dibromide, on nicotine self-administration and hyperactivity in rats. *Psychopharmacology (Berl)*. 2006;184: 426–434.
362. Rauhut AS, Mullins SN, Dwoskin LP, et al. Reboxetine: attenuation of intravenous nicotine self-administration in rats. *J Pharmacol Exp Ther*. 2002;303:664–672.
363. Rahman S, Neugebauer NM, Zhang Z, et al. The effects of a novel nicotinic receptor antagonist N,N-dodecane-1,12-diyl-bis-3-picolinium dibromide (bPiDDB) on acute and repeated

nicotine-induced increases in extracellular dopamine in rat nucleus accumbens. *Neuropharmacology.* 2007;52:755–763.
364. Ikemoto S, Qin M, Liu ZH. Primary reinforcing effects of nicotine are triggered from multiple regions both inside and outside the ventral tegmental area. *J Neurosci.* 2006;26:723–730.
365. Singer G, Wallace M, Hall R. Effects of dopaminergic nucleus accumbens lesions on the acquisition of schedule induced self injection of nicotine in the rat. *Pharmacol Biochem Behav.* 1982;17:579–581.
366. Corrigall WA, Franklin KB, Coen KM, et al. The mesolimbic dopaminergic system is implicated in the reinforcing effects of nicotine. *Psychopharmacology (Berl).* 1992;107:285–289.
367. Corrigall WA, Coen KM. Selective dopamine antagonists reduce nicotine self-administration. *Psychopharmacology (Berl).* 1991; 104:171–176.
368. Corrigall WA, Coen KM, Adamson KL. Self-administered nicotine activates the mesolimbic dopamine system through the ventral tegmental area. *Brain Res.* 1994;653:278–284.
369. Laviolette SR, van der Kooy D. The neurobiology of nicotine addiction: bridging the gap from molecules to behaviour. *Nat Rev Neurosci.* 2004;5:55–65.
370. Mansvelder HD, McGehee DS. Cellular and synaptic mechanisms of nicotine addiction. *J Neurobiol.* 2002;53:606–617.
371. Fattore L, Cossu G, Martellotta MC, et al. Baclofen antagonizes intravenous self-administration of nicotine in mice and rats. *Alcohol Alcohol.* 2002;37:495–498.
372. Paterson NE, Vlachou S, Guery S, et al. Positive modulation of GABA(B) receptors decreased nicotine self-administration and counteracted nicotine-induced enhancement of brain reward function in rats. *J Pharmacol Exp Ther.* 2008;326:306–314.
373. Fadda P, Scherma M, Fresu A, et al. Baclofen antagonizes nicotine-, cocaine-, and morphine-induced dopamine release in the nucleus accumbens of rat. *Synapse.* 2003;50:1–6.
374. Corrigall WA, Coen KM, Adamson KL, et al. Response of nicotine self-administration in the rat to manipulations of mu-opioid and gamma-aminobutyric acid receptors in the ventral tegmental area. *Psychopharmacology (Berl).* 2000;149:107–114.
375. Cousins MS, Roberts DC, de Wit H. GABA(B) receptor agonists for the treatment of drug addiction: a review of recent findings. *Drug Alcohol Depend.* 2002;65:209–220.
376. Picciotto MR, Zoli M, Rimondini R, et al. Acetylcholine receptors containing the beta2 subunit are involved in the reinforcing properties of nicotine. *Nature.* 1998;391:173–177.
377. Grottick AJ, Trube G, Corrigall WA, et al. Evidence that nicotinic alpha(7) receptors are not involved in the hyperlocomotor and rewarding effects of nicotine. *J Pharmacol Exp Ther.* 2000; 294:1112–1119.
378. Watkins SS, Epping-Jordan MP, Koob GF, et al. Blockade of nicotine self-administration with nicotinic antagonists in rats. *Pharmacol Biochem Behav.* 1999;62:743–751.
379. Tessari M, Pilla M, Andreoli M, et al. Antagonism at metabotropic glutamate 5 receptors inhibits nicotine- and cocaine-taking behaviours and prevents nicotine-triggered relapse to nicotine-seeking. *Eur J Pharmacol.* 2004;499:121–133.
380. Kenny PJ, Paterson NE, Boutrel B, et al. Metabotropic glutamate 5 receptor antagonist MPEP decreased nicotine and cocaine self-administration but not nicotine and cocaine-induced facilitation of brain reward function in rats. *Ann N Y Acad Sci.* 2003;1003:415–418.
381. Paterson NE, Semenova S, Gasparini F, et al. The mGluR5 antagonist MPEP decreased nicotine self-administration in rats and mice. *Psychopharmacology (Berl).* 2003;167:257–264.
382. Kenny PJ, Chartoff E, Roberto M, et al. NMDA receptors regulate nicotine-enhanced brain reward function and intravenous nicotine self-administration: role of the ventral tegmental area and central nucleus of the amygdala. *Neuropsychopharmacology.* 2009;34:266–281.
383. Liechti ME, Lhuillier L, Kaupmann K, et al. Metabotropic glutamate 2/3 receptors in the ventral tegmental area and the nucleus accumbens shell are involved in behaviors relating to nicotine dependence. *J Neurosci.* 2007;27:9077–9085.
384. Mansvelder HD, Keath JR, McGehee DS. Synaptic mechanisms underlie nicotine-induced excitability of brain reward areas. *Neuron.* 2002;33:905–919.
385. Schilstrom B, Fagerquist MV, Zhang X, et al. Putative role of presynaptic alpha7* nicotinic receptors in nicotine stimulated increases of extracellular levels of glutamate and aspartate in the ventral tegmental area. *Synapse.* 2000;38:375–383.
386. Markou A, Paterson NE. The nicotinic antagonist methyllycaconitine has differential effects on nicotine self-administration and nicotine withdrawal in the rat. *Nicotine Tob Res.* 2001;3: 361–373.
387. Rauhut AS, Neugebauer N, Dwoskin LP, et al. Effect of bupropion on nicotine self-administration in rats. *Psychopharmacology (Berl).* 2003;169:1–9.
388. Bruijnzeel AW, Markou A. Characterization of the effects of bupropion on the reinforcing properties of nicotine and food in rats. *Synapse.* 2003;50:20–28.
389. Fu Y, Matta SG, Brower VG, et al. Norepinephrine secretion in the hypothalamic paraventricular nucleus of rats during unlimited access to self-administered nicotine: an in vivo microdialysis study. *J Neurosci.* 2001;21:8979–8989.
390. Fu Y, Matta SG, Kane VB, et al. Norepinephrine release in amygdala of rats during chronic nicotine self-administration: an in vivo microdialysis study. *Neuropharmacology.* 2003;45:514–523.
391. Coen KM, Adamson KL, Corrigall WA. Medication-related pharmacological manipulations of nicotine self-administration in the rat maintained on fixed- and progressive-ratio schedules of reinforcement. *Psychopharmacology (Berl).* 2009;201:557–568.
392. Paterson NE, Balfour DJ, Markou A. Chronic bupropion differentially alters the reinforcing, reward-enhancing and conditioned motivational properties of nicotine in rats. *Nicotine Tob Res.* 2008;10:995–1008.
393. Cohen C, Perrault G, Voltz C, et al. SR141716, a central cannabinoid (CB(1)) receptor antagonist, blocks the motivational and dopamine-releasing effects of nicotine in rats. *Behav Pharmacol.* 2002;13:451–463.
394. Shoaib M. The cannabinoid antagonist AM251 attenuates nicotine self-administration and nicotine-seeking behaviour in rats. *Neuropharmacology.* 2008;54:438–444.
395. Cryan JF, Bruijnzeel AW, Skjei KL, et al. Bupropion enhances brain reward function and reverses the affective and somatic aspects of nicotine withdrawal in the rat. *Psychopharmacology (Berl).* 2003;168:347–358.
396. Houdi AA, Pierzchala K, Marson L, et al. Nicotine-induced alteration in Tyr-Gly-Gly and Met-enkephalin in discrete brain nuclei reflects altered enkephalin neuron activity. *Peptides.* 1991;12:161–166.
397. Rukstalis M, Jepson C, Strasser A, et al. Naltrexone reduces the relative reinforcing value of nicotine in a cigarette smoking choice paradigm. *Psychopharmacology (Berl).* 2005;180:41–48.
398. Brauer LH, Behm FM, Westman EC, et al. Naltrexone blockade of nicotine effects in cigarette smokers. *Psychopharmacology (Berl).* 1999;143:339–346.

399. Liu X, Palmatier MI, Caggiula AR, et al. Naltrexone attenuation of conditioned but not primary reinforcement of nicotine in rats. *Psychopharmacology (Berl)*. 2009;202:589–598.
400. DeNoble VJ, Mele PC. Intravenous nicotine self-administration in rats: effects of mecamylamine, hexamethonium and naloxone. *Psychopharmacology (Berl)*. 2006;184:266–272.
401. Berrendero F, Kieffer BL, Maldonado R. Attenuation of nicotine-induced antinociception, rewarding effects, and dependence in mu-opioid receptor knock-out mice. *J Neurosci*. 2002;22:10935–10940.
402. Pomerleau OF, Pomerleau CS. Neuroregulators and the reinforcement of smoking: towards a biobehavioral explanation. *Neurosci Biobehav Rev*. 1984;8:503–513.
403. Picciotto MR, Addy NA, Mineur YS, et al. It is not "either/or": activation and desensitization of nicotinic acetylcholine receptors both contribute to behaviors related to nicotine addiction and mood. *Prog Neurobiol*. 2008;84:329–342.
404. Fowler CD, Arends MA, Kenny PJ. Subtypes of nicotinic acetylcholine receptors in nicotine reward, dependence, and withdrawal: evidence from genetically modified mice. *Behav Pharmacol*. 2008;19:461–484.
405. Epping-Jordan MP, Picciotto MR, Changeux JP, et al. Assessment of nicotinic acetylcholine receptor subunit contributions to nicotine self-administration in mutant mice. *Psychopharmacology (Berl)*. 1999;147:25–26.
406. Pons S, Fattore L, Cossu G, et al. Crucial role of alpha4 and alpha6 nicotinic acetylcholine receptor subunits from ventral tegmental area in systemic nicotine self-administration. *J Neurosci*. 2008;28:12318–12327.
407. Maskos U, Molles BE, Pons S, et al. Nicotine reinforcement and cognition restored by targeted expression of nicotinic receptors. *Nature*. 2005;436:103–107.

CHAPTER 6

Psychological Factors (In Determinants of Abuse and Dependence)

Steven Shoptaw

Psychological and social factors abound in the lives of individuals with substance abuse and dependence. Yet, the interplay of cultural, social and familial, individual predispositions, neurobiology, and genetic factors, though frequent, is apparently not sufficient for reliably determining substance abuse or dependence conditions. While psychological and social factors can contribute to the development and maintenance of substance abuse and dependence across the life span for many individuals, it remains that other individuals often do not develop these disorders, even given similar circumstances and biologies. Indeed, the effect sizes of psychological and social factors in determining substance abuse and dependence are modest (1). Further, once substance use disorders are established, accompanying neural changes and conditioned behaviors ascend in importance, with the roles of psychological and social factors having less impact in maintaining substance abuse or dependence. This chapter reviews the evidence regarding psychological factors and social experiences that contribute to substance abuse and dependence, with particular consideration given to various points across the life span.

SUBSTANCE ABUSE ACROSS THE LIFE SPAN

Estimates from the National Epidemiological Survey on Alcohol and Related Conditions (NESARC) show incidence of drug use disorders is low (2.0%) across the life span, with lifetime prevalence about 10% (2). Two factors, particularly gender and age reliably show differences: males are more likely than females to have drug abuse and dependence. Younger individuals also are more likely to have drug abuse or dependence, with incidence of these disorders peaking in late adolescence and being rare after age 25. Yet for the first time, Americans are not aging out of drug abuse problems, with baby boomers entering retirement with alcohol and drug use problems (2), particularly cannabis abuse.

One of the most potent predictors of substance abuse problems across the life span is a historical or current problem with another drug of abuse. Among youth, this observation took the shape of the "gateway hypothesis," the observation that use of a licit drug (e.g., alcohol and tobacco) or an illicit drug like marijuana during early adolescence predicted use of other illicit drugs (3). In a very strong prospective birth cohort study in New Zealand, development of drug abuse or dependence conditions correlated significantly with having parents who used illicit drugs, with male gender, with high needs for novelty seeking and with childhood conduct disorder (4)—associations that were mediated by marijuana use, alcohol use, and affiliation with substance using peers during ages 16 to 25. While strong evidence supporting the gateway hypothesis is provided by findings from the Virginia Twin Registry (5), the registry is comprised exclusively of White twins. For individuals from racial/ethnic groups, the buffering effects of family and culture delay of onset of illicit drug use in adolescents (6). Withdrawal of these buffering effects for youth reaching age of majority, however, contributes to comparable rates of incidence of drug and alcohol abuse. Finally, the logic of predicting substance abuse problems based on prior or current drug use is clearest among those who are already abusers of illicit drugs. Among those who are dependent on cocaine, methamphetamine, or heroin, concomitant use of alcohol, tobacco, and marijuana is highly prevalent (2). It also remains that the vast majority of adolescents who become regular daily users of nicotine and/or alcohol do not go on to become regular daily users of illicit drugs.

PSYCHOLOGICAL FACTORS

Personality

Individuals with substance abuse or dependence often complain they have an "addictive personality." The concept of the "addictive personality" frequently relates to long-standing and generalizable traits that involve inability to control indulgences with molecules or behaviors. This popular term, though descriptive, has little empirical support. By contrast, research into long-standing psychological and personality "traits" or styles shared by individuals with substance abuse or dependence shows a good deal of support for common characteristics, specifically sensation seeking, delay discounting, and other components of impulsivity (7). Behavioral scientists are likely to understand the factors that co-occur with substance abuse or dependence as constrained and limited. So while the concept of an "addictive personality" can be salient to patients and clinicians, the variance unexplained requires a more careful evaluation of stable intrapersonal styles that may be involved in determining substance abuse and dependence.

Personality Disorders

In the NESARC, a representative national sample of 43,093 individuals, those who met criteria for *any* personality disorder were 1.8 (95% confidence interval [CI]: 1.3–2.5) and 3.3 (95% CI: 2.0–5.3) times more likely to be comorbid for drug abuse or drug dependence than those who did not meet criteria for a personality disorder, respectively (2). Individuals with antisocial personality disorder, in specific, were two-and-one-half times more likely than those without antisocial personality disorder to also meet criteria for drug abuse and dependence after controlling for demographic characteristics and other psychiatric diagnoses. Antisocial, borderline, and narcissistic personality disorders (Cluster B in the DSM-IV-TR) share a defining feature: impaired capacity of individuals to inhibit impulses, which can facilitate repeated exposures to alcohol and/or illicit drugs sufficient to establish comorbid alcohol and drug use diagnoses (8). Individuals who meet criteria for drug abuse or dependence who are comorbid with personality disorders respond similarly to their peers in treatment who do not have personality disorders along drug use outcomes (9–11). Yet, there remain important ways in which patients living with personality disorders and comorbid substance dependence disorders bring significant disturbances to treatment, including criminal behaviors and overdose that require additional focus during treatment from those who do not have these disorders (12,13).

Bipolar Illness

Individuals with bipolar illness represent an important group who face genetic, neurobiologic, and environmental factors that can contribute to a high prevalence of comorbid substance abuse and dependence disorders (13). Providing evidence suggesting shared genetic pathways that explain the nearly 2.4 times greater risks for tobacco use disorders than the general public (14), three candidate genes have been shown (COMT, SLC6A3, SLC6A4) to interact in predisposing bipolar and tobacco use disorders. Individuals with bipolar illness and comorbid substance abuse and dependence share, at least partially, common neurobiologic pathways that are the biologic bases for expression of these behavioral disorders. Aspects of serious mental illness, such as bipolar disorder, share behavioral features including problems in inhibiting impulses and excessive time spent on sensation seeking. Substance abuse and dependence bring with them significant clinical distress (including independent risks for suicide), which interacts negatively with symptoms of bipolar disorder and can enhance negative individual, familial, and social consequences of either condition alone. Substance use can ameliorate these symptoms and exaggerate expansive experiences related to mania. Further, onset of substance use disorders and bipolar disorders imparts key information determining the course and severity, particularly of bipolar disease (15). About one third of comorbid individuals report substance abuse disorders preceded onset of their bipolar disorder. Among individuals whose bipolar disorder onset was earlier than or concurrent with onset of substance abuse disorders, a more unstable and severe course of bipolar disorder is noted (15). Continued substance use disorders among individuals with bipolar disorder have no impact on time to resolution of depressive phase, but can contribute to switching directly from depression to mania, hypomania, or mixed states (16). Indeed, substance abuse, particularly stimulant abuse can precipitate a manic episode or perhaps facilitate establishment of a bipolar condition that may have gone unexpressed in the absence of stimulant use (15).

Major Depression

Studies consistently document that depressive disorders co-occur with alcohol and drug abuse and dependence. Individuals with depressive disorders commonly seek out substance use to mediate depressed feelings and thoughts. A recent report noted that individuals in the general population with major depression, dysthymia, generalized anxiety disorder, or panic disorder concurrent with problem drug use are more likely than those who do not have these conditions to initiate and use prescribed opioids (17), presumably to minimize uncomfortable psychological states from those disorders. With repeated administrations, however, substance abuse or dependence conditions can develop and require treatment in their own regard. Compared to those who are not depressed, having a major depressive disorder doubles the odds for meeting criteria for alcohol and drug use disorders (18). Those with concurrent depression and substance abuse disorders are likely to be younger, male, divorced or never married, at greater current suicide risk, have an earlier age of onset of depression, have greater depressive symptomatology, report more previous suicide attempts, have anxiety disorders, and have greater functional impairment than those who are depressed only (19). Negative clinical consequences that result from alcohol and drug abuse or dependence are worsened compared to those with substance problems only, with older individuals showing stronger associations between negative consequences, depression, and substance use (20). The relationship between suicidal behaviors and substance abuse has long been recognized and particularly in individuals with comorbid depression and alcohol use disorders, risks for suicide are extremely high. Up to 7% of individuals with depression and alcohol dependence end their lives by committing suicide (21,22). Suicidal behaviors associated with alcohol dependence are also linked with higher levels of impulsive aggression, drug use, and psychiatric comorbidity, particularly personality and depressive disorders (20–22). As might be expected, depression negatively predicts success in maintaining alcohol abstinence following intensive treatment for alcohol dependence (23). Although clinical reports consistently document associations between depression and alcohol use disorders, less consistent associations are noted between depression and users of other drugs. Among injecting drug users (IDUs), co-occuring depression is associated with "concurrent" alcohol and drug use (and corresponding negative clinical consequences due to polysubstance use), needle sharing, and substance abuse treatment participation (24). Strong associations between depression and increased substance-related behaviors are not, however, universal across all substances of abuse. The same group failed to find similar substance-related behaviors in a meta-analysis of cocaine abusers with comorbid depression (25).

Thought Disorders

Individuals living with schizophrenia have one of the highest rates of comorbidities with substance use disorders. In a probability sample, 47% of respondents with schizophrenia also met criteria for lifetime diagnoses of substance abuse (13). Clinical researchers have pondered why individuals with thought disorders are prone to substance abuse and dependence and at the same time recognized that heavy use of some substances, particularly hallucinogens and stimulants, can produce experiences similar to schizophrenia in nonpsychotic individuals. As well, one report from Thailand indicates that among 445 methamphetamine-abusing individuals, those who have a first degree relative with schizophrenia were significantly more likely to develop methamphetamine psychosis than users who did not have a relative with schizophrenia (26). More, while there is some indication that dopamine dysregulation may predispose individuals with schizophrenia to abuse drugs (27), it has long been recognized that individuals living with schizophrenia engage in drug abuse behaviors because the substances help them to feel good and provide relief from the dulling effects of their antipsychotic medications and medications to treat side effects. On the other hand, there is scant evidence that even chronic abuse of substances contributes to the development of thought disorders. Among the approximately 1% of adolescents who ultimately develop schizophrenia, there is no indication that their use of marijuana or other substances differs significantly from the vast majority of adolescents who do not develop schizophrenia (28). In their review, individuals with thought disorders who abuse substances face several severe negative consequences including: (1) increased positive symptoms; (2) relapse of psychosis; (3) heightened risk of violence; (4) heightened risk of suicide; (5) increased medical comorbidities; (6) legal complications, including heightened risk of incarceration; and (7) increased propensity to antipsychotic-related side effects. The most important consequence to individuals with schizophrenia and comorbid substance abuse disorders involves disruption of psychiatric medication adherence, which ultimately erodes stability for the individual and increases the potential for negative consequences common to end stage substance abuse disorders such as homelessness and grave disability.

Anxiety Disorders/Posttraumatic Stress Disorder (PTSD)

Anxiety disorders and substance abuse disorders co-occur at substantial rates. Analyses of NESARC data (29) showed that individuals with any mood disorders were substantially more likely than those with any anxiety disorders to also meet criteria for alcohol abuse, alcohol dependence, drug abuse, or drug dependence. Still, compared to individuals who had no anxiety disorders, individuals with any anxiety disorder were 2.6 times (95% CI: 2.2–3.0) and 6.2 times (95% CI: 4.4–8.7) more likely to meet criteria of alcohol dependence and any drug dependence, respectively. Twelve-month prevalence of substance use disorders was highest for any alcohol, any drug, and cannabis use disorders. Individuals with anxiety disorders may abuse alcohol, cannabis, and prescription analgesics or sedatives in order to medicate symptoms of anxiety. The typical anxiety disorder patient with substance abuse or dependence, however, differs in presentation from other types of individuals with comorbid psychological and substance use disorders. Indeed, data from the National Comorbidity Survey-Replication study (30) indicate that presence of an anxiety disorder reduces the association between externalizing problems (such as conduct disorder, oppositional defiant disorder) and substance use disorders, possibly because fear/anxiety interferes with individuals with externalizing problems from engaging in drug-seeking behaviors.

While many Americans have experiences that meet the criterion for trauma, only a minority goes on to develop the full range of PTSD symptoms. Even so, PTSD is prevalent in alcohol and drug abusing populations in treatment. Links between PTSD and substance abuse are well recognized by clinicians and patients. Individuals with PTSD frequently report using substances in order to reduce anxiety and to block re-experiencing the traumatic event. Recent evidence that supports the self-medication rationale comes from a national multisite trial for comorbid PTSD and substance abuse. Participants who experienced reductions in PTSD symptoms correspondingly showed decreases in symptoms of substance abuse (31). By contrast, individuals who responded solely to substance abuse treatment showed no association with their experiences with PTSD symptoms.

Impulsivity

A behaviorally based definition of impulsivity focuses on the likelihood of an individual to rapidly act on an impulse rather than to act based on consideration; the failure to inhibit these impulses can include behaviors that even carry potential for self harm (32). A central psychological characteristic shared by many individuals with substance abuse and dependence involves a significant and principle deficit of inhibiting impulses linked to using substance. Impairments in inhibiting cognitive impulses can generalize beyond substance use to erode overall quality of executive functioning in substance abusers (33). Several examples of impulsive cognitive style have been noted in individuals with substance abuse or dependence, including delay discounting, that is, discounting the value of rewards that may be more valuable, but more distant, in favor of lower value rewards that are immediately available (34). Using a trait definition, impulsive sensation seeking or behavioral disinhibition traits best predicted substance use in a large sample of 457 young adults at 6-year follow-up evaluations (35). Inhibitory control deficits observed in childhood (36), inhibitory control deficits with onset during adolescence (37), and genetic variation in inhibitory control deficits (38) represent independent contributions to enhanced risks for development of substance abuse or dependence disorders across the lifetime. In specific, impulsivity most likely is a risk factor for development of stimulant abuse (39). One important component of impulsivity that can contribute to establishment of substance abuse disorders is sensation seeking, a behavioral trait that can be conceptualized on a continuum, ranging from excitement-adventure seeking (a vulnerability to boredom) to disinhibition. In her review of the topic, de Wit (7) argued convincingly that impulsive behavior is both a determinant and a consequence of drug use. Individuals who have long-standing (trait) and momentary (state) forms of impulsivity face increased risks for development of substance abuse disorders. At the same time, drug use compromises impulse inhibition and contributes to continued substance use, particularly for those who have made efforts to quit using substances. Neurobiologic studies demonstrate that drug abuse is associated with inhibitory changes not only in the reward circuitry (anterior cingulate), but also in the orbitofrontal cortex, which is a brain region involved in executive functioning (40). Initial voluntary drug use is associated with prefrontal cortical function, executive control, whereas drug dependence represents a neural shift to striatal control involving dorsal striatum dopaminergic innervation. In the absence of impulse controls, a conditioned excitatory cycle of substance-related stimuli and substance availability contributes to attentional biases that favor drug-seeking behavior (41). Dopamine levels can augment conditioned learning (42). Specifically, addictive reinforcing effects of substances are dependent on the amount and the rate of dopamine increases in the striatum (42). Again, in the absence of impulse inhibitions, drug will likely be readministered. Emphasizing that impulsivity can have circular effects on substance use over time and can compound likelihood of establishment of a substance use disorder, evidence from human and animal models is generally consistent in showing feedback loops between impulsive behaviors and substance abuse, periods of abstinence, episodic relapse, and ultimately to treatment (43).

Attention Deficit Hyperactivity Disorder (ADHD)

ADHD is a psychiatric diagnosis of childhood marked by severe behavioral disruptions from pervasive problems in controlling impulses. Children diagnosed with ADHD mature into adults who vary in the rates of continued problems in impaired inhibitory control. Among adults with substance use disorders, about one in five have ADHD diagnoses (44); between 65% and 89% of all adults who have histories of ADHD diagnoses also are diagnosed with one or more additional psychiatric disorders—most commonly with mood and anxiety disorders, substance use disorders, and personality disorders (45). Individuals diagnosed with ADHD as children who matured into adults with substance abuse disorders carry substantial genetic predisposition for both disorders (46). Interestingly, ADHD among females carries a more serious risk factor for development of substance abuse or dependence than in males. The finding is concerning when considering that a decade separates age of incidence for the two disorders, indicating females may face acute risks for developing substance use disorders as preteens (47). By contrast, while ADHD is not a significant risk factor for substance use disorders when male gender, co-occurring disruptive behavior, and socioeconomic status are controlled (48), the combination of ADHD and conduct disorder is a strong predictor (49). Danish individuals in a large cohort contacted after 40 years and who had conduct disorder and ADHD during childhood were six times more likely to develop severe alcohol dependence than those who did not have the combined disorders during childhood (50). A natural question to parents of children with ADHD is whether treating the disorder with psychostimulants might predispose their child to substance abuse or dependence in adulthood. A meta-analysis of seven studies (51) suggested that treatment had no deleterious effects and may have even extended a protective effect for children who received treatment. As children with ADHD age, treatment with psychostimulants often continues, raising the potential that these individuals may misuse or divert their medications, particularly during college years. Evidence indicates that most students use their medications as prescribed, with only a minority diverting or misusing their medications. Moreover, those who did misuse or divert their medications had co-occurring problems with impulsivity and substance abuse (52).

SOCIAL FACTORS (IN DETERMINANTS OF ABUSE AND DEPENDENCE)

Violence and Aggression

Among individuals with substance abuse and dependence, especially those who have multiple treatment and incarceration experiences, there exists a high prevalence of comorbid violence and aggression. Estimates of the incidence of violence from the NESARC sample ($N = 34,632$) showed significantly higher rates for people living with severe mental illness who are comorbid with substance abuse or dependence than those who have no comorbid conditions. Specifically, severe mental illness alone does not appear sufficient to predict future violence. Variables that correlated with violence included a significant history with violence (past violence, juvenile detention, physical abuse, parental arrest record), comorbid substance abuse, demographic variables (young age, male gender, low income), and social contexts (recent divorce, unemployment, victimization) (53). As expected, alcohol has a strong and consistent link to violence and aggression, with associations between these variables becoming most apparent as severity of alcohol use disorders increases (54). Links between alcohol and violence are so strong and consistent that some posit that at least for alcohol and violent crime, the links approach causality (55). Rationale for such thinking is based on the observations that among individuals with historical, social, and demographic factors who also have psychiatric comorbidity, chronic and heavy alcohol use diminishes inhibitions or morals against violent or antisocial behaviors, fuels feelings of rage, constrains ability to think of options, and reduces concerns over negative consequences of behaviors—culminating in aggression and criminal behaviors. While alcohol use significantly increases risks for violence and aggression in individuals with predisposing vulnerabilities, combining illicit stimulant use with alcohol, particularly cocaine and methamphetamine, further exaggerates risks for violence. When cocaine and methamphetamine are combined with alcohol use, individuals with predisposing vulnerabilities toward violence are more likely to increase the severity and aggressiveness of their violent acts (56,57). Analyses of combined national data sets (National Household Survey on Drug Abuse, Survey of Inmates in State and Federal Correctional Facilities) showed that risks for committing a homicide were nine times greater when an individual uses methamphetamine and that these risks persist after adjusting for other drug abuse histories and sociodemographic factors (58).

Intimate Partner Violence

Violence and aggression that occurs within the context of a close interpersonal relationship, intimate partner violence (IPV), is a specialized form of violence that is gaining recognition as a social problem and that frequently co-occurs with abuse of alcohol and other drugs. In a large screening trial of women in primary health care settings in Canada, risks for IPV were approximately doubled if the woman or her partner had a drug abuse problem (59). IPV also was significantly more likely to occur among married women and women with a mental health issue. Intimate relationships are the contexts in which adults typically reveal vulnerabilities to their partners, including vulnerabilities for engaging violent behaviors when one or both partners have a predisposition and comorbid substance abuse problem or mental illness. Not all aggression is physical however. Among those predisposed and who engage in heavy drinking episodes, cocaine use, and experience depressive symptoms, psychological aggression is very common (60). The results indicate that there is a small to moderate effect size for the association between alcohol use/abuse and male-to-female partner violence and a small effect size for the association between alcohol use/abuse and female-to-male partner violence (54). Estimates of the effect size for drug use and drug-related problems in promoting IPV are in the moderate range ($d = .27$). Cocaine use showed medium to large effect sizes in associating with psychological, physical, and sexual aggression ($d = .39$ to $.62$), though marijuana use also correlated significantly with partner aggression. Moderator analyses revealed that relative to other groups, married or cohabiting couples and Black participants showed significantly stronger effect sizes (61). In a descriptive study of home visits by police regarding IPV from Albuquerque, New Mexico, perpetrators were more likely to be male, to have witnessed IPV as a child, and to have used (in descending order) methamphetamine, cocaine, and alcohol during the episode of IPV (62). Though males remain statistically more likely to be the perpetrator, the prevalence of females as perpetrators in IPV is increasing, perhaps due to increased substance use (63).

Childhood Adversity and Family Factors

In retrospective reports, individuals with substance abuse and dependence commonly cite a range of early experiences with childhood adversities, including parental substance abuse, family violence, physical and sexual abuse, and poverty. Childhood adversities are typically studied as single occurrences, yet individuals with substance abuse disorders commonly mention more than one childhood adversity, and among those who do mention more than one adversity, the average number is four (64). Childhood adversities can vary in their relative strength to correlate with health outcomes in adulthood. One large sample of adult women interviewed in primary care settings showed strong associations between childhood sexual abuse and adult psychiatric functioning. Women who reported histories of childhood sexual abuse were significantly more likely to be abusing drugs, to have a history of alcohol abuse and to have significant psychiatric problems, including suicide attempts than their peers without such histories (65). Reflecting the range of associations with symptoms indicating psychiatric problems, women with experiences with childhood sexual abuse also were more likely to have more physical symptoms and higher scores for depression, anxiety, somatization, and lower self-esteem scores than women who had no such experiences. Efforts to refine assessment of associations between multiple childhood adversities, compared to single adversities, with adult psychiatric diagnoses and contextual risk factors (social and familial factors) are now yielding findings. In a large national probability sample, maladaptive family functioning types of childhood adversities, including parental substance abuse, family violence, physical and sexual abuse, predicted the development of and the persistence of substance abuse disorders (66). Moreover, the strength of associations between maladaptive family functioning-type childhood adversities and psychiatric comorbidities were observed throughout the life span, including in elderly respondents. Multivariate analyses of these retrospective data found no support for the common approach to summing the number of childhood adversities to yield a severity marker, though findings do recognize the potential consequences to psychiatric functioning later in life from early adversities involving maladaptive family functioning. In less quantitative descriptions, childhood adversities combine to make the home a chaotic, unpredictable environment for children. While a significant minority of children who grow up in maladaptive family environments will as adults develop substance abuse or dependence, a majority will avoid associated outcomes as adults.

Life Stress

Adults commonly cope with stressful life events by turning to tobacco, alcohol, or other drugs to reduce psychological discomfort that accompany those stressful life events. Yet it appears relatively uncommon for even severe life stressors to be an independent major contributor to establishing a substance use disorder or worsening an existing one. In the aftermath of the attacks on New York City, PTSD and depressive disorders were detected, particularly for individuals in proximity to the event, but with minimal impact on substance use behaviors (67). As noted, some individuals respond to stressful life events with psychological responses that include experiencing negative emotional states (e.g., depression, overwhelmed) or behavioral disruptions (e.g., destroying property, physical fights). Use of substances in these episodes can both numb negative emotional states corresponding to the life stress and can intensify behavioral disruptions by increasing their destructiveness and threat levels. In adolescents, negative life events are often mediated through "hanging out" with deviant peers and participating in peers' substance use behaviors, both of which can increase risks for development of substance abuse or dependence. Individuals with comorbid psychological disorders may be constrained in the ways in which they manage stressful life events. In a large, probability survey of community health, mental health, and well-being in Canada, women respondents living with mental disorders reportedly dealt with their stress by talking to others and eating more/less compared to men. By contrast, men with mental disorders were more likely to avoid people and drink alcohol to deal with stress than women (68). At least one example exists of stress exaggerating substance use in an analysis of data from the 2002 National Survey on Drug Use and Health. In that report, adults who reported experiencing serious psychological distress at the time of the survey had greater odds of lifetime, past month, and daily use of cigarettes and other tobacco products than adults without serious psychological distress. As well, those with serious psychological distress were more likely to be nicotine dependent and were less likely to quit or to be former smokers than those without serious psychological distress (69). Findings do not address the question, however, of whether respondents with serious psychological stress were predisposed to heavier use of tobacco products. In perhaps the only prospective test of longitudinal data in adolescents maturing to young adulthood, youth who experienced stressful life events during adolescence showed increases in both negative emotional states and externalizing symptoms (e.g., behavioral disruptions), though analyses showed that externalizing symptoms alone mediated later effects of stressors on the development of drug dependence in young adulthood (70).

Social Attachment

Development of substance abuse and dependence is less frequent in individuals who have strong social attachments to their families and their culture, including the institutions within the culture. This influence is apparent even among criminals. In an analysis of a large national sample of male arrestees drawn from 24 urban areas, individual social attachments to marriage and to the labor force represented the principal pathway for mediating substance abuse and aggression. Only a minority of the variance in explaining substance abuse and aggression was accounted for by female-headed households and by households receiving welfare support (71), which are factors popularly promoted as explanations of substance abuse and dependence in urban areas. Social attachments also appear to protect against development of substance use disorders among adolescents growing up in families in which the father is an illicit drug user. Among Hispanic adolescents in such families, the father's level of marijuana and/or methamphetamine use was unrelated to the youths' bonds with their families. Instead, family bonding was positively influenced by youths' commitment to their communities and adoption of cultural values and of respect for elders/family (72). Among adolescents, poor family attachment, poor school attachment, involvement with friends who use drugs, and a student's own use of drugs are predictors in substance use disorders. Moreover, poor family attachments appear to influence youth's drug use via poor school attachment and involvement with friends who use drugs. By contrast poor school attachment exerts its effect on drug use through involvement with friends who use drugs (73).

SUMMARY

The data presented describe many of the ways in which substance use, abuse, and dependence can be established via factors ranging from use of multiple and other substances to comorbid psychiatric conditions to psychological states to social, cultural, and familial conventions and mores. When available, effect sizes for these factors in establishing substance abuse and dependence generally ranged between weak to moderate sizes. This indicates that across our diverse populations, there are neither psychological factors nor social determinants of drug abuse and dependence that approach causality. To illustrate this heterogeneity, clients seeking treatment commonly cite many and differing reasons that they attribute to their initially becoming involved with their drug(s) of choice. Once abuse and dependence take over, and the neurobiologic and behavioral processes common to addiction predominate, the ranges of voices of clients begin to harmonize and the principle reason for seeking treatment becomes very simple and universal: "to get my life back."

ACKNOWLEDGMENTS

The author gratefully acknowledges the assistance of Noah Haas-Cohen, Psy.D. in the preparation of this chapter.

REFERENCES

1. Hser YI, Longshore D, Anglin MD. The life course perspective on drug use. *Eval Rev*. 2007;31:515–545.
2. Compton WM, Thomas YF, Stinson FS, et al. Prevalence, correlates, disability, and comorbidity of DSM-IV drug abuse and dependence in the United States: results from the national epidemiologic survey on alcohol and related conditions. *Arch Gen Psychiatry*. 2007;64:566–576.
3. Kandel DB. Stages in adolescent involvement in drug use. *Science*. 1975;190:912–914.
4. Fergusson DM, Boden JM, Horwood LJ. The developmental antecedents of illicit drug use: evidence from a 25-year longitudinal study. *Drug Alcohol Depend*. 2008;96:165–177.
5. Agrawal A, Neale MC, Prescott CA, et al. A twin study of early cannabis use and subsequent use and abuse/dependence of other illicit drugs. *Psychol Med*. 2004;34:1227–1237.
6. Wu ZH, Temple JR, Shokar NK, et al. Differential racial/ethnic patterns in substance use initiation among young, low-income women. *Am J Drug Alcohol Abuse*. 2010;36:123–129.
7. de Wit H. Impulsivity as a determinant and consequence of drug use: a review of underlying processes. *Addiction Biology*. 2008;14:22–31.
8. Lara DR, Pinto O, Akiskal K, et al. Toward an integrative model of the spectrum of mood, behavioral and personality disorders based on fear and anger traits: I. Clinical implications. *J Affect Disord*. 2006;94:67–87.
9. Ralevski E, Ball S, Nich C, et al. The impact of personality disorders on alcohol-use outcomes in a pharmacotherapy trial for alcohol dependence and comorbid Axis I disorders. *Am J Addict*. 2008;16:443–449.
10. Messina N, Farabee D, Rawson R. Treatment responsivity of cocaine-dependent patients with antisocial personality disorder to cognitive-behavioral and contingency management interventions. *J Consult Clin Psychol*. 2003;71:320–329.
11. Darke S, Ross J, Williamson A, et al. Borderline personality disorder and persistently elevated levels of risk in 36-month outcomes for the treatment of heroin dependence. *Addiction*. 2007;102:1140–1146.
12. Ciraulo DA, Piechniczek-Buczek J, Iscan EN. Outcome predictors in substance use disorders. *Psychiatr Clin North Am*. 2003;26:381–409.
13. Regier DA, Farm ME, Rae DS. Comorbidity of mental disorders with alcohol and other drug abuse: results from the Epidemiologic Catchment Area (ECA) study. *JAMA*. 1990;264:2511–2518.
14. McEachin RC, Saccone NL, Saccone SF, et al. Modeling complex genetic and environmental influences on comorbid bipolar disorder with tobacco use disorder. *BMC Med Genet*. 2010;11:14.
15. Swann AC. The strong relationship between bipolar and substance-use disorder: mechanisms and treatment implications. *Ann N Y Acad Sci*. 2010;1187:276–293.
16. Ostacher MJ, Perlis RH, Nierenberg AA, et al. Impact of substance use disorders on recovery from episodes of depression in bipolar disorder patients: prospective data from the Systematic Treatment Enhancement Program for Bipolar Disorder (STEP-BD). *Am J Psychiatry*. 2010;167:289–297.
17. Hasin DS, Goodwin RD, Stinson FS, et al. Epidemiology of major depressive disorder: results from the National Epidemiologic Survey on Alcoholism and related conditions. *Arch Gen Psychiatry*. 2005;62:1097–1096.
18. Davis L, Uezato A, Newell JM, et al. Major depression and comorbid substance use disorders. *Curr Opin Psychiatry*. 2008;21:14–18.
19. Conner KR, Pinquart M, Gamble SA. Meta-analysis of depression and substance use among individuals with alcohol use disorders. *J Subst Abuse Treat*. 2009;37:127–137.
20. Sher L. Risk and protective factors for suicide in patients with alcoholism. *Scientific World Journal*. 2006;6:1405–1411.
21. Carballo JJ, Bird H, Giner L, et al. Pathological personality traits and suicidal ideation among older adolescents and young adults with alcohol misuse: a pilot case-control study in a primary care setting. *Int J Adolesc Med Health*. 2007;19:79–89.
22. Modesto-Lowe V, Brooks D, Ghani M. Alcohol dependence and suicidal behavior: from research to clinical challenges. *Harv Rev Psychiatry*. 2006;14:241–248.
23. Kodl MM, Fu SS, Willenbring ML, et al. The impact of depressive symptoms on alcohol and cigarette consumption following treatment for alcohol and nicotine dependence. *Alcohol Clin Exp Res*. 2008;32:92–99.
24. Conner KR, Pinquart M, Duberstein PR. Meta-analysis of depression and substance use and impairment among intravenous drug users (IDUs). *Addiction*. 2008;103:524–534.
25. Conner KR, Pinquart M, Holbrook AP. Meta-analysis of depression and substance use and impairment among cocaine users. *Drug Alcohol Depend*. 2008;98:13–23.
26. Chen CK, Lin SK, Sham PC, et al. Morbid risk for psychiatric disorder among the relatives of methamphetamine users with and without psychosis. *Am J Med Genet B Neuropsychiatr Genet*. 2005;136B:87–91.
27. O' Daly OG, Guillin, Tsapakis EM, et al. Schizophrenia and substance abuse comorbidity: a role for dopamine sensitization? *J Dual Diagn*. 2005;1:11–40.
28. Buckley PF, Miller BJ, Lehrer DS, et al. Psychiatric comorbidities and schizophrenia. *Schizophr Bull*. 2009;35:383–402.
29. Grant BF, Stinson FS, Dawson DA, et al. Prevalence and co-occurrence of substance use disorders and independent mood and anxiety disorders: results from the National Epidemiologic Survey on alcohol and related conditions. *Arch Gen Psychiatry*. 2004;61:807–816.
30. Hofmann SG, Richey JA, Kashdan TB, et al. Anxiety disorders moderate the association between externalizing problems and substance use disorders: data from the National Comorbidity Survey-Revised. *J Anxiety Disord*. 2009;23:529–534.
31. Hien DA, Jiang H, Campbell AN, et al. Do treatment improvements in PTSD severity affect substance use outcomes? A secondary analysis from a randomized clinical trial in NIDA's Clinical Trials Network. *Am J Psychiatry*. 2010;167:95–101.
32. Moeller FG, Barratt ES, Dougherty DM, et al. Psychiatric aspects of impulsivity. *Am J Psychiatry*. 2001;158:1783–1793.
33. Verdejo-García A, Lawrence AJ, Clark L. Impulsivity as a vulnerability marker for substance-use disorders: review of findings

from high-risk research, problem gamblers and genetic association studies. *Neurosci Biobehav Rev*. 2008;32:777–810.
34. Rachlin H, Green L. Commitment, choice, and self control. *J Exp Anal Behav*. 1972;17:15–22.
35. Sher KJ, Bartholow BD, Wood MD. Personality and substance use disorders: a prospective study. *J Consult Clin Psychol*. 2000;68: 818–829.
36. Kreek MJ, Nielsen DA, Butelman ER, et al. Genetic influences on impulsivity, risk taking, stress responsivity and vulnerability to drug abuse and addiction. *Nat Neurosci*. 2005;8:1450–1457.
37. Iacono WG, Malone SM, McGue M. Behavioral disinhibition and the development of early-onset addiction: common and specific influences. *Annu Rev Clin Psychol*. 2008;4:325–348.
38. Ivanov I, Schulz KP, London ED, et al. Inhibitory control deficits in childhood and risk for substance use disorders: a review. *Am J Drug Alcohol Abuse*. 2008;34:239–258.
39. Moeller FG, Dougherty DM, Barratt ES, et al. Increased impulsivity in cocaine dependent subjects independent of antisocial personality disorder and aggression. *Drug Alcohol Depend*. 2002;68:105–111.
40. Lubman DI, Yücel M, Pantelis C. Addiction, a condition of compulsive behaviour? Neuroimaging and neuropsychological evidence of inhibitory dysregulation. *Addiction*. 2004;99: 1491–1502.
41. Field M, Cox WM. Attentional bias in addictive behaviors: a review of its development, causes, and consequences. *Drug Alcohol Depend*. 2008;97:1–20.
42. Volkow ND, Fowler JS, Wang GJ, et al. Dopamine in drug abuse and addiction: results of imaging studies and treatment implications. *Arch Neurol*. 2007;64:1575–1579.
43. Perry JL, Carroll ME. The role of impulsive behavior in drug abuse Aggressiveness. *Psychopharmacology (Berl)*. 2008;200: 1–26.
44. Wilens TE, Fusillo S. When ADHD and substance use disorders intersect: relationship and treatment implications. *Curr Psychiatry Rep*. 2007;9:408–414.
45. Kunwar A, Dewan M, Faraone SV. Treating common psychiatric disorders associated with attention-deficit/hyperactivity disorder. *Expert Opin Pharmacother*. 2007;8:555–562.
46. Faraone SV. Genetics of adult attention-deficit/hyperactivity disorder. *Psychiatr Clin North Am*. 2004;27:303–321.
47. Biederman J, Faraone SV. The Massachusetts General Hospital studies of gender influences on attention-deficit/hyperactivity disorder in youth and relatives. *Psychiatr Clin North Am*. 2004; 27:225–232.
48. McGough JJ, Smalley SL, McCracken JT, et al. Psychiatric comorbidity in adult attention deficit hyperactivity disorder: findings from multiplex families. *Am J Psychiatry*. 2005;162: 1621–1627.
49. Upadhyaya HP. Substance use disorders in children and adolescents with attention-deficit/hyperactivity disorder: implications for treatment and the role of the primary care physician. *Prim Care Companion J Clin Psychiatry*. 2008;10: 211–221.
50. Knop J, Penick EC, Nickel EJ, et al., Childhood ADHD and conduct disorder as independent predictors of male alcohol dependence at age 40. *J Stud Alcohol Drugs*. 2009;70:169–177.
51. Faraone SV, Wilens TE. Effect of stimulant medications for attention-deficit/hyperactivity disorder on later substance use and the potential for stimulant misuse, abuse, and diversion. *J Clin Psychiatry*. 2007;68(suppl 11):15–22.
52. Rabiner DL, Anastopoulos AD, Costello EJ, et al. The misuse and diversion of prescribed ADHD medications by college students. *J Atten Disord*. 2009;13:144–153.
53. Elbogen EB, Johnson SC. The intricate link between violence and mental disorder: results from the National Epidemiologic Survey on Alcohol and Related Conditions. *Arch Gen Psychiatry*. 2009; 66:152–161.
54. Foran HM, O'Leary KD. Alcohol and intimate partner violence: a meta-analytic review. *Clin Psychol Rev*. 2008;28:1222–1234
55. Parker RN. Alcohol and violence: connections, evidence and possibilities for prevention. *J Psychoactive Drugs*. 2004;Suppl. 2: 157–163.
56. Macdonald S, Erickson P, Wells S, et al. Predicting violence among cocaine, cannabis, and alcohol treatment clients. *Addict Behav*. 2008;33:201–205.
57. Chermack ST, Blow FC. Violence among individuals in substance abuse treatment: the role of alcohol and cocaine consumption. *Drug Alcohol Depend*. 2002;66:29–37.
58. Stretesky PB. National case-control study of homicide offending and methamphetamine use. *J Interpers Violence*. 2009;24: 911–924.
59. Wathen CN, Jamieson E, MacMillan HL. Who is identified by screening for intimate partner violence? *Womens Health Issues*. 2008;18:423–432.
60. Chermack ST, Murray RL, Walton MA, et al. Partner aggression among men and women in substance use disorder treatment: correlates of psychological and physical aggression and injury. *Drug Alcohol Depend*. 2008;98:35–44.
61. Moore TM, Stuart GL, Meehan JC, et al. Drug abuse and aggression between intimate partners: a meta-analytic review. *Clin Psychol Rev*. 2008;28:247–274.
62. Ernst AA, Weiss SJ, Enright-Smith S, et al. Perpetrators of intimate partner violence use significantly more methamphetamine, cocaine, and alcohol than victims: a report by victims. *Am J Emerg Med*. 2008;26:592–596.
63. Dowd L, Leisring PA. A framework for treating partner aggressive women. *Violence Vict*. 2008;23:249–263.
64. Green JG, McLaughlin KA, Berglund PA, et al. Childhood adversities and adult psychiatric disorders in the national comorbidity survey replication I: associations with first onset of DSM-IV disorders. *Arch Gen Psychiatry*. 2010;67:113–123.
65. McCauley J, Kern DE, Kolodner K, et al. Clinical characteristics of women with a history of childhood abuse: unhealed wounds. *JAMA*. 1997;277:1362–1368.
66. McLaughlin KA, Green JG, Gruber MJ, et al. Childhood adversities and adult psychiatric disorders in the national comorbidity survey replication II: associations with persistence of DSM-IV disorders. *Arch Gen Psychiatry*. 2010;67: 124–132.
67. Galea S, Ahern J, Resnick H, et al. Psychological sequelae of the September 11 terrorist attacks in New York City. *N Engl J Med*. 2002;346:982–987.
68. Wang J, Keown LA, Patten SB, et al. A population-based study on ways of dealing with daily stress: comparisons among individuals with mental disorders, with long-term general medical conditions and healthy people. *Soc Psychiatry Psychiatr Epidemiol*. 2009;44:666–674.
69. Hagman BT, Delnevo CD, Hrywna M, et al. Tobacco use among those with serious psychological distress: results from the national survey of drug use and health, 2002. *Addict Behav*. 2008;33: 582–592.

70. King KM, Chassin L. Adolescent stressors, psychopathology, and young adult substance dependence: a prospective study. *J Stud Alcohol Drugs*. 2008;69:629–638.
71. Valdez A, Kaplan CD, Curtis RL Jr. Aggressive crime, alcohol and drug use, and concentrated poverty in 24 U.S. urban areas. *Am J Drug Alcohol Abuse*. 2007;33:595–603.
72. Castro FG, Garfinkle J, Naranjo D, et al. Cultural traditions as "protective factors" among Latino children of illicit drug users. *Subst Use Misuse*. 2007;42:621–642.
73. Henry KL. Low prosocial attachment, involvement with drug-using peers, and adolescent drug use: a longitudinal examination of mediational mechanisms. *Psychol Addict Behav*. 2008;22:302–308.

CHAPTER 7 Behavioral Aspects

Kenneth Silverman ■ Anthony DeFulio ■ Jeffery J. Everly

Much of human behavior is maintained and modifiable by its consequences through the process of operant conditioning (1). Under this process, some consequences of behavior, called reinforcers, increase the probability that a person will repeat a behavior in the future. Reinforcement is a fundamental process that affects the behavior of a vast range of creatures, from organisms as simple as a sea slug (2) to insects, fish, reptiles, birds, and mammals (3). Sensitivity to reinforcement has clear adaptive value and has probably evolved through natural selection (4). Reinforcement is deeply involved in shaping much of human behavior, from simple activities like walking, turning a doorknob, and riding a bicycle; to complex behaviors like writing, conversing, and composing music (1,5). Early theory (1) and an extensive body of experimental research suggest that the extended pattern of behavior that we call drug addiction, like much of human behavior, is also operant behavior that is maintained by its consequences.

Evidence that the instances of drug addiction we observe in society and treat in our clinics are operant in nature is necessarily indirect. Those instances of addiction develop through some unknown and uncontrolled history of experience and are typically observed by clinicians only after they are well established. Knowing with confidence the factors that produced or currently control a specific instance of addiction may not be possible. However, extensive experimental research conducted over more than four decades provides strong evidence that drug addiction *can* be operant behavior that, like many other human behaviors, is maintained and modifiable by its consequences. This research provides a plausible basis for conceptualizing instances of drug addiction that we see in society as operant behavior. The evidence can be grouped into three broad categories: laboratory models of drug addiction showing drugs are reinforcers that can modify and maintain the behavior of animals and humans; laboratory studies demonstrating the sensitivity of drug use to nondrug consequences; and clinical studies demonstrating the sensitivity of drug addiction to its consequences. This body of laboratory and clinical research has both theoretical and clinical implications. Theoretically, the research provides a framework for understanding drug addiction. Clinically, the research suggests the types of environmental conditions that can lead to the development of drug addiction, and the types and parameters of interventions that could be effective in treating drug addiction. This chapter reviews key experimental research on the operant nature of drug addiction and discusses the theoretical and clinical implications of that research.

Operant conditioning includes four basic elements: an antecedent stimulus, a response, a consequence, and a contingency that specifies the relationship between the other three elements. In a typical laboratory arrangement with a rat as an experimental subject, the antecedent stimulus might be a green light, the response a lever press, and the consequence a food pellet. The contingency might specify that each lever press emitted when the green light is illuminated will produce a food pellet, and that lever presses emitted when the green light is not illuminated will not produce food pellets. If this contingency produces an increase in the frequency of the lever pressing, the food pellets are called reinforcers and the process is called reinforcement. With sufficient exposure to the contingency, lever presses can become common in the presence of the illuminated green light and rare when the green light is not illuminated. If, as a result of the contingency, lever pressing becomes more common when the green light is on than when it is off, then the green light is called a discriminative stimulus. The process whereby discriminative stimuli come to alter the probability of responding is called stimulus discrimination. Certain motivational variables called establishing operations (5) can alter the effectiveness of a reinforcer. In our illustrative example, food deprivation can increase the effectiveness of food pellets to reinforce lever pressing or increase the frequency of lever pressing after reinforcement has occurred; food satiation can have the reverse effects. Research conducted over the past 70 years in the experimental analysis of behavior has revealed in exquisite detail how operant processes shape and maintain behavior, as well as the broad generality of the principles of operant conditioning (5).

LABORATORY MODELS OF DRUG ADDICTION

Early laboratory research in nonhuman subjects provided strong evidence that drug addiction can be viewed as operant behavior maintained by drug reinforcement (6). These studies demonstrated that nonhuman subjects could acquire and maintain behavior that led to the administration of a variety of drugs via a variety of routes of administration. In the typical laboratory arrangement, in the presence of some discriminative stimulus (e.g., a light), a laboratory subject is required to make one or more responses (e.g., lever presses) to receive a single administration (e.g., an intravenous infusion) of a drug. Over the course of an experimental session, the subject has repeated opportunities to respond and receive drug administrations. The responses required to produce drug administrations are conceptualized as drug seeking and the administration of the drug as drug use.

Laboratory models of drug addiction in nonhumans provide a unique and rich source of information on the nature of drug addiction and the variables that affect it. This research allows investigation of drug use in drug-naive organisms, and the rigorous experimental control of key variables that might influence drug use. This body of research has added to our understanding of drug addiction and to the development of effective behavioral and pharmacologic treatments for drug addiction. One seminal study by Deneau, Yanagita, and Seevers (7) showed that drug-naive monkeys would reliably press a lever that produced infusions of any of a variety of drugs that are commonly abused by humans (morphine, codeine, cocaine, morphine-cocaine, amphetamines, pentobarbital, and ethanol), but that they would not press a lever that produced infusions of saline or drugs that are not abused by humans (nalorphine or chlorpromazine). Animals in this study could press one lever that produced drug infusions or a different lever that did not produce infusions. Drug-naive animals were given continuous access to a drug under this arrangement and were monitored over extended periods of time. Seven of ten monkeys initiated and sustained lever pressing when lever presses produced 2.5 mg/kg infusions of morphine; the remaining three monkeys began morphine-maintained lever pressing after being exposed to periodic (every 4 hours) experimenter-administered infusions of morphine. Monkeys showed progressive increases in the total daily dose administered over several weeks; they maintained regular diurnal patterns of administration, characterized by high intake during the day and low or no intake at night; none of the animals discontinued lever pressing; and the animals maintained good overall health over time. Two of four monkeys initiated and sustained lever pressing when presses produced 0.25 mg/kg infusions of cocaine, and the two who did not initiate lever pressing at that dose initiated pressing when the dose was increased to 1.0 mg/kg. The monkeys showed a rapid increase in cocaine self-administration, although the pattern of self-administration over days was erratic. Remarkably, monkeys continued self-administration of cocaine despite severe toxicity, including biting of their skin and fingers to the point of amputation, and died within 30 days. None of four monkeys initiated self-administration of nalorphine; none of six monkeys initiated self-administration of chlorpromazine and despite "frequent attempts, including the use of raisin inducements," no animals self-administered physiologic saline. This pioneering work provided an impressive outline of the nature of drug reinforcement in laboratory animals. The study showed that only some drugs are reliably self-administered (e.g., morphine and cocaine are, but nalorphine and chlorpromazine are not); that saline is not self-administered; that the daily and hourly patterns of self-administration differ across drugs; that there are individual differences across monkeys in the propensity to acquire drug self-administration; and that animals will self-administer drugs like cocaine despite severe adverse consequences, up to and including death.

Operant Analyses of Drug Use: Experimental Examinations

Experimental studies in nonhumans and humans have provided thorough analyses of the roles of the basic elements of operant conditioning in drug self-administration. These studies confirm the operant nature of drug addiction and illustrate the critical role of operant conditioning in drug use.

The Reinforcer

A classic review of laboratory research on drug reinforcement showed that animal and human subjects in laboratory settings self administer the same range of drugs that are commonly abused in society (8). Reviews published since that paper have shown that nonhumans and humans will self-administer most commonly abused drugs, including although not limited to cocaine (9,10), opiates (11), alcohol (12), benzodiazepines (13), nicotine (14), and marijuana (15).

Experimental Demonstrations of Reinforcement A central issue underlying operant laboratory models of drug addiction is whether persistent drug use is operant behavior maintained by drug reinforcement. Do drugs function as reinforcers that maintain drug seeking and drug self-administration? To determine whether reinforcement is responsible for drug self-administration, studies must experimentally manipulate the contingent relation between responding and reinforcer presentation. If responding occurs only when the drug is presented contingent on responding, it provides evidence that drug reinforcement is critical in maintaining responding and that the drug self-administration is operant in nature.

Many studies have provided strong experimental evidence that drug self-administration in laboratory animals is operant in nature. In one recent study (16), rats were studied in a chamber with two holes through which they could poke their noses. One hole was designated as active and the other inactive. Nose pokes through the active hole produced cocaine infusions during some conditions, whereas nose pokes through the inactive hole never produced cocaine infusions. Nose pokes through the inactive hole remained extremely low throughout the experiment. Initially, nose pokes in the active hole produced intravenous infusions of cocaine. Nose pokes in the active hole increased quickly for both doses, but nose pokes in the inactive hole did not increase. When cocaine was replaced with saline, nose pokes in the active hole decreased abruptly and significantly to a level that was comparable to the inactive hole. When cocaine then replaced saline, nose pokes abruptly increased again in the active hole. Finally, when saline again replaced cocaine, nose pokes in the active hole decreased again. This study showed that responding in the study rats increased only when cocaine infusions were presented contingent on nose poking and not when saline infusions were contingent, and that the topography of nose poking (i.e., poking in the active versus the inactive hole) was a product of the cocaine contingency. These data provided strong evidence that cocaine reinforcement maintained cocaine self-administration in these rats.

A particularly informative way to assess reinforcement is to compare responding when a reinforcer is presented contingent on a response to when the same reinforcer is presented according to the same rate and pattern but independent of responding. This kind of experimental design allows researchers to isolate the role of the behavioral contingency. If responding is maintained at higher rates when a reinforcer is presented contingent on responding than when it is presented independent of responding, it provides firm evidence that the responding is maintained by reinforcement, and is not simply a product of the direct pharmacologic effects of the drug. Numerous studies with nondrug reinforcers have shown that response-contingent presentation of the reinforcer is essential to increase and maintain responding (2,17). A few recent studies have provided clear demonstrations of cocaine (16,18) and morphine (16) reinforcement in rats using noncontingent control conditions. In one of those studies (18), 20 rats were randomly assigned to master and yoked groups. Reinforcement contingencies were arranged for "master" rats in which nose pokes through one (the active hole) of two holes in the chamber produced a cocaine infusion. The number of nose pokes through the active hole required for each cocaine infusion was increased from one to five. Each master rat was paired with a "yoked" rat that received cocaine infusions that were identical in pattern and amount to the infusions received by the master rat; the only difference was the cocaine infusions experienced by a yoked rat occurred independently of whether the yoked rat poked its nose through either of the two holes in the chamber. After several sessions, cocaine was replaced with saline. Figure 7.1 shows the rate of nose poking in active and inactive holes by the master and yoked rats. The figure shows that during the cocaine reinforcement period, nose pokes in the active hole by master rats increased dramatically to a level that was significantly higher than their rate of nose pokes in the inactive hole. Furthermore, when saline replaced cocaine, nose poking in the active hole decreased to a near-zero level. In marked contrast, yoked rats never showed an increase in nose poking in either the active or the inactive holes. This study showed that *contingent* cocaine infusions could reinforce nose poking: nose poking only increased in rats when cocaine infusions were presented contingent on responding, only in the active hole on which reinforcement was contingent, and not when cocaine was presented independent of responding or when cocaine was replaced by saline.

Studies in humans using some of the same control conditions have demonstrated reinforcement by a number of drugs of abuse (8,10,13–15). These studies have used a variety of controls to demonstrate reinforcement, including placebo control conditions and reinforcement of selected response topographies (e.g., left vs. right response choices).

Parameters of the Reinforcement Contingency As with nondrug reinforcers (19), key parameters of the reinforcer and its delivery can modulate drug reinforcement. Immediacy and magnitude of reinforcement are two factors that seem

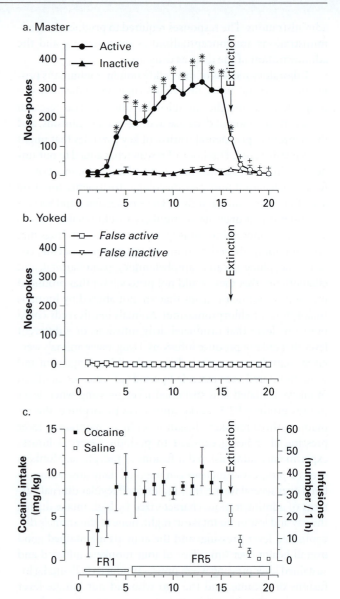

Figure 7.1. A: Cumulative responses (nose pokes) during cocaine self-administration and extinction (master rats). Results are expressed as mean ± SEM of cumulative nose pokes in the active and inactive holes of $n = 6$ master rats (1st–20th day). Asterisk denotes $p < 0.05$ versus inactive nose pokes, a plus sign denotes $p < 0.05$ versus the corresponding active nose pokes on the 15th day of cocaine SA session. ANOVA followed by Tukey post hoc test. **B:** Cumulative responses (nose pokes) during passive cocaine and saline administration in rats yoked to the self-administering ones. Results are expressed as mean ± SEM of cumulative nose pokes in the false active and inactive holes of $n = 6$ yoked rats (1st–20th day). **C:** Daily cocaine intake and number of infusions during cocaine self- and yoked administration and during extinction. Intake of cocaine, expressed as milligrams per kilogram of cocaine, during each 1-h daily 1st–15th sessions (left Y-axis filled squares). Data are also expressed as number of infusions of cocaine (filled squares) during the corresponding day session (filled squares) or saline (open squares) during the extinction phase (16th–20th days, right Y-axis). (Reproduced from Lecca D, Cacciapaglia F, Valentini V, et al. Differential neurochemical and behavioral adaptation to cocaine after response contingent and noncontingent exposure in the rat. *Psychopharmacology (Berl)*. 2007;191(3):653–667, with permission.)

particularly important. Increasing the delay between response and reinforcer typically diminishes reinforcement effects. One study compared the cocaine reinforcement effects produced when cocaine doses were administered to rhesus monkeys over varying durations (20). That study showed that the amount of responding maintained by cocaine reinforcement increased as the infusion duration decreased, suggesting the faster onset of drug effects increased drug reinforcement.

Assessing the effects of reinforcement magnitude can be complicated. In drug reinforcement, the magnitude of reinforcement can be increased by increasing the dose of the drug. Very high doses of some drugs can have aversive effects, or can lead to satiation, or performance impairment, all of which can affect measures of drug reinforcement (see the section "Regulation of Drug Intake"). However, assessments that mitigate those effects typically show that higher drug doses are more effective reinforcers than lower doses. For example, when subjects are given a choice between two doses of a reinforcing drug, they typically choose the higher over the lower dose (21). Higher doses also can sustain higher amounts of responding when the response requirement for reinforcement is increased (see the section "Drug-Seeking Response") (22).

The Discriminative Stimulus

In the lives of drug users, certain environmental events seem to serve as triggers that prompt drug seeking and drug use. In one study of methadone patients (23), over 80% of the participants said that having the drug present, being offered the drug, and having money available were likely to lead to drug use. These stimuli or events probably acquired their "triggering" function in large part through operant conditioning. These stimuli are all present when drug seeking and drug taking occurs, and they are typically less common or absent when drug taking does not occur. The availability of money, for example, frequently sets the occasion for a chain of drug seeking behaviors that leads to drug use and drug reinforcement. Thus, the money in the example may come to serve as a discriminative stimulus, whose presence increases the probability of drug seeking and drug taking. In the prototypic laboratory study, the role of discriminative stimuli in drug seeking and drug taking is modeled using arrangements in which two (or more) stimuli are presented in alternating periods. When one of the stimuli is present, drug-seeking responses (e.g., lever pressing) produce drug administrations (e.g., infusions; reinforcement), but when the other stimulus is present responses do not produce drug administrations (i.e., extinction). As with reinforcement by nondrug reinforcers (5), laboratory studies have shown that discriminative stimuli can dramatically influence drug seeking and drug taking.

Discriminative Stimuli and Drug Self-Administration The power of discriminative stimuli to influence drug seeking and drug taking was dramatically illustrated in a study in which rats' lever presses were reinforced with intravenous cocaine infusions when a tone or a light was on, but not when the tone and light were off (i.e., differential reinforcement) (24). Tests were then conducted in which the light and tone

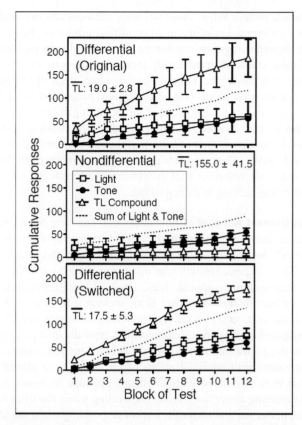

Figure 7.2. Results of stimulus-compounding tests performed in extinction for the rats originally given differential training (Differential group; *upper panel*) and for rats in the nondifferential group after nondifferential training *(center panel)* and after being switched to the differential schedule *(lower panel)*. Data presented as mean cumulative number of responses (±SEM) by blocks in tone, light, and the tone-light (TL) compound. Dotted lines represent the sum of the tone (T) and light (L) curves. Mean (±SEM) number of responses in the absence of tone and light ($\overline{TL}$) over the entire test is indicated numerically for each condition. During each block, tone, light, and tone-plus-light were each presented for 1 minute, and the ($\overline{TL}$) was presented for a total of 3 minutes. (Reproduced from Panlilio LV, Weiss SJ, Schindler CW. Cocaine self-administration increased by compounding discriminative stimuli. *Psychopharmacology (Berl)*. 1996;125(3): 202–208, with permission.)

were each presented alone and together. In tests in which cocaine infusions were not provided, the rats showed a threefold increase in the rate of lever pressing when the tone and light were presented together above the rate when either of those stimuli was presented alone (see Fig. 7.2, top panel; differential reinforcement). In subsequent tests in which cocaine infusions were provided contingent on lever pressing, the rats showed a twofold increase in the amount of cocaine intake when the tone and light were presented together compared to when either of those stimuli was presented alone (data not shown). Importantly, compounding the two stimuli did not increase lever pressing in rats who had undergone training in which the tone and light were presented at random times, unrelated to the availability of cocaine reinforcement (nondifferential reinforcement, middle panel). When those rats were subsequently exposed to a differential reinforcement condition similar to the rats in the original group, combining the tone and light had the similar effect of dramatically increasing the rate of lever pressing above the rates observed when each stimulus was presented alone (Fig. 7.2; bottom panel, differential reinforcement). Similar effects of compounding discriminative stimuli can increase heroin-maintained responding and heroin intake, as well as food-maintained responding and food intake. These studies provide clear evidence of the remarkable influence that discriminative stimuli can exert over drug seeking and drug taking.

An Operant Account of Reinstatement For over 30 years, researchers have investigated a laboratory model of relapse called the reinstatement model (25). Under this model, subjects experience self-administration sessions in which a drug-seeking response (e.g., lever pressing) produces drug administrations. After drug seeking and drug self-administration are established under this arrangement, the drug-seeking response is extinguished, typically by replacing the drug with saline or vehicle. In subsequent test sessions, noncontingent administrations of the drug (or of stimuli that were associated with the drug) produce increases in responding above the level of responding when the drug is not presented and above the level of responding when saline or vehicle is administered. In general, reinstatement of responding increases as a function of the dose of the drug tested, the similarity of the test drug to original training drug, and whether the drug is presented alone or in combination with stimuli that were associated with drug administration in the original training sessions (25).

From an operant perspective, a drug that has a reinforcing function (as a consequence) can also acquire a discriminative function (as an antecedent). In drug self-administration sessions, as in other studies of operant reinforcement, the reinforcer is presented contingent on responding on given trials, but it also precedes responding on subsequent trials. Through this arrangement, reinforcers can acquire discriminative functions for subsequent responding. Similar to the studies of drug reinstatement described above, several studies have shown that noncontingent presentation of nondrug reinforcers could reinstate extinguished responding in rats (26,27), pigeons (26), college students (26), developmentally delayed individuals (28), and baboons (29). These studies showed that the reinstated responding occurs uniquely in response to the presentation of the reinforcer, and did not occur when selected other novel stimuli are presented. One study explicitly established the reinforcers as discriminative stimuli (27). In that study, rats were exposed to sessions in which periods of availability of standard food pellets and sucrose pellets alternated. When standard food pellets were available, only left lever presses produced reinforcement, whereas when sucrose pellets were available, only right lever presses produced reinforcement. By the 35th session, the rats shifted their responses throughout the session in concert with the shifting availability of the different kinds of pellets. When food pellets were provided, the rats made more left-lever presses; when sucrose pellets were available, the rats made more right-lever presses. The results obtained in this study showed that the type of pellet acquired discriminative stimulus and reinforcing functions, and provided experimental evidence that a stimulus can simultaneously serve as a reinforcer and a discriminative stimulus.

Drug-Seeking Response

In general, drug self-administration varies as a function of the effort or price required to procure the drug. In laboratory studies with nonhuman subjects and sometimes with human subjects, this phenomenon is investigated by modulating the number of responses required for each drug administration. While the precise relationship between consumption and response requirement can differ as a function of a variety of conditions, extensive laboratory research in nonhuman and human subjects confirms that consumption of a particular reinforcer generally decreases as the number of responses required for reinforcement increases (22).

If the number of responses required for reinforcement is increased progressively, nonhuman and human subjects will typically reach a response requirement where they stop responding to drug. The point at which a particular subject stops responding is called a breaking point and has been used widely as a measure of the strength of a reinforcer. In a seminal study (30), rats could press a lever to receive sweetened condensed milk, but the number of responses required for each reinforcer increased progressively within the session. When the concentration of the sweetened condensed milk was varied in a random order across days for two rats, breaking points for both subjects increased as the concentration increased. Furthermore, when the total amount of food consumed each day for two other rats was decreased to reduce their body weight, the breaking points increased as their body weights decreased. Analyses of breaking points have been used extensively to study variables that modulate drug reinforcement (31,32).

In general, as the number of responses required for a given dose of a drug increases, intake of that drug decreases (22). Frequently, as the number of drug-seeking responses required for each drug administration increases, overall responding increases in a way that produces a relatively small decrease in the overall intake of the drug. However, at some point, progressive increases in the response requirements will produce more dramatic decreases in response rate and overall drug intake (22).

Establishing Operations

Certain motivational variables called establishing operations can affect the reinforcing effectiveness of a stimulus (5). The effects of deprivation and satiation in increasing and decreasing, respectively, reinforcement-maintained behavior have been recognized for many years and have been demonstrated for behaviors maintained by a variety of reinforcers, from food reinforcement in rats (30) to social reinforcement in children (33). As with nondrug reinforcers, drug reinforcement can be modulated by a variety of establishing operations.

Early studies of drug reinforcement in nonhuman subjects showed that chronic administration of opioids can produce physical dependence and can serve as a robust establishing operation that modulates the reinforcing effects of opioid drugs (6,11,34). While it quickly became clear that drugs can serve as reinforcers in individuals who are not physically dependent, research conducted over the past 40 years shows that self-administration of opioid drugs like heroin can be increased in opioid-dependent subjects after a period of forced abstinence or after the administration of an opioid antagonist. Provision of opioid agonists prior to self-administrations can also decrease opioid reinforcement (35). Several studies in humans have shown that the behavioral requirements following drug administration can modulate the reinforcing effects of a drug (13). In one study, for example, reinforcement by the sedative triazolam was increased when participants were required to lie down and rest following drug administration, whereas amphetamine reinforcement was increased when participants had to perform a vigilance task following drug administration.

Regulation of Drug Intake As illustrated in the study by Deneau and colleagues described above (7), when laboratory animals are given unrestricted and continuous access to drugs, patterns of drug use emerge that appear specific to the drug and frequently lead to severe toxic consequences up to and including death. However, many laboratory studies impose constraints on drug consumption by, for example, restricting the duration of study sessions or the number of drug administrations allowed. In these laboratory studies, animals and human subjects frequently show patterns of drug use that have been reasonably described as regulated. Under those conditions, animals tend to respond in ways that maintain a relatively constant overall amount of drug over time (21). Increases in the dose of the drug, for example, increases the pausing between responses and thereby increases the duration of the interval between self-administered doses. Lynch and Carroll (21) suggested that regulation of drug intake is controlled by aversive effects of high drug intake that subjects might avoid or escape; direct effects of high drug intake that might directly diminish response rates; and a satiation that occurs with high drug intake and that produces an establishing condition which might diminish the momentary reinforcing value of the drug, similar to the effects of satiation with food or other reinforcers.

Modulation of Drug Reinforcement by Nondrug Consequences

Drug use occurs in complex environments. Drug users engage in many behaviors, of which drug use is only one. These behaviors have varied consequences; and drug reinforcement is only one of those consequences. An extensive body of laboratory research in nonhuman and human subjects has shown that drug self-administration can be modulated by nondrug consequences when those consequences are arranged directly on the drug self-administration behaviors, and when those consequences are arranged contingent on other behaviors.

Punishment

Behaviors can have both positive and potentially unpleasant consequences. Sweet and bitter tastes in foods might function to increase or decrease, respectively, the eating of different foods. The discussion above has focused on reinforcers, the consequences of behavior that increase the future probability of those behaviors. Here we focus on consequences that decrease the future probability of behaviors. When an event is presented contingent on a behavior and that contingency decreases the future probability of that behavior, the event is called a punisher and the process is called punishment. Research on punishment has shown that events like electric shock can have profound and very orderly effects on operant behavior (5).

In an early study, Grove and Schuster (36) examined the effects of punishment on cocaine self-administration in rhesus monkeys. That study showed that cocaine self-administration was decreased when brief electric shocks were administered along with cocaine administrations contingent on lever pressing. Furthermore, the study showed clearly that the rate of shocked responses decreased as the shock intensity increased.

Relatively little research has been done to evaluate the effects of punishment on human drug taking; however, some classic studies were conducted by Bigelow, Griffiths, and Liebson in the 1970s that demonstrated that alcohol use is sensitive to punishment (37). In one of those studies, 10 "chronic alcoholics" were invited to participate while residing on a residential research unit. Participants were allowed to drink between 12 and 24 drinks (the maximum number differed for different participants). Using a within-subject reversal design, the study evaluated the effects of contingent isolation on alcohol drinking. After an initial baseline period, participants were exposed to a Contingent Isolation condition in which they were required to go to an isolation booth for 10 to 15 minutes immediately after receiving a drink; six of the participants were exposed to a second baseline condition. The study demonstrated clear and substantial decreases in alcohol drinking during the Contingent Isolation condition. Although there was variation in the amount of suppression, on average participants decreased drinking by 50% of the baseline period; drinking was almost completely suppressed in two participants; and only one participant showed no decrease.

Reinforcement of Alternative Behaviors

Organisms engage in a range of behaviors that are maintained by different reinforcers. Drug users, for example, may engage in behaviors to obtain and use drugs; but they also eat, sleep, talk, work, and play, all under the control of different reinforcers. Organisms continually make choices between reinforcers and distribute their behavior accordingly. A large body of research conducted in laboratory studies suggests that nondrug reinforcement for behaviors that are alternatives to drug use can decrease drug use.

Extensive research, primarily conducted in nonhuman subjects, has shown that organisms distribute their behaviors among available alternatives in ways that increase, and possibly maximize, their overall rate of reinforcement. Research conducted over the past 40 years has generally confirmed a principle proposed by Richard Herrnstein (19) called the matching law that explains how reinforcement rates for different behaviors affect choice. Highly controlled laboratory studies in which subjects have multiple response options have shown that, in general, the relative rate of responding for any response option is equal to the relative rate of reinforcement obtained for that option. Importantly, this relationship is very precise and quantitatively predictable and has been observed in diverse species, including in humans.

The matching law is relevant to understanding and treating drug addiction, because it suggests that drug use could be decreased by arranging nondrug reinforcers for behaviors that would be alternatives to drug seeking and drug use. Indeed, one study showed that when rhesus monkeys were given opportunities to respond for food or cocaine, the matching law provided a good description of how the monkeys distributed their responding across those two options (38).

In matching studies, subjects are generally free to engage in either of two (or more) responses in the same time interval, they can alternate responses continually over time, and obtaining reinforcement for one response option does not preclude obtaining reinforcement for the other option. Many related studies have been conducted in which subjects are given mutually exclusive choices between drug and nondrug reinforcers. In these studies, on repeated trials, the subject can choose to take the drug or the nondrug alternative; taking one option precludes taking the other. This research has shown that drug taking can be decreased dramatically by offering nondrug alternative reinforcers (39). In this paradigm, alternative reinforcers have been shown to decrease use of most commonly abused drugs, including alcohol, cigarettes, cocaine, opiates, benzodiazepines, and in diverse species including rats, monkeys, and humans. Importantly, drug use decreases as the magnitude of the alternative reinforcer increases (35,40).

Validity of the Laboratory Model of Drug Addiction

Are demonstrations of drug self-administration in laboratory animals and humans qualitatively similar to clinical instances of drug addiction? We probably cannot answer this question definitively, but data collected in selected studies provides some evidence of the validity of the laboratory models of drug addiction. First and probably most persuasively, several early studies showed that laboratory animals will self-administer some drugs persistently, despite serious adverse consequences. As noted above, Deneau and colleagues (7) showed that monkeys continued self-administration of cocaine despite severe toxicity, including biting of their skin and fingers to the point of amputation and death within 30 days.

More recently, researchers studying nonhuman models of addiction (41–43) have developed intriguing models that attempt to apply the clinical criteria for addiction to classify their subjects as addicted or not, including the adaptation of formal clinical criteria for drug dependence. Under one model (41), rats are given repeated opportunities over many sessions to self-administer cocaine under a simple schedule in which nose pokes through a hole in a chamber wall produce infusions of cocaine. Within each session, periods of cocaine availability are signaled by the illumination of a blue key light and alternate with periods in which nose pokes do not produce cocaine infusions; periods of nonavailability are signaled by darkening of the key light and the illumination of the chamber. To assess whether individual rats meet criteria for addiction, three tests were administered. The first test assessed whether the rat "has difficulty stopping drug use or limiting drug intake." Under this test, the experimenters measured the rats drug seeking (i.e., nose pokes) during the signaled periods within sessions when cocaine is not available. The second test assessed whether the rat had "an extremely high motivation to take the drug, with activities focused on procurement and consumption." Under this test, cocaine was available to subjects under a progressive ratio schedule in which the number of responses (nose pokes) required for each cocaine infusion increased progressively across the session; the measure of "addiction" was the breakpoint, or the maximum number of responses that the rat made before responding stopped. The third test assessed the extent to which cocaine use is "continued despite its harmful consequences." To assess this, the experimenters measured the rat's persistence of cocaine-reinforced responding when responses (nose pokes) were also punished with electric shocks. This arrangement yielded a variety of intriguing observations on the nature of drug self-administration in laboratory animals. Perhaps most interestingly, this research has shown that there is considerable variability in the amount and persistence of drug self-administration both across and within rats. In one study (41), rats were categorized based on the amount of cocaine-seeking responses emitted on the three tests of "addiction"; rats in the 66th to the 99th percentile of each test were considered to be positive for that cocaine addiction criterion. Almost half the rats (41.4%) were not positive for any of the criteria and only a minority (17%) was positive for all three criteria.

Interestingly, the presence or absence of the more extreme and persistent patterns of cocaine self-administration can also vary within individual rats, and appears to be related to a number of parameters of the drug self-administration sessions, such as the duration of cocaine self-administration sessions (42), the number of drug self-administrations sessions, and the duration of the cocaine injections (43). These individual differences in cocaine self-administration provide interesting parallels to human drug use and addiction.

The various models of addiction described in this research demonstrated that some individuals show more persistent drug use than others, and that certain environmental conditions can lead to more persistent or higher levels of drug use. These are important and interesting observations. However, it is important to note that drug use of "addicted" individuals still appears to be operant behavior that is maintained by drug reinforcement and is sensitive to nondrug consequences (41). Furthermore, in these studies, the designation of "addicted" or "compulsive" seems to convert characteristics that vary on a continuum to dichotomous groupings. While some individuals may be more sensitive to drug reinforcement than others, either due to unspecified biologic differences or due to different environmental histories, even the behavior of the most "addicted" or "compulsive" rats appears sensitive to its consequences and operant in nature.

OPERANT MODULATION OF DRUG USE IN CLINICAL POPULATIONS

Laboratory research shows that drug self-administration can be viewed as operant behavior that is maintained by drug reinforcement and modifiable by the same range of environmental events that affect other operant behavior; however, the relevance of the laboratory research to understanding human drug addiction is not certain. Importantly, clinical research on the effects of environmental interventions provides additional support that drug addiction is operant behavior and sensitive to its consequences. Two types of environmental interventions are particularly informative: (1) interventions that increase the price of a drug and (2) abstinence reinforcement interventions that provide nondrug reinforcement contingent on drug abstinence.

Population level analyses of the effects on price on cigarette smoking have shown that increases in prices can decrease cigarette smoking, particularly among low-income populations and adolescents (44). These data are consistent with studies of drug reinforcement described above that show that an increase in the number of responses required for drug reinforcement, and a laboratory analog of price, can decrease drug self-administration.

For about 40 years, researchers have studied the effectiveness of interventions that arrange for the direct reinforcement of drug abstinence (45). Under these procedures, patients receive a desirable consequence contingent on providing biologic evidence of drug abstinence (e.g., drug-free urine samples). These procedures have proven to be among the most effective behavioral or psychosocial treatments for drug addiction (46). In addition to demonstrating the clinical utility of the operant approach, these studies also show that persistent drug use is sensitive to its consequences and operant in nature.

Some of the clearest data come from research on voucher-based abstinence reinforcement. In 1991, Higgins and colleagues developed a voucher-based reinforcement intervention. In this intervention, patients received monetary vouchers exchangeable for goods and services for providing cocaine-negative urine samples (47). A recent meta-analysis showed that voucher-based abstinence reinforcement has effectively promoted abstinence from cocaine, opiates, opiates and cocaine, polydrug use, marijuana, and cigarette smoking (47).

A number of the studies reviewed in that meta-analysis compared the effects of voucher-based abstinence reinforcement to control conditions in which participants were randomly assigned to receive vouchers on a noncontingent basis, independent of their urinalysis results. In those studies, the two groups differed only in whether or not vouchers were presented contingent on drug-free urines. This kind of comparison allows for the determination of whether the presentation of vouchers *contingent* on drug-free urine samples is critical in producing the abstinence outcomes. Like the noncontingent control conditions described above in the studies of drug reinforcement, the noncontingent control conditions arranged in clinical research studies allow us to determine whether operant reinforcement is the mechanism responsible for the increase in abstinence. The meta-analysis showed that the outcomes of studies that used noncontingent control conditions were similar to the outcomes of studies that used no-voucher control conditions; and in both groups of studies, the voucher-based abstinence reinforcement produced medium effect sizes.

The first voucher study to use a noncontingent control condition evaluated the effectiveness of a voucher-based abstinence reinforcement intervention in promoting cocaine abstinence in injection drug users who were enrolled in methadone treatment in Baltimore City (48). In that study, participants were randomly assigned to an abstinence reinforcement intervention in which they could earn up to $1155 in vouchers for providing cocaine-free urine samples (Abstinence Reinforcement Group) or to a noncontingent control group (Control Group). Figure 7.3 shows that 47% of the

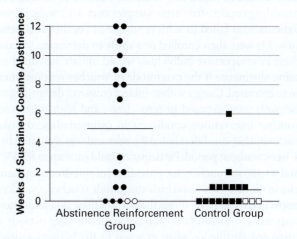

Figure 7.3. Longest duration of sustained cocaine abstinence achieved during the 12-week voucher condition. Each point represents data for an individual patient and the lines represent group means. The 19 Abstinence Reinforcement patients are displayed in the left column (circles) and the 18 control patients in the right (squares). Open symbols represent patients who dropped out of the study early. (Reproduced from Silverman K, Higgins ST, Brooner RK, et al. Sustained cocaine abstinence in methadone maintenance patients through voucher-based reinforcement therapy. *Arch Gen Psychiatry*. 1996;53(5):409–415, with permission.)

participants in the Abstinence Reinforcement Group achieved over 7 weeks of sustained cocaine abstinence, whereas only 6% of the Control Group achieved more than 2 weeks of abstinence. This study provided a vivid demonstration of the effectiveness of the voucher-based abstinence reinforcement intervention, and also showed that the contingency between voucher presentation and cocaine urinalysis was critical in producing the abstinence outcomes. These results provide additional evidence that the drug use of many drug users that we see in our clinics is sensitive to its consequences and operant in nature.

Not all individuals achieve sustained abstinence when exposed to an abstinence reinforcement intervention. As would be expected based on the research on operant conditioning described above, responsiveness to abstinence reinforcement interventions can be modulated by manipulating key parameters of operant conditioning. The meta-analysis on voucher-based reinforcement described above, for example, showed that a decreased delay to voucher reinforcement and increased voucher magnitude were associated with better effectiveness of the voucher intervention. These data provide further support for the operant nature of the persistent drug use in clinical populations.

Despite our best efforts, in virtually all (if not all) studies of abstinence reinforcement, some individuals do not achieve abstinence. Is the drug use of those nonresponsive individuals truly "out of control" and not sensitive to consequences? Silverman and colleagues conducted a study that partially addressed this issue (49). In that study, injection drug users who used cocaine persistently during methadone treatment were exposed to a voucher-based abstinence reinforcement intervention in which they could earn $1,155 in vouchers for providing cocaine-free urine samples over a 12-week period. Patients who failed to achieve sustained cocaine abstinence ($n = 22$) were then enrolled in a study to determine whether these nonresponsive individuals would initiate sustained cocaine abstinence if the magnitude of voucher reinforcement were increased. Using a within-subject crossover design, all participants were exposed to zero-, low-, and high-magnitude voucher intervention conditions in counterbalanced order. Each voucher condition lasted 9 weeks and was separated by a 4-week washout period. Participants could earn up to $0, $382, and $3,480 in vouchers for providing cocaine-free urine samples in the zero-, low-, and high-magnitude voucher conditions, respectively. Figure 7.4 shows that 45% of these previously nonresponsive individuals (10 of 22) achieved long periods of sustained abstinence when exposed to the high-magnitude voucher intervention in which they could earn up to $3,480 in vouchers over 9 weeks. This study suggests that the proportion of individuals whose cocaine use appears unresponsive to its consequences can be dwindled down by systematically manipulating familiar parameters of operant conditioning. We do not know whether further manipulations could promote abstinence in the remaining group of unresponsive individuals, but the data reviewed in this chapter provide a strong basis to expect that the persistent cocaine use of even the most refractory individuals would prove malleable given the right parameters.

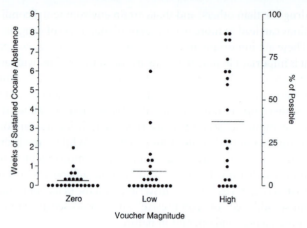

Figure 7.4. Longest duration of sustained cocaine abstinence achieved by a group of methadone maintenance patients who had failed to initiate sustained cocaine abstinence when exposed to a standard voucher intervention in which they could have earned up to $1,155 in vouchers for providing cocaine-negative urine samples. Each of these individuals was exposed to a zero (*left column*), low (*middle column*), and high (*right column*) magnitude voucher conditions, in counterbalanced order. Each *point* represents data for an individual patient ($n = 22$) and the *lines* represent condition means. Each patient was exposed to each of the three voucher conditions in counterbalanced order. The maximum possible duration of sustained abstinence was 9 weeks for each condition. (Reproduced from Silverman K, Chutuape MA, Bigelow GE, et al. Voucher-based reinforcement of cocaine abstinence in treatment-resistant methadone patients: effects of reinforcement magnitude. *Psychopharmacology (Berl)*. 1999; 146(2):128–138, with permission.)

CONCLUSIONS

The laboratory and clinical research that we have reviewed provides strong evidence that drug addiction *can* be operant behavior that is maintained and modifiable by its consequences. The laboratory research on nonhuman and human drug self-administration has provided an impressive model of drug addiction as operant behavior that is (1) maintained by drug reinforcement; (2) under the strong antecedent control of discriminative stimuli that acquire their influence through conditioning histories; (3) sensitive to the effort or price required to procure the drug; (4) modulated by a variety of establishing operations that alter the reinforcing value of drugs; and (5) profoundly modified by nondrug consequences, either through the direct punishment of drug seeking or drug use or through the reinforcement of behaviors that are alternatives to drug use. Drug self-administration in the laboratory bears important resemblances to the persistent drug use that we see in clinical populations and suggests that laboratory studies of drug reinforcement provide a valid model of drug addiction. The validity of the operant model of drug addiction is probably most impressively established in the applications of these principles to the treatment of drug addiction in clinical populations, particularly in the large number of studies that have demonstrated that persistent drug use, including drug use in some of the most refractory patients, can be decreased by the direct reinforcement of drug abstinence.

In offering this analysis, we do not intend to suggest that the principles of operant conditioning are the only factors that influence drug addiction. To say that drug addiction can be viewed as operant behavior that is maintained and modifiable by its consequences does not ignore the importance of biologic or genetic factors in understanding addiction. As emphasized in this chapter, the basic process of reinforcement that underlies addiction is a fundamental principle of behavior that is common across a vast range of organisms from the simple sea slug to humans. If nothing else, the commonality of the basic process of reinforcement across biologic species suggests that reinforcement itself is a fundamental biologic process. Furthermore, as we have described in this chapter, sensitivity to drug reinforcement is also common across a wide range of organisms, a fact that provides further evidence of the genetic basis of drug reinforcement itself. Like all genetically determined characteristics, organisms can vary in their susceptibility to drug reinforcement because of their genetic makeup.

To recognize that drug addiction is ultimately controlled by observable environmental events (reinforcers, discriminative stimuli, response requirements, contingencies, and establishing operations) does not deny the existence of private events (50). Private events can serve as discriminative stimuli, responses, and even reinforcers in a conceptual analysis. However, private events like craving or pleasure that are frequently considered internal causes of addiction have yet to be objectively measured (i.e., by two independent observers) or manipulated, and thus must remain outside of our present analysis. Importantly, the existence of private events does not diminish the value of the experimental manipulation of environmental events that have been shown to modulate drug use in laboratory models and in clinical settings. The facts related to the role of private events (or other intervening variables) in drug addiction, whatever they may be, do not alter the functional relations between behavior and environment reviewed here.

Drug addiction is frequently described as behavior that is "out of control." Yet, the operant analysis described in this chapter suggests that much of what we describe as drug addiction is orderly behavior under clear environmental control. Far from being out of control, persistent drug use in laboratory subjects and in clinical populations can be systematically modulated by manipulating key features of the operant arrangement. The operant analysis has much to contribute to our understanding of drug addiction at the conceptual level and to the treatment of this troubling clinical problem.

ACKNOWLEDGEMENTS

Preparation of this chapter was supported by grants R01DA13107, R01DA019386, R01DA019497, R01DA023864, and T32DA07209 from the National Institute on Drug Abuse, National Institutes of Health.

REFERENCES

1. Skinner BF. *Science and Human Behavior*. New York: Macmillan; 1953.
2. Brembs B, Lorenzetti FD, Reyes FD, et al. Operant reward learning in aplysia: neuronal correlates and mechanisms. *Science*. 2002;296(5573):1706–1709.
3. Grossett D, Roy S, Sharenow E, et al. Subjects used in JEAB articles: is the snark a pigeon? *Behav Analyst*. 1982;5(2):189–190.
4. Skinner BF. Selection by consequences. *Science*. 1981;213(4507): 501–504.
5. Catania AC. *Learning*. 4th interim ed. Cornwall-on-Hudson, NY: Sloan Pub.; 2007.
6. Schuster CR, Thompson T. Self administration of and behavioral dependence on drugs. *Annu Rev Pharmacol*. 1969;9: 483–502.
7. Deneau G, Yanagita T, Seevers MH. Self-administration of psychoactive substances by the monkey. *Psychopharmacologia*. 1969;16(1):30–48.
8. Griffiths RR, Bigelow GE, Henningfield JE. Similarities in animal and human drug-taking behavior. In: Mello NK, ed. *Advances in Substance Abuse*. Greenwich, CT: JAI Press, Inc.; 1980:1–90.
9. Johanson CE, Fischman MW. The pharmacology of cocaine related to its abuse. *Pharmacol Rev*. 1989;41(1):3–52.
10. Carroll ME, Bickel WK. Behavioral-environmental determinants of the reinforcing functions of cocaine. In: Higgins ST, Katz JL, eds. *Cocaine Abuse: Behavior, Pharmacology, and Clinical Applications*. San Diego, CA: Academic Press; 1998:81–106.
11. Schuster CR, Johanson CE. An analysis of drug-seeking behavior in animals. *Neurosci Biobehav Rev*. 1981;5(3):315–323.
12. Meisch RA. Oral drug self-administration: an overview of laboratory animal studies. *Alcohol*. 2001;24(2):117–128.
13. Griffiths RR, Weerts EM. Benzodiazepine self-administration in humans and laboratory animals–implications for problems of long-term use and abuse. *Psychopharmacology (Berl)*. 1997; 134(1):1–37.
14. Le Foll B, Goldberg SR. Control of the reinforcing effects of nicotine by associated environmental stimuli in animals and humans. *Trends Pharmacol Sci*. 2005;26(6):287–293.
15. Justinova Z, Goldberg SR, Heishman SJ, et al. Self-administration of cannabinoids by experimental animals and human marijuana smokers. *Pharmacol Biochem Behav*. 2005;81(2):285–299.
16. Mierzejewski P, Koros E, Goldberg SR, et al. Intravenous self-administration of morphine and cocaine: a comparative study. *Pol J Pharmacol*. 2003;55(5):713–726.
17. DeFulio A, Hackenberg TD. Combinations of response-dependent and response-independent schedule-correlated stimulus presentation in an observing procedure. *J Exp Anal Behav*. 2008;89(3): 299–309.
18. Lecca D, Cacciapaglia F, Valentini V, et al. Differential neurochemical and behavioral adaptation to cocaine after response contingent and noncontingent exposure in the rat. *Psychopharmacology (Berl)*. 2007;191(3):653–667.
19. Herrnstein RJ, Rachlin H, Laibson DI. *The Matching Law: Papers in Psychology and Economics*. New York; Cambridge, Mass.: Russell Sage Foundation; Harvard University Press; 1997.
20. Woolverton WL, Wang Z. Relationship between injection duration, transporter occupancy and reinforcing strength of cocaine. *Eur J Pharmacol*. 2004;486(3):251–257.
21. Lynch WJ, Carroll ME. Regulation of drug intake. *Exp Clin Psychopharmacol*. 2001;9(2):131–143.

22. Hursh SR, Galuska CM, Winger G, et al. The economics of drug abuse: a quantitative assessment of drug demand. *Mol Interv*. 2005;5(1):20–28.
23. Kirby KC, Lamb RJ, Iguchi MY, et al. Situations occasioning cocaine use and cocaine abstinence strategies. *Addiction*. 1995;90(9):1241–1252.
24. Panlilio LV, Weiss SJ, Schindler CW. Cocaine self-administration increased by compounding discriminative stimuli. *Psychopharmacology (Berl)*. 1996;125(3):202–208.
25. Carroll ME, Comer SD. Animal models of relapse. *Exp Clin Psychopharmacol*. 1996;4(1):11–18.
26. Reid RL. The role of the reinforcer as a stimulus. *Br J Psychol*. 1958;49(3):202–209.
27. Cruse DB, Vitulli W, Dertke M. Discriminative and reinforcing properties of two types of food pellets. *J Exp Anal Behav*. 1966;9(3):293–303.
28. Spradlin JE, Fixsen DL, Girarbeau FL. Reinstatement of an operant response by the delivery of reinforcement during extinction. *J Exp Child Psychol*. 1969;7(1):96–100.
29. Foltin RW, Evans SM. Effect of response-independent candy on responding maintained by candy using a novel model of commodity acquisition and consumption in nonhuman primates. *Pharmacol Biochem Behav*. 2002;72(3):729–739.
30. Hodos W. Progressive ratio as a measure of reward strength. *Science*. 1961;134:943–944.
31. Stafford D, LeSage MG, Glowa JR. Progressive-ratio schedules of drug delivery in the analysis of drug self-administration: a review. *Psychopharmacology (Berl)*. 1998;139(3):169–184.
32. Stoops WW. Reinforcing effects of stimulants in humans: sensitivity of progressive-ratio schedules. *Exp Clin Psychopharmacol*. 2008;16(6):503–512.
33. Gewirtz JL, Baer DM. Deprivation and satiation of social reinforcers as drive conditions. *J Abnorm Psychol*. 1958;57(2):165–172.
34. Katz JL. Drugs as reinforcers: pharmacological and behavioral factors. In: Liebman JM, Cooper SJ, eds. *The Neuropharmacological Basis of Reward*. Oxford, U.K.: Oxford University Press; 1989:164–213.
35. Donny EC, Brassier SM, Bigelow GE, et al. Methadone doses of 100 mg or greater are more effective than lower doses at suppressing heroin self-administration in opioid-dependent volunteers. *Addiction*. 2005;100(10):1496–1509.
36. Grove RN, Schuster CR. Suppression of cocaine self-administration by extinction and punishment. *Pharmacol Biochem Behav*. 1974;2(2):199–208.
37. Bigelow G, Liebson I, Griffiths H. Alcoholic drinking: suppression by a brief time-out procedure. *Behav Res Ther*. 1974;12(2):107–115.
38. Anderson KG, Velkey AJ, Woolverton WL. The generalized matching law as a predictor of choice between cocaine and food in rhesus monkeys. *Psychopharmacology (Berl)*. 2002;163(3–4):319–326.
39. Higgins ST. The influence of alternative reinforcers on cocaine use and abuse: a brief review. *Pharmacol Biochem Behav*. 1997;57(3):419–427.
40. Nader MA, Woolverton WL. Effects of increasing the magnitude of an alternative reinforcer on drug choice in a discrete-trials choice procedure. *Psychopharmacology (Berl)*. 1991;105(2):169–174.
41. Deroche-Gamonet V, Belin D, Piazza PV. Evidence for addiction-like behavior in the rat. *Science*. 2004;305(5686):1014–1017.
42. Ahmed SH, Koob GF. Transition from moderate to excessive drug intake: change in hedonic set point. *Science*. 1998;282(5387):298–300.
43. Roberts DC, Morgan D, Liu Y. How to make a rat addicted to cocaine. *Prog Neuropsychopharmacol Biol Psychiatry*. 2007;31(8):1614–1624.
44. Thomas S, Fayter D, Misso K, et al. Population tobacco control interventions and their effects on social inequalities in smoking: systematic review. *Tob Control*. 2008;17(4):230–237.
45. Higgins ST, Silverman K, Heil SH. *Contingency Management in Substance Abuse Treatment*. New York: Guilford Press; 2008.
46. Dutra L, Stathopoulou G, Basden SL, et al. A meta-analytic review of psychosocial interventions for substance use disorders. *Am J Psychiatry*. 2008;165(2):179–187.
47. Lussier JP, Heil SH, Mongeon JA, et al. A meta-analysis of voucher-based reinforcement therapy for substance use disorders. *Addiction*. 2006;101(2):192–203.
48. Silverman K, Higgins ST, Brooner RK, et al. Sustained cocaine abstinence in methadone maintenance patients through voucher-based reinforcement therapy. *Arch Gen Psychiatry*. 1996;53(5):409–415.
49. Silverman K, Chutuape MA, Bigelow GE, et al. Voucher-based reinforcement of cocaine abstinence in treatment-resistant methadone patients: effects of reinforcement magnitude. *Psychopharmacology (Berl)*. 1999;146(2):128–138.
50. Skinner BF. *About Behaviorism*. Oxford England: Alfred A. Knopf; 1974.

CHAPTER 8

Sociocultural Factors and Their Implications

Nady el-Guebaly ■ Pedro Ruiz

Mankind's relationship with substances served socially desired functions. Drugs were used as medicine, in the performance of rituals and religious functions and as recreation. Not surprisingly, sociocultural factors have played a major role in moderating or modulating the use of these substances. Sociocultural factors affect individuals either through small group effects or through the larger social environment. Each of these factors may have both risk and protective properties. They are part of the etiology as well as prevention and treatment of substance abuse. Increasingly, over the last decade the focus of research has moved from the investigation of a list of sociocultural factors in isolation to a study of their relative relevance and interdependence as well as their links with genetic influences. This chapter highlights the promises of these fields of inquiry. The following are current definitions of the concepts of society and culture, including race and ethnicity as an extension of culture.

Society refers to a group of persons regarded as forming a single community of related, interdependent individuals. Social factors are the variables affecting their dealings with one another.

Culture is the set of meanings, behavioral norms, values, every day practices, and beliefs used by members of a particular group in society as a way of conceptualizing their views of the world and during their interactions with their environment. In this context, culture includes language, nonverbal expressions, social relationships, style of expressions of emotions, conditions, and/or philosophies.

Ethnicity refers to a subjective sense of belonging to a given group of persons who are held to have a common origin and share a matrix of cultural beliefs and practices. In this context, ethnicity becomes a component of one's sense of identity; it, thus, needs to be regarded as an important source of clinical and social manifestations with respect to the person's self-image and intrapsychic life.

Race is a concept under which human beings historically chose to group themselves, based primarily on their common physiognomy; in this context, physical, biologic, and genetic connotations can also be attached to this concept (1).

SOCIAL GROUPS AND THE MICROENVIRONMENT

Small group effects may protect or facilitate an individual's drug use through one or several of the following social communities.

The Family Unit and Parenting

Family interactions may serve as protective or risk factors for drug use. Youth's first drug-related discussions and/or modeling of use occurs through the parental and older siblings' perceptions and behaviors. Examples of predictive factors for drug use include conflict-ridden versus warm family interactions, quality and quantity of family time a child experiences as well as parental monitoring of child's activities (2). Earlier general statements about family interactions are now challenged by further contextual analyses in recent research.

Parenting styles have been a focus of evaluation both as protective factors including degree of parental warmth as well as limit setting. In general, substance abusers have been described as dysfunctional parents. Addicted women's parenting has been, in prior research, characterized by a range of across the board parenting deficits including neglect, physical and emotional abuse, excessive control and punishment, inconsistent discipline, and lack of emotional involvement. This indictment uniquely attributed to the mother's drug abuse needs to be investigated against other contextual factors such as low socioeconomic status (SES) and the mother's perceptions of the children's maladaptive behavior. A study compared 120 mothers (i.e., methadone enrollees) with a child under 16 years of age demographically matched with mothers attending a primary care facility serving comparable lower SES women. While the link between maternal addiction and a lack of parental involvement was confirmed, the link between low SES and a parental style leading to a child's restricted autonomy could be an adaptive response to living in environments where children's exposure to violence, crime, drug addiction, and health hazards is more. Cohabitation with partners and having fewer children may also lead to more protective and enmeshed parenting style. This study demonstrates the importance of studying the impact of drug use against other contextual factors, such as poverty, transience, vocational instability, trauma exposure, and children's maladjustment, as well as the need to differentiate parenting effectiveness across different parenting domains (3).

Another related challenge has been the study of partner support or coping in response to the addiction (4). Initial notions about family members pathologized their reactions to disordered drinking or attributed blame for the drinking on spouses of alcoholics. Significant others are now recognized to engage in coping behaviors with substance abusers along with experiencing significant mental and physical strain resulting from their specific types of caretaking and attempts to stabilize the dyadic or family environment. Such specific behaviors have ranged from enabling, potentially reinforcing continued use of alcohol or other drugs to the more ambiguous construct of codependency with themes of caretaking, pleasing others, and association with a person who has alcohol or drug problems. The coping behaviors of wives of alcoholics have been described as a trial-and-error progression from attempts at logical persuasion, nagging, threats to leave to more "behind the scenes" manipulative approaches, many futile (5). In general, studies using control groups and psychologically oriented measures with adult children of alcoholics have not supported the codependency construct (6).

The Peer Group

Friends and peer affiliation can inhibit or promote drug use behaviors. Group members are influenced to act consistently to gain or maintain acceptance of other group members. Affiliation with deviant peer groups increase the likelihood that one will experiment with drugs as group members offer drugs to each other and role model drug use. Parental influence dominates until early adolescence, by then, peer groups act as informational source for how to behave. Parents may still exert more of an indirect influence on behavior through friendship selection (2).

The Schools

The school environment may be conducive to drug experimentation or may promote delay in exposure to drugs. Large community surveys concur that for men and women of all ages, an increased risk for alcohol use and illicit drug disorders is associated with dropping out of high school or leaving college early. Schools have been the stage of a number of educational initiatives aiming at informing children as to why drug use is bad for them. Strategies based on inducing fear or providing information, that is, if youths are frightened about the negative effects of drugs, or just know the facts, they would not want to experiment with them, have been found to be largely ineffective. An alternate assumption is a value-based model aimed at producing more global attitudinal changes including enhanced self-esteem without addressing drug use specifically; the evidence of its effectiveness is scant (7).

The Workplace

Employment, or working for pay, is also related to the prevalence of substance use. Unemployment is associated with higher risk for alcoholism and so are "blue collar" occupations and lower SES. This association may be a cause or result of substance use. Stressful work circumstances have been associated with high levels of alcohol intake. In a longitudinal study of 1010 teenagers in St. Paul, Minnesota, long hours of after school work (over 20 hrs/week) increased levels of drinking. This was possibly mediated though work-derived independence from parents and an early transition to an adult role (8). The prevention of problem drinking in the workplace can be achieved by effective controls of the work environment (9). In safety-sensitive situations, a program of urine monitoring of illegal substances can ensure the safe handling of vehicles and machines.

The Social Networks and Support Availability

Assistance provided by social support networks may include companionship (i.e., sharing time or life experiences), conformity (i.e., pressure to engage in a certain behavior), and information (i.e., contextual knowledge). It may also provide support such as attention to basic needs. Social support may be either provided by family, friends, and other acquaintances or through community agencies (10). Within these networks, role models as sports coaches and youths' support groups may act as teachers of the time and place and quantity and methods of drug use.

Social networks influence an individual's choices about those with whom they have contact or interact with. These interactions can determine behavior either through constraints to inhibit action or influences promoting action. A youth may likely be a member of a variety of networks at school, home, and other public organizations such as religious institutions and sports and recreational activities. An individual's connections may be different in different contexts and the outcome as to one's drug use may be derived from a balance of influences.

Group Identification and Deviancy

Further to the development of social networks, people also tend to identify or place themselves and others into labeled groups, which may promote or inhibit drug use behavior. Adolescence is a period when youth begins to make independent choices about life. Unsure about the life decisions they should make, an adolescent will search for a place to belong among peers they identify with and conform to their norms (11). Differential socialization may lead to group norms that serve to rationalize problem behavior or deviant subcultures. These norms include the development of beliefs, intentions, expectations, perceptions, and modeling of social behaviors. Time spent with deviant peers, their positive reactions for rule-breaking behavior, and the resulting attention earned are all components of deviancy training that may lead to exposure followed by increase in drug use (12).

LARGER SOCIAL STRUCTURES AND THE MACRO ENVIRONMENT

The larger physical and sociocultural environment will also protect from or facilitate drug use. The size, density, and configuration of a geographical area or its climate are all determinants in the availability of drugs and so is the common culture modulating individual behaviors.

Neighborhood Disorganization

A lack of centralized authority or an unstable one may result in a lack of behavioral monitoring.

Chaotic areas may be more heavily exposed to social disobedience. Access to more prosocial activities (i.e., community centers or movie theaters) is typically limited. Abandoned, dilapidated buildings and enclosed public spaces may result in greater incidence of drug exposures as one of the local gang activities (13).

Adverse Socioeconomic Conditions

The association between these adverse conditions and drug abuse is complex and can be a two-way process, that is, low status, leading to drug abuse or drug abuse resulting in a downward socioeconomic drift. Low socioeconomic conditions, often in densely populated areas, are often twinned with sparse community remedial resources or may increase the exposure to drug-related criminal activity. Disadvantaged conditions reduce the impact of the family or social fabrics resulting in self-medication with drugs. Other confounding factors may include the association with poor mental health status (14). Conversely, individuals of higher SES may be able to financially afford large quantities of drugs resulting in significant physical damage prior to a descent in social status.

In a large population survey ($n = 23,564$) carried out in Quebec, Canada, and that included smoking behavior, SES was defined as household incomes above or below Can$40,000 per year, employment status, and level of education. Smokers, as expected, reported health as poor or fair more frequently than nonsmokers, in addition this difference was significantly greater among those with low incomes and no employment (15).

Environmental Availability

Individual drug use is influenced by the local ease of distribution, access, and acquisition of drugs. Areas of drug production (i.e., cannabis or opium fields), manufacturing (i.e., cocaine or heroin creation), and distribution routes tend to equally be regions at high risk for abuse. In South America, cocaine-type drugs dominate while the majority of treatment admissions in Southeast Asia are for opioid use. In Washington DC, using geographic information systems (GIS), Mason et al. computed the linear distances between the homes of adolescent substance users and the reported "risky" (i.e., alcohol outlets) and "safe" places (i.e., boys and girls clubs). The homes of substance users were three times closer to "risky" places than "safe" places (14).

Cultural Influences

Culturally shaped life habits or rituals, normative structures, and expectations as well as beliefs about drug use and its effects all may affect drug use initiation and maintenance. The regular use of wine as food with meals in France or Italy is an example of a normed "life habit" while the use of peyote by few Native American Church groups is an example of "ritualized" belief (16).

Cross-culturally, a defining characteristic of the transition from drug use to abuse appears to be the ability to carry or not to carry a culturally specific role (17). These roles may vary by gender or ethnicity. Sex-role expectations within one's environment and differential stigma associated with use may affect drug prevalence or self-disclosure. There may be a world expectation that females do not misuse drugs and that their misuse is more stigmatizing than for males. Female drug abusers may fear seeking treatment because of reprisal such as the loss of custody of their children. Indeed, part of the stigma against female drug use may derive from the potential harm coming to the child including the risk of fetal alcohol syndrome and low birth weight from maternal cigarette smoking (18). Females are also more likely to be victims of traumatic life events such as various forms of childhood physical or sexual abuse (19).

Ethnicity also plays a role as a predictor or protective factor for drug use. In the United States, Asian groups have reported lower rates of alcohol abuse and dependence than other ethnic groups. A possible explanation has been the presence of an alcohol aldehyde deficiency resulting in a "flushing response" after consuming alcohol (20). However, Native Americans, many of whom with a flushing response but in a socially disadvantaged position, have relatively worse alcohol and drug problems than other ethnic groups. Ethnic pride may also be a strong direct protective factor among disadvantaged groups (21).

The impact of ethnicity interacts with demographics such as gender and age, as well as type of drug or SES. Methodologic challenges encountered in a review of the examination of ethnicity in 18 US-based treatment outcome studies of adolescent substance abusers involved (22):

- a general tendency to report ethnicity as defined by funding agencies such as the National Institutes of Health (i.e., American Indian/Alaska Native, Asian/Pacific Islander, Black/African American and Hispanic). These groupings do not acknowledge the heterogeneity that exists within each of these ethnic minority groups (23).
- the referral sources used to recruit study participants and particularly referrals from juvenile justice agencies, and courts could influence the reported prevalence of the predominant substances abused per ethnic group. For example, Caucasian youths report higher use of methamphetamines but are less likely to be mandated for treatment compared to African American and Hispanic/Latino youths predominantly using marihuana.
- aside from the "culture neutral" urinalysis, the validity and appropriateness of outcome measures and the caveats on the interpretation of cultural findings were not addressed. Translation of an instrument into another language does not equate with cultural appropriateness.

- based on the groups' heterogeneity involved, even family-oriented therapies compatible with the cultural values and beliefs of interdependence in some ethnic minority groups resulted in mixed findings.
- a qualitative investigation of the degree to which it was important for the person to address culture-related factors, but that investigation was lacking to tailor an individualized intervention.

Failing to address the above challenges may result in overly simplistic conclusions of limited clinical utility.

Acculturation

Acculturation has been defined as the processes whereby immigrants change their behavior and attitudes toward those of the host society. The degree to which newly exposed individuals adopt a culture may inhibit or promote drug use depending on the culture they are from and the norms of the new culture. There is still no agreement on the best way to operationalize this construct. There are at least 15 popular scales assessing acculturation among Latinos alone where particular attention has been paid to the relationship between acculturation and drinking outcomes (24). A review of 24 studies disaggregating genders and using appropriate outcomes resulted in some consistent findings among the women in particular. Higher acculturation was strongly related to a higher probability of drinking, greater consumption, and problems. Such effects were not attributable to demographic confounds. By contrast the results for Latino men were more ambiguous. There was a probability that higher acculturation was related to higher odds of drinking but not to other drinking outcomes. Rising income and SES generally seemed to be a strong candidate for explaining the relationship between higher acculturation and higher odds of drinking. The particular effect on women seemed to be more related to the more favorable drinking norms of the host culture compared to the relative discouragement from drinking in the culture of origin.

The stressors of acculturation resulting from the migration process have been pointed out, among Hispanic Americans, to lead to a range of adaptation in the context of the host culture (i.e., "integration," "assimilation," "rejection," or "marginalization"). These adaptive modalities influence the abuse of substances as well as the rate of alcoholism (25). Additionally, the first 5 years of the migration process constitute the most vulnerable ones for migrants, not only with respect to the abuse of substances including alcohol, but for suicide as well (26).

Another body of studies have investigated the relationship between drinking patterns and ethnic identity and enculturation among Native Americans. Such studies have provided inconsistent results concerning the associations between loss of ethnic identity and greater alcohol use perhaps as a result of measurement limitations (27). Earlier work also suggested that biculturality (i.e., having positive attitudes toward and involvement in both cultures) is most adaptive generally and protective against alcohol-related problems.

In studying the complex role of acculturation, it is also important to recognize that family dynamics, socioeconomic factors up to poverty levels, ethnocultural characteristics, and the role of religion, among others, have their direct and/or indirect influences in the frequency, amount, and types of drugs used and/or abused among the different ethnic groups who reside in the United States (28,29).

Media and Worldwide Electronic Information

Increasingly, the sociocultural influence of the media affects the initiation and experimentation to drug use. Media advertisement can affect an individual's preferences and behavioral options toward drug use. The glamorized portraying of rock stars' struggle with drug dependence encourage youths seeking a "cool" subculture to accept them as their role models. In a study of seventh graders in Southern California ($N = 2998$), increased exposure to televised alcohol advertisements was found to be associated with increased consumption in the eighth grade (30). Mass media disseminates quickly large amounts of information to worldwide audiences. Indeed, a concern from cultural traditionalists worldwide is the media-promoted potential dominance of Western culture on a range of local host cultures with more limited media marketing potential.

Movies glamorize various drug-related behaviors, and over the years their stars have promoted cigarette smoking and alcohol use. Smoking in movies rarely depicts negative health outcomes and smokers in movies appear to be in very good shape (31). The World Wide Web is a trove of wide ranging information about drugs. The impact of the Internet or various demographic groups remains to be systematically investigated.

MANAGEMENT IMPLICATIONS AND THEIR CHALLENGES

The sociocultural variables, just reviewed, have significant implications in every aspect of the management of the spectrum of the substance use disorders.

Diagnoses and Sociocultural Variation

Sociocultural variations may affect the meaningfulness of the diagnostic categories in the substance use disorders (32). A comparative analysis by the WHO of the Alcohol Use Disorder and Associated Disabilities Interview Schedule—Alcohol/Drug-Revised (AUDADIS-ADR) found substantial variations across sites of administration in test–retest reliability. Sydney, Australia, showed the highest reliability on seven of nine current alcohol dependence items, the results from Jebel, Romania, were close to those of Sydney while responders from Bangalore, India, had "difficulty understanding the constructs underlying the questions" (33). In the context of categorical diagnoses and criteria, cross-culturally many different thresholds may be applied. Where regular drinking is normalized, thresholds for what is problematized are set much higher than in cultures where use of substances is particularly suspect.

Social stigmatization is also built in the terms "abuse" or "dependence." A part of the diagnostic decision-making process depends on the threshold whereby family, friends, or a societal representative notices a behavior and decides that it should be brought to a professional's attention. Regarding withdrawal from alcohol, those in the "wet" wine cultures may be inclined to set relatively low thresholds and no clear distinction from hangovers. In the WHO study, graver signs were assigned in cultures where drinking was viewed as more problematic.

While the diagnostic category of dependence has fared better, both "harmful use" (the ICD category) and "abuse" (the DSM category) have not performed well in test-retest studies. Deciding on a failure in work role cannot be culture-free. Half of the diagnosis of "abuse" in the United States follows a drinking an impaired offence, a behavior that may not be equivalent to a psychiatric disorder (34).

The Need for an Individualized Sociocultural Formulation

The multiaxial assessment process in the *Diagnostic and Statistical Manual of Mental Disorders* (35) recognizes in its Axis IV the need to assess an individual's psychosocial and environmental problems that may affect the diagnosis, treatment, and prognosis. These include problems with the primary support group, social environment, and educational, occupational, housing, economic, and legal problems as well as problems with access to health care services.

The cultural dimension, by contrast, is addressed only as an appendix to supplement the multiaxial diagnostic assessment. This may unwittingly reduce the clinical perception of the importance of identifying the person's cultural identity involvement with both culture of origin and host culture as well as his or her parents' ethnicity. In a cultural formulation, the meaning and perceived severity of the symptoms, the perception of social stressors, or supports in relation to cultural norms needs also to be identified. While rare culture-bound syndromes have been identified, there are common clinical presentations where culture plays a significant part including:

- norm conflict between the person's behavior and his or her cultural standard
- normative or socially prescribed substance use involving religious rites or meal-related practices
- cultural change achieved through migration or exposure to new norms

Perceptions of similarities and differences between the clinician and patient's cultures of relevance to the therapy should conclude the formulation (36).

Social Preventive Strategies

Could people be "inoculated" against the social pressures precipitating drug trial and experimentation through social coalition building? There are many examples of evidence-based interventions targeting social units.

The Family: Prevention programs include early childhood education, social support for parents and skills acquisition in parent–child communication, crisis management, and resource networking. Examples of evidence-based programs include Strengthening Families, three 14-week courses on parenting training, children's skills training, and family life skills training (37). Another such program is Family Matters, involving four booklets, delivered to the home and follow-up telephone calls by health educators (38).

The School: Drug education programming relies on a number of mediating agents of change. These include a mix of beliefs and skills (39). Mediating beliefs include the perceived prevalence of drug use and its acceptability among peers, the consequences of use, and the potential incongruence with other future aspirations. Mediating skills include the ability to resist pressure, goal setting, and prosocial alternatives as well as stress management, self-esteem, and social skills.

In public schools, optimal cultural communication occurs when the intervention program includes cultural elements from each of the ethnic groups in the school (multicultural curriculum) rather than targeting an individual's ethnic group. A message of inclusion, rather than exclusion, followed by actions and practices that embrace diversity has been shown to be optimal for a school (40). Cultural grounding must convey inclusiveness, not exclusiveness. School-based assistance programs can also provide nonthreatening early interventions for students at risk.

The Use of Media

High-profile media campaigns "against drugs" abound, many of dubious effectiveness. Mass media campaigns targeted at youths that appear to exert the strongest effect on drug misuse depict dramatic true consequences, appeal to sensation-seeking youths through fast-paced and exciting material, take an activism stance including correction of normative misperceptions, and offer greater autonomy from nondrug lifestyles (41).

Prevention Efforts on a Global Scale

Historically, the only strategic focus of international conventions was supply reduction of illegal drugs through interdiction by authorities, crop burning, drug seizures, and so on. The results of this strategy have been limited. The globalization of trade efforts for legal drugs, that is, tobacco and alcohol, in addition to illegal drugs has necessitated the draft of international "conventions" for both seeking to coordinate a global preventative effort. A recent intervention has been the WHO Framework Convention on Tobacco Control signed by some 168 countries and encouraging an array of preventative interventions including the enaction of bans on tobacco advertising and the use of deceptive terms such as "light" and "mild" cigarettes, the placement of principally displayed health warnings on packaging, the protection from second-hand exposure to smoke in the workplace, public transport, and indoor public places, increase of tobacco taxes, and the combat of smuggling (42).

Social Treatment Strategies

Could a treatment modality targeting the social environment reduce the demand for substances? A number of socially based therapeutic interventions have been developed.

Family Therapy: The use of a family's strength and resources can help drug users minimize the negative impact of their behavior on themselves as well as their families. A safe environment is provided for the family members to express their feelings and concerns and in the process improve communication with each other.

Group Therapy: In contrast to the family, the group is composed exclusively of drug abusers providing support and corrective feedback to each other guided by a trained leader. Both approaches are cornerstones of many treatment programs (43).

Network Therapy: In this multimodal approach, specific family friends and friends are enlisted with the help of the therapist to provide ongoing support to the abuser and promote attitudinal change aiming at the prompt achievement of abstinence, relapse prevention, and a drug-free lifestyle (44).

Therapeutic Community: The community serves as the primary therapist often in a residence. In addition to a primary counselor, each resident has the responsibility to be therapist and teacher to the rest of this community. Peers often lead peer group meetings. Individuals are provided with increased responsibility and privileges as they pass through structured phases of treatment (45).

Sober Living Homes: A safe environment is provided for those who have completed residential treatment or inpatient care, or for those who need a structured living environment to maintain sobriety. Residents are expected to work or attend school or treatment sessions outside the home.

Twelve-Step Program: A worldwide network based on small group support and a basic philosophy is the cornerstone of the recovery of many considered outsiders in their community. The fellowship is established through autonomous groups, ensuring members' anonymity and a sense of belonging to anyone who wants to stop drinking or using. A blueprint for recovery is laid through the 12 steps (46).

Employee Assistance Programs (EAPs): The combined prevalence of drug-induced absenteeism and risk of mistakes and injuries has led the organized workplace to develop programs aiming at motivating employees to improve their performance rather than risk losing their jobs as well as saving corporate losses. Typical programmatic components include educational and counseling services, supervisory training, drug testing and other screening services, and eventually referral to services (47).

Prison Settings: Programs in prisons have gradually expanded to provide the gamut of prevention and treatment services as well as provision for after care. Recently, a formal diversion program from incarceration to community-based treatment through Drug Courts has gained increased recognition for its cost-effectiveness (48).

Treatment and Cultural Competence

Cultural competence consists of the capacity to make accurate assessments (devoid of stereotypes or misconceptions) and to conduct potent interventions in addressing the complex real-world issues that affect the addictive behaviors of racial/ethnic minority clients struggling to recover from substance abuse and dependence. A clinician's awareness of his or her own cultural values and biases is important. Examples of culturally relevant thematic issues in substance abuse treatment have included the following:

- For African Americans, the stressors of racial discrimination and related life challenges. Similarly gender-role obligations may pose significant burdens and barriers for African American women (50).
- For Hispanics/Latinos, issues include linguistic barriers and acculturation conflicts as well as issues of ethnic identity development, family conflicts, and family obligations. In a recent study, Spanish-Speaking Latinos/Hispanics residing in the United States were more socioeconomically stable and thus exposed to less stress than those Latinos/Hispanics who did not speak Spanish fluently. Likewise, their rates of incarceration as well as the prevalence of substance use disorders were lower among Spanish-Speaking Latinos/Hispanics than among non–English-speaking Latinos/Hispanics or Caucasian populations (51).
- For American Indians, issues include feelings of alienation and staff insensitivity, requirement of disclosure of personal feelings conflicting with traditional Indian ways (52).
- For Asian Americans, issues include culturally incongruent need to admit to antisocial behaviors or prompt to self-disclosure creating shame or "loss of face" (53).

A taxonomy of the ways programs can be made culturally sensitive has been proposed by Kreuter et al. (54), which is as follows:

- *Peripheral Strategies:* Packaging the program to reflect the intended cultural gap through appropriate colors, images, fonts, and pictures.
- *Evidential Strategies:* Enhancing the perceived relevance of a health issue for a group by presenting evidence as to how it impacts that group.
- *Linguistic Strategies:* Making the program more accessible by using the intended audience dominant or native tongue.
- *Constituent-involving Strategies:* Involving lay community members in the program's planning and decision making.
- *Sociocultural Strategies:* Discussion of the health issue in the broader context of the audience's sociocultural values and characteristics.

CONCLUDING REMARKS

1. The study of sociocultural factors in isolation may lead to simplistic stereotypes. As each factor may have both risk and protective properties, the study of their differential relevance and interdependence is important.
2. Sociocultural factors may be of particular relevance in understanding the relative risk of initiation of substance use and in the early phases of drug experimentation while the genetic and neurophysiologic influences may become more relevant in the progression to the substance-dependence stage.
3. The Acculturation Process plays a role in determining the increases in the use and abuse of substances among migrants who arrive to the United States; particularly in their first 5 years of arrival. The acquisition of language competence in the host country may act as a protective factor to substance abuse.
4. The gene–environment or nature–nurture dichotomy perception is increasingly a phase in history. The study of outcome variables for prevention and treatment activities aiming to disentangle the respective roles of the individual and that of the environment eventually unravels their effect on each other. Genetic factors significantly influence the probability that an individual will be exposed to environmental risk factors such as the occurrence of stressful life events, low levels of social support, and poor parenting. Genetic factors may also render individuals more or less vulnerable to the pathogenic effects of environmental risk factors (55). Conversely, adverse environments may lead to genetic risks. Future research will further consider how the environment gets "under the skin."
5. Statistical innovation methods such as twin studies, growth curve trajectories, and/or mediation analysis may contribute further to the understanding of the interaction between biologic and environmental causal pathways. Unreliability of measurements remains a real problem (55).
6. A comprehensive assessment requires an individualized contextual sociocultural formulation. There is huge variation in the individual response to all types of physical and psychological hazards demonstrating the interaction of individual risk and resilience.
7. Evidence-based prevention and treatment interventions targeting social and cultural units are available. Demonstrating the efficacy and effectiveness of these approaches remains however a complex endeavor.

REFERENCES

1. Gonzalez CA, Griffith EEH, Ruiz P. Cross-cultural issues in psychiatric treatment. In: Gabbard GO, ed. *Treatment of Psychiatric Disorders*. Vol. 1. 3rd ed. Washington, DC: American Psychiatric Press; 2001:47–67.
2. Flay BR, Hu FB, Siddiqui O, et al. Differential influence of parental smoking and friends' smoking on adolescent initiation and escalation of smoking. *J Health Soc Behav*. 1994;35:248–265.
3. Suchman NE, Luthar SS. Maternal addiction, child maladjustment and socio-demographic risks: implications for parenting behaviors. *Addiction*. 2000;95(9):1417–1428.
4. Rotunda RJ, Doman K. Partner enabling of substance use disorders: critical review and future directions. *Am J Fam Ther*. 2001;29:257–270.
5. Wiseman J. The "Home Treatment": the first steps in trying to cope with an alcoholic husband. *Family Relations*. 1980;29:541–549.
6. Gotham H, Sher K. Do codependent traits involve more than basic dimensions of personality and psychotherapy? *J Stud Alcohol*. 1996;57:34–39.
7. Evans RI. A historical perspective on effective prevention. In: Bukowski WJ, Evans RI, eds. *Cost-Benefit/Cost-Effectiveness Research of Drug Abuse Prevention: Implications for Programming and Policy*. NIDA Research Monograph 176. Rockville, MD: National Institute on Drug Abuse, National Institute of Health; 1998:37–58.
8. McMorris BJ, Uggen C. Alcohol and employment in the transition to adulthood. *Health Soc Behav*. 2000;41:276–294.
9. Ames GM, Grube JW, Morre RS. Social control and workplace drinking norms: a comparison of two organizational cultures. *Stud Alcohol*. 2000;61:203–219.
10. Cohen S. Psychosocial models of the role of social support in the etiology of physical disease. *J Health Psychol*. 1988;7:269–299.
11. Sussman S, Pokhrel P, Ashmore R, et al. Adolescent peer group identification and characteristics: a review of the literature. *Addict Behav*. 2007;32:1602–1627.
12. Poulin F, Dishion TJ, Burraston B. Three-year iatrogenic effects associated with aggregating high risk adolescents in cognitive behavioral preventive interventions. *Appl Dev Sci*. 2001;5:214–224.
13. Skogan WG, Lurigio AJ. The correlates of community antidrug activism. *Crime Delinq*. 1992;38:510–521.
14. Mason M, Cheung I, Walker L. Substance use, social networks and the geography of urban adolescents. *Subst Use Misuse*. 2004;39:1751–1777.
15. Birch S, Jerrett M, Eyles J. Heterogeneity in the determinants of health and illness: the example of socioeconomic status and smoking. *Soc Sci Med*. 2000;51:307–317.
16. Julien RM. A primer of drug action. 9th ed. New York: WH Freeman and Company; 2005.
17. Quintero G, Nichter M. The semantics of addiction: moving beyond expert models to lay understandings. *J Psychoactive Drugs*. 1996;28:219–228.
18. Kyskan CE, Moore TE. Global perspectives on fetal alcohol, syndrome: assessing practices, policies and campaigns in four English speaking countries. *Can Psychol*. 2005;46:153–156.
19. Felitti VJ, Anda RF, Nordenberg D, el al. Relationship of childhood abuse and household dysfunction to many of the leading causes of death in adults: the Adverse Childhood Experiences (ACE) Study. *Am J Prev Med*. 1998;4:245–258.
20. Suzuki K, Matsushita S, Ishii T. Relationship between the flushing response and drinking behavior among Japanese high school students. *Alcohol Clin Exp Res*. 1997;21:1726–1729.
21. Scheier LM, Botvin GJ, Diaz T, el al. Ethnic identity as a moderation of psychosocial risk and adolescent alcohol and marihuana use: concurrent and longitudinal analysis. *J Child Adolesc Subst Abuse*. 1997;6:21–47.
22. Strada MJ, Donahue B, Lefforge NL. Examination of ethnicity in controlled treatment outcome studies involving adolescent substance abusers: a comprehensive literature review. *Psychol Addict Behav*. 2006;1:11–27.

23. Hall NGC. Psychotherapy research with ethnic minorities: empirical, ethical and conceptual issues. *J Consult Clin Psychol.* 2001;69:502–510.
24. Zemore SE. Acculturation and alcohol among Latino adults in the United States: a comprehensive review. *Alcohol Clin Exp Res.* 2007;31(2):1968–1990.
25. Ruiz P. La Psiquiatria de las Minorias Etnicas: El Ejemplo de Estados Unidos. In: Vallejo Ruiloba J, Leal Cercos C, eds. *Tratado de Psiquiatria.* Vol II. Barcelona, Spain: ARS Medica; 2005:2273–2280.
26. Ruiz P, Langrod JG. Substance abuse among Hispanic-Americans: current issues and future perspectives. In: Lowinson JH, Ruiz P, Millman RB, Langrod JG, eds. *Substance Abuse: A Comprehensive Textbook.* 2nd ed. Baltimore, MD: Williams & Wilkins; 1992:868–874.
27. Whitbeck LB, Chen X, Hoyt DR, et al. Discrimination, historical loss and enculturation: culturally specific risk and resiliency factors for alcohol abuse among American Indians. *J Stud Alc.* 2004;65:409–418.
28. Rothe EM, Ruiz P. Substance abuse among Cuban Americans. In: Straussner SLA, ed. *Ethnocultural Factors in Substance Abuse Treatment.* New York, NY: Guilford Press; 2001:97–110.
29. Alvarez LR, Ruiz P. Substance abuse in the Mexican American population. In: Straussner SLA, ed. *Ethnocultural Factors in Substance Abuse treatment.* New York: Guilford Press; 2001: 111–136.
30. Stacy AW, Zogg JB, Unger JB, et al. Exposure to televised alcohol ads and subsequent adolescent alcohol use. *Am J Health Behav.* 2004;28:498–509.
31. Charlesworth A, Glantz A. Smoking in the movies increases adolescent smoking: a review. *Pediatrics.* 2005;116:1–13.
32. Room R. Taking account of cultural and societal influences on substance use diagnoses and criteria. *Addiction.* 2006;101(suppl 1):31–39.
33. Chatterji S, Saunders JB, Vrasti R, et al. Reliability of the alcohol and drug modules of the Alcohol Use Disorder and Associated Disabilities Interview Schedule—Alcohol/Drug Revised (AUDADIS-ADR): an international comparison. *Drug Alcohol Depend.* 1997:47:171–185.
34. Hasin D, Paykin A, Endicott J, et al. Validity of DSM-IV alcohol abuse: drunk drivers versus all others. *J Stud Alcohol.* 1999; 60:746–755.
35. American Psychiatric Association. *Diagnostic and Statistical Manual of Mental Disorders.* 4th ed., rev. Washington, DC: American Psychiatric Association; 2000.
36. Westermeyer J, Mellman L, Alarcon R. Cultural competence in addiction psychiatry. *Addict Disord Their Treat.* 2006;5:107–119.
37. Kumpfer KL, Alvarado R, Whiteside HO. Family-based interventions for substance use and misuse prevention. *Subst Use Misuse.* 2003;38:1759–1787.
38. Bauman KE, Foshee VA, Ennett ST, et al. The influence of a family program on adolescent tobacco and alcohol use. *Am J Public Health.* 2001;91:604–610.
39. Hansen WB. School-based substance abuse prevention: a review of the state of the art in curriculum, 1980–1990. *Health Educ Res Theor Pract.* 1992;7:403–430.
40. Hecht ML, Raup Krieger JL. The principle of cultural grounding in school-based substance abuse prevention: the Drug Resistance Strategies Project. *J Lang Soc Psychol.* 2006;25:301–319.
41. Slater MD, Kelly KJ, Edwards RW, et al. Combining in-school and community-based media efforts: reducing marijuana and alcohol uptake among younger adolescents. *Health Educ Res.* 2005;21:157–167.
42. Yach D, Bettcher D. Globalization of the tobacco industry influence and new global responses. *Tob Control.* 2000;9:206–216.
43. Liddle HA, Rowe CL, Dakof GA, et al. Early intervention for adolescent substance abuse: pre-treatment to post-treatment outcomes of a randomized clinical trial comparing multi-dimensional family therapy and peer group treatment. *J Psychoactive Drugs.* 2004;36:49–63.
44. Galanter M. *Network Therapy for Addictions: A New Approach.* Expanded ed. New York: Guilford; 1999.
45. DeLeon G. *The Therapeutic Community: Theory, Model, and Method.* New York, NY: Springer; 2000.
46. Alcoholics Anonymous. *Alcoholics Anonymous.* New York, NY: Alcoholic Anonymous World Services; 1976.
47. Bennett JB, Lehman WEK. Employee attitude crystallization and substances use policy: test of a classification scheme. *J Drug Issues.* 1996;26:831–865.
48. Perry A, Coulton S, Glanville J, et al. Interventions for drug-using offenders in the courts, secure establishments and the community. *Cochrane Database Syst Rev.* 2006;3:CD005193.
49. Castro FG, Garfinkle J. Critical issues in the development of culturally relevant substance abuse treatments for specific minority groups. *Alcohol Clin Exp Res.* 2003;27(8):1381–1388.
50. Locke DC. *Increasing Multicultural Understanding.* 2nd ed. Thousand Oaks, CA: Sage; 1998.
51. Ruiz P. Spanish, English and mental health services—editorial. *Am J Psychiatry.* 2007;164(8):1133–1135.
52. Moran JR, Reaman JA. Critical issues for substance abuse prevention targeting American Indian Youth. *J Prim Prev.* 2002; 22(3):201–233.
53. Ja D, Aoki B. Substance abuse treatment: cultural barriers in the Asian American community. *J Psychoactive Drugs.* 1993;25:61–71.
54. Kreuter MW, Lukwago SN, Bucholtz DC, et al. Achieving cultural appropriateness in health promotion programs: targeted and tailored approaches. *Health Educ Behav.* 2003;30:133.
55. Kendler KS, Prescott CA. *Genes, Environment and Psychopathology. Understanding the Causes of Psychiatric and Substance use Disorders.* New York: Guilford; 2006.

SECTION 3 ■ EVALUATION

CHAPTER 9 Clinical Assessment

LaVerne Hanes Stevens ■ Michael L. Dennis

A good clinical assessment is one of the fundamental elements of effective treatment planning for substance use disorders. An assessment that effectively synthesizes the patient's self-report with information from additional sources and sound clinical judgment on a wide array of patient issues will do more than provide a diagnosis; it will accurately identify the patient's needs across a broad spectrum of related life domains, consider how those needs may affect the delivery of treatment, ensure that they are the basis for the ongoing process of counselor–patient collaboration on treatment planning, and monitor the patient's progress (1).

Expert panels (2) suggest that the best assessment is a comprehensive process sensitive to a broad range of life areas and that collects information necessary for treatment planning and evaluating the patient's progress. However, for decades the field of substance use disorder treatment has been characterized by multiple service sectors (e.g., medical, legal) with disjointed and often competing approaches to treating clinical disorders. Each sector has its own model and has historically operated in a vacuum, with one-way passive referrals that tend to focus on different aspects of the patient's history (1). This has frequently resulted in an inefficient clinical process that leads to patient frustration and inefficient use of increasingly scarce treatment dollars.

In this chapter, we will discuss assessment principles for identifying multiple patient needs, synthesizing them into a cohesive picture, translating them into treatment planning, and facilitating communication between multiple service providers to address those needs. While these principles are based on our clinical interpretation training for the Global Appraisal of Individual Needs (GAIN) (3,4), they can be readily applied to any clinical assessment.

CORE PRINCIPLES

Sources of Information

The clinical assessment process is like a three-legged stool that requires three components, or "legs," to generate a solidly supported treatment plan:

- **Clinical judgment.** Before any patient's information is gathered, the clinician's knowledge is the primary factor in the assessment process. The patient's interview then informs the treatment professional's clinical judgment and treatment recommendations.

- **Patient's self-report.** The patient's self-report information is gathered in the interview itself. This is essential for successful clinical planning and treatment engagement because without patient input, treatment plans are likely to be generic, may omit important individualized treatment issues, and may include services that are unnecessary or counterproductive for the patient's progress. When treatment goals are mutually determined and targeted at real needs, they are more likely to enhance the patient's motivation.

- **Collateral reports.** The assessment should also incorporate information from the patient's family, prior treatment records, and other systems of care. This information can be significant because patients may not always recognize or be willing to share all of the salient issues in their lives. It can also be beneficial to know how others perceive the patient's problems and to note whether the patient has had trouble with other interventions.

GOALS OF A CLINICAL NEEDS ASSESSMENT

Besides providing a diagnosis for the treatment of substance use disorders, it is essential to utilize a comprehensive needs assessment process that (a) provides a report that is sharable and usable by professionals in multiple service sectors; (b) covers a broad range of life areas; (c) promotes early identification and response to co-occurring disorders and environmental or situational risk factors; (d) identifies strengths, supports, personal resources, and interpersonal resources; (e) identifies the patient's involvement with other systems; (f) identifies and addresses possible barriers to treatment; (g) provides a baseline for monitoring change in problems; (h) supports evidence-based practice (EBP); (i) has good validity and reliability; and (j) can be administered and interpreted with cultural sensitivity. Each of these is examined below.

Provide a Report That Is Sharable and Usable by Professionals in Multiple Service Sectors

Often, assessment processes are inefficient and consumer unfriendly because they ask the same questions, or slight variations, multiple times: over the phone, at intake, and again with the patient's primary counselor, social worker, nurse, and psychiatrist! Furthermore, because multiple episodes of treatment are actually the norm (5), this process can be repeated with every admission to treatment, further frustrating the patient (6). Thus, an efficient needs assessment must be sharable with professionals and with others outside the direct treatment system who may need access to the information. If the assessment report is highly transferable, it will eliminate the need for repeated assessments as the patient moves through the provider system and will allow more systematic tracking of services provided in response to the identified need.

Cover a Broad Range of Life Areas

Over 80% of the people presenting for substance abuse treatment have three or more major diagnoses or clinical conditions, and half have five or more (7–13). Thus, a good assessment process should cover multiple domains, including substance use, physical health, health risk behaviors, mental health, victimization and other sources of psychosocial stress, recovery environment, legal issues, and vocational concerns, as well as social and spiritual support systems and personal strengths. Because multiple admissions to treatment are also common, it is very important that the assessment includes questions about past treatment and service utilization. These kinds of questions can help inform level-of-care placement decisions and can also provide an important validity check on areas that may be underreported or misrepresented.

Promote Early Identification and Response to Co-occurring Disorders and Environmental or Situational Risk Factors

A competent, experienced clinician can often get to the main problem quickly with an unstructured assessment, but in doing so they also routinely miss co-occurring problems that contribute to the core problem or lead to treatment dropout if not addressed. These may include relatively common problems such as internalizing and externalizing disorders, victimization, suicidal thoughts, self-mutilation, and even problems that the patients may not recognize as posing serious threats to themselves and others, such as tobacco use or high-risk sexual activity. These kinds of issues are overlooked more often than most clinicians realize. Research suggests that 60% to 80% of people entering treatment for substance use disorders have one or more co-occurring psychiatric disorders, yet only 16% of adults and 28% of adolescents have a co-occurring disorder actually documented in their intake assessments (14,15). In a review of a hundred cases where a patient's self-report identified such major clinical problems while the staff evaluation did not, supervisors agreed that the clinical problems were present but were missed by the staff in all but one case (16). Thus, using a comprehensive needs assessment to screen for a wide range of clinical problems is essential for improving the total reliability of practice and for identifying, documenting, and addressing co-occurring disorders, abuse, victimization, and other problems that the patient might not otherwise disclose at intake.

Identify Strengths, Psycho–Social–Spiritual Supports, Personal Resources, and Interpersonal Resources

Frequently the patient's problems become the focal point of the assessment and subsequent interventions. A good assessment, however, will also assess for positive aspects of the patient's life. These positive resources can be beneficial for several reasons, two of which are described below.

First, in the case of substance use disorders, the patient's strengths and resources can easily be overlooked or disregarded by the patient. A high score on a strength-based measure indicates the presence of factors that can be further developed to assist the patient in achieving recovery goals. Strength-based questions in an assessment can help identify the patient's personal reasons for quitting, the patient's perceived self-efficacy for avoiding relapse in various high-risk situations, spiritual or faith-beliefs and support systems, recognition of the presenting problems, motivation, perceived personal strengths, social supports, and much more. The result is that the assessment process can help boost patients' morale and give them a sense of mastery over their problems. Those assets can then provide hope and promote resiliency for attaining recovery goals.

Second, when the assessment identifies the patient's strengths, those strengths can be the basis for therapeutic interventions that help the patient replace drug-related activities with more prosocial activities. Recovery typically involves significant changes and losses. The loss of the patient's relationship with the substance itself is compounded by the loss of drug-associated activities and friends. Because substance use impacts all life domains, especially as the disorder becomes more severe, it can also result in the loss of employment and educational opportunities, relationships, housing, a car or driving privileges, health, and numerous other things that will be grieved by the patient. If the patient has been institutionalized, the substance use disorder has even resulted in a loss of personal freedom. Yet by using the assessment to also identify strengths and supportive resources, the clinician can help the patient see opportunities for gaining new ground.

Identify Involvement in Other Systems and How That May Impact Treatment

Each system of care in which the patient is involved may have its own set of competing demands that have to be managed. For instance, an adult patient may not be able to spend 90 days in residential treatment without losing their job, or an adolescent patient (for whom schooling is important developmentally) may not be able to receive traditional schooling while in treatment. The role of the individual in a family system (e.g., primary caregiver, babysitter) may also be a critical issue that has to be managed to minimize conflicts and treatment dropouts. Involvement with the justice or welfare systems can be particularly complicated because they often operate on longer timelines than does a single treatment episode (e.g., a patient may have made considerable progress in treatment but still be sentenced based on a prior event). It is also important to coordinate care if someone is already being treated for co-occurring mental or physical conditions. Substance use treatment must support compliance with the requirements of these other systems, and providers and decision makers in these systems must be apprised of treatment progress. Additionally, understanding and ensuring that patients are complying with the expectations of these systems may help with treatment, if these requirements involve goals in which the patient is willing to invest.

Identify and Address Possible Barriers to Treatment

If an assessment identifies the patient's treatment needs without addressing the potential barriers to accessing needed services, the assessment is incomplete. Barriers may be physical or material, such as funding, transportation, and childcare. Or they can be psychological, such as motivation, fear of losing relationships, or fear of change. Thus, the treatment staff must have an assessment process that is comprehensive enough to help both the clinician and the patient recognize potential roadblocks to treatment.

Provide a Baseline for Monitoring Change in Problems

If patient's progress is to be measured, the needs assessment must provide a baseline for monitoring change. When a treatment provider has an empirical method for assessing the severity of a patient's problems at intake, that provider can use similar questions at selected intervals to determine the degree of progressive or regressive change in those problems. This ability to monitor and quantify the patient's progress allows for both individual and program-level outcome measurement.

Support Evidence-Based Practice

Treatment providers are increasingly facing demands from payers, policymakers, and the public at large to use EBPs that can (a) reliably produce practical and cost-effective interventions, therapies, and medications to reduce substance use and its negative consequences among those who are abusing or dependent, (b) reduce the likelihood of relapse for those who are recovering, and (c) reduce risks for initiating drug use among those not yet using. The move toward EBP involves:

- Introducing reliable and valid assessments that can be used at the individual level to immediately guide clinical judgments about diagnosis, problem severity, treatment planning, level-of-care placement, and the patient's responsiveness to treatment.

- Introducing explicit intervention protocols targeted at specific problems, subgroups, and outcomes. These protocols should have explicit quality assurance procedures to encourage protocol adherence at the individual level and implementation at the program level.
- Having the ability to pool the data to evaluate performance and outcomes for both the same program over time and relative to other interventions.

A good assessment should feed directly into the treatment plan and help a clinician match individuals to evidence-based approaches targeted to their needs. In practice, many critical needs (such as child maltreatment or suicide ideation) go unaddressed, and it is common for a program to routinely assign *all* patients to certain core services regardless of need. This results in wasted resources that could be redirected toward other gaps in services.

Additionally, a good assessment should help support the actual implementation of an EBP. One of the most common methods is to restate the information from the assessment using a personal feedback report as part of a formal process of motivational interviewing (17). Such interventions work best when relevant information from the assessment is formally passed on to the clinician in a format designed to support the specific intervention. Yet, in practice, this rarely happens because most interventions and assessments are developed separately.

It is also important to have an assessment that can be a part of the infrastructure to support program planning at a higher level. By pooling data, programs can identify the most common needs of their patients, determine where they do or do not have evidence-based programs to address them, and assess which practices work best with a given patient or particular subgroups.

Has Good Validity and Reliability

Highly standardized measures have historically been recognized as more reliable, while clinical interviews (which are often relatively unstructured) have historically been deemed more valid (4). The most useful needs assessment will integrate the best of both processes to produce results that are statistically reliable *and* clinically valid. Reliable data means that if we ask the patient the same question twice, we will get the same answer twice. Valid data is truthful, accurate, and precisely captures and describes the phenomena that we intend to measure. Neither reliability nor validity is sufficient by itself. Patients in an interview can reliably give an invalid answer because they misunderstand the question. Conversely, a clinical insight by one interviewer might lead to further clarification of a patient's response, thereby increasing its validity, but this same response may not be replicated when the same question is asked by a different interviewer.

Research has typically achieved reliability by using classical test theory or a "stimulus–response" model. The interviewer asked the question exactly as printed (stimulus), and whatever the patient answered was recorded (response). This administration style leads to the most reliable answers and typically includes instruments like a standardized intelligence test. A major advantage of this approach is the ability to produce norms and to evaluate how they compare for different subgroups (e.g., by gender, race) or over time (e.g., by age). The problem with this approach is that it does not take into account whether the patient misunderstood the item, had a question about the item, or gave an answer that did not make sense relative to other answers or information known to the interviewer. This becomes particularly problematic when we move from questions about facts to questions about symptoms, behaviors, and perceptions.

Clinical interviews, on the other hand, typically contain a series of topic areas to cover and a list of general questions. The clinical data-gathering session follows the patient's lead more like a journalist or investigator might. Follow-up questions are based on information provided by the patient, and the interviewer probes areas needing further explanation. Clinicians have found this informal clinical interview to be appealing because of its ability to immediately build patient–counselor rapport and the speed with which it often gets to a core problem. Two downsides of this approach are that the lack of structure invites room for error in the hands of less experienced staff members (common in our field), and even experienced clinicians routinely miss important co-occurring problems. It is also difficult to pool or generate norms from this kind of interview.

A *semi structured assessment* is a cross between a traditionally structured assessment and a clinical interview. It attempts to balance the reliability of a standardized assessment against the validity of a clinical interview. With a semi structured assessment like the GAIN (3), the focus is on standardization of understanding over strict standardization of administration. The goal is for patients to understand the items as the assessment intends so that they can give valid answers while allowing the interviewer to deviate from the administration guidelines if those guidelines prevent the participant from understanding an item. Rapport is still maintained by using skip-outs that mimic the process of moving on if there is not a problem or probing when there is evidence of a possible problem. The advantage of this approach is that being able to deviate from general administration guidelines results in greater validity while preserving reliability and the ability to pool data. The major disadvantage of this approach is that it requires investment in training, greater clinical experience by the interviewer (vs. a structured interview), and quality assurance to implement it well.

Administer and Interpret with Cultural Sensitivity

The importance of cultural competence in assessments cannot be overemphasized. This applies to both the interview and the interpretive phases of the process. Any assessment is only as culturally sensitive as the person who administers and interprets the assessment. Whether the interview is structured, semi structured, or unstructured, the assessor must be aware of their own potential biases related to race, ethnicity, socioeconomics, gender, religion, sexual orientation, age, disability, and other factors.

Those who administer assessments must take responsibility for their own cultural competence in asking and clarifying questions in ways that are relevant, understandable, sensitive, and unbiased. Additionally, treatment providers have an ethical obligation to undertake due diligence in recognizing and safeguarding against individual, institutional, and systemic biases in order to avoid creating a disservice or disparity. Simply stated, questions need to be framed in a reasonable cultural framework, examples should be culturally relevant, clarifications must be culturally clear to the patient, interpretation needs to be culturally contextualized, and nothing should be culturally offensive.

HALLMARKS OF A GOOD CLINICAL ASSESSMENT

Informs the Treatment Plan

Ideally, the assessment summary should flow directly into treatment planning. In practice, however, most assessments focus primarily on diagnosis and do not always take the necessary steps to facilitate treatment planning, either in general or with specific EBPs. While diagnosis is important, it should not be the only goal of the assessment. When the assessment merely categorizes the patient with a diagnostic label, then the value and intent of the assessment are lost. Additionally, if the patient believes that they were merely labeled, they may be less likely to comply with treatment recommendations. On the other hand, if the patient is assured that the assessment will be used to identify their needs, to understand and prioritize their problems, and to develop a plan for accessing appropriate services, then the patient may be more likely to provide more accurate information and to make a greater commitment to treatment goals. Throughout the assessment and debriefing, the assessor should make it clear to the patient that they are listening and understand the patient's individual situations and desires. This is an essential step in being an effective agent for change and in supporting positive treatment outcomes.

It is essential to use the assessment information to start an informal treatment plan during the very first session, even before developing a formal treatment plan. Some patients may require admission into detoxification services before they can complete the assessment or before they can enter primary treatment. Others may require immediate help with suicidal thoughts or safety issues. The clinician should be sure to assess and immediately address any other barriers to returning to treatment, such as transportation difficulties, childcare, work schedules, or lack of insurance. Even if the patient does not have major barriers, it is important for the clinician to make sure that the patient has an explicit plan for coming back for the next session. Finally, it is often desirable to provide some level of intervention or make sure that the patient has access to some kind of drug-free environment or support system, such as a sponsor or friend in recovery, to reduce the risk associated with relapse between treatment sessions. All of these areas are informal steps that provide a link to the formal treatment plan. Clearly communicating that the needs assessment will be used for treatment planning and reinforcing this perspective during the assessment will typically result in obtaining more valid information from the patient.

Cross-checks for Inconsistencies in the Patient's Self-reported Information

With any needs assessment, the clinician must know how to use the full body of self-reported and collateral information to check for the possibility of inaccurate or misreported information that might affect the report's validity. Patients may overreport or underreport information in order to achieve a desired outcome (e.g., exaggerating substance use in order to enter treatment and lessen legal consequences of their use, or understating substance use to keep a job). In other cases, the patient may have an asymptomatic self-report because of the effective use of medication, treatment, or environmental controls such as institutionalization. It is incumbent on the clinician to compare the patient's self-reported problems and severity against the report of consequences and service utilization to verify the validity of the clinical information. Where available, current self-report information should be compared to prior self-reports to check for discrepancies. Biological tests such as breath, saliva, hair, and urine tests provide another means of verifying the patient's report. Additionally, prior treatment records and input from family members, employers, teachers, social workers, doctors, and probation or parole officers can often provide valuable insight into the patient's report. Ideally, such additional information should be revealed early in the process to avoid a "gotcha" moment that makes the patient feel like they have been tricked.

Help Facilitate Patient Recall and Give the Patient "Voice"

A good needs assessment should also help address a common patient complaint: that they did not remember, know how, or even have an opportunity to articulate one or more of their problems. The assessment process must be designed to help patients define and communicate problems and desires that they might not otherwise have been able to discuss. This is very different from approaches that focus more on categorizing people based on diagnostic boxes or meeting paperwork or funding requirements. Additionally, the assessment should assist the patient in identifying the effects of substance use on their current life problems and the effects of continued harmful use or abuse.

USING THE ASSESSMENT FOR SEVERITY-BASED PROBLEM PRIORITIZATION

Assessing Recency, Breadth, and Prevalence of Clinical Problems

A thorough clinical needs assessment should show the treatment provider the severity level of the reported problems based on three concrete factors: the problem's recency, the breadth of symptoms and services, and the current rate of prevalence. This is useful for both diagnosis and placement.

Recency looks at timing, specifically the most recent occurrence of a problem. It reflects whether a clinical problem is occurring presently, occurred in the past, or has never occurred. Things that happened in the past week, past month, or past 90 days will typically play a greater role in current treatment than those that happened 3 to 12 months ago or 1 or more years ago. For any current problems, the clinician should include an appropriate treatment recommendation and a referral for further evaluation, or other ancillary services.

Breadth looks at the severity of a current problem and is measured by the extent and diversity of the presenting symptoms or the service utilization history. Characteristically, a more diverse symptom presentation and more service utilization are associated with higher severity. For clinical problems, the focus will generally be on the past year (or since the last interview when conducting follow-up assessments). For service utilization, the focus will be on the lifetime service history.

Current prevalence looks at the frequency of a current problem or service utilization and is measured by how often something has happened in the past 90 days or some other recent period. As a rule, things that happen more frequently are going to be more important than those that happened only once or twice. Even if something is common, it is also useful to understand the extent to which it interferes with responsibilities or functioning at home, work or school, or socially. Typically, things that interfere more frequently with functioning or responsibilities are more important than those that do not.

Using Scale Scores in Assessments as Measures of Problem Severity

Combining multiple questions into an index or scale, with clearly defined cut points for marking severity and clinical decisions, also helps generate more reliable, valid, and useful information. Clinicians often do this intuitively: recognizing that while one symptom or problem might be a red flag, greater priority needs to be given to areas where there is a pattern of recent problems, multiple symptoms, high prevalence, or impaired functioning.

The GAIN is an example of a clinical assessment that is widely used (over 1,200 agencies in 49 states, half the provinces of Canada, and several other countries) and known for its effective use of scales and indices (described further below). The GAIN is based on a measurement model that combines classical scales and summative indices. Classical scales are those where the items represent symptoms of a larger

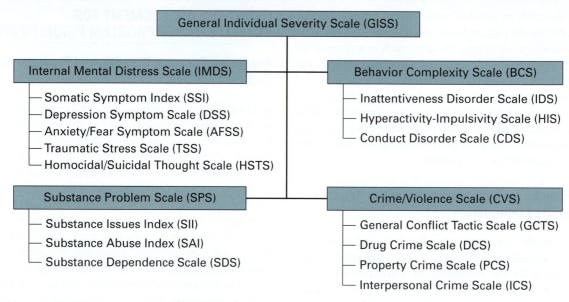

Figure 9.1. Structure of GAIN clinical scales.

underlying disorder, syndrome, or latent construct, such as dependence, depression, or violence. Indices (also known as formative or summative measures) are counts of problems that may not have the same cause but still add up to predict outcomes of interest (18). Examples of index measurements include sources of stress, sources of pressure to be in treatment, or a count of the patient's clinical diagnoses or problems. The GAIN arranges several of these scales and indices into a hierarchical system (see example in Fig. 9.1) that gives clinicians and researchers information about overall severity (the total symptom count). It also has scales representing the main dimensions of variation (substance use, internal distress, external behavior problems, crime/violence) and clinically oriented subscales within each, for problems like dependence, depression, anxiety, attention-deficit/hyperactivity disorder (ADHD), and conduct disorder. These in turn are made up of face-valid individual items that address salient issues like suicidal thoughts (19). Another notable advantage of using scales and indices is that many individual questions have slightly different meanings for key subgroups (e.g., by gender, race, age, sexual orientation, geography), but these differences average out when you look at the pattern across multiple items (20). This helps reduce bias and ensure cultural sensitivity when doing the assessment. It should be noted that many of these properties are not unique to the GAIN; there are actually compendiums of other scales, indices, and multiple domain assessment batteries available (see http://www.athealth.com/practitioner/ceduc/ health_tip31k.html; http://pubs.niaaa.nih.gov/publications/Assesing%20Alcohol/index.htm).

Treatment History and Problem History as an Indicator of Severity

The needs assessment should help treatment providers look not only at the presence of a particular problem but also at the patient's treatment history and the severity of the reported problems. Table 9.1 shows the possible combinations of problem and treatment history and the typical next clinical step. In assessing placement and treatment needs, the clinician will need to consider both problem severity and treatment. The horizontal axis in Table 9.1 represents whether the patient has a current high-severity or low-severity problem, a past history of problems, or no problem. The vertical axis represents current treatment, a history of past treatment, or no treatment history. The type of service or treatment becomes more intense from the left side of the chart to the right. Consider, for instance, a current problem. In the absence of any prior treatment history for a problem of low to moderate severity, the clinician would be more likely to recommend a less invasive treatment (e.g., buprenorphine vs. methadone, outpatient vs. residential). Reporting the same severity of problems while already in treatment, in contrast, may indicate the need to increase the intensity, level of care, or range of services.

The response to treatment (whether positive, neutral, or negative) can be one of the most clinically significant pieces of information in deciding what to do next. Past treatment requires consideration of the recency of the problem, the extent to which the patient complied with treatment recommendations, the speed with which the problem returned (if it dissipated), and the willingness of the patient to try again. The last point is important because while 60% of all people reporting substance use disorders eventually achieve sustained recovery (no use, abuse, or dependence for at least a year), most require multiple episodes of treatment before reaching at least a year of sobriety (5). Past problems and past treatment suggest the need for relapse prevention and monitoring for change. Past problems with current treatment suggest the potential readiness to step down or be discharged. If a patient reports treatment for a problem they do not endorse, it suggests that they may be mis-

CHAPTER 9 ■ Clinical Assessment

TABLE 9.1 Problem Severity and Intervention History Grid

		Problem recency			
		None	**Past**	**Current (past 90-day period)**	
				Low/moderate severity	High severity
Service/intervention history	None	1. No problem	2. Past problem *Consider monitoring and relapse prevention.*	3. Low/moderate problems; not in treatment *Consider initial or low invasive treatment.*	4. Severe problems; not in treatment *Consider a more intensive treatment or intervention strategies.*
	Past	0. Not logical *Check for misunderstanding of problem/ treatment or lying and recode.*			
	Current (Past 90 days)		5. No current problems; currently in treatment *Review for step down or discharge.*	6. Low/moderate problems; currently in treatment *Review need to continue or step up.*	7. Severe problems; currently in treatment *Review need for more intensive or assertive levels.*

understanding or misreporting their symptoms or treatment history and the problem generally should be reviewed and reclassified.

Clinicians can do this kind of evaluation for the overall need for substance abuse treatment as well as for related life domains such as withdrawal problems and detoxification services history, physical health, emotional and behavioral health, readiness for change and motivational interventions, relapse potential and relapse prevention interventions, and recovery environment factors. In each case, there is a continuum of problem severity and treatment history.

WRITING THE FINAL REPORT

After the interview, most agencies and funders require a written report summarizing the assessment. The following is the format we generate from the GAIN and generally suggest.

Presenting Concerns and Identifying Information

Include basic demographics such as age, race, gender, and marital status; number of children; physical appearance and disabilities; source and reason for referral; vocational status; and custody arrangements; and current living situation.

Evaluation Procedure and Validity Concerns

Describe the type of administration, for example, orally administered by staff; the environmental context of the assessment; the patient's behaviors during the meeting; and any other sources of information consulted as a part of evaluation, such as urine test results, records, referral letters, family assessments, and probation reports. This also includes comments on possible areas of underreporting, overreporting, and symptom suppression or other factors that may have influenced the validity of the participant's responses, such as other people within hearing range of the interview.

Diagnosis

Document the patient's diagnoses from the *Diagnostic and Statistical Manual of Mental Disorders* (21) or the *International Classification of Disease* (22) using the multiaxial system that includes Clinical Disorders/Focal Conditions (Axis I), Personality Disorders/Mental Retardation (Axis II), General Medical Conditions (Axis III), Psychosocial and Environmental Problems (Axis IV), and Ratings of Functioning (Axis V). The latter generally includes the Global Assessment of Functioning (GAF) during the past year and past 90 days. It may also include ratings of Global Assessment of Relational Function (GARF) and Social and Occupational Functioning Assessment Scale (SOFAS).

Summary of Substance Use and Treatment History

Summarize the patient's lifetime history of substance use and treatment, including age of first use, preferred substance, and other substances used; abuse and dependency diagnoses and the specific symptoms reported; recency, frequency, and peak amount of use; date and amount of last use (required by some insurance organizations); other drugs used even if diagnostic criteria are not met; and substances identified through biometric testing (e.g., urine, saliva, or hair) or collateral reports. Also include the patient's history of substance abuse treatment, including a detailed treatment history with programs, levels of care, and intake and discharge dates.

Treatment Planning

The American Society of Addiction Medicine's (ASAM) Patient Placement Criteria (PPC) outlines six treatment planning dimensions that should be considered when assessing a patient for admission, continued stay, or discharge from any level of care (23). Those treatment planning dimensions are:

1. acute alcohol or drug intoxication or withdrawal potential;
2. biomedical conditions and complications;
3. emotional, behavioral, or cognitive conditions and complications;
4. readiness to change;
5. relapse, continued use, and continued problem potential; and
6. recovery environment.

For each of these dimensions or other areas of assessment, there should be a summary of the problems, treatment history, and treatment planning recommendations. The recommendations are the most important part of the report and should address three areas.

First, the report should acknowledge specific requests for help or services from the patient. By beginning with the patient's requests, rather than the clinician's list of recommendations, the treatment plan reinforces the therapeutic alliance and shows respect for the patient's understanding of their own problems. It validates the patient and the therapeutic relationship by showing that the treatment provider has listened to them and is not minimizing the issues that the patient wants to address. This is an important step toward garnering patient buy-in of other clinical recommendations.

Second, other recommendations in the needs assessment will be represented by Table 9.1 cell placements. These "cell-specific" treatment planning options are generated based on treatment history and problem recency and severity. For example, if a patient is currently experiencing low to moderate mental health problems but is not currently receiving services for those problems, their mental health service needs would fall into cell 3. The treatment recommendations might include statements such as:

- Discussing current emotional, behavioral, or cognitive problems to review the need for services, barriers to accessing them, and accommodations needed to participate in treatment.
- Discussing how the emotional, behavioral, or cognitive problems and other problems (school, work, custody) may be related.
- Referral to specific services or specific skill-building related to emotional, behavioral, or cognitive conditions required to participate in treatment: [list].
- Help identify triggers or areas that agitate mental health or behavioral problems.

As another example, if a patient reports high-severity problems with continued use and relapse but has never been in substance abuse treatment or relapse prevention programs, the clinician would generate cell 4 treatment planning recommendations. The text might read as follows:

- Discussing situations that pose a risk of relapse, for example, who are the people, places, and things that put the patient at high risk? How can such situations be avoided? What refusal skills does the patient have or need to develop? What will be the plan for handling emergency risk situations?
- Discussing the patient's willingness to participate in a 12-step or other recovery program.
- Developing and discussing options for building or enhancing a nonusing social support network; engaging in substance-free recreational activities; building situational confidence; strengthening refusal skills; and coping with relapse.

The third type of recommendation statements reflect service needs that are not specific to any level of treatment history, that are generally expected by funding or monitoring entities, or that are so significant that they take precedence in treatment prioritization. These recommendations are based on the patient's responses to key items that generally carry an ethical, legal, or clinical responsibility. They include responses to safety issues such as suicidal ideations, homelessness, or current abuse, or responses that suggest the need for intensive case management or coordination of care with other systems.

Summary of Recommendations

This section should include a program or level-of-care placement recommendation based on the patient's needs and where the recommended services can be accessed in the available treatment system. Where ideal placement or services are not immediately available, this should be noted explicitly and interim recommendations should be given. This section should also summarize any barriers to returning to treatment, existing treatment or systems involvement, and things that need to happen before the next session.

Signatures

Most agencies and funders require multiple signatures on the summary report. Typically this includes the signatures of anyone who must read and approve the report. Most commonly these include the patient, clinician, clinical supervisor, and medical doctor.

ADOPTING A PROGRESSIVE APPROACH TO ASSESSMENT

There are numerous benefits of using a progressive approach to assessment instead of a one-size-fits-all approach. In a general population setting, it is useful to administer a 5-minute screener like the GAIN Short Screener (19) to first decide whether an assessment is warranted. In a targeted population, it is useful to use a 20- to 30-minute assessment like the GAIN-Quick (24) for screening, brief interventions, and referral to treatment for more severe cases. When patients present for more formal substance abuse treatment, they generally have multiple problems and benefit from a more extensive (60- to 120-minute) assessment like the full GAIN-Initial (3). Although each of these assessments has successively more information and opportunities for use, the principles outlined in this chapter generally apply to each of them and to the dozens of available alternatives to the GAIN.

CONCLUSION

In this chapter, we have conveyed several overarching messages. First, there is a need to shift our focus from finding the fastest way to provide patient information to one staff person at one point in time to instead, finding the most efficient and least frustrating way for information to be collected and shared with multiple staff and programs over time. Second, clinical assessment rests on good clinical judgment as well as reliable and valid information from both patients and collateral sources. Third, great clinical assessment is all about how the information is used to guide clinical decision making related to diagnosis, treatment planning, and placement at the individual level and pooling of the data to guide program planning. As these principles are incorporated into practice, the field of addiction treatment advances.

ACKNOWLEDGMENTS AND CONTACT INFORMATION

This work was supported by funds and data from CSAT contract no. 270-07-0191. The opinions are those of the authors and do not reflect official positions of the government. The authors would like to thank Tim Feeney for assistance in preparing the manuscript. Please address comments or questions to Dr LaVerne Hanes Stevens, Chestnut Health Systems, 448 Wylie Drive, Normal, Ill 61761; 404-704-2280; lhanesstevens@chestnut.org.

REFERENCES

1. Hanes-Stevens L, White M. Effective treatment planning for substance abuse and related disorders. *Counselor*. 2008;9:10–18.
2. Center for Substance Abuse Treatment. *Addiction Counseling Competencies: The Knowledge, Skills, and Attitudes of Professional Practice*. Rockville, MD: Substance Abuse and Mental Health Services Administration; 2008. Technical Assistance Publication (TAP) Series 21. DHHS Publication No. (SMA) 08-4171.
3. Dennis ML, White M, Titus JC, et al. *Global Appraisal of Individual Needs: Administration Guide for the GAIN and Related Measures (version 5)*. Bloomington, IL: Chestnut Health Systems; 2003. Available at: http://www.chestnut.org/LI/gain/ index.html#Administration%20Manual. Accessed August 7, 2009.
4. Hanes-Stevens L, Dennis ML, White M. *GAIN Clinical Interpretation Training Manual*. Bloomington, IL: Chestnut Health Systems; 2007.
5. Dennis ML, Scott CK. Managing addiction as a chronic condition. *Addict Sci Clin Pract*. 2007;4:45–55.
6. Ford JH II, Green CA, Hoffman KA, et al. Process improvement needs in substance abuse treatment: admissions walk-through results. *J Subst Abuse Treat*. 2007;33:379–389.
7. Chan YF, Dennis ML, Funk RR. Prevalence and comorbidity co-occurrence of major internalizing and externalizing disorders among adolescents and adults presenting to substance abuse treatment. *J Subst Abuse Treat*. 2008;34:14–24.
8. Angst J, Sellaro R, Ries MK. Multimorbidity of psychiatric disorders as an indicator of clinical severity. *Eur Arch Psychiatry Clin Neurosci*. 2002;252:147–154.
9. Kandel DB, Johnson JG, Bird HR, et al. Psychiatric comorbidity among adolescents with substance use disorders: findings from the MECA study. *J Am Acad Child Adolesc Psychiatry*. 1999;38: 693–699.
10. Dennis ML, White M, Ives MI. Individual characteristics and needs associated with substance misuse of adolescents and young adults in addiction treatment. In: Leukefeld CG, Gullotta TP, Staton-Tindall M, eds. *Handbook on Adolescent Substance Abuse Prevention and Treatment: Evidence-Based Practice*. New London, CT: Child and Family Agency Press; 2009:45–72.
11. Kessler RC, Chiu WT, Demler O, et al. Prevalence, severity and comorbidity of 12-month DSM-IV disorders in the National Comorbidity Survey replication. *Arch Gen Psychiatry*. 2005;62: 617–627.
12. Krueger RF, Markon KE. Reinterpreting comorbidity: a model-based approach to understanding and classifying psychopathology. *Annu Rev Clin Psychol*. 2006;2:111–133.
13. Regier DA, Farmer ME, Rae DS, et al. Comorbidity of mental disorders with alcohol and other drug abuse: results from the Epidemiologic Catchment Area (ECA) study. *JAMA*. 1990;264: 2511–2518.
14. Drug and Alcohol Services Information System (DASIS). Admissions with co-occurring disorders: 1995 and 2001. *DASIS Rep 2004*. Available at: http://www.oas.samhsa.gov/2k4/dualTX/dualTX.htm. Accessed August 7, 2009.
15. Drug and Alcohol Services Information System (DASIS). Adolescents with co-occurring psychiatric disorders: 2003. *DASIS Rep 2005*. Available at: http://www.oas.samhsa.gov/2k5/youthMH/youthMH.htm. Accessed April 1, 2008.
16. This was done for the second author as part of the planning for the Assertive Continuing Care (ACC) experiment (NIAAA grant no. AA010368, PI Mark Godley mgodley@chestnut.org).
17. Miller WS. Motivational interviewing with problem drinkers. *Behav Psychother*. 1983;11:147–172.
18. Bollen K, Lennox R. Conventional wisdom on measurement: a structural equation perspective. *Psychol Bull*. 1991;110: 305–314.
19. Dennis ML, Chan YF, Funk R. Development and validation of the GAIN Short Screener (GSS) for internalizing externalizing, and substance use disorders and crime/violence problems among adolescents and adults. *Am J Addict*. 2006;15:1–12.
20. Conrad KJ, Conrad KM, Dennis ML, et al. Validation of the Substance Problem Scale (SPS) to the Rasch Measurement Model. GAIN Methods Report 1.1. Chicago, IL: Chestnut Health Systems; 2009. Available at: http://chestnut.org/LI/gain/psychometric_reports/Conrad_et_al_2009_SPS_Report.pdf. Accessed May 19, 2010. (See also other GAIN Working Papers for each of the scales in exhibit 1 at http://www.chestnut.org/li/gain/#GAIN%20Working%20 Papers.)

21. American Psychiatric Association. *Diagnostic and Statistical Manual of Mental Disorders (DSM-IV-TR)*. 4th ed., text rev. Washington, DC: American Psychiatric Association; 2000.
22. World Health Organization. *International Statistical Classification of Disease and Related Health Problems, tenth revision (ICD-10)*. 2nd ed. Geneva: Author; 2007. Retrieved August 7, 2009, from http://apps.who.int/classifications/apps/icd/icd10online/.
23. American Society of Addiction Medicine (ASAM). *Patient Placement Criteria for the Treatment for Substance-Related Disorders.* 2nd ed. Chevy Chase, MD: American Society of Addiction Medicine; 2001.
24. Titus JC, Dennis ML, Lennox R, et al. Development and validation of short versions of the Internal Mental Distress and Behavior Complexity Scales in the Global Appraisal of Individual Needs (GAIN). *J Behav Health Serv Res.* 2008;35: 195–214.

CHAPTER 10

Diagnosis and Classification: *DSM-IV-TR* and *ICD-10*

George E. Woody ■ John Cacciola

The *Diagnostic and Statistical Manual of Mental Disorders*, 4th ed. (*DSM-IV*) (1) is the diagnostic classification system developed by the American Psychiatric Association. Although the *DSM-IV* was updated and published as the *DSM-IV-TR* (*Text Revision*), the disorders and diagnostic criteria have not changed as of this writing (2) though changes are being considered for *DSM-V*, which is tentatively scheduled for publication in 2013. The *International Classification of Disease, Tenth Revision* (*ICD-10*) (3) is the system used by the World Health Organization and has also remained unchanged though it may be modified after *DSM-V* is published. The substance use disorders sections of previous iterations of each classification system differed significantly from each other, though many of the concepts they contained were similar. As a result, considerable efforts were made to make these two systems as similar as possible and these efforts were mostly successful. *ICD-10* actually has two versions: the clinical and the research. The clinical version is the manual that is used in clinical practice and is the main focus of this chapter, although the research version of *ICD-10* is mentioned briefly in the discussion of course modifiers for dependence.

This chapter compares the sections of *ICD-10* and *DSM-IV-TR* that deal with substance-related disorders and discusses proposed changes in *DSM-IV-TR* that are being considered for *DSM-V*. Many details are only mentioned or described in very general terms so as to present an easily readable and memorable comparison of the two systems.

OVERVIEW

Psychiatric disorders attributable to abusable substances are of two general types: (a) disorders related to the pattern and/or consequences of substance use itself (i.e., dependence, abuse [in *DSM-IV-TR*], and harmful use [in *ICD-10*]) and (b) disorders produced by the pharmacologic effects of the substances themselves (i.e., intoxication, withdrawal, and substance-induced mental disorders).

The edition preceding *DSM-IV-TR*, the *Diagnostic and Statistical Manual of Mental Disorders*, 3rd ed., revised (*DSM-III-R*), organized these two general types of disorders into two areas, whereas *ICD-10* placed them in one section. In *DSM-III-R*, the substance-induced disorders were found in a section titled "Psychoactive Substance-Induced Organic Mental Disorders," whereas dependence and abuse were found in the "Psychoactive Substance Use Disorders" section. A major accomplishment of *DSM-IV* was to place all of these disorders into one section, "Substance-Related Disorders," consisting of two parts: "Substance Use Disorders," which includes dependence and abuse, and "Substance-Induced Disorders," which includes intoxication, withdrawal, and substance-induced mental disorders. This major change in the organization of *DSM-IV*, and retained in the *DSM-IV-TR*, has made their overall organization much more similar to that of *ICD-10*. Nevertheless, there still exist substance-induced disorders that are not shared by the two classification systems, and criteria-level differences still exist between disorders that are shared by the two systems.

In each classification system, abusable substances or their general drug class are listed and criteria are provided so that any of the disorders attributable to that substance can be identified and numbered. For example, "Alcohol Withdrawal" in the *DSM-IV-TR* is described and diagnostic criteria are summarized and coded as 291.8; "Amphetamine-Induced Mood Disorder" is identified and coded as 292.84; "Cocaine Dependence" is described and coded as 304.20; and so on. In general, the descriptive text for each of the diagnostic categories in *DSM-IV-TR* is more detailed than that found in *ICD-10*.

Differences remain, however, the most prominent of which is found in the use of the terms "abuse" in *DSM-IV-TR* and "harmful use" in *ICD-10*. Most importantly, each classification system is founded on the Edwards and Gross definition of the dependence syndrome (4,5), a concept that was originally developed from work with individuals having problems with alcohol but later expanded to all abusable substances.

DEPENDENCE, ABUSE, AND HARMFUL USE

Dependence

DSM-IV-TR has seven criteria items for dependence and *ICD-10* has six. In each classification system, three items are necessary to make a diagnosis of dependence. Specific items are ordered differently in each system; however, as Table 10.1 illustrates, their similarities are readily apparent when they are compared.

In *DSM-IV-TR*, dependence is specified as being either with or without physiologic features. Dependence with physiologic features is present if there is evidence of tolerance or withdrawal (i.e., criterion items 1 or 2 are present). Dependence without physiologic features is present if three or more items

TABLE 10.1 Comparison of *DSM–IV* and *ICD-10* criteria items for dependence

DSM-IV	ICD-10
Three or more of:	same
1) tolerance	iv) same
2) withdrawal	iii) same
3) the substance is often taken in larger amounts or over a longer period than was intended	ii) difficulties in controlling substance-taking behavior in terms of its onset, termination, or levels of use
4) any unsuccessful effort or a persistent desire to cut down or control substance use	no corresponding *ICD* category
5) a great deal of time is spent in activities necessary to obtain substance or recover from its effects	v) increased amounts of time necessary to obtain or take the substance or recover from its effects. Note: (v) item has two parts; this phrase represents one part
6) important social, occupational, or recreational activities given up or reduced because of substance use	v) progressive neglect of the alternative pleasures or interests. Note: (v) item has two parts; this phrase represents one part
7) continued substance use despite knowledge of having had a persistent or recurrent physical or psychological problems that are likely to be caused or exacerbated by the substance	vi) persisting with substance use despite evidence of overtly harmful problem consequences
no corresponding *DSM* category	i) a strong desire or sense of compulsion to take the substance

are present but none of these are items 1 or 2. There is no comparable subtyping of dependence in *ICD-10*.

Abuse and Harmful Use

Although the current *ICD* and the *DSM* definitions of dependence are very similar, the two systems differ sharply on the concepts of abuse and harmful use. In *DSM-IV-TR*, abuse is defined in social terms, that is, problematic use in the absence of compulsive use, tolerance, and withdrawal. *ICD* has been reluctant to accept criteria items that are defined in terms of social impairment. However, *ICD* does recognize a nondependent type of substance use disorder. In *ICD-10*, this disorder is called "Harmful Use" and involves substance use that results in actual physical or mental damage.

This difference between *DSM* and *ICD* in the acceptability of social criteria for defining a disorder is primarily because *ICD* must be applicable to a wide range of cultures. Social mores differ so markedly between countries that it is difficult to develop socially defined criteria that can be applied across cultures. For example, any use of alcohol in a Moslem country can lead to major adverse social consequences, whereas Western societies have integrated alcohol use into their social fabric. The *ICD-10* category of harmful use is one that can be applied cross-culturally, and is the closest that *ICD* comes to the *DSM* concept of abuse. However, harmful use is really a different construct because it is limited to use that causes actual physical or mental damage. Harmful use is in many ways a more restrictive category than abuse, and some persons having a *DSM-IV-TR* abuse diagnosis do not meet criteria for harmful use. Table 10.2 is a summary comparison of Abuse and Harmful Use.

In addition to pointing out the major differences between *DSM-IV-TR* and *ICD-10* in this area, Table 10.2 also reflects a major change made to the definition of abuse. Unlike *DSM-III-R* and other earlier iterations of the *DSM*, *DSM-IV-TR* separates the criteria items for abuse from those for dependence. This change was done by attempting to identify only items that signify problematic or hazardous use as abuse and by leaving only items signifying compulsive use, tolerance, or withdrawal as dependence.

Four *DSM-IV* criteria items were developed for abuse. One (hazardous use) had been part of earlier definitions.

TABLE 10.2 A comparison of abuse and harmful use

DSM-IV	ICD-10
Abuse	**Harmful use**
One or more of the following occurring over the same 12-month period:	Clear evidence that the substance use was responsible for (or substantially contributed to) physical or psychological harm, including impaired judgment or dysfunctional behavior.
1) recurrent substance use resulting in a failure to fulfill major role obligations at work, school, or home	
2) recurrent substance use in situations in which it is physically hazardous	
3) recurrent substance-related legal problems	
4) continued substance use despite having persistent or recurrent social or interpersonal problems caused or exacerbated by the effects of the substance Never met criteria for dependence	

Another (use resulting in failure to fulfill role obligations) was moved from a *DSM-III-R* dependence criterion item to abuse. The third and fourth items (recurrent substance-related legal problems; continued use despite having recurrent social or interpersonal problems) were split from one *DSM-III-R* dependence item and moved to abuse. Portions of that original item (recurrent substance-related medical or psychiatric problems) remained in a *DSM-IV* dependence item. Because diagnostic criteria did not change from *DSM-IV* to *DSM-IV-TR*, the operationalization of abuse is the same for both.

DSM-IV-TR DEPENDENCE COURSE MODIFIERS

Both *DSM-IV-TR* and *ICD-10* include course modifiers for dependence. *DSM-IV* expanded the limited number of course modifiers that were present in *DSM-III-R*, again resulting in greater consistency between *DSM-IV-TR* and *CD-10*. The course modifiers for both classification systems apply only to dependence and not to abuse or harmful use.

DSM-IV-TR organizes its course modifiers in terms of stage of remission, agonist therapy, or being in a controlled environment.

Remission

A person is not classified as being in remission until that person has been free of all criteria items for dependence and all of the "A" items for abuse (to be described later in Table 10.2) for at least 1 month. The first 12 months following cessation of problems with the substance is a period of particularly high risk for relapse; thus, it is given the special designation of "Early Remission." There are two categories:

- *Early Full Remission:* No criteria for dependence, and none of the "A" criteria for abuse, have been met for the last 1 to 12 months.
- *Early Partial Remission:* Full criteria for dependence or abuse have not been met for the last 1 to 12 months; however, one or two dependence, or one or more of the "A" abuse criteria, have been met, intermittently or continuously, during this period of Early Remission.

When 12 months of Early Remission have passed without relapse to dependence, the person is in "Sustained Remission." There are two categories in this case:

- *Sustained Full Remission:* None of the criterion items for dependence and none of the criterion items for abuse have been present in the last 12 months.
- *Sustained Partial Remission:* Full criteria for dependence have not been met for a period of 12 months or longer. However, one or two dependence, or one or more of the "A" criteria for abuse, have been met, either continuously or intermittently, during this period of Sustained Remission.

On Agonist Therapy

For the course modifier "on agonist therapy," the person is on prescribed, supervised agonist medication related to the substance, and the criteria for dependence or abuse (other than tolerance or withdrawal) have not been met for the agonist medication in the last month. This category also applies to persons being treated for dependence using an agonist/antagonist with prominent agonist properties, such as buprenorphine.

In a Controlled Environment

Another course modifier is that the person is "in a controlled environment." In this case, no criteria for dependence or abuse are met but the person has been in an environment for 1 month or longer where controlled substances are highly restricted. Examples are closely supervised and substance-free jails, therapeutic communities, or locked hospital units. Occasionally, persons will be on agonist therapy while also in a controlled environment. In such cases, both course modifiers (on agonist therapy and in a controlled environment) apply.

Just as the remission categories require a transitional month without satisfying any criteria for dependence or abuse, the 1-month period after cessation of agonist therapy or release from a controlled environment is a corresponding transition period. Thus, persons in this 1-month period are still considered dependent. They will move into an Early Remission category after being free of all criteria for dependence and of the "A" abuse criteria for 1 month.

ICD-10 DEPENDENCE COURSE MODIFIERS

The course modifiers for *ICD* are similar but not identical and are as follows:

- Currently abstinent
- Currently abstinent, but in a protected environment (e.g., hospital, therapeutic community, prison)
- Currently on a clinically supervised maintenance or replacement regime (controlled dependence) (e.g., with methadone, nicotine gum, or nicotine patch)
- Currently abstinent, but receiving treatment with aversive or blocking drugs (e.g., naltrexone [Narcan] or disulfiram [Antabuse])
- Currently using the substance (active dependence)
- Continuous use
- Episodic use (dipsomania)

After publication of the *ICD-10* clinical criteria, the *ICD-10* research criteria were published. The section on course modifiers in the research criteria were made even more similar to those of *DSM-IV-TR* by adding three subcategories to "Currently abstinent," namely, "Early Remission," "Partial Remission," and "Full Remission." Also, two subcategories were added to "Currently using the substance," "Without physical features" and "With physical features." The phrase, "The course of the dependence may be further specified, if desired, as follows:" was added before the terms "Continuous use" and "Episodic use [dipsomania]." These changes to the *ICD-10* research criteria set the stage for even more integration between *DSM-V* and the next iteration of the *ICD*.

SUBSTANCE-INDUCED DISORDERS

As described above, intoxication, withdrawal, and the wide range of substance-induced mental disorders are included in a single section in both *DSM-IV-TR* and *ICD-10*. *DSM-IV-TR* provides a brief description of the clinical manifestations of intoxication and withdrawal for each substance; exceptions are those few substances that do not have an identified withdrawal syndrome, such as lysergic acid diethylamide (LSD). *ICD-10* provides less detail about each substance but provides general criteria that allow for classification of intoxication or withdrawal according to specific substances.

DSM-IV-TR also provides considerable detail for the substance-induced mental disorders. Table 10.3 identifies and summarizes the wide range of mental disorders that can be produced by substances.

Each of the mental disorders that are listed in Table 10.3 are referenced and coded in the text accompanying that specific substance. They are also cross-referenced with the section of *DSM-IV-TR* that deals with that type of disorder. For example, psychotic disorders attributable to alcohol intoxication or withdrawal are mentioned and coded in the text dealing with alcohol, and the reader is directed to the psychotic disorders section of *DSM-IV-TR* for a more complete description of these disorders. *ICD-10* provides a more general format that allows for classification of substance-induced mental disorders, but provides much less substance-specific detail than *DSM-IV-TR*.

COMPARISONS OF DIFFERENCES IN SPECIFIC DIAGNOSTIC CATEGORIES

There are a few other important categories that are found in one system but not the other. For instance, *DSM-IV-TR* has three categories that are not specified in *ICD-10*: "Polysubstance Dependence," "Other (or Unknown) Substance-Related Disorders," and "Phencyclidine (or Phencyclidine-Like)-Related Disorders." These categories would likely be classified under the *ICD-10* heading of "Disorders Resulting from Multiple Drug Use and Use of Other Psychoactive Substances."

A number of substances have limited diagnostic possibilities in *DSM-IV-TR* but have a wider range of *ICD-10* diagnostic labels. For instance, caffeine is included in the stimulant section of *ICD-10* and thus is open to a wide range of subcategories. In contrast, "Caffeine Intoxication," "Caffeine-Induced Anxiety Disorder," and "Caffeine-Induced Sleep Disorder" are the only categories available for this substance in *DSM-IV*. Similarly, *DSM-IV-TR* has only two categories involving nicotine: dependence and withdrawal. *ICD-10* has the same wide range of diagnostic categories for nicotine that is available for all other substances.

ICD-10 has a section (listed as a subsection of "Behavioural Syndromes Associated with Physiological Disturbances and Physical Factors") that is separate from the psychoactive substance use section and that is used for classifying abuse of non–dependence-producing substances. This includes problematic use of antidepressants, laxatives, steroids, and

TABLE 10.3	Diagnoses associated with class of substances												
Alcohol	X	X	X	X	I	W P	P	I/W	I/W	I/W	I	I/W	
Amphetamines	X	X	X	X	I			I	I/W	I	I	I/W	
Caffeine			X					I		I			
Cannabis	X	X	X		I			I		I			
Cocaine	X	X	X	X	I			I	I/W	I/W	I	I/W	
Hallucinogens	X	X	X		I			I[a]	I	I			
Inhalants	X	X	X		I		P	I	I	I			
Nicotine	X			X									
Opioids	X	X	X	X	I			I	I		I	I/W	
Phencyclidine	X	X	X		I			I	I	I			
Sedatives, hypnotics, or anxiolytics	X	X	X	X	I	W	P	P	I/W	I/W			
Polysubstance	X												
Other	X	X	X	X	I	W	P	P	I/W	I/W	I/W	I	I/W

[a]Also "Hallucinogens Persisting Disorder (Flashbacks)."

Note: X, I, W, I/W, and P indicate that the category is recognized in *DSM–IV*. In addition, I indicates that the specifier "With Onset During Intoxication" may be noted for the category (except for "Intoxication Delirium"); W indicates that the specifier "With Onset During Withdrawal" may be noted for the category (except for "Withdrawal Delirium"); and I/W indicates that either "With Onset During Intoxication" or "With Onset During Withdrawal" may be noted for the category. P indicates that the disorder is persisting. Reproduced from Frances A, Pincus HA, First MB, eds. *Diagnostic and Statistical Manual of Mental Disorders*. 4th ed. Washington, DC: American Psychiatric Association Press; 1994:177, with permission.

hormones. A comparable section in *DSM-IV-TR* is found under "Other (or Unknown) Substance-Related Disorders."

CHANGES CURRENTLY UNDER CONSIDERATION FOR *DSM-V*

Several changes are under consideration for *DSM-V* though no final decisions have been made. Among the changes that appear most likely to occur are substituting "addiction" for "dependence," merging some or all of the abuse criteria with those for dependence (i.e., the new category of "addiction") so there is one disorder with varying levels of severity (6), and adding a category for marijuana withdrawal (7).

Changes that are being discussed but with less certainty are adding a category for compulsive behaviors such as gambling, and listing in the Appendix other potential nonsubstance addictions such as Internet use, eating, shopping, and sex (6); adding a category for disorders first diagnosed in infancy, childhood, or adolescence that would include conduct disorder and problematic substance use, since they often occur together and there are data showing that they share common genetic factors; adding age of onset and number of substances used to determine severity of the disorder; being more specific about terms such as "recurrent" or "continued" use in the definitions so as to improve the precision of assessments that are used to make diagnoses (8); and modifying the remission criteria so a patient can be diagnosed as in remission from opioid dependence while on medication-assisted therapy (medication to be specified). All disorders will have a dimensional component, at least for severity, and comorbidity of substance use disorder with other mental disorders will be listed though the format for such a listing has not been determined as of this writing (6).

SUMMARY

Many of the major differences between the *DSM* and *ICD* classification systems were eliminated or considerably reduced by the development of the *DSM-IV-TR* and *ICD-10*. The most prominent remaining difference is in the concepts underlying abuse and harmful use but this difference may lessen in *DSM-V*. Less-prominent differences are found in the less-detailed descriptions of the various clinical syndromes in *ICD-10* as compared to *DSM-IV-TR*, and in *ICD-10*'s ability to attach the entire range of substance-related diagnoses to any drug class, whereas *DSM-IV-TR* provides more limits on the number of diagnostic possibilities. Generally, *ICD-10* has more categories available for each substance than *DSM-IV-TR*, but some of these categories are rarely used because their existence is unclear. An example is hallucinogen withdrawal—a possible category in *ICD-10* that is not present in *DSM-IV-TR* and probably rarely used in *ICD-10* due to uncertainty about its existence.

Overall, there are many more similarities than differences between *DSM-IV-TR* and *ICD-10*, especially when one focuses on the specific categories described (with the exception of abuse and harmful use, also likely to change in *DSM-V*), and on the similarities in the ways dependence and its course modifiers are defined. It is hoped that future work will succeed in creating even more consistency between these two classification systems. A review of the two systems by Rounsaville discusses other barriers to reconciling *ICD* and *DSM* in the future (9). He concludes, as suggested by this review, that reconciliation may be most difficult for the abuse/harmful use disparity, perhaps less so for the substance-induced disorders, and most readily achieved for dependence.

REFERENCES

1. American Psychiatric Association. *Diagnostic and Statistical Manual of Mental Disorders.* 4th ed. (*DSM-IV*). Washington, DC: American Psychiatric Association; 1994.
2. American Psychiatric Association. *Diagnostic and Statistical Manual of Mental Disorders.* 4th ed., text revision (*DSM-IV-TR*). Washington, DC: American Psychiatric Association; 2000.
3. World Health Organization. *Tenth Revision of the International Classification of Disease (ICD-10).* Geneva: World Health Organization; 1992.
4. Edwards G, Gross MM. Alcohol dependence: provisional description of a clinical syndrome. *Br J Med.* 1976;1:1058–1061.
5. Edwards G. The alcohol dependence syndrome: a concept as stimulus to enquiry. *Br J Addict.* 1986;81:171–183.
6. O'Brien C. Addiction vs. dependence for DSM V. Presented at annual meeting of College on Problems of Drug Dependence, Reno, Nv, June 2009
7. Budney A. Inclusion of cannabis withdrawal and related issues. Presented at annual meeting of College on Problems of Drug Dependence. Reno, NV, June 2009.
8. Crowley TJ. Combining abuse with dependence. Presented at annual meeting of College on Problems of Drug Dependence. Reno, NV, June 2009.
9. Rounsaville B. Experience with ICD-10/*DSM-IV* substance use disorders. *Psychopathology.* 2002;35:82–88.

Diagnostic Laboratory: Screening for Drug Abuse

Karl G. Verebey ■ Gerard Meenan

Alcohol and drug abuse are two major health care problems in America. This has prompted advancement in laboratory methods diagnosing substance abuse in psychiatric patients and suspected drug abusers. Physicians are more knowledgeable today than in the past about the nature of drug abuse, yet uncertainty remains over the use of the "diagnostic laboratory." The confusion surrounding drug-abuse testing is a result of many variable technicalities. Each drug is unique, and detectability depends on the drug's chemical properties, size of the dose, frequency of use, the biologic specimen tested, differences in individual drug metabolism, sample collection time in relation to use, and sensitivity of the analytic method (1,2). All these variables make each test request unique, and there are no general rules for all drugs and all situations.

This chapter reviews drug-abuse testing from several perspectives. A brief history is followed by a section on the reasons for testing. In addition, sections on the available methodologies, testing strategies, and data interpretation are included.

HISTORY OF DRUG TESTING

The modern drug-abuse testing laboratory is a relatively recent development. Initially, drug testing was exclusively part of the pathology services in which overdose or fatal toxicity cases were investigated for the causative agents. Very large sample volumes were processed with crude, nonspecific methodology. As drugs of abuse became a major social problem, overdose cases also became more common. Hospital laboratories were called upon to perform emergency toxicology procedures to identify drug classes or specific drugs.

Another branch of testing developed when patients in drug-abuse treatment programs needed follow-up to objectively monitor whether or not the substitute drug (generally methadone) was taken. Also, testing for drugs of abuse checked if abstinence was maintained. Such testing that aided rehabilitation was performed mostly in hospitals or clinical laboratories.

The volume of drug-abuse testing has increased as a consequence of widespread employee testing by the federal government, the military, and the private industry. This has influenced the development of specific urine drug testing laboratories.

Forensic drug testing is the newest to appear on the scene, forced upon the clinical laboratories by the legal profession. The results of a drug test were used for more than clinical purposes. The results could have punitive consequences. Positive results were sometimes questioned or flatly denied, and lawyers started to scrutinize every step of the testing process from collection to reporting of results. Forensic accountability was then required to protect the "due process rights" of clients. After losing court cases, clinical laboratories that performed legally sensitive testing began to reorganize. "Chain of custody" procedures were designed, and quality control and quality assurance procedures were implemented to promote reliability and reproducibility of test results. Drug-testing procedures and instrumentation became more sophisticated, more sensitive, and more specific. As a result, extremely small quantities of drugs can be determined reliably at the nanogram and picogram range, and gas chromatography-mass spectrometry (GC-MS) and gas chromatography-tandem mass spectrometry (GC-MS-MS) provide assurance of specific drug identification (2,3). More recently LC-MS and LC-MS-MS became favored because in many cases no extraction was needed, simplifying analysis.

RATIONALE FOR TESTING

Drug abuse is characterized by impulsive drug-seeking behavior with occasional interruption and later almost certain relapses. A common feature of many drug abusers is denial. Abusers lie to themselves and the forbidding outside world to protect their continued, obsessive use of drugs and/or alcohol. For this reason, physicians are seldom given voluntarily the diagnostically important information about addictive habits.

The type of drug and the abuse pattern are important parts of the medical history. The attending physician cannot properly design treatment when kept in the dark about the patient's addiction. Symptoms of physical and/or psychiatric illness may be simulated by the presence or absence of certain drugs. The dichotomy of symptoms associated with the presence or absence of a drug is best illustrated by the opioid class of drugs (4). While under the influence of an opioid drug such as heroin, the addict experiences euphoric, anxiolytic sedation; mental clouding; sweating; and constipation. Opioid withdrawal signs and symptoms are characterized by pupillary mydriasis, agitation, anxiety, panic, muscle aches, gooseflesh, rhinorrhea, salivation, and diarrhea. Thus, the two different sets of symptoms belong to the abuse of the same drug, observed at times when opioid drugs are present and at times when opioid drugs are absent.

In predisposed individuals, drugs can trigger behavior similar or identical to psychosis. For example, phencyclidine (PCP), lysergic acid diethylamide (LSD), amphetamines, or cocaine can cause toxic psychosis that is indistinguishable from paranoid schizophrenia. These drugs can produce model psychosis in anyone given an adequate dose. Drug-induced psychosis has a different prognosis and must be treated differently from psychosis related to endogenous organic, anatomic, or neurochemical disorders (5).

Treatment of drug abusers in therapy would be extremely handicapped if testing were not used. Comprehensive drug testing is important for making precise follow-up evaluations and selecting appropriate treatment (6). Thus, the first good reason for laboratory drug testing is to provide objective identification of drug abusers and identify the substance abused.

Testing is also important after drug abusers are identified. Treatment strategies are intimately connected to frequent urinalyses to monitor recovering addicts. Negative results support the success of treatment, while positive results alert the physician to relapses. An exception is methadone treatment, where a positive result proves that the substitute drug is taken as prescribed. Objective testing, therefore, is a necessary component of modern substance abuse treatment (6).

Drug-abuse testing may also be forensic in nature. Parole officers monitor ex–drug abusers after release from incarceration. A positive drug test may signal to law enforcement the parolee's involvement with drugs and may invalidate the parole.

Often health care professionals such as doctors, dentists, and nurses are afflicted with drug-abuse problems. Once involvement with drugs is exposed, professional medical licenses are in danger of suspension. Rehabilitation of addicted health care professionals is linked to drug testing as a condition of probation. But testing must meet forensic standards because of possible legal challenges.

Professional athletes sometimes abuse drugs. Both national and international sport associations prohibit the use of performance-enhancing drugs (7). Staying drug free is a prerequisite for athletes to be allowed to compete. Forensic laboratory testing for drugs of abuse and performance-enhancing drugs is the objective technique used to enforce these rules.

Finally, workplace and public safety may be endangered by impaired or intoxicated employees. Bankers and stockbrokers who handle investors' money must not be influenced by psychoactive drugs, especially drugs that cause delusions and impulsive risk-taking behavior such as cocaine and amphetamine. Similarly, drug-abusing professionals in other fields may endanger the public. Drug and alcohol abuse has been identified among airline pilots, bus drivers, railroad engineers, and police officers. In all these professions, drug-abuse testing is helpful to the drug abuser and in protecting the general public. The abuser gets early treatment and a chance for early rehabilitation. The public is saved from potential drug-related accidents and associated damages.

A decrease in drug abuse as a result of drug testing has been demonstrated clearly in the military. Prior to the institution of mandated random testing in 1981, 48% of armed forces personnel used illegal drugs. Three years after testing began, fewer than 5% were using drugs (8). Although critics often attack testing as ineffective, drug abuse clearly decreases where effective drug testing exists. Testing is a deterrent because most people do not take chances if they know that when their drug use is identified it can result in the loss of their job.

ABUSED DRUGS TESTED

Epidemiologic studies expose the types of drugs used, new trends, and frequency of drug abuse by different populations in specific geographic regions and countries. Such information is used to help identify drug abusers in critical areas. The testing of five drugs, selected by the Department of Health and Human Services/Substance Abuse and Mental Health Services Administration (DHHS/SAMHSA), is required for accreditation by their National Laboratory Certification Program (NLCP) (Table 11.1). Panel I testing includes amphetamines, cannabinoids, cocaine, opioids, and PCP (usually referred to as the SAMHSA-5). Panel II represents other commonly abused drugs, such as barbiturates, benzodiazepines, methadone, oxycodone, methylenedioxymethamphetamine (MDMA), methylenedioxyamphetamine (MDA), and ethanol. Interestingly, some powerful hallucinogens are seldom tested routinely. LSD, psilocybin, and ketamine are listed in Panel III with club drugs and other designer drugs. Some of these drugs are psychoactive

TABLE 11.1 Panel groups of abused drugs: tests performed by laboratories

I: Required[a]	II: Commonly performed	III: Not commonly performed
Amphetamines	Barbiturates	LSD
Cannabinoids	Benzodiazepines	Fentanyl
Cocaine	Methadone	Psilocybin
Opioids	Oxycodone	Ketamine
Phencyclidine	MDMA	GHB
	MDA	Designer drugs
	Ethanol	

[a]Testing required for certification by the DHHS/SAMHSA National Laboratory Certification Program.

in very low doses. Therefore, when they are diluted in total body water, concentration is low and detection is difficult, unless large doses are taken or samples are collected shortly after drug use.

"Designer drugs" often are structurally similar to the commonly abused drugs. While they are new and structurally different, they are already regulated when sold and used. Nevertheless, "street chemists" are synthesizing new and often dangerous drugs. They will operate as long as abusers will try new drugs, and their illegal trade remains profitable. Alpha-methylfentanyl is an example of an illicit analog of fentanyl. The laboratory's role is to develop new and sensitive methods for the detection of new designer drugs in the biofluids of users.

CLUB DRUGS OF ABUSE

Gamma-hydroxybutyrate (GHB) is a central nervous system depressant. It is an endogenous substance in human and mammalian tissues at very low concentrations and thought to be a neuromodulator. It has clinical use in the treatment of cataplexy. Some of the pharmacologic effects are drowsiness, euphoria, dizziness, vomiting, respiratory depression, and death. Use of this drug as a recreational or club drug has resulted in GHB intoxication and death (9). Detection of GHB is accomplished with analysis of urine by GC-MS.

Another drug used in clubs and date rapes is flunitrazepam (Rohypnol), a member of the benzodiazepine family of drugs. Only available in Europe, it is abused in the United States as a club drug. At low doses it causes relaxation and sleepiness, and at larger doses, anesthesia. Similar to other benzodiazepines, detection is performed by screening with an immunoassay and confirmation with GC-MS or high performance liquid chromatography (HPLC) (10).

Recently, ketamine (Ketalar) or Special K has appeared in clubs. It is chemically related to PCP or angel dust (10). Both of these drugs were used as rapidly acting dissociative anesthetics. However, in some individuals, ketamine and PCP produce exit psychosis with paranoid ideation. For this reason ketamine is currently not used in humans; it is used in veterinary medicine. Abuse of ketamine results in a diverse set of reactions depending on individual predispositions: numbness, loss of coordination, sense of invulnerability and muscle rigidity in some individuals, aggressive/violent behavior, slurred speech, blank stare, and an exaggerated sense of strength in others. Immunoassays were developed for ketamine screening. Positive results are confirmed by GC-MS, GC-MS-MS, or LC-MS-MS (10).

TESTS AVAILABLE

A number of different laboratory methods are available for drug screening. When the drug-abuse habit of a patient is unknown, the physician usually requests a "comprehensive drug screen." Different laboratories have different definitions of the term "comprehensive," omitting some important but less used drugs. The physician should be familiar with laboratory menus to ensure effective use of the drug-testing laboratory.

Urine samples are most commonly sent for a "routine drug screen." But oral fluid (saliva) testing is becoming more popular because of the ease of observed collection (11). Psychiatrists and other physicians assume that a comprehensive drug test detects all abused drugs. Thin-layer chromatography (TLC), mostly used in the past, is not sensitive enough to detect drugs such as marijuana, PCP, LSD, psilocybin, mescaline, and fentanyl, among others. Thus, a negative drug screen may mean one or more of the following: the test menu doesn't contain the drug(s) of interest, the test cutoff is too high, and there is no evidence of high dose or recent abuse of drugs commonly detected by the screening method used. Low-level abuse of drugs is not likely to be detected; therefore, "false negatives" are a possible result. More sensitive enzyme immunoassays (EIA) have replaced TLC as an initial screening procedure. EIA, enzyme-linked immunoadsorbent assay (ELISA), fluorescent polarization immunoassay (FPIA), and radioimmunoassay (RIA) are routinely used for initial drug screening in serum, urine, oral fluid, sweat, and hair.

If, for example, a physician suspects marijuana abuse, he/she must specifically request that a marijuana screen be performed by an immunoassay at the lowest cutoff. Screening for an unknown drug can be performed by capillary gas–liquid chromatography (GLC). In a single GLC analysis, more than 25 drugs can be identified (Fig. 11.1). This system is advantageous when there is no clue to the identity of the

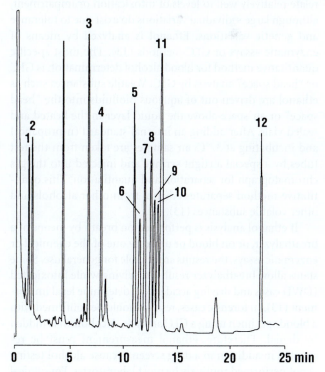

Figure 11.1. Gas–liquid chromatographic (GLC) tracing showing separation of a drug mixture. The abscissa is time in minutes; the ordinate is detector response. The different drugs are number coded on the tracing. The drugs are *1*, amphetamine; *2*, methamphetamine; *3*, meperidine; *4*, phencyclidine (PCP); *5*, methadone; *6*, amitriptyline; *7*, imipramine; *8*, cocaine; *9*, desipramine; *10*, pentazocine; *11*, codeine; and *12*, oxycodone. (Reprinted with permission from Alltech Associates, Inc., Deerfield, IL.)

abused or toxic substance. However, GLC, LC-MS, and GC-MS are all time-consuming, labor-intensive, and usually expensive procedures. LC-MS is similar to GC-MS in principle; however, sample preparation is easier. *LC-MS is preferable for the water-soluble drugs that are difficult to extract.* The EIA and ELISA tests are significantly less expensive and more practical for screening. Also, EIA procedures are easily adaptable for high-volume automated screening of drugs. In fact, most good laboratories offer a 5- or 10-drug panel, with or without alcohol, performed by EIA.

ANALYTIC METHODOLOGIES

Alcohol

Alcohol abuse is a legal version of drug abuse in the United States and most parts of the world. The addictive chemical substance in all alcoholic beverages is ethanol or ethyl alcohol. Ethanol is present in beer (3.2% to 4.5%), wine (7.11% to 14%), and distilled beverages (40% to 75%) (12). Using an average of 0.02 g% blood alcohol increase per drink, a 170-pound subject must ingest about four drinks of either 12 oz beer, 4 oz wine, or 1.5 oz whiskey in 1 hour to reach the ethanol level of 0.08 g/100 mL blood, or 80 mg/100 mL blood. The per se illegal limit to operate an automobile in most states is 0.08 g%.

Ethanol is one of the few drugs for which blood levels correlate relatively well to levels of intoxication or impairment, although large individual variations do exist due to tolerance and genetic variations. Ethanol is analyzed by means of enzymatic assays or GLC methods (13). The most specific quantitative method for blood alcohol determination is GLC or "head space" analysis by GLC. Volatile substances such as ethanol are driven out of aqueous biofluids into the "head space" or air space above the liquid layer in the heated and sealed vials. After adding an internal standard (n-propanol) and incubating at 37°C, air samples are taken from the test tubes by a special airtight syringe and injected into the gas chromatograph for separation and quantitation. This quantitative method separates ethanol from other alcohols and other volatile substances (13).

If ethanol analysis is performed on breath by means of a breathalyzer, or on blood or urine by one of the chemical or enzymatic assays, the results are reliable for general use. Some states allow breathalyzer results in driving while intoxicated (DWI) cases and driving accidents to determine legal impairment (13). In forensic cases, results should be confirmed with a blood specimen using a GLC analysis. Alcoholism is hidden by denial. Therefore, ethanol measurement must be requested in addition to a drug screen because alcohol testing is not performed routinely by most laboratories. For clinical purposes, urine alcohol levels can be converted to blood levels by a factor of 1.3 urine-to-blood ratio. In other words, the urine levels are usually 30% higher than blood levels. However, there is a great variation in the ratios shown in numerous studies. Breath alcohol analysis is widely used by law enforcement officers due to its practicality and quick noninvasive characteristic.

Alcohol Biomarkers

Alcohol biomarkers have been described as useful, objective indicators of outcome measures of pharmacologic or behavioral interventions for alcohol abuse, screening tests for people with alcohol problems, and a means of confirming abstinence in people prohibited from drinking (14). Alcohol biomarkers are either indirect or direct. Indirect biomarkers include blood chemistry analytes that demonstrate the harmful effects of alcohol. Examples of indirect biomarkers include gamma-glutamyltransferase (GGT), alanine aminotransferase (ALT), aspartate aminotransferase (AST), and carbohydrate-deficient transferrin (CDT). Direct alcohol biomarkers are metabolites of alcohol. Examples of direct biomarkers include ethyl glucuronide (EtG) and ethyl sulfate (EtS) (14).

Ethyl Glucuronide

EtG is a biomarker for recent alcohol use or exposure. Laboratory testing is performed on urine specimens, and EtG is detected for a significantly longer time after ingestion than alcohol (15). Testing for EtG includes EIA, HPLC, GC-MS, and LC-MS-MS. EIA offers a fast, inexpensive screen that can be performed on analyzers found in most clinical laboratories. EIA helps rule out alcohol consumption. All nonnegative EIA screens should be confirmed by an alternate methodology such as LC-MS-MS, which provides sensitive and highly specific results for EtG. The significant cost of an LC-MS-MS instrument and the need for a highly skilled instrument operator make EtG confirmation testing available at more specialized laboratories. LC-MS-MS can provide detection levels much lower than that of EIA. However, alcohol is ubiquitous in society; it is present in a number of commercial and household goods. Definitive data about a reliable cutoff to differentiate between alcohol abuse and accidental exposure is still under investigation.

Information in the scientific literature has reported that EtG levels greater than 500 ng/mL are extremely unlikely to be caused by accidental exposure to alcohol (15–17). Scientific studies have been made of different types of accidental exposures. One study (16) of hand sanitizer use (i.e., 20 washes per day with 60% ethanol containing handwash for 5 days) has been reported. Nine subjects' first morning urine samples, the most concentrated of the day, demonstrated levels between less than 10 and 114 ng/mL. Similarly, another study (17) of mouthwash use (i.e., three times daily with mouthwash containing 12% alcohol) demonstrated the following after 5 days. The first morning urine specimens were tested and all showed levels of less than 120 ng/mL. The risk of accidental exposure exists and must be considered in the evaluation of any patient.

An additional caution in the interpretation of a positive EtG result is the presence of glucose in a patient's urine. A study of postcollection synthesis of EtG by bacteria suggests the following: The risk of glucose in the urine of a diabetic patient is high. Microbial fermentation of the glucose to produce ethanol is likely. Bacterial contamination of the urine because of a urinary tract infection can occur. When these three factors are present, the likelihood of a positive EtG result is at least one in three (18).

Similar to the interpretation of other laboratory tests, a positive EtG result should be used as a sign—in this case a sign of possible alcoholic beverage consumption. Upon receipt of a positive EtG result, the health care professional needs to make further evaluation of the patient.

Enzyme Immunoassays and Enzyme-Linked Immunoadsorbent Assays

Figure 11.2 depicts the principle of immunoassays in drug detection. Antibodies are used to seek out specific drugs in biofluids. In samples containing one or more drugs, competition exists for available antibody-binding sites. The presence or absence of specific drugs is determined by the percent binding.

The specificity and sensitivity of the antibodies to a given drug differ depending on the particular drug assay and the assay manufacturer. Immunoassay can be very specific; however, compounds structurally similar to the drug of interest (i.e., metabolites or structural congeners) often cross-react. Interaction of the antibody with a drug plus its metabolites increases the sensitivity of the assay.

EIA, ELISA, and FPIA are commonly used for drug-abuse screening because no complicated extraction is required and the system lends itself to easy automation. EIA with specific antibodies is sensitive for most drugs and detects low drug and metabolite concentrations in biofluids (19).

ELISA offers greater sensitivity than some other screening assays (11). The sensitivity and specificity of the ELISA provide valuable utility to the clinician. A variety of biologic samples are applicable to ELISA such as urine, serum/plasma/blood, and oral fluid (saliva). Depending on the concentration of drug expected in the specimen, sample size can be adjusted accordingly. ELISA is available for manual, semiautomated, and fully automated platforms. Analysis time varies between 1 and 2 hours. ELISA cutoff levels and limits of detection (LODs) for oral fluid samples are very low: amphetamines 50 and 1 ng/mL, barbiturates 20 and 1 ng/mL, benzodiazepines 5 and 2 ng/mL, cocaine 20 and 1 ng/mL, methadone 5 and 1 ng/mL, opiates 40 and 0.25 ng/mL, PCP 10 and 0.5 ng/mL, THC 4 and 0.1 ng/mL, respectively. Also sample volumes for ELISA are as low as 10 μL per analysis (20).

As seen in the preceding paragraph, allowing for analysis of low levels of drug abuse, the LOD is in the very low nanogram range (11).

Comparative studies in the scientific literature support oral fluid as an excellent alternative to urine and blood for the identification of drug abuse. Because oral fluid collection is convenient, noninvasive, fast, and observable, sample adulteration is not likely to occur (11).

Several oral fluid sample collection devices are available. However, neat oral fluid collected in plain test tubes contained the highest concentrations of drugs when compared to collectors containing liquid buffer. Also, when collecting saliva into a liquid buffer, using a "lollipop"-type collector, one does not know if any oral fluid is actually collected (21,22). On the other hand, spitting into a tube is not as acceptable to subjects as are the "lollipop"-type collectors.

On-Site Screening Immunoassays

The increased prevalence of drug use and abuse has prompted the development of new drug screening technology that produces results in as little time as 5 minutes. Several situations require immediate results. Hospital emergency departments need rapid detection of drugs causing overdose toxicity and psychiatric reactions. In addition, quick results are useful for monitoring compliance within drug rehabilitation programs and supervising parolees released conditionally from prison. Because these tests are designed to be performed on-site, they are performed directly in front of the person being tested or, certainly, at the collection site. All presumptive positive tests must be confirmed by a laboratory-based alternate method. On-site testing is particularly useful for preemployment screening, random testing, probable cause workplace testing, and accident-related injuries. On-site screening may also be important to conduct in safety-oriented occupations, such as public transportation, aviation, and nuclear energy plants.

Visually interpreted immunoassays do not require complex instrumentation and no special technical skills. These kits are

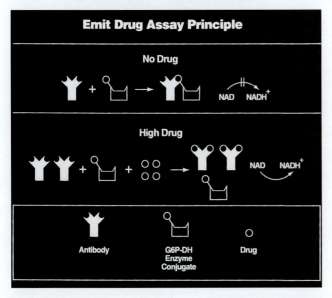

Figure 11.2. The basic principle of enzyme immunoassay (EIA) reactivity as it relates to drug detection. Molecules with similar functional groups cross-react; hence, immunoassays have less specificity than do chromatographic assays. EIA is the most popular screening procedure. G6P-DH = glucose-6-phosphate dehydrogenase; NAD = nicotinamide adenine dinucleotide; NADH = nicotinamide adenine dinucleotide (reduced form). (Reproduced with permission from Syva Company, Inc., Palo Alto, CA.)

particularly effective because there is no calibration, instrument maintenance, or downtime and no special skills needed to perform these tests. Most kits have built-in quality control zones in each panel, which ensures reagent integrity, sample validity checks, and sufficient sample size. Lastly, most on-site devices have an extended shelf life at room temperature.

There are currently many on-site kits available using simultaneous multiple drug detection capabilities. Some of the kits employ regular urine collection cups with multiple drug tests in a separate chamber in the device. Urine samples are in contact with the solid-phase, lyophilized reagents, and the reaction is allowed to continue for 5 minutes. The operator visually examines each zone for the presence or absence of a colored bar. A positive specimen produces a blank reaction in the drug detection zone. A negative specimen produces a colored bar. The method incorporates preset threshold concentrations that are set for each drug by SAMHSA.

The iScreen (Instant Technologies) in Figure 11.3 is a CLIA-waived stat screening kit, which detects 1 to 10 drugs from 15 drugs or drug classes. The device is dipped in urine and the results are visually read in 5 minutes. The iScreen also contains controls and several validity tests. It is a one-step, competitive, membrane-bound immunoassay. A urine sample can be evaluated for the presence of each of the specified classes of drugs. When one or more drugs are present or positive in a urine sample, the result window remains blank. Negative results are shown as a colored bar next to each result window. On-site screening kits have demonstrated greater than 97% agreement with confirmatory tests such as GC-MS (23). However, it must be stressed that these kits provide only preliminary test results, just as immunoassay tests run in a laboratory. A more specific alternate chemical method must be used to confirm presumptive positive screening results. GC-MS and LC-MS are the most specific confirmation methods.

An example of an on-site screening analyzer is the i-Cup (Instant Technologies, Fig. 11.4). The i-Cup performs two functions: It is a urine collection device ready to send out to a laboratory for confirmation of positive screen tests. Also, it is a one-step test for the rapid, qualitative detection of 3 to 9 drugs choosing from 14 drugs or drug classes in human urine. The choices are cannabinoids, cocaine/metabolite, opiates, amphetamines, PCP, tricyclic antidepressants, barbiturates, methadone, benzodiazepines, ecstasy (MDMA), methamphetamine, morphine, oxycodone, and propoxyphene.

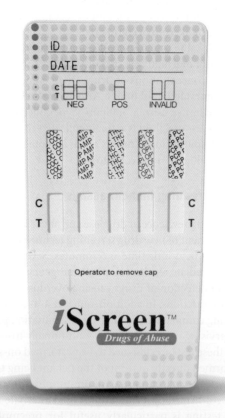

Figure 11.3. iScreen is a one-step urine drug detection card. The choice is from 15 commonly abused/used drugs. The program may choose 1 to 10 drugs to be placed on the test card. A simple dip in the urine sample and read provides results in minutes. The card also contains sample validity test zones for pH, specific gravity, oxidants, pyridinium chlorochlorate, glutaraldehyde, and creatinine. (Reproduced with permission from Instant Technologies, Norfolk, VA.)

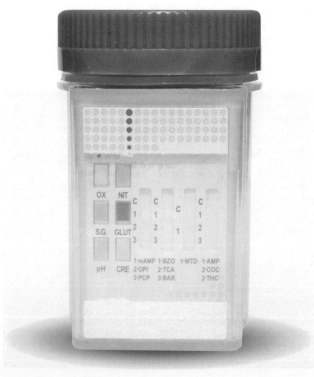

Figure 11.4. The i-Cup is an "all in one" urine sample collector and drug testing device. It detects the presence of drugs and adulterants (if present) in 5 minutes. Also, it measures the urine temperature (90°F–100°F) to prevent dilution during collection. The choice is from 14 drugs or drug classes that can be custom ordered in 3 to 10 drug panels. Positive samples can be sent directly to the laboratory for confirmation. The i-Cup also screens for adulterants: pH, specific gravity, and various oxidants. (Reproduced with permission from Instant Technologies, Norfolk, VA.)

Gas–Liquid Chromatography and Gas Chromatography-Mass Spectrometry

GLC is an analytic technique that separates molecules by migration, similar to TLC. The TLC plate is replaced by long glass or metal tubing called columns, which are packed or coated with stationary materials of variable polarity. Figure 11.1 is an example of a GLC tracing showing separation of drugs in a mixture. The extracted analyte is carried through the column to the detector by a steady flow of heated gas. The detector responds to the vaporized drugs. This response is graphically recorded and quantified as area under the peak. The peak area is proportional to the amount of drug or metabolite present in the sample. Identical compounds travel through the column at the same speed because they have identical interaction with the stationary column packing. The time between injection and the observed response of the peak at the recorder represents the retention time. Identical retention times of drugs or metabolites on two different polarity columns constitute strong evidence that the substances are identical.

Indisputable evidence can be obtained by the use of the MS detector, which identifies substances by gas chromatography separation and mass fragmentation patterns. Figure 11.5 shows a GC-MS separation and fragmentation pattern of cocaine and its major metabolite benzoylecgonine. The separation is shown at the bottom of the figure, while the fragmentation is shown in the top two panels. Cocaine has the fragments 82, 182, and 303 masses, while benzoylecgonine has 82, 240, and 361 masses.

Not all bonds in molecules are of equal strength. The weak bonds are more likely to break under stress. In the MS detector, electron beam bombardment breaks weak molecular bonds. The exact mass and quantity of the molecular fragments or breakage products are measured by the mass detector. The breakage of molecules results in a fragmentation pattern unique for a specific drug. The fragments occur in specific ratios to one another; thus, the GC-MS method is often called "molecular fingerprinting." Therefore, mass spectroscopy with either GC or LC separation is the most reliable and most definitive procedure in analytic chemistry for drug identification (3).

The fragmentation pattern of unknowns is checked against a computer library that lists the mass of drugs and related fragments. Matching a control's fragments and fragment ratios is considered absolute confirmation of a particular compound. The sensitivity of GLC for most drugs is in the nanogram range, but with special detectors some compounds can be measured at picogram levels. GLC and GC-MS can also be used quantitatively, which provides additional information helping to interpret a clinical syndrome or explain corroborating evidence in forensic cases. Tandem mass spectrometry (MS-MS) offers even greater sensitivity than GC-MS or LC-MS alone. For example, LSD confirmation by GC-MS-MS is as low as 200 pg. As the screening method's sensitivity approaches the low-nanogram range, confirmation sometimes requires picogram-level sensitivity to confirm presumptively positive samples.

Technically, samples are introduced into MS-MS detectors from gas chromatographs, liquid chromatographs, or direct insertion probes. The choice depends on sample volatility and purity. Thus, MS-MS provides a confirmation procedure for the even more sensitive screening methods (e.g., ELISA) and is used at very low drug concentrations common in alternate matrices, such as oral fluids, sweat, and hair analysis.

HPLC is used especially for drugs that are polar or not volatile and cannot be made volatile by derivatization. Some of these drugs and glucuronidated metabolites are not amenable for analysis by GC or GC-MS. Examples of drugs

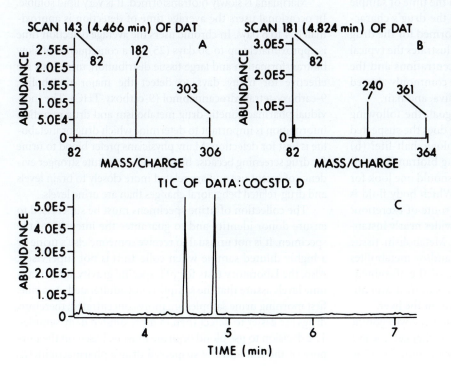

Figure 11.5. Gas chromatography-mass spectrometry showing the fragmentation pattern of cocaine (**A**) and benzoylecgonine (**B**). Total ion chromatogram (**C**) showing the chromatographic separation of cocaine (4 minutes 28 seconds) and benzoylecgonine (4 minutes 51 seconds). (Reproduced with permission from Drs. R. W. Taylor, N. C. Jain, and the *Journal of Analytical Toxicology*.)

TABLE 11.2 Performance characteristics of different assays for drugs of abuse

Assay	Sensitivity	Specificity	Accuracy	Turnaround time	Cost ($)
On-site	Moderate–high	Moderate	Qualitative[a]	Minutes	4–25
EMIT, FPIA, ELISA	Moderate–high	Moderate	Low–high	1–4 hours	5–10
GC	High	Moderate	Excellent	Day(s)	20–40
GC-MS	High	High	Excellent	Day(s)	30–100
LC-MS	High	High	Excellent	Day(s)	30–100

[a]Results are generally expressed only in qualitative terms (i.e., positive/negative); consequently, accuracy may be difficult to assess. Presumptive positive test results need confirmation by either GC-MS or LC-MS.

EMIT, enzyme-multiplied immunoassay technique; FPIA, fluorescent polarization immunoassay; GC, gas chromatography; GC-MS, gas chromatography-mass spectrometry; ELISA, enzyme-linked immunoadsorbent assay; LC-MS, liquid chromatography-mass spectrometry.

Adapted from Cone EJ. New developments in biological measures of drug prevalence. *NIDA Res Monogr Ser.* 1986;167:104–126.

or drug groups for which HPLC is the choice of analysis are the benzodiazepines, tricyclic antidepressants, and acetaminophen, among others.

When a routine toxicology screen is ordered, the physician is often not aware that options are available for more specific screening and confirmation methods. Table 11.2 shows the performance characteristics of different types of assays for drugs of abuse identification.

CHOICE OF BODY FLUIDS AND TIME OF SAMPLE COLLECTION

Some drugs are metabolized extensively and are excreted very quickly, such as cocaine (24), whereas others, such as marijuana, stay in the body for a long time (25). Thus, success of detection depends not only on the time of sample collection after the last use, but also on the drug's characteristics and whether the analysis is performed for the drug itself or for its metabolite(s). Table 11.3 illustrates the typical screening and confirmation cutoff concentrations and the expected times of detectability for some commonly abused drugs when analyzed in urine, blood, saliva, and hair.

When drug-abuse detection is the goal, the following questions should be asked: (a) How long does the suspected drug stay in the body, or what is its biologic half-life? (b) How fast and how extensively is the drug biotransformed? Based on the rate of biotransformation, should one look for the drug itself or its metabolite(s)? (c) Which body fluid is best for analysis, and what is the major route of excretion? Intravenous use or smoking of drugs provides nearly instantaneous absorption into the bloodstream. Metabolism, tissue distribution, and excretion of the drug and/or metabolites into urine occur depending on the rate of the aforementioned processes. Oral use of drugs will result in slower absorption, but greater first-pass metabolism in the liver.

Cocaine is rapidly biotransformed into benzoylecgonine and ecgonine methyl ester. Less than 10% unchanged cocaine is excreted into the urine, and it is detectable only for 12 to 18 hours after use. What does this suggest to the clinician who wants to identify a cocaine abuser? Cocaine has a short half-life; therefore, if use is suspected within hours or the patient is under the influence of cocaine at the time of sample collection, the parent compound should be present in detectable concentrations both in blood and in urine (24). Plasma enzymes continue to metabolize cocaine to benzoylecgonine even after blood is taken from the body. Therefore, blood samples must be collected into tubes containing sodium fluoride to inactivate the plasma enzymes. Benzoylecgonine is the major metabolite of cocaine; its half-life is about 6 hours and it is excreted into urine at levels totaling approximately 45% of the dose. Thus, cocaine abuse detection is best accomplished by collecting urine and analyzing it for benzoylecgonine, which is the target compound of most assays.

Marijuana is slowly biotransformed. It is very lipid soluble. In occasional users the average time of detection is approximately 4 to 6 days. In chronic users the average detection time is approximately up to 30 days (25). As a consequence of slow biotransformation and large tissue distribution, urine tests are effective for many days to detect the major metabolite, 9-carboxy-tetrahydrocannabinol (9-carboxy-THC). The individual pharmacokinetic drug metabolism and drug excretion information is important to determine which drug or metabolite is best for detection. Many physicians prefer blood to urine for drug screening because blood levels constitute stronger evidence of recent use and are related more closely to brain levels and drug-related behavioral changes than are urine levels.

The collection of urine specimens must be supervised to ensure donor identity and to guarantee the integrity of the specimen. It is not unusual to receive someone else's urine or a highly diluted sample when collection is not supervised. Also, the laboratory tests for pH, specific gravity, and creatinine levels assure that the sample is not adulterated. As a rule, first morning urine samples are more concentrated; therefore, drugs are easier to detect than in more diluted daily samples. The decision to use blood or urine must be based on the purpose of the test and the suspected drug's pharmacokinetic,

TABLE 11.3 Drugs of abuse reference guide

Substance	Urine screening cutoff concentration (ng/mL)	Urine confirmation cutoff concentration (ng/mL)	Urine detection times	Blood/oral fluid detection times	Hair detection times
Amphetamine	1000	500	1–3 days	12 hours	Up to 90 days
Barbiturates (short acting)	200	200	2–3 days	1–2 days	Up to 90 days
Barbiturates (long acting)	200	200	2–3 weeks	4–7 days	Up to 90 days
Benzodiazepines (therapeutic use)	200	200	3 days	6–48 hours	Up to 90 days
Benzodiazepines (chronic use)	200	200	4–6 weeks	6–48 hours	Up to 90 days
Cocaine (benzoylecgonine)	300	150	2–5 days	2–5 days	Up to 90 days
Codeine	300	300	2–3 days	2–3 days	Up to 90 days
Morphine	300	300	2 days	1–2 days	Up to 90 days
Heroin (6-acetylmorphine)	10	10	Up to 24 hours		
Marijuana	50	15	Casual use: 1–3 days Chronic use: up to 30 days	Up to 24 hours	Up to 90 days
Methadone	300	300	2–4 days	2–4 days	Up to 90 days
Methamphetamine	1000	500	3–5 days	1–3 days	Up to 90 days
Phencyclidine	25	25	Casual use: 2–7 days Chronic use: up to 30 days	Up to 48 hours	Up to 90 days

Adapted from *Drugs of Abuse Reference Guide* (http://www.labcorpsolutions.com/images/Drugs_of_Abuse_Reference_Guide_Flyer_3166.pdf), LabCorp Inc., retrieved online June 8, 2009.

metabolic, and excretion characteristics. Generally, drug levels in urine are higher than in blood; therefore, urine is the biofluid of choice for drug detection.

INTERPRETATION OF RESULTS

Psychoactivity of most drugs lasts only a few hours, while urinalysis can detect some drugs and/or metabolites for days or even weeks (24,25). Thus, the presence of a drug (or metabolite) in urine is only an indication of prior exposure, not a proof of intoxication or impairment at the time of sample collection. In some cases, quantitative data in blood or urine can corroborate observed behavior or action of a subject, especially when the levels are so high that it is impossible for the subject to be free of drug effects. Nevertheless, laboratory data and corroborating drug-induced behavior must be interpreted by experts in psychopharmacology and toxicology with experience in drug biotransformation and pharmacokinetics (26).

Drug analysis reports, either positive or negative, may raise questions about the meaning of the results. The usual questions are as follows: (a) What method was used? (b) Did the laboratory analyze for the drug only, or the metabolite only, or both? (c) What is the "cutoff" value for the assay? (d) Was the sample time close enough to the suspected drug exposure?

False-negative results occur more easily than false-positive results, mainly because once a test is screened negative, it is usually not tested further. If the screening method was EIA, the cutoff may have been set too high, in which case, drugs present below the cutoff concentration are reported negative. It is imperative for the physician to know the cutoff for each drug tested and, for diagnostic purposes, ask for any drug presence above the blank and below the cutoff. Another possibility for false negatives is that the sample was taken too long after the last drug exposure. Whatever the case may be, if the suspicion of drug use is strong, the clinician must repeat testing and ask the laboratory for a more sensitive cutoff level. False-positive results can also occur especially in the screening process. Most common are the so-called cross reactivity issues. This happens when drugs or chemicals with similar chemical structures react with the antibodies of the drug test. A typical example occurs with amphetamines testing. Immunoassays for amphetamine and methamphetamine may cross-react and test positive with other sympathomimetic amines, such as ephedrine or pseudoephedrine.

In general, analytic methods have improved significantly and the trend is toward further improvement. As technology advances, more drugs and chemicals will be analyzed in biofluids at the nanogram and picogram levels. However, advancement does not mean that modern methodologies are infallible or that they replace clinical judgment. Theoretically and practically, technical or human error can influence testing results. Therefore, certified laboratories, with checks and balances in their procedures, limit the occurrences of human or technical errors. With knowledge of the available analytic methods, one can interpret and scrutinize laboratory results with confidence as to their validity.

CLINICAL DRUG TESTING

Clinical drug testing has three components: emergency toxicology, rehabilitation toxicology, and diagnostic toxicology. Each has slightly different goals and requirements. Emergency toxicology requires quick analysis, responding to critical situations in overdose cases. Sometimes the clinical symptoms or the leftover drug is a sufficient clue to the laboratory for which drug to test. On-site, one-step, nontechnical kit screening is becoming more popular to provide instant results. Instrumental immunoassays are also quick and practical, but as in all screening techniques, they give only "present" or "absent" results for each drug or drug class tested. If the target drug is not on the menu, no identification is possible, and tracking down the "unknown" one by one is a slow process. However, if there is a clue to a drug's identity, immunoassays provide quick answers. Confirmation of positive results is performed by an alternate scientific methodology, usually chromatography. It is at the discretion of the physician to request confirmation or identification of the specific drug.

In rehabilitation programs, drug testing is of foremost importance. Identified ex–drug abusers need to know that the therapist or the counselor knows objectively that they are in good standing or in danger of relapsing to drug use. In this situation, drug-abuse testing is a deterrent and an important component of the treatment process. However, from the laboratory's point of view, testing is significantly different from emergency toxicology. The test results may not be available for at least 24 hours, and large numbers of samples need to be analyzed in a batch for the many rehabilitation clinics.

The laboratory usually performs a screening test rechecks and/or confirms positives by means of an alternate scientific method. The choice of method depends on assay sensitivity, specificity, expense, and practicality. Instrumental immunoassay methods, such as EIA and ELISA, are used most frequently for screening when large numbers of samples must be tested at a reasonable cost. An FDA-approved sweat patch aids rehabilitation drug testing. The patch placed on the skin is worn for several days, and it detects drugs used during that period; thus, use of short-acting drugs will also be detected (27–29). Urine testing is the most common; however, oral fluid testing is also becoming popular in drug treatment clinics. When direct observation of urine collection is not possible or collection of urine is difficult because the donor has renal disease or a shy bladder, oral fluid is an appropriate alternative.

Diagnostic drugs of abuse identification is another important testing with a slightly different goal. Denial is typical of drug abusers. Therefore, astute physicians are frequently testing their patients for drug use or abuse. A critical role of diagnostic testing is to prevent false negatives caused by poor timing of sample collection or poor sensitivity. From the laboratory's perspective, sensitive methods with the lowest cutoff and a large drug panel screening must be used. Immunoassays and GLC techniques are appropriate for ultimate sensitivity.

FORENSIC DRUG TESTING

Forensic or legal drug testing has three components: workplace testing, postmortem testing (medical examiner), and criminal justice (correctional and parole) testing.

Historically, forensic drug testing developed from clinical and pathologic testing. Laboratories had to implement numerous legally acceptable procedures, and testing also needed improvement. Certified laboratories must be able to prove that positive test results are accurate and reliable and that the tests performed were from the individual listed on the report. Weak links in external and internal chain-of-custody procedures or poor standards and/or quality control in the testing process provide sufficient ammunition to defense attorneys and expert witnesses to contradict the validity of positive results. For this reason the forensic drug-testing facility must be significantly more secure and better organized than that of a clinical drug-testing laboratory.

Workplace testing is performed on subjects at their place of employment. Many industries and governmental agencies mandate testing of individuals performing critical duties. These places of employment have strict drug policies in place, informing employees that drug abuse is not tolerated and that tests are performed to protect the public interest. The different types of tests performed are preemployment, for cause, and random drug testing. Positive tests can result in loss of job or job opportunity. The consequences of workplace testing are very serious and often disputed. People's livelihoods depend on laboratory results; therefore, sufficient safeguards must be built into the system to provide assurance that the results are reliable. In forensic testing, the usual procedure is screening with an automated immunoassay analyzer (i.e., EIA, ELISA, and FPIA) and confirmation of positive screening tests by GC-MS, LC-MS, or MS-MS for additional sensitivity.

Other forms of forensic drug testing requiring "litigation documentation" are medicolegal cases and postmortem analysis of body fluids for the presence of drugs, alcohol, and poisons. Before workplace testing became common, even the medicolegal or postmortem toxicology testing was less stringent. Currently, very strict rules and regulations govern workplace testing. More rigorous and complete chain-of-evidence documentation and more accurate methods are required in medicolegal and postmortem testing.

Another area of drug testing is in correctional institutions and testing in the prison system. A very large percentage of the prisoners' criminal activity is connected either to drug use or to drug trafficking. It is not unusual to find that drug abuse continues in the prisons. Consequently, correctional facilities have adopted a drug-abuse testing policy in prisons and also during parole. Although the consequences of testing are potentially punitive, testing of inmates in many states requires only screening without confirmation of positive results.

TESTING DRUGS IN ORAL FLUID

Although drug detection in oral fluid (saliva) is not a new idea, the last decade, from 1998 to 2009, has exploded with a large number of new research and scientific publications (30,31,32). Articles describing these technical advances have been described in O. H. Drummer's excellent review articles (30,33).

In the past, blood and urine samples were preferred for drug detection, until analytic methods, especially LC-MS-MS, increased sensitivity to a desired level. This advancement opened up the possibility for oral fluid as an alternative specimen for drug detection. There are several advantages for using oral fluid for drug screening: (a) collection of specimens is noninvasive and easily observable by the collector, (b) the introduction of LC as an analytic instrument negates the often difficult and time-consuming extraction and cleanup steps needed for GC and GC-MS analyses, (c) the sensitivity of LC-MS-MS permits identification and quantitation of drugs in relatively small oral fluid samples, and (d) water-soluble drugs, conjugated drugs, and metabolites can be easily recovered from the oral fluid without extraction.

However, there are also limitations for using oral fluid for drug detection. (a) Often the collected sample is either inadequate or too small for further analysis and confirmation, if needed. (b) The detection time of drugs or metabolites in oral fluids is about the same as in blood, but shorter than in urine (34,35). The many different oral fluid collectors available when compared to each other are better for some drugs or drug classes than for others (21,22). The fact that they are not uniformly effective for some drugs may cause contradictory results just from the choice of collector used.

Conclusively, properly validated oral fluid testing performed in certified laboratories provides a reasonable opportunity for screening and confirmation of recent drug use (30). However, urine specimens still provide longer detection times and larger sample volumes for further analysis and confirmation, if requested.

TESTING DRUGS IN SWEAT AND HAIR

Sweat is approximately 99% water and is produced by the body as a heat-regulation mechanism. Because the amount of sweat produced is dependent on environmental temperatures, routine sweat collection is difficult because of a large variation in the rate of sweat production and lack of adequate standardizations. However, cocaine, morphine, nicotine, amphetamine, ethanol, and other drugs have been identified in sweat (27,36). A "sweat patch" resembles an adhesive bandage and is applied to the skin for a period of several days to several weeks. Sweat is absorbed and concentrated on the cellulose pad, which is then removed from the skin and tested for drug content. Cone et al. (27) evaluated sweat testing for cocaine. Generally, there appeared to be a dose–concentration relationship; however, there was wide intersubject variability, which is a disadvantage of this technology. Research in this testing technology is still developing and is indicating apparent advantages of the sweat patch, such as high subject acceptability of wearing the patch for drug monitoring and the ability to monitor drug intake for a period of several weeks with a single patch (27).

Testing for drugs in hair is an alternate method to the drug-abuse detection technology (37–39). Because of the very low concentrations of drugs incorporated in hair, very sensitive methodology must be used. Screening is performed by RIA with ultrasensitive antibodies, or by ELISA, with confirmation by GC-MS, GC-MS-MS, or LC-MS-MS (40). Representatives from virtually all abused drug classes have been detected in hair (41,42). Drugs can enter the hair in various ways: (a) diffusion from blood into the hair follicle and hair cells with subsequent binding to hair strands (37) (Fig. 11.6); (b) excretion in sweat, which bathes hair follicles and hair strands; (c) excretion in oily secretions into the hair follicle and onto the skin surface; and (d) entry from the environment (37). Two controversial issues in hair drug testing are the possibility of environmental contamination that may result in false-positive test results and the difficult interpretation of dose-to-time relationships. Although it has been generally assumed that the hair strand, when sectioned, provides a long-term time course of drug-abuse history, studies with labeled cocaine have not supported this interpretation. Henderson et al. (38) concluded: "… there is not, at present, the necessary scientific foundation for hair analysis to be used to determine either the time or amount of cocaine use." On the other hand, Cone found a good dose–response relationship and time profile of morphine and codeine in human beard (43). In spite of some controversial aspects of hair testing, this technique is being used on an increasingly broad scale in a variety of circumstances (44). This technology may be used to estimate the long-term drug-abuse habit of the patient who is in denial. Self-reported drug use over a period of several months can be compared to hair test results from a hair strand (about 3.9 cm long) representative of the same time

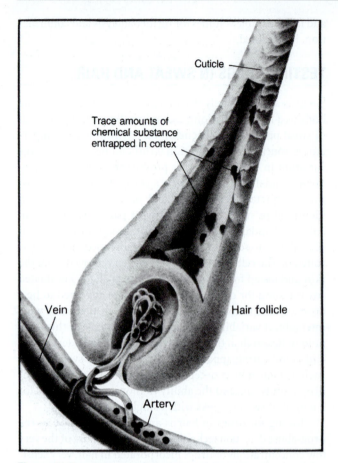

Figure 11.6. A conceptual drawing of drug transfer from the blood to hair follicle and its subsequent encapsulation in the hair shaft. (Reproduced with permission from Psychemedics, Inc., Santa Monica, CA.)

period (41,43). It is expected that this type of comparison would be more effective than urine testing because urine provides a historical record of only 2 to 4 days under most circumstances (41,43). Because denial is a major problem with drug abusers, this technology is an invaluable tool in drug-abuse diagnosis and therapy. Table 11.4 illustrates the comparison of usefulness of urine, saliva, sweat, and hair as a biologic matrix for drug detection. Advantages and disadvantages of urine, saliva, hair, and sweat are reviewed by Caplan and Goldberger (19) (Table 11.5).

ETHICAL CONSIDERATIONS

Legitimate need for drug-abuse testing in the clinical setting is indisputable. Denial makes identification of drug abuse difficult; therefore, testing is necessary both for identifying drug abusers and for monitoring of treatment outcome. Drug testing in the workplace and in sports is more controversial because positive test results may be used in termination of long-time employees or refusal to hire new ones.

Private companies believe that it is their right to establish drug- and alcohol-free workplaces and sport arenas. The opposition believes that one is ill-advised to terminate individuals for a single positive test result, even when it is confirmed by forensically acceptable procedures. A testing program is reasonable when a chance for rehabilitation is also offered. Probationary periods provide an opportunity to stop using drugs through treatment or self-help programs. Employee assistance programs, which refer employees to drug counseling, are available in larger companies and governmental organizations.

TABLE 11.4 Comparative usefulness of urine, saliva, sweat, and hair as a biologic matrix for drug detection

Biologic matrix	Drug detection time	Major advantages	Major disadvantages	Primary use
Urine	2–4 days	Mature technology; on-site methods available; established cutoffs	Detects only recent use	Detection of recent drug use
Saliva	12–24 hours	Easily obtainable; samples-"free" drug fraction; parent drug presence	Short detection time; oral drug contamination; collection methods influence pH and s/p ratios; detects only recent use; new technology	Linking positive drug test to behavior and performance impairment
Sweat	1–4 weeks	Cumulative measure of drug use	High potential for environmental contamination; new technology	Detection of recent drug use (days–weeks)
Hair	Months	Long-term measure of drug use; similar sample can be recollected	High possibility for environmental contamination; new technology	Detection of drug use in recent past (1–6 months)

From Cone EJ. New developments in biological measures of drug prevalence. *NIDA Res Monogr.* 1986;167:104–126.

TABLE 11.5	Summary of advantages and disadvantages of urine, oral fluid, hair, and sweat	
Specimen	Advantages	Disadvantages
Urine	Drugs and drug metabolites are highly concentrated Extensive scientific basis for testing methodology Performance testing is liberally practiced Results are frequently accepted in court Uniform testing criteria (e.g., cutoffs) established Easily tested by commercial screening methods	Period of detection 2–3 days No dose–concentration relationship Drug concentration influenced by the amount of water intake Susceptible to adulteration and substitution
Oral fluid	Useful in the detection of recent drug use Results may be related to behavior/performance Ready accessibility for collection Observed collection Detects parent drugs and metabolites	Detection window may be shorter Contamination following oral, smoked, and intranasal routes of drug administration Collection volume may be device dependent Performance testing under development
Hair	Provides a longer estimate of time of drug use Detects parent drugs and metabolites (e.g., 6-acetylmorphine) Observed collection Ease of obtaining, storing, and shipping specimens Second specimen can be obtained from original source	Inability to detect recent drug use Potential hair color bias Possible environmental contamination for some drug classes Susceptible to adulteration by treatment prior to collection
Sweat	Provides cumulative measure of drug exposure Ability to monitor drug intake for a period of days to weeks Detects parent drugs and metabolites (e.g., 6-acetylmorphine) Noninvasive specimen collection Collection device is relatively tamper-proof	Large variation in sweat production Specimen volume unknown Limited collection devices High intersubject variability Risk of accidental removal Risk of contamination during application/removal Cannot detect prior exposure Performance testing under development

From Caplan YH, Goldberger BA. Alternative specimens for workplace drug testing. *J Anal Toxicol.* 2001;25:396–399.

It is important that this new, powerful tool—drug testing—be used judiciously as a means of early detection, rehabilitation, and prevention. Test results must be interpreted only by individuals who understand drugs of abuse medically and pharmacologically. The federal government requires that in its drug-testing program, the results go directly to medical review officers (MROs), who are supposed to be trained to interpret such reports. Improper testing or improper interpretation of drug testing data must be prevented.

CONCLUSION

As long as illegal drug use is prevalent in our society, drug-abuse testing will have an important clinical and forensic role. Testing in the clinical setting aids the physician who treats subjects with psychiatric signs and symptoms secondary to drug abuse, monitors treatment outcome, and handles serious overdose cases. Drug testing in the forensic setting will be used for workplace testing and monitoring of parolees convicted of drug-related charges.

Civil rights must be respected to protect the innocent. Names of subjects should be known only to the medical office where the sample is collected. Testing must follow strict security and chain-of-custody procedures to ensure anonymity and prevent sample mix-up during testing. Many laboratories instituted bar-code labeling of samples and related documents to ensure confidentiality. Bar coding also improves accuracy of reporting and tracking of samples and records. This system ultimately prevents sample mix-up as a consequence of human error during accessioning and processing.

The reliability of testing procedures is of foremost importance. Good laboratories institute internal open, blind, and external quality control systems to assure high quality of testing (2). Reliability depends on three major factors: well-qualified and well-trained laboratory personnel, state-of-the-art instrumentation, and logical organization of the testing laboratory.

Before issuing certification, governmental agencies require laboratories to adhere to strict standards in personnel qualifications, experience, quality control, quality assurance programs, chain-of-custody procedures, and multiple review prior to reporting results.

Nationally recognized agencies protect the rights of government-mandated testing programs by assuring proper procedures in forensic drug testing. The DHHS/SAMHSA administers its NLCP. Similarly, the College of American Pathologists (CAP) runs its Forensic Toxicology Inspection and Proficiency Program. In addition, numerous state and city regulatory agencies, such as the New York State Health Department, inspect and certify drug-testing laboratories. Good laboratories are easily identified by having current certificates of qualification (COQ) issued by national and/or local regulatory agencies.

Drug-abuse testing has come a long way in terms of accuracy and reliability (45). Testing started in traditional "wet chemistry" laboratories, using huge sample volumes and crude methodologies of low sensitivity. Now autoanalyzers perform hundreds of tests on minute sample volumes, accurately measuring low-nanogram, and in some cases picogram, amounts of drugs. The insecurity of physicians, counselors, and forensic investigators about drug-abuse testing should not be a concern when using properly certified licensed laboratories.

REFERENCES

1. Verebey K, Martin D, Gold MS. Drug abuse: interpretation of laboratory tests. In: Hall W, ed. *Psychiatric Medicine*. Washington, DC: U.S. Government Printing Office; 1982:155–167.
2. Blanke RV. Accuracy in urinalysis. *NIDA Res Monogr*. 1986; 73: 43–53.
3. King LA, McDermott SD. Drugs of abuse. In: Moffat AC, Osselton MD, Widdop B, eds. *Clarke's Analysis of Drugs and Poisons*. 3rd ed. London, Chicago: Pharmaceutical Press; 2004.
4. Jaffee JH. Drug addiction and drug abuse. In: Gilman AS, Rall TW, Nies AS, et al., eds. *The Pharmacological Basis of Therapeutics*. 8th ed. New York: Macmillan; 1990:522–535.
5. Gold MS, Verebey K, Dackis CA. Diagnosis of drug abuse: drug intoxication and withdrawal states. *Fair Oaks Hospital Psychiatry Letter*. 1980;3(5):23–34.
6. Pottash ALC, Gold MS, Extein I. The use of the clinical laboratory. In: Sederer LI, ed. *Inpatient Psychiatry: Diagnosis and Treatment*. Baltimore: Williams & Wilkins; 1982:205–221.
7. Wadler GI, Heinline B. *Drugs and Athletes*. Philadelphia: FA Davis; 1989:195–210.
8. Willette E. Drug testing programs. *NIDA Res Monogr*. 1986;73: 5–12.
9. Mazarr-Proo S, Kerrigan S. Distribution of GHB in tissues and fluids following a fatal overdose. *J Anal Toxicol*. 2005;29: 398–400.
10. Baselt RC. *Disposition of Toxic Drugs and Chemicals in Man*. 6th ed. Foster City, CA: Biomedical Publications; 2002:441–442, 559–562, 827–830.
11. Bosker WM, Huestis MA. Oral fluid testing for drugs of abuse. *Clin Chem*. 2009;55(11):1910–1931.
12. Garriott JC. *Medical-Legal Aspects of Alcohol*. 4th ed. Tucson, AZ: Lawyers and Judges Publishing Company, Inc.; 2003:10, 149–156, 188–189.
13. Musselman J, Solanky A, Arnold W. *Increasing Accuracy of Blood-Alcohol Analysis Using Automated Headspace-Gas Chromatography. Case Study*, Shelton, CT: PerkinElmer Life and Analytical Sciences; 2006.
14. Substance Abuse Treatment Advisory. Center for Substance Abuse Treatment. The role of biomarkers in the treatment of alcohol use disorders. 2006;5(4). Available at: http://ncadistore.samhsa.gov/catalog/productDetails.aspx?ProductID=17559.
15. Kuntz DJ. EtG: urinary metabolite for monitoring alcohol ingestion. *Clinical & Forensic Toxicology News*; December 1–6, 2006.
16. Rosano TG, Lin J. Ethyl glucuronide excretion in humans following oral administration of and dermal exposure to ethanol. *J Anal Toxicol*. 2008;32:594–600.
17. Costantino A, Digregorio EJ, Korn W, et al. The effect of the use of mouthwash on ethyl glucuronide concentrations in urine. *J Anal Toxicol*. 2006;30:659–662.
18. Helander A, Olsson I, Dahl H. Postcollection synthesis of ethyl glucuronide by bacteria in urine may cause false identification of alcohol consumption. *Clin Chem*. 2007;53:1855–1857.
19. Caplan YH, Goldberger BA. Alternative specimens for workplace drug testing. *J Anal Toxicol*. 2001;25:396–399.
20. Methadone Direct ELISA Kit, Product Insert, Immunalysis Corporation, Pomona, CA, 2008.
21. Langel K, Engblom C, Pehrsson A, et al. Drug testing in oral fluid – evaluation of sample collection devices. *J Anal Toxicol*. 2008;32:393–401.
22. Crouch DJ. Oral fluid collection: the neglected variable in oral fluid testing. *Forensic Sci Int*. 2005;150:165–173.
23. Crouch DJ, Hersch RK, Cook RF, et al. A field evaluation of five on-site testing devices. *J Anal Toxicol*. 2002;26:493–499.
24. Verebey K. Cocaine abuse detection by laboratory methods. In: Washton AM, Gold MS, eds. *Cocaine: A Clinician's Handbook*. New York, London: The Guilford Press; 1987:214–228.
25. Goodwin RS, Darwin WD, Chiang CN, et al. Urinary elimination of 11-nor-9-carboxy-Δ^9-tetrahydrocannabinol in cannabis users during continuously monitored abstinence. *J Anal Toxicol*. 2008;32:562–569.
26. Verebey K, Martin D, Gold MS. Drug abuse: interpretation of laboratory tests. In: Gold MS, Pottash ALC, eds. *Diagnosis and Laboratory Testing in Psychiatry*. New York: Plenum Medical Book Company; 1986:155–166.
27. Cone EJ, Hillsgrove MJ, Jenkins AJ, et al. Sweat testing for heroin, cocaine, and metabolites. *J Anal Toxicol*. 1994;18(6):298–305.
28. Barns AJ, Smith ML, Kacinko SL, et al. Excretion of methamphetamine and amphetamine in human sweat following controlled oral methamphetamine administration. *Clin Chem*. 2008;54:172–180.
29. Schwilke EW, Barnes AJ, Kacinko SL, et al. Opioid disposition in human sweat after controlled oral codeine administration. *Clin Chem*. 2006;52(8):1539–1545.
30. Drummer OH. Drug testing in oral fluids. *Clin Biochem Rev*. 2008;27:147–159.
31. Lillsunde P. Analytical techniques for drug detection in oral fluid. *Ther Drug Monit*. 2008;30:181–187.
32. Cone EJ, Huestis MA. Interpretation of oral fluid tests for drugs of abuse. *Ann NY Acad*. 2007;1098:51–103.
33. Drummer OH. Review: pharmacokinetics of illicit drugs in oral fluid. *Forensic Sci Int*. 2005;150:133–142.
34. Verstraete AG. Detection times of drugs in blood, urine and oral fluids. *Ther Drug Monit*. 2004;26:200–205.
35. Huestis MA, Cone EJ. Methamphetamine disposition in oral fluid, plasma and Urine. *Ann NY Acad Sci*. 2007;1098:104–121.
36. Gallardo E, Queiroz JA. The role of alternative specimens in toxicological analysis. *Biomed Chromatogr*. 2008;22:795–821.

37. Baumgartner WA, Hill VA, Blahd WH. Hair analysis for drugs of abuse. *J Forensic Sci.* 1989;34:1433–1453.
38. Henderson GL, Harkey MR, Zhou C, et al. Incorporation of isotopically labeled cocaine and metabolites into human hair: 1. dose-response relationships. *J Anal Toxicol.* 1996;20:1–12.
39. Mitchell JM, ed. Hair drug testing. *Forensic Sci Rev.* 2007;19(2):50–93.
40. Moore C, Coulter C, Crompton K. Determination of cocaine, benzoylecgonine, cocaethylene and norcocaine in human hair using solid-phase extraction and liquid chromatography with tandem mass spectrometric detection. *J Chromatogr B.* 2007;859: 208–212.
41. Kinz P, Villgin M, Cirimele V. Hair analysis for drug detection. *Ther Drug Monit.* 2006;28:442–446.
42. Pragst F, Balikova MA. State of the art in hair analysis for detection of drug and alcohol abuse. *Clin Chim Acta.* 2006; 370: 17–49.
43. Cone EJ. Testing human hair for drugs of abuse. I. Individual dose and time profiles of morphine and codeine in plasma, saliva, urine, and beard compared to drug induced effects on pupils and behavior. *J Anal Toxicol.* 1990;14:1–7.
44. Spiehler V. Hair analysis by immunological methods from the beginning to 2000. *Forensic Sci Int.* 2000;107:249–259.
45. Frigs CS, Battaglia DJ, White RM. Status of drugs of abuse testing in urine under blind conditions. *Ann AACC Study Clin Chem.* 1989;35:891–944.

SECTION 4 ■ SUBSTANCES OF ABUSE

CHAPTER 12 — Alcohol Use Disorders

Carlos A. Hernandez-Avila ■ Henry R. Kranzler

INTRODUCTION

During the past three decades, there have been significant advances in the understanding of the neuronal basis of alcohol use disorders. Progress in neuropharmacology, genetics, and neuroimaging has yielded remarkable insights into the causes, pathophysiology, and treatment of these problems. Concomitantly, there have been significant advances in the understanding of environmental and psychological factors influencing the risk for alcoholism. In developed countries, these insights have translated into modest but gradual changes in the way that alcoholic patients are treated. From a public health perspective these developments have also been of significance, allowing interested governments and health agencies to implement effective policies aiming at reducing problem drinking and its devastating effects.

One important consequence of this progress is the emergence of a trend in which alcohol use disorders are gradually becoming less stigmatized, allowing a greater number of alcoholic patients to seek professional help. Another consequence is that rather than being restricted to addiction specialists as is currently the case, alcoholism treatment may potentially become more accepted into the routine work of primary care practitioners who generally are the first and only clinical contact for the majority of patients experiencing drinking problems.

HISTORICAL ASPECTS

Prehistoric Times

Throughout their evolutionary history, humans have been exposed to low levels of alcohol by eating fermented fruits and vegetables. For thousands of years, foods containing alcohol and alcoholic beverages have been a source of calories and water, micronutrients, and neurotransmitter precursors, all necessary for the survival of the human species.

Archeologic evidence suggests that purposeful fermentation of alcoholic beverages by humans was initiated approximately 12,000 years ago. Cultivation of grape vines suitable for wine making began about 8000 years ago in the Eurasian region currently known as Armenia (1,2). During this time, water supplies in population centers were often polluted with dangerous waste products causing lethal outbreaks of dysentery and other infectious diseases. Due to their acidity and the antiseptic effects of alcohol, beer and wine are generally free of pathogens. In this context, alcoholic beverages may have been an important source, and in some instances, the only source of drinkable water in early civilization (1,2).

The Ancient Eastern World

By 4000 BC, the grapevine was used in wine making by the Egyptians, who worshipped Osiris as the wine goddess. Egyptians also believed that Osiris created beer. Although ancient Egyptians were aware of the risks of excessive drinking, they did not appear to consider inebriation a problem (1).

By 2700 BC, Babylonians worshipped several wine deities and regularly offered beer and wine to them. Around 1750 BC, the Code of Hammurabi mentioned concerns about fair trade of alcoholic beverages, but inebriation was not considered an offense (1).

In ancient China, alcohol was also considered a spiritual food with an important role in religious and civil ceremonies. Ancient Chinese believed that drinking alcohol in moderation was a "prescription from heaven" (1).

The Hellenic and Roman World

By 2000 BC, wine making reached the Greek peninsula from the Middle East, and by 1700 BC, wine was widely consumed, becoming part of the daily Hellenic diet and incorporated in most religious and civil ceremonies (1,3). In ancient Greece, wine was also consumed to remedy a variety of health problems (4). Hippocrates (460–370 BC) identified numerous medicinal properties of wine and recommended different types of wine to treat different types of ailments (5). Xenophon (431–351 BC) and Plato (429–347 BC) praised the moderate use of wine as beneficial to health and happiness, and similar to Aristotle (384–322 BC) and Zeno (336–264 BC), identified excessive drinking as problematic (1,3).

In Rome, between the founding of the empire in 753 BC and the third century BC, drinking in moderation was the norm. This ended between 509 and 133 BC, after the conquest of the Italian peninsula and the rest of the Mediterranean region. By then, traditional Roman values of temperance, frugality, and simplicity were gradually replaced by heavy drinking, ambition, degeneracy, and corruption (1,3). Roman practices that encouraged excessive drinking included drinking before meals on an empty stomach, inducing vomiting to permit more food and wine consumption, and drinking games such as rapidly consuming as many cups as indicated by a throw of the dice (1,3).

By the beginning of the second century BC, wine became a valuable commodity and played an important economic role in the Mediterranean market. Spreading through Europe following the expansion of the Roman Empire, wine was brought to the north of Europe and England; however, regional dominant groups such as the Vikings, Saxons, Jutes, and Angles were more inclined to produce and consume ale and cider.

As the Roman Empire declined, Roman viniculture also declined. At that time and during the obscurantist period of the European Middle Ages, the Catholic Church was the only institution with sufficient resources to maintain wine production and Roman viniculture techniques (1).

The Era of Distilled Spirits

By AD 700–750, in the Mideast, a technical development occurred that radically changed the way in which alcoholic beverages were produced and consumed. The invention of distillation by Arab alchemists made it possible to produce alcoholic beverages with alcohol concentrations greater than that found in fermented beverages. By AD 1100, this method was adopted in Europe giving birth to the era of distilled spirits (2).

During the 13th and 14th centuries, the consumption of spirits rapidly spread to the rest of Europe, following the path of the Black Plague and other pandemic diseases. By AD 1500, the first printed book on alcohol distillation was published: *Liber de Arte Distillandi,* by the Alsatian physician Hieronymus Brunschwig. Although ineffective as a cure, the use of spirits as a remedy by medieval and Renaissance physicians was a common practice (2).

The American Continent

Discovery and early exploration of the American continent by European explorers such as Christopher Columbus was made feasible in part by the availability of wine and beer during their long voyages.

Available historical evidence suggests that before the arrival of Europeans most of the indigenous people of North America had limited exposure to alcohol. It appears that Native people of what is currently the southwestern United States, Mexico, Central America, and peoples of the Amazonian and Andes regions consumed fermented alcoholic beverages mainly in the context of religious ceremonies. The Pimas and Papagos in the southwestern United States extracted ferment from the saguaro cactus. The Tepehuanes and Tarahumaras, who inhabited territory in modern-day northern Mexico, fermented corn to produce *tesvino,* which they also consumed at ceremonies to mark important stages in an individual's life, such as the passage to adulthood. The Aztecs of Mexico drank pulque, which they fermented from the maguey or American aloe and the Mayas fermented *balche* from bark and honey. In Mexico, after the Spanish conquest, facilities were built to produce *aguardiente* (burning water), a spirit derived from sugarcane or corn, significantly expanding the amount of alcohol available for consumption.

In other parts of North America, when Europeans met Native Americans they offered them alcohol. However, systematic trading of alcohol did not begin until the mid-17th century, when British and French colonists, using sugar produced in the West Indies, initiated the large-scale distillation of spirits, and sold it as liquor in the North American colonies (4).

After the revolutionary war in the United States, the liquor trade spread farther west affecting Native and European Americans (4).

The Temperance Movement and the "Medicalization" of Alcoholism

As early as 1784, Benjamin Rush recognized that a key component of alcoholism is the inability to control the urge to drink. He launched the first health education campaign warning the public about the risks of drinking alcohol. He has been credited as the founder of the temperance movement in North America (5).

Although the temperance movement came to be dominated by religious and puritan ideology, it was originally a health promotion movement that sought to improve the human condition.

With the triumph of the enlightenment philosophy in the western hemisphere, alcoholism and madness came to be viewed as curable diseases. Benjamin Rush identified alcoholism as a disease in which alcohol serves as a causal agent and loss of control over drinking behavior is the characteristic symptom. Similar to the mentally ill, alcoholics were to be treated away from home in inebriate asylums. Samuel B. Woodward and subsequent members of the American Association for the Cure of Inebriates wrote on the physical nature of alcoholism and proposed total abstinence as the only effective cure for intemperance. Nineteenth century physicians differentiated between chronic alcoholism and alcohol addiction. Chronic alcoholism was characterized by the physical and psychological consequences of chronic alcohol drinking, whereas alcohol addiction consisted of an uncontrollable craving for alcohol, alcohol withdrawal symptoms, and loss of control (5).

It was not until 1954, in a World Health Organization report, that Griffith Edwards turned attention back to the pharmacologic effects of alcohol as the critical factor in the disease process. This notion gained ground and was expanded in the writings of Jellinek, who linked the features of tolerance and adaptation to the "craving" to drink excessively (5).

EPIDEMIOLOGY OF ALCOHOL CONSUMPTION

International Drinking Patterns

It has been estimated that approximately 2 billion people or one half of the world's adult population consume alcoholic beverages. Although the use of alcohol is distributed unevenly throughout the population, generally, consumption rates are greater among men (55%) than among women (34%) (6). Around the world most of the alcohol is consumed by a relatively small group of consumers with the top 30% of drinkers accounting for up to 75% of all consumption (6).

In most Western countries consumption rates of alcoholic beverages have remained stable and are expected to remain that way over the next two decades. However, in countries of the South-East Asian Region and the low- to middle-income countries of the Western Pacific Region, which include nearly half of the world's population, alcohol consumption is expected to increase during the same period (6,7).

The Dry/Wet Culture Dichotomy

Research examining international patterns of alcohol consumption has traditionally classified countries or cultures as dry or wet based on whether their per capita alcohol consumption is low or high.

In wet cultures, consumption of alcoholic beverages is integrated into daily life, with such beverages frequently consumed with meals and easily available with few legal restrictions. In countries with this cultural background, wine is the beverage most frequently consumed by a large segment of the population, usually in moderation. In these countries, wine is considered to have social, nutritional, and medicinal value. Although in this type of culture abstinence is infrequent, inebriation is uncommon. Mediterranean European countries such as Spain, Portugal, Italy, France, and Greece have traditionally been identified as wet cultures. Due to their high per capita alcohol consumption, however, these countries have a greater prevalence of alcohol-related health problems such as liver disease (6,8).

In dry cultures drinking is not prevalent in everyday life. In countries with this type of culture abstinence is common, but when drinking occurs it is likely to be at inebriating levels. Northern and Eastern European countries such as Norway, Sweden, Finland, Poland, and Russia have been classified as dry cultures. In these countries, drinking is not considered a key dietary component and distilled spirits are more frequently consumed than wine. Alcohol-related problems in these countries consist largely of accidents, public intoxication, and social disruption. In other dry countries such as Germany, Austria, Belgium, the United States, and the United Kingdom, beer consumption is predominant. In beer-consuming countries, per capita alcohol consumption tends to be lower than that in spirits-drinking countries but greater than that in wine-drinking countries (6,8).

One limitation of the wet/dry culture dichotomy is that it has focused primarily on differences among North American and European countries, representing a scale of extremes on which to measure drinking cultures. In recent decades, economic and globalization forces appear to be blurring the wet/dry culture distinction, especially in Europe, where a homogenization process of consumption rates and beverage preferences appears to be occurring. (8).

A different group of countries with low per capita alcohol consumption and low prevalence of alcohol-related problems are those with predominant or large Islamic populations such as Pakistan, Iraq, and Israel. Abstinence rates among adults in these countries can reach 90% of the population (6). Among other factors, the large abstinence rates found in the Middle East can be attributed to the fact that consumption of alcoholic beverages is forbidden by Islam.

The greatest prevalence of high-risk drinking, as defined by consumption of 40 g alcohol per day in men and more than 20 g in women, is found in Europe and Central Asia, followed by the sub-Saharan African and Latin American countries. The lowest prevalence of high-risk drinking on the other hand is found in the Middle East and North Africa with rates lower than 1% (6,8).

Alcohol Use Disorders around the World

In 2000, 76.4 million people worldwide suffered from an alcohol use disorder (e.g., alcohol abuse or alcohol dependence). Of this number, 63.7 million were men and 12.7 million were women. Regarding lifetime prevalence of alcohol abuse or dependence, these have been seen to vary from as low as 4.5 % in Hong Kong to a high of 22% in Korea (6–8).

Alcohol Consumption in the United States

In the United States, the majority (87.8%) of the adult population (>18 years old) has consumed alcohol in their lifetime (9). Regarding rates of current drinking, slightly more than half (51.6%) of Americans aged 12 or older reported drinking at least once during the last month (9). Among them, the majority (57.7%) was male. However, among youths aged 12 to 17, the percentage of males who were current drinkers (14.2%) was similar to that for females (15.0%).

Alcohol consumption in the United States is greatest among young men 18 to 25 years old. Among older Americans, the prevalence of current drinking decreases with increasing age (9). Regarding ethnicity, the highest prevalence of drinking is found among non-Hispanic whites, followed by Native Americans and Hispanics, whereas the lowest prevalence is seen among non-Hispanic blacks and Asians (9).

In the United States, the prevalence of alcohol consumption appears to increase as a function of education level, with college-educated individuals being almost twice as likely to be current drinkers as individuals with less than a high school education (9).

Prevalence of Alcohol Use Problems in the United States

In 2008, about one quarter (23.3%) of the U.S. population aged 12 or older reported binge drinking (i.e., the consumption of five or more drinks on an occasion) at least once during the past month. The prevalence of heavy drinking (i.e., the consumption of five or more drinks on the same occasion on each of 5 or more days) during the past month was 7% (9).

Men and young adults were more likely to report these problematic patterns of consumption than women and older adults. Among U.S. ethnic groups, Hispanics, followed by Native Americans and non-Hispanic whites had the highest frequency of problem drinking, whereas Asians and non-Hispanic blacks had the lowest rates (9).

The National Epidemiological Survey on Alcohol and Related Conditions (NESARC) (10) showed that alcohol abuse or dependence, defined by the fourth edition of the *Diagnostic and Statistical Manual of Mental Disorders* text revised (DSM-IV-TR) criteria (11) affected 8.5% of the U.S. population, with 4.7% meeting criteria for a diagnosis of alcohol abuse and 3.8% for alcohol dependence. A more recent population survey conducted in 2007 by the U.S. Substance Abuse and Mental Health Services Administration (SAMHSA) (9) showed that the past-year prevalence of DSM-IV-TR alcohol abuse or dependence among individuals 12 years old or older was 7.3%. Differences in prevalence rates between NESARC and SAMHSA studies appear to be due to differences in sampling and diagnostic methods.

The demographic predictors identified for alcohol abuse or dependence in the U.S. population are similar to those reported for heavy or binge drinking. These disorders affect men (9.7%) more frequently than women (5.1%), and are most common among adults 18 to 25 years old (9). Among ethnic groups, Hispanics, Native Americans, and non-Hispanic whites are affected more frequently than Asians and non-Hispanic blacks. The risk for alcohol use disorders is also negatively correlated with educational level and is greater among the unemployed and in urban populations (9).

CLASSIFICATION AND PHENOMENOLOGY OF ALCOHOL USE DISORDERS

Classification of Alcohol Use Disorders

The most widely used definitions for alcohol use disorders are those included in recent editions of the American Psychiatric Association DSM (11) and the International Classification of Diseases (ICD) of the World Health Organization (WHO). Studies of alcohol treatments, human genetics, and epidemiology all rely on these definitions, which constitute a near-universal reference for research and clinical practice on alcoholism.

The most recent editions of the DSM and the ICD (DSM-IV-TR and ICD-10, respectively) recognize and use similar diagnostic criteria for alcohol dependence. However, alcohol abuse is recognized only by the DSM-IV-TR. The ICD-10 includes the diagnosis of harmful drinking, which was created by the WHO to address concerns that health problems related to alcohol consumption were underreported. Harmful use is defined by alcohol consumption that causes physical and/or mental damage in the absence of alcohol dependence.

Studies consistently have showed high reliability for DSM-IV and ICD-10 alcohol dependence diagnoses but lower reliability for those of alcohol abuse/harmful use. Similarly, validity studies indicate that DSM-IV and ICD-10 alcohol dependence diagnoses have good validity, but the validity for alcohol abuse/harmful use is much lower (12).

Contrary to the notion that alcohol abuse and alcohol dependence represent two distinct disorders, recent evidence suggests that alcohol use disorder criteria may be best modeled as reflecting a unidimensional continuum of alcohol-problem severity. It is likely that changes in alcohol dependence and alcohol abuse diagnoses in future versions of the DSM-IV and ICD will reflect this conceptualization.

The alcohol dependence criteria in the DSM and subsequently in the ICD were adopted from the alcohol dependence syndrome (ADS) proposed by Edwards and Gross in 1976. In this tridimensional model, the biologic domain reflects the emergence of tolerance and withdrawal symptoms secondary to chronic alcohol consumption. The behavioral and cognitive dimensions reflect impaired control and the salience of drinking behavior.

In the DSM-IV-TR (11), the diagnosis of alcohol dependence requires that at least three criteria from a list of seven be present during a 1-year period and that they cause significant clinical impairment (Table 12.1). If the individual's drinking pattern does not meet criteria for alcohol dependence but there is a pattern of drinking that leads to clinically significant impairment as reflected by the presence of one or more alcohol abuse criteria, then the alcohol abuse diagnosis is considered.

Phenomenology and Natural Course of Alcohol Dependence

The clinical and phenomenologic presentation of alcohol dependence can be complex and multifaceted. Although it is difficult to describe a typical pattern that describes the course of this disorder, studies conducted in clinical samples suggest that certain clinical characteristics and progression patterns are prominent in the natural history of alcoholism.

In the early phases of the disorder, generally during the individual's early and mid twenties, the most prominent feature is daily heavy drinking or frequent binge drinking leading to significant intoxication. Early in the drinking career, individuals describe a rewarding sense of euphoria and elation that immediately follows the first drinks and is commonly described as the alcohol high or buzz. As heavy drinking persists, *tolerance* to alcohol's effects sets in, leading the individual to escalate alcohol consumption. Increased frequency and intensity of drinking may be associated with irresistible urges to drink or "craving" that are often triggered by environmental cues (e.g., bar scenes, celebratory gatherings, loud music) and/or internal cues (e.g., negative or positive mood states). Drinking may then become associated with "blackouts" or amnesia for events while intoxicated, and frequent "hangovers."

During an individual's early thirties, alcohol-related psychosocial problems may become prominent. Typically, the person experiences increasing days absent from work, frequent family conflicts, and other interpersonal and legal problems. Work, home, and/or motor vehicle accidents while intoxicated causing injury also become common.

From the individual's mid-to-late thirties, there may be a frank loss of control over drinking that is associated with a worsening of social and work-related problems and the onset of medical complications. Attention to personal care and hygiene may deteriorate, and despite the loss of personal relationships and employment, alcohol consumption can dominate the individual's life. Often, at this point, the individual's global level of functioning is further impaired by alcohol-induced cognitive deficits. In some cases, alcoholics may

TABLE 12.1	DSM-IV-TR criteria for alcohol dependence
A maladaptive pattern of drinking as manifested by three or more of the following during a 12-month period:	
(1)	Tolerance, that is, either: (a) a need for markedly more alcohol to achieve intoxication (b) markedly diminished effect despite continued consumption of the same amount of alcohol
(2)	Withdrawal, that is, either: (a) two or more signs or symptoms (autonomic hyperactivity, tremor, insomnia, nausea or vomiting, transient illusions or hallucinations, psychomotor agitation, anxiety, grand mal seizures) within several hours of stopping or reducing heavy, prolonged drinking (b) consuming alcohol or a related substance (e.g., benzodiazepines) to relieve or avoid withdrawal symptoms
(3)	Alcohol is often consumed in larger amounts or over a longer period than was intended
(4)	There is a persistent desire to cut down or control drinking
(5)	A great deal of time is spent in drinking or recovering from drinking
(6)	Important social, occupational, or recreational activities are given up or reduced because of drinking
(7)	Drinking is continued despite knowledge of having a persistent or recurrent physical or psychological problem that is likely to have been caused or exacerbated by alcohol.

Reprinted from the *Diagnostic and Statistical Manual of Mental Disorders*, Fourth Edition, Text Revision, with permission. Copyright 2000 American Psychiatric Association.
DSM-IV-TR Criteria 305.00.

experience feelings of remorse or guilt, which lead them to conceal their drinking. Alcoholic beverages are concealed at home or work and solitary drinking may help to avoid feelings of guilt and depression.

By the time the individual is in his or her late thirties or early forties, severe medical complications such as liver cirrhosis or chronic pancreatitis may develop, leading to frequent visits to emergency services and hospitalizations. Voluntary or involuntary efforts to stop drinking may be associated with significant symptoms of alcohol withdrawal (e.g., tachycardia, tremulousness, diaphoresis, insomnia, anxiety) that in a small group of alcoholics can be complicated by grand mal seizures and/or episodes of delirium (e.g., confusion, disorientation, hallucinations). The individual often resumes drinking to relieve or avoid withdrawal symptoms. Continued heavy drinking often exacerbates medical complications, with potentially fatal results.

Variables Influencing the Course of Alcohol Dependence

Variables that have been shown to influence the course of alcohol dependence, especially the response to treatment, include the age at onset of the disorder, severity of the disease, and presence of co-occurring psychiatric disorders. An early age at onset of alcohol dependence has shown to predict a greater severity of alcoholism and poor treatment response (13). Greater severity of alcoholism as evidenced by alcohol withdrawal symptoms is associated with a poor treatment response. A comorbid psychiatric diagnosis is also a predictor of poorer posttreatment outcomes.

In this regard, affective dysregulation may contribute to risk of alcohol dependence by promoting the use of alcohol to "self-medicate" negative affective states such as anxiety and depression. This theory is supported by research indicating an association between alcohol problems, mood disorders, and life stress. Also, deviance proneness or behavioral undercontrol, as indicated by hyperactivity, distractibility, sensation seeking, impulsivity, difficult temperament, and conduct disorder, appears to contribute to school failure and association with deviant peers, which then provide a context for heavy drinking and other substance use. Consistent with this, a diagnosis of antisocial personality disorder (ASPD), mood disorder, or another substance abuse/dependence diagnosis among alcohol-dependent individuals in general is associated with a poorer drinking outcome, more illicit drug use, and poorer social functioning during the posttreatment period than in alcoholics without these comorbidities (14,15).

Alcoholism Subtypes

A variety of typologies have been proposed to classify the diverse clinical presentations associated with alcoholism and to provide a heuristic framework to understand the complex interaction of the diverse etiologic factors. Cloninger and colleagues (16) studied adopted sons of Swedish alcoholics and developed a typology that differentiated between Type 1 and Type 2 alcoholism. In Type 1 or "milieu-limited" alcoholism the etiologic role of environmental factors is predominant. These individuals are characterized by a late initiation of problem drinking and rapid development of tolerance to alcohol. Type 1 alcoholics generally experience intense guilt and anxiety associated with drinking behavior, though it is uncommon for them to experience legal problems or be involved in fights. In Type 2 or *male-limited* alcoholism, the etiologic role of genetic factors is emphasized with transmission of the disease occurring predominantly from fathers to sons. Type 2 alcoholics characteristically experience drinking problems at a young age. These individuals do not experience substantial guilt or fear concerning their drinking though they frequently are involved in fights and experience legal problems related to drinking.

Cloninger hypothesized that differences between alcoholic subtypes could be explained by differences in three basic personality traits or temperaments: novelty seeking, harm avoidance, and reward dependence. These features in turn could be explained by specific neurochemical and genetic factors. Cloninger proposed that novelty seeking, which is characterized by frequent exploratory behavior and intense pleasurable responses to novel stimuli, was modulated by the dopaminergic neurotransmission system. He hypothesized that harm avoidance, a tendency to respond intensely to aversive stimuli and their conditioned signals, was modulated by serotonergic systems. Finally, he hypothesized that norepinephrine modulated reward dependence, which is defined as resistance to extinction of previously rewarded behavior. In Cloninger's typology, high reward dependence, high harm avoidance, and low novelty seeking are characteristic of Type 1 alcoholics, and Type 2 alcoholics are characterized by high novelty seeking, low harm avoidance, and low reward dependence. Although this tridimensional personality theory and other aspects of Cloninger's typology were attractive to researchers and clinicians, studies have failed to provide empirical support for this theory (17).

Babor and colleagues (18), using statistical clustering techniques, proposed a similar dichotomous classification of alcoholics. These authors described two homogeneous subtypes: Type A alcoholics were characterized by a late initiation of problem drinking and the absence of antisocial behaviors, and Type B alcoholics were characterized by an early initiation of problem drinking and by frequent antisocial behavior typically exacerbated by inebriation.

More recently, several multidimensional empirically derived typologies of alcohol use disorders, derived primarily for research purposes, have been described (17). Using different statistical methods, these studies have consistently found as many as four homogeneous types of alcoholics: a chronic/severe type, a depressed/anxious type, a mildly affected type, and an antisocial type (17). Further research is needed, however, in order to determine the clinical utility of these alcoholism subtypes.

DETERMINANTS OF ALCOHOL CONSUMPTION

Pharmacology of Alcohol

Absorption

After alcohol is ingested, it is rapidly absorbed in the gastrointestinal (GI) tract through the wall of the stomach and small intestine. Absorption of alcohol from the duodenum and jejunum is greater (80%) and faster than that occurring in the stomach (20%). However, when alcohol is consumed with food, gastric emptying is slowed and the stomach becomes the main site of absorption.

Alcohol absorption through the gastric and intestinal mucosa occurs by passive diffusion down a concentration gradient. The rapid removal of alcohol by efficient blood flow at the site of absorption is also necessary to maintain the alcohol concentration gradient.

The main factor governing the absorption rate of orally administered alcohol into the bloodstream is the rate of gastric emptying into the small intestine via the pyloric sphincter. This effect is due to the smaller absorptive surface area of the stomach compared with the duodenum and jejunum. Whether alcohol is consumed on an empty stomach or with food affects its rate of absorption. Food in the stomach delays gastric emptying, thereby reducing the absorption of alcohol. Foods high in fat, carbohydrate, or protein content are equally effective in retarding gastric emptying.

The amount and rate of drinking may also influence alcohol absorption. When alcohol is consumed in a single large dose rather than several smaller doses, the resulting alcohol concentration gradient is greater, potentially yielding higher peak blood alcohol concentrations. However, when alcohol-containing beverages are rapidly ingested, the irritant properties of alcohol not infrequently cause superficial erosions and hemorrhages of the mucosa, causing paralysis of the smooth muscle and reduced blood perfusion. This can reduce alcohol absorption. Other factors that influence gastric emptying and alcohol absorption include smoking, diurnal changes in blood glucose, physical activity, and medications such as ranitidine or erythromycin (19).

Due to the significant variability in rates of gastric emptying and in alcohol absorption, the time to achieve peak blood alcohol concentration is also highly variable. In one controlled study (30), the rate of absorption ranged from 14 to 130 minutes (with a mean of 57 minutes for men and 42 minutes for women) (19).

Distribution

Although alcohol shows little solubility in fat, it has the ability to cross all biologic membranes. Alcohol distributes from the bloodstream into all body tissues and fluids in proportion to their relative water content. Because of this and given that there is no binding of alcohol to plasma protein, alcohol concentration in body tissues rapidly reaches equilibrium with blood alcohol concentration.

Due to the fact that in humans there are large variations in the proportions of body fat and body water content, an equivalent alcohol dose per unit of body weight can yield different blood alcohol levels in different individuals. For example, due to lower volumes of total body water among women and the elderly, they have a smaller volume of distribution for alcohol than men and younger individuals. Thus, women and older individuals will reach greater peak blood alcohol levels than men and younger individuals when given an equivalent dose of alcohol (19).

Metabolism

First-Pass Metabolism of Alcohol Some of the alcohol that is consumed orally does not enter the systemic circulation but is oxidized in the gastric mucosa by isoforms of the enzyme alcohol dehydrogenase (ADH). This first-pass metabolism appears to be important in determining alcohol toxicity since its efficiency determines alcohol bioavailability. First-pass metabolism is reduced in women and alcoholics secondary to decreased ADH activity. This may translate into increased sensitivity to alcohol and greater blood alcohol concentrations in these populations (31). Several drugs, including histamine 2 receptor blockers such as cimetidine or ranitidine, or aspirin, decrease gastric first-pass metabolism by inhibiting gastric ADH activity. First-past metabolism also appears to occur in the liver, particularly when the delivery of alcohol into the portal vein is slow, as occurs in the fed state (19).

Nearly all (i.e., 92% to 95%) of the alcohol that is ingested is metabolized in the liver by ADH located in the cytosolic fraction of hepatocytes. Alcohol-metabolizing enzymes are also located in the microsomal fraction of the liver, specifically CYP2E1. In the most common pathway, alcohol is first oxidized to acetaldehyde by a class I ADH. Subsequently, acetaldehyde is oxidized to acetate by the enzyme aldehyde dehydrogenase (ALDH), which is localized in the mitochondria. The coenzyme nicotinamide adenine dinucleotide (NAD+) is required for these two nonreversible reactions to occur. During the hepatic oxidation of alcohol, the ratio of NADH to NAD+ in the liver cells significantly increases. The rate-limiting step in these reactions appears to be the reoxidation of NADH to NAD+. It is believed that the altered reduction–oxidation (redox) state accounts for many of the metabolic disturbances and hepatotoxic effects associated with heavy drinking. Finally, the last step in alcohol metabolism occurs when acetate is oxidized to CO_2 and water in peripheral tissues as part of the Krebs cycle (19).

Alcohol is a nutrient with a caloric value of approximately 7 kcal/g. In comparison, carbohydrates and proteins provide 4 kcal/g while fat yields 9 kcal. Unlike carbohydrates and fat, which can be stored, alcohol remains dissolved in body water until eliminated. Given that alcohol is generally oxidized preferentially over carbohydrates, fat, or proteins, calories derived from alcohol usually are produced at the expense of the metabolism of other nutrients. Alcoholics often consume 200 to 300 g of alcohol per day, the equivalent of 1400 to 2100 kcal, with consumption of normal nutrients usually neglected. Another important fact is that unlike metabolism of major nutrients, which is under complex hormonal control (involving, e.g., insulin, glucagon, leptin, catecholamines, thyroid hormones), there is little hormonal regulation of alcohol metabolism or elimination. Consequently, there is a major metabolic burden on the liver to oxidize alcohol and to remove it from the body (19).

Alcohol Dehydrogenase (ADH) ADH is an enzyme with broad substrate specificity that oxidizes many primary and secondary alcohols. It also appears to be involved in steroid and bile acid metabolism. Although found in other tissues, ADH is mainly found in the liver and GI tract. ADH is composed of two subunits (α, β, and γ subunits) or dimmers with unit composition determining enzyme's ability to oxidize alcohol. In this regard seven types of ADH have been identified and classified into five classes based on similarities in their amino acid sequence and unit composition. ADH encoded by class I genes (*ADH1A*, *ADH1B*, and *ADH1C*) account for most of the oxidizing capacity in the liver (19,20). Several mutations have been identified in the *ADH1B* and *ADH1C* genes that are differentially distributed across population groups and that produce enzymes with different pharmacokinetic properties. A further discussion of this topic is reviewed in the genetics section.

Acetaldehyde Dehydrogenase (ALDH) There are two main ALDH enzymes, ALDH1 and ALDH2, which oxidize the acetaldehyde generated during alcohol metabolism. ALDH1 is found in the cytosol and ALDH2 is found in the mitochondria. ALDH1 and ALDH2 have a similar structure being 70% identical in amino acid sequence. Gene variants coding for ALDH1 and ALDH2 are differentially distributed across populations producing enzymes with different pharmacokinetic properties (19,20). A further discussion on this topic is reviewed in the genetics section.

Elimination

As discussed earlier in this section, 90% to 95% of ingested alcohol is metabolized by the ADH–ALDH enzymatic system and eliminated as water and CO_2. A small proportion of consumed alcohol (~1%) undergoes conjugation with glucuronic acid to yield ethyl glucuronide as a by-product that can be measured in urine. The remainder of the consumed alcohol (~4%) is excreted unchanged in the breath, urine, and sweat. Because the amount of alcohol expelled in the breath is proportional and in equilibrium with the concentration in the pulmonary arterial blood, alcohol breath tests can be used as a noninvasive means to estimate the blood alcohol concentration (19).

Although alcohol elimination rates vary widely, in humans the metabolic capacity to remove alcohol is approximately 170 to 240 g/day for a person with a body weight of 70 kg. This is equivalent to an average metabolic rate of about 7 to 10 g/h, which translates to about one drink per hour (19).

Effects of Alcohol on Neurotransmission

Alcohol administration appears to have effects across major neurotransmitter systems (i.e., dopaminergic, GABAergic, glutamatergic, opioidergic, and serotonergic). These systems are affected by both acute and chronic alcohol administration and they appear to play a major role in mediating the rewarding effects of alcohol (21).

In general, alcohol has been considered to have central nervous system anesthetic or depressive properties, especially when administered in large doses. However, alcohol can elicit euphoria and stimulation when given in small doses (21).

To date, alcohol-specific binding sites or receptors on neurons have not been identified. It has been hypothesized that at large doses, alcohol may disturb the fluidity of the bilayer lipid neuronal membrane. Disturbances in membrane fluidity may indirectly modify the structure and function of neurotransmitter receptors and ion channels. It is unlikely, however, that this is the mechanism by which alcohol exerts its effects on neurons at the lower doses that normally are consumed by humans. In this regard, some evidence suggests that at blood concentrations within the range of typical human consumption, alcohol can directly affect the function of several neuronal ion channels and receptors (21).

The Dopaminergic System

The ventral tegmental area (VTA), nucleus accumbens (NAc), amygdala, and prefrontal cortex in the mesolimbic dopaminergic circuit are the major brain structures mediating the rewarding effects of alcohol (21–23). A number of studies in rodents have examined the mechanisms by which acute alcohol exposure increases dopamine tone in the mesolimbic system. Results of these reports suggest that alcohol enhances dopamine release by directly increasing the firing rate of dopamine cells in the VTA. PET imaging and MRI studies in moderate drinkers described that intoxicating doses of alcohol resulted in a significant increase of dopamine levels in the ventral striatum (21–23).

Chronic alcohol exposure and alcohol withdrawal result in profound neuroadaptive changes in dopaminergic transmission that in general are contrary to the acute effects of alcohol on this system. Using PET imaging techniques, researchers found significantly lower baseline dopamine receptor (D2/D3) density among alcoholics than controls, demonstrated by a lower binding of the D2/D3 selective ligand [^{11}C] raclopride. A significant decrease was also observed in dopamine release among alcoholic subjects after administration of the dopamine reuptake blocker methylphenidate. Together, these findings support the notion that a reduction in dopaminergic signaling among alcoholics may explain the decrease in alcohol rewarding effects during chronic alcohol consumption and the emergence of negative mood states (e.g., depression, dysphoria anhedonia) during alcohol withdrawal (21–23).

The GABAergic System

A significant involvement of GABAergic neurotransmission in the pharmacologic effects of alcohol was initially hypothesized based on observations that alcohol had effects (e.g., anxiolysis, impaired motor coordination and cognition, anticonvulsant effects) resembling those produced by drugs known to act on the GABAergic system. It was also apparent that there was significant cross-tolerance of alcohol with GABAergic agents such as benzodiazepines and barbiturates, compounds that also are highly effective in treating alcohol withdrawal.

Alcohol effects on the GABAergic system have been mainly attributed to a postsynaptic mechanism similar to that of benzodiazepines and barbiturates, compounds that allosterically enhance GABA$_A$ receptor function. More recently, however, it has been recognized that alcohol administration also enhances GABAergic inhibitory effects presynaptically by increasing GABA release in many brain regions including the hippocampus and the cerebellum (21–23).

Although many studies have suggested that alcohol specifically potentiates the function of the GABA$_A$ receptor type (Criswell et al. 1993), experiments that have directly examined the effects of alcohol on GABA$_A$ receptors-mediated ion currents have yielded conflicting results, showing wide differences in alcohol sensitivity. An explanation for these discrepancies is that there is a rich variability in GABA$_A$ receptors subunit composition and posttranslational processes (21–23). It appears that presence of the α1 subunit is critical in determining the sensitivity of GABA$_A$ receptors to alcohol. Pharmacologic manipulation of GABA$_A$α1 receptors on mesocorticolimbic neurons of alcohol preferring rodents has been shown to modify the reinforcing effects of alcohol (21–23).

Contrary to the effects of acute alcohol administration, chronic alcohol exposure and alcohol withdrawal in rodents and humans results in decreased GABAergic tone and in symptoms of anxiety, dysphoria, and alcohol craving. Reinstatement of alcohol consumption transiently relieves such negative states, negatively reinforcing drinking behavior.

A growing number of preclinical and clinical studies have shown that several compounds such as topiramate or baclofen that enhance GABAergic inhibition, are efficacious in reducing alcohol drinking and craving in alcohol-dependent subjects (21–23).

The Glutamatergic System

Alcohol administration has important effects on the glutamatergic neurotransmitter system. Acute administration of alcohol antagonizes NMDA receptors, whereas chronic administration increases the density of these receptors (21–23). This antagonist effect of acute alcohol on glutamatergic neurotransmission has been observed in the hippocampus and bed nucleus of the stria terminalis and in many other brain regions. Alcohol has also been shown significantly to reduce NMDA-evoked currents neurons, confirming the postsynaptic nature of this effect (21–23).

Recent studies have identified specific amino acids in NMDA receptor subunits that represent a putative alcohol interaction site. Generally, alcohol has relatively minimal effects on other subtypes of glutamate receptors. However, in a few specific brain regions, alcohol has been shown to have relatively potent inhibitory effects on AMPA and kainate receptor–gated synapses.

Chronic alcohol exposure and withdrawal results in significant increases in glutamatergic neurotransmission mediated by NMDA receptors in the basolateral amygdala and in the NAc (40). This increase in NMDA receptor function during alcohol withdrawal appears to be related to the emergence of significant anxiety levels (21–23). A similar increase in NMDA receptor function also appears to contribute to seizure activity observed during alcohol withdrawal. For example, treatment with NMDA receptor antagonists effectively blocked epileptiform spike patterns in the hippocampus typically seen during alcohol withdrawal (21–23).

The Opioidergic System

Alcohol administration stimulates hypothalamic synthesis, release, and binding of endogenous opioids such as β-endorphin and enkephalin to μ-opiate receptors (24). Disturbances in opioidergic neurotransmission have been described among alcoholic patients and their unaffected adult children (24).

In comparison to adult children of nonalcoholic individuals (i.e., paternal-history-negative or PHN), paternal-history-positive (PHP) subjects have lower plasma and cerebrospinal fluid levels of beta-endorphin (24). After alcohol administration, PHP individuals show a greater increase or normalization of their beta-endorphin levels (24). Based on these findings, it has been hypothesized that offspring of alcoholics have an inherited or acquired deficiency in endogenous opioid activity that leads them to drink to compensate for the deficiency (opioid deficiency hypothesis) (24). Support for the opioidergic hypothesis of alcoholism is provided by the fact that opioid antagonists reliably reduce alcohol preference and consumption in different experimental paradigms and across different animal species.

In humans, several placebo-controlled clinical studies have shown efficacy of the opioid antagonist naltrexone (23,24) in the treatment of alcohol dependence. Although the specific mechanisms responsible for these therapeutic effects in humans are not fully understood, some preclinical studies have shown that naltrexone can significantly attenuate the increase in NAc dopamine associated with alcohol consumption, thereby decreasing voluntary alcohol intake (24).

The Serotonergic System

The acute administration of alcohol to rodents increases their brain concentrations of serotonin (5-HT). Direct infusion of 5-HT activates dopaminergic neurons in the VTA (40,43). In contrast, chronic exposure to alcohol reduces 5-HT concentrations in the brain, which was associated with impulsive aggression and behavioral disinhibition (21–23). Although administration of 5-HT reuptake inhibitors to alcohol preferring rodents reduced alcohol drinking behavior, it was unclear whether these compounds specifically dampened the reinforcing effects of alcohol or produced a reduction in all consummatory behaviors (21–23).

In humans, derangements in central serotonergic activity may contribute to alcohol and drug use disorders, particularly among individuals with antisocial personality. Consistent with this interpretation, antisocial alcoholics had lower basal CSF concentrations of the serotonin metabolite 5-HIAA than normal controls (21–23). Also, antisocial alcohol and drug-dependent men exhibited blunted cortisol and prolactin responses to a challenge with the 5-HT agonist fenfluramine (21–23). Additionally, children with a parental history of substance abuse and/or criminal behavior showed a reduced density of 5-HT_{2A} receptors on platelets (21–23).

There is evidence that the 5-HT_3 receptor plays an important role in the serotonergic modulation of the mesolimbic reward circuit. This receptor is unique among the 5-HT receptors in that it directly gates an ion channel that regulates rapid depolarization, causing the rapid release of neurotransmitters and/or peptides. Preclinical findings indicate that antagonism of the 5-HT_3 receptor in the VTA, NAc, or amygdala reduces alcohol self-administration and/or alcohol-associated effects. Consistent with preclinical findings, treatment with 5-HT_3 antagonists such as ondansetron attenuates the subjective effects of low alcohol doses and reduces relapse rates among early-onset alcoholic patients (21–23).

The Cholinergic System

Neuronal nicotinic acetylcholine receptors activate the release of dopamine in the CNS (21,22). Several nicotinic receptors subtypes ($\alpha4\alpha6\beta2\beta3$, $\alpha6\beta2\beta3$, $\alpha6\beta2$, $\alpha4\beta2$, and $\alpha4\alpha5\beta2$) are expressed on dopamine nerve terminals. The nicotinic receptors located in the soma of dopaminergic neurons of the VTA activate these neurons directly, leading to release of dopamine in the NAc. Nicotinic receptors also modulate dopaminergic reward circuits indirectly by the activation of $\alpha7$ homomeric receptors on glutamatergic neurons. This $\alpha7$ activation triggers release of glutamine, which in turn stimulates NMDA receptors on dopaminergic neurons, leading to dopamine release (21,22).

Studies in rodents showed that the alcohol-induced dopamine release in the NAc can be antagonized by the central nicotinic receptor antagonist mecamylamine (40). Further, pretreatment with the partial nicotine receptor agonist varenicline antagonized the dopamine stimulatory effect of acute nicotine and of coadministration of alcohol and nicotine in rodents (21,22).

In healthy humans and social drinkers, pharmacologic manipulation of the nicotinic cholinergic receptor with mecamylamine or varenicline (21,22) appears to reduce the stimulant effects of acute alcohol administration and alcohol consumption. These findings suggest that pharmacologic treatment with compounds targeting nicotinic receptors may be a useful strategy to reduce alcohol consumption among alcoholics.

Genetics of Alcohol Dependence

Family, adoption, and twin studies strongly support the involvement of genetic factors in the etiology of alcohol dependence. Family studies have shown that there is a sevenfold risk of alcohol dependence in first-degree relatives of alcohol-dependent individuals, especially among men. The observation that the majority of alcohol-dependent individuals do not have an alcohol-dependent first-degree relative underscores the fact that risk for alcohol dependence is also determined by environmental factors that may interact in complex way with genetics (25).

Adoption studies conducted during the past three decades have examined the effects of having a biologic alcoholic parent in the context of an environment provided by a nonalcoholic adoptive family. They show that there is a greater risk of alcohol dependence in adopted-away offspring from alcoholic biologic parents than in adopted away biologic children of nonalcoholic parents. The risk ratio for alcohol problems described in these studies has ranged from 1.6 to 3.6 in men and from 0.5 to 6.3 in women (25).

Twin studies have shown that the proportion of risk attributable to genetic factors (i.e., the heritability) of alcohol dependence ranges from 0.52 to 0.64 with no significant differences between men and women. Despite a rapidly changing social environment, a study conducted in Sweden that examined four birth cohorts showed that estimates of heritability remained stable over a five-decade period (25).

Linkage Studies

Linkage studies are family-based studies in which markers spaced throughout the genome are used to identify regions of chromosomes that are likely to harbor genes contributing to risk of a disorder. Linkage studies of alcohol dependence by the Collaborative Study on the Genetics of Alcoholism (COGA) group and by investigators at the National Institute on Alcohol Abuse and Alcoholism (NIAAA) have implicated a region on the long arm (q) of chromosome 4 where an ADH gene cluster has been identified. More recently, similar findings were obtained for the phenotype of alcoholism severity on chromosome 4 in a sample of 474 Irish families and among 243 Mission Native Americans from the southwest United States (25).

Among African Americans (AAs), a significant linkage between alcohol dependence and markers in chromosome 10 was also reported. This region contains numerous genes potentially relevant to alcohol dependence, such as those encoding the synaptic vesicular amine transporter and the 5-HT$_7$ receptor. Consistent with this finding, suggestive linkages were found on chromosomes 10, 11, and 22 for a low level of response to alcohol in a predominantly European American sample of college students (25). This trait has shown prospectively to predict an increased risk of alcohol dependence.

Other chromosomal regions of interest are those reported on chromosomes 6, 12, 15, and 16, which showed suggestive linkages with alcoholism severity and with alcohol withdrawal symptoms among Mission Native Americans (25).

Candidate Gene Studies

Candidate gene studies are population-level investigations in groups of unrelated individuals, in which genetic loci that encode proteins believed to be important in the etiology of a disorder are examined. In this approach, a statistical comparison of allele or haplotype frequencies at a candidate locus is made between affected individuals and control subjects.

ALDH Genes The influence of genetic variants encoding ADHs and ALDHs on risk of alcohol dependence in some populations is well established (20,25).

ALDH1A1 and *ALDH2* are the genes that encode ALDH1 and ALDH2. These genes have been mapped to chromosomes 9 and 12, respectively. A well-known coding variant of the *ALDH2* gene, *ALDH2*2*, encodes a substitution of lysine for glutamate at position 504. This mutation results in the coding of an ALDH2 enzyme with very little oxidizing activity (i.e., a null mutation). People with one copy of the *ALDH2*2* allele have almost no detectable ALDH2 activity in their liver, whereas people who are homozygous have no detectable activity (20,25). The inactive *ALDH2*2* variant is relatively frequent among people of Chinese, Japanese, and Korean origin but is almost absent in people of European or African descent (20,25). People with an *ALDH2*2* allele experience a typical reaction when alcohol is consumed, which is characterized by severe skin flushing, nausea, and tachycardia. This reaction among *ALDH2*2* carriers is due to the rise in the blood concentration of unmetabolized acetaldehyde. This *ALDH* gene variant that reduces or inactivates completely ALDH function has shown to be protective against alcohol dependence especially among Asians. It is known that subjects heterozygous for the inactive ALDH2 variant have only one fourth the risk for alcohol dependence as those with two functional alleles (20,25).

ADH Genes To date, there are seven known human ADH genes: *ADH1A*, *ADH1B*, *ADH1C*, *ADH4*, *ADH5*, *ADH6*, and *ADH7*. These genes have been mapped to a small region on chromosome 4. The ADH enzymes that they encode are composed of two subunits or dimers. The seven ADH types have been divided into five classes based on similarities in their amino acid sequence and their ability to oxidize alcohol. The class I genes, *ADH1A*, *ADH1B*, and *ADH1C*, encode the α, β, and γ subunits, which can form homodimers or heterodimers that account for most of the oxidizing capacity in the liver. Several mutations have been identified in the *ADH1B* and *ADH1C* genes that are differentially distributed across population groups and that produce enzymes with different pharmacokinetic properties (20,25). There are three different *ADH1B* variants that modify the amino acid sequence of the encoded β subunit. The *ADH1B*1* allele encodes a β1 subunit that has arginine (Arg) at positions 48 and 370. The β2 subunit is coded by *ADH1B*2* and has the amino acid histidine (His) at position 48. This variant is frequently found among Asians. *ADH1B*3* is commonly found among individuals of African descent and encodes the β3 subunit with cysteine (Cys) at position 370. The amino acid substitutions in both the β2 and β3 subunits occur at a site of the amino chain that directly interacts with NAD+, resulting in a faster release of NAD+ at the end of the reaction. In comparison to the β1 subunit, the enzymes with these amino acid substitutions have a 70- to 80-fold greater turnover rate (20,25).

There also are three variants of the *ADH1C* gene. *ADH1C*1* encodes the γ1 subunit with Arg at position 272 and isoleucine (Ile) at position 350. *ADH1C*2* encodes the γ2 subunit, which has a glutamine (Gln) at position 272 and a valine (Val) at position 350. *ADH1C*Thr352* encodes a subunit with threonine at position 352. The homodimeric γ2γ2 enzyme has a turnover rate that is approximately 70% greater than the γ1γ1 ADH enzyme (20,25). The functional significance of the *ADH1C*Thr352* is still unknown.

The differences in the amino sequence encoded by *ADH1B* and *ADH1C* translate in differential rates of alcohol oxidation by the liver. It was estimated that in a person homozygous for the *ADH1B*1* and *ADH1C*2* variants, the total alcohol-metabolizing capacity would be approximately 20% lower than that of a person homozygous for both *ADH1B*1* and *ADH1C*1*. In a person homozygous for the *ADH1B*2* and *ADH1C*1* alleles, the alcohol oxidizing capacity would be eight times greater than that of the person homozygous for both reference alleles. For a person homozygous for the *ADH1B*3* and *ADH1C*1* variants, the metabolizing capacity would be almost twice than that of the person homozygous for both reference alleles (20,25).

One *ADH4* variant, the -75A allele, is a promoter polymorphic site that has twice the level of activity than the -75C allele. A strong association between alcohol dependence diagnosis and *ADH4* alleles has been reported (20,25).

GABAergic Genes A variety of loci encoding proteins that play a role in GABAergic neurotransmission have been associated with alcohol dependence and related phenotypes. In a sample of families with multiple alcohol-dependent members, EEG frequency, a quantitative high-risk trait linked to chromosome 4p, was associated to *GABRA2*, which encodes the α-2 $GABA_A$ subunit. Other groups, using case-control samples, independently replicated this finding. Although this association has been reported many times, there are studies that have failed to replicate this association and no specific causative variant or mechanism of action has been identified (25).

Interestingly, there have also been reported associations of a *GABRA2* allele with the subjective response to alcohol among healthy subjects and with drinking outcomes and the response to psychotherapeutic treatment of alcoholism (25).

Acetylcholine Receptor Genes Initial evidence that variation in the gene encoding the muscarinic acetylcholine receptor M2 (*CHRM2*) contributes to risk for alcohol dependence was independently reported. *CHRM2* maps to chromosome 7q and like the regions of chromosome 4p and 4q, it was identified by the COGA alcohol dependence linkage study as a region of interest (25).

Serotonergic Genes Genes encoding proteins in the serotonergic system have also been targeted as candidates for alcohol dependence risk. An insertion–deletion polymorphism consisting of a repetitive sequence of base pairs in the promoter region of the serotonin transporter protein (genetic locus *SLC6A4*) has been of particular interest. Compared with the "long" (L) allele, the allele with the smallest number of repeats, commonly called the "short" (S) allele, has lower transcriptional activity, leading to marked reductions in messenger ribonucleic acid (mRNA) levels, serotonin binding, and serotonin uptake in both platelets and lymphoblast. In a meta-analysis of data from 17 studies that included 3489 alcoholics and 2325 controls, presence of the S allele increased the risk for alcohol dependence by almost 20%. Moreover, the greatest association with the S allele was seen among individuals with alcohol dependence complicated by either a comorbid psychiatric condition or early-onset or more severe alcohol dependence (25,26).

Gene by environment studies have also shown that the S allele moderates the effects of various environmental stressors to increase alcohol consumption in children, adolescents, and college students. However, findings from COGA failed to replicate this moderating effect on risk of alcohol dependence. In a study examining a cohort of children at risk who were followed from birth into young adulthood, men homozygous for the higher expression L allele, when exposed to high psychosocial stressors, reported more hazardous drinking than those with the S allele or than those without exposure to stressors (25).

Opioidergic Genes A meta-analysis of studies focusing on the gene encoding the μ-opioid receptor (genetic locus *OPRM1*) failed to provide convincing evidence of association to alcohol dependence (27). Some evidence suggests, however, that an A118G polymorphism that encodes an Asn40Asp amino acid substitution in *OPRM1* may moderate the response to treatment with the opioid antagonist naltrexone (25). Healthy individuals with one or two Asp40 alleles who were pretreated with naltrexone, reported lower levels of alcohol craving and greater alcohol-induced "high" than Asn40 homozygotes after intravenous alcohol administration. Further, pretreatment with naltrexone blunted the positive response to alcohol, an effect that was stronger among individuals with the Asp40 allele.

Among alcoholic subjects treated with naltrexone, effects of the *OPRM1* Asp40Asn polymorphism on drinking behavior have varied. Several treatment studies (25) showed that naltrexone-treated patients with one or more Asp40 alleles were significantly less likely to relapse to heavy drinking than Asn40 homozygotes. However, other studies have failed to replicate this finding (25).

In addition to the Asn40Asp polymorphism, investigators (25) have studied two other *OPRM1* SNPs, three markers in *OPRD1* (which encodes the δ-opioid receptor), and one marker in *OPRK1* (which encodes the κ-opioid receptor). No significant interaction between any of these markers and the response to naltrexone treatment was detected (25). In summary, the available evidence shows that the risk of alcohol dependence is determined by multiple genes that interact with environmental factors. To date, variants in genes encoding proteins that metabolize alcohol (ADH and ALDH genes) and GABAergic neurotransmission have consistently been found to influence the risk for alcohol dependence. Although the mechanism of the effects of genetic variation on alcohol metabolism appears to be related to the aversive effects of acetaldehyde, the mechanism of other genetic effects that have been identified remains unclear. Despite substantial evidence that a genetic component is operative in the development of alcohol dependence, the disorder is etiologically complex, with a variety of other vulnerability factors playing a substantial role (25).

EVALUATION AND TREATMENT

Conducting a detail, systematic evaluation of alcohol dependent patients allows clinician to develop an individualized plan of treatment. To determine the most appropriate level of care and the type and intensity of therapeutic interventions, clinicians should determine the severity of the disorder, the nature of co-occurring conditions, the extent of social support available, and a history of previous responses to treatment.

To build a therapeutic alliance and increase the chance of accurate reporting, it is crucial for the clinician to avoid communicating judgments that he or she may have regarding the patient's drinking behavior, remaining neutral and empathetic.

A complete drinking history should be obtained, including specific questions on typical quantity and frequency of alcohol consumption, maximal number of drinks per drinking occasion, frequency of heavy drinking episodes, and history of alcohol-related problems such as family and interpersonal problems. Other areas of inquiry include work and legal problems, psychiatric symptoms and the nature of their relationship with alcohol consumption (e.g., precipitation or exacerbation), and history of medical complications (e.g., alcohol withdrawal, alcoholic gastritis or pancreatitis, alcoholic liver disease).

Screening

Diverse clinical settings, including primary care practices or general hospitals, provide an opportunity to identify persons at risk for alcohol-related problems, as well as those who are already experiencing adverse effects of drinking. Evidence suggests that screening in conjunction with brief interventions (discussed below) can be very effective in prompting people whose alcohol consumption is risky or harmful to cut back on their drinking and/or to seek treatment (28). In addition to clinical settings, screening can take place in community agencies, colleges, churches, etc.

A number of self-report screening tests have been developed to identify alcoholics and individuals at risk for alcohol problems. One of the most frequently used is the CAGE, which includes four questions: (1) Have you ever felt you ought to *cut* (the "C" in CAGE) down on your drinking? (2) Have people *Annoyed* (A) you by criticizing your drinking? (3) Have you ever felt bad or *Guilty* (G) about your drinking? (4) Have you ever had a drink first thing in the morning to steady your nerves or get rid of a hangover that is, an *Eye* opener (E)?

A total CAGE score of 2 or greater (i.e., at least two of the items are endorsed as being positive) is considered highly suggestive of an alcohol use disorder.

The CAGE has shown to have a high test–retest reliability (0.80–0.95) and to adequately correlate (0.48–0.70) with other screening instruments. This is a valid screening tool for detecting alcohol use disorders in medical and surgical populations, and in psychiatric inpatients with an average sensitivity 0.71 and specificity of 0.90. However, the CAGE has not performed well among nonpregnant, pregnant women, and college students. Also, this questionnaire appears to have a poor screening efficiency in detecting low severity drinking problems (29).

Another commonly used screening instrument is the Alcohol Use Disorders Identification Test (AUDIT), which consists of 10 items. In addition to being sensitive and specific in the identification of hazardous or harmful drinkers, the AUDIT can identify alcohol-dependent individuals and may be used as the first step in a comprehensive alcohol use history (30). The AUDIT includes items examining the frequency and intensity of alcohol consumption, symptoms of alcohol dependence, and alcohol-related consequences. Using an AUDIT's cutoff score of 8 or more yields a sensitivity ranging from 61% to 97% and a specificity from 78% to 90% in detecting alcohol use disorders (30).

A brief version of the AUDIT that includes only the first three consumption questions (AUDIT-C) has been evaluated and found to have an acceptable sensitivity (54% to 98%) and specificity (57% to 93%) in detecting drinking problems (30).

Because alcoholic patients commonly abuse or become dependent on other addictive substances, screening should include questions concerning the use of other psychoactive substances, including tobacco products, marihuana, cocaine and other stimulants, and opioids.

Psychiatric History

Given the lack of reliability in unstructured clinical diagnoses, it is highly recommended that clinicians treating patients with alcohol dependence use a structured or semistructured interview to conduct and report their diagnostic evaluations. If it is not possible to use a complete psychiatric interview, such as the Composite International Diagnostic Interview (CIDI) or the Structured Clinical Interview for DSM-IV (SCID), then the alcohol sections of these interviews can be used.

To obtain an estimate of illness severity, the number of DSM symptoms obtained during a structured interview with the SCID can be tallied. Alternatively, the total scores on the AUDIT screening test can be used to assess past-year or lifetime severity, respectively. Another useful measure of substance dependence severity is the Composite Score from the Drug and Alcohol (CSDA) section of the Addiction Severity Index (ASI).

The ASI also includes a subscale that provides an overall estimate of psychiatric severity, including the number of inpatient and outpatient treatment episodes, medication status, and lifetime and current symptoms.

It is important to obtain estimates of psychological function such as measures of depression, anxiety, and more global psychological distress. Instruments such as the Beck Depression Inventory and the Symptom Checklist 90-Revised are reliable, valid, and acceptable in a variety of health care settings.

Other measures that are useful in treatment planning for alcoholic patients include estimates of motivation and the patient's readiness to change. The 32-item University of Rhode Island Change Assessment Scale (URICA) and the 12-item Readiness to Change Questionnaire (RCQ) are instruments designed to evaluate the stages of change across diverse problem behaviors including alcohol drinking. In some studies, the URICA and RCQ scores have shown to predict treatment outcome among alcoholics.

Physical Examination and Laboratory Findings

Physical Examination

Medical complications are a common consequence of heavy drinking and clinicians should be aware that such complications often develop in the absence of an alcohol dependence diagnosis. Conversely, early in the course of alcohol dependence, alcoholics may show no physical or laboratory abnormalities, but as the disorder progresses, most organ systems are adversely affected.

The physical examination provides essential information about the presence and extent of alcohol-induced organ damage most commonly in the GI system, the central and peripheral nervous system, and the cardiovascular system. The clinician should be alert to frequent acute alcohol-related signs, including alcohol withdrawal or delirium, intoxication or withdrawal from other drugs, and the acute presentation of psychiatric symptoms. Other systemic or nonspecific health problems associated with alcoholism include malnutrition and vitamin deficiencies, polyneuropathy, immune suppression and infectious diseases such as tuberculosis, viral hepatitis and other sexually transmitted diseases, and trauma secondary to fights and accidents.

Laboratory Tests

Laboratory testing is a valuable tool in the assessment of the effects of alcohol consumption on organ systems. Laboratory assessments can also be helpful in assessing individuals who deny or minimize their alcohol consumption or in resolving diagnostic dilemmas in patients whose self-report information and physical findings are inconclusive. Test results can also be used by the clinician to provide objective, nonjudgmental feedback to alcoholic patients on the negative medical consequences of excessive drinking, thereby enhancing the patient's motivation to reduce or stop drinking.

Another goal of laboratory testing is the early detection of relapse. Detection of relapse allows clinicians to modify the treatment plan and to implement more intensive therapeutic interventions.

Initially during the assessment phase, and during treatment, laboratory determinations should be obtained every other week, and subsequently, once a month during the follow-up period. To help patients appreciate changes in laboratory indexes, it is recommended that results be presented to them in an easy-to-comprehend graphic format that enables them to compare their findings with normal values.

Carbohydrate Deficient Transferring (CDT) The most sensitive and specific laboratory test for the identification of heavy alcohol consumption is the determination of CDT concentrations in blood. Transferrin is a globular protein that is responsible for iron transport in plasma. CDT is a collective term for a group of transferrins that lack sialic acid residues. An increase in CDT concentration is induced by heavy drinking. To date, CDT is the only laboratory test approved by the FDA for the detection of heavy alcohol consumption (31).

In differentiating heavy drinking individuals from light drinkers or abstainers, CDT has shown a sensitivity ranging from 82% to 91% and a specificity of 97% to 100% (31). CDT values also correlate significantly ($r = 0.64$) with the amount of alcohol consumed during the preceding month. Although the sensitivity of CDT appears to be comparable to that of another heavy drinking marker (gamma-glutamyl-transpeptidase—see below), CDT appears to be more specific in detecting heavy drinkers without liver disease. In this regard, CDT elevations are associated with fewer confounding conditions such as nonalcoholic liver disease or the effects of medications (31). The accuracy of this marker is poorer, however, among younger alcoholics and women. Generally, CDT concentrations return to normal levels after 1 to 2 weeks of abstinence from drinking. Among patients in alcohol treatment, CDT appears to detect relapse to heavy drinking more accurately than other laboratory tests (31).

Gamma-glutamyl-transpeptidase (GGTP) The hepatic enzyme GGTP is the most widely employed marker of heavy drinking. GGTP is a biliary canalicular enzyme, the concentration of which can be elevated as a consequence of its induction by heavy alcohol consumption. GGTP concentrations are also increased as a consequence of its release into the bloodstream during acute hepatocellular damage. GGTP levels are particularly elevated in patients with severe alcoholic liver disease, though these may be decreased during the later stages of liver cirrhosis. After the cessation of heavy drinking, the concentration of serum GGT gradually falls by approximately 50% within 2 weeks, usually returning to the reference range over a 6- to 8- week period (31). The normalization of GGTP levels may be delayed or incomplete if there is underlying alcoholic liver disease or other medical disorders. GGTP concentrations are also elevated in a variety of nonalcoholic liver diseases such as hepatobiliary disease and in subjects consuming barbiturates or other enzyme-inducing agents. Nonetheless, elevations of GGTP occur in approximately three fourths of alcoholics before there is clinical evidence of liver disease. In comparison to CDT, an abnormal GGTP level appears to be more specific in detecting alcoholics with hepatic damage secondary to heavy drinking (31).

Whenever possible, CDT and GGTP should be used together to detect heavy drinking individuals. This approach has been shown to increase the likelihood of correctly identifying individuals with alcohol use disorders (31) and may be especially useful in diagnostically complex cases (e.g., alcoholics with a primary liver disease, those with iron metabolic abnormalities, and those being treated with anticonvulsants).

Liver Function Tests Other laboratory tests related to hepatic function, such as serum transaminases, bilirubin, prothrombin time, and partial thromboplastin time, have been used by clinicians to identify or evaluate severity of alcohol dependence. As with GGTP, elevations of the transaminases serum glutamic oxaloacetic transaminase (SGOT) and serum glutamic pyruvic transaminase (SGPT) are frequently observed when heavy drinking affects the liver. However these enzymes can also be elevated in nonalcoholic liver disease. Consequently, transaminase elevations are less sensitive indicators of heavy drinking. SGOT is elevated in 32% to 77% of alcoholics while elevations in SGPT have been observed in 50% of alcoholics. The ratio of SGPT to SGOT may provide a more accurate indicator of heavy drinking than the absolute values. Heavy alcohol consumption is more likely to be present when the ratio of these two enzymes exceeds 1.5, whereas other liver pathologies are more commonly associated with a lower ratio (31).

Mean Corpuscular Volume (MCV) Erythrocyte MCV can also be used as an objective indicator of heavy drinking. The MCV may be most useful when used in combination with GGTP or CDT. An elevation of MCV, which is caused by folate deficiency in alcoholics, is more prominent among alcoholics who are smokers. Because there is a 2- to 4- month period of abstinence required for MCV to normalize, this marker is not an efficient indicator of relapse (31).

The Alcohol Breath Test and Blood Alcohol Level (BAL) The alcohol breath test can be helpful in clinical settings such as emergency departments, or in circumstances such as driving while drinking, in which it is important to obtain a rapid estimate of the circulating alcohol concentration. This test measures the amount of alcohol in expired air, providing an indirect estimate of the venous BAL. Although its accuracy is contingent upon the patient's cooperation in exhaling into the instrument, which is commonly limited in intoxicated patients, the alcohol breath test can be a reliable and inexpensive method to assess recent alcohol consumption. When the patient is comatose and dangerously high levels of intoxication are suspected, or for medical–legal purposes, a direct venous BAL can also be obtained. A BAL greater than 150 mg/dL in a patient showing no signs of intoxication (i.e., no dysarthria, motor incoordination, gait ataxia, nystagmus, or impaired attention) can be interpreted to reflect physiologic tolerance. In nontolerant individuals, a BAL in excess of 400 mg/dL can result in death, and 300 mg/dL indicates a need for emergency care.

Miscellaneous Laboratory Tests Another laboratory evaluation that is indicated in alcoholics is the urine toxicology screen, a test that is potentially helpful in identifying drug use among patients who may not recognize it or who deny it as a problem. The screen should include opioids, cocaine, cannabis, and benzodiazepines. Urinalysis, blood chemistries, viral hepatitis profile, complete blood count, serologic test for syphilis, and other sexually transmitted diseases, and a serum pregnancy test among women, should also be obtained routinely.

Treatment

The first step in treatment planning for a patient diagnosed with an alcohol use disorder is to determine the appropriate type, setting, and intensity of the therapeutic intervention. The clinical needs of patients affected by alcohol use disorders differ widely, so the nature and intensity of interventions must be chosen to match the patient presentation. For example, a brief intervention that provides feedback on negative consequences of excessive drinking and recommends a specific goal for reducing alcohol consumption may be sufficient to curb excessive drinking among hazardous drinkers who do not have alcohol dependence (32). However, these interventions may have a limited affect on alcohol-dependent individuals (32).

Consequently, alcohol-dependent individuals need multiple and more intensive interventions addressing both heavy drinking and associated psychosocial and medical complications. These interventions should include both psychosocial and pharmacologic interventions. An important step in developing a treatment plan for patients with a diagnosis of alcohol dependence is to establish treatment goals. Generally, the stabilization of acute medical and psychiatric conditions (e.g., severe alcohol withdrawal symptoms) has priority over other treatment goals.

Alcohol-dependent patients often have limited motivation to stop drinking, so that an important objective early in treatment is to enhance the patient's motivation for recovery. Generally, this goal can be achieved by building a therapeutic alliance, which provides the context within which recovery can occur. The presence of a trusting and encouraging relationship with a clinician can facilitate the patient's acknowledgement of alcohol-related problems and promotes motivation for treatment.

Early in treatment, clinicians should also advise patients who are alcohol dependent to establish a goal of complete abstinence. One approach to achieving this goal is through the provision of coping and relapse prevention skills training, which can include social skills training and the identification and avoidance of high-risk situations. Once established, the clinician should aim to promote the maintenance of abstinence through ongoing participation in structured treatment and/or self-help groups. In this regard, the patient should be made aware of the widespread availability of Alcoholics Anonymous (AA) and the wide diversity of its membership. A goal of moderate drinking may be appropriate for individuals who have not had multiple prior attempts to reduce their drinking to sensible limits. Such individuals may be less amenable to participation in AA, where the orientation is primarily one of abstinence.

Patients who need to change their living circumstances (e.g., to avoid frequent exposure to situations that are high-risk for drinking) may benefit from the clinician's assistance in achieving this goal. Finally, clinicians should assist patients in dealing with dysfunctional family or couples dynamics and in rebuilding supportive relationships that may help to sustain the patient's recovery efforts.

Treatment Setting

In patients with a diagnosis of alcohol dependence, it is critical to determine the severity of the disorder and whether the patient is in need of medical detoxification. Outpatient nonpharmacologic treatment is indicated when risk of withdrawal symptoms is low; however, when risk of withdrawal is moderate or high, outpatient or inpatient pharmacologic detoxification is indicated.

Several medical complications of alcoholism indicate the need for immediate admission into an inpatient treatment setting for acute stabilization. These include conditions that create a high risk for complicated alcohol withdrawal, including severe medical or surgical diseases such as hepatic insufficiency, acute pancreatitis, and bleeding esophageal varices, and severe comorbid psychiatric conditions (e.g., psychosis, suicidal intent) and/or drug dependence disorders (e.g., benzodiazepines, barbiturates) where there is a potential for serious withdrawal reactions. Psychosocial problems that commonly interfere with the completion of detoxification and/or rehabilitation such as homelessness and/or the lack of a social support network also may warrant admission into an inpatient or residential treatment setting to provide an opportunity to remediate these complicating social problems.

Research suggests that alcoholism outpatient treatment is equally effective and less expensive than more intensive inpatient treatment. However, patients who choose to be treated in outpatient settings are generally less severely alcohol dependent, less physically ill, less psychiatrically impaired, or more motivated for recovery. In this regard, patients with severe alcohol dependence and medical and psychosocial complications appear to benefit from inpatient treatment (33). Also, long-term residential treatment appears to be the only suitable option for recidivist alcoholics who frequently utilize emergency departments and/or medical or psychiatric wards, and who do not respond to more limited rehabilitation efforts.

Treatment of Alcohol Withdrawal

An important initial intervention in treating alcohol-dependent patients is the management of alcohol withdrawal symptoms (i.e., detoxification). The objectives in detoxification are the relief of discomfort, prevention or treatment of complications, and preparation for rehabilitation.

There are two approaches to the management of alcohol withdrawal. One is a nonpharmacologic approach known as social detoxification, which is indicated in patients experiencing mild symptoms. Medical detoxification, on the other hand, is indicated for patients experiencing moderate-to-severe or complicated alcohol withdrawal.

Social detoxification consists of frequent reassurance, reality orientation, monitoring of vital signs, personal attention, and general nursing care. Medical detoxification involves the use of one or more of a variety of agents that act predominantly on the GABAergic neurotransmitter system. Due to their favorable side effect and safety profile, benzodiazepines are the drugs of first choice in the pharmacologic treatment of this condition (34). Although all benzodiazepines will control alcohol withdrawal symptoms, diazepam and chlordiazepoxide appear to have a slight advantage over compounds such as lorazepam and oxazepam in preventing seizures and delirium tremens. This effect is explained by the fact that as a result of being metabolized to long-acting compounds, diazepam and chlordiazepoxide appear to self-taper. However, because metabolism of these drugs is predominantly hepatic, impaired liver function may complicate their use. Oxazepam and lorazepam, on the other hand, are not oxidized to long-acting metabolites and thus carry less risk of accumulation.

Anticonvulsants such as carbamazepine, gabapentin, topiramate, and valproate appear to be useful in the treatment of alcohol withdrawal (35). However, these medications have not shown greater efficacy, safety, or cost-effectiveness than benzodiazepines for this indication.

Although antipsychotics are not indicated for the treatment of withdrawal, these compounds can be added to benzodiazepine in cases where hallucinosis or severe agitation are present. Clinician should be aware, however, that in addition to extrapyramidal side effects, antipsychotics lower the seizure threshold, which may be particularly risky in patients experiencing alcohol withdrawal symptoms.

The prevention, detection, and treatment of common co-occurring or complicating medical conditions in alcoholics are important clinical considerations during detoxification. Good supportive care is also essential. Administration of thiamine (50 to 100 mg by mouth or intramuscularly) and multivitamins is a low-cost, low-risk intervention for the prophylaxis and treatment of alcohol-related neuropsychiatric complications such as Wernicke–Korsakoff syndrome.

Psychosocial Treatment of Alcoholism

In both residential and outpatient settings, the most commonly utilized psychosocial treatments include group or individual cognitive-behavioral psychotherapies, self-help groups (AA), family therapy, and recreational and occupational therapy. In many programs, these interventions are combined and delivered as components of an integrated rehabilitation plan under the notion that multimodal treatment potentially has a greater therapeutic effect on the multiple therapeutic needs commonly experienced by alcoholic patients.

Cognitive-Behavioral Therapies Empirical studies have consistently demonstrated the efficacy of cognitive-behavioral therapies and 12-step facilitation, which is based on the principles of AA, in the treatment of alcohol dependence (36).

Effective techniques most commonly used by cognitive-behavioral therapists are relapse prevention, social skills and assertiveness training, motivational enhancement, contingency management, cognitive restructuring, cue exposure therapy, and behavioral marital therapy (36).

Cognitive-behavioral therapies emphasize the teaching of adaptive skills aimed at changing precipitants and reinforcers (internal or external) of drinking behavior. Also, these interventions emphasize learning alternative interpersonal skills, and coping skills to deal with events, feelings, and thoughts that promote alcohol consumption (36).

Alcoholics Anonymous (AA) With more than 100,000 groups in 150 countries, AA is the most widely used source of help for people experiencing drinking problems around the world. AA and other self-help organizations are more numerous than alcohol outpatient treatment programs, particularly in developing countries, where they may constitute the only source of help for alcoholic persons. Although these self-help groups are not considered formal treatment, they are often used as an adjunct to or as a substitute for formal treatment.

Providing a strong social support for recovery, AA emphasizes the notion of the alcoholic's powerlessness over drinking and the need to endorse the existence of a higher power as a means to restore sanity and maintain sobriety. In addition to this spiritual emphasis, AA promotes the disease concept of alcoholism, in which lifelong abstinence is the only means to recovery. However, not all people with drinking problems are willing to endorse these principles.

Clinicians working with alcohol-dependent patients should be familiar with the AA philosophy and organization, taking the time to identify patients who may benefit from participation in AA. When referring patients to AA, clinicians should also take the time to follow up with the patients, monitoring their attendance at meetings and their drinking behavior. Despite the fact that AA is regarded as one of the most useful recovery resources, the empirical evidence supporting the efficacy of AA is somewhat limited.

A few large, methodologically sound studies, however, showed that participation in AA after formal alcohol treatment was associated with a greater chance of abstinence during the following 6 months (37–39). In multisite studies, patients who attended more self-help group meetings had better outcomes after 1year than did patients who were less involved in such groups (37–39). Patients who attended more self-help groups in the first year after acute treatment were more likely to be in remission at 2 years and 5 years. Similarly, in a longitudinal naturalistic study (38), irrespective of having received formal alcohol treatment, alcoholics who participated in AA groups for an average of 27 weeks during an initial follow-up period of 3 years showed better drinking outcomes after 16 years than did alcoholics who did not participate in AA. Interestingly, in the subgroup of alcoholics who were formally treated, the effects of treatment appeared to be enhanced by AA participation. Taken together these studies indicate that participation in 12-step self-help groups and the number of meetings attended is associated with a greater likelihood of abstinence and remission in the short and long term.

It has been argued that beneficial effects of AA may be due to greater motivation for recovery or lower disease severity among alcoholics who attend these groups. Relevant to this question is a study that assessed 2319 male alcohol-dependent veterans during a 2-year follow-up period after alcohol treatment (39). In this study, AA attendance was associated with improved outcomes but neither motivation levels nor psychopathology explained the relationship between AA involvement and outcome.

Behavioral Family Therapy Despite the fact that alcoholism has severe consequences in families, there are few studies documenting the efficacy of family interventions aimed at reducing drinking problems and/or improving family functioning. Available reports have mainly examined the effects of couples rather than family therapy interventions in alcoholics. In a meta-analysis of 12 available studies including 754 individuals, behavioral couples therapy showed to be superior than control conditions in yielding greater relationship satisfaction, greater reductions in alcohol consumption, and greater reductions in drinking consequences (40).

Self-help groups for relatives of alcohol-dependent individuals have also been integrated in many alcohol treatment programs. Although not formally affiliated with AA, Al-Anon and Alateen groups, which are for the families and the teenage children of alcoholics, respectively, have a similar structure and philosophy as AA, and they frequently hold concurrent meetings with AA.

Pharmacotherapy of Alcoholism

During the past decade, the use of medications in the rehabilitation treatment of alcohol dependence has gained increasing importance. Progress in this field has been fueled by an increased understanding of specific neurotransmitter systems involved in the modulation of alcohol consumption.

In the following section, we will discuss pharmacologic interventions that aim to reduce drinking directly by targeting specific neurotransmitter systems (e.g., the opioidergic, glutamatergic, GABAergic, and serotonergic systems), and medications such as disulfiram, which act by sensitizing individuals to alcohol, resulting in aversive effects associated with drinking. We will also discuss some medications, the use of which is intended to reduce symptoms associated with common psychiatric disorders that are thought to maintain heavy drinking, so as to reduce alcohol consumption by indirect effects.

Naltrexone Opioidergic neurotransmission plays an important role in drinking behavior (24). In rodents and humans, alcohol intake increases beta-endorphin release in brain regions such as the nucleus accumbens, an effect that is blocked by the opioid antagonist naltrexone (24). Naltrexone and naloxone (another opioid antagonist) also suppress alcohol intake across a wide range of animal paradigms (24).

Among alcoholic patients naltrexone has shown to be more effective than placebo in delaying the time to relapse, in reducing the rate of relapse to heavy drinking, and in reducing the risk of relapse to heavy drinking in individuals who had consumed alcohol (41–43). To this date more than 20 clinical trials examining the efficacy of naltrexone in the treatment of alcoholism have been conducted (41,42). Some, but not all, of these studies (41–43) have shown that naltrexone is superior to placebo in reducing drinking. Bouza et al. (41) and Srisurapanont et al. (42) conducted meta-analyses showing that naltrexone treatment was associated with a 36% to 38% ($p \leq 0.0001$) reduction in the likelihood of relapse to heavy drinking and with a 26% greater chance, at the level of a nonsignificant trend ($p = 0.08$), of complete abstinence (41). Additionally, naltrexone treatment delayed the time to relapse and reduced the number of drinking days, drinks per drinking day, and total alcohol consumption. Such reductions in drinking were mirrored by reductions in concentrations of the liver enzymes GGT and AST (41).

Also, in a large multicenter clinical trial ($n = 1383$) (44), naltrexone in combination with medical management was as effective in reducing heavy drinking as when it was combined with a more intensive behavioral intervention. Findings from this study suggest that naltrexone may be effective when prescribed by primary care physicians to alcoholic patients. This is important because many alcoholics seek help in primary care settings.

Clinical characteristics that appear to predict a therapeutic response among alcoholics treated with naltrexone include high levels of craving, a family history of alcoholism, and medication adherence. On the other hand, increased severity of alcohol dependence and the presence of significant medication side effects were associated with a lack of treatment response (41–43). Poor adherence to naltrexone treatment commonly results from adverse effects of the medication, including nausea, which is reported by up to 15% of patients. This adverse effect is most common at the initiation of treatment and may reflect the rapid rise in plasma concentrations that occurs following the oral administration of naltrexone.

In 2006, a sustained-release (i.e., depot) formulation of naltrexone that yields detectable plasma concentrations of the drug for more than 30 days following an intramuscular (IM) injection was approved by the FDA. The relatively constant plasma naltrexone levels produced by a slow but regular release from a depot formulation may help to prevent side effects such as nausea that can lead to poor adherence and discontinuation of treatment. A monthly naltrexone depot injection could enhance medication adherence since it obviates the patient's need to remember to take the medications daily. Additionally, steady naltrexone plasma concentrations during the month following the depot injection may translate to greater exposure to this compound thereby enhancing its beneficial effects.

The FDA approval was based on the study reported by Garbutt et al. (45), who showed that patients receiving 380 mg of depot naltrexone (Vivitrol) in a large, 24-week, multicenter clinical trial had a lower percentage of heavy drinking days than those getting an intramuscular injection of placebo ($p = 0.02$). A lower naltrexone dosage of long-acting naltrexone (190 mg) was also associated with a greater reduction than those receiving placebo, but this difference did not reach statistical significance. In this study, secondary analysis showed that the beneficial effect of the 380 mg dose was limited to men. Although no clear mechanism could be determined for the lack of efficacy of the naltrexone formulation in women, since the study was not designed to test the effects in women, it likely was due to chance. Additional research is needed to determine whether there are sex differences in the effects of this formulation.

Summarizing, naltrexone appears to produce a modest but clinically significant effect on drinking behavior among alcoholics. Given the modest overall effect of the medication, a variety of other factors, including medication adherence, family history of alcoholism, severity of alcohol dependence, and presence of adverse effects, have to be considered so as to optimize the treatment response to this medication.

Topiramate In an initial 12-week clinical trial, topiramate (up to 300 mg/day) was more effective than placebo in reducing heavy drinking and alcohol craving and in improving alcohol-dependent patients' quality of life. Reductions in self-reported heavy drinking in the topiramate group were confirmed by reductions in GGT plasma concentrations. Subsequently, in a 14-week, multicenter clinical trial in 371 patients, topiramate treatment, up to 300 mg/day, was more effective than placebo in reducing self-reported drinking and GGT concentrations and in increasing quality of life among alcoholics who concomitantly received a weekly brief compliance enhancement intervention (23,46). From this study, it was estimated that the magnitude of topiramate's treatment effect in reducing the percentage of heavy drinking days ranged from 0.52 to 0.63 (46), a moderate effect size and one that is greater than that estimated for naltrexone treatment (43).

In general, topiramate has a favorable adverse effect profile, with most adverse events described as mild to moderate in severity. The most frequent adverse effects include paresthesia, anorexia, difficulty with memory or concentration, and taste disturbances. Topiramate treatment is also associated with uncommon visual adverse events such as myopia, angle-closure glaucoma, and increased intraocular pressure. Generally, these problems resolve within a few days of discontinuing topiramate. To prevent or reduce topiramate's adverse effects, a slow titration to a maximal dose of 300 mg/day for 8 weeks is recommended. However, regardless of the titration schedule or final dosage, approximately 1 in 10 patients taking this medication may experience cognitive disturbances.

Among other actions that may explain the reductions in alcohol drinking associated with topiramate is the ability of this compound to antagonize alpha-amino-3-hydroxy-5-methylisoxazole-4-propionic acid (AMPA) receptors and kainate glutamate receptors (23). Topiramate also facilitates inhibitory $GABA_A$-mediated currents at nonbenzodiazepine sites on the $GABA_A$ receptor (23). Studies in rodents have shown that a high-dose (50 mg/kg) but not a low-dose (1, 5, and 10 mg/kg) of topiramate suppressed alcohol intake in C57BL/6 mice (23). Topiramate also has been shown to reduce alcohol drinking in both alcohol preferring (P) and Wistar rats (23) and to reduce alcohol withdrawal symptoms in rodents (23).

In summary, although more research is needed to establish the efficacy of topiramate's effects on heavy drinking, available evidence strongly supports its efficacy in the treatment of alcohol dependence.

Acamprosate This amino acid derivative (calcium acetyl homotaurinate) has effects on both gamma-aminobutyric acid (GABA) and excitatory amino acid (i.e., glutamate) neurotransmission. Acamprosate appears to antagonize NMDA glutamate receptors (22,23), potentially restoring the balance between excitatory and inhibitory neurotransmission, which is dysregulated after chronic alcohol drinking. Specifically, acamprosate may modulate glutamate neurotransmission by affecting metabotropic-5 glutamate receptors (mGluR5) (22,23).

Results from human laboratory studies in healthy volunteers and alcohol-dependent individuals (23) showed no risk of liver toxicity and no interaction with alcohol. Acamprosate is not metabolized by the liver, rather it is excreted unchanged by the kidney. It is safe and well tolerated, with the most common adverse effects associated with its administration being diarrhea, nervousness, and fatigue.

A meta-analysis of the literature (47) that examined data from 17 published acamprosate clinical trials involving 4087 alcohol-dependent patients showed that continuous abstinence rates at 6 months were greater in acamprosate-treated patients (36.1%) than in those treated with placebo (23.4%) ($p < 0.001$). However, the effect size of acamprosate treatment has been shown to be small (0.14 for increasing the percentage of nonheavy drinking days and 0.23 for reducing the risk of relapse to heavy drinking) (43).

The majority of studies showing a therapeutic effect of acamprosate have been conducted in Europe, where this medication has been used for many years. In 2004, the FDA approved the use of acamprosate in the United States for the treatment of alcohol dependence, based on the evidence of the medication's efficacy provided by these studies. However, multicenter trials in the United States, Europe, and Australia have failed to detect beneficial effects of acamprosate compared with placebo in the treatment of alcohol dependence (22,23,44).

Discrepancies in the results of different studies have been attributed to differences in the use of standardized psychosocial interventions and in the severity of alcohol dependence, cognitive dysfunction, and psychological problems, as well as the prevalence of co-occurring drug abuse in most European studies compared with those conducted in the United States and Australia. Also, the small therapeutic effect of acamprosate can be difficult to detect in heterogeneous samples that are typically examined in multicenter studies.

Predictors of a favorable response to acamprosate among alcohol-dependent individuals appear to include greater levels of anxiety and physiologic dependence, a negative family history of alcoholism, a late age of alcoholism onset, and female sex. Although there is evidence suggesting that acamprosate is helpful in the treatment of alcohol dependence, effects of this compound in reducing alcohol consumption appear to be small and difficult to replicate in more recent clinical trials (47).

Serotonergic Medications Another group of medications that has been examined for the treatment of alcohol dependence are serotonergic compounds. In rodent models, pharmacologic manipulation of this system has consistently shown to influence alcohol consumption, with an inverse relationship between serotonergic activity and drinking behavior (21–23). In humans, however, evidence supporting beneficial effects of serotonergic compounds on drinking behavior is less consistent (22,23).

Although several investigators have reported that treatment with the selective serotonin reuptake inhibitor (SSRI) fluoxetine (at a dosage of 40–80 mg/day) or citalopram (at a dosage of 40 mg/day) reduced alcohol consumption among nondepressed alcoholics, subsequent placebo-controlled trials showed no overall advantage of these medications on drinking outcomes (22,23).

More recent trials described that treatment with sertraline reduced the frequency of drinking only among a subset of patients with lower vulnerability/later onset of alcoholism (Babor's type A alcoholics). In contrast, among high-risk/early-onset alcoholics (Babor's type B or Cloninger's type II alcoholics) treatment with fluoxetine or fluvoxamine appeared to be associated with greater rates of relapse (22,23).

Ondansetron, a 5-HT$_3$ antagonist, has been found to reduce drinking among alcoholics whose onset of problem drinking occurred before age 25 (23). In this regard, early-onset alcoholics treated with low-dose ondansetron (i.e., 1, 4, or 16 μg/kg/day) had significantly more abstinent days and significantly less alcohol consumption than a control group. Among alcoholics with a later onset of problem drinking, the effects of ondansetron on drinking did not differ from those of placebo (23).

In summary, the use of SSRIs to treat alcohol dependence requires that alcoholism risk/vulnerability and age of onset be considered in evaluating treatment effects. Beneficial effects of SSRIs appear to be limited to alcoholics with lower vulnerability/later onset of alcoholism. The beneficial effects of treatment with the 5-HT$_3$ antagonist ondansetron, on the other hand, appear to be greatest in early-onset alcoholics. Further research examining a matching strategy based on age at onset or subtype of alcoholism is needed before these compounds can be recommended for the treatment of alcohol dependence.

Baclofen Experiments in rodents and in humans have shown that the GABA$_B$ receptor agonist baclofen decreases voluntary alcohol consumption (21–23). Among alcoholics, open label and placebo-controlled studies have shown a therapeutic effect of baclofen (up to 30 mg/day), reducing craving and drinking and increasing abstinence rates from pretreatment levels (23,48). In one of these trials, 70% of the baclofen-treated patients remained abstinent, compared with 21.1% in the placebo group ($p < 0.005$). In addition, baclofen reduced anxiety symptoms and craving. In general, baclofen was well tolerated with no evidence of abuse liability (23,48). Reported side effects were mild and included nausea, vertigo, sleepiness, and abdominal pain (23,48). These findings suggest that baclofen is safe and potentially effective in treating alcohol-dependent patients. More studies with larger sample size and longer treatment duration are warranted.

Disulfiram For many years, alcohol-sensitizing medications (i.e., those that induce an unpleasant reaction when alcohol is consumed) such as disulfiram have been used in the clinic. Disulfiram (Antabuse) was the first medication and is the only alcohol-sensitizing medication approved in the United States for the treatment of alcoholism.

Disulfiram binds irreversibly to ALDHs, the enzymes that metabolize the alcohol metabolite acetaldehyde, increasing acetaldehyde concentrations when alcohol is consumed. The increased acetaldehyde concentration causes the aversive reaction known as the disulfiram-ethanol reaction (DER), which is characterized by flushing of the skin, nausea, vomiting, and headache. Disulfiram also inactivates other enzymes such as dopamine-beta-hydroxylase, an effect that has been linked to reduced rewarding effects of alcohol and cocaine among individuals addicted to both drugs.

Common side effects of disulfiram independent of its alcohol-sensitizing effects include drowsiness, lethargy, and fatigue. More serious (though rare) adverse effects are optic neuritis, peripheral neuropathy, hepatotoxicity, and when prescribed in large dosages, exacerbation of psychotic and depressive symptoms in patients with schizophrenia or mood disorders.

In the United States, disulfiram approved daily dosage is 250 mg orally. However, to achieve blood concentrations sufficient to elicit the DER, some patients may need a disulfiram dosage in excess of 1 g/day. The need for greater dosages in some patients may be explained by the fact that disulfiram undergoes extensive bioactivation before it is capable of inhibiting ALDH (22,23). At the dosage that is generally used in the clinic, a reduced bioactivation of disulfiram in some individuals may yield an inadequate concentration of the active metabolite.

There are few placebo-controlled studies of the efficacy of disulfiram for the treatment of alcohol dependence. In an early placebo-controlled study, disulfiram was prescribed concomitantly with stimulus control training, role playing, communication skills training, and recreational and vocational counseling. In this context, the medication was superior to placebo in reducing drinking (22,23). However, in a multicenter trial that involved more than 600 male alcoholic veterans randomly assigned to receive disulfiram 1 or 250 mg/day, or a placebo (22,23), there were no differences in abstinence rates among treatment groups. However, patients who showed good adherence to the treatment were more likely to remain abstinent during the 1-year treatment period. Also, among patients who resumed drinking, those in the group receiving 250 mg of disulfiram had significantly fewer drinking days than patients in either of the other two groups. When disulfiram treatment was supervised to enhance adherence during outpatient alcohol treatment, patients receiving disulfiram had more abstinent days and consumed fewer drinks on drinking days than those taking placebo. These findings support the contention that supervised adherence is an important element in the successful use of disulfiram (22,23). Due to the limited evidence of the efficacy of disulfiram for the prevention of alcoholic relapse, this medication is not recommended as a first-line treatment for alcohol dependence and should be prescribed only to patients who have not responded to other pharmacologic treatments and/or to patients in whom treatment adherence can be supervised.

Patients who are prescribed disulfiram should be warned to avoid over-the-counter preparations and food preparations that contain alcohol and medications that may interact with disulfiram. Given that substantial efforts are generally necessary to assure adherence with disulfiram treatment, this medication should be prescribed only to patients participating in treatment programs or by practitioners who make a systematic effort to enhance medication adherence.

Pharmacotherapy of Psychiatric Comorbidity in Alcoholics

Clinically significant anxiety, depression, insomnia, and general distress induced by chronic alcohol consumption are common complaints among alcohol-dependent patients after detoxification. Frequently, these symptoms represent a diagnostic challenge since they are usually indistinguishable from psychiatric disorders with onset prior to the initiation of heavy drinking. Regardless of the cause, when untreated, these problems can increase the likelihood of relapse in alcoholic patients, whereas attempts to relieve emotional symptoms can translate into reduced drinking.

Pharmacotherapy of Depressed Alcoholics During the early phases of alcohol withdrawal, depressive symptoms are common; however, they tend to improve spontaneously with sustained sobriety. However, for depressive symptoms that last longer than the acute withdrawal period (which for practical purposes might best be considered 2 to 4 weeks), antidepressant treatment may be beneficial (49).

Nunes and Levin (50) reviewed data from 15 published clinical trials that examined antidepressant treatment of depressed patients with alcohol and/or other substance use disorders. Nine studies showed a moderate beneficial effect of antidepressants and six studies showed no evidence of efficacy. In the studies in which antidepressant treatment was effective in improving mood, there were reductions in alcohol and drug use. However, abstinence rates were low even in the studies in which a robust antidepressant response was seen. Seven of these clinical trials examined the effects of the selective serotonin reuptake inhibitors (SSRIs) fluoxetine and sertraline, among alcoholics with a major depression diagnosis. In these studies, patients who received the active medication generally showed a greater reduction in depressive symptoms than those receiving placebo. However, treatment with SSRIs appeared to be less effective than treatment with a tricyclic or other antidepressant such as nefazodone. Despite this, due to their favorable safety and side effect profile and lack of interactions with alcohol, SSRIs are considered the first-line antidepressant treatment among alcoholics. In summary, although it is believed that most cases of alcohol-induced depression spontaneously remit with abstinence, a significant proportion of patients continue to experience severe and persistent depression. Given the favorable safety profile of SSRIs, particularly in relation to risk of suicide by medication overdose, use of these compounds is preferable to the use of tricyclic antidepressants.

Pharmacotherapy of Anxious Alcoholics Due to the potential of benzodiazepines to produce dependence and additive CNS depressant effects when ingested concurrently with alcohol, the use of these and other brain depressants in alcoholics is probably best limited to the detoxification phase of treatment.

Buspirone, a nonbenzodiazepine anxiolytic without sedative effects or abuse potential that does not interact with alcohol, has shown to be effective in the treatment of anxious alcoholics. Although no effects on drinking were reported, initial placebo-controlled clinical trials reported greater retention in treatment and greater reductions in alcohol craving, depression, and anxiety measures among alcoholics treated with buspirone (49,51). Subsequent studies described that irrespective of a specific anxiety disorder diagnosis, a greater severity of pretreatment anxiety symptoms predicted a greater response to treatment with buspirone (49,51). Interestingly in these studies, buspirone treatment was also associated with a longer retention in treatment and longer time to relapse to heavy drinking.

In reports that failed to find differences in anxiety or alcohol consumption between buspirone-treated patients and those treated with placebo, lack of patient involvement in a psychosocial intervention program and greater severity of alcoholism appeared to explain the lack of buspirone effects (49,51).

In summary, buspirone treatment appears to be useful in the treatment of anxious alcoholics in the context of appropriate psychosocial interventions.

COMORBIDITIES AND COMPLICATIONS OF ALCOHOL CONSUMPTION

Alcoholism Comorbidity with Other Psychiatric Disorders

Community and clinical epidemiology studies suggest that in comparison to nonalcoholics, individuals diagnosed with an alcohol use disorder have a greater likelihood of having a mental health problem. Conversely, patients suffering from certain mental illnesses are more likely to experience alcohol abuse or dependence. Antisocial personality disorder, mood disorders, anxiety disorders, and another substance use disorder are the most commonly comorbid psychiatric problems in alcoholics.

Recent data from a large representative community survey examining comorbidity of past-year prevalence of alcohol use disorders and other mental health problems have been provided by the National Epidemiological Survey on Alcohol and Related Conditions (NESARC), survey that examined 43,093 household respondents residing in the United States, including Alaska and Hawaii using the DSM-IV diagnostic criteria (15,52–54).

The NESARC survey showed that among those in the community diagnosed with a current alcohol use problem, one third experienced at least another axis I disorder. This prevalence rate is two times greater than the prevalence rate of psychiatric problems observed among nonalcoholic respondents. The NESARC survey also described that in comparison to those with no diagnosis of a mental illness, those with a psychiatric diagnosis had a three times greater risk of experiencing an alcohol use disorder.

Comorbidity with Other Substance Use Disorders

NESARC described that 13.05% of persons diagnosed with an alcohol use disorder experienced a drug use disorder (OR = 9.0), whereas among persons diagnosed with drug abuse or dependence more than half (55.2%) were diagnosed with an alcohol use problem. Individuals with cocaine dependence appeared to be at the greatest risk for this comorbidity (OR = 43.0), with 89.4% of them also experiencing an alcohol use disorder. Similarly, persons who were diagnosed with hallucinogens, amphetamines, opioid, cannabis, tranquilizers, or a sedative use disorder had a greater increase in the risk for alcohol problems (52).

NESARC also described that more than half of the persons with an alcohol use disorder (58.2%) use tobacco, a rate two times higher than the prevalence observed for the use of this substance in the community. Additionally, patients with a diagnosis of alcohol abuse or dependence were more frequently found to be heavy smokers (53).

Comorbidity with Mood Disorders

In NESARC, mood disorders were diagnosed in 18.9% of alcoholics (OR = 2.6). Conversely, among individuals diagnosed with a mood disorder, 17.3% also experienced an alcohol problem. Individuals diagnosed with a mania or hypomania had the greatest risk (OR = 3.5%), with 24.0% diagnosed with a comorbid alcohol use disorder. Other mood disorders such as major depression were relatively common among alcoholics (13.7%) and were significantly associated with drinking problems (OR = 2.3) (54).

Comorbidity with Anxiety Disorders

The NESARC showed that 17.1% of persons diagnosed with alcohol abuse or dependence experienced an anxiety disorder (OR = 1.7) while in those diagnosed with an anxiety disorder, 13.0% had an alcohol use disorder. In NESARC, panic disorder with agoraphobia was the anxiety disorder with the strongest association with alcoholism (OR = 2.5), followed by generalized anxiety (OR = 1.9) and social phobia (OR = 1.7) (54).

Comorbidity with Antisocial Personality Disorder (ASPD)

The NESARC also showed that 12.3% of individuals with an alcohol use disorder met criteria for ASPD (OR = 4.8), whereas 28.7% of persons diagnosed with ASPD also had alcohol abuse or dependence (15). It is important to mention that the strong association observed between these two disorders may reflect in part substantial overlap in diagnostic criteria since antisocial behavior may be caused by alcohol intoxication.

Psychiatric Complications of Alcohol Use

Alcohol Intoxication

This condition is characterized by behavioral disturbances such as aggression or inappropriate sexual behavior, or psychological changes such as labile mood and impaired judgment that begin shortly after heavy drinking. Other clinical signs suggestive of alcohol intoxication include slurred speech, lack of coordination, unsteady gait, nystagmus, impairment of attention and memory, and in the most severe cases, stupor and coma. After large amounts of alcohol have been ingested, severe disturbances in consciousness and cognition can occur. This is known as alcohol intoxication delirium, a problem that generally subsides after blood alcohol concentrations decline. During the assessment of patients presumed to be intoxicated with alcohol, the clinician must rule out general medical conditions or other substance use or psychiatric disorders.

Alcohol Withdrawal

Among alcohol-dependent individuals, alcohol withdrawal occurs following a substantial reduction in drinking (among individuals who have severe physical dependence) or the abrupt cessation of alcohol consumption (in the majority of physically dependent individuals). Uncomplicated alcohol withdrawal is characterized by signs and symptoms of autonomic hyperactivity including increased heart rate, diaphoresis, tremor, nausea, vomiting, insomnia, and anxiety. The symptoms of alcohol withdrawal generally begin 4 to 12 hours after the last drink, and symptom severity generally reaches its peak after 48 hours, subsiding after 4 to 5 days of sobriety. Less severe anxiety, insomnia, and autonomic hyperactivity may last for a few weeks, though in some cases they can persist for up to 6 months in what is known as protracted alcohol withdrawal.

Approximately 10% of alcohol-dependent patients can experience episodes of alcohol withdrawal complicated by delirium and/or grand mal seizures. Alcohol withdrawal delirium, also known as *delirium tremens,* is seen in approximately 5% of the cases. This condition is characterized by severe signs of autonomic hyperactivity accompanied by a fluctuating level of consciousness and disorientation generally occurring 36 to 72 hours after the last drink. During alcohol withdrawal, patients can also experience vivid illusions and hallucinations of an auditory, visual, or tactile nature, which can also occur in a clear sensorium. Alcohol withdrawal seizures occur in approximately 3% to 5% of cases, generally within the first 48 hours after drinking cessation. A failure or delay in instituting treatment in patients with complicated alcohol withdrawal is associated with an elevated mortality risk. Predictors of complicated alcohol withdrawal include older age, poor nutritional status, co-occurring medical or surgical conditions, a history of high tolerance to alcohol, and a history of previous episodes of delirium tremens and/or alcohol withdrawal seizures.

Alcohol-Induced Cognitive Disorders

Chronic heavy alcohol drinking can result in severe folate and thiamine deficiency leading to severe neurocognitive problems such as Wernicke encephalopathy, which is characterized by confusion and disorientation, ataxia, nystagmus, and gaze palsies. Generally, this disorder responds promptly to thiamine repletion and sustained sobriety; however, if heavy drinking persists, repeated episodes of Wernicke encephalopathy can lead to a persistent alcohol-induced amnestic disorder known as Korsakoff psychosis. Although not a true psychotic disorder, a prominent characteristic of this condition is confabulation that stems from profound deficits in anterograde and retrograde memory that prevent the retention of previously learned information and/or the acquisition of new information. Despite a profound disorientation to time and place, Korsakoff's patients are unaware of their deficits.

With sobriety, improvement in the cognitive impairments usually occurs in 20% of cases of Korsakoff syndrome. However, memory deficits may remain unchanged or can be exacerbated by continued heavy drinking, resulting in an alcohol-induced persisting dementia. In addition to memory impairment, this complication is characterized by apraxia, agnosia, and disturbances in executive functioning. In addition to heavy drinking, a history of head trauma is frequently seen among individuals with this condition. Repeated episodes of Wernicke encephalopathy may also result in alcohol-induced persisting dementia. Typical neurologic findings in this condition include atrophy of the frontal lobes and increased ventricular size. As with patients with Korsakoff psychosis, continuous drinking exacerbates the dementia, whereas sobriety may improve the deficits.

Alcohol-Induced Mood and Anxiety Disorders

Chronic heavy alcohol drinking can also result in mood and/or anxiety disorders, characterized by depressed mood and anhedonia, elevated, expansive, and/or irritable affect or in the case of anxiety symptoms, indistinguishable from a primary generalized anxiety, panic, or a phobic disorder. Mood and anxiety disturbances are common, affecting up to 90% of alcoholic patients entering treatment. Alcohol-induced mood and anxiety disorders can occur during alcohol intoxication or episodes of alcohol withdrawal, and may be indistinguishable from a primary mood or anxiety disorder. Typically, the severity and duration of alcohol-induced mood and anxiety symptoms are greater than the symptoms usually attributable to alcohol withdrawal (e.g., dysphoria, insomnia, and lack of energy). However, alcohol-induced mood and anxiety symptoms generally subside fully within 2 to 4 weeks following alcohol cessation.

In the assessment of these conditions, the clinician should seek evidence that the mood or anxiety disturbances are not better explained by a primary mood or anxiety disorder. Such evidence includes the initiation of mood or anxiety symptoms before the onset of alcoholism and the persistence of symptoms during extended periods of sobriety. Given that suicide is highly prevalent among depressed and anxious alcoholics, clinicians should closely monitor the patient for emerging suicidal thoughts and/or behaviors.

Alcohol-Induced Psychotic Disorder

Hallucinations or delusions induced by chronic heavy alcohol consumption generally occur within 30 days of alcohol intoxication or a withdrawal episode. Although alcohol-induced psychosis can occur during or shortly after an episode of alcohol intoxication or delirium, hallucinations and/or delusions do not occur exclusively during the course of these conditions. However, alcohol-induced psychotic symptoms tend to subside within a few weeks of abstinence.

During the mental status exam, the patient experiencing this condition is fully alert and oriented, unaware that the symptoms are alcohol related. Evidence supporting a diagnosis of an alcohol-induced psychotic disorder include an atypical or a late age at onset of psychotic symptoms, heavy drinking preceding the onset of delusions and/or hallucinations, and improvement in the psychotic symptoms during extended periods of sobriety.

Alcohol-Induced Sleep Disorder

Heavy drinking commonly produces disturbances of sleep architecture. Acute alcohol intoxication is associated with an increase in the density of nonrapid eye movement (NREM) sleep and a reduction in the density of rapid eye movement (REM) sleep. However, chronic heavy drinking results in a reduction in NREM sleep and a rebound in REM sleep density. These effects are clinically reflected by increased wakefulness, restless sleep, and vivid dreams, or nightmares. Alcohol withdrawal is also characterized by sleep fragmentation and an increase in REM sleep. Even after months or years of sobriety, some patients can continue to experience fragmented and unsatisfying sleep. However, generally speaking, sleep tends to improve during periods of sustained sobriety. An alcohol-induced sleep disorder is characterized by an initiation of drinking before the onset of the sleep disturbance. Although sleep problems can occur during alcohol intoxication or alcohol withdrawal, alcohol-induced sleep disorder has a longer duration and a greater severity than that typically seen during these conditions. Persistence of sleep disturbances for more than 4 weeks and/or a history of a previous sleep problem are highly suggestive of a primary sleep disorder.

Finally, it is important to notice that heavy alcohol consumption can also exacerbate other psychiatric disorders that present with sleep disturbances such as mood or anxiety disorders, or other sleep problems such as narcolepsy or breathing-related sleep disorders.

Morbidity and Mortality Associated with Alcohol Use

The World Health Organization (6) has identified heavy drinking as an important risk to global health. In 2002, 2.3 million deaths (3.7% of global mortality) were attributable to alcohol. Although there is evidence that nonhazardous drinking (which according to the National Institute on Alcohol Abuse and Alcoholism consists of ≤1 drink/day for women and ≤2 drinks/day for men) protects against cardiovascular disease, this effect appears to be confined to men 45 years old or older and postmenopausal women. Conversely, greater levels of drinking have been shown to increase mortality risk due to cardiovascular disease and other health problems. In this regard, the number of years of life lost due to drinking appears to outweigh saved years attributed to the protective effects of moderate alcohol consumption.

After accounting for its health protective effects and without considering other adverse consequences it was estimated that alcohol drinking accounts for 4.4% of the global burden of disease. Alcohol drinking is known to be associated with more than 60 health problems, most frequently alcoholic liver disease, cancer of the upper gastrointestinal track, breast cancer, fetal alcohol syndrome, immunologic impairments resulting in increased incidence of infectious diseases, seizures, and neuropsychiatric disorders.

In the United States, excessive drinking is the third leading preventable cause of death (55). In 2001, an estimated 75,766 deaths and 2.3 million years of potential life lost were attributable to the harmful effects of excessive alcohol consumption. Of the alcohol-attributable deaths, 46% resulted from chronic complications such as alcoholic liver cirrhosis and pancreatitis, whereas 54% resulted from acute complications such as injury from motor vehicle crashes and violence (55). Overall, 72% of all alcohol-attributable deaths involved men, with 75% of these involving men aged ≥35 years. Despite the fact that the frequency of fatal car accidents related to alcohol intoxication has declined during recent years, alcohol intoxication is still a common risk factor for motor vehicle related injuries. Also, alcohol intoxication is associated with other risky behaviors and their adverse effects, as well as to deaths attributable to suicide and homicide.

In addition to medical morbidity and mortality, heavy drinking also contributes to financial, social, and family problems. Reduced productivity and unemployment, increased criminality, and increased health care cost are highly prevalent problems related to heavy drinking. It was estimated that globally, the cost of heavy drinking amounted to more than 1% of the gross national product in high-income and middle-income countries, with the cost of social harm constituting the major proportion, exceeding those related to health care (55).

In the United States, the cost of alcohol-related problems, including hospitalization and institutionalization, motor vehicle crashes, and crime more than tripled during the past two decades, going from $70.3 billion in 1985 to an estimated $220 billion in 2005. In 2005, this cost was greater than that associated with other health problems such as obesity ($133 billion) and cancer ($196 billion).

REFERENCES

1. Lucia SP. *A History of Wine as Therapy*. Philadelphia, PA: Lippincott; 1963.
2. Blue AD. *The Complete Book of Spirits: A Guide to Their History, Production, and Enjoyment*. New York, NY: HarperCollins Publishers; 2004.
3. Babor T. *Alcohol: Customs and Rituals*. New York, NY: Chelsea House; 1986.
4. Coyhis DL, White WL. *Alcohol Problems in Native America: The Untold Story of the Resistance and Recovery—The Truth about the Lie*. Colorado Springs, CO: White Bison; 2006.
5. Meyer RE. Overview of the concept of alcoholism. In: Rose RM, Barret JE, eds. *Alcoholism: Origins and Outcome*. New York, NY: Raven Press; 1987:1–13.
6. Rehm J, Room R, Monteiro M, et al. Alcohol. In: Ezzati M, Lopez AD, Rodgers A, et al., eds. *Comparative Quantification of Health Risk: Global and Regional Burden of Disease due to Selected Major Risk Factors*. Geneva: World Health Organization; 2004:959–1108.
7. Anderson P. Global use of alcohol, drugs and tobacco. *Drug Alcohol Rev*. 2006;25(6):489–502.
8. Bloomfield K, Stockwell T, Gmel G, et al. International comparisons of alcohol consumption. *Alcohol Res Health*. 2003;27:95–109.
9. *National Household Survey on Drug Use and Health, Office of Applied Studies, Substance Abuse and Mental Health Services Administration*. Rockville, MD: Unites States Department of Health and Human Services; 2008.
10. Grant BF, Dawson DA, Stinson FS, et al. The 12-month prevalence and trends in DSM-IV alcohol abuse and dependence: United States, 1991–1992 and 2001–2002. *Drug Alcohol Depend*. 2004;74:223–234.
11. American Psychiatric Association. *Diagnostic and Statistical Manual of Mental Disorders* DSM-IV-TR (Text Revision). Washington, DC: American Psychiatric Association; 2000.
12. Hasin D. Classification of alcohol use disorders. *Alcohol Res Health*. 2003;27:5–17.
13. Grant BF, Stinson FS, Harford TC. Age at onset of alcohol use and DSM-IV alcohol abuse and dependence: a 12-year follow-up. *J Subst Abuse*. 2001;13:493–504.
14. Grant BF, Stinson FS, Dawson DA, et al. Prevalence and co-occurrence of substance use disorders and independent mood and anxiety disorders: results from the National Epidemiologic Survey on Alcohol and Related Conditions. *Arch Gen Psychiatry*. 2004;61:807–816.
15. Grant BF, Stinson FS, Dawson DA, et al. Co-occurrence of 12-month alcohol and drug use disorders and personality disorders in the United States: results from the National Epidemiologic Survey on Alcohol and Related Conditions. *Arch Gen Psychiatry*. 2004;61:361–368.
16. Cloninger CR, Bohman M, Sigvardsson S. Inheritance of alcohol abuse. Cross-fostering analysis of adopted men. *Arch Gen Psychiatry*. 1981;38:861–868.
17. Hesselbrock VM, Hesselbrock MN. Are there empirically supported and clinically useful subtypes of alcohol dependence? *Addiction*. 2006;101(S1): 97–103.
18. Babor TF, Hofmann M, DelBoca FK, et al. Types of alcoholics, I. Evidence for an empirically derived typology based on indicators of vulnerability and severity. *Arch Gen Psychiatry*. 1992;49: 599–608.
19. Norberg A, Jones AW, Hahn RG, et al. Role of variability in explaining ethanol pharmacokinetics: research and forensic applications. *Clin Pharmacokinet*. 2003;42:1–31.
20. Edenberg HJ. The genetics of alcohol metabolism: role of alcohol dehydrogenase and aldehyde dehydrogenase variants. *Alcohol Res Health*. 2007;30: 5–13.
21. Vengeliene V, Bilbao A, Molander A, et al. Neuropharmacology of alcohol addiction. *Br J Pharmacol*. 2008;154:299–315.
22. Ross S, Peselow E. Pharmacotherapy of Addictive Disorders. *Clin Neuropharmacol*. 2009;32:277–289.
23. Johnson BA. Update on neuropharmacological treatments for alcoholism: scientific basis and clinical findings. *Biochem Pharmacol*. 2008;75:34–56.
24. Gianoulakis C, de Waele JP, Thavundayil J. Implication of the endogenous opioid system in excessive ethanol consumption. *Alcohol*. 1996;13:19–23.
25. Gelernter J, Kranzler HR. Genetics of alcohol dependence. *Hum Genet*. 2009;126:91–99.
26. Feinn R, Nellissery M, Kranzler HR. Meta-analysis of the association of a functional serotonin transporter promoter polymorphism and alcohol dependence. *Am J Med Genet B Neuropsychiatr Genet*. 2005;133B:79–84.
27. Arias A, Feinn R, Kranzler HR. Association of an Asn40Asp (A118G) polymorphism in the μ-opioid receptor gene with substance dependence: a meta-analysis. *Drug Alcohol Depend*. 2006;83:262–268.
28. McCambridge J, Day M. Randomized controlled trial of the effects of completing the Alcohol Use Disorders Identification Test

questionnaire on self-reported hazardous drinking. *Addiction.* 2008;103:241–248.
29. Dhalla S, Kopec JA. The CAGE questionnaire for alcohol misuse: a review of reliability and validity studies. *Clin Invest Med.* 2007;30:33–41.
30. Reinert DF, Allen JP. The alcohol use disorders identification test: an update of research findings. *Alcohol Clin Exp Res.* 2007;31: 185–199.
31. Das SK, Dhanya L, Vasudevan DM. Biomarkers of alcoholism: an updated review. *Scand J Clin Lab Invest.* 2008;68:81–92.
32. Kaner E, Beyer F, Dickinson H, et al. Effectiveness of brief alcohol interventions in primary care populations. *Cochrane Database Syst Rev.* 2007;2:CD004148. DOI:004110.001002/14651858. CD14654148.
33. Rychtarik RG, Connors GJ, Whitney RB, et al. Treatment settings for persons with alcoholism: evidence for matching clients to inpatient versus outpatient care. *J Consult Clin Psychol.* 2000;68: 277–289.
34. Ntais C, Pakos E, Kyzas P, et al. Benzodiazepines for alcohol withdrawal. *Cochrane Database Syst Rev.* 2005;3:CD005063.
35. Ait-Daoud N, Malcolm Jr RJ, Johnson BA. An overview of medications for the treatment of alcohol withdrawal and alcohol dependence with an emphasis on the use of older and newer anticonvulsants. *Addict Behav.* 2006;31:1628–1649.
36. McCaul ME, Petry NM. The role of psychosocial treatments in pharmacotherapy for alcoholism. *Am J Addict.* 2003;12(S1): 41–52.
37. Tonigan JS, Connors GJ, Miller WR. Participation and involvement in alcoholics anonymous. In: Babor TF, DelBoca FK, eds. *Matching Alcoholism Treatments to Client Heterogeneity: The Results of Project MATCH.* New York, NY: Cambridge University Press; 2003:184–204.
38. Moos RH, Moos BS. Participation in treatment and alcoholics anonymous: a 16-year follow-up of initially untreated individuals. *J Clin Psychol.* 2006;62:735–750.
39. McKellar J, Stewart E, Humphreys K. Alcoholics anonymous involvement and positive alcohol-related outcomes: cause, consequence, or just a correlate? A prospective 2-year study of 2,319 alcohol-dependent men. *J Consult Clin Psychol.* 2003;71:302–308.
40. Powers MB, Vedel E, Emmelkamp PM. Behavioral couples therapy (BCT) for alcohol and drug use disorders: a meta-analysis. *Clin Psychol Rev.* 2008;28:952–962.
41. Bouza C, Angeles M, Muñoz A, et al. Efficacy and safety of naltrexone and acamprosate in the treatment of alcohol dependence: a systematic review. *Addiction.* 2004;99:811–828.
42. Srisurapanont M, Jarusuraisin N. Opioid antagonists for alcohol dependence. *Cochrane Database Syst Rev.* 2005;25:CD001867.
43. Kranzler HR, Van Kirk J. Efficacy of naltrexone and acamprosate for alcoholism treatment: a meta-analysis. *Alcohol Clin Exp Res.* 2001;25:1335–1341.
44. Anton RF, O'Malley SS, Ciraulo DA, et al. COMBINE Study Research Group. Combined pharmacotherapies and behavioral interventions for alcohol dependence: the COMBINE study: a randomized controlled trial. *JAMA.* 2006;295:2003–2017.
45. Garbutt JC, Kranzler HR, O'Malley SS, et al. Ehrich EW for the Vivitrex® Study Group. Efficacy and tolerability of long-acting injectable naltrexone for alcohol dependence. *JAMA.* 2005;293: 1617–1625.
46. Johnson BA, Rosenthal N, Capece JA, et al. Topiramate for Alcoholism Advisory Board; Topiramate for Alcoholism Study Group. Topiramate for treating alcohol dependence: a randomized controlled trial. *JAMA.* 2007;298:1641–1651.
47. Mann K, Lehert P, Morgan MY. The efficacy of acamprosate in the maintenance of abstinence in alcohol-dependent individuals: results of a meta-analysis. *Alcohol Clin Exp Res.* 2004;28: 51–63.
48. Addolorato G, Leggio L, Ferrulli A, et al. Effectiveness and safety of baclofen for maintenance of alcohol abstinence in alcohol-dependent patients with liver cirrhosis: randomised, double-blind controlled study. *Lancet.* 2007;370:1915–1922.
49. Kranzler HR, Rosenthal RN. Dual diagnosis: alcoholism and comorbid psychiatric disorders. *Am J Addict.* 2003;12(S1):26–40.
50. Nunes EV, Levin FR. Treatment of depression in patients with alcohol or other drug dependence: a meta-analysis. *JAMA.* 2004;291:1887–1896.
51. Tiet QQ, Mausbach B. Treatments for patients with dual diagnosis: a review. *Alcohol Clin Exp Res.* 2007;31:513–536.
52. Stinson FS, Grant BF, Dawson DA, et al. Comorbidity between DSM-IV alcohol and specific drug use disorders in the United States: results from the National Epidemiologic Survey on Alcohol and Related Conditions. *Drug Alcohol Depend.* 2005;80:105–116.
53. Falk DE, Yi H, Hiller-Sturmhöfel S. An epidemiologic analysis of Co-occurring alcohol and tobacco use and disorders: findings from the national epidemiologic survey on alcohol and related conditions. *Alcohol Research & Health.* 2006;29:162–171.
54. Centers for Disease Control and Prevention. Alcohol-Attributable Deaths and Years of Potential Life Lost—United States, 2001. *MMWR Morb Mortal Wkly Rep.* 2004;53:866–870.
55. Rehm J, Mathers C, Popova S, et al. Global burden of disease and injury and economic cost attributable to alcohol use and alcohol-use disorders. *Lancet.* 2009;373:2223–2233.

CHAPTER 13 Opioids

David H. Epstein ■ Karran A. Phillips ■ Kenzie L. Preston

INTRODUCTION

Terminology: Opioids and Opiates

The term *opiates* refers to two of the psychoactive alkaloids (morphine and codeine) that occur in opium and to the many similarly psychoactive compounds that can be derived from them (such as heroin and oxycodone) (1). *Opioid* is a superset of *opiates*: it additionally includes fully synthetic compounds (such as methadone and fentanyl) and endogenous compounds (such as endorphins, enkephalins, and dynorphins) that share the actions and effects of opiates (1).

Classification of Opioids through Their Actions at Receptors

Decades of behavioral research led to what might be called the classic view of the opioid analgesics, expressed here by the director of the Addiction Research Center (ARC) in 1963: "All strong analgesics clinically employed are essentially morphine-like, differing only from morphine in such characteristics as rate of onset and duration of action, routes by which they can be administered, potency, analgesic ceiling, and side effects" (2). Although this statement almost certainly needs qualification, it remains difficult to say along what lines one should split the opioids it lumps together. The classification described above—natural opi*ates*, semisynthetic opi*ates*, and fully synthetic opi*oids*—is commonly encountered in textbooks, but is rarely useful. Opioids can be also classified as "long-acting" or "short-acting"; this distinction can be useful for prescribers choosing an opioid for a specific indication, although many of the available prescription opioids have fairly similar durations of analgesic action (typically 4 to 6 hours, despite differences in plasma half-life) (1).

A more "carved at the joints" classification of opioids is likely to emerge from increased understanding of their actions at receptors. The four known types of opioid receptor are mu, delta, kappa, and nociceptin/orphanin FQ peptide (NOP) receptors. Each type is G protein coupled, and although each has been suggested to have further subtypes, such variation seems to reflect posttranslational modifications (3). There are at least 20 endogenous opioid ligands, most with preferential but promiscuous affinities for receptor types (4).

Mu receptors are preferentially activated by beta-endorphin (3) and are largely responsible for the constellation of effects classically associated with morphine-like drugs: analgesia, euphoria, cough suppression, respiratory suppression, pupillary constriction, and (via receptors in the gut) constipation. Studies of mu-knockout mice suggest that mu receptors are necessary for morphine-induced analgesia and for development of tolerance to morphine (5,6).

Delta receptors are preferentially activated by enkephalins (3). Delta agonists are self-administered by laboratory animals and produce conditioned place preference (4), but the extent to which this represents delta activity is unclear: seemingly selective delta agonists have turned out to be less selective than initially thought when tested in delta-knockout mice (3). Delta agonists do produce effects distinct from those of mu agonists; in laboratory animals, these include anxiolytic and antidepressant-like effects, along with proconvulsant effects (7) and only limited efficacy for analgesia (8) (though a recently developed selective delta agonist appears to be highly efficacious in rodent models of allodynia (9)). Mu but not delta antagonists produce conditioned place aversions (4), suggesting that some basal level of mu but not delta activation modulates hedonic tone. However, chronic antagonism of delta receptors reduces self-administration of mu agonists such as morphine (without reducing analgesia) (4); this and other findings suggest that delta receptors contribute to the abuse liability of opioids (10,11). This contribution may be mediated by the ability of delta receptors to dimerize or oligomerize with mu receptors—that is, to link together into complexes of two or more receptors—and such dimers or oligomers may also play important roles in tolerance and withdrawal (4,8). The clinical implication is that delta ligands might help prevent tolerance to and abuse of mu agonists without reducing their analgesic efficacy; the ligands could be delta antagonists (such as naltrindole) or bivalent ligands (which have two binding sites and a connecting spacer so that they bind specifically to dimers) (4,11–13).

Kappa receptors are preferentially activated by dynorphin A (14). Kappa agonists, such as pentazocine, cyclazocine, and salvinorin A, are not self-administered by laboratory animals; the agonists produce analgesia, but also produce a distinct profile of other effects, most notably "prodepressant" and aversive effects (15) that presumably correspond to what human users experience as dysphoria and psychotomimesis (16). (Another signature effect of kappa agonists is micturition (17).) The aversive effects of kappa agonism may be at least partly mediated by reduction of dopamine release in the nucleus accumbens. This action might make kappa agonists clinically useful as "antagonists" of abused psychostimulants (15), or it might make kappa antagonists clinically useful to counteract the dysphoria associated with cocaine withdrawal (18). One commonly used opioid with kappa-antagonist properties is buprenorphine, though its effectiveness against cocaine use disorders is still debated (19,20). Finally, like delta receptors, kappa receptors can dimerize with other opioid receptors, and the dimers can be targeted with bivalent ligands (21).

NOP receptors (also called opioid receptor like-1 [ORL-1] receptors) are preferentially activated by nociceptin (also called orphanin FQ) (22). They are considered part of the family of opioid receptors due to structural similarities, but they appear to represent a separate branch of the family, in terms of both their pharmacology and their effects when activated. For example, in rodents, NOP agonists induce *hyperalgesia* when administered intracerebroventricularly (22), block expression of cocaine-conditioned place preference (23), and prevent behavioral sensitization to cocaine (24). NOP receptors have little or no affinity for most of the prototypical endogenous opioids (endorphins, enkephalins, and dynorphins), analgesic opioids, or the prototypical antagonist naloxone (3). One seeming exception is buprenorphine, whose partial agonism at NOP receptors may account for some of its effects at high doses, such as inhibition of ethanol drinking in rats (25). However, some investigators have been unable to confirm that buprenorphine activates NOP receptors with adequate selectiveness or efficacy to support that idea (26).

Thus, the three receptor types most relevant to a classification of abused or prescribed opioids are mu, delta, and kappa. But classification in these terms is often not straightforward: a given opioid can interact with all three types of receptors and be an agonist, partial agonist, or antagonist at each (1). This complexity is reflected in the term *mixed agonist–antagonist*, which has sometimes been used interchangeably with *partial agonist*, but now typically describes a drug that is an agonist or partial agonist at one type of receptor while being an antagonist at another type.

The existence of multiple types of opioid receptors was predicted long before the tools of molecular biology were available, based both on knowledge of the structures of opioids (27) and on behavioral data (28). Nonetheless, human laboratory studies had supported the classic view cited at the beginning of this chapter, in which mu-preferring analgesics were lumped into a single category. For example, when heroin and morphine were administered intravenously to experienced users in a double-blind fashion, the users could identify no clear qualitative differences between the two drugs—though they could discriminate between them, a finding attributed to peripheral effects such as the "pins and needles" feeling that accompanied morphine injection (29). Common wisdom was that heroin, morphine, and the mu-preferring synthetic analgesics all exerted the same pharmacodynamic effects (primarily mu agonism, with some contribution of delta agonism later recognized) once they reached the brain.

This view leaves some clinical observations unaccounted for. For example, ostensibly similar prescription opioids do not produce complete cross-tolerance (30); in fact, practitioners treating chronic pain often rely on "opioid rotation," switching one opioid to an equianalgesic dose of another to prevent or counteract the development of tolerance (31,32). (It seems, however, that the effectiveness of this practice has been tested only in open-label trials.) Anecdotally, clinicians sometimes find that a patient's pain responds to only one of two similar opioids (such as oxycodone and hydrocodone) at presumably equianalgesic doses (Pasternak, personal communication, March 31, 2009). These observations could be explained by genetic variations in metabolism (as described below in the section "Differences among Users.") or by several aspects of opioid-receptor function that are only beginning to be fully appreciated.

One such aspect is the existence of splice variants, which has been shown in mice, rats, and humans. For example, the classic mu receptor, transcribed from exons 1–4 of the 16-exon MOR-1 gene, coexists in the human brain with at least 10 alternatively spliced mu receptors; different opioids bind with equal affinity across these variants, but each opioid's potency and efficacy at a given variant are uncorrelated with its affinity and with each other (33). In mice, disruption of exon 1 blocks the analgesic effect of morphine, but not the analgesic effect of heroin or the morphine metabolite M6G (30); disruption of exon 11 blocks the analgesic effect of heroin, M6G, and fentanyl, but not the analgesic effect of morphine or methadone (34). Thus, splice variants of the mu receptor appear to respond preferentially to morphine and methadone on the one hand versus fentanyl, M6G, and heroin (presumably acting through its active metabolite 6-acetylmorphine) on the other. In both rats and mice, these splice variants are differentially distributed in specific brain regions (30), perhaps helping to account for subtle differences in the effects of analgesic opioids. Genetic differences in expression of splice variants could help account for idiosyncratic responses to specific opioids.

Another recently appreciated aspect of opioid-receptor function is that ligands can display functional selectivity—that is, they can induce different responses at the same receptor (35). For example, mu agonists differ in the degree to which they induce responses associated with development or avoidance of tolerance, such as phosphorylation (which desensitizes mu receptors) and internalization (which protects mu receptors from desensitization, prevents compensatory superactivation of the cAMP second-messenger system, and is typically followed by receptor relocation to the cell surface (36)). In rat-brain slices, mu receptors are desensitized by morphine, methadone, M6G, DAMGO, fentanyl, etorphine, and [Met]^{5}enkephalin, but, unexpectedly, not by oxycodone (37). Differences among splice variants come into play here as well: the splice variant mMOR-1C is internalized by morphine, but the splice variant mMOR-1 is not (38).

All of these findings suggest that the classification of opioids is in transition between the classic "lumping" (especially of the mu-preferring agonists) and a new "splitting" whose exact contours are not yet known.

HISTORY

History of Opioid Use

The use of opium for intoxicant purposes (including religious purposes) and analgesia appears to date back at least to ancient Greece and Sumer, where typical routes of administration were oral ingestion of opium or inhalation of its vapors from heated vessels (39). By the 8th century CE Arab traders had brought opium to China and India; between 1000 and 1300, opium use spread to Europe, and the first surviving accounts of opium addiction began to appear in all these regions. Use of opium via smoking apparently first became popular in China in the 1600s after a ban on tobacco smoking (39).

Morphine was isolated and named by the German pharmacist Friedrich Sertürner in 1806 (39); the other naturally occurring opiate, codeine, was isolated in 1832 by the French chemist Pierre Jean Robiquet (40). Heroin (diacetylmorphine, i.e., an acetylated analog of morphine) was initially synthesized in 1874 by Charles Wright in London and was tested in frogs and rabbits at the University of Edinburgh in the 1880s, but only as part of a series of studies on structure–activity relationships (41). The now-famous (re)synthesis of heroin at Friedrich Bayer and Company in 1898 occurred in the midst of the "acetylation mania" that had included Felix Hoffman's synthesis of aspirin (42). In fact, Hoffman synthesized heroin just 2 weeks after first synthesizing aspirin; its effects were then assessed in rabbits and humans by Heinrich Dreser, head of pharmacology at Bayer (41,42). Dreser's primary interest was in finding a cough suppressant with a more benign side-effect profile than morphine's; his spirometry studies in rabbits quickly led him to the intriguing—and wildly erroneous—conclusion that heroin stimulated and strengthened the lungs (41,42). One historian contends that this mistaken finding led Bayer to market heroin, which otherwise seemed to have no advantages over morphine (41). Another historian notes that between 1898 and 1911, scientific and medical controversy surrounding heroin focused almost exclusively on its respiratory effects, not on its addictiveness—cases of iatrogenic heroin addiction apparently having been rare due to the use of low doses and oral administration (42).

During those same years, however, heroin became a staple ingredient in the plethora of unregulated patent medicines that already included morphine (and had probably done so since the very early 1800s) (43). Opiate-containing patent medicines were sold in nearly every conceivable dosage form for nearly every conceivable indication, including, for gynecologic problems, heroin-impregnated tampons (42). In the medical literature, the first explicit warning about heroin abuse and addiction was probably a 1912 *JAMA* article by physician John Phillips of Cleveland, Ohio, who described three individuals' "habits" of insufflating heroin; two of the users had initially been attempting to relieve coughs, while the other seemed to have sought out heroin for its psychoactive effects. Two of the users had also told Philips that heroin was frequently used for euphoriant effects "in the tenderloin districts" of Ohio cities or among soda-fountain employees with daily workplace access to it (44). These patterns of use were especially notable in light of heroin's reputation (among both laypeople and physicians) as a nonaddictive drug (44). Phillips's article marked the start of wide public concern about heroin abuse and addiction in the United States (41). In December 1913, fully 3 years after President Taft had declared to Congress that cocaine was "more appalling in its effects than any other habit-forming drug used in the United States" (45)[1] and the *Chicago Tribune* had featured a headline about "The War Against Cocaine" (46), an article in the *New York Times* was introducing the word *heroin* to a readership still presumed to be unfamiliar with it:

> Dr. C.J. Douglas of Boston ... described the ravages of the new drug which, he said, was making victims by the hundred in his own city. This is a new product of opium and its discovery has been so recent that no existing State law may be made to apply against it. This new chemical is called heroin. Its effects are like those of morphine, and it is sold so openly in one district of Boston that the vicinity of the drug store which markets it has become known as "heroin square." The victims, who have increased by the hundreds within the last few months, hold regularly what are known as "sniffing parties," when the drug is passed around occasionally as the chief means of entertainment (47).

The lurid tone of the *New York Times* article suggests that heroin was becoming the center of what sociologists call a "moral panic." The moral panic may also have been stoked by growing public antipathy toward Germany in the years leading up to World War I (41).

With the 1914 passage of the Harrison Narcotic Act, access to heroin in the United States was restricted to those whose physicians would prescribe it (in federally regulated amounts), and as of 1924, heroin could no longer legally be prescribed, either (though it always remained available by prescription in the United Kingdom). By many accounts, the criminalization of heroin caused a demographic shift in the profile of those who abused or were addicted to it, whereby the middle-class misuser of patent or prescribed medicines gave way to the marginalized, "deviant" seeker of euphoriant effects. However, as the 1913 *New York Times* article suggests,

---

[1] Several textbooks and scholarly articles add the irresistible factoid that Taft had called cocaine "public enemy number one." There is no evidence that Taft used this phrase, which did not enter common parlance until the 1930s (Joseph F. Spillane, personal communication, July 1, 2009). The misquotation may have arisen from a misreading of David Musto's 1989 summary of the *gist* of Taft's statement.

the Harrison Act may have been a *reaction* to—though also an exacerbating influence on—an already present trend in that direction (48).

History of Behavioral Research on Human Opioid Use and Addiction

Human behavioral research[2] on opioids in the 1900s can be considered in terms of at least three major strands: the psychiatric and clinical-pharmacology approaches taken at the ARC in Lexington, Kentucky from 1930s to the 1970s (48–50); the behavioral-pharmacology approach taken by experimental psychologists at Johns Hopkins and other universities from the 1950s onward (50); and the sociologic approaches taken by Chicago School theorists and others, beginning in the 1930s and becoming influential from the 1950s onward (48).

Psychiatry and Clinical Pharmacology at the Addiction Research Center (ARC)

The ARC was established as an independent entity within a unique federal narcotics hospital/prison in which inmates had access to ostensibly therapeutic farm work and were asked to participate in research studies (50). The published output of the ARC from the 1930s through the 1950s shows the movement of addiction research from psychodynamic concepts to behavioral ones (49). Lawrence Kolb, the ARC's first medical director (48), organized some aspects of the program with a psychodynamic typology of addicts he had developed in the 1920s (50). In 1948, Abraham Wikler, associate director of the ARC, developed a theory of addiction through a study consisting of psychoanalytic interviews with one especially articulate user during readdiction to and withdrawal from morphine (50,51). Yet the theory, which Wikler called a "pharmacodynamic" theory, was ultimately more behavioral than psychodynamic: although Wikler ascribed the initial misuse of opiates largely to personality defects, he ascribed ongoing addiction to "factors of little or no symbolic significance"—specifically, the avoidance or termination of withdrawal symptoms (52). Later, Wikler would discuss the theory in exclusively behavioristic terms (53,54), but even in 1953, Wikler invoked processes and concepts that remain important to current scientific thinking about addiction:

> ... a "conditioning" process may play a role in relapse, particularly in the case of addiction to opiate drugs. A number of opiate addicts have stated that experiences akin to that of the opiate abstinence syndrome, including intensified "craving" for such drugs, may occur long after "cure," when opportunities to obtain narcotics present themselves (52).

Harris Isbell, director of the ARC from 1945 to 1962, discussed Wikler's conditioning theory in terms that comport even more closely with current thinking:

> The instantaneous relief of this [withdrawal-related] suffering afforded by opiates serves to heighten the addict's esteem for this class of drugs and causes him to use the drug for the relief of discomfort from any cause. In a sense, the addict becomes "conditioned"—any unpleasant situation calls for an injection. A pleasurable experience, such as meeting an old friend, also requires a celebration, using drugs as a means of heightening the pleasure already experienced (55).

In the same article, Isbell endorsed a harm-based definition of addiction to which physical dependence was not essential, and acknowledged that personality dysfunction could be either a cause or consequence of opiate addiction (55). Isbell had also published the first findings indicating that withdrawal from methadone could be preferable to withdrawal from morphine (56); methadone was thereafter used at the ARC to manage withdrawal symptoms (50), though maintenance treatment was apparently not discussed, except insofar as to point out that the Harrison Act seemed to forbid it (57). Treatment with mu antagonists such as nalorphine was discussed (58).

Other important advances during the early days of the ARC occurred in a laboratory directed by Clifton Himmelsbach, where careful characterization of the opiate-withdrawal syndrome (59) was used to develop methods for addiction-liability testing of new drugs (50,60,61).

From 1963 to 1977, ARC research was directed by William Martin (50). As mentioned in the previous section, Martin used behavioral and physiologic data to infer that there were multiple types of opiate receptors (28). Martin also postulated a syndrome of "protracted abstinence" lasting up to 30 weeks, characterized by subtle physiologic signs and, he hypothesized, associated with vulnerability to relapse (62); this syndrome continues to be investigated. Martin, and later Donald Jasinski, continued to test opioid antagonists as maintenance treatments (63–65). Charles Haertzen developed the Addiction Research Center Inventory (ARCI), a subjective-drug-effects questionnaire refined by factor analysis in the tradition of personality inventories (66). The ARCI has become a standard measure for characterizing experimental drugs in terms of their resemblance to known classes of drugs.

In the 1970s, as the ethical acceptability of research with prisoners was increasingly called into question, the ARC moved to a medical campus in Baltimore, becoming part of the National Institute on Drug Abuse (NIDA) (50). The campus was already home to the Behavioral Pharmacology Research Unit (BPRU) of Johns Hopkins University; this geographical proximity led to an entwinement of the ARC's research traditions with those of another strand of research: behavioral pharmacology.

Behavioral Pharmacology

Although views of opioid addiction at the ARC became less psychodynamic and more behavioral over the decades, the branch of behaviorism embraced at the ARC (as in Wikler's conditioned-withdrawal theory) was largely Pavlovian. In the 1950s and 1960s, investigators primarily interested

---

[2] For a brief review of the history of molecular research on opioids and their receptors, see Ref. 39.

in Skinnerian (operant) conditioning established the field of behavioral pharmacology. Among the clearest contrasts between the two schools of thought was that behavioral pharmacologists tended to doubt the value of the kinds of self-report data collected by clinical pharmacologists at ARC (67). Behavioral pharmacologists also favored single-subject designs in which the individual's behavior was intensively analyzed (50)—this at a time when ARC director Harris Isbell was stating, at a 1963 conference, that "all new suggested programs for opiate addiction should be evaluated by rigidly controlled clinical trials" (49). Human research at the ARC relied heavily on what was uniquely human—the ability to provide self-report data—whereas research in behavioral pharmacology usually involved applying a given methodology across species (and was thus necessarily oriented toward nonverbal behavior). Thus, even this brief summary of human research needs to include some discussion of laboratory-animal research.

The first major achievement for behavioral pharmacology in the study of opioid addiction occurred in the late 1950s at the University of Maryland, where Joseph Brady had been developing high-throughput behavioral screens with rats to study the effects of new drugs (68). Brady's students, Charles Schuster and Travis Thompson, fortuitously discovered that monkeys would self-administer morphine (68; 69). Although self-administration research helped confirm Wikler's assertion that morphine use could be induced by cue-induced withdrawal (70), some ARC investigators initially doubted that such work was relevant to addiction (68). Perhaps this reflected their awareness of its implications: self-administration work allowed addiction to be conceptualized in terms of principles of behavior analysis (a point made by Fischman and Schuster (71)). This meant that causal attribution for drug use and misuse began to change from antecedents (such as users' psychiatric defects) to consequences (68)—which could be similar for anyone in a given environment.[3]

From 1963 to 1968, Schuster ran a behavioral-pharmacology laboratory at the University of Michigan that came to include James Woods, Chris-Ellyn Johanson, and Maxine Stitzer. Schuster and Woods showed that morphine self-administration (in monkeys) could be maintained at doses that did not require physical dependence (73); such findings are reflected in the current criteria for opioid addiction, which hold that physical dependence is neither necessary nor sufficient for the diagnosis (74).

From 1968 to 1974, Schuster and Marian Fischman ran a behavioral-pharmacology laboratory at the University of Chicago (75), where self-administration techniques began to be more frequently applied to human research. One project completed there was a study of human self-administration of methadone, codeine, and pentazocine, showing that pentazocine's abuse liability was lower than those of methadone and codeine (76). During approximately the same years, Travis Thompson ran a behavioral-pharmacology laboratory at the University of Minnesota, where his trainees included George Bigelow and Roland Griffiths; Thompson and Bigelow continued the self-administration work with monkeys (67).

In the 1970s, many of these investigators converged back in Maryland, this time at Johns Hopkins University. By 1974, Bigelow, Griffiths, and Stitzer had named their Hopkins laboratory the Behavioral Pharmacology Research Unit (BPRU) (77). Bigelow and Ira Liebson studied the effects of behavioral treatments in methadone patients (78); this and related work at BPRU (79) were the genesis of contingency-management treatment. As mentioned, in 1974 the ARC (by then part of NIDA) moved from Lexington to BPRU's Hopkins campus; by 1986, the former gulf between the ARC and behavioral pharmacologists had been eradicated in a more than symbolic way, as NIDA's director was now Charles Schuster.

Also in 1974, behavioral pharmacologists Jack Mendelson and Nancy Mello established the Alcohol and Drug Abuse Research Center at McLean Hospital in Boston (80). Mendelson had attended Johns Hopkins and the University of Maryland (80), but was not directly associated with the investigators who formed the BPRU. At the Mendelson and Mello laboratory in Boston, investigators did further work with heroin self-administration in humans, showing that sequential self-administrations of heroin produced ever smaller phasic increases in euphoria against a tonic background of increasingly intense dysphoria (81). This observation—that self-administration continued despite demonstrably diminishing reward—presaged the idea of a dissociation between wanting and liking (82), which would become an influential hypothesis in addiction research.

Mendelson and Mello also showed that human self-administration of heroin is suppressed by buprenorphine (86); this finding was instrumental in the development of buprenorphine for treatment. Perhaps reflecting the blurring of the lines between clinical and behavioral pharmacology, the abstract from the report of this study includes a distinctly un-Skinnerian emphasis on subjective responses to the test medication: "The subjects liked buprenorphine and indicated that it was preferable to methadone or naltrexone."

Sociology and Ethnography

A third strand of human research on opioid use and addiction consists of work done by sociologists and ethnographers. These investigators have been more geographically disparate

---

[3] By the 1970s, the social implications of these findings were being openly expressed by behavioral pharmacologists and neuropharmacologists. For example, the neuropharmacologist Avram Goldstein wrote: "This [opioid self-administration] is not the anomalous behavior of a few, but the predictable behavior of all. Thus, on fundamental biologic grounds, we may infer that were it not for countervailing influences in human society, narcotic addiction might well be the norm rather than an aberration" (72).

than the ARC and BPRU investigators, and it is accordingly more difficult to summarize their history in a few paragraphs.[4]

The roots of this body of work can be traced to a doctoral dissertation completed in the 1930s by University of Chicago sociologist Bingham Dai, who conducted in-depth interviews with heroin addicts in order to supplement epidemiologic data; although his conclusions placed heroin addiction in a social context, he still emphasized the etiologic role of individual addicts' psychiatric pathologies, much like his contemporaries at the ARC such as Kolb (48). Dai's fellow student Alfred Lindesmith, who completed similar fieldwork at the same time, explicitly rejected Kolb's conceptualization of heroin addiction as a manifestation of psychopathology (48), formulating a "sociologic theory of addiction"—but Lindesmith's sociologic theory was in many ways a cognitive theory, stressing the etiologic importance of recognizing and labeling one's own withdrawal symptoms (43).

In the 1950s, a "second Chicago School" emerged, including Howard Becker, whose studies of deviance in drug users influenced later sociologists such as Dan Waldorf (86,87), Bruce Johnson (88), and Charles Faupel (89). Each of the latter three discussed heroin addicts' long-term trajectories of use in terms of "using careers," implying that addicts function (often adaptively) within a particular social system and have some degree of mobility within that system. Becker has stated that he and Lindesmith were hostile or indifferent toward most of the accounts of addiction emerging from the ARC and from behaviorists and that the feeling seemed reciprocal (90).

Nonetheless, the intellectual descendents of the first and second Chicago Schools produced work that has radically reshaped scientific thinking about addiction in general. Probably the most celebrated example is the work of Lee Robins, who showed that heroin-addicted U.S. soldiers returning from Vietnam defied expectations by overwhelmingly reverting to abstinence (or moderate use) without treatment or participation in self-help programs (94–98). Following up on Robins' surprising findings on natural recovery from heroin addiction, ethnographers Dan Waldorf and Patrick Biernacki suggested that the seemingly uncontrollable pull of addiction can be defeated by "the pulls of 'the good life', as exemplified by the dominant value system—work, stable life, and high levels of consumption" (96). Another implication of Robins' findings—that addiction is determined largely by social setting—was fleshed out in the work of psychiatrist Norman Zinberg, whose in-depth interviews provided evidence that certain subcultural norms can support chipping, the long-term recreational use of heroin or other opiates in the absence of addiction (97–99).

History of Methadone Maintenance

For opioid addicts who did need treatment, the early 1960s saw what remains the major breakthrough: methadone maintenance, pioneered largely by Vincent Dole and Marie Nyswander at Rockefeller University Hospital in New York City.[5] Their initial report on methadone maintenance included data from only 22 patients (101), yet remains a remarkably informative primer. Their follow-up work with a larger sample of methadone-maintained patients showed multiple indicators of treatment success, including reductions in criminality (102).

Methadone maintenance and other agonist treatments, despite being surprisingly straightforward approaches to a problem of such theoretical complexity, have never existed in isolation from the research that preceded and followed them. The theoretical roots of methadone maintenance can arguably be traced back to laboratory-animal self-administration studies done by behavioral pharmacologists (this argument was made by Fischman and Schuster (71)). Once methadone maintenance was established, it was used as a platform for behavioral studies, such as a study of self-regulation of methadone doses (103).

Dole and Nyswander themselves did not present methadone maintenance in a theoretical vacuum. They argued that the unexpectedly good psychosocial outcomes of their first few hundred patients militated against notions of inherent and intractable psychiatric dysfunction (104). Dole and Nyswander did state that methadone maintenance should be accompanied by psychotherapy or psychosocial case management, but when they discussed how those aspects of treatment should be individualized, they wrote in terms that might have come from the Chicago School–influenced sociologists:

> [T]he social problems of the street addict will continue to disable him unless effective social helps are also given. The slum-born, minority-group addict was underprivileged before he became addicted, and these social problems remain with him after his heroin use is stopped …. This may not be true of the middle-class addict who presents psychiatric rather than social problems (105).

This idea—that opioid addiction might be a different "disease" for addicts of different socioeconomic classes—is rarely stated so plainly in current research literature.

---

[4] One criminologist, John Ball, worked at the ARC in the early 1960s, characterizing the population there, but he worked more from an epidemiologic standpoint than an ethnographic one; for example, he compiled statistics on all Asian patients, all patients who died, and all patients whose primary addiction was to methadone (84). He later coauthored a classic book on correlates of outcome in methadone programs (85).

[5] This breakthrough was not without precedent. Between 1919 and 1923, the Shreveport Morphine Maintenance Clinic successfully maintained 762 patients until state and federal pressure caused its closing (100).

The success of Dole and Nyswander's work helped to change U.S. federal policy toward addiction, though in some ways the change was transient. Under President Nixon, federal funding for addiction treatment came to exceed federal funding for enforcement, but this change had already been reversed before Nixon's administration ended, long before the emergence of the better-known punitive drug policies of the 1980s (48). Similarly, Don Des Jarlais (who in the 1970s had published treatment-outcome research with Dole and Nyswander) provided evidence in the 1980s for the effectiveness of needle exchange and community outreach (106), yet most of his findings have not been incorporated into federal policy (48).

A more encouraging interaction among research, treatment, and policy can be seen in the history of buprenorphine treatment; this is discussed in Section 6 of this book.

EPIDEMIOLOGY OF OPIOID USE AND DEPENDENCE

Prevalence and incidence of opioid use in the United States can be gleaned from the National Survey on Drug Use and Health (NSDUH), which reports on the use of illicit drugs, alcohol, and tobacco in respondents aged 12 and older (107). In 2007, the most recent year for which data are available, the survey included interviews from a sample of 67,870 people, selected to be representative of the civilian, noninstitutionalized population of the United States, with demographic minorities oversampled to facilitate reliable extrapolation. Opioid use is reported under two categories, "heroin" and "pain relievers"; the latter is a subset of the "prescription-type psychotherapeutics used nonmedically."

Heroin Use

Prevalence

The number of current heroin users (defined as those who have used in the past month) in the United States is not trivial in absolute terms, but is small as a proportion of the general population: extrapolation from NSDUH data suggests that in 2007, 153,000 persons 12 years or older were current heroin users (107). This is a decrease from the 2006 number of 338,000 and corresponds to a decrease in current heroin use prevalence from 0.14% to 0.06% of the U.S. population. The decrease from 2006 to 2007 was consistent across most demographic groups: among females 12 years or older, the rate decreased from 0.06% to 0.02%; among adults 26 years and older, from 0.14% to 0.05%; and among youth, from 0.06% to 0.01%.

Incidence

In 2007, an estimated 106,000 persons aged 12 or older had used heroin for the first time within the last 12 months. The average age of first use was 21.8 years, which was unchanged from 2006 (107).

Nonmedical Use of Pain Relievers

Prevalence

In 2007, an estimated 5.2 million persons aged 12 or older (2.1% of the U.S. population) had used prescription-type pain relievers nonmedically in the past month; this rate was similar to the rate seen in 2006. Sources of the drug (among those who used nonmedically in the past 12 months) often included a friend or relative, either through free access (56.5%), purchase (8.9%), or theft (5.2%); in addition, the drug was obtained from doctors (18%, who reported that they got the drug from just one doctor), drug dealers or other strangers (4.1%), and Internet sources (0.5%). Rates of past-month use of OxyContin were similar among males (0.2%) and females (0.1%).

Incidence

Among past-year illicit drug initiates, 19% initiated with nonmedical use of pain relievers. Pain relievers tied with marijuana as the two illicit drug categories with the largest number of past-year initiates among persons aged 12 or older; each had an estimated 2.1 million. These estimates were not significantly different from those seen in 2006. The number of new nonmedical users of OxyContin aged 12 or older was 554,000, and 24 years was their average age at first use.

Opioid Use among Youth

Trends in drug use among youth can be gleaned from Monitoring the Future, a long-term study of American adolescents, college students, and adults through age 50 (108). The 2008 national sample included approximately 16,300 8th graders, 15,500 10th graders, and 14,600 12th graders, for a total of approximately 46,000 students in 386 secondary schools.

Youth Prevalence

In 2008, the lifetime prevalence of heroin use with a needle was 0.9%, 0.7%, and 0.7% in grades 8, 10, and 12 respectively; without a needle, the corresponding prevalences were 0.9%, 0.8%, and 1.1%. Lifetime prevalence of use of narcotics other than heroin (assessed in 12th graders only) was substantially greater: 13.2%. The annual prevalence of heroin use for all three grades (8th, 10th, and 12th) fluctuated between 0.7% and 0.9% from 2005 through 2008. During this same time period, the annual prevalence of use of narcotics other than heroin by 12th graders fluctuated between 9.0% and 9.2%. The annual prevalence of use of OxyContin and Vicodin specifically among 12th graders between 2005 and 2008 fluctuated between 4.3% and 5.5% (OxyContin) and between 9.5% and 9.7% (Vicodin) (108).

Youth Attitudes

Perceived Risk and Disapproval of Opioid Use In 2008, a small majority (55.5%) of 12th graders perceived trying heroin once or twice as a "great risk," and a larger majority (86.4%) perceived taking heroin regularly as a "great risk." Among 12th graders, 93.3% "disapproved" of trying heroin once or twice, and 94.2% "disapproved" of trying heroin once or twice without using a needle; these percentages were not appreciably different from those seen in 2007 (108).

Almost 60% of youth reported that they had talked in the past year with a parent about the dangers of drug, tobacco, or alcohol use (108).

Opioid Availability Heroin was said to be "fairly easy" or "very easy to get" by 25.4% of 12th graders in 2008; this was a modest but statistically significant decrease from 2007 (29.7%). Similar decreases in availability were seen with some other opioids (including methadone and excluding heroin), which were said to be "fairly easy" or "very easy to get" by 37.3% of 12th graders in 2007 and 34.9% in 2008 (108).

Opioids and Emergency Department (ED) Visits

Drug-related ED visits in the United States are monitored by a public health surveillance system called the Drug Abuse Warning Network (DAWN) (109). DAWN estimates for 2006, based on a national sample of general, nonfederal hospitals operating 24-hour EDs, suggest that 113 million ED visits occurred, and that just over 1.5% of these (1,742,887; Confidence Interval (CI): 1,451,086 to 2,034,688) were drug related. Of these drug-related visits, approximately 11% (189,780; CI: 119,525 to 260,035) were related to heroin; this is likely an underestimate, because some heroin use is misclassified as an "unspecified opiate" use. Accounting for population size and margin of error, ED visits involving heroin were higher for males than females and highest in patients aged 21 to 54. There were no significant changes in rates or proportions of heroin-related ED visits between 2004 and 2006. Of the ED visits made by patients seeking detoxification, 29% were specifically for heroin detoxification.

The DAWN data include a separate category for "nonmedical use of prescription or over-the-counter pharmaceuticals or dietary supplements"; there were approximately 741,425 (CI: 674,198 to 808,652) such visits, of which approximately 33% involved opioid analgesics. From 2004 to 2006, visits involving opioid analgesics increased 43%, with some of the largest increases seen in visits involving "hydrocodone/combinations" (44% increase), "oxycodone/combinations" (56% increase), and "unspecified opiates" (60% increase). Of the ED visits made by patients seeking detoxification, 26% were specifically for detoxification from opioid analgesics.

Opioid Abuse or Dependence and Treatment

In 2007, 213,000 persons aged 12 or older met *Diagnostic and Statistical Manual of Mental Disorders, Fourth Edition* (*DSM-IV*) criteria for heroin abuse or dependence (74). A much larger number—1.7 million—met *DSM-IV* criteria for pain-reliever abuse or dependence; this was second only to cannabis (3.9 million). The estimate for pain relievers has remained unchanged between 2002 and 2007. These diagnoses (the criteria for which are discussed in the Section Phenomenology of use and withdrawal, and criteria for opioid-use disorders of this chapter) reflect not merely physical dependence, but patterns of use with broad adverse psychological or interpersonal consequences.

Past-Year Treatment for an Opioid-Use Problem

In 2007, an estimated 335,000 aged 12 or older had received treatment in the past year for drug problems involving heroin, and an estimated 558,000 people had received treatment in the past year for drug problems involving pain relievers. The latter figure represents a substantial increase over the preceding 5 years (2002: 360,000 persons) (107).

An estimated 21 million people (8.4% of the U.S. population aged 12 or older) needed but did not receive treatment for a problem with illicit drugs or alcohol in 2007. An estimated 1 million people perceived a need to be treated, but only 28.5% of them made an effort to get treatment. The most commonly reported reasons for not receiving treatment (combining data from respondents who did and did not seek treatment, from 2004 to 2007) were: lack of health coverage or ability to pay (35.9%), not being ready to stop using (26.6%), ability to handle the problem without treatment (12.5%), lack of transportation or convenient access (10.5%), concerns about negative opinions from neighbors/community (8.9%), lack of type of treatment needed (8.1%), concerns about negative effects on employment (7.0%), and lack of knowledge of where to go for treatment (6.9%).

Treatment Admissions for Opioid Problems

Treatment facilities that are licensed or certified by state substance-abuse agencies provide data for the Treatment Episode Data Set (TEDS) (110). TEDS data from 2007 show that 13.6% of all treatment admissions for substance abuse were related to heroin and 5% were related to other opioids. Of the individuals admitted for heroin-related problems, 68.5% were male, 52.3% were white (non-Hispanic), 22.1% black (non-Hispanic), 22.4% Hispanic, and 6.6% of other races/ethnicities; the average age at admission was 36 years. Of the individuals admitted for problems related to other opioids, 53.4% were male, 88.6% were white (non-Hispanic), 3.7% black (non-Hispanic), 4.1% Hispanic, and 3.5% of other races/ethnicities; the average age at admission was 32 years. The plurality of those admitted for heroin problems had had five or more prior treatment episodes, while the plurality of those admitted for other opioid problems had had no prior treatment episodes. Admissions for opioids other than heroin increased from 1% of all admissions in 1997 to 5% in 2007.

Longitudinal Course of Opioid Dependence

Given that heroin use disorders are relatively rare among substance use disorders (107), heroin users seem to be overrepresented among treatment admissions for substance use disorders (110). The high treatment numbers almost certainly reflect the fact that agonist maintenance is among the most effective addiction treatments ever developed. Nonetheless, there has long been a relatively hidden population of individuals who recover from addiction to heroin or other opioids without formal treatment (or attendance at self-help groups).

In 1962, Charles Winick reviewed official records from the Federal Bureau of Narcotics and found that by age 35 to 40 years, individuals tended to drop out of the files, a phenomenon he attributed to their "maturing out" of their substance use problems (111). The "maturing out" hypothesis has received only partial empirical support: a recent review concluded that there is "no particular age at which the probability of becoming abstinent either increases or decreases" and that periods of use and abstinence tend to be cyclical (112). Users who do achieve long-term abstinence tend to be those who, as ethnographer Dan Waldorf had suggested (96), have or establish hallmarks of a conventional lifestyle, such as employment, good social relationships, and a variety of leisure activities (112,113).

For users who do not achieve abstinence, health consequences seem to be cumulative over decades (114). A 33-year longitudinal study of 581 male heroin addicts, with a mean age of 25 years at enrollment, showed a mortality rate of nearly 49% (115). This statistic would be easier to interpret if it had been accompanied by data on the expected mortality rate in demographically matched men without heroin addiction. One clear aspect of the findings, however, was that 45 (8%) of the men had died of heroin overdose.

PHENOMENOLOGY OF USE AND WITHDRAWAL, AND CRITERIA FOR OPIOID USE DISORDERS

Phenomenology of Use

A study by Mirin and colleagues, mentioned in the "History" section of this chapter, evocatively describes the behavioral sequelae of *ad libitum* heroin use in a laboratory setting:

> With the onset of heroin use, behavior typical of addicts in a more natural setting was clearly in evidence. Quarreling, sarcasm, verbal hostility, and threats of assault were more frequent, both among themselves and with staff. Complaints about the quality of the heroin were voiced even while subjects were "nodding out." ... When asked if their attitudes or behavior differed in any way from previous cycles of addiction, most volunteered that "this is the way I get." Despite the negative clinical and social effects of prolonged heroin use, the subjects continued to work for and self-administer increasingly larger doses of the drug (80).

A first-person description of heroin effects notes that heroin can initially be a social lubricant and euphoriant, at least for some users:

> The unglamorous truth is that it's not that pleasurable or interesting a drug—except at the beginning .... The first time I snorted heroin, I couldn't believe it had such bad press: I felt absolutely wonderful and consummately able to conduct all essential life activities—talk, write, listen to music. Sex, it turned out, wasn't so great, but you can't have sex all the time anyway. I liked heroin much better than alcohol and didn't notice a physical downside: my coordination was okay and nothing was blurred or confused. The high felt ... like nothing so much as happiness itself (116).

On chronic use, these positive effects become unreliable: "Sometimes you can do dope all night and function the next day; other times hours of vomiting replace the evening partying you had in mind" (116). Eventually, the effects of heroin use may become, at best, emotionally numbing:

> What passes for interaction is so much more minimal on dope .... A non-drug-using friend called some of my junkie pals "holograms," as in: "they're not really there, you can't talk to them." But that's just the point; heroin may not warm a cold world, but it lowers your comfort zone to the reptilian average. Heroin loses its savor once you start seeing this numbing effect as a negative rather than an advantage. Used regularly, heroin is mainly a way of lowering one's expectations .... Among users, heroin is proverbially what you do when you really must organize your files or your house; it lends itself to cushioning activity that's deadening and inherently repetitious (116).

Phenomenology of Withdrawal

Withdrawal from opioids produces a flu-like syndrome that is not life threatening (117). The syndrome has been described in medical literature as either "subjectively severe but objectively mild" or "objectively mild but subjectively severe," presumably depending where the writer wanted to place the emphasis. For users, the subjective severity tends to be paramount. Even an objective onlooker would be unlikely to describe the behavioral manifestations of unaided withdrawal as "mild." Isbell and Harris (118) noted that even prodromal symptoms of withdrawal are sufficient to drive ongoing use of morphine. In our own treatment-research clinic, we have noted that anticipatory anxiety about an eventual dose taper (sometimes called "detoxification phobia" (119)) can hinder patients' acceptance of a sufficiently high maintenance dose of methadone.

Abrupt discontinuation of relatively short-acting mu agonists such as heroin (but not methadone) typically leads to onset of symptoms in 6 to 8 hours; the most prominent are yawning, watery eyes, runny nose, chills, muscle aches, nausea/vomiting, diarrhea, and fever. Eating is disrupted for approximately 7 days; sleeping is increased on the first day, but disrupted for at least 15 days; fever peaks on the third day and may persist for approximately 15 days (120).

Abrupt discontinuation of methadone leads to symptoms that are slower in onset (usually starting after 24 hours), longer in duration, and possibly milder (117). In clinical practice, methadone is typically tapered over 8 to 24 weeks, depending on the maintenance dose. Some patients state that methadone withdrawal (even during a taper) is at least as severe as heroin withdrawal, and there is some evidence to support this contention, at least when street-methadone addicts were compared with heroin addicts in a 10-day open-label taper from methadone (121). A double-blind, double-dummy study would be needed to resolve the issue.

Ten patients' perceptions of lengthy individualized methadone tapers (11 months on average) were described in detail by Eklund and colleagues (122):

Among the individual psychological symptoms, sleeping disturbances, fatigue, and insecurity were judged to be the most discomforting. Various forms of sleeping disturbances are ... the symptom the patients mention as being the most discomforting. Insecurity was reported high, and several of the subjects say that they particularly experience a general feeling of insecurity in different social situations, for example when they run errands in town, go out shopping, or meet acquaintances (122).

Eklund and colleagues noted that insecurity had not been specifically reported in other studies of methadone withdrawal, but "nervousness" had. Proneness to other psychological symptoms, such as depression, varied across individuals. As for physiological symptoms:

only excessive sweating, yawning, diarrhea, and muscular aches increased significantly from the first to the second half of the withdrawal process. Of these, the greatest change is noted for excessive sweating and yawning. These symptoms thus escalate in later parts of the dose reduction process and have caused considerable problems for a couple of the subjects. For example, Subject 7 ... suffered from excessive sweating mainly in the face and armpits for a long time after conclusion of withdrawal, which can be very embarrassing, particularly on the job .... Two years after the last methadone dose, Subject 7 still reports abnormal sweating, although the problem has gradually diminished. Regarding yawning, this is also a common sign of abstinence and can be discomforting owing to the fact that it is deeper and more frequent than ordinary yawning (122).

Eklund and colleagues also noted an "almost total absence of cramps"; abdominal cramps seem to be much more common during abrupt withdrawal of shorter-acting opioids than during a methadone taper. Finally, Eklund and colleagues noted some potentially positive changes: "Many methadone patients during withdrawal report that they become more awake, alert, and active, their senses are intensified, and they are more in touch with their emotions" (122).

Some of the clinically observable signs of opioid withdrawal (such as increased blood pressure, increased metabolic rate, and lowered body weight) may take approximately 6 months to resolve (123), an observation that has been discussed in terms of a subtle "protracted abstinence syndrome" (62) in which such signs are accompanied by dysphoria and vulnerability to relapse. There is evidence that the severity of cue-induced craving for heroin in a laboratory setting becomes and remains elevated for at least 6 months after a methadone taper (123).

Criteria for Opioid Use Disorders

In both of the major diagnostic systems for substance use disorders—the *DSM-IV* (74) and the *ICD-10* (124)—the criteria are generic, applying across substances. These criteria are discussed in Chapter 10. What bears emphasis here is that, in either system, physical dependence (tolerance or withdrawal) is neither necessary nor sufficient for diagnosis of an opioid use disorder. This is consistent with observations made as long ago as 1949 by ARC investigators: "[A]ddicts repeatedly relapse to the use of morphine long after withdrawal, not because they are suffering with any physical distress, but because they desire the euphoria produced by the drug or the relief of the psychic and emotional discomfort which it gives. This is simply another way of saying that habituation is more important in addiction than in physical dependence" (117).

The *DSM-IV* provides for diagnoses of dependence (a term intended to replace *addiction*) or abuse. The intended distinction between dependence and abuse is that dependence reflects adverse psychological or medical consequences of use, while abuse reflects adverse social, legal, or interpersonal consequences; in other words, the two categories are meant to be logically independent of each other (125). Nonetheless, a diagnosis of abuse is not made if criteria for dependence are met. In either case, the pattern of use must be "maladaptive"; thus, criteria for a disorder will not be met by chronic-pain patients for whom opioids improve quality of life, nor by occasional users whose use remains nonproblematic.

The *ICD-10* provides for diagnoses of dependence and harmful use. The dependence diagnosis reflects mostly the same set of criteria as the *DSM-IV* dependence diagnosis, though it also incorporates a "sense of compulsion" as one possible (not required) criterion. The "harmful use" diagnosis reflects patterns of use that damage physical or mental health without otherwise meeting criteria for dependence (124).

DETERMINANTS OF USE

Drug-Related Determinants

Receptor Activity

Among the numerous factors that determine the degree to which a given drug is abused, the most fundamental is the interaction between the drug and endogenous receptors. Upon binding to a receptor, a drug may be a *full agonist* (fully activating the receptor), a *partial agonist* (activating the receptor to a lesser degree than a full agonist), or an *antagonist* (blocking the receptor). In the presence of a full agonist, a partial agonist can produce the behavioral effects of an antagonist. Some drugs, termed *mixed agonist–antagonists*, can act at more than one receptor with differing degrees of agonist and antagonist activities. Small differences in structure can result in substantial differences in receptor activity (126,127).

Drugs that act as full agonists at the mu-opioid receptor are more likely to be abused than those with activity at other opioid receptors. In fact, all of the most highly abused opioids are mu agonists, including morphine, heroin, hydrocodone, oxycodone, hydromorphone, fentanyl, and methadone (1,128). When administered to experienced drug users, these drugs produce positive mood effects, described as euphoria, along with a wide range of other subjective and physiologic effects such as nausea, vomiting, itching, dry mouth, and respiratory depression. With repeated administration of mu agonists, tolerance and physical dependence develop. Development of tolerance to the positive mood effects of mu agonists may play a role in the dose escalation that frequently occurs during opioid dependence. On abrupt discontinuation of use of mu agonists following repeated administration, there is a characteristic abstinence syndrome, characterized by muscle cramps, chills, vomiting, and malaise (59).

Drugs with kappa-agonist activity, such as cyclazocine, ketocyclazocine (after which the kappa receptor is named), and enadoline, produce a different profile of subjective effects, including sedation and effects described as psychotomimetic or dysphoric (16,129–131). Abrupt discontinuation of repeated administration of kappa agonists produces an abstinence syndrome distinct from that of mu agonists (132,133). Kappa-agonist activity is associated with low abuse liability. In fact, although kappa agonists have been investigated for analgesia and other potential benefits such as neuroprotection in ischemia, their unpleasant subjective effects have so far prevented their successful development as medications.

The group of drugs that act at multiple-opioid receptors are often referred to as the agonist–antagonist opioids. Some of these are marketed as analgesics, such as pentazocine, butorphanol, nalbuphine, and buprenorphine. Pentazocine, butorphanol, and nalbuphine have varying degrees of mu- and kappa-agonist activities (1,134,135). Each of these three drugs can be distinguished from mu agonists such as morphine using subjective-effect questionnaires (cf. 133) and human drug-discrimination procedures (137–140). In fact, the differences in subjective effects between prototypic mu-opioid agonists and the agonist–antagonist opioids, respectively, described as morphine-like and nalorphine-like in early work, were a partial basis for the development of the multiple-opioid-receptor theory (28). Nalorphine was one of the first agonist–antagonists studied in animals and humans. It was originally marketed as an antagonist to treat opioid overdose until the more selective opioid antagonist naloxone became available. Pentazocine, butorphanol, and nalbuphine precipitate withdrawal when administered to individuals who are physically dependent on mu agonists (141–143), an attribute that limits abuse. In general, agonist–antagonist opioids have been less abused than prototypic mu agonists (128), though, as noted below, they have been abused under some circumstances.

Buprenorphine differs from the other agonist–antagonists in having partial mu-agonist activity without kappa-agonist activity; its activity at the kappa receptor is as an antagonist. Buprenorphine's subjective effects are very similar to those of the full mu agonists (144–146). Without the abuse-limiting kappa-agonist effects of the other agonist–antagonists, buprenorphine has some history of diversion and abuse (147). However, its abuse by chronic users of full mu agonists (such as heroin, oxycodone, or methadone) is naturally limited because it blocks the acute effects of full mu agonists and can thereby precipitate withdrawal in individuals who are physically dependent on them (144,148). Also, because buprenorphine is only a partial agonist at mu receptors, it is relatively unlikely to produce respiratory depression, even at high doses (145,146). However, deaths have occurred with buprenorphine, especially when it is taken in combination with benzodiazepines (149).

Opioid antagonists that lack agonist effects, such as the opioid antagonists naloxone and naltrexone, are generally devoid of subjective effects except at high doses (64), although one early study in healthy volunteers suggested that intravenous naloxone (10 mg/mL) can block "thrills" elicited by nondrug stimuli such as music (150). These drugs have little or no abuse liability. Indeed, although naltrexone has been available for the treatment of opioid dependence for several decades, its clinical utility is severely limited by low adherence by patients (151).

Some opioids have additional activity at nonopioid sites, which can affect their abuse liability. Examples include tramadol, which produces analgesia through both mu-agonist activity and blockade of noradrenergic reuptake transporters (152), and meperidine, which has both mu-agonist and anticholinergic activities (153). Meperidine has a long history of abuse, sharing many subjective effects with more selective mu agonists, but it also has a distinctive profile of adverse effects that appear to limit its abuse relative to those drugs (128,154,155). Tramadol has not been widely abused despite its wide availability in a variety of dosage forms (156,157), perhaps because it is less potent in producing positive mood effects than in producing analgesia (158).

Overall, opioids with selective mu-agonist activity have somewhat higher abuse liability than those with mixed actions and much higher abuse liability than those without any mu-agonist activity.

Pharmacokinetics

The abuse liability of opioids is influenced by the numerous factors that determine their bodily distribution, metabolism, and excretion. One important factor is the speed with which the drug is delivered to the central nervous system. In general, abuse potential is enhanced by speeding the delivery of drug to the brain, thus shortening the interval between drug administration and the perceived onset of pharmacodynamic effects (159). One likely reason for the popularity of heroin over morphine is that its onset is faster than that of morphine. Also relevant, of course, is the fact that heroin is approximately twice as potent as morphine (and can thus be transported at a lower volume per unit dose) (160).

Although the pharmacokinetic profile of a particular opioid is largely determined by its physical/chemical attributes, the route of administration can also have a substantial impact on speed of delivery. For most drugs, the rank order for routes of administration from slowest to fastest delivery is typically as follows: oral < intranasal < intramuscular ≈ subcutaneous <<< intravenous ≤ inhalation (e.g., smoking). Opioids that can be inhaled or injected intravenously will likely have greater liability for abuse than those than can be used only orally. Methadone is typically dispensed as a liquid (e.g., cherry-flavored syrup) in maintenance programs in part to reduce the likelihood that it will be used by a parenteral route of administration.

Nonpharmacological Drug-Related Factors

The abuse liability of opioids is also affected by at least two nonpharmacological factors that are nonetheless related to the drug itself: availability and formulation.

The availability of heroin is not evenly distributed around the world, and rates of use and abuse can follow changes in availability. For example, India, the largest producer of licit raw opium, also has the highest illicit opium use, a fact attributed in part to diversion of licit opium production (161). Heroin trafficking from the point of production to major markets can also increase local heroin use (and the attendant adverse consequences such as HIV infection) along the route (162,163). Temporary decreases in heroin supply can decrease the rate of initiation of new heroin users (164).

Abuse of prescription opioids has been increasing somewhat disproportionately to the number of licit opioid prescriptions (165). Availability partly determines which specific opioids are abused. For example, when availability is limited to hospitals, the opportunity for abuse of even highly abusable opioids will obviously be reduced; even within hospitals, availability and opportunity play a role in rates of abuse, as evidenced by the greater prevalence of substance abuse among anesthesiologists than among other physician groups (166,167). In contrast, even the least desirable opioid may be abused if it is widely available. An example of this is the over-the-counter cough suppressant dextromethorphan, with activity at sigma and PCP receptors. Early studies of dextromethorphan showed that it did not produce morphine-like subjective effects and was not liked by experienced opioid users (168,169). Nevertheless, dextromethorphan has been abused, mostly by teenagers either specifically seeking a dissociative/hallucinogenic experience or simply seeking any intoxicating effect (170).

Increasing the availability of a medication with a low rate of abuse can substantially increase the incidence of abuse. For example, abuse of both fentanyl (a potent mu agonist with high abuse liability) and butorphanol (a mixed agonist–antagonist with moderate abuse liability) increased when each drug was approved for prescribed use in outpatients, despite the use of formulations that might have been expected to minimize abuse liability (170). In the case of fentanyl, until 1990, reports of abuse usually involved health care providers with access to the intravenous formulation in hospital settings. After 1990, when fentanyl became available to outpatients (in a transdermal-patch formulation), abuse spread to a much broader population, mostly individuals who were not legitimate patients. Butorphanol was an unscheduled, injectable analgesic available primarily for acute administration in hospitals with only sporadic reports of abuse until another (intranasal) dosage form was approved for outpatient use in 1991. Reports of overuse and physical dependence began to appear soon afterward, leading to the scheduling of butorphanol by the DEA in 1997. In contrast to the pattern seen with fentanyl, many of those who overused butorphanol were patients taking the medication for treatment of migraine headaches and trying to avoid rebound of migraine symptoms, despite not liking the subjective effects of the butorphanol (170).

Formulation changes were probably not the direct culprit in increases in fentanyl or butorphanol abuse, given that a transdermal or intranasal formulation is generally less reinforcing than an intravenous formulation. The role of formulation becomes clearer when users devise a way to self-administer a drug by a route other than that intended by the manufacturer. For example, sustained-release formulations designed to deliver a low, constant dosage of medication over an extended period should have lower abuse liability than immediate-release formulations. However, if the slow-release formulation can be defeated, making the entire contents of the product rapidly available, abuse liability can be increased, particularly if the preparation contains large quantities of drug. The best-known example is that of OxyContin, a time-release formulation of oxycodone hydrochloride, which abusers found that they could crush to release the medication rapidly. Abuse of OxyContin became widespread; at least one study found the prevalence of its abuse greater than that of other formulations of oxycodone, methadone, morphine, hydromorphone, fentanyl, or buprenorphine (171). There is also evidence that buprenorphine tablets intended for sublingual administration are abused intravenously (172). Transdermal systems developed to deliver medication slowly for extended periods of time have been prime targets for subversion and misuse (173).

Formulation-based strategies have sometimes been used to decrease the abuse liability of prescription opioids. Naloxone, which is far more bioavailable when injected than when taken orally, has been added to pentazocine and buprenorphine tablets to decrease the likelihood that they will be dissolved and injected by opioid-dependent individuals. Sustained-release products that resist manipulation are also being considered. Further development of abuse-deterrent formulations must meet criteria for both risk-benefit and cost-effectiveness. Meeting patients' pain treatment needs while suppressing illicit use is a complex problem that is under investigation (174,175).

Work is also underway to devise early detection monitoring systems for drug diversion problems (156,171). The goal of these systems is to prevent epidemics of abuse of prescription medications through rapid detection and intervention.

Differences among Users

Genetics

The role of common allelic variants in modifying opioid effects was recently reviewed in depth by Rollason and colleagues (176); the review focused on implications for individualized prescription of analgesics. The variants of interest occur in genes coding for the following: a drug-clearing cell-membrane transporter (P-glycoprotein), phase I drug-metabolizing enzymes (specifically, cytochrome P450 enzymes in the liver), phase II drug-metabolizing enzymes (such as UDP-glucuronosyltransferase, which facilitates urinary excretion of drugs), and opioid receptors. Rollason and colleagues noted that a given allelic variant—for example, duplication of the CYP2D6 allele, resulting in an "ultrarapid metabolizer" phenotype—could increase sensitivity to one opioid (such as oxycodone) while decreasing sensitivity to another opioid (such as methadone). Genetic differences could also have implications for nonmedical use of opioids.

A recent case-control study of single-nucleotide polymorphisms at sites representing 130 candidate genes suggested small associations between heroin addiction and several variants in noncoding regions of genes for mu, delta, and kappa receptors (177). Genetic differences like these might lead to individual differences in splice variants of opioid receptors, the significance of which is discussed in the section Classification of Opioids through Their Actions at Receptors of this chapter.

Cognitive Factors

The process of social learning, initially described by Becker (178) to explain how seemingly unpleasant effects of marijuana or LSD could be reinterpreted by users as desired effects, can apply to opioids as well. For example, a user's first nonmedical experience with an opioid often includes nausea and vomiting, but the user may learn from experienced peers that these symptoms are an intrinsic part of a desirable experience (43,89). Thus, the phrase "pleasant sick" is among the standard clinical descriptors for opioid effects; one user in an ethnographic study described her early heroin experiences by saying, "The more I puked, the higher I got" (89).

Social learning may also play a role in defining oneself as an addict and behaving accordingly: some addicted users report that they had initially interpreted their withdrawal symptoms as flu symptoms until experienced users told them otherwise, leading them to seek more opioids for relief (179). We have heard similar reports from patients in our treatment-research clinic.

As discussed below, environment is a strong determinant of patterns of opioid use—yet not everyone in a high-risk environment uses opioids or becomes addicted to them. One possible explanation is that individuals' differing *perceptions* of identical environments lead to different outcomes. To address this issue, Nurco and colleagues (180) interviewed adult heroin addicts about their perceptions of deviance in their neighborhoods of origin and compared their responses to those of two never-addicted control groups: the addicts' childhood peers and nonpeers, all from the same neighborhoods of origin. The neighborhoods were perceived as having been more deviant by the addicts than by their nonpeer controls. However, perceptions were fairly similar between the addicts and their peer controls. Thus, perceptions of the neighborhood seemed to explain only a small amount of variation in outcome among childhood peers. Perhaps such variation will be better explained by some combination of peer interactions and genetic predispositions, as has been argued for personality development in general (181).

Environmental Determinants

Peers and General Environmental Setting

As mentioned in the section History of Behavioral Research on Human Opioid Use and Addiction, addiction to opioids in exceptional circumstances, such as war, often resolves when the circumstances change (94–98). In this section, we discuss opioid use and addiction in more typical circumstances.

The archetypal pusher who distributes free samples of heroin to snare nonusers is largely a myth (182). Ethnographic studies indicate that initiation of heroin use typically occurs with peers, is often serendipitous, and is attributed retrospectively to curiosity (89,179). However, in some recent small studies, addicts report having been tricked into their first use of heroin by peers who said that the heroin was cocaine or referred to it with unfamiliar slang (179). These claims are difficult to dismiss, because some addicts have acknowledged perpetrating such tricks (183). It is not clear whether being tricked into heroin use is common; it was first described in a study of a rural area, where high heroin prices had led many users to sell heroin to support their own use and to seek buyers proactively (183). It remains likely that the modal circumstance of first exposure involves a combination of availability and curiosity.

Initiation of opioid use is sometimes said to be causally related to prior use of marijuana or other drugs; this is the strong version of the gateway hypothesis. This hypothesis would be difficult to prove or disprove, but is not necessary to explain epidemiological data. The observations that underlie the gateway hypothesis—association and temporal sequencing of marijuana use and opioid use—can be fully accounted for in a computer model incorporating only two rules: differing individual propensities to use drugs in general, and temporally staggered availabilities of different drugs (184).

Once nonmedical opioid use is established, environmental factors seem to be prime determinants of whether it progresses to addiction or remains at the level of chipping (regular but nonproblematic, noncompulsive use). For illicit drugs in general, the likelihood of addiction, given use, increases with low educational background (185,186), low income, and minority-group membership (185), but the surveys from which these statistics were drawn do not disaggregate opioid addiction from other drug addiction. The classic work on determinants of opioid addiction, given use, is ethnographic rather than epidemiological: Norman Zinberg (99) interviewed 61 opioid (mostly heroin) chippers and 30 addicts, all of whose patterns of use had been stable for several years. The modest size of Zinberg's sample limits the ability to draw negative conclusions from it, but permits large effects to be observed. Zinberg found few or no differences between chippers and addicts in terms of opioid of choice, route of administration, initial responses to opioids, neighborhood availability of opioids, family background, or personality. The clearest differences were these: the chippers had more friends than the addicts; the chippers chose to remain friends with other chippers and to shun former friends who became addicts (whereas the addicts had frequently been shunned by former friends); and the chippers tended to adhere to specific rules about opioid use, such as planning use in advance, budgeting funds for use, and buying opioids only under certain circumstances (for example, only from personally known sellers). Zinberg interpreted these findings as evidence of a healthy form of social learning in which subcultural rules and rituals keep continued drug use under control, much as societal norms regarding drunkenness keep most adults' drinking under control despite the legality and ubiquity of alcohol (99). Unfortunately, for most nonmedical opioid users, social networks tend to become increasingly narrow (179)—so even if selection of the right peer group can facilitate nonproblematic use of opioids, most nonmedical users may have difficulty finding such a peer group.

Specific Opioid-Associated Cues

General aspects of the environment affect individuals' overall propensities toward opioid use, abuse, and addiction. Specific opioid-associated cues seem to contribute to ongoing use, and to lapses and relapses, among established users. As described above, Wikler (184) theorized that environmental cues associated with past use of opioids (or with opportunities to obtain opioids) induce conditioned responses that can occur long after the last use of opioids, can include withdrawal symptoms and craving, and can play a role in relapse. Wikler's theory was based largely on anecdotal reports from users. Later laboratory work by Charles O'Brien and colleagues showed that signs and symptoms of opioid withdrawal could be induced in five of eight users by cues (an auditory tone and the odor of peppermint) that had been paired with a prior experience (187). The prior experience in this case was not opioid use, but naloxone-precipitated withdrawal. The clinical relevance of this phenomenon—exposure to cues associated with prior withdrawal—was not supported by opioid users' retrospective accounts of relapse, despite interviewers' specific probes (188). However, further work by Anna Rose Childress (in collaboration with O'Brien and Tom McLellan at the University of Pennsylvania) demonstrated that cues previously paired with opioid *use* could induce craving and "high-like feelings" as well as withdrawal symptoms and that each cue-induced response could occur independently of the others (189). The conditioned responses occurred in a variety of settings (laboratory, clinic, and home), but their exact precipitants and manifestations varied across users and across occasions. Childress and colleagues suggested that the variability of the responses hampers users' ability to recognize cue-elicited opioid seeking as a general phenomenon in daily life (189). The daily-life relevance of opioid cues was supported by findings from an ecological momentary assessment study by our group, in which opioid-dependent patients maintained on methadone reported on their heroin use and surroundings: the results showed a significant linear increase in cue-exposure reports in the 5 hours preceding episodes of heroin craving in daily life (190). The increase in cue-exposure reports was much less robust in the hours preceding episodes of actual use; our speculative explanation for this was that methadone maintenance partly decoupled craving from use (190).

If cue-elicited craving and withdrawal do contribute to relapse, it might seem encouraging to note that they can be extinguished in a laboratory setting (188,191). Unfortunately, efforts to parlay this finding into an extinction-based treatment have been thwarted by the failure of extinction to generalize outside the environment in which it occurs (192,193). In fact, the context-specific nature of extinction is the basis of an animal model of relapse (194).

COMPLICATIONS OF OPIOID USE AND COMORBID DISORDERS

History and Physical Examination in Patients with Opioid Use Disorders

History

Like all clinical medicine, evaluation and treatment of opioid use disorders requires the development of a therapeutic relationship based on trust and a two-way exchange of information. Patients with opioid use disorders should undergo all elements of a basic medical history (chief complaint, history of present illness, past medical history, medications, allergies, and review of systems). Additionally, special attention should be paid to the patient's social history; this should include a complete assessment of substance use and HIV risk factors (Table 13.1).

The medical history in patients with opioid use disorders should also include a screening for depression and anxiety and an assessment for personal safety in regard to both living situation and personal relationships.

Physical Examination

A complete physical examination is warranted in all patients with opioid use disorders. In addition to the standard elements, the physical examination should include special attention to signs and symptoms related to opioid use and its complications (Table 13.2).

Complications of Opioid Use

Chronic use of pure opioid analgesics does not produce frank signs of toxicity in any major bodily organ, though it may be immunosuppressant to a degree whose clinical significance is not clear (195). Nonetheless, chronic misuse of opioids usually has considerable medical sequelae, many of them attributable to the associated lifestyle and to the routes of administration employed.

Heroin is most often taken by sniffing, intravenous injection, or "skin popping" (subcutaneous injection); these routes are also sometimes used for other opioids (such as crushed OxyContin tablets). Each route of administration has accompanying complications (Table 13.3). Injection can result in the entry of organisms from the skin, injection works, or perhaps the drug itself (197) into the surrounding soft tissue and the bloodstream. This can result in a localized infection such as cellulitis, abscess, wound botulism, or necrotizing fasciitis. It can also result in more widespread systemic infection such as endocarditis and septic emboli. Injection drug users are more likely than nondrug users to be admitted to the hospital for infection (198). Treatment should be driven by culture and sensitivity of the offending organism, with incision and drainage or debridement as necessary. Of note, "classic" findings are not always evident

TABLE 13.1 Elements of a substance use and HIV risk factor assessment

Sexual practices
- Number of sexual partners
- Kinds of sexual contacts (one-time, anonymous, groups, exclusively with one partner, etc.)
- Type of sexual activity (receptive or insertive, vaginal or anal intercourse, oral–genital, oral–anal, manual–anal, etc.)
- Condom/barrier use and negotiation of safe-sex practices with partner
- Use of drugs or alcohol to enhance sexual encounters
- Sex in exchange for money, drugs, or shelter
- Sex with someone known or suspected to have HIV/AIDS
- History of sexually transmitted infections

Drug practices
- Drugs used
- Routes of drug administration (smoking, huffing, sniffing, injecting, etc.)
- Source of needles (pharmacy, needle exchange, street, shooting gallery, etc.)
- Sharing of needles, works, cottons, cookers, rinse water, or any other injection equipment
- Sharing of straws or other material to sniff drugs, etc.
- Cleaning injection equipment with bleach

Data from CDC Drug-Related HIV Risk and Preventive Behaviors (CDPB), version 4. US CDC HIV/STD Behavioral Surveillance Working Group (2001). Core Measures for HIV/STD Risk Behavior and Prevention: Questionnaire-Based Measurement for Surveys and Other Data Systems.

TABLE 13.2 Focused physical examination in patients with opioid-use disorders

Organ system/area examined	Signs/symptoms (and rationale)
General	- Height - Weight - Calculated BMI; assessment of nutritional status
Skin and soft tissues (include between toes, groin and genital area, etc.)	- Injection-site infections
Head, eyes, ears, nose, and throat	- Dental decay related to neglect and xerostomia - Erosion of nasal cavity and septum from sniffing drugs - Signs of opioid withdrawal—lacrimation, rhinorrhea
Cardiovascular	- Cardiac murmurs (concern for endocarditis)
Abdominal	- Liver examination (possible medication- or hepatitis-induced effects)
Lymphatic	- Cervical, axillary, supraclavicular, and inguinal lymphadenopathy
Laboratory	- Complete blood count - Chemistry panel, including liver function tests - Urinalysis - Fasting lipid profile

TABLE 13.3	Complications of injection drug use (intravenous and subcutaneous)
Cardiovascular	■ Arrhythmia
Endocrine	■ Impaired gonadotropin release ■ Impaired sperm motility ■ Menstrual irregularities
Gastrointestinal	■ Mechanical obstruction (due to concealment of drugs by "body packing")
General	■ Sleep disturbances
Infections (skin and soft tissue)	■ Cellulitis (usually staphylococci and streptococci) ■ Abscess (*Staphylococcus aureus*) ■ Necrotizing fasciitis ■ Septic thrombophlebitis ■ Gas gangrene ■ Pyomyositis ■ Localized Fournier gangrene ■ Botulism
Infections (other)	■ Septic emboli (to brain, spleen, heart, etc.) ■ Sexually transmitted infections (STIs) ■ HIV-related (Aspergillosis, etc.) ■ Hepatitis B and C ■ Endocarditis ■ Epidural or vertebral infection ■ Osteomyelitis ■ Meningitis ■ Mycotic aneurysms (subclavian, carotid, and pulmonary arteries) ■ Endophthalmitis ■ Septic arthritis (sternoclavicular, sacroiliac) ■ Tetanus (now rare due to childhood vaccination) ■ Malaria (foreign travel-related)
Neurologic	■ Peripheral neuropathies (compression, plexopathy, polyradiculopathy, mononeuropathy, etc.)
Respiratory	■ Bacterial pneumonia ■ Talc or starch granulomatosis ■ Pulmonary hypertension (granulomatous disease, vasoconstriction) ■ Pulmonary emphysema ■ Pneumothroax/hemothorax (large central vein injections) ■ Respiratory depression with pulmonary edema ■ Bronchospasm with pulmonary edema ■ Tuberculosis ■ HIV-related opportunistic infections (Nocardia, etc.)
Renal	■ HIV-related nephropathy (diffuse sclerosing glomerulonephritis) ■ Amyloidosis ■ Nephrotic syndrome (due to chronic skin infections) ■ Interstitial nephritis ■ Glomerulonephritis (from hepatitis C) ■ Rhabdomyolysis/acute renal failure ■ Factitious hematuria
Trauma	■ Gunshot wounds, stab wounds ■ Head injury (due to impaired coordination or risky situations)
Vascular	■ Arterial embolus injection and digital ischemia ■ Pseudoaneurysm ■ Venous valve damage (↑ risk of deep venous thrombosis (DVT), edema, ulcers) ■ Hemorrhagic cerebrovascular accident (CVA; coagulopathy from renal and liver disease) ■ Lymphedema

Data from Cherubin CE, Sapira JD. The medical complications of drug addiction and the medical assessment of the intravenous drug user: 25 years later. *Ann Intern Med.* 1993;119(10):1017–1028. (196)

in physical examination or laboratory tests of injection drug users, so providers should have a low threshold for initiating workup and treatment when otherwise clinically indicated.

Sniffing opioids can result in pulmonary complications including granulomatous responses, hemoptysis from airway irritation, and emphysema. There may also be nasal irritation, chronic sinusitis, and septal perforation.

As might be expected, overdose is a common adverse event among opioid misusers; it has been estimated that for every fatal overdose involving opioids, there are roughly 30 nonfatal ones (199). Most opioid misusers acknowledge having witnessed a nonfatal overdose, many acknowledge having witnessed a fatal one, and many also acknowledge having experienced a nonfatal overdose themselves (200,201). The mechanisms of overdose death are unclear (202); it has been argued that most such deaths involved synergistic effects of opioids and other drugs (203).

Because opioid misusers are often reluctant to summon help for peers who have overdosed in their presence, and because many also hold inaccurate beliefs about resuscitation methods (204), a case has been made for providing take-home naloxone with appropriate training for emergency use. Initial arguments against take-home naloxone included an anecdotal report of recreational "flatlining," a practice in which "one drug user stands guard with naloxone while another uses opiates in a dose that far exceeds tolerance" (205). This fear was not borne out in any of several subsequent pilot programs in several different cities (206–210). In one of the programs, bystander-administered naloxone was shown to be effective when administered as a nasal spray, eliminating the risks associated with injection (209).

Primary Care and Substance Use–Related Comorbidities

All patients with opioid use disorders should undergo the age-appropriate preventive health measures that are recommended for the general population (screening for breast, cervical, colon, and prostate cancer and for elevated cholesterol) as outlined by the United States Preventive Services Task Force. In addition, these patients should be screened for the following substance use–related comorbidities: hepatitis, HIV, sexually transmitted infections (STIs), and tuberculosis (TB). Treatment and management of comorbidities should be undertaken as indicated.

Hepatitis C Virus (HCV)

Hepatitis C is the most common bloodborne infection in the United States, with a prevalence of almost 2% (211). In some case series, HCV infection is seen in more than 80% of injection drug users (212,213). In HIV-infected injection drug users, the prevalence of HCV is 50% to 90% (214). HCV is primarily spread by contact with infected blood or blood products. In the United States, the main routes of transmission are blood transfusions and shared, unsterilized injection equipment.

All individuals with substance use disorders should be tested for HCV. The initial screening test is the anti-HCV enzyme immunoassay (EIA). False positives are possible, so confirmatory testing of positive EIAs should be performed for HCV RNA with polymerase chain reaction or transcription-medicated amplification. In immunocompromised individuals, anti-HCV EIA tests may produce false negatives due to lack of antibody production, so in these individuals, testing for HCV RNA is recommended if clinical suspicion is high (215).

Among individuals with chronic HCV, 50% report chronic fatigue and abdominal discomfort and over 40% have elevated serum transaminases either intermittently or persistently. Treatment of HCV in injection drug users should be based on individual risk-benefit assessments (216).

Other Hepatidides

Injection drug users have elevated rates of hepatitis A, and approximately 50% of injection drug users have serological evidence of exposure to hepatitis B. Individuals with opioid use disorders who test negative for hepatitis A and/or hepatitis B should be vaccinated against them.

HIV

Current guidelines from the Centers for Disease Control and Prevention (CDC) are that HIV screening should be performed routinely for all patients aged 13 to 64 years and that screening should be annual in patients at high risk for HIV infection, including patients with substance use disorders (217).

Rapid HIV tests have been FDA approved and facilitate early detection. These tests can detect antibodies in blood obtained by venipuncture or finger stick or in oral fluid in about 20 minutes. All positive HIV screening tests should be confirmed with supplemental HIV testing.

A study in our treatment-research clinic (218) is among many that have shown decreases in drug-related and sex-related risk behaviors during methadone maintenance treatment.

Sexually Transmitted Infections (STIs)

In a study by Sullivan and Fiellin (219), individuals who inject drugs were found to be at higher risk for STIs, probably due to increased involvement in trading sex for drugs and also due to the disinhibition caused by drug use. The authors recommended that all drug-injecting patients receive syphilis screening and that women and symptomatic men receive screening for gonorrhea and Chlamydia. CDC Guidelines for screening and treatment of STIs can be found at http://www.cdc.gov/std/treatment/2006/toc.htm.

Syphilis—Testing for syphilis is done with the rapid plasma reagin test or the Venereal Disease Research Laboratory (VDRL) test. However, these tests are often falsely positive in injection drug users due to increased immune activation and should therefore be confirmed by a treponemal test (fluorescent treponemal antibody test, FTA-Abs) or microhemagglutination test. Positive syphilis tests need to be followed by patient education and appropriate antibiotic treatment (http://www.cdc.gov/std/syphilis/default.htm).

Gonorrhea and Chlamydia—*Neisseria gonorrhoeae* and *Chlamydia trachomatis* can be detected with a urethral culture in men, a cervical culture in women, or urine testing in either (first 10 to 30 mL for nucleic acid amplification test). Testing should be done annually in all sexually active patients, and more often as indicated in high-risk patients such as injection drug users (220). Positive results are a marker for high-risk behavior and warrant-enhanced counseling, treatment, and contact tracing (http://www.cdc.gov/std/chlamydia/default.htm and http://www.cdc.gov/std/Gonorrhea/default.htm).

Tuberculosis (TB)

Rates of TB are high in injection drug users (221) and the emergence of multidrug resistant strains is rising. Patients with opioid use disorders should be screened for TB annually with a purified protein derivative (PPD) skin test. Known or suspected cases of active TB must be reported to the U.S. Public Health Service, and state and federal laws require follow-up and treatment in individuals with known exposure to an active TB case. A positive PPD test (>10 mm in general population and >5 mm in HIV positive individuals) requires follow-up with a chest radiograph. Providers should be aware of the signs and symptoms of TB including fever, weight loss, fatigue, night sweats, and persistent cough, and should be prepared to follow up, assess, and manage as appropriate. Complete guidelines for TB screening, classification, and management are available from the CDC (http://www.cdc.gov/tb/).

Other Medical Comorbidities

In a cross-sectional study of substance-dependent patients without primary care, De Alba and colleagues (220) found that such patients had a significantly lower mean score on the physical component summary from the short-form health survey (SF-36) than the U.S. general-population norm (44.1 vs. 50, $p < 0.001$). Furthermore, 47% of study participants reported at least one chronic medical condition, 20% reported two or more, and 35% had had an episodic medical condition in the last 6 months. Eighty percent of study participants had been hospitalized for medical reasons one or more times (mean 3.9 times per patient), 21% were being prescribed medications for a chronic medical illness, and 61% had experienced a medical problem in the last 30 days.

In a study of methadone-maintained patients over the age of 50, 58% of respondents reported fair to poor physical health, with high rates of past-year health problems, including arthritis (54%), hypertension (45%), heart conditions (18%), chronic lung conditions (22%), stomach ulcers or irritable bowel syndrome (21%), cirrhosis (14%), hepatitis C (49%), diabetes (11%), and tobacco use (87%) (223). Heroin use has also been shown to be independently associated with greater insulin resistance, and methadone maintenance has been shown to be independently associated with previously diagnosed diabetes (224).

These findings show that the opioid abusers develop chronic medical comorbidities much like those of the general population in addition to more specific comorbidities. Management and treatment of these chronic medical comorbidities should be addressed in the primary-care setting and, if possible, incorporated into substance-abuse treatment.

Polysubstance Use

Polysubstance use is common in patients with opioid use disorders. For example, at the most recent time point in a 33-year longitudinal study of heroin-dependent individuals, past-year prevalence of drug use was 67% for tobacco, 22% for daily alcohol, 36% for marijuana, 19% for cocaine, 10% for crack, and 12% for amphetamines. Even in the subset of individuals who had been heroin-abstinent for 5 or more years, past-year prevalences were 50% for tobacco, 15% for daily alcohol, 25% for marijuana, 4% for cocaine, 3% for crack, and 4% for amphetamines (115). Issues concerning these drugs are addressed more completely in the other chapters of Section 4 in this book.

In patients with polysubstance use disorders, assessment of medical complications needs to include consideration of each substance and of possible interactions. Special attention should be paid to use of alcohol and sedative-hypnotics such as benzodiazepines or barbiturates: these substances are sometimes used by opioid abusers in an effort to minimize opioid withdrawal or enhance a high (225). In addition to presenting more serious withdrawal complications than opioids do, they can synergistically exacerbate the respiratory depression and sedation induced by opioids.

Co-occurring Disorders (CODs)

"Co-occurring disorders" (CODs) refers to the co-occurrence of substance use disorders with mental-health disorders. CODs are common: among adults aged 18 or older in the United States, an estimated 5.4 million have a co-occurring serious psychological disorder and substance use disorder (107). CODs also entail elevated medical risks: when compared to individuals with only one or the other type of disorder, individuals with CODs had the highest adjusted odds for heart disease, asthma, gastrointestinal disorders, skin infections, and acute respiratory disorders (226). Additionally, individuals with COD have higher rates of hospitalization and inefficient use of health care services (227). For a detailed discussion of CODs, see Section 7 of this book.

EVALUATION APPROACHES

Overview of Screening and Evaluation

In January 2008, the United States Preventive Services Task Force concluded that there are reliable and valid standardized questionnaires for screening the use and misuse of illicit drugs, but also warned that there is not yet sufficient evidence to assess the "balance of benefits and harms" associated with such screening, whether in adolescents, pregnant women, or a general population of adults. Nonetheless, some of these questionnaires are widely used in primary-care settings (228).

There is no standard tool for the evaluation of candidates for opioid-addiction treatment. A consensus panel convened by the Center for Substance Abuse Treatment had recommended that treatment programs develop their own tools and methods for assessment based on their patient population and their own infrastructure (225). We will review some of the available tools.

Tools for Screening and Evaluation

Addiction Severity Index (ASI)

The fifth edition of the Addiction Severity Index (ASI) is a 161-item multidimensional clinical and research instrument administered as a semistructured face-to-face interview. It addresses two timeframes—lifetime and past 30 days—and assesses functioning in seven domains: Medical, Employment/Support Status, Alcohol, Drug, Legal, Family/Social, and Psychological. The ASI is designed to provide basic diagnostic information on an individual before, during, and after treatment for substance use–related problems, and is thus useful for assessment of treatment outcome (229). The numeric summary data generated by the ASI—the composite scores and especially the interviewer severity ratings—have been criticized in terms of their reliability, validity, and suitability for clinical decision making (230); examination of individual items from the ASI may be of greater value.

Drug Abuse Screening Test (DAST)

The DAST is a 28-question self-report measure used to screen and evaluate individuals in both clinical and research settings. Each question is dichotomous (yes/no) and valued at one point, resulting in a score from 0 to 28. A cutoff of 6 is generally used to indicate drug abuse or dependence (231). The DAST has been found to have moderate-to-high levels of test–retest, interitem, and item-total reliabilities, moderate-to-high sensitivity and specificity, and acceptable criterion, construct, and discriminative validity (232).

ICD-10 Symptom Checklist for Mental Disorders

ICD-10 Symptom Checklist for Mental Disorders Psychoactive Substance Use Syndromes Module is a 10-question instrument that asks about symptoms associated with heroin or other opioid use in the time period immediately before admission to current treatment. The symptom list corresponds to the ICD-10 criteria for substance dependence or harmful use (233).

NIDA-Modified ASSIST

The NIDA-Modified ASSIST (Alcohol, Smoking and Substance Involvement Screening Test) was introduced in April of 2009 as part of NIDAMED, a collection of research-based screening tools and resources (available at: http://www.drugabuse.gov/NIDAMED). The package also includes a reference guide and a resource guide for clinicians. The NIDA-Modified ASSIST is based on the World Health Organization ASSIST, Version 3.0 (available at: http://www.wo.int/substance_abuse/activitiea/assist_v3_english.pdf) that has been shown to have good concurrent, discriminative, and construct validity (234).

Severity of Dependence Scale (SDS)

The SDS is a 5-item questionnaire that takes less than a minute to complete. Each question is scored on a 4-point scale (0–3); the total score is an opioid dependence severity score (the higher the score, the higher the level of dependence). The SDS has been shown to satisfy several criteria for reliability and criterion validity (235).

TREATMENT APPROACHES

Overview of Treatment Approaches

Opioid addiction, like all addiction, is considered a chronic relapsing disorder, and as such, its treatment is a long-term process. Detoxification (the management of opioid-withdrawal symptoms that occur when an individual discontinues use) addresses the "physical" component of addiction (we use quotation marks here to avoid suggesting that psychological factors have no physical basis) and can be an initial step in treatment. However, detoxification should be followed by long-term treatment to address the full syndrome of addiction. Maintenance therapy, when administered correctly, addresses the full syndrome by providing long-term opioid replacement and supportive psychosocial treatments. Combining several treatment modalities is more effective than giving stand-alone treatment, but no specific combination has been shown to be superior to all other possible combinations, so treatment approaches should be individualized based on the patient's needs. The best approach is the one that works for that particular patient at that particular time. Of paramount importance is respecting that abstinence is achieved in different ways by different individuals (96,236).

Detoxification

The goal of detoxification is safe management of withdrawal symptoms while the patient adjusts to an opioid-free state. Gerstein and colleagues (237) demonstrated that repeated detoxifications in the absence of subsequent treatment are neither cost-effective nor helpful. This is because detoxification addresses only the acute physiological effects of opioid withdrawal, not the emotional, cognitive, behavioral, and social aspects of recovery. Detoxification in and of itself does not constitute treatment for opioid dependence (238–240). Rather, it should be considered a precursor to treatment, or a first stage of treatment, and should be followed by formal assessment and referral (241).

Detoxification has high utilization rates because it is quick and comparatively inexpensive, qualities that appeal to patients and third-party payers alike. Detoxification can occur in several settings and with various approaches. Some individuals attempt detoxification on their own without specialized treatment assistance. Self-detoxification methods include abrupt cessation of opioids (going "cold turkey"), detoxification with benzodiazepines, detoxification with opioids, avoidance, and distraction—and all of these methods have low success rates (118). Detoxification with assistance can occur in inpatient settings (either psychiatric or medical), residential settings, or outpatient settings (such as substance-abuse clinics, primary-care offices, and prisons). Use of detoxification programs is associated with increased rates of initiation of long-term treatment for addiction (including methadone maintenance and other forms of addiction treatment) (242).

Traditional Detoxification Methods

Traditionally, opioid detoxification consisted of a methadone taper. This method has been criticized by providers and patients alike for the long duration of withdrawal symptoms associated with it. The method has been improved with the use of adjunctive medications for symptomatic relief; these include alpha-2 adrenergic agonists such as clonidine and lofexidine. An alternative to methadone-assisted detoxification emerged when the FDA approved buprenorphine for the same indication ("medically supervised withdrawal"). Buprenorphine tapers over 7 days appear to be safe and well-tolerated (243).

Comparison of Traditional Detoxification Methods

Methadone and buprenorphine have been shown to be comparable in suppressing signs and symptoms of opioid withdrawal and in their adverse-event profiles and rates of treatment completion (244,245). In a systematic review comparing buprenorphine to clonidine, buprenorphine was found more effective in decreasing signs and symptoms and was associated with greater treatment retention and fewer adverse events (245). When given as a stand-alone treatment for opioid withdrawal, clonidine provides considerably less reduction of subjective symptoms than of autonomic signs (246); given that the problematic aspect of opioid withdrawal is the distress associated with symptoms rather than any medical risk associated with autonomic signs, clonidine is probably best used as an adjunct to a methadone-assisted or buprenorphine-assisted taper.

Detoxification under Anesthesia

For approximately 20 years, detoxification under anesthesia has been advertised as a quick and painless way of opioid withdrawal. However, this approach is expensive, generally not covered by insurance, carries significant medical risks, and lacks evidence of effectiveness. Collins et al. (247) conducted a randomized controlled trial of 106 treatment-seeking heroin-dependent patients comparing three detoxification methods: anesthesia-assisted rapid opioid de-toxification with naltrexone induction, buprenorphine-assisted rapid opioid detoxification with naltrexone induction, and clonidine-assisted opioid detoxification with delayed naltrexone induction. Results showed that mean withdrawal-severity scores, rates of inpatient detoxification completion, and treatment retention over 12 weeks were comparable across the three treatments—but that in the anesthesia group, there were three potentially life-threatening adverse events not seen in the other two groups. The authors concluded that the anesthesia procedure conveys "no benefit ... over a safer, cheaper, and potentially outpatient alternative using buprenorphine as a bridge to naltrexone treatment" and that "general anesthesia for rapid antagonist induction does not currently have a meaningful role to play in the treatment of opioid dependence."

Detoxification and Coordination of Care

Chutuape and colleagues (248) found that after a 3-day hospital-based inpatient detoxification, patients had significant decreases in drug use and drug-related activities over three follow-up evaluations (1, 3, and 6 months). There was a significant decrease in mean days of use of heroin, cocaine, alcohol, and multiple drugs in the last 30 days, and a decline in the percentages of opioid-positive and cocaine-positive urines. At the three follow-ups, 15% to 24% of patients reported current enrollment in treatment; their self-reported days of heroin and alcohol use, and their percentages of opioid-positive and cocaine-positive urines, were significantly lower than those of the patients who were not in treatment. This and other studies highlight that detoxification is most successful when followed by additional treatment. Efforts to coordinate aftercare following detoxification are of paramount importance.

Maintenance

Maintenance combines pharmacologic therapy with psychosocial interventions and support services and has the greatest likelihood of success in most patients. The pharmacological therapies include methadone, buprenorphine, and naltrexone and are described more fully in Section 6 of this book.

Methadone Maintenance

Methadone is a long-acting synthetic opioid that blocks the effects of heroin and other opioids by binding with mu receptors found in the brain and periphery. It is dispensed as an oral solution, liquid concentrate, tablet/diskette, or powder. Treatment with methadone is usually conducted in specialized settings (e.g., methadone-maintenance clinics). The goal of methadone maintenance is to find a methadone dose that balances positive effects (such as preventing opioid withdrawal and decreasing heroin use and craving) with possible negative effects (such as constipation and sedation). Determination of the appropriate methadone dose is patient-specific. Like most medications, methadone requires especially careful monitoring and dosage adjustment in patients who are taking other medications or who have other chronic medical conditions (249).

LAAM (Levo-Alpha Acetyl Methadol) Maintenance

LAAM is a full mu-opioid agonist that, like methadone, blocks the euphoric effect of opioids while controlling opioid craving. When it was in clinical use, it was dispensed as an oral solution that was noted for its long duration of action, suppressing opioid-withdrawal symptoms for up to 72 hours (250). However, due to reported LAAM-related disturbances in cardiac function, Roxane Laboratories withdrew LAAM from the U.S. market in 2004 (251).

Buprenorphine Maintenance

Buprenorphine received FDA approval for the treatment of opioid addiction in October 2002. Buprenorphine has two sublingual formulations: one with buprenorphine alone and another that is a combination of buprenorphine and naloxone; the addition of naloxone is intended to deter abuse by injection but to be of no consequence when the medication is taken sublingually. In maintenance treatment, buprenorphine is as effective as, but no more effective than, methadone; however, it may be better tolerated than methadone or clonidine in detoxification (252). From a legal standpoint in the United States, buprenorphine differs from methadone in that it can be prescribed in a specially licensed physician's private office rather than only in a counselor-staffed addiction-treatment clinic.

Abuse rates for buprenorphine in the United States are low. Smith et al. (253) counted abuse cases of sublingual buprenorphine and sublingual buprenorphine/naloxone in 18 regional poison-control centers for 2003 to 2005 and found 77 reported cases, an average quarterly ratio of abuse cases per 1000 prescriptions dispensed of 0.08 (SD ±0.09) for buprenorphine and 0.16 (SD ±0.08) for buprenorphine/naloxone.

Naltrexone Maintenance

Naltrexone is a pure opioid antagonist that comes in an oral tablet and was approved for opioid dependence treatment by the FDA in 1984. Naltrexone has a higher affinity for mu receptors than heroin, morphine, or methadone and will displace these drugs from the receptors, blocking their effects. This action precipitates withdrawal symptoms in individuals who have not been abstinent from short-acting opioids for 7 days and longer-acting ones for at least 10 days (254). Naltrexone has no abuse potential and produces no withdrawal symptoms when discontinued. The main barrier to its effectiveness as a maintenance treatment is poor adherence by patients (148).

Heroin Maintenance

Heroin maintenance is the provision of prescribed heroin as a harm-reduction mechanism to chronic heroin-dependent individuals who have failed other treatments. In a 2006 systematic review of four randomized controlled trials of heroin maintenance, the findings were inconclusive in regards to retention in treatment, relapse to street-heroin use, criminal activities, and social functioning, due to the heterogeneity of interventions and measures (255). A multisite randomized trial in Canada was substantially compromised by political and regulatory barriers (256). Nonetheless, the results from that trial showed that heroin maintenance produced better outcomes than methadone maintenance in terms of nondrug criminal behavior, employment, family and social relationships, and medical and psychiatric status (257). This finding is surprising considering that oral methadone requires less frequent dosing than intravenous heroin and is far less likely to produce acute intoxication. However, the trial was conducted in patients for whom at least two prior attempts at treatment (including at least one attempt at methadone maintenance) had been unsuccessful; heroin maintenance may be indicated in such cases.

Other Pharmacological Approaches

Montoya and Vocci (258) reviewed novel antiaddiction medications, including new formulations of already FDA-approved medications such as buprenorphine and naltrexone, off-label uses of FDA-approved medications such as clonidine and tramadol, and not-yet-FDA-approved medications such as antagonists at N-methyl-D-aspartic acid (NMDA) receptors or corticotropin-releasing hormone (CRH) receptors.

Long-acting formulations of buprenorphine, such as subcutaneous depot injections, provide effective buprenorphine delivery for several weeks, with therapeutic effects persisting even at fairly low plasma concentrations of buprenorphine (259). Sustained-release injectable formulations of naltrexone are also being studied and are showing promise in regard to treatment retention and prolonged opioid abstinence (260). Also under study is an implant formulation of naltrexone; individuals given a naltrexone implant in a Norwegian study had naltrexone blood levels above 1 ng/mL for at least 6 months and less heroin and opioid use than controls, with a low rate of adverse events (261).

The alpha-2 adrenergic agonists lofexidine and clonidine are not FDA-approved as treatments for opioid withdrawal but have been shown to be effective (262). The mixed-action opioid tramadol produces some suppression of withdrawal symptoms, but further studies are needed to determine what role, if any, it might play in treatment (263).

NMDA-receptor antagonists such as memantine, ketamine, dextromethorphan, and phencyclidine have been shown in laboratory-animal studies to suppress the development of tolerance and dependence to the analgesic effects of morphine, and may be useful in treating opioid craving in humans (264). Antagonists at receptors for CRH have been shown in animal models to lessen opioid withdrawal (265), block withdrawal-induced conditioned place aversion (266), and prevent stress-induced reinstatement of opioid seeking (267); thus, they may have a role in treatment.

Another treatment approach being tested is the use of oral naltrexone at ultralow doses for a seemingly para-doxical effect: although naltrexone is an antagonist, ultralow doses eased withdrawal symptoms during a methadone-assisted taper (268), perhaps by preventing or counteracting some of the receptor changes associated with chronic agonist use.

Vaccines

Immunotherapies are appealing for their lack of addiction liability, minimal side effects, and potential for long-lasting protection against drug use (269). Immunotherapies can also potentially be combined with existing pharmacological interventions and behavioral therapies for a multipronged approach to addiction treatment. Vaccines against morphine were first created and tested in the early 1970s (270), around the same time that methadone maintenance was becoming more widespread. In the developing world, where methadone treatment is expensive and often not well accepted, there has been a recent resurgence of interest in vaccine development (271).

Anton and Leff (272) described the initial development of a bivalent vaccine against morphine/heroin. The vaccine produced a high-titer antibody response with equivalent specificities for heroin and morphine but not other opioids. In an animal self-administration model, vaccinated rats developed antibodies against heroin that blocked its reinforcing effects. To date, research with this vaccine has been conducted in rodents and rhesus macaques, but not in humans. Even a successful antidrug vaccine will not be sufficient as a stand-alone treatment for addiction, because it will not address the problems that initially led to the addiction, nor the problems that resulted from the addiction.

Behavioral Therapies

Behavioral therapies encourage cessation of opioid use and teach patients to function without drugs, handle cravings, avoid drug-using people and drug-associated places, and cope with lapses and relapses. They are most effective when used in conjunction with pharmacological treatments, but when this is not possible, they are also effective alone. Behavioral treatment can be delivered in both residential and outpatient settings and may include individual counseling, group or family counseling, contingency management, and cognitive-behavioral therapies, among others. Below is a quick overview of a few behavioral therapies utilized in the treatment of opioid addiction; more detail is provided in Section 6 of this book.

Contingency Management

Contingency management—that is, clinician control of the contingencies (consequences) associated with patients' behaviors—is typically implemented as a voucher-based approach in which patients earn credit for achieving treatment goals. These goals could be opioid-negative urine-toxicology results, meeting goals for clinic attendance or counseling attendance, attending job training, and so on. The earned vouchers can be exchanged for goods and services in the community consistent with treatment goals. The goods and services might include workplace-appropriate clothes, bus passes, payment of utility bills, a down payment on a car, or a security deposit for an apartment. Much of the clinical research underlying contingency management for treatment of opioid dependence was performed with patients maintained on opioid agonists, and the results have shown that contingency management has an important place in treatment of opioid addiction, although barriers involving cost and social acceptance need to be surmounted (273).

Cognitive-Behavioral Therapy (CBT)

In CBT, the patient and counselor work to identify problems related to drug use and practice coping skills to modify drug use behaviors. Specific techniques include exploring the positive and negative consequences of continued use, self-monitoring to recognize drug cravings early on and to identify high-risk situations for use, and developing strategies for avoiding or coping with high-risk situations and the desire to use (274). In cocaine addicts, the benefits of CBT have been shown to emerge months after completion of treat-ment (275).

Needle Exchange

Access to needle-exchange programs (NEPs) in the United States is inadequate. Wodak and Cooney (276) conducted an international review of the literature and concluded that NEPs are both clinically effective and cost-effective in reducing HIV, and that there is no convincing evidence for unintended negative consequences (e.g., increases in the initiation, duration, or frequency of illicit drug use or injection). Furthermore, there is evidence that NEPs might increase entry into drug-treatment programs and contact with primary health care (277). Given the evidence, NEPs should be seen as an important component of an evidence-based approach to reducing the spread of HIV and other bloodborne infections.

Access to Treatment

Methadone maintenance, which is available only through highly regulated methadone clinics, reaches only an estimated 15% to 20% of the people needing treatment for opioid addiction (225). The Drug Addiction Treatment Act of 2000, signed into law by President Clinton, eased access to treatment by legalizing office-based opioid maintenance treatment by physicians in private practice (278).

In 2008, the Paul Wellstone and Pete Domenici Mental Health Parity and Addiction Equity Act was passed by Congress and signed into law by President George W. Bush. This law is intended to improve access to treatment for behavioral and psychiatric problems, including addiction, by prohibiting treatment limits and other discriminatory restrictions.

Linkage of Care

Despite the high prevalence of comorbidities in individuals with opioid use disorders, treatment for comorbid conditions often occurs in an uncoordinated, parallel fashion. This parallel approach interferes with communication between the players in what should be a multidisciplinary collaboration (279). The resultant fragmentation of care may result in premature treatment termination, relapse, criminal involvement, and preventable use of high-cost resources such as EDs and inpatient admissions (280,281).

A 2005 report from the Institute of Medicine advocated coordination of care among primary-care providers, mental-health specialists, and addiction specialists. Such coordination, which should emphasize a patient-centered approach, can occur on a spectrum from straightforward formal agreements among providers to clinically integrated practices (282).

Linking substance-abuse care and primary care has many benefits, such as broadening access to both types of care, reducing the stigma associated with addiction medicine among some medical providers, and creating support for reimbursement parity for substance-abuse services (279). To some degree, linkage can also reduce health care costs by increasing efficiency. For example, on-site delivery of primary care reduced use of EDs and hospitals among methadone-maintenance patients and long-term residential-facility patients (though not among nonmethadone patients) (283). Off-site referral for primary care reduced use of EDs (though not hospitalizations) in long-term residential patients (283).

Reimbursement for Treatment

In January 2008, two new American Medical Association Current Procedural Terminology codes for screening and brief intervention (99408 and 99409) went into effect. These codes afford health care providers a mechanism to report and receive reimbursement for structured screening and brief intervention for substance use disorders (http://www.whitehousedrugpolicy.gov/dfc/files/sbi_codes.pdf).

CONCLUSIONS

Opioids, and the use and misuse of opioids, are more complex than they might seem. For example, as we have discussed, opioids that could once be mentioned in the same breath as mu-preferring analgesics with differing pharmacokinetics (morphine, heroin, oxycodone, methadone) might act quite differently from each other at different mu-receptor variants, with behaviorally and therapeutically significant consequences. Newly selective agonists may disaggregate aspects of opioid-induced analgesia (for example, delta agonists may relieve allodynia without producing more general analgesia). New types of mixed or bivalent ligands, or new ways of administering antagonists (such as ultralow-dose regimens with seemingly paradoxical effects), may open new possibilities for prevention or treatment of physical dependence. At the same time, physical dependence is increasingly understood not to be the defining feature of opioid addiction. And opioid addiction, given use, is increasingly understood to be determined in large part by cognitive and sociocultural factors, despite lore that emphasizes the irresistibility of intoxication and the hellishness of withdrawal.

These insights have emerged from disciplines as remote from each other as ethnography and molecular biology, as well as the behavioral sciences that in some respects bridge the two. Continued work in all of those disciplines should increase the proportion of good outcomes from therapeutic use of opioids, and should also expand the already good range of treatments available for opioid use disorders. One important challenge is to ensure that these treatments, most of which were developed in the context of heroin addiction, are applied effectively to the growing problem of addiction to prescription opioids.

ACKNOWLEDGEMENTS

This review was supported by the Intramural Research Program (IRP) of the National Institute on Drug Abuse (NIDA), National Institutes of Health.

REFERENCES

1. Jaffe JH, Martin WR. Opioid analgesics and antagonists. In: Gilman AG, Rall TW, Nies AS, eds. *The Pharmacological Basis of Therapeutics.* 8th ed. New York: Pergamon Press; 1991.
2. Martin WR. Strong analgesics. In: Root WS, Hofmann FG, eds. *Physiol Pharmacol.* New York: Academic Press; 1963:275–305.
3. Cox BM, Borsodi A, Caló G, et al. Opioid receptors, IUPHAR database (IUPHAR-DB). 2009. Available at: http://www.iuphar-db.org/GPCR/ChapterMenuForward?chapterID=1295. Accessed June 2, 2009.
4. Shippenberg TS, LeFevour A, Chefer VI. Targeting endogenous mu- and delta-opioid receptor systems for the treatment of drug addiction. *CNS Neurol Disord Drug Targets.* 2008;7(5):442–453.
5. Matthes HW, Maldonado R, Simonin F, et al. Loss of morphine-induced analgesia, reward effect and withdrawal symptoms in mice lacking the mu-opioid-receptor gene. *Nature.* 1996; 383(6603):819–823.
6. Sora I, Takahashi N, Funada M, et al. Opiate receptor knockout mice define mu receptor roles in endogenous nociceptive responses and morphine-induced analgesia. *Proc Natl Acad Sci USA.* 1997;94(4):1544–1549.
7. Jutkiewicz EM, Baladi MG, Folk JE, et al. The convulsive and electroencephalographic changes produced by nonpeptidic delta-opioid agonists in rats: comparison with pentylenetetrazol. *J Pharmacol Exp Ther.* 2006;317(3):1337–1348.
8. Ananthan S. Opioid ligands with mixed mu/delta opioid receptor interactions: an emerging approach to novel analgesics. *AAPS J.* 2006;8(1):E118–E125.
9. Codd EE, Carson JR, Colburn RW, et al. JNJ-20788560 [9-(8-azabicyclo[3.2.1]oct-3-ylidene)-9H-xanthene-3-carboxylic acid diethylamide], a selective delta opioid receptor agonist, is a potent and efficacious antihyperalgesic agent that does not produce respiratory depression, pharmacologic tolerance, or physical dependence. *J Pharmacol Exp Ther.* 2009;329(1):241–251.
10. Bie B, Zhu W, Pan ZZ. Rewarding morphine-induced synaptic function of delta-opioid receptors on central glutamate synapses. *J Pharmacol Exp Ther.* 2009;329(1):290–296.
11. Chefer VI, Shippenberg TS. Augmentation of morphine-induced sensitization but reduction in morphine tolerance and reward in delta-opioid receptor knockout mice. *Neuropsychopharmacology.* 2009;34(4):887–898.
12. Daniels DJ, Lenard NR, Etienne CL, et al. Opioid-induced tolerance and dependence in mice is modulated by the distance between pharmacophores in a bivalent ligand series. *Proc Natl Acad Sci USA.* 2005;102(52):19208–19213.
13. Lenard NR, Daniels DJ, Portoghese PS, et al. Absence of conditioned place preference or reinstatement with bivalent

ligands containing mu-opioid receptor agonist and delta-opioid receptor antagonist pharmacophores. *Eur J Pharmacol.* 2007; 566(1-3):75–82.
14. Chavkin C, James IF, Goldstein A. Dynorphin is a specific endogenous ligand of the kappa opioid receptor. *Science.* 1982; 215(4531):413–415.
15. Shippenberg TS, Zapata A, Chefer VI. Dynorphin and the pathophysiology of drug addiction. *Pharmacol Ther.* 2007; 116(2):306–321.
16. Pfeiffer A, Brantl V, Herz A, et al. Psychotomimesis mediated by kappa opiate receptors. *Science.* 1986;233(4765):774–776.
17. Leander JD. A kappa opioid effect: increased urination in the rat. *J Pharmacol Exp Ther.* 1983;224(1):89–94.
18. Shippenberg TS. The dynorphin/kappa opioid receptor system: a new target for the treatment of addiction and affective disorders? *Neuropsychopharmacology.* 2009;34(1):247.
19. Montoya ID, Gorelick DA, Preston KL, et al. Randomized trial of buprenorphine for treatment of concurrent opiate and cocaine dependence. *Clin Pharmacol Ther.* 2004;75(1):34–48.
20. Vigezzi P, Guglielmino L, Marzorati P, et al. Multimodal drug addiction treatment: a field comparison of methadone and buprenorphine among heroin- and cocaine-dependent patients. *J Subst Abuse Treat.* 2006;31(1):3–7.
21. Peng X, Neumeyer JL. Kappa receptor bivalent ligands. *Curr Top Med Chem.* 2007;7(4):363–373.
22. Meunier JC, Mollereau C, Toll L, et al. Isolation and structure of the endogenous agonist of opioid receptor-like ORL1 receptor. *Nature.* 1995;377(6549):532–535.
23. Kotlinska J, Wichmann J, Legowska A, et al. Orphanin FQ/nociceptin but not Ro 65-6570 inhibits the expression of cocaine-induced conditioned place preference. *Behav Pharmacol.* 2002; 13(3):229–235.
24. Lutfy K, Khaliq I, Carroll FI, et al. Orphanin FQ/nociceptin blocks cocaine-induced behavioral sensitization in rats. *Psychopharmacology.* 2002;164(2):168–176.
25. Ciccocioppo R, Economidou D, Rimondini R, et al. Buprenorphine reduces alcohol drinking through activation of the nociceptin/orphanin FQ-NOP receptor system. *Biol Psychiatry.* 2007; 61(1):4–12.
26. Spagnolo B, Calo G, Polgar WE, et al. Activities of mixed NOP and mu-opioid receptor ligands. *Br J Pharmacol.* 2008;153(3):609–619.
27. Portoghese PS. A new concept on the mode of interaction of narcotic analgesics with receptors. *J Med Chem.* 1965;8(5):609–616.
28. Martin WR. Opioid antagonists. *Pharmacol Rev.* 1967;19(4): 463–521.
29. Martin WR, Fraser HF. A comparative study of physiological and subjective effects of heroin and morphine administered intravenously in postaddicts. *J Pharmacol Exp Ther.* 1961;133:388–399.
30. Pasternak GW. Molecular biology of opioid analgesia. *J Pain Symptom Manage.* 2005;29(suppl 5):S2–S9.
31. Cherny N, Ripamonti C, Pereira J, et al. Strategies to manage the adverse effects of oral morphine: an evidence-based report. *J Clin Oncol.* 2001;19(9):2542–2554.
32. Smith MT. Differences between and combinations of opioids re-visited. *Curr Opin Anaesthesiol.* 2008;21(5):596–601.
33. Pan L, Xu J, Yu R, et al. Identification and characterization of six new alternatively spliced variants of the human mu opioid receptor gene, Oprm. *Neuroscience.* 2005;133(1):209–220.
34. Pan YX, Xu J, Xu M, et al. Involvement of exon 11-associated variants of the mu opioid receptor MOR-1 in heroin, but not morphine, actions. *Proc Natl Acad Sci USA.* 2009;106(12):4917–4922.
35. Simmons MA. Let's go rafting: ligand functional selectivity may depend on membrane structure. *Mol Interv.* 2008;8(6): 281–283.
36. Koch T, Hollt V. Role of receptor internalization in opioid tolerance and dependence. *Pharmacol Ther.* 2008;117(2):199–206.
37. Virk MS, Williams JT. Agonist-specific regulation of mu-opioid receptor desensitization and recovery from desensitization. *Mol Pharmacol.* 2008;73(4):1301–1308.
38. Abbadie C, Pasternak GW, Aicher SA. Presynaptic localization of the carboxy-terminus epitopes of the mu opioid receptor splice variants MOR-1C and MOR-1D in the superficial laminae of the rat spinal cord. *Neuroscience.* 2001;106(4):833–842.
39. Brownstein MJ. A brief history of opiates, opioid peptides, and opioid receptors. *Proc Natl Acad Sci USA.* 1993;90(12):5391–5393.
40. Brunton TL. On the use of codeine to relieve pain in abdominal disease. *BMJ.* 1888;1(1432):1213–1214.
41. Sneader W. The discovery of heroin. *Lancet.* 1998;352(9141): 1697–1699.
42. de Ridder M. Heroin: new facts about an old myth. *J Psychoactive Drugs.* 1994;26(1):65–68.
43. Faupel CE, Horowitz AM, Weaver GS. *The Sociology of American Drug Use.* New York: McGraw-Hill; 2004.
44. Phillips J. Prevalence of the heroin habit: especially the use of the drug by "snuffing". *JAMA.* 1912;59(24):2146–2147.
45. Musto DF. America's first cocaine epidemic. *Wilson Q.* 1989; 13(3):59–64.
46. The war against cocaine. *Chicago Tribune.* April 18, 1910:8. Available at: http://pqasb.pqarchiver.com/chicagotribune/access/387308641.html?dids=387308641:387308641&FMT=CITE&FMTS=CITE:AI&date=Apr+18%2C+1910. Accessed June 30, 2009.
47. Say drug habit grips the nation. *New York Times.* December 5, 1913:8. Available at: http://query.nytimes.com/gst/abstract.html?res=9F01E5DD173DE633A25756C0A9649D946296D6CF. Accessed June 30, 2009.
48. Acker CJ. *Creating the American Junkie: Addiction Research in the Classic Era of Narcotic Control.* Baltimore: Johns Hopkins University Press; 2002.
49. Addiction Research Center. *Annotated Bibliography of Papers from the Addiction Research Center 1935-1975.* Rockville, MD: US Department of Health, Education, and Welfare; 1978.
50. Campbell ND. *Discovering Addiction: The Science and Politics of Substance Abuse Research.* Ann Arbor: University of Michigan Press, 2007.
51. Wikler A. A psychodynamic study of a patient during experimental self-regulated re-addiction to morphine. *Psychiatr Q.* 1952;26(2):270–293.
52. Wikler A, Rasor RW. Psychiatric aspects of drug addiction. *Am J Med.* 1953;14(5):566–570.
53. Wikler A. On the nature of addiction and habituation. *Addiction.* 1961;57(2):73–79.
54. Wikler A. Dynamics of drug dependence: implications of a conditioning theory for research and treatment. *Arch Gen Psychiatry.* 1973;28(5):611–616.
55. Isbell H. Medical aspects of opiate addiction. *Bull NY Acad Med.* 1955;31(12):886–901.
56. Isbell H, Wikler A, Eddy NB, et al. Tolerance and addiction liability of 6-dimethylamino-4-4-diphenylheptanone-3 (methadon). *JAMA.* 1947;135(14):888–894.
57. Fraser HF, Grider JA Jr. Treatment of drug addiction. *Am J Med.* 1953;14(5):571–577.

58. Fraser HF. Human pharmacology and clinical uses of nalorphine (N-allylnormorphine). *Med Clin North Am.* 1957;41(2): 393–403.
59. Himmelsbach CK. The morphine abstinence syndrome, its nature and treatment. *Ann Intern Med.* 1941;15(5):829–839.
60. Himmelsbach CK. Clinical studies of drug addiction I: the absence of addiction liability in "perparin". *Public Health Rep.*1937; (suppl 122):1–4.
61. Himmelsbach CK, Andrews HL. Studies on modification of the morphine abstinence syndrome by drugs. *J Pharmacol Exp Ther.* 1943;77(1):17–23.
62. Martin WR, Jasinski DR. Physiological parameters of morphine dependence in man—tolerance, early abstinence, protracted abstinence. *J Psychiatr Res.* 1969;7(1):9–17.
63. Martin WR, Gorodetzky CW, and McClane TK. An experimental study in the treatment of narcotic addicts with cyclazocine. *Clin Pharmacol Ther.* 1966;7(4):455–465.
64. Jasinski DR, Martin WR, Sapira JD. Antagonism of the subjective, behavioral, pupillary, and respiratory depressant effects of cyclazocine by naloxone. *Clin Pharmacol Ther.* 1968;9(2):215–222.
65. Martin WR, Sandquist VL. A sustained release depot for narcotic antagonists. *Arch Gen Psychiatry.* 1974;30(1):31–33.
66. Haertzen CA, Hill HE, Belleville RE. Development of the addiction research center inventory (ARCI): selection of items that are sensitive to the effects of various drugs. *Psychopharmacologia.* 1963;4:155–166.
67. Griffiths RR. Oral-history interview. 2007. Available at: http://sitemaker.umich.edu/substance.abuse.history/oral_history_interviews&mode=single&recordID=2154551. Accessed July 10, 2009.
68. Brady JV. Oral-history interview. 2007. Available at: http://sitemaker.umich.edu/substance.abuse.history/oral_history_interviews&mode=single&recordID=2207461. Accessed July 10, 2009.
69. Thompson T, Schuster CR. Morphine self-administration, food-reinforced, and avoidance behaviors in rhesus monkeys. *Psychopharmacologia.* 1964;5:87–94.
70. Goldberg SR, Woods JH, Schuster CR. Morphine: conditioned increases in self-administration in rhesus monkeys. *Science* 1969;166(910):1306–1307.
71. Fischman MW, Schuster CR. Drug seeking: a behavioral analysis in animals and humans. *NIDA Res Monogr* 1978;(20):4–23.
72. Goldstein A. Heroin addiction: sequential treatment employing pharmacologic supports. *Arch Gen Psychiatry.* 1976;33(3):353–358.
73. Woods JH, Schuster CR. Reinforcement properties of morphine, cocaine, and SPA as a function of unit dose. *Subst Use Misuse.* 1968;3(1):231–237.
74. American Psychiatric Association. *Diagnostic and Statistical Manual of Mental Disorders, Fourth Edition, Text Revision.* Washington, DC: American Psychiatric Association; 2000.
75. Schuster CR. Oral-history interview. 2007. Available at: http://sitemaker.umich.edu/substance.abuse.history/oral_history_interviews&mode=single&recordID=1894364. Accessed July 10, 2009.
76. Schuster CR, Smith BB, Jaffe JH. Drug abuse in heroin users: an experimental study of self-administration of methadone, codeine, and pentazocine. *Arch Gen Psychiatry.* 1971;24(4):359–362.
77. Stitzer ML. Oral-history interview. 2007. Available at: http://sitemaker.umich.edu/substance.abuse.history/oral_history_interviews&mode=single&recordID=2252708. Accessed July 10, 2009.
78. Liebson I, Bigelow G, Flamer R. Alcoholism among methadone patients: a specific treatment method. *Am J Psychiatry.* 1973; 130(4):483–485.
79. Stitzer ML, Bigelow G, Lawrence C, et al. Medication take-home as a reinforcer in a methadone maintenance program. *Addict Behav.* 1977;2(1):9–14.
80. Jaffe JH. Obituary: Jack Harold Mendelson 1929–2007. *Addiction.* 2008;103(3):509–510.
81. Mirin SM, Meyer RE, McNamee HB. Psychopathology and mood during heroin use: acute vs chronic effects. *Arch Gen Psychiatry.* 1976;33(12):1503–1508.
82. Robinson TE, Berridge KC. The neural basis of drug craving: an incentive-sensitization theory of addiction. *Brain Res Rev.* 1993;18:247–291.
83. Mello NK, Mendelson JH. Buprenorphine suppresses heroin use by heroin addicts. *Science.* 1980;207(4431):657–659.
84. Waldorf D. *Careers in Dope.* Englewood Cliffs, NJ: Prentice-Hall; 1973.
85. Waldorf D. Misadventures in the drug trade. *Subst Use Misuse.* 1998;33(9):1957–1991.
86. Johnson BD, Goldstein PJ, Preble E, et al. *Taking Care of Business: The Economics of Crime by Heroin Abusers.* Lexington, MA: Lexington Books; 1985.
87. Faupel CE. *Shooting Dope: Career Patterns of Hard-core Heroin Users.* Gainsville, FL: University of Florida Press; 1991.
88. Becker HS. Oral-history interview. 2005. Available at: http://sitemaker.umich.edu/substance.abuse.history/oral_history_interviews&mode=single&recordID=2287158. Accessed July 14, 2009.
89. Robins LN, Davis DH, Goodwin DW. Drug use by U.S. Army enlisted men in Vietnam: a follow-up on their return home. *Am J Epidemiol.* 1974;99(4):235–249.
90. Robins LN, Helzer JE, Davis DH. Narcotic use in southeast Asia and afterward: an interview study of 898 Vietnam returnees. *Arch Gen Psychiatry.* 1975;32(8):955–961.
91. Robins LN. The natural history of drug abuse. *Acta Psychiatr Scand Suppl.* 1980;284:7–20.
92. Robins LN. Vietnam veterans' rapid recovery from heroin addiction: a fluke or normal expectation? *Addiction.* 1993;88(8): 1041–1054.
93. Robins LN, Slobodyan S. Post-Vietnam heroin use and injection by returning US veterans: clues to preventing injection today. *Addiction.* 2003;98(8):1053–1060.
94. Waldorf D, Biernacki P. Natural recovery from heroin addiction: a review of the incidence literature. *J Drug Issues.* 1979; 9(2):281–289.
95. Zinberg NE, Jacobson RC. The natural history of "chipping". *Am J Psychiatry.* 1976;133(1):37–40.
96. Harding WM, Zinberg NE, Stelmack SM, et al. Formerly-addicted-now-controlled opiate users. *Int J Addict.* 1980;15(1): 47–60.
99. Zinberg NE. *Drug, Set, and Setting: The Basis for Controlled Intoxicant Use.* New Haven, CT: Yale University Press, 1984.
100. Waldorf D, Orlick M, Reinarman C. *Morphine Maintenance: The Shreveport Clinic 1919-1923.* Washington, DC: Drug Abuse Council; 1974.
101. Dole VP, Nyswander M. A medical treatment for diacetylmorphine (heroin) addiction: a clinical trial with methadone hydrochloride. *JAMA.* 1965;193:646–650.
102. Dole VP, Nyswander ME, Warner A. Successful treatment of 750 criminal addicts. *JAMA.* 1968;206(12):2708–2711.

103. Stitzer M, Bigelow GE. Drug abuse research in outpatient clinics. *NIDA Res Monogr.* 1978;(20):59–67.
104. Dole VP, Nyswander ME. Heroin addiction—a metabolic disease. *Arch Intern Med.* 1967;120(1):19–24.
105. Nyswander M, Dole VP. The present status of methadone blockade treatment. *Am J Psychiatry.* 1967;123(11):1441–1442.
106. Des Jarlais DC. Oral-history interview. 2009. Available at: http://sitemaker.umich.edu/substance.abuse.history/oral_history_interviews&mode=single&recordID=2834166. Accessed July 14, 2009.
107. SAMHSA. *Results from the 2007 National Survey on Drug Use and Health: National Findings (NSDUH Series H-34, DHHS Publication No. SMA 08-4343).* Rockville, MD: Department of Health and Human Services; 2008.
108. Johnston LD, O'Malley PM, Bachman JG, et al. *Monitoring the Future—National Results on Adolescent Drug Use: Overview of Key Findings 2008 (NIH Publication No. 09-7401).* Bethesda, MD: National Institute on Drug Abuse; 2009.
109. SAMHSA. *Drug Abuse Warning Network, 2006: National Estimates of Drug-Related Emergency Department Visits. DAWN Series D-30, DHHS Publication No. SMA-08-4339.* Rockville, MD: Department of Health and Human Services; 2008.
110. SAMHSA. Treatment Episode Data Set (TEDS) data received through October 6, 2008. 2009. Available at: http://drugabusestatistics.samhsa.gov?TEDS2k7highlights.htm. Accessed August 4, 2009.
111. Winick C. Maturing out of narcotic addiction. *Bulletin on Narcotics.* 1962;14(1):1–7.
112. Scherbaum N, Specka M. Factors influencing the course of opiate addiction. *Int J Methods Psychiatr Res.* 2008;17(suppl 1):S39–S44.
113. Klingemann KH, Efionayi-Mader D. How much treatment does a person need? Addiction, spontaneous remission and "family" as biographical as leitmotiv. *Schweiz Rundsch Med Prax.* 1994;83(34):937–949.
114. Darke S, Mills KL, Ross J, et al. The ageing heroin user: career length, clinical profile and outcomes across 36 months. *Drug Alcohol Rev.* 2009;28(3):243–249.
115. Hser YI, Hoffman V, Grella CE, et al. A 33-year follow-up of narcotics addicts. *Arch Gen Psychiatry.* 2001;58(5):503–508.
116. Marlowe A. Listening to heroin: what dope says about pleasure, poison, and keeping score. *Village Voice.* 1994;25–30.
117. Glaser FB, Ball JC. Death due to withdrawal from narcotics. In: Ball JC, Chambers CD, eds. *The Epidemiology of Opiate Addiction in the United States.* Springfield, IL: Charles C. Thomas, 1970:263–287.
118. Isbell H, Vogel VH. The addiction liability of methadon (amidone, dolophine, 10820) and its use in the treatment of the morphine abstinence syndrome. *Am J Psychiatry.* 1949;105(12):909–914.
119. Milby JB, Gurwitch RH, Wiebe DJ, et al. Prevalence and diagnostic reliability of methadone maintenance detoxification fear. *Am J Psychiatry.* 1986;143(6):739–743.
120. Himmelsbach CK. Clinical studies of drug addiction. *Arch Intern Med.* 1942;69(5):766–772.
121. Gossop M, Strang J. A comparison of the withdrawal responses of heroin and methadone addicts during detoxification. *Br J Psychiatry.* 1991;158:697–699.
122. Eklund C, Hiltunen AJ, Melin L, et al. Patient perceptions of psychological and physiological withdrawal symptoms and positive factors associated with gradual withdrawal from methadone maintenance treatment: a prospective study. *Subst Use Misuse.* 1997;32(11):1599–1618.
123. Shi J, Zhao LY, Epstein DH, et al. Long-term methadone maintenance reduces protracted symptoms of heroin abstinence and cue-induced craving in Chinese heroin abusers. *Pharmacol Biochem Behav.* 2007;87(1):141–145.
124. World Health Organization. *The ICD-10 Classification of Mental and Behavioural Disorders.* Geneva: World Health Organization; 1992.
125. Helzer JE. Psychoactive substance abuse and its relation to dependence. In: Widiger TA, Frances AJ, Pincus HA, et al. eds. *DSM-IV Sourcebook.* Washington, DC: American Psychiatric Association; 1994:21–32.
126. Bertha CM, Flippen-Anderson JL, Rothman RB, et al. Probes for narcotic receptor-mediated phenomena. 20. Alteration of opioid receptor subtype selectivity of the 5-(3-hydroxyphenyl)morphans by application of the message-address concept: preparation of delta-opioid receptor ligands. *J Med Chem.* 1995;38(9):1523–1537.
127. Xu H, Hashimoto A, Rice KC, et al. Opioid peptide receptor studies. 14. Stereochemistry determines agonist efficacy and intrinsic efficacy in the [(35)S]GTP-gamma-S functional binding assay. *Synapse.* 2001;39(1):64–69.
128. Dasgupta N, Kramer ED, Zalman MA, et al. Association between non-medical and prescriptive usage of opioids. *Drug Alcohol Depend* 2006;82(2):135–142.
129. Martin WR, Eades CG, Thompson JA, et al. The effects of morphine- and nalorphine-like drugs in the nondependent and morphine-dependent chronic spinal dog. *J Pharmacol Exp Ther.* 1976;197(3):517–532.
130. Walsh SL, Strain EC, Abreu ME, et al. Enadoline, a selective kappa opioid agonist: comparison with butorphanol and hydromorphone in humans. *Psychopharmacology.* 2001;157(2):151–162.
131. Preston KL, Umbricht A, Schroeder JR, et al. Cyclazocine: comparison to hydromorphone and interaction with cocaine. *Behav Pharmacol.* 2004;15(2):91–102.
132. Young GA, Khazan N. Comparison of abstinence syndromes following chronic administration of mu and kappa opioid agonists in the rat. *Pharmacol Biochem Behav.* 1985;23(3):457–460.
133. Gmerek DE, Dykstra LA, Woods JH. Kappa opioids in rhesus monkeys. III. Dependence associated with chronic administration. *J Pharmacol Exp Ther.* 1987;242(2):428–436.
134. Su TP. Further demonstration of kappa opioid binding sites in the brain: evidence for heterogeneity. *J Pharmacol Exp Ther.* 1985;232(1):144–148.
135. Emmerson PJ, Clark MJ, Mansour A, et al. Characterization of opioid agonist efficacy in a C6 glioma cell line expressing the mu opioid receptor. *J Pharmacol Exp Ther.* 1996;278(3):1121–1127.
136. Preston KL, Jasinski DR. Abuse liability studies of opioid agonist-antagonists in humans. *Drug Alcohol Depend.* 1991;28(1):49–82.
137. Preston KL, Bigelow GE. Subjective and discriminative effects of drugs. *Behav Pharmacol.* 1991;2(4–5):293–313.
138. Preston KL, Bigelow GE. Drug discrimination assessment of agonist-antagonist opioids in humans: a three-choice saline-hydromorphone-butorphanol procedure. *J Pharmacol Exp Ther.* 1994;271(1):48–60.
139. Preston KL, Bigelow GE. Opioid discrimination in humans: discriminative and subjective effects of progressively lower training dose. *Behav Pharmacol.* 1998;9(7):533–543.
140. Jones HE, Bigelow GE, Preston KL. Assessment of opioid partial agonist activity with a three-choice hydromorphone dose-discrimination procedure. *J Pharmacol Exp Ther.* 1999;289(3):1350–1361.

141. Preston KL, Bigelow GE, Liebson IA. Butorphanol-precipitated withdrawal in opioid-dependent human volunteers. *J Pharmacol Exp Ther.* 1988;246(2):441–448.
142. Preston KL, Bigelow GE, Liebson IA. Antagonist effects of nalbuphine in opioid-dependent human volunteers. *J Pharmacol Exp Ther.* 1989;248(3):929–937.
143. Strain EC, Preston KL, Liebson IA, et al. Precipitated withdrawal by pentazocine in methadone-maintained volunteers. *J Pharmacol Exp Ther.* 1993;267(2):624–634.
144. Jasinski DR, Pevnick JS, Griffith JD. Human pharmacology and abuse potential of the analgesic buprenorphine: a potential agent for treating narcotic addiction. *Arch Gen Psychiatry.* 1978;35(4):501–516.
145. Walsh SL, Preston KL, Stitzer ML, et al. Clinical pharmacology of buprenorphine: ceiling effects at high doses. *Clin Pharmacol Ther.* 1994;55(5):569–580.
146. Umbricht A, Hoover DR, Tucker MJ, et al. Opioid detoxification with buprenorphine, clonidine, or methadone in hospitalized heroin-dependent patients with HIV infection. *Drug Alcohol Depend.* 2003;69(3):263–272.
147. Aitken CK, Higgs PG, Hellard ME. Buprenorphine injection in Melbourne, Australia—an update. *Drug Alcohol Rev.* 2008;27(2):197–199.
148. Strain EC, Preston KL, Liebson IA, et al. Buprenorphine effects in methadone-maintained volunteers: effects at two hours after methadone. *J Pharmacol Exp Ther.* 1995;272(2):628–638.
149. Megarbane B, Hreiche R, Pirnay S, et al. Does high-dose buprenorphine cause respiratory depression?: possible mechanisms and therapeutic consequences. *Toxicol Rev.* 2006;25(2):79–85.
150. Goldstein A. Thrills in response to music and other stimuli. *Physiol Psychol.* 1980;8(1):126–129.
151. Johansson BA, Berglund M, Lindgren A. Efficacy of maintenance treatment with naltrexone for opioid dependence: a meta-analytical review. *Addiction.* 2006;101(4):491–503.
152. Raffa RB. Basic pharmacology relevant to drug abuse assessment: tramadol as example. *J Clin Pharm Ther.* 2008;33(2):101–108.
153. Latta KS, Ginsberg B, Barkin RL. Meperidine: a critical review. *Am J Ther.* 2002;9(1):53–68.
154. Isbell H, White WM. Clinical characteristics of addictions. *Am J Med.* 1953;14(5):558–565.
155. Harmer M, Slattery PJ, Rosen M, et al. Comparison between buprenorphine and pentazocine given i.v. on demand in the control of postoperative pain. *Br J Anaesth.* 1983;55(1):21–25.
156. Schneider MF, Bailey JE, Cicero TJ, et al. Integrating nine prescription opioid analgesics and/or four signal detection systems to summarize statewide prescription drug abuse in the United States in 2007. *Pharmacoepidemiol Drug Saf.* 2009;18(9):778–790.
157. Inciardi JA, Cicero TJ, Munoz A, et al. The Diversion of ultram, ultracet, and generic tramadol HCL. *J Addict Dis.* 2006;25(2):53–58.
158. Epstein DH, Preston KL, Jasinski DR. Abuse liability, behavioral pharmacology, and physical-dependence potential of opioids in humans and laboratory animals: lessons from tramadol. *Biol Psychol.* 2006;73(1):90–99.
159. Nelson RA, Boyd SJ, Ziegelstein RC, et al. Effect of rate of administration on subjective and physiological effects of intravenous cocaine in humans. *Drug Alcohol Depend.* 2006;82(1):19–24.
160. Jasinski DR, Preston KL. Comparison of intravenously administered methadone, morphine and heroin. *Drug Alcohol Depend.* 1986;17(4):301–310.
161. Paoli L, Greenfield VA, Charles M, et al. The global diversion of pharmaceutical drugs. India: the third largest illicit opium producer? *Addiction.* 2009;104(3):347–354.
162. Sarkar K, Panda S, Das N, et al. Relationship of national highway with injecting drug abuse and HIV in rural Manipur, India. *Indian J Public Health.* 1997;41(2):49–51.
163. Beyrer C, Razak MH, Lisam K, et al. Overland heroin trafficking routes and HIV-1 spread in south and south-east Asia. *Aids.* 2000;14(1):75–83.
164. Day C, Degenhardt L, Hall W. Changes in the initiation of heroin use after a reduction in heroin supply. *Drug Alcohol Rev.* 2006;25(4):307–313.
165. Zacny J, Bigelow G, Compton P, et al. College on Problems of Drug Dependence taskforce on prescription opioid nonmedical use and abuse: position statement. *Drug Alcohol Depend.* 2003;69(3):215–232.
166. Alexander BH, Checkoway H, Nagahama SI, et al. Cause-specific mortality risks of anesthesiologists. *Anesthesiology.* 2000;93(4):922–930.
167. Booth JV, Grossman D, Moore J, et al. Substance abuse among physicians: a survey of academic anesthesiology programs. *Anesth Analg.* 2002;95(4):1024–1030.
168. Fraser H, Isbell H. Human pharmacology and addictiveness of certain dextroisomers of synthetic analgesics. *Bulletin on Narcotics* 1962:25–35.
169. Jasinski DR, Martin WR, Mansky PA. Progress report on the assessment of the antagonists nalbuphine and GPA-2087 for abuse potential and studies of effects of dextromethorphan in man. *Committee on Problems of Drug Dependence.* 1971;33:143–178.
170. Preston KL, Epstein DH, Schmittner J, et al. Abuse of marketed medications. In: Karch SB, ed. Drug Abuse Handbook. 2nd ed. Boca Raton, FL: CRC Press, 2006.
171. Cicero TJ, Inciardi JA, Munoz A. Trends in abuse of Oxycontin and other opioid analgesics in the United States: 2002-2004. *J Pain.* 2005;6(10):662–672.
172. Vidal-Trecan G, Varescon I, Nabet N, et al. Intravenous use of prescribed sublingual buprenorphine tablets by drug users receiving maintenance therapy in France. *Drug Alcohol Depend.* 2003;69(2):175–181.
173. Roberge RJ, Krenzelok EP, Mrvos R. Transdermal drug delivery system exposure outcomes. *J Emerg Med.* 2000;18(2):147–151.
174. Fudala PJ, Johnson RE. Development of opioid formulations with limited diversion and abuse potential. *Drug Alcohol Depend.* 2006;83(suppl 1):S40–S47.
175. Katz NP, Adams EH, Chilcoat H, et al. Challenges in the development of prescription opioid abuse-deterrent formulations. *Clin J Pain.* 2007;23(8):648–660.
176. Rollason V, Samer C, Piguet V, et al. Pharmacogenetics of analgesics: toward the individualization of prescription. *Pharmacogenomics.* 2008;9(7):905–933.
177. Levran O, Londono D, O'Hara K, et al. Genetic susceptibility to heroin addiction: a candidate gene association study. *Genes Brain Behav.* 2008;7(7):720–729.
178. Becker HS. History, culture and subjective experience: an exploration of the social bases of drug-induced experiences. *J Health Soc Behav.* 1967;8(3):163–176.
179. Best D, Manning V, Strang J. Retrospective recall of heroin initiation and the impact on peer networks. *Addict Res Theory.* 2007;15(4):397–410.
180. Nurco DN, Kinlock T, O'Grady K, et al. Perceptions of social pathology in the neighborhood and the etiology of narcotic

180. addiction. A retrospective study. *J Nerv Ment Dis.* 1996; 184(1):35–42.
181. Harris JR. *The Nurture Assumption: Why Children Turn Out the Way They Do.* New York: Simon & Schuster; 1998.
182. Coomber R. There's no such thing as a free lunch: "freebies" and "credit" operate as part of rational drug market activity. *J Drug Issues.* 2003;33(4):939–962.
183. Furst RT, Herrmann C, Leung R, et al. Heroin diffusion in the mid-Hudson region of New York State. *Addiction.* 2004; 99(4):431–441.
184. Morral AR, McCaffrey DF, Paddock SM. Reassessing the marijuana gateway effect. *Addiction.* 2002;97(12):1493–1504.
185. Warner LA, Kessler RC, Hughes M, et al. Prevalence and correlates of drug use and dependence in the United States: results from the National Comorbidity Survey. *Arch Gen Psychiatry.* 1995;52(3):219–229.
186. Swendsen J, Conway KP, Degenhardt L, et al. Socio-demographic risk factors for alcohol and drug dependence: the 10-year follow-up of the National Comorbidity Survey. *Addiction.* 2009;104(8): 1346–1355.
187. O'Brien CP, O'Brien TJ, Mintz J, et al. Conditioning of narcotic abstinence symptoms in human subjects. *Drug Alcohol Depend.* 1975;1(2):115–123.
188. McAuliffe WE. A test of Wikler's theory of relapse: the frequency of relapse due to conditioned withdrawal sickness. *Int J Addict.* 1982;17(1):19–33.
189. Childress AR, McLellan AT, O'Brien CP. Conditioned responses in a methadone population: a comparison of laboratory, clinic, and natural settings. *J Subst Abuse Treat.* 1986;3(3): 173–179.
190. Epstein DH, Willner-Reid J, Vahabzadeh M, et al. Real-time electronic diary reports of cue exposure and mood in the hours before cocaine and heroin craving and use. *Arch Gen Psychiatry.* 2009;66(1):88–94.
191. O'Brien CP, Childress AR, McLellan AT, et al. Use of naltrexone to extinguish opioid-conditioned responses. *J Clin Psychiatry.* 1984; 45(9 pt 2):53–56.
192. McLellan AT, Childress AR, Ehrman R, et al. Extinguishing conditioned responses during opiate dependence treatment: turning laboratory findings into clinical procedures. *J Subst Abuse Treat.* 1986;3(1):33–40.
193. Conklin CA, Tiffany ST. Applying extinction research and theory to cue-exposure addiction treatments. *Addiction.* 2002; 97(2):155–167.
194. Bossert JM, Gray SM, Lu L, et al. Activation of group II metabotropic glutamate receptors in the nucleus accumbens shell attenuates context-induced relapse to heroin seeking. *Neuropsychopharmacology.* 2006;31(10):2197–2209.
195. Sacerdote P. Opioid-induced immunosuppression. *Curr Opin Support Palliat Care.* 2008;2(1):14–18.
196. Cherubin CE, Sapira JD. The medical complications of drug addiction and the medical assessment of the intravenous drug user: 25 years later. *Ann Intern Med.* 1993;119(10): 1017–1028.
197. McLauchlin J, Mithani V, Bolton FJ, et al. An investigation into the microflora of heroin. *J Med Microbiol.* 2002;51(11): 1001–1008.
198. Weintraub E, Dixon L, Delahanty J, et al. Reason for medical hospitalization among adult alcohol and drug abusers. *Am J Addict.* 2001;10(2):167–177.
199. Darke S, Mattick RP, Degenhardt L. The ratio of non-fatal to fatal heroin overdose. *Addiction.* 2003;98(8):1169–1171.
200. Cullen W, Bury G, Langton D. Experience of heroin overdose among drug users attending general practice. *Br J Gen Pract.* 2000;50(456):546–549.
201. Sherman SG, Cheng Y, Kral AH. Prevalence and correlates of opiate overdose among young injection drug users in a large U.S. city. *Drug Alcohol Depend.* 2007;88(2–3):182–187.
202. White JM, Irvine RJ. Mechanisms of fatal opioid overdose. *Addiction.* 1999;94(7):961–972.
203. Darke S, Zador D. Fatal heroin "overdose": a review. *Addiction.* 1996;91(12):1765–1772.
204. Beswick T, Best D, Bearn J, et al. From salt injection to naloxone: accuracy and myths in peer resuscitation methods for opiate overdose. *J Drug Issues.* 2002;32(4):1103–1114.
205. Ashworth AJ, Kidd A. Take home naloxone for opiate addicts: apparent advantages may be balanced by hidden harms. *BMJ.* 2001;323(7318):935.
206. Piper TM, Rudenstine S, Stancliff S, et al. Overdose prevention for injection drug users: lessons learned from naloxone training and distribution programs in New York City. *Harm Reduct J.* 2007;4:3.
207. Piper TM, Stancliff S, Rudenstine S, et al. Evaluation of a naloxone distribution and administration program in New York City. *Subst Use Misuse.* 2008;43(7):858–870.
208. Strang J, Manning V, Mayet S, et al. Overdose training and take-home naloxone for opiate users: prospective cohort study of impact on knowledge and attitudes and subsequent management of overdoses. *Addiction.* 2008;103(10):1648–1657.
209. Doe-Simkins M, Walley AY, Epstein A, et al. Saved by the nose: bystander-administered intranasal naloxone hydrochloride for opioid overdose. *Am J Public Health.* 2009;99(5):788–791.
210. Kim D, Irwin KS, Khoshnood K. Expanded access to naloxone: options for critical response to the epidemic of opioid overdose mortality. *Am J Public Health.* 2009;99(3):402–407.
211. Alter MJ, Kruszon-Moran D, Nainan OV, et al. The prevalence of hepatitis C virus infection in the United States, 1988 through 1994. *N Engl J Med.* 1999;341(8):556–562.
212. Hagan H. Hepatitis C virus transmission dynamics in injection drug users. *Subst Use Misuse.* 1998;33(5):1197–1212.
213. Patrick DM, Tyndall MW, Cornelisse PG, et al. Incidence of hepatitis C virus infection among injection drug users during an outbreak of HIV infection. *CMAJ.* 2001;165(7):889–895.
214. Sulkowski M, Brinkley-Laughton S, Thomas D. Prevalence, genotype distribution and severity of liver disease in an urban HIV clinic. *Hepatology.* 2000;32(4 pt 2):212a.
215. National Institute of Diabetes and Digestive and Kidney Diseases. *Chronic Hepatitis C: Current Disease Management.* NIH Publication No. 07-4230. Bethesda, MD: National Institutes of Health; 2006.
216. Edlin BR, Seal KH, Lorvick J, et al. Is it justifiable to withhold treatment for hepatitis C from illicit-drug users? *N Engl J Med.* 2001;345(3):211–215.
217. Branson BM, Handsfield HH, Lampe MA, et al. Revised recommendations for HIV testing of adults, adolescents, and pregnant women in health-care settings. *MMWR Recomm Rep.* 2006;55(RR-14):1–17; quiz CE11-14.
218. Willner-Reid J, Belenduik KA, Epstein DH, et al. Hepatitis C and human immunodeficiency virus risk behaviors in poly-drug users on methadone maintenance. *J Subst Abuse Treat.* 2008;35(1): 78–86.
219. Sullivan LE, Fiellin DA. Hepatitis C and HIV infections: implications for clinical care in injection drug users. *Am J Addict.* 2004;13(1):1–20.

220. Workowski KA, Berman SM. Sexually transmitted diseases treatment guidelines. *MMWR Recomm Rep.* 2006;55(RR-11):1–94.
221. Batki SL, Gruber VA, Bradley JM, et al. A controlled trial of methadone treatment combined with directly observed isoniazid for tuberculosis prevention in injection drug users. *Drug Alcohol Depend.* 2002;66(3):283–293.
222. De Alba I, Samet JH, Saitz R. Burden of medical illness in drug- and alcohol-dependent persons without primary care. *Am J Addict.* 2004;13(1):33–45.
223. Howard AA, Floris-Moore M, Lo Y, et al. Abnormal glucose metabolism among older men with or at risk of HIV infection. *HIV Med.* 2006;7(6):389–396.
224. Rosen D, Smith ML, Reynolds CF 3rd. The prevalence of mental and physical health disorders among older methadone patients. *Am J Geriatr Psychiatry.* 2008;16(6):488–497.
225. Center for Substance Abuse Treatment. *Medication-Assisted Treatment for Opioid Addiction in Opioid Treatment Programs: Treatment Improvement Protocol (TIP) Series 43. DHHS Publication No. (SMA) 06-4214.* Rockville, MD: Substance Abuse and Mental Health Services Administration; 2005.
226. Dickey B, Normand SL, Weiss RD, et al. Medical morbidity, mental illness, and substance use disorders. *Psychiatr Serv.* 2002;53(7):861–867.
227. Coffey R, Graver L, Schroeder D, et al. *Mental Health and Substance Abuse Treatment: Results from a Study Integrating Data from State Mental Health, Substance Abuse, and Medicaid Agencies. DHHS Publication No. SMA- 01-3528.* Rockville, MD: Department of Health and Human Services; 2001.
228. United States Preventive Services Task Force. Screening for illicit drug use. 2008. http://www.ahrq.gov/clinic/uspstf/uspsdrug.htm. Accessed August 13, 2009.
229. McLellan AT, Kushner H, Metzger D, et al. The fifth edition of the addiction severity index. *J Subst Abuse Treat.* 1992;9(3):199–213.
230. Makela K. Studies of the reliability and validity of the Addiction Severity Index. *Addiction.* 2004;99(4):398–410; discussion 411–398.
231. Skinner HA. The drug abuse screening test. *Addict Behav.* 1982;7(4):363–371.
232. Yudko E, Lozhkina O, Fouts A. A comprehensive review of the psychometric properties of the Drug Abuse Screening Test. *J Subst Abuse Treat.* 2007;32(2):189–198.
233. Janca A, Ustun TB, van Drimmelen J, et al. *ICD-10 Symptom Checklist for Mental Disorders, Version 1.1.* Geneva: Division of Mental Health, World Health Organization; 1994.
234. Humeniuk R, Ali R, Babor TF, et al. Validation of the alcohol, smoking and substance involvement screening test (ASSIST). *Addiction.* 2008;103(6):1039–1047.
235. Gossop M, Darke S, Griffiths P, et al. The severity of dependence scale (SDS): psychometric properties of the SDS in English and Australian samples of heroin, cocaine and amphetamine users. *Addiction.* 1995;90(5):607–614.
236. Waldorf D. Natural recovery from opiate addiction: some social-psychological processes of untreated recovery. *J Drug Issues.* 1983;13(2):237–280.
237. Gerstein D, Harwood H. *Treating Drug Problems: A Study of Effectiveness and Financing of Public and Private Drug Treatment Systems.* Washington, DC: National Academics Press; 1990.
238. Lipton DS, Maranda M. *Detoxification from Heroin Dependency: An Overview of Method and Effectiveness.* New York: Haworth Press; 1983.
239. Mattick RP, Hall W. Are detoxification programmes effective? *Lancet.* 1996;347(8994):97–100.
240. Gowing LR, Ali RL. The place of detoxification in treatment of opioid dependence. *Curr Opin Psychiatry.* 2006;19(3):266–270.
241. National Institute on Drug Abuse. *Principles of Drug Addiction Treatment: A Research-Based Guide, 2nd Edition. NIH Publication No. 09-4180.* Bethesda, MD: National Institutes of Health; 2009.
242. Wood E, Tyndall MW, Zhang R, et al. Rate of detoxification service use and its impact among a cohort of supervised injecting facility users. *Addiction.* 2007;102(6):916–919.
243. Ling W, Hillhouse M, Domier C, et al. Buprenorphine tapering schedule and illicit opioid use. *Addiction.* 2009;104(2):256–265.
244. Mattick RP, Kimber J, Breen C, et al. Buprenorphine maintenance versus placebo or methadone maintenance for opioid dependence. *Cochrane Database Syst Rev.* 2008; Apr 16;(2):CD002207.
245. Gowing L, Ali R, White JM. Buprenorphine for the management of opioid withdrawal. *Cochrane Database Syst Rev.* 2009; Jul 8;(3):CD002025.
246. Jasinski DR, Johnson RE, Kocher TR. Clonidine in morphine withdrawal. Differential effects on signs and symptoms. *Arch Gen Psychiatry.* 1985;42(11):1063–1066.
247. Collins ED, Kleber HD, Whittington RA, et al. Anesthesia-assisted vs buprenorphine- or clonidine-assisted heroin detoxification and naltrexone induction: a randomized trial. *JAMA.* 2005;294(8):903–913.
248. Chutuape MA, Jasinski DR, Fingerhood MI, et al. One-, three-, and six-month outcomes after brief inpatient opioid detoxification. *Am J Drug Alcohol Abuse.* 2001;27(1):19–44.
249. Moolchan ET, Umbricht A, Epstein D. Therapeutic drug monitoring in methadone maintenance: choosing a matrix. *J Addict Dis.* 2001;20(2):55–73.
250. Jaffe JH, Senay EC, Schuster CR, et al. Methadyl acetate vs methadone. A double-blind study in heroin users. *JAMA.* 1972; 222(4):437–442.
251. Jaffe JH. Can LAAM, like Lazarus, come back from the dead? *Addiction.* 2007;102(9):1342–1343.
252. Sung S, Conry JM. Role of buprenorphine in the management of heroin addiction. *Ann Pharmacother.* 2006;40(3):501–505.
253. Smith MY, Bailey JE, Woody GE, et al. Abuse of buprenorphine in the United States: 2003–2005. *J Addict Dis.* 2007;26(3):107–111.
254. O'Connor PG, Fiellin DA. Pharmacologic treatment of heroin-dependent patients. *Ann Intern Med.* 2000;133(1):40–54.
255. Ferri M, Davoli M, Perucci CA. Heroin maintenance treatment for chronic heroin-dependent individuals: a Cochrane systematic review of effectiveness. *J Subst Abuse Treat.* 2006;30(1):63–72.
256. Oviedo-Joekes E, Nosyk B, Marsh DC, et al. Scientific and political challenges in North America's first randomized controlled trial of heroin-assisted treatment for severe heroin addiction: rationale and design of the NAOMI study. *Clin Trials.* 2009;6(3):261–271.
257. Oviedo-Joekes E, Brissette S, Marsh DC, et al. Diacetylmorphine versus methadone for the treatment of opioid addiction. *N Engl J Med.* 2009;361(8):777–86.
258. Montoya ID, Vocci F. Novel medications to treat addictive disorders. *Curr Psychiatry Rep.* 2008;10(5):392–398.
259. Sigmon SC, Moody DE, Nuwayser ES, et al. An injection depot formulation of buprenorphine: extended bio-delivery and effects. *Addiction.* 2006;101(3):420–432.

260. Comer SD, Sullivan MA, Hulse GK. Sustained-release naltrexone: novel treatment for opioid dependence. *Expert Opin Investig Drugs*. 2007;16(8):1285–1294.
261. Kunøe N, Lobmaier P, Vederhus JK, et al. Naltrexone implants after in-patient treatment for opioid dependence: randomised controlled trial. *Br J Psychiatry*. 2009;194(6):541–546.
262. Carnwath T, Hardman J. Randomised double-blind comparison of lofexidine and clonidine in the out-patient treatment of opiate withdrawal. *Drug Alcohol Depend*. 1998;50(3):251–254.
263. Carroll CP, Walsh SL, Bigelow GE, et al. Assessment of agonist and antagonist effects of tramadol in opioid-dependent humans. *Exp Clin Psychopharmacol*. 2006;14(2):109–120.
264. Bisaga A, Comer SD, Ward AS, et al. The NMDA antagonist memantine attenuates the expression of opioid physical dependence in humans. *Psychopharmacology*. 2001;157(1):1–10.
265. Heinrichs SC, Menzaghi F, Schulteis G, et al. Suppression of corticotropin-releasing factor in the amygdala attenuates aversive consequences of morphine withdrawal. *Behav Pharmacol*. 1995;6(1):74–80.
266. Stinus L, Cador M, Zorrilla EP, et al. Buprenorphine and a CRF1 antagonist block the acquisition of opiate withdrawal-induced conditioned place aversion in rats. *Neuropsychopharmacology*. 2005;30(1):90–98.
267. Shaham Y, Funk D, Erb S, et al. Corticotropin-releasing factor, but not corticosterone, is involved in stress-induced relapse to heroin-seeking in rats. *J Neurosci*. 1997;17(7):2605–2614.
268. Mannelli P, Patkar AA, Peindl K, et al. Very low dose naltrexone addition in opioid detoxification: a randomized, controlled trial. *Addict Biol*. 2009;14(2):204–213.
269. Kosten T, Owens SM. Immunotherapy for the treatment of drug abuse. *Pharmacol Ther*. 2005;108(1):76–85.
270. Bonese KF, Wainer BH, Fitch FW, et al. Changes in heroin self-administration by a rhesus monkey after morphine immunisation. *Nature*. 1974;252(5485):708–710.
271. Kinsey BM, Jackson DC, Orson FM. Anti-drug vaccines to treat substance abuse. *Immunol Cell Biol*. 2009;87(4):309–314.
272. Anton B, Leff P. A novel bivalent morphine/heroin vaccine that prevents relapse to heroin addiction in rodents. *Vaccine*. 2006;24(16):3232–3240.
273. Epstein DH, Preston KL. Contingency management in the treatment of opiate-use disorders. In: Higgins ST, Silverman K, Heil SH, ed. *Contingency Management in the Treatment of Substance Use Disorders: A Science-Based Treatment Innovation*. New York: Guilford;2008:42–60.
274. Carroll K. *A Cognitive-Behavioral Approach: Treating Cocaine Addiction*. Rockville, MD: US Department of Health and Human Services; 2007.
275. Carroll KM, Rounsaville BJ, Nich C, et al. One-year follow-up of psychotherapy and pharmacotherapy for cocaine dependence: delayed emergence of psychotherapy effects. *Arch Gen Psychiatry*. 1994;51:989–997.
276. Wodak A, Cooney A. Do needle syringe programs reduce HIV infection among injecting drug users: a comprehensive review of the international evidence. *Subst Use Misuse*. 2006;41(6-7):777–813.
277. Burris S. Needle Exchange Knowledge Assist: website created by the Robert Wood Johnson Foundation's Substance Abuse Policy Research Program. 2009. Available at: http://saprp.org/knowledgeassets/Knowledge_Detail.cfm?KAID=15. Accessed August 14, 2009.
278. Sullivan LE, Fiellin DA. Narrative review: buprenorphine for opioid-dependent patients in office practice. *Ann Intern Med*. 2008;148(9):662–670.
279. Samet JH, Friedmann P, Saitz R. Benefits of linking primary medical care and substance abuse services: patient, provider, and societal perspectives. *Arch Intern Med*. 2001;161(1):85–91.
280. Saitz R, Mulvey KP, Samet JH. The substance abusing patient and primary care: linkage via the addiction treatment system? *Subst Abuse*. 1997;18(4):187–195.
281. Mangrum LF, Spence RT, Lopez M. Integrated versus parallel treatment of co-occurring psychiatric and substance use disorders. *J Subst Abuse Treat*. 2006;30(1):79–84.
282. Institute of Medicine. *Improving the Quality of Healthcare for Mental and Substance-Use Conditions: The Quality Chasm Series*. Washington, DC: National Academics Press; 2005.
283. Friedmann PD, Hendrickson JC, Gerstein DR, et al. Do mechanisms that link addiction treatment patients to primary care influence subsequent utilization of emergency and hospital care? *Med Care*. 2006;44(1):8–15.
284. Ball J, Ross A. *The Effectiveness of Methadone Maintenance Treatment: Patients, Programs, Services, and Outcome*. New York: Springer-Verlag; 1991.
285. Ball JC. Oral-history interview. 2008. http://sitemaker.umich.edu/substance.abuse.history/oral_history_interviews&mode=single&recordID=2544008. Accessed July 14, 2009.

CHAPTER 14

Cocaine and Crack

Richard P. Paczynski ■ Mark S. Gold

INTRODUCTION

Viewed as a gift from the gods, the coca leaf was to the Incas of ancient Peru both mood and performance enhancing—it could lift spirits and increase stamina over long days of back-breaking labor. Today our lives are more sedentary, our age has been described as self-indulgent, and rather than a gift cocaine is seen by many as a curse from the devil. In this chapter we will address many aspects of cocaine abuse and addiction, prominently including discussion of crack cocaine. The following key points are emphasized throughout:

- Cocaine addiction results frequently from exposure to the highly concentrated, potent forms of cocaine now available on the streets of most American cities and towns, and it is difficult to treat successfully; partial responses to treatment and lifelong morbidity are common.
- Cocaine addiction is a particularly virulent disease because it involves a potentially lethal combination of sensitization of the brain's primary "pleasure centers" (to which the cocaine molecule has direct access) *and* powerful reinforcement of drug pursuit behaviors. Together these effects greatly increase the likelihood of use despite catastrophic consequences. Ironically, the pleasure associated with continued use often decreases.
- The mainstay of cocaine treatment is an integrative approach with thorough consideration of all medical, psychological, and social factors that may be per-petuating active addiction; cognitive–behavioral therapy (CBT) and other forms of "psychological" intervention, including tried and true 12-step programs, feature prominently.
- Better understanding of the neurobiology of cocaine addiction is opening up new possibilities for pharmacologic interventions which target different facets of the disease, greatly increasing the prospects for long-term treatment success.
- Prolonged use of cocaine frequently results in severe medical and neurologic complications that lead to deterioration of health, disintegration of personality, and lost integrity of the higher cognitive centers necessary for full recovery. Early, effective intervention is therefore imperative.

HISTORY: FROM COCA LEAVES TO CRACK

The amount of cocaine ingested by the Incas was probably quite low. It is estimated that the average user chewed 60 g of coca leaves in a day. Given that the cocaine alkaloid content of a coca leaf is approximately 0.5% and that only a portion of the alkaloid is absorbed in digestion, the total dosage would probably have been 200 to 300 mg over a 24-hour period (1). In contrast, a similar or greater dose may be delivered to the brain after just a few "hits" from a crack pipe.

Word about cocaine spread from the Andes to Europe through reports first by explorers and later by naturalists and botanists. By 1860, essays and medical testimonies inspired makers of various tonics to add the newly isolated active ingredient of coca leaves to their formulations. The French chemist Angelo Mariani produced inexpensive Bordeaux fortified with coca leaves, a product so popular that it was endorsed by none other than Pope Leo XIII, who is reported to have carried around a supply of the elixir in a hipflask. Within 15 years people could also buy snuff that contained pure cocaine, touted as a remedy for asthma and hay fever. Cocaine was also a common ingredient in "toothache drops." These new cocaine preparations, the much higher daily doses, and routes of administration marked the first change in the pattern of cocaine use in more than 4000 years.

Prominent medical men of the late 19th century fraternized with cocaine, often with tragic results. A famous essay by Sigmund Freud published in 1884 ("Uber Coca") advocated therapeutic use of cocaine as a stimulant, an aphrodisiac and virtual tonic for a variety of disorders. Freud prescribed it to alleviate the symptoms of withdrawal from alcohol and morphine addiction. Not surprisingly, some patients who used cocaine as a substitute for alcohol or morphine became dependent on it, as did Freud. Likewise, the brilliant American surgeon William Stewart Halsted, who pioneered the use of cocaine as a local anesthetic, became seriously addicted.

Atlanta druggist John Pemberton devised a patent medicine during the mid-1880s that contained two naturally occurring stimulants, cocaine and caffeine. Pemberton advertised his product as an "intellectual beverage," a "brain tonic," and a "temperance drink" due to the fact that it contained no alcohol. This product eventually became known as Coca-Cola and until 1903, contained approximately 60 mg of cocaine per 8-ounce serving. In response to public pressure and news reports about the dangers of cocaine, the maker voluntarily removed cocaine from the formulation. The Coca-Cola Company still uses an extract of the coca leaf, minus the active ingredient.

The beginning of the 20th century thus marked a turn in public and professional attitudes about cocaine. The American Medical Association, seeking to raise the standards of medical practice, lobbied to curb the sales of patent medicines, including those containing cocaine. The Harrison Narcotic Act of 1914 (which mistakenly listed cocaine as a narcotic) banned the use of cocaine in proprietary medications and tightened the restrictions on the manufacture and distribution of coca products. As a result of these restrictions, and for other reasons, drug users turned to amphetamines and other centrally stimulating drugs, a trend documented abundantly in the beatnik literature of the 1950s. These drugs were easily substituted for cocaine because they cost less, were more widely available, and induced a sense of euphoria that lasted longer. They were also more deadly. By the late 1960s, the drug-using subculture recognized the danger in amphetamines, as reflected in the contemporary slogan "speed kills." Eventually amphetamines were listed as Schedule II drugs (drugs with a high abuse potential and prescription limitations), making them much more difficult to obtain.

Stimulant abusers searching for a "safer" recreational euphoria soon rediscovered cocaine in the mid- to late 1970s. As described in detail in the following section, cocaine abuse skyrocketed well into the 1980s, especially among middle- and upper middle–class populations, trendsetters, and disco queens, where it became known as "the champagne of pharmaceuticals." The warnings of cocaine's dangers from past generations had been forgotten. During the 1970s, cocaine was usually administered intranasally in a powder form, and individual doses were usually moderate. A typical user bought 1 g of cocaine for approximately $150 and insufflated (snorted) the drug from a tiny "coke spoon," a "tooter," or even a fingernail cultivated for the purpose. A "line" of cocaine inhaled through a straw or rolled bill delivered approximately 25 mg and typical users would repeat the dose in both nostrils. The general perception among users was that cocaine was safe and nonaddictive, and the medical literature of the time did little to contradict this false perception. Writing in the 1980 edition of the *Comprehensive Textbook of Psychiatry*, Grinspoon and Bakalar stated: "Chronic cocaine abuse usually does not appear as a medical problem" (2). People willing or prone to misuse drugs interpreted these and other similar statements from medical "experts" as a license to try, and then to use, cocaine freely.

A newer method called "freebasing" began in the late 1970s, became popular in the mid-1980s, and was made notorious by the late comedian Richard Pryor who was severely burned when the ether used to extract cocaine alkaloid ignited. Freebasing made cocaine "smokable," allowing rapid self-administration of much higher doses than ever before in the form of a dense vapor, often dozens of times greater than that achieved by snorting. Another form of smokable cocaine appeared in the United States in the mid-1980s and opened a particularly tragic chapter in the history of the drug. Essentially mass-produced freebase cocaine, crack was low priced (as little as $2 per dose), making it available to younger and poorer users and sending the average age of the user spiraling down. Crack is named after the characteristic crackling sound that the "rock" makes when heated. This newest and most deadly formulation of cocaine is remarkably addictive.

The association between cocaine, and crack in particular, and violence is compelling. Just being shot appears to be associated with the presence of cocaine in the blood. Commission of a felony is highly associated with the presence of cocaine in the body of the perpetrator. Our report from 1995 correlated illicit drug use with carrying weapons and violence among 6th through 12th grade students, and there is little to indicate that this has changed much over the past 15 years (3). For example, in 2001, cocaine was the most frequently reported drug in emergency room visits nationwide, with 76 visits per 100,000 population; 24% of the emergency mentions in the report were attributed to crack. Rates in some metropolitan areas far exceeded the national rates. In 2006, the Drug Abuse Warning Network (DAWN) survey estimated 548,608 emergency department (ED) visits involving cocaine, which was by far the most common illicit drug to be involved in emergency care presentations (57% of all illicit drug-related ED visits); a greater number of these 2006 presentations appeared to be linked with crack cocaine than in 2001 (4). Cocaine is consistently among the top three drugs mentioned in mortality data from DAWN, and cocaine or cocaine in combination with alcohol is extremely common in association with suicides (5).

In summary, dramatic changes in the patterns of cocaine use, the typical dosage, and the route of administration have combined to produce deadly epidemics of addiction to a drug once touted by medical experts as "safe." Despite declines in the percentage of the population initiating cocaine use, the percentage of adults who are chronically using cocaine on a regular basis, a large percentage of whom are addicted to crack, is staggering. Approximately 75% of these individuals are likely to meet the *Diagnostic and Statistical Manual of Mental Disorders, Fourth Edition (DSM-IV)* criteria for cocaine dependence. There are high rates of recidivism and tens of thousands of Americans seeking rehabilitation at any given time.

EPIDEMIOLOGY: THE EVOLVING COCAINE "EPIDEMICS"

To be most effective in clinical practice, it is essential to understand the "cocaine problem" from the widest possible perspective. Fortunately, a number of valuable information resources are available to the clinician (6–9). Cocaine abuse in the United States had reached truly epidemic proportions by the late 1970s. When at its peak in the mid-1980s, over 6 million Americans, about 20% of whom were under the age of 18, were using cocaine repeatedly, and many more had tried it at least once. It is estimated that in 1980 alone, nearly 1.5 million Americans were initiated to cocaine use, and that as many as 30 out of every 1,000 young adults were using cocaine. Fortunately, by 1990 the National Household Survey on Drug Abuse (NHSDA) found cause for hope, documenting a dramatic decline in the number of current cocaine users—people who had used the drug within the past 30 days—from 5.8 million in 1985 to 1.6 million in 1990 (6). By 1993, the rate of initiation of cocaine use had dropped to less than half the rate in 1980 and because of increased awareness of the dangers of cocaine, interdiction efforts, or a combination of factors, the rapid "infective" phase of America's worse cocaine epidemic seemed to have subsided. However, the dramatic decline in overall cocaine use from the peak years of the early 1980s should not be viewed as a decrease in the seriousness of the cocaine problem for the following reasons:

1. Although casual experimental use of powder cocaine undoubtedly decreased from the mid-1980s, the introduction of "crack" cocaine around the same time, a much more addictive smokable form of the drug, marked the beginning of a trend in which a core population of frequent, heavy, persistent users began to appear, initially in major urban centers. Obviously, not all compulsive cocaine users are addicted to crack, but it is now well established that even though "only" about 25% of regular cocaine users smoke crack, this comparative minority represents the majority, perhaps as much as 75%, of those entering some form of treatment for cocaine abuse or addiction. With the advent of the crack subepidemic there has been a protracted wave of violence and crime, a burgeoning of serious medical complications, child neglect, increased demand for treatment and, tragically, jail space.

2. By the late 1990s current overall use of cocaine among Americans 12 years and older appeared to be increasing again, with the NHSDA estimating 1.7 million cocaine users, 406,000 of whom (about 23%) were current users of crack in 2001. The best available evidence suggests that this second wave of the cocaine epidemic mostly reflected a moderate increase in use mainly among 18 to 25 year olds. In our 2006 surveillance report on cocaine use in Florida, there was evidence of a renewed epidemic among students and the more affluent, with striking increases in per capita cocaine-related deaths (7).

3. On the one hand, the most recent data from the national surveys suggest that overall use of illicit drugs (other than marijuana) has not continued to increase significantly in the young adult demographic, and in children may have decreased somewhat over the years since 2001. For example, the percentage of 8th and 10th graders reporting lifetime, past year, and past month use of any illicit drug—other than marijuana—has decreased substantially since 2001, according to the most recent reports from the National Institute of Drug Abuse, "Monitoring the Future Survey" (8); if this trend is sustained, it may represent the beginning of a welcome new phase of the cocaine epidemic. However, it should be kept in mind that the rates of initiation and current use of cocaine among youths still remain much higher than those estimated from the 1970s. Furthermore, abuse of prescription and illicit manufactured psychostimulants (e.g., methylphenidate and methamphetamine) by youths and young adults has clearly increased over the past 10 or so years, representing to some extent a "substitute epidemic." Figure 14.1 shows a timeline of usage.

Another important phenomenon to note is that, unlike other drugs of abuse, where rates are highest among adolescents and very young adults, a remarkably high rate of regular (past month) use of cocaine in individuals 26 years and older has been well documented in recent years. Record numbers of middle-aged and even elderly patients are appearing in treatment centers with cocaine abuse as their chief problem. Illicit drug use in general has increased rather dramatically in persons aged 50 to 59 in recent years, with an uncertain contribution from persistent or reinitiated use in aging baby boomers. In 1995, only 37% of drug treatment admissions primarily for problems with smoked cocaine

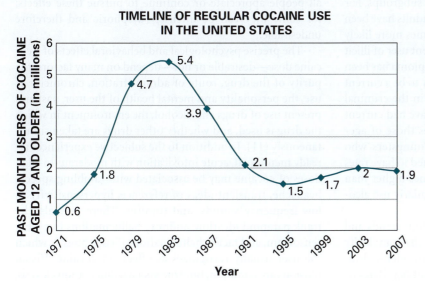

Figure 14.1. Timeline of regular cocaine use in the United States. Estimates of regular cocaine use (number of past month users aged 12 and older in millions) abstracted from the NHSDA and NSDUH reveal striking changes over the past four decades. Although cocaine use has decreased dramatically since the mid-1980s, between 1.5 and 2 million Americans have continued to use frequently in recent years, a substantial percentage of whom are addicted to crack cocaine.

were over the age of 35, but by 2005 68% were in this age group (9).

Beginning in 2002 the National Survey on Drug Use and Health (NSDUH) replaced the NHSDA and, applying more rigorous methodology and much larger sample sizes, brought forward more fine-grained demographic data focusing on current use of cocaine. A brief review of the highlights of the NSDUH-reported trends from 2002 to 2007—the most recent analyzed data set available—is instructive (6). Current cocaine use appears to have been holding steady over most of the past decade at between 0.8% and 1.0% of Americans aged 12 years and older, with approximately 2% of 18 to 25 year olds using cocaine currently. The most recent NSDUH suggested the possibility of a decline in current cocaine use in young adults (from 2.2% in 2006 to 1.7% in 2007), but it will take several more years to see if this, as with the data from the youth surveys noted above, is the beginning of a persistent downward trend. To place current cocaine use in context, current use of marijuana in the young adult demographic has held steadily at a rate six to eight times that of cocaine use over the same time period, while current use of heroin was about half as frequent, the latter perhaps declining slightly. A consistent 20% to 25% of current cocaine users have been identified as users of crack and, although precise estimates are not currently available, most instances of frequent cocaine use—persons using cocaine more than 51 days out of the past year—and most daily or nearly daily use appears to be crack related. In 2007, the NSDUH estimated that there were 610,000 current users of crack ages 12 and up (approximately 0.23% of that demographic), a figure that has not changed appreciably over the past decade. As noted above, crack cocaine users represent a disproportionately high percentage—approximately 75%—of those cocaine users entering treatment. However, from a clinician's perspective it is important to note that a large number of court-sanctioned referrals skew these treatment figures.

The stable rates of overall cocaine use belie the dramatically elevated rates of current use in certain subgroups. For example, over the past decade, unemployed adults have been shown consistently to be about 1.5 to 2.0 times more likely than a full-time employed adult to be a current user of illicit drugs, and an adult without a high school diploma has been shown consistently to be about twice as likely to be a current user than a college graduate. Young adults in the criminal justice system (parolees or on probation) have had current illicit drug use rates as much as four times those of age-matched adults over the past 10 years. Youngsters who smoke cigarettes regularly are well documented to have rates of current illicit drug use as much as 15 times higher than that of nonsmokers, even higher if they regularly use alcoholic beverages.

In summary, a nuanced view of the various trends and subtrends of the cocaine epidemics exposes the complexity of the social factors that the clinician must consider in dealing effectively with the addict or potential addict. Rates of initiation of use and rates of compulsive, regular use vary across age groups, and within any one age group there is considerable variation depending on social status, race, educational achievement, contact with the criminal justice system, and concurrent use of other mind- or mood-altering substances.

PHENOMENOLOGY

Most people try cocaine out of curiosity but those who pursue it seek the unique experience of cocaine intoxication. Although chronic addicts will often relate that they never quite obtain the same subjective "highs" that they did when they first started using, there is nonetheless anecdotal evidence that the typical cocaine user experiences with reasonable consistency a combination of intense, brief pleasure and related enhancements of sensation and perception that are generally outside the scope of normal everyday human experience (10). Patients may develop brisk speech, strained facial expressions, darting eyes, fidgeting, and pacing. Sexual interest and sensitivity is often piqued, and some users describe the experience as akin to a "full body orgasm." The feeling of increased alertness reported subjectively with cocaine can be confirmed by electroencephalographic recordings, which show a general desynchronization of brain waves after cocaine administration. Such desynchronization, which indicates arousal, reveals widespread involvement of the cerebral hemispheres through brainstem and thalamic relays which mediate conscious awareness, attention, and wakefulness. Despite the feeling of arousal, individuals using cocaine usually do not gain superior ability or greater knowledge. Their sense of omnipotence is a temporary delusion; they tend to misinterpret their enhanced confidence and lowered inhibitions as signs of enhanced physical or mental acuity. Taken together, these symptoms, signs, and sensations can be referred to as the euphorigenic and psychostimulant effects of cocaine, and they can be characterized in human functional imaging studies and sometimes inferred in animal models of addiction. Not all people appreciate or continue to pursue these effects; for some they can be intensely dysphoric and therefore undesirable.

The precise psychological and behavioral effects of a cocaine dose—desirable or not—depend on many factors: the purity of the drug, route of administration, chronicity of use, the personality and mental health of the user, past and present use of drugs and alcohol, the environment in which the drug is used, and whether other drugs are taken simultaneously (11). In addition to the subjective experiences already mentioned, acute intoxication with moderate-to-high doses of cocaine may be associated with rambling speech, headache, transient ideas of reference, hypersensitivity to low frequency sounds, and tinnitus. There may also be frank paranoid ideation, auditory hallucinations in a clear sensorium, and tactile hallucinations ("coke bugs"), which the user usually recognizes as effects of cocaine. Visual illusions are common, but true visual hallucinations less so, and when they do occur this is usually indicative of very high or protracted dosing, often in combination with sleep deprivation. Extreme anger with threats or acting out of aggressive behavior may occur. Mood changes such as depression, suicidal ideation, irritability, anhedonia, emotional lability, or disturbances in attention and concentration are common.

The initial experience of cocaine differs widely between people. Interestingly, clinical surveys in both the United States and Europe suggest that only about 10% to 20% of persons who use cocaine become dependent on it, but precise data as to how many of the remainder of those who have tried cocaine subsequently remain casual abusers over long periods of time (as opposed to "turned off" and fully abstinent) are not available. Durable features of personality such as a tendency toward risk taking have been linked with greater likelihood of cocaine abuse and dependence, as have specific psychiatric disorders, including but not limited to attention-deficit hyperactivity disorder (ADHD), schizophrenia, and affective disorders (especially bipolar disorder). In schizophrenics, where tobacco abuse is almost the rule, concurrent use of cocaine may represent a form of self-treatment as, paradoxically, the user may report a temporary calming effect on the psyche, not unlike the calming effect of prescription psychostimulants (e.g., methylphenidate and dextroamphetamine) in persons with ADHD. However, despite the high coincidence of enduring psychopathology in cocaine abusers compared to the general population, it is important to note that many people seeking help will not have identifiable major psychiatric illness or personality disorders; behavioral, cognitive, and emotional abnormalities may resolve dramatically with long-term abstinence and successful treatment.

Not long ago many medical experts assumed that cocaine was not addictive; however, *DSM-IV* now acknowledges that cocaine use can most definitely lead to addiction and establishes criteria for dependence (see Table 14.1). Self-motivated or externally imposed abstinence in cocaine-dependent individuals may or may not be accompanied by signs of withdrawal, although cocaine rarely, if ever, produces physiologic dependence, as is common with addiction to opiates, alcohol, and barbiturates. At the extreme ends of the spectrum cocaine withdrawal may manifest with minimal degrees of dysphoria or produce frank anhedonia with psychomotor retardation (12). Patients may have limited interest in the environment, limited ability to experience pleasure, and severely decreased energy. Elopement from treatment and relapse are very common within the first several days postcessation of use.

TABLE 14.1 Clinical criteria for cocaine dependence

The ***DSM-IV-TR*** defines cocaine dependence as "a maladaptive pattern of use leading to clinically significant impairment or distress." Three or more of the following clinical features, occurring within a 1-year period, are needed to make the diagnosis:

1. Tolerance. There is a need for more cocaine to achieve the desired effect or the experiences markedly diminished effect with continued use of the same amount.
2. Withdrawal. After cessation of heavy or prolonged cocaine use, the patient may experience pronounced dysphoric mood and one or more of the following: fatigue, unpleasant dreams, insomnia or hypersomnia, increased appetite, psychomotor retardation, or agitation. The symptoms above cause clinically significant impairment of functioning and are not accounted for by another mental disorder.
3. Loss of control over use. Large amounts of cocaine are taken or it is used over a longer period of time, especially when the person did not "intend" to use as much as they actually did.
4. Persistent desire to change or control use, including unsuccessful or aborted efforts to quit.
5. Preoccupation with obtaining or securing supply; inordinate time using the substance or recovering from intoxication.
6. Reduction or elimination of important social, occupational, or recreational activities because of use.
7. Continued use despite serious adverse consequences. Ongoing use despite major physical, psychological, or social consequences.

Criteria 3 through 7 are highlighted. The emphasis is on lack of control over use and continued use despite what are often devastating consequences. According to revisions in the *DSM-IV*, it is not necessary to manifest (1) tolerance or (2) withdrawal in order to be diagnosed with substance dependence. With this modified definition, cocaine is recognized as addictive even though there are often no major physical withdrawal symptoms, and tolerance is quite variable.

The *DSM-IV-TR* formally acknowledges this change in diagnostic criteria by specifying the following modifiers:

- Dependence with Physiological Dependence—evidence of tolerance or withdrawal (i.e., item 1 or item 2 is present).
- Dependence without Physiological Dependence—no evidence of tolerance or withdrawal (i.e., neither item 1 nor item 2 is present).

DETERMINANTS OF USE

Elements that influence susceptibility to cocaine addiction include the speed of onset and duration of elevated blood levels, genetically determined differences in pharmacodynamic response, postdrug effects and social–environmental setting. The particular roles of each of these factors have been elucidated at various levels of detail and certainty over the past 30 years, and animal models of addiction have been of tremendous value in parsing them. A full account of each is well beyond the scope of this chapter, but a few of the more important considerations most relevant to clinical practice are briefly addressed.

Pharmacologic Considerations

Cocaine—benzoylmethylecgonine—is a naturally occurring crystalline alkaloid of the tropane family that also includes atropine and scopolamine. It does not exert notable anticholinergic effects. As described in more detail in the following section, cocaine's primary neuropharmacologic effect is to block the uptake of monoamines released into synapses of the central nervous system. However, cocaine also has sympathomimetic actions in peripheral tissues and quinidine-like anesthetic/type I antidysrhythmic properties. As a local anesthetic, cocaine's main effect is to block sodium channels in excitable tissues, and in high doses it can also interfere with certain potassium channels and induce a profound failure of electrical transmission in the heart and central nervous system, as may be seen with accidental massive overdoses (e.g., a smuggler who "bodypacks," or "bodystuffing" during a police raid).

Cocaine is a relatively small (molecular weight 303) lipophilic molecule that is well absorbed through mucous membranes and alveoli. About one-third of an oral or nasal dose of powder cocaine, and up to 95% of an inhaled dose of freebase or crack cocaine may be bioavailable. Once in the blood, it readily penetrates the blood–brain barrier. Binding of cocaine to plasma proteins is minimal and volume of distribution is low; blood to plasma concentration ratios are typically close to unity. At the doses typically seen in clinical practice, ingestion of cocaine can be viewed as a multitoxic exposure because enzymatic and nonenzymatic hydrolysis produce a number of metabolites, some of which have the same or greater effects as cocaine. Active metabolites may intensify or prolong cocaine euphoria. As a testimony to the desperation that may accompany compulsive use of cocaine, there are case reports of addicts injecting cholinesterase-inhibiting insecticides to attempt to enhance their highs. Benzoylecgonine, a neuropharmacologically active and cardiotoxic agent, is produced rapidly by enzymatic (hepatic carboxyesterases) and nonenzymatic hydrolysis and is usually the major metabolite of cocaine, but when cocaine is smoked there may be relatively greater production of ecgonine methylester. The latter is generally considered the least toxic of the major metabolites and is formed readily by the action butyrylcholinesterases in plasma, brain, and lung. Bacterially derived choline esterases and mutant forms of human butyrylcholinesterase, both of which have orders of magnitude greater activities than native enzymes, are under active investigation as "antidotes" for the emergency management of life-threatening overdose situations. These modified enzymes can facilitate rapid metabolism of cocaine to the less toxic ecgonine methylester. Under conditions that inactivate butyrylcholinesterases or activate hepatic N-demethylation, benzoylecgonine and norcocaine may be produced in considerably larger metabolic amounts than their usual 50% and 5%, respectively. Inactivation conditions may be extremes of age or presence of medications with cholinesterase inhibitory action; examples of activation conditions are pregnancy or elevated progesterone and testosterone. The latter is neuropharmacologically active and is also a potent vasoconstrictor. Tiny quantities of several other metabolites are produced to varying extents under varying conditions, but these are usually of no clinical significance. Very little cocaine is passed unchanged in the urine and stool.

The purer the drug, the greater its effects, but as a rule, pure cocaine is unavailable on the street. Cocaine is typically heavily adulterated with other substances such as mannitol, lactose, or glucose to add weight, and caffeine, lidocaine, amphetamines, quinine, or even heroin to add taste and to provide additional central nervous system stimulant effects. The typical concentration of cocaine in street preparations ranges from 10% to 50%; rarely, samples can contain as much as 70% cocaine. Both the cocaine concentration and the adulterants affect the user's response to the drug and the potential complications of use, particularly venous irritation and pulmonary insults in intravenous (IV) and smoked cocaine users, respectively.

Routes of administration that deliver drug rapidly to the brain are intensely euphoric, most rapidly addicting, and also the most sensitizing to the effects of future cocaine use (11,13). In other words, a person who has used crack in the past is more likely to experience pronounced psychological and physical effects to even moderate future dosing than a person who has used a comparable dose of cocaine through insufflation. Rate of administration appears to influence the extent to which long-lasting changes in brain cell function, including expression of immediate early genes and neurotransmitter receptor populations, may occur (14). Generally, cocaine tends to be less addictive if the dose is small, the peak plasma levels low, the onset of activity slow, the duration of action long, and the unpleasant withdrawal effects absent or very mild. If cocaine is taken by means of chewed coca leaves, through oral ingestion, or through nasal insufflation, consequences are generally slow to develop. The latter consideration is part of the justification for the not unreasonable but controversial suggestion that oral cocaine in the form of tablets or tea may be used to treat people who have become addicted to cocaine delivered more rapidly to the brain.

IV cocaine use ranks high on the addiction potential scale. The onset of the IV cocaine "rush" is within 30 to 45 seconds, and the drug's effects last for 10 to 20 minutes. One hundred percent of an IV dose is delivered to the circulatory system, compared with perhaps 20% to 30% of a relatively poorly absorbed oral or intranasal dose, and peak blood levels after an injection can be more than twice those that occur following intranasal ingestion. Nevertheless, for many reasons—pain of injection, difficulty of finding and using needles and syringes, risk of infectious disease—IV administration is less appealing to most cocaine abusers than other administration methods and is considerably less common than insufflation or smoking. When it is seen in clinical practice, patients often concurrently use opiates such as heroin ("speedballing"), in part to enhance the high, in part to offset the undesirable adrenergic effects and paranoia that can attend IV injection of cocaine.

Cocaine in any smokable form, whether coca paste, freebase, or crack, probably has the highest addictive potential. The resulting high is intense and the onset is extremely rapid (15). Only 8 to 10 seconds elapse before the user experiences the high, and peak brain concentrations occur more rapidly than following IV use since the venous side of the circulation is bypassed. Anecdotal data suggest that cocaine smokers are twice as likely to fail to complete their treatment program as are intranasal abusers. Crack cocaine is frequently used in combination with alcohol. As with coadministration of an opiate in the IV cocaine user, the effects of alcohol tend to blunt the undesirable effects and may prolong the high. People who simultaneously abuse cocaine and alcohol may be susceptible to heightened morbidity related to cocaethylene, a cardiotoxic metabolite that also possesses some stimulant effect. Also contributing to the high addiction potential of crack is the fact that the effects of the drug last only 5 to 10 minutes. After the high is over, the crack user feels extremely anxious and depressed. Such a rapid shift between the drug's positive and negative effects makes users immediately crave the euphoria they felt just moments before. Most troubling to the addict (and clinician) is the dysphoria and drive for a cocaine remedy that they know can be achieved by a "hit." The intellectual knowledge that the resolution of dysphoria will not last is often overwhelmed by the intensity of the cravings that form a distinct part of the cocaine withdrawal syndrome.

One of the enduring mysteries of addiction medicine is the extent to which different people, apparently with similar initial drug exposures and opportunities for ongoing drug use, will respond so differently to those experiences. In the past, the differences between an experimenter who promptly quits, a chronic abuser, and an addict may have been attributed more to social and moral factors than to biologic ones. While the former may play some role in the broad scheme of things, 30 years of medical research unquestionably points to a powerful biologic foundation of cocaine addiction and addictions more generally (16,17). Animal models, including those involving nonhuman primates reared in naturalistic settings, clearly indicate that genetic and social–environmental factors dramatically alter the biology of brain regions intimately involved in establishing and perpetuating addictions (18,19). There is compelling evidence that animals—and presumably also humans—inclined to self-administer cocaine may have both quantitative and qualitative differences in receptor populations and, perhaps even more interestingly, apparent differences in the fundamental intracellular signaling events that proceed from receptor binding (20). Some of these changes appear to be fixed features of the genetic endowment, and others may actually reflect changes in brain cell function induced by the social environment, including the social context of cocaine use. The following subsection provides a brief overview of some of the compelling themes from recent research into the neurobiology of addiction.

Neurobiology

Cocaine addiction has been described as a disease of the brain's "pleasure centers"—neural networks subserved primarily by the monoamine neurotransmitter dopamine (DA) (16). However, recent insights have broadened the concept of pleasure center to include not only the dopaminergic connections between the brainstem and the structures of the basal forebrain (prominently including the nucleus accumbens [NAcc]), but several frontal cortical regions, and an increasingly important role for nondopaminergic neurotransmission. The latter prominently includes but is certainly not limited to amino acid neurotransmitters (both excitatory [glutamate] and inhibitory [gamma-aminobutyric acid, GABA]), serotonin, endogenous opioids, endocannibanoids, and proximal components of the hypothalamic–pituitary–adrenal (HPA) axis. The hippocampal formations, amygdalae, prefrontal cortex, and anterior cingulate regions—all components of the limbic system—play prominent roles in this enriched and more differentiated view of pleasure center circuitry and are the current focus of intensive research (Fig. 14.2).

There is also growing appreciation of the extent to which the brainstem's DA centers and their projections are anatomically differentiated and profoundly influenced by other neurotransmitter and neuromodulatory molecules. For example, more lateral groupings of DA-producing cells in the ventral tegmental area (VTA) of the midbrain project mainly to the more superficial shell of the NAcc. The shell region mediates reinforcement effects that increase the efficiency of acquisition behavior after initial exposure to cocaine. Cells of the NAcc core appear to be more intimately involved in the long-term plasticity that appears to underlie craving and cue-sensitive relapse behaviors. The magnitudes and patterns of release of DA from neurons originating in the VTA are in turn modulated by reciprocal, largely GABA-inhibitory projections from the NAcc and by excitatory glutamate projections from limbic prefrontal cortex (21). DA neurotransmission is generally facilitated by the effects of endocannabinoid receptor activation (22), and endogenous opioids produce mixed effects (23,24). Compounds that activate kappa-opioid receptors

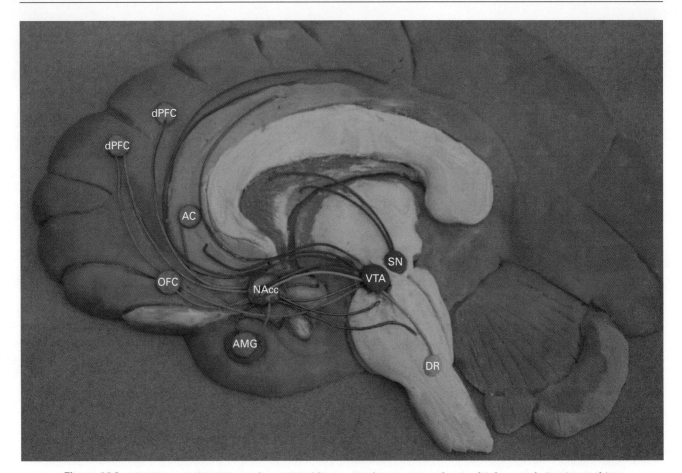

Figure 14.2. The functional anatomy of cocaine addiction can be represented as multiple neural circuits working in conjunction, providing both positive and negative feedbacks at key points of interaction. Dopamine-producing cells in the ventral tegmental area (*VTA*) and substantia nigra (*SN*) project to the nucleus accumbens (*NAcc*; part of ventral striatum) and to the dorsal-motor striatum, respectively. Serotonin-producing cells of the dorsal raphe nuclei (*DR*) also project to NAcc. In turn, GABA-producing medium spiny neurons of the NAcc project back to brainstem dopamine and serotonin centers, completing the negative feedback loop of a mesoaccumbal circuit. Dopamine projections to the ventral and dorsal striatum exert excitatory (mostly through D1 receptors) and inhibitory (mostly through D2 receptors) effects, with D3 receptors also abundantly expressed in the NAcc. GABAergic cells of the NAcc frequently coexpress the neuromodulatory peptide dynorphin. GABA-dopamine interactions are now also thought to be powerfully modulated by the hypothalamic-pituitary-adrenal axis and by endocannibanoids acting through CRF-1 and CB-1 receptors, respectively (not shown in figure).

A second circuit comprises direct projections from dopamine-producing cells of the midbrain to the amygdala (*AMG*) and multiple limbic cortical sites, prominently including dorsal prefrontal cortex (*dPFC*), orbitofrontal cortex (*OFC*), and anterior cingulate (*AC*). Cortical and AMG neurons in turn project back to the VTA and NAcc primarily using the excitatory neurotransmitter glutamate completing a mesocortical circuit. Glutamate-producing cells, which also frequently coexpress dynorphin and other neuromodulatory peptides, act through a multitude of ionotropic and metabotropic glutamate receptor subtypes that are expressed throughout the basal ganglia and brainstem. Metabotropic glutamate receptors in particular have been implicated in the long-term plasticities that accompany chronic use of cocaine.

A third integrating circuit establishes connections in a series from limbic cortex to VTA, VTA to NAcc, NAcc to discrete regions of the ventral pallidum, and thenceforth to the dorsomedial nucleus of the thalamus, which in turn projects to prefrontal cortical regions, completing a corticostriatopallidal circuit. In addition to ventral pallidum, medium spiny cells in the NAcc also send GABAergic projections to the hypothalamus, lateral preoptic area, and more caudal regions of the brainstem.

Recent data also support an important role for the dorsal-motor striatum in cocaine addiction. Acting through polysynaptic connections between the shell region of the NAcc and midbrain dopamine centers, the dorsal striatopallidal system may prominently influence the transition from conscious pursuit of cocaine to more automated habit-like behaviors. (Illustration by RP Paczynski and Jennifer Koller.)

(most notably dynorphin) tend to counteract mesolimbic DA neurotransmission, while those that activate mu-opioid receptors tend to facilitate it. Subjects with robust brain dynorphin expression in the setting of cocaine use may be at less risk of addiction. In contrast, there is strong evidence that long-term reinforcement of cocaine self-administration is difficult to induce in experimental animals with deficient mu-opioid receptor functions.

A receptor for cocaine has been identified, a high-affinity binding site on the DA transporter (DAT) in presynaptic elements of dopaminergic nerve terminals. By attaching to and reversibly inactivating these membrane-bound transport proteins, cocaine blocks the reuptake of DA when it is released and thereby produces an acute but *relatively* sustained increase in synaptic DA availability. Increased DA receptor binding occurs as a consequence. In contrast, most other drugs of abuse and many nondrug pleasure-producing stimuli appear to influence DA availability indirectly by modulating the excitability and firing patterns of DA-producing cells in the VTA. Cocaine is not a selective DAT blocker, however, and it is well established that it also impairs reuptake of serotonin and norepinephrine. It is interesting to note that in DAT "knockout" mice, cocaine may still induce increases in DA levels in the brain and still produce its primary reinforcing effects; it is believed that in these genetically altered brain serotonin reuptake transporters may in a sense "takeover" the interplay of presynaptic DA release and reuptake. The acute surpluses of monoamine neurotransmitters produced by cocaine also activate responses within the sympathetic nervous system, producing such effects as pupillary dilation, vasoconstriction, and acute increases in heart rate and blood pressure, addressed in greater detail in the discussion of comorbidities and complications of use.

Some of the best evidence for a general theory of addiction centering on DA comes from classic experiments utilizing animal models of cocaine self-administration (25). Kalivas and Duffy placed dialysis probes in the VTA projections that terminate within the NAcc, providing direct evidence for specific roles of these structures in sensitization to cocaine's effects in self-administration paradigms; Petit and Justice, using microdialysis in the NAcc, demonstrated that extracellular DA levels are increased during cocaine self-administration, with behaviors directed toward attaining specific, almost optimal, DA levels. DA levels attained were dose dependent and correlated with increased cocaine intake. However, DA projections from the VTA to NAcc are certainly not the only elements involved in increasing DA neurotransmission in response to cocaine. The pleasurable effects of cocaine are probably also related to increases in DA and serotonin in the cerebral cortex through extensive mesocortical projections (26). In addition to the relatively sustained increase in DA levels related to transporter blocking effects, it has recently been demonstrated that cocaine induces phasic surges in DA release within the NAcc and other structures on a subsecond timescale. These phasic changes are highly dynamic and have been related by Cheer et al., and other investigators, to the links between cocaine self-administration, environmental cues, and other contextual information (27).

Acute administration of cocaine clearly results in increased levels of synaptic DA. However, it is superficial to imagine that brain DA levels remain elevated in the wake of repeated cocaine exposure; the opposite may be the case (28). Using binge administration paradigms, some investigators have found significantly reduced basal DA levels after chronic self-administration, and chronic exposure to cocaine may significantly alter the patterns but not the magnitude of the acute DA response to cocaine. Dopaminergic neurons appear to demonstrate tolerance and diminished responses to chronic self-administration consistent with the notion of a functional DA deficit developing over time, as suggested in our landmark work (29). There is strong evidence that postsynaptic DA receptor availability (and probably the actual density of DA receptors) changes in response to prolonged, repeated exposure to cocaine. This has been conceived as another aspect of an evolving hypodopaminergic state, but the interactions between basal DA levels, acute presynaptic responses to cocaine, DA receptor density, and receptor responsiveness are highly complex. An interesting paradox is presented by the fact that reductions in DA receptor populations, an evident feature of cocaine tolerance, may coexist with heightened sensitivity to some of the psychomotor stimulant effects of cocaine administration after chronic self-administration. A possible explanation for sensitization phenomena in the setting of reduced receptor numbers is differential expression and/or activation of subpopulations of DA receptors that may be more specifically linked with the behaviors of sensitization behaviors. These differential effects may have important therapeutic implications (30).

Environmental and Social Features

Some of the more interesting research findings in recent years address the long-standing question of why some individuals in particular circumstances seem more inclined to psychostimulant addiction. In experiments involving drug-naive monkeys, Nader et al. have provided evidence that individuals with lower D2-type dopamine receptor levels have heightened vulnerability to the reinforcing effects of cocaine (18,19). Similarly, Volkow and colleagues have reported that nonaddict human subjects with lower levels of D2 receptors were more likely to report a euphoric response to IV methylphenidate (31). In contrast, subjects with higher levels of these receptors tended to state that methylphenidate not only did not appeal to them, but made them feel awful. It is therefore difficult to distinguish between the possibilities of increased vulnerability to psychostimulant addiction stemming from DA deficiency, and relative protection from addiction based on a generous DA receptor endowment. The situation is further complicated by the fact that, at least in subhuman primates, brain DA receptor levels may change according to position in a dynamic social hierarchy (up in dominant animals, down in submissive animals). Do these findings reflect a genetic predisposition to addiction or a vulnerability induced by social environment? The work of Nader and others demonstrate that both may be the case, raising the possibility of a "vicious cycle" of addiction risk. The suggested pathophysiology is analogous to the postulated deficit of endogenous opiate receptor functioning in heroin addicts, and the clinical implications are fascinating. Evidence of social and environmental influences on patterns of drug use is an important reminder of the dynamic nature of receptor biology.

In most animal models of cocaine dependence, drug pursuit behaviors seem to be powerfully reinforcing themselves. Brain DA levels and rapidity of reinforcement are increased in self-administration paradigms compared with circumstances where the same dose of drug is administered by the experimenter. Recent studies have tried to separate addiction from neural adaptation by comparing volitional self-administration from passive (involuntary) drug injections. Not only does addiction develop in the former, but neurochemical changes *appear to be maximized* with self-administration models. In studies of nonhuman primates, cocaine self-administration rapidly produces a progressive, spreading pattern of increased metabolic activity in the upper brainstem, mediodorsal nucleus of the thalamus, and several areas of the prefrontal cortex (26).

Pavlovian conditioned responses to environmental cues (e.g., placement preference paradigms in animal models of cocaine dependence) seem to be a major "source" of relapse. In autoradiographic studies in animals, and using positron emission tomography and functional magnetic resonance imaging in humans, a subject's perception of drug-related cues causes limbic-connected neocortical regions to "light up." For example, the sight of drug paraphernalia or a street corner where drugs were frequently purchased might elicit powerful craving that is accompanied by increased cerebral metabolism, particularly in the orbitofrontal cortex and portions of the anterior cingulate region (32). In fact, these cue-sensitive changes in regional metabolism provide some of the best evidence for a critical role of neocortical structures in mediating hallmark features of full-blown addiction: anticipation and craving as preludes to relapse, even after long periods of abstinence. Glutamatergic projections from prefrontal cortex and amygdalae to both NAcc and VTA likely play a key role in these aspects of addiction (21). Nondependent subjects exhibit metabolic changes in subcortical structures when they are exposed to the cocaine, but recent studies suggest that only addicts develop robust increases in regional metabolism in prefrontal and anterior cingulate cortex; these changes occur during periods of craving, with intoxication, and with compulsive use (binging), strongly suggesting that recruitment and sensitization of these higher brain centers are essential aspects of the addiction process (32).

On the other hand, in persons with established addiction to cocaine, or other psychostimulants, frontal lobe metabolism may be substantially *decreased* from baseline *during withdrawal* from a period of binge use. This finding does not necessarily conflict with the suggestion that phasic cortical activation is essential to the behaviors leading up to relapse. Perhaps not unexpectedly, withdrawal-related hypometabolism appears to correlate with decreased dopamine receptor availability, as judged by radiotraced DA receptor studies, consistent with the aforementioned concept of a hypodopaminergic state in the chronic abuser (28). Unfortunately, frontal deficits may not always be reversible functional changes. Certain cognitive deficits and impairments of affect, particularly those related to impulse control and assignment of circumstance-appropriate salience to stimuli, may be permanent in some people. These observations from the neuropsychology literature are consistent with some of the grim findings from gross neuropathologic studies going back several decades.

There are extensive communications between the NAcc and the amygdala. While the NAcc clearly plays a critical role in the aforementioned reinforcing properties of cocaine and other stimulants, the amygdala has extensive connections with other portions of the limbic system and integrates emotional experiences—elation, fear, anger—with specific visual, auditory, tactile, olfactory, and gustatory memories. In the mind of the user, strong associations form between cocaine and the internal and external environments from the very beginning of cocaine use. The danger, allure, and sense of the streets increase the reinforcing potency of cocaine. In the setting of functional or anatomic impairment of prefrontal cortex, the amygdala may drive a less flexible, more stimulus-bound behavioral repertoire. Environmental information and memories appear to be coupled to reinforcement of cocaine self-administration through the effects of endocannabinoids, endogenous opioids, and other neuro-modulatory proteins (22–24).

EVALUATION AND TREATMENT APPROACHES

Initial Evaluation and Management

A comprehensive assessment of the pharmacologic, medical, psychological, and social aspects of the patient's substance abuse problem is needed in all cases. For many patients, cocaine use has become the focus of their entire life. They may have become so accustomed to the mood changes, constant pursuit of supply, and the various risks involved in their lifestyle that they have all but forgotten what life without drugs is like. Thus, they come to regard the drugged state as normal and may not believe treatment is necessary (33). Consequently, many patients enter treatment only under pressure from family, friends, employers, or the judicial system. In some cases the patient may become extremely paranoid and perceive the machinations of "enemies." Therefore, families often need guidance from medical professionals in staging an intervention on a cocaine-abusing relative.

Initial contact with a patient may occur while the patient is still intoxicated, but is more often after the "cocaine crash" and during the withdrawal phase, which may last from hours to weeks. The physician should take a complete medical, family, and forensic history to include a history of *all* drug use. However, information obtained from chemically dependent people is notoriously unreliable, and there is no substitute for obtaining collateral information from family or other close contacts. A thorough physical and dental examination should include assessment for occult trauma. Patients ideally will have already been screened by medical personnel prior to arrival at a rehabilitation facility, but under many conditions this service may not have been afforded. In the patient with altered sensorium it is always best to assume the worst, namely that they may be under the escalating influence of one or more mind-altering drugs, manifesting an organic brain disorder, or both. One particular concern is that patients about to enter a hospital or other rehabilitation unit may have ingested large and potentially lethal doses of one or more drugs, often as part of an ill-conceived "last hurrah." Laboratory tests, electrocardiograms, and chest x-rays may supply useful information and may help to reassure both staff and patients as to medical stability and general state of health. Any severe conditions or impending medical emergencies may necessitate transfer to the medical floor of a hospital.

Having established medical stability, the first step in treatment is, of course, to diagnose the patient's condition accurately. Table 14.1 lists the clinical criteria of cocaine dependence and some of the features of cocaine withdrawal, based on the *DSM-IV-TR*. Importantly, the withdrawal syndrome following even heavy, frequent cocaine use may not be particularly prominent, is rarely life-threatening, and generally not the focus of the specialist in addiction medicine. It is often said that withdrawal from cocaine is primarily psychological, as opposed to the prominent physical withdrawal syndromes seen commonly with dependence to alcohol, opiates, benzodiazepines, and barbiturates. The symptoms of cocaine withdrawal syndrome are certainly of concern, however, because withdrawal-related dysphoria and intense craving increase the chances of elopement from treatment. Using the Cocaine Selective Severity Assessment (CSSA), some investigators have identified intensity of withdrawal symptoms as one of the most, if not the most, powerful predictors of treatment failure. The CSSA has also been suggested as a means to quickly identify the so-called "Type B" patients (those with more severe withdrawal symptoms and other poor prognostic indicators) for more intensive monitoring and management. Medical treatment that helps relieve withdrawal symptoms *may* therefore improve the initial prognosis, but some of the earliest clinical trials indicated that successful amelioration of withdrawal alone appears to be of limited significance *for long-term success*. Painless and symptomless cocaine withdrawal was often followed by relapse and return to active addiction, just as in the past clonidine detoxification was followed by opiate relapse, and initial success with the nicotine patch is frequently followed by return to smoking. It is a vestige of old ways of thinking about addiction within the medical community to place too much attention on "management of withdrawal" often to the detriment of long-term treatment of the addiction process. One of the clinician's most important roles is to assure the person in withdrawal from cocaine that their symptoms are common, transitory, not usually of major medical concern, and, perhaps for some, part of the process of recovery.

Regardless of the initial (provisional) diagnosis, toxicologic analysis of body fluids should be made. Testing confirms the clinical impression and may help identify concomitant use of other drugs. Negative testing may help identify numerous other disorders that can mimic all or most of the features of cocaine intoxication, cocaine withdrawal, cocaine delirium, and cocaine delusional disorder, all of which are detailed in the *DSM-IV*. Laboratory testing's main value, however, is to eliminate the need to continually question the patient about current drug use and uncover occult use in the therapeutic setting. As a therapeutic relationship is established, "trust but verify" is the operative principle, and this attitude can provide a strong motivation for the patient to remain drug free. Excellent recent discussions of forensic evaluation of cocaine dependence by Liberty et al. and others are available (34). Here, we will limit comments to a few key points the importance of which cannot be over-stated: immediately following the initial physical examination, blood and/or supervised urine samples should be collected and sent for analysis; if possible, a sample of the cocaine used by the patient should also be submitted to the laboratory; all subsequent urine collections should be supervised and taken first thing in the morning; temperature and/or specific gravity should be measured to confirm that the sample has not been adulterated.

In addition to the standard urine tests for cocaine (typically an inexpensive immunochromatographic assay for cocaine and its major metabolite benzoylecgonine), analytical methods for the simultaneous determination of cocaine and its major metabolites in oral fluid and hair and in the case of crack even sweat (captured under tamperproof patches) have been developed. Hair samples provide a long window of opportunity with each half inch of hair representing approximately 1 week of history. When the distinction is clinically important, unique pyrolysis products of crack (burned cocaine) can now be detected through gas chromatography–mass spectrometry. Although expensive, gas chromatography–mass spectrometry testing is many times more sensitive and specific than either thin-layer chromatography or immunoassay drug screens.

Characterization of the patient's pattern of use is important in assessing the extent to which the patient has progressed along the path that leads from experimental or occasional use (initiation) to compulsive, often more frequent use. The severity of withdrawal symptoms may be estimated from the pattern of use, and the chronicity of use is frequently an indirect indicator of the extent to which the patient's life may be in disarray. Unlike the so-called functioning alcoholic, it is relatively rare for a regular cocaine user to maintain anything resembling functionality. Cocaine dependence is associated with either of two patterns of self-administration: episodic or daily (or almost daily) use. Cocaine use separated by 2 or more days of nonuse is considered episodic. Binges are a form of episodic use characterized by continuous high-dose use over a period of hours or days. Binges usually terminate only when cocaine supplies are depleted, or the user becomes so exhausted that they "pass out." With chronic daily use, there are generally no wide fluctuations in dose on successive days; rather, it is an increase in dose over time that indicates the development of dependence. With continuing use there is often diminution of pleasure as a consequence of tolerance, increase in dysphoric effects, and accumulation of adverse consequences. Despite these realities, with cocaine dependence use persists or may even accelerate.

Inpatient versus Outpatient Care

An accepted method for recommendations of level of intensity of treatment is provided by the American Society of Addiction Medicine (ASAM) in its Patient Placement Criteria 2-R (PPC-2R). Two sets of guidelines are provided by the ASAM PPC-2R, one for adults and one for adolescents with five broad levels of care for each group. Information from six dimensions—(a) acute intoxication and/or withdrawal potential, (b) biomedical conditions and complications, (c) emotional/behavioral/cognitive conditions and complications, (d) readiness to change (formerly treatment acceptance/resistance), (e) relapse/continued use/continued problem potential, and (f) recovery environment—is used to determine the recommended level of care. The levels of care are Level 0.5, Early Intervention; Level I, Outpatient Treatment; Level II, Intensive Outpatient/Partial Hospitalization; Level III, Residential/Inpatient Treatment; and Level IV, Medically Managed Intensive Inpatient Treatment. A range of specific types of care are found within these broad levels of service.

For several reasons, outpatient treatment is the preferred modality of care if circumstances permit. First, as noted above, use of cocaine can usually be stopped abruptly without medical risk or major discomfort, so many cocaine abusers can be treated as outpatients. Second, the goal of treatment is always to return the patient to a normal life. Third, the cost of outpatient treatment is in general lower (although some insurance companies may refuse to pay for care delivered in the outpatient setting). Fourth, many patients—particularly women with parenting responsibilities—are more willing to accept help on an outpatient basis because it carries less of a social stigma and is less disruptive to daily life. Given the lifelong risk of relapse and the need for ongoing support, all cases of substance abuse will eventually need outpatient care and this is perhaps the most important consideration of all. On the other hand, recommending treatment in a hospital or residential rehabilitation center clearly conveys the impression of imminent danger. When drug use is severe, or if outpatient care is not possible or has failed in the past, treatment in a hospital or residential rehabilitation center is called for. Commonly recognized indications for inpatient care include chronic cocaine use with history of multiple relapses, comorbid dependence on another drug, serious comorbid psychiatric or medical illness, or major lack of social support. An important advantage of a treatment facility is removing patients from the environment—the home, the street—that may be contributing to their drug use. Patients under round-the-clock supervision are unable (in most cases) to obtain illicit drugs. They can take daily advantage of the many types of therapy the inpatient or residential facility offers. Another advantage is that patients are available for full medical and psychiatric evaluations, which will reveal whether any coexisting problems exist, such as cognitive impairment, clinical depression, HIV infection, hepatitis, and so on. Suspected cognitive impairments and psychiatric problems in particular can only be confirmed after detoxification and substantive observation. Successful initial treatment in a residential setting may improve retention by facilitating the integration of the patient into self-help and social support networks. Indeed, inpatient or residential treatment may provide an ideal transition from active addiction to abstinence and daily meetings.

Current and Future Treatment

In this section we endeavor to provide a concise overview of both nonpharmacologic and pharmacologic approaches to the treatment of cocaine dependency. Nonpharmacologic approaches are discussed first because despite impressive recent advances in the neurobiology of cocaine addiction, "psychosocial" treatments are the mainstay of management of cocaine dependence in 2010. Remarkably, with the notable exception of opiate addiction, use of medicines in the day-to-day management of addictions remains quite limited when compared to the prominent role of drugs in the other two most prevalent categories of psychiatric illness, namely affective and anxiety disorders. Addictions are currently the third most prevalent psychiatric illness. Nonpharmacologic therapies play a central role in the current standard of care and they must be included in drug trials as part of the therapeutic background against which drug effects are measured. Even the most promising biological and pharmaceutical approaches to cocaine addiction are unlikely to *replace* nonpharmacologic approaches. Indeed, drugs are more likely to be used as bridge therapies during early recovery and in periods of high risk of relapse.

Most treatment facilities have adopted the chemical dependency model, which regards drug dependence as a primary condition—a disease unto itself—not a secondary problem arising from some other underlying psychopathology. Such programs take a multidisciplinary approach to drug treatment and provide a range of behavioral, cognitive, educational, and self-control techniques aimed at reducing drug cravings and the potential for relapse. The multidisciplinary/multimodal approach has evolved in light of the highly challenging, multifaceted nature of the disease of addiction. Most persons who enter treatment do so with many aspects of their lives disrupted; the multidisciplinary approach therefore seems very appropriate.

Different treatment modalities for cocaine addiction have their advocates and detractors, but some of the more durable and commonly used include the 12-step programs, CBT, the so-called contingency management, and the matrix model. These and related therapies are discussed in depth in Part 2 of this book. Recent reviews have demonstrated that psychological and cognitive behavioral approaches to addiction have response/success rates that are generally moderate, but otherwise quite comparable to nonpharmacologic interventions for other mental health problems (35). The 12-step programs emphasize coming to terms with and "owning" addiction as a chronic disease process which is managed, never completely cured. Adherents to a 12-step program accept the individual's powerlessness over addiction, pursue ongoing social support from people in the same boat, and maintain vigilant watch over a disease process that is as much a spiritual as a physical problem. CBT is a time-tested approach that is often used in comparison with ("control group") or in addition to pharmacologic treatments in clinical trials. CBT emphasizes identification of factors that tend to trigger relapses, psychosocial barriers to sustained abstinence, and development of a rational plan of action steps that a patient can realistically employ. Reports of mixed results with CBT may reflect the fact that this form of treatment is highly "operator dependent." In the opinion of the authors there is no substitute for highly motivated, socially engaging therapists (as opposed to manual-oriented provision of CBT) in achieving favorable outcomes. The "matrix model" can be described as a holistic approach that strives to provide general supportive psychotherapy while balancing positive and negative reinforcement of sober behavior, and documented abstinence. Self-help participation, drug education, and family/group therapies are emphasized. Most treatment centers offer some form of the matrix model, either as inpatient or outpatient therapy.

In some studies contingency management or the "community reinforcement approach" has shown more efficacy than traditional counseling or pharmacotherapies (36). Literally, paying for abstinence by focusing on drug- and cocaine-free urine tests rather than a more amorphous outcome can succeed where standard drug-abuse counseling has failed to retain cocaine-dependent individuals in outpatient treatment. In one early study, a surprising 85% of patients completed 12 weeks of incentive treatment (earning vouchers exchangeable for retail items) and 65% to 70% achieved 6 or more weeks of continuous cocaine abstinence across the two trials. By contrast, less than 45% of patients assigned to standard counseling completed 12 weeks of treatment.

In recent studies the effectiveness and frequency of CBT counseling sessions have been evaluated in cocaine-dependent patients. Twelve weeks of CBT has been shown to decrease cocaine craving and use, and may be effective even when used on a less intensive schedule. Efrat, Aharonovich, and colleagues have used the MicroCog computerized battery to assess cognitive performance at treatment entry and to compare cognitive functioning between completers (patients remaining in treatment at least 12 weeks) and dropouts. The results indicated that treatment completers had demonstrated significantly better cognitive performance at baseline than had patients who dropped out of treatment. Cognitive domains that significantly distinguished between treatment completers and dropouts were attention, mental reasoning, and spatial processing.

As in relapse paradigms involving experimental animals, many cocaine-dependent individuals respond powerfully to environmental cues. In extreme cases, seemingly trivial stimuli such as the sight of talcum powder, bread crumbs, or snow may be potent reminders of cocaine. Many individuals respond with increased craving for cocaine and demonstrable physiologic arousal. Arthur Margolin and colleagues have described cue-reactivity protocols that conclude with relaxation exercises. Patients who remain abstinent often report a reduction in cue-elicited craving to below baseline levels, while in those who do not succeed in treatment, drug cues continue to produce intense craving. Cue-induced cravings are one of the most difficult challenges in weaning addicts from cocaine, and simple nonpharmacologic interventions such as relaxation exercises and acupuncture deserve in-depth study as both response markers and potential treatment modalities.

Psychosocial treatments also attempt to help patients understand their ambivalence to give up cocaine and clarify the importance of cocaine in their present life problems. At the same time, the treatment program is designed to reduce cocaine availability by encouraging patients to avoid people, places, and things associated with their addictions. The addict is encouraged to identify high-risk environments, feelings, and attitudes, and to prescribe a sponsor or group meeting rather than a relapse. The patient learns that an impulse to use need not result in an action. Just coming to a regular treatment program is a lifestyle modification that can have a very positive impact on recovery. Meetings provide an opportunity to learn and share with others and to develop new associates and coping skills. Finally, a slip does not automatically become a relapse and many intensive treatment programs manage such events by learning from them to prevent others.

Pharmacologic Treatment

Development of medications that deny the brain access to cocaine or diminish its rewarding and reinforcement effects has marked the beginning of a dramatic change in the field of addiction medicine. The National Institute of Drug Abuse's Cocaine Rapid Efficacy Screening Trial (CREST) has recently brought attention to promising drugs that influence glutamatergic and GABAergic systems. Perhaps the greatest challenge of pharmacologic treatment is to match the robust reinforcement mechanisms outlined above with equally robust yet safe therapies that can be tolerated over the course of a chronic, relapsing disease. The most realistic approaches will likely involve targeted, relatively short-term interventions with drugs that can disrupt specific aspects of the disease process while natural "extinction" of reinforcement occurs, and new life skills and healthy habits accrue in strength. The unfortunate propensity for cocaine addicts to relapse after long periods of abstinence greatly increases the challenge of effective pharmacologic therapy (32,37).

Table 14.2 highlights pharmacologic treatments for cocaine addiction. Some of these drugs are in advanced clinical testing and many more are in earlier stages of development. Pharmacologic classes and individual agents are related to broader therapeutic goals. Although there is considerable overlap in putative mechanisms of action and beneficial

TABLE 14.2	Highlights of pharmacologic Rx for cocaine addiction	
Therapeutic goal	**Pharmacologic class (agents)**	**Comments/caveats**
Reduce brain exposure to ingested cocaine ■ Increase metabolism of cocaine ■ Prevent passage across blood–brain barrier	■ "Super" cholinesterases derived from bacterial species. ■ Mutant human butyrylcholinesterases with increased activities. ■ Immunotherapy(ies): passive (autocatalytic antibodies) and active immunization (norcocaine linked with cholera B toxin)	■ Modified enzymes seem promising for emergency management of overdoses/immunologic risks appear minimal. ■ Immunotherapies show great promise because they have no abuse potential, but the immunologic response is variable and can be overcome by increased dosing; ethical concerns.
Agonist (replacement) therapies retain some aspects of cocaine's effects using drugs with reduced abuse potential or less toxicity	■ Oral cocaine (tea, tablets) ■ Available psychostimulants, DA and 5-HT augmenting agents (methylphenidate, dextroamphetamine, disulfiram, modafinil, levodopa, PLA287, ondansetron) ■ DA selective and nonselective monoamine uptake inhibitors (RTI-336 and NS2359, bupropion)	■ Reported beneficial effects in clinical trials have been highly variable, often contradictory; interpretation of results, confounded by impact on comorbid psychiatric and psychological issues ■ Even in the case of drugs with apparently low abuse potential there is concern that DA augmenting agents may perpetuate or prevent extinction of reinforcement effects of cocaine
Relapse prevention ■ Reduce perception of cocaine euphoria ■ Relapse triggered by drug-associated environmental cues ■ Relapse triggered by reintroduction of a "priming" dose of cocaine ■ Relapse triggered by stressful conditions	■ Cannabinoid-1 (CB-1) receptor antagonists (rimonabant; AM 251) ■ DA (D1) receptor agonists (dihydrexidine and benzazepine derivatives) ■ DA (D2) antagonists (olanzapine, aripiprazole) ■ DA (D3) receptor agonists (BP897) and antagonists (NGB2904) ■ GABA receptor agonists (baclofen, topiramate) ■ GABA uptake inhibitors and other GABA system modulators (tiagabine, vigabatrin) ■ Glutamate antagonists, partial agonists and other GLU-modulators (JNJ16567083, MTEP, disulfiram, N-acetyl cysteine) ■ Kappa-opioid receptor agonists (dynorphin; U62066) ■ Opiate-like receptor (ORL-1) agonists (nociceptin) ■ CRF-1 receptor antagonists (CP154,526 and DMP695) ■ Orexin receptor antagonists	■ Available CB-1 receptor antagonists are promising but may have limited tolerability given widespread effects on mechanisms of pleasure perception (e.g., the anorexant rimonabant). ■ D1 receptor agonists show promising preclinical results, but poor bioavailability, lack of receptor selectivity, and short t½ are significant challenges ■ Antipsychotic class D2 antagonists have produced unconvincing benefits in clinical trials with instances of worsening reported ■ D3 receptor modulators of great interest given selective expression of D3 in the limbic system. ■ Several GABA system modulators have entered advanced clinical trials with results that are generally moderate and contradictory; these drugs may have additional benefits as anxiolytics. ■ GLU receptor modulators are in early clinical testing; selectivity issues are a major challenge given the fact the GLU is the predominant excitatory neurotransmitter of the CNS ■ Study of genetically determined differences in endogenous opioid receptors, components of the HPA axis, and other neuromodulatory peptides have been fertile sources of potential therapeutic intervention
Treat psychiatric comorbidity	■ Antidepressants (SSRIs) ■ Anxiolytics ■ Psychostimulants for ADHD	■ Pharmacologic treatment of comorbid psychiatric conditions undertaken with caution in early stages of recovery

The table highlights pharmacologic treatments for cocaine addiction. Some of these therapies are in advanced clinical testing and many more are in earlier stages of development. Pharmacologic classes and examples of individual agents are related to broader therapeutic goals. SSRI, selective serotonin reuptake inhibitor; ADHD, attention-deficit hyperactivity disorder. DA, dopamine; GLU, glutamate; MTEP, 3-[(2-methyl-1,3-thiazol-4-yl)ethynyl-pridine)]; 5-HT, 5-hydroxytryptamine effects, the following discussion is divided into drugs that may be used for reducing brain exposure to ingested cocaine, as agonist or replacement therapies, and for relapse prevention more generally. Drugs used in treating psychiatric comorbidity are beyond the scope of this chapter and are addressed in Part 2 of this book.

Reducing Brain Exposure to Ingested Cocaine

Two of the more exciting developments of recent years have the common goal of reducing brain exposure to cocaine when cocaine is ingested. Modified enzymes capable of degrading cocaine to nonactive or less toxic metabolites include genetically engineered high-activity variants of human butyrylcholinesterase, and high-activity cholinesterases derived from bacterial species. Some of these enzymes can metabolize cocaine at rates that are orders of magnitude higher than normal, and may be useful in acute treatment of massive overdoses. The so-called immunotherapies have been designed to prevent or reduce passage of cocaine across the blood–brain barrier. The immunotherapies furthest along in development involve attachment of cocaine to larger molecules capable of stimulating an immune response, such as the inactivated cholera B toxin. In animal models, immunotherapies have reduced the behavioral reinforcement effects of cocaine and in clinical trials some subjects have reported diminished cocaine-induced euphoria. There have been promising indicators of reduced desire to pursue further use in immunized individuals. Immunotherapies have no known direct psychoactive effects and therefore no abuse liability. However, there are several important shortcomings worth noting. First, with currently available agents, mounting an effective immune response may take several weeks or even months. Second, given the variability in immune response and often low antibody titers, a dedicated addict may readily overcome the immune response by simply using more cocaine. Third, there have been concerns raised about the ethics of using a long-term immune response in socially vulnerable patient populations. Nevertheless, judicious use of cocaine immunotherapy in highly motivated addicts holds great promise.

Agonist Therapies

The so-called agonist or replacement therapies have dominated the development of drugs for cocaine addiction over the past several decades. As a general approach, agonist therapies replace some aspect(s) of the dopaminergic reinforcement mechanisms described in preceding sections, but using drugs that for pharmacokinetic or pharmacodynamic reasons may not have the same abuse potential as cocaine. In this respect they can be thought of as analogous to methadone or buprenorphine therapies for opiate addiction. A recurring concern with nearly all agonist therapies is that they may perpetuate psychostimulant reinforcement and hence prevent natural extinction of the core mechanisms of the addiction process. Some agonist therapies such as modafinil have produced modestly encouraging results in clinical trials, but abuse potential is a substantial concern as more is learned about its effects on brain chemistry. Like cocaine, modafinil appears to bind dopamine transporter proteins, among other possible mechanisms of action (39). Illicit use of psychostimulants as performance-enhancing drugs, including many agents that have been tested as agonist therapies for psychostimulant addiction, has led to the development of an underground world of "cosmetic psychiatry."

There are often no clear lines of demarcation that separate agonist therapies and the multifaceted agents under development for relapse prevention, but drugs that alter reuptake of dopamine or interact directly with dopamine receptors have been involved in most of the clinical trials for cocaine addiction to date. Major agonist therapy subgroups and individual agents, ranging from coca tea to methylphenidate, are listed in Table 14.2. Some of the more interesting developments are drugs such as RTI-336, a selective dopamine reuptake inhibitor, that appear to have a slower onset (and longer duration) of action than cocaine and so may limit rewarding effects. Drugs that exert selective agonist effects on D1 dopamine receptors—as opposed to D2 receptors—have been quite effective in reducing ongoing cocaine use and reinstatement of cocaine self-administration in animal models, highlighting the observation that D1 and D2 receptor systems may exert opposing effects, at least under certain conditions (26). Preadministration of D2 agonists may potentiate subsequent cocaine reinforcement, while preadministration of D1 agonists may substantially block it. Partial agonists and antagonists of the D3 dopamine receptor, expressed abundantly in the ventral striatum, also show promise in reducing responses to drug-associated cues and other aspects of drug-seeking in experimental animals. These latter compounds are in early stages of clinical development.

Relapse Prevention

There are a wide range of chemicals that interfere with one or more aspects of experimental cocaine self-administration and show substantial promise as relapse prevention agents. Animal models have focused on three aspects of the relapse process that realistically simulate clinical situations: relapse triggered by stressful conditions that activate the HPA axis, relapse triggered by drug-associated environmental cues, and relapse triggered by reintroduction of a "priming" dose of cocaine. These models are highly relevant to patient management at all stages of recovery. Drug therapies that could increase the threshold for slips or prevent full-blown relapses would be developments of enormous clinical importance. Drugs that reduce the euphorigenic impact of cocaine would also certainly fall into that framework.

A variety of drugs that show promise in relapse prevention are listed in Table 14.2. We have included those agents that have had disappointing results in early clinical trials in recognition of the fact that many of these studies have been small and inconclusive. Major themes include GABA receptor agonists or GABA reuptake inhibitors, certain glutamate receptor modulators, HPA axis antagonists, endocannabinoid system antagonists, and kappa-opioid system agonists.

Relating new drugs (or new indications for old drugs) to specific neurochemical mechanisms of action is often fraught with contradictions. For example, agents that increase synaptic availability of GABA (e.g., vigabatrin and tiagabine) or modulate GABA receptors (e.g., baclofen and topiramate) may augment the naturally occurring negative feedback of GABAergic neurons on brainstem DA centers. However, the same drugs may produce deleterious inhibition of functions elsewhere in the brain. Likewise, a glutamate receptor antagonist may show promise in one experimental system and a glutamate agonist or partial agonist in another. Given the lack of specificity of many available agents, and the likelihood of countervailing mechanisms at the molecular level, only long-term clinical trials with clinically meaningful outcome measures (urine tests and psychosocial data) or robust surrogate markers can prevent premature acceptance or rejection of promising agents.

Disulfiram is a drug that has been available for decades as an adjunct in the treatment of alcoholism. More recently, it has shown some promise in relapse prevention in cocaine addiction independent of effects on alcohol consumption, but the data are mixed. The purported mechanisms of action and clinical features are of considerable interest. In addition to its well-known blocking effect on aldehyde dehydrogenase, disulfiram may also inhibit dopamine B-hydroxylase and one of its metabolites may influence NMDA-subtype glutamate receptors. Theoretically, disulfiram may have the properties of a functional DA agonist and a neuroprotectant. Several randomized, placebo-controlled clinical trials have demonstrated at least moderate effects on cocaine use in patients with or without concurrent opiate dependence. However, in the event of a relapse to cocaine and/or alcohol, disulfiram may increase cocaine plasma level and compound the cardiovascular effects associated with increased blood acetaldehyde.

The story of N-acetyl cysteine provides an opportunity to discuss a novel therapeutic approach as it relates to the important role of corticofugal glutamate projections to brainstem and basal forebrain in chronic cocaine addiction. Used for decades as a mucolytic agent and antidote Tylenol poisoning, N-acetyl cysteine also appears to reverse impaired cysteine–glutamate exchange within neurons and glia. Since intact cysteine–glutamate exchange is needed to maintain normal extracellular glutamate levels (which may be low in the cocaine-addicted brain), a therapeutic effect is suggested. How cocaine impairs the functioning of cysteine–glutamate exchange is complex and not fully understood, but may involve changes in the scaffolding functions of Homer proteins that maintain amino acid exchangers as functional units (21). Regardless of the molecular details, a key principle is that low basal glutamate levels can result in amplified responses to glutamate "signals" from corticofugal projections that are triggered by cocaine; the net result may be long-term potentiation of cocaine-associated reinforcement and relapses. Restoring low basal glutamate may offset this series of events and possibly also improve baseline cortical functioning. Pilot studies with N-acetyl cysteine have been promising and controlled trials are underway. Remarkably, deletion of Homer genes in experimental animals can produce a cocaine-addicted phenotype, including complex behaviors typical of cocaine sensitization.

Numerous glutamate system modulators, and in particular group 1 metabotropic glutamate receptor antagonists, are being tested in relapse prevention paradigms. Glutamate receptor modulators will likely play a preeminent role in addiction-related pharmaceutical discovery over the coming decade. Use of a glutamate antagonist to prevent or diminish reinforcement of cocaine-seeking behavior may seem to contradict the statements above pertaining to restoration of basal glutamate levels with N-acetyl cysteine. However, the chief therapeutic target is pathologic glutamate signaling, not glutamate levels per se. A major challenge will be to develop compounds with sufficient specificity so that interference with normal glutamate-dependent brain functions may be avoided.

Recent Cochrane group meta-analyses have not found interventions involving either antiepileptic drugs or antidepressants promising enough to support their routine use in treating cocaine addiction. Recent clinical trials involving topiramate, an anticonvulsant that is also used in treating migraine headaches and bipolar disorder, have provided only weak evidence of a beneficial effect in cocaine addiction. Nevertheless, anticonvulsants are often reasonably used off-label with a rationale similar to that which justifies testing of novel GABA agonists and glutamate antagonists. The hope is that these drugs will dampen DA neurotransmission and thereby block cocaine reinforcement. D2 receptor antagonists, including commercially available antipsychotic agents, would seem to be a logical therapeutic approach, but clinical trials have been disappointing and in some cases (e.g., olanzapine), clinical decompensation of cocaine addicts has been reported. Some investigators contend that aripiprazole, with its unusual combination of dopamine receptor blocking and serotonin receptor mixed agonist properties, may have some potential in treating cocaine addiction. SSRIs, selective dopamine transport inhibitors, nonselective monoamine inhibitors, and dopamine receptor partial agonists are all under investigation as treatments for depression and restoration of cognitive deficits in patients recovering from chronic cocaine dependence. Screening for deficits and early identification of subgroups more likely to benefit from focused treatment of psychiatric comorbidity are a reasonable approach that is being pursued in many treatment centers.

The complex modulatory effects of neuropeptides relevant to addiction are beyond the scope of this chapter and are covered in other chapters of this book. However, a few comments are in order. GABA-producing cells of the NAcc often coexpress or act in parallel with cells that manufacture the important kappa-opioid receptor ligand dynorphin. Cortical components of the limbic system express dynorphin abundantly. Chronic cocaine use upregulates the kappa-opioid receptor system, and in some experimental paradigms this appears to counteract the chemistry of reinforcement. There is some evidence from human genetic material that people possessing a "multiple-copy" version of the dynorphin gene may be less prone to develop cocaine dependence after exposure to cocaine (23,24). Dynorphin and other kappa-opioid system agonists are under intensive investigation as therapeutic agents. Cannabinoid receptors are also heavily expressed throughout the limbic system and their activation can powerfully facilitate DA release in the NAcc. According to Cheer and colleagues, cannabinoid receptors may be instrumental in the fundamental process of mesoaccumbal dopamine release (27). The cannabinoid receptor (CB-1) antagonist rimonabant can block the ability of conditioned cues to trigger reinstatement of cocaine use in experimental animals with "extinguished" drug-seeking behavior. Unfortunately, rimonabant is an anorexant with nonspecific effects on pleasure-producing stimuli that may limit its tolerability. The study of CB-1 receptor interactions more generally is an important area of pharmaceutical development.

Drugs that may diminish the impact of stress on relapse (e.g., corticotrophin-releasing factor antagonists and orexin receptor antagonists) are another example of a therapeutic approach with great promise, but because of their broad actions on the HPA axis currently available compounds are not likely to be tolerated long term. Short-term interventions along these lines during periods of peak vulnerability may nonetheless be appropriate, given the importance of social–environmental stress in predicting early relapse.

COMORBIDITIES AND COMPLICATIONS OF COCAINE ABUSE

Associated Psychiatric Disorders

Depending upon diagnostic criteria and methods of data acquisition, the lifetime prevalence of psychiatric comorbidity with cocaine abuse may exceed 75%. On the other hand, psychiatric symptoms and signs at the time of presentation for treatment will be exaggerated by the various manifestations of cocaine toxicity and withdrawal (40). The clinician must therefore be wary of overdiagnosing primary psychiatric pathology while at the same time not missing opportunities to intervene in ways that may improve long-term outcome. It is important to weigh the risk of treating newly suspected psychiatric comorbidity with psychoactive prescription drugs, potentially confounding diagnosis and patient compliance with treatment for cocaine addiction, against the risk of relapse when comorbid psychopathology goes untreated. Management philosophies and medical resources vary widely. There are no straightforward guidelines in this regard, and clinical judgment is used on a case by case basis. The heterogeneity inherent in this area of addiction medicine may account for poor outcomes in certain patient populations, and in others reports of positive responses to treatment that are tantalizing but difficult to replicate.

Certain conditions, particularly anxiety disorders and major depression with prominent anxiety symptoms, may drive the reinforcing effects of cocaine and increase the risk of relapse. In animal models of relapse, there are numerous well-established correlates between resumption or acceleration of use and exaggerated primary HPA responses. These may reflect increased adrenergic inputs from brainstem centers or impaired inhibitory control of responses to stress by higher brain centers. Pharmacologic antagonists at various levels of the HPA response have been shown to reduce cocaine reinforcement and relapse. In a survey conducted by a national helpline, 50% of callers reported experiencing cocaine-induced panic attacks. Treatment facilities specializing in panic and anxiety disorders also report that onset of panic attacks frequently begins with cocaine use. Cocaine may increase the risk of panic through the process of kindling—lowering the stimulation threshold of the brain. Over time, and following ingestion of large amounts of the drug, such reactions may occur spontaneously, without drug-induced stimulation. Panic reactions may persist long after use of cocaine has stopped.

Some people with depression will experiment with cocaine, amphetamines, or even excessive caffeine and tobacco to lift themselves out of their fatigue, low energy, and disinterest in activities. Although cocaine may act temporarily like an antidepressant, people with major depression are likely to experience severe, often devastating dysphoria after cocaine use. Increased levels of serotonin in key brain regions may be part of the cocaine-induced high, but recurrent cocaine use may lead to long-lasting, selective disruptions of serotonin systems. This is likely to be a major part of the neurochemical basis for the mood changes that are commonly reported during cocaine withdrawal. Some surveys of people undergoing treatment for cocaine abuse reveal that half or more meet current diagnostic criteria for mood disorders. Lifetime major depression is diagnosed in approximately 50% of patients, whereas dysthymia is diagnosed in another 25% to 50%; a similar incidence of depression can be seen among opiate addicts. However, as much as 20% of cocaine abusers experience cyclothymic or bipolar disorder (manic depressive illness); the incidence of these conditions in opiate addicts is only about 1%. Such findings suggest that people who experience mood swings may prefer stimulants over other illicit drugs, as if seeking out a familiar, if unstable, comfort zone.

Another commonly seen condition among adult cocaine addicts is residual ADHD, occurring in up to 30% in some series. In both adolescents and adults with histories consistent with ADHD, it is often reported that cocaine ingestion may result in paradoxical relaxation comparable to the calming and focusing effects of therapeutic doses of methylphenidate and dextroamphetamine. However, these generalizations are harder to confirm in structured longitudinal studies, and destabilization of the patient with ADHD on cocaine is not uncommon. Methylphenidate has been used as a "substitution" therapy in cocaine addiction, similar to how "methadone maintenance" is used in heroin addiction. The predominant finding has been that the majority of the modest benefits attributable to methylphenidate occurs in those individuals who displayed moderate to severe ADHD symptoms.

Chronic cocaine abusers frequently cultivate "superstitions," and may even experience feelings of suspiciousness and esoteric thinking as a source of pleasure or entertainment that can play into their systems of denial. In more extreme cases, persecutory delusions may provoke violent or aggressive behavior. Acute, subacute, and chronic paranoia are commonly seen products of cocaine abuse. In its ability to induce a state resembling functional paranoid psychosis, cocaine is similar to other central stimulants, most notably methamphetamine. Like a person with schizophrenia, a person in the throes of cocaine delirium may lose contact with reality and become confused and disoriented. When the pharmacologic effects of cocaine have worn off, the delirium usually disappears. Typically, cocaine delirium with or without frank psychotic features resolves within 3 to 5 days of cessation of use; if it persists for a longer period, or if the patient becomes increasingly difficult to manage, a reevaluation of the diagnosis is indicated and an antipsychotic medication may be considered.

Perhaps more than those with any other personality disorder, people diagnosed as having antisocial personality disorder are prone to use mood-altering drugs. Alcohol is often the drug of choice in such individuals, but many also use cocaine or amphetamines or a combination of several drugs. People with this disorder are distressed, tense, unable to tolerate boredom, and agitated to the point of discomfort. Their use of drugs often removes any remaining inhibitions, increasing the risk of anger, violence, and actions that violate the rights or property of others. Because cocaine is by definition an illicit substance, use of the drug in itself constitutes a form of antisocial behavior. People with borderline personality disorder are likely to turn to mood-altering drugs for relief. They may use stimulants to induce feelings of pleasure, or depressants to reduce internal distress. Because these people are already on the edge, use of stimulants and depressants may trigger a flare-up of anger or violence.

The combined use of cocaine and alcohol is common, with reports of up to 90% of cocaine abusers also being concurrent ethanol abusers, and as many as 60% having lifetime diagnoses of alcoholism. Cocaethylene, the ethyl ester of benzoylecgonine, is produced abundantly when cocaine and alcohol are used together. Like cocaine it binds to the DA transporter and increases extracellular concentrations of DA in the NAcc, but seems to have little effect on the serotonin transporter. While similar to cocaine in producing stimulant effects, there are reports of longer half-life and increased lethality, particularly increased cardiovascular morbidity. Concurrent marijuana use is also common, and may enhance the cocaine high, not only by offsetting the anxiety and agitation of cocaine intoxication but also by altering the drug's pharmacokinetics and metabolism. In some studies marijuana pretreatment significantly reduces the latency to peak cocaine euphoria, decreases the duration of dysphoric or bad effects, and increases bioavailability of cocaine. Marijuana-induced vasodilatation of the nasal mucosa also attenuates the vasoconstrictive effects of cocaine and may thus increase its absorption.

Medical Complications

The medical complications associated with cocaine use are so numerous and complex that it would take volumes to describe them adequately. Many of the classic descriptions of cocaine toxicity produced by internists and emergency medical physicians in the 1970s and 1980s remain highly relevant, and the literature expands considerably each year. With the relatively large and rapid dose deliveries typical of today's regular user, cocaine is a frequent form of serious morbidity and mortality (41,42). However, serious medical complications, including sudden cardiac death, fatal intracranial hemorrhages, malignant hyperthermia with rhabdomyolysis, and renal failure, among others, have all been documented in association with first time use, even of moderate doses. There are obviously wide interindividual variations in both initial response and tolerance to the effects of cocaine, and the occurrence of serious medical complications does not correlate well with plasma levels of the drug at the time of presentation for emergency care.

Cardiovascular System and Pulmonary Syndromes

Cocaine rapidly triggers the physiologic responses that make up the natural "fight or flight" response to an impending threat. By affecting the release and reuptake of epinephrine and norepinephrine, cocaine causes a shift in the blood supply from the skin and the viscera into the skeletal musculature. Oxygen levels rise, as do concentrations of sugar in the blood. Tachycardia, increased cardiac contractility (beta-1 adrenergic effects), and hypertension (alpha-adrenergic effects) may be pronounced and increases in myocardial oxygen demand may outstrip supply, particularly in the presence of cocaine-induced spasm of epicardial or penetrating vessels. Persistent cocaine use has also been linked to acceleration of atherosclerotic coronary artery and renal arterial disease. Apart from the consequences of cocaine-related violence, chest pain is the most common issue prompting presentation for emergency care, 50% or more in some series.

The first detailed reports of cocaine abuse–associated cardiac toxicity appeared over 30 years ago. A review of the medical literature produced by the American Heart Association in 2008 indicates that cocaine use has been linked to virtually every type of cardiac disease imaginable, including a range of supraventricular and ventricular arrhythmias (43). Atrioventrivular nodal conduction block and QTc interval widening are common; premature ventricular depolarization, ventricular tachycardia degenerating to defibrillation, and asystole are not uncommon causes of death. Some studies have found a greater acceleration in heart rate and blood pressure associated with cocaine smoking than with IV cocaine use. Direct stimulation of vagal centers in the brainstem by cocaine or indirect stimulation of baroreceptor responses may also result in severe bradyarrhythmias.

Cocaine abusers often present with atypical, sometimes bizarre presentations of chest pain, and there may be unusual electrocardiographic findings, including those suggestive of "centrally mediated" ST segment elevations in more severe cases of cocaine toxicity. In addition to acute vasospasm or blood supply–demand mismatch in the setting of preexisting coronary artery disease, other causes of chest pain include in situ coronary embolism and coronary arterial dissections. Chronically developing myocardial fibrosis, inflammatory lesions, and other direct toxic effects on myocytes also occur and these likely contribute to the development of congestive heart failure. Cocaine toxicity should always be considered until proven otherwise when a young adult presents with chest pain or signs of congestive heart failure, with or without the presence of other risk factors. Cocaine use is also associated with acute renal failure, often in association with hyperthermia and rhabdomyolysis, and with insidious forms of chronic renal failure. An increasingly common and tragic presentation of cocaine-related vascular pathology is the middle-aged or even elderly patient who presents for emergency care with end-stage renal disease, accelerated hypertension, and positive urine tests for cocaine.

The actual incidence of myocardial infarction associated with cocaine has been controversial, but the recent Cocaine Associated Chest Pain trial, the largest prospective study of its kind ever performed, indicates that the incidence may be less than 10%, according to reports from the American Heart Association (43). The take-home message is that atypical chest pain syndromes, including a number of noncoronary ischemic presentations, need to be considered in the differential diagnosis. Mechanisms to consider, all well documented in case reports or case series, include aortic dissection in the setting of cocaine-induced hypertension, aortic thrombosis, cardiac contusions, pneumothorax, pneumopericardium, and other forms of pulmonary barotrauma. The occurrence of frank barotrauma is infrequent but by no means uncommon, and presumably relates to vigorous insufflations, Valsalva, and abnormal ventilatory patterns in smokers, with or without ischemic necrotic changes and perforations of the bronchial passages.

Shortness of breath is thought to be the second most common cocaine-related medical symptom in emergency care settings. It is well established that cocaine inhalation can cause or exacerbate asthma. The *"crack lung"* syndrome entered the medical literature in the late 1980s; people typically present with the symptoms of pneumonia: shortness of breath, atypical chest pain, high temperatures, and a negative or nonspecifically abnormal chest X-ray pattern. An eosinophilic pneumonitis may be diagnosed via bronchoscopy and biopsy, and adulterants in smoked cocaine (e.g., talc and baking soda) may be responsible for at least some of the pathology. In addition, chronic cocaine inhalation may interfere with breathing by causing telltale destruction of the nasal septum, nasal cartilage, and hard or soft palate. However, rather than pathognomonic syndromes, breathing difficulties in cocaine abusers should be thought of from the standpoint of broad differential diagnosis, as with chest pain.

Neuropathology

The spectrum of neuropathologic changes encountered in the brains of cocaine abusers is broad, but some of the most common catastrophic events include global cerebral hypoxic–ischemic insults secondary to cardiopulmonary failure, hypertensive encephalopathy, intractable seizures, thromboembolic stroke, lobar hemorrhages, and subarachnoid hemorrhages, the latter particularly in those with preexisting intracranial aneurysms or arteriovenous malformations (44). Large retrospective reviews from the neurosurgical literature indicate that concurrent use of cocaine so negatively affects outcome after a subarachnoid hemorrhage that it should be considered equal in effect to the presence of a major systemic illness such as congestive heart failure or renal disease. Accelerated atherosclerosis may occur in the cerebrovasculature just as it does in coronary, renal, and gastrointestinal vascular beds, and in some cases frank vasospasm may produce ischemic brain lesions. The relevance of cerebral vasculitis to cocaine-induced stroke has been debated in the neurologic literature for years, but postmortem pathologic studies supporting this possibility certainly exist.

Cocaine is an epileptogenic agent that can provoke generalized seizures, even after a single dose. These convulsions are typically brief and self-limited, but rare instances of status epilepticus, including difficult-to-recognize nonconvulsive status epilepticus masquerading as a toxic-metabolic encephalopathy, have been reported. Recurrent convulsions are well recognized as a poor prognostic indicator and may trigger a downward cascade including hyperpyrexia, metabolic acidosis, and rhabdomyolysis. When a witnessed or suspected seizure occurs and there is a possibility of cocaine toxicity, then appropriate diagnostic tests, vigorous hydration, and close monitoring are called for. When interictal periods are accompanied by extreme psychomotor agitation, neuroleptics should be avoided because they all, to some extent, lower seizure threshold. IV phenytoin should also be used with caution owing to its potential to induce cardiac dysrhythmias, and in most circumstances benzodiazepenes (e.g., lorazepam or midazolam) would be the anticonvulsants of choice. A rapidly deteriorating syndrome featuring premonitory signs consistent with a typical cocaine delirium, followed by seizures and cardiac arrest has been reported, sometimes within hours of first-time use of only moderate amounts. Early distinguishing features from cocaine delirium may be diminished sensorium and fever.

In addition to potentially reversible functional deficits in frontal brain regions, Volkow et al. have reported the common occurrence of multiple, small, often silent, "Swiss cheese" infarcts and neural change associated with cocaine and crack use. Our work with methamphetamine suggests reversibility should not be taken for granted and neurotoxic consequences of use may be expected. Other researchers' work supports these findings and raises concern that persisting cerebral perfusion deficits and prefrontal cortical dysfunction may result even in patients who appear to be asymptomatic (45). In landmark studies by Tony Strickland

and colleagues, single-photon emission computed tomography, magnetic resonance imaging, and selected neuropsychological measures were used to study cerebral perfusion, brain morphology, and cognitive functioning. Widespread regions of cerebral hypoperfusion in the frontal, periventricular, and temporoparietal areas, and deficits in attention, concentration, and memory were observed. Remarkably, many of these patients were drug free for 6 months or more before their evaluations.

Following chronic cocaine use the body's reservoirs of neurotransmitters and hormones may be depleted. In addition, the drug may compromise the body's ability to regenerate these biochemicals. As a result, the chronic user may experience symptoms of withdrawal and even frank dopamine depletion. As demonstrated in our work describing the dopamine depletion syndrome, chronic cocaine abuse can result in dopamine disinhibition phenomena including increased release of prolactin; in fact, hyperprolactinemia is the endocrine abnormality most often reported in clinical studies of cocaine abusers (29). Extrapyramidal dysfunction including akathisia, dystonias, choreiform movements, bruxism, and a peculiar combination of stereotyped movements and disordered gait (sometimes referred to as "crack dancing") may occur. These symptoms and signs are functionally analogous to the syndromes seen after exposure to dopamine antagonists (e.g., neuroleptics).

Cocaine potently stimulates the HPA axis. As noted previously, activation of corticotrophin-releasing factor (CRF) and increased glucocorticoid response to stressors have both been linked to acceleration of cocaine reinforcement in some animal models. Blocking CRF receptors, and other branch points of the HPA, may efficiently reduce reinitiation of cocaine use (46). Similar findings implicating HPA overdrive in relapse have been reported in humans. By inactivating the feeding center located in the lateral hypothalamus, cocaine also supersedes the primary drive to eat, thus leading to severe loss of appetite and loss of body weight, the latter sometimes a justification for sporadic use. Many people with eating disorders—anorexia and bulimia—take diet pills containing amphetamines or use cocaine to suppress the appetite. Some of these people progress to cocaine dependence. Muscle wasting, often associated with low-grade elevation of CPK (creatine phosphokinase), and often without clear etiology but possibly linked with central dopamine dysregulation, is common. The cocaine user's decreased need for sleep may result from the drug's effects on regulation of brainstem neurotransmitters, particularly serotonin, which plays a major role as modulator of the sleep cycle.

Impact on Sexual Function and Sexuality

Many users, particularly men, claim that cocaine is an aphrodisiac. Indeed, as mentioned earlier, the feeling of sexual excitement that sometimes accompanies cocaine use may be the result of its impact on the DA system and may produce spontaneous orgasm. Nonetheless, chronic cocaine abuse causes derangements in reproductive function, and loss of interest in sex and poor sexual performance noted by chronic addicts may be related in part to increased prolactin release in the setting of a chronic hypodopaminergic state. These symptoms may persist for long periods after use of cocaine has stopped. In women, cocaine abuse has adverse effects on reproductive function, including derangements in the menstrual cycle function, galactorrhea, amenorrhea, and infertility. Some women who use cocaine report having greater difficulty achieving orgasm.

Infections with hepatitis B, hepatitis C, and human immunodeficiency virus (HIV) are associated with cocaine dependence as a result of promiscuous sexual behavior. HIV seropositivity seems clearly associated with crack smoking, independent of concurrent IV use. The clear association between the smoking of crack and high-risk sexual practices has been reported and linked to acceleration in the spread of the HIV virus. A recent study by Theall et al. indicated that HIV seropositivity was at least three times higher among crack smokers than noncrack smokers (47), and recent analyses of women who had sex in exchange for money or crack showed that over 30% were infected with HIV. Cuts and burns on the lips from smoking crack cocaine are also associated with positive HIV serostatus, even after controlling for the amount of oral sex. Other sexually transmitted diseases, hepatitis, and tuberculosis are also seen in cocaine abusers.

Cocaine, Pregnancy, and Fetal Development

One of the most troubling aspects of the cocaine epidemic is its use by pregnant women. "Crack babies" are not just a tragedy of American inner cities; recent reports from Australia, Europe, and South America suggest growing problems with cocaine abuse during pregnancies and at the time of deliveries. It is important to remember that many historical accounts likely underestimate fetal exposure. This "denial" is demonstrated by a recent study of over 3,000 neonates. Although 11% of the women reported using illicit drugs during pregnancy, 31% of infants' meconium tested positive for cocaine alone, plus some additional multidrug positives. Cocaine's effects on the unborn and newborn may also be related to poor nutrition, poor hygiene, and neglect. Cocaine compromises the mother or any caregiver's ability to respond to the new baby through talking, eye contact, and tactile stimulation. Such disconnection and indifference to the infant's behavioral cues create additional problems because nurturing responses are necessary for optimal intellectual and emotional development.

The available data pertaining to cocaine's teratogenicity and obstetric complications are very complex and sometimes conflicting. The least controversial findings involve impaired somatic growth. Gestational age at birth, birth weight, head circumference, and length are often decreased. Placental abruption, or premature separation of a normally implanted placenta, is thought to occur in approximately 1% of pregnancies in women who use cocaine, making the drug a significant cause of maternal morbidity as well as of fetal mortality. Women who use cocaine during pregnancy have a high rate of spontaneous abortion, higher than that of heroin users. Pregnancy also appears to increase a woman's susceptibility to the toxic cardiovascular effects of cocaine, at least in part by the shift in hepatic metabolism of cocaine from relatively nontoxic ecgonine methylester to highly toxic norcocaine, a potent vasoconstrictor.

Neurodevelopmental consequences of exposure to cocaine in utero are heterogeneous and may be common (48). A growing experimental literature demonstrates defects of neuronal migration and dysregulation of "programmed cell death" in cortical maturation, among other effects of cocaine. Clinical and animal studies also support the concept of postnatal HPA axis hypersensitivity resulting from exposure to cocaine in utero and in early postnatal life, phenomenon with ominous implications for long-term psychological and social development.

CONCLUSIONS: REASON FOR HOPE

Recidivism among cocaine-addicted patients is high and most treatment specialists acknowledge that they offer treatment, not a cure, for addiction. Many contradictory data, some showing new therapeutic approaches with great promise, contrast with reports of abysmal relapse rates (49). Researchers have not exactly agreed on what can be termed recovery. Without long-term outcome studies that include forensic tests and rigorously collected psychosocial data, "cures" often seem based more on fashion and investigator charisma than science. Cures are a fantasy. However, there are strong reasons for hope, and as knowledge of the natural history of the relapse process and the sophistication of clinical trials increase, major breakthroughs in treatment success seem more realistic than ever. Perhaps a decade ago, only 10% to 20% of drug addicts were reported as having recovered following treatment. Some programs today report success rates of 60% to 70%, depending on definition of treatment failure (it is debatable whether brief recurrences of use—so-called slips—should constitute a relapse).

One of the major success stories of recent years has come from the management of cocaine and other addictions in health professionals. Our group has had long-standing involvement with these programs and related clinical studies. Mandatory, monitored treatment of drug addiction for health professionals can have strikingly positive long-term results and may serve as a model for treatment in the general adult population (50). The state of Florida's Professionals Resource Network (PRN) identifies, intervenes, and provides appropriate referral and case management for all physicians who are affected by chemical dependency/abuse. PRN follows individuals from evaluation through treatment and then monitors their aftercare for 5 or more years. We have recently examined outcome data from randomly selected Florida physicians who were monitored by PRN for substance abuse and dependence. Five-year recovery was documented by counselor reports, physician/psychiatrist evaluations, AA/NA attendance, return to work, and regular random urinalysis. We found that after 5 years, 92% were drug free, had attended weekly meetings, had positive counselor and physician assessments, and had returned to work. Similarly, impressive results have been reported in evaluations of various state Physician Health Programs (PHPs). Treatment settings varied widely, but the overall results from cocaine addicts, opioid addicts, and alcoholics were comparable. None were treated with methadone or other maintenance. Recent studies extending observations over several state PHPs have confirmed the importance of 12-step programs, positive and negative reinforcement, and lengthy aftercare. These PHP results are very encouraging, but it should be kept in mind that recovering health professionals often have greater material resources and access to intensive treatment modalities that may not be available to the average person.

Treatment for cocaine addiction certainly seems to be on an upward trajectory, but preventing initiation of cocaine use should remain in the forefront, and prevention ideally begins before conception. The tragedies associated with cocaine use during pregnancy and in youth are hard to fully appreciate. While it has become fashionable to scoff at the "Just Say No" campaign of the 1980s, the prevention efforts of the federal and state governments and the Partnership for a Drug-Free America brought many of this country's best scientific, advertising, and marketing minds to the awesome task of "unselling" drugs. These educational programs and ads have helped to reduce drug use in general, but they have had an especially significant effect upon adolescents and children.

At the time of publication of this book, horrendous violence and official corruption in high places have become the calling cards of cocaine trafficking in South America and more recently through Mexico. Similar violence devastates the streets of many American cities. Faced with these realities, organizations such as Law Enforcement Against Prohibition (LEAP) have forcefully argued that legalization of drugs would reduce drug-associated violence and make addictions easier to manage. However, cocaine use is a medical problem; legal or illegal, cocaine is extremely dangerous. It is difficult to justify legalization and government control over the use of a drug such as cocaine, which is so powerfully reinforcing and fundamentally linked with escalating use, impulsive behavior, and deaths (7). Cocaine-associated violence stems from the greed and conflict of illicit drug trade, and also from activation of the "fight or flight" reaction and the disinhibitions that result from impairment of higher brain centers. Legalization and bureaucratic control of supply do not seem likely to work, at least not for cocaine.

Most organizations with responsibility for drug control policy currently advocate flexible understanding and flexible approaches to cocaine addiction/abuse. A flexible approach takes into consideration the fact that there are different phases of cocaine epidemics and that they may vary considerably on a regional basis. For example, in the rapid "infective" stages of an epidemic, initiation of use may increase exponentially as established users bring friends and associates not otherwise predisposed to use above a certain socially reinforced threshold. Interdiction operations led by law enforcement may be uniquely effective in reducing spread under these circumstances. In contrast, established users may obtain supply and perpetuate their illnesses more or less regardless of the legal and other social consequences of continuing use. Yet, these same individuals are the most in need of medical treatment and the most likely to benefit from it.

Ideally, in the earliest stages of chemical dependency patients should have access to well-trained specialists in addiction medicine and/or addiction psychiatry. Addiction specialists are more likely to be aware of the pitfalls of early recovery, less likely to harbor judgmental attitudes and able to appreciate that recovery is a long, hard road. Cocaine abusers have often engaged in convoluted, dangerous lifestyles and have made many poor choices. It is wholly unrealistic to expect a quick turnaround from this tragic state of affairs, just as it is unrealistic for most diabetics to rapidly obtain lasting control over a chronic disease of metabolism. Most experienced clinicians have seen examples of impressive long-term success in addition to the many failures, and the medical community now seems ready to move beyond anecdotal experience to greater participation in rationally designed, fully integrated treatment programs.

REFERENCES

1. Gold MS. "*Drugs of Abuse: A Comprehensive Series for Clinicians*". Vol III: Cocaine. New York and London: Plenum Medical Book Company; 1993.
2. Grinspoon L, Bakalar JB. Drug dependence: nonnarcotic agents. In: Kaplan HI, Freedman AM Sadock BJ, eds. *Comprehensive Textbook of Psychiatry*. 3rd ed. Baltimore: Williams & Wilkins; 1980:1621.
3. Gold MS, Gleaton TJ. Cocaine, marijuana, alcohol, violence. Results of annual high school survey. *Biol Psychiatry*. 1995; 37:627.
4. Drug Abuse Warning Network. National Estimates of Drug-Related Emergency Department Visits. US Department of Health and Human Services, SAMSHA; 2006. Available at: http: //DAWNinfo.samsha.gov/. Accessed February 25, 2009
5. Stephens BG, Jentzen JM, Karch S, et al. National Association of Medical Examiners Position paper on the certification of cocaine-related deaths. *Am J Forensic Med Pathol*. 2004;25(1): 11–17.
6. DHHS. Results from the 2007 National Survey on Drug Use and Health: National Findings. (NSDUH Series H-34, DHHS Publication No. SMA 08-4343). Rockville, MD. Available at: http: //www.oas.samhsa.gov/NSDUH/2k7NSDUH/2k7results.cfm. Accessed April 1st, 2009
7. Goldberger BA, Graham NA, Nelson SJ, et al. A marked increase in cocaine-related deaths in the state of Florida: precursor to an epidemic? *J Addict Dis*. 2007;26(3):113–116.
8. National Institute on Drug Abuse. Monitoring the Future Survey, Overview of Findings, National Institute on Drug Abuse; 2008. Available at: http://www.drugabuse.gov/newsroom/08/MTF08Overview.html. Accessed May 19th, 2009
9. Drug and Alcohol Services Information System. The DASIS Report. Drug and Alcohol Services Information System. September 13, 2007. Available at: http://www.oas.samhsa.gov/dasis.htm. Accessed May 19th, 2009
10. Roehrich H, Gold MS. Cocaine. In: Ciraulo DA, Shader RI, eds. *Clinical Manual of Chemical Dependence*. Washington, DC: American Psychiatric Press; 1991:195–231.
11. Verebey K, Gold MS. From coca leaves to crack: the effects of dose and routes of administration in abuse liability. *Psychiatr Ann*. 1988;18:513–521.
12. Krystal JH, Gawin F, Charney DS, et al. Clinical phenomenology and neurobiology of cocaine abstinence: a prospective inpatient study. *Am J Psychiatry*. 1991;148:1712–1716.
13. Samaha A-N, Li Y, Robinson TE. The rate of intravenous cocaine administration determines susceptibility to sensitization. *J Neurosci*. 2002;22(8):3244–3250.
14. Samaha A-N, Mallet N, Ferguson SM, et al. The rate of cocaine administration alters gene regulation and behavioral plasticity: implications for addiction. *J Neurosci*. 2004;24(28):6362–6370.
15. Jenkins AJ, Keenan RM, Henningfield JE, et al. Correlation between pharmacologic effects and plasma cocaine concentrations in after smoked administration. *J Anal Toxicol*. 2002;26:382–392.
16. Dackis CA, Gold MS. Biological aspects of cocaine addiction. In: Volkow ND, Swann AC, eds. *Cocaine in the Brain*. New Brunswick, NJ: Rutgers University Press; 1988.
17. Hiroi N, Agatsuma S. Genetic susceptibility to substance dependence. *Mol Psychiatry*. 2005;10:336–344.
18. Nader MA, Czoty PW. PET Imaging of Dopamine D2 Receptors in monkey models of cocaine abuse: genetic predisposition versus environmental modulation. *Am J Psychiatry*. 2005;162: 1473–1482.
19. Nader MA, Morgan D, Gage HD, et al. PET imaging of dopamine D2 receptors during chronic cocaine self-administration in monkeys. *Nat Neurosci*. 2006;9(8):1050–1056.
20. Szumlinski KK, Dehoff MH, Kang SH, et al. Homer proteins regulate sensitivity to cocaine. *Neuron*. 2004;43:401–413.
21. Kalivas PW. Glutamate systems in cocaine addiction. *Curr Opin Pharmacol*. 2004;4:23–29.
22. Pan B, Hilliard CJ, Liu Q-S. Endocannabinoid signaling mediates cocaine-induced inhibitory synaptic plasticity in midbrain dopamine neurons. *J Neurosci*. 2008;28(6):1385–1397.
23. Kreek MJ, Bart G, Lilly C, et al. Pharmacogenetic and human molecular genetics of opiate and cocaine addictions and their treatments. *Pharmacol Rev*. 2005;57:1–26.
24. Shippenberg TS, Zapata A, Chefer VI. Dynorphin and the pathophysiology of drug addiction. *Pharmacol Ther*. 2007;116: 306–321.
25. Wise RA. Catecholamine theories of reward: a critical review. *Brain Res*. 1978;152:215–247.
26. Porrino LJ, Lyons D, Miller MD, et al. Metabolic mapping of the effects of cocaine during the initial phases of self-administration in the nonhuman primate. *J Neurosci*. 2002;22(17):7687–7694.
27. Cheer JF, Wassum KM, Sombers LA, et al. Phasic dopamine release evoked by abused substances requires cannabinoid receptor activation. *J Neurosci*. 2007;27(4):791–795.
28. Volkow ND, Fowler JS, Wolf AP, et al. Effects of chronic cocaine abuse on postsynaptic dopamine receptors. *Am J Psychiatry*. 1990;147:719–724.
29. Dackis CA, Gold MS. New concepts in cocaine addiction: the dopamine depletion hypothesis. *Neurosci Biobehav Rev*. 1985; 9:469–477.
30. Self DW, Barnhart WJ, David A, et al. Opposite modulation of cocaine-seeking behavior by D_1- and D_2-like dopamine receptor agonists. *Science*. 1996;271(5255):1586–1589.
31. Volkow ND, Wang G-J, Ma Y, et al. Activation of orbital and medial prefrontal cortex by methylphenidate in cocaine-addicted subjects but not in controls: relevance to addiction. *J Neurosci*. 2005;25(15):3932–3939.

32. Goldstein RZ, Volkow ND. Drug addiction and its underlying neurobiological basis: neuroimaging evidence for the involvement of the frontal cortex. *Am J Psychiatry.* 2002;159:1642–1652.
33. Dackis CA, Gold MS, Estroff TW. Inpatient treatment of addiction. *Treatments of Psychiatric Disorders: A Task Force Report of the American Psychiatric Association.* Washington, DC: American Psychiatric Association; 1989:1359–1379.
34. Liberty HJ, Johnson BD, Fortner N, et al. Detecting crack and other cocaine use with fastpatches. *Addict Biol.* 2003;8(2):191–200.
35. Dutra L, Stathopoulou G, Basden SL, et al. A meta-analytic review of psychosocial interventions for substance use disorders. *Am J Psychiatry.* 2008;168:179–187.
36. Carroll KM, Onken LS. Behavioral therapy for drug abuse. *Am J Psychiatry.* 2005;162:1452–1460.
37. Acri JB, Chiang N, McCann DJ, et al. Summary of NIDA medications workshop: new opportunities for chemists and pharmacologists. *Drug Alcohol Depend.* 2008;92:307–311.
38. Kinsey BM, Jackson DC, Orson FM. Anti-drug vaccines to treat substance abuse. *Immunol Cell Biol.* 2009;87:309–314.
39. Volkow, ND. Modafinil. *JAMA.* 2009;301:1148–1154.
40. Shaffer HJ, Eber GB. Temporal progression of cocaine dependence symptoms in the US National Comorbidity Survey. *Addiction.* 2001;97:543–554.
41. Hollander JE, Hoffman RS. Cocaine. In: Goldfrank LR, Flomenbaum NE, Lewin NA, et al., eds. *Goldfrank's Toxicologic Emergencies.* 7th ed. New York: McGraw Hill; 2002;1004–1019.
42. Estroff TW, Gold MS. Chronic medical complications of drug abuse. *Psychiatr Med.* 1987;3:267–286.
43. McCord J, Hani J, Hollander JE. Management of cocaine-associated chest pain and myocardial infarction: a scientific statement from the American Heart Association acute cardiac care committee of the council on clinical cardiology. *Circulation.* 2008;117:1897–1907.
44. Buttner A, Mall G, Penning R, et al. The neuropathology of cocaine abuse. *Leg Med (Tokyo).* 2003;5(suppl 1):S240–S242.
45. Bolla K, Ernst M, Kiehl K, et al. Prefrontal cortical dysfunction in abstinent cocaine abusers. *J Neuropsych Clin Neurosci.* 2004; 16(4):456–464.
46. Goeders NE. The HPA axis and cocaine reinforcement. *Psychoneuroendocrinology.* 2002;27(1–2):13–33.
47. Theall KP, Sterk CE, Elifson KW, et al. Factors associated with positive HIV serostatus among women who use drugs: continued evidence for expanding factors of influence. *Public Health Rep.* 2003;118(5):415–424.
48. Bellini C, Massocco D, Serra G. Prenatal cocaine exposure and the expanding spectrum of brain malformations. *Arch Intern Med.* 2000;160:2393.
49. Simpson DD, Joe GW, Broome KM. A national 5-year follow-up of treatment outcomes for cocaine dependence. *Arch Gen Psychiatry.* 2002;59(6):538–544.
50. Dupont RL, McClellan AT, White WL, et al. Setting the standard for recovery: physicians' health programs. *J Subst Abuse Treat.* 2009;36:159–171.

CHAPTER 15 Cannabis

Alan J. Budney ■ Ryan G. Vandrey ■ Stephanie Fearer

Cannabis is the generic and most appropriate scientific term for the psychoactive substance(s) derived from the plant, *Cannabis sativa*, and used by humans to alter their consciousness or physical state. It contains over 500 distinct chemical compounds, but the one of primary interest related to substance abuse is delta-9-tetrahydrocannabinol (THC). THC has been identified as the predominant substance in cannabis that produces the subjective "high" associated with smoking the plant. Marijuana and hashish are the most common names for cannabis used by the general population. Over the years, however, cannabis has accumulated many names (e.g., weed, pot, herb, grass, reefer, Mary Jane, dagga, dope, bhang, Aunt Mary, skunk, boom, gangster, kif, ganja, hashish, and hash oil.). In this chapter, we will use the term *cannabis* to refer generally to all the various derivatives of the *Cannabis sativa* plant used by humans, except when otherwise designated.

Cannabis is the most widely used illegal substance in the United States and most other developed countries that regulate its use. Controversy regarding its legal status, addictive potential, health consequences, and medical use has pervaded the lay and scientific communities for centuries (see below). A large component of such controversy has been skepticism regarding the dependence or addictive potential of cannabis and the perception that adverse consequences of its use are limited and relatively inconsequential. Fortunately, advances in clinical and basic science address many of these controversial aspects of cannabis use. Epidemiologic, laboratory, and clinical studies have demonstrated the existence, increasing prevalence, and clinical significance of cannabis abuse and dependence disorders (cannabis use disorders [CUDs]). Treatment research studies indicate that abstinence and relapse rates observed following treatment for CUDs are highly similar to those observed with other substance use disorders.

Scientists identified an endogenous cannabinoid system in the late 1980s that prompted research exploring the biologic underpinnings of CUD, and the potential mechanisms by which it may impact physical health and psychiatric disorders. Remarkably, such findings provide clear illustrations of similarities in the neurobiological processes involved in cannabis use and the development of CUD and other types of substance dependence (e.g., alcohol or heroin). The clinical, behavioral, and neurobiological data accumulated over the past 20 years suggest that the debate over whether or not cannabis is addictive has become obsolete. Clearly cannabis misuse and addiction are real and relatively common phenomena that pose a significant public health issue requiring continued attention by health service providers, policy makers, and families.

This chapter will provide a comprehensive overview of cannabis and its status as a psychoactive substance with potential for misuse and addiction. A brief synopsis of the long history of cannabis use by man and its ever changing status in our society will be followed by epidemiologic data illustrating trends in cannabis use among different age, gender, ethnic, and racial groups. Description of the behavioral and cognitive experiences associated with cannabis use will precede brief reviews of the pharmacologic, neurobiological, behavioral, and environmental factors related to initiation and maintenance of cannabis use and misuse. A succinct review of the treatment outcome literature will illustrate recent progress in the development and testing of psychosocial and pharmacologic interventions and discuss their effectiveness for CUDs. An overview of specific health and psychosocial consequences associated with cannabis misuse together with a review of comorbid disorders common among those with cannabis use problems will further demonstrate the broad range of issues that warrant attention when evaluating cannabis use and the severity of CUDs.

HISTORY

Many historic accounts of the use of the cannabis plant for its fiber, as medicine, and as a mind-altering substance have appeared in the literature. For those most interested in a detailed accounting of the ancient history of cannabis, we refer you to Abel's classic text, *Marihuana: The First Twelve Thousand Years* (1). Cannabis likely first appeared in Chinese culture 4000 to 5000 years ago and was grown primarily for its fiber (a.k.a. hemp) and used to make clothing, paper, and rope. Eventually, inhabitants of Central Asia, India, and the Middle East, and the Greeks and Romans began to use cannabis as a medicine to heal and ameliorate various ailments, as well as for its spiritual and mind-altering properties. Spiritual and religious uses of cannabis are described in ancient writings of these cultures. Indeed, over the years a number of cultures have deemed cannabis a "holy" plant because of its psychoactive and medicinal potential. Nonetheless, use of cannabis to change consciousness and its potential for misuse has repeatedly engendered controversy within most cultures, even in ancient China. The intermingling of three issues, cannabis' value as highly utilitarian fiber, its potential for medicinal use, and its mind- and behavior-altering effects (addictive potential and consequences), has generated debate and legislation across cultures for many centuries.

Of most relevance to those interested in current perspectives on cannabis as a substance of abuse are the more recent (past 100 to 150 years) history and controversy related to science and policy. During the mid- to late 1800s many "medical papers" were written, mostly expounding the potential of cannabis for varying medical (physical and mental) conditions. Cannabis became part of the U.S. Pharmacopeia in 1870 where it remained listed as a useful medicine until 1941. Although reports from government-sponsored "studies" on cannabis (e.g., Ohio State Medical Society, 1860 and the Indian Hemp Drug Commission, 1895) suggested that cannabis was not "addictive" and had potential health benefits, the call for such studies indicated growing societal concerns about adverse effects. During the early 1900s, cannabis became a source of public controversy in the United States when the mainstream culture became concerned that "reefer" or "marijuana," purportedly being used primarily by African Americans and Mexican Americans, was negatively influencing children of the White middle and upper classes. International concerns also became apparent at this time as annual reports from the International Opium Conference and the League of Nations indicated discussion of the need to place controls on cannabis use by multiple countries and the resistance of such controls by others. In 1924, the International Opium Conference labeled cannabis a "narcotic" and called for strict controls. Yet in 1925 a U.S. report, issued in response to high rates of soldiers' cannabis use in the Panama Canal Zone, concluded that cannabis was not addictive or harmful, and recommended no restrictions on use.

By 1941, cannabis was dropped from the U.S. Pharmacopeia, the United States legislated a Marijuana Transfer Tax in response to concerns about cannabis, and Britain officially made cannabis an illegal substance. In 1944, a "scientific" report from the New York Academy of Sciences commissioned by the Mayor of New York City indicated that the public concerns about cannabis were exaggerated and that cannabis does not lead to "addiction" in the medical sense of the word. However, the report also described multiple negative aspects of marijuana smoking and associated consequences. The increase in use in the United States during the 1960s and 1970s rekindled public and scientific interest and concerns. The Transfer Tax was declared unconstitutional, but in Britain cannabis remained classified as a Class B drug, meaning any use, including use for medical reasons, was specifically banned. In reaction to the long prison terms being imposed for possession, the U.S. National Commission on Marihuana and Drug Abuse recommended in 1972 that cannabis possession be decriminalized. In that decade a number of states replaced prison terms with either civil penalties or misdemeanor fines. Also during the 1970s, the White House Administration banned medical research on cannabis, while at the same time the state of New Mexico passed a law allowing cannabis for medical use. Similar contradictory reports, federal administrative and legislative directives, and "scientific" reports continued to appear during the 1980s. Legalization and decriminalization discussions evolved internationally with still no consensus and a resultant wide range of national and regional policies. In 1999, the Institute on Medicine released a comprehensive report acknowledging the potential negative effects of cannabis including addiction, but also provided a clear statement regarding its potential for medical benefits.

Finally, in the first decade of the 21st century, Britain downgraded cannabis to Class C status, but at the same time revised the consequences associated with possession or sale of Class C substances rendering the status of cannabis highly similar to its previous categorization. In 2009 cannabis was moved back to Class B status. Currently in the United States, cannabis remains classified under federal law as having high risk and no accepted medical use. However, approximately 13 states have passed laws "legalizing" the medical use of cannabis.

Current perception and policy in the United States and Britain reflect the history of the world's longstanding ambivalence and enduring controversy regarding cannabis use. Unfortunately, this lack of resolution has likely contributed to (a) lax attitudes toward use of cannabis increasing the probability of use and misuse; (b) reluctance of the public, scientists, and intervention specialists to consider cannabis a significant drug of abuse which may impede treatment seeking and the allocation of resources for development of effective treatment services; (c) overly severe penal consequences for possession and use of cannabis; and (d) the delay of science directed toward exploration of the potential of cannabis and/or its active compounds for treatment of physical and psychiatric disorders (2). Advances in our understanding of the addictive nature of cannabis and the mechanisms of its active compounds (to be discussed below) have provided a much clearer picture of cannabis' potential for harm, leading to a renewed emphasis on educating the public about its consequences, while continuing to explore the therapeutic potential of its chemical components. Continued debate over appropriate legal status and policy related to cannabis use will likely continue into the foreseeable future.

EPIDEMIOLOGY

Prevalence of Cannabis Use

The National Survey on Drug Use and Health (3) indicates that cannabis is the most commonly used illicit substance in the United States, with an estimated 41% of U.S. persons aged 12 and older having used it at least once in their lifetime, 10% having used it at least once in the past year, 6% having used it at least once in the past month, and approximately 2%

reported having using cannabis almost every day. These rates are similar to those seen in other developed countries, with approximately 34% of Australians and 20% of Europeans reporting lifetime use of cannabis (4). Among developing countries, use rates also appear to be increasing. Globally, an estimated 166 million people (4%) had used cannabis as of 2006 (5).

Males are more likely than females to use cannabis, with 45% versus 36% reporting lifetime use and 8% versus 4% reporting past month use (3). Use is most common among those 18 to 25 years old, with 28% reporting past-year use. Data from the Monitoring the Future Study, a survey of adolescents in the United States, indicate that 29% of 10th graders and 37% of 12th graders report having used cannabis in the past year (5). In the United States an estimated 7000 to 8000 individuals start using cannabis each day with the highest rates of initiation among those 12 to 25 years old (6). In the last decade, the risk of initiation has increased for 12 to 17 year olds, while remaining stable for those 18 years and older.

Among ethnic groups, those who identify themselves as being multiracial (two or more races) have the highest rates of use in the past year and past month, followed by African Americans, Whites, and Hispanics, respectively. Interestingly, rates of past-year and -month use among 18- to 25-year-old African Americans are lower than those of Whites, but among those 26 years and older rates are higher among African Americans, accounting for the overall disparity in use (7).

Prevalence of Cannabis Use Disorders

A review of several surveys from multiple countries estimated rates of lifetime cannabis dependence at 1% to 4% (4). The rate of abuse or dependence in the past year among those 12 years and over in the United States has remained close to 2% over the past 5 years (3), with the rate of cannabis dependence alone being 1%. The National Epidemiologic Survey on Alcohol and Related Conditions (NESARC) study observed prevalence rates of lifetime and 12-month CUD of 8.5% and 1.5%, respectively (8). Although this rate of cannabis dependence may seem a minimal percentage of the population, it is more than double the dependence rate for any other illicit drug. The high prevalence of cannabis dependence reflects the much more widespread use of cannabis relative to other illicit drugs of abuse rather than greater addictive potential.

With regard to potential demographic differences in CUD prevalence rates in the United States, compared to Whites, the risk of abuse and dependence appears to be higher among Native Americans and lower among African Americans, Asian Americans, and Hispanic Americans (8). Individuals in the Western region of the country tend to have higher rates of CUD, but there do not appear to be any differences between urban and rural areas.

Conditional Dependence

When comparing the percentage of persons who ever use a substance that then go on to develop dependence (i.e., conditional dependence), cannabis use is less likely to lead to dependence than use of most other common illicit drugs. In the United States, approximately 9% of those who try cannabis become dependent, while 17% of those who try cocaine and 23% of those who try heroin develop dependence (6). Although lower in relative terms, the 9% conditional dependence rate observed for cannabis is still alarming given the relatively large number of people who try cannabis compared with the number who try other illicit substances. Risk of dependence is also greater for those who use cannabis more frequently, for younger individuals, for those who initiate cannabis use at an earlier age, and for those who have a family history of substance abuse (4).

Increase in Prevalence

Over the past 10 to 15 years, the prevalence of CUD has increased across adults in the United States despite stabilization of rates of use, while the rates of both use and CUD have increased among adolescents (9). Such increased prevalence of CUD may be a result of several contributing factors. First, analysis of confiscated cannabis suggests that the potency of cannabis available has increased by over 60% during the past decade, which may increase its addictive potential. Second, cannabis use is being initiated at a younger age, which is clearly related to risk of developing CUD. Of note is an observed increase in prevalence of CUD among young adult African American and Hispanic males and African American females (9). The reasons for this increased rate in CUD among minority youth are not clear, but some speculate factors such as (a) deleterious effects of acculturation on Hispanic youth; (b) growing numbers of minority youth attending college where they may experience increased exposure to cannabis use; and (c) environmental and economic factors, such as higher prices and stricter policies related to alternative substances such as tobacco products and alcohol, which may impact minority youth more than Whites.

Increase in Treatment Admissions for CUD

Paralleling the rise in CUD, treatment admissions for a primary CUD have increased both in absolute numbers and as a percentage of total admissions, from 12% in 1996 to 16% in 2007 (10). Cannabis ranks a close third, behind only alcohol (40%) and opiates (18%), among primary substances reported by individuals seeking treatment. The number of adolescents receiving treatment for CUD more than tripled from 1992 to 2002, and approximately 50% of all adolescents in substance abuse treatment report cannabis as their primary substance (Fig. 15.1).

This increase may reflect a number of factors. First, the growing number of individuals experiencing CUD simply may increase the demand for treatment, although the increase in admissions far exceeds the magnitude of the increase in prevalence of CUD. Second, it may be that, as more cannabis-specific treatments become available, the "acceptability" of seeking and providing treatment for cannabis may have increased, resulting in more individuals presenting for treatment. More generally, raised awareness of cannabis' addictive potential may have increased the probability that users or

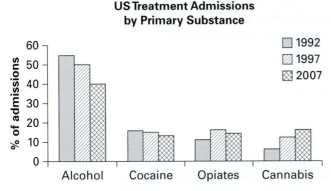

Figure 15.1. The relative increase in treatment seeking for cannabis compared with other substances over the past 15 years. (Data from SAMHSA. *Treatment Episode Data Set (TEDS) 1995–2007: National Admissions to Substance Abuse Treatment Services.* Rockville, MD: US Department of Health and Human Services; 2008.)

treatment referral sources consider the possibility that cannabis use is causing substantial problems that warrant intervention; this is most likely true among adolescents and young adults, who make up over 40% of admissions for CUD. Another factor likely contributing to the overall increase in treatment admissions is the recent advent of drug courts and other initiatives that encourage referral to treatment over incarceration for first-time or small-quantity offenders in the criminal justice system. Nonetheless, the percentage of individuals with a CUD who seek treatment remains low. Only an estimated 9.8% of individuals with a lifetime cannabis abuse diagnosis and 34.7% of those with a lifetime cannabis dependence diagnosis have ever received treatment (8).

ADMINISTRATION AND PHENOMENOLOGY

Cannabis use is associated with a myriad of behavioral, physiologic, and cognitive effects. This section reviews methods of cannabis administration and subsequent acute and chronic effects, with an emphasis placed on effects that are most likely to cause clinical concern. More detailed review of behavioral and cognitive consequences of cannabis is provided in the section "Nonpsychiatric Health Effects of Cannabis." Tolerance and withdrawal, common features of substance abuse and dependence, are also briefly discussed.

Cultivated cannabis is sold in several different preparations that encompass a range of potency (% THC concentration). The most commonly used form of cannabis is the dried plant material which can be subdivided into preparations that include whole-plant material and those that only contain the unfertilized flowers of the female plant (often referred to as sinsemilla). Whole-plant cannabis typically ranges in potency from 1% to 5% THC (v/v), and sinsemilla typically ranges from 7% to 15% THC (v/v). Hashish refers to the resin of the cannabis plant, which typically contains 10% to 20% THC (v/v). Hash oil is derived from concentrated resin extract and usually contains approximately 20% THC (v/v), but may reach as high as 60% THC (v/v). During the past few decades a steady increase in the potency of seized cannabis has been observed with mean % THC concentration (v/v) increasing from 3.4% in 1990 to 8.5% in 2008, but there has been little change in the range of potency encountered. Preference for type of cannabis preparation and method of smoking tends to vary by geographic region.

In most instances of acute cannabis use, the plant material is burned and the smoke emitted from the cannabis is inhaled. Methods of smoking cannabis are varied and include, but are not limited to, use of pipes, water pipes (bongs or hookahs), cigarette paper (joints), and the paper from hollowed-out cigars (blunts). Cannabis is also sometimes ingested orally, most often by dissolving cannabis or concentrated by-products of the cannabis plant into food (typically baked goods). More recently, devices have been developed in which cannabis is "vaporized." Vaporization involves heating the plant material at a temperature high enough to release psychoactive cannabinoids for inhalation, but low enough that combustion of the plant material does not occur. The bioavailability of THC and the time course of intoxication are similar when cannabis is smoked and vaporized. Following these routes of administration, THC bioavailability is approximately 18% and cannabis intoxication typically occurs within 1 minute, reaches peak in 15 to 30 minutes, and persists for approximately 4 hours. Following oral ingestion, THC bioavailability is approximately 6% and intoxication occurs approximately 30 minutes after administration, peaks in 2 to 3 hours, and persists for 6 hours or longer.

There are several reliable effects of acute cannabis use. Subjectively, the user feels a euphoric effect or "high" that is typically characterized by a sense of relaxation or drowsiness and an increased propensity for laughter. Sense of perception is also affected such that time seems to slow down and many report an increased appreciation for music and other mediums of art. Potentially related to the latter effect, cannabis users tend to prefer engaging in nonverbal social activities (watching a movie or listening to music) while under the influence of cannabis. Feelings of anxiety, paranoia, fear, or panic may also be experienced. These effects most often occur in less experienced users or following use of higher than usual doses. In rare cases, usually involving particularly high doses, users may experience hallucinations. These effects are not life threatening, dissipate with time, and may be reduced with comfort and reassurance.

Acute administration of cannabis produces several reliable physiologic effects. The mouth becomes dry and appetite is stimulated which typically results in an increase in the consumption of food and drink, particularly high-calorie products. At low-to-moderate doses, cannabis typically has antiemetic effects (reduces nausea), but can induce nausea or vomiting at higher doses or among less experienced users.

Acute cannabis use has a broad range of effects on cardiovascular function. Specifically, cannabis administration is associated with a significant (20% to 100%) increase in resting heart rate, slight increase in supine blood pressure, and increased orthostatic hypotension (dizziness or lightheadedness that results from a sudden drop in blood pressure after

TABLE 15.1	Cannabis withdrawal: signs and symptoms
■ Irritability or anger	
■ Nervousness or anxiety	
■ Sleep difficulty (insomnia)—may include disturbing or strange dreams	
■ Decreased appetite or weight loss	
■ Restlessness	
■ Depressed mood	
■ Physical discomfort or symptoms (e.g., headache, shakiness/tremors, sweating, stomach pain, and chills)	

Note: Cannabis withdrawal is not designated in the *DSM-IV*, but recent clinical research indicates that many chronic cannabis users experience a significant withdrawal syndrome when they abruptly stop using.

standing) (11). The increased cardiac output also causes a dilation of small blood vessels, which typically results in a redness of the eyes. Case reports have been published suggesting that the acute cardiovascular effects of cannabis can contribute to myocardial infarction or acute cardiac-related fatalities, but research and epidemiologic reports suggest this is a very rare occurrence. Despite the magnitude of the acute effects of cannabis use on cardiovascular function, tolerance develops rapidly and chronic use is not clearly associated with significant cardiovascular health risks.

Controlled laboratory studies in which cannabis or oral THC has been administered indicate that cannabis can impair focused and divided attention, short-term and episodic memory, some types of complex cognitive processing, and some aspects of motor ability (12). The research on this topic is discussed in more detail below. Many of these effects are not highly robust, have not been observed consistently across studies, are dose-related, and are moderated by cannabis use history (tolerance). Generally, moderate doses of cannabis appear to have comparable effects to moderate doses of alcohol (BAC approximately 0.05%) on measures of motor ability, attention, and episodic memory.

Studies of chronic cannabis users suggest that sustained use of cannabis may impair attention, memory, and complex cognitive abilities such as problem solving and mental flexibility (13,14). Consistent with these observations, neuroimaging studies indicate that long-term cannabis users have altered brain function in the prefrontal cortex, cerebellum, and hippocampus. Chronic cannabis users have also exhibited a greater propensity for risky decision making compared with matched controls. Most research suggests that impairments associated with chronic cannabis use are likely reversed following extended abstinence. These issues are discussed in more depth in the section "Nonpsychiatric Health Effects of Cannabis."

Pharmacologic and behavioral tolerance is fairly reliable and robust across most observed effects of cannabis (15). The severity of behavioral and cognitive impairments resulting from acute cannabis exposure is associated with the use history of the individual. Note that some have questioned whether tolerance develops to the typical euphoric effects of cannabis, and instead have suggested that increased sensitivity to such effects occurs. However, experimental studies suggest that tolerance likely develops to these euphoric effects of cannabis, and that the perception of increased sensitivity may reflect learning to discriminate and label the effects of cannabis and learning to better titrate the dose to obtain the desired effect. In general, tolerance is lost when cannabis use is discontinued for a significant period of time.

Abrupt cessation of daily or near-daily cannabis use often results in the onset of a cannabis withdrawal syndrome. Common symptoms of withdrawal in humans include: anger and aggression, anxiety, depressed mood, irritability, restlessness, sleep difficulty and strange dreams, decreased appetite, and weight loss (16). Chills, headaches, physical tension, sweating, stomach pain, and general physical discomfort have also been observed during cannabis withdrawal, but are less common. Most symptoms onset within the first 24 hours of cessation, peak within the first week, and last approximately 1 to 2 weeks. Clinical reports and survey studies suggest that cannabis withdrawal contributes to relapse among cannabis users trying to quit. Note that a Cannabis Withdrawal Disorder is not included in the *Diagnostic and Statistical Manual for Mental Disorders, 4th Edition* (*DSM-IV*); however, clinical research findings over the past 15 years suggest that withdrawal is likely to be included in the next version of the manual (Table 15.1).

DETERMINANTS OF USE

Pharmacology

The defining pharmacologic constituents of the cannabis plant are a family of compounds referred to as cannabinoids. Ninety different cannabinoids have been identified in the cannabis plant, of which THC has been identified as the primary compound responsible for the psychoactive effects of cannabis. Smoking cannabis results in rapid absorption and wide distribution of THC throughout the body, including the brain (17). Peak plasma levels of THC are achieved within minutes of smoked cannabis administration, but are delayed to 1 to 2 hours when administered orally. THC is metabolized into 11-hydroxytetrahydrocannabinol (11-OH-THC) and 11-nor-9-carboxy-tetrahydrocannabinol (THC-COOH), which are then excreted through feces and urine. Though the subjective effects of cannabis typically last a few hours, because THC is highly lipophilic it is rapidly absorbed and stored in fatty tissues and the elimination half-life can extend for as long as 4 days. There is no indication that the presence or release of cannabinoids in fat stores results in perceptible intoxication in the user.

Neurobiology

Cannabis exerts its effects on human function primarily through an endogenous cannabinoid receptor system (18). This endogenous system has only recently been discovered, and, to date, two receptor subtypes (CB1 and CB2) and five endogenous ligands (N-arachidonylethanolamide [anandamide], 2-arachidonoylglycerol [2-AG], 2-arachidonylglycerylether [noladin ether], O-arachinoyl-ethanolamine [virodhamine], and N-arachydonyl-dopamine [NADA]) have been identified. The psychoactive and reinforcing effects of cannabis are primarily mediated by activation of the CB1 receptor by THC. The CB1 receptor is a presynaptic G protein-coupled receptor, activation of which inhibits adenylyl cyclase and voltage-dependent Ca^{2+} channels, and activates K^+ channels and MAP kinase. The CB1 receptor is abundant throughout the CNS, but is expressed in the brain at the highest concentrations in the basal ganglia (reward, learning, motor control), cerebellum (sensorimotor coordination), hippocampus (memory), and cortex (planning, inhibition, higher order cognition). Changes in brain activity following administration of THC are localized mostly in these areas, which are consistent with the behavioral effects of cannabis, and imaging studies indicate that these brain activity changes are THC dose- and time-dependent effects.

A number of studies have been conducted to specifically demonstrate the neurobiological basis for cannabis abuse by focusing on the effects of THC and synthetic CB1 agonists in brain areas and systems associated with reward, reinforcement, and addiction (19). THC appears to enhance dopamine (DA) neuronal firing and synaptic DA levels in the reward pathway of the brain, and also enhances electrical brainstimulation reward. These are hallmark neurobiological features of abused drugs. Concordant with these findings, abrupt cessation of chronic THC exposure increases corticotrophin-releasing factor (CRF), decreases DA, and inhibits electrical brain-stimulation reward in the brain reward pathway. These effects have been linked to the dysphoric effects associated with withdrawal from drugs such as alcohol, opiates, and cocaine, and are thought to contribute significantly to relapse.

The pharmacologic specificity of the rewarding effects of cannabis has also been demonstrated using behavioral research. Models of human drug reward in non human species include studies in which animals are trained to (1) self-administer THC or similar synthetic cannabinoids, (2) demonstrate drug-seeking behavior by spending time in contexts associated with drug exposure (conditioned place preference), or (3) discriminate the effects of THC from other drugs for rewards. Using these models, researchers have demonstrated that THC and similar synthetic compounds are reliably self-administered, show conditioned place preference, and are discriminated from other drugs of abuse for which the pharmacologic mechanism of action is different than cannabis (e.g., cocaine, ethanol, and ketamine). These effects can be reversed or prevented either in animals pretreated with a specific CB1 receptor antagonist or in knockout mice genetically bred to lack CB1 receptors (20).

While the reinforcing effects of cannabis are primarily mediated by the CB1 receptor, there is also evidence that the opioid receptor system is involved with these effects (21). Specifically, studies with nonhuman animals have shown that administration of the mu-opioid antagonists naloxone and naltrexone can attenuate the reinforcing effects of cannabinoids and precipitate withdrawal in animals chronically exposed to THC. Cannabinoid withdrawal effects have been shown to be attenuated in opioid receptor knockout mice. Chronic administration of THC or other CB1 agonists also has been shown to affect opioid receptor function and expression. However, the effects of naltrexone have not been replicated in humans and the functional significance of cannabis and opioid system interactions on cannabis use in humans is as yet not well understood.

Genetics

Multiple studies have firmly established that genetic influences contribute to the development of CUDs. Heritable factors contributing between 30% and 80% of the total variance in risk of CUD have been reported and genetic linkage studies of CUD and earlier stages of cannabis use (including frequency of use) further establish a genetic link to cannabis use problems (22). That said, multivariate behavioral genetic analyses suggest common genetic and shared environmental influences between cannabis and other types of drug dependence, and genome-wide research suggests a common genetic basis for adolescent substance abuse and conduct problems. These studies provide evidence for not only genetic influences, but also environmental contributions, of either the shared or unique types indicating that CUD and other substance use disorders are likely best understood as being influenced by both genetic and environmental factors, and their interaction.

In the case of adolescent substance abuse, the most common of which is CUD, genetic causality is complex. At least three sources of genotypic risk (substance specific, substance nonspecific, and environmentally modifiable) have been identified. First, substance-specific genes may impact vulnerability to the general addictive potential or the pre- and post-metabolitic effects of cannabis. Second, specific genes may increase or decrease genetic vulnerability to externalizing behavior problems in general, including adolescent experimentation and misuse of psychoactive substances. Third, certain genes may impact an individual's reactivity to environmental variables such as stress, which may influence risk for substance misuse. The contribution of genetics to substance abuse in general and cannabis use and CUD in particular remains a complex issue that will hopefully provide important contributions to the advancement of prevention and intervention in the future.

Environment

A number of different environmental factors contribute to the use and abuse of cannabis. Foremost of these is the availability of cannabis, especially considering its illicit status in most countries. Cannabis is the most widely available illicit drug in the world with a conservatively estimated 88,000 to 110,000 metric tons of cannabis being cultivated to meet market demand each year. One reason for the wide availability of cannabis is that it can be cultivated outdoors in most climates, and the development of specialized equipment and genetic strains of cannabis has also allowed for substantial production using indoor facilities.

Recently there has been a trend toward the adoption of drug enforcement policies by which cannabis remains illegal, but the law is not enforced for possession of small quantities of the drug. The most notable and liberal example of this policy is that adopted by the Netherlands where use of cannabis by adult citizens and sale of limited amounts of cannabis in registered and zoned "coffee shops" is tolerated. There is no evidence that this apparent increased availability of cannabis contributes to greater use among Dutch citizens relative to places where cannabis has not been decriminalized. This may reflect the fact that cannabis remains widely available in countries where cannabis use is not tolerated. For example, in a 2008 survey of school-aged youth in the United States, 39%, 67%, and 84% of students in the 8th, 10th, and 12th grades, respectively, indicated that cannabis was either "fairly easy" or "very easy" to obtain (23). These reports of cannabis availability are substantially higher than availability ratings for other illicit drugs of abuse (e.g., cocaine, LSD, and sedatives) and approached availability ratings for alcohol by the same cohort.

Several other important environmental and demographic factors predict cannabis use and CUD (24,25). The strongest and most consistent population-based predictors of cannabis use are (1) use of other licit or illicit drugs, (2) use of cannabis by others within one's peer network, and (3) use of cannabis by immediate family members. Delinquent/rebellious behavior, unstable or abusive home life, low socioeconomic status, other types of psychopathology, and less perceived risk of harm associated with cannabis are also associated with increased risk of cannabis use and CUD.

EVALUATION

Assessment and evaluation of CUDs should not differ remarkably from that of other substance use disorders. The important clinical features of CUDs are similar to those of other substances of abuse (26). Guidelines and criteria for CUD diagnoses are found in the *DSM* of the American Psychiatric Association and the International Classification of Diseases (ICD) developed by the World Health Organization. Of note, the *DSM-IV* and ICD-10 use nonspecific criteria to diagnose substance use disorders, and these criteria may not discriminate cases in a manner consistent with the underlying constructs of abuse and dependence, or illustrate differences in severity level or specific symptom profiles. However, these diagnostic guidelines capture all aspects of CUD as well as they do most other substance use disorders, with the exception being that a formal characterization of cannabis withdrawal is omitted from the *DSM-IV*. Recent laboratory and clinical findings strongly suggest that cannabis withdrawal can be a clinically important phenomenon for many cannabis users, and as such should be assessed and evaluated as part of the clinical dependence syndrome (27). Structured or semi-structured *DSM-IV* diagnostic interviews (e.g., SCID or CIDI-SAM) are most appropriate for determining CUD diagnoses.

Screening and Assessment Tools

Cannabis-specific instruments for screening and assessment have been developed, and are slowly developing support as psychometrically valid instruments. The Cannabis Use Disorder Identification Test provides a short method for making a *DSM* diagnosis of abuse or dependence (28). Adult and adolescent versions of the Cannabis Problems Questionnaire provide a general measure of severity of cannabis-related problems (29,30). The Marijuana Screening Inventory (31) provides assessment of cannabis patterns and identification of clinical cases requiring more in-depth assessment and intervention. The Substance Dependence Severity Scale, a five-item scale designed to measure dependence severity across most classes of substances, has been validated for assessing dependence in cannabis users (32). Each of these measures has limitations and all are in need of additional testing to better evaluate and maximize their clinical utility.

Additional measures have been developed for use in treatment evaluation research settings such as the Marijuana Problem Inventory, which provides a summary score of specific cannabis-related consequences reported by the individual (33). This Inventory is sensitive to changes over time so as to be a useful index of response to treatment. A measure of cannabis withdrawal severity, the Marijuana Withdrawal Checklist, has been developed in the context of studies designed to characterize the syndrome (16). This measure can provide a useful list of signs and symptoms of withdrawal as well as an overall severity score, and short and longer versions have been developed. Although the Checklist is sensitive to changes in withdrawal severity over time, it has yet to undergo careful evaluation and psychometric testing to guide its use in clinical settings.

Biologic testing for evidence of recent cannabis use is a very useful screening and treatment outcome tool. In many screening and treatment settings, some individuals have multiple reasons to be less than forthcoming about their cannabis use. The standard method of biologic screening is detection of THC metabolites in urine specimens. There are multiple methods for reliable and valid urine testing for cannabis. Rapid dipstick-type methods yield results in approximately 2 minutes, can be administered with little to no training, are inexpensive (less than $10 USD), and provide a qualitative (positive/negative) result. Other urine toxicology methods (e.g., GC–MS and EMIT) can provide quantitative levels of THC metabolites in the urine; These methods either require access to expensive equipment and trained personnel or must be contracted to private companies. Generally, these tests are more expensive than the rapid tests, with the price varying considerably (approximate range $3 to $75). It is also important to note that the reliability and validity of urine toxicology testing with any of these methods for screening and evaluation is only adequate if (1) the urine specimen collection is performed under conditions that ensure the integrity of the sample, (2) the testing includes temperature check and measures of concentration and possible contaminants, and (3) the personnel have adequate training to properly interpret the test results. For example, a urine toxicology test may yield a cannabis-positive result for approximately 2 to 30 days following the last use of cannabis depending on the cutoff level used to detect the cannabinoid metabolite, the frequency, amount and duration of cannabis use prior to testing, the activity level of the individual prior to the test, and individual differences in metabolism and rate of elimination of cannabinoids (34). Many misconceptions exist surrounding the validity and interpretation of urinalysis testing for cannabis, and thus it is important that appropriate protocols are developed and adequate training provided prior to implementing a testing program for screening or treatment evaluation.

Other types of biologic screening include use of saliva and hair specimens. The technology for saliva testing is relatively new, and is continuously being improved; however, significant limitations related to the accuracy of the results and the time frame in which they can be obtained relative to cannabis use remain to be resolved. Hair testing for cannabis also has significant limitations related to determination of the time cannabis was used and the potential for false positives caused by passive cannabis smoke. In summary, to date, urine testing remains the gold standard for screening and evaluation of cannabis use. Use of any of these biologic screening methods requires comprehensive knowledge to facilitate appropriate interpretation of toxicology results.

PSYCHOSOCIAL TREATMENT APPROACHES

Systematic research on behavioral treatments for CUD began approximately 20 years ago; however, only a limited number of controlled studies have been conducted. Behavioral treatments developed and validated for the treatment of other disorders have been modified for use with CUD and shown much promise in the treatment of both adults and adolescents. Motivational enhancement therapy (MET), cognitive-behavioral therapy (CBT), contingency management (CM), and family-based treatments have been carefully evaluated and have consistently demonstrated superior treatment outcomes (reduction of cannabis use) relative to control conditions. The cumulative findings with adults indicate that (1) each of these interventions represents a reasonable and efficacious treatment approach; (2) combining MET and CBT is probably more potent than providing MET alone; and (3) an intervention that integrates all three approaches, MET/CBT/CM, is most likely to produce positive outcomes, especially as measured by rates of abstinence from cannabis. Following is a brief description of each approach as well as a brief review of studies evaluating their effectiveness.

Interventions for Adults

MET, based on the motivational interviewing theory and technique, addresses ambivalence about quitting and seeks to strengthen motivation to change. Therapists use a nonconfrontational, empathic style of counseling to guide the patient toward commitment to and action toward change. MET is typically delivered in 45- to 90-minute individual sessions and usually involves one to four sessions. One session often focuses on providing personalized feedback on use patterns, costs and benefits of using and of quitting, and level of self-efficacy, each of which can be used as a springboard for increasing motivation for change.

CBT focuses on teaching skills relevant to quitting marijuana and to avoiding or coping with other problems that might interfere with good outcomes. Sessions involve analysis of recent cannabis use or cravings, planning for coping with situations that might trigger use or craving, brief trainings on various coping skills, role-playing or other interactive exercises, and practice assignments. CBT is typically delivered in 45- to 60-minute, weekly individual or group counseling sessions; tested CBT interventions have ranged from 6 to 14 sessions.

CM involves the systematic use of positive and negative consequences (reward and punishment) to modify a target behavior (e.g., cannabis use). The type of CM that has been tested with CUD is an abstinence-based incentive intervention adapted from a similar program for cocaine dependence (35). This program provides tangible incentives contingent on cannabis abstinence documented via once- or twice-weekly urine testing. Participants receive vouchers worth a specific monetary value for abstaining from cannabis, which are then exchanged for prosocial retail items or gift cards that can serve as alternative reinforcers to cannabis use.

Efficacy Studies

A series of four trials have demonstrated the efficacy of CBT and MET for adults with CUD (cf. 36). An initial trial showed promising results for a CBT group intervention and a social support group intervention. This trial was followed by a second trial comparing a 14-session group CBT intervention, a 2-session individual MET, and a delayed treatment control (DTC) condition. Days of use, number of uses per day, dependence symptoms, and problems related to use also decreased significantly in the CBT and MET groups compared with the

DTC group, and gains were generally maintained throughout the 16-month follow-up. No significant differences were observed between CBT and MET conditions on any outcome measures, suggesting that brief motivational interventions may be as effective as longer CBT interventions. A similar study showed that a six-session CBT and a one-session MET treatment, both delivered in individual therapy sessions, produced greater rates of abstinence than DTC, but again little difference was observed between the active treatment groups.

The largest efficacy trial ($n = 450$) was a multisite study of MET and CBT comparing nine sessions of combined MET/CBT with two sessions of MET-only and a DTC (33). MET/CBT and MET-only produced better abstinence outcomes than DTC, and MET/CBT engendered significantly greater long-term abstinence and greater reductions in frequency of use compared with MET-only, suggesting better outcomes with the longer CBT intervention. Findings generalized across three sites and were not dependent on ethnicity or gender.

Recognizing that many people overcome substance use problems only after multiple treatment exposures, one research group developed and tested a creative, chronic care model of treatment termed "marijuana dependence treatment PRN" (37). Following an initial four sessions of MET/CBT, participants could choose to attend more sessions as desired over a 28-month period. Unfortunately, enthusiasm for this PRN intervention was limited because only a relatively small percentage of participants (25%) made use of the continuing care sessions, and the PRN group did not show increased abstinence rates compared with a fixed-session comparison condition. Encouraging, however, was the observation that the individuals who did attend numerous PRN sessions showed high levels of abstinence (60%) at follow-up.

Another effort to further enhance outcomes has been to integrate CM with MET/CBT to increase rates of abstinence. An initial 14-week trial compared MET/CBT/CM with MET/CBT only, and a four-session MET intervention (38). Individuals could earn up to $570 in abstinence-based incentives if they provided all negative urine samples throughout treatment. MET/CBT/CM clearly produced the highest abstinence rate during the 14-week treatment period. In a second trial 90 adults received MET/CBT/CM, MET/CBT, or CM alone (no counseling) (39). MET/CBT/CM and CM alone engendered equivalent abstinence rates during treatment, and both showed greater rates for abstinence than MET/CBT. During the post treatment period, MET/CB/CM evidenced greater abstinence rates than the two comparison treatments, and CM alone and MET/CBT did not differ. These findings highlight the efficacy of adding CM to MET/CBT and the importance of MET/CBT to longer term maintenance of abstinence. A third trial conducted by a different research group replicated these findings in a more diverse and larger treatment sample using a less frequent and lower magnitude reinforcement schedule (40). Again, during treatment MET/CBT/CM and CM alone produced continuous abstinence outcomes that were similar to each other and greater than MET/CBT, and, during the post treatment year, MET/CBT/CM group sustained overall positive outcomes better than the CM group.

Two additional studies tested CM with probation-referred young adults with CUDs. Those who received a three-session MET plus an *attendance-based* incentive CM program were more likely to complete treatment (64% vs. 39%), attend sessions (2.3 vs. 1.8), and continue with treatment after completing the three sessions than those receiving only MET (41). However, no concomitant positive effects were observed on cannabis use. A second study compared MET/CBT/CM, MET/CBT alone, Drug Counseling (DC) alone, and DC+CM (42). The CM groups received incentives for attendance *and* cannabis abstinence. CM engendered higher rates of attendance, with the best attendance and completion rates observed with the combination MET/CBT/CM. Across conditions MET/CBT engendered higher rates of attendance than DC. The CM treatments engendered greater cannabis abstinence during treatment, with no difference observed between MET/CBT and DC. MET/CBT/CM showed the highest rates of abstinence throughout the post treatment period, but these rates were not significantly different from those in the other treatment groups.

In summary, MET, CBT, and CM each have empirical support for their efficacy, and CM in combination with MET/CBT has demonstrated the greatest potency in outpatient treatment for adult CUD, particularly for engendering longer periods of abstinence. Although these interventions are clearly efficacious, many individuals do not improve substantially or achieve enduring abstinence, even with the most potent treatments. As with all types of substance dependence, there remains a strong need to develop more effective treatments for CUD (Table 15.2).

Interventions for Adolescents

In clinical trials of adolescents with CUD, empirical support for the efficacy of group or individual CBT and family-based treatments has emerged (43). The CBT interventions studied are similar to CBT for adults in scope and duration. Specific forms of family-based treatment that have been tested include Functional Family Therapy (44), Multidimensional Family Therapy (MDFT; 45), Multisystemic Therapy (46), Brief Strategic Family Therapy (BSFT; 47), Family Support Network intervention (48), and Family Behavior Therapy (49). These family-focused interventions take advantage of social networks that are unique to adolescents in an effort to provide a treatment intervention that extends beyond the client–therapist relationship. These generally include efforts to address and alter maladaptive family patterns that contribute to substance use (e.g., parent drug use, parent–child relationships, and parent supervision), make use of resources in the school and criminal justice system, and address problems that might be associated with the child's peer network. These interventions have demonstrated promise in reducing cannabis and other substance use across multiple clinical trials (43). Note however that, as with the adult CUD treatment studies, reductions in use have typically been modest and effects on

TABLE 15.2	Effective treatments for cannabis abuse or dependence
Adults (18 years and older)	
■ Cognitive–behavioral therapy (CBT) (6 to 14 sessions)	
■ Motivational enhancement therapy (MET) (1 to 4 sessions)	
■ Contingency management (abstinence-based reinforcement)	
Adolescents	
■ Assertive continuing care	
■ Brief Strategic Family Therapy	
■ CBT (individual or group)	
■ Contingency management	
■ Community Reinforcement Approach	
■ Functional Family Therapy	
■ Family Behavior Therapy	
■ MET combined with CBT (5 to 12 sessions)	
■ Multidimensional Family Therapy	
■ Multisystemic Therapy	

Note: These treatments have been manualized and tested in randomized clinical trials.

abstinence rates have been difficult to demonstrate. Below we describe one study that illustrates the strengths and limitations of these outcome findings.

The Cannabis Youth Treatment study included 600 adolescents aged 12 to 18 referred for substance abuse treatment who endorsed at least one criterion for cannabis abuse or dependence and had used cannabis in the previous 90 days (48). Adolescents received one of the following five treatments across four clinical sites: MET/CBT5 (2 individual and 3 group sessions), MET/CBT12 (2 individual and 10 group sessions), MET/CBT12 plus Family Support Network, the Adolescent Community Reinforcement Approach, and MDFT. Significant decreases in drug use and symptoms of dependence were observed following each of the treatments. However, robust between-treatment differences in outcomes were *not* observed, which unfortunately precludes drawing strong conclusions about their efficacy. Although results were promising compared with prior treatment studies, two thirds of the youth continued to experience significant substance-related symptoms. These findings, combined with the similarly modest effects demonstrated in prior studies with the family-focused and individual therapies mentioned above, suggest a need for continued exploration and development of more potent adolescent treatment models and interventions.

As with the interventions for adults, adding CM to "standard" therapies is currently being tested with adolescents with CUD. Although a number of the aforementioned family-based interventions incorporate teaching parents to use behavioral procedures that reflect CM principles, such procedures have not been well specified, isolated, or independently evaluated. The only published randomized trial of a CM-based treatment focused on cannabis examined an intervention with multiple CM components (50). The intervention included (a) an abstinence-based voucher incentive program of the same schedule and magnitude as that used in adult CUD trials (although incentives were earned only for documented abstinence from *all* substances), (b) a behavioral parenting intervention that focused on the development and implementation of an abstinence-based contract directing parents to provide tangible incentives for drug abstinence and to deliver negative consequences for evidence of continued use, and (c) a fishbowl incentive procedure that reinforced parents for adhering to each aspect of the parent training and CM contract. These CM components were integrated with weekly individual MET/CBT counseling and compared with an intervention that included MET/CBT, weekly educational parent sessions, and an attendance-based incentive program. Both treatments included twice-weekly urine testing with results provided immediately to the parents and the teen.

The MET/CBT/CM group demonstrated greater rates of continuous abstinence during treatment than the comparison intervention, but this effect did not clearly extend to post treatment assessments. Overall, rates of cannabis abstinence in both treatment conditions were relatively high compared with those reported in previous studies suggesting that the comparison condition might also warrant further evaluation to determine its efficacy. The twice-weekly urine testing program received in both treatment conditions, which systematically reported results to parents, was unique to this study and may be an active treatment component in its own right.

A final intervention of note involving adolescents is assertive continuing care (ACC), which was designed to maintain treatment gains (reduce relapse) achieved during residential treatment (51). This intervention consists of adolescents being assigned a case manager for 90 days after discharge from an inpatient treatment facility. Adolescents were assigned a case manager who made weekly home visits with goals of engaging in other identified services, development of a new social support system involving prosocial activities, and generally reinforcing strategies to maintain abstinence. In a randomized trial comparing ACC to usual continuing care, the ACC intervention was more effective in increasing adolescents' engagement and retention in continuing care and resulted in longer term abstinence from cannabis (51).

In summary, a number of behavior- and family-based interventions appear effective for treating adolescents with CUD. As with adults, combining CM strategies with these interventions may enhance their efficacy. Yet it remains that many youth do not respond to even the most potent interventions tested to date including the multicomponent CM program discussed above. There remains a clear and pressing need for continued treatment development research and testing.

SECONDARY PREVENTION

"Check-up" (CU) interventions have been developed that are designed to reach cannabis users who have not sought treatment but are ambivalent about stopping or do not perceive their use to be a problem that warrants treatment (52). Such interventions have typically involved adaptations of MET approaches. In an initial trial, adult cannabis users responded to advertisements stating that up-to-date information on cannabis use and its effects was available. Those who responded were near-daily cannabis users, and ambivalent about changing their use. They received an assessment followed by either one personalized CU session, one multimedia session (providing information on cannabis and its effects), or a delayed session (choice of CU or multimedia delayed by 7 weeks). CU resulted in greater reductions in cannabis use and associated problems over the course of 12 months than the multimedia condition; however, absolute levels of change were relatively small. A second study sought to enhance outcomes by adding four sessions of MET/CBT following two CU sessions. The six-session intervention successfully engaged participants, but unfortunately did not result in greater reductions in cannabis use. These studies demonstrated that this intervention model attracted a "unique" sample of ambivalent cannabis users who may be ideal candidates for secondary interventions like the CU, but alternative CU models are needed to obtain more robust effects.

A similar CU model was tested with adolescents in grades 9 to 12 who had used cannabis at least nine times in the past month (53). Volunteers recruited with posters and health education lectures were randomized to either a two-session CU intervention or a 3-month delayed treatment condition. CU consisted of a computerized assessment and two 30-minute MET sessions. Teens in both conditions significantly reduced their cannabis use over 3 months; however, no significant between-group differences were observed. This study showed that cannabis-using adolescents will volunteer to participate in a cannabis intervention provided at their school, which provides an important opportunity to explore alternative methods for early intervention on cannabis use. Indeed, two other interventions using brief MET/CBT have shown some promise in reducing cannabis use with adolescents outside a treatment setting (54,55).

In summary, a variety of effective psychosocial interventions have been developed to treat CUD in both adults and adolescents. Unfortunately, as with treatment for other substance use disorders, the rates of "success" are modest. Even with MET/CBT/CM, the most highly efficacious treatment for adults, only about half of those who enroll in treatment achieve an initial 2-week period of abstinence, and among those who do, approximately half return to use or relapse within a year (39,40). The treatment outcome data for adolescents paint a similar picture. Clearly, continued development of effective treatments for CUD will be required to better meet the needs of those who experience cannabis use-related problems.

PHARMACOTHERAPY

In an attempt to address the need for more effective treatments, researchers have recently sought to identify medications that could be used in conjunction with psychosocial treatments to improve outcomes for CUD. Use of medications to assist in the treatment of substance use disorders is common for the treatment of other drugs of abuse (e.g., opiates, tobacco, and alcohol). In these instances, the majority of the medications used are those known to either reduce the occurrence or severity of withdrawal symptoms or attenuate the reinforcing effects of a specific substance. Generally, evidence from other substance use disorders suggests that treatment approaches that combine pharmacotherapy and psychosocial therapy can enhance outcomes compared with use of either approach alone.

Laboratory Analog Studies

Multiple controlled laboratory studies with non-treatment-seeking daily cannabis users have been conducted to assess whether medications might have potential for clinical application. Inpatient and outpatient laboratory models have examined medication effects on cannabis withdrawal, the effects of smoked cannabis, and relapse. Here we provide a brief review of this research.

Laboratory studies of buproprion, valproate, nefazodone, clonidine, and naltrexone have not shown robust effects across multiple outcome measures that would suggest potential therapeutic efficacy, and in some cases had effects opposite of those desired (56–60). Positive laboratory findings have been observed with a few other medications. The most promising of these comes from studies targeting cannabis withdrawal with the oral preparation of THC, dronabinol, a CB1 receptor agonist. In three laboratory studies, dronabinol significantly reduced multiple symptoms of cannabis withdrawal compared with placebo (57,61,62). This effect was dose dependent, and higher doses demonstrated almost complete suppression of withdrawal effects. Dronabinol alone, however, has not been shown to reduce laboratory models of relapse or cannabis self-administration, but did show positive effects when combined with lofexidine in a laboratory model of relapse (61). Lofexidine, an α_2-adrenergic receptor agonist used to treat opioid withdrawal, significantly reduced ratings of chills, restlessness, and upset stomach, and improved sleep, and reduced the likelihood of relapse during a period of cannabis abstinence compared with placebo (61).

Two studies have evaluated rimonabant, a CB1 receptor partial agonist/antagonist, hypothesizing that it would block the effects of cannabis administration. Indeed in an initial study it reduced the subjective effects of smoked cannabis by approximately 40%, but the subsequent study failed to replicate this finding (63,64). Last, preliminary findings targeting sleep difficulty, a common and significant symptom of cannabis withdrawal, reported that extended-release zolpidem, an approved hypnotic, attenuated abstinence-induced sleep disturbance as measured by polysomnography in a placebo-controlled study (65).

Clinical Trials

Only three controlled clinical trials of medications for CUD have been reported. In one 6-week study, 25 participants were randomly assigned to receive either CBT plus valproate (a mood stabilizer) or CBT plus placebo (66). No effect of valproate was observed on any measures of cannabis use. A 13-week randomized trial ($n = 106$) compared individual counseling combined with one of the two antidepressant medications, nefazodone and sustained-release buproprion, or placebo (67). No effect of either medication was observed on measures of cannabis use, or on self-reported measures of cannabis withdrawal, and more than half of the participants dropped out prior to treatment completion. Last, a 12-week trial ($n = 50$) compared MET combined with either buspirone, an anti anxiety medication, or placebo (68). Nonsignificant positive findings were observed for buspirone on the number of THC-positive urine specimens and shorter time to first THC-negative urine specimen; however, again less than half of those enrolled completed the study. Buspirone appeared to be fairly well tolerated, but participants reported a higher frequency of dizziness, dry mouth, flushing/sweating, and cold-like symptoms.

One open-label clinical report evaluating dronabinol in two patients who had previously failed multiple quit attempts observed a period of sustained abstinence associated with dronabinol (initial dose, 30 mg/day) treatment (69). One patient was tapered off dronabinol without relapse, the other required long-term dronabinol maintenance (5 mg two to three times daily), and both received adjunct medications.

In summary, no medications have been approved for the treatment of CUD, and of the few published, controlled clinical trials, none have reported encouraging results. That said, several medications have been identified that hold some promise. Dronabinol (oral THC) appears to be the best candidate medication, and follows the agonist (substitution) therapy model that has been successful in the treatment of opioid (methadone) and nicotine (patch and gum) dependence. Controlled clinical trials are needed to determine the efficacy of dronabinol (alone and in combination with lofexidine) for treating CUDs. The attenuation of sleep dysfunction with zolpidem during the initial period of abstinence from cannabis is also positive, but additional research is needed to determine whether or not improved sleep translates to less overall withdrawal severity and reduced relapse in clinical samples.

Last, preclinical studies suggest that compounds other than THC that directly affect CB1 receptor function or endogenous endocannabinoid levels (e.g., the FAAH inhibitor URB597) may have potential as effective pharmacotherapies for CUD (70). Note, however, the only one of these compounds previously approved for clinical use, the CB1 receptor antagonist rimonabant, was removed from several markets following approval as a weight loss medication, and failed to be approved in the United States, due to the occurrence of significant psychiatric adverse events. Medicinal chemistry focusing on the development of a newer generation of CB1 receptor partial agonists, antagonists, or endocannabinoid modulators holds promise for medication development for CUD.

COMORBIDITY

Chronic cannabis use has generally been associated with impaired psychological functioning, and those with a CUD are at increased risk for concurrent substance use and nonsubstance use psychiatric disorders. The relation between cannabis use and psychotic disorders has engendered particular interest among basic and clinical scientists, with rekindled research and speculation prompted by the discovery of the endocannabinoid system. In this section, we review the literature on comorbidity of cannabis use and misuse and other psychiatric disorders with special attention to the question of causality. That is, does cannabis misuse lead to other psychopathology or do existing psychiatric problems increase risk for cannabis use or CUD?

CUD and Other Drug Use Disorders

Large general population studies indicate that individuals with past-year or lifetime CUD diagnoses have high rates of alcohol abuse (18%), alcohol dependence (40%), and nicotine dependence (53%) (e.g., 8). These rates of comorbid substance use problems are clearly much greater than observed among those without a CUD. Rates of substance abuse other than alcohol or nicotine are also likely to be greater among cannabis abusers, but have not been estimated independently.

Among those seeking treatment for a CUD, other types of substance use are also common. For example, data from the U.S. Treatment Episode Data Set (TEDS) indicate that among adults seeking treatment in 2007 who reported cannabis to be their primary drug of concern, 74% reported problematic use of a secondary or tertiary substance: alcohol (40%), cocaine (12%), methamphetamine (6%), and heroin or other opiates (2%) (10). Among those younger than 18 years, 61% reported problematic use of a secondary substance: alcohol (48%), cocaine (4%), methamphetamine (2%), and heroin or other opiates (2%).

Prevalence of having a secondary substance use disorder diagnosis of abuse or dependence appears to be much lower than the rates of comorbid substance use listed above (10). For adults seeking treatment for a primary CUD, rates of abuse or dependence are 5% for alcohol, 7.5% for cocaine, 1% for opiates, and 7% for other substances. Most clinical trials for primary CUD have excluded participants dependent on other substances leaving few other sources to assess prevalence of comorbid secondary substance use disorders among treatment seekers. One early study, however, reported that among adults responding to advertisements offering assessment and treatment services for cannabis users, 19% reported past 90-day problematic use of any other substance, and an additional 40% reported a lifetime history of other substance abuse or dependence (71).

The TEDS data for adolescents with primary CUD indicate 2007 prevalence rates for secondary substance use disorders at 2.5% for alcohol, 5% for cocaine, 0.3% for opiates, and 5% for other substances (10). Reports from clinical trials suggest much higher rates of comorbidity among adolescents. For example, the large multisite Cannabis Youth Treatment study reported 37% of participants had an alcohol use disorder and 12% had some other substance use disorder. Differences in the prevalence of other substance use disorders across reports are likely caused by the inclusion/exclusion criteria of the various studies. For example, most clinical studies have included adolescents with cannabis abuse or dependence symptoms regardless of whether they considered cannabis their primary substance or not, while the TEDS data on secondary substance use disorders reflect only those who indicated cannabis as their primary substance.

Cannabis is also the most common, illegal secondary substance used by those seeking treatment for other types of substance dependence. Among those in treatment for primary cocaine use disorders, 35% report cannabis as a secondary or tertiary substance use problem; among primary alcohol use disorder patients, 28% report cannabis as a secondary or tertiary problem substance; and among primary heroin abusers, 16% report cannabis as a secondary or tertiary problem (10). Note that the rate of cannabis use among heroin abusers is likely much higher than the 16% who reported cannabis as a problem substance in the TEDS. These patients report high rates of alcohol and cocaine problems, and unfortunately the TEDS limits assessment to only secondary and tertiary problem substances. Thus, the cannabis use of many of the heroin abusers may not be captured in these TEDS data because these patients are likely to use cocaine and alcohol as well and likely consider them more problematic than cannabis. Clinical trials attest to this as 50% to 85% of those seeking treatment for heroin/opiates (or cocaine) typically report regular cannabis use (72).

In summary, CUDs are experienced as significant primary problems warranting treatment intervention both with and without concurrent use or abuse of other substances. CUDs are also often observed as a secondary problem among those with a primary diagnosis of other types of substance dependence. Although such observations may appear obvious, we highlight this information here because historically many have perceived cannabis abuse to only exist as a secondary problem, typically occurring among those with other substance dependence disorders. Actually, cannabis use problems are more ubiquitous than originally believed.

Causality and the Gateway Effect

Cannabis has been designated a "gateway" drug because its use almost always precedes use of "harder" drugs such as cocaine and heroin, and frequent cannabis users have much greater probability than nonusers of using heroin or cocaine in their lifetime. Such data, in addition to the high comorbidity rates of CUD and other substance use disorders, raise the question of whether cannabis use or development of a CUD is causally related to misuse of other substances. Explanatory hypotheses for this relationship include: (a) the neurobiological effects of cannabis increase sensitivity to the reinforcing effects of other substances, (b) cannabis use increases opportunity for other substance use through increased contact with persons who use or sell other substances, and (c) common characteristics (e.g., externalizing psychopathology, neurobiological sensitivity, or environmental risk factors) exist for use of cannabis and other substances. It is likely that all of these factors contribute to a link between cannabis and other substance use. Longitudinal and genetic studies demonstrate that genes and environmental factors, and common preexisting risk factors account for much, but not all of the relations between early initiation of cannabis use and future other substance use, supporting potential influences consistent with all three of these hypotheses (73). Thus, cannabis use does frequently precede and statistically predict use and abuse of other illicit substances, but so do tobacco use and alcohol use. More evidence is emerging that the order of initiation of substance use can vary depending on culture and geography, suggesting that substance availability may drive these relations. Cannabis use may affect neurobiological reward systems modifying effects of future substance use such that continued use of a "new" substance may be more likely. Or cannabis' acute or chronic effects on cognitive functioning may impact decision making such that one is more likely to try a new substance. Note, however, that these possibilities are also likely true of most substances that are abused. Whether or not one can designate these relations as "causal" because the cannabis use occurs before the other substance use is debatable.

CUD and Other Psychiatric Disorders

Cross-sectional and longitudinal studies have reported a clear association between chronic cannabis use and impaired psychological functioning (14). In particular, cannabis use has been associated with poorer life satisfaction, increased mental health treatment and hospitalization, higher rates of depression, anxiety disorders, suicide attempts, and conduct disorder.

Large general population studies also indicate that individuals with past-year or lifetime diagnoses of cannabis abuse or dependence diagnoses also have high rates of concurrent psychiatric disorders other than substance use disorders (8). Major Depressive Disorder (11%), any anxiety disorder (24%), and Bipolar I disorder (13%) appear to be the most prevalent *DSM-IV* Axis I disorders, and Antisocial (30%), Obsessive Compulsive (19%), and Paranoid (18%) are the most prevalent Axis II personality disorders among those with a past-year diagnosis of a CUD. As with other substance use disorders, the prevalence rates of these other psychiatric disorders are greater among those with CUD than those without. Clinical trials for adult cannabis treatment seekers support the observations from general population observations. Symptom Checklist 90, Brief Symptom Inventory, and Beck Depression Inventory assessments collected from these clinical samples indicate that the great majority would meet criteria for various psychiatric diagnoses, but *DSM* or *ICD* diagnoses were not obtained in most studies.

More comprehensive data are available from clinical trials assessing concurrent psychiatric disorders among adolescents enrolled in treatment for CUD. In the Cannabis Youth Treatment study, 33% of teens enrolled in treatment reported internalizing disorders (anxiety, depression, PTSD) and 61% externalizing disorders (Conduct Disorder and ADHD). Other clinical studies have reported similarly high rates of internalizing and externalizing disorders in the adolescent treatment population (74).

Cannabis is also the most common type of illicit drug used among individuals with schizophrenia and other chronic psychotic disorders, and its prevalence in this population may be even greater than those with other psychiatric diagnoses (75). Moreover, cannabis has been linked to cases of acute psychosis, typical symptoms including some combination of hallucinations, delusions, confusion, amnesia, paranoia, hypomania, and labile mood. Prevalence data on acute psychosis are limited and range from it being very rare to occurring in over 15% of cannabis users (cf. 76).

Causality and Other Psychiatric Disorders

Self-medication is a common explanatory hypothesis for the etiology of substance use disorders, including CUD, that is, persons may use the substance to self-medicate existing psychiatric disorders and symptoms. Persons with certain psychological problems or those in current mood states may experience the initial direct effects of cannabis as either more or less reinforcing (e.g., may feel temporary relief from depressed mood or may cause increased anxious feeling in formal social situations). However, evidence from longitudinal studies particularly for the relation between cannabis and mood disorders has not supported a causal self-medication hypothesis (77,78). Whether mental health problems contribute to development of CUD, or the converse, remains equivocal. Controlling for risk factors common to both mental health and cannabis problems appears to reduce but not eliminate the positive associations between the two. Some data suggest that age of onset may relate to the direction of influence. Early onset of cannabis use is a strong predictor of later mental health problems, but such early onset also may be predicted from prior mental health problems. Psychiatric problems and early cannabis use appear to share a pathway predicted by socioeconomic disadvantage and child behavior problems; moreover, cannabis use may contribute directly to poor psychosocial outcomes.

The types of mental health problems that remain associated with cannabis use in longitudinal studies, once common etiologic factors are adequately controlled for, are primarily externalizing problems such as conduct/antisocial disorder or other drug dependence disorders. The notion that cannabis is used to "medicate" externalizing disorders is not highly tenable. Rather, the conceptualization of cannabis use and abuse as part of an externalizing syndrome that includes nondrug externalizing disorders has gathered increasing attention and support (79). In summary, cannabis use, particularly early initiation of use, can be considered a risk factor for nonpsychotic mental health problems and, as such, is a reasonable target for prevention and intervention of psychological problems.

Whether or not cannabis use can induce acute psychosis or contribute to the development of more chronic psychotic disorders (e.g., schizophrenia) also remains controversial, although data supporting such a causal relationship are emerging. Increased understanding of the actions of cannabis on the central nervous system and the functioning of the endocannabinoid system has generated increased study and concern about cannabis and its contribution to severe psychiatric disorder.

Suggestive evidence for a causal relationship between cannabis use and *acute* psychosis is primarily of two types. Clinical case reports frequent the literature with examples of patients with psychotic symptoms whose onset closely follows ingestion of cannabis; whose symptoms remit within days or, at most, a few weeks of abstinence from cannabis; and many with no previous psychiatric history. Second, experimental studies have demonstrated that cannabis administration (albeit intravenous dosing of THC) can produce psychotic-type symptoms in those without risk factors for psychotic disorders (80). Nonetheless, the literature linking cannabis use and acute psychosis includes only uncontrolled studies; thus, other causes for the psychosis cannot be ruled out. One could reasonably conclude that high doses of cannabis can precipitate psychosis in some individuals, but whether or not a predisposition to psychotic illness or some other baseline factor is necessary for acute psychosis to occur remains unknown.

Literature reviews relying on findings from longitudinal studies and laboratory studies have posed similar conclusions regarding the relationship of cannabis use and *chronic* psychotic disorders (77,78,80). The term "component cause" has been increasingly used to describe how cannabis contributes to causing psychosis in the presence of other risk factors. Moreover, human and nonhuman basic research has established biologic plausibility related to the impact of cannabis on the DA system and the possible psychotogenic role of the endogenous cannabinoid system. Suggestive but strong evidence has emerged that cannabis use can induce a psychotic disorder in at least a subpopulation of those who have other risk factors for developing psychotic symptoms or disorders. Epidemiologic and longitudinal designs can never eliminate all confounding factors and measurement issues, but causality, defined as an increased risk for experiencing a psychotic disorder, appears to be an appropriate term to use given the current data. This said, one must be cognizant of the degree of risk. Most regular cannabis users do not experience psychotic symptoms or develop psychotic disorders, and cannabis cannot be designated the cause of most cases of psychosis. Estimates of attributable risk suggest that cannabis may play a role in approximately 1 of 10 cases (78).

Cannabis Use and the Course of Psychiatric Disorder

How cannabis use may influence the course of psychiatric disorders has obvious implications for treatment. Significant associations between drug use in general and increased use of treatment resources (hospitalizations and emergency room visits) and poor treatment compliance have been reported in general psychiatric patients. Unfortunately, the impact of cannabis use in this population has not been isolated from the impact of other types of drugs. Cannabis use has been associated with increased rates of recurrent and more severe psychiatric symptomatology and relapse among schizophrenics, but again, effects of other drug use cannot be completely ruled out in these studies. Cannabis use may also result in a misdiagnosis of cannabis-related psychosis resulting in a concomitant delay of a diagnosis and treatment of schizophrenia. As with the data on cannabis use and the development of psychotic disorders, a strong association exists between cannabis use and a negative outcome in schizophrenics. Thus, cannabis use can be considered a risk factor for schizophrenia and a predictor of poor outcome in schizophrenic patients, but its role as an etiologic factor remains uncertain.

NONPSYCHIATRIC HEALTH EFFECTS OF CANNABIS

Cannabis use impacts multiple aspects of normal human functioning including the cardiovascular, immune, neuromuscular, ocular, reproductive, and respiratory systems, appetite, and cognition/perception. Cannabinoid receptors (CB1 and CB2), ubiquitous in the central nervous system and the periphery, suggest a broad functional role of endogenous cannabinoids in human functioning as well as possible influences of exogenous cannabinoids such as cannabis. As discussed earlier, this potential for pros and cons of cannabis use has engendered lively discussion and controversy for many years. Here we will briefly comment on the literature addressing the impact of cannabis consumption on a number of physiologic systems.

Respiratory System

Perhaps the most significant health effects of cannabis involve the respiratory system (cf. 81 for review). Chronic cannabis smoking has the potential for respiratory consequences comparable to tobacco cigarette smoking. Of concern, a large subpopulation of cannabis users smokes a combination of cannabis and tobacco in the form of blunts or cones and almost half of daily cannabis users also smoke tobacco concurring obvious additional risk for consequences on the respiratory system (3). The smoke of cannabis and tobacco contains similar respiratory toxic chemicals. Cannabis smoke can contain up to 50% more carcinogens and results in substantially greater tar deposits in the lungs than filtered tobacco cigarettes. Cannabis users smoke unfiltered material, inhale the smoke more deeply, and hold the smoke longer in their lungs than tobacco smokers, which likely contributes to the resultant high level of toxins entering the lungs.

The most significant acute effect of smoking cannabis is its action as a bronchodilator, which increases vulnerability to the smoke by decreasing airway resistance and increasing specific airway conductance. Cannabis smoking also increases absorption of carbon monoxide, resulting in elevated levels of blood carboxyhemoglobin (COHb). Increased COHb leads to reduced oxygen in the blood and impairment in oxygen release from hemoglobin that can stress a number of organs including the heart. Other short-term aspects of respiration such as breathing rate, breath depth, CO_2 production, respiratory exchange ratio, and arterial blood gases appear to not be significantly affected by cannabis smoking.

Chronic cannabis smoking increases the likelihood of outpatient visits due to respiratory illness and cannabis smokers exhibit respiratory symptoms of bronchitis at comparable rates to tobacco smokers. Airway obstruction and symptoms of chronic cough, sputum production, shortness of breath, and wheezing characterize chronic bronchitis. The cause of these symptoms, airway inflammation and tissue damage resulting in increased fluid production, cellular abnormalities, and reduced alveolar permeability, occurs before cough or wheezing begin. Cannabis smokers have substantially higher bronchitis index scores than non-smokers, and comparable scores to tobacco smokers, even at young ages and after only short histories of regular cannabis use (81).

Investigations of chronic obstructive pulmonary disease (COPD) in chronic cannabis smokers have been inconclusive. Cannabis smokers exhibit almost identical degrees of histopathologic and molecular abnormalities associated with progression to COPD as seen in tobacco smokers but large-scale studies of COPD in chronic users do not clearly show increased risk (82).

The functional significance of cannabis smoking on the respiratory system should be taken seriously. Chronic cannabis smoking is clearly associated with similar processes and patterns of disease that lead to aerodigestive cancers among tobacco smokers, although a causal link to cannabis has not been established definitively (see the next section). Cannabis smokers tend to smoke significantly less material per day than tobacco smokers, which may slow down its comparative impact on the lungs. Individuals who began smoking cannabis in the late 1960s are now approaching the ages that are likely to be associated with aerodigestive cancers; hence, future epidemiologic studies should clarify better the risk of cancer associated with chronic cannabis use. Chronic bronchitis can be moderately debilitating and increases the risk of additional infections. Because cannabis may suppress immune system function, recurrent bronchitis may further increase the risk of opportunistic respiratory infections such as pneumonia and aspergillosis. This may be of particular concern for those individuals with already compromised immune functions such as cancer and AIDS patients.

Immune System and Cancer

The high carcinogen levels observed in cannabis smoke lead to concern of increased risk of multiple types of cancers. Chronic cannabis smoking appears to compromise the immune system, with most available information focused on its impact on the lungs as described above (82). The immunosuppressive effect occurs in a variety of immune cells including killer cells, T cells, and macrophages. Compared with tobacco smokers and nonsmokers, pulmonary alveolar macrophages of chronic cannabis smokers exhibit a reduced ability to kill tumor cells and many microorganisms, including fungi and bacteria. Cannabis smoking also appears to impair phagocytosis and cytokine function of these macrophages. Additional concern has been raised that THC may have direct cancer-fostering properties related to acceleration or increased replication of viruses related to certain cancers (e.g., herpes virus), cancer cell proliferation, and tumor growth. Note that data and arguments for potential anti cancer impact of cannabis have also appeared in the literature. For example, cannabidiol, a nonpsychoactive constituent of cannabis, has demonstrated tumor-reducing effects in rodents (83).

The functional consequences (development of cancers or other immunosuppressive-related diseases) of cannabis' effects on the suppression of the immune system in humans are not well understood. Epidemiologic, cohort, and case control studies have yielded mixed findings regarding associated risk with head and neck, lung, oropharyngeal, and testicular cancer (cf. 84,85). Nonetheless, clinical findings suggest that such effects warrant some concern. Chronic cannabis smoking is associated with increased bronchitis and other respiratory illnesses (see the section 'Respiratory System'). Chronic use may also increase risk of exposure to infectious organisms, as cannabis and tobacco plants are often contaminated with a variety of fungi and molds including aspergillus (86). Lung illnesses in cannabis smokers have been attributed to fungal infection. Decreased immune system response could increase the vulnerability and risk of developing these respiratory illnesses and lung diseases. A better understanding of the functional significance of cannabis' effects on the immune system is imperative as attempts are made to develop safe and effective models for the medical use of cannabis and cannabinoids.

Reproductive System and Perinatal Effects

Cannabis smoking can affect some female and male reproductive hormones, but the functional significance of these effects is unclear. Unfortunately, research examining the effects of cannabis use on reproductive function in women or men has been sparse.

Pregnant women who use cannabis expose the fetus to THC, as it is known to cross the placenta. Ten to 20% of women may use cannabis during pregnancy, yet studying cannabis use during pregnancy has proven difficult, as pregnant users generally have many additional risk factors for adverse effects such as tobacco smoking, alcohol use, other illicit drug use, poorer nutrition, and lower socioeconomic status, and the validity of self-reports of cannabis use in this population is suspect. Risk of major congenital anomalies does not appear to be increased by cannabis use in pregnant women; however, some reports suggest there may be some risk associated with developing minor anomalies related to the visual system, but such data are not robust (87). Studies have reported mixed findings regarding the effects of cannabis use during pregnancy on birth weight, length, and duration of gestation (88).

Cognitive and behavioral effects of prenatal exposure to cannabis are perhaps best gleaned from the Ottawa Prenatal Prospective Study (OPPS) that has produced multiple reports over the past 20 years (89). This study collected birth data on 700 women and has periodically assessed the children of a subsample of 150 to 200 comparing those who used cannabis during pregnancy with controls who did not. Adverse effects of prenatal cannabis use were observed during the first month, with important signs including increased tremors, decreased visual habituation, exaggerated startle, and increased hand-to-mouth behavior. However, at 1, 2, and 3 years of age, no cannabis-related effects were observed. Age 4 assessments revealed performance decrements on verbal and memory tasks, which are similar findings to those reported in a separate study of 3 year olds with prenatal exposure to cannabis (90).

The OPPS group suggests that these "delayed" effects of prenatal cannabis might reflect difficulty in detection of subtle effects on complex processes in young children. However, assessment at 5 and 6 years did not reveal these same deficits, but did show deficits in sustained attention in the 6 year olds. At 9 and 12 years deficits were observed in higher order or executive functioning involving visual analysis, problem solving, hypothesis testing, and impulse control. Continued deficits were observed at ages 14 to 16 years on tests of visual memory, analysis, and integration, which are similar to deficits in chronic adolescent and adult cannabis users (see the section "Brain Function and Cognitive Performance"). Another research group has observed similar effects at age 10 with these youth showing increased hyperactivity, impulsivity, inattention, and delinquency (91).

In summary, the effects of prenatal cannabis use on cognitive functioning appear subtle, and determining causality is difficult since genetic predispositions and multiple environmental factors cannot be ruled out. The functional importance of the observed deficits is also unclear. The types of impairment observed could impact behavioral and cognitive performance of various tasks. Such data indicate that concern is warranted regarding prenatal cannabis use and its effects on human offspring.

Cardiovascular System

Most research examining cannabis and the cardiovascular system has focused on acute effects that occur when cannabis is ingested, and suggest a limited cardiovascular health impact. The primary acute effect is tachycardia with an observed dose-dependent increase in heart rate that diminishes when tolerance develops (92). Cannabis can also produce small increases in supine blood pressure and impair vascular reflexes. Note that the inhalation of carbon monoxide associated with smoking cannabis and subsequent increase in COHb in combination with tachycardia increases the work required of the heart.

Although these findings show clear changes in cardiovascular functioning due to cannabis use, the effects have not been associated with short- or long-term cardiovascular or cerebrovascular injury or disease. Case reports suggest that regular cannabis smoking may increase risk for some potentially serious cardiovascular events or disorders, but no controlled studies support these reports. For most healthy young cannabis smokers, the stress to the heart does not appear clinically detrimental. However, for individuals with cardiovascular or cerebrovascular disease, the additional cardiac stress may increase the risk for chest pain, heart attack, or stroke. Additional research is needed to elucidate the effects of chronic cannabis use on cardiovascular health, including interactions with other risk factors.

Brain Function and Cognitive Performance

A large literature has accumulated examining the effects of cannabis on cognitive functioning and performance (93). Cannabis acts on the endogenous cannabinoid system in the central nervous system and cannabinoid receptors are located in areas of the brain that suggest impact on memory, attention, and other cognitive functions. A growing neuroimaging literature suggests that chronic use of cannabis alters the cannabinoid system, but structural damage and serious impairment is not apparent. Administration of cannabis or THC increases activation in frontal, prefrontal, and paralimbic regions and the cerebellum, which is consistent with some of the behavioral and cognitive effects associated with cannabis (cf. 94,95). In chronic cannabis users, fMRI studies show alterations in the activation of brain areas involved in higher cognitive (executive) functions. Early initiation of cannabis use has been linked to a number of brain structure abnormalities and brain function patterns during performance of cognitive tasks (cf. 96). Such findings have increased concern regarding adolescent cannabis use and its impact on brain development. However, more research is needed to better understand and interpret the functional and long-term significance of these observations.

This literature generally indicates that cannabis use can lead to selective cognitive impairments, although the magnitude and functional significance of such deficits is difficult to assess. The ability to organize and integrate complex information appears compromised, most likely due to effects of cannabis on memory and attentional processes. Here we provide a brief review and discussion of both acute (direct or intoxicating) effects and chronic (long-term use) effects of cannabis use. Most controversial and difficult to assess has been the long-term effects of cannabis use and the extent to which deficits are recovered following cessation of use.

Acute Use

Demonstrating acute effects of cannabis on *psychomotor performance* has proven more elusive than might be expected. THC-induced effects on response speed and accuracy, tracking ability, body sway, and reaction time have been observed in some studies, but not in others (14,97). As one would expect, THC dose accounts for some of the variation in findings with dose–response effects observed in some studies, and moderately strong evidence that cannabis (THC) can impair performance on some psychomotor tasks at higher doses (e.g., 98,99). Tolerance (cannabis use history) also impacts the degree of impairment from acute doses of cannabis with regular heavy users showing less performance decrements than novice or less frequent users (100). This literature does not indicate a pervasive response slowing, such as decrements on simple reaction time tasks. Rather, affected tasks appear to be those that require more attention, motivation, and impulse control.

The literature also indicates that acute cannabis or THC ingestion, dose dependently, produces adverse effects on a number of *cognitive functions*, which are likely moderated by cannabis use history (tolerance). Effects have consistently been observed on short-term memory, particularly immediate memory and recall and retrieval following a lapse of time. Note, however, that when retrieval cues are available, these deficits may be obviated, suggesting that adverse effects on attentional or learning processes are likely involved. Cannabis has been shown to disrupt the ability to learn novel tasks, and adversely impacts performance on divided and sustained attention tasks. Cannabis intoxication also affects the subjective perception of time. Time estimates are shorter and time productions are longer in subjects after smoking cannabis.

Experimental studies have also demonstrated that cannabis can adversely impact decision-making and executive function, although findings have produced somewhat mixed results. Increases in response perseveration, and impairment in motor impulse control, divided attention, response adaptation, and working memory have been demonstrated with higher doses (99–101).

Chronic Use

The cognitive impairments observed in acute administration studies of cannabis have also been observed when studying long-term or chronic use of cannabis. Although these chronic effects have been difficult to pinpoint and replicate due to numerous methodological difficulties in studying long-term effects, multiple reports strongly suggest that cannabis users show cognitive and behavioral performance deficits even when not under the influence of cannabis. A series of studies showed that regular cannabis users' performance on an auditory selective-attention task was significantly worse than that of matched controls, suggesting compromised ability to filter out complex irrelevant information (102). Severity of the deficits was associated with years of cannabis use and reduction in event-related potentials (P300 amplitude), a purported marker of cognitive processing. Other studies suggest significant deficits such as increased perseveration, decreased verbal learning and memory, and deficits in complex reaction time, complex reasoning, and short-term memory (103–105). These effects have been characterized as deficits of the attentional/executive system involving mental flexibility, working memory, learning, and sustained attention. Similar to the recent findings on the impact of cannabis on brain function, a number of studies suggest more impairment in those who initiated cannabis use at an early age suggesting the possibility of increased vulnerability during early adolescence (104).

Permanent or Temporary Deficits

Evidence addressing the permanence of the cognitive impairments observed in chronic cannabis use has been mixed (93). One report indicated that ex–cannabis smokers continued to show impairment in their ability to filter out irrelevant information, although some evidence of partial recovery was noted (102). Another study observed continued impairment on multiple measures following 28 days of abstinence that was positively related to the severity of their cannabis use (106). In contrast, a similar study reported that heavy cannabis users showed signs of impairment for at least 7 days post-abstinence, but observed no cannabis-associated deficits by day 28 of abstinence (107). Much of the research on the chronic effects of cannabis use is limited by multiple confounding variables such as possible acute intoxication, testing during cannabis withdrawal states, variable use histories, unknown cognitive abilities prior to cannabis exposure, concurrent use of other drugs, demographic influences, and comorbidity with other mental or physical illnesses. Although recent studies have made strong efforts to control for many of these variables, important limitations remain.

Notwithstanding the methodological issues inherent to this research, the literature strongly suggests that chronic cannabis use can impair performance on various types of cognitive tests, specifically those thought to involve complex cognitive processes. These deficits may increase in form and severity in relation to the duration of exposure to cannabis, and early initiation of cannabis use may increase the adverse consequences. Future research is needed to better elucidate the processes that cause performance deficits and to determine their functional significance. Because most cognitive and performance tests are affected by attentional and motivational processes, understanding how cannabis affects these factors is necessary for understanding its influence on cognitive processing.

Functional Significance

The functional significance of the cannabis-associated cognitive and behavioral performance deficits discussed above is of most concern to the individual and society at large. Here we briefly discuss three potential areas of impact: driving performance, academic achievement, and motivation.

Driving The literature on the impact of cannabis intoxication on driving performance and risk of accident has been difficult to interpret, but some are concerned that it has become as great a public health risk as driving after drinking alcohol (108). Studies using driving simulators and road tests have produced mixed results (e.g., 109,110). Cannabis intoxication has been shown to adversely affect performance in emergency situations perhaps due to an increase in brake latency and worsened ability to attend to extraneous stimuli. Some have suggested that cannabis adversely impacts more well-learned, automatic driving behavior rather than skills that require more attention and conscious action. Interestingly, cannabis use appears to decrease risk-taking behavior in simulated and on-road driving situations, perhaps suggesting some awareness of and compensation for impairment. In summary, adverse effects on driving skills and behavior seem most evident when assessed in close temporal proximity to cannabis ingestion, are dose dependent, and are moderated by the individual's history of cannabis use (tolerance).

Of additional importance is the impact on driving of the combination of cannabis and alcohol, a common pattern of use among youth and young adult populations. This combination clearly increases risk of unsafe, risky driving performance (109,110). Although impaired cannabis smokers may try to compensate by using risk reduction strategies, use of alcohol likely obviates such efforts. Alcohol and cannabis use produces greater deficits than using either substance alone; even inconsequential doses of each substance can produce impairment when combined.

Epidemiologic studies also show somewhat mixed findings, but the results tend to support observations from the laboratory. Some culpability studies have reported a reduced risk of *fatal* accidents with cannabis alone (no other substances) compared to alcohol-alone or drug-free accidents, but an increased risk with the combination of alcohol and cannabis. Failure to find that use of cannabis alone increases risk of automobile crashes in these types of studies has been attributed to the method of cannabis detection. Studies that rely on indicators of very recent use of cannabis rather than simply indicating cannabis use at some time in the past show a clear increased risk of crash compared with drug-free drivers (109). The probability of being responsible for an accident increases with greater plasma levels of THC. Case control studies have been fewer in number, but have provided more clear evidence for an association between cannabis use and increased risk of crash. A recent longitudinal study reported an increased risk of crash related to self-reported cannabis use among young adults aged 21 to 25 after controlling for multiple potential confounding factors (108).

Unfortunately, epidemiologic studies have several important limitations. Measurement of cannabis levels is difficult to relate to recency of use and behavioral impairment. Also, some studies exclude cases that involve cannabis and another illicit substance, yet the combination of cannabis and other substances, including alcohol, is the most common finding in accident reviews. Moreover, when these cases are assessed, the relative contribution of cannabis to the accidents cannot be readily determined. Last, most studies do not consider the base rates of cannabis use in comparable populations (young adults) and the concomitant accident rates in that population. Overall, the data from experimental and epidemiologic studies strongly suggest a positive relationship among acute cannabis use, driving performance impairments, and accidents. Although these data are not without limitations, driving under the influence of cannabis warrants caution and much concern, particularly for younger users who may have less tolerance, greater cognitive impairment, less driving experience, and more driving distractions (e.g., peer passengers) than adults.

Academic Achievement Although one would expect that the adverse effects of cannabis use on attentional and complex cognitive processing would have direct influence on optimal academic performance, the extent of this influence is unknown. Cannabis use has been linked to low grade-point averages, decreased academic satisfaction, negative attitudes toward school, poor overall performance in school, and absence from school (111,112), with early cannabis use (prior to age 16) associated with dropping out of high school and failure to complete college. Studies that have statistically controlled for the multiple confounding influences have reported mixed results (113). Because cannabis users tend to have multiple risk factors that are associated with poor academic performance, it is most difficult to demonstrate causality. Of note, in addition to its impact on cognitive performance, cannabis may also adversely affect motivation (see section below). A negative impact on motivation to achieve in an academic setting evidenced through decreased efforts directed toward school work (see below) would likely have an even greater impact on academic performance than the subtle cannabis-related deficits in complex processing observed in the laboratory studies. Both influences are probable. In addition, poor academic performance in the early school years is also a risk factor for initiation of cannabis.

Motivation Cannabis use has long been associated with an "amotivational syndrome" reflecting lethargy, inactivity, loss of motivation, and decreased goal-directed behavior. Evidence for this amotivational syndrome comes primarily from case studies and clinical reports. Some chronic cannabis users attribute impaired vocational or academic performance and loss of ambition to their cannabis use, and procrastination and impaired motivation are commonly reported as the consequences of using cannabis and as reasons for quitting. Controlled field studies have failed to provide clear evidence of an amotivational syndrome although this research is weakened by limitations relating to sample selection and definitions of motivation. For example, many chronic users appear to be underemployed based on their education and abilities, yet well integrated with their families and community. Many of these cannabis users attribute these circumstances to a lifestyle choice rather than an adverse effect of cannabis use on motivation.

Laboratory studies examining the effect of cannabis on work performance demonstrate what could be termed amotivational behavior. These studies suggest that cannabis affects sensitivity to reinforcement, and that motivational effects of cannabis intoxication are determined by environmental context and contingencies (114). That is, performance deficits operationalized as decreased rates of working and decreased earnings are observed when participants are under the influence of cannabis; however, these effects can be countered when monetary rewards are strategically arranged (115). Adults, given a choice to work on a high-demand task that earned monetary reinforcement or switch to a no-demand task that earned a lower level of reinforcement, chose to spend less time working on the high-demand task when under the influence of cannabis than when given placebo. This effect appeared dose dependent and was partially reversed by increasing the magnitude of the reinforcement in the high-demand task. This suggests that the amotivational effects of cannabis intoxication may occur by impacting the effects of reinforcement on various types of operant behavior (e.g., change sensitivity). A similar amotivational effect of cannabis has also been observed in an experimental study with adolescents (114). Adolescents who regularly used cannabis chose to switch to a nonwork option more quickly than matched controls that were not cannabis smokers, which resulted in earning less money suggesting reduced motivation. Moreover, quicker switching to the nonwork option was related to measured cannabinoid levels in these adolescents. The interaction among the behavioral effects of cannabis and environmental variables needs further study to better understand the relation between cannabis and motivation.

Although laboratory studies indicate that acute cannabis use can engender what appears to be less motivated behavior, the link between chronic cannabis use and an *amotivational* syndrome that is unrelated to acute cannabis intoxication has not been clearly established. Additional laboratory studies that compare chronic users with nonusers on performance of various work-related tasks, while controlling for acute intoxication effects, may provide more important information and address the validity of an enduring effect of cannabis on motivational processes. Of note, the acute effects of cannabis on operant performance observed in the laboratory indicate that motivation (i.e., effort) should be considered when interpreting studies that examine the effects of cannabis on any cognitive or behavioral performance tasks.

SPECIAL CONSIDERATIONS AND CONCLUSIONS

Two commonly discussed issues related to cannabis, its potential for medicinal use and legalization, warrant comment prior to concluding this chapter. Regarding the medical use of cannabis debate, the 1999 comprehensive report from the Institute on Medicine (116) acknowledged the importance of initiating additional scientific study of the risks and benefits of the use of cannabis and cannabinoids for specific medical conditions, and in particular mentioned investigation of smoked cannabis. The compounds in cannabis clearly have potential beneficial effects for a number of medical conditions. The oral form of THC is approved by the U.S. Food and Drug Administration and by regulatory bodies in other countries for AIDS wasting syndrome and cancer patients receiving chemotherapy. Likewise, the synthetic cannabinoid, nabilone, is approved for use in cancer patients undergoing chemotherapy, and the oromucosal form of a cannabis extract, which contains cannabidiol in addition to THC, is approved to manage spasticity and neuropathic pain in multiple sclerosis.

The interest in the benefits of smoked cannabis in contrast to oral THC arises primarily from differences in the pharmacokinetics of these two routes of administration. Through the oral route, THC absorption is slow and variable, and therefore clinical effects have a slower onset and longer duration than smoked cannabis. In addition, smoked cannabis not only delivers delta-9-THC, but also other compounds (e.g., delta-8-THC and cannabidiol) are absorbed that may have direct or interactive effects of therapeutic interest. That said, smoked cannabis also has multiple disadvantages when considering it for use as a prescribed medication. The adverse effects of smoked cannabis on the respiratory system and its carcinogenic impact have been reviewed earlier. Determination and administration of therapeutic doses through smoking the plant material also poses many hurdles. In addition, its psychoactive effects and multiple adverse consequences associated with its use raise additional concerns. These issues have limited the amount of research completed on smoked cannabis, and to date, there remains very limited controlled clinical research about its efficacy and side-effect profile for medical indications.

The burgeoning of science directed toward understanding of the endocannabinoid system has greatly increased optimism for the use of cannabinoids (cannabis-like compounds) as medicine. Efforts are underway to develop alternative cannabinoid medications that could reproduce the desired effects of cannabis, without the potentially problematic effects of smoked cannabis such as abuse potential, sedation, disruption in psychomotor performance, problems with memory and other cognitive processes, carcinogenicity, and respiratory system complications. Positive findings from studies evaluating the therapeutic potential of such cannabinoid-like compounds or from compounds that can manipulate the endogenous cannabinoid system clearly indicate growing promise of medicinal value in areas such as treatment of pain, neuromuscular and neurodegenerative disorders, eating or appetite disorders, autoimmune diseases, and other psychiatric disorders (2). As such, it is likely that these novel compounds that interact with the endocannabinoid system, and not smoked cannabis, will eventually be determined effective and safe for medical use. Unfortunately such scientific advances in medicine are sometimes slowed down by certain advocates, the lay public, and legislators who are concerned that demonstrating the therapeutic potential of a class of drugs might diminish the perceived risk of a drug's addictive potential and potential for harm, and lead to increased misuse of a drug. The error of this perspective is evident in the case of the opioids, which have provided both a large and important medical benefit to society and are recognized as a class of drugs that poses a significant drug problem.

The issue of legalization of cannabis is tied closely to concerns about perceived harm, and concerns about increased availability of substances with potential for abuse and harm. As discussed above, cannabis is the most widely used illegal substance in the United States and most other developed countries that regulate its use. Controversy regarding its legal status has proliferated since the early part of the 20th century. Procannabis groups have led an ongoing effort to decriminalize or legalize cannabis use, and many respected scientists and medical professionals have joined the argument by calling for the legalization of cannabis for medical use. Anti-cannabis legalization proponents raise the concerns about the psychosocial, health, and psychiatric consequences associated with cannabis misuse and addiction reviewed earlier in this chapter.

Many who argue for the legalization of cannabis point to the data showing that alcohol use and abuse is clearly more detrimental to the individual and society than cannabis use. Like all other substances including alcohol that have addictive potential, most individuals who initiate cannabis use do not experience significant consequences, but others misuse, abuse, or become dependent and experience adverse outcomes. The argument that cannabis has legitimate medical benefits has also been used to support the call for legalization and decriminalization, but one must recognize that "medical potential" could be claimed for most other substances that are abused and currently illegal. In addition, arguments abound related to the impact of changing its legal status on issues such as: cost and availability of cannabis, tax benefits to society, prevalence rates of abuse and dependence, effects of advertising and marketing, costs related to criminal prosecution and prison housing, and the impact of criminal records related to cannabis possession on the individual.

Of course elements of the arguments proposed by both sides of the legalization debate have merit. The task of creating policy that balances protection of civil liberties and protection of the public (including children) is most difficult and requires much speculation. Currently, many U.S. states have reduced penalties for possession of small amounts of cannabis and have legislation legalizing the medical use of cannabis under very stringent conditions. At the same time, many schools and work places have adopted mandatory drug testing policies that include cannabis in the list of drugs that are not tolerated, and federal regulations remain strict.

Unfortunately, the ongoing debate over the medical use and legalization of cannabis has spawned distrust and confusion regarding the scientific data that inform our understanding of cannabis and its consequences. A reasonable perspective is to acknowledge that some level of cannabis use can and does result in harmful effects. However, while we have much to learn about the parameters of cannabis use that result in adverse consequences, a wealth of new knowledge has accumulated during the past two decades. Cannabis misuse, abuse, dependence, and withdrawal are real and relatively common phenomena with significant associated consequences that reflect a clear public health problem. In addition, scientific discoveries related to the endocannabinoid system have revealed the ubiquitous nature of cannabinoids and their complex interactions with other neuro-biologic systems, suggesting multiple avenues by which they might be used to treat clinical disorders in the future. Our hope is that this chapter provides the reader with an informed and thoughtful understanding and appreciation of cannabis and its impact on human functioning.

REFERENCES

1. Abel EL. *Marihuana: The First Twelve Thousand Years*. New York: Plenum; 1980.
2. Budney AJ, Lile JA. Moving beyond the cannabis controversy into the world of the cannabinoids. *Int Rev Psychiatry*. 2009; 21:91–95.
3. SAMHSA. *National Survey on Drug Use and Health*. 2009. Available at: http://www.oas.samhsa.gov/nsduh.htm.
4. Copeland J, Swift W. Cannabis use disorder: epidemiology and management. *Int Rev Psychiatry*. 2009;21:96–103.
5. UNODC. *2008 World Drug Report*. Vienna: United Nations Office on Drugs and Crime; 2008.
6. Anthony JC. The epidemiology of cannabis dependence. In: Roffman RA, Stephens RS, eds. *Cannabis Dependence: Its Nature, Consequences and Treatment*. Cambridge, UK: Cambridge University Press; 2006:58–95.
7. SAMHSA. *Treatment Episode Data Set (TEDS) 1995–2007: National Admissions to Substance Abuse Treatment Services*. Rockville, MD: US Department of Health and Human Services; 2008.
8. Stinson FS, Ruan WJ, Pickering R, et al. Cannabis use disorders in the USA: prevalence, correlates and co-morbidity. *Psychol Med*. 2006;36:1447–1460.
9. Compton WM, Grant BF, Colliver JD, et al. Prevalence of marijuana use disorders in the United States: 1991–1992 and 2001–2002. *JAMA*. 2004;291:2114–2121.
10. SAMHSA. *Treatment Episode Data Set*. 2009. Available at: http://www.oas.samhsa.gov/2k2/TEDS/TEDS.cfm.
11. Jones RT. Cardiovascular system effects of marijuana. *J Clin Pharmacol*. 2002;42:58S–63S.
12. Vandrey R, Mintzer MZ. Performance and cognitive alterations. In: Cohen L, Collins FL, Young AM, et al., eds. *The Pharmacology and Treatment of Substance Abuse: An Evidence-based Approach*. Mahwah, NJ: Lawrence Erlbaum Associates, Inc.; 2009: 41–62.
13. Solowij N, Stephens RS, Roffman RA, et al. Cognitive functioning of long-term heavy cannabis users seeking treatment. *JAMA*. 2002;287:1123–1131.
14. Kalant H. Adverse effects of cannabis on health: an update of the literature since 1996. *Prog Neuropsychopharmacol Biol Psychiatry*. 2004;28:849–863.
15. Jones RT, Benowitz NL, Herning RI. Clinical relevance of cannabis tolerance and dependence. *J Clin Pharmacol*. 1981; 21:143S–152S.
16. Budney AJ, Hughes JR, Moore BA, et al. A review of the validity and significance of the cannabis withdrawal syndrome. *Am J Psychiatry*. 2004;161:1967–1977.
17. Huestis MA. Human cannabinoid pharmacokinetics. *Chem Biodivers*. 2007;4:1770–1804.
18. Howlett AC, Breivogel CS, Childers SR, et al. Cannabinoid physiology and pharmacology: 30 years of progress. *Neuropharmacology*. 2004;47:345–358.
19. Gardner EL. Endocannabinoid signaling system and brain reward: emphasis on dopamine. *Pharmacol Biochem Behav*. 2005;81:263–284.
20. Beardsley PM, Thomas BF, McMahon LR. Cannabinoid CB1 receptor antagonists as potential pharmacotherapies for drug abuse disorders. *Int Rev Psychiatry*. 2009;21:134–142.
21. Corchero J, Oliva JM, Garcia-Lecumberri C, et al. Repeated administration with delta9-tetrahydrocannabinol regulates mu-opioid receptor density in the rat brain. *J Psychopharmacol*. 2004;18:54–58.
22. Agrawal A, Lynskey MT. Candidate genes for cannabis use disorders: findings, challenges and directions. *Addiction*. 2009; 104:518–532.
23. Johnston LD, O'Malley PM, Bachman JG, et al. *Monitoring the Future National Results on Adolescent Drug Use*. 2009. Available at: http://www.monitoringthefuture.org/pubs.html.
24. Brook JS, Brook DW, Arencibia-Mireles O, et al. Risk factors for adolescent marijuana use across cultures and across time. *J Genet Psychol*. 2001;162:357–374.
25. von Sydow K, Lieb R, Pfister H, et al. What predicts incident use of cannabis and progression to abuse and dependence? A 4-year prospective examination of risk factors in a community sample of adolescents and young adults. *Drug Alcohol Depend*. 2002; 68:49–64.
26. Budney AJ. Are specific dependence criteria necessary for different substances: how can research on cannabis inform this issue? *Addiction*. 2006;101:125–133.
27. Budney AJ, Hughes JR. The cannabis withdrawal syndrome. *Curr Opin Psychiatry*. 2006;19:233–238.
28. Annaheim B, Rehm J, Gmel G. How to screen for problematic cannabis use in population surveys: an evaluation of the

28. Cannabis Use Disorders Identification Test (CUDIT) in a Swiss sample of adolescents and young adults. *Eur Addict Res.* 2008;14:190–197.
29. Copeland J, Gilmour S, Gates P, et al. The Cannabis Problems Questionnaire: factor structure, reliability, and validity. *Drug Alcohol Depend.* 2005;80:313–319.
30. Martin G, Copeland J, Gilmour S, et al. The Adolescent Cannabis Problems Questionnaire (CPQ-A): psychometric properties. *Addict Behav.* 2006;31:2238–2248.
31. Alexander D, Leung P. The Marijuana Screening Inventory (MSI-X): concurrent, convergent and discriminant validity with multiple measures. *Am J Drug Alcohol Abuse.* 2006;32:351–378.
32. Miele GM, Carpenter KM, Smith Cockerham M, et al. Substance Dependence Severity Scale (SDSS): reliability and validity of a clinician-administered interview for DSM-IV substance use disorders. *Drug Alcohol Depend.* 2000;59:63–75.
33. Marijuana Treatment Project Research Group. Brief treatments for cannabis dependence: findings from a randomized multisite trial. *J Consult Clin Psychol.* 2004;72:455–466.
34. Cary PL. The marijuana detection window: determining the length of time cannabinoids will remain detectable in urine following smoking. A critical review of relevant research and cannabinoid detection guidance for drug courts. *Drug Court Practitioner Fact Sheet.* 2006;IV:1–16.
35. Budney AJ, Higgins ST. *A Community Reinforcement Plus Vouchers Approach: Treating Cocaine Addiction.* Bethesda, MD: National Institute on Drug Abuse; 1998.
36. Budney AJ, Roffman R, Stephens RS, et al. Marijuana dependence and its treatment. *Addict Sci Clin Pract.* 2007;4:4–16.
37. Stephens RS, Roffman RA. *Marijuana Dependence Treatment PRN.* Orlando, FL: College of Problems of Drug Dependence; 2005.
38. Budney AJ, Higgins ST, Radonovich KJ, et al. Adding voucher-based incentives to coping-skills and motivational enhancement improves outcomes during treatment for marijuana dependence. *J Consult Clin Psychol.* 2000;68:1051–1061.
39. Budney AJ, Moore BA, Rocha HL, et al. Clinical trial of abstinence-based vouchers and cognitive-behavioral therapy for cannabis dependence. *J Consult Clin Psychol.* 2006;74:307–316.
40. Kadden RM, Litt MD, Kabela-Cormier E, et al. Abstinence rates following behavioral treatments for marijuana dependence. *Addict Behav.* 2007;32:1220–1236.
41. Sinha R, Easton C, Renee-Aubin L, et al. Engaging young probation-referred marijuana-abusing individuals in treatment: a pilot trial. *Am J Addict.* 2003;12:314–323.
42. Carroll KM, Easton CJ, Nich C, et al. The use of contingency management and motivational/skills-building therapy to treat young adults with marijuana dependence. *J Consult Clin Psychol.* 2006;74:955–966.
43. Waldron HB, Turner CW. Evidence-based psychosocial treatments for adolescent substance abuse. *J Clin Child Adolesc Psychol.* 2008;37:238–261.
44. Waldron HB, Slesnick N, Brody JL, et al. Treatment outcomes for adolescent substance abuse at 4- and 7-month assessments. *J Consult Clin Psychol.* 2001;69:802–813.
45. Liddle HA, Dakof GA, Parker K, et al. Multidimensional family therapy for adolescent drug abuse: results of a randomized clinical trial. *Am J Drug Alcohol Abuse.* 2001;27:651–688.
46. Henggeler SW, Halliday-Boykins CA, Cunningham PB, et al. Juvenile drug court: enhancing outcomes by integrating evidence-based treatments. *J Consult Clin Psychol.* 2006;74:42–54.
47. Szapocznik J, Kurtines WM, Foote FH, et al. Conjoint versus one-person family therapy: some evidence for the effectiveness of conducting family therapy through one person. *J Consult Clin Psychol.* 1983;51:889–899.
48. Dennis M, Godley SH, Diamond G, et al. The cannabis youth treatment (CYT) study: main findings from two randomized trials. *J Subst Abuse Treat.* 2004;27:197–213.
49. Azrin NH, Donohue B, Besalel VA, et al. Youth drug abuse treatment: a controlled outcome study. *J Child Adolesc Subst Abuse.* 1994;3:1–16.
50. Stanger C, Budney AJ, Kamon J, et al. A randomized trial of contingency management for adolescent marijuana abuse and dependence. *Drug Alcohol Depend.*, 2009;105:240–247.
51. Godley MD, Godley SH, Dennis ML, et al. The effect of assertive continuing care on continuing care linkage, adherence and abstinence following residential treatment for adolescents with substance use disorders. *Addiction.* 2007;102:81–93.
52. Stephens RS, Roffman RA, Fearer SA, et al. The marijuana check-up: promoting change in ambivalent marijuana users. *Addiction.* 2007;102:947–957.
53. Walker DD, Roffman RA, Stephens RS, et al. Motivational enhancement therapy for adolescent marijuana users: a preliminary randomized controlled trial. *J Consult Clin Psychol.* 2006;74:628–632.
54. Winters KC, Leitten W. Brief intervention for drug-abusing adolescents in a school setting. *Psychol Addict Behav.* 2007;21:249–254.
55. Martin G, Copeland J. The adolescent cannabis check-up: randomized trial of a brief intervention for young cannabis users. *J Subst Abuse Treat.* 2008;34:407–414.
56. Haney M, Ward AS, Comer SD, et al. Bupropion SR worsens mood during marijuana withdrawal in humans. *Psychopharmacology (Berl).* 2001;155:171–179.
57. Haney M, Hart CL, Vosburg SK, et al. Marijuana withdrawal in humans: effects of oral THC or divalproex. *Neuropsychopharmacology.* 2004;29:158–170.
58. Haney M, Hart CL, Ward AS, et al. Nefazodone decreases anxiety during marijuana withdrawal in humans. *Psychopharmacology (Berl).* 2003;165:157–165.
59. Cone EJ, Welch P, Lange WR. Clonidine partially blocks the physiologic effects but not the subjective effects produced by smoking marijuana in male human subjects. *Pharmacol Biochem Behav.* 1988;29:649–652.
60. Haney M. Opioid antagonism of cannabinoid effects: differences between marijuana smokers and nonmarijuana smokers. *Neuropsychopharmacology.* 2007;32:1391–1403.
61. Haney M, Hart CL, Vosburg SK, et al. Effects of THC and lofexidine in a human laboratory model of marijuana withdrawal and relapse. *Psychopharmacology (Berl).* 2008;197:157–168.
62. Budney AJ, Vandrey RG, Hughes JR, et al. Oral delta-9-tetrahydrocannabinol suppresses cannabis withdrawal symptoms. *Drug Alcohol Depend.* 2007;86:22–29.
63. Huestis MA, Gorelick DA, Heishman SJ, et al. Blockade of effects of smoked marijuana by the CB1-sective cannabinoid receptor antagonist SR141716. *Arch Gen Psychiatry.* 2001;58:322–328.
64. Huestis MA, Boyd SJ, Heishman SJ, et al. Single and multiple doses of rimonabant antagonize acute effects of smoked cannabis in male cannabis users. *Psychopharmacology (Berl).* 2007;194:505–515.
65. Vandrey R, McCann U, Smith M, et al. *Sleep dysfunction during cannabis withdrawal.* Paper presented at the College on Problems of Drug Dependence, Reno, NV; June 2009.

66. Levin FR, McDowell D, Evans SM, et al. Pharmacotherapy for marijuana dependence: a double-blind, placebo-controlled pilot study of divalproex sodium. *Am J Addict.* 2004;13:21–32.
67. Carpenter KM, McDowell D, Brooks DJ, et al. A preliminary trial: double-blind comparison of nefazodone, bupropion-SR, and placebo in the treatment of cannabis dependence. *Am J Addict.* 2009;18:53–64.
68. McRae-Clark AL, Carter RE, Killeen TK, et al. A placebo-controlled trial of buspirone for the treatment of marijuana dependence. *Drug Alcohol Depend.*, 2009;105:132–138.
69. Levin FR, Kleber HD. Use of dronabinol for cannabis dependence: two case reports and review. *Am J Addict.* 2008;17:161–164.
70. Clapper JR, Mangieri RA, Piomelli D. The endocannabinoid system as a target for the treatment of cannabis dependence. *Neuropharmacology.* 2009;56(suppl 1):235–243.
71. Stephens RS, Roffman RA, Simpson EE. Adult marijuana users seeking treatment. *J Consult Clin Psychol.* 1993;61:1100–1104.
72. Budney AJ, Bickel WK, Amass L. Marijuana use and treatment outcome among opioid-dependent patients. *Addiction.* 1998;93:493–503.
73. Lynskey MT, Vink JM, Boomsma DI. Early onset cannabis use and progression to other drug use in a sample of Dutch twins. *Behav Genet.* 2006;36:195–200.
74. Kamon JL, Stanger C, Budney AJ. Relations between parent and adolescent problems among adolescents presenting for family-based marijuana abuse treatment. 2006;85:244–255.
75. Koskinen J, Lohonen J, Koponen H, et al. Rate of cannabis use disorders in clinical samples of patients with schizophrenia: a meta-analysis. *Schizophr Bull.* 2009.
76. Johns A. Psychiatric effects of cannabis. *Br J Psychiatry.* 2001;178:116–122.
77. Hall W, Degenhardt L. Cannabis use and the risk of developing a psychotic disorder. *World Psychiatry.* 2008;7:68–71.
78. Fergusson DM, Poulton R, Smith PF, et al. Cannabis and psychosis. *BMJ.* 2006;332:172–175.
79. Krueger RF, Markon KE, Patrick CJ, et al. Linking antisocial behavior, substance use, and personality: an integrative quantitative model of the adult externalizing spectrum. *J Abnorm Psychol.* 2007;116:645–666.
80. Sewell RA, Ranganathan M, D'Souza DC. Cannabinoids and psychosis. *Int Rev Psychiatry.* 2009;21:152–162.
81. Taylor DR, Fergusson DM, Milne BJ, et al. A longitudinal study of the effects of tobacco and cannabis exposure on lung function in young adults. *Addiction.* 2002;97(8):1055–1061.
82. Tashkin DP, Baldwin GC, Sarafian T, et al. Respiratory and immunologic consequences of marijuana smoking. *J Clin Pharmacol.* 2002;42:71S–81S.
83. Mechoulam R, Peters M, Murillo-Rodriguez E, et al. Cannabidiol—recent advances. *Chem Biodivers.* 2007;4:1678–1692.
84. Hashibe M, Straif K, Tashkin DP, et al. Epidemiologic review of marijuana use and cancer risk. *Alcohol.* 2005;35:265–275.
85. Berthiller J, Lee YC, Boffetta P, et al. Marijuana smoking and the risk of head and neck cancer: pooled analysis in the INHANCE consortium. *Cancer Epidemiol Biomarkers Prev.* 2009;18:1544–1551.
86. Verweij PE, Kerremans JJ, Voss A, et al. *Fungal Contamination of Tobacco and Marijuana* [Research Letter]. *JAMA.* 2000;284(22). December 13, 2000. Available at: http://jama.ama-assn.org/issues/current/ffull/jlt1213-8.html.
87. O'Connell CM, Fried PA. An investigation of prenatal cannabis exposure and minor physical anomalies in a low risk population. *Neurotoxicol Teratol.* 1984;6:345–350.
88. Day N, Richardson GA. *Prenatal Marijuana Use: Epidemiology, Methodological Issues and Infant Outcome.* Philadelphia: W.B. Saunders; 1991.
89. Fried P, Watkinson B, Gray R. Differential effects on cognitive functioning in 13- to 16-year olds prenatally exposed to cigarettes and marihuana. *Neurotoxicol Teratol.* 2003;25:427–436.
90. Day N, Richardson GA, Goldschmidt L, et al. The effect of prenatal exposure on the cognitive development of offspring at age three. *Neurotoxicol Teratol.* 1994;16:169–176.
91. Richardson GA, Ryan C, Willford J, et al. Prenatal alcohol and marijuana exposure: effects on neuropsychological outcomes at 10 years. *Neurotoxicol Teratol.* 2002;24:309–320.
92. Jones RT, Benowitz N. The 30-day trip: clinical studies of cannabis tolerance and dependence. In: Braude MC, Szara S, eds. *Pharmacology of Marihuana.* New York: Raven Press; 1976:627–642.
93. Grant I, Gonzalez R, Carey CL, et al. Non-acute (residual) neurocognitive effects of cannabis use: a meta-analytic study. *J Int Neuropsychol Soc.* 2003;9:679–689.
94. Chang L, Chronicle EP. Functional imaging studies in cannabis users *Neuroscientist.* 2007;13:422–432.
95. Martin-Santos R, Fagundo AB, Crippa JA, et al. Neuroimaging in cannabis use: a systematic review of the literature. *Psychol Med.* 2010;40:383–398.
96. Jacobus J, Bava S, Cohen-Zion M, et al. Functional consequences of marijuana use in adolescents. *Pharmacol Biochem Behav.* 2009;92:559–565.
97. Budney AJ, Vandrey RG, Hughes JR, et al. Comparison of cannabis and tobacco withdrawal: severity and contribution to relapse. *J Subst Abuse Treat.* 2008;35:362–368.
98. Ramaekers JG, Moeller MR, van Ruitenbeek P, et al. Cognition and motor control as a function of delta9-THC concentration in serum and oral fluid: limits of impairment. *Drug Alcohol Depend.* 2006;85:114–122.
99. Weinstein A, Brickner O, Lerman H, et al. A study investigating the acute dose–response effects of 13 mg and 17 mg delta 9-tetrahydrocannabinol on cognitive-motor skills, subjective and autonomic measures in regular users of marijuana. *J Psychopharmacol.* 2008;22:441–451.
100. Ramaekers JG, Kauert G, Theunissen EL, et al. Neurocognitive performance during acute THC intoxication in heavy and occasional cannabis users. *J Psychopharmacol.* 2009;23:266–277.
101. Lane SD, Cherek DR, Lieving LM, et al. Marijuana effects on human forgetting functions. *J Exp Anal Behav.* 2005;83:67–83.
102. Solowij N. Long-term effects of cannabis on the central nervous system. In: Kalant H, Corrigall WA, Hall W, et al., eds. *The Health Effects of Cannabis.* Toronto: Centre for Addictions and Mental Health; 1999:195–266.
103. Lane SD, Cherek DR, Tcheremissine OV, et al. Response perseveration and adaptation in heavy marijuana-smoking adolescents. *Addict Behav.* 2007;32:977–990.
104. Pope HG, Jr., Gruber AJ, Hudson JI, et al. Early-onset cannabis use and cognitive deficits: what is the nature of the association? *Drug Alcohol Depend.* 2003;69:303–310.
105. Whitlow CT, Liguori A, Livengood LB, et al. Long-term heavy marijuana users make costly decisions on a gambling task. *Drug Alcohol Depend.* 2004;76:107–111.
106. Bolla KI, Brown K, Eldreth D, et al. Dose-related neurocognitive effects of marijuana use. *Neurology.* 2002;59:1337–1343.
107. Pope HG, Jr., Gruber AJ, Yurgelun-Todd D. Residual neuropsychologic effects of cannabis. *Curr Psychiatry Rep.* 2001;3:507–512.

108. Fergusson DM, Horwood LJ, Boden JM. Is driving under the influence of cannabis becoming a greater risk to driver safety than drink driving? Findings from a longitudinal study. *Accid Anal Prev.* 2008;40:1345–1350.
109. Ramaekers JG, Berghaus G, van Laar M, et al. Dose related risk of motor vehicle crashes after cannabis use. *Drug Alcohol Depend.* 2004;73:109–119.
110. Sewell RA, Poling J, Sofuoglu M. The effect of cannabis compared with alcohol on driving. *Am J Addict.* 2009;18:185–193.
111. Lynskey M, Hall W. The effects of adolescent cannabis use on educational attainment: a review. *Addiction.* 2000;95:1621–1630.
112. Hall W, Degenhardt L. Prevalence and correlates of cannabis use in developed and developing countries. *Curr Opin Psychiatry.* 2007;20:393–397.
113. Fergusson DM, Horwood LJ, Beautrais AL. Cannabis and educational achievement. *Addiction.* 2003;98:1681–1692.
114. Lane SD, Cherek DR, Pietras CJ, et al. Performance of heavy marijuana-smoking adolescents on a laboratory measure of motivation. *Addict Behav.* 2005;30:815–828.
115. Cherek DR, Lane SD, Dougherty DM. Possible amotivational effects following marijuana smoking under laboratory conditions. *Exp Clin Psychopharmacol.* 2002;10:26–38.
116. Joy JE, Watson SJ, Benson JA. (Eds.) *Marijuana and Medicine; Assessing the Science Base.* Washington, DC: National Academy Press; 1999.

CHAPTER 16
Amphetamines and Other Stimulants

Kevin P. Hill ■ Roger D. Weiss

The number of Americans meeting *Diagnostic and Statistical Manual of Mental Disorders, 4th Edition* (*DSM-IV*) criteria for amphetamine abuse and dependence has increased substantially in recent years due to the popularity of methamphetamine, a derivative of amphetamine made from readily accessible chemicals. Communities across the United States are working to prevent additional growth in methamphetamine use while trying to treat those already dependent on the drug.

In this chapter, we review the use and abuse of amphetamines. Amphetamines may be used as medications or as drugs of abuse. First, we will review the history of amphetamine use and its importance to particular population groups who have viewed amphetamines as performance-enhancing agents. Next, we will explore the epidemiology of amphetamine use in the United States and abroad while discussing the public health implications of amphetamine dependence. We then discuss the pharmacology of amphetamines, from the literature on preclinical studies that suggest future clinical treatment targets for amphetamine dependence to the physiology of these drugs that makes them appealing yet potentially harmful to users, to current clinical indications for amphetamines as medications. A significant portion of the chapter is devoted to the treatment of those with amphetamine dependence. We review the evidence addressing the effectiveness of popular behavioral interventions as treatments for amphetamine dependence. We then cover the array of medications that have been studied as treatments for amphetamine dependence. A discussion of pharmacogenetics as a new tool that may improve the effectiveness of treatments for amphetamine dependence follows. Finally, we summarize our findings and look to the future of amphetamines and treatment of amphetamine dependence.

HISTORY OF AMPHETAMINES

Stimulants have been used as medications for thousands of years. Ma-huang, or ephedra, is a stimulant that has been used as a herbal remedy in Chinese medicine for the past 5000 years (1). In 1887, Nagayoshi Nagai determined that the active agent in Ma-Huang was ephedrine. That same year in Berlin, amphetamine was synthesized by Lazar Edeleanu (2). Amphetamines' actions on the central nervous system (CNS)—euphoria, heightened alertness, increased energy, and intensified emotions—were described in 1933, when an amphetamine inhaler was marketed as a decongestant (3). Feelings of euphoria, improved performance, and anorexia were key factors in the reports of abuse that soon followed; these effects continue to be important reasons for the widespread abuse of stimulants today.

Amphetamine abuse peaked in the United States in the late 1960s. Stimulant pills were readily accessible; at that time, far more stimulant pills were manufactured than were prescribed. The U.S. government shifted its philosophy in response to this oversupply. From 1969 to 1971, the government oversaw an 80% reduction in production of amphetamines, alerted physicians to the addictive potential of these agents, and reclassified amphetamines as Schedule II drugs through the Food and Drug Administration, in order to closely monitor their distribution (2). Since amphetamines became Schedule II drugs, physicians have been more cautious about their clinical use.

Amphetamine-type stimulants (ATS) fall into three main groups: amphetamine, methamphetamine, and methylphenidate (Table 16.1). Amphetamine formulations are often prescribed for attention-deficit hyperactivity disorder (ADHD) but have high abuse potential because of their powerful effects. Methamphetamine can be synthesized from readily available chemical components and is the most commonly abused ATS. Methylphenidate formulations are the most commonly prescribed ADHD medications, although, like amphetamine formulations, they are sometimes misused, usually by those for whom they are prescribed. When misused, ATS are highly addictive; amphetamine-dependent individuals require increasing amounts of amphetamine to achieve the desired effect, they are often unable to stop using on their own, and consequences result in multiple spheres of their lives including their relationships and work.

While there have been surges in amphetamine use in general, the appeal of amphetamines has remained consistent among three groups: the military, athletes, and students. Amphetamines appeal to these groups primarily because of the increased energy and improved performance associated with amphetamine use. Amphetamines have been used by members of the military since World War II to enhance alertness and to combat fatigue. After amphetamines were distributed by the United States and Great Britain to its military and the German and Japanese military supplied methamphetamine during World War II, use by military forces continued to grow (4).

TABLE 16.1 Common types of stimulants

Stimulant	Street names	Form	Route of administration	Duration of action	Detection	Common false positives
Amphetamine (dexedrine, adderall)	Speed, uppers, bennies, black beauties	Tablets, capsules	Snorted, swallowed	4 to 12 hours	Urine: 1 to 3 days Blood: 12 hours Hair: ≤90 days	Cold medications containing pseudoephedrine, phenylpropanolamine, phenylephrine; herbal supplements containing ephedra
Methamphetamine (desoxyn)	Chalk, crank, glass, ice, meth	Tablets, powder, crystals	Swallowed, smoked, snorted, injected	8 to 12 hours	Urine: 3 to 5 days Blood: 1 to 3 days Hair: ≤90 days	Same as amphetamine
Methylphenidate (Ritalin, Concerta)	MPH, r-ball, vitamin R	Tablets, capsules	Swallowed, snorted, injected	2 to 12 hours	Urine: 1 to 3 days Blood: 12 hours Hair: ≤90 days	Not common as methylphenidate; requires a specific test

Bower and Phelan (5) characterized the effects of amphetamines on military performance into two categories: performance enhancement and performance maintenance. Performance enhancement occurs when amphetamines are thought to improve one's maximum performance level for a given task. Performance maintenance is the use of amphetamines to restore skills that may have degraded as a result of sleep deprivation or normal circadian rhythm–associated decrements. Military units and pilots who work long hours with little sleep have relied on amphetamines to perform at a high level without fulfilling their biological sleep requirements. Because of concerns about side effects of amphetamines such as hypertension and tachycardia as well as adverse reactions including paranoia, military forces are evaluating nonamphetamine stimulant drugs such as modafinil as possible alternatives to amphetamines in combat settings (6).

Athletes have used amphetamines to improve performance for many years, dating back in the United States to the 1940s for football and the 1950s for other sports (7). An early study by Smith and Beecher (8) showed that administration of amphetamine improved the performance of college swimmers when they were fatigued. While these findings were not supported by other studies, athletes often are willing to pay more attention to positive rather than negative results when considering risks and benefits, especially if they believe that they will gain a competitive advantage by using amphetamines. Thus, although evidence supporting positive effects of amphetamine or naturally occurring ephedra alkaloids on athletic performance is equivocal, ATS continue to be used because of their perceived positive effects on attention, energy, self-confidence, mood, and aggression (9).

Amphetamines have been used by athletes in a variety of sports, from contests requiring speed and power to those requiring prolonged concentration. In the 1960s and 1970s, amphetamine use in professional football and baseball was noted to be rampant (10). Deaths of athletes have been attributed to amphetamine misuse by (1) an increase in blood pressure caused by increased exercise and peripheral vasoconstriction that hampers the body's ability to cool itself, leading to heatstroke, and (2) cardiac arrest (11). Amphetamines may mask the warning signs of fatigue that usually result in athletes' decreasing their effort; as a result, injury may occur. Adverse events resulting from amphetamine use led to its presence on the first list of substances banned by the International Olympic Committee in 1968 (12). As with the military, athletes use nonamphetamine drugs with stimulant properties like modafinil and adrafinil in an attempt to receive the perceived competitive advantage received from taking stimulants; this can unfortunately be accompanied by the hypertension and tachycardia that result from amphetamines (9,13). Increased use of modafinil and adrafinil by athletes has led to its ban by the World Anti-Doping Agency as a performance-enhancing drug (14).

Students and professionals also use amphetamines to increase productivity. Many students believe that amphetamines and other stimulants improve concentration, increase alertness, and assist with studying (15). Prescription amphetamine and methylphenidate formulations are commonly misused by this group. The National Survey on Drug Use and Health

(2009) demonstrated that full-time college students aged 18 to 22 were twice as likely as their age-matched counterparts who were not full-time college students to abuse amphetamines (16). Students report improved academic performance stemming from an ability to work at a high level for an extended period of time (17). Along with risk for developing dependence on these stimulants, students who use these medications in an attempt to improve performance report higher rates of binge alcohol consumption, cannabis use, and cocaine use (18). Students or professionals who use amphetamines and other stimulants in this context also are at increased risk for heart attack and stroke (19). In an effort to identify potentially safer alternative medications with more favorable side-effect profiles, these population groups have also used stimulant-like medications such as modafinil to prolong alertness and reduce their need for sleep. Interestingly, despite increased use and abuse of modafinil in such settings, Randall et al. (20) demonstrated that modafinil has limited effect on mood, bodily symptoms, or cognitive performance in individuals without sleep disorders.

EPIDEMIOLOGY OF AMPHETAMINES: SCOPE OF THE PROBLEM

Amphetamine misuse remains an enormous problem worldwide. The United Nations Office on Drugs and Crime (UNODC) *World Drug Report 2009* estimates that as many as 51 million people around the world regularly use amphetamines, in comparison to approximately 21 million users each of cocaine and opioids (21). Methamphetamine is the most widely available and most commonly misused type of amphetamine; the UNODC estimates that methamphetamine users comprise 54% to 59% of amphetamine users globally. The UNODC estimated that between 230 and 640 metric ton of ATS was manufactured in 2007. The spread of illicit manufacture to new countries each year suggests that amphetamine use disorders (AUDs) will remain a problem in the coming years. Different use patterns of ATS are evident in different regions of the world. Smart and Osborne (22) compared drug use in 36 countries and found that, after cannabis, ATS are the illicit drugs most likely to be used by high-school students, suggesting that amphetamine misuse will remain a concern in the coming decades.

Diversion of prescribed amphetamines is a concern. While the prevalence of AUDs has remained steady globally, amphetamine consumption and prescription rates are increasing at a proportion that suggests that diversion may be occurring. Consumption estimates in the United States from 1995 to 2006 by the World Health Organization (WHO) and prescription rates during the same time period have both increased linearly (23). The WHO estimates that consumption of amphetamines has more than tripled, from approximately 5 to 18 daily doses per 1000 persons. The number of prescriptions per year, in contrast, has only doubled, from 15 to 30 million. The larger increase in consumption in comparison to number of prescriptions suggests that prescribed amphetamines may be diverted to meet the consumption demand.

Methamphetamine dependence remains an important problem in the United States in particular. Most of the reported methamphetamine production operations globally occur within the United States, with the United States accounting for 82% of the methamphetamine laboratories seized in 2007 (21). Methamphetamine production laboratories are increasing in size, sophistication, and production yields, as organized crime groups see methamphetamine as a source of income (21). While methamphetamine use was focused primarily in the western part of the United States in the early 1990s, the problem has spread across the country in the past 15 years (24). As a result, the United States has enacted several policies aimed at suppressing production of methamphetamine by restricting access to precursor chemicals. Policies have targeted precursor chemicals in forms used by those producing methamphetamine on both large and small scales. Regulations affecting large-scale producers of methamphetamine, such as improved monitoring of bulk purchases of ephedrine and pseudoephedrine, have been beneficial by contributing to a reduction in purity of methamphetamine available in the United States (25). Policies designed to combat small-scale methamphetamine production, however, such as the limitation and tracking of pharmacy purchases of ephedrine and pseudoephedrine, have had little or no effect (25).

The prevalence of methamphetamine use has remained relatively constant since 2002, with 1.3 million Americans using methamphetamine in 2007. However, severity of use is increasing (26); the number of methamphetamine users in the past month meeting criteria for drug abuse or dependence during the past year more than doubled from 27.5% in 2002 to 59.3% in 2004 (27). Similarly, methamphetamine users progress more quickly than cocaine users from first use to regular use to entrance into substance use disorder treatment (28). In the United States, emergency room visit diagnoses mentioning amphetamine or methamphetamine increased 54% between 1995 and 2002 (29). Despite efforts to reduce access to the chemical precursors of methamphetamine, it is likely methamphetamine will remain accessible and inexpensive, and public health costs associated with increased use will continue to rise (30).

AUDs are associated with other psychiatric disorders. Those who use methamphetamine chronically are more likely to experience psychiatric symptoms including drug-induced psychotic symptoms that may persist over time (31). Zweben et al. (32) found that 27% of treatment-seeking methamphetamine users reported a previous suicide attempt, and 43% reported violent behavior problems. Those who misuse stimulants are more likely to misuse other illicit drugs as well. Wu et al. (33) showed that the lifetime prevalence of cocaine/crack and heroin use in a representative sample of youths and young adults aged 16 to 25 who regularly use amphetamines was several times higher than the prevalence in the general population.

Psychosis resulting from amphetamine use is similar to psychoses resulting from cocaine use or other psychotic disorders such as schizophrenia. McKetin et al. (34) found that 13% of 309 Australians actively using amphetamines screened positive for acute psychosis. Acute amphetamine psychosis is difficult to distinguish from acute schizophrenia (35), with hallucinations, ideas of reference, paranoia, and agitation (36,37). Amphetamine-induced psychoses usually resolve quickly with removal of the amphetamine, while psychotic symptoms resulting from schizophrenia do not. Amphetamine psychoses may be chronic, though, with some individuals experiencing persistent psychotic symptoms even after removal of amphetamine. Others have recurrence of the psychotic state with even minimal re-exposure to amphetamine. Psychotic symptoms resulting from amphetamines are treated with antipsychotic medications just like psychotic symptoms of other etiologies (38).

AUDs have significant public health effects as well. Clandestine in-home methamphetamine laboratories have resulted in environmental costs as well as increased pediatric deaths and emergency room visits from burns and poisoning (39,40). Fetal exposure to methamphetamine leads to multiple prenatal complications (41). Methamphetamine use has also been associated with higher rates of hepatitis C and HIV (42,43). AUDs are associated with criminal justice costs as well. Cartier et al. (44) demonstrated that methamphetamine use is highly predictive of violent criminal behavior and recidivism among parolees; 82% of methamphetamine uses returned to custody with 12 months, as opposed to 54% of nonusers.

DETERMINANTS OF USE

Pharmacology

Amphetamines activate the CNS, by increasing synaptic concentrations of the monoamines dopamine (DA), serotonin (5-hydroxytryptamine [5-HT]), and norepinephrine (NE) (45,46). ATS are known as "releasers" because they bind to transporter proteins and increase monoamine levels by a transporter-mediated exchange or the disruption of neurotransmitter storage in vesicles via vesicular monoamine transporter (VMAT)-2 (45,47). The rapid efflux of intravesicular monoamines results in high concentrations of cytosolic monoamines. High levels of intracellular monoamines reverse monoamines in the cell membrane, ultimately causing a movement of monoamines into the extracellular space.

Considerable evidence suggests that the mesocorticolimbic dopaminergic system mediates the rewarding effects of amphetamines (48–50). This system, which originates from the ventral tegmental area (VTA) of the midbrain and targets a number of limbic and cortical structures, including the nucleus accumbens, amygdale, and prefrontal cortex, has been shown to play an essential role in stimulant reward (50). The noradrenergic system helps to mediate the cardiovascular effects of amphetamines, and mounting evidence also suggests that the noradrenergic system is critical in mediating amphetamine's rewarding effects in preclinical models of addiction (51). The noradrenergic system, together with the dopaminergic system, may also contribute to withdrawal symptoms that occur with stimulant discontinuation (52,53).

Changes in mood associated with stimulants result in part from activation of the serotonergic system, but 5-HT may also play a role in modulating the rewarding effects of stimulants through its impact on the DA system (54).

Preclinical Target Systems

Extensive preclinical work has played an integral role in developing ATS as medications for the aforementioned indications. Researchers hope that ongoing preclinical work will identify additional clinical indications for ATS as treatments. In addition, several potential therapeutic target systems for the treatment of amphetamine dependence have been identified using preclinical models of drug dependence, including amphetamine self-administration, reinstatement of amphetamine use, and both behavioral and locomotor sensitization to amphetamines. We will provide a brief overview of relevant preclinical studies in the study of these target systems (Table 16.2).

Dopaminergic

The dopaminergic system plays a critical role in mediating the reinforcing effects of amphetamines. Both D_1- and D_2-like receptors have been proposed to mediate acute and chronic effects of stimulants. The D_1-like family of receptors, including the D_1 and D_5 receptors, stimulates cyclic AMP formation. The D_2-like family of receptors, including the D_2, D_3, and D_4 receptors, inhibits cyclic AMP formation. The D_2-like receptors also function as autoreceptors reducing DA release (55). As a result, agents modulating DA release have been studied in several behavioral models. Tyrosine, an amino acid precursor of both DA and NE, has been shown to decrease amphetamine self-administration in rats exposed to amphetamine for 4 to 6 months (56). The dopamine transporter (DAT) inhibitor GBR 12909 nearly eliminates the DA-releasing effects of methamphetamine in rats (57). Izzo et al. (58) studied terguride, a partial D_2 agonist, due to the variations in dopaminergic tone that result from the use of psychostimulants like amphetamine. In a progressive ratio schedule, terguride acted as a functional DA receptor antagonist, attenuating intravenous self-administration in rats in a similar fashion as the D_2 antagonist eticlopride. The D_3 receptor antagonist U99194 was shown to inhibit the development of locomotor sensitization to amphetamine (59). Finally, the D_1 agonist SKF-38393 reversed the stereotypy associated with behavioral sensitization (60). Behavioral sensitization, in which repeated exposure to amphetamine produces increasingly robust motor responses and stereotyped behavior, is thought to underlie drug craving and relapse (61).

GABAergic

Dopaminergic effects are modulated by gamma-aminobutyric acid (GABA) and glutamate, the main inhibitory and excitatory neurotransmitters in the brain. Dopaminergic activity is decreased by GABA and increased by glutamate, suggesting that alteration of either GABA or glutamate

TABLE 16.2　Preclinical investigations of potential treatments for amphetamine dependence

Drugs	Year	Authors	Effect on primary outcome
Dopaminergic			
■ Tyrosine	1986	Geis et al. (56)	Attenuated amphetamine self-administration
■ Terguride, eticlopride	2001	Izzo et al. (58)	Attenuated amphetamine self-administration in a progressive ratio schedule
■ D_3 receptor antagonist U99194A	2003	Chiang et al. (59)	Attenuated amphetamine-induced behavioral sensitization
■ D_1 receptor agonist SKF-38393	2007	Moro et al. (60)	Reversed stereotypy associated with behavioral sensitization
GABAergic			
■ Gamma-vinyl GABA	1999	Gerasimov et al. (71)	Attenuated methamphetamine-induced increases of dopamine
■ Baclofen	2002	Ranaldi and Poeggel (66)	Attenuated methamphetamine self-administration
■ Baclofen	2005	Brebner et al. (63)	Attenuated amphetamine self-administration
■ Baclofen	2005	Bartoletti et al. (69)	Attenuated amphetamine-induced behavioral sensitization
Glutamatergic			
■ Riluzole	2000	Itzhak and Martin (75)	Attenuated amphetamine-induced behavioral sensitization
■ Agonist LY379268	2005	Kim et al. (72)	Attenuated amphetamine self-administration
Adrenergic			
■ Prazosin	2003	Auclair et al. (83)	Attenuated amphetamine-induced behavioral sensitization if coadministered with $5-HT_{2A}$ antagonist SR46349B
■ Atipamezole	2005	Juhila et al. (85)	Attenuated amphetamine-induced behavioral sensitization
■ Timolol	2005	Colussi-Mas et al. (190)	Attenuated amphetamine-induced behavioral sensitization
Serotonergic			
■ Amitriptyline, imipramine	1980	Kokkinidis et al. (88)	Restored amphetamine-induced self-stimulation
■ Fluoxetine	1984	Leccesse and Lyness (86)	Attenuated amphetamine self-administration
Cannabinoid			
■ CB1 receptor antagonist SR14176A	2004	Anggadiredja et al. (93)	Attenuated reinstatement of drug-seeking behavior
■ CB1 receptor antagonist AM 251	2008	Thiemann et al. (94)	Attenuated amphetamine-induced behavioral sensitization
Acetylcholinergic			
■ Lobeline	2001	Harrod et al. (96)	Attenuated amphetamine self-administration
■ Mecamylamine	2004	Hiranita et al. (95)	Antagonized nicotine's attenuation of methamphetamine-seeking behavior
■ Nicotine Donepezil	2006	Hiranita et al. (188)	Attenuated reinstatement of drug-seeking behavior
Opioid			
■ Naltrexone	2004	Anggadiredja et al. (105)	Attenuated reinstatement of drug-seeking behavior
■ Naltrexone	2005	Chiu et al. (104)	Attenuated methamphetamine-induced behavioral sensitization
■ Naltrexone	2009	Haggkvist et al. (107)	Attenuated amphetamine self-administration
Nitrergic			
■ Minocycline	1993	Kofman et al. (113)	Attenuated amphetamine-induced psychomotor activity
■ 7-Nitroindazole	1997	Itzhak and Ali (108)	Attenuated methamphetamine-induced behavioral sensitization
Other			
■ N-Acetyl-L-cysteine	2004	Fukami et al. (189)	Attenuated methamphetamine-induced behavioral sensitization

transmission is a possible strategy in the development of a new medication for stimulant dependence (62,63). GABA effects are mediated through two types of GABA receptors: $GABA_A$ and $GABA_B$. $GABA_A$ receptors increase chloride influx and mediate the fast inhibitory responses to GABA. In contrast, $GABA_B$ receptors, found both pre- and postsynaptically, mediate the slow inhibitory response to GABA (64). Thus, both $GABA_A$ and $GABA_B$ receptors are potential treatment targets for new medications for stimulant dependence (63,65). Baclofen, a $GABA_B$ agonist, has been shown to produce a dose-dependent reduction in intravenous self-administration of both methamphetamine and D-amphetamine (66,67). Similarly, baclofen also attenuates the development of both conditioned place preference and behavioral sensitization following administration of D-amphetamine (68,69). The ability of 2-hydroxysaclofen, a $GABA_B$ antagonist, to reverse the effects of baclofen on the discriminative stimulus effects of D-amphetamine in the conditioned taste aversion procedure also supports a role for GABA in modulating the effects of stimulants (70). The irreversible GABA-transaminase inhibitor, gamma-vinyl GABA, which increases synaptic GABA levels, reduced metham-phetamine-induced increases of DA in the nucleus accumbens (71).

Glutamatergic

Glutamate acts on two varieties of highly specialized receptors: ionotropic and metabotropic receptors. *N*-Methyl-D-aspartate (NMDA), kainite, and alpha-amino-3-hydroxy-5-methylisoxazole-4-propionic acid (AMPA) receptors are called "ionotropic" receptors due to their action as ion channels. While ionotropic glutamate receptors are widespread and mediate fast synaptic transmission, metabotropic receptors are coupled to G-proteins and mediate the slow, neuromodulatory effects of glutamate. Pharmacological antagonism of glutamate transmission has been shown to block stimulant effects in preclinical paradigms of addiction. Glutamatergic drugs that act on the VTA block stimulant sensitization and reward (62). The metabotropic glutamate agonist LY379268 also prevented the enhanced self-administration associated with amphetamine sensitization (72). Consistent with these findings, riluzole, which decreases glutamate release, has been used in several preclinical paradigms to underscore the role of glutamate in amphetamine addiction. It blocks amphetamine-induced conditioned place preference, moderately attenuates amphetamine-induced locomotion, and attenuates the expression of amphetamine-induced behavioral sensitization (73–75). Although preclinical evidence for sensitization may outweigh research in humans currently, sensitization to amphetamine may be important clinically (76). Chronic amphetamine use may make it more difficult to maintain abstinence, increase the likelihood of amphetamine-induced psychosis, and worsen prognosis (77,78). These behavioral findings are supported by cellular studies demonstrating riluzole's effectiveness in blocking DA release in the striatum and other brain areas involved in dependence (79).

Adrenergic

Noradrenergic axons project widely throughout the brain and the noradrenergic system contributes to an array of psychological processes including affective regulation, learning, memory, sleep, and reinforcement, as well as physiological responses including regulation of heart rate and blood pressure (80). These functions are mediated by α- and β-adrenergic receptors and their subtypes (53,81). Multiple preclinical studies have demonstrated that adrenergic receptors are critical in development of amphetamine dependence. Drouin et al. (82) showed that pretreatment with the $α_1$-antagonist prazosin reduced the acute locomotor effects of D-amphetamine in rats, and concomitant administration of prazosin and the $5-HT_{2A}$ antagonist SR46349B produced a complete blockade of these effects along with the development of behavioral sensitization. The $α_{2A}$-antagonist atipamezole attenuated both locomotor hyperactivity and behavioral sensitization following D-amphetamine administration (83,84). Similarly, treatment with a β-antagonist timolol prevented the development of behavioral sensitization to amphetamines in rats (85). These studies suggest that α- and β-adrenergic antagonists may have promise as medications for amphetamine dependence.

Serotonergic

Neurons containing 5-HT project from the raphe nuclei to nigrostriatal and mesolimbic neurons containing DA, prompting study of the relationship of 5-HT to DA-mediated amphetamine effects. Multiple preclinical models have demonstrated the role of serotonergic neurons in amphetamine self-administration, indicating that 5-HT may attenuate the reinforcing effects of methamphetamine (54,86,87). Tricyclic antidepressants (TCAs), which affect monoamine reuptake and have anticholinergic activity as well, restore hypoactive intracranial self-stimulation in rats exposed to chronic amphetamine administration (88). Acute injection of fluoxetine, a selective serotonin reuptake inhibitor (SSRI), attenuates the self-administration of D-amphetamine in rats (86,87). Other studies have built upon these findings to investigate the relationship between serotonergic and noradrenergic systems. Salomon et al. (89) demonstrated that both the $α_1$-antagonist prazosin and the $5-HT_{2B}$ antagonist SR46349B attenuate the development of amphetamine-induced behavioral sensitization. Repeated administration of D-amphetamine produced a hyperactivity of NE and 5-HT neurons that was blocked by antagonist pretreatment, suggesting an uncoupling of NE and 5-HT that occurs with chronic amphetamine dependence administration. Recent studies also suggest that reduced serotonergic neurotransmission may contribute to amphetamine withdrawal states. In rats, the serotonin selective reuptake inhibitor paroxetine, combined with a $5-HT_{1A}$ antagonist, p-MPPI, attenuated the reward deficit associated with amphetamine withdrawal (90). These findings suggest that the serotonergic system, by modulating both amphetamine reinforcement and withdrawal, may prove to be a promising target for new treatments for amphetamine dependence.

Cannabinoid

Evidence linking the endocannabinoid system to the reward circuit has encouraged study of the effects of this system on amphetamine-induced behaviors (91). A link between the cannabinoid and dopaminergic systems is suggested by the induction of sensitization to amphetamine-induced hyperlocomotion by Δ^9-tetrahydrocannabinol, the psychoactive ingredient of marijuana (92). Similarly, the cannabinoid CB1 receptor antagonist SR14176A blocked the reinstatement of methamphetamine-seeking behavior induced by drug-priming and drug-associated cues (93). In this study, Δ^8-tetrahydrocannabinol attenuated methamphetamine-induced reinstatement. Another CB1 receptor antagonist, AM251, was shown to attenuate amphetamine-induced behavioral sensitization (94). These findings suggest that cannabinoid antagonists may be developed as potential medications for amphetamine dependence.

Acetylcholinergic

Nicotinic and muscarinic cholinergic receptor types mediate acetylcholinergic effects. While few studies have examined a possible role for cholinergic receptors in treatments for amphetamine dependence, some studies have yielded promising results. Hiranita et al. (95) showed that systemic nicotine and donepezil, an acetylcholinesterase inhibitor, attenuated the reinstatement of methamphetamine-seeking behavior. Additional experiments by this group using muscarinic and nicotinic antagonists indicated that donezepil's effects were mediated by the nicotinic, not muscarinic receptors (95). Lobeline, a nicotine agonist that decreases DA release via inhibition of VMAT-2, also attenuates intravenous self-administration in rats (96). Additionally, lobeline reduces the DA-releasing effects of methamphetamine, suggesting that lobeline has unique properties at the DAT and VMAT-2. These studies suggest that nicotinic receptors may be promising targets for the treatment of amphetamine addiction (97,98).

Opioid

Opioid and dopaminergic neurons interact in the VTA, substantia nigra, striatum, and limbic areas of the brain (99,100). In addition, the endogenous opioid release following acute administration of amphetamines suggests a functional connectivity between dopaminergic and the opioid system (101). This connectivity has been illustrated in multiple behavioral studies as well. The opioid antagonist naloxone attenuated the locomotor response to amphetamine as well as the corresponding increase in extracellular DA (102). Similarly, pretreatment with naloxone decreased methamphetamine-induced conditioned place preference (103). Chiu et al. (104) demonstrated that naltrexone, the nonselective opioid antagonist, attenuated methamphetamine-induced behavioral sensitization. Naltrexone also inhibited reinstatement of drug-seeking behavior by methamphetamine-associated cues (105). It is important to note, however, that naltrexone did not affect reinstatement induced by priming with methamphetamine in this study, and earlier work has already documented that naltrexone has no effect on methamphetamine self-administration (106). Another recent study, however, showed that naltrexone attenuated reinstatement of amphetamine self-administration (107).

Nitrergic

Nitric oxide (NO) is a lipid-soluble, short-lived second messenger that plays a role in diverse functions including learning and memory, neurotransmitter release, and cell death (108). NO serves as a second messenger for NMDA receptors and is released by neuronal nitric oxide synthase (nNOS) following NMDA-type glutamate receptor activation (109). Several studies have supported the role of NO in mediating the psychomotor sensitization and reinforcing effects of stimulants. Pretreatment with 7-nitroindazole, an NOS inhibitor previously shown to attenuate signs of opioid withdrawal, attenuated the development of methamphetamine-induced behavioral sensitization in mice (110–112). Acute minocycline treatment attenuated amphetamine-induced psychomotor activity and striatal (DA) release in rats (113,114). Consistent with these findings, a recent positron emission tomography imaging study in monkeys demonstrated that minocycline treatment protected against methamphetamine-induced neurotoxicity by attenuating the reduction of DAT in the striatum of monkeys pretreated with methamphetamine (115). The mechanism by which minocycline interacts with dopaminergic and glutamatergic neurotransmission has not been clarified, but it may be due to minocycline's capacity to inhibit inducible NOS and the resultant inhibition of NO release (116). These studies suggest that NO might be a significant treatment target for the development of medications for amphetamine addiction.

In summary, studies that focus on preclinical models of amphetamine will continue to serve an important purpose in the identification of new treatment targets for pharmacotherapies for amphetamine dependence. In addition, preclinical studies of medications acting on DA, GABA, glutamate, cannabinoid, nicotinic, and opioid receptors all have produced findings warranting further study.

Physiology

Amphetamines have a long duration of action. They produce an initial "rush" of euphoria, heightened alertness, increased energy, decreased appetite, and intensified emotions (117). Euphoria may be experienced in as little as 5 minutes with intravenous or smoked amphetamine and lasts 8 to 12 hours (118). Amphetamine half-lives range from 4 to 5 hours for methamphetamine to 7 to 31 hours for amphetamine (119,120). Amphetamines, therefore, produce powerful, long-lasting effects that many people find appealing; this allows amphetamines to compare favorably to other illicit drugs in terms of cost (121).

Not all effects of amphetamines are desirable, however. Acute adverse effects of amphetamines include insomnia, restlessness, hyperthermia, and even seizures. In addition to abuse and dependence, chronic use can result in agitation, paranoia, mood disturbances, psychosis, and cognitive impairment (122). After prolonged use of amphetamines, some users experience unpleasant physical side effects or a withdrawal syndrome marked by depression, irritability, anxiety, fatigue, and aggression (123). Unpleasant withdrawal symptoms during the initial days of abstinence from chronic amphetamine use can contribute to relapse or even suicidal ideation (124). Finally, the safety of prescribed stimulants was called into question recently, as Gould et al. (125) demonstrated an association between the use of stimulants and sudden unexplained death among children and adolescents. The potential for abuse and the side-effect profile of ATS underscores the prescribing clinician's responsibility to educate patients about these medicines.

AMPHETAMINES AS MEDICATIONS

Clinical Indications

Amphetamines and ATS have proven to be effective treatments in a variety of clinical situations. They are FDA-approved as pharmacotherapy ADHD and narcolepsy (126,127). ATS such as methylphenidate, mixed amphetamine salts, dextroamphetamine, and lisdexamfetamine are first-line treatments for ADHD. Amphetamines can also be used to augment antidepressant medications in treatment-resistant depression (128,129). Other uses of ATS include treatment of symptoms associated with traumatic brain injury and stroke (130). There is also evidence supporting the use of ATS as treatment for HIV-related neuropsychiatric symptoms (130). Use of ATS for weight loss is not encouraged by physicians largely due to the potential for dependence.

AMPHETAMINES AS DRUGS OF ABUSE

Evaluation and Treatment Approaches

A variety of evidence-based psychotherapies and pharmacotherapies have been used for amphetamine dependence. We will briefly summarize the support for these treatments in the following section.

Behavioral Interventions for Amphetamine Dependence

Trials of behavioral interventions for amphetamine dependence have produced promising results warranting further study. Both cognitive behavioral therapy (CBT) and contingency management (CM) have been shown to reduce methamphetamine use. CBT involves examining learning processes in order to reduce amphetamine use. The patient receiving CBT becomes skilled at recognizing situations associated with use, avoiding them when possible, or coping with them when necessary. CM provides tangible incentives like money-based vouchers or prizes, based on objective measures of drug abstinence. CBT is a prominent component of the Matrix Model, a 4-month, manualized, intensive outpatient therapy that combines CBT, psychoeducation, 12-step program participation, and positive reinforcement for behavioral change and treatment adherence (131). In a multisite clinical trial of 978 methamphetamine-dependent subjects, Rawson et al. (131) found that the Matrix Model was more effective as a 16-week treatment for methamphetamine dependence than standard treatments, as evidenced by increased treatment retention, methamphetamine-free urine drug screens, and periods of abstinence.

Four recent clinical trials suggest that CM has promise as a behavioral intervention for amphetamine dependence. CM, using voucher-based reinforcers, was shown to improve treatment retention and increase periods of continuous abstinence when compared to standard CBT in a 16-week trial of 162 methamphetamine-dependent gay and bisexual men, demographic groups affected by methamphetamine's recent surge in popularity (132). In another study of methamphetamine-dependent subjects that evaluated CM in conjunction with CBT and sertraline, subjects in the CM arm were significantly more likely than those not receiving CM to achieve a 3-week period of in-treatment abstinence (133). In a large 12-week study of 415 subjects dependent on methamphetamine or cocaine, CM outperformed treatment as usual with respect to treatment retention and abstinence in a community treatment setting (134). Similarly, in a 16-week study of a group of 171 subjects dependent on methamphetamine or cocaine, CM was shown to be more effective than CBT with respect to treatment retention and abstinence (135). Interestingly, the combination of CM and CBT did not produce an additive effect. This study demonstrated the potential of CM for engaging methamphetamine-dependent patients and helping them stay in treatment while achieving abstinence. The aforementioned clinical trials have produced intriguing results that necessitate further study.

Pharmacotherapy

Despite promising results from preclinical studies, clinical studies have not produced reliably efficacious treatments for amphetamine dependence. Translation of preclinical models for amphetamine dependence into effective treatments has proven difficult, and the positive signals seen in animals have, for the most part, not been reproduced in humans. In addition, the inability to develop effective pharmacotherapies for amphetamine dependence makes it difficult to assess the validity of preclinical models. Many research groups have worked to develop medications for amphetamine dependence since methamphetamine use surged in the 1980s following the cocaine epidemic. Thus far, randomized controlled trials (RCTs) of multiple classes of medications have generated inconclusive results. The classes of medications evaluated in these trials were influenced, perhaps, by previous trials of medications studied for cocaine dependence. In addition to RCTs, open-label studies have been done with a variety of medications; these studies provide hope for the eventual identification of an effective medication for amphetamine dependence. We briefly summarize the results from clinical trials of medications for amphetamine dependence.

Antidepressants

Antidepressants, including SSRIs and TCAs, have been studied as potential pharmacotherapies for amphetamine dependence for two important reasons. First, preclinical studies of amphetamine self-administration suggest that medications blocking the reuptake of 5-HT may attenuate the reinforcing effects of amphetamine (58,87). Second, blockade of the 5-HT and NE reuptake can combat some of the depressive symptoms experienced in amphetamine withdrawal such as depressed mood, fatigue, and anhedonia, which may lead to relapse (136). Other medications with effects on 5-HT, NE, and DA have been studied as well. Although antidepressants have not been shown to be efficacious as medications for cocaine dependence, several studies evaluating this class as treatments for amphetamine dependence have been done.

Unfortunately, trials of both SSRIs and TCAs have had limited success in identifying an effective medication for amphetamine dependence. The SSRIs fluoxetine, paroxetine, and sertraline failed to distinguish themselves from placebo as treatments for methamphetamine use (133,137,138). Galloway et al. (139) showed that treatment with 150 mg imipramine improved treatment retention in 32 methamphetamine-dependent subjects attending an outpatient detoxification program, but did not differ from a 10 mg imipramine control group in negative urine drug screens, depression scores, days since last use of methamphetamine, attendance of study visits, or craving. This study followed a case series showing increased treatment retention in two subjects taking desipramine for amphetamine dependence (140).

Antidepressants with mild stimulant properties have been studied as well. Amineptine, a DA reuptake inhibitor, alleviated symptoms of depressed mood, decreased energy, increased appetite, and craving for sleep in patients experiencing amphetamine withdrawal (141,142). Bupropion, a DA and NE reuptake inhibitor, has been shown to be safe in methamphetamine users (143) but was no more effective than placebo in two studies whose primary outcomes were proportion of subjects having a methamphetamine-free week (144,145). Post hoc analyses, however, suggest that bupropion may be effective as a treatment for methamphetamine dependence in at least a subgroup of men using low-to-moderate amounts of methamphetamine (144,145). The monoamine oxidase B inhibitor selegiline has been shown to be safe for use as a treatment for methamphetamine dependence, producing minimal changes in the subjective responses of subjects to methamphetamine (146). Serotonergic antagonists have also been examined; mirtazapine, a $5-HT_2$ and $5-HT_3$ antagonist, was shown to be more effective than treatment as usual for methamphetamine withdrawal (147), and ondansetron, a $5-HT_3$ blocker but not an antidepressant, has been shown thus far to be safe as a treatment for methamphetamine dependence (148).

GABA Enhancers

Preclinical studies showing the ability of GABA agents to attenuate drug-seeking behavior have prompted clinical investigations of these medications (149). These results led to positive studies of GABAergic agents as medications for cocaine dependence and provided a rationale for trials of these agents as medications for amphetamine dependence (150,151).

Clinical trials of GABAergic agents have provided preliminary evidence that such medications may be useful in the treatment of amphetamine dependence. Topiramate, a GABAergic anticonvulsant, did not have an adverse effect on cognitive processes in 10 methamphetamine-dependent subjects in a 27-day crossover study. Topiramate's effects on cognitive processes were mixed; it improved attention and concentration in subjects while worsening psychomotor retardation (152). In a 16-week, randomized, placebo-controlled, double-blind trial, neither gabapentin, a GABA-transaminase inhibitor, nor the $GABA_B$ agonist baclofen produced significant differences relative to placebo on standard treatment outcome measures (153). Post hoc analyses, however, showed a significant treatment effect for baclofen versus placebo in a subgroup that was highly compliant in taking study medication. Another GABA-transaminase inhibitor, gamma vinyl-GABA (GVG), was shown to be a safe treatment for methamphetamine dependence in an open-label, 9-week safety study (154). In this study, 15 of 27 methamphetamine-dependent subjects completed the study and at least two-thirds of these subjects were drug-free for at least 4 weeks of the study. In a separate placebo-controlled study, GVG did not alter amphetamine levels or cardiovascular effects of amphetamine, nor did it attenuate the positive subjective effects of methamphetamine in nontreatment-seeking methamphetamine-dependent volunteers (155). Thus, further investigations of these medications, or longer acting or more potent GABA agents, have potential to identify an effective treatment for amphetamine dependence.

Antipsychotics

Atypical antipsychotic medications have been investigated as treatments for methamphetamine dependence in part due to the effects of DA and, to a lesser extent, 5-HT on amphetamines. Medications with dopaminergic and serotonergic function, such as risperidone and aripiprazole, have been shown to block some of the behavioral effects of amphetamines that contribute to their abuse (156,157). Preliminary studies of these medications have been conducted. A 4-week open-label trial demonstrated that treatment with risperidone, a D2 and $5-HT_{2A}$ antagonist, produced significant reductions in episodes of methamphetamine use and psychiatric symptoms (158). A human laboratory study of the D2 and $5-HT_{1A}$ partial agonist and $5-HT_{2A}$ antagonist aripiprazole demonstrated moderate reductions in abstinence-related and cue-induced methamphetamine craving (159). These studies provide a basis for additional investigations of medications with dopaminergic and serotonergic action for amphetamine dependence.

Calcium Channel Blockers

Dopamine's role in the rewarding effects of stimulants has led to the study of medications that modulate midbrain DA systems. The ability of calcium channel blockers to attenuate cocaine-induced DA output in the striatum has led to investigation of this class of medications in models of amphetamine dependence (160). The calcium channel blocker isradipine, for example, has been shown in preclinical studies to suppress amphetamine-induced conditioned place preference and locomotor activity in rats (161).

Two clinical studies have followed this promising preclinical finding. Isradipine attenuated some of the subjective effects of and craving for D-methamphetamine in a human laboratory study of 18 healthy volunteers (162). However, a double-blind, randomized, placebo-controlled trial of another calcium channel blocker, amlodipine, did not produce positive results. Eight weeks of amlodipine treatment was not significantly different from placebo on measures methamphetamine use, depressive symptoms, and craving (163).

Stimulant-Like Medication

Another strategy for treating stimulant dependence is to employ medications that produce some of the same positive effects as the stimulant being abused. Modafinil, for example, is a wakefulness-promoting agent that is approved by the FDA for the treatment of narcolepsy. It has some pharmacological effects similar to amphetamines, such as increases in heart rate and blood pressure, but it is marketed as having less abuse potential than amphetamines (164–166). A small open-label trial has reported preliminary findings on modafinil as a pharmacotherapy for methamphetamine withdrawal. Treatment with modafinil attenuated subjective and observer-reported withdrawal severity when compared to treatment as usual (148). Subjects in the modafinil group reported less hypersomnia, fewer night-time awakenings, and deeper sleep than subjects receiving treatment as usual during methamphetamine withdrawal. Sofuoglu et al. (167) evaluated the effects of the NE transporter inhibitor atomoxetine on acute physiological and subjective responses to D-amphetamine in healthy volunteers. Atomoxetine, which is FDA-approved for the treatment of ADHD, attenuated some of the standard physiological responses to amphetamine and some of the positive subjective effects as well.

In summary, preliminary clinical trials of several classes of medications have yielded mixed results (Table 16.3). However, findings from some of these studies warrant additional investigation.

Agonist Pharmacotherapy

Another therapeutic approach, the replacement of amphetamine with agonist pharmacotherapy, has not been studied extensively, perhaps due to the lack of an established agonist pharmacotherapy for cocaine dependence (168). Several studies of amphetamine substitution, using retrospective and uncontrolled designs, describe promising results (169–172). In the lone randomized, controlled trial of amphetamine substitution treatment, Shearer et al. (173) showed the feasibility of urine toxicology screens for distinguishing between medication compliance with a prescribed amphetamine and changes in illicit methamphetamine use. The treatment group received dextroamphetamine, in addition to counseling, and improved on several outcome measures, but failed to distinguish itself from the control group that received only counseling.

Genetic Mechanisms Underlying Differences in Amphetamine Response among Animals

Although progress has been made in the development of psychotherapeutic and pharmacological treatments of amphetamine dependence, the efficacy of available treatments is limited. One possible explanation for the lack of success of these treatments is the heterogeneity of populations dependent on amphetamine. This heterogeneity likely results from a variety of factors, including genetics and psychosocial factors such as addiction severity, treatment history, and chronicity of use. Genotypes, the specific composition of genes coding for the phenotype, may offer information about patients' potential response to treatment.

Preclinical work has supported the concept of functional polymorphisms. Animals with risk polymorphisms display increased amphetamine effects compared to wild-type (WT) organisms, while those with protective polymorphisms show decreased amphetamine effects compared to WT organisms. Spielewoy et al. (174) showed that knockout mice lacking the DAT demonstrated a decreased locomotor response to amphetamine; this locomotion was decreased in a dose-dependent manner by the SSRI fluoxetine as well. In an investigation targeting the DA second messenger pathway, a quantitative trait locus (QTL) for methamphetamine-induced activity was identified in a region of chromosome 15 containing the casein kinase 1 epsilon gene (Csnk1e) (175). The casein kinase 1 gene positively regulates the activity of dopamine-and-cAMP-regulated-phosphoprotein-32 kDa (DARPP-32), a prominent component of the dopaminergic second messenger pathway that regulates the locomotor response to stimulants (176). A 10-fold difference in the expression of this gene in the high-activity mouse line compared to the low-activity line was shown. They identified an expression QTL that comapped to both the QTL for methamphetamine-induced activity and physical location of Csnk1e in the mouse genome, suggesting that this expression locus was responsible for differences in methamphetamine-induced activity. Mice without the α_{2A}-adrenoreceptor exhibited greater acute amphetamine-induced hyperactivity after administration of D-amphetamine than WT mice (85). However, the knockout mice displayed less amphetamine-induced hyperactivity after repeated administration of D-amphetamine than WT mice. These findings point to a complex interaction of α_{2A}-adrenoreceptor subtypes in the regulation of amphetamine-induced hyperactivity and the development of behavioral sensitization to repeated amphetamine administration.

Human Gene Polymorphisms and Associations with Amphetamine Dependence and Treatment Outcome

Pharmacogenetics may be a useful tool in the development of treatments for amphetamine dependence by helping to individualize therapies. This approach has been applied in

TABLE 16.3 Randomized controlled clinical trials of medications for amphetamine dependence

Drugs	Year	Author	Dose (mg/day)	N	Controls	Effects on primary outcome
Antidepressants						
■ Imipramine	1996	Galloway et al. (139)	150	22	10	Improved retention in treatment. No differences in urine toxicology, depressive symptoms, or craving
■ Fluoxetine	2000	Batki et al. (137)	40	NR	NR	No improved outcomes
■ Paroxetine	2003	Piasecki et al. (138)	20	20	NR	Only 15% completed study; no statistical analyses performed
■ Ondansetron[a]	2004	Johnson et al. (148)	Maximum 4 mg bid	152	NR	Safety study only
■ Bupropion	2005	Newton et al. (143)	300	10	10	Attenuated subjective effects of MA and craving
■ Bupropion	2008	Elkashef et al. (144)	300	79	72	No difference from PLA on primary outcomes. Post hoc analyses suggest increased MA-free urine screens for light users
■ Bupropion	2008	Shoptaw et al. (145)	300	36	37	No difference from PLA on primary outcomes. Post hoc analyses suggest increased MA-free urine screens for light users
■ Selegiline	2005	Newton et al. (146)	10	5	4	Slightly increased methamphetamine-associated "bad effects"
■ Sertraline	2006	Shoptaw et al. (133)	100	120	109	No improved outcomes
GABA enhancers						
■ Baclofen	2006	Heinzerling et al. (153)	60	25	37	No main effects, but significant treatment effect for baclofen in group most compliant with medication
■ Gabapentin			2400	26		
Calcium channel blockers						
■ Amlodipine		Batki et al. (163)	Up to 10	51	26	No improved outcomes

[a]Not an antidepressant but has effects on the serotonergic system (5-HT$_3$ receptor antagonist).
Bid: twice daily; NR: not reported.

several other clinical areas, primarily in two ways (177,178). First, pharmacogenetics can be used to identify new treatment targets for medications, such as particular neurotransmitter systems. Second, these studies may improve the efficacy of pharmacotherapies currently being used, either by describing subgroups of patients more likely to respond to a given treatment or by providing improved dosing recommendations.

Progress made in using functional polymorphisms to inform treatment in other substance use disorders and studies employing these polymorphisms in relation to amphetamine dependence continue to be described. Several studies have documented genetic effects on the subjective responses to amphetamine. Following the aforementioned DAT variable number tandem repeat (VNTR) studies, Lott et al. (179) showed variations in subjective responses to D-amphetamine in 101 healthy controls. Those with the nine-repeat DAT allele had decreased subjective responses to acute amphetamine administration on the Drug Effects Questionnaire (DEQ), the Profile of Mood States (POMS), and the Addiction Research Center Inventory (ARCI), suggesting less of a risk of amphetamine dependence in these individuals. In addition, the promoter-region gene-linked polymorphic region (5-HTTLPR) and the VNTR in the second intron of the serotonin transporter gene (5-HTT) were shown to contribute to the acute subjective responses to D-amphetamine in this cohort. The same group showed that a single-nucleotide polymorphism (SNP) in the Csnk1e region was associated with increased feeling of drug effect on the DEQ (180). Similarly, Dlugos et al. (181) showed that healthy volunteers with certain polymorphisms in the NE transporter (SLC6A2) gene had increased mood and elation responses after receiving 20 mg of D-amphetamine. Brain-derived neurotrophic factor (BDNF) potentiates neurotransmitters strongly linked to substance abuse. Flanagin et al. (182) showed that healthy adult volunteers homozygous for the val allele of the BDNF G196A gene experienced more pronounced subjective responses and a less pronounced physiological response from a single moderate dose of amphetamine than genotypic groups. A functional polymorphism for the catechol-O-methyl transferase (COMT) gene has also been demonstrated in a functional magnetic resonance imaging (fMRI) study; amphetamine enhanced efficiency of prefrontal function during a working memory task in those with val/val genotype, but had no effect on those with met/met genotype, suggesting this group may be at increased risk for adverse response to amphetamine (183). Finally, increased feelings of anxiety on the POMS after amphetamine administration are associated with the 1976C/T and the 2592C/T$_{ins}$ polymorphisms of the adenosine receptor gene in 99 healthy volunteers (184). Stimulation of adenosine receptors antagonizes DA function, providing another potential substance abuse treatment target.

Other studies describe vulnerability to adverse drug effects, such as psychosis resulting from amphetamine use. Ujike et al. (185) studied four exonic polymorphisms of the DAT gene and did not find a difference in genotypic and allelic distribution of the four polymorphisms between methamphetamine-dependent subjects and healthy volunteers. However, those experiencing methamphetamine psychosis on discontinuation of methamphetamine were significantly more likely to possess excess nine or fewer repeat alleles of the DATVNTR, supporting the findings of Gelernter et al. (186). Similarly, the met allele frequency of the COMT gene is associated with patients who experience methamphetamine psychosis and relapse into methamphetamine use, suggesting that patients with a met allele appear to be at increased risk of an adverse response to methamphetamine. Another polymorphism associated with extended methamphetamine psychosis has been found in the promoter region of the quinone oxidoreductase (NQO2) gene in a Japanese sample (187). This gene is involved in protection from methamphetamine-induced oxidative stress and neurotoxicity, suggesting a role for the NQO2 gene in prolonged methamphetamine psychosis.

CONCLUSIONS

Around the world, people continue to abuse amphetamines, often with significant negative consequences. Although there is variation in patterns of use in different parts of the world, amphetamine dependence can be associated with great personal and societal costs. Methamphetamine dependence, for example, is exacting a tremendous toll on many communities within the United States. While there are currently no effective pharmacotherapies for amphetamine dependence, strides are being made in multiple areas of research directed toward this goal, from preclinical studies to randomized, controlled clinical trials. Preliminary findings in a variety of areas require additional investigation. Although progress has been made in the development of behavioral treatments for amphetamine dependence, the need for effective medications has propelled exciting preclinical and clinical research.

Pharmacogenetics research appears to be a promising new approach that may speed the development of treatments for amphetamine dependence. Ultimately, genotypic information may allow clinicians to tailor treatment to each individual through consideration of polymorphisms affecting treatment response. Effective pharmacotherapies may become integral components of successful comprehensive treatment strategies for amphetamine dependence.

ACKNOWLEDGMENT

The authors have no conflicts of interest that are directly related to the content of this chapter.

This work has been supported in part by NIDA K24DA022288 to Dr. Weiss.

REFERENCES

1. Abourashed E, El-Alfy A, Khan I, et al. Ephedra in perspective—a current review. *Phytother Res.* 2003;17:703–712.
2. Caldwell J. The metabolism of amphetamines and related stimulants in animals and man. In: Caldwell J, ed. *Amphetamines and Related Stimulants: Chemical, Biological, Clinical, and Social Aspects.* Boca Raton, FL: CRC Press; 1980.

3. Rasmussen N. Making the first antidepressant: amphetamine in American medicine, 1929–1950. *J Hist Med Allied Sci.* 2006;61: 288–323.
4. Rasmussen N. America's first amphetamine epidemic 1929–1971: a quantitative and qualitative retrospective with implications for the present. *Am J Public Health.* 2008;98:974–985.
5. Bower EA, Phelan JR. Use of amphetamines in the military environment. *Lancet.* 2003;362:S18–S19.
6. Eliyahu U, Berlin S, Hadad E, et al. Psychostimulants and military operations. *Mil Med.* 2007;172:383–387.
7. Jones AR, Pinchot JT. Stimulant use in sports. *Am J Addict.* 1998; 7:243–255.
8. Smith GM, Beecher HK. Amphetamine sulfate and athletic performance. *JAMA.* 1959;170:542–557.
9. McDuff DR, Baron D. Substance use in athletics: a sports psychiatry perspective. *Clin Sports Med.* 2005;24:885–897.
10. Wadler GI, Hainline B. *Drugs and the Athlete.* Philadelphia, PA: F.A. Davis; 1989.
11. Avois L, Robinson N, Saudan C, et al. Central nervous system stimulants and sport practice. *Br J Sports Med.* 2006; 40(suppl I): i16–i20.
12. Puffer JC. The use of drugs in swimming. *Clin Sports Med.* 1986;5:77–89.
13. Ballon JS, Feifel D. A systematic review of modafinil: potential clinical uses and mechanisms of action. *J Clin Psychiatry.* 2006; 67:554–566.
14. World Anti-Doping Agency. *The 2009 Prohibited List: International Standard.* Available at: http://www.wada-ama.org/rtecontent/document/2009_Prohibited_List_Eng_Final_20_Sept_08.pdf. Accessed August 8, 2009.
15. Teter CJ, McCabe SE, LaGrange K, et al. Illicit use of specific prescription stimulants among college students: prevalence, motives, and routes of administration. *Pharmacotherapy.* 2006; 1501–1510.
16. Substance Abuse and Mental Health Services Administration. (2009). *Results from the 2008 National Survey on Drug Use and Health: National Findings* (Office of Applied Studies, NSDUH Series H-36, HHS Publication No. SMA 09-4434). Rockville, MD.
17. Substance Abuse and Mental Health Services Administration, Office of Applied Studies. *The NSDUH Report: Nonmedical Use of Adderall among Fulltime College Students.* Rockville, MD; April 7, 2009. Accessed August 10, 2009.
18. McCabe SE, Knight JR, Teter CJ, et al. Non-medical use of prescription stimulants among US college students: prevalence and correlates from a national survey. *Addiction.* 2005;100: 96–106.
19. National Institute on Drug Abuse. *NIDA InfoFacts: Stimulant ADHD Medications—Methylphenidate and Amphetamines;* June 2008. Available at: http://www.drugabuse.gov/Infofacts/ADHD.html.
20. Randall DC, Fleck NL, Shneerson JM, et al. The cognitive-enhancing properties of modafinil are limited in non-sleep-deprived middle-aged volunteers. *Pharmacol Biochem Behav.* 2004;77:547–555.
21. United Nations Office for Drug Control and Crime Prevention. *World Drug Report 2009.* Available at: http://www.unodc.org/documents/wdr/WDR-2009/ WDR2009_eng_web.pdf. Accessed August 16, 2009.
22. Smart RG, Osborne AC. Drug use and drinking among students in 36 countries. *Addict Behav.* 2000;25:455–460.
23. Swanson JM, Volkow ND. Increasing use of stimulants warns of potential abuse. *Nature.* 2008;453:586.
24. Durell TM, Kroutil LA, Crits-Christoph P, et al. Prevalence of nonmedical methamphetamine use in the United States. *Subst Abuse Treat Prev Policy.* 2008;3:19.
25. Cunningham JK, Liu LM, Callaghan R. Impact of US and Canada precursor regulation on methamphetamine purity in the United States. *Addiction.* 2009;104:441–453.
26. Substance Abuse and Mental Health Services Administration. *Results from the 2007 National Survey on Drug Use and Health: National Findings.* Rockville, MD: Office of Applied Studies; 2008. NSDUH series H-34, DHHS publication no. SMA08-4343. Accessed August 10, 2009.
27. Office of Applied Studies. *Results from the 2004 National Survey on Drug Use and Health: National Findings.* Rockville, MD: Substance Abuse and Mental Health Services Administration; 2005. DHHS publication no. SMA 05-4062, NSDUH series H-28.
28. Gonzalez Castro F, Barrington EH, Walton MA, et al. Cocaine and methamphetamine: differential addiction rates. *Psychol Addict Behav.* 2000;14:390–396.
29. Office of Applied Studies, Substance Abuse and Mental Health Services Administration. *Amphetamine and Methamphetamine Emergency Department Visits 1995–2002 [DAWN Report];* 2004. Available at: http://dawninfo.samsha.gov/old_dawn/pubs_94_02/shortreports/. Accessed November 21, 2006.
30. Rawson RA, Anglin MD, Ling W. Will the methamphetamine problem go away? *J Addict Dis.* 2002;21:5–19.
31. Yui K, Goto K, Ikemoto S, et al. Susceptibility to subsequent episodes of spontaneous recurrence of methamphetamine psychosis. *Am J Addict.* 2001;64:133–142.
32. Zweben JE, Cohen JB, Christian D, et al. Psychiatric symptoms in methamphetamine users. *Am J Addict.* 2004;13:181–190.
33. Wu LT, Pilowsky DJ, Schlenger WE, et al. Misuse of methamphetamine and prescription stimulants among young adults in the community. *Drug Alcohol Depend.* 2007;89:195–205.
34. McKetin R, McLaren J, Lubman DI, et al. The prevalence of psychotic symptoms among methamphetamine users. *Addiction.* 2006;101:1473–1478.
35. Sato M, Numachi Y, Hamamura T. Relapse of paranoid psychotic state in methamphetamine model of schizophrenia. *Schizophrenia Bull.* 1992;18:115–122.
36. Dore G, Sweeting M. Drug-induced psychosis associated with crystalline methamphetamine. *Australas Psychiatry.* 2006;14:86–89.
37. Srisurapanont M, Ali R, Marsden J, et al. Psychotic symptoms in methamphetamine psychotic in-patients. *Int J Neuropsychopharmacol.* 2003;6:347–352.
38. Shoptaw SJ, Kao U, Ling W. Treatment for amphetamine psychosis. *Cochrane Database Syst Rev.* 2009;1:CD003026.
39. National Drug Intelligence Center. *Information Bulletin: Children at Risk.* Available at: http://www.usdoj.gov/ndic/pubs1/1466. Accessed November 21, 2006.
40. Kolecki P. Inadvertent methamphetamine poisoning in pediatric patients. *Pediatr Emerg Care.* 1998;14:385–387.
41. Plessinger MA. Prenatal exposure to amphetamines. Risks and adverse outcomes in pregnancy. *Obstet Gynecol Clin North Am.* 1998;25:119–138.
42. Blumenthal RN, Kral AH, Gee L, et al. Trends in HIV seroprevalence and risk among gay and bisexual men who inject drugs in San Francisco, 1988 to 2000. *J Acquir Immune Defic Syndr.* 2001;28:264–269.
43. Harris NV, Thiede H, McGough JP, et al. Risk factors for HIV infection among injection drug users: results of blinded surveys in drug treatment centers, King County, Washington 1988–1991. *J Acquir Immune Defic Syndr.* 1993;6:1275–1282.

44. Cartier J, Farabee D, Prendergast ML. Methamphetamine use, self-reported violent crime, and recidivism among offenders in California who abuse substances. *J Interpers Violence*. 2006;21:435–445.
45. White FJ, Kalivas PW. Neuroadaptations involved in amphetamine and cocaine addiction. *Drug Alcohol Depend*. 1998;51:141–153.
46. Rothman RB, Partilla JS, Dersch CM, et al. Methamphetamine dependence: medication development efforts based on the dual deficit model of stimulant addiction. *Ann N Y Acad Sci*. 2000;914:71–81.
47. Partilla JS, Dempsey AG, Nagpal AS, et al. Interaction of amphetamines and related compounds at the vesicular monoamine transporter. *J Pharmacol Exp Ther*. 2006;319:237–246.
48. Bardo MT. Neuropharmacological mechanisms of drug reward: beyond dopamine in the nucleus accumbens. *Crit Rev Neurobiol*. 1998;12:37–67.
49. Koob GF. Neural mechanisms of drug reinforcement. *Ann N Y Acad Sci*. 1992;654:171–191.
50. Tzschentke TM, Schmidt WJ. Functional relationship among medial prefrontal cortex, nucleus accumbens, and ventral tegmental area in locomotion and reward. *Crit Rev Neurobiol*. 2000;14:131–142.
51. Steketee JD. Neurotransmitter systems of the medial prefrontal cortex: potential role in sensitization to psychostimulants. *Brain Res Rev*. 2003;41:203–228.
52. Robbins TW, Everitt BJ. Central norepinephrine neurons and behavior. In: Bloom FE, Kupfer DJ, eds. *Psychopharmacology: The Fourth Generation of Progress*. New York: Raven Press; 1988:363–372.
53. Aston-Jones G, Harris GC. Brain substrates for increased drug seeking during protracted withdrawal. *Neuropharmacology*. 2004;47:167–179.
54. Lyness WH, Friedle NM, Moore KE. Increased self-administration of D-amphetamine after destruction of 5-hydroxytryptaminergic neurons. *Pharmacol Biochem Behav*. 1980;12:937–941.
55. Missale C, Walsh SR, Robinson SW, et al. Dopamine receptors: from structure to function. *Pharmacol Rev*. 1998;78:189–225.
56. Geis LS, Smith DG, Smith FL, et al. Tyrosine influence on amphetamine self-administration and brain catecholamines in the rat. *Pharmacol Biochem Behav*. 1986;25:1027–1033.
57. Baumann MH, Ayestas MA, Sharpe LG, et al. Persistent antagonism of methamphetamine-induced dopamine release in rats pretreated with GBR12909 decanoate. *J Pharmacol Exp Ther*. 2002;301:1190–1197.
58. Izzo E, Orsini C, Koob GF, et al. A dopamine partial agonist and antagonist block amphetamine self-administration in a progressive ratio schedule. *Pharmacol Biochem Behav*. 2001;68:701–708.
59. Chiang YC, Chen PC, Chen JC. D_3 dopamine receptors are down-regulated in amphetamine sensitized rats and their putative antagonists modulate the locomotor sensitization to amphetamine. *Brain Res*. 2003;972:159–167.
60. Moro H, Sato H, Ida I, et al. Effects of SKF-38393, a dopamine D1 receptor agonist on expression of amphetamine-induced behavioral sensitization and expression of immediate early gene arc in prefrontal cortex of rats. *Pharmacol Biochem Behav*. 2007;87:56–64.
61. Steketee JD. Cortical mechanisms of cocaine sensitization. *Crit Rev Neurobiol*. 2005;17:69–86.
62. Tzschentke TM, Schmidt WJ. Glutamatergic mechanisms in addiction. *Mol Psychiatry*. 2003;8:373–382.
63. Brebner K, Childress AR, Roberts DCS. A potential role for $GABA_B$ agonists in the treatment of psychostimulant addiction. *Alcohol Alcohol*. 2002;37:478–484.
64. Blein S, Hawrot E, Barlow P. The metabotropic GABA receptor: molecular insights and their functional consequences. *Cell Mol Life Sci*. 2000;57:635–650.
65. Sofuoglu M, Kosten TR. Emerging pharmacological strategies in the fight against cocaine addiction. *Expert Opin Emerg Drugs*. 2006;11:91–98.
66. Ranaldi R, Poeggel K. Baclofen decreases methamphetamine self-administration in rats. *Neuroreport*. 2002;13:1107–1110.
67. Brebner K, Ahn S, Phillips AG. Attenuation of D-amphetamine self-administration by baclofen in the rat: behavioral and neurochemical correlates. *Psychopharmacology (Berl)*. 2005;177:409–417.
68. Li SM, Yin LL, Ren YH, et al. $GABA_B$ receptor agonist baclofen attenuates the development and expression of D-amphetamine-induced place preference in rats. *Life Sci*. 2001;70:349–356.
69. Bartoletti M, Gubellini C, Ricci F, et al. Baclofen blocks the development of sensitization to the locomotor stimulant effect of amphetamine. *Behav Pharmacol*. 2005;16:553–558.
70. Miranda F, Jimenez JC, Cedillo LN, et al. The GABA-B antagonist 2-hydroxysaclofen reverses the effects of baclofen on the discriminative stimulus effects of D-amphetamine in the conditioned taste aversion procedure. *Pharmacol Biochem Behav*. 2009; 93:25–30.
71. Gerasimov MR, Ashby CR Jr, Gardner EL, et al. Gamma-vinyl GABA inhibits methamphetamine, heroin, or ethanol-induced increases in nucleus accumbens dopamine. *Synapse*. 1999;34:11–19.
72. Kim JH, Austin JD, Tanabe L, et al. Activation of group II mGlu receptors blocks the enhanced drug taking induced by previous exposure to amphetamine. *Eur J Neurosci*. 2005;21:295–300.
73. Tzschentke TM. Measuring reward with the conditioned place preference paradigm: a comprehensive review of drug effects, recent progress and new issues. *Prog Neurobiol*. 1998;56:613–672.
74. da Silva AL, Hoffman A, Dietrich MO, et al. Effect of riluzole on MK-801 and amphetamine-induced hyperlocomotion. *Neuropsychobiology*. 2003;48:27–30.
75. Itzhak Y, Martin JL. Effect of riluzole and gabapentin on cocaine- and methamphetamine-induced behavioral sensitization in mice. *Psychopharmacology (Berl)*. 2000;151:226–233.
76. Bradberry CW. Cocaine sensitization and dopamine mediation of cue effects in rodents, monkeys, and humans: areas of agreement, disagreement, and implications for addiction. *Psychopharmacology*. 2007;191:705–717.
77. Pierce RC, Kalivas PW. A circuitry model of the expression of behavioral sensitization to amphetamine-like psychostimulants. *Brain Res Rev*. 1997;25:192–216.
78. Ujike H, Sato M. Clinical features of sensitization to methamphetamine observed in patients with methamphetamine dependence and psychosis. *Ann N Y Acad Sci*. 2004;1025:279–287.
79. Boireau A, Meunier M, Imperato A. Ouabain-induced increase in dopamine release from mouse striatal slices antagonized by riluzole. *J Pharm Pharmacol*. 1998;50:1293–1297.
80. Sofuoglu M, Sewell RA. Norepinephrine and stimulant addiction. *Addict Biol*. 2009;14:119–129.
81. Cooper JR, Bloom FE, Roth RH. *The Biochemical Basis of Neuropharmacology*. New York: Oxford University Press; 2003.
82. Drouin C, Blanc G, Villegier AS, et al. Critical role of α_1-adrenergic receptors in acute and sensitized locomotor effects of D-amphetamine, cocaine, and GBR 12783: influence of preexposure conditions and pharmacological characteristics. *Synapse*. 2002;43:51–61.
83. Auclair A, Drouin C, Cotecchia S, et al. 5-HT_{2A} and $\alpha 1b$-adrenergic receptors entirely mediate dopamine release, locomotor response and behavioural sensitization to opiates and psychostimulants. *Eur J Neurosci*. 2004;20:3073–3084.

84. Juhila J, Haapalinna A, Sirvio J, et al. The α_2-adrenoreceptor antagonist atipamezole reduces the development and expression of D-amphetamine-induced behavioural sensitization. *Arch Pharmacol.* 2003;367:274–280.
85. Juhila J, Honkanen A, Sallinen J, et al. α_{2A}-Adreno-receptors regulate D-amphetamine-induced hyperactivity and behavioural sensitization in mice. *Eur J Pharmacol.* 2005;517:74–83.
86. Leccesse AP, Lyness WH. The effects of putative 5-hydroxytryptamine active agents on D-amphetamine self-administraion in controls and rats with 5,7-dihydroxytryptamine median forebrain bundle lesions. *Brain Res.* 1984;303:153–162.
87. Yu DSL, Smith FL, Smith DG. Fluoxetine-induced attenuation of amphetamine self-administration in rats. *Life Sci.* 1986;39:1383–1388.
88. Kokkinidis L, Zacharko RM, Predy PA. Post-amphetamine depression of self-stimulation responding from the substantia nigra: reversal by tricyclic antidepressants. *Pharamacol Biochem Behav.* 1980;13:379–383.
89. Salomon L, Lanteri C, Glowinski J. Behavioral sensitization to amphetamine results from an uncoupling between noradrenergic and serotonergic neurons. *Proc Natl Acad Sci U S A.* 2006;103: 7476–7481.
90. Markou A, Harrison AA, Chevrette J. Paroxetine combined with a 5-HT$_{1A}$ receptor antagonist reversed reward deficits observed during amphetamine withdrawal in rats. *Psychopharmacology.* 2005;178:133–142.
91. Gardner EL, Schiffer WK, Horan BA, et al. Gamma vinyl GABA, an irreversible inhibitor of GABA transaminase, alters the acquisition and expression of cocaine-induced sensitization in male rats. *Synapse.* 2002;46:240–250.
92. Gorriti MA, de Fonseca FR, Navarro M, et al. Chronic (−)-Δ^9-tetrahydrocannabinol treatment induces sensitization to the psychomotor effects of amphetamines in rats. *Eur J Pharmacol.* 1999;365:133–142.
93. Anggadiredja K, Nakamichi M, Hiranita T, et al. Endocannabinoid system modulates relapse to methamphetamine seeking: possible mediation by the arachidonic acid cascade. *Neuropsychopharmacology.* 2004;29:1470–1478.
94. Thiemann G, Di Marzo V, Molleman A, et al. The CB(1) cannabinoid receptor antagonist AM 251 attenuates amphetamine-induced behavioural sensitization while causing monoamine changes in nucleus accumbens and hippocampus. *Pharmacol Biochem Behav.* 2008;89:384–391.
95. Hiranita T, Nawata Y, Sakimura K, et al. Suppression of methamphetamine-seeking behavior by nicotinic agonists. *Proc Natl Acad Sci U S A.* 2006;103:8523–8527.
96. Harrod SB, Dwoskin LP, Crooks PA, et al. Lobeline attenuates D-amphetamine self-administration in rats. *J Pharmacol Exp Ther.* 2001;298:172–179.
97. Siegal D, Erickson J, Varoqui H, et al. Brain vesicular acetylcholine transporter in human users of drugs of abuse. *Synapse.* 2004;52:223–232.
98. Hikida T, Kitabatake Y, Pastan I, et al. Acetylcholine enhancement in the nucleus accumbens prevents addictive behaviors of cocaine and morphine. *Proc Natl Acad Sci U S A.* 2003;100: 6169–6173.
99. Sesack SR, Pickel VM. Dual ultrastructural localization of enkephalin and tyrosine hydroxylase immunoreactivity in the rat ventral tegmental area: multiple substrates for opioid–dopamine interactions. *J Neurosci.* 1992;12:1335–1350.
100. Kubota Y, Inagaki S, Kito S, et al. Ultrastructural evidence of dopaminergic input to enkephalinergic neurons in rat neostriatum. *Brain Res.* 1986;367:374–378.
101. Olive MF, Koenig HN, Nannini MA. Stimulation of endorphin neurotransmission in the nucleus accumbens by ethanol, cocaine, and amphetamine. *J Neuroscience.* 2001;21(RC184):1–5.
102. Hooks MS, Jones GH, Liem BJ, et al. Sensitization and individual differences to IP amphetamine, cocaine, or caffeine following repeated intracranial amphetamine infusions. *Pharmacol Biochem Behav.* 1992;43:815–823.
103. Trujillo KA, Belluzzi JD, Stein L. Naloxone blockade of amphetamine place preference conditioning. *Pharmacology.* 1991;104: 265–274.
104. Chiu CT, Ma T, Ho IK. Attenuation of methamphetamine-induced behavioral sensitization in mice by systemic administration of naltrexone. *Brain Res Bull.* 2005;67:100–109.
105. Anggadiredja K, Sakimura K, Hiranita T, et al. Naltrexone attenuates cue- but not drug-induced methamphetamine seeking: a possible mechanism for the dissociation of primary and secondary reward. *Brain Res.* 2004;1021:272–276.
106. Harrigan SE, Downs DA. Continuous intravenous naltrexone effects on morphine self-administration in rhesus monkeys. *J Pharmacol Exp Ther.* 1978;204:481–486.
107. Haggkvist J, Lindholm S, Franck J. The opioid receptor antagonist naltrexone attenuates reinstatement of amphetamine drug-seeking in the rat. *Behav Brain Res.* 2009;197:219–224.
108. Itzhak Y, Ali SF. Role of nitrergic system in behavioral and neurotoxic effects of amphetamine analogs. *Pharmacol Ther.* 2006; 109:246–262.
109. Garthwaite J, Charles SL, Chess-Williams R. Endothelium-derived relaxing factor release on activation of NMDA receptors suggest role as intercellular messenger in the brain. *Nature.* 1988;336:385–388.
110. Itzhak Y. Modulation of cocaine- and methamphetamine-induced behavioral sensitization by inhibition of brain nitric oxide synthase. *J Pharmacol Exp Ther.* 1997;282:521–527.
111. Vaupel DB, Kimes AS, London ED. Comparison of 7-nitroindazole with other nitric oxide synthase inhibitors as attenuators of opioid withdrawal. *Psychopharmacology (Berl).* 1995;118: 361–368.
112. Vaupel DB, Kimes AS, London ED. Nitric oxide synthase inhibitors. Preclinical studies of potential use for treatment of opioid withdrawal. *Neuropsychopharmacology.* 1995;13:315–322.
113. Kofman O, van Embden S, Alpert C, et al. Central and peripheral minocycline suppresses motor activity in rats. *Pharmacol Biochem Behav.* 1993;44:397–402.
114. Kofman O, Klein E, Newman M, et al. Inhibition by antibiotic tetracyclines of rat cortical noradrenergic adenylate cyclase and amphetamine-induced hyperactivity. *Pharmacol Biochem Behav.* 1990;37:417–424.
115. Hashimoto K, Tsukada H, Nishiyama S, et al. Protective effects of minocycline on the reduction of dopamine transporters in the striatum after administration of methamphetamine: a positron emission tomography study in conscious monkeys. *Biol Psychiatry.* 2007;61:577–581.
116. Du Y, Ma Z, Lin S, et al. Minocycline prevents nigrostriatal dopaminergic neurodegeneration in the MPTP model of Parkinson's disease. *Proc Natl Acad Sci U S A.* 2001;98:14669–14674.
117. Gawin FH, Ellinwood EH Jr. Cocaine and other stimulants. Actions, abuse, and treatment. *N Engl J Med.* 1988;318:1173–1182.
118. National Institute on Drug Abuse. *Methamphetamine abuse and addiction [Research Report series].* Bethesda, MD: National Institutes of Health; 1998 January Publication 02-4210.
119. *Product Information: Desoxyn(R), Methamphetamine.* North Chicago, IL: Abbott Laboratories; 1996.

120. *Product Information: ADDERALL(R) Oral Tablets, Amphetamine Aspartate Monohydrate, Amphetamine Sulfate, Dextroamphetamine Saccharate, Dextroamphetamine Sulfate Oral Tablets.* Wayne, PA: Shire US Inc; 2006.
121. Rawson RA, Huber A, Brethen P. Methamphetamine and cocaine users: differences in characteristics and treatment retention. *J Psychoactive Drugs.* 2000;32:233–238.
122. Simon SL, Domier C, Carnell J, et al. Cognitive impairment in individuals currently using methamphetamine. *Am J Addict.* 2000;9:222–231.
123. Newton T, Kalechstein A, Duran S, et al. Methamphetamine abstinence syndrome: preliminary findings. *Am J Addict.* 2004;13:248–255.
124. Scott JC, Woods SP, Matt GE, et al. Neurocognitive effects of methamphetamine: a critical review and meta-analysis. *Neuropsychol Rev.* 2007;17:275–297.
125. Gould MS, Walsh BT, Munfakh JL, et al. Sudden death and use of stimulant medications in youths. *Am J Psychiatry.* 2009; AiA:1–10.
126. Rappley MD. Attention deficit-hyperactivity disorder. *N Engl J Med.* 2005;352:165–173.
127. Woodworth T. Statement of Terrance Woodworth, Deputy Director, Office of Diversion Control, Drug Enforcement Administration, before the Committee on Education and the Workforce, Subcommittee on Early Childhood, Youth, and Families; May 16, 2000.
128. Fawcett JF, Busch KA. Stimulants in psychiatry. In: Schatzberg AF, Nemeroff CB, eds. *The American Psychiatric Press Textbook of Psychopharmacology.* Washington, DC: American Psychiatric Press; 1995:417–435.
129. Carvalho AF, Cavalcante JL, Castelo MS, et al. Augmentation strategies for treatment-resistant depression: a literature review. *J Clin Pharm Ther.* 2007;32:415–428.
130. Ng B, O'Brien A. Beyond ADHD and narcolepsy: psychostimulants in general psychiatry. *Adv Psychiatric Treat.* 2009;15:297–305.
131. Rawson RA, Marinelli-Casey P, Anglin MD, et al. A multi-site comparison of psychosocial approaches for the treatment of methamphetamine dependence. *Addiction.* 2004;99;708–717.
132. Shoptaw S, Reback CJ, Peck JA, et al. Behavioral treatment approaches for methamphetamine dependence and HIV-related sexual risk behaviors among urban gay and bisexual men. *Drug Alcohol Depend.* 2005;78:125–134.
133. Shoptaw S, Huber A, Peck JA, et al. Randomized, placebo-controlled trial of sertraline and contingency management for the treatment of methamphetamine dependence. *Drug Alcohol Depend.* 2006;85:12–18.
134. Petry NM, Peirce JM, Stitzer ML, et al. Effect of prize-based incentives on outcomes in stimulant abusers in outpatient psychosocial treatment programs. *Arch Gen Psychiatry.* 2005;62: 1148–1156.
135. Rawson RA, McCann MJ, Flammino F, et al. A comparison of contingency management and cognitive-behavioral approaches for stimulant-dependent individuals. *Addiction.* 2006;101:267–274.
136. Peck JA, Reback CJ, Yang X, et al. Sustained reductions in drug use and depression symptoms from treatment for drug abuse in methamphetamine-dependent gay and bisexual men. *J Urban Health.* 2005;82:100–108.
137. Batki SL, Moon J, Bradley M, et al. Fluoxetine in methamphetamine dependence—a controlled trial: preliminary analysis. In: Harris LS, ed. *Problems of Drug Dependence 1999.* Proceedings of the 61st Annual Scientific Meeting of the College on Problems of Drug Dependence, Inc (NIDA Research Monograph 180, NIH Publication No. 00-4737). Washington, DC, US: Government Printing Office; 2000:235.
138. Piasecki MP, Steinagel GM, Thienhaus OJ. An exploratory study: the use of paroxetine for methamphetamine craving. *J Psychoactive Drugs.* 2003;34:301–304.
139. Galloway GP, Newmeyer J, Knapp T, et al. A controlled trial of imipramine for the treatment of methamphetamine dependence. *J Subst Abuse Treat.* 1996;13:493–497.
140. Tennant RS Jr, Tarver A, Pumphrey E, et al. Double-blind comparison of desipramine and placebo for treatment of phenicyclidine or amphetamine dependence. *NIDA Res Monogr.* 1986; 67:310–317.
141. Jittiwutikan J, Srisurapanont M, Jarusuraisin N. Amineptine in the treatment of amphetamine withdrawal: a placebo-controlled, randomised, double-blind study. *J Med Assoc Thai.* 1997;80:587–591.
142. Srisurapanont M, Jarusuraisin N, Jittiwutikan J. Amphetamine withdrawal: II. A placebo-controlled, randomised, double-blind study of amineptine treatment. *Aust N Z J Psychiatry.* 1999; 33:94–98.
143. Newton TF, Roache JD, De La Garza II R. Safety of intravenous methamphetamine administration during treatment with bupropion. *Psychopharmacology.* 2005;182:426–435.
144. Elkashef AM, Rawson RA, Anderson AL, et al. Bupropion for the treatment of methamphetamine dependence. *Neuropsychopharmacology.* 2008;33:1162–1170.
145. Shoptaw S, Heinzerling KG, Rotheram-Fuller E, et al. Bupropion hydrochloride versus placebo, in combination with cognitive behavioral therapy, for the treatment of cocaine abuse/dependence. *J Addict Dis.* 2008;27:13–23.
146. Newton TF, De La Garza R 2nd, Fong T, et al. A comprehensive assessment of the safety of intravenous methamphetamine administration during treatment with selegiline. *Pharmacol Biochem Behav.* 2005;82:704–711.
147. McGregor C, White JM, Srisurapanont M, et al. *Open-label Pilot Trials of Mirtazapine and Modafinil in Inpatient Methamphetamine Withdrawal: Symptoms and Sleep Patterns.* Poster Presentation at the 67th Annual Scientific Conference of the College on Problems of Drug Dependence; 2005.
148. Johnson BA, Rawson RA, Elkashef A, et al. *Ondansetron for the Treatment of Methamphetamine Dependence.* Poster Presentation at the 66th Annual Scientific Conference of the College on Problems of Drug Dependence; 2004.
149. Cousins MS, Roberts DC, Harriet de Wit GABA(B) receptor agonists for the treatment of drug addiction: a review of recent findings. *Drug Alcohol Depend.* 2002;65:209–220.
150. Shoptaw S, Yang X, Rotheram-Fuller EJ, et al. Randomized placebo-controlled trial of baclofen for cocaine dependence: preliminary effects for individuals with chronic patterns of cocaine use. *J Clin Psychiatry.* 2003;64:1440–1448.
151. Haney M, Hart C, Collins ED, et al. Smoked cocaine discrimination in humans: effects of gabapentin. *Drug Alcohol Depend.* 2005;80:53–61.
152. Johnson BA, Roache JD, Ait-Daoud N, et al. Effects of topiramate on methamphetamine-induced changes in attentional and perceptual-motor skills of cognition in recently abstinent methamphetamine-dependent individuals. *Prog Neuropsychopharmacol Biol Psychiatry.* 2007; 31:123–130.
153. Heinzerling KG, Shoptaw S, Peck JA, et al. Randomized, placebo-controlled trial of baclofen and gabapentin for the treatment of methamphetamine dependence. *Drug Alcohol Depend.* 2006;85:177–184.
154. Brodie JD, Figueroa E, Laska EM, et al. Safety and efficacy of gamma-vinyl GABA (GVG) for the treatment of the treatment

of methamphetamine and/or cocaine addiction. *Synapse.* 2005; 50:261–265.
155. La Garza RD 2nd, Zorick T, Heinzerling KG, et al. The cardiovascular and subjective effects of methamphetamine combined with gamma-vinyl-gamma-aminobutyric acid (GVG) in non-treatment seeking methamphetamine-dependent volunteers. *Pharmacol Biochem Behav.* 2009;94(1):186–193.
156. Rush CR, Stoops WW, Hays LR, et al. Risperidone attenuates the discriminative-stimulus effects of D-amphetamine in humans. *J Pharmacol Exp Ther.* 2003;306:195–204.
157. Lile JA, Stoops WW, Vansickel AR, et al. Aripiprazole attenuates the discriminative-stimulus and subject-rated effects of D-amphetamine in humans. *Neuropsychopharmacology.* 2005; 30:2103–2114.
158. Meredith CW, Jaffe C, Yanasak E, et al. An open-label pilot study of risperidone in the treatment of methamphetamine dependence. *J Psychoactive Drugs.* 2007;39:167–172.
159. Reid MS, Palamar J, Falmmino F, et al. *A Double-blind, Placebo-controlled Assessment of Aripiprazole Effects on Methamphetamine Craving: Inpatient Longitudinal and Cue Reactivity Studies.* Oral Presentation at the 68th Annual Scientific Conference of the College on Problems of Drug Dependence; 2006.
160. Pani L, Carboni S, Kusmin A, et al. Nimodipine inhibits cocaine-induced dopamine release and motor stimulation. *Eur J Pharmacol.* 1990;176:245–246.
161. Pucilowski O, Plaznik A, Overstreet DH. Isradipine suppresses amphetamine-induced conditioned place preference and locomotor stimulation in the rat. *Neuropsychopharmacology.* 1995;12:239–244.
162. Johnson BA, Roache JD, Bordnick PS, et al. Isradipine, a dihydropyridine-class calcium channel antagonist, attenuates some of D-methamphetamine's positive subjective effects: a preliminary study. *Psychopharmacology.* 1999;144:295–300.
163. Batki SL, Moon J, Delucchi K, et al. Amlodipine treatment of methamphetamine dependence, a controlled outpatient trial: preliminary analysis. *Drug Alcohol Depend.* 2001;63(suppl 1):12.
164. Taneja I, Diedrich A, Black BK, et al. Modafinil elicits sympathomedullary activation. *Hypertension.* 2005;45:612–618.
165. Jasinki DR. An evaluation of the abuse potential of modafinil using methylphenidate as a reference. *J Psychopharmacol.* 2000;14:53–60.
166. Rush CR, Kelly TH, Hays LR, et al. Acute behavioral and physiological effects of modafinil in drug abusers. *Behav Pharmacol.* 2002;13:105–115.
167. Sofuoglu M, Poling J, Hill K, et al. Atomoxetine attenuates dextroamphetamine effects in humans. *Am J Drug Alcohol Abuse.* 2009;35:412–416.
168. Grabowski J, Shearer J, Merrill J, et al. Agonist-like, replacement pharmacotherapy for stimulant abuse and dependence. *Addict Behav.* 2004;29:1439–1464.
169. Fleming PM, Roberts D. Is the prescription of amphetamine justified as a harm reduction measure? *J R Soc Health.* 1994; 114:127–131.
170. Pates R, Coombes N, Ford N. A pilot programme in prescribing dexamphetamine for amphetamine users (part 1). *J Subst Misuse Nurs Health Soc Care.* 1996;1:80–84.
171. McBride AJ, Sullivan G, Blewett AE, et al. Amphetamine prescribing as a harm reduction measure: a preliminary study. *Addict Res.* 1997;5:95–112.
172. Klee H, Wright S, Carnath T, et al. The role of substitute therapy in the treatment of problem amphetamine use. *Drug Alcohol Rev.* 2001;20:417–429.
173. Shearer J, Wodak A, Mattick RP, et al. Pilot randomised controlled study of dexamphetamine for amphetamine dependence. *Addiction.* 2001;96:1289–1296.
174. Spielewoy C, Biala G, Roubert C, et al. Hypolocomotor effects of acute and daily D-amphetamine in mice lacking the dopamine transporter. *Psychopharmacology.* 2001;159:2–9.
175. Palmer AA, Verbitsky M, Suresh R, et al. Gene expression differences in mice divergently selected for methamphetamine sensitivity. *Mamm Genome.* 2005;16:291–305.
176. Greengard P. The neurobiology of slow synaptic transmission. *Science.* 2001;294:1024–1030.
177. Berrettini WH, Lerman CE. Pharmacotherapy and pharmacogenetics of nicotine dependence. *Am J Psychiatry.* 2005;162: 1441–1451.
178. Wolf CR, Smith G, Smith RL. Science, medicine, and the future: pharmacogenetics. *BMJ.* 2000;320:987–990.
179. Lott DC, Kim SJ, Cook EH Jr. Serotonin transporter genotype and acute subjective response to amphetamine. *Am J Addict.* 2006;15:327–335.
180. Veenstra-Vanderweele J, Qaadir A, Palmer AA, et al. Association of the casein kinase 1 epsilon gene and subjective response to D-amphetamine. *Neuropsychopharmacology.* 2006; 31:1056–1063.
181. Dlugos A, Freitag C, Hohoff C, et al. Norepinephrine transporter gene variation modulates acute response to D-amphetamine. *Biol Psychiatry.* 2007;61:1296–1305.
182. Flanagin BA, Cook EHJ, de Wit H. An association study of the brain-derived neurotrophic factor Val66Met polymorphism and amphetamine response. *Am J Med Genet B Neuropsychiatr Genet.* 2006;14:1056–1073.
183. Mattay VS, Goldberg TE, Fera F, et al. Catechol O-methyltransferase val[158]-met genotype and individual variation in the brain response to amphetamine. *Proc Natl Acad Sci U S A.* 2003;100: 6186–6191.
184. Hohoff C, McDonald JM, Baune BT, et al. Interindividual variation in anxiety response to amphetamine: possible role for adenosine A_{2A} receptor gene variants. *Am J Med Genet.* 2005; 139:42–44.
185. Ujike H, Harano M, Inada T, et al. Nine- or fewer repeat alleles in VNTR polymorphism of the dopamine transporter gene is a strong risk factor for prolonged methamphetamine psychosis. *Pharmacogenomics J.* 2003;3:242–247.
186. Gelernter J, Kranzler HR, Satel RA, et al. Genetic association between dopamine transporter protein alleles and cocaine-induced paranoia. *Neuropsychopharmacology.* 1994;11: 195–200.
187. Ohgake S, Hashimoto K, Shimizu E. Functional polymorphism of the NQO2 gene is associated with methamphetamine psychosis. *Addict Biol.* 2005;10:145–148.
188. Hiranita T, Anggadiredja K, Fujisaki C, et al. Nicotine attenuates relapse to methamphetamine-seeking behavior (craving) in rats. *Ann N Y Acad Sci.* 2006;1025:504–507.
189. Fukami G, Hashimoto K, Koike K, et al. Effect of antioxidant N-acetyl-L-cysteine on behavioral changes and neurotoxicity in rats after administration of methamphetamine. *Brain Res.* 2004;1016:90–95.
190. Colussi-Mas J, Panayi F, Scarna H, et al. Blockade of β-adrenergic receptors prevents amphetamine-induced behavioural sensitization in rats: a putative role of the bed nucleus of the stria terminalis. *Int J Neuropsychopharmacol.* 2005;8:1–13.

CHAPTER 17 Sedative–Hypnotics

Domenic A. Ciraulo ■ Clifford M. Knapp

INTRODUCTION

The defining characteristic of sedative–hypnotics is their ability to inhibit neurotransmission in the nervous system, primarily, but not exclusively, through their action on γ-aminobutyric acid (GABA) receptor systems. Most have an established role in medical practice, although their liability for abuse, tolerance, and toxicity may restrict their use. The risk for dependence on these agents varies substantially among different agents, with those used commonly in clinical practice having relatively lower potential for misuse than those agents used purely for their hedonic effects. Abuse liability of these agents is best viewed on a continuum that takes into account the characteristics of the individual using the drug, even in a therapeutic context. This chapter first presents an overview of the sedative–hypnotics and then discusses individual agents and chemical classes in greater detail.

HISTORY

In the early 1900s barbital and phenobarbital were the first barbiturates introduced into medical practice. These drugs are derivatives of barbituric acid, which was synthesized by von Baeyer in 1864. The barbiturates are still used in modern medicine as general anesthetics, anticonvulsants, and sedatives, and in combination with other medications in products used to treat headaches, asthma, and gastrointestinal disorders. Barbiturates have a risk of lethality in overdose, tolerance, dependence, abuse, drug interactions, and a life-threatening withdrawal syndrome after abrupt discontinuation of high doses.

Given the limitations of the barbiturates, the introduction of meprobamate in 1955 and the benzodiazepine, chlordiazepoxide, in 1957 was embraced by clinicians. Meprobamate was widely prescribed as an antianxiety agent but its use declined as practitioners found that it was more likely than barbiturates to lead to a withdrawal syndrome on discontinuation, which was often severe in nature and associated with seizures. The therapeutic index also proved unfavorable, with fatalities associated with doses as low as 12 g (typical therapeutic doses are between 1.2 and 1.6 g daily, with a maximum of 2.4 g daily). Chlordiazepoxide and other benzodiazepines became the dominant antianxiety agents and hypnotics with established efficacy and less risk of lethal overdose or drug interactions. The use and availability of other sedative–hypnotics such as chloral hydrate, ethchlorvynol, glutethimide, and methprylon also declined, because they were more toxic and less effective than the benzodiazepines. Newly developed nonbenzodiazepine hypnotics, commonly referred to as the "Z-drugs," were introduced in the 1990s. These include zopiclone, eszopiclone, zolpidem, and zaleplon. These hypnotics may have subtle differences from the benzodiazepine hypnotics, although clinical experience is limited compared to benzodiazepines. The Z-drugs are associated with abuse liability, dosage escalation above recommended levels, and associated toxicity, including seizures and a withdrawal syndrome. On the other hand, some studies suggest a low risk for tolerance, physical dependence, and rebound insomnia when Z-drugs are administered as hypnotics in therapeutic doses. Another type of sedative–hypnotic is gamma-hydroxybutyrate (GHB). In the United States GHB is marketed as Xyrem and approved by the FDA for the treatment of cataplexy and excessive daytime sleepiness in narcolepsy. Its abuse liability is equivalent to ethanol and flunitrazepam (one of the most reinforcing benzodiazepines). Administration of GHB at high doses for prolonged periods in animals produces physical dependence. Human cases of dependence and life-threatening withdrawal syndromes have been reported. Most GHB use appears to be limited to intermittent use by individuals between 16 and 23 years old in social settings, although regular use may be common in other countries and specific subgroups in the United States.

EPIDEMIOLOGY

While public concern about benzodiazepine dependence has declined over the past decade, clinicians remain divided about appropriate prescribing practices. On the one hand, there is a substantial database suggesting that abuse of benzodiazepines is not a significant health problem. Supporting this position are the results of the 2008 SAMSHA National Survey of Drug Use and Health. Figures 17.1 to 17.4 from the NSDUH demonstrate that sedatives (1) are rarely the first drug abused by an individual, (2) have the lowest rate of abuse compared to other commonly misused drugs, (3) are rarely responsible for initiation of a treatment episode, and (4) when compared to marijuana (56.6%), pain relievers (22.5%), and even inhalants (9.7%), the sedatives (3.8%), and tranquilizers (3.2%) are very rarely the specific drug used when initiating illicit drug use. Benzodiazepines

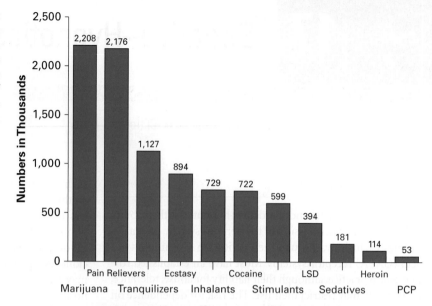

Figure 17.1. Past-year initiates for specific illicit drugs among persons aged 12 or older: 2008. (Data from Substance Abuse and Mental Health Services Administration. *Results from the 2008 National Survey on Drug Use and Health: National Findings.* Office of Applied Studies, NSDUH series H-36, HHS publication no. SMA 09-4434. Rockville, MD; 2009.)

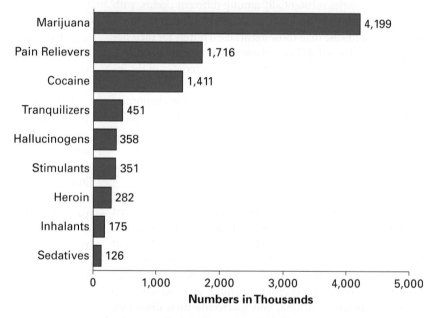

Figure 17.2. Dependence on abuse of specific illicit drugs in the past year among persons aged 12 or older: 2008. (Data from Substance Abuse and Mental Health Services Administration. *Results from the 2008 National Survey on Drug Use and Health: National Findings.* Office of Applied Studies, NSDUH series H-36, HHS publication no. SMA 09-4434. Rockville, MD; 2009.)

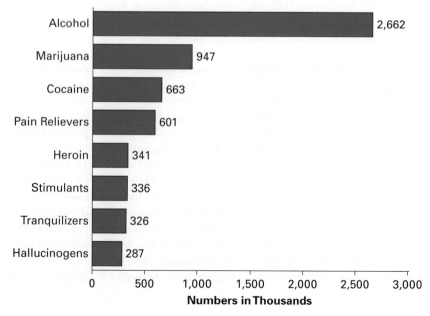

Figure 17.3. Substances for which most recent treatment was received in the past year among persons aged 12 or older: 2008. (Data from Substance Abuse and Mental Health Services Administration. *Results from the 2008 National Survey on Drug Use and Health: National Findings.* Office of Applied Studies, NSDUH series H-36, HHS publication no. SMA 09-4434. Rockville, MD; 2009.)

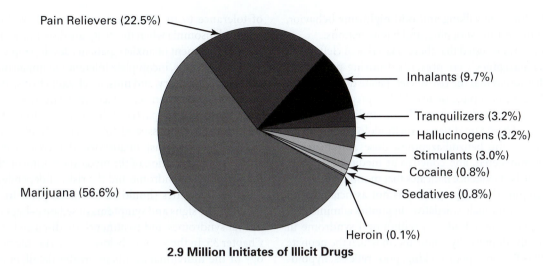

Figure 17.4. Specific drug used when initiating illicit drug use among past year initiates of illicit drugs aged 12 or older: 2008. (Data from Substance Abuse and Mental Health Services Administration. *Results from the 2008 National Survey on Drug Use and Health: National Findings.* Office of Applied Studies, NSDUH series H-36, HHS publication no. SMA 09-4434. Rockville, MD; 2009.)

are not often the primary drug of abuse leading to treatment, and when they are involved it is usually in combination with other drugs such as marijuana, opioids, and alcohol.

In addition to SAMSHA data, other survey data and expert reports show that the number of U.S. prescriptions for benzodiazepines has steadily declined from a peak of 87 million in 1973. As expected, the "Z-drugs" have increased numbers of U.S. prescriptions, but remain at relatively modest levels. The percentage of the U.S. population taking a benzodiazepine at least once during a given year varies from 7.4% to 17.6%. More consistent rates are found when duration of treatment is included. Only about 1% of the U.S. population takes prescription benzodiazepines for longer than 1 year, which is consistent with European studies reporting 1 year of medical use of 1.7% and 6-month use of approximately 3%. Long-term medical use is more common among the elderly, women, and individuals with chronic health problems or psychological disorders.

The highest rates of use and misuse occur in patients with comorbid addictions such as opioid or alcohol dependence. Approximately 15% to 20% of alcoholics presenting for treatment are also taking benzodiazepines. This is partially explained by self-medication of alcohol withdrawal and the high prevalence of substance-induced anxiety disorder in this population. Methadone patients also have very high rates of urine samples positive for nonprescribed benzodiazepines (30% to 90%). About 30% of psychiatric patients are prescribed benzodiazepines, most commonly those with long duration of illness, affective disorders, and who are frequent users of medical services. Anxiety disorder patients, as a group, do not misuse benzodiazepines, and tend to decrease the dose over time. Benzodiazepine prescriptions for anxiety disorders have declined, supplanted by the use of selective serotonin reuptake inhibitors as a first-line treatment in several types of anxiety. Patients with chronic pain also tend to use prescribed benzodiazepines in higher amounts than the general population.

COMORBIDITIES AND COMPLICATIONS OF USE

The toxicities of benzodiazepines and barbiturates differ more in severity than in the pattern of adverse consequences. All agents are CNS depressants, which at low doses produce sedation and at the highest doses may result in obtundation, coma, and death. At typical initial therapeutic doses problems with oversedation, motor impairment, slowed cognition, and amnesia may occur. At higher therapeutic doses slurred speech, ataxia, and impaired gag reflex may be observed. As a general rule when doses are kept within a therapeutic range, tolerance to many of these adverse effects occurs. For example, while initial treatment with a benzodiazepine may produce anterograde amnesia, learning difficulties, and impairment of attention and concentration, tolerance usually occurs with continued treatment. The scientific literature in this area is contradictory. Some studies have found that long-term benzodiazepine treatment does not impair cognitive function while others have seen persistent problems in learning, psychomotor function, concentration, and motor skills. Some of these contradictory findings are attributable to studies of populations taking different doses, various benzodiazepines, unknown duration of treatment, and heterogeneity of risk factors in the group studied (e.g., young vs. elderly). Elderly patients may be at risk for both cognitive difficulties and falls, although it is unclear whether these drugs present greater risks to the elderly than other sedative psychotherapeutic agents. Cognitive impairment is likely to persist in the elderly although most patients do not recognize it or feel that it does not impair their daily functioning. A somewhat unusual adverse effect has been seen with high doses of the Z-drugs. There have been several reports of Z-drug-related amnesia associated with sleepwalking and odd nighttime behavior, such as driving, eating, shopping, and hallucinations.

Early studies suggested that there was a risk of cleft palate when benzodiazepines were prescribed during pregnancy. These studies found that the risk of cleft palate doubled from 0.06% in the general population to 0.12% in pregnant woman exposed to the benzodiazepines. These studies have been highly criticized based on different methodologies, failure to control for specific benzodiazepines, dose administered, duration administered, and concurrent medications used. At present, the best evidence indicates that monotherapy with a benzodiazepine during pregnancy is not associated with major congenital anomalies. Sedative–hypnotics administered during pregnancy may lead to a withdrawal syndrome in newborns or the floppy baby syndrome, in which the neonate has low APGAR scores, poor sucking, poor reflexes, hypotonia, and apnea. Congenital abnormalities resulting from barbiturates are difficult to distinguish from those associated with other anticonvulsants because phenobarbital is usually not given as a monotherapy. When phenobarbital is given alone or in combination with other anticonvulsants, higher rates of major malformations are reported compared to mothers with a history of epilepsy who took no anticonvulsants during pregnancy.

OVERVIEW OF DETERMINANTS OF ABUSE

Sedative–hypnotics have a potential for misuse if the agent has strong euphoric or mood-altering effects, tolerance develops to its primary therapeutic effect, or the severity of the withdrawal syndrome is such that discontinuation of the drug is difficult.

Among the commonly used sedative–hypnotics, barbiturates produce the greatest pleasant mood alterations, although others, such as flunitrazepam and GHB, may be similar. Among the benzodiazepines, there are differences in the ability to induce mood enhancement associated with abuse. Theories that attempt to explain differing effects are not entirely satisfactory. The most common explanation is that drugs with a rapid onset of action, followed by a rapid termination of single-dose effects, are associated with higher abuse liability *in vulnerable populations*, such as recovering alcoholics and methadone maintenance patients. It is unlikely that pharmacokinetics explains the acute mood effects of benzodiazepines entirely; we know that binding to subtypes of the alpha subunit of the receptor may influence a variety of actions, including sedation, anxiety, memory, anticonvulsant, and perhaps hedonic effects. With respect to acute euphoric effects, immediate-release alprazolam and flunitrazepam are consistently rated by experienced substance abusers as producing a high that they like. This is consistent with clinical experience, but any sedative–hypnotic may be abused by high-risk individuals.

Tolerance to barbiturates and benzodiazepines is well established. Some evidence suggests that temazepam and the Z-drug, eszopiclone, are not associated with the development of tolerance to their hypnotic effect and have low risk of rebound insomnia when the drugs are discontinued. With respect to treatment of anxiety, patients develop rapid tolerance to sedative effects, incomplete tolerance to impairment of coordination, memory, and muscle relaxant effects, and little or no tolerance to antianxiety effects. In the treatment of seizures with clonazepam, partial tolerance develops. Clinicians should discuss the issue of tolerance with all patients, and caution them against unauthorized increases in dose or abrupt discontinuation of the medication. Information about the withdrawal syndrome and the risks of dependence on all sedative–hypnotics should be discussed prior to initiating therapy. The signs and symptoms of sedative–hypnotic withdrawal syndromes and treatments are discussed in detail in Chapter 35. In the sections below we describe the pharmacology of the individual agents in greater detail, emphasizing mechanisms of action that produce clinical effects, tolerance, and dependence.

BENZODIAZEPINES

Pharmacology

$GABA_A$ receptors act as the primary mediator of inhibition of neurotransmission in the mammalian brain. The $GABA_A$ receptor systems play a major role in mediating the actions of most of the sedative–hypnotic agents in current use. $GABA_A$ receptors are ligand-gated chloride channels that are commonly formed by five subunits. The subunit composition of these receptors, in conjunction with their precise location in the neuronal tissues, determines their functional and pharmacologic properties. Nineteen types of $GABA_A$ subunits have been identified and can be divided into seven distinct families. The α, β, δ, and λ families combine to form the receptors that are the primary targets of the sedative–hypnotic agents. There are six members of the α family (α_1 to α_6), four members of the β family, and three of the λ family. The subunit composition of $GABA_A$ receptors in the brain most frequently consists of two α subunits and two β subunits that exist in association with a γ or δ subunit. Receptors with the $\alpha_1\beta_2\gamma_2$ mix of subunits occur with the greatest frequency in the brain.

GABA binds at the interface between the α and β subunits of the $GABA_A$ receptors. Benzodiazepines bind at the interface of α and γ subunits. Binding of GABA to the $GABA_A$ receptor opens a chloride channel, which results in most instances in hyperpolarization of the neuron. The binding of benzodiazepine produces an allosteric modification in the GABA binding site. This modification usually leads to an increase in the frequency of the opening of the chloride channel.

$GABA_A$ receptors that are sensitive to the benzodiazepines contain α subunits 1, 2, 3, or 5, combined with two β subunits and a γ subunit. $GABA_A$ receptors containing the α_4 and α_6 subunits may be insensitive to the effects of benzodiazepines (1). This may be of significance because the α_4 and α_6 subunits in combination with δ subunit may localize primarily in extrasynaptic regions of the neuron, and may consequently act to regulate the tonic inhibitory as opposed to the synaptic phasic inhibitory effects of GABA (2). There is now increasing evidence that tonic currents play a major role in controlling neuronal excitability. The ability of drugs to interact with receptors that regulate tonic currents may determine the extent to which they can influence seizures, sleep, and other brain activity.

Data from animal studies suggest that $GABA_A$ receptors containing different types of the α subunit appear to mediate distinct behavioral effects of benzodiazepines and other benzodiazepine receptor agonists. Receptors containing the α_1 subunit have been implicated in the production of sedation, amnesia, antiseizure effects, and ataxia (3). The presence of the α_2 and α_3 subunits is associated with the anxiolytic and muscle relaxant-inducing effects of the benzodiazepine receptor agonists (4). The behavioral effects of benzodiazepine agonist stimulation of the α_5 subunit containing receptors remain to be elucidated. However, it has been shown that learning and memory functions appear to be enhanced in animals missing the α_5 subunit suggesting that benzodiazepine might produce impairment of cognition by interacting with receptors that have this subunit (5).

Determinants of Abuse

Abuse liability of benzodiazepines has been assessed in animal models, human laboratory studies, and surveys of substance abusers, patients, and the general population. With respect to animal models, the most consistent finding indicating abuse liability is produced by models using continuous drug access, that is, drug self-administration models. Other models such as place preference show weaker signals; however, diazepam and barbiturates do exhibit reinforcing effects in these models. Human laboratory studies rely on two basic models: (1) self-administration of sedative–hypnotics and placebo by individuals with a history of substance abuse and (2) determination of subjective mood effects such as "high" or "liking" after a single dose of drug. In addition, surveys of clinical populations of individuals being treated for addictive disorders ask subjects to rate the abuse liability of a variety of drugs. In general, all of these models consistently show that the benzodiazepines have a moderate potential for abuse that is substantially lower than that of methaqualone, barbiturates, and older sedative–hypnotics, such as chloral hydrate. Among the benzodiazepines themselves the preponderance of evidence suggests that flunitrazepam, diazepam, lorazepam, alprazolam, and triazolam have higher abuse potential than chlordiazepoxide or oxazepam. It is unclear whether these research findings have practical clinical significance because the abuse of this class of drugs depends more on patient characteristics than benzodiazepine-induced acute subjective effects. Individuals at high risk include alcoholics, opioid addicts, and individuals with mixed substance abuse problems. In clinical situations, tolerance to the therapeutic action may result in unauthorized dosage escalation.

Evidence of tolerance to the benzodiazepines includes the observation that diazepam-induced chloride influx into cortical membrane vesicles is reduced after chronic exposure to this drug (6). Several mechanisms have been implicated in the development of tolerance to the benzodiazepines. Exposure to these benzodiazepines leads to uncoupling between the benzodiazepine and GABA receptor sites, that is, there is a decrease in the allosteric interactions between these sites (7). This, in part, may be the result of the internalization of $GABA_A$ receptors originally located on the surface of neurons.

Chronic treatment with benzodiazepines may result in the modification of the subunit composition of brain $GABA_A$ receptors. For example, animal studies suggest that proteins for the hippocampal and cortical α_1 and β_3 subunits may be reduced by chronic benzodiazepine treatment (8). Hippocampal α_5 subunits may decrease in density following prolonged treatment with benzodiazepines (9), but increases in the messenger RNA (mRNA) for this subunit have been observed in the cortical tissues of rats treated chronically with diazepam (10). Withdrawal from chronic diazepam exposure, in contrast, results in the upregulation of α_4 subunit mRNA in rat cerebellar tissue (11). Changes in $GABA_A$ receptor subunit composition may be one of the factors that contribute to development of tolerance to benzodiazepines.

In addition to effects on $GABA_A$ receptor systems, chronic benzodiazepine exposure alters the activity of other systems that are involved in the regulation of neuronal activity. Voltage-gated calcium channels help to regulate the influx of calcium ions into the neuron, which serve as major signaling ion within these cells. Prolonged exposure to benzodiazepines may lead to the upregulation of L-type high voltage-gated calcium channel subunits and voltage-gated channel currents are increased during chronic benzodiazepine treatment (12). Coadministration of the L-type calcium channel antagonist, nimodipine, with benzodiazepines blocks the development of tolerance in $GABA_A$-mediated synaptic currents (12).

Prolonged treatment with benzodiazepines also alters the activity of amino-3-hydroxy-5-methyl-4-isoxazole (AMPA), which mediates the effects of the excitatory neurotransmitter glutamate. Chronic benzodiazepine exposure also increases hippocampal AMPA receptor currents and AMPA receptor binding sites (13), an effect that is blocked by pretreatment with nimodipine (12). These increases are correlated with increases in anxiety during withdrawal from benzodiazepines. Benzodiazepine-induced increases in AMPA receptor currents and withdrawal anxiety can be attenuated by the concurrent administration of nimodipine.

Most benzodiazepines undergo rapid and extensive absorption after being administered orally. Up to 50% of midazolam, however, may be metabolized in the liver by the cytochrome P450 enzyme CYP 3A5 following oral administration of this drug. The highly lipophilic benzodiazepines, such as diazepam, readily cross the blood–brain barrier to exert their effects in the brain, but then may quickly redistribute into other tissues. The onset of action of less lipophilic agents, such as lorazepam, may be somewhat delayed.

TABLE 17.1 — Benzodiazepine and Z-drugs, active metabolites of these drugs, $T_{1/2}$ (half-life in hours) of parent drugs, and known major P450 cytochromes implicated in mediating the hepatic metabolism of these agents

Drug	$T_{1/2}$	Active metabolites	p450 cytochrome
Benzodiazepines			
■ Alprazolam	12 to 15	α-Hydroxy-alprazolam	CYP3A4&A5
■ Clonazepam	19 to 60	Inactive only	CYP3A4
■ Chlordiazepoxide	10 to 30	Desmethylchlordiazepoxide, demoxepam, nordazepam, oxazepam	
■ Clorazepate	Prodrug	Nordazepam, oxazepam	
■ Diazepam	20 to 70	Nordazepam, oxazepam	CYP2C19, CYP3A4
■ Estazolam	16	1-Oxo-estazolam	
■ Flurazepam	74	N-Hydroxyethyl-flurezapam, N-Desalkyflurazepam	
■ Lorazepam	10 to 20	Inactive only	
■ Midazolam	1 to 4	α-Hydroxy-midazolam	CYP3A4&A5
■ Oxazepam	5 to 10	Inactive only	
■ Quazepam	39	2-Oxo-quazepam, N-Desalkyflurazepam	CYP2C19, CYP3A4
■ Temazepam	10 to 15	Oxazepam	
■ Triazolam	2 to 4	α-Hydroxy-triazolam	CYP3A4
Z-drugs			
■ Eszopiclone	6	(S)-N-Desmethyl zopiclone	CYP3A4, CYP2E1
■ Zaleplon	1	Inactive only	CYP3A4
■ Zolpidem	2.1	Inactive only	CYP3A4, CYP1A2, CYP2C9

Most of the benzodiazepines in use undergo biotransformation in the liver in reactions catalyzed by a variety of cytochrome P450 enzymes. Active metabolites of the benzodiazepines are shown in Table 17.1 as are the known cytochrome enzymes implicated in their metabolism. Because a variety of drugs can alter the activity of the cytochrome P450 enzymes, the pharmacokinetic properties of the benzodiazepines that undergo hepatic metabolism have the potential of being involved in adverse drug–drug interactions. There is also a possibility that impairment of liver function as may occur in aging or a number of hepatic disorders may place patients at risk for developing benzodiazepine toxicity.

Benzodiazepines and their metabolites are frequently conjugated with glucuronide prior to their being excreted in the urine. A few benzodiazepines including lorazepam and oxazepam only undergo glucuronidation prior to being excreted. These drugs offer the advantage being unlikely to interact with other drugs and of being safer to use in individuals with compromised hepatic function.

Alprazolam, midazolam, and triazolam are hydroxylated prior to being conjugated with glucuronide. In addition to hydroxylation benzodiazepine metabolites may also be the product of demethylation and nitroreduction. Clonazepam undergoes nitroreduction, catalyzed by CYP 3A4 to form inactive metabolites. Some of the older benzodiazepines including chlordiazepoxide, diazepam, and flurazepam may be transformed into a variety of active metabolites that may greatly extend the duration of action of these drugs. Diazepam, for example, is converted to nordazepam, which has a half-life of between 50 and 180 hours.

Z-DRUGS

Several nonbenzodiazepine drugs have been developed that share many of the pharmacologic actions of the benzodiazepines. These agents include the cyclopyrrolones, zopiclone and its S-enantiomer, eszopiclone, the imidazopridine, zolpidem, and the pyrazolopyrimidine, zaleplon. Although these agents do not form a single specific class of drugs, for convenience this group of drugs can be designated as being the "Z-drugs." These drugs are able to induce sleep at doses that produce lower levels of residual sedation and residual functional impairment in cognitive and psychomotor tasks versus barbiturate or benzodiazepine hypnotic agents. As compared to the barbiturates and the benzodiazepines, the Z-drugs do not produce marked undesirable changes in sleep architecture (14). There is, however, some evidence that zopiclone may produce modest suppression of REM sleep (15), but this drug did not significantly alter REM sleep when used in a therapeutic dose in a clinical trial (16). In addition to sedative–hypnotic effects, these drugs have amnesic effects, anticonvulsant actions, anxiolytic activity, motor-impairing effects, and muscle relaxant effects (17,18). The Z-drugs show less pronounced amnesic and antianxiety effects than do the benzodiazepines (17).

Zaleplon and zolpidem may produce alterations in vision that may include altered color perception, pulsating of light, and room spinning. Common adverse effects associated with the use of zolpidem include headache, somnolence, dizziness, and nausea. This drug may produce hallucinations when administered concurrently with serotonin reuptake inhibitors. Eszopiclone and zopiclone, in addition to sedation, may produce dry mouth and a metallic taste (14). Complex behaviors during sleep including sleepwalking, driving, eating, and cooking have been reported to occur in patients being treated with Z-drugs.

Pharmacology

The Z-drugs may activate the benzodiazepine receptor site located on the $GABA_A$ receptor complex. The actions of these drugs are antagonized by the administration of the benzodiazepine receptor antagonist flumazenil. Eszopiclone, zopiclone, and zolpidem have been demonstrated to bind in the region of the benzodiazepine binding site, but they may differ from the benzodiazepines and from each other with respect to precisely which amino acid residues within this site are essential for their activity.

The Z-drugs all potentiate GABA-mediated currents in neurons containing $GABA_A$ receptors. This action produces an increase in chloride ion conductance. Binding studies, however, suggest that these agents may differ in their affinity for $GABA_A$ receptors with different α subunit compositions than do the benzodiazepines (19). Electrophysiologic studies indicate these differences may have functional significance. Like the benzodiazepines, the Z-drugs have a low affinity for $GABA_A$ receptors that contain the α_4 and α_6 subunits. Zolpidem is between 5 and 10 times more selective for α_1-containing $GABA_A$ receptors than it is for α_2- and α_3-containing receptors, while having extremely low selectivity for receptors containing the α_5 subunit. Zaleplon has two- to threefold greater selectivity for α_1-containing receptors as compared to those having α_2 and α_3 subunits. This drug has minimal actions on $GABA_A$ receptors that have α_5 subunits. In contrast to zolpidem and zaleplon, zopiclone has almost equal selectivity for α_1- and α_5-containing receptors, while having between four and eight times less selectivity for those receptors with α_2 and α_3. Compared to benzodiazepines, then, the Z-drugs have modest degree of selectivity for receptors containing α_1 subunits as compared to those with α_2 or α_3 subunits.

Evidence from animal studies is consistent with the idea that zolpidem acts selectively on $GABA_A$ receptors containing α_1 subunits to produce its behavioral effects. These findings include the observations that the hypnotic, sedative, motor-impairing, and anticonvulsant effects of this drug are attenuated by either selective genetic deletion of the α_1 subunits or the administration of select α_1 subunit antagonists (3).

Animal studies indicate that zolpidem and, to a lesser degree, zaleplon have greater potency as hypnotic agents than as muscle relaxants (19). Zopiclone, in contrast, produces its hypnotic and muscle relaxant effects at similar doses. The modest differences in the selectivity of the Z-drugs for $GABA_A$ receptors containing α_1 subunits may not be great enough to completely explain the minimal residual adverse effects seen after these agents have been used to treat insomnia.

The effects of the Z-drugs on receptor systems other than the $GABA_A$ systems have not been extensively explored. Zaleplon has been shown to have little affinity for dopamine, muscarinic, noradrenergic, opioid, and serotoninergic receptors. Zopiclone can inhibit the activity of both nicotinic receptor and N-methyl-D-aspartate (NMDA) receptors, which mediate the effects of excitatory amino acids, such as glutamate (20).

The receptor changes that occur after chronic Z-drug treatment have not been thoroughly studied. In the rat repeated zolpidem administration is associated with an increase in cortical mRNA levels for the α_4 and β_1 $GABA_A$ receptor subunits after 7 days and a decrease in mRNA for the α_1 subunit after 14 days (21). Chronic exposure to either zaleplon or zolpidem of cell cultures containing rat cerebellar granule cells results in an elevation in mRNA for the α_4 subunit and a reduction in mRNA for α_1 and γ_2 subunits during withdrawal from either zolpidem or zaleplon (22).

Animals treated chronically with flurazepam show tolerance to the inhibitory effects of zolpidem in the hippocampus (12). Administration of the L-type calcium channel blocker, nimodipine, did not block the development of flurazepam-induced tolerance to the inhibitory effects of zolpidem in the hippocampus. This suggests that in contrast to the benzodiazepines, L-type voltage-gated calcium channels may not be implicated in the development of tolerance to zolpidem.

The pharmacokinetic properties of the Z-drugs may be one of the factors that explain the lower incidence of residual adverse effects that are associated with their use. The elimination half-life of zolpidem is approximately 2 hours while that of zaleplon is 1 hour (see Table 17.1) (17). Eszopiclone has comparatively longer half-life of 4 hours, which can reach up to 7 hours in elderly individuals (14). Both zolpidem and zaleplon are metabolized in the liver into inactive metabolites (17). Zopiclone is metabolized to N-oxide zopiclone and desmethylzopiclone. The N-oxide metabolite has some activity. The oxide metabolite of eszopiclone, (S)-zopiclone-N-oxide, does not bind to $GABA_A$ receptors while the (S)-desmethylzopiclone metabolite of this drug may have anxiolytic effects.

Because zopiclone and eszopiclone are more slowly eliminated than are zolpidem or zaleplon, they can help to maintain sleep throughout the night. Zopiclone has been shown to produce psychomotor impairment 7 hours following its administration. A sustained-release formulation of zolpidem is currently being marketed and a sustained-release formulation of zaleplon is in development. These sustained-release formulations are designed to allow patients to maintain sleep throughout the night when being treated with either zaleplon or zolpidem for insomnia.

Determinants of Abuse

There are a number of case reports of Z-drug-related abuse and dependence. In many instances extremely high doses of drugs may be self-administered. Doses of zolpidem in cases of abuse are often in the range of hundreds of milligrams being administered daily. This is in comparison with a therapeutic dose of zolpidem of about 10 mg daily.

Many individuals who misuse zolpidem have reported using the drug not for its sedative effects, but rather for its anxiolytic, euphoric, or stimulant effects. Human laboratory studies of the effects of Z-drugs indicate that these drugs may produce stimulus effects that present some risk for abuse. In social drinkers zolpidem administration increased ratings of drug liking, but did not elevate scores on the Addiction Research Center Inventory-Morphine Benzedrine Group subscale (ARCG-MBG), a subscale that is sensitive to drug-induced euphoria (23). The drug-liking effects of zolpidem in these subjects were not found to be additive with those of alcohol. Subjects with a history of sedative abuse reported greater liking of triazolam and zolpidem than placebo (24). In subjects with a history of alcohol and drug abuse, higher doses of zolpidem produced elevations in scores for drug-liking and good effects (25). Zolpidem administration also resulted in elevations in rating of drug high and good effects in healthy subjects, who found triazolam and pentobarbital to have similar stimulus effects to those of zolpidem (25).

The results of several studies suggest that the risk for the development of tolerance, physical dependence, and withdrawal is low when therapeutic doses of the Z-drugs are used to treat insomnia. For example, no tolerance to the sleep-inducing effects of either zaleplon or zolpidem was seen when administered for several weeks. Tolerance was not observed to the hypnotic effects of eszopiclone or a sustained formulation of zolpidem when subjects were treated with this agent for primary insomnia over a 6-month period (26,27). Several studies also indicate that no rebound insomnia was observed after discontinuation of the Z-drugs. In contrast, there are some studies that indicate that modest increases in anxiety and reduced sleep were observed in subjects treated with immediate-release formulations of zaleplon, zopiclone, or zolpidem (28,29). This has also been observed in individuals being treated with a sustained-released formulation of zolpidem (30). Overall, results from sleep trials suggest that dependence and withdrawal may not be problematic for patients being treated for insomnia with therapeutic doses of Z-drugs.

Animal studies have been conducted to determine whether Z-drugs can produce physical dependence with prolonged administration of these agents. Chronic administration of zolpidem did not result in physical dependence in mice (31). In contrast, work in primates has demonstrated that Z-drugs can produce physical dependence. In monkeys, the discontinuation of chronic zopiclone administration resulted in symptoms of withdrawal including apprehension, hyperirritability, and motor impairment (32). Flumazenil-induced withdrawal from zolpidem produced withdrawal signs that were moderate in severity in baboons that included tremor, jerk, and rigid posture (33).

Several case reports have been published that suggest that problems of dependence and withdrawal may occur in humans receiving Z-drugs (34). Seizures have been observed after the discontinuation of zolpidem in individuals using extremely high doses of this agent (34), as have other signs of withdrawal including tremor, agitation, and anxiety.

BARBITURATES

Barbiturates are barbituric acid derivatives. Prior to the introduction of the benzodiazepines, the barbiturates were extensively used as sedative–hypnotic agents. They also have been administered for their anticonvulsant effects and as anesthetic agents. The therapeutic indices of the barbiturates are comparatively low and toxic reactions, sometimes resulting in death, were frequent occurrences associated with the use of these agents. It, also, has been evident since the early 1950s that the use of these drugs is associated with a high risk of abuse and forms of dependence that can lead to severe, sometimes lethal episodes of withdrawal.

As with the benzodiazepines, barbiturates have been used in the treatment of insomnia, seizure disorders, and anxiety disorders and to produce sedation and to induce anesthesia. Barbiturates with short to intermediate ranges of duration of action, that is, from 3 to 12 hours, including amobarbital, butabarbital, pentobarbital, and secobarbital, are currently used as sedative–hypnotic agents. Butalbital is used as a sedative component of antimigraine combination agents that also contain caffeine and either aspirin or acetaminophen. Long-acting, less lipophilic barbiturates such as mephobarbital and phenobarbital are used primarily as anticonvulsant agents. The highly lipophilic, ultrashort-acting barbiturates, methohexital and thiopental, are used in the induction of anesthesia.

The barbiturates produce depression of central nervous system activity that can range from sedation to sleep, anesthesia, and finally coma. These agents are not selective in their actions and their antianxiety effects are not separable from their other depressant effects. The barbiturates will reduce slow wave and REM sleep. Respiratory depression produced by the barbiturates, often in combination with other CNS depressants, may be a major contributory factor to death in cases of barbiturate overdoses.

Adverse effects of the barbiturates include sedation and disruption of motor coordination. In some patients, for example, in elderly individuals, the administration of a barbiturate may lead to the appearance of paradoxical excitement. Allergic reactions may occur in some patients receiving barbiturates and exfolative dermatitis may sometimes be caused by phenobarbital administration.

Chronic barbiturate intoxication may produce somnolence, confusion, ataxia, nystagmus, coarse tremor, and emotional instability. Severe barbiturate toxicity may lead to coma and respiratory depression. Respiratory depression can cause respiratory acidosis and cerebral hypoxia. Fatal complication of barbiturate toxicity may include pulmonary complications such as pulmonary edema and renal failure.

Pharmacology

With respect to their actions at the $GABA_A$ receptor complex, low concentrations of barbiturates act as positive allosteric modulators of GABA action at the receptor. At higher concentrations the barbiturates may directly activate the $GABA_A$ receptor. Millimolar concentrations of barbiturates appear to block the $GABA_A$ receptor. The extent of activation of the $GABA_A$ receptor system by barbiturates is dependent on the subunit composition of the receptor. The type α subunit contained in the $GABA_A$ receptor may be a major determinant of the degree of receptor activation by barbiturates. For example, pentobarbital produces greater potentiation of the effects of GABA in receptors containing the α_6 as compared to the α_1 subunit (35). The maximum direct effect of this drug on $GABA_A$ receptors was greatest in those receptors with α_6 as compared with those containing α_2 or α_5 subunits. In contrast to the benzodiazepines, pentobarbital also strongly activates $GABA_A$ receptors containing the α_4 subunit.

Actions of the barbiturates may not be limited to their effects on $GABA_A$ receptors. Ionotropic glutamate receptors may be subject to inhibition produced by barbiturate administration. Thiopental may decrease the activity of NMDA excitatory glutamate receptors, while phenobarbital appears to be ineffective in blocking the effects of NMDA (36,37). Thiopental and pentobarbital when administered may have inhibitory actions on AMPA receptors (38). In vitro, the sensitivity of AMPA receptors to pentobarbital is increased when these receptors contain the AMPA GluR2 subunit (38). Genetic deletion of the GluR2 subunit, however, results, paradoxically, in enhanced sensitivity of mice to the anesthetic effects of pentobarbital (39).

Barbiturates have inhibitory effects on voltage-gated calcium ion channels (40). This effect may lead to the inhibition of the stimulated release of noradrenaline and dopamine produced by thiopental, pentobarbital, and phenobarbital (41). Pentobarbital may also block calcium-dependent release of other neurotransmitters including GABA, glutamate, and acetylcholine (42,43).

The barbiturates are inactivated by hepatic metabolism, with oxidation being an important step in the biotransformation of most of these drugs. Approximately 25% of a dose of phenobarbital is excreted in the urine in unchanged form. Phenobarbital and other barbiturates induce cytochrome P450 enzymes in the liver. Cytochrome enzymes induced by phenobarbital exposure include CYP2B6, CYP2C9, and CYP3A4. Consequently, the chronic administration of phenobarbital has the potential to reduce the plasma concentrations of a large number of drugs.

Determinants of Abuse

While barbiturates may present a high risk for the development of dependence in many patient populations, this may not always be the case. The risk of developing dependence in seizure patients being treated with barbiturates may be low, but a small percentage of these patients do report feelings of craving and may use higher than prescribed doses of their medication (44).

In the laboratory setting the positive effects of pentobarbital have been shown to be greater than those of benzodiazepines (45). Healthy subjects rated a 100-mg dose of pentobarbital as producing greater "high" and "good effects" than placebo (46). This occurred in conjunction with larger pentobarbital-induced increases in ratings of drowsiness, sleepiness, and performance impairment.

Long-term use of the barbiturates can result in physical dependence characterized by a severe, sometimes life-threatening withdrawal syndrome. Delirium and seizures may appear during withdrawal. Withdrawal can be a problem for seizure patients who have discontinued treatment with phenobarbital. Migraine patients receiving butalbital containing combination drugs for extended periods of time are also at risk of developing withdrawal symptoms, which can include the onset of generalized seizures.

Tolerance to the barbiturates may result from both pharmacokinetic and pharmacodynamic factors. The ability of barbiturates such as phenobarbital to induce hepatic metabolic enzymes may lead to an increase in the rate of their own elimination, thus producing "pharmacokinetic" tolerance. Chronic exposure to pentobarbital can lead to the decrease in the interaction between the barbiturate and GABA recognition sites producing pharmacodynamic tolerance (7).

Prolonged exposure to pentobarbital results in the upregulation of cerebellar δ $GABA_A$ receptor subunit mRNA in tolerant rats, and downregulation of this subunit mRNA occurs during withdrawal from this agent (47). Pentobarbital tolerant rats show an increase in mRNA for α_6 subunit. The subunit composition of NMDA receptors, which mediate the excitatory effects of glutamate, may also change in response to chronic barbiturate exposure. NMDA receptor subunits also may be altered by chronic pentobarbital treatment. NMDA NR2B subunit mRNA is decreased in the parietal cortex and hippocampus, in animals made tolerant to pentobarbital and in animals withdrawn from this drug, while the opposite result was seen for cortical NR2A subunit (48).

γ-HYDROXYBUTYRATE (OXYBATE)

GHB is a short-chain fatty acid that is found in both the brain and peripheral tissues (49). Endogenous GHB may act as either a neurotransmitter or a neuromodulator. Synthetic GHB is used as a therapeutic agent and as a drug of abuse, but at doses that produce concentrations that are several orders of magnitude greater than those produced endogenously.

GHB is approved in the United States for the treatment of cataplexy and excessive daytime sleepiness in narcolepsy patients (49). This drug is used in Europe in the management of alcohol dependence and withdrawal. GHB has been abused, often in nightclub settings, sometimes in combination with other "club" drugs such as 3,4-methylenedioxymethamphetamine (MDMA) and ketamine. It also has been administered to women prior to sexual assault as a so-called "date-rape" drug.

GHB was available in the 1980s and early 1990s as a natural supplement, but is now classified as a controlled substance in the United States (50). Other designations for GHB include γ-hydroxybutyric acid, 4-hydroxybutanoic acid, and oxybate. The sodium salt of oxybate is marketed under the trade name Xyrem. GHB is called a variety of street names including "G," GHB, Georgia Home Boy, Grievous Bodily Harm, "liquid ecstasy," and "liquid X." Precursors of GHB, γ-butyrolactone and 1,4-butanediol may be used as substitutes for GHB, because they can produce the same range of effects. This may sometimes occur when products sold as GHB contain precursors of this drug.

Exogenously administered GHB undergoes rapid absorption from the gastrointestinal tract and then readily crosses the blood–brain barrier. This agent can cause sedation and induce sleep, and at higher doses produce anesthesia. Subjects who abuse GHB report that this drug can cause euphoria, disinhibition, and increased libido. Other pharmacologic effects of this agent include impairment of motor coordination.

GHB has a low therapeutic index (49). Toxic doses of GHB can produce coma, respiratory depression, myoclonus, seizures, bradycardia, and death. Respiratory depression, pulmonary edema, and positional asphyxia may be contributory factors to death resulting from GHB. Intoxication with GHB frequently occurs while other abused substances are being used, such as ethanol, that act synergistically to enhance the toxicity of GHB.

Pharmacology

In the brain, GHB is the product of the transformation of succinic semialdehyde, a GABA metabolite with the conversion reaction being mediated by the enzyme semialdehyde reductase (49,50). GABA is converted into succinic semialdehyde by the enzyme GABA transaminase. This reaction is reversible and succinic semialdehyde can then undergo biotransformation into GABA. Semialdehyde reductase is found in GABA-containing neurons. GABA and GHB may colocalize in inhibitory nerve terminals.

The precise physiologic role of endogenous GHB remains unclear. Specific high-affinity binding sites have been found in the brain for this substance including in hippocampus, cortex, and thalamus. Selective GHB receptors have been isolated and cloned. They appear to be orphan G-protein-coupled receptors. The behavioral effects of activation of selective GHB receptors remain to be elucidated. GHB-induced excitation of neurons in the prefrontal cortex is blocked by the administration of the selective GHB receptor antagonist NCS-382 (50).

GHB acts as a partial agonist at $GABA_B$ receptors. Millimolar concentrations of GHB are required to activate these receptors (50). Consequently, the activity of GHB at the $GABA_B$ receptor is of most relevance to the actions of this compound when it is exogenously administered. Behavioral manifestations of GHB-induced sedation include decreased locomotor activity, catalepsy, and loss of righting reflex. The administration of $GABA_B$ antagonists can block these effects (50). Reductions in locomotor activity produced by treatment with either GHB or γ-butyrolactone are not observed in mice who do not express the $GABA_B$ receptor (51).

The administration of GHB has an overall effect of producing a mild stimulatory effect on the firing of dopamine neurons in the ventral tegmental area (52). The activity of neurons in the nucleus accumbens is decreased by the administration of GHB. The activation of VTA dopamine neurons and the inhibition of nucleus accumbens neurons are characteristic changes in the mesolimbic system produced by a variety of abused substances.

GHB is readily absorbed when administered orally. Peak concentrations of this drug are attained in less than an hour following oral ingestion. The primary route of metabolism of GHB is oxidation to succinic semialdehyde by succinic semialdehyde dehydrogenase. GHB is rapidly eliminated with its half-life being in the range of 20 to 40 minutes. The rapid elimination of this compound makes it difficult to detect its use by utilizing chemical assays. Also, as a consequence of its short half-life, rapid reversal of the effects of GHB may occur, with rapid transitions from a state of unconsciousness to being alert in users being seen following ingestion of a large dose of this compound.

γ-Butyrolactone and 1,4-butanediol are biotransformed in humans into GHB. Both of these agents have been abused (49). Circulating lactonases mediate the conversion of γ-butyrolactone into GHB. Alcohol dehydrogenase and aldehyde dehydrogenase catalyze the conversion of 1,4-butanediol into GHB (49). Concurrent use of ethanol with 1,4-butanediol may result in competition between these compounds for alcohol dehydrogenase.

Determinants of Abuse

GHB is self-administered by rodents, but has not been consistently self-administered by monkeys. Clearer evidence of the high likelihood of GHB being abused is provided by human laboratory studies. In the human laboratory setting, GHB administration leads to responses in both abusers of sedative–hypnotics and GHB club users that include elevated ratings of drug-liking and good effects (45). Club users of this drug show elevations in ARCI-MBG scores and stimulation following GHB administration. The positive effects of GHB were at least comparable to those of ethanol and flunitrazepam in club users. In contrast to these two other agents,

GHB also produced bad effects including dizziness, confusion, and dysphoria as measured by the ARCI-LSD subscale. Sedative–hypnotic users also indicated experiencing nausea and other symptoms of gastrointestinal distress after the ingestion of GHB. GHB also produced impairments in memory function and psychomotor performance. At high doses GHB had a sedative effect in sedative–hypnotic users.

Tolerance to the sedative effects of GHB and signs of dependence during discontinuation of this agent were not observed in subjects receiving therapeutic doses of this drug (53). Case reports indicate that daily administration of high doses of either GHB (in the range of 20 g/day) or γ-butyrolactone may produce physical dependence (54). Experimental studies in baboons support the idea that the prolonged administration of high doses of either GHB or γ-butyrolactone can result in physical dependence (55).

CONCLUSION

Barbiturates have been used to treat a variety of disorders but possess the highest abuse liability of the sedative–hypnotics presently in common medical use. Their low therapeutic index poses high risks of toxicity, including lethal overdoses and severe withdrawal syndromes on drug discontinuation. In contrast, benzodiazepines are characterized by large margins of safety. Benzodiazepines are associated with moderate levels of risk for abuse and dependence, particularly in certain substance-using populations. Toxicity and rates of abuse for benzodiazepines are dramatically less than the barbiturates.

The Z-drugs appear to be an incremental advance over the benzodiazepines with regard to the safety of their use in the treatment of insomnia. There seems to be some, but comparatively lower risk of the development of problems related to abuse and dependence with these agents than the benzodiazepines, but more extensive prescribing experience is required to establish if these are clinically relevant differences.

GHB produces subjective effects that are similar to those produced by other sedative–hypnotic agents. It is interesting that in contrast to the other sedative–hypnotic agents, the effects of GHB appear not be mediated by the $GABA_A$ receptor complex. With respect to its abuse liability, there is clear reason for concern regarding misuse because it produces positive stimulus effects that are at least equal to those of flunitrazepam and ethanol.

REFERENCES

1. Gunnersen D, Kaufman CM, Skolnick P. Pharmacological properties of recombinant "diazepam-insensitive" GABAA receptors. *Neuropharmacology*. 1996;35(9–10):1307–1314.
2. Belelli D, Harrison NL, Maguire J, et al. Extrasynaptic GABAA receptors: form, pharmacology, and function. *J Neurosci*. 2009;29(41):12757–12763.
3. Kralic JE, O'Buckley TK, Khisti RT, et al. GABA(A) receptor alpha-1 subunit deletion alters receptor subtype assembly, pharmacological and behavioral responses to benzodiazepines and zolpidem. *Neuropharmacology*. 2002;43(4):685–694.
4. Morris HV, Dawson GR, Reynolds DS, et al. Both alpha2 and alpha3 GABAA receptor subtypes mediate the anxiolytic properties of benzodiazepine site ligands in the conditioned emotional response paradigm. *Eur J Neurosci*. 2006;23(9):2495–2504.
5. Collinson N, Kuenzi FM, Jarolimek W, et al. Enhanced learning and memory and altered GABAergic synaptic transmission in mice lacking the alpha 5 subunit of the GABAA receptor. *J Neurosci*. 2002;22(13):5572–5580.
6. Marley RJ, Gallager DW. Chronic diazepam treatment produces regionally specific changes in GABA-stimulated chloride influx. *Eur J Pharmacol*. 1989;159(3):217–223.
7. Friedman LK, Gibbs TT, Farb DH. Gamma-aminobutyric acid A receptor regulation: heterologous uncoupling of modulatory site interactions induced by chronic steroid, barbiturate, benzodiazepine, or GABA treatment in culture. *Brain Res*. 1996;707(1):100–109.
8. Chen S, Huang X, Zeng XJ, et al. Benzodiazepine-mediated regulation of alpha1, alpha2, beta1–3 and gamma2 GABA(A) receptor subunit proteins in the rat brain hippocampus and cortex. *Neuroscience*. 1999;93(1):33–44.
9. Li M, Szabo A, Rosenberg HC. Down-regulation of benzodiazepine binding to alpha 5 subunit-containing gamma-aminobutyric acid(A) receptors in tolerant rat brain indicates particular involvement of the hippocampal CA1 region. *J Pharmacol Exp Ther*. 2000;295(2):689–696.
10. Holt RA, Bateson AN, Martin IL. Chronic treatment with diazepam or abecarnil differently affects the expression of GABAA receptor subunit mRNAs in the rat cortex. *Neuropharmacology*. 1996;35(9–10):1457–1463.
11. Follesa P, Cagetti E, Mancuso L, et al. Increase in expression of the GABA(A) receptor alpha(4) subunit gene induced by withdrawal of, but not by long-term treatment with, benzodiazepine full or partial agonists. *Brain Res Mol Brain Res*. 2001;92(1–2):138–148.
12. Xiang K, Earl DE, Davis KM, et al. Chronic benzodiazepine administration potentiates high voltage-activated calcium currents in hippocampal CA1 neurons. *J Pharmacol Exp Ther*. 2008;327(3):872–883.
13. Allison C, Pratt JA, Ripley TL, et al. α-Amino-3-hydroxy-5-methylisoxazole-4-propionate receptor autoradiography in mouse brain after single and repeated withdrawal from diazepam. *Eur J Neurosci*. 2005;21(4):1045–1056.
14. Hair PI, McCormack PL, Curran MP. Eszopiclone: a review of its use in the treatment of insomnia. *Drugs*. 2008;68(10):1415–1434.
15. Yoshimoto M, Higuchi H, Kamata M, et al. The effects of benzodiazepine (triazolam), cyclopyrrolone (zopiclone) and imidazopyridine (zolpidem) hypnotics on the frequency of hippocampal theta activity and sleep structure in rats. *Eur Neuropsychopharmacol*. 1999;9(1–2):29–35.
16. Nakajima T, Sasaki T, Nakagome K, et al. Comparison of the effects of zolpidem and zopiclone on nocturnal sleep and sleep latency in the morning: a cross-over study in healthy young volunteers. *Life Sci*. 2000;67(1):81–90.
17. Drover DR. Comparative pharmacokinetics and pharmacodynamics of short-acting hypnosedatives: zaleplon, zolpidem and zopiclone. *Clin Pharmacokinet*. 2004;43(4):227–238.
18. Fahey JM, Grassi JM, Reddi JM, et al. Acute zolpidem administration produces pharmacodynamic and receptor occupancy changes at similar doses. *Pharmacol Biochem Behav*. 2006;83(1):21–27.
19. Sanger DJ. The pharmacology and mechanisms of action of new generation, non-benzodiazepine hypnotic agents. *CNS Drugs*. 2004;18(suppl 1):9–15 (discussion 41, 43–45).
20. Fleck MW. Molecular actions of (S)-desmethylzopiclone (SEP-174559), an anxiolytic metabolite of zopiclone. *J Pharmacol Exp Ther*. 2002;302(2):612–618.

21. Holt RA, Bateson AN, Martin IL. Chronic zolpidem treatment alters GABA(A) receptor mRNA levels in the rat cortex. *Eur J Pharmacol*. 1997;329(2–3):129–132.
22. Follesa P, Mancuso L, Biggio F, et al. Changes in GABA(A) receptor gene expression induced by withdrawal of, but not by long-term exposure to, zaleplon or zolpidem. *Neuropharmacology*. 2002;42(2):191–198.
23. Wilkinson CJ. The abuse potential of zolpidem administered alone and with alcohol. *Pharmacol Biochem Behav*. 1998;60(1):193–202.
24. Evans SM, Funderburk FR, Griffiths RR. Zolpidem and triazolam in humans: behavioral and subjective effects and abuse liability. *J Pharmacol Exp Ther*. 1990;255(3):1246–1255.
25. Rush CR, Baker RW, Wright K. Acute behavioral effects and abuse potential of trazodone, zolpidem and triazolam in humans. *Psychopharmacology (Berl)*. 1999;144(3):220–233.
26. Krystal AD, Walsh JK, Laska E, et al. Sustained efficacy of eszopiclone over 6 months of nightly treatment: results of a randomized, double-blind, placebo-controlled study in adults with chronic insomnia. *Sleep*. 2003;26(7):793–799.
27. Krystal AD, Erman M, Zammit GK, et al. Long-term efficacy and safety of zolpidem extended-release 12.5 mg, administered 3 to 7 nights per week for 24 weeks, in patients with chronic primary insomnia: a 6-month, randomized, double-blind, placebo-controlled, parallel-group, multicenter study. *Sleep*. 2008;31(1):79–90.
28. Elie R, Rüther E, Farr I, et al. Sleep latency is shortened during 4 weeks of treatment with zaleplon, a novel nonbenzodiazepine hypnotic. Zaleplon Clinical Study Group. *J Clin Psychiatry*. 1999;60(8):536–544.
29. Voderholzer U, Riemann D, Hornyak M, et al. A double-blind, randomized and placebo-controlled study on the polysomnographic withdrawal effects of zopiclone, zolpidem and triazolam in healthy subjects. *Eur Arch Psychiatry Clin Neurosci*. 2001;251(3):117–123.
30. Roth T, Soubrane C, Titeux L, et al. Efficacy and safety of zolpidem-MR: a double-blind, placebo-controlled study in adults with primary insomnia. *Sleep Med*. 2006;7(5):397–406.
31. Perrault G, Morel E, Sanger DJ, et al. Lack of tolerance and physical dependence upon repeated treatment with the novel hypnotic zolpidem. *J Pharmacol Exp Ther*. 1992;263(1):298–303.
32. Yanagita T. Dependence potential of zopiclone studied in monkeys. *Pharmacology*. 1983;27(suppl 2):216–227.
33. Weerts EM, Ator NA, Grech DM, et al. Zolpidem physical dependence assessed across increasing doses under a once-daily dosing regimen in baboons. *J Pharmacol Exp Ther*. 1998;285(1):41–53.
34. Cimolai N. Zopiclone: is it a pharmacologic agent for abuse? *Can Fam Physician*. 2007;53(12):2124–2129.
35. Thompson SA, Whiting PJ, Wafford KA. Barbiturate interactions at the human GABAA receptor: dependence on receptor subunit combination. *Br J Pharmacol*. 1996;117(3):521–527.
36. Liu H, Dai T, Yao S. Effect of thiopental sodium on N-methyl-D-aspartate-gated currents. *Can J Anaesth*. 2006;53(5):442–448.
37. Zhan RZ, Fujiwara N, Yamakura T, et al. Differential inhibitory effects of thiopental, thiamylal and phenobarbital on both voltage-gated calcium channels and NMDA receptors in rat hippocampal slices. *Br J Anaesth*. 1998;81(6):932–939.
38. Yamakura T, Sakimura K, Mishina M, et al. The sensitivity of AMPA-selective glutamate receptor channels to pentobarbital is determined by a single amino acid residue of the alpha 2 subunit. *FEBS Lett*. 1995;374(3):412–414.
39. Joo DT, Xiong Z, MacDonald JF, et al. Blockade of glutamate receptors and barbiturate anesthesia: increased sensitivity to pentobarbital-induced anesthesia despite reduced inhibition of AMPA receptors in GluR2 null mutant mice. *Anesthesiology*. 1999;91(5):1329–1341.
40. Ffrench-Mullen JM, Barker JL, Rogawski MA. Calcium current block by (−)-pentobarbital, phenobarbital, and CHEB but not (+)-pentobarbital in acutely isolated hippocampal CA1 neurons: comparison with effects on GABA-activated Cl-current. *J Neurosci*. 1993;13(8):3211–3221.
41. Hirota K, Kudo M, Kudo T, et al. Barbiturates inhibit K(+)-evoked noradrenaline and dopamine release from rat striatal slices—involvement of voltage sensitive Ca(2+) channels. *Neurosci Lett*. 2000;291(3):175–178.
42. Miao N, Nagao K, Lynch C 3rd. Thiopental and methohexital depress Ca2+ entry into and glutamate release from cultured neurons. *Anesthesiology*. 1998;88(6):1643–1653.
43. Waller MB, Richter JA. Effects of pentobarbital and Ca2+ on the resting and K+-stimulated release of several endogenous neurotransmitters from rat midbrain slices. *Biochem Pharmacol*. 1980;29(16):2189–2198.
44. Uhlmann C, Froscher W. Low risk of development of substance dependence for barbiturates and clobazam prescribed as antiepileptic drugs: results from a questionnaire study. *CNS Neurosci Ther*. 2009;15(1):24–31.
45. Carter LP, Richards BD, Mintzer MZ, et al. Relative abuse liability of GHB in humans: a comparison of psychomotor, subjective, and cognitive effects of supratherapeutic doses of triazolam, pentobarbital, and GHB. *Neuropsychopharmacology*. 2006; 31(11): 2537–2551.
46. Rush CR, Madakasira S, Goldman NH, et al. Discriminative stimulus effects of zolpidem in pentobarbital-trained subjects: II. Comparison with triazolam and caffeine in humans. *J Pharmacol Exp Ther*. 1997;280(1):174–188.
47. Lin LH, Wang LH. Region-specific changes in GABAA receptor delta subunit mRNA level by tolerance to and withdrawal from pentobarbital. *Neurosci Lett*. 1996;202(3):149–152.
48. Jang CG, Oh S, Ho IK. Changes in NMDAR2 subunit mRNA levels during pentobarbital tolerance/withdrawal in the rat brain: an in situ hybridization study. *Neurochem Res*. 1998; 23(11):1371–1377.
49. Snead OC 3rd, Gibson KM. Gamma-hydroxybutyric acid. *N Engl J Med*. 2005;352(26):2721–2732.
50. Wong CG, Gibson KM, Snead OC 3rd. From the street to the brain: neurobiology of the recreational drug gamma-hydroxybutyric acid. *Trends Pharmacol Sci*. 2004;25(1):29–34.
51. Kaupmann K, Cryan JF, Wellendorph P, et al. Specific gamma-hydroxybutyrate-binding sites but loss of pharmacological effects of gamma-hydroxybutyrate in GABA(B)(1)-deficient mice. *Eur J Neurosci*. 2003;18(10):2722–2730.
52. Pistis M, Muntoni AL, Pillolla G, et al. Gamma-hydroxybutyric acid (GHB) and the mesoaccumbens reward circuit: evidence for GABA(B) receptor-mediated effects. *Neuroscience*. 2005; 131(2):465–474.
53. Mamelak M, Scharf MB, Woods M. Treatment of narcolepsy with gamma-hydroxybutyrate. A review of clinical and sleep laboratory findings. *Sleep*. 1986;9(1 Pt 2):285–289.
54. Miotto K, Darakjian J, Basch J, et al. Gamma-hydroxybutyric acid: patterns of use, effects and withdrawal. *Am J Addict*. 2001; 10(3):232–241.
55. Goodwin AK, Griffiths RR, Brown PR, et al. Chronic intragastric administration of gamma-butyrolactone produces physical dependence in baboons. *Psychopharmacology (Berl)*. 2006; 189(1): 71–82.

CHAPTER 18 Hallucinogens

Robert N. Pechnick ■ Kathryn A. Cunningham

INTRODUCTION

This chapter focuses on the major current and past hallucinogens: the prototype ergot hallucinogen lysergic acid diethylamide (LSD); other indolealkylamines such as psilocybin, psilocin, and dimethyltryptamine (DMT); and the phenethylamines, including mescaline and dimethoxymethylamphetamine (DOM). Cannabis, phencyclidine (PCP), and designer drugs such as methylenedioxymethamphetamine (MDMA or ecstasy), which are sometimes classified as hallucinogens, are covered in other chapters in this volume (see Chapters 15 and 19).

The term *hallucinogen* means "producer of hallucinations." A hallucination is defined as a profound distortion in the perception of reality, frequently described as a sensory experience of something that is not there. Many drugs, when taken in sufficient quantity, can cause auditory and/or visual hallucinations. Such hallucinations can be present as part of a delirium, accompanied by disturbances in judgment, orientation, intellect, memory, emotion, and level of consciousness (e.g., organic brain syndrome). Delirium also can result from drug withdrawal (e.g., sedative–hypnotic withdrawal or delirium tremens in alcohol). However, hallucinogen generally refers to compounds that alter consciousness without producing delirium, sedation, excessive stimulation, or intellectual or memory impairment as prominent effects. This label actually is inaccurate because true LSD-induced "hallucinations" are rare; what are commonly seen are illusory phenomena. An illusion is a perceptual distortion of an actual stimulus in the environment: to see someone's face seeming to be melting is an illusion; whereas, to see a melting face when no face is present is a hallucination. There are a variety of widely accepted synonyms for the hallucinogens, including the term psychedelic (1). The term *psychotomimetic*, meaning "a producer of psychosis," also has been widely used. For a review of the original terminology and a classification system for the hallucinogenic drugs, see Shulgin (2).

Over the last 2 decades, a number of features regarding the study and use of hallucinogens have changed. First, the Internet has become a widely used source of information on hallucinogens (3). Second, during the 1980s little clinical research was carried out, but beginning in 1990s there was a resurgence of clinical studies carried out under highly controlled conditions (4–13). The results obtained from these clinical studies provided important and unbiased information, in contrast to much of the earlier anecdotal information that came from limited first-person accounts (14), "street pharmacologists," and from hospital emergency room reports. Third, this resurgence in clinical research has taken place at the same time that there have been major advances regarding mechanisms of action of the hallucinogens. For example, much more is now known about the effects of hallucinogens on the synthesis, release, and metabolism of indoleamines and catecholamines, and their interactions with specific pre- and postsynaptic receptor subtypes; we now might be reaching a point where we can begin to develop a unified conceptual framework regarding the fundamental mechanisms underlying their pharmacologic effects in humans.

HISTORY

To a large degree, the attention to drug abuse that began in the United States in the mid-1960s and continues today initially came from concern over the use of hallucinogens, particularly LSD. In the early 1960s, Timothy Leary, then a young psychology instructor at Harvard, began experimenting with hallucinogens, particularly LSD. He claimed that LSD provided instant happiness, enhanced creativity in art and music, facilitated problem-solving ability in school and at work, increased self-awareness, and might be useful as an adjunct to psychotherapy. Leary popularized this on college campuses, coining the phrase "turn on, tune in, drop out." When he was not reappointed to the faculty at Harvard, he became a highly publicized, self-proclaimed martyr to his cause, and his followers began to proselytize for LSD. Leary's advocates organized their lifestyle around LSD and developed a subculture of fellow LSD users who shared this common interest. Furthermore, they would not use other classes of drugs; they would not smoke tobacco, use amphetamine or amphetamine-like psychostimulants or barbiturates, or even drink alcohol. Thus, very little polydrug abuse occurred among these LSD users.

The lay press repeatedly "discovered" LSD and, in effect, advertised the LSD experience. As publicity increased, subcultures experimenting with LSD began to emerge in many east and west coast cities. Other hallucinogenic compounds, such as mescaline and psilocybin, began to be taken as well, although LSD remained the most widely used hallucinogen due to its ready availability on the street. Musicians, rock music, the hippie lifestyle, and "flower children" were loosely joined with Leary's philosophy. There were highly publicized festivals celebrating LSD, such as "The Summer of Love" in the Haight-Ashbury district of San Francisco. Later, its use began to increase in all socioeconomic groups, particularly among middle-class and affluent youth. Moreover, many of these individuals also became active in various "protest" movements, speaking out against such government policies as the war in Vietnam, and about other national issues, such as civil rights and "free speech." About this time, various adverse reactions to LSD (and other hallucinogens) began to be reported from medical centers around the country. The whole phenomenon continued to be widely publicized, and in many cases sensationalized (15), by the press. The populace reacted with anxiety and fear, worrying that many of the young would soon become "acidheads."

Many of the LSD users eventually became involved in polydrug abuse, using other drugs besides hallucinogens. This included the extensive use of marihuana, hashish, and, in some cases, methamphetamine or even heroin. Various "street" substances, whose identity was frequently unknown, as well as combinations of drugs were consumed. In addition, in the search for new drugs with different and improved characteristics, such as more or less euphoria, hallucinogenic activity or stimulant properties, longer or shorter duration of action, literally hundreds of so-called designer drugs were synthesized (e.g., DOM, MDMA, DMT). Concern about drug abuse rose to the point of becoming perceived as one of the nation's most pressing problems, along with the economy and the war in Vietnam. The nation geared up to declare the "war on drugs," and the national drug abuse effort expanded from a relatively small research-oriented program under the National Institute of Mental Health (NIMH) to the then newly created National Institute on Drug Abuse (NIDA) and the National Institute on Alcohol Abuse and Alcoholism (NIAAA). Eventually, a new "superagency," the Alcohol, Drug Abuse, and Mental Health Administration (ADAMHA) was established to oversee NIDA, NIAAA, and NIMH. ADAMHA subsequently merged into the National Institutes of Health (NIH), only to be desolved in later years. Yet, these NIH institutes, the Drug Enforcement Agency (DEA), the Bureau of Alcohol, Tobacco, and Firearms (BATF), the Office of the National Drug Control Policy (ONDCP), and local law enforcement agencies continue to be involved in the "war on drugs."

By the mid-1960s, more than a 1000 articles on LSD had appeared in the medical literature. Sandoz Laboratories stopped distributing the drug in late 1966 because of the reported adverse reactions and the resulting public outcry. At that time, all of the existing supplies of LSD were turned over to the government, which was to make the drug available for legitimate and highly controlled research; however, research on humans essentially was discontinued. Although some of the hallucinogens originally were developed and studied for use in chemical warfare, the results of these experiments remain classified. Today, LSD, along with heroin, marihuana, and other psychoactive drugs, remains classified as a Schedule I drug according to the Comprehensive Drug Abuse Prevention and Control Act of 1970. Legally, LSD is regarded as having no currently accepted medical use in the United States, a high potential for abuse, and to be unsafe even when administered by a physician. Nevertheless, "black market" LSD remains widely available on the street. The therapeutic potential of LSD as an adjunct to psychotherapy, in the management of the dying patient, and in the treatment of alcoholism and neuropsychiatric illness such as obsessive–compulsive disorder remains unresolved (16–18), but there has been a resurgence in interest in carrying out hallucinogen research in humans (19–22).

EPIDEMIOLOGY

The available epidemiologic data on the use of hallucinogens center on the use of LSD and primarily come from the Monitoring The Future studies (23,24). Many studies have lumped hallucinogens and "club drugs" (e.g., MDMA) together, making the data very difficult to interpret. The use of LSD peaked in 1995 among college students and young adults and in 1996 among 8th, 10th, and 12th graders, after which it gradually declined, then dropped sharply in 2002 (23). This might have been due to, at least in part, the closing of a major LSD lab by the DEA. In 2008, 4% of 12th graders reported lifetime use of LSD, whereas approximately 20% of adults aged 29 to 30 reported lifetime use (24). A survey among club-going young adults indicated that 25% had used LSD (25). Among White, African American, and Hispanic 12th graders, Whites have the highest rate of LSD use (23). In 2008, approximately 28% of 12th graders indicated that LSD was fairly easy or very easy to get (23). More than 85% of 12th graders disapproved of trying LSD once or twice but only 34% felt trying LSD presented a risk (23).

PHENOMENOLOGY

In the 1960s, LSD was used primarily by those interested in its ability to alter perceptual experiences (sight, sound, taste, and feeling states). Much attention was paid to *set*, the expectation of what the drug experience would be like, and *setting*, the environment in which the drug was used. The early drug missionaries promulgated the erroneous notion that only good LSD "trips" would result if the prospective user established a number of preconditions before his or her drug experience. The preconditions relating to set included: being relaxed and largely stress/anxiety free; having no major resentment or anger and no recent arguments at home, school, or work; and freeing up several days, often an entire weekend, for the drug experience and its aftermath. The preconditions relating to setting included: having a close friend present as a sitter or guide for the experience; being in quiet, comfortable surroundings, particularly outdoors, or sitting on soft, thick carpeting; listening to pleasant sounds or music (originally, the sitar music of Ravi Shankar); and reading reassuring passages (originally, from the *Tibetan Book of the Dead*). In more recent years, users often attend concerts, dances ("raves"), or films (particularly psychedelic or brightly colored ones) during the drug experience. Use is rarely more than once weekly because tolerance to LSD and other hallucinogens occurs so rapidly (see below).

CHEMICAL CLASSIFICATION

The commonly abused hallucinogenic substances can be classified according to their chemical structure. Figure 18.1 shows the structures of these hallucinogens. Note that all of these drugs are organic compounds and some occur naturally.

Indolealkylamines

All of the indole-type hallucinogens have structural similarities to the neurotransmitter serotonin (5-hydroxytryptamine [5-HT]), suggesting that their mechanism of action could involve the alteration of serotonergic neurotransmission.

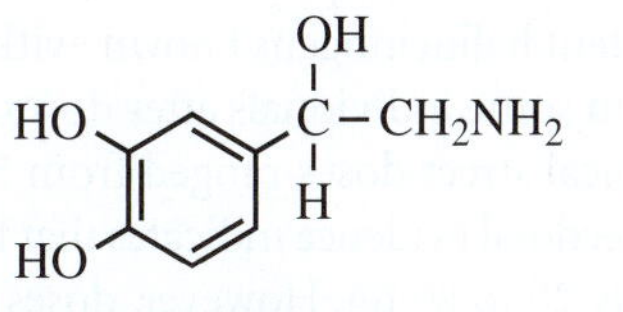

NOREPINEPHRINE
(neurotransmitter)

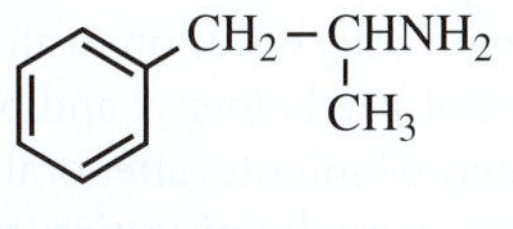

AMPHETAMINE
(psychostimulant)

PHENETHYLAMINE HALLUCINOGENS

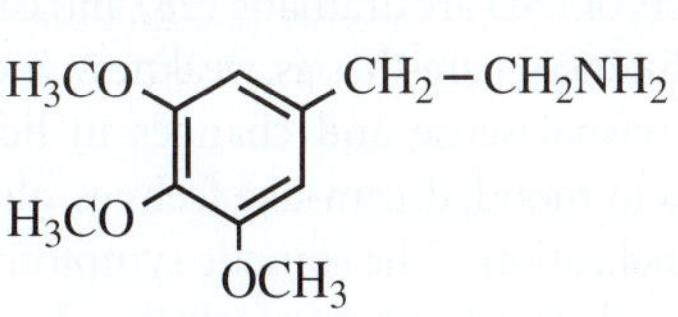

MESCALINE

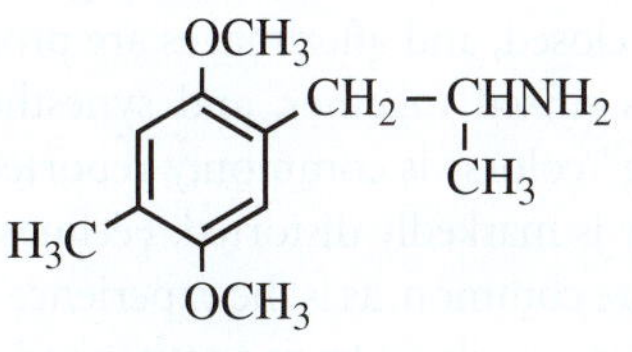

DOM

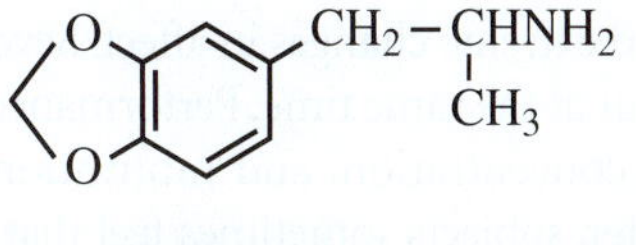

MDA

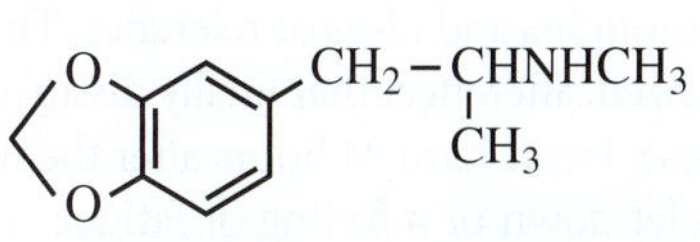

MDMA

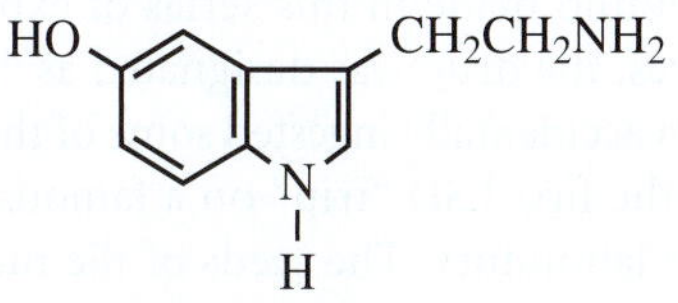

SEROTONIN
(neurotransmitter)

INDOLEALKYLAMINE HALLUCINOGENS

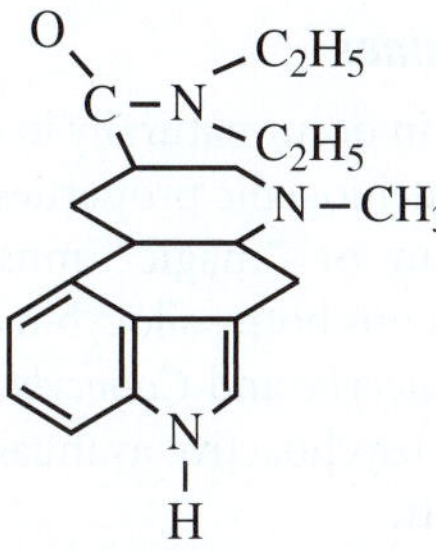

LSD

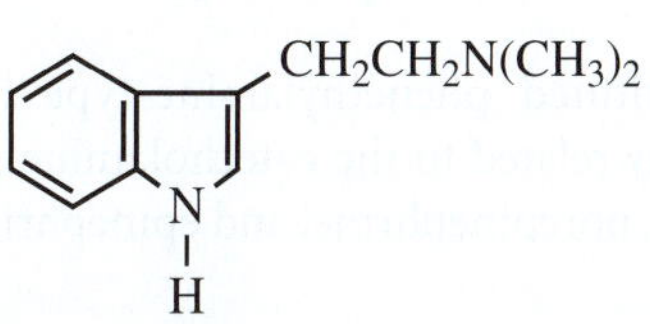

DMT

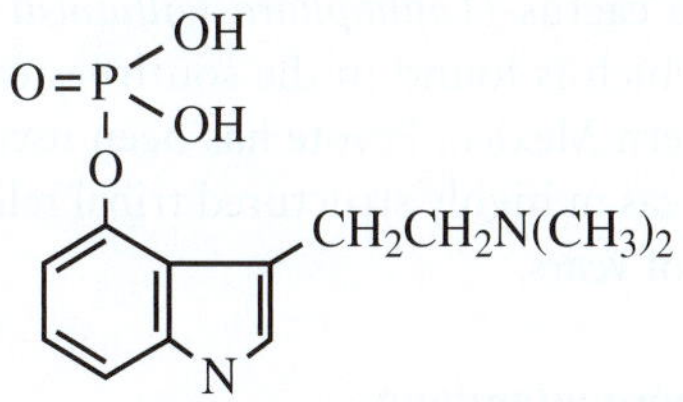

PSILOCYBIN

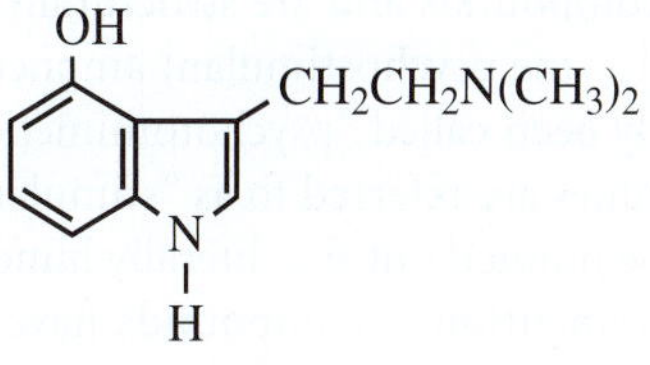

PSILOCIN

Figure 18.1. Structures of phenethylamine- and indolealkylamine-type hallucinogens.

Lysergic Acid Derivatives

Lysergic acid is one of the constituents of the ergot fungus that grows on rye. Inadvertently baked into bread, ergot intake has been associated with profound mental changes (26). Because the presence of the diethylamide group is a prerequisite for hallucinogenic activity, it is not clear whether these reported epidemics actually were caused by ergot in the bread, or by some other related substances or (psychological) phenomena. LSD was first synthesized by Hofmann in 1938; as the 25th compound made in this series of experiments on ergot derivatives, the drug was designated as "LSD-25." In 1943, Hofmann accidentally ingested some of the compound and soon had the first LSD "trip" on a famous bicycle ride home from his laboratory. The seeds of the morning glory (*Ipomoea*) contain lysergic acid derivatives, particularly lysergic acid amide. Although they are packaged commercially, many varieties have been treated with insecticides, fungicides, and other toxic chemicals.

Substituted Tryptamines

Psilocybin and psilocin occur naturally in a variety of mushrooms that have hallucinogenic properties. The most publicized is the Mexican or "magic" mushroom, *Psilocybe mexicana*, which contains both psilocybin and psilocin, as do some of the other *Psilocybe* and *Conocybe* species. DMT, although found in the psychoactive ayahuasca (13), is usually produced synthetically.

Substituted Phenethylamines

The substituted phenethylamine-type hallucinogens are structurally related to the catecholamine neurotransmitters dopamine, norepinephrine, and epinephrine.

Mescaline

Mescaline is a naturally occurring hallucinogen present in the peyote cactus (*Lophophora williamsii* or *Anhalonium lewinii*), which is found in the southwestern United States and northern Mexico. Peyote has been used by the Indians in these areas in highly structured tribal religious rituals for hundreds of years.

Phenylisopropylamines

The phenylisopropylamine hallucinogens DOM (or STP, from "serenity, tranquility, and peace"), MDA (methylenedioxyamphetamine or "Eve"), and MDMA (or ecstasy) are synthetic compounds and are structurally similar to mescaline as well as the psychostimulant amphetamine. They have inaccurately been called "psychotomimetic amphetamines," and sometimes are referred to as "stimulant hallucinogens." It should be pointed out that literally hundreds of analogues of the aforementioned compounds have been synthesized (14) and sometimes are found on the street, the so-called designer drugs (see Chapter 19).

ACUTE EFFECTS

The overall psychological effects of many of the hallucinogens are quite similar; however, the rate of onset, duration of action, and absolute intensity of the effects differ among the drugs. Moreover, the various hallucinogens vary widely in potency and the slope of the dose–response curve. Thus, some of the apparent qualitative differences among hallucinogens may be partly a result of the amount of drug ingested relative to its specific dose–response characteristics. LSD is one of the most potent hallucinogens known, with behavioral effects occurring in some individuals after doses as low as 20 μg. In the past, typical street doses ranged from 50 to 300 μg; however, some anecdotal evidence indicates that today's street LSD contains only 20 to 80 μg. However, doses reported on the street are often highly inaccurate. Because of its high potency, LSD can be applied to paper blotters or the backs of postage stamps. The absorption of LSD from the gastrointestinal tract occurs rapidly, with drug diffusion to all tissues, including the brain. The onset of psychological and behavioral effects occurs approximately 60 minutes after oral administration and peaks 2 to 4 hours after administration, with a gradual return to the predrug state in 10 to 12 hours. Both Hofmann (27) and Hollister (28) have described the effects of LSD in great detail.

The first 4 hours are sometimes called a "trip." The subjective effects of LSD are dramatic (28) and can be divided into somatic (dizziness, paresthesias, weakness, and tremor), perceptual (altered visual sense and changes in hearing), and psychic (changes in mood, dream-like feelings, altered time sense, and depersonalization). The somatic symptoms usually occur first. Later, visual alterations are marked and sounds are intensified. Visual distortions and illusory phenomena occur, but true hallucinations are rare. Dream-like imagery may develop when the eyes are closed, and afterimages are prolonged. Sensory input becomes mixed together, and synesthesia ("seeing" smells, "hearing" colors) is commonly reported. Touch is magnified and time is markedly distorted. Feelings of attainment of true insight are common, as is the experience of delusional ideation. Separating one object from another and self from environment becomes difficult, and depersonalization can develop. Emotions become intensified, and extreme lability may be observed, with rapid and extreme changes in affect. Several emotional feelings may occur at the same time. Performance on tests involving attention, concentration, and motivation is impaired. Several hours later, subjects sometimes feel that the drug is no longer active, but later they recognize that at that time they had paranoid thoughts and ideas of reference. This is a regular, but little publicized, aftereffect that finally dissipates 10 to 12 hours after the dose. From 12 to 24 hours after the trip, there may be some slight let down or a feeling of fatigue. There is no immediate craving to take more drug to relieve this boredom; one trip usually produces "satiation" for some time. Memory for the events that occurred during the trip is quite clear.

Effects produced by DMT are similar to those produced by LSD, but DMT is inactive after oral administration and must be injected, sniffed, or smoked. It has a rapid onset, almost immediately after intravenous administration, and a short duration of action, about 30 minutes (8). Because of its short duration of action, DMT was once known as the "businessman's LSD" (i.e., one could have a psychedelic experience during the lunch hour and be back at work in the afternoon). However, the sudden and rapid onset of a period of altered perceptions that soon terminates is disconcerting to some. DMT has never been a widely, steadily available or popular drug on the streets. The effects of ayahuasca, a psychoactive beverage that contains DMT, last about 4 hours (13). In contrast to DMT, a very slow onset and a long duration (longer than 24 hours) of effects are reported for DOM. Mescaline is approximately two to three orders of magnitude less potent than LSD, and its effects last about 6 to 10 hours, whereas the effects of psilocybin last about 2 hours (11).

The hallucinogens also possess significant autonomic activity. LSD produces marked pupillary dilation, hyperreflexia, increases in blood pressure and body temperature, tremor, piloerection, and tachycardia. Some of these autonomic effects of the hallucinogens are variable and might be partly a result of the anxiety state of the user. DMT and ayahuasca also increase heart rate, pupil diameter, and body temperature (7,13). LSD can cause nausea, and nausea and vomiting are especially noteworthy after the ingestion of mescaline or peyote. The hallucinogens also alter neuroendocrine function. For example, in humans, DMT elevates plasma levels of adrenocorticotropic hormone (ACTH), cortisol, and prolactin (7). Similarly, the hallucinogen 1-(2,5-dimethoxy-4-iodophenyl)-2-aminopropane (DOI) (29) increases plasma glucocorticoids in the rat.

EFFECTS OF CHRONIC USE

A high degree of tolerance develops to the behavioral effects of LSD after repeated administration. Such behavioral tolerance develops very rapidly, after only several days of daily administration, and tolerance is also lost rapidly after the individual user stops taking the drug for several days. Because of this rapid development of tolerance, LSD users typically self-usually limit themselves the use of taking the drug to once or twice weekly (30). Cross-tolerance develops between LSD and other hallucinogens, such as mescaline and psilocybin, suggesting a similar mechanism of action. However, cross-tolerance does not develop to other classes of psychotropic agents that are thought to have different underlying mechanisms of action, such as amphetamine, PCP, and marihuana. It should be pointed out that little tolerance develops to the various autonomic effects produced by the hallucinogens. There is no withdrawal syndrome after the cessation of the chronic administration of the hallucinogens.

MECHANISMS OF ACTION

Hallucinogenic drugs interact with multiple neurotransmitter systems (31) and the mechanisms of action to evoke their physiologic and psychological effects are complex. However, the ability of LSD and other hallucinogens to alter serotonin neurotransmission is of critical importance (32). Many hallucinogens, including LSD, were identified to be structurally similar to serotonin (see Fig. 18.1) and, in 1961, Freedman (33) was the first to provide direct evidence that LSD acted upon serotonergic systems within the central nervous system. He found that LSD increased the levels of serotonin in rat brain, but decreased the levels of serotonin metabolites, whereas the nonhallucinogenic analogue bromo-LSD failed to have the same effects. But, bromo-LSD does not produce hallucinatory phenomena, suggesting that the hallucinogenic effects of LSD might be caused by LSD-induced decreases in serotonin turnover (synthesis and release) in the brain. Other evidence supporting the interaction of hallucinogens with serotonergic systems: (a) the chronic administration of monoamine oxidase inhibitors decreased the density of serotonin receptors and reduced the behavioral effects of LSD (34) and (b) treatments that decreased brain levels of serotonin (e.g., lesions, reserpine, parachloroamphetamine, or other neurotoxins), upregulated postsynaptic serotonin receptors, and increased the behavioral effects of LSD (32).

Serotonin released from nerve terminals is available to interact with multiple receptors that transduce serotonin actions in the brain and periphery. Early studies demonstrated that LSD blocked the contractile effects of serotonin in isolated smooth muscle preparations, suggesting that LSD might produce its psychic effects by having similar antagonist activity at central serotonergic synapses. However, the LSD analogue bromo-LSD was identified as a potent peripheral serotonin antagonist that did not evoke an LSD-like psychopharmacologic profile. Thus, the mechanism of the hallucinogenic activity of LSD could not be explained solely by its direct serotonergic antagonist activity. Rather, evidence accumulated rapidly to support an agonist-like action for LSD and other hallucinogens at serotonin receptors in the brain. It is important to note that serotonin acts at multiple receptor subtypes (5-HTXR) found in the brain and periphery. These receptors have been identified and grouped into seven families (5-HT$_1$R to 5-HT$_7$R) according to their structural and functional characteristics, including 13 distinct G-protein coupled receptors, coupled to various effector systems, and two subtypes of the 5-HT$_3$R which is a pentameric ligand-gated ion channel (35). Our understanding of the serotonin system emerged rapidly as new receptor subtypes were cloned during the 1980s to 1990s, and several receptors were renamed and/or reclassified as functional information became available; thus, caution must be used in comparing results and conclusions drawn from older studies with the nomenclature currently used.

LSD binds to most serotonin receptor subtypes, except the 5-HT$_3$R and 5-HT$_4$R; however, its affinity for most of these receptors is too low to predict receptor activation at the brain levels achieved after ingestion of psychoactive doses. The receptors thought to contribute predominantly to its effects include the 5-HT$_{1A}$R, 5-HT$_{2A}$R, 5-HT$_{2C}$R, 5-HT$_{5A}$R, and 5-HT$_6$R. Aghajanian and coworkers found that LSD inhibits the firing of serotonergic neurons in the dorsal raphe nucleus, most likely by interacting with presynaptic autoreceptors (36), termed the

5-HT_{1A}R. Other indole-type hallucinogens, such as psilocin and DMT, also produce this effect (36). However, strong evidence refutes a direct linkage between the presynaptic effects of LSD and its hallucinogenic activity: (a) phenethylamine hallucinogens, such as mescaline, do not have the same inhibitory effects on the firing of serotonergic neurons (37); (b) there is no correlation between the activity of drugs at the presynaptic 5-HT_{1A}R and their hallucinogenic activity (38); and (c) tolerance does not develop to the effects of the hallucinogens on neuronal firing, but behavioral tolerance rapidly develops after the repeated administration of hallucinogens (37). These findings suggest that interactions with the presynaptic 5-HT_{1A}R cannot be the sole mechanism of action of the hallucinogens, and other factors must be involved.

Both indole- and phenethylamine-type hallucinogens bind with varying affinities to the three members of the serotonin 5-HT_2R which is composed of the 5-HT_{2A}R, 5-HT_{2B}R, and 5-HT_{2C}R; its actions at these receptors are characterized as either full or partial agonists (39). There is compelling evidence that an agonist action at the 5-HT_{2A}R is a key component underlying the mechanisms of action of the hallucinogens. For example: (a) there are very high correlations between the binding affinities of both indolealkylamine- and phenethylamine-type hallucinogens for the 5-HT_{2A}R and their hallucinogenic activity in humans and their potency in behavioral studies in laboratory animals (39); (b) the chronic administration of LSD, but not the nonhallucinogenic analogue bromo-LSD, decreases the density of 5-HT_{2A}R, an effect associated with the development of tolerance to the behavioral effects of LSD (40); and (c) preclinical studies found that many of the effects of hallucinogens are blocked by 5-HT_{2A}R antagonists (39).

Even though the interaction of hallucinogens with the 5-HT_{2A}R appears to be critical, other serotonergic receptor subtypes also might be involved. For example, interactions with the closely related 5-HT_{2C}R (formerly called 5-HT_{1C}R) might contribute to the psychoactive effects of hallucinogens (41). Although apparently not critical for hallucinogenic activity, interactions with presynaptic 5-HT_{1A}R might contribute to the effects of some hallucinogens. LSD has recently been reported to act as an agonist at the 5-HT_5R (5-HT_{5A}R and 5-HT_{5B}R) and 5-HT_6R; however, a full appreciation of how these receptors contribute to the myriad of effects of hallucinogens awaits a full characterization of the receptors. The differential interactions of the various hallucinogens with numerous sites and systems might underlie the qualitative differences between the subjective experiences of the class of hallucinogenic drugs. However, the commonality of interactions with 5-HT_{2A}R suggests that drugs that possess 5-HT_{2A}R antagonist activity might be useful in blocking the behavioral effects of the hallucinogens in humans.

ADVERSE REACTIONS

Strassman (42) has characterized adverse reactions according to the temporal relationship between drug exposure and symptomatology, with acute and chronic reactions at the end of the continuum, and delayed (subsequent panic attacks) and intermittent (flashback phenomena) between the ends of the continuum. Although the existence of some of the acute adverse reactions is clear-cut and not subject to debate, some of the purported long-term adverse effects remain controversial. One of the problems is that many of the studies reporting long-term adverse reactions lack adequate knowledge concerning baseline levels of state prior to self-administration of the hallucinogen.

Acute Adverse Reactions

Social factors, media presentations, and public fear have all shaped perceptions of the effects of LSD and other hallucinogens. A person's reaction to the effects of a drug may be felt to be either a pleasant or an unpleasant experience; a perceptual distortion or illusion may cause intense anxiety in one user and be a pleasant and amusing interlude for another user. Individuals who place a premium on self-control, advance planning, and impulse restriction may do particularly poorly on LSD. Traumatic and stressful external events can precipitate an adverse reaction (e.g., being arrested and read one's rights in the middle of a pleasant experience may precipitate an anxiety reaction). Predictions of who will have an acute (or other) adverse reaction are unreliable (43), and the occurrence of multiple previous pleasurable LSD experiences renders no immunity from an adverse reaction. Adverse reactions have occurred after doses of LSD as low as 40 µg, and no adverse effects have been observed in some individuals after ingesting 2000 µg, although in general the hallucinogenic effects are dose dependent. Thus, acute adverse behavioral reactions generally are not dose related, but a function of personal predisposition, setting, and circumstance. Because of the perceptual distortions (and subsequent deficits in judgment), there is always the risk of self-destructive behavior. Some of the adverse reactions that occur after ingesting hallucinogens can be caused by other contaminants in the product, such as strychnine, PCP, or amphetamine. Once commonly reported by medical facilities, acute adverse LSD reactions are rarely seen today, yet the drug remains in use. Moreover, the paucity of users seeking emergency medical treatment may reflect increased knowledge of how to deal with such situations on the part of the "drug-using community," a decrease in the doses of LSD currently used compared to those used in the past, and the availability of drugs to reduce the adverse effects (e.g., benzodiazepines for anxiety reactions).

Acute anxiety or panic reactions, the so-called "bad trip," are the most commonly reported acute adverse reactions. They usually wear off before medical intervention is sought; most LSD is metabolized and excreted within 24 hours, and acute panic reactions usually subside within this time frame. Depression with suicidal ideation can occur several days after LSD use. Paranoid ideation, "hallucinations," and a confusional state (organic brain syndrome) are other commonly reported acute adverse reactions (44). Initially, it was thought that LSD could replicate the signs and symptoms of schizophrenia in some subjects, and the induction of such a model psychosis could be used to study and potentially find a cure for this major psychiatric illness. These hopes did not materialize, as major differences have been found between hallucinogen-induced psychosis and the schizophrenic state (45). Using single-photon emission computed tomography (SPECT), it has been found that the administration of mescaline to controls produced a "hyperfrontal" pattern, whereas "hypofrontality" has been observed in schizophrenics (6). However, using positron emission tomography, Gouzoulis-Mayfrank et al. (10) found that psilocybin produced changes in glucose metabolism similar to those in acute schizophrenic patients.

The differential diagnosis between LSD psychosis and paranoid schizophrenia is an important distinction to be made clinically, particularly because patients, who in fact are paranoid, now often complain of being poisoned with LSD. A history of prior mental illness, a psychiatric examination that reveals the absence of an intact or observing ego, and auditory (rather than visual) hallucinations all suggest schizophrenia. Other drug-induced psychoses, including those from psychostimulants or PCP, must be ruled out. An organic brain syndrome in general speaks against LSD, especially when obtunded consciousness is present. Toxicologic analysis of body fluids can be helpful in making the ultimate diagnosis, but supportive treatment must not be withheld. Atropine poisoning can be differentiated by the presence of prominent anticholinergic effects such as dry mouth and blurred vision. Patients with amphetamine psychosis often fail to differentiate their perceptual distortions from reality, whereas LSD users are aware of the difference.

In terms of adverse physiologic effects, LSD has a very high therapeutic index. An elephant was killed after the experimental administration of a massive dose relative to brain weight, 0.15 mg/kg, or approximately 300,000 µg of LSD (46). The lethal dose in humans has not been determined, and fatalities that have been reported usually are secondary to perceptual distortions with resultant accidental death (e.g., "flying" off a roof, merging with an oncoming automobile on the freeway) (47). Posterior reversible encephalopathy syndrome with accompanying seizures occurred after ingesting LSD (48). A fibrotic inflammatory mass located in the mesentery was reported in a chronic LSD user (49), and multifocal cerebral demyelination was reported after the use of "magic mushrooms" (50). Although LSD has prominent effects on the serotonin system, there is no evidence of association of its use with the serotonin syndrome, a potentially life-threatening reaction to some serotonergic drugs (51). DMT and ayahuasca have been reported to be relatively safe (52). Although mescaline is often viewed as posing a minimal health risk (53), a case of fatal peyote ingestion associated with Mallory–Weiss lacerations, probably as a result of peyote-induced vomiting, has been reported (54).

Treatment of Acute Adverse Reactions

Treatment of the acute adverse reactions to hallucinogens first must be directed toward preventing the patient from physically harming self or others. Anxiety can be handled by means of interpersonal support and reassurance. Psychotherapeutic intervention consists of reassurance, placing the patient in a quiet room, and avoidance of physical intrusion until the patient begins to calm down. The use of a benzodiazepine, such as lorazepam, also can be effective. The oral route can be used for administering such medication in mildly agitated patients; however, it can be difficult to convince severely agitated and/or paranoid patients to swallow a pill, in which case parenteral administration might be necessary. Severely agitated patients who fail to respond to a benzodiazepine may be given a neuroleptic agent. Caution must be used in administering neuroleptics because they can lower the seizure threshold and elicit seizures, especially if the hallucinogen has been cut with an agent that has convulsant activity, such as strychnine. Phenothiazine-type antipsychotics, such as chlorpromazine given orally or intramuscularly can end an LSD trip and are effective in treating LSD-induced psychosis. Because anticholinergic crises can develop with chlorpromazine in combination with other drugs with anticholinergic activity (PCP and DOM), haloperidol is a safer therapeutic choice when the true nature of the drug ingested is unknown. It has been suggested that a combination of intramuscular haloperidol and lorazepam is particularly effective in treating acute adverse reactions (55). Theoretically, selective 5-HT$_{2A}$R antagonists should block the effects of hallucinogens; however, other drugs with significant 5-HT$_{2A}$R antagonist activity such as atypical antipsychotics (e.g., olanzapine and risperidone) also might be effective. Vollenweider et al. (11) found that the psychotomimetic effects of psilocybin are blocked by the 5-HT$_{2A}$R antagonists ketanserin and risperidone; however, haloperidol *increased* the psychotomimetic effects. It should be noted that there is some indication that risperidone might exacerbate flashbacks (56).

Long-Term Adverse Effects

There is no generally accepted evidence of brain cell damage, chromosomal abnormalities, or teratogenic effects after the use of the indole-type hallucinogens and mescaline (42). Chronic adverse reactions include psychoses, depressive reactions, acting out, paranoid states, and flashbacks. The use of LSD has been found to coincide with the onset of depression, suggesting its possible role in the etiology of some depression in the young (57). Flashbacks are a well-publicized adverse reaction that can occur after taking hallucinogens. They now have been renamed "hallucinogen persisting perception disorder" (58), and have specific diagnostic criteria (59). In the past, the use of variable definitions of what constitutes a flashback was a major problem; hopefully, the establishment of specific diagnostic criteria will facilitate the study and understanding of this problem. Only a small proportion of LSD and other hallucinogenic users experiences flashbacks. They can occur spontaneously a number of weeks or months after the original drug experience, appear not to be dose related, and can develop after a single exposure to the drug (60). During a flashback, the original drug experience is recreated complete with perceptual and reality distortion. Even a previously pleasant drug experience may be accompanied by anxiety when the person realizes that he or she has no control over its recurrence. In time, flashbacks decrease in intensity, frequency, and duration (although initially they usually last only a few seconds), whether treated or not. Flashbacks may or may not be precipitated by stressors or the subsequent use of other psychoactive drugs, such as psilocybin or marihuana. The administration of selective serotonin reuptake inhibitor antidepressants (61) and risperidone (56) is reported to initiate or exacerbate flashbacks in individuals with a history of LSD use. Flashbacks usually can be handled with psychotherapy. An anxiolytic or neuroleptic may be indicated but probably is as much for the reassurance of the therapist as for the patient. Various pharmacologic agents, such as clonidine or clonazepam (62), or drug combinations (e.g., fluoxetine and olanzapine) (63), have been found to be useful in the treatment of flashbacks. The exact mechanism underlying this phenomenon remains obscure. Individuals with flashbacks have a high lifetime incidence of affective disorder when compared to non–LSD-abusing substance abusers (64). LSD users have long-term changes in visual function (65). For example, a visual disturbance consisting of prolonged afterimages (palinopsia) has been found in individuals several years after the last reported use of LSD (66). Such changes in visual function might underlie flashbacks.

Psychosis can develop and persist after hallucinogen use, but it remains unclear whether hallucinogen use can "cause" long-term psychosis, or if it has a role in precipitating the onset of illness. For example, hallucinogens may have a variety of effects in a person who is genetically predisposed to schizophrenia: they may cause the psychosis to manifest at an earlier age; they may produce a psychosis that would have remained dormant if drugs had not been used; or they may cause relapse in a person who has previously suffered a psychotic disorder (45). Although there is some evidence that prolonged psychotic reactions tend to occur in individuals with poor premorbid adjustment, a history of psychiatric illness and/or repeated use of hallucinogens, severe and prolonged illness has been reported in individuals without such a history (42).

There are few, if any, long-term neuropsychological deficits attributable to hallucinogen use (67). Chronic personality changes with a shift in attitudes and evidence of magical thinking can occur after the use of hallucinogens. There is always the risk that such thinking can lead to destructive behavior, in acute as well as chronic reactions. The effects of the chronic use of LSD must be differentiated from the effects of personality disorders, particularly in those who use a variety of drugs in polydrug abuse patterns. In some individuals with well-integrated personalities and with no previous psychiatric history, chronic personality changes have resulted from repeated LSD use. Personality changes that result from LSD use can occur after a single experience, unlike other classes of drugs (except PCP, perhaps). In addition, the hallucinogenic drugs interact in a variety of nonspecific ways with the personality, which may particularly impair the developing adolescent. The suggestibility that may come from many experiences with LSD may be reinforced by the social values of a particular subculture in which the drug is used. For example, if some of these subcultures embrace withdrawal from society, that is to say, a noncompetitive approach toward life, the person who "withdraws" after the LSD experience may be suffering from a side effect that represents more of a change in social values than a true drug effect. Treatment of chronic hallucinogen abuse can include psychotherapy on a long-term basis to determine what needs are being fulfilled by the use of the drug for this particular person. Twelve-step meetings also might be useful for reinforcement of the decision to remain abstinent.

Drug Interactions

Drug interactions involving the hallucinogens do not appear to be an important source of adverse reactions. There are reports that the effects of LSD are reduced after the chronic administration of monoamine oxidase inhibitors or selective serotonin reuptake inhibitor antidepressants such as fluoxetine (68,69), whereas the effects of LSD are increased after the chronic administration of lithium or tricyclic antidepressants (69).

ACKNOWLEDGMENTS

The authors would like to thank Dr. Michael P. Bova for preparing the figure. R.N.P. is supported in part by NIDA grants R01 DA021249 and R21 DA021805; K.A.C is supported in part by NIDA grants R01 DA06511, P20 DA024157, and K05 DA020087.

REFERENCES

1. Osmond H. A review of the clinical effects of psychotomimetic agents. *Ann N Y Acad Sci.* 1957;66:418.
2. Shulgin AT. Psychotomimetic drugs: structure-activity relationships. In: Iversen LL, Iversen SD, Snyder SH, eds. *Handbook of Psychopharmacology*. Vol 11. New York, NY: Plenum Press; 1978:243–333.
3. Halpern JH, Pope HG Jr. Hallucinogens on the Internet: a vast new source of underground drug information. *Am J Psychiatry.* 2001;158:481–483.
4. Hermle L, Fünfgeld M, Oepen G, et al. Mescaline-induced psychopathological, neuropsychological, and neurometabolic effects in normal subjects: experimental psychosis as a tool for psychiatric research. *Biol Psychiatry.* 1992;32:976–991.
5. Hermle L, Spitzer M, Borchardt D, et al. Psychological effects of MDE in normal subjects. *Neuropsychopharmacology.* 1993;8:171–176.
6. Gouzoulis E, von Bardeleben U, Rupp A, et al. Neuroendocrine and cardiovascular effects of MDE in healthy volunteers. *Neuropsychopharmacology.* 1993;8:187–193.
7. Strassman RJ, Qualls CR. Dose-response study of N, N-dimethyltryptamine in humans. I. Neuroendocrine, autonomic and cardiovascular effects. *Arch Gen Psychiatry.* 1994;51:85–97.
8. Strassman RJ, Qualls CR, Uhlenhuth EH, et al. Dose-response study of N, N-dimethyltryptamine in humans. II. Subjective effects and preliminary results of a new rating scale. *Arch Gen Psychiatry.* 1994;51:98–108.

9. Strassman RJ. Hallucinogenic drugs in psychiatric research and treatment. Perspectives and prospects. *J Nerv Ment Dis.* 1995; 183:127–138.
10. Gouzoulis-Mayfrank E, Schreckenberger M, Sabri O, et al. Neurometabolic effects of psilocybin, 3,4-methylene-dio-xyethylamphetamine (MDE) and *d*-methamphetamine in healthy volunteers. *Neuropsychopharmacology.* 1999;20:565–581.
11. Vollenweider FX, Vollenweider-Scherpenhuyzen MFI, Babler A, et al. Psilocybin induces schizophrenia-like psychosis in humans via a serotonin-2 agonist action. *Neuroreport.* 1998;9:3897–3902.
12. Vollenweider FX, Vontobel P, Hell D, et al. 5-HT modulation of dopamine release in basal ganglia in psilocybin-induced psychosis in man—a PET study with [^{11}C]raclopride. *Neuropsychopharmacology.* 1999;20:424–433.
13. Riba J, Rodriguez-Fornells A, Urbano G, et al. Subjective effects and tolerability of the South American psychoactive beverage ayahuasca in healthy volunteers. *Psychopharmacology (Berl).* 2001;154:85–95.
14. Shulgin A, Shulgin A. *PIHKAL: A Chemical Love Story.* Berkeley, CA: Transform Press; 1991.
15. Weil A. *Natural Mind.* Boston, MA: Houghton Mifflin; 1972:10.
16. Magini M. Treatment of alcoholism using psychedelic drugs: a review of the program of research. *J Psychedelic Drugs.* 1998; 30:381–418.
17. Delgado PL, Moreno FA. Hallucinogens, serotonin and obsessive-compulsive disorder. *J Psychedelic Drugs.* 1998;30:359–366.
18. Grob CS. Psychiatric research with hallucinogens: what have we learned. In: Grob CS, ed. *Hallucinogens, A Reader.* New York, NY: Jeremy P. Tarcher/Putnam; 2002:263–291.
19. Gouzoulis-Mayfrank, Heekeren K, Neukirch A, et al. Psychological effects of (s)-ketamine and N,N-dimethyltryptamine (DMT): a double-blind, cross-over study in healthy volunteers. *Pharmacopsychiatry.* 2005;38:301–311.
20. Griffiths RR, Richards WA, McCann U, et al. Psilocybin can occasion mystical-type experiences having substantial and sustained personal meaning and spiritual significance. *Psychopharmacology (Berl).* 2006;187:268–283.
21. Johnson MW, Richards WA, Griffiths RR. Human hallucinogen research: guidelines for safety. *J Psychopharmacol.* 2008;22: 603–620.
22. Sessa B. Is it time to revisit the role of psychedelic drugs in enhancing human creativity? *J Psychopharmacol.* 2008;22:821–827.
23. Johnston LD, O'Malley PM, Bachman JG, et al. *Monitoring the Future National Survey Results on Drug Use, 1975–2008: Volume I, Secondary School Students* (NIH Publication No. 09-7402). Bethesda, MD: National Institute on Drug Abuse; 2009.
24. Johnston LD, O'Malley PM, Bachman JG, et al. *Monitoring the Future National Survey Results on Drug Use, 1975–2008: Volume II, College Students and Adults Ages 19–50* (NIH Publication No. 09-7403). Bethesda, MD: National Institute on Drug Abuse; 2009.
25. Kelly BC, Parsons JT, Wells BE. Prevalence and predictors of club drug use among club-going young adults in New York City. *J Urban Health.* 2006;83:884–895.
26. Fuller JG. *The Day of St. Anthony's Fire.* New York, NY: Macmillan; 1968.
27. Hofmann A. Chemical, pharmacological and medical aspects of psychotomimetics. *J Exp Mend Sci.* 1961;5:31–51.
28. Hollister LE. Psychotomimetic drugs in man. In: Iversen LL, Iversen SD, Snyder SH, eds. *Handbook of Psychopharmacology.* Vol 11. New York, NY: Plenum Press; 1978:389–424.
29. Nash FJ, Meltzer HY, Gudelsky GA. Selective cross-tolerance to 5-HT$_{1A}$ and 5-HT$_2$ receptor-mediated temperature and corticosterone responses. *Pharmacol Biochem Behav.* 1989;33:781–785.
30. Ungerleider JT, Fisher DD. The problems of LSD and emotional disorders. *Calif Med.* 1967;106:49–55.
31. Hamon M. Common neurochemical correlates to the action of hallucinogens. In: Jacobs BL, ed. *Hallucinogens: Neurochemical, Behavioral and Clinical Perspectives.* New York, NY: Raven Press; 1984:143–169.
32. Freedman DX. Hallucinogenic drug research–if so, so what? Symposium summary and commentary. *Pharmacol Biochem Behav.* 1986;24:407–415.
33. Freedman DX. Effects of LSD-25 on brain serotonin. *J Pharmacol Exp Ther.* 1961;134:160–166.
34. Lucki I, Frazer A. Prevention of the serotonin syndrome in rats by repeated administration of monoamine oxidase inhibitors but not tricyclic antidepressants. *Psychopharmacology (Berl).* 1981;77:205–211.
35. Hannon J, Hoyer D. Molecular biology of 5-HT receptors. *Behav Brain Res.* 2008;16:198–213.
36. Aghajanian GK, Sprouse JS, Rasmussen K. Physiology of the midbrain serotonin system. In: Meltzer HY, ed. *Psychopharmacology: The Third Generation of Progress.* New York: Raven Press; 1987:141–149.
37. Trulson ME, Heym J, Jacobs BL. Dissociations between the effects of hallucinogenic drugs on behavior and raphe unit activity in freely moving cats. *Brain Res.* 1981;215:275–293.
38. Aghajanian GK. Serotonin and the action of LSD in the brain. *Psychiatr Ann.* 1994;24:137–141.
39. Glennon RA. Do classical hallucinogens act as 5-HT$_2$ agonists or antagonists? *Neuropsychopharmacology.* 1990;3:509–517.
40. Buckholtz NS, Zhou D, Freedman DX, et al. Lysergic acid diethylamide (LSD) administration selectively downregulates serotonin receptors in rat brain. *Neuropsychopharmacology.* 1990;3:137–148.
41. Burris KD, Breeding M, Sanders-Bush E. (+)Lysergic acid diethylamide, but not its nonhallucinogenic congeners, is a potent serotonin 5-HT$_{1C}$ receptor agonist. *J Pharmacol Exp Ther.* 1991; 258:891–896.
42. Strassman RJ. Adverse reactions to psychedelic drugs: a review of the literature. *J Nerv Ment Dis.* 1984;172:577–595.
43. Ungerleider JT, Fisher DD, Fuller MC, et al. The bad trip: the etiology of the adverse LSD reaction. *Am J Psychiatry.* 1968; 125:1483–1490.
44. Ungerleider JT. The acute side effects from LSD. In: Ungerleider JT, ed. *The Problems and Prospects of LSD.* Springfield, IL: Charles C Thomas; 1972:61–68.
45. Bowers MB Jr. The role of drugs in the production of schizophreniform psychoses and related disorders. In: Meltzer HY, ed. *Psychopharmacology: The Third Generation of Progress.* New York: Raven Press; 1987:819–823.
46. Cohen S. A quarter century of research with LSD. In: Ungerleider JT, ed. *The Problems and Prospects of LSD.* Springfield, IL: Charles C Thomas; 1972:20–45.
47. Ungerleider JT, Fisher DD, Fuller MC. The dangers of LSD: analysis of seven months' experience in a university hospital's psychiatric service. *JAMA.* 1966;197:389–392.
48. Legriel S, Bruneel F, Spreux-Varoquaux O, et al. Lysergic acid amide-induced posterior reversible encephalopathy syndrome with status epilepticus. *Neurocrit Care.* 208;9:247–252.
49. Berk SI, LeBlond RF, Hodges KB, et al. A mesenteric mass in a chronic LSD user. *Am J Med.* 1999;107:188–198.

50. Spengos K, Schwartz A, Hennerici M. Multifocal cerebral demyelination after magic mushroom abuse. *J Neurol.* 2000; 247;224–225.
51. Gillman PK. Triptans, serotonin agonists, and serotonin syndrome (serotonin toxicity): a review. *Headache.* 2009;50: 264–272.
52. Gable RS. Risk assessment of ritual use of oral dimethyltryptamine (DMT) and harmala alkaloids. *Addiction.* 2007;102:24–34.
53. Carstairs SD, Cantrell FL. Peyote and mescaline exposures: a 12-year review of a statewide poison center database. *Clin Toxicol.* 2010;48:350–353.
54. Nolte KB, Zumwalt, RE. Fatal peyote ingestion associated with Mallory-Weiss lacerations. *West J Med.* 1999;170:328.
55. Miller PL, Gay GR, Ferris KC, et al. Treatment of acute, adverse reactions: "I've tripped and I can't get down." *J Psychoactive Drugs.* 1992;24:277–279.
56. Lerner AG, Shufman E, Kodesh A, et al. Risperidone-associated, benign transient visual disturbances in schizophrenic patients with a past history of LSD abuse. *Isr J Psychiatry Relat Sci.* 2002; 39:57–60.
57. Abraham HD, Fava M. Order of onset of substance abuse and depression in a sample of depressed outpatients. *Compr Psychiatry.* 1999;40:44–50.
58. Halpern JH, Pope HG Jr. Hallucinogen persisting perception disorder: what do we know after 50 years? *Drug Alcohol Depend.* 2003;69:109–119.
59. American Psychiatric Association. *Diagnostic and Statistical Manual of Mental Disorders.* 4th ed. Washington, DC: Author; 1994.
60. Levi L, Miller NR. Visual illusions associated with previous drug abuse. *J Clin Neuroophthalmol.* 1990;10:103–110.
61. Markel H, Lee A, Holmes RD, et al. LSD flashback syndrome exacerbated by selective serotonin reuptake inhibitor antidepressants in adolescents. *J Pediatr.* 1994;125:817–819.
62. Alcantara AG. Is there a role of alpha-2 antagonism in the exacerbation of hallucinogen-persisting perception disorder with risperidone. *J Clin Psychopharmacol.* 1998;18:487–488.
63. Lerner AG, Gelkopf M, Skladman I, et al. Flashback and hallucinogen persisting perception disorder: clinical aspects and pharmacological treatment approach. *Isr J Psychiatry Relat Sci.* 2002;39:92–99.
64. Abraham HD, Aldridge AM. LSD: a point well taken. *Addiction.* 1994;89:763.
65. Abraham HD, Aldridge AM. Adverse consequences of lysergic acid diethylamide. *Addiction.* 1993;88:1327–1334.
66. Kawasaki A, Purvin V. Persistent palinopsia following ingestion of lysergic acid diethylamide (LSD). *Arch Ophthalmol.* 1996; 114:47–50.
67. Halpern JH, Pope HG Jr. Do hallucinogens cause residual neuropsychological toxicity. *Drug Alcohol Depend.* 1999;53: 247–256.
68. Strassman RJ. Human hallucinogen interactions with drugs affecting serotonergic neurotransmission. *Neuropsychopharmacology.* 1992;7:241–243.
69. Bonson KR, Murphy DL. Alterations in responses to LSD in humans associated with chronic administration of tricyclic antidepressants, monoamine oxidase inhibitors or lithium. *Behav Brain Res.* 1996;73:229–233.

CHAPTER 19: PCP/Designer Drugs/MDMA

Una D. McCann

Certain drugs of abuse do not fall under any readily categorized drug class. Among these are phencyclidine (phenylcyclohexylpiperidine, PCP) and 3,4- methylenedioxymethamphetamine (MDMA), which are both sometimes referred to as "designer drugs" because they are manufactured in a chemical laboratory, rather than being derived from natural substances. This chapter reviews the history, psychopharmacology, epidemiology, and neurotoxicity of PCP and MDMA, and briefly discusses several of the other more common "designer drugs" that continue to be used and abused on an international basis.

PCP

History

The original chemistry that led to the development of PCP took place in 1926 (1,2). However, it took approximately an additional 30 years for PCP's anesthetic properties to be noted, initially in animals (3). In 1953, it was patented by Parke-Davis under the trade name of Sernyl in a research program targeting general anesthetics. Initial studies were promising and described the development of complete analgesia without respiratory or cardiovascular depression within a few minutes following intravenous administration of a relatively low dose (4). However, at higher doses that were necessary to achieve full surgical levels of anesthesia, undesirable adverse reactions were noted, including the requirement of pentobarbital for control of an "excited state" (4).

Other early experiments involving the use of PCP for general anesthesia in humans also reported untoward side effects, including the development of apparent trance-like ecstatic states during anesthesia, and hallucinations, visual distortions, dizziness, slurred speech, and manic behavior upon emergence from anesthesia (5,6). According to some reports, nearly half of the patients who received PCP for anesthesia went on to develop psychotic reactions, some of which persisted for more than a week after surgery (5,4,7). Qualitatively similar, but less severe adverse effects were seen following administration of lower doses of PCP (7). The trance-like states that occurred in patients undergoing anesthesia with PCP, without full loss of consciousness, led to its classification as a "dissociative" anesthetic, along with the related compounds, cyclohexamine and ketamine.

Despite early promise and potential advantages over traditional general anesthetics, PCP's adverse effects and long half-life in the human body made it unsuitable for medical applications and it was removed from the market in 1965. In 1967, it was given the trade name *Sernylan* and marketed as a veterinary anesthetic, but was again discontinued. Ironically, the ability of PCP to produce hallucinations and an altered sense of consciousness appeared to fuel, rather than deter, the first PCP epidemic in the 1970s (2).

Psychopharmacology

The existence of PCP receptors in the brain of rats was first demonstrated in 1979 (8,9). Subsequent research in the 1980s demonstrated that PCP's primary mechanism of action was as a potent inhibitor of neurotransmission mediated by N-methyl-D-aspartate (NMDA) receptors, one of several receptor sites for the excitatory amino acid, glutamate (10). At 10-fold higher dosages, PCP also blocks presynaptic monoamine reuptake, resulting in increased synaptic levels of dopamine (DA), norepinephrine, and serotonin. Although activity at NMDA receptors occurs at much lower dosages of NMDA than required to influence monoaminergic activity, monoaminergic inhibition may be achieved at doses abused recreationally that lead to intoxication (10). At levels of extreme intoxication, PCP blocks sodium and potassium channels and can interact with cholinergic, opiate, and γ-aminobutyric acid (GABA)/benzodiazepine receptors. These interactions are minor and not likely to occur at doses typically used in recreational settings (10).

PCP is highly lipid soluble and is primarily metabolized through hepatic pathways. It is stored in fatty body tissues (11), and it is believed that mobilization of fat stores of PCP is responsible for waxing and waning states of intoxication that can last for weeks, "flashbacks," and persistent "positive drug tests" that persist days to weeks after PCP ingestion (12). Hepatic recirculation of PCP may also explain fluctuating levels of intoxication seen following PCP use.

The behavioral effects of PCP are dose related but highly variable among individuals. In a classic National Institute on Drug Abuse research monograph published during the peak of the first PCP epidemic in the United States, Domino (13) described the major central nervous system effects of the drug as follows:

1. **Small doses** lead to a "drunken" state with numbness of the extremities and in some species, excitation.
2. In **moderate doses**, analgesia and anesthesia is observed.
3. A psychic state somewhat resembling sensory isolation is produced. Sensory impulses in grossly distorted form do reach the neocortex.

4. Cataleptiform motor responses occur.
5. *Large doses* may produce convulsions.

These early observations have largely borne out. Lower doses of PCP typically lead to a giddy euphoria that resembles alcohol intoxication, although anxiety, paranoia, and emotional outbursts can be seen (14,15). Higher dosages can lead to dysarthria, ataxia, increased deep tendon reflexes, decreased pain sensation, tachycardia, hypertension, and, as previously mentioned, altered perception (16). Malignant hyperthermia after PCP intoxication has been reported, and PCP intoxication can progress to stupor and coma (17). PCP is one of only a few drugs that can cause vertical nystagmus (horizontal nystagmus can also occur), the combination of nystagmus and hypertension in an otherwise healthy young adult should alert the physician to the possibility of PCP intoxication.

PCP-induced psychosis has been put forth as a model for schizophrenia (18,19), and a number of authors have hypothesized, based on clinical experience and available epidemiologic evidence, that individuals with previous psychiatric problems who use PCP are at the highest risk for developing persistent psychotic symptoms following PCP use (16,10).

Epidemiology

PCP is sold as tablets, capsules, or as white or colored powder. It is odorless and water soluble. It is often misrepresented as being more expensive substances (e.g., lysergic acid diethylamide, tetrahydrocannabinol, mescaline, and cocaine) and is often used to lace inferior batches of other drugs (e.g., marijuana). There are literally hundreds of street names for PCP (20), but commonly used names include angel dust, killer weed, PeaCe Pill, ozone, wack, and power fuel. Because of the large number of names for PCP and the fact that it is often used as an adulterant of other illicit substances, many people are unaware that they have used PCP. Epidemiologic data, therefore, are obtained using a variety of methods, including reports from emergency room visits, deaths, drug abuse treatment facilities, and national surveys.

Using these sources for data, it has been suggested that there was an epidemic of phencyclidine use between 1973 and 1979 and again, perhaps, between 1981 and 1984 (10). Although there are regional differences in the mode of ingestion, in more than 85% of the cases PCP is smoked (21), followed by inhalation or oral ingestion. Less than 2% of individuals use PCP intravenously. Usually, smoked PCP is in conjunction with marijuana, tobacco, or parsley (10). Individuals report developing a tolerance to PCP, with experienced users needing higher dosages of PCP to achieve the same effect.

Current Trends in PCP Use

According to the most recent data from the National Survey on Drug Use and Health (22), 53,000 individuals in the United States over the age of 12 initiated use of PCP during 2008. This is significantly lower than the numbers in 2002, 2003, and 2004, when the number of new users of PCP were estimated to be 123,000, 105,000, and 106,000, respectively. To put this number in perspective, the number of new users of marijuana in 2008 was estimated at 2.2 million, and new users of MDMA were estimated at 894,000. An estimated 6,631,000 individuals reported that they had used PCP at some point during their life in 2008, with approximately 99,000 individuals having used PCP within the past year (22). These numbers are not significantly different from those reported in 2007.

Neurotoxicity

In 1989, Olney and colleagues (23) reported that single doses of PCP and related compounds (MK-801 and ketamine) led to neuronal damage of cortical neurons in rats. In particular, neurons located in layers III and IV of the posterior cingulate and retrosplenial cortices were observed to have abnormal cytoplasmic vacuolization that was directly correlated with the potency of noncompetitive NMDA blockade. More recent studies (24) indicate that PCP induces neuronal degeneration in a variety of cerebrocortical and limbic regions, although the mechanism of degeneration is not well understood. It is also not known whether PCP-induced neuronal injury is related to lasting psychiatric and cognitive changes that have been reported in some PCP users.

MDMA

History

MDMA (sometimes also known as "ecstasy") was synthesized and patented by Merck in 1914 but was never used for commercial purposes (25). Although it is an amphetamine analog, it is also structurally related to mescaline, the classic hallucinogen. MDMA received little attention from the pharmaceutical or scientific communities until the 1970s when, as part of a larger study of mescaline analogs, Hardman and colleagues (26) evaluated MDMA's behavioral effects (and determined lethal dosages) in several animal species. A report by Shulgin and Nichols (27) indicated that MDMA produced "an easily controlled altered state of consciousness with emotional and sensual overtones" and further suggested that MDMA may have potential as psychotherapeutic adjunct. Little was written about MDMA following this report until 1985, when the Drug Enforcement Administration (DEA) in the United States moved to severely restrict MDMA use by placing it on Schedule I of controlled substances (28). The DEA indicated that their decision was based on reports that recreational use of MDMA was on the rise, as well as concerns that MDMA might pose a public health threat, since a closely related congener of MDMA, 3,4-methylenedioxyamphetamine (MDA), had recently been found to produce toxic effects on brain serotonin neurons in rodents (29). The DEA also argued that MDMA had no medical utility, a statement that was disputed by a number of mental health specialists who asserted that it had utility in psychotherapeutic settings (30–32).

At roughly the same time that the DEA placed MDMA on Schedule I, MDMA's popularity was increasing on college campuses (33). Interestingly, this increase in popularity took place despite growing preclinical evidence that MDMA, like MDA, had the potential to damage brain serotonin neurons (34–36).

Psychopharmacology

The most prominent acute pharmacologic effect of MDMA is calcium-independent release of brain serotonin (5-HT) from brain serotonin neurons (37,38) via vesicular and plasma membrane monoamine transporters (39). To a lesser degree, MDMA also induces release of DA (40–42). Like other amphetamines, the most prominent effects of MDMA are mediated indirectly, via release of monoamines, rather than by directly interacting with monoaminergic receptors (43). This primary indirect action of MDMA is in contrast with hallucinogenic amphetamines that act primarily by activating serotonergic receptors (43).

Although MDMA's primary effects are indirect, it does bind to a several postsynaptic receptor sites (44,45). These include, in order of affinity, the $5-HT_{2A}$ receptor, the α-2 adrenergic receptor, the $5-HT_2$ receptor, the histamine H_1 receptor, and the muscarinic M_1 receptor. Binding at other 5-HT and adrenergic receptors, DA receptors, opioid receptors, and benzodiazepine receptors only occurs at very high concentrations (44).

As might be predicted by its acute pharmacologic effects, in animals MDMA administration leads to typical signs of sympathomimetic stimulation (26,46,47). However, some behavioral studies suggest that MDMA can be distinguished from typical stimulants (48,49). In drug discrimination studies, MDMA substitutes for D-amphetamine in rats (50), pigeons (51), and monkeys trained to discriminate D-amphetamine from saline (52). Results from testing with hallucinogens are less clear-cut. In particular, MDMA does not substitute for the hallucinogen, DOB (53,54), but does substitute with the alpha-ethyl derivative of the hallucinogen, DOM, as well as the alpha-ethyl derivative alpha-methyltryptamine (55). Several animal models suggest that MDMA has abuse liability. In particular, both baboons and monkeys self-administer MDMA (56,57). Further, in intracranial self-stimulation models, MDMA consistently lowers the threshold for rewarding electrical stimulation delivered via electrodes stereotaxically implanted in the medial forebrain bundle region (58).

Knowledge regarding the behavioral effects of MDMA in humans has been derived from both retrospective clinical reports (59,60) and reports from research subjects who receive MDMA in controlled research settings (61–69). As might be anticipated by MDMA's acute pharmacology and behavioral effects in animals, both sources indicate that, as in animals, MDMA has prominent acute stimulant effects. In addition, human MDMA users also report effects that are commonly associated with hallucinogens. Shortly after drug ingestion, stimulant effects of MDMA that have been reported include increased heart rate and blood pressure, increased core body temperature, dry mouth, decreased appetite, increased alertness, decreased speech fluency, jaw clenching, increased sleep latency, and altered sleep architecture. Associated with these physiologic effects of MDMA is an increased sense of well-being and, occasionally, euphoria. Most MDMA users do not report hallucinations, but often report increased emotional sensitiveness, a feeling of "oneness," depersonalization or sense that certain body parts are "other," derealization, and altered time perception.

There continues to be interest by some mental health practitioners in the utility of MDMA as a potential psychotherapeutic adjunct. In particular, in 2002, a plan to investigate the utility of MDMA in the treatment of posttraumatic stress disorder (PTSD) in the United States was announced (70). No results have yet been reported. A brief report describing a pilot study that was stopped prematurely "because of political pressures" was published, but insufficient subjects took part to determine the safety or efficacy of MDMA for the treatment of PTSD (71).

Epidemiology

The best epidemiologic data on MDMA use in the United States is derived from the Monitoring the Future (MTF) Survey, which has measured trends in drug use among 8th, 10th, and 12th graders since 1975 (72), and the National Survey on Drug Use and Health (22), which measures trends in drug use among individuals who are 12 years and older. According to MTF data, MDMA use peaked among adolescents in 2001 and has been relatively stable since 2006. Although use of MDMA is not currently rising, the perceived risk associated with MDMA use has been in decline for the past 6 years, which is considered a concern. In 2009, 4.3% of high school seniors reported having used MDMA in the past year, with 3.7% and 1.3% of 10th and 8th graders reporting past-year use.

The most recent National Survey on Drug Use and Health data indicate that in 2008, an estimated 555,000 individuals (0.2% of the population) in the United States over the age of 12 had used MDMA in the month prior to the survey. Lifetime use in this same demographic group was significantly increased from 4.3% (10.2 million individuals) in 2002 to 5.2% (12.9 million) in 2008; however, past-year use of MDMA decreased from 1.3% to 0.9% during the same period. Approximately 894,000 Americans used MDMA for the first time in 2008, which is a significant increase from the 615,000 first-time users reported in 2005 (22).

Toxicity

Toxic effects of MDMA are, in large part, an exaggeration of acute pharmacologic actions and can include anxiety, agitation, confusion, insomnia, nausea, and palpitations (73). More serious adverse effects include potentially fatal malignant hypertension, severe hyperthermia, cardiac arrhythmias, myocardial infarction, strokes (both ischemic and hemorrhagic), cerebral edema, and seizures. Less well understood adverse effects of MDMA that have been reported are the development of a syndrome of inappropriate antidiuretic hormone secretion, marked elevation in serum creatine kinase in the absence of muscle injury, and persistent neuropsychiatric complications (73,74).

Neurotoxicity

In addition to its use as a recreational drug, MDMA is also a well-documented brain serotonin (5-HT) neurotoxin in animals (75). In particular, MDMA causes dose-related reductions of brain serotonin (5-HT) and 5-hydroxyindoleacetic acid (5-HIAA) concentrations (34–36,76), the density of 5-HT uptake sites (36,77,78), and the activity of tryptophan hydroxylase activity (35,79,80). Neurochemical deficits, which have been documented up to 7 years after drug administration in nonhuman primates, are associated with a loss of 5-HT axon terminals, as measured using immunocytochemical methods (81–83), indicating that they are related to a distal axotomy. Although MDMA-induced 5-HT neurotoxicity is dose related, even single oral dosages that produce plasma levels on the order of those seen following human recreational use (84) have been shown to produce neurotoxic injury (85).

There are also significant data indicating that some humans who use MDMA, like animals with documented MDMA-induced 5-HT lesions, develop a persistent reduction in brain 5-HT axonal markers (86–93). The duration of these lesions and their functional consequences are still a matter of debate, but it has been hypothesized that the MDMA-induced 5-HT neurotoxicity may underlie cognitive and sleep abnormalities that have been documented in abstinent MDMA users (94,95).

Miscellaneous Designer Drugs

As noted previously, designer drugs are drugs that are synthesized making minor modifications to the chemical structure of an existing drug. The goal of this enterprise is to circumvent laws (e.g., create a substance that is not illegal or scheduled) or to save money (create more potent or cheaper analogs of an existing, expensive product). In an effort to prevent the legal distribution and sale of "look alike" designer drugs, the U.S. government amended the Controlled Substances Act in 1986 to include the Controlled Substances Analogues Enforcement Act. This law states that a substance is classified as illegal if it is "substantially similar" to the chemical structure of an already controlled substance in Schedule I or II. Despite this action, there is sufficient ambiguity in the definition of "substantially similar" that some argue that the law is imprecise and essentially useless (96).

As might be concluded by the definition of designer drugs, the possibilities for such compounds are virtually endless. Indeed, in a classic book about "designer" phenethylamine analogs (97), Alexander Shulgin and Ann Shulgin describe the synthesis and subjective effects of 179 designer drugs, including MDMA.

In addition to MDMA and related compounds, the most important designer compounds in terms of public health and substance abuse have been drugs that have been used as substitutes for opiates. Alpha-methylfentanyl, also known as China White, was first manufactured in clandestine laboratories in Orange County, California in 1979, and was the first synthetically produced fentanyl; it resulted in at least 15 overdose deaths. Over the next 5 years, at least three other analogs were identified in street drug samples and in the bodily fluids of overdose victims: α-methylacetylfentanyl, 3-methylfentanyl, and parafluorofentanyl (98,99). In 1988, 3-methylfentanyl was identified in 16 unintentional overdose deaths in Allegheny County, Pennsylvania.

Designer analogs of meperidine (marketed as Demerol) have also appeared periodically in the illicit drug market. Two meperidine analogs that have appeared on the streets include MPPP (1-methyl-4-phenyl-4-propionoxypiperidine) and PEPAP (1-[2-phenylethyl]-4-acetyloxypiperdine). In 1983, there was an unusual outbreak of parkinsonism among young intravenous heroin abusers in California (100). These cases were reminiscent of an earlier similar case that had been identified at the National Institute of Health campus in Bethesda, Maryland (101). It was subsequently determined that the illicitly manufactured MPPP was tainted with 1-methyl-4-phenyl-1,2,3,6-tetrahydropyridine (MPTP), a potent neurotoxin that destroys DA-containing cells in the pars compacta of the substantia nigra, the chief site of pathology in Parkinson disease (101–103). These cases underscore the potential disastrous results from even minor modifications to the chemical structure of drugs with known safety and efficacy profiles.

CONCLUSION

MDMA and PCP are illicit drugs that have the potential to damage brain cells, in addition to their risks as drugs of abuse. The functional consequences of MDMA- and PCP-induced neurotoxicity are not fully understood but may include lasting cognitive disturbance. Although other "designer drugs" are not used by large percentages of the population, they periodically appear in the drug market, particularly during periods when the parent drug is scarce or expensive. In the case of designer opioids, deaths from unintentional overdose related to increased drug potency, and the development of parkinsonism related to drug contamination, underscore the fact that even minor chemical modifications to a drug structure can lead to profound pharmacologic and toxicologic changes.

REFERENCES

1. Kotz A, Merkel P. Hydroaromatic alkamines. *J Prakt Chem.* 1926; 113:49.
2. Shulgin AT, MacLean DE. Illicit synthesis of phencyclidine (PCP) and several of its analogs. *Clin Toxicol.* 1976;9(4):553–560.
3. Chen G, Ensor CR, Russel D, et al. The pharmacology of 1-(1-Phencyclidine) piperidine HCL. *J Pharm Exp Ther.* 1959;127: 241–250.
4. Greifenstein FE, Yoskitake J, DeVault M, et al. A study of 1-arylcyclohexylamine for anesthesia. *Anesth Analg.* 1958;37:

283–294.
5. Johnstone M, Evans V, Baigel S. Sernyl (Cl-395) in clinical anesthesia. *Br J Anaesth.* 1958;31:433–439.
6. Riffin, IM. An appraisal of new induction agents. *J Med Soc New J.* 1960;57:15–19.
7. Meyer JS, Greifenstein F, DeVault M. A new drug causing symptoms of sensory deprivation. *J Nerv Ment Dis.* 1959;129:54–61.
8. Vincent JP, Kartalouski B, Geneste P, et al. Interaction of phencyclidine ("angel dust") with a specific receptor in rat brain membranes. *Proc Natl Acad Sci U S A.* 1979;76:4678–4682.
9. Zukin SR, Zukin RS. Specific ^{3}H-phencyclidine binding in rat central nervous system. *Proc Natl Acad Sci U S A.* 1979;76:5372–5376.
10. Zukin SR, Sloboda Z, Javitt DC. Phencyclidine (PCP). In: Lowinson JH, Ruiz P, Millmann B, et al., eds. *Substance Abuse: A Comprehensive Textbook.* Philadelphia, PA: Lippincott Williams & Wilkins; 1994:324–335.
11. James SH, Schnoll SH. Phencyclidine: tissue distribution in the rat. *Clin Toxicol.* 1976;2:573.
12. Misra AL, Pontani RB, Bartolemeo J. Persistence of phencyclidine (PCP) and metabolites in brain and adipose tissue and implications for long-lasting behavioural effects. *Res Commun Chem Pathol Pharmacol.* 1979;24:431–445.
13. Domino EF. Neurobiology of phencyclidine: an update. In: Petersen RC, Stillman RC, eds. *Phencyclidine (PCP) Abuse: An Appraisal.* NIDA Research Monographs. Washington DC: National Institute on Drug Abuse; 1978;21:44.
14. Sioris LJ, Krenzelok EP. Phencyclidine intoxication: a literature review. *Am J Hosp Pharm.* 1978;35:1362.
15. McCarron MM, Schulze BW, Thompson GA, et al. Acute phencyclidine intoxication: incidence of clinical findings in 1000 cases. *Ann Emerg Med.* 1981;10:237.
16. Aniline O, Pitts FN. Phencyclidine (PCP): a review and perspectives. *Crit Rev Toxicol.* 1982;10(2):145–177.
17. Baldridge EB, Bessen HA. Phencyclidine. *Emerg Med Clin North Am.* 1990;8:541.
18. Luby ED, Cohen BD, Rosenbaum F, et al. Study of a new schizophrenomimetic drug Sernyl. *Arch Neurol Psychiatry.* 1959; 81: 363–369.
19. Domino EF, Luby E. Abnormal mental states induced by phencyclidine as a model of schizophrenia. In: Domino EF, ed. *PCP (phencyclidine): Historical and Current Perspectives.* Ann Arbor, MI: NPP Books; 1981:37–50.
20. Office of National Drug Control Policy. Street terms database 2010. Available at: http://www.whitehousedrugpolicy.gov/streetterms.
21. Substance Abuse and Mental Health Services Administration, Office of Applied Studies. *Treatment Episode Data Set (TEDS): 1996-2006. National Admissions to Substance Abuse Treatment Services,* 2008. Rockville, MD: DASIS Series: S-43, DHHS Publication No. (SMA) 08-4347.
22. Substance Abuse and Mental Health Services Administration. Results from the 2008 National Survey on Drug Use and Health: National Findings, 2010. Rockville, MD: Office of Applied Studies, NSDUH Series H-36, HHS publication No. SMA 09-4434.
23. Olney J, Labruyere J, Price M. Pathological changes induced in cerebrocortical neurons by phencyclidine and related drugs. *Science.* 1989;244:1360.
24. Corso TD, Sesma MA, Tenkova TI, et al. Multifocal brain damage induced by phencyclidine is augmented by pilocarpine. *Brain Res.* 1997; 752:1–2.
25. Shulgin AT. The background and chemistry of MDMA. *J Psychoactive Drugs.* 1986;18(4):291–304.
26. Hardman HF, Haavik CO, Seevers MH. Relationship of the structure of mescaline and seven analogs to toxicity and behavior in five species of laboratory animals. *Toxicol Appl Pharmacol.* 1973;25:299–309.
27. Shulgin AT, Nichols DE. Characterization of three new psychotomimetics. In: Stillman RC, Willette RE, eds. *The Psychopharmacology of Hallucinogens.* New York: Pergamon Press; 1978:74–83.
28. Lawn, JC. Schedules of controlled substances scheduling of 3,4-methylenedioxymethamphetamine (MDMA) into Schedule I of the Controlled Substances Act. *Fed Regist.* 1986;51:36552–36560.
29. Ricaurte GA, Bryan G, Strauss L, et al. Hallucinogenic amphetamine selectively destroys brain serotonin nerve terminals. *Science.* 1985;229:986.
30. Greer G. Using MDMA in psychotherapy. *Advances.* 1985;2(2):57–59.
31. Greer G, Tolbert R. Subjective reports of the effects of MDMA in a clinical setting. *J Psychoactive Drugs.* 1986;18(4):319–327.
32. Greer G, Strassman RJ. Information on "Ecstasy." *Am J Psychiatry.* 1985;142(11):1391
33. Peroutka SJ. Incidence of recreational use of 3,4-methylenedioxymethamphetamine (M13MA, "Ecstasy") on an undergraduate campus. *N Engl J Med.* 1987;317:1542–1543.
34. Schmidt CJ, Wu L, Lovenberg W. Methylenedioxymethamphetamine: a potentially neurotoxic amphetamine analogue. *Eur J Pharmacol.* 1986;124(1–2):175–178.
35. Stone DM, Stahl DC, Hanson GR, et al. The effects of 3,4-methylenedioxymethamphetamine (MDMA) and 3,4 methylenedioxyamphetamine (MDA) on monoaminergic systems in the rat brain. *Eur J Pharmacol.* 1986;128(1–2):41–48.
36. Commins DL, Vosmer G, Virus RM, et al. Biochemical and histological evidence that methylenedioxymethylamphetamine (MDMA) is toxic to neurons in the rat brain. *J Pharmacol Exp Ther.* 1987;241(1):338–345.
37. Johnson MP, Hoffman AH, Nichols DE. Effects of the enantiomers of MDA, MDMA and related analogues on [3H]-serotonin and [3H]-dopamine release from superfused rat brain slices. *Eur J Pharmacol.* 1986;132:269–276.
38. McKenna DJ, Peroutka SJ. Neurochemistry and neurotoxicity of 3,4-methylenedioxymethamphetamine (MDMA, "ecstasy"). *J Neurochem.* 1990;54(1):14–22.
39. Rudnick G, Wall SC. The molecular mechanism of "ecstasy" [3,4-methylenedioxymethamphetamine (MDMA)]: serotonin transporters are targets for MDMA-induced serotonin release. *Proc Natl Acad Sci U S A.* 1992;89:1817–1821.
40. Yamamoto BK, Spanos LJ. The acute effects of methylenedioxymethamphetamine on dopamine release in the awake-behaving rat. *Eur J Pharmacol.* 1988;148:195–203.
41. Hiramatsu M, Cho AK. Enantiomeric differences in the effects of 3,4-methylenedioxymethamphetamine on extracellular monoamines and metabolites in the striatum of freely-moving rats. *Neuropharmacology.* 1990;29:269–275.
42. Nash JF, Meltzer HY, Gudelsky GA. Effect of 3,4-methylenedioxymethamphetamine on 3,4-dihydroxyphenylalanine accumulation in the striatum and nucleus accumbens. *J Neurochem.* 1990;54:1062–1067.
43. Titeler M, Lyon RA, Glennon RA. Radioligand binding evidence implicates the brain 5-HT$_2$ receptor as a site of action for LSD and central phenylisopropylamine hallucinogens. *Psychopharmacology.* 1988;94:213–216.
44. Battaglia G, Brooks BP, Kulsakdinum C, et al. Pharmacologic profile of MDMA (3,4-methylenedioxymethamphetamine) at various brain recognition sites. *Eur J Pharmacol.* 1988;149:159–163.

45. Pierce PA, Peroutka SJ. Ring-substituted amphetamine interactions with neurotransmitter receptor binding sites in human cortex. *Neurosci Lett.* 1988;95(1–3):208–212.
46. Gordon CJ, Watkinson WP, O'Callaghan JP, et al. Effects of 3,4-methylenedioxymethamphetamine on autonomic thermoregulatory responses of the rat. *Pharmacol Biochem Behav.* 1991; 38(2):339–344.
47. Frith CH, Chang LW, Lattin DL, et al. Toxicity of methylenedioxymethamphetamine (MDMA) in the dog and the rat. *Fundam Appl Toxicol.* 1987;9(1):110–119.
48. Gold LH, Koob GF, Geyer, MA. Stimulant and hallucinogenic behavioral profiles of 3,4-methylenedioxymethamphetamine and N-ethyl-3,4-methylenedioxyamphetamine in rats. *J Pharmacol Exp Ther.* 1988;247:547–555.
49. Spanos LJ, Yamamoto BK. Acute and subchronic effects of methylenedioxymethamphetamine (±-MDMA) on locomotion and serotonin syndrome in the rat. *Pharmacol Biochem Behav.* 1989; 32:835–840.
50. Glennon RA, Young RY. Further investigations of the discriminative stimulus properties of MDA. *Pharmacol Biochem Behav.* 1984;20:501–505.
51. Evans SM, Johanson CE. Discriminative stimulus properties of (+/−)-3,4-methylenedioxymethamphetamine and (+/−)-3,4-methylenedioxyamphetamine in pigeons. *Drug Alcohol Depend.* 1986;18(2):159–164.
52. Kamien J B, Johanson CE, Schuster CR, et al. The effects of (+)-methylenedioxymethamphetamine and (+)-methylenedioxyamphetamine in monkeys trained to discriminate (+)-amphetamine from saline. *Drug Alcohol Depend.* 1986;18:139–147.
53. Glennon RA, Young R, Rosecrans JA, et al. Discriminative stimulus properties of MDA and related agents. *Biol Psychiatry.* 1982;17:807–814.
54. Nichols DE. Differences between the mechanism of action of MDMA, MBDB, and the classic hallucinogens. Identification of a new therapeutic class: Entactogens. *J Psychoactive Drugs.* 1986; 18:305–313.
55. Glennon RA. MDMA-like stimulus effects of alphaethyltryptamine and the alpha-ethyl homolog of DOM. *Pharmacol Biochem Behav.* 1993;46(2):459–462.
56. Lamb RJ, Griffiths RR. Self-injection of 3,4-methylenedioxymethamphetamine (MDMA) in the baboon. *Psychopharmacology.* 1987;91:268–272.
57. Beardsley PM, Balster RL, Harris LS. Self-administration of methylenedioxymethamphetamine (MDMA) by rhesus monkeys. *Drug Alcohol Depend.* 1986;18:149–157.
58. Hubner CB, Bird M, Rassnick S, et al. The threshold lowering effects of MDMA (ecstasy) on brain-stimulation reward. *Psychopharmacology.* 1988;95(1):49–51.
59. Downing, J. The psychological and physiological effects of MDMA on normal volunteers. *J Psychoactive Drugs.* 1986;18: 335–340.
60. McCann UD, Ricaurte GA. Reinforcing Subjective Effects of (±) 3,4-methylenedioxymethamphetamine (MDMA;"Ecstasy") may be separable from its neurotoxic actions: clinical evidence. *J Clin Psychopharmacol.* 1993;13(3):214–217.
61. Grob CS, Poland RE, Chang L, et al. Psychobiologic effects of 3,4-methylenedioxymethamphetamine in humans: methodological considerations and preliminary observations. *Behav Brain Res.* 1996;73:103–107.
62. Vollenweider FX, Gamma A, Liechti M, et al. Psychological and cardiovascular effects and short-term sequelae of MDMA ("Ecstasy") in MDMA-naïve healthy volunteers. *Neuropsychopharmacology.* 1998;19:241–251
63. Mas M, Farre M, de la Torre R, et al. Cardiovascular and neuroendocrine effects and pharmacokinetics of 3, 4-methylenedioxymethamphetamine in humans. *J Pharmacol Exp Ther.* 1999; 290(1):136–145.
64. Tancer ME, Johanson CE. The subjective effects of MDMA and mCPP in moderate MDMA users. *Drug Alcohol Depend.* 2001; 65(1):97–101.
65. Tancer M, Johanson CE. Reinforcing, subjective, and physiological effects of MDMA in humans: a comparison with d-amphetamine and mCPP. *Drug Alcohol Depend.* 2003;72(1):33–44.
66. Freedman RR, Johanson CE, Tancer ME. Thermoregulatory effects of 3,4-methylenedioxymethamphetamine (MDMA) in humans. *Psychopharmacology (Berl).* 2005;183(2):248–256.
67. Johanson CE, Kilbey M, Gatchalian K, et al. Discriminative stimulus effects of 3,4-methylenedioxymethamphetamine (MDMA) in humans trained to discriminate among D-amphetamine, meta-chlorophenylpiperazine and placebo. *Drug Alcohol Depend.* 2006;81(1):27–36.
68. Randall S, Johanson CE, Tancer M, et al. Effects of acute 3,4-methylenedioxymethamphetamine on sleep and daytime sleepiness in MDMA users: a preliminary study. *Sleep.* 2009;32(11): 1513–1519.
69. Marrone GF, Pardo JS, Krauss RM, et al. Amphetamine analogs methamphetamine and 3,4-methylenedioxymethamphetamine (MDMA) differentially affect speech. *Psychopharmacology (Berl).* 2010;208(2):169–177.
70. Doblin R. A clinical plan for MDMA (Ecstasy) in the treatment of posttraumatic stress disorder (PTSD): partnering with the FDA. *J Psychoactive Drugs.* 2002;34(2):185–194.
71. Bouso JC, Doblin R, Farré M, et al. MDMA-assisted psychotherapy using low doses in a small sample of women with chronic posttraumatic stress disorder. *J Psychoactive Drugs.* 2008;40(3): 225–236.
72. Johnston LD, O'Malley PM, Bachman, JG, et al. Monitoring the future national results on adolescent drug use: overview of key findings 2008. Bethesda, MD: National Institute on Drug Abuse; 2009. NIH Publication No. 09-7401.
73. McCann UD, Slate SO, Ricaurte GA. Adverse reactions with 3,4-methylenedioxymethamphetamine (MDMA; 'ecstasy'). *Drug Saf.* 1996;15(2):107–115.
74. Ricaurte GA, McCann UD. Recognition and management of complications of new recreational drug use. *Lancet.* 2005;365 (9477):2137–2145.
75. Green AR, Mechan AO, Elliott JM, et al. The pharmacology and clinical pharmacology of 3,4-methylenedioxymethamphetamine (MDMA, "ecstasy"). *Pharmacol Rev.* 2003;55(3):463–508.
76. Schmidt CJ. Neurotoxicity of the psychedelic amphetamine, methylenedioxymethamphetamine. *J Pharmacol Exp Ther.* 1987; 240(1):1–7.
77. Battaglia G, Yeh SY, O'Hearn E, et al. 3,4-Methylenedioxymethamphetamine and 3,4-methylenedioxyamphetamine destroy serotonin terminals in rat brain: quantification of neurodegeneration by measurement of [3H]paroxetine-labeled serotonin uptake sites. *J Pharmacol Exp Ther.* 1987;242(3): 911–916.
78. Battaglia G, Yeh SY, Desouza EB. MDMA-induced neurotoxicity: parameters of degeneration and recovery of brain serotonin neurons. *Pharmacol Biochem Behav.* 1998;29:269–274.
79. Schmidt CJ, Taylor VL. Depression of rat brain tryptophan hydroxylase activity following the acute administration of methylenedioxymethamphetamine. *Biochem Pharmacol.* 1987;36 (23): 4095–4102.

80. Stone DM, Johnson M, Hanson GR, et al. A comparison of the neurotoxic potential of methylenedioxyamphetamine (MDA) and its N-methylated and N-ethylated derivatives. Eur J Pharmacol. 1987;134(2):245–248.
81. O'Hearn E, Battaglia G, De Souza EB, et al. Methylenedioxyamphetamine (MDA) and methylenedioxymethamphetamine (MDMA) cause selective ablation of serotonergic axon terminals in forebrain: immunocytochemical evidence for neurotoxicity. J Neurosci. 1988;8(8):2788–2803.
82. Molliver ME, Berger UV, Mamounas LA, et al. Neurotoxicity of MDMA and related compounds: anatomic studies. Ann N Y Acad Sci. 1990;600:649–661; discussion 661–664.
83. Wilson MA, Ricaurte GA, Molliver ME. Distinct morphologic classes of serotonergic axons in primates exhibit differential vulnerability to the psychotropic drug 3,4-methylenedioxymethamphetamine. Neuroscience 1989;28 (1):121–137.
84. Irvine RJ, Keane M, Felgate P, et al. Plasma drug concentrations and physiological measures in 'dance party' participants. Neuropsychopharmacology. 2006;31(2):424–430.
85. Mechan A, Yuan J, Hatzidimitriou G, et al. Pharmacokinetic profile of single and repeated oral doses of MDMA in squirrel monkeys: relationship to lasting effects on brain serotonin neurons. Neuropsychopharmacology. 2006;31(2):339–350.
86. McCann UD, Szabo Z, Scheffel U, et al. Positron emission tomographic evidence of toxic effect of MDMA ("Ecstasy") on brain serotonin neurons in human beings. Lancet. 1998;352 (9138): 1433–1437.
87. McCann UD, Szabo Z, Seckin E, et al. Quantitative PET studies of the serotonin transporter in MDMA users and controls using [11C]McN5652 and [11C]DASB. Neuropsychopharmacology. 2005;30(9):1741–1750.
88. McCann UD, Szabo Z, Vranesic M, et al. Positron emission tomographic studies of brain dopamine and serotonin transporters in abstinent (+/−)3,4-methylenedioxymethamphetamine ("ecstasy") users: relationship to cognitive performance. Psychopharmacology (Berl). 2008;200(3):439–450.
89. Semple DM, Ebmeier KP, Glabus MF, et al. Reduced in vivo binding to the serotonin transporter in the cerebral cortex of MDMA ('ecstasy') users. Br J Psychiatry. 1999;175:63–69.
90. Reneman L, Lavalaye J, Schmand B, et al. Cortical serotonin transporter density and verbal memory in individuals who stopped using 3,4-methylenedioxymethamphetamine (MDMA or "ecstasy"): preliminary findings. Arch Gen Psychiatry. 2001; 58: 901–906.
91. Buchert R, Thomasius R, Nebeling B, et al. Long-term effects of "ecstasy" use on serotonin transporters of the brain investigated by PET. J Nucl Med. 2009;44:375–384.
92. Buchert R, Thomasius R, Wilke F, et al. A voxel-based PET investigation of the long-term effects of "Ecstasy" consumption on brain serotonin transporters. Am J Psychiatry. 2004;161: 1181–1189.
93. Thomasius R, Zapletalova P, Petersen K, et al. Mood, cognition and serotonin transporter availability in current and former ecstasy (MDMA) users: the longitudinal perspective. J Psychopharmacol. 2006;20:211–225.
94. Kalechstein AD, De La Garza R II, Mahoney JJ III, et al. MDMA use and neurocognition: a meta-analytic review. Psychopharmacology (Berl). 2007;189(4):531–537.
95. McCann UD, Ricaurte GA. Effects of (+/−) 3,4-methylenedioxymethamphetamine (MDMA) on sleep and circadian rhythms. Scientific World Journal. 2007;7:231–238.
96. Shulgin AT. How similar is substantially similar? J Forensic Sci. 1990;35:10–12.
97. Shulgin A, Shulgin A. PIHKAL: A Chemical Love Story. Berkeley, CA: Transform Press; 1991.
98. Morgan JP. Designer drugs. In: Lowinson JH, Ruiz P, Millmann B, eds. Substance Abuse: A Comprehensive Textbook. Baltimore, MD: Lippincott Williams & Wilkins; 2004:367–373.
99. Henderson GL. Blood concentrations of fentanyl and its analogs in overdose victims. Proc West Pharmacol Soc. 1983;26: 287–290.
100. Langston JW, Ballard P, Tetrud JW, et al. Chronic parkinsonism in humans due to a product of meperidine-analog synthesis. Science. 1983;219:979–980.
101. Davis GC, Williams AC, Markey SP, et al. Chronic Parkinsonism secondary to intravenous injection of meperidine analogues. Psychiatry Res. 1979;1:249.
102. Langston JW. The etiology of Parkinson's disease with emphasis on the MPTP story. Neurology. 1996;47:S153.
103. Smeyne RJ, Jackson-Lewis V. The MPTP model of Parkinson's disease. Mol Brain Res. 2005;134:57.

CHAPTER 20 Inhalants

Charles W. Sharp ■ Matthew O. Howard ■ Wynne K. Schiffer

Volatile substances are ubiquitous and varied. Thus, *Inhalant Abuse* includes a variety of drug-using behaviors that cannot be easily classified by their pharmacology or toxicology but are grouped based on their primary mode of administration. Other substances can be inhaled (e.g., tobacco, marijuana, and even heroin or crack). Natural vaporization of these latter substances is not the primary mode of administration; therefore, they do not fall into the "inhalant" classification of abused "drugs." The available products containing volatile solvent mixtures, gaseous products, and aerosols that are "inhalable" are variable from one region to another within the United States and throughout the world and over time. These products include a variety of chemical mixtures that can be found everywhere, in industry, in the workplace, and in the home. Thus, it is not surprising that anyone can find a favorite intoxicating vapor to be used to "get high." These substances are a bargain when one compares the going price of a "toke" or a "hit" of marihuana or cocaine. This chapter reviews the use and the resulting toxicities of many of those substances now known to be commonly abused through inhalation of "unheated" vapors by various groups, many youth, those with psychoses, and various professional groups (dry cleaners, painters, medical personnel, everyday workers, and novices from all walks of life). The chemical mixtures present in the products inhaled (Table 20.1) present a pharmacologic challenge to understand, both from a toxicologic view and more importantly from an understanding of preference and dependence for any one substance. Both these issues will be addressed in this chapter. Categorization or grouping of any products using any specific chemical can only be accomplished through an understanding of physiologic actions of specific compounds. Where possible, the clinical toxicologic findings of different products are correlated with the "key" substance, contained in the product predominately being inhaled, through studies on animals. Those results have recently provided more valuable data to help interpret clinical findings and are discussed herein. These "disease states" will then be partially explained through the knowledge gained by these laboratory studies on small animals and primates. The DSM criteria of "inhalants," still in flux, and limited treatment approaches of this condition are also discussed.

HISTORICAL EVENTS

Substances

Inhalation to produce euphoria can be traced to the ancient Greeks (1). Faraday was the first to report the effects of inhaling ether in 1818 (2). With the advent of the use of anesthetics in the mid-1800s, chloroform and ether parties occurred; these substances are still abused (3–5). The term "laughing gas" accurately describes one of the recreational uses of another anesthetic, nitrous oxide, which also originated in the late 1800s. It is stated that the use of ether and nitrous oxide at parties initiated the use of these compounds as anesthetics (2). With the increased use of gasoline at the turn of the 20th century, many more volatile substances became available through the process of petroleum "cracking" and distillation.

Little attention was given to the deliberate inhalation of these substances until the 1950s, when reporters (6) and judicial action focused on what was then called "glue sniffing." One of the first reports on the inhalation of vapors (gasoline) to get high came in 1951 (7). Glue sniffing is still widely used today to describe a myriad of substances that now include special polishes, glue, gasoline, thinners, other solvents, aerosols (paint spray, cooking lubricant spray, deodorant and hair sprays, and others), cleaning fluids, refrigerant gases (e.g., fluorocarbons and the newer partially hydrogenated–halogenated replacements (8)), anesthetics, primarily nitrous oxide (commercially available in whipped cream aerosols as the propellant and often referred to as "whippets"), organic nitrites (often called room "odorizers"), cooking or lighter gases, and in recent years, head cleaners/electronic "dusters" (9). There are also clinical reports of other substances (e.g., mothballs Ref. (10)). For many years it has been common for Mexican street children to sell "toluene-type" solvents on the street. This practice of selling fairly pure toluene from commercial drums in coke bottles is practiced even in the United States.

Nitrous oxide also has a more unique history. In the late 1970s, head shops sold a device for releasing the gas from little cylinders of nitrous oxide to facilitate its use. Since then, the selling of nitrous oxide from tanks dispersed in balloons has become a profitable venture before it became illegal in some locales. Also, more ambitious vendors took a tank to outdoor

TABLE 20.1 Chemicals commonly found in inhalants

Inhalant	Chemicals
Adhesives	
Airplane glue	Toluene, ethylacetate
Other glues	Hexane, toluene, methyl chloride, acetone, methyl ethyl ketone, methyl butyl ketone
Special cements	Trichloroethylene, tetrachloroethylene
Aerosols	
Paint sprays	Butane, propane, hydrochlorofluorocarbons, toluene,
Hair sprays	Butane, propane, hydrogenated chlorofluorocarbons, vinyl Cl
Deodorants, air fresheners	Butane, propane, hydrogenated chlorofluorocarbons
Analgesic spray	Hydrogenated chlorofluorocarbons
Asthma spray	Hydrogenated chlorofluorocarbons
Fabric spray	Butane, trichloroethane
Personal computer cleaners	Fluorohydrocarbons (fluoroethane), Dimethyl ether
Anesthetics	
Gaseous	Nitrous oxide
Liquid	Halothane, enflurane
Local	Ethyl chloride
Cleaning agents	
Dry cleaners	Tetrachloroethylene, trichloroethane
Spot removers	Xylene, petroleum distillates, chlorohydrocarbons
Degreasers	Tetrachloroethylene, trichloroethane, trichloroethylene
Solvents and gases	
Nail polish remover	Acetone, ethyl acetate, (toluene)
Paint remover	Methylene chloride, methanol, acetone, ethyl acetate
Paint thinners	Petroleum distillates, esters, acetone
Magic markers, permanent markers	Isopropanol, other alcohols
Correction fluids (fast drying)	Trichloroethylene, trichloroethane
Fuel gas	Butane, isobutane, isopropane
Cigar-type gas	Butanes
Lighter fluid (cigarette)	Petroleum distillates, liquid hydrocarbons
Fire extinguisher propellant	Bromochlorodifluoromethane
Carburetor cleaner	Volatile hydrocarbons (mineral spirits)
Food products	
Whipped cream aerosols	Nitrous oxide
Whippets	Nitrous oxide
Room odorizers	
Poppers, fluids (Rush, Locker Room)	Isoamyl, isobutyl, isopropyl, or butylnitrite (now illegal) or cyclohexyl

music festivals of young people and sold balloons-full from a tank. Still today, vendors distribute information on the Internet about grades of nitrous oxide and "crackers," a term used to describe implements that release "nitrous" from the "whippet" cartridges.

It is important to keep in mind that there are many different chemicals in most of the different products being abused. All have different dependence/reinforcing properties as well as different toxicities and are present in many different concentrations. Sometimes, the "desired" substances are listed on the container with or without the proportion of each; many times these substances come under the label of "nontoxic" substances, especially the propellants. It is important to focus on these propellants used in "aerosols," as they are most often the undefined substance that is the most desired chemical in these products. *Freons* were one of the most popular propellants until the early 1980s when they became illegal to use due to atmospheric environmental concerns. Then butane/propane combinations became the propellant of choice. Although some thought this would no longer make aerosols a reinforcing product, it became apparent very early that these "new" aerosols, even without another dependence-producing substance in the product, were highly abused. "Glue sniffing" was the term early identified with inhalant abuse in the 1950s, but it is now most often referred to as "inhalant" or "volatile solvent" abuse. Along with glue, fluorocarbons and gasoline were prominently noted as abused substances (11); then cleaning/correction-type fluids became popular, then bottled-type nonhalogenated gases in propane tanks or butane cigar lighters, and most recently, other types of halogenated chemicals present in electronic head cleaners are abused. These are often referred to as "AIR" (Table 20.1). Because of the diversity and complex composition of many of the products, the primary substance(s) are often not readily recognized (e.g., aerosol spray paints often contain toluene as a solvent and butane/propane as the propellant). Hydrogenated fluorocarbons may now become more commonly used as the propellant.

Toluene is often quoted as the substance involved, when other substances are also present, that may contribute to or be the primary substance being studied. This can be put in perspective by the following example: Transmission fluid was reportedly abused in Florida and stated to contain toluene. However, there is no toluene in transmission fluid. There is toluene in "Transgo," a wax stripper, which is a substance of abuse in the Florida area where transmission fluid is reportedly abused. When users are asked what substances they are abusing, it is easy to see how the above misnomer could easily occur, and a reporting error result. Also, one of the more toxic agents, hexane, a peripheral nervous system toxicant, was identified, after the fact, in products that did not list it on the product's label. Only through careful analysis of the product, and verification by the formulator, was the characterized syndrome in those subjects abusing the product correlated with hexane exposure, instead of toluene. The best corroboration of the causative substance is a measure, when possible, of the substance present in body fluids. Only through an analysis of the products used (e.g., by quantitative gas chromatography) is it possible to determine most of the volatile solvents and their proportion in a product (if the product can be readily obtained). Even then, the identification of all chemicals in one product used by the inhalant abuser may be very difficult due to the myriad of products included in the abuser's repertoire that should be considered in the diagnosis of the health problem, or the dependence of the abuser on the product.

These substances are widely available, readily accessible, cheap, and legally obtained. The intoxicating effects of the toluene in airplane glue were accidentally discovered by a number of adolescents while working on their model airplane kits (12). In a specific case nearly 40 years ago, Knox and Nelson (13) described a man who felt euphoric while working with paint thinner at an aircraft-manufacturing company. His initial and insistent requests to continue working in the capacity that employed the paint thinner went unnoticed. Eventually, he developed a habit that escalated to deep inhalations of concentrated vapors from a small container more than 10 times per hour throughout the day, including meal times. This behavior persisted for over 14 years. In other places during those early years, articles appeared in the lay and scientific press about model airplane glue sniffing. These substances provide a quick high, with a rapid dissipation of the high. Subjects who use inhalants heavily over short periods often complain of headaches. The practice of "sniffing," "snorting," "huffing," "bagging," or inhaling to get high describes various forms of inhalation. If the substance is glue or some other form of dissolved solid, the users will empty the can's contents (or a gas) into a plastic bag and then hold the bag to the nose/mouth and inhale (bagging). Another method is to soak a rag with the mixture and then stick the rag in the mouth and inhale the fumes (huffing). A simple but more toxic approach is to spray the substance directly into the oral orifices. These modes of administration allow abusers to be identified by various telltale clues; for example, *chemical* odors on the breath or clothes, stains on the clothes or around the mouth, empty spray paint or solvent containers, and other unusual paraphernalia. These clues may enable one to identify inhalant users before they suffer serious health problems or death.

Toxicities/Deaths

Historically, arrhythmia, cardiac arrest, and anoxia are the most serious consequences of inhalant abuse. *Death* is often the result of either anoxia or arrhythmia and can occur on the *first use or after many inhalation episodes*. Youth of the *very affluent, often well-educated as well as of the impoverished/indigent and troubled families fall victim* to the toxic actions of these substances. It has always been difficult to gather quantitative data on the number of deaths associated with inhalant use. In 1970, Bass studied

110 cases of "sudden sniffing deaths" resulting from intentionally inhaling fluorocarbons, gasoline, and other substances (14,15). There were noted "preponderance (of deaths) in the suburban middle-income white" families (14). Although there were no "bag-related" suffocations noted, hyperactivity was, and this preceded death in 18 of the youth. In many cases, the causes of several deaths were withheld and only in conversations with family or friends was a solvent identified as the cause of death. Since then, reports of deaths caused by different products (often identifying the primary chemical substance) have been an alarm for more critical intervention in "inhalant abuse" cases. Many of these deaths were reported (in the mid-1990s, more than 100 cases were reported in the U.S. newspapers as counted by different groups) and included detailed case histories. Many deaths are also noted in the yearly Annual Report of the American Association of Poison Control Centers (as reviewed in Ref. (15)). In these reports, deaths include accidental deaths brought to the attention of these centers, as well as those caused by the subject using the product to get high, or to commit suicide. It lists many deaths caused by many household products; the route of administration is also noted in the list of reported deaths. The number of tabulations of deaths noted in this report guides the field in understanding this issue.

Progression/Timing of These Events

In the years following Bass's investigation of medical examiners' records, many articles and medical reports have noted other types of inhalants (chemicals and/or products) as the major contributor to lethality. By following reports of death of different substances one can see some order of popularity of products shift from one substance to another. Thus, another halocarbon, trichloroethylene (TCE), present in typewriter correction fluid became popular and reports of deaths emerged in 1985 in Britain (16) and in the United States (17). The correction fluids, containing chlorocarbons, were often inhaled in the period of the 1970s till the 1990s and often resulted in death (18). The products have had formula changes and are, also, much less commonly available today in the desirable formulation needed for getting "high."

Soon after that, butane gas inhalation was identified, in 1990 in the Cincinnati region by Siegel and Wason (19), as a serious and deadly practice. About that time, butane/propane mixtures replaced fluorocarbons as the main aerosol propellant in the early 1980s and may have contributed to many more deaths. England began tabulating butane deaths in the late 1970s and included butane and other aliphatic hydrocarbons. Many reports are still documenting deaths due to inhalant abuse of "butane/propane" on a regular basis (19–23). It is indeed unusual that these very dangerous substances are still inhaled, and it is often hard to tell whether some deaths are a result of intentional or accidental "overexposure." Fire is an additional problem associated with butane when used as an inhalant (21). To reduce these serious outcomes resulting from any undesired exposure to cooking gases, it is now mandatory in the United States to add thiols to some portable gas containers, such as propane tanks, and it has been suggested that thiols (a substance that is added to our natural gas supplied for cooking) be added to even smaller gas containers (e.g., cigar lighter gases).

The restriction of the use of fluorocarbons in aerosols in 1980 has not abolished fluorocarbon-type abuse (24). Current use of "partially hydrogenated fluorocarbons" (25) instead of the fully halogenated hydrocarbons still "entices" abuse. Early abuse of fluorocarbons was noted by the theft of the refrigerant (fluorocarbon) gases from air conditioning units to be used for inhalation purposes. The addictive nature of fluorocarbons is also exemplified by cases of asthma inhalers, when the "inhaler" uses these products at levels exceeding the level of medication (26). This specific problem was also studied in antisocial youth where high inhalant abuse prevalence occurs (27). This use of a "freon" as the propellant is being changed, but its replacement may still be a substance that would produce dependence. This is one of the few marketable forms of fluorocarbons present in substances used medicinally by the public.

The use of nitrous oxide became more prominent in the 1980s when whipped cream dispensers, nonclinical grade cylinder tanks (dispersing the gas by the balloon), and medical-grade tanks of nitrous oxide (most common in dentist's offices) were used. Although some deaths were reported for nitrous oxide by 1978 (28), most reports started appearing a decade later and sill are being published (29,30).

As often said, history repeats itself. With less "freon" available, electronic cleaner sprays, (containing simple fluoro- or chloro-carbons (often dihalo-ethane) and often referred to as "AIR") have been discovered and abused (15), with numerous reports of death (31,32). Other problems occur with the abuse of "AIR Dusters." One reports an occurrence of burns (33); others correlate different toxicities with the abuse of these products (34). Calling these products AIR misleads the user into believing these materials are nontoxic and do not contain any "chemical" other than nitrogen. Additional case reports of death continue to be printed and include toluene-type products (35–37), gasoline (38), and halocarbons (18,26, 39,40).

Tracking

Drug-related deaths are always of concern. Inhalants produce additional problems in the identification of those deaths that may be attributable to these substances compared to other drugs. First, due to rapid elimination, they are not easily identifiable in tissues or excrements. Although hippuric acid is readily measured in urine, it is also a natural product of body elimination. Thus, the level in urine must be very high to associate its presence with solvent abuse. Even the frequently occurring acetone breath may be the result of diabetes and may mislead emergency personnel. Deaths, occurring after inhalant exposure, leave even fewer clues. Because of this, medical examiner death certificates are many times not associated with "inhalants," especially as only relatives/friends know them as an inhalant abuser. Those death certificates identifying anoxia or cardiac arrest/arrhythmia as the cause of death often need to be followed up to identify if "inhalant abuse" was involved. In three local/statewide studies, they examined death certificates to measure the impact of "inhalant abuse," one in Virginia (41) and others in Texas (42). The identified abused substances include butane/propane gases (Virginia), as well as halogenated (fluoro- or chloro-hydrocarbons) propellants/solvents (both states), as the causes of death. However, there is no indication that deaths with "no cause noted" were even accounted for in the number of possible deaths that could be linked to inhalant use. Thus, many deaths related to inhalants are missed.

One country, Great Britain, thoroughly tracks the cause of death by following up each case to identify and record the most likely cause for every death. In the continuing reporting of these causes of deaths in Great Britain, Field-Smith et al. annually record the number of deaths caused by butane/propane gases, aerosols, and other volatile solvents (16). This group in England has been accumulating data on deaths related to inhalant abuse for three decades (for solvents and gases, but excluding nitrous oxide deaths). The English are much more thorough in delineating almost all causes of death. They diligently pursue every case to determine this; very few are listed "cause unknown." The number of these deaths increased from 50 in 1981 to 152 in 1990 (the highest number), and then dropped to a current value around 50 in 2006. Gas fuels generally accounted for approximately 50% of the inhalant abuse deaths throughout. Aerosols were over 20% at the peak level of cases, but their use has dropped; the use of glues has dropped most dramatically, possibly related to the pursuit of a strong prevention program in Great Britain over the last decade (16). Also, adoption of legislation banning the sale of butane lighter refills to minors was considered a major deterrent (16). Most deaths are attributed to direct toxic effects, which include the cardiotoxic actions of butane, fluorocarbons, and other solvents/gases, inhalation of gastric contents, trauma, and suffocation.

There are also other causes of death related to intoxication resulting from the inhalation of these substances (e.g., running in front of a car during or after intoxication). Garriott et al. documented such occurrences in their compilation of similar data for the Dallas and San Antonio areas (43). There is also an Australian report on numerous "inhalant deaths" attributed to or derived from inhalant gas exposure (44). They identified only "solvents" as the cause of death. The size of the population in the United States is five times that of Great Britain. If the United States pursued the cause of death more diligently, as do the Britons, the death rate in the United States related to inhalant abuse could well be well over a hundred per year and most of these are children. Hopefully, as there are some indications that fewer deaths per year occur now than a decade ago, due to efforts to educate the public, these tragic events may have diminished. Although the United States has an annual reporting system of deaths identified by medical examiners related to abused substances, the Drug Abuse Warning Network (DAWN), the system is not set up to clearly identify many "inhalant-related" deaths. For example, in the past year only Massachusetts, of eight states listed, noted any deaths due to inhalants (45).

EPIDEMIOLOGY

Surveys

The prevalence of inhalant use continues to be a relatively underresearched drug abuse issue, especially among adults. The United States, England (16), and many other countries are systematically evaluating the abuse of solvents. Studies in Spain, Japan, Brazil, Canada, Australia, New Zealand, South Africa, Tunisia, and other nations underscore the global significance of inhalant use as a problem of serious proportions (46–48). Medina-Mora and Real recently reviewed studies relevant to the international epidemiology of inhalant use and inhalant use disorders (IUDs) (46). In the United States, the pattern of inhalant use is exemplified by national studies, including the National Institute on Drug Abuse: Monitoring the Future (MTF) (49) survey, which includes interviews of secondary school and college students, the Substance Abuse and Mental Health Services Administration: National Survey on Drug Use and Health (NSDUH) (50), and the Centers for Disease Control and Prevention's Youth Risk Behavior Survey (YRBS) (51), a survey of 9th- to 12th-grade students. These surveys approach a national representation of youth; however, the MTF and YRBS are school based and do not include youth who are absent during survey administration due to truancy, expulsion, having dropped out, incarceration, or institutionalization. The NSDUH involves interviews of persons 12 and older that are conducted in households but does not include institutionalized or homeless populations. The failure of these large studies to survey incarcerated, institutionalized, or homeless populations is a particularly important limitation, because prior reports suggest that these groups may have disproportionately high levels of inhalant abuse (52). Other concerns with these surveys have to do with the validity of self-reported inhalant use, cross-sectional nature of the data (which does not allow causal inferences to be drawn regarding reported associations between inhalant use and other factors), and use of a single omnibus inhalant assessment item to assess use of chemically distinct classes of agents (e.g., nitrites, toluene, butane, and nitrous oxide).

Although one often looks at large state or national surveys, these surveys do not clearly delineate many regions where there is a higher proportion of inhalant use, such as in some inner cities that include impoverished or ethnic minorities or other isolated communities, especially those of Native Americans (53) or Latinos. In some surveys, there appears to be an underrepresentation of African Americans in the solvent-abusing populations, but inhalants *are* abused by African Americans (54). Although Hispanic groups are often considered to be overrepresented in the solvent-abusing population, the large surveys generally do not find a much greater proportion of Hispanics than of the larger "Anglo-American" population using inhalants. The extent of use in these groups is difficult to evaluate properly, because many of the inhalant-using individuals are not accessed by survey systems. To look at the regional problems of solvent abuse, Beauvais and Oetting extensively studied many Native American groups (53). Howard et al. (55) studied urban Native Americans; others have studied Hispanic communities (56). Another study observed a lifetime prevalence of inhalants by the household population in the state of New York to be 2% to 4%, whereas the lifetime rate of use by the homeless was 15% to 18% (54). Poly-inhalant use appears to be the norm for many inhalant users. More than one third of adults with a history of inhalant use participated in the NSDUH reported lifetime use of two or more inhalants. Poly-inhalant use was even more prevalent among 12- to 17-year-old NSDUH inhalant users, with nearly one third reporting use of three or more inhalants and over one half reporting lifetime use of two or more inhalants (50). Studies of delinquent inhalant users have identified even higher rates of poly-inhalant use than those identified in the general population (52). The U.S. national government began to evaluate the extent of the problem of inhalant use in the mid-1970s. Annual or semi-annual surveys of the problem are now available online (http://www.monitoringthefuture.org/; http://www.oas.samhsa.gov/nsduh.htm). Inhalant abuse has also been recently studied in the U.S. military, as it had become identified as an unrecognized threat (57).

Abuse Patterns

The extent of use of inhalants can be compared to that of other drugs. In the national surveys, it is interesting to note that the prevalence of inhalant lifetime (ever use) use is highest in junior high students, but below that of marijuana, cigarettes, and alcohol. Although this measure of lifetime use of inhalants is often higher for youths younger than age 16, the drop in lifetime use beyond this age raises several questions. Are some "heavy" users lost to the survey? Are the questions misinterpreted by young respondents (at either the 8th- or 12th-grade levels)? For example, could very young children think that "liking the smell" is the equivalent of "getting high?" Is there a "forgetfulness" about this type of behavior or a downgrading of this event in the conscious thinking as they mature? Some assign this change to a diminished "remembrance" of this event as "getting high" for a number of reasons.

For that reason, the discontinuance of use of substances is now being studied. The so-called desistance or noncontinuation rates for inhalant use were the highest reported among 23 drug classes assessed in the MTF survey (49). MTF investigators defined noncontinuation rates as the proportion of people who "ever used a drug (once or more) and who did not use it in the twelve months preceding the survey."

Of those drugs measured, lifetime (ever) use of inhalants shows the largest percentage of subjects reporting discontinuance of use, especially in the 12th graders. Inhalant discontinuation rates for 8th, 10th, and 12th graders were 47%, 52%, and 65% in 2007, respectively. For comparison purposes, discontinuation rates for alcohol use (the least discontinued drug) for 8th, 10th, and 12th graders were 18%, 9%, and 8%, respectively (Table 20.2). Factors that increase the risk for continuation of inhalant use, at least in high-risk antisocial youth, include younger age, prior problems with inhalants, greater psychiatric distress, more severe personal substance abuse problems, and friends/siblings who use inhalants (58).

A very recent study measured "the recantation" of inhalant use (59). The investigators compared self-reported responses of seventh graders and their responses again in the eighth grade. They also queried the use of cigarettes and alcohol. The observed validation of a positive response to inhalant lifetime use dropped to about half, whereas tobacco use diminished by only 5%. They noted denial of ever reporting this use as well as erroneous reporting as the bases of this "recanting." From this study, they believe that 67% of those who reported earlier use was the likely *true* value. This further indicates a high overreported "ever use" of inhalants and, especially in very young children, may indicate they first report more of a curiosity "sniff" than actual use of the product to "get high."

This lifetime use issue can be examined by comparing the use of inhalants and alcohol; two substances abused early by young people. These substances, plus cigarettes and marijuana, are the earliest and most frequently used drugs of addiction. This comparison of drug-use patterns is enhanced by examining the incidence/frequency of the use of these drugs; few surveys have examined the multiple or "chronic" use of most drugs. It is now becoming more common to ask about the frequency of drug use, especially in relation to use in the past month. The use of inhalants can be compared to that of alcohol; these two substances are seldom compared by prevalence but are both known to be depressants (Table 20.2). The lifetime inhalant use (especially when "corrected" for "recantation") is about one fourth that of alcohol use. A comparison of use in "past year" or "past month" of inhalants by the 12- to 17-year-old group is about one tenth that of alcohol. Also, the number of subjects who repeatedly use each of these substances shows a 20- to 30-fold preference for alcohol (looking at number of respondents). These findings accentuate the difference in the "real" addictive nature of inhalants, as compared to alcohol, even at a young age, is not very high. One must additionally consider that the pharmacologic effects of inhalants are of much shorter duration (rapidly eliminated) than is alcohol, making these substances even weaker reinforcing agents than most other drugs.

SAMHSA has provided yearly data on the lifetime prevalence of various groups of inhalants for mind-altering purposes for several years. In 2007, inhalation of aerosol sprays, nitrous oxide, and toluene- or butane/propane-containing products were the most prevalent forms of

TABLE 20.2 Percentages of adolescents reporting lifetime, annual, last month, and daily use of inhalants or alcohol in the Monitoring the Future (MTF) (2007) and NSDUH (2007)

Grade/age	Percent inhalant use in 2007					Percent alcohol use in 2007				
	Life	Ann	30 days	Daily	Discontinuance[a]	Life	Ann	30 days	Daily	Discontinuance[a]
MTF										
8th	15.6	8.3	3.9		47	38.9	31.8	15.9	0.6	18
10th	13.6	6.6	2.5		52	61.7	56.3	33.4	1.4	9
12th	10.5	3.7	1.2		65	72.2	66.4	44.4	3.1	8
NSDUH										
8th	12	6	2.1			28.2	20.9	8.7		
10th	10.7	4.3	1.4			54.4	45.4	21.9		
12th	8.2	2.3	0.3			70	61.2	38.1		
By age										
12–17 yr olds	9.6	3.9	1.2	0.1		39.4	31.8	15.9		
12–17 yr olds[b]	2422	994	295			9949	8016	4021		
12–17 yr olds[c]										
a		59.1	57.5				47.9	49.5		
b		21.7	24.2				27.2	26.6		
c		9.4	10.6				12.7	20.9		
d		9.9	7.6				12.2	3.0		

[a]Rate of Discontinuation of reported lifetime use.
[b]This is the number of 12–17 year olds using inhalants or alcohol in those surveyed.
[c]The data from this group were subdivided into percent use (4 categories) as follows: Number days of use in "annual" response: a = 1–11, b = 12–49, c = 50–99, d = 100 +. Percent responding for each group (i.e., a, b, c, or d).
Number days use in "last month" response: a = 1–2, b = 3–5, c = 6–19; d = 20+.

TABLE 20.3 Trends in the percentages of adolescents aged 12 to 21 reporting lifetime use of different inhalant groups: 2007 National Survey of Drug Use and Heath (NSDUH) findings

Inhalant	Age									
	12	13	14	15	16	17	18	19	20	21
Nitrous oxide	0.1	0.4	0.6	1.2	1.9	3.1	3.7	6	6.5	7.4
Glue, shoe polish, or toluene	3.3	4.8	4.5	5	3.6	2.8	2.1	1.4	1.7	1.5
Gasoline or lighter fluid	2.7	4.2	4.7	4.2	2.8	2.7	2.2	1.8	1.8	1.5
Spray paints	2.3	3.6	4.2	4.1	2.8	2.1	1.7	1.5	1.3	1
Correction fluid, degreaser, or cleaning fluid	1.5	2.8	2.7	3.1	1.9	1.6	1.5	1.2	1	1
Lacquer thinner or other paint solvent	1	1.8	1.7	2.3	1.8	1.4	1.7	1.3	1.1	0.9
Aerosol sprays other than spray paints	1.2	1.7	2.4	3	2.7	2.6	2.3	2	1.6	1.6
Nitrites	1.1	1.8	2.3	2.5	1.6	1.4	1.6	1.5	1.4	1.6
Lighter gases such as butane or propane	0.7	1.3	1.4	1.5	0.8	1	1	0.6	0.6	0.5
Halothane, ether, or other anesthetics	0.1	0.2	0.4	0.7	0.6	0.5	0.6	0.8	0.5	0.7

Data retrieved from NSDUH (2007) household survey. Substance Abuse and Mental Health Services Administration. *Results from the 2007 National Survey on Drug Use and Health: National Findings.* NSDUH Series H-34, Publication No. SMA 08-4343. Rockville, MD: Office of Applied Studies, DHHS. Available at: http://oas.samhsa.gov.
Number of respondents (in thousands): all groups = 22,676. Percentage responding to all categories is 9.2%.

"lifetime use" of inhalants for 12- to 17-year-olds. In younger children, use of spray paint, glue/toluene, gas/lighter fluid, and correction fluid was highest (Table 20.3). By age 14, these agents plus other sprays, lighter gas, nitrites, and thinner were becoming more prevalent. By age 16, nitrous oxide was nearly as popular. There is a great concern about the inhalation of gases/solvents by younger age groups (e.g., seventh and eighth graders) because of their lack of understanding of the problem, both what is meant by "getting high" and the resulting consequences of this use. This emphasizes the need for increased education for children, especially their parents, about the nature and dangers of this problem.

No study to date answers the perplexing question: What attracts young people to certain specific substances/products? Although some may consider the odor, color, or type of product to be important, the reinforcement and feeling one gets after inhalation is most important for continuing use of any inhalant. Even then, it is difficult to say what products/substances are preferred. Howard et al. (52) were among the first to assess preference for specific inhalants in a group of subjects. They asked 723 adolescents in residential care for behavior problems about their use of 65 inhalants, including 55 volatile solvents/gases, and 10 additional inhalants. The prevalence of use, numbers of those getting high, and frequency of use are presented in Table 20.4. Of the 55 volatile products used, gasoline, permanent markers, computer duster spray and other fluorocarbons, spray paint (and other products containing toluene); nitrous oxide, paint thinner, air freshener, correction fluid, butane, permanent markers, and Freon rated high in all these categories. Each youth reporting use of an inhalant was also asked if they "got high" when they inhaled the substance. Between 80% and 90% of users of gasoline, computer duster spray, paint thinner, "Freon," ether and carburetor cleaner reported they became intoxicated when they used these products. Comparatively large percentages of butane (14%), computer duster spray (13%), gasoline (12%), liquid paint (11%), air freshener (10%), paint thinner or nitrous oxide (10%), and spray paint (8.4%) users reported 100 or more lifetime days of use of those substances. Conversely, most users of gun cleaning products, waxes, mothballs, cooking gases, other cleaning agents, plaster and gum remover, insecticide spray, shoe shine/polish, other glues/cements, and balsa wood cement reported less than 5 lifetime days of use of these inhalants, respectively. The high percentage who "got high" on nail polish is perplexing as many "like it's smell," but it is not very volatile. Garland, Howard, and Perron (60) reported that 16% of the 723 adolescents had used nitrous oxide, most of who reported intoxication following use of the agent. Thus, findings indicated that the most prevalently and frequently used volatile solvents were those that were perceived as generally producing intoxication; these results suggest that many adolescent inhalant users are purposively seeking out inhalants that reliably produce intoxication/reinforcement and were repeatedly searched for and used. A very recent analysis of cases reported to the National Poison Data System (16) is unique in identifying the products (including primary substances present) that were abused.

Modalities

In terms of modalities of use, more than half of all inhalants were usually sniffed from a container such as a jar or bottle. Sniffing from a container was particularly common among nail polish, correction fluid, gasoline, and paint pen users. Spraying the inhalant into the nose or mouth was uncommon and associated with use of computer duster spray and butane. Inhaling from a cloth saturated with a substance was prevalent among users of paint thinner, air freshener, hair spray, paint remover, deodorant spray, ether, and carburetor cleaner. Mixed modes of administration were common across inhalants. Another inhalant-specific study was published using the sample described above. Hall and Howard (61) found that only 1.7%, of the 723 youth they studied, reported lifetime use of nitrites; however, most (83%) nitrite users reportedly became intoxicated when they used nitrites. A similarly low rate of nitrite use was recently reported in a nationally representative sample of adolescents (62).

SOCIALCULTURAL ISSUES

Many solvent abusers, more than other drug users, are poor, come from broken homes, have lower self-esteem, and do poorly in school (63,64). They have difficulty with acculturation and strong peer influence that enhances their entrance into inhalant use, as well as other drug use (64), although findings are not wholly supportive of an acculturation stress–inhalant use relationship (65). The family atmosphere is often disruptive for the abusers and has been identified as less adjusted or more conflictual than for controls (66). Relatively few rationally based or empirically derived typologies of inhalant users have been developed. Schemes proposed include McSherry's (67) description of experimental abusers (14- to 17-year-olds with less than 2 years' experience with inhalants and only sporadic use), acute abusers (17- to 21-year-old youth with 2 to 4 years of inhalant use at least three times weekly), and chronic abusers (ages 20 to 28 who have used inhalants for 5 to 15 years and who are dependent on them). Oetting et al. (68) distinguished between inhalant-dependent adults, polydrug abusers, and young adult users. Inhalant-dependent adults have the most serious health problems, because they have used heavily for a long time; the young inhalant users are those for whom treatment is most desirable to keep them from progressing to the other groups and for whom there may be hope for successful intervention. Although all inhalant abusers use other drugs (both illegal drugs, tobacco and alcohol), the first group predominately uses inhalants, even though other drugs are available. The second group infrequently uses inhalants primarily because they cannot get their drug of choice; their problems arise more from the use of other drugs and are less related to

TABLE 20.4 Inhalant use in a sample of 723 antisocial youth in residential care in Missouri: The lifetime prevalence of use and proportions of users who got high, reported 100 or more lifetime occasions of use, and who reported weekly or more frequent inhalant use in the prior year are presented for specific inhalants including volatile solvents, gases, nitrites, and nitrous oxide

Inhalant[5]	[1]Prevalence N (%)	Got high[2] N (%)	[3]100+ occasions of use	[4]Past-year weekly use
Gasoline[g]	159 (22.0)	130 (81.8)	19 (11.9)	21 (13.2)
Computer duster spray[f]	106 (14.7)	96 (90.6)	14 (13.2)	22 (21.0)
Freon[f]	44 (6.1)	41 (93.2)	2 (4.5)	5 (11.4)
Spray paint[t,b]	83 (11.5)	65 (78.3)	7 (8.4)	12 (14.5)
Paint thinner[g]	60 (8.3)	54 (90.0)	6 (10.0)	10 (16.7)
Carburetor cleaner[g]	17 (2.4)	14 (82.4)	3 (17.6)	6 (35.3)
Lighter fluid[g]	14 (1.9)	9 (64.3)	1 (7.1)	1 (7.1)
Air freshener[b]	58 (8.0)	41 (70.7)	6 (10.3)	7 (12.1)
Deodorant spray[b]	20 (2.8)	14 (70.0)	1 (5.0)	4 (20.0)
Hairspray[b]	29 (4.0)	15 (51.7)	1 (3.4)	1 (3.4)
Nitrous oxide[n]	65–80	55+	10+	9+
Butane[b]	50 (6.9)	29 (58.0)	7 (14.0)	9 (18.0)
Propane[b]	21 (2.9)	15 (71.4)	1 (4.5)	2 (9.5)
Permanent markers[a]	106 (14.7)	45 (42.5)	11 (10.4)	15 (14.2)
Airplane/model glue[t]	39 (5.4)	22 (56.4)	0 (0.0)	0 (0.0)
Rubber cement[a,c]	35 (4.8)	17 (48.6)	2 (5.7)	2 (5.7)
Other glues/cements[g,h]	29 (4.0)	17 (58.6)	2 (6.9)	2 (6.9)
Nail polish remover[g]	63 (8.7)	30 (47.6)	3 (4.8)	3 (4.8)
Paint remover/stripper[t,g]	25 (3.5)	19 (76.0)	1 (4.0)	0 (0.0)
Amyl, butyl nitrites	7 (1.0)?	5 (100)	1	0
Ether	20 (2.8)	18 (90.0)	1 (5.0)	2 (10.0)
Any other cleaner	18 (2.5)	9 (50.0)	0 (0.0)	1 (5.6)
Nail polish	61 (8.4)	25 (41.0)	3 (4.9)	4 (6.6)
Correction fluid[c]	52 (7.2)	18 (34.6)	1 (1.9)	0 (0.0)
PAM	7 (1.0)	3 (42.9)	0 (0.0)	1 (14.3)

Only reason for different "liking" of amyl versus butyl is availability; differences are less than for sucrose and glucose.
[1]Lifetime prevalence of inhalant use; all figures in table are N's followed by percentages in parentheses.
[2]Number and percentage of users of each inhalant who reported having "gotten high" while using that inhalant.
[3]Number of inhalant users who reported 100 or more lifetime occasions of use of that inhalant.
[4]Weekly or more frequent use of that inhalant over the year prior to assessment.
[5]The Products in which the most likely primary reinforcing chemicals are noted by type of chemical likely present in high concentrations: a is for isopropanol or other alcohols, b is for low-molecular-weight gaseous hydrocarbons, pure butane/propane alone or if used as a propellant; c is for chlorinated hydrocarbons; f is for products with fluorocarbons; g is for gasoline and other liquid fuels with medium to high molecular weight hydrocarbons; h is for hexane, a very specific neurotoxin; n is for all forms of products containing only nitrous oxide gas; t is for products containing toluene. See Table 20.1.

those discussed in this chapter. The young inhalant users, however, are in the experimentation period with inhalants, having started with tobacco, alcohol, or possibly even marihuana, as well as inhalants. Before any of this group matures into the first group, inventing behavioral modifications are very important. May and Del Vecchio (69) also developed a tripartite classification scheme, identifying young inhalant users involved in experimental use of inhalants, adolescent polydrug users who use inhalants frequently, and adult chronic users of inhalants.

Vaughn et al. (70) identified one class of inhalant users with high levels of inhalant use in response to social contextual influences. This class evidenced significantly greater psychiatric distress and substance use problems than two other classes of adolescent inhalant users differing in frequency of social contextual inhalant use. Additional taxonomic studies are needed that empirically identify types of inhalant users. Recent findings in adolescents (71) and adults (72) suggest that inhalant users, particularly girls, women, and persons with *DSM-IV* IUDs, are at substantial risk for suicidal ideation and perhaps suicide itself. Studies have associated inhalant use early in life with later injection drug use (73). Additional findings in samples of inhalant users include significant academic problems such as high rates of dropout, suspension, and expulsion, parental alcoholism and criminality, histories of physical or sexual abuse, deviant peers including inhalant users, impulsive, sensation seeking and fearless temperaments, and involvement in criminal and antisocial conduct (52,71–73).

One trait that is often associated with "sniffers" is disruptive behavior. Some report them to be more violent. In one carefully controlled study, the only aggressive feature that stood out was self-directed aggression (63). Another recent study of a national sample of adult inhalant users identified significantly elevated rates of interpersonal violence in inhalant users compared to inhalant nonusers, with especially high rates of such violence observed among persons with lifetime inhalant abuse or dependence (74). Early aggressiveness, antisocial attitudes, and involvement in criminal behavior (52,55,64) were also found to be characteristic of inhalant users in longitudinal and cross-sectional studies. Two recent reports identified significant associations between serious behavior problems and inhalant use (75).

Cognitive measures support the antisocial and self-destructive nature of inhalant abusers. At least two major studies found these groups to have lower Wechsler verbal scores; it remains unanswered as to whether these groups self-selected inhalant abuse because of these predilections or whether the deficiencies came about as the result of inhalant abuse (66). In some instances, school records indicate that cognitive deficits probably occurred before inhalant use began. Although it is uncertain how they became dysfunctional, it is very likely that inhalants prevent their continued growth and development (64,68). For further reading on the nature of the problem, especially the social–cultural conditions, we refer the reader to other reviews of this area (64,68).

TOXICOLOGY OF INHALANT ABUSE

Criteria for Defining Inhalant Toxicity

High-level exposure occurs in the inhalant abuse setting at levels several thousandfold higher than the usual occupational setting. Also, most abusers inhale several distinctly different solvents as well as use other illicit "drugs." These are hardly ever noted by "history" profiles on entry into hospital, doctor's office, or in coroner's reports, except when an "incident" identifies this as an issue. The majority of either "novices" or "very experienced" inhalant abusers never reach a hospital or an outpatient facility with inhalant abuse identified as a "health problem." Basically the solvent abuser may appear as a "drunk or in an intoxicated state," as many of the symptoms resemble alcohol intoxication. An initial excitation turns to drowsiness, disinhibition, lightheadedness, and agitation. With increasing intoxication, individuals may develop ataxia, dizziness, and disorientation. In extreme intoxications, they may show signs of sleeplessness, general muscle weakness, dysarthria, nystagmus, and, occasionally, hallucinations or disruptive behavior. Several hours after, especially if they have slept, they are likely to be lethargic, or hung over with mild to severe headaches. At lower levels (just over 200 parts per million [ppm]), fatigue, headache, paresthesia, and slowed reflexes appear (76). Exposure at levels approaching 1000 ppm causes confusion or delirium, and euphoric effects appear at or above that level. Physical symptoms include weight loss, muscle weakness, general disorientation, inattentiveness, and lack of coordination. Too many times, death can occur during the course of primary intoxication. When it does occur, it is usually the result of asphyxia, ventricular fibrillation, or induced cardiac arrhythmia following high exposures to various solvents. The concentration of toluene in the body that causes death has been estimated based on data from the deaths of painters by Hobara et al. (77).

Although most cases of inhalant abuse occur in the general population, anesthetics are an abuse problem of medical personnel (3,78,79), especially nitrous oxide (30) as well as other anesthetics. It is well known that oxygen should be administered using specific devices. However, in some instances (e.g., homes, food services, or the ophthalmologist's office where it may be used as a cryogen), there are usually no masks available for those receiving nitrous oxide, and death may occur. Also, these and other expand from the "condensed" state causing the lips to freeze.

Neurotoxic disorders have a nonfocal presentation and may be confused with metabolic, degenerative, nutritional, or demyelinating diseases (80). Thus, chronic toluene abuse may clinically resemble the multifocal demyelinating disease, multiple sclerosis (MS), in the findings on neurologic examination (81). Mild cases of intoxication may be very difficult to diagnose. The most reliable information comes from documented cases of long-term heavy exposure; details of low-level exposure and presymptomatic diagnoses are vague at best. In general, inhalant-related neurotoxic

TABLE 20.5	Major neurologic syndromes produced by organic solvents
Encephalopathy	
Acute encephalopathy—nonspecific; high-level exposure	
Chronic encephalopathy—seen with repeated high-level exposure over years	
Cerebellar ataxia	
Peripheral neuropathy—distal axonopathy	
Cranial neuropathy—primarily cranial nerves V and VII	
Parkinsonism	
Visual loss—optic neuropathy	
Multifocal	
Central nervous system (e.g., toluene)	
Central and peripheral	

injuries rarely have specific identifying features on diagnostic tests such as computed tomography (CT), magnetic resonance imaging (MRI), or nerve conduction studies (80). Because many neurotoxic effects are reversible and some chronic neurotoxic injuries of the brain may not be associated with structural damage sufficiently large to be detected within the spatial resolution of current MRI scanners and imaging sequences, brain imaging studies are primarily used to rule out other disorders. However, recent studies of chronic solvent inhalant abusers suggests that MRI may be the most sensitive and specific method of detecting the brain injury associated with the high dose setting of the inhalant abuser. Chronic neurotoxic injury related to solvent abuse is slowly and incompletely reversible, and usually does not progress after cessation of exposure (81). In addition, acute neurotoxicities and clinical manifestations of a substance may *not* be attributable to the parent compound, but may be associated with a metabolite of this compound. In addition, in several known cases, a solvent was reported to either diminish or potentiate the neurotoxic potency of a second solvent (82). Some acute incidents that are irreversible probably act by producing secondary systemic effects such as cerebral hypoxia or a metabolic acidosis (83). Table 20.5 lists those syndromes associated with organic solvent exposure. Major neurotoxic syndromes occurring in individuals chronically exposed to select organic solvents include a peripheral neuropathy, ototoxicity, and an encephalopathy. Less commonly, a cerebellar ataxic syndrome or a myopathy may occur alone or in combination with any of these clinical syndromes.

This section reviews several important issues: (a) the different physiologic and psychologic medical effects, as demonstrated by case reports and by the use of toluene or nitrous-oxide-containing products in contrast to products that contain other substances such as butane, fluorocarbons, or acetone; (b) the use of PET studies of radiolabeled solvents locating different sites of action in the brain; and (c) the toxic manifestations of several different inhalants as reflected in the cognitive and neuropsychologic consequences measured in animals.

CLINICAL NEUROTOXICOLOGY

Encephalopathy

In 1961, Grabski (84) reported the first patient with persistent neurologic consequences of chronic toluene self-maintained inhalation. Many of these case studies reporting persistent central CNS effects involved adults whose initial experience with the euphoric effects of abused solvents occurred in the occupational setting, unrecognizable by these exposed workers as being associated with the chemical effects of the solvent. Since then, many reports of neurotoxicity, often of a severe nature, have appeared in the literature (13,83,85–95). The neurologic pattern is very clearly delineated, with effects primarily on the CNS. Syndromes of persistent and often severe neurotoxicity include cognitive dysfunction (13,81,87,90,94,95), cerebellar ataxia (81,84–88,94,96), optic neuropathy (86,94,97–99), sensorineural hearing loss (86), and an equilibrium disorder (92). The encephalopathy has been characterized using CT (100) and, more extensively, using MRI (91,94,95,101–105). Most commonly, toluene neurotoxicity includes several of the above syndromes and with multifocal CNS involvement (81,89–91). There are many instances of "persistent" neurologic deficits. However, the enduring nature of these deficits has been difficult to capture and it is possible that brain structural changes measured with MRI or CT persist despite a return in cognitive function. For example, abstinence has been documented prior to clinical evaluation and appears to relate to the degree of structural damage (81,105). Although longitudinal experiments where several brain scans are obtained over time with abstinence are lacking, most chronic solvent abusers represent the severe end of the spectrum, and the issue is further complicated by equivocal evidence concerning impairment of cognitive function in solvent abusers: reports have provided evidence both for (85,106) and against (85) recovery of cognitive impairment with prolonged abstinence.

Also, microencephalopathy has emerged as a possible embryopathic syndrome in infants of women exposed during pregnancy to solvents containing toluene (107). Recently, encephalopathies have been observed following inhalation of butane-type products (a fluorocarbon-152A was also present in one case) and low-molecular-weight chlorohydrocarbons. One study of butane exposure showed increasing cerebral atrophy by MRI after 3 weeks (95); another was unremarkable as measured by MRI 3 days after admission (96). Chloro-methane/ethane-type products (often from head cleaner aerosols) are also possibly encephalitic.

Twenty chronic abusers of spray paint, containing toluene, and with documented abstinence for at least 1 month prior to evaluation (81) were some of the early studies. In those chronic solvent abusers, 65% showed neurologic impairment. This was a small and unselected sample, so the findings probably do not reflect the true prevalence of neurologic damage. However, there was a fairly consistent pattern of neurologic abnormality. As has been suggested, the CNS is selectively vulnerable. In fact, no peripheral neuropathy has been correlated with toluene exposure. Intoxication with some aliphatic hydrocarbons, for example, *n*-hexane, in humans has been associated with diminished vision and memory (108).

Neurologic abnormalities varied from mild cognitive impairment to severe dementia, associated with elemental neurologic signs such as cerebellar ataxia, corticospinal tract dysfunction, oculomotor abnormalities, tremor, deafness, and hyposmia. Cognitive dysfunction was the most disabling and frequent feature of chronic toluene toxicity and may be the earliest sign of damage. Dementia, when present, was typically associated with cerebellar ataxia and other signs (81). One patient had pyramidal and cerebellar signs without cognitive impairment. Oculomotor dysfunction, deafness, and tremor were seen only in severely affected individuals. Cranial nerve abnormalities were confirmed for olfactory and auditory dysfunction. Toluene-induced optic neuropathy was not substantiated by larger studies (81,91). However, visual-evoked potential abnormalities were found in chronic toluene abusers. Studies from Japan and Turkey have identified visual-evoked latencies/amplitudes resulting from toluene exposure due to inhalation abuse and from occupational exposure (109). Abstinence from exposure commonly brought restoration of function. This type of toxicity also occurs following hexane exposure (see below), which is expressed more extensively in peripheral neuropathic conditions. Other investigators have found a similar syndrome after chronic exposure to toluene (85,88). Although some investigators emphasized the cerebellar disorder, they noted that most cases also showed impairment in a variety of cerebral functions.

The clinical data suggest that the cognitive, cerebellar, corticospinal, and brainstem signs are caused primarily by diffuse effects of toluene on the CNS. In one prior report of an autopsy of a chronic solvent abuser, there was prominent degeneration and gliosis of ascending and descending long tracts with cerebral and cerebellar atrophy (110). Unfortunately, as in most reports of toluene neurotoxicity, this patient was abusing many solvents contained in several different product mixtures, so the effects of individual solvents could not be determined.

Clinical Neuropathology

The first report of neuropathologic changes was in an individual who was primarily an abuser of paint thinner containing toluene (84). In the late 1980s, the first reports were published that began to look more closely at the pathophysiology of toluene inhalation (87,90). These studies used MRI and demonstrated for the first time that chronic abuse of toluene-containing substances caused diffuse CNS white matter changes (87,90). This has been thoroughly reviewed by Filley (113). The first published report was based on the MRI findings of the brain in six individuals and the neuropathologic changes in one abuser not studied by MRI (90). All individuals abused the same toluene-containing mixture, which contained primarily toluene (61%) and methylene chloride (10%). MRI of the six individuals revealed the following abnormalities: (a) diffuse cerebral, cerebellar, and brainstem atrophy; (b) loss of differentiation in the gray and white matter throughout the CNS; and (c) increased periventricular white matter signal intensity on T2-weighted images. These findings were supported in a more recent neuropathologic study (103). In this latter report, the neuropathologic and biochemical changes seen in the brains of chronic toluene abusers were identical with those seen in adrenoleukodystrophy (ALD). ALD is a rare X-linked disorder associated with accumulation of very-long-chain fatty acids in certain tissues, including brain (111). More recent MRI studies support these original observations (86,87,93,95,101,102).

These latter studies come from the United States (104), Japan (112), and Turkey (102). In adults, toluene precipitates an organic mental syndrome characterized by personality change and intellectual decline with mild dysfunction of the peripheral nervous system (113). Acute toluene intoxication produces a reversible neurologic syndrome characterized by encephalopathy and cerebellar ataxia (81). Chronic inhalation abuse induces a more severe white matter leukoencephalopathy characterized by a profound reduction in brain white matter regions along with cerebellar, brainstem, and pyramidal tract dysfunction (113). White matter changes have been reported as an increased signal in white matter areas such as corpus callosum, internal capsule, centrum semiovale, brainstem, and cerebellar peduncles in T2-weighted images along with many reports of enlarged ventricles (90,98,114). These changes most likely arise from a relative increase in the water content of white matter caused by demyelination (90,93,94). Specifically, MRI results (93) suggest a possible mechanism for the abnormalities in the basal ganglia and thalamus.

An important clinical feature of white matter disorders is that the potential for recovery may be greater than in gray matter disorders (115). Recent reports indicate a full recovery of cognitive function in adult abusers of petrol (106). Cerebral white matter pathology may not be as complete or permanent as is usually the case with primary neuronal disorders. For example, white matter may be damaged without neuronal loss, and recovery of function appears more likely. Spontaneous remission is well known in MS, a disease similar in loss of neuronal function and possibly related to remyelination (116). Remyelination also may restore axonal conduction after traumatic and compressive lesions (117).

Recent MRI studies of these and other cortical areas (102,105) confirmed the above as well as observed changes in the ratios of choline/creatine in the basal ganglia in "toluene" abusers. Only the U.S. study had a comparison group of other drug abusers (primarily chronic cocaine abusers), which also exhibited significant neuropsychological abnormalities but fewer MRI abnormalities. Of interest in the U.S. study, there was a dose–response relationship between the degree of inhalant abuse and the MRI changes, but no relationship was observed with neuropsychological measures. Additional studies using state-of-the-art MRI techniques may help to further delineate the pathophysiology of the neurologic effects of toluene abuse, and the degree of recovery of these pathophysiologic effects with abstinence.

While MRI has been very useful in attempting to understand the central nervous system effects of toluene abuse, an additional study using the imaging technique of brain SPECT (single-photon emission CT) to measure brain perfusion (or blood flow) in boys aged 16 to 18 was recently published (100). Multifocal abnormalities were seen in all 10 patients studied, but no distinct pattern of abnormalities emerged among the subjects. This may be due to the wide range of abstinence observed within the relatively small cohort (from 1 to 11 months abstinent). In a single case study, brain glucose metabolism (a measure of brain function) was measured using positron emission tomography (PET) after high-dose exposure to tetra-bromo-ethane. Compared to a large control group, this case study documented reduced glucose uptake in frontal and temporal cortical areas and subcortically in the hippocampus, basal ganglia, amygdala, thalamus, and putamen (118). These deficits were consistent with decrements in neuropsychological function, underscoring the notion that even relatively brief exposures can cause significant functional impairments reflected in both brain function and neuropsychological measures. Recovery of metabolic or cognitive function was not studied in this patient. Clearly, more controlled studies of brain function using these types of functional biologic measures are necessary, due to the many equivocal findings regarding cognitive deficits associated with inhalant abuse described above.

Although an exact dose–effect relationship cannot be drawn yet for chronic toluene exposure, it is clear that all severely affected individuals have had heavy and prolonged exposure. The lack of correlation between the type or duration of exposure and neurologic impairment may be a result of unreliable histories or other factors, such as genetic predisposition (unlikely) or hypoxemia resulting from "huffing" or "bagging." Nutritional factors and other concomitantly used substances may also be involved. Gradual resolution of acute toxicity and absence of withdrawal symptoms were probably due to slow elimination of "significant amounts" of toluene from the CNS.

Myelopathy (Nitrous Oxide)

This type of inhalation abuse can be evaluated prospectively and not rely on retrospective evaluation (119). This is only possible because nitrous oxide is an approved anesthetic, as is sevoflurane. In human laboratory studies, Zacny and colleagues have evaluated over several years the pleasurable inhalation of nitrous oxide by humans, exposed to various concentrations of oxygen and nitrous oxide (119,120). The investigators measured moods over time at different doses resembling those of the "recreational" user. They noted that the effects lasted only a couple of minutes, and word tests demonstrated that memory retention within 5 minutes of the event was reduced. Some users liked the effect, whereas others did not. Subjects preferred different levels of exposure to obtain the preferred dose of nitrous oxide to satisfy them. This group has also compared this anesthetic, although not at the same time, to another, sevoflurane (120) and in combination with alcohol self-administration (121). Moderate drinkers preferred nitrous oxide (at levels 20–40% nitrous oxide) more than light drinkers, showing an enhanced desire for nitrous oxide in the presence of significant levels of alcohol. Other studies have measured the neuropsychological effects of nitrous oxide on humans after lower 1-hour doses (122) or after anesthesia (123). Other reports discuss the use of nitrous oxide for anxiety reduction, especially for children in dental treatment (124); another report even suggests use of nitrous oxide for treatment of alcoholism, an untested and unapproved treatment.

Nitrous oxide is not an organic solvent but has been noted to cause some unusual toxicities. A neuropathy was first observed in medical personnel (125). Recently, three other cases of myelopathy were reported (125). In the early studies, both central and peripheral nerve damage resulted following high levels of N_2O exposure, which occurred even in the presence of adequate oxygen and even after short-term use when nitrous oxide was used as an anesthetic

(126). This is consistent with recent case reports documenting numbness and weakness in the limbs, loss of dexterity, sensory loss, and loss of balance with the clinical use of nitrous oxide (127). The neurologic examination indicates sensorimotor polyneuropathy. Patients with vitamin B_{12} deficiencies are especially sensitive (128), and a combined degeneration of the posterior and lateral columns of the cord has been observed that resembles vitamin B_{12} deficiency. Studies focusing on the mechanism of action indicate that cobalamins (vitamin B_{12}) are inactivated by N_2O; more recent studies show an inactivation of the methionine synthase, an enzyme that needs vitamin B_{12} to function (129). There was no recovery using vitamin B_{12} (or folinic acid) in some patients (129); however, recovery was documented in others (130). In this regard, a report of a neuropathy in an undiagnosed "cobalamin-deficient" infant exposed to nitrous oxide (131) is of interest. Another treatment approach, the use of dietary methionine, might be helpful as indicated by studies in rats (132). Rehabilitation proceeds with abstinence from nitrous oxide exposure and is relative to the extent of neurologic damage. Recent reviews cover the medical aspects of the pros and cons of using nitrous oxide (129), most recently by Sanders, Weimann and Maze (133). Despite the widespread distribution of this information to the medical community (134) and the reduced availability of pressurized cylinders, cases are still being observed (30). A recent report even identifies inflammation as a result of nitrous oxide exposure (135).

Laboratory Studies

There are new important imaging techniques increasingly used to elucidate human toxicology through use of animal studies. PET and other imaging approaches, such as MRI, combined with behavioral measures evaluates/identifies those volatile solvents/gases with mild to strong abuse potential. The physiologic consequences of inhalant abuse and the capacity of neural systems to rebound upon cessation of inhalant exposure are also being studied. Also reviewed are electrophysiologic and behavioral studies used to elucidate functional and morphological changes in the brain associated with inhalant exposure, especially as they relate to inhalant abusing subjects.

It is especially important to understand the complexities of human toxicology of inhalants in the developing brain. Primates begin myelination at birth; then, there is a period of increased myelination in adolescence and periadolescence as the brain remodels to ensure efficient communication between cortical and subcortical brain regions (136). Similarly, rodents begin myelination around postnatal day (PND) 15, with a surge in the number of myelinated axons between 25 and 60 days (137). In view of the potent toxicity of volatile solvents, the impact of inhalant abuse in this age group on the structural genesis of the brain and on brain function could be severe and lasting. Neuropsychological deficits observed in adult inhalant abusers have been directly related to the degree of white matter pathology (90,91). However, it is not known how this is manifested, especially in adolescent brains.

The reinforcing properties and CNS effects of inhalants are related chemically and pharmacologically. For years, studies of animals have explored the relative abuse potential of different organic solvents using models describing the stimulus properties of these chemicals. Nonhuman primates, for example, will self-administer vapors of toluene (138), mice will intravenously self-administer toluene (139), and develop a preference for environments in which they previously inhaled toluene (140,141). In addition, nonhuman primate PET studies were established to measure the uptake and distribution of several potentially abused inhalants (142).

Case reports (13,84) of occupational overexposure were the basis for animal models of inhalant abuse. Conditioned place preference (CPP) paradigms utilize a drug-free animal that has previously received pairings of an inhaled solvent in a particular environment and subsequently become conditioned to favor a drug environment over a neutral environment. In fact, it has been observed that adults at risk for solvent abuse include those whose work brings them into contact with these substances, such as shoemakers, painters, people working with gas and jet fuel, in addition to aircraft manufacturing (143). These case reports are a guide not only for establishing the CPP technique but also to the ubiquity of addictive and surprisingly toxic substances that are generally considered "safe" by the average user.

Traditional radioligand competition assays have facilitated the identification and comparison of widely abused drugs, for example, cocaine and heroin, with few common chemical features. However, inhalant pharmacology has been clouded by the absence of a potently bound initial protein target in the brain. The net effect of most abused compounds is to increase brain dopamine concentrations, whether through direct mechanisms (e.g., binding to dopamine receptors or stimulating dopamine synthesis in the mesolimbic reward system) or indirect pathways (inhibition of inhibitory GABA tone and subsequent disinhibition of dopamine). Yet the impact of inhalants on mesolimbic dopamine has yet to be unequivocally demonstrated (144–146). Different strengths of reinforcement of different inhalants related to site-directed actions had to be approached differently (147). An understanding of the protein-specific nature of inhalant effects has been indirectly inferred based on the lipophilicity hypothesis (144): (a) the ability of specific compounds (e.g., benzodiazepines and barbiturates) (148) to block or substitute for behavioral aspects of inhalant reinforcement (148,149) and (b) specific protein mutations that affect inhalant action on cell membranes and ion channels (150).

The uptake and distribution of inhalants can be attributed to factors including tissue lipid content and blood perfusion rates (142). The identification of the "target systems" is enhanced by the ability of specific compounds to block or substitute for behavioral aspects of inhalant reinforcement

(148,149) and specific protein mutations that affect inhalant action on cell membranes and ion channels (150). Also, the reversal of toluene-induced place preference by prior treatment with a drug that increases brain GABA (149) indicates another route.

Toluene

The measure of radioactive binding in PET studies, using radiotracers of toluene, most likely reflects both specific and nonspecific binding. However, these measures indicate high uptake and rapid clearance of [^{11}C]toluene from the brains of anesthetized baboons (151), consistent with clinical observations that toluene intoxication lasts approximately 5 minutes and takes 30 minutes to subside (35). Primate studies are more relevant to human toxicology than are rodents. Toluene metabolites are formed quickly and include benzoic and hippuric acids, which are excreted in urine, and benzaldehyde. There is also a clear redistribution of the labeled compound to brain regions of high white matter content (149,151), such as the corpus callosum and central semiovale (Fig. 20.1), in agreement with molecular resonance (MR) measures of pathology observed in human abusers. Thus, the enduring effects of toluene and other abused inhalants as measured by MRI techniques need further exploration in suitable animal models to understand these "white matter" manifestations. In this respect, toluene and other inhalants resemble alcohol, focusing on metabolic parameters instead of a "drug-binding" site.

As in primate studies, toluene uptake was greatest in pons, colliculi, and the internal capsule of the rodent brain (see Fig. 20.2; 152). At 20 minutes, histologic examination of coronal slices of the striatum (a), internal capsule (b), mammillary bodies (c), and cerebellar white matter (d and e) of rat brain shows very little uptake of toluene in gray matter (i.e., cortical regions). MTR scans revealed enlarged ventricles in these animals. White matter changes and thalamic hypointensity were observed, as well as a strong decrease in MTR signal in the pons, medulla, corpus callosum, and midbrain. On the other hand, hyperintensity was present in the frontal, sensory/motor cortex, and the amygdala. These studies of rats (152) demonstrate that brain regions where toluene accumulates are also the most vulnerable to structural damage, as measured by MRI. There is a strong correlation between toluene uptake and regional decline in the MTR MRI signal. Therefore, PET may be a useful tool to predict which areas of the brain are vulnerable to insult with the abuse of different inhalants.

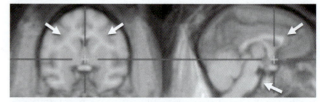
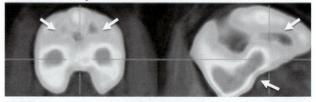
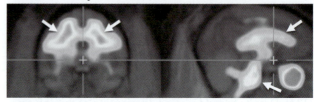

Figure 20.1. Redistribution of ^{11}C-toluene from gray matter to white matter regions of the baboon brain. White arrows indicate white-matter-rich regions of the brain, including the corpus callosum and brainstem.

FDG PET Studies of Toluene-Induced Changes in Brain Glucose Metabolism

Toluene alters brain metabolic function in adolescent animals, and these alterations are reproducible, regionally specific, and to some extent, reversible with abstinence. Analysis of region-specific effects indicates that the thalamus and hippocampus are particularly sensitive to toluene-induced changes in FDG uptake and that the temporal cortex is particularly resistant to recovery (Fig. 20.3). However, light microscopic analysis of myelin integrity showed no gross morphological differences between toluene and air-exposed animals.

The highest decreases in FDG uptake in rats were in cortical regions, including the temporal and somatosensory cortices (153). The white matter appears more predominantly in areas such as the pons, where neural tracts are bundled together. The gray matter more predominantly

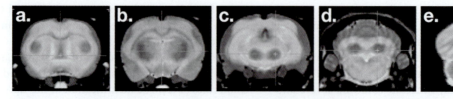

Figure 20.2. Distribution of ^{11}C-toluene in the rat brain. The brain has been separated into coronal slices showing uptake in the septum at the level of the striatum (a), internal capsule (b), mammilary bodies (c), and cerebellar white matter (d and e).

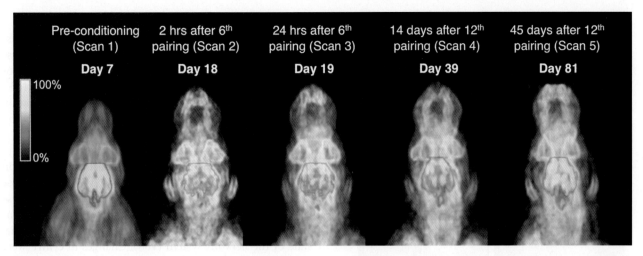

Figure 20.3. Impact of CPP to 5000 ppm toluene on 18FDG uptake. Serial data obtained from the same animal in adolescence prior to, throughout, and following a course of conditioning in which this animal expressed a significant preference (CPP) for toluene.

occupies regions such as cortex and thalamus and consists mainly of neuronal cell bodies and unmyelinated fibers. Because white matter regions are responsible for transmission of neural signals between gray matter regions, it is feasible that the impact of toluene on white matter could be reflected by alterations in gray matter as well as white matter function. This is evident in the high uptake of toluene itself in lipophilic, typically white matter-rich regions, while the functional consequences of toluene exposure are largely in gray matter regions such as the cortex. Thus, solvent or toxin-induced changes in morphology and metabolism ultimately raise the question of whether changes in morphology lead to functional decline or whether functional (i.e., metabolic) deterioration produces morphological damage. Taken together with clinical findings, it is possible that initially reinforcing doses of toluene produce functional changes resulting from metabolic disturbances which after years of abuse, alter brain structure and contribute to the well-established leukoencephalopathy described by Filley and colleagues (113). In addition, affected areas with less lipid content, such as the frontal and temporal cortices, reflect alterations in neurochemical transmission after repeated toluene exposure. The degree to which the regional distribution and mechanism of action of toluene and other abused inhalants are mediated by a receptor- or enzyme-driven mechanism is an area of active investigation (144). Early studies observed toluene-produced changes on brain dopamine concentrations, with more of an effect in the frontal cortex than in the striatum (152). More recently, studies of frontal areas appear more susceptible to the consequences of toluene exposure than striatal regions.

Butane/Propane

Very little is known about the mechanism of action through which these gases affect brain function. For example, butane is the prototypical aliphatic hydrocarbon abused and even high concentrations of butane or cyclopropane fail to alter the function of GABAA receptors (156). Unlike toluene, butane and cyclopropane do not act directly through GABA-mediated mechanisms (150,154–156,158). Instead, psychoactive concentrations of these gases appear to inhibit N-methyl-D-aspartate (NMDA)–sensitive glutamate channels and neuronal nicotinic acetylcholine receptors, a mechanism also shared by toluene and TCE (150,156,157).

Clinical reports and preclinical behavioral studies support the observed differences in the mechanism of action between toluene and butane. A butane-induced "high" is known to be extremely short-lasting (of the order of minutes) and of different quality (more pronounced visual hallucinations and distorted perception of body form) than the "high" experienced after toluene inhalation, where users report that thoughts are slowed, time appears to pass more quickly, and tactile hallucinations are experienced (35,155). Toluene is much more soluble in tissues, and butane is excreted rapidly through the lungs. Furthermore, the aliphatic hydrocarbon with the shortest chain length, methane, is rarely abused because it does not induce the desired pharmacologic effects (35). Evidence such as this supports the notion that the pharmacokinetics and pharmacodynamics of individual inhaled solvents greatly impact their rewarding or reinforcing properties. The link between pharmacokinetics and behavioral features of these inhalants related to their abuse liability remains to be established.

Acetone

Acetone is present in nail polish removers and some paint thinners. Acetone is not metabolized (158). It is a less potent CNS depressant than toluene or butane and less toxic. Radiolabeled metabolic PET studies support this conclusion (Fig. 20.4) (142). Acetone diffuses more slowly into the CNS than toluene (159,160). The acetone brain/blood ratio is 0.82; the

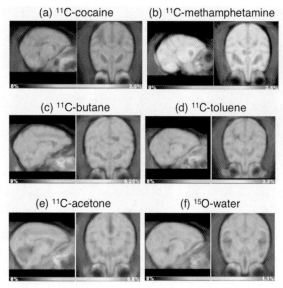

Figure 20.4. Radioactivity distribution of abused or potentially abused compounds in the primate brain. The distribution of two compounds with established abuse liability, ^{11}C-cocaine (a) and ^{11}C-methamphetamine (b), can be compared to compounds with lower abuse liability such as ^{11}C-butane (c), ^{11}C-toluene (d), ^{11}C-acetone (e), control (f).

toluene brain/blood ratio is 2.7, indicating that toluene passes from the blood into the brain much faster and at much lower concentrations. It is possible that, unlike toluene, which distributes to specific regions of the brain and other lipid-rich regions of the body, acetone prefers more aqueous regions. In fact, DiVincenzo (161) observed that the slow rate of disappearance of acetone from the blood of humans and animals followed zero-order kinetics, a characteristic of water-soluble anesthetics. The initial distribution of acetone in the primate brain resembles that of water, whereas toluene and butane distribute immediately from the blood into lipid-rich regions of the brain (142).

The abuse potential of acetone is low, since it is highly soluble in blood and solute areas and will poorly diffuse into the brain (160). These authors determined the LD_{50} for acetone to be 55,700 ppm while that for toluene was only 8600 ppm. In sum, it seems unlikely that solvent abusers would select acetone because of its slow onset and prolonged duration of action. Although early behavioral studies (161,162) suggest that acetone is reinforcing, more recently no effect at all was observed (162). Other studies of a wide range of inhaled acetone concentrations failed to produce a place preference in rodents (141). Inasmuch as toluene is the prototypical abused solvent, acetone should be at the other end of the spectrum—that of the prototypical nonabused solvent. Nevertheless, acetone is ubiquitous in commercial products in combination with other solvents and likely plays a role in the overall effect experienced by the person who abuses these toxicants.

Chlorohydrocarbons

Trichloroethane and TCE (common in dry cleaning fluids) share a profile of acute behavioral effects similar to those of CNS depressants and reproducibly substitute for benzodiazepines in drug discrimination studies (148,163). Other similarities include the development of sensitization (148,163) and tolerance (164), and biphasic effects on locomotor activity (165) and operant responding (166).

Limited ex vivo studies of these chlorohydrocarbons in rats provide evidence for a unique regional brain distribution (167). They also observed a decrease in cGMP (cyclic glucose monophosphate) production after administration of these chemicals. cGMP is a second messenger for excitatory (glutamatergic) transmission and reflects the general functional state of the nervous system (168). Changes in cGMP were noted to be regionally specific after inhalation of trichloroethane (169). While other compounds were not studied in these experiments, several neurochemical consequences of trichloro-ethane/ethylene exposure are thought to distinguish these inhaled solvents from other volatile chemicals such as toluene or halothane. Differences/similarities between toluene, styrene, and trichloro-ethane/ethylene actions on the cerebellar–vestibular circuit (170) are discussed below. Also, trichloroethane, but not florothyl, inhibits NMDA receptor function (157).

Nitrous Oxide

Nitrous oxide (N_2O) is an abused inhalant as well as an anesthetic, used primarily in dentistry for analgesia. This inhalant differs from most small hydrocarbons; it has a well-defined site(s) of action. Recent reports discuss the mechanisms of actions of nitrous oxide (125,171,172). Opioids have been known to alter the antinociceptive effect by the release of an opioid peptide in the brain stem, activating the descending noradrenergic inhibitory neurons and thereby modulating pain processing in the spinal cord. These authors studied the involvement of the brain stem opioidergic and γ-aminobutyric acid–mediated (GABAergic) neurons in the N_2O-induced antinociceptive effect. These results support the hypothesis that both opioidergic and GABAergic neurons mediate the antinociceptive effect of N_2O at the periaqueductal gray area and A7 in the brain stem. The authors postulate that N_2O-induced opioid peptide release leads to the inhibition of GABAergic neurons via opioid receptors. The descending noradrenergic inhibitory pathways, which are tonically inhibited by these γ-aminobutyric acid neurons, are thereby activated (disinhibited) and modulate pain processing in the spinal cord.

Other groups have focused on the action of nitrous oxide through the NMDA system (171,172). One group observed a reversible neurotoxic reaction in neurons of the posterior cingulate/retrosplenial cortex exposure of adult rats exposed to nitrous oxide (N_2O) and resembles that caused by low doses of NMDA antagonists (172). They consider N_2O to also be an NMDA antagonist. Prolonged exposure to other NMDA antagonists can cause neurons to die. They also noted that prolonged N_2O exposure also causes neuronal cell death in adult rats. After termination of N_2O exposure and following concurrently administered GABAergic agents (e.g., diazepam or isoflurane) prevented this cell death. Also, an increased binding of MK801, an NMDA antagonist, occurred with nitrous oxide administration (172).

Ketamine is another anesthetic acting on the NMDA glutamate receptors, and clinically, induces a psychotomimetic reaction in humans and pathomorphological changes in the rat brain. They found a combination of ketamine and N_2O caused an apparent neurotoxic reaction in young adult rat brain. In another study, they compared the neurotoxicity of ketamine and/or N_2O in 18- and 24-month-old rats to 6-month-old rats. Here, they observed a greater neurotoxic reaction in the older rats induced by either ketamine alone or the ketamine plus N_2O combination, but an equal neurotoxicity in either age group induced by N_2O alone (172).

With regard to the dependency of nitrous oxide, animal studies on selectively bred mice for alcohol dependence showed a cross-dependency on nitrous oxide (173). They also observed handling-induced convulsions shortly after cessation of nitrous oxide, which could be prevented by either alcohol or nitrous oxide. This might indicate a physical dependence on nitrous oxide that needs to be dealt with in the treatment of patients in this drug abuse state. Almost all solvents produce anesthesia if sufficient amounts are inhaled; some of them are described in a detailed study (174). Although this is an important property of the agent, the ability to produce anesthesia has not been correlated with the extent of abuse of any given substance. Eger and colleagues have measured different anesthetic neuronal responses for years, especially nitrous oxide (175).

PERIPHERAL NEUROPATHIES

Ototoxicity

Clinical

The clinical nature of ototoxicity was evaluated in 11 chronic toluene abusers by measures of brainstem auditory-evoked responses (BAERs) and MRI (90). Neurologic abnormalities, including cognitive, pyramidal, cerebellar, and brainstem findings, were seen in 4 of 11 individuals. MRI of the brain was abnormal in 3 of 11 individuals, and all 3 also had abnormalities on neurologic examination. Abnormalities on MRI were the same as those reported previously (91). BAERs were found to be abnormal in 5 of 11 individuals and were similar to those previously reported in toluene abusers (89). In this study (90), all three individuals with abnormal MRI scans and neurologic examinations also had abnormal BAERs. Of the five individuals with abnormal BAERs; however, two had normal neurologic examinations and MRI scans. This study suggests that BAERs may detect early CNS injury from toluene inhalation even at a time when neurologic examination and MRI scans are normal. These results suggested that BAERs could be a screening test to monitor individuals at risk from toluene exposure for early evidence of CNS injury.

Laboratory Studies

Laboratory-based studies have clarified some of the "toluene-type" neurotoxicities (176). Early studies of Pryor et al. (176) were the first to demonstrate persistent irreversible mid-frequency hearing loss by cued behavioral responses, BAERs, and pathology. Other studies (170,177) extended these findings. Hearing deficits are produced after as little as 2 weeks of exposure to 1200 ppm or 1400 ppm of toluene. This is attributed to cochlear dysfunction rather than the central conduction pathology found in the human studies noted above. After the initial studies on toluene were observed, Pryor et al. conducted a broad ranged structure–activity study on other related solvents. This group was also the first to identify a mid-frequency hearing loss in rats after exposure to TCE similar to that observed for toluene exposure (178). Others have since corroborated these studies (179). Pryor has published a list (Table 20.6) of several solvents that produce this hearing loss, including TCE, ethylbenzene (but not benzene), and styrene (180). Recently, ethylbenzene has been recommended to be defined as "ototoxic" in occupational settings (181). The exposure of rats to TCE produces a loss of spinal ganglion cells in the middle turn of hair cells (182). Other than ototoxicity, studies on rats have identified a toluene-induced motor syndrome that is characterized by a widened landing foot splay and a short and widened gait that may relate to the cerebellar syndrome in humans (183).

The common chemical structure feature of the most hazardous compounds is the presence of a vinyl-type unsaturation, not dissimilar to that occurring in some fatty acids. Further work needs to be done to clarify the chemical and molecular basis of this toxicity. Niklasson and colleagues (170) also analyzed the effects of some of these compounds on the vestibular function and correlated the changes with nystagmus. In a related area, Mergler and Beauvais (184) studied olfactory responses to toluene.

Hexane augments toluene toxicities, presumably through a reduction in the metabolism of toluene. Toluene causes age-related hearing loss in various inbred mice populations (185). This may result from different rates of metabolism in C57, but not CBA mice. In addition, noise has been thought to contribute to ototoxicity in the presence of toluene. A recent study of rats demonstrated that only "impulse" noise augmented auditory toxicity, not "low-level" noise (186). Also, toxicities in workers exposed to solvents were measured (187). They did not observe any changes in the amplitude of the auditory P300-evoked potential but did observe abnormal latencies in these subjects. A recent report discusses the difference between toluene

TABLE 20.6 Hearing loss produced (or not) by different solvents

Solvent	Hearing loss
Benzene	No
Toluene	Yes
Ethylbenzene	Yes
n-Propylbenzene	Yes
Isopropylbenzene (cumene)	No
Methoxybenzene	Yes
1,4-Dimethylbenzene (p-xylene)	Yes
1,2-Dimethylbenzene (o-xylene)	No
1,3-Dimethylbenzene (m-xylene)	No
Styrene	Yes
Monochlorobenzene	Yes
Carbon disulfide	Yes
Dichloromethane	No
Trichloroethane	No
Trichloroethylene	Yes
Tetrachloroethylene	No
Acetone	No
Methyl ethyl ketone	No
Ethyl alcohol	No
n-Hexane	No

type and excessive noise impairment of auditory function (188). As hearing loss has been identified in humans exposed to high levels of toluene, inhalant abusers of these types of chemicals should be provided good auditory evaluations.

n-Hexane and Methyl Butyl Ketone

These two organic solvents are classified together because both n-hexane and methyl butyl ketone (MBK) are metabolized to the same neurotoxin, 2,5-hexanedione (2,5-HD), and produce an identical clinical syndrome characterized by a peripheral neuropathy. MBK had limited industrial use until the 1970s when it became more widely used as a paint thinner, clearing agent, and a solvent for dye printing. Soon afterward, numerous outbreaks of polyneuropathy associated with chronic exposure to MBK were reported (189). Originally, methyl isobutyl ketone had been used. When methyl isobutyl ketone was replaced by MBK, reports of polyneuropathy began to appear in the literature.

The clinical syndrome is characterized by the insidious onset of an initially painless sensorimotor polyneuropathy, which begins several months after continued chronic exposure.

Even following cessation of exposure, the neuropathy may develop or may continue to progress for up to 3 months. In severe cases, an unexplained weight loss may be an early symptom. Sensory and motor disturbance begins initially in the hands and feet, and sensory loss is primarily a small fiber (i.e., light touch, pinprick, and temperature) with relative sparing of large-fiber sensation (i.e., position and vibration). Electrophysiologic studies reveal axonal polyneuropathy, pathologically multifocal axonal degeneration and multiple axonal swellings, and neurofilamentous accumulation at paranodal areas (190). Overlying the axonal swellings, thinning of the myelin sheath occurs. These findings are typical of a distal axonopathy or "dying-back" neuropathy described in other toxic and metabolic causes of peripheral neuropathy. Prognosis for recovery correlates directly with the intensity of the neurologic deficit before removal from toxic exposure, with mild to moderate residual neuropathy seen in the most severely affected individuals up to 3 years after exposure.

In related incidents in the 1970s, peripheral neurotoxicities were correlated with n-hexane, a solvent used in printing, in the extraction of vegetable oils, as a diluent in the manufacture of plastics and rubber, in cabinet finishing, and as a solvent for glues and adhesives. Cases of n-hexane polyneuropathy have been reported both after occupational exposure (191) and after deliberate inhalation of vapors from products containing n-hexane, such as glues (108,192). When glues have been analyzed in some reports of a polyneuropathy occurring after glue sniffing, n-hexane has been a major component of the products' composition. Another major component of glues has been toluene. However, polyneuropathy does not occur from inhalation of glues containing only toluene without the presence of n-hexane. In contrast to toluene, n-hexane does not usually induce significant signs of CNS dysfunction, except with high-level exposures where an acute encephalopathy may occur. Many cases of peripheral neuropathies still occur in industry (191). Both sensory and sensory-motor peripheral neuropathies have resulted in a shoe factory using glues with up to 50% hexane (191). Altered subclinical visual-evoked responses were also reported for some of these workers. In this study, 18 patients had sustained altered motor and sensory responses; 83% did have complete recovery 12 months later. Although the United States limits the use of hexane in many products, glues and other products (including some non-U.S. products) still contain this chemical in sufficient amounts to cause neuropathies in "glue sniffers."

2,5-HD is responsible for most, if not all, of the neurotoxic effects that follow exposure to n-hexane or MBK (193,194). Chemical structure may predict, but not invariably, the neurotoxic effects. This is exemplified by studies of two closely related compounds: 2,5-HD (the toxic metabolite of n-hexane) and 2,4-HD. A fixed dose of 2,5-HD produces axonal degeneration in a particular species that is very similar to that produced by hexane, whereas 2,4-HD never produces these changes. Thus, a small but important change in the compound's structure elicits a change from a positive to a nonpharmacologic action. Methyl ethyl ketone (MEK) alone produces neither clinical nor pathologic evidence of a peripheral neuropathy in experimental animals (193). The importance of MEK is related to a synergistic effect between MEK and MBK and between MEK and *n*-hexane detected in experimental animals and probably in humans (82). This potentiation of toxicity of one compound (MBK or *n*-hexane) by an otherwise nontoxic compound (MEK) underscores the difficulty with sorting out toxic effects of individual solvents contained within a mixture and suggests that any human exposure to solvent mixtures should be carefully monitored and kept to extremely low levels.

Both clinical and experimental animal studies provide some evidence of CNS effects from *n*-hexane. Experimental animal studies show *n*-hexane to cause axonal degeneration in the CNS (195). Clinically, cranial neuropathy, spasticity, and autonomic dysfunction occasionally occur (193). Abnormalities on electrophysiologic tests of CNS function, including electroencephalography, visual-evoked responses, color vision testing, and somatosensory-evoked responses, are also seen (196). In spite of these findings, clinically chronic low-level exposure to *n*-hexane primarily affects the peripheral nervous system.

Methylene Chloride (Dichloromethane)

Methylene chloride is widely used for paint stripping, as solvent for degreasing, in rapidly drying paints, and in aerosol propellants. As with other solvents, methylene chloride is a CNS depressant at high levels of exposure and may lead rapidly to unconsciousness and death (197,198). This has been reported both in industrial settings (197) and as a result of solvent inhalation abuse (198). A similar problem has also resulted from deliberate inhalation of the higher homologue dichloroethane. Methylene chloride is metabolized to carbon monoxide (199); consequently, both its hypoxic effect and its narcotic actions must be considered together with regard to its CNS-depressant effects. Carbon monoxide, at high levels, and other forms of cerebral hypoxia are known to cause permanent neurologic sequelae.

The effects of methylene chloride exposure on three tests of cognitive function (reaction time, short-term memory, calculation ability) were tested in 14 normal subjects (200). Three different exposures of methylene chloride showed no statistically significant impairment in performance. Methylene chloride may not be a choice inhalant if it is the only chemical present. However, inhalant abusers do inhale large quantities of methylene chloride from paint stripper solutions (90). In this regard, a recent report on the oral ingestion of this material identifies the problems that may occur after deliberate excess inhalation of methylene chloride (201). These include CNS depression, tachypnea, gastrointestinal injury, and high carboxyhemoglobin. In summary, the evidence suggests that methylene chloride does not produce permanent neurologic sequelae except with massive acute exposures that are associated with hypoxic encephalopathy. No evidence exists that chronic low-level exposure causes any serious long-term CNS injury.

1,1,1-Trichloroethane

1,1,1-Trichloroethane is widely used as an industrial degreasing solvent and, compared with other solvents, is less toxic. However, several reports of severe toxicity and deaths exist in the literature (202). Its acute toxicity has made it unsuitable as a volatile anesthetic, and its use as a carrier in aerosols was abandoned in the United States in 1973. In those cases where postmortem examination of the brain was undertaken, the pathologic changes suggested cerebral hypoxia occurred either primary to CNS depressant effect (202) or secondary to cardiac or respiratory arrest (202). 1,1,1-Trichloroethane is postulated to act on the autonomic nervous system and to cause sleep apnea (203). Cardiac toxicity is also a possible toxicity related to chronic 1,1,1-trichloroethane exposure (204). It appears that 1,1,1-trichloroethane is not associated with either acute or chronic neurotoxicity at levels below 1000 ppm and that the only permanent neurologic sequelae are related to cerebral hypoxia after massive exposure. In contrast to TCE, equivalent doses of trichloroethane do not produce hearing loss when administered to rats (180).

Gasoline

Gasoline is a complex mixture of organic solvents and other chemicals and metals. The inhalation of gasoline is common among various solvent abusers, especially on some remote Native American reservations. Leaded gasoline is not now readily available in the United States but still may present a problem in some areas. Although some CNS or peripheral neuropathies may occur as a result of the solvents in gasoline, there have been toxicities that resulted from tetraethyllead (or its metabolite triethyllead) (106). In cases where high lead levels were observed, various disorders occurred, including hallucinations and disorientation, dysarthria, chorea, and convulsions. The symptoms include moderate to severe ataxia, insomnia, anorexia, slowed peripheral nerve conduction, limb tremors, dysmetria, and sometimes limb paralysis. In most cases, the electroencephalogram (EEG) is normal, but in severe states, an abnormal to severely depressed cortical EEG is observed. In only one lethal case was any kidney damage noted; electrolytes are usually in the normal range. Because many of these symptoms in the early stages of the disease can be reversed by parenteral chelation therapy with ethylenediaminetetraacetic acid (EDTA), British anti-Lewisite (BAL) (dimercaprol), and/or penicillamine. It is important to check the serum lead levels in any chronic inhalant abuser to see whether this treatment should be prescribed. This type of therapy has recently been reviewed

(205). It was considered generally effective and the complications surrounding the treatment of these individuals were discussed (206).

Alcohol Alone or with Other Solvents

Methanol neurotoxicity is well known and exemplified by one case (207), where necrosis of the putamen region of the brain was noted. Recent studies of rats exposed to methanol have described the damage done to the retina and optic nerve (208). Methanol intoxication was identified in an individual intoxicated on a spray can of carburetor cleaner containing toluene (42%), methanol (23%), and methylene chloride (20%) (209). Although mild acidosis did occur, the main concern was the high blood level of methanol. Ethanol therapy was used to prevent formation of high levels of formic acid from methanol. The above mixture is abused and is very similar in composition to paint thinner; yet the repercussions of prolonged use are unclear.

One interesting phenomenon has been observed following the exposure to two or more solvents. Degreaser's flush was ascribed to a flushing of the face when occupational workers left their degreasing vats and drank alcohol after leaving work (210). Heavy drinking has been associated with toluene exposure (211). More recently, both humans and rats have been noted to be thirsty when exposed to toluene and alcohol (212,213). Also, animal studies have shown that solvents alter the metabolism of alcohol and prolong its action (214). This might explain the "flushing phenomenon" but may or may not relate to the psychological dependence of solvents or to the development of thirst. An attempt to study the acute effects of alcohol and toluene, at low exposures in human volunteers, failed to produce any interaction as measured by their behavior. This may be indicative that the interaction takes some time and/or high levels of exposure to develop. Another alcohol–drug interaction was recently reported. Campo et al. (215) showed an enhanced hearing loss in rats when ethanol was combined with toluene exposure. Again, both solvents given together are more hazardous following dual administration rather than with only one solvent.

NONNERVOUS SYSTEM TOXICITY OF INHALANT ABUSE

Most of the known adverse clinical effects of inhalant abuse involve the nervous system. There are, however, other adverse effects on other organ systems.

Renal Toxicity

Currently, spray paints are widely abused substances, at least in the United States. The abuse of these substances occurs not only among polydrug users but also by painters. Metallic spray paints contain large quantities of toluene; also, thinner and glue contain high levels of toluene noted in a study of street children in Turkey (216). The exposure to these and similar substances has resulted in the hospitalization of inhalant abusers for various kidney disorders (217–234). A recent report of diminished electrolytes occurred in a worker overexposed to paint thinner in a poorly ventilated room. He died after several days of corrective treatment for these low electrolytes and for hyposmia (219). A 32-year-old woman, identified as having renal distal acidosis after sniffing spray paint (220), presented to the hospital with severe quadriparesis. These subjects often have associated gastrointestinal involvement, including nausea, vomiting, and severe abdominal cramps. Lauwerys et al. (221) reviewed the early reports on nephrotoxicity in humans.

In one of the early reports, Streicher et al. (217) examined several cases and described them in detail, eliciting the nature of distal renal acidosis in groups of paint and/or glue sniffers from the southwestern United States and Hawaii. Streicher et al. and others have noted the recurrence of renal dysfunction associated with solvent abuse: the disease state reappears in many individuals who return to their habit after release from the hospital. Their symptoms include hyperchloremic metabolic acidosis, hypokalemia, hypocalcemia, and other electrolyte imbalances. A recent case included quadriparesis and respiratory failure (218). Solvents usually cause a unique distal-type tubular acidosis, but proximal tubules are also affected. Although the distal tubule is responsible for the known electrolyte and metabolic imbalance, the proximal type is responsible for the wasting of amino acids and other proteins. In spite of this tubular damage being reversible, other organs, particularly brain, are the target of repetitive acidosis, plus a depletion of important amino acids. A slightly different kidney dysfunction, glomerulonephritis, has also been identified in workers using solvents, especially painters, and reviewed by Daniell et al. (222). In addition, an interstitial nephritis leading to renal failure has been reported by Taverner et al. (223). Rhabdomyolysis is also observed after exposure to solvents (224). All of these reports indicate that kidney dysfunction is a common toxicity noted for solvent abusers. Even of greater concern might be the diabetic patient who presents after an overdose of solvents. Solvent odors might cover up the "acetone breath" of the diabetic patients and prevent the identification of the condition and/or the basis of that acidosis if the patient is unconscious (225). In a recent study of renal function in street children in Turkey, pyria, hematuria, and proteinuria were common (216), and glomerulopathy and tubulopathy were apparent. No acute or chronic renal failure indicators were evident. Glomerular filtration rate was in the lower range of normal, but urinary output of protein was higher, including urinary NAG (*N*-acetyl-glucoseamidase). These could be early indicators of renal toxicity and failure in these children. Toluene content of the thinner and glue that were abused was reported and appears to be the predominant solvent present.

There are also reports that halohydrocarbons—chloroform and others (226), methylene chloride (227), TCE (228), methoxyflurane (229), and dichloropropane (230)—may contribute to, if not cause, renal damage. The nephrotic pathologic changes reported include tubular necrosis and calcification. Studies of humans occupationally exposed to high levels of TCE, compared to nonexposed individuals, had elevated levels of alpha-microglobin excretion. This relates to an increased reported incidence of renal cell cancer incidence in these TCE-exposed individuals (231), reviewed by Lock et al. (226). Others (232) observed signs of Goodpasture syndrome; also, bladder changes are correlated to toluene exposure (233).

Although toluene is often proposed as the toxic agent and is present in most of the substances abused by these subjects, there has been no animal data to verify that toluene is a causative agent for renal dysfunction. Recently, Batlle et al. (234) exposed the turtle bladder to high concentrations of toluene and observed a diminished hydrogen ion transport that had no affect on the sodium transport. Also, toluene did not reduce the pH gradient across the bladder. Efforts to reproduce these nephrotic changes in rodents have met with limited success. Acute solvent exposure of liver cells determined an induced activation of cytochrome P4502E1 as the cause of proximal tubular cell necrosis by oxidative stress (235). Animal studies have also shown mild nephrotic changes following exposure to hydrocarbons (236). In most cases, more than one substance is present; this may indicate that the most severe nephrotic changes occur in the presence of two or more of these solvent compounds.

Thus several kinds of solvent mixtures are associated with glomerulonephritis, distal renal tubular acidosis, or other nephrotic changes. Usually, these different kidney disorders do not occur in the same individual and may be related to individual and/or other environmental factors. Although metallic spray paints are frequently used by these subjects, they also use paint thinners, glue vapors, and other solvents. It would appear reasonable to conclude that toluene may account for some but not all of these renal abnormalities. Renal toxicity may also be due to the metals contained in the spray paint, such as cadmium and lead, which are known to be nephrotoxic (237), or concurrent alcohol use and/or infections (238,239). As cases of renal toxicity continue to be reported, it is important that individuals exposed to high doses of solvents be checked for renal changes and metabolic imbalance. Correction of salt and electrolyte imbalance, including potassium, calcium, magnesium, and chloride, should be considered in the treatment of solvent abusers for muscle fatigue, even in the absence of more severe kidney disorders. However, one has cautioned the use of bicarbonate early for the treatment of these subjects.

Renal Toxicity in Pregnancy

One must especially be alert for nephrotoxicity in pregnant women who abuse solvents (also see the "Neonatal Syndrome" section). Pregnant women have presented with renal tubular acidosis. In one report (240), three of the five infants showed growth retardation. A similar case was reported where no known causative agent was identified (241). These women often, but not always, respond to treatment for their metabolic imbalance after 72 hours of treatment and abstinence of solvent abuse.

Hepatotoxicity

Chlorohydrocarbons (e.g., TCE, chloroform, halothane) have been known for years to produce hepatotoxicities. Several reports describe solvent-related toxicities (3,229, 239,242–244). Any individual who is chronically exposed to these compounds would expect hepatorenal insults, depending on the dose and length of exposure (242). Buring et al. (245) evaluated the effects of low levels of exposure measured retrospectively by several investigators. They concluded an increased risk exists for operating room personnel using chlorohydrocarbon anesthetics: however, Brown and Gandolfi (229) questioned whether liver toxicity occurs very often after use of halothane as an anesthetic.

The inhalation of correction fluids for "pleasure," which did, and may still, contain TCE, and trichloroethanes or tetrachloroethanes (246), did lead to toxicities in inhalant abusers (247). Even during occupational use, exposure to chlorohydrocarbons in poorly ventilated areas is considered to lead to hepatotoxicity. A recent paper describes an occurrence of hepatitis for a shoemaker working with a glue containing TCE in his basement for several years (244). He presented with anorexia, fatigue and upper abdominal discomfort. Marked elevation of liver enzyme and bilirubin levels could only be related to the TCE exposure. Although there was no knowledge that this excessive exposure occurred due to self-directed inhalation, this type exposure of these halohydrocarbons by inhalant abusers does occur and may have resulted in hepatic damage in some unreported individuals.

A refrigerant gas, HCFC-123, was identified as hepatotoxic in a hospital worker (248). This is more readily metabolized than the previously used fully halogenated fluorocarbons and has been compared in toxicity to an analogue, halothane, which is used for anesthesia (249,250). Hepatocellular and other carcinomas are observed at high doses of TCE (228) and halothane (251). Anesthetic chlorinated hydrocarbons (halothane, TCE, and chloroform) are also considered to be carcinogenic (252). Increased availability of TCE for dry-cleaning purposes could present more cases of nephrotic and hepatotoxic diseases, including cancer (253).

Pulmonary Toxicity

The trachea and lungs are the primary organs affected by inhalants; yet, there are few cases noted where the pulmonary system is severely compromised. As mentioned earlier, asthmatics excessively administer the very medication that they need (27). These products have been reported to cause pulmonary hypertension, acute respiratory distress, increased airway resistance, and residual volume and restricted ventilation. One "outbreak of respiratory illness" was associated with changes in solvents/propellants of a leather conditioner (254). This product produced tachypnea, pulmonary edema, and hemorrhage in rats. Respiratory problems would therefore be expected in inhalant abusers using these or similar products. In addition, increased airway resistance or residual volume may be more clearly noted following an exercise challenge (255). Additionally, response to an aerosolized bronchodilator is suggestive of an airway involvement perhaps induced by habitual inhalation of hydrocarbons. Smoking may have been a contributory factor in one study (256) and was not ruled out in the others. In studies of workers using waterproofing aerosols containing trichloroethane (257) or using a paint stripper (258), acute respiratory distress has been correlated with the chlorinated hydrocarbon exposure. Although solvents irritate the pulmonary system, it is not at all clear from the limited case studies reported, to date, how extensive or what types of pulmonary damage occur that can be primarily caused by solvent exposure and not to other inspired substances that are dissolved in the solvents. For example, a report of a homicidal case (a spray paint "sniffer") noted metallic deposition alongwith hemorrhagic alveolitis (259). It is uncertain how to generalize the impact of dual exposure of solvent and infection, but an animal study showed decreased pulmonary bacteriocidal activity after exposure to dichloroethylene (260). Injury of trachea mucosa was recently observed following spray paint exposure (261). This case, however, was not associated with self-abuse.

Cardiotoxicity

It is not as evident, but the results of several cases link fibrillation and other cardiac insufficiencies to the use of halocarbons (4,18,202–204) and numerous others. These types of products range from anesthetics (halothane) used by hospital and other medical personnel to the more common solvents/propellants and fluorocarbons (dichloroethanes, trichloroethanes, tetrachloroethanes, and TCE) contained in cleaning fluids and other products. Most interestingly, the resuscitation of inhalant abusers following cardiopulmonary arrest does not usually occur; yet, a successful resuscitation from fluorocarbon cardiac arrhythmia has been reported (262); also, another patient who suffered nonfatal respiratory arrest (twice) after "sniffing glue" was resuscitated (263). In another report, cardiopulmonary complications resulted from paint thinner (containing toluene and benzene derivatives) overexposure for several hours (219). Cardiac arrest occurred on day 2, he was resuscitated, but remained unconscious till death 9 days later.

Many solvent abusers may die from direct or indirect cardiotoxic actions of solvents without note in any public or private record. Several cases of the abuse of different products have been reported (204,262). Some of the subjects had inhaled TCE- (264) or trichloroethane-containing solvents (204) and some subjects were additionally compromised by anesthesia (e.g., halothane) (204). Fluorocarbons cause arrhythmias in animals (265). Chenoweth and colleagues showed that butane, hexane, heptane, gasoline, some anesthetics, and toluene also produce these arrhythmias (266). Reports have linked glue sniffing to arrhythmias, myocarditis, and cardiac arrest. Glues usually do not contain halocarbons but do contain toluene and other hydrocarbons. A very recent report identifies a cardiomyopathy following paint thinner and glue (containing toluene) inhalation (267). Recent studies, conducted on oocytes (268), measured sodium or potassium channel currents to partially explain the cardiotoxic actions of toluene. Therefore, where heavy solvent exposure is suspected, strenuous exercise or anesthesia should be avoided.

Hematologic Toxicity

There are three areas of concern with regard to solvent inhalation and the hematopoietic system. First, methylene chloride exposure can increase the carboxyhemoglobin levels (198), a change that also occurs with cigarette smoking. The levels of carboxyhemoglobin may become sufficiently high to cause brain damage (269) or death (270). In one case, inhalation of methylene chloride prompted a sustained (at 24 hours postexposure) elevation of carboxyhemoglobin (199). A second substance, benzene, causes aplastic anemia, acute myelocytic leukemia, and other hematopoietic cancers (221,271). Benzene is present in thinners, varnish removers, and other solvents, and in varying proportions in gasoline, sometimes at high concentrations that will produce "toxic" levels following episodes of inhalant abuse. A third group of substances, the organic nitrites, produce methemoglobinemia and hemolytic anemia (272).

The latter group, the volatile liquid isoamyl (amyl), isobutyl or butyl nitrites, propyl nitrites, cyclohexyl nitrites, and maybe other organic nitrites deserve a special discussion. During the late 19th and early 20th centuries, amyl nitrite was used in clinical practice as a vasodilator to treat angina pectoris. Although this use of the drug is uncommon today, it is sometimes used for diagnostic purposes in echocardiogram examinations (273) and for cyanide poisoning (274). These abused drugs do *not* produce the typical solvents/gases neurologic actions described above; however, they are often included in the "inhalant abuse" category. Different adult individuals (predominately homosexuals) are the primary abusers of these organic nitrites. Subjects may use them for sphincter dilation and penile engorgement. Use by others for nonsexual purposes is unclear. One study could not correlate changes in regional blood flow with any psychological measures or somatic changes (275); also, isoamyl nitrite did not substitute for barbiturates, as do toluene and other solvents (276). These studies do not offer any explanation for why individuals become dependent on nitrites. However, the finding by Mathew et al. (275) that nitrites reduce anger, fatigue, and depression may offer a clue.

The nitrites are usually not considered acutely toxic during inhalation because of syncope (fainting). However, Guss et al. (277) noted a dangerously high 37% methemoglobin level in a normal subject who had used isobutyl nitrite. This methemoglobinemia is the major identified toxicity and is the cause of several deaths. There is a specific treatment for nitrite overdose. The high and slowly reversible reduction of methemoglobin can be aided by the use of methylene blue (278).

Heavy organic nitrite has been considered a risk factor for the development of acquired immune deficiency syndrome (AIDS) (279) and of Kaposi sarcoma (KS) (280). Thus, the use of organic nitrites became an issue when KS (now considered to be caused by the virus HHV-8 (281) was linked with nitrite use in homosexual populations (282). A recent study (283) of HIV-negative men showed that abuse of nitrite inhalants was an independent risk factor for infection with HHV-8, the etiologic agent of KS. The potential use of nitrites has also been studied in the U.S. military (57).

To understand the actions of these nitrites, animal studies were conducted to evaluate their actions on the immune system (284). Soderberg reviews the potential for nitrites to impair the immune system (285). Earlier studies reported that exposure to isobutyl nitrite inhibited several acquired immune responses, including the induction of T-dependent antibodies (285). B cells and isolated T cells, however, had normal functions. In their studies, after inhalation exposure of mice for 14 days to isobutyl nitrite, there is a reduced capacity for the concanavalin A (but not lipopolysaccharide) stimulation of T-cell functions, an induction of cytotoxic T cells, a reduced tumoricidal activity, and an increased tumor incidence (285). Recent data suggest that at least some innate immune mechanisms were also impaired by inhalant exposure, that is, a reduction in important AIDS factors, the chemokines. IL-1 has been reported to inhibit HIV replication through the induction of chemokines, MIP-1α, MIP-1β, and RANTES (286). Abusers of nitrite inhalants could be more susceptible to HIV infection and to KS tumor growth in multiple ways if the inhalants impair both acquired and innate immune responses. In this manner, the factors leading to or augmenting KS, including the organic nitrites, are discussed in Refs. (281,285). In other reports from Fung's laboratory, isobutyl nitrite stimulated the hepatic mRNA and protein expression of vascular endothelial growth factor (VEGF) (287). Isobutyl nitrite reduces several hepatic enzymes, including cytochrome-mediated deethylation (288). They discussed the issue of KS related to some of these findings.

Neonatal Syndrome

There is evidence that solvent inhalation during pregnancy produces a "fetal solvent syndrome." There are numerous cases of infants of mothers who chronically abuse solvents (107,240,241,289–292) diagnosed with this syndrome. The mothers inhaled paint reducer, solvent mixtures from paint sprays, and drank various quantities of alcohol. Whether toluene alone (often noted as the major solvent), other solvent components, and/or these components in combination with alcohol or other environmental factors are responsible is still unsubstantiated by laboratory studies. Toluene still appears to be a major contributor. This toluene embryopathy has been compared to the better recognized fetal alcohol syndrome (107). The infants present with growth retardation, some dysmorphic features, including microcephaly, as well as distal renal acidosis, aminoaciduria (290), ataxia, tremors, and slurred speech (291). Toluene has been considered a human teratogen (292). This inhalant "fetal syndrome" has recently been evaluated in a study of pregnant women who used toluene-based solvents and/or alcohol (293). In this study, only the babies of mothers who abused alcohol were observed to have a "fetal alcohol syndrome." However, some of the newborns of solvent abusers presented with renal acidosis.

Some of these abnormalities related to toluene and other solvents were also observed in rodents exposed to toluene (294); however, the extent and severity of the effects are unclear. It is difficult to produce these abnormalities in rodents (295). Growth retardation occurs in rats with doses of toluene that produce fetal mortality without producing malformations (296). Weight loss, altered motor activity, renal abnormalities, and some neurologic insults were also recently reported (297–299).

Nitrous oxide has been reported to produce some "major visceral and minor skeletal (fetal) abnormalities" (300). Surprisingly, these abnormalities are reportedly protected against by 0.27% halothane, but not by folinic acid. Also, animal fetal liver toxicities occur after administration of carbon tetrachloride (301) or malformations following chloroform (302). With so little knowledge and yet with all the potential dangers, it is very important that pregnant women not be exposed to very high concentrations of solvents/gases.

DSM EVALUATIONS OF INHALANT ABUSE

DSM-IV and Inhalant Use Disorders

Inhalant use and IUDs are defined by the *Diagnostic and Statistical Manual of Mental Disorders*, 4th Edition (*DSM-IV-TR*, American Psychiatric Association [APA], 2000). *DSM-IV* inhalant abuse and dependence criteria parallel the generic *DSM-IV* substance abuse and dependence diagnostic criteria, except that the withdrawal criterion included in the generic substance dependence criteria set is not included in the inhalant dependence criteria set. One of four criteria must be met to receive a *DSM-IV* inhalant abuse diagnosis (e.g., legal trouble due to inhalant use) and at least three of six criteria (e.g., tolerance to inhalants) must be met to receive a diagnosis of inhalant dependence, the most serious of the inhalant disorders. Inhalant-induced disorders include inhalant use-precipitated delirium and dementia, among other clinically important conditions, but specifically exclude use of nitrite vasodilators such as amyl or isobutyl nitrite and the anesthetic gas nitrous oxide.

The estimated prevalence of IUDs depends to some extent on the nosology employed to assign diagnoses and the characteristics of the sample under investigation. For example, Howard, Cottler, Compton, and Ben-Abdallah (303) found a substantially smaller proportion of lifetime inhalant users, who participated in the *DSM-IV* Field Trial for Substance Use Disorders, met *DSM-IV* IUD criteria than met comparable *DSM-III-R* or ICD-10 criteria. Rates of formal IUDs are also often higher in samples of antisocial or delinquent youth and in other high-risk populations than in the general population.

Few studies of the natural history of IUDs have been conducted. Perron, Howard, Maitra, and Vaughn (304) recently reported that 19%, who initiated inhalant use in the NESARC (National Survey on Alcohol and Related Conditions) study, developed a *DSM-IV* IUD. Most of these transitions were to inhalant abuse rather than inhalant dependence and that risk for transition was substantially greater in the first year following initiation of inhalant use and low thereafter. The presence of a mood or anxiety disorder or alcohol use disorder antedating initiation of inhalant use predicted significantly elevated risk for IUD, whereas being married lowered risk for onset of IUDs. Nationally representative data from the NESARC survey also reveal high rates of *DSM-IV* mood, anxiety, and personality disorders (305) and prevalent noninhalant substance use disorders (306) among adult inhalant users.

Adolescents

Relatively few studies have examined the prevalence of IUDs in national samples of adolescents. Wu, Pilowsky, and Schlenger (307) examined the prevalence of IUDs in 36,850 12- to 17-year-olds who participated in the 2000–2001 National Household Survey on Drug Abuse. Overall, 0.4% of adolescents aged 12 to 17 years met past-year inhalant abuse or dependence criteria. Alternatively, 10.6% of past-year inhalant users met past-year inhalant abuse or dependence criteria. Similar figures were reported for 15- to 24-year-olds participating in the National Comorbidity Survey (NESARC); 8% of participants reported inhalant use, the proportion of overall respondents ($N = 8,098$) with a history of inhalant dependence was 0.6%, and the proportion of inhalant users with a lifetime history of dependence was 8% (308).

Ridenour, Bray, and Cottler (309)[1] reported much higher rates of *DSM-IV* IUDs in a community sample of 162 adolescents/young adult inhalant users (medium age = 20; SD = 2.4) who were recruited via community flyers or referral. Approximately, 28% of respondents met criteria for inhalant abuse, whereas 12% met inhalant dependence criteria. Overall, use of inhalants in hazardous situations (29%) was the most prevalent inhalant abuse criterion, whereas inhalant-related legal problems (1.9%) was the least prevalent inhalant abuse criterion. The most prevalent dependent criteria were inhalant use despite a known physical or psychological problem related to such use (59%) and using inhalants in a greater quantity over a longer time than was planned (30%). Sakai et al. (310) examined IUDs in 847 youth aged 13 to 19 who were treated at a university-based program for behavior or substance misuse problems. Although approximately 19% of youth had used inhalants, only 3.3% met criteria for lifetime inhalant abuse or dependence. In another study, high rates of inhalant abuse (19%) and dependence (28%) were observed among 279 inhalant users who were in residential care for antisocial behavior in Missouri (311). Overall, 18.1% of youth in the Missouri Division of Youth Services residential treatment system met criteria for Inhalant Use Disorders and 5 of 10 *DSM-IV* IUD criteria were met by <10% of the total sample of 723 current residents.

Adults

Drawing upon data from the 2002–2003 administrations of the NSDHU, Wu and Ringwalt (312) estimated that approximately 10% of U.S. adults had used inhalants and that 4.8% of this group had used inhalants within the prior year. Among past-year inhalant users, approximately 8% met criteria for past-year IUDs. Among participants aged 15 to 54 in the NESARC, the proportion of overall respondents with a history of inhalant dependence was 0.3%, and 3.7% of inhalant users developed inhalant dependence (62). Only 2% of adult respondents in the NESARC reported lifetime inhalant use, but of this proportion nearly one in five (19%) met criteria for a lifetime IUD (305). Taken together, surveys of adolescents and adults suggest that inhalant use is far more prevalent than IUDs in the general population. However, signs and symptoms of IUDs and associated criteria may be prevalent among some high-risk groups such as antisocial youth, which are commonly excluded from large surveys of noninstitutionalized populations.

TREATMENT

There is no accepted treatment approach for inhalant abusers. There are a variety of treatment programs for inhalant abusers used by educators, drug treatment clinics, and physicians, but there are a relatively few drug abuse treatment "professionals," who focus primarily on inhalant "abusers." The available programs range from basic and limited behavioral modification to medical pharmacologic clinics (which do not usually segregate inhalant abusers from other drug abusers), but little is evidence-based treatment.

---

[1] The subdividing of various "inhalant abusers" in this paper into different groups uses overlapping chemical/physical criteria that place some of the abused compounds in more than one "class."

Many drug treatment facilities refuse treatment of the inhalant abuser, as some believe that inhalant abusers are resistant to treatment. Some programs use models that range from short-term to longer periods of treatment. Longer periods of treatment are needed to be able to address the complex psychosocial, economic, and biophysical issues of the "heavy" inhalant user. Many environmental stimuli are associated with these "drug" effects and include family problems, poverty, environment, and associations. When brain injury in a very limited number of subjects occurs, mostly in the form of cognitive dysfunction, the rate of progression in recovery is even slower.

The diagnostic criteria, which measure signs of compulsive drug seeking, are the same for all drug categories, even though the mechanisms for activating the reward system are quite different (313). Also, when psychiatric disorders co-occur with addiction, these disorders must be treated concomitantly and preferably by the same treatment team. Use of many addictive drugs may be diminished by pharmacologic action, and thus, treatment may benefit by medication. No specific, well-documented pharmacologic agent has been reported, although case studies of the use of different drugs have been sporadically reported noting limited success. The primary addictive disorder may also benefit through combination of counseling with medication (313). However, no pharmacologic treatment is known for "inhalants." The "serious" inhalant abuser typically does not respond to any usual drug rehabilitation treatment modality. Several factors may be involved, particularly in situations of the chronic or "heavy" abuser, where significant psychosocial problems may coexist. Treatment becomes slower and progressively more difficult when the severity of brain injury worsens as abuse progresses from transient social use (experimenting in groups) to chronic use in isolation. Specific drug treatment may also be difficult to evaluate largely due to the weak tolerance or physiologic dependence that occurs with inhalants.

Sakai et al. (310) have published studies on the clinical treatment of inhalant abuse. This is one of few studies of patients, which measures various disorders associated with inhalant abuse. In this program, few are "chronic inhalant users." They describe an association between inhalant use and antisocial behavior, which has long been noted in cross-sectional studies (310). Also, some adolescents in this study had been in a jail, detention center, prison, hospital, or treatment program prior to follow-up assessment. It was stated that inhalant intoxication in this sample of drug abusers accounted for the high severity of relapse at follow-up. It may be that inhalant use serves as a marker for severity of impulsivity, risk taking propensity, and poor decision-making ability. Interestingly, only one adolescent in this group reported using inhalants in the previous 30 days at the 2-year follow-up. This is characteristic of most "inhalant abusers" in these treatment programs; they are not current chronic users of inhalants and may never have been. As a corollary, the physicians did not observe neuropsychological impairment associated with inhalant use (310).

Beauvais queried several associated treatment groups they worked with (314). This study assessed the attitudes and success of drug user treatment program directors toward the problem of inhalant "abuse." Areas covered included treatment success and prognosis for inhalant users, level of neurologic damage incurred by users, availability of treatment resources, their program's policies toward admission of users, and staff training needs for inhalant use including their assessment of barriers to treatment and subjective feelings about the topic of inhalant use. Five hundred and fifty responses were received. The responses were general in nature with limited details. Reidel, Herbert and Byrd (315) have published a more substantive report regarding the effects of and approaches to treatment of some of these inhalant users. These authors are associated with one of the few treatment programs in the country dedicated to "primary" inhalant users. They detected significant improvement in neuropsychological functioning among patients at the end of treatment (using Halstead–Reitan scores).

Dinwiddie et al. (316) studied treatment of eleven "primary" inhalant users, who were mostly in their twenties. The data came from subject records of those admitted for treatment and which were reviewed for medical and psychiatric illness and other substance abuse. Antisocial personality disorder and narcotics abuse were commonly associated factors; also symptoms suggesting neurologic or gastrointestinal dysfunction were noted. The patients' response to treatment was poor. Those patients, using solvents chronically, had associated behavioral patterns that contribute to poor social adjustment. Ten entered treatment, but only half finished, and all relapsed within 6 months.

Drug screening may be useful in monitoring inhalant abusers (317). Routine urine screens for hippuric acid, the major metabolite of toluene (219), performed two to three times weekly, will detect the high level of exposure to toluene usually seen in "chronic" inhalant abusers. However, analysis must always take into account the average background level of hippuric acid resulting from general metabolism. It should be noted that the metabolism of any one compound may be modified by the presence of another, either increased (following inducement by drugs, e.g., barbiturates) or decreased (benzene metabolism reduced in the presence of toluene) (219).

Neuroleptics and other forms of pharmacotherapy are usually not useful in the treatment of inhalant abusers. However, as alcohol is a common secondary drug of abuse among inhalant abusers, a monitored program for alcohol abuse may be necessary in any treatment. Other medication has been used but seldom evaluated, especially in any large population samples. Also, "oil of mustard" has been considered and sometimes used to prevent abuse. Its presence in "correction fluids" often irritated secretaries and others who use the product correctly, but it does not appear to stop those who really want to "sniff." Risk perception is a frequent question on national surveys (NUSDUH and MTF). However, it has seldom been evaluated. See discussion in the "Epidemiology" section.

Neuroimaging studies in inhalant-exposed animals could reveal the role of a number of molecular targets in solvent-induced white matter degeneration, narrowing possible treatment options for stimulating remyelination in animal models of treatment (318). For example, if toluene's rewarding effects are mediated by dopamine, then this dopamine site becomes a therapeutic target for its addictive liability. Similarly, if toluene selectively damages white matter, then remyelinating agents that have been successful in the treatment of relapse-remitting MS might facilitate recovery. Some examples are interferon beta 1b (319), copolymer 1 (320), and interferon beta 1a (321).

ACKNOWLEDGMENTS

The authors acknowledge the support of the National Institute on Drug Abuse, NIH, DHHS. The authors also acknowledge the excellent assistance of Dr. James Colliver (SAMHSA), the excellent technical support of Betty Sharp, without whom this chapter would not have been completed, and the excellent previous contributions of Dr. Neil Rosenberg, who passed away suddenly in 2003. His contribution is still part of this chapter. Dr. Rosenberg, as an active neurologist, was concerned about young people's drug habits causing dementia prematurely. He focused not only on excessive voluntary exposure to solvents but also on the use of other neurotoxic substances such as methamphetamine. He was a pioneer in the field of defining the neurologic manifestations of solvent abuse. To assist those in need, he and his wife, Cathy, founded the International Institute on Inhalant Abuse. He also devoted his energies through academic groups, including NIH and the American Academy of Neurology. He traveled throughout the United States and Central and South America educating people about the dangers of inhaling chemicals and did extensive humanitarian work with poor people in Peru and other countries in Latin America, as well as with Native Americans in the northern hemisphere, always with the prime goal of diminishing solvent and other drug use. He is sorely missed.

REFERENCES

1. Carroll E. Notes on the epidemiology of inhalants. In: Sharp CW, Brehm ML, eds. *NIDA Research Monograph, Review of Inhalants: Euphoria to Dysfunction*. Number 15. Rockville, MD: National Institute on Drug Abuse, U.S. Public Health Service; 1977: 14–22.
2. Faraday M. *Quart J Sc Arts*. 1818;4:158–159, in Smith TC, Cooperman LH, Wollman H. History and principles of anesthesiology. In: Goodman GA, Goodman LS, Gilman A, eds. *Goodman and Gilman's the Pharmacological Basis of Therapeutics*. 6th ed. New York: Macmillan; 1980:258.
3. Hutchens KS, Kung M. "Experimentation" with chloroform. *Am J Med*. 1985;78:715–718.
4. Kringsholm B. Sniffing-associated deaths in Denmark. *Forensic Sci Int*. 1980;15:215–225.
5. Krenz S, Zimmermann G, Kolly S, et al. Ether: a forgotten addiction. *Addiction*. 2003;98:1167–1168.
6. Kerner K. Current topics in inhalant abuse. In: Crider RA, Rouse BA, eds. *NIDA Research Monograph, Epidemiology of Inhalant Abuse: An Update*. Rockville, MD: National Institute on Drug Abuse, U.S. Public Health Service; 1988;85:8–29.
7. Clinger OW, Johnson NA. Purposeful inhalation of gasoline vapors. *Psychiatr Q*. 1951;25(4):557–567.
8. Trochimowicz HJ. Development of alternative fluorocarbons. In: Sharp CW, Beauvais F, Spence R, eds. *NIDA Research Monograph. Inhalant Abuse: A Volatile Research Agenda*. Rockville, MD: National Institute on Drug Abuse, US Public Health Service; 1992;129:287–300.
9. Finch CK, Lobo BL. Acute inhalant-induced neurotoxicity with delayed recovery. *Ann Pharmacother*. 2005;39:169–172.
10. Kong JT, Schmiesing C. Concealed mothball abuse prior to anesthesia: mothballs, inhalants, and their management. *Acta Anaesthesiol Scand*. 2005;49:113–116.
11. Bass M. Death from sniffing gasoline. *N Engl J Med*. 1978; 299:203.
12. Cohen S. Inhalant abuse: an overview of the problem. In: Sharp CW, Brehm ML, eds. *NIDA Research Monograph, Review of Inhalants: Euphoria to Dysfunction*. Rockville, MD: National Institute on Drug Abuse, U.S. Public Health Service; 1977;15: 2–11.
13. Knox JW, Nelson JR. Permanent encephalopathy from toluene inhalation. *N Engl J Med*. 1966;275:1494–1496.
14. Bass M. Sudden sniffing death. *JAMA*. 1970;212:2075–2079. [110 cases]
15. Marsolek MR. Inhalant abuse: monitoring trends by using poison control data, 1993–2008. *Pediatrics*. 2010;125:905–913.
16. Field-Smith ME, Butland BK, Ramsey JD, et al. *Trends in Deaths Associated with Abuse of Volatile Substances, 1971–2007. Report 22*. London: St. George's Hospital Medical School; 2009. Available at: http://www.vsareport.org/.
17. National Institute for Occupational Safety and Health. *Special Occupational Hazard Review with Control Recommendations: Trichloroethylene*. 1978;78–130. Washington, DC: Department of Health, Education, and Welfare.
18. Troutman WG. Additional deaths associated with the intentional inhalation of typewriter correction fluid. *Vet Hum Toxicol*. 1988;30:130–132.
19. Siegel E, Wason S. Sudden death caused by inhalation of butane and propane. *N Engl J Med*. 1990;323:1638.
20. Rohrig TP. Sudden death due to butane inhalation. *Am J Forensic Med Pathol*. 1997;18:299–302.
21. Wheeler MG, Rozycki AA, Smith RP. Recreational propane inhalation in an adolescent male. *J Toxicol Clin Toxicol*. 1992;30:135–139.
22. Pfeiffer H, Al Khaddam M, Brinkmann B, et al. Sudden death after isobutane sniffing: a report of two forensic cases. *Int J Legal Med*. 2006;120:168–173.
23. Sugie H, Sasaki C, Hashimoto C, et al. Three cases of sudden death due to butane or propane gas inhalation: analysis of tissues for gas components. *Forens Sci Int*. 2004;143:211–214.
24. Suwaki H. Addictions: what's happening in Japan. *Int Rev Psychiatry*. 1989;1:9–11.
25. Fitzgerald RL, Fishel CE, Bush LL. Fatality due to recreational use of chlorodifluoromethane and chloropenta-fluoroethane. *J Forensic Sci*. 1993;38:477–483.
26. Thompson PJ, Dhillon P, Cole P. Addiction to aerosol treatment: the asthmatic alternative to glue sniffing. *BMJ*. 1983;287:1515–1516.

27. Perron BE, Howard MO. Endemic asthma inhaler abuse among antisocial adolescents. *Drug Alcohol Depend.* 2008;96: 22–29.
28. DiMaio VJM, Garriott JC. Four deaths resulting from abuse of nitrous oxide. *J Forensic Sci.* 1978;23:169–172.
29. Winek CL, Wahba WW, Rozin L. Accidental death by nitrous oxide inhalation. *Forensic Sci Int.* 1995;73:139–141.
30. Wagner SA, Clark MA, Wesche DL, et al. Asphyxial deaths from the recreational use of nitrous oxide. *J Forensic Sci.* 1992; 37:1008–1015.
31. Avella J, Wilson JC, Lehrer M. Fatal cardiac arrhythmia after repeated exposure to 1,1-difluoroethane (DFE). *Am J Forens Med Path.* 2006;27:58–60.
32. Sasaki C, Shinozuka T, Irie W, et al. A fatality due to inhalation of 1,1-difluoroethane (HFC-152a) with a peculiar device. *Forensic Toxicol.* 2009;27:45–48.
33. Moreno C, Beierle EA. Hydrofluoric acid burn in a child from a compressed air duster. *J Burn Care Res.* 2007;28:909–912.
34. Schloneger M, Stull A, Singer JI. Inhalant abuse a case of hemoptysis associated with halogenated hydrocarbons abuse. *Pediatr Emer Care.* 2009;25:754–757.
35. Evans AC, Raistrick D. Patterns of use and related harm with toluene-based adhesives and butane gas. *Br J Psychiatry.* 1987;150:773–776; and Phenomenology of intoxication with toluene-based adhesives and butane gas; 769–773.
36. Shu LR, Tsai, SJ. Long-term glue sniffing: report of six cases. *Int J Psychiatry Med.* 2003;33:163–168.
37. Yajima, Y, Funayama M, Niitsu H, et al. Concentrations of toluene in the body killed by an injury to the head shortly after ingesting thinner. *Forensic Sci Int.* 2005;147:9–12.
38. Martinez MA, Ballesteros, S. Investigation of fatalities due to acute gasoline poisoning. *J Anal Toxicol.* 2005;29:643–651.
39. Clark MA, Jones JW, Robinson JJ, et al. Multiple deaths resulting from shipboard exposure to trichlorotrifluoroethane. *J Forensic Sci.* 1985;30:1256–1259.
40. Groppi A, Polettini A, Lunetta P, et al. A fatal case of trichlorofluoromethane (Freon 11) poisoning. Tissue distribution study by gas chromatography-mass spectrometry. *J Forensic Sci.* 1994;39:871–876.
41. Bowen SE, Daniel J, Balster RL. Deaths associated with inhalant abuse in Virginia from 1987 to 1996. *Drug Alcohol Depend.* 1999;53(3):239–245.
42. Maxwell JC. Deaths related to the inhalation of volatile substances in Texas: 1988–1998. *Am J Drug Alcohol Abuse.* 2001;27(4):689–697.
43. Garriott J. Death among inhalant abusers. In: Sharp CW, Beauvais F, Spence R, eds. *NIDA Research Monograph. Inhalant Abuse: A Volatile Research Agenda.* Vol 129. Rockville, MD: National Institute on Drug Abuse, US Public Health; 1992:181–192.
44. Wick R, Gilbert JD, Felgate P, et al. Inhalant deaths in South Australia: a 20-year retrospective autopsy study. *Am J Forensic Med Pathology.* 2007;28(4):319–322.
45. Substance Abuse and Mental Health Services Administration. Office of Applied Sciences, Department of Health and Human Services. *Mortality Data from the Drug Abuse Warning Network, 2000.* Available at: http://www.aasamhsa.gov/oas/DAWN/mortality2k.pdf.
46. Medina-Mora M, Real T. Epidemiology of inhalant use. *Cur Opin Psychitr.* 2008;3:247–251.
47. McMorris BJ, Hemphill SA, Toumbourou JW, et al. Prevalence of substance use and delinquent behavior in adolescents from Victoria, Australia and Washington State, United States. *Health Ed Behav.* 2007;34(4):634–650.
48. Patrick ME, Collins LM, Smith E, et al. A prospective longitudinal model of substance use onset among South African adolescents. *Subst Use Misuse.* 2009;44(5):647–662.
49. Johnston LD, O'Malley PM, Bachman JG, et al. Monitoring the future national results on adolescent drug use, 1975–2008. Volume 1, *Secondary School Students.* Publication No. 08-6418A. Bethesda, MD: NIDA; 2008.
50. Substance Abuse and Mental Health Services Administration. *Results from the 2007 National Survey on Drug Use and Health: National Findings.* NSDUH Series H-34, Publication No. SMA 08-4343. Rockville, MD: Office of Applied Studies, DHHS. Available at: http://oas.samhsa.gov.
51. Centers for Disease Control and Prevention. Youth risk behavior surveillance, United States, 2007. *MMWR* 2008;57.
52. Howard MO, Balster RL, Cottler LB, et al. Inhalant use among incarcerated adolescents in the United States: prevalence, characteristics, and correlates of use. *Drug Alcohol Depend.* 2008; 93:197–209.
53. Beauvais F, Wayman JC, Thurman PJ, et al. Inhalant abuse among American Indian, Mexican American, and non-Latino white adolescents. *Am J Drug Alcohol Abuse.* 2002;28(1):171–187.
54. Johnson BD, Frank B, Marel R, et al. *Statewide Household Survey of Substance Abuse, 1986: Illicit Substance Use Among Adults in New York State's Transient Population.* New York: New York State Division of Substance Abuse Services; 1988, and Rainone GR, Marel R. *The OASAS School Survey; Alcohol and Other Drug Use Among 5th–12th Grade Students, 1998.* New York: New York State Division of Substance Abuse Services; 1998.
55. Howard MO, Walker RD, Walker PS, et al. Inhalant use among urban American Indian youth. *Addiction.* 1999;94:83–95.
56. Bernal B, Ardila A, Bateman JR. Cognitive Impairments in adolescent drug-abusers. *Int J Neurosci.* 1994;75:203–212.
57. Lacey BW, Ditzler TF. Inhalant abuse in the military: an unrecognized threat. All inhalant use and problems. *Mil Med.* 2007;172:388–392.
58. Perron BE, Howard MO. Perceived risk of harm and intentions of future use among adolescent inhalant users. *Drug Alcohol Depend.* 2008;97:185–189.
59. Martino SC, McCaffrey DF, Klein DJ, et al. Recanting of life-time inhalant use: how big a problem and what to make of it. *Addiction.* 2009;104:1373–1381.
60. Garland EL, Howard MO, Perron BE. Nitrous oxide inhalation among adolescents: prevalence, correlates, and co-occurrence with volatile solvent inhalation. *J Psychoactive Drugs.* 2009; 41(4):337–347.
61. Hall MT, Howard MO. Nitrite inhalant abuse in antisocial youth: prevalence, patterns, and predictors. *J Psychoactive Drugs.* 2009;41:135–143.
62. Wu LT, Schlenger WE, Ringwalt CL. Use of nitrite inhalant ("poppers") among American Youth. *J Adolesc Health.* 2005; 37:52–60.
63. Korman M, Matthew RW, Lovitt R. Neuropsychological effects of abuse of inhalants. *Percept Mot Skills.* 1981;53:547–553.
64. Howard MO, Jenson JM. Inhalant use among antisocial youth: prevalence and correlates. *Addict Behav.* 1999;24:59–74.
65. Barrett ME, Joe GW, Simpson DD. Acculturation influences on inhalant use. *Hispanic J Behav Sci.* 1991;13(3):276–296.
66. Matthews RW, Korman M. Abuse of inhalants: motivation and consequences. *Psychol Rep.* 1981;49:519–526.

67. McSherry TM. Program experiences with the solvent abuser in Philadelphia. In: Crider RA, Rouse BA, eds. *NIDA Research Monograph. Epidemiology of Inhalant Abuse: An Update.* Rockville, MD: NIDA, NIH, U.S. Public Health Service; 1988;85:106–120.
68. Oetting ER, Edwards RW, Beauvais F. (1988) Social and psychological factors underlying inhalant abuse. In: Crider RA, Rouse BA, eds. *NIDA Research Monograph. Epidemiology of Inhalant Abuse: An Update.* Rockville, MD: NIDA, U.S. Public Health Service; 1988;85:172–203.
69. May PA, Del Vecchio AM. The three common behavioral patterns of inhalant/solvent abuse: selected findings and research issues. In: Beauvais F, Trimble JE, eds. *Drugs and Society.* 1997;10(1/2):3–38.
70. Vaughn MG, Perron BE, Howard MO. Variations in social contexts and their effect on adolescent inhalant use: a latent profile investigation. *Drug Alcohol Depend.* 2007;91:129–133.
71. Freedenthal S, Vaughn MG, Jenson JM, et al. Inhalant use and suicidality among incarcerated youth. *Drug Alcohol Depend.* 2007;90:81–88.
72. Howard MO, Perron BE, Sacco P, et al. Suicide ideation and attempts among inhalant users: results from the national epidemiologic survey on alcohol and related conditions. *Suicide Life Threat Behav.* 2010;40(3):276–286.
73. Wu LT, Howard MO. Is inhalant use a risk factor for heroin and injection drug use among adolescents in the United States? *Addict Behav.* 2007;32:265–281.
74. Howard MO, Perron BE, Vaughn MG, et al. Inhalant use, inhalant use disorders, and antisocial behavior: findings from the National Epidemiologic Survey on Alcohol and Related Conditions. *J Studies Alcohol Drugs.* 2010;71(2):201–209.
75. Storr CL, Accornero VH, Crum RM. Profiles of current disruptive behavior: association with recent drug consumption among adolescents. *Addict Behav.* 2007;32:248–264.
76. Benignus VA. Health effects of toluene: a review. *Neurotoxicology.* 1981;2:567–588.
77. Hobara T, Okuda M, Gotoh M, et al. Estimation of the lethal toluene concentration from the accidental death of painting workers. *Ind Health.* 2000;38:228–231.
78. Krause JG, McCarthy WB. Sudden death by inhalation of cyclopropane. *J Forensic Sci.* 1989;34:1011–1012.
79. Jacob B, Heller C, Daldrup T, et al. Fatal accidental enflurane intoxication. *J Forensic Sci.* 1989;34:1408–1412.
80. Schaumburg HH, Spencer PS. Recognizing neurotoxic disease. *Neurology.* 1987;37:276–278.
81. Hormes JT, Filley CM, Rosenberg NL. Neurologic sequelae of chronic solvent vapor abuse. *Neurology.* 1986;36:698–702.
82. Altenkirch H, Wagner HM, Stoltenburg-Didinger G, et al. Potentiation of hexacarbon-neurotoxicity by methyl-ethyl-ketone (MEK) and other substances: clinical and experimental aspects. *Neurobehav Toxicol Teratol.* 1982;4:623–627.
83. Rosenberg NL. Neurotoxicology. In: Sullivan JB, Krieger GR, eds. *Medical Toxicology of Hazardous Materials.* Baltimore: Williams & Wilkins; 1992:145–153.
84. Grabski DA. Toluene sniffing producing cerebellar degeneration. *Am J Psychiatry.* 1961;118:461–462.
85. Boor JW, Hurtig HI. Persistent cerebellar ataxia after exposure to toluene. *Ann Neurol.* 1977;2:440–442.
86. Ehyai A, Freemon FR. Progressive optic neuropathy and sensorineural hearing loss due to chronic glue sniffing. *J Neurol Neurosurg Psychiatry.* 1983;46:349–351.
87. King MD. Neurological sequelae of toluene abuse. *Hum Toxicol.* 1982;1:281–287.
88. Malm G, Lying-Tunell U. Cerebellar dysfunction related to toluene sniffing. *Acta Neurol Scand.* 1980;62:188–190.
89. Metrick SA, Brenner RP. Abnormal brainstem auditory evoked potentials in chronic paint sniffers. *Ann Neurol.* 1982;12:553–556.
90. Rosenberg NL, Spitz MC, Filley CM, et al. Central nervous system effects of chronic toluene abuse—clinical, brainstem evoked response and magnetic resonance imaging studies. *Neurotoxicol Teratol.* 1988;10:489–495.
91. Rosenberg NL, Kleinschmidt-DeMasters BK, Davis KA, et al. Toluene abuse causes diffuse central nervous system white matter changes. *Ann Neurol.* 1988;23:611–614.
92. Sasa M, Igarashi S, Miyazaki T, et al. Equilibrium disorders with diffuse brain atrophy in long-term toluene sniffing. *Arch Otorhinolaryngol.* 1978;221:163–169.
93. Unger E, Alexander A, Fritz T, et al. Toluene abuse: physical basis for hypointensity of the basal ganglia on T2-weighted MR images. *Radiology.* 1994;193:473–476.
94. Kamran S. Bakshi R. MRI in chronic toluene abuse: low signal in the cerebral cortex on T2-weighted images. *Neuroradiology.* 1998;40:519–521.
95. Kile SJ, Camilleri CC, Latchaw R, et al. Bithalamic lesions of butane encephalopathy. *Pediatric Neurol.* 2006;35:439–441.
96. Harris D, Mirza Z. Butane encephalopathy. *Emer Med J.* 2005;22:676–677.
97. Ojanpaa H, Nasanen R, Pallysaho J, et al. Visual search and eye movements in patients with chronic solvent-induced toxic encephalopathy. *NeuroToxicology.* 2006;27:1013–1023.
98. Poblano A, Ishiwara K, Ortega P, et al. Thinner abuse alters optokinetic nystagmus parameters. *Arch Med Res.* 2000;3:182–185.
99. Kiyokawa M, Mizota A, Takasoh M, et al. Pattern visual evoked cortical potentials in patients with toxic optic neuropathy caused by toluene abuse. *Jpn J Ophthalmol.* 1999;43:438–442.
100. Kucuk NO, Kilic EO, Aysev A, et al. Brain SPECT findings in long-term inhalant abuse. *Nucl Med Commun.* 2000;21:769–773.
101. Doring G, Baumeister FA, Peters J, et al. Butane abuse associated encephalopathy. *J Klinische Padiatrie.* 2002;214:295–298.
102. Aydin K, Sencer S, Ogel K, et al. Single-voxel proton MR spectroscopy in toluene abuse. *Magn Reson Imaging.* 2003;21:777–785.
103. Kornfeld M, Moser AB, Moser HW, et al. Solvent vapor abuse leukoencephalopathy comparison to adrenoleukodystrophy. *J Neuropathol Exp Neurol.* 1994;53:389–398.
104. Rosenberg NL, Grigsby J, Dreisbach J, et al. Neuropsychologic impairment and MRI abnormalities associated with chronic solvent abuse. *J Toxicol Clin Toxicol.* 2002;40(1):21–34.
105. Takebayashi K, Sekine Y, Takei N, et al. Metabolite alterations in basal ganglia associated with psychiatric symptoms of abstinent toluene users: a proton MRS study. *Neuropsychopharm.* 2004;29:1019–1026.
106. Cairney S, Maruff P, Burns CB, et al. Neurological and cognitive recovery following abstinence from petrol sniffing. *Neuropsychopharmacology.* 2005;30:1019–1027.
107. Pearson MA, Hoyme HE, Seaver LH, et al. Toluene embryopathy: delineation of the phenotype and comparison with fetal alcohol syndrome. *Pediatrics.* 1994;93:211–215.
108. Towfighi J, Gonatas NK, Pleasure D, et al. Glue sniffer's neuropathy. *Neurology.* 1976;26:238–243.
109. Gundogan FC, Oz O, Gorgun E, et al. Toluene related toxic optic neuropathy. *Neuro-Ophthalmology.* 2009;33:248–252.

110. Escobar A, Aruffo C. Chronic thinner intoxication: clinicopathologic report of a human case. *J Neurol Neurosurg Psychiatry*. 1980;43:986–994.
111. Poser C. The dysmyelinating diseases. In: Joynt RJ, ed. *Clinical Neurology*. Philadelphia: Lippincott-Raven; 1983:31–36.
112. Uchino A, Kato A, Yuzuriha T, et al. Comparison between patient characteristics and cranial MR findings in chronic thinner intoxication. *Eur Radiol*. 2002;12:1338–1341.
113. Filley CM, Halliday W, Kleinschmidt-DeMasters BK. The effects of toluene on the central nervous system. *J Neuropath Exper Neurol*. 2004;63:1–12.
114. Aydin K, Kircan S, Sarwar S, et al. Smaller gray matter volumes in frontal and parietal cortices of solvent abusers correlate with cognitive deficits. *AJNR*. 2009;30:1922–1928.
115. Filley CM. Toxic leukoencephalopathy. *Clin Neuropharmacol*. 1999;22:249–260.
116. Ghatak NR, Leshner RT, Price AC. et al. Remyelination in the human central nervous system. *J Neuropath Exper Neurol*. 1989;48:507–518.
117. Smith KJ, Blakemore WF, McDonald WI. The restoration of conduction by central remyelination. *Brain*. 1981;104:383–404.
118. Morrow LA, Callender T, Lottenberg S, et al. PET and neurobehavioral evidence of tetrabromoethane encephalopathy. *J Neuropsychiatry Clin Neurosci*. 1990;2(4):431–435.
119. Kangas BD, Walker DJ. An adjusting-dose procedure for assessing the reinforcing effects of nitrous oxide with humans. *Pharmacol Biochem Behavior*. 2008;91:104–108.
120. Beckman NJ, Zacny JP, Walker DJ. Within-subject comparison of the subjective and psychomotor effects of a gaseous anesthetic and two volatile anesthetics in healthy volunteers. *Drug Alcohol Depend*. 2006;81:89–95.
121. Zacny JP, Walker DJ, Derus LM. Choice of nitrous oxide and its subjective effects in light and moderate drinkers. *Drug Alcohol Depend*. 2008;98:163–168.
122. Fagan D, Paul DL, Tiplady B, et al. A dose-response study of the effects of inhaled nitrous oxide on psychological performance and mood. *Psychopharmacology (Berl)*. 1994;116:333–338.
123. Cheam EW, Dob DP, Skelly AM, et al. The effect of nitrous oxide on the performance of psychomotor tests. A dose-response study. *Anaesthesia*. 1995;50:764–768.
124. Stach DJ. Nitrous oxide sedation: understanding the benefits and risks. *Am J Dent*. 1995;8:47–50.
125. Butzkueven H, King JO. Nitrous oxide myelopathy in an abuser of whipped cream bulbs. *J Clin Neurosci*. 2000;7:73–75.
126. Kinsella LJ, Green R. "Anesthesia paresthetica": nitrous oxide-induced cobalamin deficiency. *Neurology*. 1995;45:1608–1610.
127. Toohey JI. Vitamin B-12 and methionine synthesis: a critical review. Is nature's most beautiful cofactor misunderstood? *Bio Factors*. 2006;26:45–57.
128. Flippo TS, Holder WD Jr. Neurologic degeneration associated with nitrous oxide anesthesia in patients with vitamin B_{12} deficiency. *Arch Surg*. 1993;128:1391–1395.
129. Nunn JF. Clinical aspects of the interaction between nitrous oxide and vitamin B_{12}. *Br J Anaesth*. 1987;59:3–13.
130. Vishnubhakat SM, Beresford HR. Reversible myeloneuropathy of nitrous oxide abuse: serial electrophysiological studies. *Muscle Nerve*. 1991;14:22–26.
131. Felmet K, Robins B, Tilford D, et al. Acute neurologic decompensation in an infant with cobalamin deficiency exposed to nitrous oxide. *J Pediatr*. 2000;137:427–428.
132. Fujinaga M, Baden JM. Methionine prevents nitrous oxide-induced teratogenicity in rat embryos grown in culture. *Anesthesiology*. 1994;81:184–189.
133. Sanders RD, Weimann J, Maze M. Biologic effects of nitrous oxide - A mechanistic and toxicologic review. *Anesthesiol*. 2008;109:707–722.
134. Schwartz RH, Calihan M. Nitrous oxide: a potentially lethal euphoriant inhalant. *Am Family Pract*. 1984;30:171–172.
135. Lehmberg J, Waldner M, Baethmann A, et al. Inflammatory response to nitrous oxide in the central nervous system. *Brain Res*. 2008;246:88–95.
136. Paus T. Mapping brain maturation and cognitive development during adolescence. *Trends Cogn Sci*. 2005;9:60–68.
137. Nunez JL, Nelson J, Pych JC, et al. Myelination in the splenium of the corpus callosum in adult male and female rats. *Brain Res Dev Brain Res*. 2000;120:87–90.
138. Wood RW. Stimulus properties of inhaled substances. *Environ Health Perspect*. 1978;26:69–76.
139. Blokhina EA, Dravolina OA, Bespalov AY, et al. Intravenous self-administration of abused solvents and anesthetics in mice. *Eur J Pharmacol*. 2004;485:211–218.
140. Gerasimov MR, Collier L, Ferrieri A, et al. Toluene inhalation produces a conditioned place preference in rats. *Eur J Pharm*. 2003;477:45–52.
141. Lee DE, Gerasimov MR, Schiffer WK, et al. Concentration-dependent conditioned place preference to inhaled toluene vapors in rats. *Drug Alcohol Depend*. 2006;85:87–90.
142. Gerasimov MR, Ferrieri RA, Pareto D, et al. Synthesis and evaluation of inhaled [(11)C]butane and intravenously injected [(11)C]acetone as potential radiotracers for studying inhalant abuse. *Nucl Med Biol*. 2005;32:201–208.
143. Rosenberg NL, Sharp CW. Solvent toxicity: a neurological focus. In: Sharp CW, Beauvais F, Spence R, eds. *NIDA Research Monograph. Inhalant Abuse: A Volatile Research Agenda*. Rockville, MD: National Institute on Drug Abuse; 1992;129:117–127.
144. Balster RL. Neural basis of inhalant abuse. *Drug Alcohol Depend*. 1998;51:207–214.
145. Gerasimov MR, Schiffer W, Marstellar D, et al. Toluene inhalation produces regionally specific changes in extracellular dopamine. *Drug Alcohol Depend*. 2002;65:243–251.
146. Riegel AC, French ED. Abused inhalants and central reward pathways: electrophysiological and behavioral studies in the rat. *Ann NY Acad Sci*. 2002;965:281–291.
147. Eckenhoff RG, Johansson JS. Molecular interactions between inhaled anesthetics and proteins. *Pharmacol Rev*. 1997;49:343–367.
148. Bowen SE, Wiley JL, Jones HE et al. Phencyclidine- and diazepam-like discriminative stimulus effects of inhalants in mice. *Exp Clin Psychopharmacol*. 1999;7:28–37.
149. Lee DE, Schiffer WK, Dewey SL. Gamma-vinyl GABA (vigabatrin) blocks the expression of toluene-induced conditioned place preference (CPP). *Synapse*. 2004;54:183–185.
150. Bale AS, Tu Y, Carpenter-Hyland EP, et al. Alterations in glutamatergic and gabaergic ion channel activity in hippocampal neurons following exposure to the abused inhalant toluene. *Neuroscience*. 2005;130:197–206.
151. Gerasimov MR, Ferrieri RA, Schiffer WK, et al. Study of brain uptake and bio-distribution of [11C]toluene in non-human primates and mice. *Life Sci*. 2002;70:2811–2828.
152. Schiffer WK, Lee DE, Carrion J, et al. Brain distribution of 11C-toluene predicts structural changes in an adolescent model of toluene abuse. *Synapse*. (In press)

153. Schiffer WK, Lee DE, Alexoff DL, et al. Metabolic correlates of toluene abuse: decline and recovery of function in adolescent animals. *Psychopharm.* 2006;186(2):159–167.
154. Meulenberg CJ, Vijverberg HP. Selective inhibition of gamma-aminobutyric acid type A receptors in human IMR-32 cells by low concentrations of toluene. *Toxicology.* 2003;190:243–248.
155. Tohhara S, Tani N, Nakajima T, et al. Clinical study of butane gas abuse: in comparison with toluene-based solvent and marihuana. *Arukoru Kenkyuto Yakubutsu Ison.* 1989;24:504–510.
156. Raines DE, Claycomb RJ, Scheller M, et al. Nonhalogenated alkane anesthetics fail to potentiate agonist actions on two ligand-gated ion channels. *Anesthesiology.* 2001;95:470–477.
157. Cruz SL, Gauthereau MY, Camacho-Munoz C, et al. Lopez-Rubalcava C, Balster RL. Effects of inhaled toluene and 1,1,1-trichloroethane on seizures and death produced by N-methyl-D-aspartic acid in mice. *Behav Brain Res.* 2003;140:195–202.
158. Ernstgard L, Gullstrand E, Johanson G, et al. Toxicokinetic interactions between orally ingested chlorzoxazone and inhaled acetone or toluene in male volunteers. *Toxicol Sci.* 1999;48:189–196.
159. Haggard HW, Greenberg LA, Turner JM. The physiological principles governing the action of acetone together with determination of toxicity. *J Ind Hyg Toxicol.* 1984;26:133–151.
160. Bruckner JV, Peterson RG. Evaluation of toluene and acetone inhalant abuse. I. Pharmacology and pharmacodynamics. *Toxicol Appl Pharmacol.* 1981;61:27–38.
161. DiVincenzo GD, Yanno FJ, Astill BD. Exposure of man and dog to low concentrations of acetone vapor. *Am Ind Hyg Assoc J.* 1973;34:329–336.
162. Bespalov A, Sukhotina I, Medvedev I, et al. Facilitation of electrical brain self-stimulation behavior by abused solvents. *Pharmacol Biochem Behav.* 2003;75:199–208.
163. Wiley JL, Bale AS, Balster RL. Evaluation of toluene dependence and cross-sensitization to diazepam. *Life Sci.* 2003;72:3023–3033.
164. Wiley JL, Fagalde RE, Buhler KG, et al. Evaluation of 1,1,1-trichloroethane and flurothyl locomotor effects following diazepam treatment in mice. *Pharmacol Biochem Behav.* 2002;71:163–169.
165. Bowen SE, Balster RL. A direct comparison of inhalant effects on locomotor activity and schedule-controlled behavior in mice. *Exp Clin Psychopharmacol.* 1998;6:235–247.
166. Warren DA, Reigle TG, Muralidhara S, et al. Schedule-controlled operant behavior of rats during 1,1,1-trichloroethane inhalation: relationship to blood and brain solvent concentrations. *Neurotoxicol Teratol.* 1998;20:143–153.
167. You L, Dallas CE. Regional brain dosimetry of trichloroethane in mice and rats following inhalation exposures. *J Toxicol Environ Health A.* 1998;54:285–299.
168. Wood PL, Rao TS. A review of in vivo modulation of cerebellar cGMP levels by excitatory amino acid receptors: role of NMDA, quisqualate and kainate subtypes. *Prog Neuropsychopharmacol Biol Psychiatry.* 1991;15:229–235.
169. You L, Dallas CE. Effects of inhaled 1,1,1-trichloroethane on the regional brain cyclic GMP levels in mice and rats. *J Toxicol Environ Health A.* 2000;60:331–341.
170. Niklasson M, Tham R, Larsby B, et al. Effects of toluene, styrene, trichloroethylene, and trichloroethane on the vestibulo-and opto-oculo motor system in rats. *Neurotoxicol Teratol.* 1993;15:327–334.
171. Ohashi Y, Tianzhi Guo T. et al. Brain stem opioidergic and GABAergic neurons mediate the antinociceptive effect of nitrous oxide in fischer rats. *Anesthesiology.* 2003;99:947–954.
172. Sommer N, Romano C, Jevtovic-Todorovic V. Chronic exposure to nitrous oxide increases [3H]MK801 binding in the cerebral cortex, but not in the hippocampus of adult mice. *Ann NY Acad Sci.* 2005;1053:301–308.
173. Belknap JK, Laursen SE, Crabbe JC. Ethanol and nitrous oxide produce withdrawal-induced convulsions by similar mechanisms in mice. *Life Sci.* 1987;41:2033–2040.
174. Eger EI II, Liu J, Koblin DD, et al. Molecular properties of the ideal inhaled anesthetic: studies of fluorinated methanes, ethanes, propanes, and butanes. *Anesth Analg.* 1994;79:245–251.
175. Antognini JF, Atherley RJ, Dutton RC, et al. The excitatory and inhibitory effects of nitrous oxide on spinal neuronal responses to noxious stimulation. *Anesth Analg.* 2007;104:829–835.
176. Pryor GT, Dickinson J, Howd RA, Rebert CS. Transient cognitive deficits and high-frequency hearing loss in weanling rats exposed to toluene. *Neurobehav Toxicol Teratol.* 1983;5:53–57.
177. McWilliams ML, Chen GD, Fechter LD. Low-level toluene disrupts auditory function in guinea pigs. *Toxicol Appl Pharm.* 2000;167(1):18–29.
178. Rebert CS, Day VL, Matteucci MJ, et al. Sensory-evoked potentials in rats chronically exposed to trichloroethylene: predominant auditory dysfunction. *Neurotoxicol Teratol.* 1991;13:83–90.
179. Lataye R, Campo P, Pouyatos B, et al. Solvent ototoxicity in the rat and guinea pig. *Neurotox Teratol.* 2003;25:39–50.
180. Pryor GT. Solvent-induced neurotoxicity: effects and mechanisms. In: Chang LW, Dyer RS, eds. *Principles of Neurotoxicity.* New York: Marcel Dekker; 1995:377–400.
181. Vyskocil A, Leroux T, Truchon G, et al. Ethyl benzene should be considered ototoxic at occupationally relevant exposure concentrations. *Toxicol Ind Health.* 2008;24:241.
182. Fechter LD, Liu Y, Herr DW, et al. Trichloroethylene ototoxicity: evidence for a cochlear origin. *Toxicol Sci.* 1998;42:28–35.
183. Pryor GT. A toluene-induced motor syndrome in rats resembling that seen in some solvent abusers. *Neurotoxicol Teratol.* 1991;13:387–400.
184. Mergler D, Beauvais B. Olfactory threshold shift following controlled 7-hour exposure to toluene and/or xylene. *Neurotoxicology.* 1992;13:211–215.
185. Li HS, Johnson AC, Borg E, et al. Auditory degeneration after exposure to toluene in two genotypes of mice. *Arch Toxicol.* 1992;66:382–386.
186. Lund SP, Kristiansen GB. Hazards to hearing from combined exposure to toluene and noise in rats. *Internat J Occupat Med Environ Health.* 2008;21:47–57.
187. Keski-Santti P, Holm A, Akila R, et al. P300 of auditory event related potentials in occupational chronic solvent encephalopathy. *Neuro Toxi.* 2007;28:1230–1236.
188. Fuente A, McPherson B. Organic solvents and hearing loss: the challenge for audiology. *Intern J Audiol.* 2006;45:367–381.
189. Allen N, Mendell JR, Billmaier DJ, et al. Toxic polyneuropathy due to methyl *n*-butyl ketone: an industrial outbreak. *Arch Neurol.* 1975;32:209–218.
190. Spencer PS, Schaumburg HH, Raleigh RL, et al. Nervous system degeneration produced by the industrial solvent methyl *n*-butyl ketone. *Arch Neurol.* 1975;32:219–222.

191. Kutlu G, Gomceli YB, Somnez T, et al. Peripheral neuopathy and visual evoked potential changes in workers exposedto n-hexane. *J Clin Neurosci*. 2006;16:1296–1299.
192. Shirabe T, Tsuda T, Terao A, et al. Toxic polyneuropathy due to glue-sniffing: report of two cases with a light and electron-microscopic study of the peripheral nerves and muscles. *J Neurol Sci*. 1974;21:101–113.
193. Spencer PS, Schaumburg HH, Sabri MI, et al. The enlarging view of hexacarbon neurotoxicity. *Crit Rev Toxicol*. 1980;7:279–356.
194. Ludolph AC, Spencer PS. Toxic neuropathies and their treatment. *Baillieres Clin Neurol*. 1995;4(3):505–527.
195. Frontali N, Amantini MC, Spagnolo A, et al. Experimental neurotoxicity and urinary metabolites of the C5-C7 aliphatic hydrocarbons used as glue solvents in shoe manufacture. *Clin Toxicol*. 1981;18:1357–1367.
196. Issever H, Malat G, Sabuncu HH, et al. Impairment of colour vision in patients with *n*-hexane exposure-dependent toxic polyneuropathy. *Occup Med*. 2002;52(4):183–186.
197. Tariot PN. Delirium resulting from methylene chloride exposure: case report. *J Clin Psychiatry*. 1983;44:340–342.
198. Horowitz BZ. Carboxyhemoglobinemia caused by inhalation of methylene chloride. *Am J Emerg Med*. 1986;4:48–51.
199. Stewart RD, Fisher TN, Hosko MJ, et al. Experimental human exposure to methylene chloride. *Arch Environ Health*. 1972;25:342–348.
200. Gamberale F, Annwall G, Hultengren M. Exposure to methylene chloride. II. Psychological functions. *Scand J Work Environ Health*. 1975;1:95–103.
201. Chang YL, Yang CC, Deng JF, et al. Diverse manifestations of oral methylene chloride poisoning: report of 6 cases. *J Toxicol Clin Toxicol*. 1999;37(4):497–504.
202. Gresham GA, Treip CS. Fatal poisoning by 1,1,1-trichloroethane after prolonged survival. *Forensic Sci Int*. 1983;23:249–253.
203. Wise MG. Trichloroethane (TCE) and central sleep apnea: a case study. *J Toxicol Environ Health*. 1983;11:101–104.
204. McLeod AA, Marjot R, Monaghan MJ, et al. Chronic cardiac toxicity after inhalation of 1,1,1-trichloroethane. *BMJ*. 1987;294:727–729.
205. Tenenbein M. 1997. Leaded gasoline abuse: the role of tetraethyllead. *Human Exper Toxicol*. 16:217–222.
206. Burns CB, Currie B. The efficacy of chelation therapy and factors influencing mortality in lead intoxicated petrol sniffers. *Aust N Z J Med*. 1995;25:197–203.
207. Kuteifan K, Oesterle H, Tajahmady T, et al. Necrosis and haemorrhage of the putamen in methanol poisoning shown on MRI. *Neuroradiology*. 1998;40(3):158–160.
208. Eells JT, Henry MM, Lewandowski MF, et al. Development and characterization of a rodent model of methanol-induced retinal and optic nerve toxicity. *Neurotoxicology*. 2000;21:321–330.
209. McCormick MJ. Methanol poisoning as a result of inhalational solvent abuse. *Ann Emerg Med*. 1990;19:639–642.
210. Stewart RD, Hake CL, Peterson JE. "Degreasers' flush," dermal response to trichloroethylene and ethanol. *Arch Environ Health*. 1974;29:1–5.
211. Antti-Poika M, Juntunen J, Matikainen E, et al. Occupational exposure to toluene: neurotoxic effects with special emphasis on drinking habits. *Int Arch Occup Environ Health*. 1985;56:31–40.
212. Kira S, Ogata M, Ebara Y, et al. A case of thinner sniffing: relationship between neuropsychological symptoms and urinary findings after inhalation of toluene and methanol. *Ind Health*. 1988;26:81–85.
213. Pryor GT, Howd RA, Uyeno ET, et al. Interactions between toluene and alcohol. *Pharmacol Biochem Behav*. 1985;23:401–410.
214. Cunningham J, Sharkawi M, Plaa GL. Pharmacological and metabolic interactions between ethanol and methyl *n*-butyl ketone, methyl isobutyl ketone, methyl ethyl ketone, or acetone in mice. *Fundam Appl Toxicol*. 1989;13:102–109.
215. Campo P, Lataye R, Cossec B, et al. Combined effects of simultaneous exposure to toluene and ethanol on auditory function in rats. *Neurotoxicol Teratol*. 1998;20:321–332.
216. Olgar S, Oktem F, Dindar A, et al. Volatile solvent abuse caused glomerulopathy and tubulopathy in street children. *Hum Exp Toxicol*. 2008;27:477.
217. Streicher HZ, Gabow PA, Moss AH, et al. Syndromes of toluene sniffing in adults. *Ann Intern Med*. 1981;94:758–762.
218. Kao KC, Tsai YH, Lin MC, et al. Hypokalemic muscular paralysis causing acute respiratory failure due to rhabdomyolysis with renal tubular acidosis in a chronic glue sniffer. *Clin Toxicol*. 2000;38(6):679–681.
219. Zaidi SA, Shaw AN, Patel MN, et al. Multi-organ toxicity and death following acute unintentional inhalation of paint thinner fumes. *Clin Toxicol (Phila)*. 2007;45(3):287–289.
220. Patel R, Benjamin J Jr. Renal disease associated with toluene inhalation. *Clin Toxicol*. 1986;24:213–223.
221. Lauwerys R, Bernard A, Viau C, et al. Kidney disorders and hematotoxicity from organic solvent exposure. *Scand J Work Environ Health*. 1985;11(suppl 1):83–90.
222. Daniell WE, Couser WG, Rosenstock L. Occupational solvent exposure and glomerulonephritis. *JAMA*. 1988;259:2280–2283.
223. Taverner D, Harrison DJ, Bell GM. Acute renal failure due to interstitial nephritis induced by "glue-sniffing" with subsequent recovery. *Scott Med J*. 1988;33:246–247.
224. Anetseder M, Hartung E, Klepper S, et al. Gasoline vapors induce severe rhabdomyolysis. *Neurology*. 1994;44:2393–2395.
225. Brown JH, Hadden DR, Hadden DS. Solvent abuse, toluene acidosis and diabetic ketoacidosis. *Arch Emerg Med*. 1991;8:65–67.
226. Lock EA. Mechanism of nephrotoxic action due to organohalogenated compounds. *Toxicol Lett*. 1989;46:93–106.
227. Rioux JP, Myers RA. Methylene chloride poisoning: a paradigmatic review. *J Emerg Med*. 1988;6:227–238.
228. Kimbrough RD, Mitchell FL, Houk VN. Trichloroethylene: an update. *J Toxicol Environ Health*. 1985;15:369–383.
229. Brown BR, Gandolfi AJ. Adverse effects of volatile anaesthetics. *Br J Anaesth*. 1987;59:14–23.
230. Pozzi C, Marai P, Ponti R, et al. Toxicity in man due to stain removers containing 1,2-dichloropropane. *Br J Ind Med*. 1985;42:770–772.
231. Bolt HM, Lammert M, Selinski S, et al. Urinary alpha(1)-microglobulin excretion as biomarker of renal toxicity in trichloroethylene-exposed persons. *Int Arch Occup Environ Health*. 2004;77:186–190.
232. Keogh AM, Ibels LS, Allen DH, et al. Exacerbation of Goodpasture's syndrome after inadvertent exposure to hydrocarbon fumes. *Br Med J*. 1984;288:188.
233. Yamamoto S, Mori NYH, Miyata M, et al. Neurogenic bladder caused by toluene abuse. *Acta Urol Jpn*. 1992;38:459–462.

234. Batlle DC, Sabatini S, Kurtzman NA. On the mechanism of toluene-induced renal tubular acidosis. *Nephron.* 1988;49:210–218.
235. Al-Ghamdi SS, Raftery MJ, Yaqoob MM. Acute solvent exposure induced activation of cytochrome P4502E1 causes proximal tubular cell necrosis by oxidative stress. *Toxicol in Vitro.* 2003;17:335–341; Organic solvent-induced proximal tubular cell toxicity via caspase-3 activation. *J Toxicol-Clin Toxicol.* 2003;41:941–945.
236. Short BG, Burnett VL, Cox MG, et al. Site-specific renal cytotoxicity and cell proliferation in male rats exposed to petroleum hydrocarbons. *Lab Invest.* 1987;57:564–577.
237. Wedeen RP. Occupational renal disease. *Am J Kidney Dis.* 1984;111:241–257.
238. Yamaguchi K, Shirai T, Shimakura K, et al. Pneumatosis cystoides intestinalis and trichloroethylene exposure. *Am J Gastroenterol.* 1985;80:753–757.
239. Farrell G, Prendergast D, Murray M. Halothane hepatitis. Detection of a constitutional susceptibility factor. *N Engl J Med.* 1985;313:1310–1314.
240. Goodwin TM. Toluene abuse and renal tubular acidosis in pregnancy. *Obstet Gynecol.* 1988;71:715–718.
241. Seoud M, Adra A, Khalil A, et al. Transient renal tubular acidosis in pregnancy. *Am J Perinatol.* 2000;17:249–252.
242. Benjamin SB, Goodman ZD, Ishak KG, et al. The morphologic spectrum of halothane-induced hepatic injury: analysis of 77 cases. *Hepatology.* 1985;5:1163–1171.
243. McIntyre AS, Long RG. Fatal fulminant hepatic failure in a "solvent abuser." *Postgrad Med J.* 1992;68:29–30.
244. Anagnostopoulos G, Sakorafas GH, Grigoriadis K, et al. Hepatitis caused by occupational chronic exposure to trichloroethylene. *Acta GastroEnterologica Belgicu.* 2004;67:355–357.
245. Buring JE, Hennekens CH, Mayrent SL, et al. Health experiences of operating room personnel. *Anaesthesiology.* 1985;62:325–330.
246. Ong CN, Koh D, Foo SC, et al. Volatile organic solvents in correction fluids: identification and potential hazards. *Bull Environ Contam Toxicol.* 1993;50:787–793.
247. Greer JE. Adolescent abuse of typewriter correction fluid. *South Med J.* 1984;77:297–298.
248. Takebayashi T, Kabe I, Endo Y, et al. Acute liver dysfunction among workers exposed to 2,2-dichloro-1,1,1-tryfluoroethane (HCFC-123): a case report. *Appl Occup Environ H.* 1999;14(2):72–74.
249. White INH, Matteis FD. The role of CYP forms in the metabolism and metabolic activation of HCFCs and other halocarbons. *Toxicol Lett.* 2001;124:121–128.
250. Keller DA, Lieder PH, Brock WJ, et al. 1,1,1-Trifluoro-2,2-dichloroethane (HCFC-123) and 1,1,1-trifluoro-2-bromo-2-chloroethane (halothane) cause similar biochemical effects in rats exposed by inhalation for five days. *Drug Chem Toxicol.* 1998;21(4):405–415.
251. Redfern N. Morbidity among anaesthetists. *Br J Hosp Med.* 1990;43:377–381.
252. Cohen EN. Inhalation anesthetics may cause genetic defects, abortions and miscarriages in operating room personnel. In: Eckenhoff JE, ed. *Controversy in Anesthesiology.* Philadelphia: WB Saunders; 1979:47–57.
253. Mirza T, Gerin M, Begin D, et al. A study on the substitution of trichloroethylene as a spot remover in the textile industry. *Am Ind Hyg Assoc J.* 2000;61:431–438.
254. Hubbs AF, Castranova V, Ma JYC, et al. Acute lung injury induced by a commercial leather conditioner. *Toxicol Appl Pharmacol.* 1997;143:37–46.
255. Reyes de la Rocha S, Brown MA, Fortenberry JD. Pulmonary function abnormalities in intentional spray paint inhalation. *Chest.* 1987;92:100–104.
256. Schikler KN, Lane EE, Seitz K, et al. Solvent abuse associated pulmonary abnormalities. *Adv Alcohol Subst Abuse.* 1984;3:75–81.
257. Woo OF, Healey KM, Sheppard D, et al. Chest pain and hypoxemia from inhalation of a trichloroethane aerosol product. *J Toxicol Clin Toxicol.* 1983;20:333–341.
258. Buie SE, Pratt DS, May JJ. Diffuse pulmonary injury following paint remover exposure. *Am J Med.* 1986;81:702–704.
259. Engstrand DA, England DM, Huntington RW III. Pathology of paint sniffers' lung. *Am J Forensic Med Pathol.* 1986;7:232–236.
260. Sherwood RL, O'Shea W, Thomas PT, et al. Effects of inhalation of ethylene dichloride on pulmonary defenses of mice and rats. *Toxicol Appl Pharmacol.* 1987;91:491–496.
261. Bolukbasi S, Habesoglu TE, Habesoglu M, et al. Histopathological changes of rat larynx mucosa with exposure to chronic thinner inhalation. *Otolaryngol–Head Neck Surg.* 2009;141:75–80.
262. Brilliant LC, Grillo A. Successful resuscitation from cardiopulmonary arrest following deliberate inhalation of freon refrigerant gas. *Del Med J.* 1993;65:375–378.
263. Cronk SL, Barkley DEH, Farrell MF. Respiratory arrest after solvent abuse. *BMJ.* 1985;290:897–898.
264. Mee AS, Wright PL. Congestive (dilated) cardiomyopathy in association with solvent abuse. *J R Soc Med.* 1980;73:671–672.
265. Taylor GJ, Drew RT, Lores EM Jr, et al. Cardiac depression by haloalkane propellants, solvents, and inhalation anesthetics in rabbits. *Toxicol Appl Phamacol.* 1976;38:379–387.
266. Chenoweth MB. Abuse of inhalation anesthetics. In: Sharp CW, Brehm ML, eds. *Research Monograph, Review of Inhalants: Euphoria to Dysfunction.* Number 15. Rockville, MD: National Institute on Drug Abuse, U.S. Public Health Service; 1977:102–111.
267. Vural M, Ogel K. Dilated cardiomyopathy associated with toluene abuse. *Cardiology.* 2006;105:158–161.
268. Cruz SL, Orta-Salazar G, Gauthereau MY, et al. Inhibition of cardiac sodium currents by toluene exposure. *Brit J Pharmacol.* 2003;140:653–660.
269. Barrowcliff DF, Knell AJ. Cerebral damage due to endogenous chronic carbon monoxide poisoning caused by exposure to methylene chloride. *J Soc Occup Med.* 1979;29:12–14.
270. Manno M, Chirillo R, Daniotti G, et al. Carboxyhaemoglobin and fatal methylene chloride poisoning [Letter]. *Lancet.* 1989;2(8657):274.
271. Snyder R, Kalf GF. A perspective on benzene leukemogenesis. *Crit Rev Toxicol.* 1994;24:177–209.
272. Edwards RJ, Ujma J. Extreme methaemoglobinaemia secondary to recreational use of amyl nitrite. *J Accident Emerg Med.* 1995;12:138–142.
273. Marwick TH, Nakatani S, Haluska B, et al. Provocation of latent left ventricular outflow tract gradients with amyl nitrite and exercise in hypertrophic cardiomyopathy. *Am J Cardiol.* 1995;75:805–819.
274. Klimmek R, Krettek C. Effects of amyl nitrite on circulation, respiration and blood homeostasis in cyanide poisoning. *Arch Toxicol.* 1988;62:161–166.
275. Mathew RJ, Wilson WH, Tant SR. Regional cerebral blood flow changes associated with amyl nitrite inhalation. *Br J Addict.* 1989;84:293–299.

276. Rees DC, Knisely JS, Balster RL, et al. Pentobarbital-like discriminative stimulus properties of halothane, 1,1,1-trichloroethane, isoamyl nitrite, flurothyl and oxazepam in mice. *J Pharmacol Exp Ther.* 1987;241:507–515.
277. Guss DA, Normann SA, Manoguerra AS. Clinically significant methemoglobinemia from inhalation of isobutyl nitrite. *Am J Emerg Med.* 1985;3:46–47.
278. Smith M, Stair T, Rolnick MA. Butyl nitrite and a suicide attempt. *Ann Intern Med.* 1980;92:719–720.
279. Ostrow DG, DiFranceisco WJ, Chmiel JS, et al. A case-control study of human immunodeficiency virus type 1 seroconversion and risk-related behaviors in the Chicago MACS/CCS Cohort, 1984–1992 Multicenter AIDS Cohort Study. *Am J Epidemiol.* 1994;142:875–883.
280. Chesney MA, Barrett DC, Stall R. Histories of substance abuse and risk behavior. Precursors to HIV seroconversion in homosexual men. *Am J Public Health.* 1998;88:113–116.
281. Haverkos HW. Viruses, chemicals and co-carcinogenesis. *Oncogene.* 2004;23:6492–6499.
282. Haverkos HW, Kopstein AN, Wilson H, et al. Nitrite inhalants: history, epidemiology, and possible links to AIDS Kposi's sarcoma. *Envmn Health Perspect.* 1994;102:858–861.
283. Pauk J, Huang ML, Brodie SJ, et al. Mucosal shedding of human herpesvirus 8 in men. *N Engl J Med.* 2000;343:1369–1377.
284. Dunkel VC, Rogers-Back AM, Lawlor TE, et al. Mutagenicity of some alkyl nitrites used as recreational drugs. *Environ Mol Mutagen.* 1989;14:115–122.
285. Soderberg LSF, Ponnappan U, Roy A, et al. Production of macrophage IL-1b was inhibited both at the levels of transcription and maturation by caspase-1 following inhalation exposure to isobutyl nitrite. *Toxicol Lett.* 2004;152:47–56.
286. Lokensgard JR, Gekker G, Ehrlich LC, et al. Proinflammatory cytokines inhibit HIV-1SF162 expression in acutely infected human brain cell cultures. *J Immunol.* 1997;158:2449–2455.
287. Fung H-L, Tran DC. Effects of inhalant nitrites on VEGF expression: a feasible link to Kaposi's sarcoma? *J Neuroimmune Pharmacol.* 2006;1:317–322.
288. Turowski SG, Jank KE, Fung H-L. Inactivation of hepatic enzymes by inhalant nitrite—in vivo and in vitro studies. *AAPS J.* 2007;9(3):E298–E305.
289. Costa LG, Guizzetti M, Burry M, et al. Developmental neurotoxicity: do similar phenotypes indicate a common mode of action? A comparison of fetal alcohol syndrome, toluene embryopathy and maternal phenylketonuria. *Toxicol Lett.* 2002;127:197–205.
290. Arnold GL, Kirby RS, Langendoerfer S, et al. Toluene embryopathy: clinical delineation and developmental follow-up. *Pediatrics.* 1994;93:216–220.
291. Hersh JH. Toluene embryopathy: two new cases. *J Med Genet.* 1989;26:333–337.
292. Wilkins-Haug L. Teratogen update: toluene. *Teratology.* 1997;55:145–151.
293. Tenenbein M. Fetal and neonatal effects of inhalant abuse. Presented at the Inhalant Abuse Among Children and Adolescents: Consultation on Building an International Research Agenda. Nov. 7–9, 2005. Rockville, MD: National Institute on Drug Abuse, National Institutes of Health.
294. Donald JM, Hooper K, Hopenhayn-Rich C. Reproductive and developmental toxicity of toluene: a review. *Environ Health Perspect.* 1991;94:237–244.
295. Bowen SE, Batis JC, Paez-Martinez N, et al. Last decade of solvent research in animal models of abuse: mechanistic and behavioral studies. *Neurotox Teratol.* 2006;28:636–647.
296. Ono A, Sekita K, Ohno K, et al. Reproductive and developmental toxicity studies of toluene. I. Teratogenicity study of inhalation exposure in pregnant rats. *J Toxicol Sci.* 1995;20:109–134.
297. Hougaard KS, Andersen MB, Hansen AM, et al. Effects of prenatal exposure to chronic mild stress and toluene in rats. *Neurotox Teratol.* 2005;27:153–167.
298. Jarosz PA, Fata E, Bowen SE, et al. Effects of abuse pattern of gestational toluene exposure on metabolism, feeding and body composition. *Physiol Behav.* 2008;93:984–993.
299. Warner R, Ritchie HE, Woodman P, et al. The effect of prenatal exposure to a repeat high dose of toluene in the fetal rat. *Reprod Toxicol.* 2008;26:267–272.
300. Mazze RI, Fujinaga M, Baden JM. Halothane prevents nitrous oxide teratogenicity in Sprague-Dawley rats; folinic acid does not. *Teratology.* 1988;38:121–127.
301. Cagen SZ, Klaassen CD. Hepatoxicity of carbon tetrachloride in developing rats. *Toxicol Appl Pharmacol.* 1979;50:347–354.
302. Murray FJ, Schwetz BA, McBride JG, et al. Toxicity of inhaled chloroform in pregnant mice and their offspring. *Toxicol Appl Pharmacol.* 1979;50:515–522.
303. Howard MO, Cottler LB, Compton WM, et al. Diagnostic concordance of DSM-III-R, DSM-IV, and ICD-10 inhalant use disorders. *Drug Alcohol Depend.* 2001;61:223–228.
304. Perron BE, Howard MO, Maitra S, Vaughn MG. Prevalence, timing, and predictors of transitions from inhalant use to Inhalant Use Disorders. *Drug Alcohol Depend.* 2009;100(3):277–284.
305. Wu L, Howard MO. Psychiatric disorders in inhalant users: results from the National Survey on Alcohol and Related Conditions. *Drug Alcohol Depend.* 2007;88:145–155.
306. Wu L, Howard MO. Substance use disorders among inhalant users: findings from the national epidemiologic survey on alcohol and related conditions. *Addict Behav.* 2008;33: 968–973.
307. Wu L, Pilowsky DJ, Schlenger WE. Inhalant abuse and dependence among adolescent in the United States. *J Am Acad Child Adolesc Psychiatry.* 2004;43:1206–1214.
308. Anthony JC, Warner LA, Kessler RC. Comparative epidemiology of dependence on tobacco, alcohol, controlled substances, and inhalants: basic findings from the National Comorbidity Survey. *Exp Clin Psychopharmacol.* 1994;2:244–268.
309. Ridenour TA, Bray BC, Cottler LB. Reliability of use, abuse, and dependence of four types of inhalants in adolescents and young adults. *Drug Alcohol Depend.* 2007;91:40–49.
310. Sakai JT, Hall SK, Mikulich-Gilbertson SK, et al. Inhalant use, abuse, and dependence among adolescent patients: commonly comorbid problems. *J Am Acad Child Adolesc Psychiatry.* 2004; 43:1080–1088.
311. Perron BE, Howard MO. Adolescent inhalant use, abuse and dependence. *Addiction.* 2009;104:1185–1192.
312. Wu L, Ringwalt CL. Inhalant use and disorders among adults in the United States. *Drug Alcohol Depend.* 2006;85:1–11.
313. O'Brien CP. Evidence-based treatments of addiction. *Phil Trans R Soc B.* 2008;363:3277–3286.
314. Beauvais F, Jumper-Thurman P, Plested B, et al. A survey of attitudes among drug user treatment providers toward the treatment of inhalant users. *Subst Use Misuse.* 2002;37(11):1391–1410.
315. Reidel S, Herbert T, Byrd P. Inhalant abuse: confronting a growing challenge. In: Center for Substance Abuse Treatment. *Treating Alcohol and Other Drug Abusers in Rural and Frontier Areas: 1994 Award for Excellence Papers.* Technical Assistance

Publication 17. DHHS Pub. No. (SMA) 95-3054. Rockville, MD: Substance Abuse and Mental Health Services Administration; 1995:1–12.
316. Dinwiddie SH, Zorumski CF, Rubin EH. Psychiatric correlates of chronic solvent abuse. *J Clin Psychiatry.* 1987;48:334–337.
317. Selden A, Hultberg B, Ulander A, et al. Trichloroethylene exposure in vapour degreasing and the urinary excretion of N-acetyl-beta-D-glucosaminidase. *Arch Toxicol.* 1993;67:224–226.
318. Schiffer WK, Liebling CNB, Patel V, et al. Targeting the treatment of drug abuse with molecular imaging. *Nucl Med Biol.* 2007;34(7):833–847.
319. Group IM. Interferon beta-1b in the treatment of multiple sclerosis: final outcome of the randomized controlled trial. *Neurology.* 1995;45:1277–1285.
320. Johnson KP, Brooks BR, Cohen JA, et al. Copolymer 1 reduces relapse rate and improves disability in relapsing-remitting multiple sclerosis: results of a phase III multicenter, double-blind, placebo-controlled trial. *Neurology.* 1995;57:S16–S24.
321. Jacobs LD. Intramuscular interferon beta-1a for disease progression in relapsing multiple sclerosis. The Multiple Sclerosis Collaborative Research Group (MSCRG). *Ann Neurol.* 1996;39: 285–294.

CHAPTER 21 Nicotine

Joy M. Schmitz ■ Angela L. Stotts

INTRODUCTION

Nicotine causes tobacco addiction, which in turn causes serious health problems, including heart disease, lung disease, and cancer, and increased susceptibility to a variety of infectious diseases. Most of the nearly 45 million adults in the United States who smoke indicate an interest in quitting, but rates of successful cessation remain disappointingly low. The chronicity and relapsing characteristics of nicotine can be largely explained by the actions of nicotine on the brain. This chapter provides a review of the clinical neuropharmacology of nicotine, with a focus on new discoveries since the previous edition of the textbook. Topics include the latest findings on individual differences in vulnerability to nicotine addiction, mechanisms associated with nicotine dependence, evaluation and treatment considerations, and current efforts to regulate nicotine delivery products.

HISTORY

Nicotine is named after *Nicotiana tabacum*, the tobacco plant, which is named after Jean Nicot de Villemain, a French ambassador who sent tobacco and seeds from Brazil to Paris in 1560 and promoted their medicinal use. Nicotine was first isolated from tobacco by German chemists Posselt and Reimann in 1828, who thought it was a poison (1). Thus, nicotine has long been considered a toxic chemical and has even been used previously as an insecticide (2). It is one of the most toxic chemicals in tobacco, significantly contributing to tobacco-related disease. Not until 1964, however, did the landmark 1964 Surgeon General's Report on Smoking and Health definitively indicate nicotine use via smoking to be extremely harmful, causing lung cancer and other diseases.

EPIDEMIOLOGY

Prevalence

There are about 1.2 billion smokers in the world, with the prevalence varying greatly by country from less than 5% (e.g., women in China and India) to more than 55% (e.g., men in Indonesia and Russia) (3). It is estimated that smoking causes 5 million deaths per year worldwide, and if present trends continue 10 million smokers are projected to die per year by 2025 (3). In the United States, recent data from the January–June 2009 National Health Interview Survey conducted by Centers for Disease Control and Prevention (CDC) indicate that 20.4% of adults aged 18 years and older were current smokers (4). Prevalence varies by gender and race and thus needs to be evaluated separately for a more accurate picture.

Recent Trends and Patterns

The percentage of adult smokers has not changed significantly over the past 5 years, hovering around 20%. However, these rates are substantially decreased from the late 1960s, at which time about 40% of adults reportedly were current smokers (see Fig. 21.1).

Prevalence rates vary greatly between men and women. Currently, in the United States the percentage of smokers is higher for men (23.3%) than for women (17.7%). Smoking rates also vary by age. For both sexes combined, the percentage of adults who report being current smokers is lower among adults aged 65 years and older (9.5%) compared to adults aged 18 to 44 years (22.9%) and 45 to 64 years (22.1%). For the age groups 18 to 44 and 45 to 64 years, men were more likely than women to be current smokers. With regard to race and ethnicity, the January–June 2009 CDC National Health Interview Survey indicates, adjusting for age and sex difference, that approximately 13.2% of Hispanic persons, 22.4% of non-Hispanic white persons, and 22.0% of non-Hispanic black persons are current smokers.

Public Health Impact

To assess the economic and public health burden from smoking, the CDC calculates smoking-attributable mortality (SAM), years of potential life lost (YPLL), and productivity losses in the United States from smoking. The most recent data from 2000 to 2004 indicate that cigarette smoking and exposure to tobacco smoke resulted in at least 443,000 premature deaths, approximately 5.1 million YPLL, and $96.8 billion in productivity losses annually. The premature death rate is higher than the average annual estimate of approximately 438,000 deaths during 1997–2001. Further, although smoking prevalence has declined dramatically since its peak in the 1960s, the number of smoking-attributable deaths has remained unchanged, primarily because of increases in population size (particularly among older age groups). Cohorts of smokers with the highest peak prevalence have now reached the ages with the highest incidence of smoking-attributable diseases.

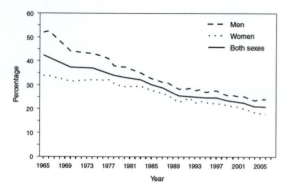

Figure 21.1. Estimated percentage of persons aged >18 years who were current smokers, by sex—National Health Interview Survey, United States, 1965–2006. During 1965–1991, current smokers were defined as persons who reported smoking at least 100 cigarettes during their lifetimes and who, at the time of interview, reported smoking ("Have you smoked at least 100 cigarettes in your entire life?" and "Do you smoke cigarettes now?"). In 1992, the definition changed to more accurately assess intermittent smoking (i.e., smoking on some days) and included persons who reported they smoked either every day or some days ("Do you now smoke cigarettes every day, some days, or not at all?"). Centers for Disease Control and Prevention. Cigarette Smoking Among Adults—United States, 2006. MMWR 2007; 56(44):1161.

NICOTINE DEPENDENCE AND TOBACCO ADDICTION

It is primarily the pharmacologic effects of nicotine that produce dependence and tobacco addiction. Indeed, non–nicotine-containing cigarettes do not sustain addiction. DSM-IV criteria for nicotine dependence include evidence of the following: (1) tolerance, (2) withdrawal or smoking to avoid or reduce withdrawal, (3) smoking in larger amounts or longer than intended, (4) persistent desire or unsuccessful efforts to cut down, (5) great deal of time spent to obtain, use or recover from smoking, (6) activities given up or reduced because of smoking, and (7) smoking despite physical or psychological problems caused or exacerbated by smoking. An individual is classified as dependent if he or she reports experiencing at least three of these criteria associated with their smoking behavior. Research findings from the SAMHSA 2006 National Survey on Drug Use and Health (NSDUH) show that among cigarette smokers aged 12 or older, 57% met criteria for nicotine dependence. Those who were nicotine dependent were more likely to engage in alcohol use and to experience serious psychological distress in the past year than those who were not nicotine dependent (5).

The likelihood of dependence does not correspond directly with the duration and quantity of nicotine use. Nicotine dependence can occur in smokers who report low (nondaily) levels of use (6). Conversely, some heavy daily cigarette smokers do not meet criteria for nicotine dependence (7). Thus, factors in addition to cigarette consumption are critical in the development of nicotine dependence.

Predictors of Nicotine Dependence

Smoking onset takes place in adolescence with most smokers trying their first cigarette before age 18. Following initial tobacco use, progression to daily smoking and development of nicotine dependence is very rapid. In one recent study, 25% of young tobacco users progressed to full dependence syndrome within 23 months following onset of smoking (8). Of note, however, is the fact that most adolescents who experiment with tobacco do not become dependent on nicotine (9). Factors associated with increased risk of transitioning to nicotine dependence are listed in Table 21.1, along with recent supporting evidence.

Racial and gender differences in risk of nicotine dependence have been identified. Rates of nicotine dependence are higher among whites than minorities and among females than males. Rates of nicotine dependence are inversely related to level of education and income (14). Age of onset has been identified as a risk factor. Animal studies have shown that early exposure to nicotine, including in utero exposure, predicts greater neurochemical changes, higher nicotine self-administration as adults, and more severe levels of dependence (24). Vulnerability to development of nicotine dependence is higher in people with psychiatric disease and/or substance abuse disorders. Some studies (14,20), but not all (15), have found that offspring of parents who smoke have an increased risk of becoming regular smokers or nicotine dependent. Association with peers who smoke has been shown to increase risk of dependence (14,15,21). Another risk factor is prenatal maternal smoking, which predicts offspring nicotine dependence (20,25). There is also evidence that sensitivity to the initial smoking experience predicts continued smoking and perhaps nicotine dependence. The most sensitive individuals, that is, those who initially experience more positive or both more positive and negative effects, may be most likely to become dependent (14,15,18).

Determining which adolescents are more susceptible to the addictive nature of nicotine has been a major area of research. A number of environmental and individual factors play a role in the development of nicotine dependence. Many of these factors may result from preexisting genetic vulnerabilities, as described in the following section.

Genetic Influences on Nicotine Dependence

Approximately 50% of the variance in risk for nicotine dependence is attributable to genetic factors (26,27). Attempts to identify specific genes are complicated by the fact that nicotine dependence is complex and polygenic, involving several chromosomes that are functionally overlapping and interactive (28). A variety of plausible candidate genes have been examined, primarily in two main areas: genes involved in the neurotransmitter pathways for the brain reward system and genes altering nicotine metabolism.

Nicotine's addictive properties are a result of the activation of nicotinic acetylcholine receptors (nAChRs) in the

TABLE 21.1	Predictors of nicotine dependence
Factors associated with higher rates of nicotine dependence in adolescents	**Supporting evidence**
White race/ethnicity; female gender	Andreski and Breslau, 1993 (10); Breslau et al., 2001 (7); DiFranza et al., 2002 (11); Kandel and Chen, 2000 (12); O'Loughlin et al., 2002 (13)
Lower education level; lower income level	Hu et al., 2006 (14)
Earlier age of smoking onset	Audrain-McGovern et al., 2007 (15); Breslau et al., 1994 (16)
Shorter latency between onset and daily smoking	Hu et al., 2006 (14)
Use of other substances	Audrain-McGovern et al., 2007 (15); Timberlake et al., 2007 (17)
Comorbidity with psychiatric disorders (e.g., depressive mood, anxiety, personality disorders)	DiFranza et al., 2004 (18); Isensee et al., 2003 (19)
Parental smoking	Hu et al., 2006 (14); Lieb et al., 2003 (20)
Peer smoking	Audrain-McGovern et al., 2007 (15); Baker et al., 2004 (21); Ellickson et al., 2004 (22); Hu et al., 2006 (14)
Prenatal maternal smoking	Abreu-Villaca et al., 2004 (23); Lieb et al., 2003 (20)
Greater sensitivity to the reinforcing effects of nicotine	Audrain-McGovern et al., 2007 (15); DiFranza et al., 2004 (18); Hu et al., 2006 (14)

brain and the impact this has on certain neurotransmitter systems (e.g., dopamine, serotonin, and GABA). Thus, genes that encode nAChR proteins have been investigated as likely candidate genes (29). Several nAChR subunit genes have been identified (e.g., CHRNA3–CHRNA6 and CHRNB2–CHRNB4 gene clusters) and shown to be associated with smoking-related phenotypes (30,31), including linkage for nicotine dependence (20). Gene association studies have also identified variation in dopamine receptor subtypes (D_1–D_5). In particular, the A1 allele of the *DRD2* gene (Taq1 A) polymorphisms has been associated with smoking initiation (32), cigarette consumption (33), and craving (34). One interpretation is that individuals with DRD2 A1 genotypes exhibit lower dopamine D2 receptor density and, therefore, may have lower levels of neuronal dopamine-dependent activity compared to individuals with DRD2*A2 genotypes (35). In an effort to compensate for deficiencies in the dopaminergic system, carriers of the DRD A1 allele use more nicotine to increase brain dopamine levels.

Allele frequencies have also been examined in studies of the *CYP2A6* gene. Nicotine is almost wholly metabolized by the CYP2A6 enzyme. Dependent smokers regulate the amount they smoke to maintain plasma and brain nicotine levels, thus smoking behavior is increased when renal nicotine clearance (metabolism) is high. The hypothesis that genetically poor metabolizers (i.e., people with variant *CYP2A6* genes associated with substantially reduced enzyme activity) smoke fewer cigarettes and are less dependent on nicotine has been supported in some (36), but not all (37), studies.

Although considered a relatively new field of study, pharmacogenetics research in smoking has shown promise, with evidence that genetic variation is related to differential outcome to nicotine cessation pharmacotherapies. In studies of the U.S. Food and Drug Administration (FDA)-approved medications, including nicotine replacement and bupropion, candidate alleles at the D2 dopamine receptor gene and μ-opioid receptor gene have been shown to predict therapeutic response (38–40). Response to bupropion has also been studied in a preliminary manner, with evidence of an association with the CYP2B6 genotype and the dopamine DRD2 gene (41).

In summary, there is convincing evidence that smoking behavior and nicotine dependence are strongly influenced by genetic and environmental factors. Research has been productive in identifying genes that alter sensitivity to nicotine and potentially predict response to specific pharmacotherapies. Further development of genetics-based methods and models is underway.

DETERMINANTS OF USE

Nicotine Pharmacology

Nicotine is the main psychoactive ingredient in cigarettes, readily crossing the blood–brain barrier and targeting the nAChRs (42). The nAChR complex is diverse, consisting of five subunits. It is the α-4 and β-2 subunit receptors that account for 90% of high-affinity binding in the brain. The β-2 subunit is critical for dopamine release and for the behavioral effects of nicotine, while the α-4 subunit is an important determinant of nicotine sensitivity (43).

Activation of presynaptic nAChRs facilitates release of neurotransmitters. Dopamine release in particular is critical to the reinforcing effects of nicotine and other drugs of abuse. Other neurotransmitters are released and mediate various behaviors in smokers, including norepinephrine (arousal, appetite suppression), acetylcholine (arousal, cognitive enhancement), serotonin (mood modulation, appetite suppression), GABA (reduction of anxiety and tension), glutamate (learning, memory enhancement), and endorphins (reduction of anxiety and tension) (43). It is primarily through its effects on dopamine release that acute nicotine administration increases brain reward function.

Chronic nicotine exposure results in neuroadaptation or the development of tolerance to some of the effects of nicotine (44). Neuroadaptation is characterized by an increase in the number of nAChR binding sites in the brain, which in turn leads to upregulation in response to nicotine-mediated desensitization of receptors (45). This process has been linked to key aspects of nicotine dependence, including nicotine withdrawal (46). Symptoms of nicotine withdrawal due to deficient dopamine responses include craving and inability to experience pleasure. These neural plasticity changes appear to be long lasting and responsible for persistent craving and risk of relapse long after stopping smoking.

Nicotine Pharmacokinetics and Pharmacodynamics

Smoking is a highly efficient form of drug administration. Compared to absorption through mucous membranes (e.g., chewing tobacco, snuff, or nicotine gum), inhaled nicotine enters the circulation rapidly through the lungs and moves into the brain within seconds. This increased speed of absorption and entry of the drug into the brain corresponds with greater concentrations and reinforcing effects of the drug. The smoking process allows for precise dose titration. Smokers have fingertip control of the dose, on a puff-by-puff basis, so that topographic features of smoking, such as number, volume, duration, and depth of inhalation, can predict the exact level of nicotine intake. Regular smokers become very consistent in self-administering nicotine to a level that produces desired effects.

Nicotine is metabolized to cotinine, primarily by the liver enzyme CYP2A6 (47). Cotinine is subsequently metabolized to *trans*-3-hydroxycotinine (3HC) by CYP2A6 (43). It is the ratio of 3HC to cotinine that has been used as a phenotypic marker for defining rate of nicotine metabolism (i.e., CYP2A6 activity). As mentioned above, recent findings show that slower metabolizers are at lower risk to develop nicotine dependence and may have lower risk for certain cancers (48,49). In general, Asians and African Americans metabolize nicotine more slowly than do Caucasians or Hispanics (50). In addition, the rate of nicotine metabolism is faster in women than men (51,52).

At low doses, nicotine acts like a stimulant, producing arousal, increased heart rate, and blood pressure. In contrast, high doses of nicotine produce ganglionic blockade, leading to bradycardia, hypotension, and depressed mental state (43). Tolerance to many of the acute subjective effects and physiologic effects of nicotine develops within a day for most smokers. That means that for a daily smoker the positive rewards of smoking diminish throughout the day, and smoking becomes driven primarily by efforts to maintain a threshold level of nicotine to keep withdrawal symptoms at bay.

Environmental Factors

Cigarette smoking is maintained, in part, by conditioning. The behavior of smoking is paired, repeatedly, with specific situations (e.g., with coffee and after a meal), settings (e.g., bar), or mood states (e.g., stress and frustration). Over time, these associations cause environmental situations to become strong cues for smoking or the urge to smoke. In similar fashion, other aspects of the smoking behavior (handling the cigarette, the taste and smell of smoking) become associated with the pleasurable effects of nicotine and further strengthen the conditioning process. Functioning imaging studies have shown that just the exposure of smoking-related cues can activate cortical regions of the brain (53).

Conditioning develops from pairing the pharmacologic actions of nicotine with associated behaviors and environmental situations. At the same time, however, conditioning factors appear to maintain nicotine use during periods of receptor desensitization, that is, when there is a loss or decrease in the biologic response to nicotine due to prior exposure to nicotine. Thus, environmental conditioning plays a critically important role in the reinstatement or relapse to smoking in abstinent smokers. To be effective, therapies for nicotine dependence need to address the role of conditioned stimuli and conditioned reinforcers in maintaining smoking behavior.

EVALUATION AND TREATMENT

Screening and Identification

According to the *Clinical Practice Guideline on Treating Tobacco Use and Dependence* (hereafter referred to as the *Guideline*) at least 70% of smokers see a physician each year, and almost one third see a dentist (54). Other smokers are likely to come in contact with physicians, nurse practitioners, pharmacists, counselors, and other clinicians. These various clinicians are in prime position to intervene with patients on their tobacco use. Many smokers report wanting to quit smoking and cite that physician's advice to quit smoking is an important motivator for attempting to stop smoking. Unfortunately, clinicians and health care systems do not capitalize on this opportunity consistently. According to the National Committee for Quality Assurance's "State of Health Care Quality Report," improvements have been made in increasing tobacco use interventions for patients with some form of private insurance, including Medicare; 71% to 75% of these patients received cessation advice. By contrast, however, only 25% of Medicaid patients reported any assistance with their smoking habits. In addition, only about one third of adolescents who visited a physician or dentist reported receiving counseling regarding the dangers of using tobacco, according to the 2000 National Youth Tobacco Survey. Another study indicated that while 71% of 4207 patients reported that they had been advised to quit smoking at least once over the past year, 56% were assessed for nicotine dependence, 49% received some form of assistance, only 38% were offered pharmacotherapy, and only 9% received a recommendation for follow-up (55). Clearly, improvements are needed in screening and intervention with tobacco users in health care settings.

The *Guideline* put forth compelling reasons why members of a busy clinical team should make the screening and treatment of tobacco use a priority: (1) clinicians can make a difference with even a minimal (less than 3 minutes) intervention; (2) a relation exists between the intensity of intervention and tobacco cessation outcome (higher intensity = better outcomes); (3) even when patients are not willing to make a quit attempt, clinician-delivered brief interventions enhance motivation and increase the likelihood of future quit attempts; (4) tobacco users are being primed to consider quitting by a wide range of societal and environmental factors (e.g., public health messages, policy changes, cessation marketing messages, and family members); (5) there is growing evidence that smokers who receive clinician advice and assistance with quitting report greater satisfaction with their health care than those who do not; (6) tobacco use interventions are highly cost effective; and (7) tobacco use has a high case fatality rate (up to 50% of long-term smokers die of a smoking-related disease).

Identifying tobacco users is, of course, the first step in this process. Formal screening instruments exist that can be used to identify smokers and their nicotine dependence severity. The most well-known is the Fagerström Test for Nicotine Dependence (FTND) (56). The FTND is a standardized questionnaire for assessing level of physical dependence on nicotine. FTND scores may assist in tailoring treatment, for example higher scores suggest more intensive treatment versus lower scores, and can be used to track progress over time. Many clinicians are not accustomed to using standardized instruments, however, and therefore may be reluctant to incorporate this measure. An alternative is to simply ASK the patient about tobacco use at each clinical encounter. Repeated tobacco-use screening and brief intervention is one of the top three most important and cost-effective preventive services that can be provided in medical practice (57,58).

Treatment

There are many treatment options to promote smoking cessation, both pharmacologic and behavioral. Pharmacologic therapies fall into two main categories: (1) nicotine replacement therapies (NRTs) and (2) non-nicotine medications.

A brief summary of these treatments is provided in Table 21.2 and the following section. The reader is referred to Chapter 6 of this textbook for a more comprehensive review.

Nicotine Replacement Therapies

The primary aim of NRT is to reduce the physiologic and psychomotor withdrawal symptoms often experienced during smoking cessation attempts, which theoretically should increase the likelihood of abstinence. Nicotine replacement products are formulated for absorption through oral mucosa (chewing gum, lozenges, sublingual tablets, inhaler) or skin (transdermal patches). Across multiple studies, the various forms of NRT in general are associated with a 50% to 70% increase in the rate of long-term abstinence when compared to placebo treatment (59). Evidence that NRT helps people to stop smoking is now well accepted, and many clinical guidelines recommend NRT as the first-line treatment for people amenable to pharmacologic assistance with quitting smoking (e.g., Ref. 54).

The choice of which form of NRT depends upon the patients' preferences, needs, tolerability, and cost considerations. The nicotine patch is distinct from the other forms of NRT in that nicotine is delivered slowly and passively throughout the day, with some brands designed for 24-hour use and some for 16-hour use; wearing the patch during daytime only has been found to be as effective as wearing it for 24 hours/day (59). With the patch, plasma levels tend to be similar to the trough levels seen in heavy smokers (59). Patches are likely to be easier to use than gum, nasal spray, or inhaler, but patches cannot be used for relief of acute cravings, nor do they replace the behavioral activities of smoking. There is evidence of benefit from combining the nicotine patch with an acute dosing NRT (e.g., gum) compared to use of a single form (59).

Non-nicotine Medications

Bupropion Bupropion sustained release (SR) (Zyban) is the first non-nicotine FDA-approved medication for smoking cessation. Its mechanism of action is presumed to relate to its ability to block the reuptake of dopamine and norepinephrine, with no clinically significant effects on serotonin (60). Thirty-one studies with almost 10,000 participants comparing bupropion SR to placebo confirm the benefit of this medication, indicating that it approximately doubles long-term (>5 months) abstinence rates compared to placebo (54,61). Other studies also support its efficacy. Gonzales et al. (62) evaluated smokers ($n = 450$) who had previously used bupropion in a smoking cessation attempt. Subjects received either bupropion SR 300 mg per day or placebo for 12 weeks. The bupropion group exhibited significantly higher continuous abstinence rates at 6 months postquit (12%) than did the placebo group (2%). While the recommended dose is 300 mg daily, at least two studies have documented no evidence of a significant difference in the odds of being quit at 12 months for 150 mg daily compared to 300 mg.

With regard to relapse prevention, Hays and colleagues (63) examined 429 smokers who had recently quit smoking.

TABLE 21.2 Mayo clinic NDC tobacco dependence treatment medication

Description & examples	Pros & cons	Comments	Dosing recommendations
Combination nicotine replacement therapy (NRT)	**Pros** ■ Permits sustained levels of nicotine with rapid adjustment for acute needs ■ More efficacious than monotherapy **Cons** ■ May increase risk of nicotine toxicity ■ Cost	**Comments/limitations** ■ Providing two types of delivery system, one passive and one active, appears to be more efficacious. ■ Should be considered for those who have failed single therapy in the past and those considered highly tobacco dependant. ■ Not an FDA approved strategy.	**Dosing**** Dose the patch as described. Prescribe 2 mg gum, 2 mg lozenge, nicotine inhaler or nicotine nasal spray on an as needed basis when acute withdrawal symptoms and urges to use tobacco occur. Adjust dose of patch if frequent use of other NRTs: goal is to minimize need for short-acting NRT dosing.
Nicotine patch (OTC) 24 hour delivery systems 21, 14, 7 mg/24 hr 16 hour delivery systems 15 mg/16 hr (Generic available)	**Pros** ■ Achieve high levels of replacement ■ Easy to use ■ Only needs to be applied once a day ■ Few side effects **Cons** ■ Less flexible dosing ■ Slow onset of delivery ■ Mild skin rashes and irritation	**Comments/limitations** ■ Patches vary in strengths and the length of time over which nicotine is delivered. ■ Depending on the brand of patch used, may be left on for anywhere from 16 to 24 hours. Patches may be placed anywhere on the upper body—including arms and back. Rotate the patch site each time a new patch is applied. ■ May purchase without a prescription	**Dosing** (24 hour patch)** ≥40 cpd = 42 mg/day 21–39 cpd = 28–35 mg/day 10–20 cpd = 14–21 mg/day <10 cpd = 14 mg/day ■ If a dose > 42 mg/day may be indicated, contact the patient's prescriber. ■ Adjust based on withdrawal symptoms, urges, and comfort. After 4–6 weeks of abstinence, taper every 2–4 weeks in 7–14 mg steps as tolerated.
Nicotine lozenge (OTC) Delivers nicotine through the lining of the mouth while the lozenge dissolves. 2 mg, 4 mg	**Pros** ■ Easy to use ■ Delivers doses of nicotine approximately 25% higher than nicotine gum **Cons** ■ Should not eat or drink 15 minutes before use or during use ■ Should not be chewed or swallowed ■ Nausea frequent (12–15%)	**Comments/limitations** ■ Use at least 8–9 lozenges/day initially. ■ Efficacy and frequency of side-effects related to amount used. ■ May purchase without a prescription	**Dosing as monotherapy** Based on time to first cigarette of the day: <30 minutes = 4 mg ≥30 minutes = 2 mg Based on cigarettes/day (cpd) >20 cpd: 4 mg 20 cpd: 2 mg Initial dosing is 1–2 lozenges every 1–2 hours (minimum of 9/day). Taper as tolerated

Nicotine gum (OTC)

2mg, 4mg

Flavors: Orange, Mint, Regular

The term "gum" is misleading. It is not chewed like regular gum but rather is chewed briefly and then "parked" between cheek and gum. The nicotine is absorbed through the lining of the mouth

(Generic Available)

Pros
- Convenient/flexible dosing
- Faster delivery of nicotine than the patches

Cons
- May be inappropriate for people with dental problems and those with temporomandibular joint (TMJ) syndrome
- Should not eat or drink 15 minutes before use or during use
- Frequent use during the day required to obtain adequate nicotine levels

Comments/limitations

Many people use this medication incorrectly. Review package directions carefully to maximize benefit of product

May purchase without a prescription

Dosing as monotherapy**

Based on cigarettes/day (cpd)
- \>20 cpd: 4 mg gum
- 20 cpd: 2 mg gum

Based on time to first cigarette of the day:
- <30 minutes = 4 mg
- \>30 minutes = 2 mg

Initial dosing is 1–2 pieces every 1–2 hrs (10–12 pieces/day).

Taper as tolerated.

Nicotine nasal spray

Delivers nicotine through the lining of the nose when sprayed directly into each nostril.

Pros
- Flexible dosing
- Can be used in response to stress or urges to smoke
- Fastest delivery of nicotine of currently available products but not as fast as cigarettes

Cons
- Nose and eye irritation is common, but usually disappears within 1 week.
- Frequent use during the day required to obtain adequate nicotine levels

Comments/limitations

Unlike nasal sprays used to relieve allergy symptoms, the nicotine spray is not meant to be sniffed. Rather, it is sprayed against the lining of each nostril once or twice an hour (maximum of five times in one hour).

Prescription required for purchase

Dosing as monotherapy

1 spray in each nostril 1–2 times/hr (up to 5 times/hr or 40 times/day)

Most average 14–15 doses/day initially

Taper as tolerated

Nicotine inhaler

A plastic cylinder containing a cartridge that delivers nicotine when puffed. The inhaler delivers nicotine to the oral mucosa, not the lung, and enters the body much more slowly than the nicotine in cigarettes.

Pros
- Flexible dosing
- Mimics the hand-to-mouth behavior of smoking
- Few side effects

Cons
- Frequent use during the day required to obtain adequate nicotine levels
- May cause mouth or throat irritation

Comments/limitations

Puffing must be done frequently, far more often than with a cigarette.

Each cartridge designed for 80 puffs over 20 minutes of use. Patient does not need to inhale deeply to achieve an effect.

Prescription required for purchase

Dosing as monotherapy

Minimum of 6 cartridges/day, up to 16/day

Taper as tolerated

Continued

TABLE 21.2 Mayo clinic NDC tobacco dependence treatment medication (*Continued*)

Description & examples	Pros & cons	Comments	Dosing recommendations
Non-nicotine medication **Bupropion SR** (Generic available)	**Pros** ■ Easy to use ■ Pill form ■ Few side effects ■ May be used in combination with NRT (nicotine patches, spray, gum and inhaler)** **Cons** ■ Contraindicated with certain medical conditions and medications	**Comments/limitations** A slight risk of seizure (1:1000) is associated with use of this medication. Seizure risk should be assessed. Risk of seizure is increased if: ■ Personal history of seizures ■ Significant head trauma/brain injury ■ Anorexia nervosa or bulimia ■ Concurrent use of medications that lower the seizure threshold Prescription required for purchase	**Dosing: Take doses at least 8 hours apart** Start medication 1 week prior to the Target Quit Date (TQD) 150 mg once daily for 3 days, then 150 mg twice daily for 4 days, then **On TQD STOP SMOKING** Continue at 150 mg BID 12 weeks, or longer if necessary. May stop abruptly; no need to taper.
Non-nicotine medication **Varenicline**	**Pros** ■ Easy to use ■ Pill form ■ Generally well tolerated ■ No known drug interactions **Cons** ■ Nausea is common	**Comments/limitations** ■ Nausea is common. Taking the medication with food and titrating the dose as directed will help ■ It appears that varenicline can be safely used in combination with bupropion and/or NRT. However, efficacy of these combinations has not been shown ■ Dose must be adjusted if kidney function is impaired Prescription required for purchase	**Dosing: TAKE WITH FOOD** Start medication 1 week prior to the Target Quit Date (TQD) 0.5 mg once daily X3 days, then 0.5 mg twice daily X 4 days, then **ON TQD STOP SMOKING AND** Take 1.0 mg twice daily X 11 weeks If not smoking at the end of 12 weeks, may continue at 1.0 mg twice daily for an additional 12 weeks May stop abruptly. No need to taper.

SMOKELESS TOBACCO (ST) Treatment recommendations	24 hour nicotine patch:	Other NRTs:	Non-nicotine pharmacotherapy
	>3 cans or pouches/week = 42 mg/day 2–3 cans or pouches/week = 21 mg/day <2 cans or pouches/week = 14 mg/day Adjust based on withdrawal symptoms, urges, and comfort. After 4–6 weeks of abstinence, taper every 2–4 weeks in 7–14 mg steps as tolerated	Nicotine lozenge: 4 mg if >3 tins/week 2 mg if 3 tins/week Nicotine gum or nicotine lozenge may be combined with nicotine patch as described for cigarette smokers. Nicotine inhaler and nicotine nasal spray are *not* recommended for use in ST users.	Empiric evidence suggests that bupropion and varenicline may be of benefit in this population of tobacco users, using the dosing guidelines recommended for cigarette smokers.

The table is a summary of recommendations for use of medication in the treatment of tobacco dependence. The most effective dose varies by individual. Costs will vary depending on retailer. (Adapted from Ebbert JO, et al. *J Thorac Oncol.* 2007;2: 249–256; Fiore, et al. U.S. Public Health Service Guideline, June 2000; Shiffman et al., *Arch Intern Med.* 2002; 162: 1267–1276. Varenicline Product Information profile (May 2006). Revised November 2007.)

All participants received bupropion SR 300 mg per day for the initial 7 weeks of the trial, then the same dosage or placebo for the next 38 weeks. Although there was an initial benefit from continued therapy at 1 year from the quit date, no significant differences were found at 2 years. Other studies have also noted bupropion's lack of effect for preventing relapse (64,65).

Nortriptyline Typically used as an antidepressant (tricyclic), nortriptyline does not have FDA approval for smoking cessation. It remains a second-line medication because of potential side effects and limited evidence to support its efficacy. Several studies have demonstrated benefit for nortriptyline over placebo for smoking cessation, while several have not (66,67). Comparisons of bupropion and nortriptyline have favored bupropion, but no significant differences between the two have been found (66–68).

Varenicline In 2006 a new medication, Varenicline (Chantix), was approved by the FDA for smoking cessation. Varenicline is a highly selective partial agonist that also displays antagonist properties, that is, it prevents full stimulation of the nicotine receptor that ensues when nicotine is coadministered. Thus, varenicline has the potential to provide relief from withdrawal (agonist effect) and block the rewarding effects of nicotine (antagonist effect) (69). It is well tolerated in most patients, although there have been recent reports of increased psychiatric symptoms associated with varenicline administration. In February 2008, the FDA added a warning indicating that depressed mood, agitation, changes in behavior, suicidal ideation, and suicide have been reported in patients attempting to quit smoking while using varenicline.

A randomized, double-blind clinical trial comparing varenicline (2 mg), buproprion (300 mg), and placebo showed overall continuous abstinence rates through 1 year posttreatment of 23%, 14.6%, and 10.3% (70). Further, varenicline nearly tripled the odds of quitting over placebo during the last 4 weeks of treatment (70). A recent review of nicotine receptor partial agonists for smoking cessation concluded that varenicline increased odds of quitting over Bupropion SR with a minimal to moderate side effect profile (71). In a separate study, an additional 12 weeks of varenicline (24 total weeks) was shown to reduce the risk of relapse among smokers who were abstinent at the end of the first 12 weeks, suggesting a relapse prevention benefit as well (72). Smokers taking varenicline have reported significantly less craving and withdrawal symptoms.

The FDA-approved dosing of varenicline is 2 mg/day (1 mg twice daily), however there is evidence that 1 mg daily is also effective. A meta-analysis of four studies with five study arms was conducted to evaluate the effects of the dose (73). Results indicated that compared to placebo, the 1 mg daily dose approximately doubles a smoker's likelihood of long-term abstinence from tobacco, while the 2 mg daily dose approximately tripled the likelihood of abstinence. Thus, the 1 mg dose is an acceptable alternative for smokers who experience intolerable, dose-related side effects.

Combination Smoking Treatments

Clinical practice guidelines for tobacco treatment state that some combinations of first-line medications have been found effective for smoking cessation. Only the nicotine patch + bupropion combination has been approved by the FDA for smoking cessation; however, other combinations have been tested. A 2008 meta-analysis revealed that the nicotine patch + bupropion SR, nicotine patch + inhaler, and long-term nicotine patch + ad libitum NRT have all been shown effective relative to placebo, and are recommended for use as first-line treatments (54,74). At least one study is underway to evaluate combination therapy with bupropion and varenicline (by PI [P. Cinciripini]). The presumed differences in mechanisms of action may afford a broader range of biologic targets identified as important in smoking cessation.

Behavioral Therapies

The characteristics of behavioral interventions for smoking cessation vary widely. The *Guideline* examined four of these characteristics: advice to quit, intensity, treatment format, and type of clinician, as well as specific elements of various types of counseling and therapy.

Overall results revealed a strong dose–response relationship between treatment intensity (i.e., session length, total contact time, and number of sessions) and treatment effectiveness. However, evidence also indicated that physician advice to quit smoking significantly increases long-term abstinence rates, even with a modal intervention length of 3 minutes or less. Analysis of different treatment formats demonstrated that telephone and group and individual counseling all improve smoking abstinence rates compared to no intervention; further, using multiple treatment formats increases abstinence rates as compared to use of a single format. A comparison of the effectiveness of different clinician types (e.g., physician, psychologist, nurse, and dentist) revealed no significant differences in abstinence rates based on this factor. Also studied was the effectiveness of including multiple clinicians from different disciplines. Although nonsignificant statistically, findings suggest that the involvement of a variety of clinicians in treatment may be more effective than that of a single clinician.

Brief Clinician Interventions There are five main components of a brief intervention for smoking cessation that are often referred to as "the 5 A's" and are particularly useful in a health care setting (see Table 21.3). As mentioned earlier in this chapter, the first step is to ASK the patient at each visit if he or she uses tobacco. This can be done in either written or oral fashion with the primary goal of systematically identifying all tobacco users at every visit. Second, once a smoker has been identified, the health care provider should ADVISE the patient to quit. The provider should present the advice clearly and strongly. For example, "As your clinician, I need you to know that quitting smoking is the most important thing you can do to protect your health now and in the future." The advice should also be personalized. Tobacco use should be tied to current symptoms and health concerns, and/or social and economic costs, and/or the impact of tobacco use on children or others in the household. For example, "Continuing to smoke will make your asthma worse, while quitting smoking would make it better."

The next step is to ASSESS the patient's willingness to make a quit attempt. If the patient is willing to try to quit, the

TABLE 21.3	The "5 A's" for brief intervention
Ask about tobacco use	Identify and document tobacco use status for every patient at every visit
Advise to quit	In a clear, strong, and personalized manner urge every tobacco user to quit
Assess willingness to make a quit attempt	Is the tobacco user willing to make a quit attempt at this time?
Assist in quit attempt	For the patient willing to make a quit attempt, use counseling and pharmacotherapy to help him or her quit
Arrange follow-up	Schedule follow-up contact, preferably within the first week after quit date

From Fiore MC, Jaen CR, Baker TB, et al. *Treating Tobacco Use and Dependence: 2008 Update*. Clinical Practice Guidelines. Rockville, MD: U.S. Department of Health and Human Services, Public Health Service; 2008:40.

physician should ASSIST the patient with a plan. This plan should include first-line medications such at NRTs, bupropion or varenicline, and smoking cessation counseling. Free telephone counseling is available through various federal agencies or organizations such as the American Cancer Society. For the patient who is not interested in quitting, strategies are available to increase motivation and the likelihood of future quit attempts. Finally, the physician should ARRANGE follow-up. For patients willing to set a quit date, arrange a subsequent appointment for 1 week after that date. Multiple contacts are encouraged. For patients unwilling to make a quit attempt, be sure to repeat the 5 A's at their next clinic visit.

For patients who are unwilling to attempt to quit smoking, motivational strategies can be employed that may increase the likelihood of later quitting. These strategies have been adopted from motivational interviewing (MI) (75), a directive yet patient-centered counseling method. There is evidence that MI is effective in increasing future quit attempts (76,77), although positive abstinence outcomes have been elusive, particularly for those already motivated to quit (78). As summarized in the *Guideline*, the general strategies involve exploring feelings, beliefs, ideas, and values that result in abstinence about using tobacco. The clinician selectively elicits, supports, and strengthens the patient's "change talk" (e.g., reasons, ideas, and needs for eliminating tobacco use) and commitment language (e.g, intentions to take action to change smoking behavior). Eliciting ideas about change from patients is more effective than lectures or arguments for change presented by the physician (79).

Based on a meta-analysis of 64 studies, more intensive counseling and behavioral interventions with demonstrated effectiveness include: (1) providing smokers with practical problem-solving skills, (2) providing support and encouragement during a smoker's direct contact with a clinician, (3) intervening to increase social support in the smoker's environment, and (4) using aversive smoking procedures (rapid smoking, rapid puffing, other smoking exposure). However, the authors of the *Guideline* in reviewing multiple studies decided not to recommend extra-treatment social support as well as aversive smoking based on questionable effectiveness and side effects from the latter.

In summary, there is a myriad of smoking cessation treatments available, both pharmacologic and behavioral, with proven effectiveness. Thus, health care providers have the luxury of tailoring their treatment to patients' needs and preferences. If one method fails, there are many more, including combination pharmacotherapy, that can be utilized. Establishing clinic-wide policies among multiple health care providers to promote smoking cessation with every patient at every visit has the potential for major impact on smoking rates.

SPECIAL CONSIDERATIONS

Nicotine and Psychiatric Comorbidities

Tobacco smoking is highly prevalent and more intense in psychiatric patients. Comorbidity rates are particularly high for schizophrenia and depression, where smoking rates of 70% to 90% have been reported (80) compared to <25% in the general population. Those who have a psychiatric diagnosis and are nicotine dependent (7%) consume 34% of all cigarettes. Early onset of tobacco use has been associated with greater risk of later psychiatric problems (81).

It is commonly assumed that psychiatric patients use tobacco for self-medication. For example, the actions of nicotine on nAChRs improve attention in schizophrenia by normalizing several deficits in sensory processing. Moreover, a genetic link between the α-7 nAChR subunit and schizophrenia has been found (82). Nicotine improves attention in ADHD patients likely through its effects on dopamine release (similar to stimulant ADHD medications).

Increased smoking and nicotine dependence in schizophrenics may represent an attempt to overcome the potentially dysphoric and unwanted side effects of traditional neuroleptic medications caused by dopamine blockade (83). A related hypothesis is that neuroleptic medications may block the aversive properties of nicotine, thereby increasing sensitivity to the dependence producing rewarding properties of nicotine (84).

Some clinical evidence suggests that smoking may be associated with reduced symptoms of parkinsonism (85) but increased tardive dyskinesia (86). Studies of patients with schizophrenia who are treated with atypical (e.g., clozapine, olanzapine) rather than conventional antipsychotics have reported lower frequency of smoking and higher cessation rates (87,88).

Smokers with depression are less likely to quit and more likely to experience severe withdrawal symptoms, including depressed mood. Depressed smokers themselves often perceive smoking as a self-medicating strategy, reporting an increased likelihood of smoking during negative emotional situations than nondepressed smokers. In terms of antidepressant effects, nicotine has been shown to improve psychomotor retardation, sleep, and overall depressive symptomatology (89,90). The release of serotonin and norepinephrine in the brain by nicotine is similar to the neurochemical effects of certain antidepressant medications. Additionally, cigarette smoking inhibits MAOA and MAOB, similar to the antidepressant effect of MAO inhibitors (91).

Tobacco smoke activates the cytochrome P450 1A2 (CYP1A2) enzyme that is responsible for the metabolism of many commonly used psychiatric drugs. This increased CYP1A2 activity by tobacco smoke can result in substantially lower serum concentrations of psychiatric drugs in smokers compared with nonsmokers. Cigarette smoking has been shown to be associated with increased clearance of fluphenazine, haloperidol, olanzapine, and tiotixene, as well as some benzodiazepines (92). Faster metabolism of these drugs can result in need for higher dosages, which can increase side effects, cost, adherence, and efficacy. It is important that plasma levels of psychiatric drugs be carefully monitored in patients who are attempting to stop smoking.

In summary, understanding how psychiatric comorbidities contribute to smoking and vice versa is increasingly important, especially as this represents a growing subpopulation of difficult-to-treat smokers (93). The literature to date highlights key mechanisms explaining this comorbidity. The reader is referred to Chapter 6 of this textbook and Ziedonis et al. (94) for a more complete review of tobacco cessation strategies in psychiatric disorders.

Nicotine and Other Drug Dependence

The prevalence of tobacco use among individuals who use alcohol and/or other illicit drugs is high (~75%). Compared with nonsubstance abusing populations, substance abusers tend to smoke more heavily, report more symptoms of nicotine dependence, experience more severe withdrawal symptoms, and have greater difficulty quitting smoking. Substance abusers who smoke are at higher risk of health consequences due to the synergistic effects of smoking and alcohol/drugs on the development of cardiovascular disease and cancers.

The comorbidity of nicotine with other substance use disorders may be due to a common genetic vulnerability. Support for this idea comes from classic genetic studies showing that polygenic genetic variants influence risk of addiction to substances in general, rather than to specific substances (95,96). One approach has been to identify genetic variants associated with personality-related phenotypes. Impulsivity, for example, defined as a predisposition toward rapid, unplanned reactions to internal or external stimuli without regard to the negative consequences of these reactions to themselves or others (97), is highly associated with addictive disorders. Not surprisingly, candidate genes with variants for impulsivity have been associated with alcoholism and other addictions (98). Other studies have identified genetic variants associated with risk-taking traits and addiction (99). Genetic linkage studies have also identified genetic variants of stress responsivity, that is, HPA axis function, with addiction risk (100,101). Thus, multiple genetic variants that influence vulnerability to addiction in general might explain the high rates of nicotine dependence in people with other drug dependence disorders.

Pharmacologic mechanisms may explain the strong comorbidity. Combined drug effects may be additive, that is, producing enhanced rewarding effects, or modulatory. Both nicotine and alcohol, for example, have anxiolytic and antidepressant effects, which appear to be additive when the drugs are used together (102). At the same time, alcoholic individuals may use nicotine to offset or delay the sedative and cognition-impairing effects of alcohol (103). Nicotine effects have been shown to modulate alcohol withdrawal symptoms and mitigate some of alcohol's neurotoxic effects (104,105). Finally, the direct actions of nicotine on cholinergic systems, that is, nAChRs, appear to be involved in the development and maintenance of psychostimulant-rewarded behaviors. From this, it has been proposed that exposure to nicotine may facilitate dependence on cocaine and other stimulants (106).

From a behavioral perspective, environmental cues present during combined drug use acquire strong motivating and controlling properties. Models of young adult peer influence also offer possible explanations for the concurrent use of cigarettes and other drugs. In a recent study of young adults aged 19 to 25, both concurrent and prospective analyses found that peer use predicted young adult cigarette use and other substance use (107). The "gateway" theory of substance use predicts that use of a less dangerous drug (e.g., nicotine) increases the risk of starting to consume other more harmful drugs, in a so-called "staircase" fashion. In general, research on patterns of onset of substance use among adolescents show typical progression through initiation of tobacco, alcohol, and marijuana before use of other illicit drugs (108,109). Substance use progression appears to be influenced not only by causal biologic mechanisms, but also by variables such as drug availability and attitudes (109).

In summary, co-occuring use of nicotine and other substances is highly prevalent and associated with harmful consequences. Most patients seek treatment for a single drug problem, despite their codependence. A better understanding of the genetic, neurochemical, and behavioral factors that underlie comorbid addictions will improve prevention and treatment efforts.

Nicotine Regulation

It is fitting to close this chapter with a brief discussion of current events regarding nicotine and tobacco regulation efforts. As a result of an unequivocal evidence regarding the

TABLE 21.4 The Family Smoking Prevention and Tobacco Control Act, H.R. 1256

The Family Smoking Prevention and Tobacco Control Act
- Grants the Food and Drug Administration (FDA) power to regulate tobacco products.
- Requires tobacco product manufacturers to disclose all ingredients in its products, the form and delivery method of nicotine, and any research into the health, toxicologic, behavioral, or physiologic effects of tobacco products to the FDA and notify the FDA of any future changes to any of the above.
- Requires tobacco manufacturers to release all marketing research documents to the FDA.
- Requires tobacco manufacturers to notify the FDA of any future changes to the ingredients of their products.
- Requires all owners and operators of companies manufacturing or processing tobacco products to register with the Secretary of Health and Human Services and to be inspected once every 2 years.
- Prohibits the FDA from banning existing tobacco products or requiring that they eliminate nicotine.
- Requires FDA review of new tobacco products before they can go to market unless they are similar to products marketed before February 15, 2007.
- Bans companies from promoting products as lower-risk alternatives to traditional tobacco unless the FDA certifies that its sale is likely to improve public health.
- Establishes a mechanism to assess fees on tobacco companies and traders to finance FDA oversight of the industry.
- Orders a study on the public health implications of raising the minimum age to purchase tobacco products.
- Requires the Secretary of Health and Human Services to create a plan relating to enforce restrictions on the advertising and promotion of menthol and other cigarettes to minors.
- Mandates larger more varied and more prominent warning labels on tobacco products.

addictiveness and harmfulness of cigarette smoking, a truly historic event occurred on June 22, 2009 when President Obama signed into law the Family Smoking Prevention and Tobacco Control Act, H.R. 1256, giving the FDA the authority to effectively regulate the manufacturing, marketing, labeling, distribution, and sale of tobacco products. In essence, this law ends the special protections enjoyed by the tobacco industry and instead begins to protect the nation's health (Table 21.4). Thus, this legislation represents the strongest action that the federal government has ever taken to reduce tobacco use, the leading preventable cause of death in the United States.

The new law will take several steps toward restricting tobacco marketing and sales to youths. In addition, it will empower the FDA authority to require changes in tobacco products, such as the removal or reduction of harmful ingredients. The reader is reminded that modern cigarettes are uniquely designed to enable relatively easy inhalation of nicotine and other substances deep into the lung. New tobacco products that offer reduced exposure or risk are currently being marketed to smokers as alternatives to conventional cigarettes. "Quest" (Vector Tobacco Inc., Durham, NC; http://www.questcigs.com) cigarettes, for example, use genetically modified tobacco with substantially lower nicotine levels compared to regular brands. Whether such products produce meaningful health benefit or, as some have argued, actually increase tobacco use (amount and frequency) because of their perceived "safer" profile remains to be determined and has become an important topic of study (110,111).

CONCLUSIONS

The intent of this chapter is to review the latest research on nicotine, including how the pharmacologic effects of nicotine influence smoking behavior and promote development of dependence. Approximately 20% of American adults are cigarette smokers, with rates of smoking two- to fourfold higher in patients with comorbid psychiatric and other substance use disorders. Prevalence rates vary by gender, with men smoking more than women. Rates differ by race as well. Hispanic persons are less likely to smoke than non-Hispanic white or non-Hispanic black persons.

Research has shown that nicotine dependence produces numerous changes to behavioral and neural functioning, and these changes can be modulated by environmental and genetic factors. Certain individuals appear to be more vulnerable to nicotine dependence, with new evidence that genetic factors contribute significantly to this vulnerability. As researchers continue to identify specific genes involved in nicotine dependence, the findings are likely to have important implications for improving existing smoking cessation treatments.

The first step in treatment is identifying tobacco users and characterizing the degree to which the patient is physically dependent on nicotine, either formally using the FTND or informally during a clinical interview. All smokers should be provided with a recommendation to quit and offered behavioral and/or pharmacologic treatment. Various NRT products, bupropion SR, varenicline, and combination therapy are all effective first-line tobacco treatments. Brief clinician interventions for smoking should also be implemented by all health care providers to every patient at every visit. More intensive behavioral treatments are also available if warranted.

New federal regulation of nicotine products offers the promise of a nicotine-reducing strategy to make cigarettes less addictive. Studies on the feasibility of nicotine reduction will need to address the concern that smokers will smoke more cigarettes to compensate for lower nicotine levels. Current knowledge about the clinical pharmacology of nicotine will be critical in future decisions about harm reduction and federal regulatory strategies.

REFERENCES

1. Henningfield JE, Zeller M. Nicotine psychopharmacology research contributions to United States and global tobacco regulation: a look back and a look forward. *Psychopharmacology*. 2006;184:286–291.
2. Benowitz NL. *Nicotine Safety and Toxicity*. New York, NY: Oxford University Press; 1998.
3. Hatsukami DK, Stead LF, Gupta PC. Tobacco addiction. *Lancet*. 2008;371(9629):2027–2038.
4. Centers for Disease Control. Early Release of Selected Estimates Based on Data From the January–June 2009 National Health Interview Survey: Current Smoking 2009. Available at: http://www.cdc.gov/nchs/data/nhis/earlyrelease/200912_08.pdf. Accessed on January 14, 2010.
5. Substance Abuse and Mental Health Services Administration, OAS. The NSDUH Report: Nicotine Dependence: 2006. Rockville, MD.
6. Rose JS, Dierker LC, Donny E. Nicotine dependence symptoms among recent onset adolescent smokers. *Drug Alcohol Depend*. 2010;106(2–3):126–132.
7. Breslau N, Johnson EO, Hiripi E, et al. Nicotine dependence in the United States: prevalence, trends, and smoking persistence. *Arch Gen Psychiatry*. 2001;58(9):810–816.
8. Kandel DB, Hu MC, Griesler PC, et al. On the development of nicotine dependence in adolescence. *Drug Alcohol Depend*. 2007;91(1):26–39.
9. Rubinstein ML, Benowitz NL, Auerback GM, et al. Rate of nicotine metabolism and withdrawal symptoms in adolescent light smokers. *Pediatrics*. 2008;122(3):e643–e647.
10. Andreski P, Breslau N. Smoking and nicotine dependence in young adults: differences between blacks and whites. *Drug Alcohol Depend*. 1993;32(2):119–125.
11. DiFranza JR, Savageau JA, Fletcher K, et al. Measuring the loss of autonomy over nicotine use in adolescents: the DANDY (Development and Assessment of Nicotine Dependence in Youths) study. *Arch Pediatr Adolesc Med*. 2002;156(4):397–403.
12. Kandel DB, Chen K. Extent of smoking and nicotine dependence in the United States: 1991–1993. *Nicotine Tob Res*. 2000;2(3):263–274.
13. O'Loughlin J, DiFranza J, Tarasuk J, et al. Assessment of nicotine dependence symptoms in adolescents: a comparison of five indicators. *Tob Control*. 2002;11(4):354–360.
14. Hu MC, Davies M, Kandel DB. Epidemiology and correlates of daily smoking and nicotine dependence among young adults in the United States. *Am J Public Health*. 2006;96(2):299–308.
15. Audrain-McGovern J, Al Koudsi N, Rodriguez D, et al. The role of CYP2A6 in the emergence of nicotine dependence in adolescents. *Pediatrics*. 2007;119(1):e264–e274.
16. Breslau N, Kilbey MM, Andreski P. DSM-III-R nicotine dependence in young adults: prevalence, correlates and associated psychiatric disorders. *Addiction*. 1994;89(6):743–754.
17. Timberlake DS, Haberstick BC, Hopfer CJ, et al. Progression from marijuana use to daily smoking and nicotine dependence in a national sample of U.S. adolescents. *Drug Alcohol Depend*. 2007;88(2–3):272–281.
18. DiFranza JR, Savageau JA, Fletcher K, et al. Recollections and repercussions of the first inhaled cigarette. *Addict Behav*. 2004;29(2):261–272.
19. Isensee B, Wittchen HU, Stein MB, et al. Smoking increases the risk of panic: findings from a prospective community study. *Arch Gen Psychiatry*. 2003;60(7):692–700.
20. Lieb R, Schreier A, Pfister H, et al. Maternal smoking and smoking in adolescents: a prospective community study of adolescents and their mothers. *Eur Addict Res*. 2003;9(3):120–130.
21. Baker TB, Brandon TH, Chassin, L. Motivational influences on cigarette smoking. *Annu Rev Psychol*. 2004;55:463–491.
22. Ellickson PL, Orlando M, Tucker JS, et al. From adolescence to young adulthood: racial/ethnic disparities in smoking. *Am J Public Health*. 2004;94(2):293–299.
23. Abreu-Villaca Y, Seidler FJ, Tate CA, et al. Prenatal nicotine exposure alters the response to nicotine administration in adolescence: effects on cholinergic systems during exposure and withdrawal. *Neuropsychopharmacology*. 2004;29(5):879–890.
24. Levin ED, Lawrence SS, Petro A, et al. Adolescent vs. adult-onset nicotine self-administration in male rats: duration of effect and differential nicotinic receptor correlates. *Neurotoxicol Teratol*. 2007;29(4):458–465.
25. Buka SL, Shenassa ED, Niaura R. Elevated risk of tobacco dependence among offspring of mothers who smoked during pregnancy: a 30-year prospective study. *Am J Psychiatry*. 2003;160(11):1978–1984.
26. Lessov-Schlaggar CN, Pergadia ML, Khroyan TV, et al. Genetics of nicotine dependence and pharmacotherapy. *Biochem Pharmacol*. 2008;75(1):178–195.
27. Li MD, Cheng R, Ma JZ, et al. A meta-analysis of estimated genetic and environmental effects on smoking behavior in male and female adult twins. *Addiction*. 2003;98(1):23–31.
28. Ho MK, Tyndale RF. Overview of the pharmacogenomics of cigarette smoking. *Pharmacogenomics J*. 2007;7(2):81–98.
29. Portugal GS, Gould TJ. Genetic variability in nicotinic acetylcholine receptors and nicotine addiction: converging evidence from human and animal research. *Behav Brain Res*. 2008;193(1):1–16.
30. Swan GE, Hops H, Wilhelmsen KC, et al. A genome-wide screen for nicotine dependence susceptibility loci. *Am J Med Genet B Neuropsychiatr Genet*. 2006;141B(4):354–360.
31. Loukola A, Broms U, Maunu H, et al. Linkage of nicotine dependence and smoking behavior on 10q, 7q and 11p in twins with homogeneous genetic background. *Pharmacogenomics J*. 2008;8(3):209–219.
32. Audrain-McGovern J, Lerman C, Wileyto EP, et al. Interacting effects of genetic predisposition and depression on adolescent smoking progression. *Am J Psychiatry*. 2004;161(7):1224–1230.
33. Morley KI, Medland SE, Ferreira MA, et al. A possible smoking susceptibility locus on chromosome 11p12: evidence from sex-limitation linkage analyses in a sample of Australian twin families. *Behav Genet*. 2006;36(1):87–99.
34. Erblich J, Lerman C, Self DW, et al. Stress-induced cigarette craving: effects of the DRD2 TaqI RFLP and SLC6A3 VNTR polymorphisms. *Pharmacogenomics J*. 2004;4(2):102–109.

35. Noble EP. Addiction and its reward process through polymorphisms of the D2 dopamine receptor gene: a review. *Eur Psychiatry*. 2000;15(2):79–89.
36. Munafo MR, Flint J. Meta-analysis of genetic association studies. *Trends Genet*. 2004;20(9):439–444.
37. Carter B, Long T, Cinciripini P. A meta-analytic review of the CYP2A6 genotype and smoking behavior. *Nicotine Tob Res*. 2004;6(2):221–227.
38. Cinciripini P, Wetter D, Tomlinson G, et al. The effects of the DRD2 polymorphism on smoking cessation and negative affect: evidence for a pharmacogenetic effect on mood. *Nicotine Tob Res*. 2004;6(2):229–239.
39. Johnstone EC, Yudkin PL, Hey K, et al. Genetic variation in dopaminergic pathways and short-term effectiveness of the nicotine patch. *Pharmacogenetics*. 2004;14(2):83–90.
40. Lerman C, Wileyto EP, Patterson F, et al. The functional mu opioid receptor (OPRM1) Asn40Asp variant predicts short-term response to nicotine replacement therapy in a clinical trial. *Pharmacogenomics J*. 2004;4(3):184–192.
41. Lerman C, Shields PG, Wileyto EP, et al. Effects of dopamine transporter and receptor polymorphisms on smoking cessation in a bupropion clinical trial. *Health Psychol*. 2003;22(5):541–548.
42. Lockman PR, McAfee G, Geldenhuys WJ, et al. Brain uptake kinetics of nicotine and cotinine after chronic nicotine exposure. *J Pharmacol Exp Ther*. 2005;314(2):636–642.
43. Benowitz NL. Clinical pharmacology of nicotine: implications for understanding, preventing, and treating tobacco addiction. *Clin Pharmacol Ther*. 2008;83(4):531–541.
44. Wang H, Sun, X. Desensitized nicotinic receptors in brain. *Brain Res Rev*. 2005;48(3):420–437.
45. Benowitz NL. Pharmacology of nicotine: addiction, smoking-induced disease, and therapeutics. *Annu Rev Pharmacol Toxicol*. 2009;49:57–71.
46. Vallejo YF, Buisson B, Bertrand D, et al. Chronic nicotine exposure upregulates nicotinic receptors by a novel mechanism. *J Neurosci*. 2005;25(23):5563–5572.
47. Hukkanen J, Jacob P III, Benowitz NL. Metabolism and disposition kinetics of nicotine. *Pharmacol Rev*. 2005;57(1):79–115.
48. Derby KS, Cuthrell K, Caberto C, et al. Nicotine metabolism in three ethnic/racial groups with different risks of lung cancer. *Cancer Epidemiol Biomarkers Prev*. 2008;17(12):3526–3535.
49. Kadlubar S, Anderson JP, Sweeney C, et al. Phenotypic CYP2A6 variation and the risk of pancreatic cancer. *JOP*. 2009;10(3):263–270.
50. Haiman CA, Stram DO, Wilkens LR, et al. Ethnic and racial differences in the smoking-related risk of lung cancer. *N Engl J Med*. 2006;354(4):333–342.
51. Ben-Zaken Cohen S, Pare PD, Man SF, et al. The growing burden of chronic obstructive pulmonary disease and lung cancer in women: examining sex differences in cigarette smoke metabolism. *Am J Respir Crit Care Med*. 2007;176(2):113–120.
52. Benowitz NL, Lessov-Schlaggar CN, Swan GE, et al. Female sex and oral contraceptive use accelerate nicotine metabolism. *Clin Pharmacol Ther*. 2006;79(5):480–488.
53. Franklin TR, Wang Z, Wang J, et al. Limbic activation to cigarette smoking cues independent of nicotine withdrawal: a perfusion fMRI study. *Neuropsychopharmacology*. 2007;32(11):2301–2309.
54. Fiore MC, Jaen CR, Baker TB, et al. *Treating Tobacco Use and Dependence: 2008 Update*. Clinical Practice Guidelines. Rockville, MD: U.S. Department of Health and Human Services, Public Health Service; 2008.
55. Quinn VP, Stevens VJ, Hollis JF, et al. Tobacco-cessation services and patient satisfaction in nine nonprofit HMOs. *Am J Prev Med*. 2005;29(2):77–84.
56. Heatherton TF, Kozlowski LT, Frecker RC, et al. The Fagerström Test for Nicotine Dependence: a revision of the Fagerström Tolerance Questionnaire. *Br J Addict*. 1991;86(9):1119–1127.
57. Maciosek MV, Coffield AB, Edwards NM, et al. Priorities among effective clinical preventive services: results of a systematic review and analysis. *Am J Prev Med*. 2006;31(1):52–61.
58. Solberg LI, Maciosek MV, Edwards NM, et al. Repeated tobacco-use screening and intervention in clinical practice: health impact and cost effectiveness. *Am J Prev Med*. 2006;31(1):62–71.
59. Stead LF, Perera R, Bullen C, et al. Nicotine replacement therapy for smoking cessation. *Cochrane Database Syst Rev*. 2008;(1):CD000146.
60. Hurt RD, Sachs DP, Glover ED, et al. A comparison of sustained-release bupropion and placebo for smoking cessation. *N Engl J Med*. 1997;337(17):1195–1202.
61. Hughes JR, Stead LF, Lancaster T. Antidepressants for smoking cessation. *Cochrane Database Syst Rev*. 2007;(1):CD000031
62. Gonzales DH, Nides MA, Ferry LH, et al. Bupropion SR as an aid to smoking cessation in smokers treated previously with bupropion: a randomized placebo-controlled study. *Clin Pharmacol Ther*. 2001;69(6):438–444.
63. Hays JT, Hurt RD, Rigotti NA, et al. Sustained-release bupropion for pharmacologic relapse prevention after smoking cessation: a randomized, controlled trial. *Ann Intern Med*. 2001;135(6):423–433.
64. Hurt RD, Krook JE, Croghan IT, et al. Nicotine patch therapy based on smoking rate followed by bupropion for prevention of relapse to smoking. *J Clin Oncol*. 2003;21(5):914–920.
65. Killen JD, Fortmann SP, Murphy GM Jr, et al. Extended treatment with bupropion SR for cigarette smoking cessation. *J Consult Clin Psychol*. 2006;74(2):286–294.
66. Haggstram FM, Chatkin JM, Sussenbach-Vaz E, et al. A controlled trial of nortriptyline, sustained-release bupropion and placebo for smoking cessation: preliminary results. *Pulm Pharmacol Ther*. 2006;19(3):205–209.
67. Wagena EJ, Knipschild PG, Huibers MJ, et al. Efficacy of bupropion and nortriptyline for smoking cessation among people at risk for or with chronic obstructive pulmonary disease. *Arch Intern Med*. 2005;165(19):2286–2292.
68. Hall SM, Humfleet GL, Reus VI, et al. Extended nortriptyline and psychological treatment for cigarette smoking. *Am J Psychiatry*. 2004;161(11):2100–2107.
69. Coe JW, Brooks PR, Vetelino MG, et al. Varenicline: an alpha4beta2 nicotinic receptor partial agonist for smoking cessation. *J Med Chem*. 2005;48(10):3474–3477.
70. Jorenby DE, Hays JT, Rigotti NA, et al. Efficacy of varenicline, an alpha4beta2 nicotinic acetylcholine receptor partial agonist, vs placebo or sustained-release bupropion for smoking cessation: a randomized controlled trial. *JAMA*. 2006;296(1):56–63.
71. Cahill K, Stead LF, Lancaster T. Nicotine receptor partial agonists for smoking cessation. *Cochrane Database Syst Rev*. 2007;(1):CD006103.
72. Tonstad S, Tonnesen P, Hajek P, et al. Effect of maintenance therapy with varenicline on smoking cessation: a randomized controlled trial. *JAMA*. 2006;296(1):64–71.
73. Oncken C, Gonzales D, Nides M, et al. Efficacy and safety of the novel selective nicotinic acetylcholine receptor partial agonist, varenicline, for smoking cessation. *Arch Intern Med*. 2006;166(15):1571–1577.

74. Shah SD, Wilken LA, Winkler SR, et al. Systematic review and meta-analysis of combination therapy for smoking cessation. *J Am Pharm Assoc (2003)*. 2008;48(5):659–665.
75. Miller WR, Rollnick S. *Motivational Interviewing: Preparing People for Change*. 2nd ed. New York, NY: Guilford Press; 2002.
76. Chan SS, Lam TH, Salili F, et al. A randomized controlled trial of an individualized motivational intervention on smoking cessation for parents of sick children: a pilot study. *Appl Nurs Res*. 2005;18(3):178–181.
77. Curry SJ, Ludman EJ, Graham E, et al. Pediatric-based smoking cessation intervention for low-income women: a randomized trial. *Arch Pediatr Adolesc Med*. 2003;157(3):295–302.
78. Hettema J, Steele J, Miller WR. Motivational interviewing. *Ann Rev Clin Psychol*. 2005;1:91–111.
79. Amrhein PC, Miller WR, Yahne CE, et al. Client commitment language during motivational interviewing predicts drug use outcomes. *J Consult Clin Psychol*. 2003;71(5):862–878.
80. Dani JA, Harris RA. Nicotine addiction and comorbidity with alcohol abuse and mental illness. *Nat Neurosci*. 2005;8(11):1465–1470.
81. McGue M, Iacono WG. The association of early adolescent problem behavior with adult psychopathology. *Am J Psychiatry*. 2005;162(6):1118–1124.
82. Stephens SH, Logel J, Barton A, et al. Association of the 5′-upstream regulatory region of the alpha7 nicotinic acetylcholine receptor subunit gene (CHRNA7) with schizophrenia. *Schizophr Res*. 2009;109(1–3):102–112.
83. Dalack GW, Healy DJ, Meador-Woodruff JH. Nicotine dependence in schizophrenia: clinical phenomena and laboratory findings. *Am J Psychiatry*. 1998;155(11):1490–1501.
84. Laviolette SR, van der Kooy D. Blockade of mesolimbic dopamine transmission dramatically increases sensitivity to the rewarding effects of nicotine in the ventral tegmental area. *Mol Psychiatry*. 2003;8(1):50–59.
85. Decina P, Caracci G, Sandik R, et al. Cigarette smoking and neuroleptic-induced parkinsonism. *Biol Psychiatry*. 1990;28(6):502–508.
86. Yassa R, Lal S, Korpassy A, et al. Nicotine exposure and tardive dyskinesia. *Biol Psychiatry*. 1987;22(1):67–72.
87. McEvoy JP, Freudenreich O, Levin ED, et al. Haloperidol increases smoking in patients with schizophrenia. *Psychopharmacology (Berl)*. 1995;119(1):124–126.
88. Rohsenow DJ, Tidey JW, Miranda R, et al. Olanzapine reduces urge to smoke and nicotine withdrawal symptoms in community smokers. *Exp Clin Psychopharmacol*. 2008;16(3):215–222.
89. Picciotto MR, Brunzell DH, Caldarone BJ. Effect of nicotine and nicotinic receptors on anxiety and depression. *Neuroreport*. 2002;13(9):1097–1106.
90. Malpass D, Higgs S. Acute psychomotor, subjective and physiological responses to smoking in depressed outpatient smokers and matched controls. *Psychopharmacology (Berl)*. 2007;190(3):363–372.
91. Lewis A, Miller JH, Lea RA. Monoamine oxidase and tobacco dependence. *Neurotoxicology*. 2007;28(1):182–195.
92. Desai HD, Seabolt J, Jann MW. Smoking in patients receiving psychotropic medications: a pharmacokinetic perspective. *CNS Drugs*. 2001;15(6):469–494.
93. Warner KE, Burns DM. Hardening and the hard-core smoker: concepts, evidence, and implications. *Nicotine Tob Res*. 2003;5(1):37–48.
94. Ziedonis D, Hitsman B, Beckham JC, et al. Tobacco use and cessation in psychiatric disorders: National Institute of Mental Health report. *Nicotine Tob Res*. 2008;10(12):1691–1715.
95. Uhl GR, Drgon T, Johnson C, et al. Addiction genetics and pleiotropic effects of common haplotypes that make polygenic contributions to vulnerability to substance dependence. *J Neurogenet*. 2009;23(3):272–282.
96. Kendler KS, Aggen SH, Tambs K, et al. Illicit psychoactive substance use, abuse and dependence in a population-based sample of Norwegian twins. *Psychol Med*. 2006;36(7):955–962.
97. Moeller FG, Barratt ES, Dougherty DM, et al. Psychiatric aspects of impulsivity. *Am J Psychiatry*. 2001;158(11):1783–1793.
98. Kreek MJ, Nielsen DA, Butelman ER, et al. Genetic influences on impulsivity, risk taking, stress responsivity and vulnerability to drug abuse and addiction. *Nat Neurosci*. 2005;8(11):1450–1457.
99. Schinka JA, Letsch EA, Crawford FC. DRD4 and novelty seeking: results of meta-analyses. *Am J Med Genet*. 2002;114(6):643–648.
100. Bart G, Heilig M, LaForge KS, et al. Substantial attributable risk related to a functional mu-opioid receptor gene polymorphism in association with heroin addiction in central Sweden. *Mol Psychiatry*. 2004;9(6):547–549.
101. Oswald LM, McCaul M, Choi L, et al. Catechol-O-methyltransferase polymorphism alters hypothalamic-pituitary-adrenal axis responses to naloxone: a preliminary report. *Biol Psychiatry*. 2004;55(1):102–105.
102. Little HJ. Behavioral mechanisms underlying the link between smoking and drinking. *Alcohol Res Health*. 2000;24(4):215–224.
103. Ceballos NA, Tivis R, Lawton-Craddock A, et al. Nicotine and cognitive efficiency in alcoholics and illicit stimulant abusers: implications of smoking cessation for substance users in treatment. *Subst Use Misuse*. 2006;41(3):265–281.
104. Tizabi Y, Al-Namaeh M, Manaye KF, et al. Protective effects of nicotine on ethanol-induced toxicity in cultured cerebellar granule cells. *Neurotox Res*. 2003;5(5):315–321.
105. Butt CM, King NM, Stitzel JA, et al. Interaction of the nicotinic cholinergic system with ethanol withdrawal. *J Pharmacol Exp Ther*. 2004;308(2):591–599.
106. Hansen ST, Mark GP. The nicotinic acetylcholine receptor antagonist mecamylamine prevents escalation of cocaine self-administration in rats with extended daily access. *Psychopharmacology (Berl)*. 2007;194(1):53–61.
107. Andrews JA, Tildesley E, Hops H, et al. The influence of peers on young adult substance use. *Health Psychol*. 2002;21(4):349–357.
108. Young SE, Corley RP, Stallings MC, et al. Substance use, abuse and dependence in adolescence: prevalence, symptom profiles and correlates. *Drug Alcohol Depend*. 2002;68(3):309–322.
109. Grau LE, Dasgupta N, Harvey AP, et al. Illicit use of opioids: is OxyContin a "gateway drug"? *Am J Addict*. 2007;16(3):166–173.
110. Parascandola M, Augustson E, O'Connell ME, et al. Consumer awareness and attitudes related to new potential reduced-exposure tobacco product brands. *Nicotine Tob Res*. 2009;11(7):886–895.
111. Parascandola M, Augustson E, Rose A. Characteristics of current and recent former smokers associated with the use of new potential reduced-exposure tobacco products. *Nicotine Tob Res*. 2009;11(12):1431–1438.

CHAPTER 22 Caffeine

Laura M. Juliano ■ Britta L. Anderson ■ Roland R. Griffiths

Caffeine (1,3,7-trimethylxanthine) is the most widely used mood-altering drug in the world. Caffeine is found in more than 60 species of plants and is the best-known member of the methylxanthine class of alkaloids. The dimethylxanthines, which include theophylline and theobromine, are structurally related compounds that are also found in various plants.

Caffeine is a nonselective A_1 and A_{2A} adenosine receptor antagonist and mild central nervous system (CNS) stimulant that produces various physiologic and psychological effects. It has long been recognized for its mild stimulating effects and has been consumed in one form or another for thousands of years despite repeated attempts throughout history to ban its use on moral, medical, economic, or political grounds. Today caffeine use remains ubiquitous. In fact, caffeine ingestion is so intricately tied to social customs and daily rituals that it is often not perceived as a drug, despite its well-documented pharmacologic effects. Moreover, common foods and other products often contain significant amounts of caffeine, although they may not be labeled as such. Thus, it is possible to significantly underestimate caffeine consumption and the role that it may play in one's daily experiences.

Behaviorally active doses of caffeine are consumed daily by a majority of adults in the United States. Caffeine is generally considered to be safe relative to classic drugs of dependence, and research suggests that it may even offer protective effects against certain diseases (e.g., Parkinson disease). However, caffeine is not a completely innocuous drug. Although there is a lack of agreement on whether caffeine should be formally considered a drug of clinical dependence, some behavioral features of caffeine use closely resemble those associated with classic drugs of dependence. Caffeine can produce tolerance and a characteristic withdrawal syndrome, and heavy use (>400 mg/day) is associated with increased risk for various health problems. Caffeine functions as a reinforcer and many habitual caffeine consumers report an inability to quit or reduce caffeine use despite a desire to do so. Caffeine can cause discrete psychopathology (e.g., caffeine intoxication, caffeine-induced anxiety disorder), exacerbate existing psychopathology (e.g., anxiety, insomnia), and interfere with the efficacy of some medications (e.g., benzodiazepines). There is also evidence that caffeine may interact with classic drugs of dependence. This chapter will review empirical data on the pharmacologic, behavioral, and clinical effects of caffeine. The review will conclude with a discussion of the clinical implications of caffeine use and practical guidelines for modifying caffeine use.

HISTORY

Caffeine was first isolated from coffee in 1820 and tea in 1827, and its chemical structure was first characterized in 1875. Caffeine has been ingested in one form or another throughout various parts of the world for thousands of years. Tea was first cultivated in China; coffee in Ethiopia; guarana, cacao, and maté in South America; and kola nut in West Africa. The word coffee is believed to have been derived from the Arabic word "qahwa," which historically referred to wine. According to legend, coffee was discovered after an Arabian goatherd observed his goats eating berries and subsequently behaving in an energetic manner. The technique of roasting and grinding coffee beans for beverage preparation was developed in Arabia by the 14th century. With the development of worldwide trade routes during the 17th and 18th centuries, caffeinated products spread rapidly from their indigenous environments to other parts of the world. The introduction of caffeine into societies, not unlike the introduction of other drugs such as tobacco, has sometimes provoked moral outrage and attempts to ban use. Failed efforts to suppress the use of caffeine-containing foods, usually in the form of coffee or tea, have been documented worldwide (including Arabia, Turkey, Egypt, England, France, and Prussia). In the late 1700s America protested a British tax on tea resulting in the "Boston Tea Party" in which shipments of tea were thrown into the Boston Harbor. The Continental Congress subsequently passed a resolution against tea consumption, and over the course of a few years coffee became the caffeinated beverage of choice in America. Today coffee is second only to oil as the largest import in the United States.

In the late 1800s, entrepreneurs began selling flavored carbonated beverages with added caffeine. Soft drink consumption has increased steadily over the last century and has become a significant source of caffeine use among individuals of all ages. Over the past decade energy drinks, which typically contain significantly higher concentrations of caffeine than soft drinks, have been growing in popularity in the United States and elsewhere. Some countries presently ban the sale of energy drinks or require health warnings on them due to concerns about negative health effects.

SOURCES OF CAFFEINE

Caffeine occurs naturally in a variety of plant-based products including coffee, tea, cocoa, kola nut, guarana, and maté. In addition to beverages made from these plants, significant

TABLE 22.1 Caffeine content of common foods and medications			
Product	Serving size (volume or weight)	Typical caffeine content (mg)	Range (mg)
Coffee			
Brewed/drip	6 oz	100	54–210
Starbucks hot brewed coffee	16 oz	330	
Espresso	1 oz	70	60–95
Starbucks espresso (solo)	1 oz	75	
Instant	6 oz	70	20–130
Decaffeinated	6 oz	4	0–10
Tea			
Brewed	6 oz	40	30–90
Instant	6 oz	30	10–35
Canned or bottled	12 oz	20	8–32
Soft drinks			
Typical caffeinated soft drink	12 oz	40	22–69
Mountain Dew/Diet Mountain Dew	12 oz	55	
Pepsi One	12 oz	55	
Mellow Yellow/Diet Mello Yellow	12 oz	51	
Diet Coke	12 oz	47	
RC Cola	12 oz	43.2	
Diet Sunkist	12 oz	42	
Sunkist	12 oz	41	
Dr. Pepper/Diet Dr. Pepper	12 oz	41	
Mr. Pibb/Diet Mr. Pibb	12 oz	40	
Pepsi-Cola	12 oz	38	
Diet Pepsi	12 oz	36	
Coke Classic	12 oz	35	
Coke Zero	12 oz	35	
Cherry Coke	12 oz	34	
A&W Cream Soda	12 oz	29	
Barq's Root Beer	12 oz	23	
A&W Diet Cream Soda	12 oz	22	
Cocoa/hot chocolate	6 oz	7	2–10
Chocolate milk	6 oz	4	2–7
Chocolate			
Hershey's Chocolate Bar	1.55 oz	9	
Hershey's Special Dark	1.45 oz	18	
Hershey's Baking Chocolate	1.0 oz	30	
Caffeinated water			
Typical amount	16.9 oz	60	60–200
Water Joe	16.9 oz	60	
Buzzwater	16.9 oz	100 or 200	
Energy drinks			
Typical amount	varies	varies	50–505
Wired-X-505	23.5 oz	505	
FIXX	20 oz	500	
Cocaine	8.2 oz	280	
Rockstar	16 oz	160	
Full Throttle	16 oz	144	

Product	Serving size (volume or weight)	Typical caffeine content (mg)	Range (mg)
Red Bull	8.3 oz	80	
Coffee ice cream or yogurt	8 oz (one cup)	50	8–85
Dannon Coffee Yogurt	6 oz	30	
Starbucks Coffee Ice Cream	8 oz	60	
Miscellaneous foods and beverages			
Stay Alert Caffeinated Gum	1 stick	100	
Starbucks bottled Frappuccino	9.5 oz	85	
Extreme Sport Beans Jelly Beans	1 oz	50	
Powerbar Tangerine Powergel	41 g	50	
Jolt Caffeinated Gum	1 stick	33	
Penguin Peppermints	1 mint	7	
Stimulants			
Typical	1 tablet	100 or 200	100–200
Vivarin	1 tablet	200	
NoDoz	1 tablet	100 or 200	
Analgesics (OTC and prescription)			
Typical	2 tablets	64 or 130	64–130
Anacin Advanced Headache	2 tablets	130	
Excedrin Extra Strength	2 tablets	130	
Goody's Headache Powder	1 powder packet	32.5	
Fiorinal	2 tablets	80	
Darvon	1 tablet	32.4	
Weight-loss products/sports nutrition			
Typical	1 or 2 tablets	Varies	50–300
Metabolife Ultra	2 caplets	150	
Dexatrim Max	1 caplet	50	
Leptopril	2 capsules	220	
Stacker 3	1 caplet	254	
Swarm Extreme Energizer	1 capsule	300	

1 fluid oz = 30 mL; 1 oz weight = 28 g; serving sizes are based on commonly consumed portions, typical container sizes, or pharmaceutical instructions. Caffeine values for brand name products were obtained from product labels, or the manufacturer's Web site or customer service department.

amounts of caffeine are found in foods such as coffee ice cream, coffee yogurt, and dark chocolate. Caffeine is added to cola and noncola soft drinks as well as to other common food items such as energy drinks, water, candy bars, mints, and gum. Caffeine is also added to hundreds of prescription and over-the-counter (OTC) medications including stimulants, analgesics, weight-loss supplements, and nutritional supplements. Table 22.1 lists the caffeine content of many common foods and medications.

In the United States, coffee and soft drinks are the major dietary sources of caffeine. The Food and Drug Administration limits the amount of caffeine that can be added to soft drinks to 0.2 mg/ml or 71.5 mg for a 12-oz serving. It is noteworthy that energy drinks often contain significantly higher levels of caffeine than those permitted in soft drinks with levels ranging from 50 to over 500 mg per can or bottle (1).

Also, manufacturers are not required to list caffeine as an ingredient in products made with naturally occurring sources of caffeine (e.g., coffee, guarana, kola nut, maté). Products made from some of the less well-recognized sources of caffeine can be a significant hidden source of caffeine. Manufacturers are also not required to provide the amount of caffeine added to beverages and other food products; however, some of the larger soft drink manufacturers have begun to label the amount of caffeine in their products in recent years.

EPIDEMIOLOGY

Estimating actual caffeine exposure in the population is challenging because caffeine is present in a vast number of products, and many consumers are completely unaware of

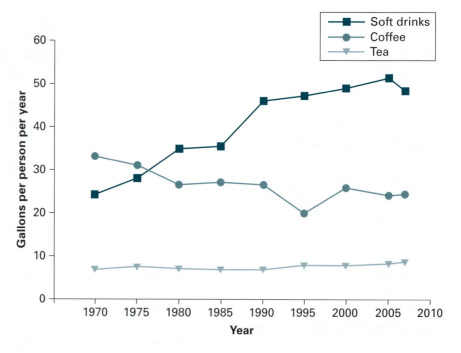

Figure 22.1. Annual per capita consumption of the three major dietary sources of caffeine in the United States. Data from the USDA/Economic Research Service 2009. U.S. Food Supply Data (1970–2007).

whether or not a given product contains caffeine. Furthermore, for many types of caffeinated products both the caffeine concentration and the serving sizes can vary over a wide range. For example, the amount of caffeine in a serving of coffee can range from 17 mg for a small 5-oz cup of instant coffee to 500 mg for a large 20-oz cup of drip coffee.

The most recent large-scale published epidemiologic data on caffeine consumption in the United States was collected more than 10 years ago. Based on the Continuing Survey of Food Intakes by Individuals in 1994 to 1996 and in 1998, it is estimated that 87% of the population in the United States 2 years and older regularly consume caffeine with an average daily consumption of about 193 mg (2). Caffeine use tends to increase with age with the highest consumption observed among adults aged 35 to 64 years (2). Caffeine consumption among adult consumers in the United States is estimated to be about 280 mg with higher daily intakes estimated for some European countries (3). Subgroups that have been identified as being heavy caffeine consumers include psychiatric patients, prisoners, smokers, alcoholics, and individuals with eating disorders. Coffee is the major source of caffeine for adults, followed by soft drinks and tea, whereas soft drinks are the major source of caffeine among children and adolescents (2). More than 50% of adults consume coffee every day, and drink just over three cups per day. Caffeinated soft drinks account for the vast majority of soft drink sales.

Figure 22.1 displays trends in annual per capita consumption of coffee, tea, and soft drinks, the three major sources of caffeine consumption in the United States. Over the nearly four decades shown, use of carbonated soft drinks has more than doubled, while coffee consumption has decreased by about 25%. Tea consumption has increased only slightly over this time period. Since the introduction of Red Bull in the United States in 1997, the energy drink market has grown exponentially, with hundreds of different brands of energy drinks now available to consumers. Sales of energy drinks have increased an average of 55% each year and sales are expected to continue on this trajectory in the coming years (1).

GENETICS

There is evidence that genetic factors account for some of the variability in the use and effects of caffeine (for citations see (4)). Large-scale twin studies have shown that relative to dizygotic twins, monozygotic twins have higher concordance rates for total caffeine consumption, heavy caffeine consumption, coffee and tea intake, caffeine tolerance, caffeine withdrawal, caffeine intoxication, and caffeine-related sleep disturbances with heritabilities ranging between 34% and 77% (5). Findings from twin studies have also suggested that there may be common genetic factors that underlie the use of caffeine, cigarette smoking, and alcohol. One large-scale twin study found that caffeine and nicotine dependence were substantially influenced by genetic factors that appeared to be unique to these licit drugs and distinct from genetic factors found to be common among illicit drugs (6).

Association studies have also been conducted to evaluate how specific gene variations are related to individual differences in the use and effects of caffeine. Because caffeine's primary mechanism of action is adenosine receptor antagonism, one particular gene that has been the focus of attention is the A_{2A} receptor gene (ADORA2A). Another gene of interest is the CYP1A2 gene, which is linked to enzymes responsible for caffeine metabolism. It has been posited that understanding variability in the CYP1A2 gene across individuals could explain variability in caffeine consumption. It has also been proposed as a method of elucidating dose-response associations between actual caffeine consumption and various effects, and health and pregnancy outcomes, by taking differences in caffeine metabolism into account. For example, recent studies have indicated that individuals who carry the CYP1A2 genotype associated with slow caffeine metabolism are at greater risk for coffee-associated hypertension and myocardial infarction (7,8). In another large-scale study, genetic variability in the ADORA2A receptor gene, but not the CYP1A2 gene, was associated with caffeine consumption (9). Variability in the ADORA2A gene has also predicted differential effects of a specific caffeine dose on anxiety (10) and sleep (11).

PHARMACOKINETICS

After oral consumption, caffeine is rapidly and completely absorbed. Caffeine rapidly passes through the blood–brain barrier and enters the brain, which accounts for the quick onset of mood-altering effects (12). Peak caffeine blood concentration (C_{max}) is generally reached in 30 to 45 minutes (13). Caffeine is highly lipid soluble and is rapidly and widely distributed throughout all body tissues and fluids including breast milk and semen. There is no placental barrier to caffeine, and thus the levels of caffeine in the fetus approach the levels of the mother (14). Saliva caffeine concentrations are highly correlated with plasma caffeine concentrations and are often used as a noninvasive alternative to measuring serum levels.

Caffeine metabolism is complex, and more than 25 caffeine metabolites have been identified in humans (15). The primary metabolic pathways involve the cytochrome P-450 liver enzyme system (primarily the CYP1A2 isoenzyme), which carries out the demethylation of caffeine to three pharmacologically active dimethylxanthines: paraxanthine, theophylline, and theobromine (16). These active metabolites need to be considered in understanding the pharmacologic actions of caffeine, especially the primary metabolite paraxanthine. The half-life of caffeine is typically 4 to 6 hours; however, the rate of caffeine metabolism is quite variable across healthy adults and can range from 2 to 12 hours (12). Due to impaired enzyme functioning, caffeine metabolism is significantly slowed among individuals with liver disease (17) as well as women in the second and third trimesters of pregnancy, who show about a threefold increase in the half-life of caffeine (18). Fetuses and newborns lack the liver enzymes needed to metabolize caffeine. Thus, caffeine metabolism in infants prior to 6 months of age is very slow, with a half-life of 80 to 100 hours (18). Tobacco smoking increases the rate of metabolism of caffeine due to stimulation of the CYP1A2 enzyme, with smokers metabolizing caffeine about twice as fast as nonsmokers.

An implication of the central role of cytochrome P-450 liver enzymes in metabolizing caffeine is that other therapeutic drugs may pharmacokinetically interact with caffeine. Inhibition of caffeine metabolism via competition for liver enzymes could lead to caffeine intoxication symptoms that could be misattributed to the effects of the drug. Furthermore, caffeine can impair the metabolism of other drugs, thus interfering with their safety and therapeutic effectiveness. Because the large majority of the population consumes caffeine, knowledge of potential caffeine–drug interactions is desirable when treating various types of psychological and physical conditions. Numerous compounds have been shown to significantly inhibit the metabolism of caffeine including but not limited to oral contraceptives, quinolone antibiotics (e.g., Enoxicin), and some selective serotonin reuptake inhibitors (SSRIs) (e.g., Luvox), reducing the clearance of caffeine by 40% to 80% (15). Some medications used to treat gastroesophageal reflux disease (GERD; e.g., cimetidine) and heart arrhythmias (e.g., propafenone) also interfere with the metabolism of caffeine (15). Caffeine has been shown to interfere with the metabolism of the sleep medication zolpidem, the antipsychotic clozapine, and bronchodilator theophylline (15).

NEUROPHARMACOLOGY

Adenosine

The primary mechanism of action of caffeine is nonselective antagonism at adenosine receptors. Adenosine is an endogenous nucleoside that plays a role in a number of central and peripheral nervous system functions. Although four adenosine receptor subtypes have been identified, A_1 and A_{2A} receptors are the major targets of caffeine (19). A_1 and A_{2A} receptors are both g-protein coupled receptors that produce a variety of downstream cellular effects via multiple mechanisms including inhibition and activation of adenylyl cyclase, respectively, and inhibition and activation of various ion channels (e.g., Ca^{2+}) (14). A_1 receptors are widely expressed in the brain with the highest densities in the hippocampus, cerebellum, cerebral cortex, and areas of the thalamus. A_{2A} receptors tend to be concentrated in dopamine-rich areas of the brain including the striatum, nucleus accumbens, and the olfactory tubercle (14). Adenosine receptors are also colocalized and functionally interact with each other as well as with dopamine receptors and glutamate receptors in various brain regions (19). A detailed analysis of the respective functions of adenosine receptors and their heteromers in physiologic and behavioral processes is presented elsewhere (14,19).

In general, adenosine has inhibitory effects on the CNS. Adenosine inhibits the release of excitatory neurotransmitters, reduces the spontaneous rate of neuron firing, and has anticonvulsant effects (14). There is also evidence that the accumulation of adenosine, triggered by energy depletion, functions as a sleep-promoting factor (20). Adenosine also suppresses motor activity and operant response rates. In the periphery, adenosine causes cerebral vasodilation, constricts bronchial smooth muscle, produces negative inotropic/chronotropic effects on the heart, and inhibits gastric secretions, lipolysis, and renin release (21).

Caffeine, which is structurally similar to adenosine, binds with adenosine receptors and produces effects that are consistent with reversal of the inhibiting effects of adenosine on the aforementioned systems. For example, in the CNS, caffeine increases spontaneous neuronal firing, increases the turnover or levels of various neurotransmitters (e.g., acetylcholine, norepinephrine, dopamine, serotonin, glutamate, and GABA), has convulsant activity, increased motor activity, and inhibits sleep (20,21). Some of the peripheral nervous system effects of caffeine include cerebral vasoconstriction, relaxation of bronchial smooth muscle, and increased gastric secretions.

Dopamine

Similar to classic stimulants such as amphetamine and cocaine, there is evidence that some of the motor and reinforcing effects of caffeine are mediated by dopaminergic mechanisms. Caffeine antagonizes adenosine at receptors that are colocalized and that functionally interact with dopamine receptors (i.e., adenosine–dopamine heteromers). Functionally, caffeine produces its motor and reinforcing effects in part by releasing the pre- and postsynaptic brakes imposed by antagonistic adenosine–dopamine interactions (19). In animal studies, caffeine produces behavioral effects similar to classic dopaminergically mediated stimulants such as increased locomotor activity, increased rotational behavior, stimulant-like discriminative stimulus effects, and self-injection. Caffeine potentiates the behavioral effects of dopaminergically mediated stimulants on these same behaviors, effects that can be diminished or abolished by the blockade or depletion of dopamine receptors (14,22).

Dopamine release in the shell of the nucleus accumbens appears to be a neuropharmacologic mechanism underlying the abuse potential of many drugs (23). In vivo microdialysis studies demonstrate that caffeine increases dopamine release in the dorsal shell of the nucleus accumbens (24,25).

Other Mechanisms

Caffeine can also inhibit phosphodiesterase activity and mobilize intracellular calcium release (21). However, these effects are generally observed at levels much higher than typical dietary doses. Nevertheless, it remains possible that these nonadenosine mechanisms may mediate some of the effects produced by high doses of caffeine such as those associated with caffeine intoxication. For example, there are preclinical data that suggest that some of the cardiac and respiratory effects of caffeine may be mediated via inhibition of phosphodiesterase activity (21).

PHYSIOLOGIC EFFECTS

Caffeine produces effects on a variety of organ systems as has been reviewed elsewhere (4,12). At moderate dietary doses, caffeine increases blood pressure and tends to have no effect or to reduce heart rate. Caffeine constricts cerebral blood vessels and reduces cerebral blood flow. Caffeine dilates bronchial pathways, although not as effectively as theophylline (12), and increases the rate of respiration. Caffeine stimulates gastric acid secretion (12) and colonic activity. Caffeine produces dose-related thermogenic effects, lipolysis (12), and has been shown to be ergogenic during exercise (26,27). Caffeine increases plasma epinephrine, norepinephrine, rennin, and free fatty acids. Caffeine increases diuresis and the urinary excretion of calcium, magnesium, potassium, sodium, and chlorides. Caffeine also increases adrenocorticotropic hormone (ACTH) and cortisol levels. Caffeine increases insulin levels and reduces insulin sensitivity in healthy individuals, and increases postprandial glucose and insulin responses among patients with type 2 diabetes who are habitual coffee drinkers (28). Not all of the observed physiologic effects of caffeine necessarily have clinical significance (see the section "Caffeine and Health" in this chapter), and the development of tolerance needs to be considered in understanding the physiologic effects of caffeine consumption.

THERAPEUTIC USES

As a mild central nervous stimulant, caffeine is commonly used to increase energy and alertness and ward off fatigue. A number of OTC caffeine preparations are marketed as energy aids (e.g., Vivarin, NoDoz). Studies demonstrate that caffeine can enhance cognitive and motor performance, especially under conditions of fatigue, sleep deprivation, or caffeine withdrawal. Caffeine is also used to enhance athletic performance due to its ergogenic effects (26,27), and has been restricted by some major athletic governing bodies. Caffeine can enhance the analgesic effects of certain medications, and it is currently added to a variety of OTC and prescription analgesics (e.g., Excedrin, Cafergot) used to treat various types of pain including headache. Not surprisingly, caffeine is the most effective treatment for caffeine withdrawal headaches, which are likely caused by rebound cerebral vasodilation in response to acute caffeine abstinence. Likewise, caffeine can prevent postsurgical caffeine withdrawal headaches when administered prophylactically to habitual caffeine consumers (29). As a respiratory stimulant, caffeine is one of the standard treatments for apnea of prematurity in neonates. Because of its lipolytic and thermogenic effects, caffeine is also used to promote weight loss and can be found in many weight-loss products. Caffeine has also been used to treat postprandial hypotension, although its therapeutic effectiveness for this indication is unclear.

CAFFEINE AND HEALTH

The possibility that caffeine may pose health risks is of great interest to the general public and scientific community, and has been the focus of numerous studies and scholarly reviews (30–32). Though associations between caffeine consumption and various health conditions have been found, there is no evidence for nonreversible pathologic consequences of caffeine use (e.g., cancer, congenital malformations). However, there are some groups of individuals who are considered to be at higher risk for caffeine-related problems including pregnant women, children, adolescents, and the elderly (31). Furthermore, individuals with medical problems such as hypertension, diabetes, cardiac problems, urinary incontinence, insomnia, and anxiety may be more vulnerable to the adverse effects of caffeine. As discussed in more detail throughout this chapter, caffeine use can also be associated with several distinct psychiatric syndromes: caffeine intoxication, caffeine withdrawal, caffeine dependence, caffeine-induced sleep disorder, and caffeine-induced anxiety disorder. Recent epidemiologic research also suggests that caffeine and/or coffee consumption may offer some protective effects against specific diseases (31). The associations between caffeine and specific health issues are briefly outlined below.

Negative Health Effects

Research has shown that caffeine can increase blood pressure by 5 to 15 mg Hg systolic and 5 to 10 Hg diastolic for several hours in healthy adults (32). It has been argued that, even after taking the effects of tolerance into account, the hypertensive effects of caffeine represent an important cardiovascular risk factor (33,34). A recent longitudinal genetic association study found that variability in the CYP1A2 gene predicted the later development of hypertension, with those carrying the allele associated with slow metabolism of caffeine having a much greater risk of developing coffee-associated hypertension (7). Caffeine can influence heart rate variability and increase arterial stiffness with peak effects about 60 minutes after ingestion, but the clinical significance of these findings is not clear (35). Both caffeinated and decaffeinated coffees contain lipids that significantly raise serum total and low-density lipoprotein (LDL) cholesterol (31). The highest levels of lipids are delivered from espresso (a component of many popular coffee drinks such as cappuccino and latte), French press, Turkish, and boiled coffee. Instant coffees and those prepared by paper filtration contain much lower levels of these lipids. Epidemiologic studies examining the relationship between coffee consumption and risk of myocardial infarction (MI) on the whole have been equivocal; however a recent analysis suggests that coffee-associated risk of MI is much greater among coffee drinkers who have the CYP1A2 genotype associated with slow caffeine metabolism (8). Some studies suggest that coffee can exacerbate gastroesophageal reflux (GERD); however, it is not clear if it is due specifically to caffeine or other coffee constituents.

Caffeine also increases detrusor instability (i.e., unstable bladder) in patients with complaints of urinary urgency and detrusor instability. Chronic caffeine consumption has been shown to contribute to urinary incontinence in psychogeriatric patients, and caffeine reduction can improve urinary incontinence symptoms (36). Caffeine increases the urinary excretion of calcium. Thus, it has been suggested that caffeine may negatively affect overall calcium balance; however, the amount of increased calcium loss due to caffeine is likely not clinically significant in individuals with adequate calcium intake (32). Associations between high caffeine consumption and bone fractures have been observed in some epidemiologic studies, particularly among women with low calcium intake (37); however, a direct effect of caffeine on the increased likelihood of fractures has not been observed. Caffeine has also been shown to impair glucose metabolism and insulin sensitivity among individuals with type 2 diabetes (28) and among pregnant women with gestational diabetes (38).

The degree to which maternal caffeine consumption affects pregnancy outcomes has been given considerable research attention. Caffeine readily crosses the placental barrier and is distributed to all fetal tissues including the CNS. Fetuses lack the necessary enzyme systems to metabolize caffeine, and caffeine metabolism slows considerably in the later stages of pregnancy allowing for substantial fetal exposure (18). Research suggests that maternal caffeine use increases the likelihood of spontaneous abortion in a roughly dose-dependent fashion (39,40). Associations between high caffeine use and decreased fecundity and reduced fetal growth have also been observed (31,32), including a recent study that showed that reduced fetal growth was predicted by as little as one to two cups of coffee consumption per day (41). Comprehensive scientific reviews of research on caffeine and pregnancy have concluded that reproductive aged women should consume no more than 300 mg of caffeine per day (31,32).

There is no evidence that caffeine has negative effects on cancer risk, fibrocystic breast disease, peptic or duodenal ulcers, or risk of stroke.

Positive Health Effects

Case control and epidemiologic studies have suggested a relationship between caffeine consumption and reduced risk of Parkinson disease (42). Epidemiologic studies have also reported an association between coffee drinking and reduced incidence of chronic liver disease (43), although the potential mechanisms are unclear, and may be unrelated to caffeine. Additionally, epidemiologic studies have reported a protective effect of coffee drinking for risk of developing type 2 diabetes with the effects attributed to coffee constituents other than caffeine (44).

SUBJECTIVE AND DISCRIMINATIVE STIMULUS EFFECTS

Acute doses of caffeine in the typical dietary dose range (i.e., 20 to 200 mg), produce a number of positive subjective effects including increased well-being, happiness, energy, alertness, and sociability (4,45). These effects are qualitatively similar to those produced by other stimulants such as amphetamine and cocaine (46). In habitual caffeine consumers positive subjective effects are most reliably demonstrated when caffeine is administered after a period of caffeine abstinence and thus may in part represent a reversal of withdrawal (47,48). However, positive subjective effects of caffeine have also been demonstrated in caffeine consumers under conditions of minimal caffeine abstinence as well as among light nonhabitual caffeine consumers.

Negative subjective effects typically emerge at higher caffeine doses. Acute doses of caffeine greater than 200 mg are more likely to produce increased reports of anxiety, jitteriness, tense negative mood, upset stomach, insomnia, and "bad effects." Individual differences in caffeine sensitivity and tolerance seem to play an important role in the likelihood and severity of negative subjective effects. For example, individuals with panic disorder or generalized anxiety disorder tend to be particularly sensitive to the anxiogenic effects of caffeine.

The negative subjective effects of caffeine tend to be relatively mild and short-lived, consistent with its half-life of 4 to 6 hours. However, very high doses of caffeine have been associated with clinically significant distress and psychopathology (e.g., caffeine intoxication), as discussed in the section "Caffeine Intoxication."

Several studies have demonstrated that most individuals can reliably discriminate caffeine (100 to 320 mg) from placebo (4). Some individuals are able to discriminate very low doses of caffeine (e.g., 10 mg) after training (45), which is consistent with findings that low doses of caffeine (e.g., 9 to 12.5 mg) can produce improvements in behavioral performance (49). Subjects in these studies generally report making the discrimination based on the subjective effects of caffeine, with positive subjective effects typically providing the basis for low caffeine dose discrimination and negative subjective effects providing the basis for high dose discrimination.

Drug discrimination studies have demonstrated both similarities and differences between caffeine and other stimulant drugs. For example, both caffeine and d-amphetamine produced cocaine-appropriate responding in a cocaine versus placebo discrimination study (50). Other studies showed that caffeine produced dose-related partial generalization to d-amphetamine in d-amphetamine-trained subjects (46) and that subjects can be trained to reliably discriminate between caffeine and d-amphetamine (51). In caffeine-trained subjects methylphenidate and theophylline produced caffeine-appropriate responding (4).

PERFORMANCE

Many studies have examined the effects of caffeine on human performance (for citations see (4)). In general, caffeine at normal dietary doses can restore performance that has been degraded by sleep deprivation, fatigue, prolonged vigilance, or caffeine withdrawal (52,53). Specifically, caffeine improves sustained attention (or vigilance), reaction time, and tapping speed relative to placebo, although results are variable across studies and the effects are often small. The effect of caffeine on memory has also been investigated, but there is little evidence for an association. A number of recent studies using military personnel have demonstrated that caffeine can improve performance relative to placebo on military-type cognitive (e.g., vigilance) and physical tasks (e.g., running times) after periods of prolonged wakefulness (53).

The great majority of studies claiming to demonstrate performance-enhancing effects of caffeine are difficult to interpret because they do not account for the effects of caffeine withdrawal. That is, many studies compare the effects of caffeine versus placebo in regular caffeine consumers who have abstained from caffeine, usually overnight. Under these conditions, improvements in performance after caffeine relative to placebo may reflect restoration of performance deficits caused by withdrawal, rather than a performance-enhancing effect of caffeine per se (47). However, some studies have shown caffeine-related performance enhancements among light nondependent caffeine consumers and nonconsumers. It seems likely that caffeine enhances human performance on some types of tasks (e.g., vigilance), especially among nontolerant individuals. Performance enhancements beyond withdrawal reversal effects are likely to be modest among high-dose habitual caffeine consumers (47).

There is a growing body of research on the effects of caffeine on exercise performance. In general, controlled studies show that relative to placebo, caffeine can enhance performance during endurance exercise (e.g., 30 to 120 minutes) (26,54), can reduce ratings of perceived exhaustion or effort, and can improve speed and/or power output in simulated race conditions. Some studies have also demonstrated a beneficial effect of caffeine during short-term high-intensity exercise and anaerobic resistance training, but these effects are generally more difficult to demonstrate and smaller than effects observed during endurance activities (54). A number of nonindependent mechanisms have been proposed to explain caffeine's ergogenic effects including increased fatty acid oxidation, increased availability of muscle glycogen, mobilization of intracellular calcium, increased muscle contractile force, and direct CNS effects via adenosine antagonism (26). There is also some evidence that caffeine may increase muscle contractile force during endurance exercise (27).

Studies have directly compared the effects of caffeine, modafinil, and d-amphetamine on vigilance performance after an extended period of sleep restriction (44 to 64 hours) and showed that the three stimulants were equally effective at restoring vigilance performance, with caffeine having the shortest duration of action and d-amphetamine having the longest (55).

CAFFEINE AND SLEEP

It is well documented that caffeine increases wakefulness and inhibits sleep onset. The mechanism of action is hypothesized to be antagonism of endogenous adenosine, which is believed to be a homeostatic sleep factor that mediates sleepiness following prolonged wakefulness (20). Perhaps the most widely accepted therapeutic use of caffeine is to increase wakefulness and alertness, and reverse performance decrements produced by sleep deprivation (56). There is also abundant evidence that caffeine has disruptive effects on planned sleep (i.e., insomnia). Caffeine ingested throughout the day or before bedtime has been shown to interfere with sleep onset, total time slept, sleep quality, and sleep stages (56). Because of caffeine's ability to disrupt sleep, caffeine is used as a challenge agent to study insomnia in healthy volunteers. Caffeine's effects on sleep appear to be determined by a number of factors including dose, the time between caffeine ingestion and attempted sleep, and individual differences in sensitivity and/or tolerance to caffeine. Caffeine's effects on sleep appear to be dose dependent, with greater amounts of caffeine causing greater sleep difficulties. The closer caffeine is taken to bedtime, the more likely it is to produce disruptive effects. However, 200 mg of caffeine taken early in the morning has been shown to produce small but significant effects on the following night's total sleep time, sleep efficiency, and EEG power spectra (57). Caffeine-induced sleep disturbance is greatest among nonconsumers of caffeine; however, it is not clear whether this difference is due to an absence of acquired tolerance or to a preexisting population difference in sensitivity to caffeine. Genetic factors appear to explain some of the individual differences in sensitivity to the sleep-disruptive effects of caffeine. For example, variation in the ADORA2A gene has been shown to be associated with individual differences in caffeine's effects on sleep, measured both subjectively and objectively (11). Although there is evidence for tolerance to the sleep-disrupting effects of caffeine, tolerance appears to be incomplete, and thus regular caffeine consumers may still be vulnerable to caffeine-related sleep problems. A recent study concluded that the sleep-disruptive effects of caffeine are more pronounced during daytime recovery sleep than nocturnal sleep, perhaps due to an interaction of caffeine pharmacology and circadian rhythms (58).

In addition to caffeine's ability to disrupt sleep, there have been case reports of caffeine causing hypersomnia. Furthermore, acute abstinence after chronic caffeine consumption has been shown to increase daytime sleepiness as well as to increase nighttime sleep duration and quality (59).

The *DSM-IV-TR* includes a diagnosis of caffeine-induced sleep disorder, which is characterized by a prominent sleep disturbance that is etiologically related to caffeine use (60). It is not necessary to meet full criteria for a *DSM-IV-TR* sleep disorder to qualify for a diagnosis of caffeine-induced sleep disorder. Caffeine is most often associated with insomnia; however, the *DSM-IV-TR* also recognizes hypersomnia due to caffeine withdrawal. Caffeine-induced sleep disorder is diagnosed when symptoms of a sleep disturbance (e.g., insomnia) are greater than would be expected during caffeine intoxication or caffeine withdrawal. There are no specific data on the prevalence or incidence of caffeine-induced sleep disorder.

REINFORCEMENT

A number of carefully controlled research studies over the past 20 years provide substantial evidence for the reinforcing effects of caffeine (for citations see (4)). Controlled laboratory studies demonstrate that subjects will choose caffeine over placebo in double-blind choice procedures, as well as perform work or forfeit money in exchange for caffeine. When multiple self-administration opportunities are available within a day, doses as low as 25 mg have been shown to be reinforcing (61). When self-administration is limited to once a day, then doses of 100 and 200 mg are reinforcing, while doses of 400 mg and greater tend to be avoided.

There is quite a bit of individual variability in the reinforcing effects of caffeine. Across studies, the overall incidence of caffeine reinforcement in normal caffeine users is approximately 40%, with a higher incidence (i.e., 80% to 100%) of reinforcement under conditions of repeated caffeine exposure. In choice studies, subjects who choose caffeine tend to report positive subjective effects, whereas those who choose placebo are more likely to report negative subjective effects (e.g., jitteriness) at low to moderate caffeine doses (62).

Caffeine physical dependence potentiates the reinforcing effects of caffeine. For example, caffeine consumers were more than twice as likely to show caffeine reinforcement if they reported caffeine withdrawal symptoms after drinking decaffeinated coffee (63). In studies in which caffeine physical dependence has been experimentally manipulated, subjects are more than twice as likely to choose caffeine over placebo when they are physically dependent (64). There is also evidence that avoidance of caffeine withdrawal determines caffeine consumption to a greater extent than the positive effects of caffeine (64). Caffeine reinforcement also appears to be influenced by task requirements. That is, in a double-blind study subjects chose caffeine over placebo when required to perform a vigilance task, but chose placebo over caffeine when required to engage in relaxation (65).

A series of studies have used a conditioned flavor preference paradigm to provide indirect evidence of caffeine reinforcement (66). In these studies, subjects who were repeatedly exposed to a novel flavored drink paired with caffeine tended to show increased ratings of drink pleasantness, while subjects receiving placebo-paired drinks showed decreased ratings of drink pleasantness (67). Among habitual caffeine consumers, the ability of caffeine to produce increases in flavor liking appears to be primarily determined by the alleviation of withdrawal symptoms (i.e., negative reinforcement) (67). It seems plausible that such conditioned flavor preferences in the natural environment play an important role in the development of consumer preferences for different types of caffeine-containing beverages.

Caffeine reinforcement has also been observed in animals using self-administration, conditioned place preference, and conditioned taste aversion procedures. In contrast to classic abused stimulants such as amphetamine and cocaine, caffeine self-administration is observed in animals under a relatively narrow range of conditions (4).

TOLERANCE

The degree of caffeine tolerance depends on a number of factors including the challenge and maintenance doses, frequency of administration, and individual differences in caffeine elimination. High doses of caffeine (400 to 1200 mg/day) administered throughout the day have been shown to produce "complete" tolerance to some, but not all of the effects of caffeine. However, typical dietary doses of caffeine do not usually produce complete tolerance to caffeine's central and peripheral effects.

Controlled human laboratory studies have demonstrated tolerance to the subjective effects of caffeine. Complete tolerance (i.e., no difference between placebo and caffeine after prolonged caffeine administration) to subjective effects (e.g., energetic) has been demonstrated after 300 mg t.i.d. for 18 days (62) and 200 mg b.i.d for 14 days (68), but not after lower doses or shorter exposure periods (69). Substantial but incomplete tolerance has been shown to the sleep-disruptive effects of high doses of caffeine (e.g., 400 mg t.i.d. for 7 days) (4).

Some studies have shown complete tolerance to blood pressure and other physiologic effects (plasma norepinephrine and epinephrine and plasma rennin activity) after high doses of caffeine (e.g., 600 to 750 mg/day) (33). However, about half of the subjects fail to show complete tolerance to the hypertensive effects of caffeine even after maintenance dosing with 600 mg/day (70). Doses in the range of typical daily caffeine consumption (i.e., 300 to 400 mg/day) produce only incomplete tolerance to hypertensive and other physiologic effects of caffeine (e.g., cerebral blood flow velocity, EEG) (33,68,69).

PHYSICAL DEPENDENCE AND WITHDRAWAL

The caffeine withdrawal syndrome has been well-characterized. A 2004 comprehensive review of caffeine withdrawal evaluated 57 experimental studies and 9 survey studies to validate individual symptoms of caffeine withdrawal and identify other important parameters of the caffeine withdrawal syndrome (71). That review identified 13 caffeine withdrawal symptoms that were reliably observed across carefully controlled studies (Table 22.2). Headache is a hallmark feature of caffeine withdrawal with approximately 50% of regular caffeine users reporting headache by the end of the first day of abstinence. Such headaches have been described as diffuse, throbbing, gradual in development, and sensitive to movement. Caffeine constricts cerebral blood vessels via antagonism of adenosine. Caffeine abstinence produces rebound cerebral vasodilatation and increased cerebral blood flow, and such vascular changes are a likely mechanism underlying caffeine withdrawal headache (68,72). Other commonly observed caffeine withdrawal symptoms include fatigue, decreased energy/activeness, decreased alertness, drowsiness, decreased contentedness, depressed mood, difficulty concentrating, irritability, and foggy/not clearheaded. In addition, flu-like symptoms, nausea/vomiting, and muscle pain/stiffness can be present (71). These symptoms can be conceptually clustered into five categories: (a) headache, (b) fatigue or drowsiness, (c) dysphoric mood, depressed mood or irritability, (d) difficulty concentrating, and (e) flu-like somatic symptoms of nausea, vomiting, and muscle pain/stiffness (71), but empirical studies are needed to statistically determine how symptoms cluster together. Changes in EEG, increased cerebral blood flow, and cognitive and behavioral performance deficits have also been observed during acute caffeine abstinence (68,71).

Withdrawal symptoms typically emerge 12 to 24 hours after the last dose of caffeine and tend to peak within the first 2 days. Symptoms usually persist anywhere from 2 to 9 days (71), although there are reports of caffeine withdrawal headache lasting for up to 3 weeks (71).

The severity of caffeine withdrawal can range from mild to incapacitating. There is variability in withdrawal severity both within and across individuals. The incidence of caffeine withdrawal–related impairment or distress to the point of significantly interfering with normal functioning is about 13%. For example, caffeine withdrawal can produce severe headaches that are described as the worst ever experienced (73). Some individuals experiencing caffeine withdrawal have reported that they cannot continue to perform their normal daily activities such as caring for children or going to work (74).

Although there is wide variability across individuals, in general the likelihood and severity of caffeine withdrawal increases as daily caffeine dose increases (75). The daily caffeine dose necessary to produce withdrawal is surprisingly low, with significant withdrawal symptoms observed in individuals consuming as little as 100 mg caffeine per day—the amount in a small cup of brewed coffee (75,76). Caffeine withdrawal can occur after relatively short-term exposure to daily caffeine. Significant withdrawal symptoms have been observed after just three consecutive days of 300 mg/day caffeine, with more severe withdrawal symptoms manifesting after 7 and 14 consecutive days of caffeine (75). In individuals who normally abstain from caffeine, withdrawal headache has been observed in individuals after just a week of prescribed heavy caffeine consumption (i.e., 600 to 750 mg) (73).

Caffeine withdrawal symptoms are usually alleviated quickly after caffeine re-exposure (i.e., 60 minutes or less). Caffeine withdrawal can be suppressed by caffeine doses well below the usual daily dose (e.g., 25 mg caffeine suppressed withdrawal after daily doses of 300 mg) (75). An implication of these findings is that a substantial decrease in caffeine consumption is necessary to manifest the full caffeine withdrawal syndrome.

TABLE 22.2 Empirically validated symptoms of caffeine withdrawal

Headache
Tiredness/fatigue
Drowsiness/sleepiness
Irritability
Depressed mood
Difficulty concentrating
Muzzy/foggy/not clearheaded
Flu-like symptoms
Nausea/vomiting
Muscle pain/stiffness
Decreased energy/activeness
Decreased alertness/attentiveness
Decreased contentedness/well-being

Source: Juliano LM, Griffiths RR. A critical review of caffeine withdrawal: empirical validation of symptoms and signs, incidence, severity, and associated features. *Psychopharmacology (Berl)*. 2004;176:1–29.

Retrospective survey studies have also been conducted to determine the frequency of caffeine withdrawal in the general population. In one population-based random digit dialing survey study, 44% of caffeine users reported having stopped or reduced caffeine use for at least 24 hours in the past year. Of those, over 40% reported experiencing one or more withdrawal symptoms. Interestingly, over 70% of those who stopped or reduced caffeine as part of a permanent quit attempt reported withdrawal symptoms, and 24% reported headache and other symptoms that interfered with performance (77). In another study, 11% of caffeine users who were making an inquiry about participation in a clinical research trial reported that they had "problems or symptoms on stopping caffeine in the past," of which 25% reported that the problems were severe enough to interfere with normal activity (78). The number of individuals who actually experienced a period of caffeine abstinence was not ascertained.

Although most withdrawal research has been with adults, there is evidence that children and adolescents who use caffeine also experience caffeine withdrawal symptoms upon abstinence (79). It is possible that children may be even more susceptible to experiencing withdrawal episodes as they likely have less control over the regular availability of caffeine-containing products. Caffeine withdrawal has also been documented in neonates born to mothers who have had recent caffeine exposure.

The observations that caffeine withdrawal can cause clinically significant distress or functional impairment have resulted in the inclusion of caffeine withdrawal as an *ICD-10* diagnosis (80) and as a proposed diagnosis in *DSM-IV-TR* (60,81). The 1994 *DSM* Work Group included caffeine withdrawal as a proposed diagnosis rather than an official diagnosis to encourage further research on the range and specificity of caffeine withdrawal symptoms (81). Carefully controlled research on caffeine withdrawal has more than doubled since 1994, now providing a sound empirical basis for a diagnosis of caffeine withdrawal (71). The *DSM-IV-TR* criteria are conservative in that it excludes cases in which other withdrawal symptoms occur in the absence of headache. It also excludes symptoms that have been documented in recent studies including dysphoric mood, difficulty concentrating, and irritability, and includes a symptom for which there is little empirical support (i.e., anxiety). To date, only one study has evaluated the incidence of caffeine withdrawal using *DSM-IV-TR* criteria (77). This population-based survey found that 11% of those who had given up or reduced caffeine use in the past year met criteria for caffeine withdrawal. Among individuals who reported trying to stop caffeine use permanently, 24% met criteria for caffeine withdrawal.

Caffeine withdrawal symptoms overlap with various psychological and physical ailments. Caffeine withdrawal should be considered when patients present with headaches, fatigue, mood disturbances, impaired concentration, and flu-like symptoms. Patients are often asked to stop food and fluids before certain blood tests, surgery, or medical procedures (e.g., colonoscopies, fasting blood sugar tests) and may experience adverse effects that could go unrecognized as caffeine withdrawal. Caffeine withdrawal has been identified as a significant cause of postoperative headaches, the risk of which can be reduced if habitual caffeine consumers are administered caffeine on the day of the surgical procedure (29).

A recent study directly compared periods of abstinence from either caffeine or nicotine among habitual users of both drugs and found no differences between the two in the psychosocial manifestations of withdrawal as measured by subjective well-being, social functioning, and drug craving (82).

CAFFEINE INTOXICATION

Caffeine intoxication is currently defined by the *DSM-IV-TR* by a number of symptoms and clinical features that emerge in response to excessive consumption of caffeine (Table 22.3) (60). The most common features of caffeine intoxication include nervousness, restlessness, insomnia, gastrointestinal upset, muscle twitching, tachycardia, and psychomotor agitation. Fever, irritability, tremors, sensory disturbances, tachypnea, and headaches have also been reported in response to excess caffeine use (4).

DSM-IV-TR diagnostic guidelines require that the diagnosis be dependent on recent consumption of at least 250 mg of caffeine, but much higher doses (>500 mg) are usually associated with the syndrome. High-dose intoxicating effects of caffeine are very unpleasant and are not usually sought out by users. Individual differences in sensitivity to caffeine and tolerance likely play a role in vulnerability to caffeine intoxication. Although caffeine intoxication can occur in the context of habitual chronic consumption of high doses of caffeine, it most often occurs after consumption of large doses in infrequent caffeine users, or in regular users who have substantially increased their intake. There are generally no long-lasting consequences of caffeine intoxication, although caffeine can be lethal at very high doses (e.g., 5 to 10 g), and there are documented cases of accidental death and suicide by caffeine overdose, usually in the form of pills (4).

Few studies have assessed the prevalence of caffeine intoxication, and most have evaluated selected populations (e.g., psychiatric inpatients) and used ambiguous criteria. One general population survey found that 7% of respondents met *DSM-IV* criteria for caffeine intoxication (77). The occurrence of individual symptoms of caffeine intoxication appears to be fairly common (e.g., nervousness). For example, a study involving more than 3600 twins found that 29% reported having felt ill or shaky or jittery after consuming caffeinated beverages (83). In a survey of college students, 19% reported experiencing heart palpitations after consuming energy drinks (1).

A recent study evaluated 265 cases of caffeine overuse that were reported to a local area poison center between 2001 and 2004 after ingestion of caffeinated products other than coffee or tea (1). They found that caffeine was in the

TABLE 22.3	Diagnostic criteria for caffeine intoxication (*DSM-IV-TR*)
A)	Recent consumption of caffeine, usually in excess of 250 mg (e.g., more than two to three cups of brewed coffee)
B)	Five (or more) of the following signs, developing during, or shortly after, caffeine use: 1) Restlessness 2) Nervousness 3) Excitement 4) Insomnia 5) Flushed face 6) Diuresis 7) Gastrointestinal disturbance 8) Muscle twitching 9) Rambling flow of thought and speech 10) Tachycardia or cardiac arrhythmia 11) Periods of inexhaustibility 12) Psychomotor agitation
C)	The symptoms in Criterion B cause clinically significant distress or impairment in social, occupational, or other important areas of functioning.
D)	The symptoms are not due to a general medical condition and are not better accounted for by another mental disorder (e.g., an anxiety disorder).

From American Psychiatric Association. *The Diagnostic and Statistical Manual of Mental Disorders, Fourth Edition Text Revision.* Washington, DC: American Psychiatric Association; 2000, with permission.

form of a medication in 77% of the cases, a caffeine-enhanced beverage in 16% of cases, and a dietary supplement in 14% of cases. Patients were typically young (21 years old on average), half were male, and 12% required hospitalization. Caffeine was implicated in 4656 reports to poison control centers in the United States in 2005, with half warranting treatment in a health care facility (1). Caffeinated gum and energy capsules have also been implicated in published case reports of caffeine intoxication in teenagers requiring medical attention.

It appears that reports of caffeine intoxication may be increasing with the growing popularity of highly caffeinated energy drinks (1). It has been postulated that the potential for caffeine intoxication to occur from consumption of energy drinks may be greater than other dietary sources of caffeine because of the absence of caffeine content labeling and appropriate health warnings, and their appeal and marketing to young and perhaps nontolerant individuals (1). For example, a recent series of case reports based on poison control center data found that a particular energy drink containing 250 mg of caffeine was implicated in a number of reports of caffeine intoxication. The most common symptoms were hypertension, jitteriness, agitation, tremors, nausea, vomiting, and dizziness (84). Consumption of about eight cans of energy drinks (or 640 mg caffeine) was implicated in the cardiac arrest suffered by a 28-year-old male motocross racer (1). There have also been numerous media reports of children becoming sick after consuming energy drinks (1).

CAFFEINE AND ANXIETY

The anxiogenic effects of caffeine are well established (for citations see (4)). Acute doses of caffeine generally greater than 200 mg have been shown to increase anxiety ratings in nonclinical populations, with higher doses sometimes inducing panic attacks (85). Individuals with anxiety disorders tend to be particularly sensitive to the effects of caffeine. Experimental studies have demonstrated that caffeine exacerbates anxiety symptoms in individuals with panic disorder and generalized anxiety disorder to a greater extent than healthy control subjects. Genetic factors can predict variability among individuals to the anxiolytic effects of caffeine. Genetic polymorphisms on the A_{2A} receptor gene (ADORA2A) were shown in two studies to be associated with anxiogenic responses to 150-mg dose of caffeine among low caffeine consumers (10). Furthermore, first-degree relatives of patients with panic disorder show a greater anxiogenic response to a high dose of caffeine (85). It has been suggested that individuals with anxiety disorders may find the stimulus effects of caffeine aversive and therefore may naturally limit their caffeine intake. Laboratory studies have demonstrated that lower baseline anxiety levels predict caffeine consumption using drug choice procedures under double-blind conditions (62). Some correlational studies have found that individuals with anxiety disorders, such as panic disorder, report consuming less caffeine than healthy controls. However, other studies have shown a positive relationship between anxiety disorders or greater anxiety levels and caffeine use, or no relationship. In light of this mixed data, it seems reasonable to conclude that some but not all highly anxious individuals will limit caffeine, and it is possible that some may fail to recognize the role that caffeine plays in their anxiety.

Abstention from caffeine has been shown to produce improvements in anxiety symptoms among individuals seeking treatment for an anxiety disorder. Interestingly, individuals with high caffeine consumption have been shown to have greater rates of minor tranquilizer use (e.g., benzodiazepines) relative to those with low to moderate caffeine consumption (86), although the mechanism underlying this association has not been established.

The *DSM-IV-TR* includes a diagnosis of caffeine-induced anxiety disorder (60). Caffeine-induced anxiety disorder is characterized by prominent anxiety, panic attacks, obsessions, or compulsions etiologically related to caffeine use. It is not necessary to meet full criteria for a *DSM-IV-TR* anxiety disorder to qualify for a diagnosis of caffeine-induced anxiety disorder. The prevalence and incidence of caffeine-induced anxiety disorder is not known.

CAFFEINE DEPENDENCE

Substance dependence is defined by a cluster of cognitive, behavioral, and physiological symptoms indicating that an individual continues to use a substance despite experiencing significant substance-related problems (60). The *DSM-IV-TR* does not presently include caffeine in its diagnostic schema for substance dependence. In contrast, the World Health Organization's *ICD-10* includes a diagnosis of substance dependence on caffeine, using very similar diagnostic criteria as the *DSM-IV-TR*. The rationale for excluding substance dependence on caffeine during the last major revision of the *DSM* in 1994 was that although it had been established that caffeine produces physical dependence, there was a lack of information pertaining to other features of substance dependence such as the inability to stop caffeine use and continued caffeine use despite knowledge of negative health consequences (81).

Since that time a number of published studies have described adults and adolescents who report problematic caffeine consumption and fulfill *DSM-IV-TR* substance dependence criteria on caffeine (Table 22.4) (74,77,79,87,88). For example, one investigation found that 16 of 99 individuals who self-identified as having psychological or physical dependence on caffeine met *DSM-IV* criteria for substance dependence on caffeine, when only a restrictive set of four of the seven *DSM-IV* criteria that seemed most appropriate to problematic caffeine use were assessed (use despite harm, desire, or unsuccessful efforts to stop, withdrawal, and tolerance) (74). Using the same four criteria, another study identified adolescents who fulfilled diagnostic criteria for caffeine dependence (79). A study of pregnant women found that 57% of caffeine users fulfilled *DSM-IV* criteria for lifetime substance dependence on caffeine by endorsing three or more of the seven criteria (87).

The one population-based survey to date suggests that when individuals in the general population are surveyed about their caffeine use, a surprisingly large proportion endorse substance dependence criteria. In a random digit dialing telephone survey in which all seven *DSM-IV* criteria for substance dependence were assessed, 30% of caffeine users fulfilled diagnostic criteria by endorsing three or more

TABLE 22.4 Prevalence of endorsement of *DSM-IV* criteria for substance dependence among caffeine users (in %)

	General population		DSM-IV defined caffeine dependent individuals		
	Adults[a] (Ref. 77)	Pregnant women[a] (Ref. 87)	Adults[b] (Ref. 74)	Adolescents[b] (Ref. 79)	College students[a] (Ref. 88)
Used despite harm	14	43	94	58	57
Desire or unsuccessful efforts to stop	56	45	81	83	60
Withdrawal	18	77	94	100	73
Tolerance	8	50	75	92	70
Used more than intended	28	45	–	–	83
Give up activities to use	<1	0	–	–	20
Great deal of time with the drug	50	25	–	–	77
Endorsed three or more criteria	30	57	100	100	100

[a] Assessed all seven *DSM-IV* criteria for substance dependence.
[b] Assessed four *DSM-IV* criteria thought to be most pertinent to a meaningful assessment of problematic caffeine use.

dependence criteria. When the more restrictive set of four criteria were used, as in the studies described above, 9% met criteria for substance dependence. The most commonly reported symptom (56%) was persistent desire or unsuccessful efforts to cut down or control caffeine use (77).

As shown in Table 22.4, the rates of endorsement of the individual criteria vary widely across samples and data collection methodologies. The five *DSM-IV-TR* criteria for substance dependence that appear to be most pertinent to a meaningful assessment of problematic caffeine use are: (a) continued use despite knowledge of a persistent or recurrent physical or psychological problem that is likely to have been caused or exacerbated by the substance; (b) persistent desire or unsuccessful efforts to cut down or control substance use; (c) characteristic withdrawal syndrome or use of the substance to relieve or avoid withdrawal symptoms; (d) tolerance as defined by a need for markedly increased amounts of the substance to achieve desired effect, or markedly diminished effect with continued use of same amount of substance; and (e) substance is often taken in larger amounts or over a longer period than was intended. The remaining two criteria would not seem to be relevant to a widely available, culturally accepted drug like caffeine: (f) important social, occupational, or recreational activities are given up or reduced because of substance use and (g) a great deal of time is spent in activities necessary to obtain the substance, use the substance, or recover from its effects. Furthermore, inclusion of the last criterion could trivialize the diagnosis of caffeine dependence (e.g., sipping soft drinks throughout the day).

Individuals meeting criteria for caffeine dependence have shown a wide range of daily caffeine intake and have been consumers of various types of caffeinated products (e.g., coffee, soft drinks, tea, medications). A diagnosis of caffeine dependence has been shown to prospectively predict a greater incidence of caffeine reinforcement (89) and more severe withdrawal (74). Furthermore, among a sample of pregnant women advised by their physician to eliminate all caffeine throughout pregnancy, a caffeine dependence diagnosis predicted greater use of caffeine during pregnancy and a history of daily cigarette smoking (87). In that study, those with a caffeine dependence diagnosis and a family history of alcoholism used potentially problematic amounts of caffeine during pregnancy (i.e., half used more than 300 mg/day). Caffeine dependence has also been shown to be associated with a past history of alcohol abuse or dependence (74).

Available research and case reports suggest that a clinically meaningful caffeine dependence syndrome does exist. Additional research is needed to determine the prevalence of the disorder, the utility and clinical significance of the diagnosis, its relationship with other drug dependencies, and effective treatment strategies. Therapeutic assistance should be made available for those who feel that their caffeine use is problematic and have been unable to quit on their own. The Composite International Diagnostic Interview–Substance Abuse Module (CIDI-SAM), a well-regarded structured interview focused on substance-use disorders, contains a section for caffeine dependence according to *DSM-IV-TR* and *ICD-10* criteria.

CAFFEINE AND OTHER DRUGS OF DEPENDENCE

Alcohol

Heavy use and clinical dependence on caffeine is associated with heavy use and clinical dependence on alcohol (90). In one study, almost 60% of individuals fulfilling *DSM-IV* diagnostic criteria for substance dependence on caffeine had a history of alcohol abuse or dependence (74). Despite common lore that caffeine reverses the impairing effects of alcohol, controlled research suggests that such effects are generally of small magnitude and highly inconsistent across different types of behavioral and subjective measures. There is suggestive evidence that individuals consuming caffeine with alcohol tend to underestimate their levels of intoxication and impairment and may be more prone to injury (1). The popular practice of combining caffeinated energy drinks and alcohol, presumably to counteract the sedative effects of alcohol, suggests there is a need for research in this area.

Benzodiazepines

Benzodiazepines and benzodiazepine-like drugs (e.g., zolpidem) are widely used in the treatment of anxiety disorders and insomnia. Animal and human studies suggest a mutually antagonistic relationship between caffeine and benzodiazepines. An important clinical implication is that caffeine use should be evaluated when treating anxiety or insomnia with benzodiazepines. One study reported that a greater percentage of heavy caffeine consumers also use benzodiazepine minor tranquilizers; however, in general, rates of caffeine intake are similar among benzodiazepine users and nonusers.

Nicotine and Cigarette Smoking

Epidemiologic studies have shown that cigarette smokers consume more caffeine than nonsmokers (91), a finding that is consistent with the observation that cigarette smoking increases caffeine metabolism. Several studies have shown that cigarette smoking abstinence results in significant increases in caffeine blood levels among heavy caffeine consumers, presumably due to a reversal of smoking-induced increased caffeine metabolism. Although it has been posited that this effect could make smoking cessation attempts more difficult, the clinical significance has not been demonstrated (91). Some human and animal studies have demonstrated that caffeine can increase the reinforcing and discriminative stimulus effects of intravenous nicotine (92). Some studies have failed to show that caffeine administration reliably increases cigarette smoking or nicotine self-administration (93,94).

Cocaine

There is little epidemiologic data on the co-occurrence of caffeine and cocaine use. One study reported that the prevalence of caffeine use among cocaine abusers is lower than the general population (95). Interestingly, in that same study, cocaine users who consumed caffeine reported using less cocaine than those who do not regularly consume caffeine.

In animal studies caffeine increases the acquisition of cocaine self-administration, reinstates responding previously maintained by cocaine, and potentiates the stimulant and discriminative stimulus effects of cocaine (22). Caffeine was shown to produce cocaine-appropriate responding in a cocaine versus placebo discrimination study (50). The subjective effects of intravenous caffeine have been reported as cocaine-like in one study (96), but not another (97). Intravenous caffeine administration has been shown to produce a significant increase in craving for cocaine in cocaine abusers (96); however, oral administration of caffeine has not produced this effect (98). Although the documented interactions between caffeine and cocaine are interesting, the clinical importance has not been established.

CLINICAL IMPLICATIONS

Given the wide range of symptoms produced by excessive caffeine use and withdrawal, as described throughout this chapter, caffeine use should be routinely assessed during medical and psychiatric evaluations. Caffeine use or intoxication should be assessed in individuals with complaints of anxiety, insomnia, headaches, palpitations, tachycardia, or gastrointestinal disturbance. Caffeine intoxication should be considered in the differential diagnosis of amphetamine or cocaine intoxication, mania, medication-induced side effects, hyperthyroidism, and pheochromocytoma. Likewise, caffeine withdrawal should be considered when patients present with headaches, fatigue, mood disturbances, or difficulty concentrating. Caffeine withdrawal should be considered in the differential diagnosis of migraine or other headache disorders, viral illnesses, and other drug withdrawal states.

Caffeine users who are instructed to refrain from all food and beverages prior to medical procedures may be at risk for experiencing caffeine withdrawal. Caffeine withdrawal has been identified as a cause of postoperative headaches, and caffeine supplements during surgery have been shown to be effective in preventing withdrawal (29).

Caffeine interacts with a number of medications. Caffeine and benzodiazepine-like drugs (e.g., diazepam, alprazolam, triazolam) are mutually antagonistic, and thus caffeine use may interfere with the efficacy of benzodiazepines (4). Caffeine may also interfere with the metabolism of the antipsychotic clozapine as well as the bronchodilator theophylline to an extent that may be clinically significant (15). Case studies have suggested that caffeine withdrawal may be associated with increased serum lithium concentrations and lithium toxicity (15). Numerous compounds have been shown to decrease the rate of elimination of caffeine including oral contraceptive steroids, cimetidine, and fluvoxamine (15).

TREATMENT

Reduction or elimination of caffeine is advised for individuals who have caffeine-related psychopathology or when it is believed that caffeine is causing or exacerbating medical or psychiatric problems, or interfering with medication efficacy. A surprisingly large percentage of caffeine users in the general population (56%) report a desire or unsuccessful efforts to stop or reduce caffeine use (77). Fourteen percent of adults with a lifetime history of caffeine use report stopping caffeine completely, usually due to health concerns or unpleasant side effects (99).

There are no published reports of treatment interventions designed to assist individuals who would like to completely eliminate caffeine. Several reports suggest the efficacy of a structured caffeine reduction regimen (i.e., caffeine fading) for achieving substantial reductions of caffeine intake (4). A study of patients recruited from a urinary continence clinic found that a 4-week reduction program with a consumption goal of <100 mg/day was effective at reducing caffeine intake as well as urinary frequency and urgency outcomes (36).

Given the limited number of treatment strategies that have been evaluated for reducing or eliminating caffeine consumption, a reasonable approach is to adapt validated behavioral techniques used to treat dependence on other drugs (e.g., tobacco dependence). Effective behavior modification strategies include coping response training, self-monitoring, social support, and reinforcement for abstinence. Substance abuse treatment strategies including motivational interviewing and relapse prevention could also be readily applied to the treatment of caffeine dependence. Providing a list of caffeine-containing products may help to increase awareness of sources of caffeine and should facilitate self-monitoring efforts (Table 22.1). Some individuals may not readily accept the idea that caffeine is contributing to their problems (e.g., insomnia, anxiety). Such individuals should be encouraged to engage in a caffeine-free trial. There is some evidence that withdrawal symptoms may thwart quit attempts. Gradually reducing caffeine consumption may help attenuate withdrawal symptoms, although there has been no systematic research to determine the most efficacious reduction schedule. In general, reduction schedules over the course of 3 to 4 weeks have been shown to be effective. No data about the probability of relapse is currently available, although relapse after caffeine reduction has been reported (4). Table 22.5 lists practical guidelines for reducing or ceasing caffeine use.

TABLE 22.5	Guidelines for reducing or eliminating caffeine
1) *Education* Patients should be educated about potential sources of caffeine. It may be useful to provide patients with a list of common caffeinated products (see Table 22.1). Some individuals may not be aware that caffeine is present in noncola beverages such as lemon-lime soft drinks and products made with guarana, maté, or kola nut.
2) *Self-monitoring* Caffeine use should be self-monitored using a food diary for 1–2 weeks to determine a baseline level. If a self-monitoring period is not feasible, treatment providers can determine a rough estimate of total caffeine consumption via self-report. Self-monitoring should also be continued during the caffeine reduction phase of treatment.
3) *Calculate total daily caffeine consumption (mg)* Calculate daily caffeine exposure in milligrams, taking into account the caffeine content of specific products, the serving sizes, and the number of servings.
4) *Determine a caffeine modification goal* Decide on a caffeine modification goal with the patient. Some individuals may be interested in completely eliminating caffeine, whereas others may want to reduce their caffeine consumption. Individuals who would like to continue to consume some amount of caffeine, but who want to avoid experiencing withdrawal symptoms if they omit caffeine for a day, should be advised to consume no more than 50 mg/day.
5) *Generate a gradual reduction schedule* A gradual reduction schedule should help to prevent or alleviate caffeine withdrawal symptoms. A reasonable decrease would be 10–25% of the baseline dose every few days until the caffeine moderation or cessation goal is achieved. Patients should identify a noncaffeinated substitute for their usual caffeine-containing beverage. Caffeinated beverages can either be omitted to achieve the desire amount or can be mixed with decaffeinated beverages.
6) *Employ behavior modification techniques* Patients may benefit from behavior modification techniques shown to be effective in the treatment of dependence on other substances (e.g., nicotine). Such strategies may include self-monitoring, coping response training, reinforcement for abstinence, identifying barriers to change, social support, and reframing withdrawal as a temporary inconvenience.
7) *Follow-up* Schedule a follow-up contact with the patient to check on the patient's progress.

ACKNOWLEDGMENTS

Preparation of this chapter was supported, in part, by the United States Public Health Service grant R01 DA03890 from the National Institute on Drug Abuse.

REFERENCES

1. Reissig CJ, Strain EC, Griffiths RR. Caffeinated energy drinks—a growing problem. *Drug Alcohol Depend.* 2009;99:1–10.
2. Frary CD, Johnson RK, Wang MQ. Food sources and intakes of caffeine in the diets of persons in the United States. *J Am Diet Assoc.* 2005;105:110–113.
3. Barone JJ, Roberts HR. Caffeine consumption. *Food Chem Toxicol.* 1996;34:119–129.
4. Juliano LM, Ferre S, Griffiths RR. Caffeine: Pharmacology and clinical effects. In: Graham AW, Schultz TK, Mayo-Smith M, et al., eds. *Principles of Addiction Medicine.* 4th ed. Chevy Chase, MD: American Society of Addiciton Medicine, Inc.; 2009:159–178.
5. Vink JM, Staphorsius AS, Boomsma DI. A genetic analysis of coffee consumption in a sample of Dutch twins. *Twin Res Hum Genet.* 2009;12:127–131.
6. Kendler KS, Myers J, Prescott CA. Specificity of genetic and environmental risk factors for symptoms of cannabis, cocaine, alcohol, caffeine, and nicotine dependence. *Arch Gen Psychiatry.* 2007;64:1313–1320.
7. Palatini P, Ceolotto G, Ragazzo F, et al. CYP1A2 genotype modifies the association between coffee intake and the risk of hypertension. *J Hypertens.* 2009;27:1594–1601.
8. Cornelis MC, El-Sohemy A, Kabagambe EK, et al. Coffee, CYP1A2 genotype, and risk of myocardial infarction. *JAMA.* 2006;295:1135–1141.
9. Cornelis MC, El-Sohemy A, Campos H. Genetic polymorphism of the adenosine A2A receptor is associated with habitual caffeine consumption. *Am J Clin Nutr.* 2007;86:240–244.
10. Childs E, Hohoff C, Deckert J, et al. Association between ADORA2A and DRD2 polymorphisms and caffeine-induced anxiety. *Neuropsychopharmacology.* 2008.
11. Retey JV, Adam M, Khatami R, et al. A genetic variation in the adenosine A2A receptor gene (ADORA2A) contributes to individual sensitivity to caffeine effects on sleep. *Clin Pharmacol Ther.* 2007;81:692–698.

12. Benowitz NL. Clinical pharmacology of caffeine. *Annu Rev Med.* 1990;41:277–288.
13. Liguori A, Hughes JR, Grass JA. Absorption and subjective effects of caffeine from coffee, cola and capsules. *Pharmacol Biochem Behav.* 1997;58:721–726.
14. Fredholm BB, Battig K, Holmen J, et al. Actions of caffeine in the brain with special reference to factors that contribute to its widespread use. *Pharmacol Rev.* 1999;51:83–133.
15. Carrillo JA, Benitez J. Clinically significant pharmacokinetic interactions between dietary caffeine and medications. *Clin Pharmacokinet.* 2000;39:127–153.
16. Denaro CP, Benowitz NL, Caffeine metabolism: Disposition in liver disease and hepatic-function testing. In: Watson RR, ed. *Drug and Alcohol Abuse Reviews, Liver Pathology and Alcohol.* Vol. 2. Totowa, NJ: The Human Press, Inc; 1991:513–539.
17. Frye RF, Zgheib NK, Matzke GR, et al. Liver disease selectively modulates cytochrome P450-mediated metabolism. *Clin Pharmacol Ther.* 2006;80:235–245.
18. Anderson BA, Juliano LM, Schulkin J. Caffeine's implications for women's health and survey of obstetrician–gynecologists' caffeine knowledge and assessment practices. *J Womens Health.* 2009;18:1457–1466.
19. Ferre S. An update on the mechanisms of the psychostimulant effects of caffeine. *J Neurochem.* 2008;105:1067–1079.
20. Basheer R, Strecker RE, Thakkar MM, et al. Adenosine and sleep–wake regulation. *Prog Neurobiol.* 2004;73:379–396.
21. Daly JW, Mechanism of action of caffeine. In: Garattini S, ed. *Caffeine, Coffee, and Health.* New York: Raven Press; 1993:97–150.
22. Garrett BE, Griffiths RR. The role of dopamine in the behavioral effects of caffeine in animals and humans. *Pharmacol Biochem Behav.* 1997;57:533–541.
23. Di Chiara G, Bassareo V. Reward system and addiction: what dopamine does and doesn't do. *Curr Opin Pharmacol.* 2007;7:69–76.
24. Solinas M, Ferre S, You ZB, et al. Caffeine induces dopamine and glutamate release in the shell of the nucleus accumbens. *J Neurosci.* 2002;22:6321–6324.
25. Borycz J, Pereira MF, Melani A, et al. Differential glutamate-dependent and glutamate-independent adenosine A1 receptor-mediated modulation of dopamine release in different striatal compartments. *J Neurochem.* 2007;101:355–363.
26. Ganio MS, Klau JF, Casa DJ, et al. Effect of caffeine on sport-specific endurance performance: a systematic review. *J Strength Cond Res.* 2009;23:315–324.
27. Tarnopolsky MA. Effect of caffeine on the neuromuscular system—potential as an ergogenic aid. *Appl Physiol Nutr Metab.* 2008;33:1284–1289.
28. Lane JD, Feinglos MN, Surwit RS. Caffeine increases ambulatory glucose and postprandial responses in coffee drinkers with type 2 diabetes. *Diabetes Care.* 2008;31:221–222.
29. Weber JG, Klindworth JT, Arnold JJ, et al. Prophylactic intravenous administration of caffeine and recovery after ambulatory surgical procedures. *Mayo Clin Proc.* 1997;72:621–626.
30. James JE. *Caffeine and Health.* San Diego, CA: Academic Press, Inc.; 1991.
31. Higdon JV, Frei B. Coffee and health: a review of recent human research. *Crit Rev Food Sci Nutr.* 2006;46:101–123.
32. Nawrot P, Jordan S, Eastwood J, et al. Effects of caffeine on human health. *Food Addit Contam.* 2003;20:1–30.
33. Farag NH, Vincent AS, Sung BH, et al. Caffeine tolerance is incomplete: persistent blood pressure responses in the ambulatory setting. *Am J Hypertens.* 2005;18:714–719.
34. James JE. Blood pressure effects of dietary caffeine are a risk for cardiovascular disease. In: Smith BD, Gupta U, Gupta BS, eds. *Caffeine and Activation Theory: Effects on Health and Behavior.* Boca Raton, FL: Taylor & Francis; 2007:133–153.
35. Smith BD, Aldridge K, Acute cardiovascular effects of caffeine: hemodynamics and heart function. In: Smith BD, Gupta U, Gupta BS, eds. *Caffeine and Activation Theory: Effects on Health and Behavior.* Boca Raton, FL: Taylor & Francis; 2007:81–91.
36. Bryant CM, Dowell CJ, Fairbrother G. Caffeine reduction education to improve urinary symptoms. *Br J Nurs.* 2002;11:560–565.
37. Hallstrom H, Wolk A, Glynn A, et al. Coffee, tea and caffeine consumption in relation to osteoporotic fracture risk in a cohort of Swedish women. *Osteoporos Int.* 2006;17:1055–1064.
38. Robinson LE, Spafford C, Graham TE, et al. Acute caffeine ingestion and glucose tolerance in women with or without gestational diabetes mellitus. *J Obstet Gynaecol Can.* 2009;31:304–312.
39. Weng X, Odouli R, Li DK. Maternal caffeine consumption during pregnancy and the risk of miscarriage: a prospective cohort study. *Am J Obstet Gynecol.* 2008;198:279 e271–e278.
40. Fernandes O, Sabharwal M, Smiley T, et al. Moderate to heavy caffeine consumption during pregnancy and relationship to spontaneous abortion and abnormal fetal growth: a meta-analysis. *Reprod Toxicol.* 1998;12:435–444.
41. The Care Study Group. Maternal caffeine intake during pregnancy and risk of fetal growth restriction: a large prospective observational study. *BMJ.* 2008;337:a2332.
42. Ross GW, Abbott RD, Petrovitch H, et al. Association of coffee and caffeine intake with the risk of Parkinson disease. *JAMA.* 2000;283:2674–2679.
43. Ruhl CE, Everhart JE. Coffee and tea consumption are associated with a lower incidence of chronic liver disease in the United States. *Gastroenterology.* 2005;129:1928–1936.
44. van Dam RM. Coffee and type 2 diabetes: from beans to beta-cells. *Nutr Metab Cardiovasc Dis.* 2006;16:69–77.
45. Griffiths RR, Evans SM, Heishman SJ, et al. Low-dose caffeine discrimination in humans. *J Pharmacol Exp Ther.* 1990;252:970–978.
46. Chait LD, Johanson CE. Discriminative stimulus effects of caffeine and benzphetamine in amphetamine-trained volunteers. *Psychopharmacology (Berl).* 1988;96:302–308.
47. James JE, Rogers PJ. Effects of caffeine on performance and mood: withdrawal reversal is the most plausible explanation. *Psychopharmacology (Berl).* 2005;182:1–8.
48. Griffiths RR, Bigelow, GE, Liebson IA. Human coffee drinking: reinforcing and physical dependence producing effects of caffeine. *J Pharmacol Exp Ther.* 1986;239:416–425.
49. Haskell CF, Kennedy DO, Milne AL, et al. Caffeine at levels found in decaffeinated beverages is behaviourally active. *Appetite.* 2008;50:559.
50. Oliveto AH, McCance-Katz E, Singha A, et al. Effects of d-amphetamine and caffeine in humans under a cocaine discrimination procedure. *Behav Pharmacol.* 1998;9:207–217.
51. Heishman SJ, Henningfield JE. Stimulus functions of caffeine in humans: relation to dependence potential. *Neurosci Biobehav Rev.* 1992;16:273–287.
52. James JE. *Understanding Caffeine.* Thousand Oaks, CA: Sage Publications, Inc.; 1997.
53. McLellan TM, Kamimori GH, Voss DM, et al. Caffeine effects on physical and cognitive performance during sustained operations. *Aviat Space Environ Med.* 2007;78:871–877.

54. Doherty M, Smith PM. Effects of caffeine ingestion on exercise testing: a meta-analysis. *Int J Sport Nutr Exerc Metab.* 2004;14: 626–646.
55. Killgore WD, Rupp TL, Grugle NL, et al. Effects of dextroamphetamine, caffeine and modafinil on psychomotor vigilance test performance after 44 h of continuous wakefulness. *J Sleep Res.* 2008;17:309–321.
56. Roehrs T, Roth T. Caffeine: sleep and daytime sleepiness. *Sleep Med Rev.* 2008;12:153–162.
57. Landolt HP, Werth E, Borbely AA, et al. Caffeine intake (200 mg) in the morning affects human sleep and EEG power spectra at night. *Brain Res.* 1995;675:67–74.
58. Carrier J, Fernandez-Bolanos M, Robillard R, et al. Effects of caffeine are more marked on daytime recovery sleep than on nocturnal sleep. *Neuropsychopharmacology.* 2007;32:964–972.
59. Sin CW, Ho JS, Chung JW. Systematic review on the effectiveness of caffeine abstinence on the quality of sleep. *J Clin Nurs.* 2009; 18:13–21.
60. American Psychiatric Association. *Diagnostic and Statistical Manual of Mental Disorders.* 4th ed. text revision. Washington, DC: American Psychiatric Press; 2000.
61. Liguori A, Hughes JR, Oliveto AH. Caffeine self-administration in humans: 1. Efficacy of cola vehicle. *Exp Clin Psychopharmacol.* 1997;5:286–294.
62. Evans SM, Griffiths RR. Caffeine tolerance and choice in humans. *Psychopharmacology (Berl).* 1992;108:51–59.
63. Hughes JR, Oliveto AH, Bickel WK, et al. Caffeine self-administration and withdrawal: incidence, individual differences and interrelationships. *Drug Alcohol Depend.* 1993;32:239–246.
64. Garrett BE, Griffiths RR. Physical dependence increases the relative reinforcing effects of caffeine versus placebo. *Psychopharmacology (Berl).* 1998;139:195–202.
65. Silverman K, Mumford GK, Griffiths RR. Enhancing caffeine reinforcement by behavioral requirements following drug ingestion. *Psychopharmacology (Berl).* 1994;114:424–432.
66. Rogers PJ, Richardson NJ, Elliman NA. Overnight caffeine abstinence and negative reinforcement of preference for caffeine-containing drinks. *Psychopharmacology (Berl).* 1995;120: 457–462.
67. Yeomans MR, Jackson A, Lee MD, et al. Expression of flavour preferences conditioned by caffeine is dependent on caffeine deprivation state. *Psychopharmacology (Berl).* 2000;150:208–215.
68. Sigmon SC, Herning RI, Better W, et al. Caffeine withdrawal, acute effects, tolerance, and absence of net beneficial effects of chronic administration: cerebral blood flow velocity, quantitative EEG, and subjective effects. *Psychopharmacology (Berl).* 2009; 204:573–585.
69. Watson J, Deary I, Kerr D. Central and peripheral effects of sustained caffeine use: tolerance is incomplete. *Br J Clin Pharmacol.* 2002;54:400–406.
70. Farag NH, Vincent AS, McKey BS, et al. Hemodynamic mechanisms underlying the incomplete tolerance to caffeine's pressor effects. *Am J Cardiol.* 2005;95:1389–1392.
71. Juliano LM, Griffiths RR. A critical review of caffeine withdrawal: empirical validation of symptoms and signs, incidence, severity, and associated features. *Psychopharmacology (Berl).* 2004;176:1–29.
72. Jones HE, Herning RI, Cadet JL, et al. Caffeine withdrawal increases cerebral blood flow velocity and alters quantitative electroencephalography (EEG) activity. *Psychopharmacology (Berl).* 2000;147:371–377.
73. Driesbach RH, Pfeiffer C. Caffeine-withdrawal headache. *J Lab Clin Med.* 1943;28:1212–1219.
74. Strain EC, Mumford G, Silverman K, et al. Caffeine dependence syndrome: evidence from case histories and experimental evaluations. *JAMA.* 1994;272:1043–1048.
75. Evans SM, Griffiths RR. Caffeine withdrawal: a parametric analysis of caffeine dosing conditions. *J Pharmacol Exp Ther.* 1999;289: 285–294.
76. Griffiths RR, Evans SM, Heishman SJ, et al. Low-dose caffeine physical dependence in humans. *J Pharmacol Exp Ther.* 1990; 255:1123–1132.
77. Hughes JR, Oliveto AH, Liguori A, et al. Endorsement of DSM-IV dependence criteria among caffeine users. *Drug Alcohol Depend.* 1998;52:99–107.
78. Dews PB, Curtis GL, Hanford KJ, et al. The frequency of caffeine withdrawal in a population-based survey and in a controlled, blinded pilot experiment. *J Clin Pharmacol.* 1999;39: 1221–1232.
79. Oberstar JV, Bernstein GA, Thuras PD. Caffeine use and dependence in adolescents: one-year follow-up. *J Child Adolesc Psychopharmacol.* 2002;12:127–135.
80. World Health Organization. *The ICD-10 Classification of Mental and Behavioural Disorders: Clinical Descriptions and Diagnostic Guidelines.* Geneva, Switzerland: World Health Organization; 1992.
81. Hughes JR, Caffeine withdrawal, dependence, and abuse. In: *American Psychiatric Association: Diagnostic and Statistical Manual of Mental Disorders.* 4th ed. Washington, DC: American Psychiatric Association; 1994:129–134.
82. Miyata H, Hironaka N, Takada K, et al. Psychosocial withdrawal characteristics of nicotine compared with alcohol and caffeine. *Ann N Y Acad Sci.* 2008;1139:458–465.
83. Kendler KS, Myers J, Gardner CO. Caffeine intake, toxicity and dependence and lifetime risk for psychiatric and substance use disorders: an epidemiologic and co-twin control analysis. *Psychol Med.* 2006;36:1717–1725.
84. Walsh MJ, Marquardt KA, Albertson TE. Adverse effects from the ingestion of redline energy drinks. *Clin Toxicol.* 2006;44:642.
85. Nardi AE, Valenca AM, Lopes FL, et al. Caffeine and 35% carbon dioxide challenge tests in panic disorder. *Hum Psychopharmacol.* 2007;22:231–240.
86. Greden JF, Procter A, Victor B. Caffeinism associated with greater use of other psychotropic agents. *Compr Psychiatry.* 1981;22: 565–571.
87. Svikis DS, Berger N, Haug NA, et al. Caffeine dependence in combination with a family history of alcoholism as a predictor of continued use of caffeine during pregnancy. *Am J Psychiatry.* 2005;162:2344–2351.
88. Jones HA, Lejuez CW. Personality correlates of caffeine dependence: the role of sensation seeking, impulsivity, and risk taking. *Exp Clin Psychopharmacol.* 2005;13:259–266.
89. Liguori A, Hughes JR. Caffeine self-administration in humans: 2. A within-subjects comparison of coffee and cola vehicles. *Exp Clin Psychopharmacol.* 1997;5:295–303.
90. Istvan J, Matarazzo JD. Tobacco, alcohol, and caffeine use: a review of their interrelationships. *Psychol Bull.* 1984;95: 301–326.
91. Swanson JA, Lee JW, Hopp JW, et al. The impact of caffeine use on tobacco cessation and withdrawal. *Addict Behav.* 1997;22:55–68.
92. Jones HE, Griffiths RR. Oral caffeine maintenance potentiates the reinforcing and stimulant subjective effects of intravenous nicotine in cigarette smokers. *Psychopharmacology (Berl).* 2003; 165:280–290.
93. Chait LD, Griffiths RR. Effects of caffeine on cigarette smoking and subjective response. *Clin Pharmacol Ther.* 1983;34:612–622.

94. Perkins KA, Fonte C, Stolinski A, et al. The influence of caffeine on nicotine's discriminative stimulus, subjective, and reinforcing effects. *Exp Clin Psychopharmacol.* 2005;13:275–281.
95. Budney AJ, Higgins ST, Hughes JR, et al. Nicotine and caffeine use in cocaine-dependent individuals. *J Subst Abuse.* 1993;5:117–130.
96. Rush CR, Sullivan JT, Griffiths RR. Intravenous caffeine in stimulant drug abusers: subjective reports and physiological effects. *J Pharmacol Exp Ther.* 1995;273:351–358.
97. Garrett BE, Griffiths RR. Intravenous nicotine and caffeine: subjective and physiological effects in cocaine abusers. *J Pharmacol Exp Ther.* 2001;296:486–494.
98. Liguori A, Hughes JR, Goldberg K, et al. Subjective effects of oral caffeine in formerly cocaine-dependent humans. *Drug Alcohol Depend.* 1997;49:17–24.
99. Hughes JR, Oliveto AH. A systematic survey of caffeine intake in Vermont. *Exp Clin Psychopharmacol.* 1997;5:393–398.

CHAPTER 23: Anabolic–Androgenic Steroids

Laurence M. Westreich

INTRODUCTION

This chapter reviews the anabolic–androgenic steroids (AAS), the much-maligned molecules which, in addition to their legitimate uses, have engendered a clandestine industry of advisors, purveyors, and drug-test manipulators. All of the AAS are analogs of testosterone, and all promote muscle growth (anabolic) and masculinizing (androgenic) effects to greater or lesser degrees. As opposed to the corticosteroids and female gonadotrophic steroids like estrogen and progesterone, athletes and others may use the AAS illicitly in the supraphysiologic doses necessary for increasing lean body mass, shortening muscle recovery time, and increasing strength, thereby enhancing athletic performance and muscle size.

The historical development of the AAS began with the observation that the testes produced a substance—the hormone testosterone—which controlled masculinization, and proceeded through increasingly sophisticated attempts to understand, control, and eventually replicate the hormone's effect. Those scientific efforts have resulted in the present day's wide availability of various AAS, on both the licit and illicit markets. They are perhaps the most sought-after substances on the Internet, usually by those seeking their muscle-building effects. The political, legal, and cultural contexts for AAS use provide a fascinating example of science used for societally approved uses and for uses that are forbidden—and the sometimes confusing boundary between with two.

There remains little doubt that the AAS do enhance muscle growth, strength, and in some cases athletic performance, although the side effect profile of the drugs limits their nonclinical use to those willing to risk significant harm, in addition to legal jeopardy and disqualification from legitimate sports competitions. The excess levels of testosterone which all of the AAS elicit in the nonhypogonadic user stimulate muscle growth as long as the user exercises those muscles, but also provoke ligament rupture, cardiac lipoprotein abnormalities, virilizing effects in women, feminizing effects in men, and psychiatric abnormalities.

Since illicit use of the AAS is both illegal and banned by sports organizations, a significant amount of science has developed around testing and avoiding detection of AAS use. A large criminal industry has arisen to manufacture and deliver these drugs illicitly, often leading to the same sorts of illegal dangerous behaviors usually associated with more conventional drugs of abuse. The ethical issues surrounding the use of drugs for performance enhancement present a variety of conundrums for the thinking person, best addressed with the scientific facts in hand and a full understanding of the variety of approaches already in place.

HISTORY OF THE AAS

Although farmers have known for centuries that castration of livestock promoted domestication of their farm animals, and human beings have created eunuchs and castratos for specific reasons, it was not until 1849 that Dr. Arnold Berthold demonstrated the effects of castration on roosters and the reversal of those effects when the testis were surgically returned to the abdominal cavity. This elegant experiment showed that some factor in the testis, later named testosterone, controls male sexual characteristics (1). In 1889 Dr. Charles Brown Sequard trumped Berthold by injecting himself with an extract of dog and guinea pig testicles, and documented an increase in his own physical strength, intellectual functioning, and appetite. This self-injection instigated a boom in the injection of testis derivatives and the transplantation of both animal and human testicles, advertised as an "Elixir of Life" and promoted by "… physicians uneducated in the techniques and inherent risk of animal injection … putting many patients at risk for infection and inflammation" (2).

As Figure 23.1 shows, testosterone was first synthesized in 1935; despite hints and suppositions, no conclusive evidence exists of performance-enhancing use of steroids by competitive athletes until the 1950s. Although records are understandably sparse, AAS use by the Soviet National Weightlifting teams of the mid-1950s has been deemed quite likely, and the U.S. Olympic team physician at the time, Dr. John Ziegler, acknowledged learning from the Soviets to prescribe testosterone to the U.S. weightlifters. Dr. Ziegler later prescribed the first commercially available AAS, Dianabol (methandrostenolone) to his charges. The obvious masculinized appearance of female track and field athletes from the Eastern European countries in the late 1950s and early 1960s raised suspicions, which were ultimately confirmed, that the women were taking testosterone and/or AAS (3).

An article written by a German scientist collaborating with a former German Democratic Republic (GDR) Olympic Team discus thrower (4) reveals the facts about the GDR's well-coordinated use of performance-enhancing drugs—mostly AAS—during the years 1966 to 1989. That country's elite sports establishment, assisted by physicians and other scientists, encouraged the use of AAS by several generations of athletes, including minors and women who were given

AAS Time line

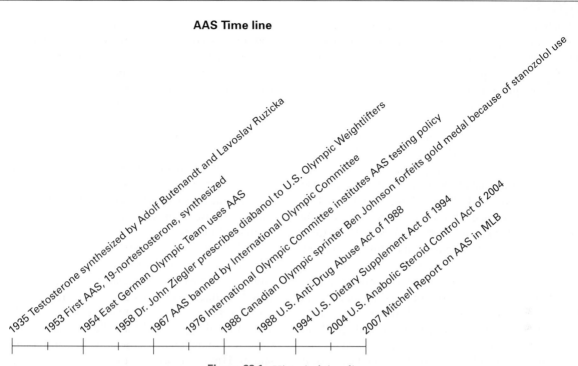

Figure 23.1. Historical time line.

1935 Testosterone synthesized by Adolf Butenandt and Lavoslav Ruzicka
1953 First AAS, 19-nortestosterone, synthesized
1954 East German Olympic Team uses AAS
1958 Dr. John Ziegler prescribes diabanol to U.S. Olympic Weightlifters
1967 AAS banned by International Olympic Committee
1976 International Olympic Committee institutes AAS testing policy
1988 Canadian Olympic sprinter Ben Johnson forfeits gold medal because of stanozolol use
1988 U.S. Anti-Drug Abuse Act of 1988
1994 U.S. Dietary Supplement Act of 1994
2004 U.S. Anabolic Steroid Control Act of 2004
2007 Mitchell Report on AAS in MLB

large dosages of testosterone and other AAS. In their pursuit of Olympic medals, the coaches and scientists foisted high doses of AAS on athletes who were initially unknowing, and many of whom were coerced into consenting to ongoing use of the drugs that were so obviously damaging their bodies while enhancing their athletic achievements.

The GDR athletic/medical establishment kept careful records of the substances athletes took, as well as the improvement in athletic performances attributable to the drugs. Using an "On-Off Protocol," the scientists were able to prove that a particular athlete's 2-m improvement in her shot-put score was attributable to the Oral-Turbinol she took, and not to other variables like additional training, nutrition, or coaching. In order to avoid detection, the athletes' testosterone:epitestosterone (T:E) levels were closely monitored, and they were given the biologically inert epitestosterone with the purpose of passing the increasingly frequent drug tests. The GDR scientists also dutifully recorded the AAS sequelae both acutely and over the years: hirsutism, acne, amenorrhea, ovarian cyst formation, voice changes, libido disturbance, hepatomegaly, and bile duct damage.

In response to the increasing use of performance-enhancing drugs by these and other elite athletes, the International Olympic Committee banned the use of the AAS in 1967, began general drug testing in 1968, and started specifically testing for AAS in 1976. The Olympics were eventually followed by the U.S. National Collegiate Athletic Association (NCAA) and professional sports organizations in banning and testing for the AAS and other performance-enhancing drugs, although a cursory look at the sports pages over the last several years will reveal that testing has hardly rid sports, amateur or professional, of illicit AAS use (5).

American societal viewpoints about drug-related performance enhancement and the AAS specifically have been ambiguous, with organized medicine expressing a certain ambivalence about the use of AAS. As late as 1977 the American College of Sports Medicine, while acknowledging the dangers of AAS use, still formally believed that the AAS were not particularly effective in normals, or in high dosages for athletes: "The administration of anabolic–androgenic steroids to healthy humans below age 50 in medically approved therapeutic doses often does not of itself bring about any significant improvements in strength, aerobic endurance, lean body mass, or body weight. There is no conclusive evidence that extremely large doses of anabolic–androgenic steroids either aid or hinder athletic performance …" (6).

However, when Canadian sprinter Ben Johnson was disqualified several days after his gold medal race in the 1988 Olympic 100-m dash, a sea change occurred in worldwide public attitudes toward the AAS, and performance-enhancing drugs in general (7). In addition to catalyzing the Olympic drug-testing program, other sports organizations and the U.S. government began taking AAS use seriously.

The Anabolic Steroids Control Act of 1990 (8) added the AAS to schedule III of the Schedule of Federal Controlled Substances. Schedule III drugs, which include the barbiturates and ketamine, are defined as follows:

A. The drug or other substance has a potential for abuse less than the drugs or other substances in schedules I and II.
B. The drug or other substance has a currently accepted medical use in treatment in the United States.
C. Abuse of the drug or other substance may lead to moderate or low physical dependence or high psychological dependence (9).

Interestingly, the American Medical Association (AMA) opposed the scheduling of the AAS on the grounds that the health effects of the AAS were unclear, there was no good evidence of physical or psychological dependence, and the change side-stepped the usual process of drug scheduling change via the U.S. Attorney General's office (10). The rescheduling listed the common AAS used by athletes, provided jail time for any advisor who induced another person to take AAS, and even included human growth hormone (HGH) in the same category of illegal substances.

In contrast to the Anabolic Steroids Control Act of 1990, the Dietary Supplement Health and Education Act of 1994 (DSHEA) (11) weakened—however unintentionally—the prevention and enforcement efforts directed at the AAS. In essence, DSHEA eliminated the Food and Drug Administration's ability to regulate the myriad products considered herbs, nutritional supplements, or dietary supplements: basically anything not a medication for a specific illness. The broad definition of these "nondrug" substances was intended to include substances like "ginseng, garlic, fish oils, psyllium, glandulars, and mixtures of these ..." (11) and placed the burden of proving safety and efficacy on the manufacturers. In the DSHEA legislation, the manufacturers were forbidden from making any claims of medical effectiveness and admonished to adhere to good manufacturing practices, but were allowed to provide "third party" educational materials, as long as the materials presented a (undefined) balanced view of the science underlying whatever claims were actually made about the supplement. Substances like DHEA and melatonin were specifically protected by DSHEA from FDA oversight.

The result of DSHEA's deregulation of the supplement industry was a concomitant looseness in the production, packaging, and labeling of nonpharmaceutical supplements. In a 2001 study of over-the-counter (OTC) supplements (12), researchers found that of the 12 brands of (then-legal) AAS supplements they bought at health-food stores, 11 did not even meet the DSHEA labeling requirements. One brand contained 10 mg of testosterone, an illegal additive not listed on the label, and the others contained inaccurate amounts of their active ingredient based on the labeling. In light of a more recent apparent mislabeling case—in which a professional athlete claimed to have bought an androstenedione-tainted supplement at a GNC store in Florida (13), the mislabeling and contamination of nutritional supplements continues. Even more worrisome than a sports-related suspension is a recent case series (14) of liver and kidney damage due to contaminated dietary supplements. According to the gastroenterologists who first documented these cases, OTC nutritional supplements containing AAS were inadvertently taken by their patients, two of whom evidenced hepatotoxic reactions, and one who suffered a nephrotoxic reaction.

EPIDEMIOLOGY OF AAS USE

The epidemiology of AAS use in the United States is complicated by several definitional, scientific, and practical variables. The fluidity of boundaries between testosterone, the synthetic AAS, and nutritional supplements makes for a nightmare in constructing surveys, and often the survey takers are reluctant to disclose their illicit behavior. Individuals coming from various perspectives—users, drug testers, sports officials, and legislators—have vested interests in promoting a high or low estimates of those who are actually taking AAS. The surveys and studies mentioned below reflect the self-acknowledged use of mostly illicit AAS by athletes and young people who, at least when they were using the AAS, must have hidden that use. So, the veracity of their reports is suspect, and the reader must remember that past and present AAS users may answer survey questions inaccurately, refuse to answer at all, or evade even the best surveying techniques.

In his memorable *Sports Illustrated* cover story of 2002 (15), former major league baseball (MLB) player Ken Caminiti estimated that "at least half" of MLB players were actively using steroids, while his similarly retired former competitor Jose Canseco estimated that "85%" of MLB players use AAS, although he himself did not take the illicit substances. Washington Redskins tackle Jon Jansen subsequently said on HBO's *Costas Now* that "maybe 15–20 percent" of NFL players took HGH, but quickly (though not very convincingly) recanted by saying that no one he knew on his team took HGH, "but other guys have talked about what goes on in other places" (16). Caminiti later died from a drug overdose (17) and Canseco published a book chronicling widespread use of AAS in MLB, including his own (18). But elite athletes who speak publicly often have obvious biases: showing that his or her own use is the norm, salving a conscience, or looking for personal publicity or book sales.

In an attempt to more rigorously quantify, among other things, AAS use and attitudes among professional athletes, all 3683 members of the National Football League's retired Player's Association were sent a survey about their AAS use, and 2552 former players responded (19). Of those admittedly self-selected former players, 9.1% admitted using AAS during their careers. The average age of the responders was 53.8 (±13.4) years, with an average career length of 6.6 (±3.6) years. Predictably, those who had played positions requiring the most size and strength reported the highest use of AAS, with offensive and defensive linemen admitting rates of 16.3% and 14.8%, respectively. Also predictably, among those players who were active in the 1980s, a total of 20.3% admitted that they had used AAS during their careers. The study authors also note a significant correlation between AAS use and joint/cartilage injures, disc herniations, meniscus injuries, elbow injuries, spine injuries, and foot/toe/ankle injuries, but no association between self-reported AAS use and muscle/tendon injuries.

Data supplied by government agencies and universities provide more accurate, if less pungent, assessments of drug use. For the last 33 years, the Survey Research Center in the University of Michigan's Institute for Social Research has published a yearly assessment of the drug-related behaviors, attitudes, and values of U.S. high school and college students (20). "Various stimulant drugs show continuing grad-

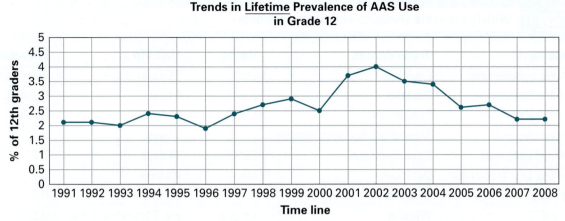

Figure 23.2. Use among high school students. Data from http://www.monitoringthefuture.org/data/08data/pr08t1/pdf.

ual declines among teens in 2008, most illicit drugs hold steady" (21). Since 1991 the surveyors have asked about the AAS, and have therefore been able to track the usage and attitudes behind that usage of a generation of American young people.

As Figures 23.2 and 23.3 show, there was a sharp increase in the use of AAS by high school students in the late 1990s, and then a decrease in use up until the present. The past five years have seen an increase in those 12th graders who say that they see "great risk" in using steroids, which likely caused the concomitant decrease in use.

A smaller but more sophisticated study protocol on the subject of athlete's attitudes toward the AAS (22) asked two groups of male athletes—one with the average age of 22 years old and one with the average age of 53—why they chose *not* to use AAS. The younger group mentioned power, control, body image, and narcissism as reasons they avoided the AAS, while the older group focused on the (unfair) enhancement of athletic performance as a reason to avoid the AAS. Both the older and younger men agreed that media representations of the male physique were simply "unattainable without chemical means."

AAS users choose their particular substances using a variety of criteria, including availability, anabolic:androgenic effect ratio, cost, reputation, and sometimes simply fashion. The Internet provides many sources of advice for which AAS to use, along with convenient links to buy those drugs, and books like "The Steroid Bible" (23)—a 126-page wire-bound manual which retails for $49.95—provide comprehensive, if illegal, advice on how to use the AAS safely and effectively. Table 23.1 shows some of the more widely available AAS, along with their routes of use, half-lives, and provenance.

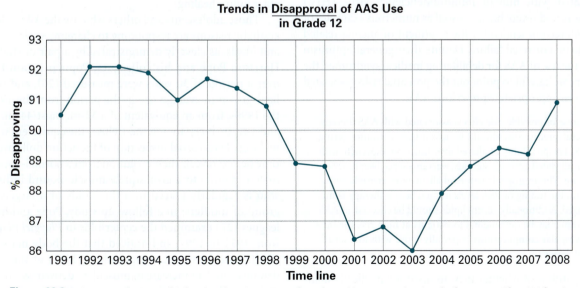

Figure 23.3. Disapproval among high school seniors. Data from http://www.monitoringthefuture.org/data/08data/pr08t1/pdf.

TABLE 23.1 Widely available anabolic–androgenic steroids

Generic name	Trade names	Route	Half-life	Provenance
Boldenone undecanoate	Equipoise	i.m.	14 days	Veterinary
Methandrostenolone	Dianabol	p.o.	6 hours	Non-U.S.
Methenolone enathane	Primobolan	i.m.	10.5 days	Non-U.S.
Methyltestosterone	Metandren, Testomet, Android	p.o.	4 days	U.S.
Nandrolone decanoate	Deca-Durobolin	i.m.	14 days	U.S.
Nandrolone phenpropionate	Durobolin	i.m.	4.5 days	U.S.
Oxandrolone	Oxandrin	p.o.	9 hours	U.S.
Stanozolol	Winstrol	i.m./p.o.	p.o. 9 hours/i.m. 1 day	U.S.
Testosterone	Androgel	Cutaneous	1.5 hours	U.S.
Testosterone cypionate	Depo-testosterone	i.m.	12 days	U.S.
Trenbolone	Finaplix-H	s.c./i.m.	3 days	Veterinary

INDICATIONS FOR AAS USE

Although the AAS have now become synonymous with cheating in athletic competition, they were initially prescribed for legitimate medical conditions, and continue to have well-defined indications for the treatment of various chronic diseases and medical conditions. Treatment of both hypogonadism and growth hormone deficiency (GHD) in males can include the use of testosterone or the AAS (24).

One review paper (25) looked at the legitimate uses for the AAS documented in the medical literature between 1966 and 2000, and found that the majority of recommendations were for the palliation of the cachexia and muscle wasting associated with chronic disease. The authors found consistent documentation of AAS use for the treatment of muscle loss associated with human immunodeficiency virus (HIV) infection, and severe burns, as well as numerous examples of the AAS recommended for the treatment of anemia related to leukemia or renal failure. Despite their general optimism about the use of AAS for debilitating medical syndromes, the authors are careful to point out the potential risks associated with even appropriately prescribed AAS:

> Because of possible side effects associated with AAS therapy, several precautions should be taken before administering AAS. The possibility of altered liver function, especially with 17α-alkylated anabolic steroids, warrants serial liver function testing. The androgenic nature of all anabolic steroids necessitates the testing of PSA levels in men before therapy is initialized. Additionally, serum lipids should be checked, as AAS therapy may be detrimental to patients at high risk for cardiovascular complications, especially those with low serum HDL levels (25).

Regardless of whether they are used for medically managed and legitimate purposes, or ad hoc and illegitimately, the anabolic effects of the AAS do not necessarily confer functional strength. Even with necessary weight-bearing exercise as a concomitant, muscle growth derived from the AAS improves size of the muscle more than function: the earliest widespread use of AAS by nonelite athletes was in the bodybuilding community, where the desired end result was muscle size and definition, rather than actual strength. Of course, some AAS use obviously does promote functional strength, as evidenced by the hordes of amateur and professional athletes who use them for performance enhancement purposes, despite the drugs' dangers, cost, legal risks, and risks of disqualification. Although in many sports an overabundance of muscle can degrade necessary agility and range of motion, many athletes have learned to titrate their dosages to promote more modest muscle growth while enhancing muscular injury healing.

Those adolescents and others who use the AAS solely for aesthetic reasons are responding to changing societal norms and ideals, as cleverly demonstrated by a pair of studies by Harrison Pope and his colleagues. Popular action figures over a period of 30 years were measured (26), and seen to have grown in average size in the period from the 1960s to the 1990s, from an equivalent of a 32-in. waist/44-in. chest, and a 12-in. bicep to—in the 1990s—the equivalent of a 55-in. bicep. Even casual inspection of the action dolls over that time period reveals their evolution from a normal-appearing male physique to a grotesquely muscle-bound individual who is regularly placed into the hands of a largely male group of toddlers. In a follow-up study, Pope and his colleagues (27) examined the centerfolds in *Playgirl* magazine from 1973 to 1997, and noticed that the body mass index (BMI) and the fat-free mass index (FFMI) of the models demonstrated an increase in muscular "denseness" and general muscularity over the study period, demonstrating again our society's increasing fascination with muscularity as a prized aesthetic value, if not necessarily as an avenue for athletic performance.

Pope terms this male obsession with a perfect—and muscular—body "The Adonis Complex" (28), and compares it to "anorexia in reverse" for men. Although he can cite multiple descriptive research studies by his group and others, Pope does not attempt to define one singular cause for this societal body dysmorphic disorder, but rather points to a variety of psychological and cultural phenomena which provoke and then support the unrealistic expectations that both men and women have of their own bodies.

The proliferation of "antiaging" clinics presents a dilemma for the competent clinician and organized medicine in general since these clinics often make promises and deliver therapies far beyond the accepted standard of care, but mimic accepted medical practice. The antiaging clinics merely expand upon the reasonable health habits promoted for aging people, and the cosmetic medications and surgical procedures that mainstream medicine promotes for the baby boomer generation struggling against old age. The aging male who would never consider buying drugs on the street or visiting a shaman is much more amenable to consultation with a clinic which advertised in an airline magazine, yellow pages, or the Internet.

An organization called "The American Academy of Anti-Aging Medicine" (29), founded in 1992, claims 22,000 members worldwide, 85% of whom are physicians. The organizations stated goals are to "… (serve) as an advocate for the new clinical specialty of anti-aging medical science and (act) as a conduit to the physicians, scientist, and the educated public who wish to benefit from the almost daily breakthrough in biotechnology which promise both a greater quality as well as quantity of life." In addition to facilitating referrals to members of the organization, the Web site features books for sale such as "Grow Young with HGH," and "Cellular Phones: Medical Menaces of a Modern-Day Convenience."

One Internet advertisement for an antiaging clinic (30) promotes "hormone replacement therapy" with "testosterone pellet therapy" and promises, among other things, that the treatment for men "increases muscle, improves sexual libedo (sic) and performance, increases energy, reduces depression, improves memory & concentration, reduces sleep disturbances, protects against heart disease, improves the skin's elasticity, encourages bone growth, improves blood flow…." While some of the above responses might indeed occur for the truly hypogondal male, many of the clinics do not even test testosterone levels or other relevant indices, or support the treatment of testosterone values which are merely in the lower range of normal.

Although the range of clinics which call themselves "antiaging" is certainly broad and contains some legitimate medical providers, the industry itself has become notorious for providing useless, illicit, and sometimes dangerous preparations. In his report to the Commissioner of Major League Baseball on AAS and other performance-enhancing substances (PES) (31), former Senator George Mitchell wrote about a criminal justice investigation "… including several so-called 'rejuvenation centers,' exposing another source of illegal performance enhancing substances. Some businesses that describe themselves as anti-aging or rejuvenation centers sell steroids or human growth hormone and arrange for buyers to obtain prescriptions for those substance from corrupt or suspended physicians, or even, in some cases, a dentist. The prescriptions are then filled by a compounding pharmacy affiliated with the center and delivered to the buyer whether through the mail or at the 'clinic.'"

Although the provision of HGH is a standard treatment at many antiaging clinics, HGH is usually combined with testosterone or the AAS in order to achieve appreciable results. Do these interventions have a favorable risk:benefit ratio for the aging, but healthy, individual?

One early study done in 1996 (32) assigned 43 normal men to one of four groups: placebo with no exercise, testosterone with no exercise, placebo and exercise, and testosterone plus exercise. The subjects received 600 mg of testosterone enanthate injection or a placebo weekly for 10 weeks, and the exercise groups did standardized weightlifting exercises three times per week. The outcome variables were fat-free mass, muscle size, and arm strength, as well as endocrine responses and mood/behavior.

Those individuals, given the massive dosages of testosterone, had markedly elevated testosterone levels at 10 weeks, 2828 ng/dl in the no-exercise groups and 3244 ng/dl in the exercise groups, while the placebo groups did not change from their normal baseline testosterone levels. The no-exercise subjects given testosterone had statistically significant increases over baseline in triceps size, quadriceps size, bench-press strength, and squatting strength, and the exercise subjects given testosterone had improvements on all parameters when compared to either no-exercise group. Exercise combined with testosterone, not surprisingly, improved both muscle strength and function. There were no observed negative effects on cardiovascular lipid profiles or mood and behavior, despite the authors' diligent attempts to monitor for any such side effects. The 10-week time frame probably prevented the emergence of any such side effects, and even the supraphysiologic dosage of testosterone given is far below that taken by many illicit users. In their conclusions, the authors opine that while the AAS might be clinically useful for immobilized patients, cancer- or HIV-related cachexia, or other wasting disorders, but point out that "…(our) results in no way justify the use of anabolic–androgenic steroids in sports, because, with extended use, such drugs have potentially serious adverse effects on the cardiovascular system, prostate and lipid metabolism, and insulin sensitivity. Moreover the use of any performance-enhancing agent in sports raises serious ethical issues. …"

A later (2002) randomized and placebo controlled study (33) of 27 women and 34 men, all older than 68 years, examined the effects of HGH and testosterone in an aging population and found that although HGH with or without testosterone or AAS did in fact increase lean body mass and decreased fat mass, and HGH and testosterone together slightly increased muscle strength and VO_2 max in men; both sets of results came at the expense of frequent adverse effects. Although the study lasted only 26 weeks, these statistically significant side effects—tied to both HGH and the testosterone/AAS use—included edema, carpal tunnel syndrome, arthralgias, glucose intolerance, and frank diabetes. The authors note that the improvements in lean body mass and decreased fat after the hormonal treatments were about the same as those reported after three times per week exercise training for six months, but less than the improvements found in subjects exercising once per week.

AAS METABOLISM

Males produce about 95% of their testosterone, the endogenous analog for all the AAS, in testicular Leydig cells, with the rest produced in the adrenal glands. Females produce relatively small amounts of testosterone in the ovaries. Most circulating testosterone is bound to sex hormone binding protein (SHBP); only the free testosterone is biologically active (34). The hormone's *androgenic* effects are mediated by the metabolism of testosterone to the more-potent 5α-dihydrotestosterone (DHT) by the 5α-reductase, which resides in specifically male target tissue like the prostate gland, seminal vesicles, and external genitalia. These androgenic, or virilizing, effects occur in the male fetus, adolescent, and adult, to varying degrees according to the level of circulating testosterone. In some other tissues, like adipose and brain, aromatase converts circulating testosterone to estradiol, a fact of great importance to those who ingest exogenous testosterone or AAS (35).

The *anabolic* effects of testosterone and its AAS mimickers are promotion of bone and muscle growth, as the hormone promotes protein synthesis, decreases protein catabolism, and increases erythropoiesis. Although AAS with pure anabolic effects in the absence of any androgenic side effects would be ideal for athletes, no such compound has yet been developed. However, testosterone and the various AAS vary widely in the ratio of anabolic to androgenic effects. Testosterone and methyltestosterone (Android and others) have about a 1:1 ratio of androgenic to anabolic effects, fluoxymesterone (Halotestin and others) has a 1:3 ratio and oxandrolone (Oxandrin) can have a 1:13 ratio (36). The androgenic activity of any compound is most accurately determined by using a variant of the Hershberger assay, in which lab animals are exposed to AAS, sacrificed, and have their androgen-sensitive tissue like bulbocavernosus muscle, ventral prostate, and seminal vesicles weighed (37). Of course, the Hershberger assay suffers from being a laboratory-derived procedure using an animal model, and illicit AAS users, of course, simply look up Internet estimates or listen to word of mouth in the gyms.

As Figure 23.4 demonstrates in simplified form, all endogenous testosterone derives from (noncirculating) cholesterol, the basic steroid molecule that is metabolized to androstenedione and pregenenolone, and then to testosterone. Testosterone is eventually broken down into 5α-DHT and estradiol in peripheral tissue. Modification of the basic four-ringed steroid structure—three cyclohexane rings and a cyclopentane ring—confers varying degrees of oral availability, serum half-life, and side effect profile.

For instance, substitution of a methyl or ethyl group for the hydrogen at the 17th position of the cyclopentane ring confers oral availability on the resultant AAS by reducing hepatic first-pass metabolism. Paradoxically, these orally available compounds—like stanozolol (Winstrol)—have turned out to confer more adverse effects than the injectable compounds, because of their hepatotoxicity. Esterification at the 17-β position allows for longer serum half-life of the molecule because of increased lipophilicity and a resultant slower release from the oily injection vehicle into the blood stream. Testosterone cypionate (Depo-testosterone) and nandrolone decanoate (Deca-Durobolin) both have longer half-lives than their nonesterified building-block molecules, with that half-life directly related to the length of the ester chain (35).

Cynthia Kuhn (38) nicely reviewed the four basic ways in which structural and pharmacokinetic properties can be expressed from the basic testosterone structure. First, the standard testosterone molecule can be utilized parenterally, as a skin patch, skin cream, or alternatively in a micronized oral preparation. Secondly, esterification at the 17-β site (as noted above) promotes lipophilicity on the testosterone cypionate, propionate, enanthate, and undecanoate preparations. Thirdly, manipulation at the 17-α site produces methyltestosterone, danazol, and oxandrolone, which resist hepatic first-pass metabolism and become orally available, but therefore have increased liver toxicity. Finally, various modifications at the A, B, or C rings (as with mesterolone, nortestosterone, and nandrolone) provide (variously) slowed metabolism, enhanced androgen receptor affinity, resistance to aromatization to estradiol, and decreased metabolite binding to androgen receptors.

AAS-related "dietary supplements" are simply prohormones that have the same or similar biologic effects as the AAS themselves, but remained available long after the AAS were placed on the Federal Schedule. For instance, the prohormone supplements dehydroepiandrosterone (DHEA) and androstenedione were legal and available OTC when baseball superstar Mark McGuire was famously noticed by a news reporter to display a bottle of "Andro" in his clubhouse locker (39). DHEA, though banned by most major sports organizations, still remains available as a dietary supplement, reportedly because of an intervention by a U.S. senator with many supplement manufacturers in his home state (40). Although these supplements usually are less potent than the AAS, they nonetheless are converted to testosterone and cause measurable androgenic and anabolic effects.

In addition, some substances marketed as dietary supplements actually contain AAS, and on July 28, 2009 the U.S. FDA issued a consumer advisory (41), along with a warning to one of the manufacturers, American Cellular Laboratories, which advised consumers to avoid the most obvious culprits, those substances which are marketed as AAS or with names that sound like AAS. The advisory made the point that these products may contain synthetic AAS or AAS-like active ingredients and are therefore not dietary supplements, and specifically mentioned Tren-Tren-Streme, MASS Xtreme, Estro Xtreme,

Figure 23.4. Biosynthesis and metabolism of testosterone.

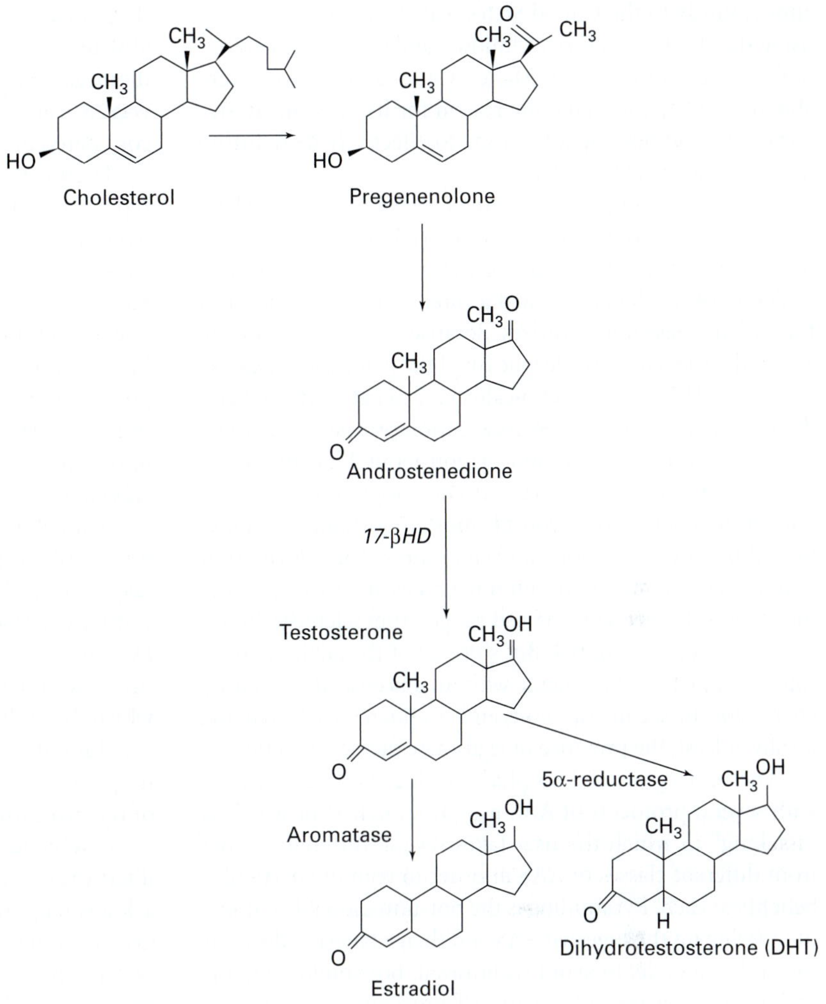

and substances marketed as "similar to Stanozolol," "similar to Boldenone," or "very similar to 1-testosterone."

The advisory's statement on health risks of these products was detailed and quite worrisome:

> Adverse event reports received by FDA for body building products that are labeled to contain steroids or asteroid alternatives involve men (ages 22 to 55) and include cases of serious liver injury, stroke, kidney failure and pulmonary embolism (blockage of an artery in the lung). Acute liver injury is known to be a possible harmful effect of using anabolic steroid-continuing products. In addition, anabolic steroids may cause other serious long-term adverse health consequences in men, women, and children. These include shrinkage of the testes and male infertility, masculinization in women, breast enlargement in males, short stature in children, adverse effects on blood lipid levels, and increased risk of heart attack and stroke.

DESIGNER AAS

A variety of AAS—the "designer steroids"—have been designed specifically to evade drug testing and provide a high anabolic–androgenic profile. Although epitestosterone was used by the GDR to evade drug tests and is still prescribed by some physicians despite its biologic inertness and ineffectuality for any purpose other than evading drug testing, other more sophisticated strategies have been developed for evading those tests. For instance, Norbolethone, which was initially packaged as "The Clear" by notorious AAS purveyor Victor Conte of San Francisco's BALCO laboratory (42) was developed in the 1960s, never marketed because of concerns about potential toxicity, but came to light as a present day illicit AAS when U.S. cyclist Tammy Thomas was found to have an elevated T:E ratio at the 2000 World Cycling Championships in Belgium. Thomas was eventually found to have been using norbolethone provided by Victor Conte and chemist Patrick Arnold at BALCO labs (43).

After the exposure of norbolethone as "The Clear," Arnold, newspaper accounts allege (44), changed the active ingredient in "The Clear" to tetrahydrogestrinone (THG), a previously unknown molecule structurally related to two AAS already banned by the World Anti-Doping Association (WADA), gestrinone and trenbolone. In his 2004 report on the discovery of the new substance THG (45), AAS expert Don Catlin described his work identifying the unknown substance provided to him in "a spent syringe that had allegedly contained an anabolic androgenic steroid undetectable by sport doing control urine tests (which had been) provided anonymously to the United States Anti-Doping Agency." By using standard laboratory techniques and some educated hypotheses about the new substance, Catlin and his team were able to identify the THG, the reason for its previous undetectability, and develop a lab assay to effectively deny future illicit AAS users THG, at least.

In an interesting legal side note to the discovery of THG, four NFL players were found to have THG in their urine samples—which had been collected before a test for THG was available (46). The NFL tested a total of 4000 samples and found only these four positives. Because retrospective testing found the substance, the league fined the players for AAS use although THG was not technically banned before it had been discovered. The NFL Players Association protested the fines.

AAS users obtain their information about these substances from a large variety of sources: friends, suppliers, easily obtainable manuals, and—probably most importantly—sophisticated Internet sites, blogs, and chatrooms. The information that users get, both on optimum regimens and managing the inevitable side effects of AAS use, ranges from scientifically accurate to frankly criminal. But since all of the advice constitutes the practice of medicine without a license, there is little chance for the second opinions and considered trials that are, ideally at least, the province of legitimate medical practice.

The underground AAS pharmacologists have come up with several protocols of AAS use (47), the first of which is "stacking" in which the user takes several different agents from different classes of AAS in order to reap the particular benefits of each. Pyramiding is the not-unreasonable pattern of tapering up the ingested AAS and then a tapering down at the end of a cycle, to avoid withdrawal. Bodybuilding gyms and the Internet are replete with self-proclaimed experts who offer to guide the novice through a bodybuilding regimen, which often enough reveals substantial results within a few months, leading to increased faith in the "coach."

COMPLICATIONS OF AAS USE

Use of the AAS has been associated with numerous medical problems, some more serious than others. Since the supraphysiologic dosages used illicitly cannot be prescribed ethically to research study participants, researchers often rely on convenience samples of AAS users who present with medical problems, as well as animal models, to determine and characterize these complications. Given the usually clandestine nature of AAS use, the population of AAS users who experience no side effects or subclinical side effects remains unknown since they neither seek nor receive medical attention. Keeping these caveats in mind, however, there exists a convincing literature of well-documented medical problems attributable to the AAS.

Most dramatic is the occasional cardiac death attributed to the AAS, including a well-documented case report of two AAS-using athletes who died from sudden cardiac arrhythmias (48). Two bodybuilders, one aged 29 and the other aged 30, collapsed and died without any obvious reasons, and were found to have been using stanozolol, nandrolone, and testosterone, but no drugs of abuse or ethanol. Cardiac pathology revealed that the athletes had normal gross cardiac pathology, so simple cardiomegaly was not the cause of death. The T:E ratio in one case was 28.7, and in the second was 42, far above the 6 commonly considered the upper limit of normal.

Despite the absence of gross cardiomegaly, the pathology report did show focal myocardial fibrosis and contraction band necrosis, which the authors attribute to the use of AAS combined with exercise, rather than simply exercise itself. Since the cardiac vessels and conduction systems appeared free of pathology, the authors were convinced that this "direct injury" to the heart was the likely cause of death. They hypothesized that "…the combined effects of vigorous weight training, anabolic steroid use, and androgen sensitivity may have predisposed these young men to myocardial injury and subsequent sudden cardiac death."

A small study of 6 AAS-using bodybuilders compared to 9 non-AAS-using bodybuilders and 16 age-matched sedentary controls showed by Doppler echocardiography of the left ventricular (LV) myocardium that there was no increase in LV wall thickness in the AAS users (49). However, the AAS users exhibited a smaller passive component to LV filling, which the authors speculate was related to their AAS use, and conclude that "… the decrease in LV relaxation properties might have been due to an alteration in the active properties of the myocardium, but that has yet to be confirmed."

In a broader review of the cardiac arrhythmias linked to illicit drug use by athletes, Furlanello and colleagues (50) acknowledge the more significant clinical ramifications of the QTc prolongation associated with the use of ephedra and caffeine products, as well as the myocardial infarction and ventricular tachycardia experienced by athletes using amphetamines. However, they point out that the AAS are often taken with diuretics to avoid detection, and HGH to enhance anabolic effects, both of which potentiate cardiac problems such as myocardial hypertrophy and hypotension.

In a less dramatic, though arguably more common way, AAS users consistently suffer from serum lipoprotein abnormalities caused by their AAS use. Given the cardiac pathology associated with low high-density lipoprotein (HDL) values, it is worth considering the AAS well-documented effects on serum lipoproteins. AAS users consistently experience falling levels of HDL after a few days of AAS use, probably related to stimulation of hepatic triglyceride lipase, which is responsible for modulating HDL-2 and apolipoprotein-A1. Interestingly, the 17-alkylated AAS reduce HDL by about half, while nandrolone and testosterone esters have little effect, probably because testosterone does not induce triglyceride lipase. Total cholesterol often remains stable in AAS users, because LDL is increased by AAS use (51).

Kuipers and his colleagues (52) injected 100 mg of nandrolone decanoate into a cohort of bodybuilders each week for 8 weeks, and compared various physical parameters to a control group of bodybuilders 8 weeks later. They found that the nandrolone-using bodybuilders experienced a 25% to 27% decreases in HDL, which reverted to normal 6 weeks after they stopped using the nandrolone. Like many such studies, this one is hampered by the ethical imperative to give research subjects the usual dosages prescribed for legitimate medical problems, although AAS users probably use more, as evidenced by one Web-based information source (53) which also contains advertisements for nandrolone decanoate: "Standard dosage of Nandrolone is 2 mg per pound of body weight. For Example, a 90 kg (200 pound) athlete should take 400 mg per week. Maximum dosages can be as high as 1000–1500 mg per week." Had the Kuipers study injected their subjects with 1500 mg/week of nandrolone decanoate (15 times higher than their study dosage!) they might well have found more or longer-lasting damage to lipid profiles.

One naturalistic study (54) that did not quantify the actual dosage of the AAS used nonetheless found valuable information about the differential effects of the AAS when compared to weightlifting or running. When compared to recreational weightlifters, heavyweight lifters, and runners, the small group of seven AAS users had significantly lower HDL levels and significantly higher LDL levels, but no difference in blood pressure. Not surprisingly, the runners had significantly lower body mass index (5% as compared to 11% for the recreational weightlifters, 10% for the heavyweight lifters, and 11% for the steroid users). The AAS users did have elevated LV mass, not explained by the fact that the steroid users were heavier in general, since this effect had been factored out.

Despite the clear evidence that AAS use causes perturbations in serum lipid profiles, and the uncontested connection between lowered HDL levels and heart disease, there is as yet little convincing evidence that AAS users suffer clinically significant lipid profile abnormalities. One study of the reversibility of AAS-related side effects (55) found that HDL decreases in fact resolved after the 12 to 43 months in which the subjects had not been taking AAS, after their long-term use. Fifteen athletes who were former AAS users were compared to 17 still-using athletes on a variety of parameters including hemoglobin, platelets, ALT, AST, testosterone, LH, and FSH. After more than a year of abstinence by the 15 ex-users, many still had increased ALT levels and depressed testosterone synthesis, and their HDL cholesterol and other parameters had normalized, although of course the clinical ramifications are not necessarily clear, even with this return to normal values.

Musculoskeletal injuries related to AAS use by adults are usually related to tendon and ligament damage caused by AAS-mediated muscle growth, without concomitant connective tissue growth. In addition, the AAS combined with exercise may interact with tendon collagen fibrils, decreasing the tensile strength of the tendon, just when it is needed to handle the newly enlarged musculature (56). One case report (57) of a 32-year-old professional bodybuilder describes his acute pain at attempting to squat-lift 400 lbs: he was found to have ruptured both quadriceps tendons. History revealed a 10-year history of multiple PES, including AAS. His use of testosterone was estimated at six times the recommended daily dose, and he had already suffered from gynecomastia, acne, and loss of his libido. Children and adolescents also experience specific musculoskeletal side effects of AAS use; this will be reviewed below.

Although hepatic pathology is often cited as one of the most worrisome potential side effects of AAS use, the literature reveals several relatively inconsequential hepatic conditions associated with AAS, and only a few serious maladies. Pelioisis hepatitis—blood-filled cysts in the liver—has been associated with tuberculosis, the use of oral contraceptives by women, and AAS use by men. Despite the understandable concern about having any sort of liver pathology, peliosis hepatitis is itself usually considered a benign finding, and is usually discovered only incidentally (58).

Similarly, liver function tests (LFTs) are often elevated in those who are presently using AAS or have recently stopped (59), but the LFTs usually normalize after a relatively short period of time, with systemic damage to the liver unclear. In an animal study which sheds light on the mechanism of hepatic changes caused by the AAS, Vieira and colleagues (60) compared, over 5-weeks' time, four groups of Westar rats: a control group, a group receiving low dose of nandrolone decanoate, intermediate doses, and supraphysiologic doses. The nandrolone caused a dose-dependent increase in LFTs (although all remained within the normal range), and an increase in collagen deposition to the liver parenchyma and portal space. They also noted an increase in the Kuppfer macrophage cells, presumably deployed to defend liver tissue against collagen deposition. The Kuppfer cells are implicated in some models of liver fibrosis and cirrhosis. The 5-week time span of the study, as well as the lack of a comparable human model detract from the study's clinical relevance, but the mechanism does seem quite similar to observations in human AAS users.

The most worrisome hepatic side effect linked with the AAS is hepatocellular carcinoma, a tumor whose prevalence has been increasing over the last two decades (61). This tumor occurs mostly in those over 65 years of age, has about a 3:1 male to female prevalence ratio, a poor prognosis, and few distinct risk factors: previous hepatitis C infection, heavy alcohol consumption, and diabetes/obesity. However, between 15% and 50% of new cases have none of these risk factors, leading to a search for other associations or etiologies. Since the disease is more prevalent in men—who have higher endogenous testosterone levels than women—AAS use should be one possible line of inquiry. But the reports on hepatocellular carcinoma in AAS users are case reports that suggest (62,63) but do not prove a connection between the sometimes massive use of AAS by the subjects and their subsequent cancer diagnoses.

The most common sex-specific side effects of the AAS in men, testicular atrophy and gynecomastia, are caused by downregulation of testicular production of testosterone and aromatization to estrogen, respectively. Although the AAS certainly cause testicular atrophy and subsequent impotence, loss of libido, and decreased sperm count, it is less clear that the AAS actually cause permanent infertility. In men, the AAS apparently directly damage sperm via altered meiotic segregation, but this effect usually resolves after cessation of AAS use (64).

Deca-Durabolin (nandrolone decanoate) is quite popular among AAS users because it has little liver toxicity and a high anabolic:androgenic effect ratio. However, the molecule

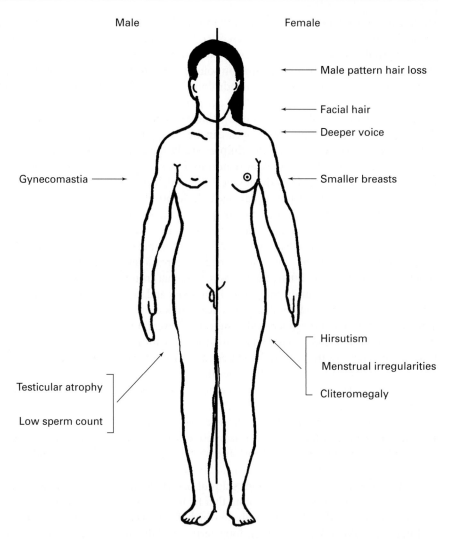

Figure 23.5. Sex-specific effects of AAS use.

is a progestin and can incite gynecomastia, suppression of the hypothalamic–pituitary–testicular axis, and complete cessation of endogenous testosterone production. The subsequent impotence—termed "Deca-Dick" by amateur pharmacologists—can be addressed by the use of testosterone production stimulants like HCG both during and after the Deca-Duroblin cycle, but there is no guarantee of any salutary effect. Many Deca-Duroblin users complain of impotence long after they have stopped using the drug, and even after attempts at stimulation of testosterone production.

Women who ingest AAS experience the effects of an abnormally high testosterone level, and therefore show easily predictable effects: increase in muscle size, deepening of the voice, increased facial hair, clitoral enlargement, and menstrual problems (65). Sex-specific effects of AAS are presented in Figure 23.5.

In one survey of AAS use patterns that suggests the relative prevalence of specific side effects, 21 gyms in Great Britain were surveyed (66), and although only 59% of individuals questioned responded, the responses were clearly segregated by sex. Fifty-five percent of the men reported testicular atrophy, 52% had gynecomastia, 36% had elevated blood pressure, and 26% reported tendon injuries. Among the women who responded to the questionnaire, 8 out of 13 (61%) reported menstrual problems and fluid retention, 4 had clitoral enlargement, and 3 complained of a decrease in breast size.

The damaging physical effects of the AAS on children and adolescents are even more marked and well described than on adults. Even those who advocate for the legitimization of AAS use would deny the drugs to children. A long list of risks specific to children and adolescents who use AAS is topped by potential abnormalities in pubertal sexual development modulated by testosterone. An animal model predicts (67) that exogenous testosterone (and therefore AAS) will increase aggression, cause permanent damage to neurotransmitter systems, and provoke a reinforcing effect distinct from that caused by the androgen receptors themselves. Even more worrisome are those proven maladies that demonstrably occur in adolescents who use AAS, most prominently psychiatric effects and musculoskeletal problems.

Although adolescents, like adults, face the danger of tendon rupture from accelerated muscle growth, adolescents have the unique added problem of premature epiphyseal plate closure (68). The epiphyseal plate cartilage presents the obvious place for a break when pressure is applied to the entire system, which results in premature closure of the plate, and resultant short stature.

PSYCHIATRIC COMPLICATIONS OF AAS USE

The AAS also cause behavioral and psychiatric phenomena, the most distinctive of which is known popularly as "roid rage." As in the case of World Wrestling Entertainment wrestler Chris Benoit, the popular media may exaggerate the effects of steroids on complex human behaviors (69), but the horrific nature of Benoit's act—strangling his wife and suffocating his 7-year-old son before hanging himself—lends itself to hyperbole and a search for causes. Benoit's stage moniker as "The Canadian Crippler" and the reported deliveries of AAS, HGH, and testosterone to his home lent decisive, if circumstantial, weight to the notion that "roid rage" caused the Benoit tragedy. However, the peer-reviewed literature contains multiple case series and literature reviews documenting AAS-related hostility, aggression, hallucinations, and delusions (70,71).

AAS-related mood perturbations may be even more prominent in children. In one preliminary report, researchers at the University of Iowa (72) surveyed 86,000 6th, 8th, and 11th graders about their use of drugs and alcohol and their attitudes toward school, family, and their community. Not surprisingly, the percentage of AAS users increased as the students aged, with 0.8% of the 6th grade boys acknowledging ever using steroids, as did 2% and 4.5% of the 8th grade and 11th grade boys. For the girls, the percentages were lower but still substantial: 0.7%, 1.8%, and 2.9%, respectively. Aggressive behavior toward others was admitted by 64.1% of the boys who had ever used AAS, as compared to 22.6% who had never used AAS. And of the boys who used AAS, 36.9% of the 11th grade boys and 53.5% of the 11th grade girls had experienced suicidal ideation, compared to 10.6% and 16.8% of the non-AAS-using boys and girls. Although these data show association, not causation, the clear connection between AAS and emotional abnormalities in high school students deserves closer scrutiny.

For adults also, AAS-related affective symptoms are much more common than psychosis, and the affective symptoms are generally experienced by unsophisticated AAS users who are taking dosages at the high end of the spectrum, far beyond the dosages for performance enhancement. Mood symptoms can include depression, hypomania, and frank mania (73). One manifestation of withdrawal from AAS can be a profound depression (74), which has been implicated in the completed suicide of some users, although another school of thought within psychology makes the point that normal developmental changes, as well as substances *in general* predispose adolescents to impulsive behaviors like suicide (75).

Although the very existence of true physiologic dependence and withdrawal from AAS has been questioned, careful analysis shows that both phenomena occur, especially in the heavy AAS user. An early case study of an AAS user who stopped abruptly revealed typical correlates of withdrawal,

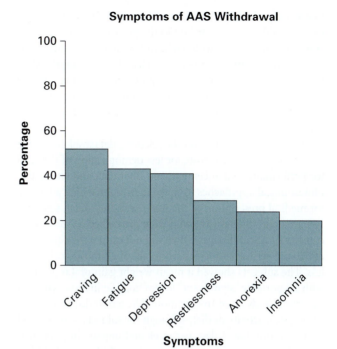

Figure 23.6. Symptoms of AAS withdrawal. Adapted from Brower KJ, Blow FC, Young JP, et al. Symptoms and correlates of anabolic–androgenic steroid dependence. *Br J Addict.* 1991;86:759–768.

including the sudden onset of dysphoria, fatigue, psychomotor retardation, impaired concentration, along with suicidal ideation (76). This symptom picture disappeared after 4 days. The same authors later reported a case series of 49 AAS-using competitive weightlifters (77) and found that 94% endorsed at least one symptom of *DSM-III-R* dependence, with 84% experiencing physiologic withdrawal, 51% using more AAS than intended, and 49% spending more time then they had intended on substance-related activities (77) (Fig. 23.6).

When compared to cocaine and heroin, the AAS are decidedly less likely to cause addiction problems like tolerance, withdrawal, and continued use despite the user's awareness of adverse consequences. However, researchers have put the "addictiveness" of the AAS on the spectrum closer to mild reinforcers like caffeine, nicotine, and benzodiazepines (78).

Perhaps more important than the peer-reviewed research about the addictive aspects of the AAS are the statements of AAS users and their loved ones. In a Web site (79) developed to commemorating the life of Taylor Hooton, a high school athlete whose suicide at the age of 16 was associated with his abrupt cessation of AAS, his parents and coaches discuss their initial ignorance about the effects of AAS. In addition, they review the apparent psychiatric effects of his use, and the apparent catastrophic and self-destructive effects of his decrease in AAS usage. Although NFL linebacker Lyle Alzado's belief that his use of AAS caused his ultimately-fatal CNS lymphoma tumor has no scientific support, his description of the AAS's profound compulsive hold on him is both heartfelt and consistent with what people say about other addictive substances: "… I started taking anabolic steroids in 1969, and I never stopped. Not when I retired from the NFL in 1985. Not ever. I couldn't …. According to the guys around the gym, if you go on steroids for six to eight weeks, then you're supposed to stop for the same number of weeks. Me, I'd be on the stuff for 10 or 12 weeks, and then I'd go off for only two, maybe three weeks, and I'd feel that was enough. It was addicting, mentally addicting. I just didn't feel strong unless I was taking something …" (80).

Despite user reports and the scientific data available, some writers continue to advocate for less demonization of the AAS for performance enhancement, and offer data and alternative philosophical approaches to make their points. One advocate for medical prescription of the AAS, Anthony Millar, followed 169 amateur athletes (81) who were prescribed a 7 to 9 week course of AAS, at dosages which did not exceed the equivalent of 500 mg per week of testosterone, although most received far less. The subjects showed a mean weight gain of 4.6 pounds, with a reportedly "significant" loss of body fat in those who had a prestudy body fat of 16% or more. The report does not quantify physical activity or diet, although the subjects were advised to train more than 4 days per week and ingest a high protein diet. Observed side effects were elevation of LFTs, total cholesterol, and lowering of HDL, as well as instances of decreased libido, all of which resolved after the study period. Three instances of gynecomastia were treated with Tamoxifen at 20 mg/day over a 4-week period, which, the author reports, "settled down" the breast inflammation, though again no data are given. From this mostly observational study, Dr. Millar concludes that small doses of the AAS can be used safely, and that ending the prohibition of AAS use would reduce overall harm from the drugs because of the present situation in which, unfairly (to his mind) "… more side effects and catastrophic events are attributed to the *use* of anabolic steroids rather than their *abuse*."

In a more-favorable-than-not review article, Hoffman and Ratamess (82) opined that some AAS side effects are exaggerated in attempts to prevent use, and that drug-testing programs do not necessarily decrease use of the AAS. They note the difficulty in studying, under laboratory conditions, AAS dosages and patterns used in the "real world" of gyms and bedrooms, and make the point that contributing factors such as genetic predisposition and diet might account for some effects now attributed to the AAS. Rather than a polemic for or against AAS use, the authors write that they merely advocate for more accurate information about AAS effect and side effects.

In a nonscientific but provocative documentary about AAS use in the United States (83), actor Chris Bell examines use of the AAS by his own brothers, as well American icons like Sylvester Stallone and Hulk Hogan. In true documentary fashion, Bell highlights the profound inconsistency in public discourse about the AAS, and notes the acceptance of other potentially dangerous modes of enhancement, like laser eye surgery, the injection of corticosteroids, and β-blockers for stage fright. The movie is not one-sided, however, skewering the supplement industry and anti-AAS crusader Congressman Henry Waxman, along with those who warn about catastrophic if unproven side effects for the AAS.

SUBSTANCES USED CONCOMITANTLY WITH THE AAS

A variety of other substances are often used along with the AAS, some to augment the effects of AAS, and some to counteract AAS side effects. One of the most commonly used adjuncts to the AAS is HGH and, starting in 1985, recombinant human growth hormone (rHGH). Native HGH is produced by the anterior pituitary, and the most common form of the hormone contains 191 amino acids. It is only available in injectable form, has a short circulating half-life (about 20 minutes) as well as a biologic half-life of 9 to 17 hours. HGH has been available commercially for 40 years, and has well-defined pediatric indications for GHD, idiopathic short stature, Turner syndrome, Prader–Willi syndrome, Noonan syndrome, and chronic renal insufficiency, with investigational use for cystic fibrosis, juvenile idiopathic arthritis, and inflammatory bowel disease (84).

Athletes taking HGH hope for the anabolic and lipolytic effects seen in patients with GHD and others with genuine HGH deficiencies, although the data supporting any sustained good effects in normals who take nothing but HGH is not particularly convincing. And reported side effects of HGH include insulin resistance, increases in very low density lipoproteins (VLDLs), arthralgia, myalgia, hypertension, cardiac failure, and an increased rate of malignancies (85).

Although the illicit use of HGH is banned by all sports organizations, despite some hopeful media reports (86), no widely available test procedure to detect HGH has been found. Although serum HGH tests were conducted at the 2004 Athens, 2006 Turin, and 2008 Beijing Olympic Games, the results were never announced, leaving some skeptical of the test's efficacy.

In addition to the AAS, stimulants are often used by athletes trying to gain a competitive advantage. Doping athletes can use commonly prescribed attention-deficit hyperactivity disorder (ADHD) remedies like amphetamine (Adderall and others); methylphenidate (Ritalin and others); OTCs like caffeine, guarana, or pseudoephedrine; or banned but previously available supplements such as ephedra. On occasion athletes will even try highly toxic drugs of abuse like cocaine for performance enhancement, although this strategy usually leads to disaster very quickly. One commonly abused stimulant is clenbuterol, a β_2 adrenergic agonist prescribed as a decongestant but used by athletes as a partitioning agent.

In attempts to "flush their system" and obtain a false-negative urine toxicology results, athletes sometimes use diuretics such as loop diuretics (e.g., hydrochlorothiazide), various herbal preparations, and simple overingestion of water (87). Consequently, loop diuretics are banned by most sports organizations unless the athlete has a documented therapeutic use exemption (TUE, as described later in this chapter). Since diuretics are perceived as relatively benign, athletes often significantly underestimate the potential risks they face of dehydration, heat stroke, kidney failure, hyponatremia, and hypokalemia with their use.

Human chorionic gonadotropin (HCG) can be used by AAS users to counteract the AAS-stimulated down-regulation of androgen production by the interstitial cells of the testes. HCG stimulates the testes to again produce testosterone, even in the ex-AAS user who may have stopped using AAS, but whose testicular function did not return. In addition, HCG is reputed to raise testosterone levels without affecting the T:E ratio, another reason athletes might use the substance. A 1995 survey of male AAS users found that 32% of the 52 users questioned had used HCG in their attempts to negate the effects of their AAS use (88). A high-profile professional baseball player recently suspended for his use of HCG (89) presumably demonstrates the ongoing use of HCG as an adjunctive treatment for those who use AAS, with the resultant testicular atrophy and shutdown.

ETHICS OF AAS USE

Any consideration of the ethics of PES use in sports necessitates an understanding of the meaning of sport, and some definition of what actually constitutes a PES, seemingly obvious concepts which become murkier when critically examined. For instance, the main focus of most sports—intense competition—lends itself to whatever sort of enhancement an athlete can muster, substances included. A swimmer choosing to wear a speed-enhancing suit, a bicyclist training at high altitude, or a skier using expensive waxes are all normative events in competitive sport, but all are also regulated by authorities within the sport. What if an athlete wants to avoid traveling to the mountains, and simply use a hypoxic chamber? Or take a substance like erythropoietin (EPO), which also raise hemoglobin levels?

And what about prosthetic devices? In one closely watched case, South African sprinter Oscar Pistorius (90) had bilateral below-the-knee amputations requiring the use of prostheses to walk, much less run. In order to compete at the Olympic level using the J-shaped prosthesis called the "Cheetah," Pistorius had to bring his case before the International Association of Athletics Foundations (IAAF) where his lawyers asserted, based on comparison studies of Pistorius' running with the endurance, fatigability, and sprinting mechanics of able-bodied athletes, that the prostheses conferred no advantage. The study data showed that Pistorius had a sprinting gait markedly dissimilar from other athletes, that he took 34% less time in the air between steps, and that he exhibited considerably less force on ground in relation to his body weight. So, although the authors concluded that Pistorius' abilities were generally similar to able-bodied athletes, this was clearly an opinion judgment call rather than an exact comparison. The IAAF accepted the reasoning of the investigators and allowed Pistorius to compete with his prostheses. Certain swimsuits can be banned, rules can be modified, and new technologies can be accepted or rejected, but all of these decisions require thoughtful and ultimately subjective judgments about the meaning of sport itself.

The use of substances to improve performance seems to many a separate case, but the same sorts of ambiguities exist in this category. Some substances, like protein powders, are allowed by all major sports, while others, like the AAS, are banned by all sports organizations. Some legitimate medications, like the β-agonists used to treat asthma, are banned by some sports organizations and not others, while other medications like the β-blockers used to treat hypertension are banned in some sports (biathlon) but not others (boxing). Just to confuse the picture, all major sports organizations must allow for the possibility that some banned substances—most notably stimulants and diuretics—may be medically necessary for a particular athlete and therefore undeniable for those who meet clinical criteria for taking that particular medication. Separating out those athletes who merely *want* the medication as opposed to those who both *want* and *need* the medications is the difficult task faced in the granting of sports TUEs, as described below.

Antidoping programs and the necessary testing often appear to be unnecessarily paternalistic, with paternalism defined by ethicist Thomas Murray as "… doing something to or for another person for their benefit but without regard for that individual's preferences" (91). This certainly seems to be an incongruity in athletics: if society allows adults to smash into opposing linebackers and drive race cars at 180 miles/h for the sake of sport, how can society forbid those same individuals from taking another acknowledged risk involving the PES? As Dr. Murray points out, however, there is an important difference between the risks inherent in a sport, and those that the athlete chooses to take on, and the athletes' choices are hardly unconstrained. If unregulated, the enormous pressures put on athletes—even those who are not professional—results in potentially self-destructive behaviors with the PES that could lead to grotesquely dangerous drug use which would surely spread to other athletes who wish to compete. Each sport has the right and obligation to regulate the boundaries of competition, from the distance between the pitching mound and home plate, to the weight of the hockey puck, all the way to what substances the players may ingest.

As one antidoping expert pointed out, the choices presented to an athlete are excruciatingly simple: "If you compete in a sport where everyone is using performance-enhancing drugs, then you have three choices: compete at a disadvantage, quit the sport, or go against your principles and take the drugs … all three are poor ethical choices" (92).

Dr. Murray, the ethicist, sets out five elements for an ethically successful and fair antidoping program, the first of which is adequate analytic capacity. That is, the scientific basis of the testing devices, laboratory procedures, and staff certification must all be as close to unquestionable as possible. Second, the sampling strategy must be tailored to the sport at hand, as well as the substances that are usually used in that sport. Testing only during competition when competitors can stop their substance of choice just before competition and come out clean makes no sense, and newer techniques—including access to serum samples and ongoing comparison of sequential lab values—are potential necessities in future drug testing. Third, the program must have an adjudication process that is "fair, open and reliable." Fourth, research into doping and drug testing must continue to provide strategies and laboratory techniques to handle the inevitable challenges in antidoping strategies. Finally, Murray recommends that the antidoping community set forth a clear set of principles as to why doping is wrong, and have a uniform and fair process for banning or allowing various substances.

Another ethical conundrum within sports doping is the role of physicians in providing treatment for athletes at all levels. Although some physicians and others provide clearly illegal services and substances to athletes, others function at the boundary between legitimate medicine and banned/illegal protocols. In the words of one sports medicine specialist quoted in the UNESCO Courier:

> Sport presents doctors with a paradox. Most of them believe physical activity makes for a balanced life. But they are also well aware that competition upsets the balance, and those chemical-based treatments can be prescribed to supplement deficiencies. If they respond to such demands, they are only reinforcing the alienating emphasis put on performance at all costs, of which sport is just the most striking example ... Sport medicine is a forerunner of the medicine of the future—a medicine at the behest of institutions in the business of boosting efficiency. It runs the risk of ushering in a common norm dictating people's appearance (though cosmetic surgery), character (through prenatal diagnosis) and social behavior, namely through the demand for performance in all fields, be it professional, sexual, or sporting (93).

THERAPEUTIC USE EXEMPTIONS (TUES)

All major sports organizations, both professional and amateur, have policies in place that contemplate the use of banned substances by athletes who take the medications for legitimate medical reasons: the TUE. The Olympics (94), the NCAA (95), the National Football League (96), Major League Baseball (97), the Professional Golf Association (98), and the National Hockey League (99), all have appeal processes for evaluating TUE requests.

While the idea is simple—in the words of the ethicist Murray: "Therapy is good, enhancement is suspect" (100), Murray points out that the line between the two often becomes blurred, changeable, and entirely indefinable. The World Anti-Doping Association publishes criteria (101) for TUEs, which attempt to clarify the four salient points:

> "... The four criteria that must be fulfilled before a TUE is granted are set forth in the International Standard for TUEs:
>
> 1. The *Athlete* would experience a significant impairment to health if the *Prohibited Substance* or *Prohibited Method* were to be withheld in the course of treating an acute or chronic medical condition ...
> 2. The *therapeutic Use* of the *Prohibited Substance* or *Prohibited Method* would produce no additional enhancement of performance other than that which might be anticipated by a return to a state of normal health following the treatment of a legitimate medical condition. The *Use* of any *Prohibited Substance* or *Prohibited Method* to increase 'low-normal' levels of any endogenous hormone is not considered an acceptable *therapeutic* intervention ... Enhancement of performance should be taken to mean the return by the athlete to his/her level of performance prior to the onset of the medical condition requiring treatment. This means that there may be some enhancement of individual performance as a result of the efficacy of the treatment. Nevertheless, such enhancement must not exceed the level of performance of the athlete prior to the onset of his/her medical condition.
> 3. There is no reasonable *therapeutic* alternative to the *Use* of the otherwise *Prohibited Substance* or *Prohibited Method* ...
> 4. The necessity for the *Use* of the otherwise *Prohibited Substance* or *Prohibited Method* cannot be a consequence, wholly or in part, of prior non-*therapeutic Use* of any substance from the *Prohibited List* ..."

Most TUEs in sport are for stimulants used to treat ADHD, β-adrenergic agonists to treat COPD, and β-blockers to treat asthma, although the NCAA itself (102) granted appeals in 2007 for players who had taken testosterone and the synthetic AAS Danazol and Madol (desoxymethyltestosterone), presumably on the basis of legitimate therapeutic use.

LEGAL ISSUES IN THE USE OF AAS

Despite the widespread nature of antiaging clinics who advertise and prescribe HGH with the veneer of legitimacy, and the clandestine pharmacies that provide the substance to athletes, those prescriptions are, contrary to most off-label prescriptions, specifically banned by the Food and Drug Administration (FDA) (103). In a warning alert published in January 2007, the FDA noted that HGH is not a dietary supplement, and specifically *banned* its use for "anti-aging, body-building, or athletic enhancement."

The AAS are on the Federal Schedule III list, putting them in the same category as the following (quite dissimilar) substances: codeine, ketamine, and buprenorphine, all of which have well-accepted medical uses. Schedule III substances are categorized as having the following characteristics (104):

> "1. The drug or other substance has less potential for abuse than the drugs or other substances in schedules I and II.
> 2. The drug or other substance has a currently accepted medical use in treatment in the United States.
> 3. Abuse of the drug or other substance may lead to moderate or low physical dependence or high psychological dependence.
> 4. Anabolic steroids, codeine and hydrocodone with aspirin or Tylenol®, and some barbiturates are examples of Schedule III substances."

Clearly, then, the AAS were placed on the Schedule III list as an acknowledgment that they have some therapeutic uses and may have to be prescribed to certain individuals. But practically speaking, most AAS are provided illegally, and have high degrees of criminal activity associated with them.

A 2007 DEA operation code-named "Raw Deal" (105) revealed much about the criminal and highly dangerous provenance of many of the AAS purchased over the Internet by U.S. citizens. In a worldwide sting operation, agents from the FDA's Office of Criminal Investigations, the U.S. Postal Inspection Service, the IRS, and other federal law-enforcement agencies, coordinated by the DEA, executed 143 federal search warrants in entering 56 steroid labs. In addition to the 11.4 million steroid dosage units and 242 kg of raw steroid powder found in China, the agents also seized $6.5 million, along with 25 vehicles, 3 boats, and 71 weapons. Although the operation was focused on the AAS and HGH, they also found conversion kits for sale to individuals who could then convert raw materials in steroids, as well as ketamine, fentanyl, ephedrine, pseudoephedrine, and GHB.

"Raw Deal" displayed the criminal infrastructure of AAS production, distribution, and sales over the Internet, not unlike drug cartels that supply users with drugs of abuse like cocaine and heroin. In addition, the operation demonstrated the haphazard and unhygienic conditions in which the drugs for sale were produced: "many of the underground labs seized in Operation Raw Deal are extremely unsanitary, further illustrating the danger in buying these products illegally. For example, recent lab seizures uncovered huge amounts of raw materials being mixed in bathtubs and bathroom sinks." This description of the illicit and criminal industry that provides AAS to users certainly correlates with clinical experience. AAS users often complain that the substances they receive do not appear to contain what the Internet advertisements claim.

TESTING FOR AAS

Testing for the use of AAS is fraught with technical, legal, and practical difficulties, not least of which is the inherent difficulty in designing testing programs that provide accurate and timely results while fairly treating those athletes being tested. Although the science of drug testing is growing by leaps and bounds, collection procedures and laboratory protocols remain imperfect both because of scientific realities and sometimes due to efforts by athletes to fake testing results.

In the most common test for AAS, exogenous use of testosterone or AAS can be detected by checking the urinary T:E ratio using high-resolution gas chromatography/mass spectroscopy (GC/MS). Since epitestosterone is unaffected by exogenous testosterone, the usual 1:1 ratio will shift upwards if the user ingests testosterone. Because some individuals have naturally elevated T:E ratios, sports organizations define an upper limit of normal for this ratio, usually 4:1 or 6:1. If an athlete claims to have a naturally elevated T:E ratio, sequential testing over several months can prove or disprove the claim because T:E ratios are stable unless manipulated by exogenous administration of testosterone. Epitestosterone has no physiologic effect, so the only reason to ingest epitestosterone would be to deceive a drug test, as demonstrated by the GDR teams of the 1960s, as described above.

GC/MS testing works by separating the various molecules in a sample by their chromatographic retention time, and breaking each one down to its characteristic ions (106). Isotope ratio mass spectroscopy (IRMS) testing can be used later, if necessary, to differentiate endogenous testosterone and epitestosterone from the exogenous varieties. IRMS identifies the carbon isotope ratio. Endogenous testosterone contains about 98.8% ^{12}C and only 1.1% ^{13}C, while pharmaceutically produced testosterone has a much lower percentage of the ^{13}C isotope.

Although laboratory protocols are vital in obtaining an accurate result, so is the forensic quality of the collection, packaging, transport, and laboratory handling of the samples. The World Anti-Doping Agency (WADA) for instance, published a 22-page protocol for urine collection alone (107), which assigns a "Doping Control Officer" who arranges a chaperone to accompany the athlete from the moment the athlete is notified of the required drug test until he or she arrives to a "Doping Control Station." The document describes the right of the athlete being tested to have a representative accompany him or her, provisions for (very minimal) privacy and confidentiality, and defines target testing for specific athletes or categories of athletes, weighted selections, and random selections. The code goes on to mandate that a witness of the same gender as the athlete observe the athlete "… Remove all clothing between the waists and midthigh, in order that the Witness has an unobstructed view of the sample provision … The Witness shall directly observe the Athlete provide the sample, adjusting his/her body position so as to have a clear view of the sample leaving the athlete's body …"

In addition, a valid "Chain of Custody" between the donating athlete, the collector, and the laboratory must be in place. Usually collecting agencies immediately split the donated urine sample into an "A" and "B" sample for later separate testing if one sample is found to contain a banned substance (108). Immediate testing at the collection site for pH, temperature, and specific gravity can increase the likelihood that a sample is valid. These sorts of carefully planned routines and procedures are absolutely necessary, both in order to provide accurate results, and to address the inevitable legal challenges that arise when a positive result causes loss of income and/or public announcement of a player's name.

TREATMENT OF AAS USERS

Treatment of AAS use must begin with a comprehensive evaluation focused on the actual effects of the substances used, any withdrawal if the substance is stopped or decreased, and concomitant substance use or mental illness. Many AAS users who have used small amounts of AAS or used AAS for a short period of time stop without any untoward effects. Often they must stop their use to avoid sanctions or detection, or because of parental disapproval. However, some AAS users find it difficult to stop their use, some experience withdrawal, and an even smaller percentage show classic signs of addiction: continued use despite knowledge of adverse consequences, compulsive use, and sustained withdrawal.

For those AAS users who require treatment, the evaluating clinician should be knowledgeable about AAS, addiction in general, and the particular ethos of the culture within which the user resides (109).

As with all addiction, the clinician should advise that the user avoid—in Alcoholics Anonymous parlance—the people, places, and things associated with the AAS use. For the athlete using AAS, this often means eschewing the gyms and practice fields where he or she had obtained the substance and isolating himself or herself from teammates, both difficult but necessary tasks in avoiding further use. The necessary paradigm shift, away from intense competition and toward a healthy lifestyle, can be managed with the help of a therapist or counselor knowledgeable about competitive athletics, and in the best situation, knowledgeable about the athlete's particular sport.

The affective syndromes like depression and anxiety that can arise from stopping AAS may have catastrophic consequences, including self-harm and completed suicide. The clinician assisting a person stopping AAS should therefore monitor the user carefully for incipient affective symptoms, and aggressively treat any symptoms that do arise. Antidepressant medications such as fluoxetine and venlafaxine may be used in treating persistent dysphoria, but since their response time is 2 to 6 weeks, the depressed AAS users should remain under closely monitored psychotherapy during (at least) that time.

Similarly, AAS withdrawal can be treated symptomatically with hormonal treatment (110) under the care of an endocrinologist knowledgeable and experienced in working with AAS users, who in order to have engendered their withdrawal symptoms most likely use supraphysiologic dosages far beyond what any physician would recommend for the treatment of any medical condition. Endocrinologists may recommend gradually tapering dosages of testosterone, the AAS that the individual was using, and even attempt stimulation of the hypothalamic–pituitary–testis axis via hormonal manipulation. The treating endocrinologist and psychiatrist should collaborate closely to render optimum care while keeping the patient as free as possible of AAS withdrawal symptomatology, both physical and psychiatric.

CONCLUSIONS

The science around the use of AAS for performance enhancement is relatively meager for easily understandable reasons; most use is illicit and therefore hidden from scientific inquiry, and the large doses of AAS used by many users could not be ethically prescribed to study subjects, because of potential danger associated with such use. This justifiably sparse body of scientific knowledge about AAS effects and side effects does, however, engenders discourse on the subject which is long on opinion and philosophy, but short on fact.

Some argue that the AAS present reasonable risks that should be assessed not by legal authorities or sports organizations, but by the users themselves. They argue that reasonable adults should make their own choices, as with other substances, and point out that allowing legitimate use of the AAS would eliminate the criminal manufacturing and distribution practices now in place, as well as allow legitimate physicians to give advice to athletes using the AAS. Despite the lack of ultimate clarity on the side effect profiles of the AAS, it is clear that they cause physical as well as psychiatric morbidity far in excess of any benefit. But in fact legitimate avenues are already available for those patients with a legitimate need for the AAS: physicians who treat HIV and other wasting disease may prescribe the AAS without concern about censure.

The Internet remains a vast repository of information combined with misinformation, most obviously when there is something to sell, in this case the AAS. The Internet user can be easily led astray by even well-meaning and apparently legitimate Web sites that purport to educate the reader. For instance, one Web site "About.com" (111) gives information about the AAS, but includes advertisements for buying AAS over the Internet, and lists as the first "Risk" for AAS users the following: "Increased Liver Function." This sounds like a good thing: who wouldn't want one's internal organs to increase in their functioning? But of course the risk is "Increased Liver Function *Tests*" and the casual or naïve reader would not see the error, and would hardly be put off by the suggested "Risk."

The use of AAS for legitimate medical purposes deserves more inquiry into present uses, and investigations of potential beyond the relatively small group of wasting diseases for which those medications are now indicated. And the use of AAS for performance enhancement, anathema though it is to most of the medical world, deserves ongoing research if only to further clarify the dangers of illicit use and develop better strategies for prevention, testing, and treatment.

REFERENCES

1. Kochakian, CD. History of anabolic–androgenic steroids. In: Lin GC, Erinoff L, eds. *Anabolic Steroid Abuse, Research Monograph 102*. Rockville, MD: National Institute on Drug Abuse; 1990:29–53.
2. Freeman ER, Bloom DA, McGuire EJ. A brief history of testosterone. *J Urol*. 2001;165(2):371–373.
3. Yesalis CE, Courson SP, Wright JE. History of Anabolic steroid use in sport and exercise. In: Yesalis CE, ed. *Anabolic Steroids in Sport and Exercise*. 2nd ed. Champaign, IL: Human Kinetics; 2000:51–72.
4. Franke WW, Berendonk B. Hormonal doping and androgenization of athletes: a secret program of the German Democratic Republic government. *Clin Chem*. 1997;43:1262–1279.
5. Goldberg L, Elliot DL. Prevention of anabolic steroid use. In: Yesalis CE, ed. *Anabolic Steroids in Sport and Exercise*. 2nd ed. Champaign, IL: Human Kinetics; 2000:117–135.
6. American College of Sports Medicine. Position statement on the use and abuse of anabolic-androgenic steroids in sports. *Med. Sci. Sports Exerc*. 1977;9:11–13.
7. Bryant H. *Juicing the Game*. New York: Viking; 2005:90.
8. http://thomas.loc.gov/cgi-bin/query/C?c101:./temp/~c101 kgDf86, accessed 7/5/09.
9. http://www4.law.cornell.edu/uscode/html/uscode21/usc_sec_21_00000812----000-.html, accessed 7/5/09.
10. Kleinman CC, Petit CE. Legal aspects of anabolic steroid use and abuse. In: Yesalis CE, ed. *Anabolic Steroids in Sport and Exercise*. 2nd ed. Champaign, IL: Human Kinetics; 2000:344–345.

11. http://vm.cfsan.fda.gov/~dms/dietsupp.html, accessed 7/5/09.
12. Green GA, Catlin DH, Starcevic B. Analysis of over the counter dietary supplements. *Clin J Sport Med*. 2001;11:254–259.
13. Crasnick J. Mitre found to have ingested Andro. ESPN.com, January 5, 2009.
14. Krishnan PV, Feng ZZ, Gordon SC. Prolonged intrahepatic cholestasis and renal failure secondary to anabolic androgenic steroid-enriched dietary supplements. *J Clin Gastroenterol*. 2009:43(7):672–675.
15. Verducci T. Totally juiced. *Sports Illustrated*, June 03, 2002.
16. CBS Sportsline.com wire reports, Sept. 7, 2006.
17. Litsky F. Report says overdose killed Caminiti. *New York Times*, November 2, 2004.
18. Canseco, J. *Juiced/Wild Times, Rampant Roids, Smash Hits, and how Baseball Got Big*. New York: HarperCollins; 2005.
19. Horn S, Gregory P, Guskiewicz K. Self-reported anabolic androgenic steroids use and musculoskeletal injuries: findings from the center for the study of retired athlete's health survey of retired NFL players. *Am J Phys Med Rehab*. 2009;88(3):192–200.
20. Johnston LD, O'Malley PM, Bachman PJ, et al. *Monitoring the Future National Results on Adolescent Drug Use, Overview of Key Findings. Bethesda, Maryland:* The University of Michigan Institute for Social Research, 2009.
21. University of Michigan News Service: Ann Arbor, MI. Retrieved 10/04/2009 from http://www.monitoringthefuture.org.
22. Leone JE, Fetro JV. Perception and attitudes toward androgenic–anabolic steroid sue among two age categories: a qualitative inquiry. *J Strength Cond Res*. 2007;21(2):532–537.
23. Gallaway S. *The Steroid Bible*. 3rd ed. Honolulu: Belle International; 1997.
24. Ranke MB, Bierich JR. Treatment of growth hormone deficiency *Clin Endocrinol Metab*. 1986;15(3):495–510.
25. Basaria S, Wahlstrom JT, Dobs AS. Anabolic androgenic steroid therapy in the treatment of chronic diseases. *J Clin Endocrinol Metab*. 2001;11:5108–5117.
26. Pope HG, Olivardia R, Gruber A, et al. Evolving ideals of male body image as seen through action toys. *Int J Eat Disord*. 1999;26(1):65–72.
27. Leit RA, Pope HG, Gray JJ. Cultural expectations of muscularity in men: the evolution of playgirl centerfolds. *Int J Eat Disord*. 2001;29(1):90–93.
28. Pope HG, Phillips KA, Olivardia R. *The Adonis Complex*. New York: Simon and Schuster; 2000.
29. http://a4minfo.net/id2.htm, accessed 10/9/09.
30. http://www.hormonewizard.com/, accessed 10/4/09.
31. Mitchell GJ. Report to the Commissioner of Baseball of an independent investigation into the illegal sure of steroids and other performance enhancing substances by players of major league baseball. Office of the commissioner of Major League Baseball, 2007:SR-22.
32. Bhasin S, Storer TW, Berman N, et al. The effect of supraphysiologic doses of testosterone on muscle size and strength in men. *N Engl J Med*. 1996;335(1):1–7.
33. Blackman MR, Sorkin JD, Münser T, et al. Growth hormone and sex steroid administration in healthy aged women and men. *JAMA*. 2002:288(18):2282–2292.
34. Mottram DR, George AJ. Anabolic steroids. *Baillières Best Price Res Clin Endocrinol Metab*. 2000;14:55–69.
35. Kicman AT. Pharmacology of anabolic steroids. *Br J Pharmacol*. 2008;154:502–521.
36. Chrousos GP. The gonadal hormones and inhibitors. In: Katzung BG, ed. *Basic and Clinical Pharmacology*. 10th ed. New York: McGraw-Hill Professional; 2007:674–675.
37. Yamada T, Kunimatsu T, Sako H, et al. Comparative evaluation of a 5-day Hershberger assay utilizing mature adult rats and a pubertal male assay for detection of flutamide's androgenic activity. *Toxicol Sci*. 2000;53:289–296.
38. Kuhn C. Anabolic steroids. *Recent Prog Horm Res*. 2002;57:411–434.
39. Hepp C. Androstenedione sharing center stage with Mark McGuire. *Knight Ridder/Tribune News Service*. August 25, 1998.
40. Kornblut E, Wilson D. How one pill escaped the list of controlled steroids. *The New York Times*, April 17, 2005.
41. http://www.fda.gov/ForConsumers/ConsumerUpdates/ucm173739.htm, accessed 8/4/09.
42. Fainaru-Wada M, Williams L. *Game of Shadows*. New York: Gotham Books; 2006:560.
43. Tammy Thomas verdict doesn't bode well for Barry Bonds, *ESPN.com*, April 4, 2008.
44. Lee H. Inventor of 'clear steroid' gets 3 months in prison. SFGate.com, August 4, 2006.
45. Catlin DH, Sekera MH, Ahrens BD, et al. Tetrahydrogestrinone: discovery, synthesis, and detection in urine. *Rapid Commun Mass Spectrom*. 2004;18:1245–1249.
46. Soliday, Bill. Robbins, Cooper face fines for use of THG. *Oakland Tribune*, July 15, 2004.
47. Hall RW, Hall RC. Abuse of supraphysiologic doses of anabolic steroids. *South Med J*. 2005;98(5)550–555.
48. Fineschie V, Riezzo I, Centini F, et al. Sudden cardiac death during anabolic steroid abuse: morphologic and toxicology findings in two fatal cases of bodybuilders. *Int J Legal Med*. 2007;121:48–53.
49. Nottin S, Nguyen LD, Terbah M, Obert P. Cardiovascular imaging. *Am J Cardiol*. 2006;97(6):912–915.
50. Furlanello F, Serdoz LV, et al. Illicit drugs and cardiac arrhythmias in athletes. *Eur J Cardiovasc Prev Rehabil*. 2007;14:487–494.
51. Friedl KE. Effects of anabolic steroids on physical health. In: Yesalis CE, ed. *Anabolic Steroids in Sport and Exercise*. 2nd ed. Champaign, IL: Human Kinetics; 2000:51–72.
52. Kuipers H, Wijnern JA, Hartgens F, et al. Influence of anabolic steroids on body composition, blood pressure, lipid profile, and liver functions in body builders. *Int J Sports Med*. 1991;12(4): 413–418.
53. http://www.ecplaza.net/product/194232_1125127/deca_300_nandrolone_decanoate.html, accessed 8/9/09.
54. Yeater R, Reed C, Ullrich I, et al. Resistance trained athletes using or not using anabolic steroids compared to runners: effects on cardio respiratory variables, body composition, and plasma lipids. *Br J Sports Med*. 1996;30:11–14.
55. Urhausen A. Reversibility of the effects on blood cells, lipids, liver function and hormones in former anabolic–androgenic steroid abusers. *J Steroid Biochem Mol Biol*. 2003;84:369–375.
56. Laster JT, Russell JA. Anabolic steroids-induced tendon pathology: a review of the literature. *Med Sci Sports Exerc*. 1990;23:1–3.
57. David HG, Green JT, Grant AJ, et al. Simultaneous bilateral quadriceps rupture: a complication of anabolic steroid abuse. *J Bone Joint Surg Br*. 1995;77(1):159–160.
58. Erpecum KJ, Jannssens AR, Kreuning J, et al. Generalized peliosis hepatitis and cirrhosis after long term use of oral contraceptives. *Am J Gastroenterol*. 2008;83(5):572–575.
59. O'Connor JS, Baldini FD, Skinner JS, et al. Blood chemistry of current and previous anabolic steroid users. *Mil Med*. 1990; 155(2):72–75.
60. Vieira RP, Franca RF, Dasmagceno-Rodriguez NR, et al. Dose-dependent hepatic response to sub chronic administration of nandrolone decanoate. *Med Sci*. 2009;40(5):842–847.

61. El-Serag H. Hepatocullular carcinoma: recent trends in the United States. *Gastroenterology*. 2009;127:S27–S34.
62. Socas L, Zumbad M, Perez-Luzardo OP, et al. Hepatocellular adenomas associated with anabolic steroid abuse in bodybuilders: a report of two cases and a review of the literature. *Br J Sports Med*. 2005;39(5):e27.
63. Gorayski P, Thompson CH, Subhash HS, et al. Hepatocellular carcinoma associated with recreational anabolic steroid use. *Br J Sports Med*. 2008;42:74–75.
64. Moretti E, Collodel G, La Marca A, et al. Structural sperm and aneuploides studies in a case of spermatogenesis recovery after the use of androgenic anabolic steroids. *J Assist Reprod Genet*. 2007;24:195–198.
65. Strauss RH, Liggett MT, Lanese RR. Anabolic steroid use and perceived effects in ten weight-trained women athletes. *JAMA*. 1985;253:2871–2873.
66. Korkia P, Stimson GV. Indications of prevalence, practice, and effects of anabolic steroid use in Great Britain. *Int J Sports Med*. 1997;18(7):557–562.
67. Sato SM, Schulz KM, Sisk CL, et al. Adolescents and androgens, receptors and rewards. *Horm Behav*. 2008;53:647–658.
68. Casavant MJ, Blake K, Griffith J, et al. Consequences of use of anabolic steroids. *Pediatr Clin North Am*. 2007;54;677–690.
69. Espn.com. June 27, 2007.
70. Perry PJ, Andersen KH, Yates WR. Illicit anabolic steroid use in athletes, a case series analysis. *Am J Sports Med*. 1990;18(4);422–428.
71. Pope HG, Katz DL. Affective and psychotic symptoms associated with anabolic steroid use. *Am J Psychiatry*. 1988;145(4):487–490.
72. Gaffney GA. Overview of anabolic steroid use and athletic doping with case presentations. *56th Annual Meeting of the American Academy of Child & Adolescent Psychiatry*, November 1, 2008.
73. Trenton AJ, Currier GW. Behavioral manifestations of anabolic steroid use. *CNS Drugs*. 2006;19(7):571–595.
74. Brower KJ, Eliopulos GA, et al. Evidence of physical and psychological dependence on anabolic androgenic steroids in weight lifters. *Am J Psychiatry*. 1990;147(4):510–512.
75. Spear LP. Neurobehavioral changes in adolescence. *Curr Dir Psychol Sci*. 2000;9:111–114.
76. Brower KJ, Blow FC, Beresford TP, et al. Anabolic–androgenic steroid dependence. *J Clin Psychiatry*. 1989;50(1);31–32.
77. Brower KJ, Blow FC, Young JP, et al. Symptoms and correlates of anabolic–androgenic steroid dependence. *Br J Addict*. 1991;86: 759–768.
78. Wood RI. Reinforcing aspects of androgens. *Physiol Behav*. 2004;83:58–64.
79. http://www.taylorhooton.org/home, accessed 6/12/09.
80. Alzado L. I'm sick and I'm scared. *Sports Illustrated*, July 8, 1991.
81. Millar AP. Licit steroid use – hope for the future. *Br J Sports Med*. 1994;28(2):79–82.
82. Hoffman JR, Ratamess NA. Medical issues associated with anabolic steroid use: are the exaggerated? *J Sports Sci Med*. 2006;4: 182–183.
83. Bell C. Bigger stronger faster. *Magnolia Pictures*; 2008.
84. Denson LA. Growth hormone therapy in children and adolescents: pharmacokinetic/pharmacodynamic considerations and emerging indications. *Exp Opin. Drug Metab Toxicol*. 2008; 4(12):1569–1580.
85. Segura J, Gutiérrez-Gallego R, Ventura R, et al. Growth hormone in sport: beyond Beijing 2008. *Ther Drug Monit*. 2009;31(1):3–13.
86. Perez AJ. Scientists say breakthrough urine test for HGH developed. *USA Today*, July 23, 2008.
87. Cone EJ. Lange R, Darwin WD. In vivo adulteration: excess fluid ingestion causes false-negative marijuana and cocaine urine test results. *J Anal Toxicol*. 1998;22(6):460–473.
88. Nilson S. Androgenic anabolic steroid use among male adolescents in Falkenberg. *Eur J Clin Psychopharmacol*. 1995;48: 9–11.
89. Schmidt MS. Manny Ramirez is banned for 50 games. *The New York Times*; 2009.
90. Oscar Pistorius: Amputee sprinter runs differently. *ScienceDaily*, August 4, 2009. 15 October 2009; http://www.sciencedaily.com/releases/2009/06/090629132200.htm.
91. Murray T. Doping in sport: challenges for medicine, science, and ethics. *J Int Med*. 2008;264:95–98.
92. Green G. Performance-enhancing drug use. *Orthopedics*. 2009; 32;647–649.
93. Liotard P. Sport medicine: to heal or to win? UNESCO Courier, September 2000, http://www.unesco.org/courier/2000_09/uk/ethique.htm, accessed 10/16/09.
94. http://www.wada-ama.org/en/exemptions.ch2, accessed 11/3/08.
95. http://www.ncaa.org/wps/ncaa?ContentID=481, accessed 11/3/08.
96. http://sports.espn.go.com/espnmag/story?section=magazine&id= 3636294, accessed 12/13/08.
97. Major League Baseball/Major League Baseball Player Association Press release; MLB, players association modify joint drug agreement. April 11, 2008.
98. Professional Golf Association Tour, *Anti-Doping Program Manual*; 2008. pp. 27–32.
99. http://www.nhl.com/nhlhq/cba/drug_testing072205.html accessed 11/5/08.
100. Murray TH. Sports enhancement. In: Crowley M. *From Birth to Death and Bench to Clinic: The Hastings Center Bioethics Briefly Book for Journalist, Policymakers, and Campaigns*. Garrison, NY: The Hastings Center; 2008:153–158.
101. World Anti-Doping Association TUE criteria http://stage.wada-ama.org/Documents/World_Anti-Doping_Program/WADP-IS-TUE/WADA_TUE_Guidelines_2009_EN.pdf accessed 10/30/09.
102. http://www.ncaa.org/wps/wcm/connect/38e412004e3edbc7bae8bf9a33b0421a/2007_08+NCAA+Drug+Testing+Results.pdf?MOD=AJPERES&CACHEID=38e412004e3edbc7bae8bf9a33b0421a accessed 9/21/09.
103. Olshansky SJ, Perls TT. New developments in the illegal provision of growth hormone for "anti-aging" and bodybuilding. *JAMA*. 2008;299(23):2792–2794.
104. DEA Website, Controlled Substances Chapter, http://www.justice.gov/dea/pubs/abuse/1-csa.htm#Formal accessed 10/30/09.
105. DEA announces largest steroid enforcement action in US History, DEA News Release September 24, 2007, http://www. usdoj.gov/dea/pubs/pressrel/pr092407.html, accessed 10/18/09.
106. Green GA. Doping control for the team physician. *Am J Sports Med*. 2006;34(10):1690–1698.
107. World Anti-Doping Agency, Guidelines for Urine Sample Collection. Version 4, June 2004, http://www.wada-ama.org/rtecontent/document/urine_testing_guideline.pdf, accessed 10/15/09.
108. Jaffee WB, Trucco E, Teter C, et al. Focus on alcohol & drug abuse: ensuring validity in urine drug testing . *Psychiatr Serv*. 2008;59:140–142.
109. Center for Substance Abuse Treatment. Anabolic steroids. *Substance Abuse Treatment Advisory* 2006;5(3).
110. Brower KJ. Withdrawal from anabolic steroids. *Curr Ther Endocrinol Metab*. 1997;6:338–343.
111. http://bodybuilding.about.com/od/supplementationbasics/a/steroiddangers_2.htm, accessed 8/9/09.

SECTION 5 ■ COMPULSIVE AND ADDICTIVE BEHAVIORS

CHAPTER 24: Eating Disorders and Substance Use Disorders

Harry A. Brandt ■ Steven F. Crawford ■ Katherine A. Halmi

INTRODUCTION

Eating disorders (EDs) and substance use disorders (SUDs) share several common elements. Both groups of illnesses are characterized by high rates of morbidity and mortality. Both pose substantial clinical challenges to the highly experienced clinician. Both have high rates of relapse and recidivism. Additionally, both sets of illnesses commonly co-occur with each other and with a number of other Axis I and Axis II diagnoses, further complicating assessment and treatment. Because of the frequent co-occurrence of SUDs and EDs, investigators have long searched for common etiologic factors in the development and perpetuation of these illnesses. To date, no single link or factor has emerged, yet the high rate of co-occurrence itself holds important implications for appropriate diagnostic assessment and treatment, and will likely guide future directions of investigation. This chapter will provide an update on ED and SUD comorbidity with applicability to those working in the substance abuse disorder and ED fields. Possible etiologic vulnerabilities underlying both sets of illnesses including a conceptual allostatic model for EDs and some general treatment recommendations for patients with co-occurring illness will be presented.

BRIEF DESCRIPTIONS OF MAJOR EATING DISORDER SYNDROMES

The EDs described in the current classification system are anorexia nervosa (AN), bulimia nervosa (BN), eating disorder not otherwise specified (EDNOS), and, in a research category, binge-eating disorder (BED).

Anorexia Nervosa (AN)

The *Diagnostic and Statistical Manual of Mental Disorders, Fourth Edition, Text Revision (DSM-IV-TR)* (1) criteria for AN are shown in Table 24.1. The current diagnostic schema also includes a subtyping designation for those who do not regularly engage in purging behaviors (restricting subtype) and those who regularly engage in binge-eating or purging behavior (binge–purge subtype).

Bulimia Nervosa (BN)

The *DSM-IV-TR* criteria for BN are presented in Table 24.2. These criteria include a subtype designation for those who engage in self-induced vomiting or the misuse of laxatives, diuretics, or enemas (purging type) and those who use other compensatory behaviors such as fasting or excessive exercise, but do not engage in self-induced vomiting or laxative, diuretic, or enema use (nonpurging type).

Eating Disorder Not Otherwise Specified (EDNOS)

According to the *DSM-IV-TR*, individuals presenting with "disorders of eating that do not meet the criteria for any specific eating disorder" (p. 550), that is, individuals not meeting criteria for AN or BN, are classified as having an EDNOS. The most commonly noted EDNOS variant is BED, for which research criteria are included in the appendix to *DSM-IV-TR*. The criteria for EDNOS can be found in Table 24.3.

Persons in the EDNOS group fail to meet the criteria for one of the specific EDs but have significant symptoms and problems. Indeed, many in the field have questioned the significance for an individual patient of failing to meet a specific criterion, such as the necessity that amenorrhea be present for a diagnosis of AN to be made in females (2). In addition to the specific BED criteria, investigators have proposed diagnostic criteria for additional forms of EDNOS, including purging disorder (PD) (3), characterized by patients with a consistent pattern of purging as a compensatory behavior, and night-eating syndrome (4).

GENERAL EPIDEMIOLOGY OF EATING DISORDER SYNDROMES

Estimates suggest that 0.5% to 2.0% of girls and women are affected by AN across their lifetime (5–7). While a 1:10 male-to-female ratio in diagnosis has been frequently cited, recent epidemiologic work reflects a less dramatic but still highly significant gender difference (6). A review of incidence studies further suggests that the number of new cases per 100,000

TABLE 24.1	**DSM-IV-TR criteria for anorexia nervosa (AN)**

A) Refusal to maintain body weight at or above a minimally normal weight for age and height (e.g., weight loss leading to maintenance of body weight less than 85% of that expected, or failure to make expected weight gain during periods of growth, leading to body weight less than 85% of that expected).

B) Intense fear of gaining weight or becoming fat, even though underweight.

C) Disturbance in the way in which one's body weight or shape is experienced; undue influence of body weight or shape.

D) In postmenarcheal females, amenorrhea, i.e., the absence of at least three consecutive menstrual cycles. (A woman is considered to have amenorrhea if her periods occur only following hormone [e.g., estrogen] administration.)

Adapted from American Psychiatric Association. *The Diagnostic and Statistical Manual of Mental Disorders, Fourth Edition. Text Revision.* Washington, DC: American Psychiatric Association; 2000.

TABLE 24.2	**DSM-IV-TR criteria for bulimia nervosa (BN)**

A) Recurrent episodes of binge eating. An episode of binge eating is characterized by both of the following:
  1) Eating, in a discrete period of time (e.g., within any 2-hour period), an amount of food that is definitely larger than most people would eat during a similar period of time and under similar circumstances.
  2) A sense of lack of control over eating during the episode (e.g., a feeling that one cannot stop eating or control what or how much one is eating).

B) Recurrent inappropriate compensatory behavior in order to prevent weight gain, such as self-induced vomiting; misuse of laxatives, diuretics, enemas, or other medications; fasting; or excessive exercise.

C) The binge eating and inappropriate compensatory behaviors both occur, on average, at least twice a week for 3 months.

D) Self-evaluation is unduly influenced by body shape and weight.

E) The disturbance does not occur exclusively during episodes of AN.

Adapted from American Psychiatric Association. *The Diagnostic and Statistical Manual of Mental Disorders, Fourth Edition. Text Revision.* Washington, DC: American Psychiatric Association; 2000.

TABLE 24.3	**DSM-IV-TR criteria for eating disorder not otherwise specified (EDNOS)**

A) Recurrent episodes of binge eating. An episode of binge eating is characterized by both of the following:
  1) Eating, in a discrete period of time (e.g., within any 2-hour period), an amount of food that is definitely larger than most people would eat during a similar period of time and under similar circumstances.
  2) A sense of lack of control over eating during the episode (e.g., a feeling that one cannot stop eating or control what or how much one is eating).

B) The binge-eating episodes are associated with three or more of the following:
  1) Eating much more rapidly than normal.
  2) Eating until feeling uncomfortably full.
  3) Eating large amounts of food when not feeling physically hungry.
  4) Eating alone because of being embarrassed by how much one is eating.
  5) Feeling disgusted with oneself, depressed, or very guilty after overeating.

C) Marked distress regarding binge eating is present.

D) The binge eating occurs, on average, at least 2 days a week for 6 months.

E) The binge eating is not associated with the regular use of inappropriate compensatory behaviors (e.g., purging, fasting, and excessive exercise) and does not occur exclusively during the course of anorexia nervosa or bulimia nervosa.

Adapted from American Psychiatric Association. *The Diagnostic and Statistical Manual of Mental Disorders, Fourth Edition. Text Revision.* Washington, DC: American Psychiatric Association; 2000.

population has increased over the 20th century, although the size of the increase was modest (8).

The prevalence estimates of BN have varied widely since its inclusion as a diagnostic category in the *DSM* in 1979. This variation may relate to changes in definitions, populations examined, and possibly, prevalence over time. A review of epidemiologic studies suggests that approximately 2% to 3% of young women meet *DSM-IV-TR* criteria for BN, with a lifetime prevalence of 1.5% for females and 0.5% for males (6). For both AN and BN, studies of incidence and prevalence have struggled to explain whether variances in prevalence are due to actual change, recall bias, growing awareness of the syndromes, or changes in media attention to the illnesses over time (9).

A number of studies indicate that BED is more common than either AN or BN in the general population. Using data from the National Comorbidity Survey Replication, Hudson and colleagues (6) reported lifetime prevalence estimates for BED of 3.5% in women and 2.0% in men (6). This was nearly double the rates reported for AN and BN combined in that survey. The prevalence of BED is noted to be even higher among the obese and in those seeking bariatric surgery or other weight loss interventions (10).

DEMOGRAPHICS OF EATING DISORDER SYNDROMES

While most commonly developing during the adolescence and young adulthood, EDs can occur at any point in the life cycle. The peak in age of onset for AN occurs between ages 13 and 17, although some patients develop anorexia earlier in childhood and some in later adulthood (5). The peak in age of onset for BN ranges from late adolescence through young adulthood. Although less is known about the onset and natural course of BED, it appears that a majority of individuals develop this illness in young-to-middle adulthood. Unlike AN and BN, severe dieting behaviors and profound concern about weight are not necessarily present prior to the onset of binge-eating behavior. Although AN and BN and, to a lesser extent, BED are all more common in females, it is important not to neglect these EDs in men (11). Few gender differences in the specific features, symptoms, morbidity, and mortality of the disorders have been found by researchers (12).

COMORBIDITY OF EATING DISORDERS AND SUBSTANCE ABUSE

SUDs and EDs commonly co-occur in both clinical populations and research samples. The overall prevalence of drug and alcohol abuse in ED patients is approximately 50%, compared with a prevalence of approximately 9% in the general population (13). Conversely, over 35% of individuals with SUDs report having EDs compared with a rate of 1% to 3% in the general population (13,14). Lifetime prevalence studies have reported rates of SUD of up to 27% in populations with AN, with significantly higher rates in the binge–purge subtype; up to 55% in those with BN; and 23% of those with BED (15,6). A recent meta-analysis of 16 studies confirmed higher prevalence rates of drug use in eating-disordered individuals than in controls. In particular, the analysis showed elevated levels of opiate abuse, cannabis abuse, and general illicit drug use. Risk was shown to be higher in individuals with BN, somewhat less in those with BED, and negligible in those with restrictive AN (16). The clinical course of development of substance use problems in ED patients is highly variable with onset at various stages of illness, suggesting that clinicians should remain attentive to the potential emergence of substance use problems long after initial presentation (17).

CONCEPTUAL ISSUES AND CONFOUNDING FACTORS IN ASSESSING COMORBIDITY

In addition to many of the usual confounding factors in studies (recruitment methods, population selection, standardized interviews vs. self reports, etc.), there are numerous complexities in evaluating the relationship between SUDs and EDs. This perhaps reflects the underlying heterogeneity in the definition of comorbidity. Various studies of comorbidity have used alternate definitions including co-occurrence of disorders that are random and independent, co-occurrence of disorders that share common etiologic underpinnings, or different disorders that may have a shared causal relationship. Overlapping diagnostic criteria may lead to falsely elevated rates of comorbidity. For example, the impulsivity criterion of borderline personality disorder can be met by binge behavior in AN, BN, and BED, or the substance use in SUD. Another study initially found higher rates of various psychiatric problems in women with BN and alcoholism than in a comparison group with BN without alcoholism; however, it was ultimately revealed through multivariate analysis that borderline personality disorder was the sole distinguishing variable between the two groups (18). Carefully designed trials have suggested that some of the apparent co-occurrence between EDs and SUDs may be, at least in part, related to other psychiatric comorbidities. The relationship between BN and alcohol use disorder reported by the National Women's Study may have been the result of associations with other psychiatric disorders such as major depressive disorder and posttraumatic stress disorder (19).

A number of investigators have pointed out the critical importance of selecting appropriate control groups to allow for correct interpretation of patterns of comorbidity. These control groups might include psychiatric populations without the ED and/or SUD (20). Several studies with relevant control groups have shown that, although EDs and SUDs co-occur, the co-occurrence is less dramatic in the relevant comparison group as opposed to the frequently used "normal" control group. For example, Grilo and colleagues found that although EDs are frequently diagnosed among inpatients with SUDs, they are also commonly seen in other psychiatric inpatients (21,22). In this properly controlled study, the frequency of AN and BN was not greater in patients with SUDs than in those without SUDs. As mentioned previously, some studies have also elucidated that patients with restrictive or nonpurging AN may be less likely to develop SUDs. This factor needs to be considered when interpreting earlier work that did not take into consideration the importance of the subtyping of AN patients. A further limitation in some studies is the lack of inclusion of rates of individuals with subthreshold EDs. One study reported that EDNOS (but not full AN or BN) was significantly more common in individuals with substance use diagnoses than those without it. Therefore, some studies may underemphasize the actual co-occurrence relationship. Clinically, the finding of an association between subclinical ED and SUD suggests the importance of a thorough assessment to facilitate early treatment (21,22).

RELATIONSHIP OF SUBSTANCE USE TO BINGE EATING

It is of clinical and theoretic importance that among individuals with some form of ED, nicotine, alcohol, and illicit drug use is much more common in those individuals who binge eat, regardless of whether they have AN, binge-purge-type AN, BN, or BED. This was replicated in a 10-year prospective study (23). The risk of onset of an SUD in persons hospitalized for AN was six times greater among those who reported binge eating while underweight compared with those with no history of binge eating as reported during the index hospitalization. Some epidemiologic studies have reported that alcohol use disorders were much more prevalent among women with AN with binge eating compared with those with AN without binge eating (24), although this pattern has not been consistently noted (25–28). A recent sample of ED probands from the Price Foundation Genetic Study revealed that the prevalence of SUD differed across the AN subtypes, with increased prevalence in the group with binge eating. Similarly, individuals who purged were more likely to report substance abuse than those who did not purge (29). The relationship of SUDs to binge-eating and purging behaviors raises interesting conceptual issues in relation to animal models that have generally revealed that food restriction enhances and food satiation reduces the self-administration of nearly every illicit substance with abuse potential (30).

PATTERNS OF SUBSTANCE ABUSE IN EATING DISORDERS

It is important to note that because of their drive for thinness, ED patients may be motivated to utilize appetite-suppressing substances (e.g., cocaine, amphetamines, and thyroid hormone) (24). However, it has also been noted that the use of substances that promote appetitive behavior (e.g., cannabis and opiates) is not uncommon among eating-disordered patients (17). In some cases, patients may be unaware that these agents may trigger binge behavior. Further, patients with EDs frequently misuse or abuse drugs not usually considered as drugs of abuse. These include laxatives, diuretics, thyroid hormone, and insulin.

HYPOTHESES TO EXPLAIN THE EATING DISORDER—SUBSTANCE USE DISORDER COMORBIDITY

Several hypotheses have been proposed to account for the comorbid occurrence of EDs and SUDs. These have generally been separated into those postulating a "shared etiology" versus a "causal etiology" (31). The "shared" etiology hypotheses suggest that both disorders stem from a common underlying predisposition and broadly include personality (i.e., both sets of illnesses result from a so-called addictive personality), family history (i.e., both sets of illnesses share family risk factors), developmental (i.e., both sets of illnesses result from susceptibility to external pressure such as cultural pressures to be thin in EDs and peer pressure to experiment with drugs in adolescence in SUDs), and biogenetic (i.e., both sets of disorders share a common biologic vulnerability toward addiction to substances, or to starvation or bingeing and purging). The "causal" etiology hypotheses focus on the influence one disorder may have on the development of another. These hypotheses include self-medication (i.e., individuals with EDs use drugs to diminish hunger, modify affects, increase energy, etc.) and food deprivation (i.e., individuals with restrictive food intake are prone to excessive substance use as a compensatory behavior).

Possible Shared Causation of Eating Disorders and Substance Use Disorders

Various animal models of eating behavior have been utilized in attempts to understand etiologic factors in the development of EDs. Some animals exhibit binge-like behavior when exposed to certain environmental factors (e.g., food restriction, stress, intermittent exposure to highly palatable food, etc.) thought to play a role in the development of human EDs (14). Notably, not only do these animals overeat palatable food, but they have also been shown to be more prone to develop addictive behavior when exposed to alcohol and cocaine. These studies suggest that under certain conditions, palatable food may produce oversensitivity of reward circuits as has been postulated to occur in SUDs (32,33). Some studies have focused on the endogenous opiate peptides (EOP) as likely candidates for dysregulation in both ED and SUD. The activity of the EOP has been shown in animal models to have an impact on patterns of food and alcohol consumption (34,35). Naltrexone, an opiate antagonist, has been used as a treatment in BN and in alcohol and drug addiction. Other neurochemical systems that have received research attention include the gamma-aminobutyric acid (GABA), serotonin (36), cholecystokinin, peptide YY, and dopamine systems, all of which can have an important impact on food and alcohol consumption (35).

Environmental and Social Factors

A number of studies have suggested that family conflict and parental modeling behavior are also major risk factors for both ED and SUDs. Just as some children may learn about dieting or an emphasis on weight from parents, they may also learn from parents to use substances as a way of coping with stress (37). Broader sociocultural influences may also contribute to the development of both sets of illnesses. The media, social environment, and peer social interaction all may play a significant role in the initial experimentation with dieting, bulimic behavior, and similarly, the initiation of drug use. Culture may also provide potent reinforcement as a perpetuating factor in both ED and SUDs.

Individual Factors, Personality, and Impulsivity

Some researchers have proposed that an addictive personality might predispose certain individuals to become addicted to one or multiple substances and/or behaviors such as those involved in EDs. Proponents of this theory, from both biobehavioral and dynamic perspectives, view food and substances as addictive substrates. While theoretically appealing, empirical evidence for this connection in personality is not conclusive. Efforts to isolate psychological characteristics common to ED and substance abuse patients have not been successful. Further, Fairburn and others have made cogent arguments that refute the conceptual model of food as an addictive substance (38). However, it has been commonly hypothesized that an association between SUDs and EDs reflects the influence of the underlying personality traits such as impulsivity. Borderline personality disorder and other cluster B personality syndromes are commonly present in individuals with EDs and substance abuse disorders, but are most frequently seen in women with co-occurring ED and SUD (21,22,39).

The role of childhood trauma in the etiology of EDs and SUDs has been the subject of numerous studies. Childhood sexual abuse predicts the onset of a myriad of psychiatric disorders, including but not exclusively EDs and SUDs (40–43). One study examining the differential rates of sexual abuse among the subtypes of EDs revealed that women with comorbid BN and substance dependence had the highest frequency and the most severe history of sexual abuse (44). However, some investigations suggest that sexual abuse is only one component of a larger and more complex etiologic picture (45).

Finally, the risk of co-occurring mood disorders is high in populations with EDs and SUDs. Depression has commonly been cited as a possible link between EDs and SUDs (15). A "self-medication" hypothesis suggesting that those with mood alterations and/or body dissatisfaction, coupled with impulsivity, might be predisposed to use substances in an attempt to alleviate these symptoms.

An Allostatic Model of Eating Disorders

Theoretic models for conceptualizing EDs as addictive disorders were proposed many years ago for AN by Szmukler (46) and for binge eating by Krahn et al. (47) and Lacey (48). More recently, Koob and LeMoal (32) proposed a model of dysregulation of the brain reward system for understanding drug addiction. This model has salient features applicable to conceptualizing the development of EDs. The model of Koob and LeMoal was based on the homeostasis and allostasis hypotheses. Homeostasis, a self-regulating process for multisystem coordination of an organism's response to an acute challenge, fails in alcoholism, drug addiction, and AN and BN, leading eventually to death or chronic impairment. The allostatic state as defined by McEwen and Steller (49) is a state of chronic deviation of the regulatory system from its normal homeostatic operating level. In other words, an allostatic state is a dysregulation of reward circuits with compensatory activation of brain and hormonal stress responses. The allostatic load is defined as the cost the body has to pay for adapting to adverse psychological and physical situations (49). It represents the presence of excessive demand on regulatory systems or the failure of these systems to relax when the demand is over. The latter may explain frequent relapses in both AN and BN. A vulnerable phenotype such as AN or BN may respond to various stresses by an allostatic maladaptation. The state of allostasis reflects both genetic and environmental factors and thus involves multiple brain mechanisms including dysfunction of neurotransmitters and aberrations of neuropeptides.

Examples of Neurobiologic Dysregulation in ED and SUD

Corticotropin-Releasing Factor (CRF) and Endogenous Opioid Peptides (EOPs)

There are similar characteristics in the EDs and SUDs. Individuals with SUDs have a compulsion to take drugs, and AN patients have a compulsion to exercise. SUD patients have a loss of control in limiting drug intake, and bulimics have a loss of control in limiting food intake. Individuals with both sets of diagnoses are characterized by engagement in repetitive dysfunctional behaviors without sufficient concern for the negative consequences (50,51) and are unable to change their behaviors. There are both positive psychological and physiologic reinforcements for restricting food for AN patients. Losing weight by restricting food makes those with EDs feel that they are in absolute control of themselves, and later these time-consuming weight-losing obsessions and compulsive behaviors provide a secondary reinforcement for avoiding perceived aversive or threatened environmental events (52). The physiologic reinforcement may reflect an increased secretion of CRF, which has an anorectic effect and a direct effect on the central nervous system mediating autonomic and behavioral responses to stresses (53,54). BN patients have a relief from dysphoria or anxiety with binge eating. Their purging behavior may produce a "high" related to EOPs and may actually become an addictive state (55).

Dopamine, Serotonin, and Neurobiologic Reward Systems

Dopaminergic neuronal function modulates feeding behavior, motor activity, reward-motivated behavior, and drug-seeking behavior (56). AN patients have restricted feeding, hyperactive stereotypic motor activity, anhedonic behavior, negative affect, and reduced novelty seeking. BN patients engage in binge/purge behavior and have a high comorbidity with alcoholism and drug addiction (51).

There is evidence of altered dopaminergic function in AN. Increased binding of D_2/D_3 receptors in the anteroventral striatum, a region that involves optimal responses to reward stimuli, was found in patients who had recovered from AN (57). Another study showed a significant association between the frequency of functional polymorphisms of dopamine D_2 receptor genes and AN, suggesting that the D_2 receptor gene is a susceptibility factor in the development of this disorder (58). Women who were recovered from the restricting type of AN showed greater hemodynamic activation in the caudate compared to healthy women (59). AN patients may be vulnerable to dopaminergic aberrations because they sustain a greater-than-expected number of perinatal insults (60). Prenatal stress has long-term effects on the dopaminergic system (61).

Serotonergic neuronal systems are also involved in the modulation of appetite, motor activity, mood and obsessional behaviors, and impulse control. Features of anxiety, perfectionism, and obsessionality are present in both AN and BN; however, as noted, impulsivity is associated only with binge behavior. There is evidence for disturbances in the serotonergic neurotransmitter system in EDs. Recovered AN and BN individuals have reduced postsynaptic $5\text{-}HT_{2A}$ receptor activity relative to controls in the subgenual cingulate, mesial temporal, and parietal cortical regions (57,61). Recovered bulimic-type AN patients have increased $5\text{-}HT_{1A}$ postsynaptic activity in the subgenual cingulate and mesial temporal regions as well as frontal cortical regions and increased presynaptic $5\text{-}HT_{1A}$ autoreceptor activity in the dorsal raphi nucleus. Increased $5\text{-}HT_{1A}$ postsynaptic activity has been reported in BN patients (62). $5\text{-}HT_{1A}$ and $5\text{-}HT_{2A}$ receptors coexist and interact in the frontal cortex, amygdala, and hypothalamic regions and contribute to the modulation of dopamine neuronal activity. An aberration of serotonin neuronal modulation may be a vulnerability for developing either AN or BN during adolescence in response to stressful events.

The repetitive compulsive behaviors in EDs may involve the same neural circuits of the corticostriatal–thalamic loops that maintain the allostatic state of compulsive drug taking. These most likely involve dopamine, serotonin, opioid peptides, GABA, and glutamate.

Genetic Vulnerability for Allostasis in Eating Disorders

Genetic factors can act as trait mechanisms in an organism to produce differential sensitivity in the brain reward and stress systems that interact with environmental factors to produce a state of allostasis when activated (63). Individuals may be vulnerable to developing EDs because of intrinsic specific brain neurocircuitry that interacts with environmental life events and stresses. AN is highly familial, with a relative risk of 11.3 in family members of probands with AN (64).

Eating Disorders: An Addiction?

The high comorbidity of impulsivity and drug addiction with BN indicates the possibility of some common genetic factors in BN and drug addiction. The repetitive compulsive behaviors present in AN and BN may involve the same neural circuits of the corticostriatal–thalamic loops that maintain the allostatic state of compulsive drug taking. The neurotransmitter systems involved in the allostatic state of AN and BN may be similar to those in drug addiction and include dopamine, serotonin, opioid peptides, GABA, and glutamate.

SPECIAL CONSIDERATIONS IN EATING DISORDER—SUBSTANCE USE DISORDER COMORBIDITY

Assessment of Patients

Patients with ED–SUD comorbidity require careful and thorough assessment to identify and characterize the nature, extent, and temporal relationship of the symptomatic elements of both disorders. With respect to substance use, for each substance, patients should be directly asked about the age of first use, age of first regular use, age of first problems, age of first treatment, efforts to reduce use, longest periods of abstinence, patterns and quantity of use, and triggers for relapse. The interviewer should obtain details regarding the impact of each substance use on work, school, home, as well as familial and nonfamilial relationships. A recent investigation highlighted the importance of assessing consequences, in addition to use patterns, when examining substance use in individuals with EDs (65), particularly because the combination of problematic substance use and disordered eating is potentially deadly (66). Special attention should be paid to the use of substances while driving or in other physically hazardous situations. Similar inquiries should be directed toward the use of commonly misused over-the-counter substances such as laxatives, diet pills, appetite suppressants, diuretics, and stimulants. Syrup of Ipecac, an emetic designed for use in accidental poisoning, is commonly misused by bulimic patients. The agent is toxic to smooth and striated muscle and can lead to toxic, potentially fatal, cardiomyopathy (67,68). Another important area of assessment should focus on the misuse of prescribed medication by the ED patient. Some patients may take higher- or lower-than-prescribed dosages of medications that they believe may impact weight or appetite. Some examples of prescribed medications misused by ED patients include various anticonvulsants (e.g., topiramate and memantine) and hormones (e.g., thyroid). Topiramate, in particular, should be used with caution in patients with a history of AN or weight loss, in light of its tendency to induce weight loss in some patients (69). Diabetic patients may avoid taking prescribed amounts of insulin and/or oral hypoglycemic agents as a means of avoiding incorporation of sugars or to induce polyuria and diuresis (70).

Assessment of the patient with comorbid SUD and ED illnesses should include a family history focusing on mood and anxiety disorders in addition to the primary illnesses in light of the strong heritability of both disorders. Family history should seek to obtain information about parental attitudes and behaviors in relation to weight, shape, physical appearance, and dieting. Similarly, a history of substance use (e.g., type and severity) in the family should be determined. In addition to developmental and childhood history, direct questions regarding emotional, physical, or sexual abuse should not be overlooked in light of data suggesting that childhood abuse is an extremely common antecedent of these disorders.

Treatment Delivery for Comorbid Patients

Despite the high rates of ED and SUD comorbidity discussed earlier in this chapter, there has been surprisingly little attention in the literature to the complex treatment planning and decision-making essential to effective treatment of this population. Patients must be motivated and ready to make radical changes in behavior. Patients with substance abuse must be motivated to abstain from alcohol and drugs, and patients with EDs must be motivated to abstain from bingeing and/or purging, or committed to normalizing restrictive eating behavior. The comorbid patient has the difficult task of attempting to do both. Unfortunately, to date, there has been little consensus and no clear guidelines regarding how to best manage co-occurring ED and SUD. Treatment delivery for patients with substance abuse and other psychiatric disorders is often described as sequential or integrated. Sequential treatment involves treating either the SUD or the ED first, without specific focus on and attention to treatment of the other disorder. Patients are then transferred to a different setting for treatment of the other disorder. While patients will often describe that they feel overwhelmed by simultaneous treatment of both disorders, sequential treatment can lead to a pattern of symptom replacement or substitution. Some patients describe a worsening of ED symptoms as they attempt to abstain from drugs and/or alcohol, and conversely, some patients describe exacerbation or relapse into substances as they attempt to normalize eating behavior. A second treatment delivery option would be parallel treatment in which a patient might receive treatment for both disorders concurrently, but by different providers or in different treatment settings. A third treatment delivery paradigm provides integrated, concurrent treatment of both disorders. While offering a number of potential advantages over sequential or parallel treatment, perhaps because of the resource-intensive nature of such settings, few integrated ED and SUD programs currently exist (71).

Elements of Treatment Integration

The recommended elements of independent multidisciplinary care for ED units have been described elsewhere (72). The integrated treatment of EDs and SUDs presents new challenges as well as new therapeutic opportunities. A number of forces that contribute to difficulties in treating co-occurring SUD and ED in sequenced treatments may be avoided through the use of comprehensive, integrated treatment. Assessment should include a full inventory of symptoms of both illnesses for all patients. Often patients may conceal or minimize the elements of either the ED or the SUD. In nonintegrated programs, the treatment team may focus primarily or exclusively on their more comfortable area of primary experience. In this regard, the patient and therapeutic staff may consciously or unconsciously collude to avoid focus on the substance use problem. Often, patients with co-occurring ED and SUD do not receive structured assessment or treatment for EDs in addiction treatment programs, and similarly, substance abuse assessment and treatment may be lacking in many ED programs (73). A thorough medical evaluation should not assume that weight loss or various physiologic derangements result from either the ED or the SUD. Evaluation should address the interactive effects of ED pathology and substance use on cardiovascular, gastrointestinal, hematologic, and endocrine/metabolic systems (74). Laboratory evaluation can be of use in identifying surreptitious ED and SUD. Decisions regarding whether detoxification can occur on the integrated unit should be individualized and based on the degree of medical instability.

TREATMENT APPROACHES FOR CO-OCCURRING SUBSTANCE USE AND EATING DISORDERS

Patients who are in simultaneous, integrated treatment for SUDs and EDs require multidimensional therapies. The abrupt cessation of ED behaviors coupled with abstinence from alcohol and/or substances may be terrifying, with the creation of profound psychic stress and anxiety. This creates a therapeutic crisis for many patients. A number of therapeutic interventions, both pharmacologic and psychotherapeutic, may be utilized on the integrated treatment unit to provide support, reduce resistance, and facilitate sustainable change.

Pharmacologic Treatment

Medications may be useful adjuncts in the integrated treatment of EDs and SUDs. Cyproheptadine in high doses (up to 24 mg/day) can facilitate weight gain in anorectic restrictors and also provide a mild antidepressant effect (75). Although chlorpromazine was the first drug to treat AN, no double-blind controlled studies are available to show the efficacy of this drug for inducing weight gain and reducing anxiety in anorectic patients. In open-trial observations, chlorpromazine may be helpful in the severely obsessive–compulsive or agitated anorectic patient. It may be necessary to start at a low dose of 10 mg two or three times per day and gradually increase the dosage while monitoring blood pressure. Newer antipsychotics such as olanzapine have also been shown to be useful for severely obsessive–compulsive or agitated anorectic patients (76,77). Tricyclic antidepressants and serotonin reuptake inhibitors (SSRIs) are not particularly effective and have undesirable side effects for severely emaciated anorectic patients (78).

For patients with BN and out-of-control bingeing and purging, fluoxetine has been approved by the U.S. Food and Drug Administration (79). The only other SSRI studied in a randomized, controlled trial and shown to be effective is sertraline (80). In patients who do not respond to an SSRI, topiramate may be helpful (81). Since weight loss is a side effect of this medication, it should be used only in patients in the high normal or overweight range. It is necessary to begin this drug in very low doses of 25 mg/day, gradually increasing the dose to avoid adverse side effects such as paresthesias and cognitive word-finding difficulties. As mentioned previously, this drug has some abuse potential in individuals who are convinced that higher doses at more regular intervals might lead to greater degrees of weight loss.

There has been limited research on compounds that might simultaneously reduce or alleviate eating disturbance and substance abuse. Ondansetron, a 5-HT3 antagonist, has been shown to be of potential benefit in the treatment of alcohol dependence (82) and in BN (83), but this agent has not gained widespread use in the treatment of either illness, nor has it been systematically evaluated in patients with comorbid ED and SUD, perhaps because of prominent side effects including abdominal pain. Naltrexone, an opioid antagonist approved for the treatment of alcohol and opioid dependence, has also been utilized in patients with BN despite the lack of systematic investigation. Extreme care should be undertaken in the pharmacologic treatment of patients with concurrent SUDs and EDs. The combined physiologic derangements of both illnesses render these patients even more vulnerable to cardiovascular, hepatic, gastrointestinal, and cognitive/neurologic effects than either disorder in isolation.

Psychological Treatments

Various psychotherapeutic interventions targeting motivation (e.g., motivational enhancement techniques), mood regulation and coping skills (e.g., dialectal behavior therapy and cognitive–behavioral therapy [CBT]), and relationship maintenance (e.g., interpersonal psychotherapy) benefit the patient with co-occurring ED and SUD. CBT is a well-researched and proven method for the treatment of BN (84). Although research on the effectiveness of CBT for the treatment of AN is much more limited, clinical evidence and data in support of its utility are emerging (85–87). Essentially, the cognitive–behavioral model for the treatment of EDs emphasizes the important role of both the cognitive (e.g., attitudes regarding the importance of weight, shape, and their control) and the behavioral (e.g., dietary restriction and binge eating) factors that maintain the ED and associated pathology. The treatment is presented in additive stages with an initial emphasis on stabilization of symptoms and behavioral change. As treatment progresses, the behavioral coping strategies are supplemented with cognitive restructuring techniques including work on interpersonal issues, body image, and affect regulation. The final stage of CBT concentrates on relapse prevention and maintenance planning. Many of the treatment elements provided in CBT specifically target behaviors that may underlie concurrent substance abuse disorder and ED symptoms.

Although the CBT treatment model was designed as an outpatient intervention, the treatment has been utilized in a variety of settings, including inpatient and partial hospital programs. In this regard, given the high level of symptom severity for patients entering an inpatient program, CBT stands out as one treatment model that is particularly well suited for this population (88). CBT emphasizes early behavior change in a structured and systematic way. Additionally, once the patient begins to stabilize and is more receptive to any form of psychotherapy (5), the CBT focus shifts to address salient cognitive and emotional concerns, while maintaining symptom control.

It is recommended that patients with co-occurring illness receive intensive CBT in the milieu, in groups, and during individual psychotherapy. Therapists with highly specific training provide a variety of CBT-based group therapies including the following: Standard CBT for Eating Disorders, Body Image, Skills Training, Self-Esteem, Motivation to Change, and Coping Skills Training. These groups are based on salient elements of the standard CBT treatment protocols (89). Each of these important elements of treatment is expanded (and modified for adolescents vs. adults), creating separate and independent group therapies. The overall effect is that patients receive all elements of CBT, but in a more intensive dose during integrated treatment of the SUD and ED. Additionally, other more specialized groups, such as CBT-based Trauma Recovery Group, can be offered as appropriate.

Hospitalized patients also may benefit from intensive individual CBT where they can focus in a more specific way on their particular problems and conflicts. In this regard, it is recommended that all patients work individually on stabilization of symptoms through coping skills training, problem solving, and cognitive restructuring around ED and SUD beliefs and assumptions. For some patients, however, it may be necessary to expand beyond the standard CBT protocol to address, in a more intensive way, specific areas of concern such as body image, self-esteem, perfectionism, interpersonal difficulties, and emotion regulation (90). Typically, the individual therapist will concentrate on one or two of these particular areas. The goal is to provide effective, focused, and individualized therapy. While not yet substantiated by controlled investigation, clinical experience suggests that CBT is of great utility in the treatment of co-occurring SUD and ED.

Another therapy showing promise in the integrated treatment of this population is Dialectical Behavior Therapy (DBT) (91,92). With its focus on mindfulness, awareness of problems and choices of responses to those problems, coping skills training, and mood regulation techniques, this form of treatment concurrently benefits ED and SUD, as well as commonly occurring personality elements. Finally, in light of the powerful ambivalence notable in both illnesses independently, and the co-occurring patient, the motivational enhancement techniques (93,94) have been of great therapeutic value in integrated treatment strategies. Further research into treatment strategies to address these disorders is greatly needed in light of their potential for relapse, morbidity, and mortality.

SUMMARY

The ED and SUD frequently co-occur, suggesting the possibility of shared etiologic and perpetuating factors, although this remains speculative. Regardless, the shared illnesses require diligent identification efforts through comprehensive medical and psychiatric assessment. Effective treatment should concurrently address the core vulnerabilities of each disorder. While more research is needed to identify the most efficacious treatment, integrated approaches using interventions such as CBT, DBT, and motivational enhancement strategies are currently recommended.

REFERENCES

1. American Psychiatric Association. *Diagnostic and Statistical Manual of Mental Disorders. Fourth Edition, Text Revision.* Washington, DC: American Psychiatric Association; 2000:589.
2. Attia E, Roberto C. Should ammenorhea be a diagnostic criterion for anorexia nervosa? *Int J Eating Disord.* 2009;42:581–589.
3. Keel PK, Haedt A, Edler C. Purging disorder: an ominous variant of bulimia nervosa? *Int J Eat Disord.* 2005;38:191–199.
4. Stunkard A, Allison K, Lundgren J, et al. Issues for DSM-V: night eating syndrome. *Am J Psychiatry.* 2008;164(4):424.
5. American Psychiatric Association Work Group on Eating Disorders. Practice guideline for the treatment of patients with eating disorders (third edition). *Am J Psychiatry.* 2006;163 (suppl 7):4–54.
6. Hudson J, Hiripi E, Pope HG Jr, et al. The prevalence and correlates of eating disorders in the National Comorbidity Survey replication. *Biol Psychiatry.* 2007;61:348–358.
7. Keski-Rahkonen A, Hoek H, Susser ES, et al. Epidemiology and course of anorexia nervosa in the community. *Am J Psychiatry.* 2007;164:1259–1265.
8. Keel PK, Klump KL. Are eating disorders culture-bound syndromes? Implications for conceptualizing their etiology. *Psychol Bull.* 2003;129:747–769.
9. Hoek HW. Incidence, prevalence and mortality of anorexia nervosa and other eating disorders. *Curr Opin Psychiatry.* 2006; 19(4):389–394.
10. Kalarchian MA, Marcus MD, Levine MD, et al. Psychiatric disorders among bariatric surgery candidates: relationship to obesity and functional health status. *Am J Psychiatry.* 2007;164:328–334.
11. Andersen AE, Holman JE. Males with eating disorders: challenges for treatment and research. *Psychopharmacol Bull.* 1997; 33:391–397.
12. Woodside DB, Garfinkel PE, Lin E, et al. Comparisons of men with full or partial eating disorders, men without eating disorders, and women with eating disorders in the community. *Am J Psychiatry.* 2001;158:570–574.
13. The National Center on Addiction and Substance Abuse at Columbia University (CASA). 2003. Available at: www.casacolumbia.org. Accessed May 2010.
14. Krug I, Treasure J, Anderluh M, et al. Present and lifetime comorbidity of tobacco, alcohol and drug use in eating disorders: a European multicenter study. *Drug Alcohol Depend.* 2008;97:169–179.
15. Holderness CC, Brooks-Gunn J, Warren MP. Co-morbidity of eating disorders and substance abuse review of the literature. *Int J Eat Disord.* 1994;16:1–34.
16. Calero-Elvira A, Krug I, Davis K, et al. Meta-analysis on drugs in people with eating disorders. *Eur Eat Disord Rev.* 2009;17:243–259.
17. Franko DL, Dorer DJ, Keel PK, et al. Interactions between eating disorders and drug abuse. *J Nerv Ment Dis.* 2008;196(7):556–561.
18. Bulik CM, Sullivan PF, Carter FA, et al. Lifetime comorbidity of alcohol dependence in women with bulimia nervosa. *Addict Behav.* 1997;22(4):437–446.
19. Dansky BS, Brewerton TD, Kilpatrick DG. Comorbidity of bulimia nervosa and alcohol use disorders: results from the National Women's Study. *Int J Eat Disord.* 2000;27:180–190.
20. Allison DB. A note on the selection of control groups and control variables in comorbidity research. *Compr Psychiatry.* 1993;34: 336–339.
21. Grilo CM, Becker DF, Levy KN, et al. Eating disorders with and without substance use disorders: a comparative study of inpatients. *Compr Psychiatry.* 1995;36:312–317.
22. Grilo CM, Levy KN, Becker DF, et al. Eating disorders in female inpatients with versus without substance use disorders. *Addict Behav.* 1995;20:255–260.
23. Strober M, Freeman R, Bower S, et al. Binge eating in anorexia nervosa predicts later onset of substance use disorder: a ten-year prospective, longitudinal follow-up of 95 adolescents. *J Youth Adolesc.* 1996;25:519–532.
24. Bulik CM, Klump KL, Thornton L, et al. Alcohol use disorder comorbidity in eating disorders: a multicenter study. *J Clin Psychiatry.* 2004;65(7):1000–1006.
25. Wiederman MW, Pryor T. Substance use among women with eating disorders. *Int J Eat Disord.* 1996;20(2):163–168.
26. Corcos M, Nezelof S, Speranza M, et al. Psychoactive substance consumption in eating disorders. *Eat Behav.* 2001;2(1):27–38.
27. Stock SL, Goldberg E, Corbett S, et al. Substance use in female adolescents with eating disorders. *J Adolesc Health.* 2002;31(2): 176–182.
28. Blinder BJ, Cumella EJ, Sanathara VA. Psychiatric comorbidities of female inpatients with eating disorders. *Psychosom Med.* 2006; 68:454–462.
29. Root T, Pinhero A, Thornton L, et al. Substance use disorders in women with anorexia nervosa. *Int J Eat Disord.* 2009;43: 14–21.
30. Carr KD. Chronic food restriction: enhancing effects on drug reward and striatal cell signaling. *Physiol Behav.* 2007;91:459–472.
31. Wolfe WL, Maisto SA. The relationship between eating disorders and substance use: moving beyond co-prevalence research. *Clin Psychol Rev.* 2000;20:617–631.
32. Koob GF, LeMoal M. Plasticity of reward neurocircuitry and the 'dark side' of drug addiction. *Nat Neurosci.* 2005;8(11):1442–1444.
33. Robinson TE, Berridge KC. The neural basis of drug craving: an incentive-sensitization theory of addiction. *Brain Res Rev.* 1993; 18:247–291.
34. Luby ED, Marrazzi MA, Sperti S. Anorexia nervosa: a syndrome of starvation dependence. *Compr Ther.* 1987;13(9):16–21
35. Mercer ME, Holder MD. Food cravings, endogenous opioid peptides, and food intake: a review. *Appetite.* 1997;29(3):325–352.
36. Jimerson DC, Brandt HA, Brewerton TD. Evidence for altered serotonin function in bulimia and anorexia nervosa: behavioral implications. In: Pirke KM, Vandereychen W, Ploog D, eds. *The Psychobiology of Bulimia Nervosa.* Berlin: Springer-Verlag; 1988: 83–89.

37. Wade T, Martin N, Tiggemann M, et al. Genetic and environmental risk factors for the weight and shape concerns characteristic of bulimia nervosa. *Psychol Med.* 1998;28:761–771.
38. Fairburn CG. *Overcoming Binge Eating.* New York: Guilford Press; 1995.
39. Sansone RA, Fine MA, Nunn J, et al. A comparison of borderline personality symptomatology and self-destructive behavior in women with eating, substance abuse, and both eating and substance abuse disorders. *J Personal Disord.* 1994;8:219–228.
40. Wonderlich SA, Brewerton TD, Jocic Z, et al. Relationship of childhood sexual abuse and eating disorders. *J Am Acad Child Adolesc Psychiatry.* 1997;36(8):1107–1115.
41. Folsom W, Christensen ML, Avery L, et al. The co-occurrence of child abuse and domestic violence: an issue of service delivery for social service professionals. *Child Adolesc Social Work J.* 2003;20(5):375–387.
42. Fairburn CG, Welch SL, Doll HA, et al. Risk factors for bulimia nervosa. A community-based case-control study. *Arch Gen Psychiatry.* 1997;54(6):509–517.
43. Welsh SL, Fairburn CG. Sexual abuse and bulimia nervosa: three integrated case control comparisons. *Am J Psychiatry.* 1994;151:402–407.
44. Deep AL, Lilenfeld LR, Plotnicov KH, et al. Sexual abuse in eating disorder subtypes and control women: the role of comorbid substance dependence in bulimia nervosa. *Int J Eat Disord.* 1999;25:1–10.
45. Everill JT, Waller G, Macdonald W. Dissociation in bulimic and non-eating-disordered women. *Int J Eat Disord.* 1995;17:127–134.
46. Szmukler GI, Tantam D. Anorexia nervosa: starvation dependence. *Br J Med Psychol.* 1984;57:303–310.
47. Krahn D, Kurth C, Demitrack M, et al. The relationship of dieting severity and bulimic behaviors to alcohol and other drug use in women. *J Subst Abuse.* 1992;4:341–353.
48. Lacey JH. Self-damaging and addictive behavior in bulimia nervosa: a catchment area study. *Br J Psychiatry.* 1993;163:192–194.
49. McEwen ES, Stellar E. Stress and the individual: mechanisms leading to disease. *Arch Intern Med.* 1993;153:2093–2101.
50. Childress AR, Mozley PD, McElgin W, et al. Limbic activation during cue induced cocaine craving. *Am J Psychiatry.* 1999;156:11–18.
51. Halmi KA. Anorexia nervosa and bulimia nervosa. In: Martin A, Folkmar F, eds. *Lewis's Child and Adolescent Psychiatry.* New York: Lippincott Williams & Wilkins; 2007:592–602.
52. Halmi KA. Treatment of anorexia nervosa. In: Wonderlich S, Mitchell JE, DeZwaan DM, et al., eds. *Annual Review of Eating Disorders: Part 2.* Oxford: Radcliff; 2006:157–167.
53. Gold PW, Gwirtsman H, Avgerinos TC. Abnormal hypothalamic-pituitary adrenal function in anorexia nervosa: pathophysiologic mechanisms in under and weight corrected patients. *New Eng J Med.* 1986;314:1335–1342.
54. Koob GF, Markou A, Weiss F, et al. Opponent process and drug dependence: neurobiological mechanisms. *Semin Neurosci.* 1993;5:351–358.
55. Goodman A. Neurobiology of addiction: an integrative review. *Biochem Pharmacol.* 2008;75:266–332.
56. Small D, Jones-Gotsman M, Dagagrad A. Feeding-induced dopamine released endorsal striatum correlates with meal pleasantness ratings in healthy human volunteers. *Neuroimage.* 2003;19:1709–1715.
57. Frank G, Bailer U, Henry S, Drebets W, et al. Increased dopamine D_2, D_3 receptor binding after recovery from anorexia nervosa measured by positron emission tomography and [11C] raclopride. *Biol Psychiatry.* 2005;58:908–912.
58. Bergen AW, Yeager M, Welch RA, et al. Association of multiple DR_{D2} polymorphisms with anorexia nervosa. *Neuropsychopharmacology.* 2005;30:1703–1710.
59. Wagner A, Aizenstein H, Venkatraman V, et al. Altered reward processing in women recovered from anorexia nervosa. *Am J Psychiatry.* 2007;164:1842–1849.
60. Favaro A, Tenconoi E, Santonastaso P. Peri natal factors in the risk of developing anorexia nervosa and bulimia nervosa. *Arch Gen Psychiatry.* 2006;63:82–88.
61. Bailer U, Price J, Melzer RA, et al. Altered $5HT_{2A}$ receptor binding after recovery from bulimia type anorexia nervosa. *Neuropsychopharmacology.* 2004;29:1143–1155.
62. Tiihonem J, Keski-Rahkonem A, Lopponem M, et al. Brain serotonin 1A receptor binding in bulimia nervosa. *Biol Psychiatry.* 2004;55:871–873.
63. Koob GF, LeMoal M. Drug abuse: hedonic hemostatic dysregulation. *Science.* 1997;278:52–58.
64. Strober M, Freeman R, Lampert C, et al. Controlled family study of anorexia nervosa and bulimia nervosa: evidence of shared liability and transmission of partial syndrome. *Am J Psychiatry.* 2000;157(3):393–401.
65. Dunn EC, Latimer ME, Neighbors C, et al. Alcohol and drug related negative consequences in college students with bulimia and binge eating disorders. *Int J Eat Disord.* 2002;32:171–178.
66. Keel PK, Dorer DJ, Eddy KT, et al. Predictors of mortality in eating disorders. *Arch Gen Psychiatry.* 2003;60:179–183.
67. Palmer EP, Guay AT. Reversible myopathy secondary to abuse of ipecac in patients with major eating disorders. *N Engl J Med.* 1985;23:1457–1459.
68. Silber T. Ipecac syrup abuse, morbidity, and mortality: isn't it time to repeal its over-the-counter status? *J Adolesc Health.* 2005;37:256–260.
69. Rosenow F, Knake S, Hebebrand J, et al. Topiramate and anorexia nervosa. *Am J Psychiatry.* 2002;159:2112–2113.
70. Goebel-Fabbri AE. Diabetes and eating disorders. *J Diab Sci Technol.* 2008;2(3):530–532.
71. Sinha R, O'Malley SS. Alcohol and eating disorders: implications for alcohol treatment and health services research. *Alcohol Clin Exp Res.* 2000;24:1312–1319.
72. Brandt HA, Halmi K. The eating disorder unit. In: Sharfstein S, Dickerson FB, Oldham J, eds. *Textbook of Hospital Psychiatry.* APPI: Arlington, VA. 2008:90–97.
73. Gordon SM, Johnson JA, Greenfield SF, et al. Assessment and treatment of co-occurring eating disorders in publicly funded addiction treatment programs. *Psychiatr Serv.* 2008;59:1056–1059.
74. Brandt HA, Halmi K. The eating disorder unit. In: Sharfstein S, Dickerson FB, Oldham J, eds. *Textbook of Hospital Psychiatry.* APPI: Arlington, VA. 2008:90–97.
75. Halmi KA, Eckert E, LaDu TJ, et al. Anorexia nervosa: treatment efficacy of cyproheptadine and amitriptyline. *Arch Gen Psychiatry.* 1986;43:177–181.
76. Powers PS, Santana CA, Bannon YS. Olanzapine in the treatment of anorexia nervosa: an open label trial. *Int J Eat Disord.* 2002;32:146–154.
77. Bissada H, Tasca GA, Barber AM, et al. Oanzapine in the treatment of low body weight and obsessive thinking in women with anorexia nervosa: a randomized, double blind, placebo-controlled trial. *Am J Psychiatry.* 2008;10:1281–1288.

78. Kaye W, Nagata T, Weltzin T, et al. Double-blind placebo controlled administration of fluoxetine in restricting and restricting-purging type anorexia nervosa. *Biol Psychiatry.* 2001;49:644–652.
79. Romano SJ, Halmi KA, Sarkar NP, et al. A placebo controlled study of fluoxetine in continued treatment of bulimia nervosa after successful acute fluoxetine treatment. *Am J Psychiatry.* 2002;159:96–102.
80. Milano W, Petrella C, Sabatino C, et al. Treatment of bulimia nervosa with sertraline: a randomized controlled trial. *Adv Ther.* 2004;21:232–237.
81. Hoopes SP, Reimherr FW, Hedges DW, et al. Treatment of bulimia nervosa with topiramate in a randomized, double-blind, placebo-controlled trial, part 1: improvement in binge and purge measures. *J Clin Psychiatry.* 2003;64:1335–1341.
82. Johnson BA. The role of serotonergic agents as treatments for alcoholism. *Drugs Today.* 2003;39(9):665
83. Faris PL, Kim SW. Effect of decreasing afferent vagal activity with ondansetron on symptoms of bulimia nervosa: a randomised, double-blind trial. *Lancet.* 2000;355:769–770.
84. Wade TD, Bergin JL, Martin NG, et al. A transdiagnostic approach to understanding eating disorders. *J Nerv Ment Dis.* 2006;194(7):510–517.
85. Cooper P, Fairburn C. Cognitive-behavioral treatment for anorexia nervosa: preliminary findings. *J Psychosom Res.* 1984;28: 493–499.
86. Hall A, Crisp A. Brief psychotherapy in the treatment of anorexia nervosa: outcome at one year. *Br J Psychiatry.* 1987; 151:185–191.
87. Pike KM, Walsh BT, Vitousek K, et al. Cognitive behavior therapy in the posthospitalization treatment of anorexia nervosa. *Am J Psychiatry.* 2003;160:2046–2049.
88. Bowers WA. Cognitive therapy for eating disorders. In: Wright JH, Thase ME, Beck AT, et al., eds. *Cognitive Therapy with Inpatients: Developing a Cognitive Milieu.* New York: Guilford; 1993: 337–356.
89. Fairburn, et al. 1993.
90. Fairburn CG, Cooper Z, Shafran R. Cognitive behaviour therapy for eating disorders: a "transdiagnostic" theory and treatment. Behav Res Ther. 2003;41(5):509–528.
91. Linehan MM. *Cognitive Behavioral Treatment of Borderline Personality Disorder.* New York: Guilford Press; 1993.
92. Safer DL, Telch CF, Agras WS. Dialectical behavior therapy adapted for bulimia: a case report. *Int J Eat Disord.* 2001;30(1): 101–106.
93. Miller WR, Rollnick S. *Motivational Interviewing: Preparing People to Change Addictive Behavior.* New York: Guilford Press; 1991.
94. Geller J. Mechanisms of action in the process of change: helping eating disorder clients make meaningful shifts in their lives. *Clin Child Psychol Psychiatry.* 2006;11(2):225–237.

CHAPTER 25: Pathologic Gambling

Elise E. DeVito ■ Marc Potenza

Gambling has a long history, spanning and likely extending beyond human written history. References to gambling in literature, including ancient religious texts (Old Testament, New Testament, and Mahabharata), as a common behavior as well as a potential source of moral downfall, suggest that problematic patterns of gambling have long been present alongside recreational patterns of engagement. However, there was limited research into gambling problems and possible forms of treatments until the 1970s and 1980s, with randomized clinical trials largely conducted within the past decade. Formal diagnostic guidelines for a gambling disorder (termed "pathological gambling" [PG]) were first included in the third edition of the *Diagnostic and Statistical Manual of Mental Disorders (DSM-III)* in 1980 and have been updated since. The core feature of PG is considered to be "persistent and recurrent maladaptive gambling behavior…that disrupts personal, family or vocational pursuits" (1). Increasing availability and participation in legalized gambling in the United States has been accompanied by increased interest into the factors associated with PG and the development, prevention, and treatment of the disorder.

TERMS AND DEFINITIONS

Gambling has been defined as "placing something of value at risk in the hopes of gaining something of greater value" (2). However, common perceptions of gambling typically involve either high risk, fairly rapid outcomes, or both, such that a long-term real estate or stock investment may be risky but may not be considered as gambling by the general public (2). "PG" is a clinical diagnosis in the *DSM-IV* defined by the presence of five or more inclusionary criteria related to gambling and the acknowledgment that the PG is not better accounted for by manic symptomatology (Table 25.1) (1). Other terms have been used to describe excessive patterns of gambling including the terms "compulsive gambling" or "problem gambling." The former term was not used as a diagnostic entity when PG was introduced in the *DSM*, in part in order to avoid confusion with the distinct diagnostic entity of obsessive–compulsive disorder (OCD). The term "probable pathological gambling" is sometimes used when achieving threshold scores using screening instruments (e.g., South Oaks Gambling Screen [SOGS]) (3), rather than relying on meeting *DSM* criteria (e.g., through a clinical interview). Given that estimated rates of PG are often higher when a screening instrument was used compared with a full *DSM-IV* clinical diagnoses, some cases of "probable pathological gambling" may not meet the *DSM-IV* criteria for "PG." "Problem gambling" is typically used as a broader term for a pattern of gambling that still is related to difficulties in one's life but may or may not meet the full criteria for PG (3). That is, "problem gambling" has been used at times inclusive of PG and at others exclusive of PG. In the gambling literature, problem gambling is often operationally defined as meeting three to four or, in other cases, one or more of the inclusionary diagnostic criteria for PG (4). "Disordered gambling" is a general term including both problem and PG. "Recreational gambling" describes gambling behavior that would not fall under disordered gambling, where the behavior is carried out in moderation without loss of control or marked negative consequences. However, a precise threshold for a difference between recreational and problem gambling has not been uniformly agreed upon.

DIAGNOSIS OF PATHOLOGIC GAMBLING

PG is included in the *DSM-IV* as an Impulse Control Disorder Not Elsewhere Classified (1). Impulse control disorders (ICDs) are characterized by a failure to resist performing an act that is harmful to oneself or others, increased feelings of arousal or tension prior to the act, and a feeling of pleasures or release of tension when performing the act (5).

A diagnosis of PG is made according to the *DSM-IV* based on the presence of at least 5 out of 10 indications of "persistent and recurrent maladaptive gambling behavior" which are not better accounted for by manic behavior (1). Indications of PG may include a preoccupation with gambling, repeated unsuccessful attempts to control or quit gambling, and irritability in the immediate setting of gambling cessation, attempts to recoup gambling losses with more gambling, a need over time to gamble larger amounts of money to achieve similar levels of excitement, gambling to modulate negative moods, being deceitful about one's extent of gambling, relying on others or illegal acts to financially support the gambling, and damaging or jeopardizing important relationships or opportunities as a result of gambling (1).

As gambling behavior is considered to lie along a continuum, alternative conceptualizations of (and thresholds for) PG have been discussed (6,7). Some of the *DSM* inclusionary criteria for PG were modeled after those for substance use disorders (SUDs) (1), but while the DSM criteria for SUDs explicitly distinguish between grades of severity characterized

TABLE 25.1	*DSM-IV-TR* criteria for pathologic gambling
A) Persistent and recurrent maladaptive gambling behavior as indicated by five (or more) of the following:	
1) is preoccupied with gambling	
2) needs to gamble with increasing amounts of money in order to achieve the desired excitement	
3) has repeated unsuccessful efforts to control, cut back, or stop gambling	
4) is restless or irritable when attempting to cut down or stop gambling	
5) gambles as a way of escaping from problems or of relieving a dysphoric mood	
6) after losing money gambling, often returns another day to get even	
7) lies to family members, therapist, or others to conceal the extent of involvement with gambling	
8) has committed illegal acts such as forgery, fraud, theft, or embezzlement to finance gambling	
9) has jeopardized or lost a significant relationship, job, or educational or career opportunity because of gambling	
10) relies on others to provide money to relieve a desperate financial situation caused by gambling	
B) The gambling behavior is not better accounted for by a Manic Episode.	

Adapted from American Psychiatric Association. *The Diagnostic and Statistical Manual of Mental Disorders,* 4th ed., Text Revision. Washington, DC: American Psychiatric Association; 2000.

by qualitative differences (substance abuse and substance dependence), PG is defined within the *DSM-IV* as a single diagnostic entity with no other specific gambling-related diagnosis (1). Some researchers and clinicians have cited evidence of clinically relevant factors associated with subsyndromal levels of PG to support either lowering the threshold to fewer than 5 out of 10 criteria, or formally recognizing a less severe form of gambling within the *DSM*.

EPIDEMIOLOGY OF GAMBLING: PREVALENCE

The vast majority of adults report having gambled at some point in their lives. Estimates of disordered gambling based on screening instruments suggest 2.5% of the U.S. population display problem gambling (4), while lifetime prevalence of PG is estimated to be between 0.4% and 3.4% of the U.S. adult population (1), with several large surveys using diagnostic assessments indicating past-year prevalence estimates in the United States in the range of 0.1% to 0.3% (8,9).

A study of probable PG in North America revealed that prevalence estimates for the general adult population (1.60%) were significantly lower than those for adolescent populations (3.88%). The general adult, adolescent, and college student (4.67%) rates have been found to be significantly lower than the estimated prevalence for adults who were either receiving psychiatric treatment (including treatment for SUDs) or were in prison (14.23%) (10).

Demographic variables such as sex, age, and race appear to influence gambling participation. Men are approximately two times more likely than women to develop PG (10), yet women may suffer from more physical and mental health complications than men at the same severity of disordered gambling (8). Compared to girls, boys make up a larger proportion of problematic or pathologic gamblers (estimated ratios range from 3:1 to 5:1), gamble more frequently and wager larger amounts, begin at an earlier age, and more often prefer skill-based games (11).

African Americans are disproportionately represented in populations of disordered gamblers (12). Controlling for socioeconomic status, a U.S.-based telephone survey found black youths displayed higher rates of frequent gambling than did white youths (13).

Multiple different motivations may promote gambling, and there is some evidence for demographic differences based on individuals' gambling motivations (14). Recreational gamblers who report gambling for excitement (excitement-seeking) tended to be younger with more symptoms of impaired impulse control (e.g., SUDs, incarceration, larger wins and losses) and reported engaging in more forms of gambling and experiencing more gambling problems (15). Men are more likely to cite excitement seeking as their motivation for gambling, while women are more likely to report gambling as a form of escape or relief from dysphoria or boredom (15).

Various forms of gambling exist and differ in significant ways such as the level of skill required (e.g., electronic gambling machines versus poker), timing of the gambling sequence (e.g., fast-paced electronic gambling machines versus slower lotteries), and size of the wager (14). There has been debate regarding whether features of electronic gambling machines make them more "addictive" than other forms of gambling, and although there is little systematic research on this topic, the current data are mixed and thus do not on the whole support this contention (14).

SOCIAL AND ENVIRONMENTAL FACTORS

The acceptability and accessibility of gambling in the United States and around the world has typically increased recently, and although gambling was previously illegal in all but a few regions of the United States, it is now legal in nearly every state. Gambling-related problems may increase with this greater availability of legal gambling outlets. Greater proximity and accessibility to gambling venues has been associated with increased gambling behavior, albeit not consistently, so increases in legal gambling venues should be carefully considered within a public health perspective (11,16).

The percentage of the general adult population reporting having gambled increased from 68% in 1975 to 86% in 1998 (17). Data from a meta-analysis of North American research studies between the years of 1974 and 1997 were consistent with an increase in rates of problem and PG across time within the general adult population, but not within the adolescent, college, or psychiatric treatment and prison-dwelling adult populations (10). One hypothesis is that increasing social acceptability with more legalized gambling venues relates to increasing gambling rates (10). Prevalence studies in the United States suggest that estimates of problem and PG in 12 to 17 year olds have increased from 1989 (median 10%, range 9% to 20%) to 1999 (median 14%, range 10% to 26%), while overall gambling rates rose from 45% to 66% in the juvenile population in the same time frame (11). Given the association between an earlier onset of gambling and more severe gambling problems in adulthood, increased rates of juvenile gambling have raised concerns that rates in adult populations may increase further with time (16). However, tempering these views are data that recent prevalence estimate surveys of problem and PG in the United States and Canada are similar to or lower than those reported in earlier prevalence estimate studies, despite increases in gambling availability. These findings suggest that increased availability of gambling does not alone predict rates of problematic or PG (9). Together, these findings indicate that at the population level, factors influencing engagement in gambling at multiple levels remain relatively poorly understood.

CO-OCCURRING PSYCHIATRIC DISORDERS

Gambling problems have been associated with increased odds of having Axis I psychiatric disorders (in particular depression, bipolar disorder, anxiety, and SUDs), and this association appears stronger in women as compared to men (7,8). Multiple Axis II disorders have also been associated with problem and PG (8,18). High frequencies of attempted suicide (17% to 24%) have been reported in individuals either receiving professional treatment for PG or regularly attending Gamblers Anonymous (GA) (19). Higher rates of disordered gambling are associated with psychotic disorders in community and clinical samples. Although high rates of co-occurrence have been found for multiple disorders across genders, women with PG appear more likely than men with PG to suffer from a comorbid mood disorder or to experience gambling-related anxiety while men appear more likely to suffer from comorbid SUDs (including alcohol dependence) (8). Juveniles with problem or PG appear more likely than their nonproblem gambling peers to report dissociative experiences while gambling (11). A U.S.-based telephone survey of community-dwelling subjects found a high co-occurrence between gambling problems and alcohol problems in youths (age 14 to 21) (13).

The co-occurrence of psychiatric disorders appears to be related to the number of PG criteria met, rather than an association being restricted to individuals who qualify for the clinical definition of PG (i.e., ≥5 DSM-IV criteria). However, associations with advantageous health measures appear more mixed at lesser severities of gambling pathology. For example, recreational gambling is associated with increased odds of substance abuse or dependence in most cases except in samples of older adults where recreational gambling has been associated with better ratings of subjective general health (20).

The etiologies of co-occurring psychiatric disorders with PG are not well understood but may arise from common factors, such as impulsivity or risk-taking, and may include shared genetic and environmental contributions (16). Individuals with PG and co-occurring SUDs, such as nicotine dependence, have higher estimates of other psychiatric comorbidities at each gambling severity level (4), and first-degree relatives of individuals with PG display increased rates of mood disorder and alcohol dependence, findings that suggest common vulnerability factors between the disorders.

Another nonmutually exclusive explanation is that development of PG or other psychiatric disorders could contribute to the development of the other. For instance, debts and strained interpersonal relationships related to PG could increase the risk for developing depression, anxiety, or substance abuse, or alternatively depressed individuals may turn to gambling as a means of escape. One study has found that phobias, antisocial personality disorders, and most SUDs tend to temporally precede PG, suggesting that these disorders may represent risk factors or share vulnerability factors with PG, while depression and stimulant dependence tend to develop after PG, suggesting these disorders may represent a reaction to some aspect of PG (12). Despite generally high rates of lifetime co-occurrence of PG and alcohol dependence, one large study of gambling helpline callers found frequencies of reported current alcohol use problems to be approximately equal to general adult population rates, with most alcohol use problems being reported as not being active (21). While the studies used different assessment procedures and data from the helpline study have limitations including possible self-report and recall biases, the findings appear consistent with the notions that alcohol misuse may frequently precede PG and that individuals may "switch" addictive outlets over time (12).

As compared with recreational gamblers who do not abuse substances, those who do abuse substances are more likely to be younger, unmarried males who began gambling prior to the age of 18 and gamble for excitement or to win money (22). Comorbid alcohol use problems in problem gamblers are associated with reports of more forms of gambling performed, suicide attempts, gambling-related arrests, tobacco and drug use, and family histories of alcohol and drug use, further suggesting the potential contribution of poor impulse control across a broad range of behaviors (21).

SOCIAL AND PUBLIC HEALTH COSTS OF GAMBLING

Estimates of the amount of money spent on gambling in the United States (including payouts) rose from approximately $17.4 billion in 1974 to $860 billion in 2001, and costs attributed to problem and PG in the United States have been estimated in the 1990s to be approximately $5 billion annually (17).

Gambling may have multiple personal and societal impacts. Individuals with PG typically gamble beyond their means, and may incur substantial debts and experience bankruptcies. PG may involve financial "bailouts" and the willingness to risk close relationships in order to pursue gambling. In more severe cases of PG, illegal behaviors (e.g., theft) may be committed in order to support the gambling behavior. Damaging behaviors such as domestic violence, child abuse, and child neglect may contribute to high rates of divorce and poor mental and physical health of family members of individuals with gambling problems (17).

Health problems such as hypertension, insomnia, gastrointestinal complaints, and cardiac arrests have been associated with disordered gambling (6). The presence of indicators of sustained stress in individuals with PG and indicators of acute stress during the act of gambling, such as increased salivary cortisol, hypertension, immune system changes, elevated heart rate, and higher levels of epinephrine and norepinephrine or their metabolites, suggest that stress may be a moderating factor in some of the health issues that commonly co-occur with PG (6).

Limited public education on the prevalence of and health impairments associated with excessive gambling behaviors may hinder attempts at prevention, early intervention, or treatment.

PATHOLOGIC GAMBLING AS ADDICTION OR IMPULSIVE–COMPULSIVE SPECTRUM DISORDER

Models of PG have primarily conceptualized it as a behavioral addiction, or as part of a spectrum of disorders lying along an impulsive–compulsive spectrum with such disorders as OCD (23). Evidence exists in support of both conceptualizations of PG, which are not mutually exclusive. Proposed core components of addiction including appetitive urges or cravings prior to the behavior, diminished self-control, compulsive or continued engagement in the behavior despite adverse consequences have been observed in both PG and SUDs, as have other aspects of addiction including tolerance, and withdrawal (23,24).

The phenomenology and clinical definition (according to the *DSM-IV*) of PG share similarities with both SUDs and OCD. Individuals with OCD, SUDs, or PG may experience motivations to perform behaviors (e.g., compulsive behavior, drug taking, gambling), may be preoccupied with thoughts of the behavior, and may demonstrate a diminished ability to resist drives to engage in excessive performance of the behavior.

In contrast with the individuals with OCD, individuals with PG or SUDs tend to experience the persistent thoughts about the behavior, anticipation of the behavior, and actual performance of the behavior as pleasurable or ego-syntonic, particularly in early stages of the disorders (25). In contrast, individuals with OCD tend to experience these motivations as ego-dystonic (i.e., inconsistent with the patient's self-image and distressing) and engagement in the subsequent behavior as a relief or release (5). Since individuals with PGs or SUDs experience these behaviors as ego-syntonic, they may not believe they have a problem, or may deny or minimize problems, typically unlike individuals with OCD (6). Excessive risk aversion and overestimation of risk, characteristics associated with compulsive disorders including OCD, are not regularly observed in PG; rather, individuals with PG are more likely to display excessive risk-taking and underestimation of risks associated with other ICDs and SUDs (5). PG also resembles SUDs in that the severity of behavioral engagement runs along a continuum (abstinence to PG) (7), and it is possible for problematic behavior to resolve without formal treatment (26). Women display a similar "telescoping" effect with PG that has been observed with alcoholism and drug dependence, meaning that women tend to begin the behavior later in life but tend to progress to problematic stages at a faster rate than do men (6). Whether the phenomenon of "telescoping" in part reflects a gender difference in the willingness to seek treatment earlier in the course of illness is not entirely clear. While some ICDs such as trichotillomania are associated with elevated odds of OCD, PG is not; however, PG carries elevated odds of SUDs (5).

CANDIDATE MEDIATORS OF PATHOLOGIC GAMBLING

A number of candidate factors have been proposed to contribute to the progression to and persistence of PG including aspects of cognition, specific neurotransmitter systems and regional brain functioning, and genetic factors. These domains are not independent nor are their contributions mutually incompatible.

When viewing PG as a nonsubstance or "behavioral" addiction, it may represent an important model of addiction without the potentially complicating toxic effects of exogenous substances, ones that may or may not be linked to the core processes of addiction. One complicating factor of much addiction research is determining which factors in individuals with current SUDs represent pre-existing vulnerabilities and which result from repeated substance use or reflect changes arising during the course of addiction. Since gambling does not involve the introduction of exogenous substances, abnormalities in groups of individuals with PG are sometimes interpreted as pre-existing vulnerability factors, although longitudinal studies are needed to directly parse potential influences related to the progression of addiction. Neuroadaptation, the alteration of neural circuitry, can occur in response to repeated exposure to exogenous substances (e.g., drugs of abuse), but may also occur following high frequency exposure to nonsubstance rewards (24). Tolerance and withdrawal, phenomena observed in PG as well as SUDs, are often conceived of as indications of neuroadaptation (10). As such, repeated engagement in gambling behavior may lead to the development of neuroadaptation or aberrant learning mechanisms that may themselves contribute to PG. A combination of premorbid vulnerabilities alongside changes resulting from repeated engagement in gambling behavior may account for the development of PG (10,27).

IMPAIRED COGNITION, IMPULSIVITY, AND COGNITIVE DISTORTIONS

Individuals with PG have been shown to be impaired on laboratory tasks of cognition including measures of cognitive control (e.g., Stroop), planning, attention, and timing (for review see (27)).

Individuals with PG have repeatedly been shown to report higher levels of self-rated impulsivity and to display impulsivity on laboratory measures, including impaired ability to withhold a prepotent response (impaired response inhibition reflective of response impulsivity) and steeper rates of temporal discounting of rewards (rapid delay discounting reflective of choice impulsivity) (27). Individuals with PG demonstrate less optimal decision-making on laboratory measures, for example, by showing greater preference for risky choices relative to their non-PG peers (27). Self-rated impulsivity has been associated with gambling severity in adults and juveniles, and adolescent impulsivity ratings are associated with later development of disordered gambling (for review see (27)). Poor impulse control on laboratory measures has been predictive of relapse in PG patients receiving treatment (28).

Impulsivity is a characteristic of multiple disorders associated with PG, including personality disorders, affective disorders, schizophrenia, SUDs, and neurologic diseases (16). Similarly, high rates of PG in adolescence have been proposed to be related to impulsivity, a feature of that developmental life phase (16).

Gambling-related cognitive biases or distortions have been shown in pathologic gamblers in interviews as well as during the "thinking aloud" method, where gamblers are asked to voice their thoughts aloud as they gamble. Some of these cognitive biases are based on a failure to appreciate the independence of trials or the randomness of outcomes. Many of these cognitive biases have been found in recreational as well as pathologic gamblers, raising questions regarding their centrality to PG. The "illusion of control" refers to the belief by the gambler that certain behaviors or rituals can increase their probability of success above that of the objective probability of the situation, or that one can control the outcome of a gamble. The "availability bias" occurs when individuals selectively recall large wins, which leads them to overestimate the likelihood or size of future "payouts." The "gambler's fallacy" refers to the belief that if an unlikely event has occurred that soon the reverse outcome will occur to even out the probabilities (e.g., after consecutive "heads" coin tosses, a "tails" outcome is more likely). In reality, each event (e.g., roll of dice, spin of roulette wheel) is independent, and the probability of an outcome is not influenced by prior trials. The gambler's fallacy could lead an individual to bet on a certain outcome that has not occurred in some time, believing it is "due." On the other hand, a belief that a certain outcome has repeatedly occurred may be interpreted as meaning it could happen again (certain dice being "hot" and having repeatedly good outcomes). "Loss-chasing," where an individual follows a gambling loss with continued gambling and an often riskier bet with the aim of winning back the amount lost, is observed in individuals who meet criteria for PG as well as those who do not. Interventions aimed at teaching independent odds have demonstrated that while individuals typically learn the mathematical concepts underlying gambling, impact on problem gambling behaviors have yet to be convincingly demonstrated, echoing findings in the drug abuse prevention field where education-based interventions alone appear insufficient to alter substance abuse behaviors (29).

NEUROTRANSMITTER SYSTEMS

Disruptions to several neurotransmitter systems, including those relating to norepinephrine, serotonin, dopamine, opioids, and gamma-aminobutyric acid, have been proposed to contribute to PG (30).

Physiologic arousal and excitement accompany the act of gambling, and subjective reports indicate that pathologic gamblers experience more intense gambling-related excitement than do recreational gamblers. Norepinephrine contributes to the regulation of arousal, attention, and aspects of impulsivity. Proximal measures of central norepinephrine levels (e.g., metabolites) are increased in men with PG as compared to those without (31). Pharmacologic challenge study results suggesting reduced sensitivity to postsynaptic alpha-2 adrenergic receptors in PG may be consistent with abnormally high norepinephrine secretion in PG (32). Levels of norepinephrine correlate with the gambling outcome and the urge to begin or continue gambling in problem gamblers, consistent with a role of norepinephrine in moderating gambling behavior (33). Norepinephrine and dopamine levels increase during the act of gambling to a greater extent in pathologic gamblers relative to recreational gamblers (33).

Lower levels of dopamine and higher levels of dopamine metabolites in the CSF of pathologic gamblers may indicate abnormal regulation of the dopamine system (31). PG has been observed in patients with Parkinson's disease, a neurologic disease primarily characterized by loss of nigrostriatal dopamine neurons. Multiple factors have been reported as being associated with PG and other ICDs in Parkinson's disease. These factors include ones related to clinical features of Parkinson's disease (e.g., age at Parkinson's disease onset), ones seemingly unrelated to Parkinson's disease (e.g., personal history of an ICD prior to Parkinson's disease onset), and ones related to the treatment of the disorder (e.g., dopamine agonists and other treatments for Parkinson disease, as well as the relative amount of dopamine replacement). Both drugs with prodopaminergic (amphetamine) and dopamine receptor antagonistic (haloperidol) properties have been found to promote gambling-related motivations and responses, suggesting that a role for dopamine in PG warrants additional investigation.

Serotonin has long been implicated in impulse control. Pathologic gamblers have decreased levels of serotonin metabolites and abnormal responses to serotonergic agonists like meta-chlorophenyl piperazine, in which they report a subjective "high" and demonstrate exaggerated prolactin increases, mirroring findings observed in alcoholic patients (34,35).

Casino gambling is associated with increased plasma concentrations of cortisol indicating activation of the hypothalamic-pituitary-adrenal (HPA) axis. During gambling, greater increases in heart rate and higher peripheral epinephrine and dopamine levels in problem gamblers may indicate exaggerated anticipatory autonomic arousal or increased sympathetic activity (33). Peripheral cortisol reactivity to stress has been demonstrated in problem gamblers, consistent with moderate levels of stress during gambling (33). Studies of beta-endorphin levels in problem gamblers have shown mixed results, leading to the suggestion that a role for endorphins may differ across forms of gambling (33).

GENETICS

Consistent with the studies of either central or peripheral neurotransmitter markers described above, genetic studies have preliminarily implicated genes involved in monoamine function. These genes include ones coding for dopamine D1, D2, and D4 receptors (*DRD1, DRD2, DRD4*), a tryptophan enzyme (tryptophan 2, 3-dioxygenase) involved in serotonin metabolism, and monoamine oxidase A, a protein relevant to norepinephrine, serotonin, and dopamine systems (36). One analysis indicated that genes important for norepinephrine, serotonin, and dopamine systems may contribute relatively equally to an additive risk for PG (36). An earlier study implicated the TaqA1 allele of *DRD2* in PG, but PG no longer showed an association with the TaqA1 allele after accounting for race and other DSM diagnoses (37). Additionally, more recent studies with sibling pair designs have not replicated an association with the TaqA1 allele, and the TaqA1 allele has also been shown to be in linkage disequilibrium with other genes (e.g., *ANKK1*) that might explain an association with addictive disorders (37).

Polymorphisms in the promotor region of *DRD1* have also been associated with SUDs and attention-deficit hyperactivity disorder as well as with PG, in preliminary studies, and D1 receptors have been implicated in reward processing and addiction, suggesting that *DRD1* may be important for the neurobiology of ICDs in general (16,37). Since many of the genes implicated in PG are also associated with other disorders consisting of impulsive–compulsive and addictive behaviors, this may support the concept that an individual with a combination of these risk factors has a raised vulnerability to develop impulse control or addictive disorders, but the specific form of impulsive or addictive behavior may also be influenced by environmental factors (36). Consistently, studies of male twins have found significant overlaps in the genetic and environmental contributions to PG and alcohol dependence as well as to PG and other externalizing behaviors (38). Future studies using state-of-the-art approaches (e.g., genome-wide association studies) are needed in order to better understand genetic contributions to PG.

NEUROANATOMY

Few functional brain imaging studies have been conducted in individuals with disordered gambling. The findings show abnormal activation in frontal–striatal regions, brain regions implicated in impulse control and decision making, and draw similarities with and differences from SUDs and OCD.

Decreased activation of the right ventrolateral prefrontal cortex (PFC) during monetary wins and losses in problem gamblers was associated with poor performance (i.e., perseveration) on a task of probabilistic reversal learning, measuring components of reward learning, and cognitive flexibility (39). The same individuals with problem gambling demonstrated intact performance and normal dorsal frontostriatal brain activity during an executive function task measuring planning (39). These findings could be consistent with PG resembling OCD or SUD (39) since hyporesponsiveness of the ventrolateral PFC was found in individuals with OCD on the same task of reversal learning and hyporesponsiveness of the PFC to monetary reward has been observed in cocaine-dependent individuals (39).

Initial viewing (prior to self-reported onset of gambling urges) of gambling-related cues was associated with lower regional activity in the frontal cortex (e.g., inferior frontal cortex, superior frontal gyrus), basal ganglia (e.g., caudate), and thalamus in individuals with PG relative to control comparison subjects without the disorder; these regions previously have been found to show increased regional activity in OCD subjects during symptom provocation (25). After the self-reported onset of gambling urges, while viewing arguably more provocative gambling-related cues, the PG group relative to a control comparison group demonstrated hypoactivation in the ventral anterior cingulated portion of the ventromedial prefrontal cortex (vmPFC), a region associated with hyperactivation in cocaine-dependent individuals while viewing cocaine-related cues (25). A direct comparison in a male sample of the neural correlates of craving in cocaine dependence and gambling urges in PG found shared activation differences in the affected groups (as compared to control groups) during viewing of the diagnostic group–specific material (gambling tapes for pathologic subjects, cocaine tapes for cocaine-dependent subjects) with respect to relatively diminished activations in specific brain regions including the ventral striatum and ventral PFC (30). Together, these findings suggest similarities between PG and SUDs as well as OCD (25). During a simulated gambling task, pathologic gamblers demonstrate diminished activity in the ventral striatum and vmPFC relative to healthy controls, and these regional functional magnetic resonance imaging (fMRI) BOLD signals correlated negatively with gambling severity ratings within the group with PG (40). Relative to healthy controls, pathologic gamblers displayed less brain activity in the vmPFC during performance of the Stroop task, a measure of cognitive control, selective attention and response inhibition (41), and individuals with SUDs with or without PG showed less activation of the vmPFC when performing a decision-making test (the Iowa Gambling Task). The ventral striatum is implicated in reward and salience processing and has also been shown to be hypoactive in substance-dependent individuals during reward processing, while the vmPFC has been implicated in impulse control and risky decision making (30). Pathologic gamblers watching a gambling scenario activated the dorsolateral prefrontal cortex more than did control subjects, and this regional increase in activation was associated with higher baseline and greater cue-induced increases in self-reported gambling urges (42).

Recent studies have investigated common gambling phenomena in healthy (nondisordered gambling) adults with fMRI. Loss-chasing was associated with increased activity in brain in regions including the vmPFC, while resisting the opportunity to loss-chase and quitting the gambling session was associated with activity in the ventral striatum, dorsal anterior cingulate cortex, anterior insula, and middle frontal gyrus. "Near-misses" occur when an unsuccessful outcome gives the appearance of coming close to winning, for example, when two out of three signals line up on a fruit machine and the third symbol is off by one, and have been proposed to promote gambling. Healthy individuals who felt they had more control over the situation reported near-misses as unpleasant but as increasing their desire to continue playing. Regional changes in brain activity during "near-misses" were similar to that following a monetary win (i.e., striatum, insula). Activation of the rostral anterior cingulate during near-misses was associated with healthy individuals' degree of perceived control over the situation, while insula activity related to their motivation to continue gambling after a near-miss. The authors concluded that the ability for near-misses to recruit reward circuitry may underlie their ability to promote ongoing gambling (43). However, as these studies did not involve individuals with PG, their relevance to PG requires further, direct examination.

Taken together, a relatively consistent finding across studies involves diminished activation of the vmPFC and ventral striatum in individuals with PG. The majority of the imaging studies in PG only included men and excluded individuals with comorbid psychiatric disorders. Given the difference in the clinical profile and demographics of individuals with comorbid psychiatric disorders, it will be important to directly assess brain function in women and youth with PG before generalizing the findings in adult males to all individuals with PG.

TREATMENT

Numerous treatment options exist for PG including, but not limited to, pharmacotherapy and psychotherapy.

In practice, a number of pharmacologic approaches are employed to treat PG, although there are not yet any FDA-approved drugs with an indication for PG. Selective serotonin reuptake inhibitors (SSRIs), mood stabilizers, and opioid antagonists have demonstrated efficacy in treating PG in double-blind placebo-controlled trials (for review see Ref. (44)), with the strongest evidence in support of opioid antagonists, including naltrexone and nalmefene (45). Other medications spanning a range of pharmacologic classes (e.g., lithium carbonate, N-acetyl cysteine) have also shown efficacy in the treatment of PG. It has been suggested that clinicians should consider comorbid diagnoses when choosing the pharmacotherapy option for PG. For instance, individuals with co-occurring anxiety disorders may respond well to SSRIs like escitalopram, whereas those with co-occurring bipolar disorders may respond well to mood stabilizers like lithium. Other clinical measures may be used to guide the selection of pharmacotherapies. For example, positive responses to opiate antagonist treatment have been associated with positive family histories of alcoholism and strong gambling urges (44,46).

Evidence for the efficacy of psychotherapies such as cognitive behavioral therapy, motivational enhancement therapy, and imaginal desensitization in the treatment of PG has been observed in controlled clinical trials (44,47), and other forms of nonpharmacologic treatments such as aversion therapy, cognitive restructuring (of erroneous gambling-related beliefs), and personalized feedback have had encouraging results in preliminary studies. However, the psychological mechanism by which these treatments reduce gambling behavior remains unclear (3).

In addition, the majority of states in the United States with legalized gambling operate problem gambling telephone helplines. The 12-step program, GA, has meetings throughout the world. Such self-help treatment options are widely used and often encouraged by clinicians as an adjunct to professional treatment. Many individuals report success with GA, and GA attendance in a gambling treatment program has been associated with better clinical outcome (48). However, data suggest there is frequent discontinuation after attending one or two GA meetings and low rates of long-term abstinence (7.5% at 1 year), suggesting GA may not be efficacious as a stand-alone treatment for most individuals (48).

While historically PG may have been thought to follow a chronic, persistent course, recent studies suggest high rates of natural recovery from PG. These findings suggest that many individuals can shift from exhibiting PG to demonstrating controlled gambling or abstinence without the aid of formal treatment (26).

Only a small proportion of individuals with disordered gambling seek treatment, many of whom are identified by screening when being treated for other disorders (e.g., SUDs). One contributing factor to low rates of treatment seeking may be that only a small proportion of individuals with gambling problems perceive themselves as having one. Furthermore, treatments for PG have traditionally focused solely on abstinence-based goals, which some individuals may be unwilling to pursue. However, some preliminary studies suggest a goal of controlled gambling may provide similar levels of success as abstinence-based goals (49).

Despite the wealth of treatment options for PG, the field of PG treatment lags behind treatment of SUDs in availability of empirically validated treatments with clearly demonstrated treatment efficacy. There have been relatively few controlled treatment trials or direct evaluations of the clinical efficacy of interventions like GA. Meta-analyses of PG treatment studies have shown substantial estimated effect sizes for both pharmacologic (0.78) and nonpharmacologic (2.01 posttreatment, 1.59 at longer term follow-up) treatments, yet one meta-analysis found the quality of study design to relate inversely to the effect size within cognitive and behavioral treatment studies for PG, such that the most poorly designed studies indicated the most robust treatment effects (50).

Many of the treatment trials should be interpreted with caution as they have only compared active treatments without a "no treatment" control arm, have been open-label, lacked pretreatment data, or used small samples. Of the controlled trials, many exclude patients with comorbid SUD including alcohol abuse or Axis 1 psychiatric disorders including depression and anxiety, all of which have high rates of comorbidity with PG. Many studies include solely or predominantly adult male subjects, raising questions of the generalizability of these results to women, juveniles, and patients with co-occurring disorders. Many of the longer duration clinical trials report a significant effect of time on treatment outcome, independent of treatment group, perhaps reflecting the tendency for gambling patterns to fluctuate over time and a possible influence of nonspecific factors or natural recovery in the clinical improvement.

CONCLUSION

The increased availability and social acceptance of legalized gambling throughout the world in the past few decades appears to have contributed to increased public and clinical awareness of PG. A growing body of research has furthered the understanding of neurobiologic, cognitive, and genetic factors that may contribute to the development or persistence of PG and contributed to the development of evidence-based treatments to address this potentially devastating disorder.

REFERENCES

1. APA. *Diagnostic and Statistical Manual of Mental Disorders*. 4th ed. Washington, DC: American Psychiatric Press; 2000.
2. Potenza MN. Should addictive disorders include non-substance-related conditions? *Addiction*. 2006;101(suppl 1):142–151.
3. Blaszczynski A. Conceptual and methodological issues in treatment outcome research. *J Gambl Stud*. 2005;21(1):5–11.
4. Grant JE, Desai RA, Potenza MN. Relationship of nicotine dependence, subsyndromal and pathological gambling, and other psychiatric disorders: data from the National Epidemiologic Survey on Alcohol and Related Conditions. *J Clin Psychiatry*. 2009; 70(3):334–343.
5. Dell'Osso B, Altamura AC, Allen A, et al. Epidemiologic and clinical updates on impulse control disorders: a critical review. *Eur Arch Psychiatry Clin Neurosci*. 2006;256(8):464–475.
6. Potenza MN, Fiellin DA, Heninger GR, et al. Gambling: an addictive behavior with health and primary care implications. *J Gen Intern Med*. 2002;17(9):721–732.
7. Potenza MN, Kosten TR, Rounsaville BJ. Pathological gambling. *JAMA*. 2001;286(2):141–144.
8. Desai RA, Potenza MN. Gender differences in the associations between past-year gambling problems and psychiatric disorders. *Soc Psychiatry Psychiatr Epidemiol*. 2008;43(3):173–183.
9. Kessler RC, Hwang I, LaBrie R, et al. DSM-IV pathological gambling in the National Comorbidity Survey Replication. *Psychol Med*. 2008;38(9):1351–1360.
10. Shaffer HJ, Hall MN, Vander Bilt J. Estimating the prevalence of disordered gambling behavior in the United States and Canada: a research synthesis. *Am J Public Health*. 1999;89(9): 1369–1376.
11. Jacobs DF. Juvenile gambling in North America: an analysis of long term trends and future prospects. *J Gambl Stud*. 2000;16 (2–3):119–152.
12. Cunningham-Williams RM, Cottler LB. The epidemiology of pathological gambling. *Semin Clin Neuropsychiatry*. 2001;6(3): 155–166.
13. Barnes GM, Welte JW, Hoffman JH, et al. Gambling, alcohol, and other substance use among youth in the United States. *J Stud Alcohol Drugs*. 2009;70(1):134–142.
14. Dowling N, Smith D, Thomas T. Electronic gaming machines: are they the 'crack-cocaine' of gambling? *Addiction*. 2005;100(1): 33–45.
15. Pantalon MV, Maciejewski PK, Desai RA, et al. Excitement-seeking gambling in a nationally representative sample of recreational gamblers. *J Gambl Stud*. 2008;24(1):63–78.
16. Chambers RA, Potenza MN. Neurodevelopment, impulsivity, and adolescent gambling. *J Gambl Stud*. 2003;19(1):53–84.
17. National Opinion Research Center. *Gambling impact and behavior study: Report to the National Gambling Impact Study Commission*. University of Chicago: Chicago; 1999.
18. Petry NM, Stinson FS, Grant BF. Comorbidity of DSM-IV pathological gambling and other psychiatric disorders: results from the National Epidemiologic Survey on Alcohol and Related Conditions. *J Clin Psychiatry*. 2005;66(5):564–574.
19. DeCaria CM, Hollander E, Grossman R, et al. Diagnosis, neurobiology, and treatment of pathological gambling. *J Clin Psychiatry*. 1996;57(suppl 8):80–83; discussion 83–84.
20. Desai RA, Maciejewski PK, Dausey DJ, et al. Health correlates of recreational gambling in older adults. *Am J Psychiatry*. 2004; 161(9):1672–1679.
21. Potenza MN, Steinberg MA, Wu R. Characteristics of gambling helpline callers with self-reported gambling and alcohol use problems. *J Gambl Stud*. 2005;21(3):233–254.
22. Liu T, Maciejewski PK, Potenza MN. The relationship between recreational gambling and substance abuse/dependence: data from a nationally representative sample. *Drug Alcohol Depend*. 2009;100(1–2):164–168.
23. Blanco C, Moreyra P, Nunes EV, et al. Pathological gambling: addiction or compulsion? *Semin Clin Neuropsychiatry*. 2001;6(3): 167–176.
24. Holden C. 'Behavioral' addictions: do they exist? *Science*. 2001; 294(5544):980–982.

25. Potenza MN, Steinberg MA, Skudlarski P, et al. Gambling urges in pathological gambling: a functional magnetic resonance imaging study. *Arch Gen Psychiatry.* 2003;60(8):828–836.
26. Slutske WS. Natural recovery and treatment-seeking in pathological gambling: results of two U.S. national surveys. *Am J Psychiatry.* 2006;163(2):297–302.
27. Verdejo-Garcia A, Lawrence AJ, Clark L. Impulsivity as a vulnerability marker for substance-use disorders: review of findings from high-risk research, problem gamblers and genetic association studies. *Neurosci Biobehav Rev.* 2008;32(4):777–810.
28. Goudriaan AE, Oosterlaan J, De Beurs E, et al. The role of self-reported impulsivity and reward sensitivity versus neurocognitive measures of disinhibition and decision-making in the prediction of relapse in pathological gamblers. *Psychol Med.* 2008;38(1):41–50.
29. Clayton RR, Cattarello AM, Johnstone BM. The effectiveness of Drug Abuse Resistance Education (project DARE): 5-year follow-up results. *Prev Med.* 1996;25(3):307–318.
30. Potenza MN. Review. The neurobiology of pathological gambling and drug addiction: an overview and new findings. *Philos Trans R Soc Lond B Biol Sci.* 2008;363(1507):3181–3189.
31. Bergh C, Eklund T, Södersten P, et al. Altered dopamine function in pathological gambling. *Psychol Med.* 1997;27(2):473–475.
32. Pallanti S, Bernardi S, Allen A, et al. Noradrenergic function in pathological gambling: blunted growth hormone response to clonidine. *J Psychopharmacol.* 2010; 24(6):847–853. (Epub 2008).
33. Meyer G, Schwertfeger J, Exton MS, et al. Neuroendocrine response to casino gambling in problem gamblers. *Psychoneuroendocrinology.* 2004;29(10):1272–1280.
34. Nordin C, Eklundh T. Altered CSF 5-HIAA Disposition in Pathologic Male Gamblers. *CNS Spectr.* 1999;4(12):25–33.
35. Pallanti S, Bernardi S, Quercioli L, et al. Serotonin dysfunction in pathological gamblers: increased prolactin response to oral m-CPP versus placebo. *CNS Spectr.* 2006;11(12):956–964.
36. Comings DE, Gade-Andavolu R, Gonzalez N, et al. The additive effect of neurotransmitter genes in pathological gambling. *Clin Genet.* 2001;60(2):107–116.
37. da Silva Lobo DS, Vallada HP, Knight J, et al. Dopamine genes and pathological gambling in discordant sib-pairs. *J Gambl Stud.* 2007;23(4):421–433.
38. Eisen SA, Slutske WS, Lyons MJ, et al. The genetics of pathological gambling. *Semin Clin Neuropsychiatry.* 2001;6(3):195–204.
39. de Ruiter MB, Veltman DJ, Goudriaan AE, et al. Response perseveration and ventral prefrontal sensitivity to reward and punishment in male problem gamblers and smokers. *Neuropsychopharmacology.* 2009;34(4):1027–1038.
40. Reuter J, Raedler T, Rose M, et al. Pathological gambling is linked to reduced activation of the mesolimbic reward system. *Nat Neurosci.* 2005;8(2):147–148.
41. Potenza MN, Leung HC, Blumberg HP, et al. An FMRI Stroop task study of ventromedial prefrontal cortical function in pathological gamblers. *Am J Psychiatry.* 2003;160(11):1990–1994.
42. Crockford DN, Goodyear B, Edwards J, et al. Cue-induced brain activity in pathological gamblers. *Biol Psychiatry.* 2005;58(10): 787–795.
43. Clark L, Lawrence AJ, Astley-Jones F, et al. Gambling near-misses enhance motivation to gamble and recruit win-related brain circuitry. *Neuron.* 2009;61(3):481–490.
44. Brewer JA, Grant JE, Potenza MN. The treatment of pathological gambling. *Addict Disord Treat.* 2008;7(1):1–13.
45. Potenza MN. Advancing treatment strategies for pathological gambling. *J Gambl Stud.* 2005;21(1):91–100.
46. Grant JE, Kim SW, Hollander E, et al. Predicting response to opiate antagonists and placebo in the treatment of pathological gambling. *Psychopharmacology (Berl).* 2008;200(4): 521–527.
47. Grant JE, Donahue CB, Odlaug BL, et al. Imaginal desensitisation plus motivational interviewing for pathological gambling: randomised controlled trial. *Br J Psychiatry.* 2009;195(3): 266–267.
48. Petry NM. Gamblers anonymous and cognitive-behavioral therapies for pathological gamblers. *J Gambl Stud.* 2005;21(1): 27–33.
49. Dowling N, Smith D, Thomas T. A preliminary investigation of abstinence and controlled gambling as self-selected goals of treatment for female pathological gambling. *J Gambl Stud.* 2009; 25(2):201–214.
50. Gooding P, Tarrier N. A systematic review and meta-analysis of cognitive-behavioural interventions to reduce problem gambling: hedging our bets? *Behav Res Ther.* 2009;47(7):592–607.

CHAPTER 26: Sexual Addiction

Virginia A. Sadock

INTRODUCTION

Sex addiction has been recognized implicitly by the culture in general and by the medical community in particular since classical times. The early names for sex addiction derive from Greek mythology: satyriasis for male sex addiction after the mythical satyrs who were characterized by uncontrolled sexual behavior, and nymphomania for female sex addiction, named for the nymphs who were driven by their desire for others. The problem has been portrayed through the ages in art, novels, plays, and films. The attention of psychiatrists was refocused on sex addiction in the late 1970s by James Orford's article on sexual dependency in the *British Journal of Sexual Addiction* and by the work of such clinicians as Patrick Carnes (1).

The concept of sex addiction has developed to refer to persons whose behavior is hypersexual, who compulsively seek out sexual experiences, and whose behavior becomes impaired if they are unable to gratify their sexual impulses (2). This concept derived from the model of addiction to such drugs as heroin or addiction to behavioral patterns such as gambling. Addiction implies psychological dependence, physical dependence, and the presence of a withdrawal syndrome if the substance (e.g., the drug) is unavailable or the behavior (e.g., gambling) is frustrated.

The phenomenon of a person whose entire life revolves around sex-seeking behavior and activities, who spends an excessive amount of time in such behavior, and who often tries to stop such behavior but is unable to do so in spite of adverse consequences is well known to clinicians. Such persons show repeated and increasingly frequent attempts to have a sexual experience, the deprivation of which gives rise to symptoms of distress. Compulsive sexual behavior is coupled with extreme sexual preoccupation and patients often incorporate diverse normal and abnormal practices in their sexual activities.

Awareness of this problem has been heightened by cultural changes. Accountability connected to sexual exploitation in religious, political, and business arenas has focused attention on the problem and the acquired immune deficiency syndrome (AIDS) epidemic has motivated patients to seek help in controlling self-destructive hypersexuality. The ubiquitous presence of sex on the Internet has escalated the prevalence of sex addiction and in some cases fostered the development of the pathology in vulnerable persons who otherwise might not have manifested the problem.

Other commonly used terms for this problem are hypersexuality, sexual compulsivity, and sexual impulsivity. Hypersexuality is descriptive of the behavior but not the pathology of this condition. One study found one third of participants to have no significant pathology in addition to hypersexuality (3). The researchers also found no evidence of an addictive personality in the participants. These results, however, are contrary to the experience and findings of most clinicians and researchers. There are compulsive elements in addictive behavior, but differentiations can be made in the relatively ego-dystonic nature of compulsions and the ego-syntonic nature of sex addiction to many people. More importantly, compulsive behavior does not, in and of itself, provide pleasure in the activity, while sex addiction usually does. The term "sex addiction" discerns the difference between compulsively accessing the pleasure centers of the brain and the nonpleasure behavior that is more typical of obsessive–compulsive acts. Similarly, features of impulse control disorder are present in sex addiction. Impulsive behavior often is used to relieve the tension of an arousal drive about which the person may feel ambivalence, whereas addictions serve as a palliative or escape from a painful affect such as anxiety, depression, or narcissistic injury. In the author's view, sex addiction is a useful concept heuristically in that it can alert the clinician to seek an underlying cause for the manifest behavior.

DIAGNOSIS

Sex addiction is a behavior involving significant and destructive loss of control of the sexual impulse. Sex addicts are motivated to gratify their sexual impulses regardless of interference with relationships, work, or danger to reputation, status, and even physical well-being. In one study 38% of men and 45% of women contracted a sexually transmitted disease as a result of their behavior (4). Eventually, the need for sexual activity increases and the person's behavior is driven solely by the persistent desire to experience the sex act. Although there may be feelings of guilt and remorse after the act, they are not sufficient to prevent its recurrence, and usually sex addicts cannot refrain from their behavior, even when they attempt to do so. Most acts culminate in a sexual orgasm, although a sense of excitement (a high) usually accompanies the sex-seeking behavior even in the absence of an orgasm. The patient invests a great deal of time in the behavior, including fantasy, preoccupation, and preparation as well as engaging in sexual activity. Signs of sexual addiction are listed in Table 26.1.

TABLE 26.1 Criteria for sex addiction

Criteria
Recurrent failure (pattern) to resist sexual impulses to engage in specific sexual behavior
Frequent engaging in those behaviors to a greater extent or over a longer period of time than intended
Persistent desire or unsuccessful efforts to stop, to reduce, or to control behaviors
Inordinate amount of time spent in obtaining sex, being sexual, or recovering from sexual experiences
Preoccupation with the behavior or preparatory activities
Frequent engaging in the behavior when expected to fulfill occupational, academic, domestic, or social obligations
Continuation of the behavior despite knowledge of having a persistent or recurrent social, financial, psychological, or physical problem that is caused or exacerbated by the behavior
Need to increase the intensity, frequency, number, or risk of behaviors to achieve the desired effect or diminished effect with continued behaviors at the same level of intensity, frequency, number, or risk
Giving up or limiting social, occupational, or recreational activities because of the behavior
Distress, anxiety, restlessness, or irritability if unable to engage in the behavior

Adapted from Carnes PJ: *Don't Call It Love*. New York, NY: Bantam Books; 1991:181–266.

Diagnosis is complicated by the fact that patients usually are not forthcoming about their behavior (5). Patients feel shame and defend against that feeling with repression and denial. They exaggerate their ability to control their behavior, minimize the impact it has on others, or define themselves as having a strong sex drive rather than an addiction. Some cultures, such as those that emphasize machismo, facilitate this distortion.

In Oscar Hijuelos' Pulitzer Prize winning novel "The Mambo Kings Plays Songs of Love," the main protagonist, Cesar, suffers from dual addictions to alcohol and sex. A combination of denial and his internalization of the macho culture in which he was raised leaves Cesar unable to understand his wife's unhappiness about his constant philandering. He sees it as absolutely normal male behavior. Additionally, he is unable to sustain real intimacy with her (6).

The differentiation between a healthy, strong libido and sex addiction is determined by recognizing whether the sexual activity is kept secret and leads to the creation of a double life, whether there is an exploitative element to the sexual behavior, whether it is used as a palliative to painful emotions, and whether the person has difficulty with a truly intimate relationship.

There is a strong tendency for patients to compartmentalize or dissociate themselves from their behavior. Patients may present for treatment because of threats of divorce from a spouse, threat of loss of a job because they have been caught spending work time sexually interacting on the Internet or sexually harassing work colleagues, and confrontations with the legal system. Often, the patient will present the precipitating event as an aberration or rare occurrence.

Some patients present with anxiety or depression, and some seek treatment because their behavior has intensified to a degree that causes them conscious shame and they feel they cannot continue with this way of life. The clinician should be particularly alert to the possibility of sex addiction if the patient gives a history of chronic affairs, compulsive masturbation, pervasive prostitution use, or habitual online surfing of sex sites.

ETIOLOGY

The incidence of sex addiction is unknown, but has been estimated to afflict 3% to 6% of Americans. It is more frequently seen in men in a ratio of men to women that has been reported variously as 3 to 1 and 4 to 1 (7). However, in cybersex the ratio is more equal, with more than 40% of participants being female (8). Sex addiction usually begins in adolescence when the hormonal changes of puberty and the psychological challenge of consolidating a sexual identity are normal developmental events in the course of a person's growth. The mastery of these adolescent challenges goes awry in the sex addict's development. The problem intensifies during the addicts 20s to 40s when the disorder becomes full-blown and affects the person's life in adverse ways. Some workers feel the intensity of sex addiction diminishes after age 40, but others disagree (9). The author's experience is that even if the behavior or acting out diminishes, the addict's fantasies and abnormally heightened preoccupation with sex continues. In general, the course of untreated sex addiction involves hypersexual behavior, interrupted by periods of abstention when the addict tries to control the addiction, followed by relapses, and further episodes of compulsive sexual activity.

Research into biologic substrates for sex addiction is a new field, but studies have shown that sex addicts frequently come from families with multiple addictions. Addiction researchers have noted that the Taq 1A1 allele of the D2 receptor gene is associated with increased risk of alcoholism, drug abuse, smoking, obesity, compulsive behaviors, and Tourette syndrome (7). Also, some workers hypothesize that increased orgasmic excitability or impaired orgasmic control may be a biologic contributant to sex addiction. Hypersexual activity of the type seen in sex addiction can sometimes be a symptom of organic pathology. Specifically, it can be the manifestation of a brain lesion, particularly a lesion in the medial basal–frontal, diencephalic, or septal region (10). Such behavior can also occur in the context of a seizure disorder, most often in association with temporal lobe epilepsy (11). Additionally, it can occur when cerebral functioning is impaired and normal inhibitory controls no longer function, as in the dementias.

Studies have found many families of sex addicts to be rigid or disengaged. Hypocrisy is another characteristic of these patients' families. That is, the families will proclaim a highly moral, even rigid set of values publicly, which they privately violate (12). For example, a parent may extol the sanctity of marriage while carrying on an affair. If the patient, often in adolescence, discovers the discrepancy, anger and rebellion frequently ensue. The rebellion may be covert, as in secret sexual activity, which starts the future sex addict on a path of leading a double life of which he or she is secretly ashamed. The dynamics in the families from which these patients come and the patients' resulting behavior prevent the learning and experiencing of intimacy. From a psychodynamic perspective, sex addiction can be viewed as an intimacy disorder.

Sex addicts report a disproportionately high incidence of childhood trauma and abuse; 72% report a history of physical abuse, 81% report a history of sexual abuse, and 97% report emotional abuse (5,12).

Many of the films of Francois Truffaut, the noted French director, present an excellent review of the etiology, symptoms, and effects of sex addiction, particularly if they are seen serially. For example, an early film, "The 400 Blows" is a portrayal of abuse that warps a child psychologically. Later films such as "The Man Who Loved Women" and "The Woman Next Door" portray, respectively, a man with sex addiction and a man obsessed with a former sexual partner, who ruins his current relationship by acting out his obsession. "Such a Gorgeous Kid Like Me" portrays a woman who continually seduces men for personal—sometimes criminal—gain. Finally, "Mississippi Mermaid" is an example of the destructiveness of uncontrolled sexual desire. Truffaut himself described it as "degradation by love."

It has been suggested that Truffaut's themes were informed by his personal experiences. Biographers note that his childhood was markedly unhappy, his mother having borne him illegitimately, and having remained extremely rejecting of him (13).

Some clinicians report that patients repeat significant emotional scenarios and actual behaviors from their abuse experiences in their sex addiction behaviors. Other sex addicts deal with their past traumas by indulging in high-risk behaviors. These may be looked at as a conditioned response linking sex or excitement with fear, or a counterphobic attempt to master engendered feelings of helplessness and danger.

A 44-year-old man presented for therapy after prolonged insistence by his wife that he do so. She wanted to engage in couple therapy, which he refused, but he eventually agreed to go for individual therapy. She suspected him of having an affair because of the late hours he kept and her frequent inability to get in touch with him, combined with a lack of sexual interaction between them.

He was a successful business man, prominent in his community as the head of numerous volunteer, civic activities. He was, in fact, sexually active on his many late nights, but his activities involved high-risk sex in questionable bars where he would seek out transgendered males. His preferred sexual behavior was oral sex with a man who had a penis, but had surgically or hormonally enhanced breasts.

His early history revealed an alcoholic mother and a father who was a martinet and forced him to take up boxing even though he was small for his age when he was a child and afraid of the sport. His first sexual experience was being taken with some friends at the age of 13 to a transgendered prostitute by an older, bullying schoolmate.

Aviel Goodman theorizes that vulnerability to the addictive process involves "impaired affect regulation, aberrant function of the motivational-reward system and impaired behavioral inhibition" (7). These three factors leave a person abnormally vulnerable to and easily destabilized by emotions that most people can cope with effectively. The person is prone to states of tension, emptiness, and anhedonia, and is largely incapable of resisting activities that provide immediate gratification or surcease from emotional pain, regardless of the destructive consequences of such behavior. Goodman believes that the selection of sex as the addiction of choice evolves from a combination of preference and opportunity. Other workers theorize that sex addiction is more likely to occur in an "eroticized child," defined as a child who has not been sexually abused, but has been covertly seduced. Carnes argues that the eroticized child is even more damaged than the overtly abused child (5). Patients who were eroticized children cannot clearly define parental behavior, doubt their perceptions, and often feel crazy. Sometimes, these patients through their sex addiction are identifying with a seductive mother who herself used sexualization as a defense against pain. In males, this serves the dual purpose of remaining attached to the mother from whom separation in childhood was particularly difficult, while at the same time asserting their maleness (14,15). Sex addiction sometimes has been explained as a way to deal with chronic separation anxiety and also as a way of protecting the patient from the fear of the final separation of death.

TYPES OF BEHAVIORAL PATTERNS

Carnes has developed a system of ten "archetypes" of sexual behavior that he believes help reveal the addict's arousal patterns (Table 26.2).

Half of these archetypes involve paraphilic behaviors. In fact, the paraphilias constitute the behavioral patterns most often found in the sex addict. As defined in DSM-IV-TR, the

TABLE 26.2	Sexual behavior patterns
Fantasy sex: sexually charged fantasies, relationships, and situations	
	Arousal depends on sexual possibility. Neglecting responsibilities to engage in fantasy or to prepare for the next sexual episode, or both, is common among fantasy sex addicts.
Seductive role sex: seduction of partners	
	Arousal is based on conquest and diminishes rapidly after initial contact. Arousal can be heightened by increasing risk or the number of partners, or both.
Voyeuristic sex: visual arousal	
	The use of visual stimulation to escape into an obsessive trance. Arousal may be heightened by masturbation, risk (e.g., peeping), or violation of boundaries (e.g., voyeuristic rape), but, for arousal to be maintained, it must be illicit somehow and must be visual.
Exhibitionistic sex: attracting attention to the body or sexual parts of the body	
	Sexual arousal stems from reaction to viewer shock or interest.
Paying for sex: purchase of sexual services	
	Arousal is connected to payment for sex, and, with time, the arousal actually becomes connected to money itself. Payment creates an entitlement and a sense of power over meeting needs, but the arousal starts with having money and the search for someone in the business.
Trading sex: selling or bartering sex for power	
	Arousal is based on gaining control of others by using sex as leverage.
Intrusive sex: boundary violation without discovery	
	Sexual arousal occurs by violating boundaries with no repercussions.
Anonymous sex: high-risk sex with unknown persons	
	Arousal involves no seduction or cost and is immediate. The arousal has no entanglements or obligations associated with it and often is accelerated by unsafe or high-risk environments, such as bars, beaches, parks, and restrooms.
Pain exchange sex: being humiliated or hurt as part of sexual arousal or sadistic hurting or degrading another sexually, or both	
	Arousal is built around specific scenarios or narratives of humiliation and shame.
Exploitive sex: exploitation of the vulnerable	
	Arousal patterns are based on target types of vulnerability. Certain types of vulnerable persons (e.g., clients or patients of professionals, children or adolescents, or distressed persons) become the focus of arousal.

essential features of a paraphilia are recurrent intense sexual urges or behaviors that are culturally unacceptable, including exhibitionism, fetishism, frotteurism, sadomasochism, voyeurism, cross-dressing, and pedophilia.

A 48-year-old lawyer presented for therapy because of marital problems and feelings of depression. His history revealed past alcohol abuse and a lack of sexual interaction with his wife since the birth of their youngest child 6 years previously. His current sexual activity was connected to visits to bars (which resulted in frequent lapses from his alcohol abstention), both because alcohol relieved his sexual inhibitions and because he was sexually aroused by watching women smoke. Legally, bars were the only public venue where smoking was permissible and smoking was a fetishistic component of sexual arousal for him.

His early history involved an emotionally sadistic father who would smoke in the family car with the windows closed, not caring if the children got sick. He remembered being attracted to a young aunt who smoked. His first cigarette was one he stole from a pack of cigarettes he found on his sister's bureau.

Paraphilias are associated with clinically significant distress and almost invariably interfere with interpersonal relationships, and they often lead to legal complications. In addition to the paraphilias, however, sex addiction can also include behavior that is considered normal, such as coitus and masturbation, except that is promiscuous and uncontrolled.

In the 19th century the psychiatrist Richard von Krafft-Ebing reported on several cases of abnormally increased sexual desire. One was that of a 36-year-old married teacher, the father of seven children, who masturbated repeatedly while sitting at his desk in front of his pupils, after which he was "penitent and filled with shame." He indulged in coitus three to four times a day in addition to his repeated masturbatory acts. In another case a woman masturbated almost incessantly and was unable to control her impulses. She had frequent coitus with many men, but neither coitus nor masturbation was sufficient, and she eventually was placed in an institution (16).

In nonparaphilic sex addiction, the aim is constant physical gratification that many therapists interpret as an excessive need for an "orgasmic high" to alleviate unrecognized emotional pain. Women sex addicts frequently use sexual behavior to engage addictively in romantic relationships in order to fill unmet needs for love, attachment, dependency and admiration.

Many sexual behavior patterns express anger, sometimes called eroticized anger, that is a major component of most sex addictions. However, the patient notices only the sex component of the behavior, not the anger (17). For example, intrusive sex behaviors involve patients who are frotteurs (people who press their genitalia against others, usually in crowded situations such as subways), peeping Toms, obscene phone callers, and professionals such as doctors, dentists, therapists, or clergy who touch patients or congregants under the guise of performing professional tasks. The intrusion is sexual, but anonymous or masked, and leaves the sex addict unaccountable to the victim. In these cases the sex addict is putting something over on, or stealing sex from the victim. In seductive role sex, the excitement lies in the seduction and conquest, not in the sex act itself. This behavior pattern has also been called Don Juanism. The sexual conquests are used to mask a fear of rejection and deep feelings of inferiority. Some therapists believe that Don Juanism is a defense against fears of being homosexual. Most Don Juans have no interest in a woman after they have had sex with her (2).

A 41-year-old man presented for therapy because of the sexual dysfunction of ejaculatory inhibition. He was able to climax with masturbation or when he went to a massage parlor, but never with a woman in mutual sex play, whether manual, oral, or with intercourse. This was the case whether the patient was with his wife, or on one of his many one-night stands. He had experienced only two exceptions to this pattern. He was able to ejaculate once when he was having sex with two women at the same time, and once when he invited a woman into his home for sex, and their was real danger that his wife would walk in on the scene. The patient compulsively continued his pattern of seductions in spite of his dissatisfaction with his sexual experiences, stating that what he really enjoyed was the conquest. In fact, he kept a list of all the women he seduced which he would show to friends.

Sex addicts often act out in several clusters of behavior, moving from one to the other. Carnes states that "The key for clinicians is to understand the escalation factor. Addicts act out using more of the behaviors, add risk and danger, or seek new behaviors, often with great risk and danger. Escalation is tempered with plateaus, efforts to reduce risk, and sexually aversive periods. Most addicts are able to pinpoint moments of escalation and resulting consequences" (5).

In many cases sex addiction is associated with a variety of other disorders. In addition to the paraphilias that are frequently present, there may be an associated major mental disorder such as anxiety disorder, depressive disorder, bipolar disorder, or schizophrenia. Antisocial personality disorder and borderline personality disorder are common. Paradoxically, persons with sex addiction may have a concurrent sexual dysfunction.

COMORBIDITY

Comorbidity (dual diagnosis) refers to the presence of an addiction that coexists with another psychiatric disorder such as those mentioned above. For example, about 50% of patients with substance-use disorders also have an associated psychiatric disorder. Similarly, many sex addicts have an associated psychiatric disorder (18). Dual diagnosis implies that the psychiatric illness and the addiction are separate disorders; one does not cause the other. The diagnosis of comorbidity is often difficult to make because addictive behavior (of all types) can produce extreme anxiety and severe disturbances in mood and affect, especially when addictive behavior is treated. If, after a period of abstinence, symptoms of a psychiatric disorder remain, the comorbid condition is more easily recognized and diagnosed than during the addictive period. Finally, there is a high correlation between sex addiction and substance-use disorders, up to 80% in some studies (7).

The centaur of Greek mythology is a perfect symbol of combined substance-use disorder and sex addiction. The centaur was a creature with the head, arms, and torso of a man and the lower body of a horse. Its weaknesses and downfall were lust and an inability to resist wine. When the centaurs drank, they were unable to control their impulses. Their physical depiction was reflective of their problems; the use of their human intellect and capacity for control was dissolved by wine and overpowered by their "animal" drives.

The term "fusion" is often used when two addictions are almost always indulged at the same time. For instance, cocaine use is almost always connected with sexual activity or intent, with both habits containing a compulsive element (19,20). Other instances of fusion can involve use of alcohol to enable the person to indulge in high-risk sex, or gambling to increase general excitement levels before having sex (21). An ironic comorbid diagnosis that is appropriate for a number of sex addicts is sexual aversion disorder. In these cases the patients are averse to and compulsively avoid sex with spouses or long-term partners, while addictively pursuing high-risk sex outside a relationship (22). This particular behavior transparently reflects intimacy problems, and is frequently the result of early family problems and traumas.

The classic French film, Belle de Jour, portrays this particular pattern. The main protagonist is an upper–middle class woman who has no interest in sex with her loving husband. However, she is preoccupied with masochistic fantasies in which she is whipped, reviled, and pelted with mud. Ultimately, she embarks on a double life, working a few hours each day at a small brothel. She is exposed to dangerous and sadistic men with whom she enjoys sex. We learn, during the course of the film, that she was repeatedly incestuously abused as a child.

Comorbidity not only complicates the task of diagnosis, but also complicates treatment.

CYBERSEX ADDICTION

Cybersex addiction has been called the crack cocaine of sexual addiction. The escalation of behavior that is inherent to the problem of sex addiction is exponentially increased when the Internet is used for compulsive sexual activity. Nonsex addicts may visit pornography sites on the Internet on an occasional basis, but they do not become sex addicts. However, persons already addicted to sexual behavior and persons who are vulnerable to the addictive process are quickly hooked by the Internet. Studies have shown that sex-related sites became the most profitable economic sector of the Internet in the past decade, exceeding sales of software and computers. Cybersex has become a problem in the workplace: 70% of Internet pornography surfing occurs during daytime work hours; and one in six workers is estimated to have a problem with sexual behavior online (5). The extraordinary addictiveness of cybersex is driven by what A.L. Cooper has called "the triple A engine: accessibility, affordability, and anonymity" or what other workers have called the ACE engine: anonymity, convenience, and escape (4).

A 48-year-old man, an accountant, presented for therapy after being fired from his job. He had worked for a small accounting firm for 22 years and had been a valued employee. The patient had always kept a stash of pornographic magazines, but did not give a history of excessive masturbation. However, after visiting pornography sites on the Internet, his traffic between numerous sites increased significantly and was accompanied by masturbation on a daily or twice daily basis. His risk-taking also increased. He began locking his office door frequently, sometimes not responding to knocks in order to indulge in cybersex. Although he was spoken to about locking his door, he continued the behavior. His risk-taking increased to the point that he would surf pornography sites on days spent servicing clients in the clients' offices, even though he had no private space other than a separate desk on these occasions. One of the clients complained vociferously to his employer, which led to his being terminated.

Relationships are profoundly affected by Internet addiction. Patients report that they withdraw from close interactions with spouses, other family members, and friends. Their marital sex life decreases. The sex addicts invest their time as well as their emotional energy in their online relationships. They have little left to give to the real people in their lives and additionally may withdraw due to an unconscious sense of shame. Cybersex addicts escalate the frequency, the variety, and the risk of their behavior. Patients report becoming obsessed rapidly with behaviors that they never tried or never even knew about before their Internet experiences. They quickly find numerous sites: different types of pornography; paraphilia sites; e-mail partners, and chat rooms where they conduct virtual affairs.

The effect of these affairs on partners and family is as destructive as that of an actual affair. Spouses feel betrayed, hurt, and angry. They experience a loss of self-esteem, feeling they could never compete with the online sex partners. Additionally, they report severe distress over being lied to repeatedly and experience a loss of trust. Children of the sex addict experience disillusionment. They may be exposed to objectification of women, and they may become involved in their parents' conflict or suffer the break up of their parents' marriage. One study reported a divorce rate of 28% following the discovery of an online affair, and consideration of divorce in over 60% of the couples where the sex addict's behavior had been discovered (23).

It is estimated that 1% of the population in the United States suffers from Internet sex addiction (8). Studies of cybersex addicts report the majority to be male, heterosexual and married. However, the single and dating also form a significant segment of this population, as do persons who are homosexually oriented. Women are a larger proportion of addicts on the Internet than they are in the overall category of sex addicts. Some researchers theorize that women, like homosexuals, fall into the category of people who are disenfranchised sexually, and that the anonymity of the Internet provides them with an outlet for sexual behavior forbidden to them by the culture at large. This theory requires more research.

In addition to serving as a catalyst for persons who might never have become sex addicts without the Internet, cybersex can intensify existing addictive behavior and can precipitate new compulsive off-line behavior. Carnes discusses a theory to explain the escalation, intensity of arousal, and compulsive behavior set in motion by the Internet: "... through the internet patients": "access the unresolved." All people have sexual experiences that leave them unfinished. Sexual play as a child, for example, may leave the person with unfinished experiences. As a person matures, he or she realizes that he or she no longer has an interest in that behavior or that those experiences are no longer appropriate for adults. Yet a person might experience the right image or story that is an absolute overlay of something unfinished from childhood or adolescence. The nature of marketing pornography is to bombard potential clients with a variety of images to stimulate the purchase of memberships. When that which is unfinished is accessed, the individual begins to search for more of the same genre. The marketing loops of sex sites are literally labyrinthine; each choice may bring a person closer to the types of images that most closely fit the unresolved, unfinished aspect of the sexual self. Patients often report the phenomenon of a "burned in" image—a specific scene out of Internet about which they cannot stop thinking. This phenomenon is similar to the intrusive images that Post-Traumatic Stress Disorder patients describe (5).

TREATMENT

Sex addiction is a chronic disease. It usually has a relapsing, remitting course. The aim, as with all chronic disease, is to keep it in remission. In sex addiction this means enabling patients to control the destructive behavior, to help them evolve a healthier sexuality, and to mitigate the psychological distress associated with the disorder as much as possible. Numerous treatment approaches are used in treating sex addiction, such as inpatient therapy, 12-step groups for sex addiction, other therapeutic groups, medication, psychodynamic psychotherapy, couple therapy, and sex therapy. Frequently, a combination of many of these modalities is necessary for treatment to be effective. Studies have evaluated the perceived helpfulness of a number of treatment options from the patient's perspective (Table 26.3).

The initial factor that is necessary for therapeutic engagement is the patient's recognition that there is a serious problem, whether this recognition is a result of the patient's insight, or imposed upon the patient by an intervention. The intervention can be initiated by spouse, family, colleagues, employers, or the legal system. The greater the acceptance by the patient of the presence of the pathology, the greater the chance of successful treatment. Similarly, the chances of success in treatment are paralleled by the degree of the patient's internal commitment to giving up the addiction. Even if treatment is imposed by threats of divorce, loss of job, or the law, recognition of the problem can be developed in treatment, along with a genuine desire to change.

Inpatient Therapy

Inpatient therapy involves institutionalization at a rehabilitation facility that may be freestanding or may be part of a larger psychiatric hospital or general hospital. Hospitalization as the first step in a treatment process is most appropriate for patients who are suicidal or dangerous to others. Paraphilias that involve victims such as pedophilia, frotteurism, or exhibitionism may require that the patient be hospitalized. Some nonparaphilic patients who cannot refrain from excessive sexual activity even though they are participants in outpatient programs are also good candidates for hospitalization. Certainly, if a patient continues high-risk practices, such as promiscuous sex with strangers, or sex with numerous partners without utilizing safe-sex precautions such as condoms, inpatient therapy is indicated.

Treatment in these settings involves multiple approaches. In addition to the removal of the patient from the pervasive sexual stimuli of the general culture, he or she participates in a 12-step program, similar to the program developed for Alcoholics Anonymous. Education regarding the disorder is provided didactically and in therapy. Family meetings also educate family members about the problem and provide opportunities for the families and patient to reconnect in a moderated setting. Sometimes these meetings lead family members to enter therapy as well, not for sex addiction, but for support, introspection, and increased self-knowledge. Medication may be prescribed for the patient and individual therapy is a part of most programs. A follow-up program and plan for continuing treatment after discharge is essential for the ongoing recovery of the patient (24).

Group Therapy

There are several forms of 12-step programs available: Sex Addicts Anonymous (SAA); Sex and Love Addicts Anonymous (SLAA); Sexaholics Anonymous (SA); and Sexual Compulsives Anonymous (SCA). The first step in all these

TABLE 26.3 Treatment choices of 190 persons asked to note the helpfulness of various treatment options

Type of treatment	Helpful (%)	Not helpful (%)
Higher power	87	3
Twelve-step group (for sexual addiction)	85	4
Friends' support	69	4
Individual therapy	65	12
Celibacy period	64	10
Sponsor	61	6
Exercise and nutrition	58	4
Twelve-step group (other)	55	8
Partner support	36	6
Inpatient	35	2
Outpatient group	27	7
Couples therapy	21	11
Family therapy	11	3
After care (hospital)	9	5

From Carnes PJ. *Don't Call It Love.* New York, NY: Bantam Books; 1991:181–266.

groups requires personal acceptance of the problem by the addict, which is emphasized by the public profession of one addiction to the group. The patient receives immediate support for recognizing his or her problem. The next two steps address the addict's conflicts over dependency and control as the addicts admit their powerlessness to regulate their behavior and accept the necessity of help from a "higher power." The remaining steps emphasize spirituality, require the patients to further confront the problem by making an inventory of behavior that has harmed others and, where possible, make amends for that behavior (24). The final step advocates helping others who have the same problem. All the 12-step programs follow this format; their differences lie in their definitions of sobriety.

SAA members individualize this definition; with the help of other fellowship members, the recovering addicts individually identify the sexual behaviors that are destructive or lead them into problems and define such behaviors as "out of bounds" for themselves. SLAA has a similar approach and defines any sexual behavior or emotional act that is a trigger for out of control behavior as "bottom-line sex." Any act of "bottom-line sex" violates sobriety. In SCA sobriety is also highly personalized; members are encouraged to follow sexual recovery plans that reflect their own values, although these are shared with and affected by group input. SA has a very specific definition of sobriety as sex only with a spouse; masturbation or sex with any partner other than a spouse constitutes a lapse from sobriety. All programs encourage the adoption of a sponsor; a group member to whom the newly recovering addict can turn for support and counsel between meetings and in times of stress and potential or actual relapse (7).

Twelve-step programs have been extremely effective in counteracting sexual addiction and preventing relapse. Many workers believe that they are essential to recovery, even though empirical evidence reveals that many recovering addicts do not complete all the steps of such a program. The nature of these fellowships varies from group to group, reflecting the characteristics of the individuals who attend them. There is a danger that some sex addicts will use a group setting to connect with another group member in order to act out their addiction. However, the benefits of these groups appear to far out weigh the risks and constructive rehabilitation occurs significantly more than destructive behavior.

Other Therapy Groups

Participation in a therapy group of any type is beneficial to those who are addicted to sex. Support, confrontation, breakthrough of isolation, and the counteracting of denial and rationalization all aid the recovery process. Also, group acceptance is a significant factor in reducing the shame, conscious or unconscious, which contributes to perpetuation of the sex addiction cycle. The group provides a safe forum in which the addict learns to make meaningful connections with others. Groups can be educational and informational, cognitive-behavioral, supportive or psychodynamic in orientation (25). Cognitive-behavioral groups are frequently used to treat sex addicts with paraphilias, and psychodynamic groups are useful for patients with comorbid personality disorders. Studies have shown that groups with structure are the most effective for persons with sex addiction disorder. The structure may somewhat counteract the threat of loss of self-coherence that many addicts suffer. Also group theory posits that the group ego is stronger than the ego of any individual member. In a structured group, the leader or the structure itself makes the greatest contribution to the group, which helps bolster the psychological frailties of the recovering patient. Additionally, groups function as a benign superego, providing nonshaming, nonpunitive controls for the addict who has insufficiently developed internal controls.

Pharmacotherapy

Pharmacotherapy is an important modality for reducing patient symptomology. The most commonly used medications are the antidepressants, particularly the selective serotonin reuptake inhibitors (SSRIs). Agents that have been found to be effective include fluoxetine (Prozac), sertraline (Zoloft), paroxetine (Paxil), and fluvoxamine (Luvox). The effectiveness of these medications derives from their side effect of reducing libido that has been reported in nonsex addict populations, from their use in treatment of obsessive–compulsive disorders, and also from their antidepressive effects. The last effect is important in those sex addicts who have comorbid affective disorder but also for most sex addicts who tend to respond to stress with intense feelings of dysphoria and addictive behavior. Studies report an effective response rate to these medications of 50% to 90% (26). Interestingly, a number of studies of paraphiliacs have found that SSRIs reduce the drive for pathologic sexual behavior in these persons, but not the drive for healthy sexual behavior (27). Other antidepressants that have proved effective in treating sex addiction include imipramine (Tofranil), nefazadone (Serzone), despramine (Norpramin), and clomipramine (Anafranil). However, clomipramine also has the paradoxical effect in some persons of producing spontaneous orgasms. Lithium is effective in the treatment of bipolar patients who evince hypersexuality in a manic episode. As is true in psychiatric disorders in general, pharmacotherapy is most effective when it is combined with other treatment modalities, particularly group or individual therapy.

Antiandrogens are sometimes used to treat sex addicts with paraphilic sexual behavior. This type of treatment is discussed below, in the section on paraphilias.

Cognitive-Behavioral Therapy (CBT)

Cognitive-behavioral approaches to sex addiction usually emphasize altering the maladaptive core beliefs that are thought to underlie the patient's addictive behavior. Cognitive-behavioral techniques for sex addiction are typically utilized in the context of therapy groups, although individual approaches are used as well (28–30).

A supportive, collaborative relationship is developed with the group or the therapist to keep patients engaged in therapy while they learn to correct their distorted beliefs and while they practice and master self-help skills to counter their addiction. The therapy is interactive and focuses on current problems and relapse prevention.

The goal in CBT is to have the patient recognize and stop the addictive behavior. In some cases, in addition to behavior modification, medication may be used to help the addict control hypersexual behavior. Instruction in anxiety reduction techniques, such as progressive relaxation, teaches patients to alleviate the anxiety that may precipitate the addictive behavior. In the group setting patient, recognition of the problem is publicly expressed to the group members, who similarly admit the same problem and provide support for one another. CBT requires a profession of commitment to the treatment process. This may be in the form of a promise to keep no secrets from the group members or therapist, or in the form of a contract made with therapist or the group about behavioral changes the patient wants to make. Such contracts are usually reviewed weekly and individuals share their thoughts about various successes and failures. In the group setting, members benefit from peer support and from confrontation by peers who are uniquely sensitive to manipulations by a patient who seems to be less than honest with himself or herself about addictive activities. An educational component is sometimes interwoven in the therapy with the therapist providing didactic material that informs the patient about the disorder. Members of the sex addict's family may become involved in therapy. The concept of sex addiction as a disorder rather than a lack of will helps diminish the shame felt by the addict. Patients may be instructed to keep journal entries as part of the therapy process. The journals provide a method for self-observation that keeps patients aware of impulses, fantasies, and affects, which they usually avoid by escaping into addictive behavior (31). CBT facilitates more adaptive social functioning through exercises in problem-solving and through assertiveness training (29). The compilation of factors that are significant in "triggering" a relapse is part of relapse prevention techniques. Patients are advised on how to deal with the triggers and how to deal with an episode of addictive sexual behavior should a lapse occur. Patients rehearse relapse prevention actions such as avoidance of triggering situations. For example, cybersex addicts are encouraged not to use computers. When such use is necessary for work, patients are instructed to position computers so the screens are clearly visible to others. In the group setting, contacting a group member for support when urges to act out occur is a crucial component of treatment. Rewards to prevent the addict from feeling excessively deprived are also an important part of the therapeutic process (5).

Psychodynamic Psychotherapy

Psychodynamic or insight-oriented psychotherapy to treat the sex addict is usually necessary to treat the dysfunctions of character or personality that are often comorbid with sex addiction. Psychodynamic psychotherapy involves treatment in a dyadic setting with a therapist who is skilled in the use of transference and familiar with the use of psychodynamic constructs. Therapy has an open-ended time frame and the focus is on the patient's verbal associations, dreams, and fantasies, and the transferential relationship to the therapist (32). The therapist is more interactive and directive than a traditional analytic psychotherapist.

Adding psychodynamic conceptualizations to behavioral techniques helps patients recognize affects of which they are unaware, helps them develop healthy defenses in place of the unhealthy defenses of denial, repression, dissociation or somatization, and frees them from the destructive behavior caused by unrecognized, unresolved inner conflicts, needs, and fears (33). Finally, it helps them correct distorted perceptions of themselves and others. Psychodynamic psychotherapy also provides the addict with what Franz Alexander called a corrective emotional experience (18).

An important concept in understanding the psychological development of a person's sexuality is the relationship between the child and his or her parents, particularly the mother.

Robert Stoller has explained:

> Freud told us ... that parents have the greatest possible influence on their children's development, that children create psychic structure in response, that adult sexual life can be traced back to effects in infancy, and that sexual desire and gratification find origins in infancy (34).

The first experience of intimacy occurs with the mothering person. That intimacy becomes the basis for subsequent experiences, including sexual experiences. Under positive circumstances, mothering experiences that gratify need appropriately and set boundaries on behavior are the basis on which future comfortable intimacy is established. Abusive, ambivalent, or neglectful mothering, in infancy, childhood, and later development, sets the stage for fear of hurt or loss and for reactive, retaliatory rage with subsequent, potentially intimate experiences. During their first year or recovery, many patients report painful memories from childhood that had been repressed and clarity about early wounds emerge (5). When past experiences and their associated affects become conscious, memories are expressed in words. Physiologic patterns, such as the development of psychosomatic disease, and behavioral patterns such as addiction that the patient used to cope with early hurts then become amenable to modification.

The replay of old reaction patterns, affects, and fantasies in a current time frame, and in a personalized context is the patient's expression of his or her transference. The transference resuscitates, in a moderated and safe setting, the patients unsatisfied claims for love, feelings of shame or humiliation, and prohibited aggressive feelings. This phenomenon offers an excellent opportunity for modification of distorted emotional responses and unhealthy behavior. Many sex addicts experience unrecognized, painful affects such as anxiety or unacceptable anger as the urge to act out sexually. Those affects are unconsciously translated into urges that often precipitate hypersexual behavior. Addicts, because of neglectful or abusive caretaking in early childhood, never developed the skills to cope with uncomfortable affects and react to them as overwhelming threats that may cause psychological disintegration. The addictive behavior provides the patient, not just with a hedonic escape, but is unconsciously experienced by the patient as a necessary defense for his or her emotional survival (7,14).

In the context of the therapeutic relationship patients shame about their behavior diminishes. They learn from the therapist that sex addiction is a disorder, not an inherent weakness or character flaw. At the same time they are confronted with the responsibility for dealing with it. The patients' capacity for coping with stress and for controlling hypersexual behavior develops as they internalize the therapist's caretaking functions and nonjudgmental attitude. They identify with and accept cultural standards for appropriate behavior. Goodman explains internalization as: "... a primary means by which psychotherapy promotes healing of impaired self regulation by providing new opportunities for patients to internalize self regulatory functions that they did not adequately internalize during childhood...." Self-care functions can develop through internalization of the message that the patient is valued as a person and worth taking care of. Healthy self-governance functions can develop through internalization of the therapist's integrity, respectfulness, nonjudgmental acceptance, and general stabilizing function.

In the course of therapy, patients recognize the stresses, both external and internal, that trigger addictive behavior. They learn to communicate with others more effectively as they become less ashamed and fearful, and they see themselves and the external world through a less distorted lens. Their expectations of themselves and others become more realistic, and they make greater use of such defenses as anticipation and suppression that help prevent relapse (33). Ideally these gains are used not just to deal with the sex addiction, but are applied both to the addict's personal relationships and to his or her work life.

Abstinence

Many sex addicts episodically refrain for all sexual behavior as a way of controlling their addiction. This has been called "acting in" (5). During these periods sexual impulses are dealt with by repression, which is ultimately ineffective. Without treatment the addictive pattern breaks through.

However, abstention is usually prescribed in the initial phase of recovery. In the beginning of treatment it is easier for the patient to abstain than to transition from addictive sexuality to healthy sexual behavior. Many patients report relief at not having to deal with sex at all; they feel freed from an activity that has controlled them. Some treatment programs require the patient to write an abstinence statement that usually defines sexual behaviors to be curtailed, describes sexual behaviors to be cultivated, and includes situations, or triggers, for addictive behavior to be avoided (e.g., avoiding a red-light district in a town). These statements are discussed with a therapist or support group as part of treatment.

The majority of patients report that a celibacy period is a helpful component of treatment. Eventually, the addicts leave the shelter of abstinence and work on gratifying their sexual impulses in the context of healthy, intimate, and nonexploitative relationships. Couple therapy and sex therapy can be useful in this regard.

Couple Therapy

During the course of a patient's addiction his or her relationship with a partner is hurt by secrecy and lies that clearly interfere with intimacy. When the patient is recovering, he or she must deal with shame or guilt and vulnerability while the spouse or partner must deal with feelings of betrayal, rejection, anger, and loss. Couple therapy provides a controlled forum in which one has to confront and process these feelings. The therapist, through definite types of communication, attempts to reverse or change maladaptive patterns of interaction and behavior, and to encourage personality growth in both partners. Communication exercises may include setting regular times for talking together, and using the word "I", as in "I feel", "I think", "I need," as often as possible in order to promote the sharing of feelings and thoughts. Daily letter writing in which feelings are shared is another technique to improve communication. Sometimes partners immediately repeat their communications back to each other to make sure they have accurately heard each other. Couple therapy can elucidate pathogenic factors in the marital relationship (29). The emphasis is on restructuring the couple's interaction and sometimes exploring the dynamics of each partner. Also, this type of therapy can engage the spouse and the energy in the relationship as agents of therapeutic change in the recovery process (35). Major goals of couple therapy include improving the communication skills, the conflict resolution skills, and the problem-solving skills of the couple, usually with behavioral techniques. The addition of an insight-oriented approach can lead to improvement in the fulfillment of individual needs for attachment and intimacy, and to increase trust and equitability in the relationship (36).

Sex Therapy

Sex therapy may be necessary to help the patient's transition to a healthy mode of expressing sexual impulses or to augment couple therapy. Frequently, sex addicts suffer from a particular sexual dysfunction. This is not as ironic as it seems because the same developmental factors that are prevalent in the creation of a sex addict may lead to a sexual dysfunction. Any experience that hinders the ability to be intimate, that leads to a feeling of inadequacy or distrust, or that develops a sense of being unloving or unlovable may result in a sexual dysfunction (3).

The following factors have been found to be causative in erectile disorders: fear of punishment; castration anxiety, fear of injury as a result of opening up to others; fear of harming women through intercourse; and fear of retaliation from other men at successful sexual relations. The central conflict in inhibited male orgasm frequently lies in rivalry with and fantasized retaliations from other men (34).

Biologic factors may contribute to these dysfunctions and to premature ejaculation, but psychological or mixed factors are causative in 50% of cases. Psychological issues are causative in a higher percentage of cases in young and middle adulthood, particularly if there are no physical health issues (3).

Among women, dynamic factors that have been noted in sexual dysfunction include fear of direct injury to the vagina from the penis, inability to trust a sexual partner, reluctance to make oneself vulnerable related to previous experiences of loss, separation, or abuse, and fear of loss of control if sexual feelings are let loose.

Sexual difficulties have also been ascribed to flight from masochistic fantasies associated with sexual coitus. Freud postulated that girls in the oedipal phase of development assume they have lost a penis. Such assumptions of genital damage or insufficiency may give rise to wishes for vengeance that find expression in a variety of ways—for example, vaginismus with a denial of entry, fantasies of vaginal mutilation of the penis, the wish to disappoint the man and envy of male prerogatives (37).

Regardless of etiology, the final common pathway of sexual dysfunction is performance anxiety. A behavioral approach is utilized to minimize anxiety. Specific exercises, both in communication and for sex play are prescribed for the couple. The exercises are performed in the couple's own home and discussed weekly or twice-weekly in psychotherapy sessions. The aim of therapy is to establish or re-establish communication within the marital unit. Sex is emphasized as a natural function that flourishes in the appropriate domestic climate and improved communication is encouraged toward that end. To minimize performance anxiety, the couple are prohibited from any sex play other than that prescribed by the therapist. Beginning exercises usually focus on heightening sensory awareness to touch, sight, sound, and smell. Initially, intercourse is interdicted and the couple practice giving and receiving bodily pleasure without the pressure of having to achieve penetration or orgasm.

The individuals alternately invite each other for exercise sessions and alternate in caressing one another. This structure inherently confronts inhibitions about sexual approach in an intimate relationship and reinforces the idea that a person has to "give to get." Exercises involving genital stimulation and quiet penetration (no thrusting) are added before the couple is advised to attempt intercourse. Psychotherapy sessions follow each new exercise period, and problems and satisfactions, both sexual and in other areas of the couple's lives, are discussed. The introduction of new exercises is geared toward the couple's progress.

One of the most effective treatment modalities is the use of sex therapy integrated with psychodynamic and psychoanalytically oriented psychotherapy. The material and dynamics that emerge in patients in analytically oriented sex therapy are the same as those in psychoanalytic psychotherapy, such as dreams, fear of punishment, aggressive feelings, difficulty trusting a partner, fear of intimacy, oedipal feelings, and the fear of genital mutilation. The sex therapy is conducted over an extended period that allows for the learning of sexual satisfaction in the context of the patients' day-to-day lives.

The structure of sex therapy inherently involves the formation of a small group of three or four people; the therapist or cotherapists and the couple. Group dynamics, including the support and confrontation that are more easily possible in a group setting, enhance the effectiveness of the therapy. Also, the therapist or cotherapy team serves as a benevolent superego that helps to relax the inhibitions of the patients.

PARAPHILIAS

Paraphilic sex is an integral part of the behavior of a significant number of sex addicts. Paraphilias or perversions are sexual stimuli or acts that are deviations from normal sexual behaviors, but are necessary for some person's to experience arousal or orgasm (see listing of paraphilias above).

These individuals can experience sexual pleasure, but are inhibited from responding to stimuli that are normally considered erotic. A special fantasy with its unconscious and conscious components is the core element of the paraphilia, with sexual arousal and orgasm being associated phenomena that reinforce the fantasy or impulse (38).

John Money has explained that the love map (the ideal program for experiencing sexual pleasure) of the paraphiliac is that person's only way of salvaging his or her sexuality from the inhibitions that have interfered with responsiveness to normal sexual stimuli (39). Ethel Person has described the paraphiliac as possessing an abnormally narrow range of sexual responsiveness, since he or she remains unstimulated by the variety of stimuli that can arouse normal people. Some sex addicts indulge in several paraphilias, for instance fetishes, bondage, and voyeurism, or any other combination of perversions. Freud has described such people as polymorphous perverse (38).

There are nonparaphilic sex addicts and people with a paraphilia who are not sex addicts. However, it is not surprising for one person to suffer from both disorders since they share similar epidemiologies and etiologies. As is true for sex addiction, paraphilias are seen much more frequently in males in a reported ratio of 4 to 1. More than 50% of paraphilias have their onset before age 18, and patients with paraphilias frequently have 3 to 5 paraphilias, either concurrently of at different times in their lives. The occurrence of paraphilic behavior peaks between the ages of 15 and 25 and gradually declines. Few acts of criminal paraphilia (such as exhibitionism) are seen in men of 50. Many acts of paraphilia that occur are practiced in isolation or with a cooperative partner.

Psychoanalytic theory holds that persons with a paraphilia have failed to complete the normal developmental process toward sexual adjustment. The paraphilia is the method chosen by the person (usually a male) to cope with the anxiety caused by threat of castration by the father and separation from the mother. However bizarre its manifestation, the resulting behavior provides an outlet for the sexual and aggressive drives that otherwise would have been channeled into normal sexual behavior.

Learning theory proposes that children learn paraphilias through early experiences that condition them to perform the perverse act. The first shared sexual experience can be important in that regard. Experiencing molestation, as a child, can predispose a person to accept continued abuse as an adult, or conversely, to become an abuser of others. Also, early experiences of abuse that are not specifically sexual, such as spankings, enemas, or verbal humiliation, can be sexualized by a child and form the basis for a paraphilia (38). Learning theory indicates that because the fantasizing of paraphilic interests begins at an early age and because personal fantasies and thoughts are not shared with others (who could block or discourage them), the use and misuse of paraphilic fantasies and urges continues uninhibited through adolescence and early adulthood. Eventually, when the person realizes that his or her sexual urges and behavior deviate from societal norms, the repetitive use of paraphilic fantasies already has become ingrained as have the sexual thoughts and behaviors associated with these fantasies (38).

Some studies have identified abnormal biologic findings in persons with paraphilias, such as abnormal hormonal levels, hard and soft neurologic signs, and chromosomal abnormalities. However, these studies investigated only known paraphiliacs who were referred to medical centers; they did not use control groups or random samples.

Different modalities are used to treat persons with paraphilias. These include external control, chemical reduction of sexual drives, treatment of comorbid conditions such as anxiety or depression, CBT, group therapy, aversive behavioral conditioning, and dynamic psychotherapy.

Prison is an external control mechanism for sexual crimes (e.g., pedophilia) that usually does not contain a treatment component. Institutionalization at a rehabilitation center exerts external control plus treatment elements.

The use of antiandrogenic agents is usually limited to the treatment of criminal paraphiliacs (e.g., pedophiles or exhibitionists). Antiandrogens such as cyproterone acetate, which is used in Europe, and medroxyprogesterone acetate, which is used in the United States, may decrease paraphilic behavior by decreasing serum testosterone levels to subnormal concentrations. These agents decrease the sex drive but do not alter the paraphilic fantasy that propels deviant sexual behavior. Serotonergic agents (such as Prozac) have been used with limited success in treatment of paraphilias (7,27).

CBT is used to disrupt learned paraphilic patterns and modify sexual behavior. The technique seems most effective when used in the context of group therapy, although it can also be utilized in individual therapy. The interventions include social skills training, sex education, cognitive restructuring (confronting and destroying the rationalizations used to support the victimization of others or to support the acceptability of the paraphilia), and development of victim empathy. Imaginal desensitization, relaxation techniques, and learning what triggers the paraphilic impulse so that such stimuli can be avoided are also taught. Aversive techniques include imagining or seeing pictures of paraphilic behavior and concurrently being exposed to or imagining noxious stimuli such as foul odors or vomiting (40,41). In modified aversive behavior rehearsal, patients are videotaped acting out the paraphilia with a mannequin. The patient is then confronted by a therapist and group members who ask questions about feelings, thought and motives associated with the behavior, and repeatedly try to correct cognitive distortions or point out lack of victim empathy (31).

Insight-oriented psychotherapy is particularly helpful to patients with comorbid anxiety disorders, mood disorders, or personality disorders. With this approach patients have the opportunity to understand their dynamics and the events that caused the paraphilia to develop (42). In particular, they become aware of the daily events that cause them to act on their impulses (e.g., fantasized or real rejection). Treatment helps them deal with life stresses better and enhances their capacity to relate to a life partner. Psychotherapy also allows patients to regain self-esteem, which in turn allows them to approach a partner in a more normal sexual manner. Sex therapy is an appropriate adjunct to treatment of patients who suffer from specific sexual dysfunctions when they attempt nondeviant sexual activities.

A poor prognosis for paraphilias is associated with an early age of onset, a high frequency of acts, no guilt or shame about the act, and substance abuse. The prognosis is somewhat better when patients have a history of coitus in addition to the paraphilia and when they are self-referred rather than referred by the legal system.

THE RECOVERY PROCESS

The recovery of a sex addict is a complicated, long-term process. It has been described by clinicians and researchers in terms of phases of recovery and in terms of behavioral and characterological changes seen through the spectrum of time. The phases that are defined include: recognition of the addictive problem; intervention with the aim of behavior modification; a period of stabilization that involves abstaining from addictive behavior and dealing with the affects that result from withdrawal from the addiction as well as the affects that are no longer masked or avoided by compulsive sexuality. Later phases of recovery involve focusing on underlying developmental issues including abuse, family-of-origin issues, and dealing with shame and unresolved grief. Recovery also requires addressing work, marriage, and family issues that may have arisen as a result of the addict's behavior. Relapse prevention is a necessary component throughout the recovery process (24).

Treatment methods can overlap and they can be utilized synchronously. As a rule directive, educative, chemical, and behavioral approaches such as didactic material about sex addiction, pharmacotherapy, and behavior therapies are utilized in the early phases of therapy. Psychodynamic psychotherapy that focuses on the healing of early wounds and trauma and includes goals of character change, the development of new values, and increased self-esteem is utilized in later phases of recovery, although CBT can be used for these purposes as well. Twelve-step programs are part of the therapeutic regimen throughout recovery; first for support and guidance in stopping addictive behavior, and later as a method of continued support and relapse prevention.

Stages of progress also can be defined when the patient's improvement is measured against the parameter of time in recovery. The first year is a tumultuous one for most recovering addicts. Relief at having recognized the problem and having determined to address it is significant. However, the person experiences anxiety about life without addiction, a sense of loss, and accompanying feelings of numbness, confusion, and an inability to concentrate, as well as painful physical feelings associated with withdrawal. Most slips in behavior occur in the second 6 months of the first years of recovery. During this time, patients grasp the damage that their sexual behavior has wrought in their lives. Also, without the defense of addiction, they re-experience the pain of early developmental abuse or neglect. These emotions may push them back into destructive behavior patterns. In addition to lapses, accidents and illnesses occur frequently. This is a challenging time for the recovering addict. Nonetheless, most patients report feeling better than they did before they entered therapy.

The second and third years represent a stage of greater stability for the patient. With addictive behavior under improved control, the patient focuses on psychological restructuring through family, couple, and/or individual psychodynamic psychotherapy. Belief systems about self, sex, family, and values are reshaped. This work is reflected in improvements in the patient's ability to cope with stress, improved self-esteem, greater productivity at work, the deepening of bonds with others, and the assumption of more responsibility in both work and personal areas, including the realms of finance and health. Patients also report an increased sense of spirituality.

Beyond the third year the patients feel increasing confidence in their base of recovery and devote substantial energy to their relationships. Connections with partners, family, and friends go through a period of renewal. There are some cases where relationships with family of origin cannot be restored (usually because these families continue to be destructive), or where a marriage cannot survive the recovery process. For the most part, relationships improve substantially, including the development of a healthier expression of sexuality. In studies of this stage, addicts report expressing more compassion for themselves and others, and they experience a new sense of trust in the integrity of relationships. Not surprisingly, patients report a dramatic increase in overall life satisfaction.

Fortunately, the brain demonstrates plasticity, allowing persons the possibility of adapting and growing throughout their lives. This characteristic permits therapy for sex addiction to be effective and allows the patient to recover from his or her addiction (30). However, the emotional programming of the earliest years of life, when the developing brain is laying down synaptic patterns, has the greatest effect on a person. If, as is the case with most addicts, early development was hurtful and neglectful, the recovered addict will remain more vulnerable to life's vicissitudes than a normally nurtured person. That is why we speak of the treated addict as recovered, not cured. He or she has to remain vigilant about relapsing into addictive behavior. Lifetime attendance at 12-step meetings (though with less frequency than is necessary at the onset of treatment) provides the addict with support to maintain recovery. Cognitive-behavioral techniques such as recognizing personal triggers for addictive behavior, avoiding tempting situations, and rehearsing corrective responses to small slips before they become full-blown relapses also are effective in relapse prevention. Similarly, developing an awareness of feelings of excessive stress, or developing an awareness of affects of depression or anxiety can precipitate seeking support through renewed participation in psychotherapy, use of medication, or by reaching out to sponsors.

A poor prognosis in sex addiction is associated with early age of onset, the presence of multiple addictions, a high frequency of hypersexual behavior, and an absence of anxiety or guilt about the behavior. A more favorable prognosis exists when the patient has a stable work life, good intelligence, the absence of nonsexual antisocial personality traits, and the presence of a successful adult attachment. As in therapy in general, the capacity for insight and a strong motivation to change augur a successful outcome. In spite of continued hypersensitivity to emotional stress, and vulnerability to relapse, the recovered addict can lead a productive life that includes an intimate sexual relationship and rewarding connections to others.

REFERENCES

1. Orford J. Hypersexuality: implications for a theory of dependence. *Br J Addict*. 1978;73:299.
2. Sadock BJ, Sadock VA. *Kaplan & Sadock's Synopsis of Psychiatry*. 10th ed. Baltimore, MD: Lippincott Williams & Wilkins; 2009:715–717, 214–215.
3. Reid RC, Bruce NC. Exploring relationships of psychopathology in hypersexual patients. *J Sex Martial Ther*. 2009;35:294.
4. Cooper A, Delmonico DL, Burg R. Cybersex users, abusers, and compulsives: new findings and implications. *Sex Addict Compuls J Treat Prevent*. 2009;7:5.
5. Carnes PJ. Sex addiction. In: Sadock BJ, Sadock VA, eds. *Kaplan and Sadock's Comprehensive Textbook of Psychiatry*. 8th ed. Baltimore, MD: Lippincott Williams & Wilkins; 2005: 1991.
6. Hijuelos O. *The Mambo Kings Play Songs of Love*. New York, NY: Farrar, Straus & Giroux; 1989.
7. Goodman A. Sexual addiction: nosology, diagnosis, etiology, and treatment. In: Lowinson JH, Ruiz P, Millman RB, et al., eds. *Substance Abuse: A Comprehensive Textbook*. 4th ed. Baltimore, MD: Lippincott Williams & Wilkins; 2004:504.
8. Cooper AL, Putnam D, Planchon LA, et al. Online sexual compulsivity: getting tangled in the net. *Sex Addict Compuls J Treat Prevent*. 1999;6:79.
9. Black DW. The epidemiology and phenomenology of compulsive sexual behavior. *CNS Spectr*. 2000;5:26–35.
10. Mohan KJ, Salo MW, Nagaswami S. A case of limbic system dysfunction with hypersexuality and fugue state. *Dis Nerv Syst*. 1975; 36:621.
11. Blumer D. Changes in sexual behavior related to temporal lobe disorders in man. *J Sex Res*. 1974;42:155–162.

12. Anderson N, Coleman E. Childhood abuse and family sexual attitudes in sexually compulsive males: a comparison of three clinical groups. *Am J Prev Psychiatry Neurol*. 1990;3:8–15.
13. De Baecque A, Toubiana S, Temerson C. *Truffaut: A Biography*. Berkeley, CA: University of California Press; 2000.
14. Coen SJ. Sexualization as a predominant mode of defense. *J Am Psychoanal Assoc*. 1981;29:893–920.
15. Schwartz MF. Reenactments related to bonding and hypersexuality. *Sex Addict Compuls J Treat Prevent*. 1996;3:195.
16. Krafft-Ebing R. *Psychopathia Sexualis*. New York, NY: Paperback Library; 1886:23.
17. Kernberg OF. *Aggression in Personality Disorders and Perversions*. New Haven, CT: Yale University Press; 1992:21–67.
18. Raymond NC, Coleman E, Miner NH. Psychiatric comorbidity and compulsive/impulsive traits in compulsive sexual behavior. *Compr Psychiatry*. 2003;44:370.
19. Perera B, Reece M, Monahan P, et al. Relations between substance use and personal dispositions towards out-of-control sexual behaviors among young adults. *Intern J Sexual Health*. 2009;21: 87–95.
20. Washington A. Cocaine may trigger sexual compulsivity. *US J Drug Alcohol Depend*. 1989;13:8.
21. Smith G, Toadvine J, Kennedy A. Women's perceptions of alcohol-related sexual disinhibition: personality and sexually-related alcohol expectancies. *Intern J Sexual Health*. 2009; 21:119–131.
22. Sadock VA. Normal sexuality and sexual dysfunctions. In: Sadock BJ, Sadock VA, Ruiz P, eds. *Kaplan and Sadock's Comprehensive Textbook of Psychiatry*. 9th ed. Baltimore, MD: Lippincott Williams & Wilkins; 2009:2027.
23. Schneider JP. Effects of cybersex addiction on the family. *Sex Addict Compuls J Treat Prevent*. 2009;7:31.
24. Carnes PJ. *Don't Call It Love*. New York, NY: Bantam Books; 1991:181–266.
25. Spitz HJ. Group psychotherapy. In: Sadock BJ, Sadock VA, Ruiz P, eds. *Kaplan & Sadock's Comprehensive Textbook of Psychiatry*. 9th ed. Baltimore, MD: Lippincott Williams & Wilkins; 2009:2832–2844.
26. Kafka MP. Successful antidepressant treatment of nonparaphilic sexual addictions and paraphilias in men. *J Clin Psychiatry*. 1991; 52:60.
27. Kafka MP. Sertraline pharmacotherapy for paraphilias and paraphilia-related disorders: an open trial. *Ann Clin Psychiatry*. 1994; 6:189.
28. Beck AT. The current state of cognitive therapy: a 40 year retrospective. *Arch Gen Psychiatry*. 2005;62:953.
29. Quadland MC. Compulsive sexual behavior: definition of a problem and an approach to treatment. *J Sex Marital Ther*. 1985; 11;121.
30. Newman CF, Beck AT. Cognitive therapy. In: Sadock BJ, Sadock VA, Ruiz P, eds. *Kaplan and Sadock's Comprehensive Textbook of Psychiatry*. 9th ed. Baltimore, MD: Lippincott Williams & Wilkins; 2009:2857.
31. Schwartz MF, Brasted WS. Sexual addiction. *Med Aspects Hum Sex*. 1985;19:103.
32. Freud S. The dynamic of transference. In: Strache J, ed. *Standard Edition of the Psychological Works of Sigmund Freud*. Vol. 12. London: Hogarth Press; 1953:97–108.
33. Valliant GE, Valliant CO. Normality and mental health. In: Sadock BJ, Sadock VA, Ruiz P, eds. *Kaplan & Sadock's Comprehensive Textbook of Psychiatry*. 9th ed. Baltimore, MD: Lippincott Williams and Wilkins; 2009:691–706.
34. Meyer JK. Individual psychotherapy of sexual disorders. In: Sadock BJ, Kaplan HI, Freedman AM, eds. *The Sexual Experience*. Baltimore, MD: Williams and Wilkins; 1976:439–456.
35. Wise TN. Fetishism and transvestism. In: Karasu TB, ed. *Treatment of Psychiatric Disorders: A Task Force of the American Psychiatric Association*. Washington DC: American Psychiatric Press; 1989:633.
36. Gurman AS, Lebow JL. Family and couple therapy. In: Sadock BJ, Sadock VA, eds. *Kaplan and Sadock's Comprehensive Textbook of Psychiatry*. 8th ed. Baltimore, MD: Lippincott Williams & Wilkins; 2005:2584.
37. Freud S. Three essays on the theory of sexuality. In: Strache J, ed. *Standard Edition of the Psychological Works of Sigmund Freud*. Vol. 7. London: Hogarth Press; 1953:191–206.
38. Person ES. Paraphilias. In: Sadock BJ, Sadock VA, eds. *Kaplan and Sadock's Comprehensive Textbook of Psychiatry*. 8th ed. Baltimore, MD: Lippincott Williams & Wilkins; 2005:1965.
39. Money J. *Lovemaps: Clinical Concepts of Sexual/Erotic Health and Pathology, Paraphilia, and Gender Transposition in Childhood, Adolescence, and Maturity*. New York, NY: Irvington; 1989:13–25.
40. McConaghy N, Armstrong MS, Blaszczynski A. Expectancy, convert sensitization, and imaginal desensitization in compulsive sexuality. *Acta Psychiatr Scand*. 1985;72:176.
41. Sideroff S, Jarvik ME. Conditioned responses to a videotape showing heroin-related stimuli. *Int J Addict*. 1980;15:529.
42. Herman JL, Perry JC, van der Kolk BA. Childhood trauma in borderline personality disorder. *Am J Psychiatry*. 1989;146:490.

CHAPTER 27

Internet Addiction

Philippe Weintraub ■ Thomas M. Dunn ■ Joel Yager ■ Zebulon Taintor

INTRODUCTION

A bulletin board flyer on Internet addiction posted in 2009 at Harvard's Science Center indicated that over 20% of Harvard undergraduate students report that computer or Internet use interferes with their academic performance, listed signs and symptoms of Internet addiction, and described how students could receive treatment for this condition. In South Korea, Internet addiction is considered one of the nation's major public health problems (1,2). In China, where medical experts report an epidemic of adolescent Internet addiction, involving one out of every eight youth, a total of approximately 10 million teenagers, concern about this problem led to the passage of laws in 2007 discouraging more than 3 hours of Internet use per day for playing games (2). Moreover, China is expected to become the first nation to recognize Internet addiction as a distinct disorder despite ongoing controversy about whether it merits a separate designation as a mental illness (3).

These examples illustrate that throughout the industrialized world, despite the enormous positive changes to society resulting from the Internet and other forms of electronic communication in the last 20 years, a small proportion but large number of users have experienced excessive and/or problematic involvement with these media, often associated with significant psychopathology. Although much needs to be learned about these phenomena and considerable debate exists among experts as to whether inappropriate applications of electronic media should be considered disorders in their own right, what is indisputable is that there are millions of individuals worldwide whose problematic use of these media is associated with significant psychopathology, clinical distress, and functional impairment. Mental health professionals, schools, and national governments have been inundated with the challenges of having to deal with the problems presented by such individuals, and the costs to society in lost productivity, increased morbidity, and rarely, cases of mortality resulting from the complications of Internet addiction, the most widely used term to describe these pathologic symptoms and behaviors, have been staggering. The recognition that mental health professionals are interested in this topic and are eager for information on how to properly diagnose and treat these syndromes is reflected by an emerging professional literature on topics related to Internet addiction and the fact that multiple journals such as *CyberPsychology and Behavior* and *Computers in Human Behavior* now exist, which feature research on understanding the impact of the Internet on behavior, human development, and society.

This chapter will review what is known about the clinical features of Internet addiction, beginning with a review of the relatively short history of these phenomena, how Internet addiction has come to be defined, and what is known of its epidemiology, which, for purposes of this review, will include all new types of electronic communication including not only use of the Internet but also texting, other uses of cell phones, and external device-mediated computer games, among others. This overview will show that, regardless of how one conceptualizes Internet addiction, these phenomena are associated with significant public health problems throughout the world.

Although excessive and problematic use of the Internet is most commonly labeled as an "addiction," many experts, notably those in the area of substance abuse and dependence, dispute the validity of labeling this syndrome as an "addiction." To put these concerns in context, we will examine the sparse literature that supports or refutes claims that patients with Internet addiction exhibit classic features of substance dependence such as tolerance, tachyphylaxis (the need for increasing dose to achieve the same effects) and withdrawal. In this regard, we will also describe current debates concerning whether Internet addiction might be better conceptualized as an impulse-control or compulsive disorder rather than as an addiction. In examining what is known about the determinants of Internet use in those with these syndromes and the extent to which these factors resemble and differ from those associated with other psychiatric disorders and syndromes like substance dependence, we will specifically consider neurobiologic and environmental factors.

We next review comorbid conditions frequently seen with Internet addiction. Here we grapple with the nosological confusion that surrounds various conceptualizations of Internet addiction as a "disease" process. Should Internet addiction be considered a disorder in its own right or primarily as a manifestation or symptom of another comorbid condition? For example, are individuals suffering from addiction to pornography on the Internet suffering from Internet addiction per se or using the Internet as a medium, the way a marijuana smoker uses a pipe, primarily to gain access to the substance or activity to which they are fundamentally addicted, that is a "pornography addiction"?

We then describe current evaluation techniques for these syndromes and review the very small research literature on treatment before offering our own recommendations on how to approach the evaluation and treatment of those suffering from Internet addiction. We conclude by discussing debates regarding Internet addiction as a possible diagnostic entity in the *Diagnostic and Statistic Manual* (DSM) and by suggesting areas for future research that can better clarify Internet addiction's status as a potential disorder and lead to its more successful identification and treatment.

HISTORY AND DEFINITION

As technological advances for delivering content to a mass media have evolved, so have concerns for unintended psychological consequences resulting from these advances. For example, a 1927 article warned that radio was detrimental to listeners, who would no longer congregate and be gregarious (4). In 1954, Meerloo raised concerns that the new medium of television could have addictive properties (5), and a 1981 article first described "computer addicts" as compulsive computer users on college campuses, postulating that such users spent so much time on computers that their grades plummeted, their relationships suffered, and some even had health problems (6). The term "Internet addiction" has been attributed to Dr. Ivan Goldberg, a psychiatrist who in 1995 first proposed it as a hoax in order to parody the Diagnostic and Statistical Manual, 4th Edition (DSM-IV) (7). The fact that the term has been so extensively adopted reflects that it has captured a commonly held perception about a cultural development.

But when the "Information Superhighway" emerged and became increasingly accessed by the general population in the 1990s, Kimberly Young was the first serious investigator to actually coin the term "Internet addiction" in referring to what she believed to be the emergence of a new psychiatric disorder resulting from the problematic use of this new medium (8). She indicated that those with this syndrome had "a preoccupation with the Internet, an inability to control Internet use, and restlessness or irritability when attempting to cut down on Internet use" (9). Accordingly, most experts have credited Young as the first person to use the term "Internet addiction" as the name for these phenomena (8). Her 1996 presentation to an American Psychological Association meeting regarding Internet addiction, later published as an article (9), and her subsequent writings on the subject stimulated tremendous interest in this area (10,11). Other less commonly used terms for this syndrome and related problematic use of other electronic media have included "computer addiction" (12,13), "problematic Internet use" (14), and "compulsive Internet use" (15).

Generally, the term "Internet addiction" is most commonly used to describe a variety of dysfunctional behaviors involving computer use, even if the Internet per se is not being accessed (16). However, some have cautioned against using a single label to describe a complicated array of behaviors that is just beginning to be understood (17).

Nevertheless, because of its widespread use and recognition among both professionals and the lay public, we will use the term "Internet addiction" throughout this chapter to describe problematic use of all types of new electronic media developed for the general public in the last 20 to 30 years. It should be noted, however, that an increasing number of experts have argued for either broadening its definition to one that does not presume any specific etiology or changing its name to one that better describes the full range of activities implied by the use of the label "Internet addiction". As cited by Pies, one definition of Internet addiction that does not imply any specific etiology and is consistent with the growing consensus of how to describe these phenomena is "the inability of individuals to control their Internet use, resulting in marked distress and/or functional impairment in daily life" (18,19). A more accurate term proposed by Pies, in an effort to reduce stigma and be more inclusive in describing the problems exhibited by individuals using the full range of electronic media, is "pathological use of electronic media" (PUEM) (18).

EPIDEMIOLOGY

General Population

According to Internet World Stats, a website that measures Internet usage with data supplied from the Nielsen Company and U.S. Census Bureau, 74% of the population of North America (in excess of 250 million people) were Internet users in the Spring of 2009 (20). These data suggest that even if prevalence rates for Internet addiction were small, the number of affected individuals would be quite large. The true prevalence of Internet addiction is difficult to ascertain since such great variability exists in diagnostic definitions, sampling methods, and other aspects of epidemiologic study designs (16). While more than a dozen studies have been published that address the prevalence of Internet addiction, most study samples have been restricted to a narrow demographic and/or geographical area and generally focus on students or other young people. Other studies with big sample sizes that have not oversampled young people have been criticized for gathering data exclusively online (17). Examples of these types of studies include one of the personal computer users between the ages of 16 and 24 years (so called "Net-geners") from Hong Kong, reporting that almost a third of the sample met criteria for Internet addiction (21). In China, estimates suggest that from 5 to more than 10 million of the country's 300 million Internet users have "Internet addictions" and that adolescents are especially vulnerable (2,22). Two studies from Iran yielded markedly different findings, with one study of high school students indicating a 3.7% prevalence rate of Internet addiction (23) while another, based on a sample of Northern Iranian Internet users, reported a 22.7% rate (24). An online UK study involving more than 300 university students reported an 18% prevalence rate of Internet addiction (25).

Data regarding gender differences in Internet addiction are also mixed with most studies finding a higher prevalence of affected males (26,27). In the Hong Kong-based "Net-geners" study noted earlier, however, more females than males were found to be addicted (21).

Methodologically, two studies stand out as being community based and reasonably representative, offering epidemiologic data regarding Internet addiction in the general populations of the United States and Western Europe. The first is a 2006 telephone survey of 2513 randomly selected representative U.S. adults (28). The authors employed four different symptom criteria sets for their analyses. In this sample, Internet addiction ranged from 0.3% to 0.7% depending on which criteria were used. Of note, persons under the age of 18 were excluded from participating in the study. The authors did not report gender data.

The second, a 2009 study, reported data obtained from a random and representative sample of the adult population of Norway (29). The sample contained almost 3400 people between the ages of 16 and 74, of whom 87% indicated they were Internet users. In this sample, 1% of the subjects met criteria for Internet addiction. Male gender and young age were found to put respondents at highest risk for Internet addiction; 4.1% of men aged 16 to 29 were addicted to the Internet compared to only 1.7% of women in the same age group. The percentage of men meeting criteria for at-risk Internet use jumped to almost 20% for young men aged 16 to 29.

A cautious interpretation of these studies suggests that the general population prevalence of Internet addiction may be approximately 1%, that it affects more males than females, and that it tends to be found predominantly in younger people.

Children and Adolescents

Numerous cross-sectional studies have been published regarding the problematic use of electronic media in children and adolescents. Studies of these age groups are important because today's generation of youth is the first to be raised with extensive exposure to such technologies and, collectively, spend considerably more time than adults using the Internet and other electronic media for social interaction and other types of activities. Given the recent advent of these technologies, there has been little opportunity for longitudinal research examining how their widespread uses affect normal childhood development and the risk for Internet addiction, other psychopathology, and long-term functional impairment not only in the general pediatric population but also on vulnerable youth already suffering from or at elevated risk for psychiatric illness.

Video game use has become a major focus of study, given the increasing amount of time devoted to it by youth in recent years and concerns about the potential adverse impact of violent video games as well as the risk for "addiction" to playing these games (30,31). The first published study of the prevalence of video game addiction based on a large, national sample of youth representative of the general population employed an online survey methodology and criteria for problematic video game use based on DSM-IV criteria for pathologic gambling (31). The sample included 1178 youth between the ages of 8 to 18. Approximately 88% of the sample played video games at least some of the time. Approximately 8.5% met criteria for pathologic use of video games, and those receiving this diagnosis achieved significantly worse grades in school and had significantly higher rates of attention problems than those not found to be ill. In recent years, text messaging on cellular phones has also exploded in popularity among teenagers, raising concerns about its impact on youth. According to the Nielson Corporation, in the fourth quarter of 2008 teenagers sent an average of 2272 text messages per month, close to 80 per day, a doubling of the average from just 1 year earlier (32).

Phenomenology

In recent years researchers worldwide have variably described the symptoms of Internet addiction, resulting in multiple definitions, each with its own specific diagnostic criteria. Most include some combination of excessive and/or inappropriate use of the Internet or other electronic media associated with clinical distress and functional impairment. A major challenge in defining the syndrome has been the problem of conceptualizing exactly what types of disorders Internet addiction may represent.

Much of the debate concerns disagreement surrounding whether to label Internet addiction as a disorder in its own right as opposed to considering it to be just one manifestation of another, more inclusive disorder. Among those who advocate for Internet addiction to be included as a separate disorder in DSM-V, some propose that it is best viewed as akin to disorders of substance dependence, whereas others argue that it more closely resembles an impulse-control disorder. In fact, as described below, some of the diagnostic criteria for Internet addiction have been based on those for pathologic gambling, a DSM-IV impulse-control disorder that is often also referred to as a prototype of a "behavioral addiction," accompanied by psychologic withdrawal symptoms such as irritability and agitation, suggesting that the clinical features of impulse-control disorders and substance dependence may overlap to at least some degree. Notably, some of the most heated opposition to labeling Internet addiction as a type of "addiction" resembling that seen with substance dependence comes from substance dependence experts. Based on the limited research to date, they argue that insufficient evidence of physiologic markers of intoxication and withdrawal in individuals with Internet addiction renders problematic characterizations of Internet addiction as a true addiction (18).

These distinctions are important because they focus on the fact that Internet and computer use per se is generally not the end purpose of excessive users. Most Internet addicts demonstrate high specificity in the activities in which they become overinvolved, ranging from social involvements, problem solving, novelty seeking, information gathering, shopping, day trading, video gaming (including those with violent themes), and sexual stimulation and gratification, to name just a few. Lumping together all those who spend excessive hours online, such as Internet gamblers; Internet shoppers; Internet pornography addicts; lonely-hearts seekers on dating services; Wikipedia contributors; Second-Life participants; social-networkers; bloggers; texters; users of gaming consoles, Wii, bridge, or chess players; and those finding a myriad of other Internet-mediated activities to become preoccupying, may cause researchers to miss the trees for the forest. The Internet may simply serve as a common pathway and conduit through which all these individuals can more easily access their routes to a variety of "individual behaviors of excess." (33)

Nevertheless, taking into account the variable definitions of Internet addiction, as described in more detail later in this chapter, reports of impairment as a result of excessive Internet use indicate that these syndromes exact a high cost on individuals and society. There is considerable data showing that Internet addiction is associated with substantial functional impairment in affected individuals worldwide and in all age groups (1,31).

TABLE 27.1	Young's Diagnostic Questionnaire for Internet addiction[a]
1) Do you feel preoccupied with the Internet (think about previous online activity or anticipate next online session)?
2) Do you feel the need to use the Internet with increasing amounts of time in order to achieve satisfaction?
3) Have you repeatedly made unsuccessful efforts to control, cut back, or stop Internet use?
4) Do you feel restless, moody, depressed, or irritable when attempting to cut down or stop Internet use?
5) Do you stay online longer than originally intended?
6) Have you jeopardized or risked the loss of significant relationship, job, educational or career opportunity because of the Internet?
7) Have you lied to family members, therapist, or others to conceal the extent of involvement with the Internet?
8) Do you use the Internet as a way of escaping problems or of relieving a dysphoric mood (e.g., feelings of helplessness, guilt, anxiety, depression)?

[a]Endorsing five or more items results in classification as an addicted Internet user.

Reprinted with permission from Young KS. Internet addiction: the emergence of a new clinical disorder. *CyberPsychol Behav.* 1998;1:237–244.

Evolution and Development of Diagnostic Criteria for Internet Addiction

The first formal attempt to establish identifying symptoms for addiction to the Internet was proposed by Young who in 1998 (9) modified the pathologic gambling criteria from the DSM-IV to develop an eight-item questionnaire that has been widely used to screen for Internet addiction (Table 27.1). After gathering data from clinicians who had treated the condition, Young et al. (34) in 1999 further delineated and proposed several subcategories of Internet addiction:

1. Cybersexual addiction: Compulsive Internet use to access pornographic material.
2. Cyber-relationship addiction: Maintaining online relationships to excess.
3. Net compulsions: Compulsive online gambling, shopping, or online trading.
4. Information overload: Excessive website surfing or search engine use.
5. Computer addiction: Using the computer to play games compulsively.

Young's criteria (9) have been criticized by Beard and Wolf (35), who noted that they are weighted too heavily on self-report and could also be applied to other behaviors that would appear to be more consistent with an impulse-control disorder rather than a true addiction. They also argue that Young's diagnostic criteria lack items that account for functional impairment secondary to the addictive behavior. Accordingly, Beard and Wolf (35) in 2001 expanded Young's criteria by adding three additional criteria (Table 27.2). These additional criteria

TABLE 27.2	Beard and Wolf's diagnostic criteria for Internet addiction
All of the following must be present:
1) Is preoccupied with the Internet (think about previous online activity or anticipate next online session).
2) Needs to use the Internet with increased amounts of time in order to achieve satisfaction.
3) Has made unsuccessful efforts to control, cut back, or stop Internet use.
4) Is restless, moody, depressed, or irritable when attempting to cut down or stop Internet use.
5) Has stayed online longer than originally intended.
At least one of the following:
1) Has jeopardized or risked the loss of a significant relationship, job, educational or career opportunity because of the Internet.
2) Has lied to family members, therapist, or others to conceal the extent of involvement with the Internet.
3) Uses the Internet as a way of escaping from problems or of relieving a dysphoric mood (e.g., feelings of helplessness, guilt, anxiety, depression).

Reprinted with permission from Beard KW, Wolf EM. Modification in the proposed diagnostic criteria for Internet addiction. *CyberPsychol Behav.* 2001;4:377–383.

TABLE 27.3	Shapira et al. diagnostic criteria for problematic Internet use
A)	Maladaptive preoccupation with Internet use, as indicated by at least one of the following:
	1) Preoccupations with use of the Internet that are experienced as irresistible.
	2) Excessive use of the Internet for periods of time longer than planned.
B)	The use of the Internet or the preoccupation with its use causes clinically significant distress or impairment in social, occupational, or other important areas of functioning.
C)	The excessive Internet use does not occur exclusively during periods of hypomania or mania and is not better accounted for by other Axis I disorders.

Reprinted with permission from Shapira NA, Lessig MC, Goldsmith TD, et al. Problematic Internet use. Classification and diagnostic criteria. *Depress Anxiety.* 2003;17:207–216.

tap functional impairment due to Internet use, deceptive behavior regarding use of the Internet, and going online as a means of escape from problems or mood disturbance.

Shapira et al. (14) argued that both Young's and Beard and Wolf's sets of diagnostic criteria are inadequate. These authors conceptualize the phenomena as "problematic Internet use" (14). They also consider Internet addiction to be more closely aligned with impulse-control disorders than with an addiction per se. To that end, Shapira et al. proposed a third set of criteria that identified problematic Internet use modeled on impulse-control disorders found in the DSM-IV-TR (Text Revision) (Table 27.3).

Several investigators have published psychometric instruments to assess Internet addiction (Table 27.4). Young developed the Internet Addiction Test (IAT) (11), a 20-item instrument, based on her original criteria. Subjects rate their Internet use and its consequences on a Likert scale. Most other instruments employ self-rated scales. We are unaware of any

TABLE 27.4	Psychometric instruments used to identify Internet addiction		
References	Instrument	Number of items	Theoretical framework
Meerkerk et al. (15)	Compulsive Internet Use Scale (CIUS)	14	Conceptual underpinnings include DSM-IV criteria for substance dependence, pathologic gambling; behavioral addictions; compulsive Internet use
Caplan (36)	Generalized Problematic Internet Use Scale (GPIUS)	39	Based on cognitive–behavioral theoretical framework of Internet addiction; incorporates items from other instruments
Nichols and Nicki (37)	Internet Addiction Scale (IAS)	36	Developed to reflect DSM-IV substance dependence criteria with Griffiths' (38) salience and mood modification
Young (11); Widyanto and McMurran (39)	Internet Addiction Test (IAT)	20	Young's (9) Diagnostic Questionnaire
Armstrong et al. (40), Widyanto et al. (41)	Internet Related Problem Scale (IRPS)	20	Addresses factors common to addiction and negative effects of Internet use
Morahan-Martin and Schumacher (26), Niemz et al. (25)	Pathological Internet Use scale (PIU)	13	Basis for item development unspecified
Davis et al. (42)	Online Cognition Scale (OCS)	36	Items purporting to identify problematic Internet use, such as procrastination, mood disruption, impulsivity, and pathologic gambling

commercially available measures of Internet addiction. Major drawbacks to the use of such instruments include the lack of a "gold standard" due to considerable disagreement regarding specific criteria for Internet addiction and the lack of generally accepted theoretical underpinnings for such a disorder. Indeed, one might heed the admonitions of Beard (43), who suggested that Internet addiction is best detected by a thorough clinical interview.

Determinants of Internet Use—Several features distinguish Internet use from that of other activities and from substance use that can evolve into an addiction: (a) Internet use offers a mechanism for accessing information and for various types of interactive activities, both constructive and maladaptive, and (b) Internet use constitutes an essential part of normal existence in the modern world. For those reasons, it is difficult to disentangle the extent to which spending large periods of time on the Internet represents evidence of a disorder specific to this medium, evidence of other mental illnesses, or simply variants of normal behavior. That is, how much "wheel spinning" or how many nonproductive activities manifesting distraction from primary tasks occurs when the individual is presumably engaged in an Internet-mediated functional activity is important to measure in determining whether use of such media is abnormal. Fortunately, recognizing this potential confound and the fact that, for many youth and adults, academic and occupational success is contingent on spending enormous amounts of time on the Internet, some researchers have controlled for this variable and still found that problematic Internet use is independently associated with functional impairment regardless of the amount of time engaged in a particular activity (31). Nevertheless, in contrast to syndromes of substance dependence where objective, physiologic evidence of tolerance and withdrawal can be noted with specific levels and duration of consumption, such signs and symptoms are neither as clear cut nor have they been systematically studied in Internet-related addictions.

Etiology and Predisposing Factors

Since intense debate exists about whether Internet addiction should even be considered a disorder, it is not surprising that no single cause has been identified (apart from the contributing factor of access to the Internet). However, as with most psychiatric disorders, etiologic factors are thought to be multifactorial (16).

Psychological Theories

Cognitive-Behavioral Theory—Several investigators have suggested that compulsive use of the Internet provides ultimately dysfunctional and ineffective methods for regulating negative emotions related to cognitions associated with low self-esteem and self-critical thoughts. Despite the short-term emotional alleviation and distraction, longer-term negative consequences include worsening relationships and poor school or work performance. This pattern then fuels a vicious cycle in which worsening self-esteem and poorer self-appraisal lead to further maladaptive use of the Internet, culminating in social withdrawal and greater exacerbation of the psychopathology that led to excessive Internet use in the first place (44).

Social Skills Deficit Theory—Caplan (45) and others, as summarized by Shaw and Black (16), postulate that individuals with poor social competence who may also be anxious about social interactions are drawn to the anonymity of the Internet and the opportunities it affords for developing relationships in less threatening circumstances than those occurring face-to-face. Additionally, individuals have greater control regarding their self-presentations and their ability to construct more favorable images for those they may be trying to impress. While this feature of Internet-mediated communication may help depressed or socially anxious individuals overcome social inhibitions, it may also potentially contribute to an avoidance of true intimacy.

Family History—Little research exists in this area. In one small study, all but one of 20 individuals with problematic Internet use had a positive family psychiatric history (46). In this sample, depression was present in at least 65% of first- or second-degree relatives; 50% of relatives had bipolar disorder; and 60% had substance dependence. Unfortunately, no inquiry was made as to whether any relatives suffered from problematic Internet use.

NEUROBIOLOGY

Although research in this area is in its infancy, initial reports have revealed neurobiologic differences between individuals with Internet addiction and nonaffected controls. Many of the reported findings resemble those found in individuals suffering from substance dependence. For example, one preliminary study using position emission tomography showed evidence for release of striatal dopamine release resulting from video game playing (47). In addition, the dopamine D2 receptor gene allele polymorphism, *DRD2 Taq1A1* was found more frequently among 79 adolescents who played video games excessively compared to 75 normal controls (48,49), a potentially significant finding in that this allele has been hypothesized to increase vulnerability to addictive behaviors and, for example, is more prevalent in adults with methamphetamine dependence than in controls (50).

Preliminary research has also linked excessive Internet use in adolescent males with the homozygous short allelic variant of the serotonin transporter gene (*SS-5HTTLPR*), a genetic polymorphism previously associated with vulnerability to depression. In addition, compared to controls these adolescents scored higher on the Beck Depression Inventory, suggesting that they have may have genetic characteristics and clinical features similar to those suffering from depression (51).

ENVIRONMENTAL FACTORS

Several investigators have found associations between family dysfunction and adolescent Internet addiction. In one South Korean cohort, for example, exposure to "violence" between parents or being a victim of "violence" perpetrated by the parent was associated with adolescent Internet addiction (52). Similarly, a Chinese study of middle school students found strong associations between a history of physical abuse and meeting criteria for Internet addiction (53). In a study of almost 9000 Taiwanese adolescents, low family monitoring, low feeling of connection to school, high family conflict, having friends who were habitual alcohol drinkers, and living in a rural community were each associated with an increased likelihood of meeting criteria for Internet addiction (54). Among Chinese University students, being from a single-parent family and homesickness were associated with Internet addiction (55). Of course, access to the Internet is a significant environmental factor: in a cohort of almost 900 Greek adolescents, having access to the Internet at home and accessing the Internet to play games were predictors of Internet addiction, especially among males (56).

Pre-existing and Concurrent Psychiatric Comorbidities— In a 2-year prospective study of 2293 Taiwanese adolescents (1179 boys and 1114 girls), hostility and attention-deficit hyperactivity disorder (ADHD) were found to be the leading risk factors for the occurrence of Internet addiction among males and female adolescents, and depression and social phobia predicted Internet addiction among female, but not male, adolescents (57). Several cross-sectional studies have shown that comorbidity is the rule rather than exception in individuals with Internet addiction. Block (2) has estimated that as many as 86% of patients with Internet addiction demonstrate at least one comorbid psychiatric condition, with many individuals suffering from multiple disorders. Those most commonly noted include mood disorders, anxiety disorders, impulse-control disorders, substance dependence, and ADHD (16,49). In China, which is experiencing an epidemic of Internet addiction, 30% of those diagnosed with Internet addiction have concurrent significant anxiety or depression, and 30% have ADHD (58).

Additional Complications—Abundant evidence suggests that individuals identified as suffering from Internet addiction and related disorders frequently suffer from significant psychiatric and medical complications. In 2006 the Korean government estimated that among the estimated 210,000 South Korean children and adolescents between the ages of 6 and 17 suffering from Internet addiction, about 80% required psychotropic medication and one fifth to one quarter required hospitalization (1,2). In fact, a major impetus in South Korea for identifying Internet addiction as a major public health problem was the report of 10 deaths resulting from cardiopulmonary causes, such as thromboembolism, occurring in Internet cafes among young healthy men who had played for more than 16 consecutive hours (2), and, in one case, a total of 80 hours (59). The increasing occurrence of this variant of thromboembolism has led to its being labeled "e-thrombosis" (60).

Sleep deprivation is another adverse consequence of excessive use of electronic devices. Among 100 adolescents 12 to 18 years of age, increased time using different forms of electronic devices after 9 PM significantly correlated with decreased sleep, increased consumption of caffeinated products, and greater risk for daytime sleepiness, including sleepiness in the classroom (61). By means of a multitasking index devised to measure the amount of time teens spent engaged using various electronic devices including watching TV after 9 PM, being online, talking on the phone, listening to an MP3 player, text messaging, and playing computer games, the majority of the sample reported engaging in at least one activity, with the average using four electronic devices. The total average daily time spent using electronic devices was 5.3 hours. Teens getting 8 to 10 hours of sleep on school nights, considered optimal for teenagers, spent significantly less time using electronic devices whereas those sleeping less used these devices 1.5 to 2 times longer. These patterns of reduced sleep in teenagers have been associated with a variety of psychological and physical problems as well as decreased quality of life (61). For additional perspective, in a Chinese study of more than 3000 cases of Internet addiction, 80% of whom were adolescent males, the average amount of time spent on the Internet was 9 hours per day (58).

Numerous social, psychological, academic, and occupational complications of Internet addiction have been identified. In young people, poor academic performance sometimes leading to school failure, disrupted family relationships, and social isolation are among the more common. Other serious functional impairments resulting from problematic Internet use include legal difficulties and job loss (43,62).

Concerns have been voiced that playing violent video games may be associated with increases in violent behavior. This issue became a focus of national concern after the Columbine High School shootings in Littleton, Colorado, when it was learned that the teenage assailants were fascinated by violent video games including one licensed by the U.S. Military used for training soldiers to "effectively kill" (63,64). One representative study examining the psychological and behavioral effects of increasingly graphic violent video games on users found aggressive behavior and delinquency to be positively associated with playing violent video games (65). This association was stronger in previously aggressive individuals and in males, reflecting that psychologically vulnerable individuals and males may be at greater risk to act out violently in real life after engaging in such fantasy activities. In a second study by the same group, exposure to an extremely violent video game produced increases in aggressive thoughts and behaviors (65).

Decreased work productivity has been a major cause of functional impairment in adults with problematic Internet use. One review of this topic reported that one in four employees engage in problematic Internet use and estimated the annual costs to American corporations in lost productivity to range from 1 to 54 billion dollars (66). Because these problems are so widespread, employers at most large public and private institutions have instituted employee Internet use policies to address them.

Most concerning, certain dysfunctional behaviors occurring with electronic devices are associated with increased risks of harm to self or others. The use of cell phones and texting messages while driving results in decreased reaction time and increased distractibility (67) leading to increased risks of motor vehicle accidents (68). These public health hazards have resulted in the passage by many localities of laws prohibiting hand-held cell phone use while driving. Nevertheless, despite using a methodology thought to underestimate cell phone usage and examining cell phone use only during daytime hours, the National Highway Traffic Safety Administration's 2007 annual survey of cell phone use while driving found significant increases in the use of cell phones and other handheld devices while driving compared to the previous year. At any given time approximately 6% of drivers were using handheld devices and 11% were using either handheld or hand-free devices, representing a total of more than 1 million vehicles at any given moment in which a driver was using a cell phone. The highest frequency of use, 8.8%, occurred in 16 to 24 year olds, an already high-risk group for automobile accidents (69). More disturbingly, a study of driver cell phone use at night found the highest rate of 12% to be among females 16 to 29 years old, much higher than the daytime rate among young people, especially concerning since young drivers are at most risk for having accidents at night (68).

The consequence of these worsening trends has been a public health crisis: a 2003 Harvard study estimated that there are more than 2500 traffic fatalities annually secondary to distractions caused by cell phone use (70). The U.S. Department of Transportation reported that driver distraction, mostly caused by cell phones, resulted in more than a doubling of this number of fatalities in 2008 (almost 6000), accounting for about one sixth of all fatal crashes; additionally, half a million people were injured in car crashes in 2008 as a result of driver distraction primarily caused by mobile phones (71). And research has shown that using a cell phone while driving is as dangerous as driving legally intoxicated with a blood alcohol level of 0.08% (70). Not surprisingly, the National Highway Traffic Safety Administration has officially recommended not using cell phones while driving.

Finally, the potential for exploitation and abuse by others, particularly among young people, is heightened by the increased social networking activities occurring via these media. Examples of situations that can result in unintended tragic ends include unsuspecting victims befriending sexual predators on the Internet and the perpetration of public humiliation, which has led to suicide, in the wake of a recent phenomenon called "sexting" in which typically teenagers send sexually explicit messages to friends on cell phones, sometimes including nude photos of themselves, which may then be maliciously more widely disseminated to others. In one notorious example, a teenage girl who had sent nude photos of herself to her boyfriend while they were dating was deeply humiliated when he subsequently forwarded embarrassing photos to her girlfriends after they broke up. The girlfriends responded by denigrating and "harassing" her, calling her a "slut" and a "whore," leading to her serious depression, school avoidance, and suicide by hanging (72). Notably, up to 20% of teens in surveys report sending or posting nude photographs of themselves (73). Furthermore, even teens who send and receive explicitly sexual messages about themselves and their friends have been charged and on occasion convicted of disseminating and/or possessing child pornography (73).

EVALUATION AND TREATMENT

Due to ongoing debates about the definition and diagnosis of Internet addiction, no generally agreed-upon standards for assessment exist, nor have any evidence-based treatments been formally tested (16). In contrast to their Asian counterparts, who appear sensitized to the high prevalence of these disorders and routinely screen for them, few American mental health professionals at present seem to consider this syndrome in their differential diagnosis when evaluating patients presenting with other conditions, and few routinely ask about these issues in clinical practice (2).

Nevertheless, various psychosocial treatment programs have been proposed, and numerous Internet addiction treatment counselors and centers have emerged throughout the world. In South Korea, where Internet addiction is viewed as a public health crisis, as of June 2007 more than 1000 counselors had received training for this condition and more than 190 hospitals and centers were available to provide treatment for the syndrome (1,2).

To date most of the treatment literature concerning Internet addiction consists of case reports, case series, and occasional open-label medication trials. In China, treatments employed at the General Hospital of Beijing's Military Region's Addiction Medicine Center (AMC), a major treatment and research center for Internet addiction, have included behavioral training; medication treatment for patients with psychiatric symptoms; dancing and sports; reading; karaoke; and elements of the "12-Step" programs of Alcoholics Anonymous. Family therapy has also been included as an important treatment component. Unfortunately, some notorious treatment programs have also emerged in China. One such program, the Yang Yonxin Center for Internet addiction treatment at Public Hospital Number Four in Linyi, Shandong Province, reportedly used excessive doses of sedatives and prolonged courses of electroconvulsive therapy (ECT) (22).

Escitalopram has shown some promise in treating Internet addiction. After a case report described successful treatment of a condition characterized as severe Internet addiction with 10 mg/day of escitalopram (74), an open-label study was organized involving a sample of 19 adult subjects with "Internet usage disorder," defined as use of the Internet that was time-consuming, uncontrollable, distressing, and causing social, financial, or occupational dysfunction. A 10-week trial of escitalopram, 20 mg today, resulted in significant improvement on the two primary outcomes measures, the Clinical Global Impressions-Improvement scale (CGI-I) and total time spent per week in nonessential Internet activities. At the end of treatment, 64% of subjects were considered CGI-I responders, and weekly time on the Internet was reduced from 37 to 16.5 hours. In a subsequent double-blind discontinuation phase, no differences were found between the two groups; both the escitalopram and placebo groups maintained their improvements (75).

One case report alleged to indirectly support the conceptualization of Internet addiction as an addictive disorder focused on the successful treatment of a patient with "sexual addiction" involving the Internet (76). After a 7-year period during which this patient's symptoms did not significantly improve following treatments with sertraline, individual therapy, group therapy, and involvement with Sexual Addicts Anonymous, his symptoms subsequently improved significantly following the addition of naltrexone, an FDA-approved treatment for alcohol dependence. In ongoing treatment akin to an ABA design fashion, his symptoms worsened again when the naltrexone was discontinued and improved again when treatment was resumed. Of course, this case raises several key questions: to exactly what was this patient "addicted"? Pornography? The Internet itself? Since the patient's use of the Internet seemed limited to pornography, it is likely that the Internet primarily served as the vehicle for expressing excessive preoccupation with pornography rather than reflecting an "addiction" to using the Internet per se.

Does Treating Comorbid Conditions Impact Internet Use?

Preliminary studies suggest that problematic Internet use can be reduced through successful treatment of comorbid conditions commonly associated with Internet addiction.

Attention-Deficit Hyperactivity Disorder (ADHD)

An open-label study evaluated the efficacy of stimulant treatment on ADHD symptoms and Internet usage in Korean children, aged 8 to 12, who had ADHD and were video game players (49). One of the study's aims was to assess whether improvement in ADHD symptoms correlated with a reduction of Internet addiction symptoms, since previous research has shown a high rate of comorbidity between the two syndromes and video game playing has been associated with release of dopamine, one mechanism through which stimulant medications operate. Based on the Korean version of the Young Internet Addiction Scale, YIAS-K, about 50% of the sample met criteria for Internet addiction. At the end of treatment, significant reductions were found for both ADHD and Internet addiction symptoms, and improvements in ADHD symptoms and decreased Internet use (i.e., time spent playing video games) were correlated. Of note, since playing videogames has been associated with improvements both in attention and visual spatial functioning, the authors speculate that video game playing in untreated ADHD individuals may represent attempts at "self-medication."

Recommendations for Evaluation and Treatment of Individuals with Internet Addiction

For all the reasons regarding the lack of consensus about the nature of these somewhat heterogeneous conditions noted above, highly specific recommendations regarding how to treat this large group of patients are difficult to formulate. With this caveat in mind, in our view it is prudent to use a flexible, biopsychosocial approach. Of key importance for all general psychiatric and mental health evaluations is that clinicians should routinely inquire about every patient's use of the Internet, both to assess whether Internet use (and the use of other electronic media and devices) per se poses a major source of distress and impairment and to ascertain if problems associated with Internet use represent manifestations of some other psychiatric disorder requiring treatment. Unlike in Asian countries like China, Korea, and Taiwan where routine screening for Internet addiction is now commonplace, contemporary American psychiatrists appear to not routinely inquire about Internet use, and, as a result, many Americans with Internet addiction go undetected. In addition, the diagnosis of comorbid conditions associated with Internet addiction is delayed when questions about Internet use are omitted, since the primary manifestation of the comorbid syndrome, for example addiction to pornography, may be mediated only by activity on the Internet.

A good quality assessment includes asking the patient to describe and quantify how much he or she uses the Internet and other electronic media and whether the patient or family members feel that the patient's use is a problem that interferes with relationships, school, and/or work. The inquiry should also investigate the various types of electronic activity in which the individual engages and the patient's perception of what attracts him or her to using the Internet and other electronic media and the needs that such use seems to satisfy, in order to assess whether the patient uses the Internet and e-media as a vehicle for expressing clinically concerning preoccupations and urges, for example, cravings for violence manifested by playing violent video games, which may in turn lower inhibitions against behaving violently in the real world. For depressed individuals, "surfing the Net" or playing videogames may be a manifestation of social withdrawal related to difficulties coping with painful life circumstances. For shy and socially anxious individuals, such use may offer routes for engaging in social interaction in less anxiety-provoking circumstances than face-to-face encounters, but as mentioned above, may deleteriously perpetuate avoidance of more mature intimacy. Also, since Internet addiction has been described as having many features of both addictions and impulse-control disorders, patients should be asked if they experience cravings regarding using the Internet, difficulties resisting impulses to use the Internet, and the extent to which they become extremely irritable, anxious, and/or depressed when forced to stop using it.

The evaluation should also routinely include standard assessments for the major psychiatric disorders, in particular ADHD, mood disorders, anxiety disorders, substance dependence, and impulse-control disorders, all so commonly comorbid with Internet addiction and which frequently lead to it. In addition, assessment for personality characteristics, such as shyness, which place individuals at higher risk for problematic Internet use, should be performed.

A thorough clinical interview and/or the routine use of a screening questionnaire developed for detecting Internet addiction are all reasonable methods for conducting an assessment. Administration of an Internet addiction rating scale can help determine the severity of impairment and provide a baseline against which to measure response to treatment. Obtaining collateral information from family, school personnel, and friends is necessary to complete an accurate clinical picture and assessment of severity of distress and impairment.

Treatment Approaches—An individualized approach is essential. To start, concrete behavioral interventions, including setting explicit goals for abstinence or for significant reductions of time spent in the dysfunctional activities may help alleviate the difficulties and offer opportunities for reversing the impairments they inflict. Treating common comorbid conditions such as mood and anxiety disorders and ADHD may frequently ameliorate Internet addiction. Interventions that have been efficacious for substance dependence and impulse-control disorders should be considered as well.

Gaining an understanding of the functions that problematic Internet use serve may help lead to successful interventions. For example, depressed individuals may reduce their reliance on the Internet when their mood improves and they have less need to withdraw from others. Particularly with children and adolescents, but with adults as well, addressing family problems that may be fueling the Internet addiction may help alleviate the disorder and may help support treatments to limit the patient's use of the Internet. Concerned family members may also be willing to confront the patient's problematic Internet use and encourage the patient to adhere to treatment.

Finally, outpatient and, recently, residential inpatient facilities devoted to treating this syndrome have appeared and in some locations proliferated. Clinicians dealing with patients presenting with these disorders will wish to learn about their treatment philosophies and other practical aspects of their programs and requirements.

SPECIAL CONSIDERATIONS

Should Internet Addiction Be Included as a Distinct Disorder in the DSM-V?

The debate as to whether Internet addiction should be recognized as a separate disorder in the DSM-V is unsettled at the time of this writing. Advocates for inclusion argue that Internet addiction manifests many of features of substance dependence or of impulse-control disorders (2,9). Detractors note that insufficient research data exists to support Internet addiction's legitimacy as a disorder in its own right at this time (18).

Although concepts of "tolerance" and "withdrawal" have been applied to "Internet addiction Disorder," these have referred only to psychological states. There is as of yet no research linking "cravings" to use the Internet and feelings of irritability that ensue when access to the Internet is denied to identifiable physiologic signs of tolerance and withdrawal in individuals suffering from Internet addiction (18). On the other hand, neurobiologic studies have shown that involvement with the Internet is associated with striatal dopamine release, suggesting links to mechanisms that contribute to the reinforcing effects of illicit drugs (47).

Arguments suggesting that Internet addiction should be conceptualized as an impulse-control disorder have also emerged. The DSM-IV-TR defines impulse-control disorders as conditions in which the major manifestation is "the failure to resist an impulse, drive, or temptation to perform an act that is harmful to the person or others." In addition, affected individuals frequently feel "an increasing sense of tension or arousal before the act and then experiences pleasure, gratification, and relief at the time of committing the act" (77).

Many aspects of the phenomenology of Internet addiction are consistent with this DSM-IV description of impulse-control disorders. Moreover, as summarized by Dell'Osso et al. (62), a DSM-V task force examining the impulse-control disorders for over a decade has considered creating four new disorders currently subsumed under "impulse control disorders not otherwise specified." Under the proposed nosological system, these syndromes would receive the new name of "compulsive–impulsive disorders" characterized by "… the impulsive features (arousal) that initiate the behavior, and the compulsive drive that causes the behaviors to persist over time." (62) The four new disorders identified by the task force are compulsive–impulsive (C–I) Internet usage disorder, C–I sexual behaviors, C–I skin picking, and C–I shopping.

CONCLUSIONS

Excessive and/or problematic use of the Internet and related electronic media has become a worldwide mental health problem of epidemic proportions in industrialized nations, and American pediatricians have raised concerns that Internet addiction might become a "new common chronic disease of childhood" and "major public health problem for the United States in the 21st century" (78). Although further research is needed to better define its boundaries and diagnostic criteria and to assess whether it merits inclusion in the DSM as a distinct disorder, abundant evidence exists that Internet addiction is associated with significant clinical distress, functional impairment, and high rates of comorbidity. In the 21st century, psychiatrists and other mental health professionals must consider this syndrome in the differential diagnosis of their patients' presenting problems and be able to utilize a flexible, biopsychosocial approach in understanding and treating this condition. Well-designed treatment studies of psychosocial interventions and medications are necessary to inform evidence-based practices that can reduce the considerable psychological and economic costs to society imposed by this new but rapidly proliferating syndrome.

REFERENCES

1. Ahn DH. Korean policy on treatment and rehabilitation for adolescents' Internet addiction, In: *2007 International Symposium on the Counseling and Treatment of Youth*. Seoul, Korea, National Youth Commission; 2007:49.
2. Block JJ. Issues for DSM-V: Internet Addiction. *Am J Psychiatry*. 2008;165:306–307.

3. TIMESONLINE. 2008. Available at: http://www.timesonline.co.uk/tol/news/world/ asia/article5125324.ece. Accessed October 11, 2009.
4. Beuick MD. The limited social effect of radio broadcasting. *Am J Sociol*. 1927;32:615–622.
5. Meerloo JAM. Television addiction and reactive apathy. *J Nerv Ment Dis*. 1954;120:290–291.
6. Ingber D. Computer addicts. *Science Digest* 1981; July:88–91 and 114–121.
7. http://www.nurseweek.com/features/97–8/iadct.html. Accessed October 21, 2009.
8. Murali V, George S. Lost online: an overview of internet addiction. *Adv Psychiatr Treat*. 2007;13:24–30.
9. Young KS. Internet addiction: the emergence of a new clinical disorder. *CyberPsychol Behav*. 1998;1:237–244.
10. Young KS. Psychology of computer use: XL. Addictive use of the internet: a case that breaks the stereotype. *Psychol Rep*. 1996;79:899–902.
11. Young KS. *Caught in the Net: How to Recognize the Signs of Internet Addiction and a Winning Strategy for Recovery*. New York, NY: John Wiley & Sons; 1998.
12. Shotton MA. *Computer Addiction? A Study of Computer Dependency*. New York, NY: Taylor & Francis; 1989.
13. Griffiths M. Does internet and computer "addiction" exist? Some case study evidence. *CyberPsychol Behav*. 2000;3:211–218.
14. Shapira NA, Lessig MC, Goldsmith TD, et al. Problematic Internet use. Classification and diagnostic criteria. *Depress Anxiety*. 2003;17:207–216.
15. Meerkerk GJ, Van Den Eijnden RJJM, Vermulust AA, et al. The Compulsive Internet Use Scale (CIUS): some psychometric properties. *CyberPsychol Behav*. 2009;12:1–6.
16. Shaw M, Black DW. Internet addiction. *CNS Drugs*. 2008;22:353–365.
17. Widyanto L, Griffiths M. 'Internet addiction': a critical review. *Int J Ment Health Addict*. 2006;4:31–51.
18. Pies R. Should DSM-V designate "Internet Addiction" a mental disorder? *Psychiatry*. 2009;6:31–37.
19. Ha JH, Yoo HJ, Cho IH, et al. Psychiatric comorbidity assessed in Korean children and adolescents who screen positive for Internet addiction. *J Clin Psychiatry*. 2006;67:821–826.
20. World Internet Users and Population Stats. *Internet World Stats*. Available at: http://www.internetworldstats.com/stats.htm. Accessed May 21, 2009.
21. Leung L. Net-Generation attributes and seductive properties of the Internet as predictors of online activities and Internet addiction. *CyberPsychol Behav*. 2004;7:333–348.
22. Stone R. China reins in wilder impulses in treatment of "Internet Addiction." *Science*. 2009;324:1630–1631.
23. Ghassemzadeh L, Shahraray M, Moradi A. Prevalence of Internet addiction and comparison of Internet addicts and non-addicts in Iranian high schools. *CyberPsychol Behav*. 2008;11:731–733.
24. Kheirkhah F, Ghabeli Juibary A, Gouran A, et al. Internet addiction, prevalence and epidemiological features: first study in Iran. *Eur Psychiatry*. 2008;23(suppl 2):S309.
25. Niemz K, Griffiths M, Banyard P. Prevalence of pathological Internet use among university students and correlations with self-esteem, the General Health Questionnaire (GHQ), and disinhibition. *CyberPsychol. Behav*. 2005;8:562–570.
26. Morahan-Martin J, Schumacher J. Incidence and correlates of pathological Internet use among college students. *Comput Human Behav*. 2000;16:13–29.
27. Kaltiala-Heino R, Lintonen T, Rimpelä A. Internet addiction? Potentially problematic use of the Internet in a population of 12–18 year old adolescents. *Addict Res Theory*. 2004;12:89–96.
28. Aboujaoude E, Koran LM, Gamel N, et al. Potential markers for problematic internet use: a telephone survey of 2,513 adults. *CNS Spectr*. 2006;11:750–755.
29. Bakken IJ, Wenzel HG, Götestam KG, et al. Internet addiction among Norwegian adults: a stratified probability sample study. *Scandn J Psychol*. 2009;50:121–127.
30. Anderson CA, Gentile DA, Buckley K. *Violent Video Game Effects on Children and Adolescents. Theory, Research, and Public Policy*. New York, NY: Oxford University Press; 2007.
31. Gentile DA. Pathological video game use among youth 8 to 18: a national study. *Psychol Sci*. 2009;20:594–602.
32. http://www.nytimes.com/2009/05/26/health/26teen.html?_r=1&ref=todayspaper. Accessed 21 October, 2009.
33. Mule SJ. *Behavior in Excess: An Examination of the Volitional Disorders*. New York, NY: Free Press; 1981.
34. Young KS, Pistner M, O'Mara J. Cyber disorders: the mental health concern for the new millennium. *CyberPsychol Behav*. 1999;2:475–479.
35. Beard KW, Wolf EM. Modification in the proposed diagnostic criteria for Internet addiction. *CyberPsychol Behav*. 2001;4:377–383.
36. Caplan SE. Problematic Internet use and psychosocial well-being: development of a theory-based cognitive-behavioral measurement instrument. *Comput Human Behav*. 2002;18:553–575.
37. Nichols LA, Nicki R. Development of a psychometrically sound Internet addiction scale: a preliminary step. *Psychol Addict Behav*. 2004;18:381–384.
38. Griffiths M. Internet addiction: does it really exist? In: Gackenbach J, ed. *Psychology and the Internet: Intrapersonal, Interpersonal, and Transpersonal Implication*. San Diego, CA: Academic Press, 1998;61–75.
39. Widyanto L, McMurran M. The psychometric properties of the Internet Addiction Test. *CyberPsychol Behav*. 2004;7:443–450.
40. Armstrong L, Phillips JG, Saling LL. Potential determinants of heavier internet usage. *Int J Hum–Comput Stud*. 2000;53:537–550.
41. Widyanto L, Griffiths M, Brunsden V, et al. The psychometric properties of the Internet Related Problem Scale: a pilot study. *Int J Ment Health Addict*. 2008;6:205–213.
42. Davis RA, Gordon LF, Besser A. Validation of a new scale for measuring problematic Internet use: implications for pre-employment screening. *CyberPsychol Behav*. 2002;5:331–345.
43. Beard KW. Internet addiction: a review of current assessment techniques and potential assessment questions. *CyberPsychol Behav*. 2005;8:7–14.
44. Davis R. A cognitive-behavioral model of pathological internet use. *Comput Human Behav*. 2001;17:187–195.
45. Caplan SE. Preference for online social interaction: a theory of problematic internet use and psychosocial well-being. *Comm Res*. 2003;30:625–648.
46. Shapira NA, Goldsmith TD, Keck PE Jr, et al. Psychiatric features of individuals with problematic internet use. *J Affect Disord*. 2000;57:267–272.
47. Koepp MJ, Gunn RN, Lawrence AD, et al. Evidence for striatal dopamine release during a video game. *Nature*. 1998;393:266–268.
48. Han DH, Lee YS, Yang KC, et al. Dopamine genes and reward dependence in adolescents with excessive internet video game play. *J Addict Med*. 2007;1:133–138.

49. Han DH, Young SL, Churl N, et al. The effect of methylphenidate on Internet video game play in children with attention-deficit/hyperactivity disorder. *Compr Psychiatry.* 2009;50:251–256.
50. Han DH, Yoon SJ, Sung HS, et al. A preliminary study: novelty seeking, frontal executive function, and dopamine receptor (D2) TaqI A gene polymorphism in patients with methamphetamine dependence. *Compr Psychiatry.* 2008;49:387–392.
51. Lee YS, Han DH, Yang KC, et al. Depression-like characteristics of 5HTTLPR polymorphism and temperament in excessive Internet users. *J Affect Disord.* 2008;109:165–169.
52. Park SK, Kim JY, Cho CB. Prevalence of Internet addiction and correlations with family factors among South Korean adolescents. *Adolescence.* 2008;43:895–909.
53. Zhang ZH, Hao JH, Yang LS, et al. [The relationship between emotional, physical abuse and internet addiction disorder among middle school students]. *Zhonghua Liu Xing Bing Xue Za Zi (Chin. J. Epidemiol.)* 2009;30:115–118.
54. Yen CF, Ko CH, Yen JY, et al. Multi-dimensional discriminative factors for Internet addiction among adolescents regarding gender and age. *Psychiatry Clin Sci.* 2009;63:357–364.
55. Ni X, Yan H, Chen S, et al. Factors influencing internet addiction in a sample of freshmen university students in China. *Cyberpsychol Behav.* 2009;12:327–330.
56. Tsitsika A, Critselis E, Kormas G, et al. Internet use and misuse: a multivariate regression analysis of the predictive factors of Internet use among Greek adolescents. *Eur J Pediatr.* 2009;168:655–665.
57. Ko C-H, Yen J-Y, Chen C-S, et al. Predictive values of psychiatric symptoms for internet addiction in adolescents: a 2-year prospective study. *Arch Pediatr Adolesc Med.* 2009;163:937–943.
58. http://www.sciencemag.org/cgi/content/full/324/5935/1630. Accessed October 21, 2009.
59. Lee H. A new case of fatal pulmonary thromboembolism associated with prolonged sitting at computer in Korea. *Yonsei Med J.* 2004;45:349–351.
60. Beasley R, Raymond N, Hill S, et al. eThrombosis: the 21st century variant of venous thromboembolism associated with immobility. *Eur Respir J.* 2003;21:374–376.
61. Calamaro CJ, Mason TBA, Ratcliffe SJ. Adolescents living the 24/7 lifestyle: effects of caffeine and technology on sleep duration and daytime functioning. *Pediatrics.* 2009;123:e1005–e1010.
62. Dell'Osso B, Altamura AC, Allen A, et al. Epidemiologic and clinical updates on impulse control disorders: a critical review. *Eur Arch Psychiatry Clin Neurosci.* 2006;256:464–475.
63. Anderson CA, Dill KE. Video games and aggressive thoughts, feelings, and behavior in the laboratory and in life. *J Pers Soc Psychol.* 2000;78:772–790.
64. Weintraub P, Hall HL, Pynoos RS. Columbine high school shootings: community response. In: Shaffi M, Shaffi SL, eds. *School Violence: Assessment, Management, Prevention.* Washington DC: American Psychiatric Publishing, Inc.; 2001:129–161.
65. http://psycnet.apa.org/?fa=main.doiLanding&doi=10.1037/0022-3514.78.4.772. Accessed October 18, 2009.
66. Calhoun R. Caught in the Web: Internet addiction costs add up in workplace. *San Antonio Business J.* 2005;February 11. Available at: http://sanantonio.bizjournals.com/sanantonio/stories/2005/02/14/focus6.html. Accessed October 12, 2009.
67. Caird JK, Willness CR, Steel P, et al. A meta-analysis of the effects of cell phones on driver performance. *Accid Anal Prev.* 2008;40:1282–1293.
68. Vivoda JM, Eby DW, St. Louis RM, et al. Cellular phone use while driving at night. *Traffic Inj Prev.* 2008;9:37–41.
69. National Highway Safety Traffic Administration. Driver electronic device use in 2007. *Ann Emerg Med.* 2009;53:267–268; discussion 268–269.
70. http://www.cbs19.tv/Global/story.asp?S=3599578. Accessed October 20, 2009.
71. http://www.cbsnews.com/stories/2009/09/30/national/main5352322.shtml. Accessed October 20, 2009.
72. http://www.msnbc.msn.com/id/29546030/. Accessed September 20, 2009.
73. http://www.msnbc.msn.com/id/28679588/. Accessed September 20, 2009.
74. Sattar P, Ramaswamy S. Internet gaming addiction. *Can J Psychiatry.* 2004;49:869–870.
75. Dell'Osso B, Hadley S, Allen A, et al. Escitalopram in the treatment of impulsive–compulsive internet usage disorder: an open-label trial followed by a double-blind discontinuation phase. *J Clin Psychiatry.* 2008;69:452–456.
76. Bostwick JM, Bucci JA. Internet sex addiction treated with naltrexone. *Mayo Clin.* 2008;83:226–230.
77. Impulse Control Disorders Not Elsewhere Classified. In: *Diagnostic and Statistical Manual of Mental Disorders. Text Revision. Fourth Edition. DSM-IV TR.* Washington DC: American Psychiatric Association; 2000;63.
78. Christakis DA, Moreno MA. Trapped in the net: will internet addiction become a 21st-century epidemic? *Arch Pediatr Adolesc Med.* 2009;163:959–960.

SECTION 6 ■ TREATMENT APPROACHES

PART 1 ■ Neurobiologic Treatments

CHAPTER 28 — Methadone Maintenance

Andrew J. Saxon ■ Karen Miotto

INTRODUCTION

Methadone maintenance is one of the most efficacious and cost-effective interventions in all of modern medicine. This chapter provides a comprehensive overview of methadone treatment for opioid dependence by reviewing the epidemiology, explaining the historical background, summarizing the regulations that govern methadone treatment, and describing the pharmacology and clinical use of methadone. The chapter will then cover a variety of practical issues that arise in the process of delivering methadone treatment in a licensed Opioid Treatment Program (OTP) including nonopioid substance use, management of co-occurring medical and psychiatric disorders, counseling and other behavioral interventions, urine testing, take-home medication, medication diversion reduction, managing problematic behavior, methadone in pregnancy, and medical and interim methadone maintenance.

EPIDEMIOLOGY AND HISTORY

During the early years of the 21st century, the purity of heroin sold in the United States generally remained higher than in previous decades, contributing to an increase in heroin-related emergency department visits from 33,900 in 1990 to 189,780 in 2006. Heroin users exhibit mortality rates 6 to 20 times those of age-matched populations (1,2). The past decade has also seen a surge in the illicit use of prescription opioid medications. In 2006, the number of emergency room visits related to nonmedical use of prescription opioids exceeded the number for heroin. Large numbers of overdoses on prescription opioids have also been noted. In 2007, as many people abused OxyContin in the past month (0.3 million) as used heroin, and 5.2 million abused some type of pain reliever (primarily hydrocodone and oxycodone) in the past month.

Methadone maintenance, available in the United States since the 1970s, is one of the primary treatment modalities for this burgeoning epidemic of opioid dependence. From 1919 until 1972, a ruling by the U.S. Supreme Court disallowed physicians from prescribing opioid medications to opioid-dependent individuals for "maintenance" purposes. The federal methadone regulations (21 CFR Part 291) promulgated in 1972 and the Narcotic Addict Treatment Act of 1974 created the current regulatory system for methadone maintenance, which allowed prescribing of methadone to opioid-dependent patients through OTPs, which follow specific federal regulations and are licensed by both federal and state authorities. The Food and Drug Administration (FDA) and the Drug Enforcement Agency (DEA) oversaw these OTPs until 2000. The federal regulations governing methadone-maintenance treatment were amended slightly in 1980 and again in 1993. The changes in 1993 allowed the use of levo-alpha acetyl methadol (LAAM, which has not been manufactured nor available since 2003) and mandated counseling on preventing exposure to and preventing transmission of human immunodeficiency virus (HIV).

The federal regulations were altered once again in 2001. The oversight by FDA was discontinued, and the authority passed to the Center for Substance Abuse Treatment of the Substance Abuse and Mental Health Services Administration within the Department of Health and Human Services (42 CFR Part 8). In addition, these new regulations required triennial accreditation of all licensed OTPs by approved accreditation organizations. Finally, the 2001 regulations permitted more latitude in provision of take-home medications, allowing a maximum of 30 take-home doses of medication for stable, long-term patients. In 2003, the regulations again were slightly amended to allow the dispensing of buprenorphine and buprenorphine/naloxone through licensed OTPs.

Methadone treatment has undergone considerable expansion in the United States. In 1988, 650 programs treated about 100,000 patients. As of 2009, over 1200 programs existed. In 2007, 265,217 patients were treated in OTPs, the vast majority with methadone. Licensed OTPs are situated in every state in the United States except North Dakota, South Dakota, and Wyoming. Methadone treatment for opioid dependence has spread worldwide, and methadone and buprenorphine were included in the 2005 World Health Organization List of Essential Medications.

FEDERAL OPIOID TREATMENT STANDARDS GOVERNING METHADONE TREATMENT

These regulations are readily and publicly available, and only the key points will be summarized here.

Administration

Each licensed OTP must have a sponsor responsible for adherence to all regulations and a medical director responsible for administering all medical services. The OTP must maintain quality assurance and quality control plans focusing on patient outcomes and must have a diversion control plan. All staff must be qualified and comply with the credentialing requirements of their respective professions.

Patient Admission Criteria

Documentation of current opioid addiction of at least 1 year's duration is required for admission. These requirements may be waived by a program physician for patients recently released from incarceration or previously treated within the past 2 years in an OTP, or for pregnant patients. Patients under age 18 must have had two prior failed attempts at medically supervised withdrawal and have parental or guardian permission.

Required Services

Adequate medical, counseling, vocational, educational, and other assessment and treatment services must be provided. Each patient must receive a complete, fully documented physical evaluation by an authorized health care professional before admission. Special services for pregnant patients must be available. Each patient accepted for treatment must be initially and periodically assessed by qualified personnel to determine the most appropriate combination of services and treatment including the preparation of a written treatment plan. Programs must provide adequate addiction counseling and when clinically necessary provide counseling and education on HIV transmission and prevention. Programs must obtain at least eight random yearly drug tests for patients in maintenance treatment.

Medication Administration, Dispensing, and Use

Medication must be dispensed by an appropriately licensed health care professional. The only medications permitted for use in licensed OTPs are methadone, LAAM (not currently manufactured), and buprenorphine or buprenorphine/naloxone. The initial dose of methadone cannot exceed 30 mg, and the total dose for the first day cannot exceed 40 mg unless the physician documents that 40 mg did not suppress opioid withdrawal symptoms. The number of allowable take-home doses is specifically dictated by the regulations based on continuous time in treatment and patient stability.

Interim Maintenance Treatment

Interim maintenance treatment is allowable for a maximum of 120 days when patients cannot obtain entrance to comprehensive treatment. Interim maintenance involves daily dispensing of medication with no take-homes and does not require counseling or development of a treatment plan.

EFFICACY OF METHADONE TREATMENT FOR OPIOID DEPENDENCE

Numerous studies over nearly half a century have examined methadone treatment. Evaluating methadone through the most rigorous approach, double-blind, placebo-controlled randomized trials, poses some challenges. Since opioid withdrawal does not show much placebo response, it is difficult to maintain the blind. In addition, methadone has such obvious clinical utility for a condition causing extensive morbidity that the ethics of using a placebo are questionable.

These concerns have been surmounted in two studies that randomly assigned subjects in double-blind fashion to methadone maintenance versus a control condition of a blinded methadone taper followed by placebo. These two studies are included in a recent meta-analysis (3), which surveyed the literature through 2001 and found six trials involving a total of 954 subjects published between 1969 and 1993 that compared methadone maintenance to some sort of control condition. The analysis determined that subjects receiving maintenance were three times as likely as control subjects to remain in treatment and one third as likely to have used heroin.

This meta-analysis failed to show that methadone treatment reduces engagement in criminal activity. However, another meta-analysis (4), which included 24 studies conducted between 1964 and 1994, found that methadone maintenance had a large effect on drug-related crime, a small-to-moderate effect on drug- and property-related crime, and a small effect on non–drug-related crime. Most of the studies included in this analysis compared criminal behavior prior to entering methadone treatment to such behavior during methadone treatment. A more recent study, which randomly assigned subjects to interim methadone treatment versus referral to community methadone treatment, found that the referral group was much less likely to enter comprehensive methadone maintenance and received significantly more illegal income at follow-up than did the interim maintenance group (5).

A multitude of observational studies also show that methadone treatment reduces HIV risk behavior. The meta-analysis cited above (4) analyzed eight studies that looked at changes in HIV risk behavior both before and after entering methadone treatment and found that methadone treatment had a small but significant effect in reducing such behaviors. A more recent systematic review examined the literature on this topic from its inception through 2003 and found 28 relevant studies (6). Only two of these studies were randomized clinical trials. The studies consistently observed reductions in both needle use and sexual risks during methadone treatment. Four of the studies looked at HIV seroconversion observationally and noted a protective effect of methadone treatment on seroconversion.

Opioid-dependent individuals exhibit mortality rates 6 to 20 times that of the age-matched population (2), but methadone treatment may partially reverse this risk. A controlled trial (7) that randomly assigned 34 heroin addicts to receive methadone treatment or to a control group that offered psychosocial treatment only showed a mortality rate of 11.8% in the control group within 2 years compared to 0% in the methadone group. Reduced mortality rates are also observed for opioid-dependent individuals in methadone treatment compared to those out of methadone treatment (8). A cost-effectiveness analysis found that the cost of methadone treatment per life-year gained falls well within the range of other commonly used medical treatments such as coronary artery bypass surgery or renal dialysis (1).

In summary, we have good evidence that medication-assisted treatment with methadone for opioid dependence keeps patients in treatment and reduces illicit opioid use better than does treatment without medication. We have a lower level of evidence that methadone treatment reduces HIV seroconversion, mortality, and criminal behavior.

METHADONE PHARMACOLOGY

Methadone possesses a unique and complex pharmacology. Its good oral bioavailability, gradual onset, and generally long half-life contribute to its efficacy, but the long half-life also confers risk of medication build up and inadvertent toxicity. Methadone also has several potential drug–drug interactions and effects on cardiac conduction. These safety issues moved the FDA to place a black box warning in the product label regarding respiratory depression and QT interval prolongation on the electrocardiogram (ECG).

Marketed methadone contains a racemic mixture of two stereoisomers, levo (L)-methadone and dextro (D)-methadone. The L-methadone enantiomer has the majority of pharmacologic activity, although the D-methadone has some antitussive action and may contribute to some side effects. Oral methadone is supplied as a solid tablet, a rapidly dissolving wafer, and a premixed liquid, all of which are basically bioequivalent.

Pharmacokinetics

Methadone is readily absorbed after oral ingestion (9), with an average bioavailability of about 80%, but interindividual variation ranging from 41% to 95% (10). Its initial effects can occur within 30 minutes, but peak effects and peak plasma levels occur on average about 4 hours following ingestion, with a range of 1 to 6 hours (11). Methadone has an average terminal half-life of 22 hours, with a range of 5 to 130 hours (12). The vast majority of methadone leaves the circulation and enters tissue stores in liver, kidneys, lungs, and brain. The tissue stores can be released back into the circulation typically when serum levels fall but also potentially at unanticipated times and at unexpectedly rapid rates. The methadone remaining in the blood is 60% to 90% bound to plasma proteins, mainly to α1-acid glycoproteins. The amount of free methadone available to tissues obviously varies with the amount of protein available for binding. For example, levels of α1-acid glycoproteins increase during stress, which would increase the amount of bound methadone and reduce the amount of free methadone (10).

As might be anticipated from the wide variability in half-life, the metabolism of methadone is complicated and not yet entirely understood. An array of evidence suggests that metabolism is catalyzed primarily by the liver enzyme CYP 450 3A4 (13) with possible additional contributions by other enzymes (14) including CYP2B6, CYP2D6, and possibly, but to a smaller extent, CYP1A2, CYP2C9, and CYP2C19 (12). Recently, the primary role of 3A4 has come into question (15), but the important point is that all of these enzymes exhibit wide interindividual variation in activity based largely on genetics and to a lesser extent on environmental factors. Methadone can also induce its own metabolism so that serum levels and effects may decline over time.

Methadone is metabolized primarily to the inactive metabolite, 2-ethylidene-1,5-dimethyl-3,3-diphenylpyrrolidine (EDDP). Most parent drug and EDDP elimination occurs through the kidneys with some eliminated in the feces. As with other aspects of the body's handling of methadone, interindividual variation also occurs in clearance rates. In addition, renal elimination varies based on urinary pH. More acid urine leads to faster elimination.

The key message for clinicians is to appreciate the potential for tremendous variability in methadone absorption, metabolism, storage, and elimination both across individuals and within a given individual over time.

Pharmacodynamics

The primary pharmacodynamic target for methadone is the μ-opioid receptor, but methadone, unlike most other opioids, also antagonizes the N-methyl, D-aspartate (NMDA) receptor (16) and blocks the serotonin and norepinephrine transporters. In addition, methadone inhibits the cardiac potassium channel hERG that, as noted above, can cause a prolonged QT interval (17) on the ECG. Given acutely prior to the development of tolerance, methadone has typical μ-opioid agonist effects including miosis, analgesia, sedation, possible euphoria, decrease in gut motility, release of histamine, and respiratory depression.

In preclinical paradigms, methadone serves as a substrate of the transport protein, P-glycoprotein. P-glycoprotein activity varies both by genetic predisposition and environmental effects such as the presence of other drugs. P-glycoprotein activity could affect absorption of methadone from the gut but also, importantly, could have a substantial impact on the relationship between plasma and brain levels, reducing brain levels when it is more actively transporting methadone out of the central nervous system (CNS).

CLINICAL USE OF METHADONE

Methadone's unique pharmacology confers several clinical challenges. Each patient has a different response to a given dose of methadone, so careful individual attention is required in the monitoring and management of each patient. Due to incomplete cross-tolerance, dose conversion calculators can be misleading or erroneous when used to switch patients from other opioids to methadone. In addition, given its long half-life, several days are required in most patients to achieve a steady state. Although a patient may report an inadequate response initially, the ultimate response to a given dose cannot be immediately determined. Too rapid dose escalation can lead to unanticipated medication accumulation causing adverse events including most seriously respiratory depression, respiratory arrest, and death. These fatalities can occur particularly among individuals who have not developed any tolerance to opioids (18). The highest-risk period for fatal intoxication is during the first weeks of treatment and periods of dose adjustments (18).

One of the very characteristics that makes methadone potentially dangerous, its long half-life, is also an attribute that renders it a superb treatment agent for opioid dependence. For most patients, a once-daily oral dose is sufficient to prevent emergence of opioid withdrawal, which is a strong driver for ongoing illicit opioid use. Based on preclinical evidence, methadone's antagonism of excitatory NMDA receptors could reduce opioid tolerance, decreasing the need for a constantly escalating dose to obtain the same effect once stabilization is achieved (19). Methadone's blockade of serotonin and norepinephrine transporters may leave more of these neurotransmitters in the synapse thereby providing some mood-elevating effects.

Methadone Induction

The induction period encompasses the time from the first administered dose until the point when a stable dose is reached, typically a span of 2 to 4 weeks. Prior to inducing a patient onto methadone, specific elements of assessment must be completed. A medical history and physical examination should be completed including information on past and recent illicit opioid and other substance use as well as a record of all the patient's current medications. Information on the patient's experience with tolerance and withdrawal is important in determining the induction dose. The required (syphilis serology) and any other indicated laboratory tests should be obtained as well as a urine specimen for toxicology analysis to confirm the recent substance use history given by the patient. Informed consent should be provided so that the patient understands the risks of methadone treatment particularly the fact that physiologic dependence on methadone will occur. The patient should sign a consent document that also lays out all the expectations for methadone treatment.

Prior to administering the initial dose, the responsible clinician should ascertain that the patient is not exhibiting any clinical evidence of sedation or intoxication. Federal regulations specify that the initial dose of methadone can range from 5 to 30 mg with 30 mg being the maximum allowed first dose. An additional 10 mg can be added after a period of observation if 30 mg does not adequately suppress withdrawal. The maximum allowed total dose for the first day is 40 mg unless the program physician clearly documents in the record that 40 mg did not suppress opioid withdrawal. Clinical judgment about the initial dose depends on a variety of patient-specific factors including any history of prior response to methadone and prior methadone dose, type, amount, and frequency of recent opioid use, recent use of other substances such as sedatives or ethanol that could have additive or synergistic effects with methadone on level of consciousness or respiratory drive, and current medical conditions or concomitant prescribed medications that could alter the pharmacokinetics or pharmacodynamics of methadone. The patient's age should also be taken into consideration since older individuals generally metabolize methadone more slowly. If any question exists as to the appropriate initial dose, it is wisest to err on the side of a lower dose to avoid any potential risks of intoxication or overdose. For patients who have not used any opioids for three or more days prior to induction, 5 to 10 mg is the most appropriate initial dose. For patients with extensive recent use of heroin, the initial dose of 30 or 40 mg as a split dose will reduce withdrawal symptoms.

The clinician should evaluate the patient 2 to 4 hours following the initial dose. If the patient shows no signs of withdrawal or intoxication and reports feeling comfortable, the appropriate first-day dose has been achieved. If there are signs or symptoms of withdrawal, the clinician can administer additional doses of methadone to a maximum of 40 mg total for day 1. In the exceedingly rare instance when a dose higher than 40 mg for day 1 is contemplated, it must be clearly documented that a dose higher than 40 mg was required to manage opioid withdrawal. In the rare instance, when a patient appears sedated or intoxicated, 2 to 4 hours after the initial dose, the patient should at minimum be kept in the clinic for observation until the effects have resolved, or, if necessary, emergency measures such as naloxone administration to reverse intoxication and airway preservation should be instituted.

The patient will return to the clinic on subsequent days for evaluation and observed medication administration. The patient can then be assessed for signs and symptoms of withdrawal or intoxication. It is very likely that the initial dose did not completely suppress withdrawal symptoms over a full 24-hour period. Nevertheless, with the 22-hour average half-life of methadone and the fact that it takes four to five half-lives to achieve a steady state, it will typically require 4 to 5 days on a given dose to ascertain the ultimate effect of that dose. Even though the patient may experience some withdrawal symptoms during the 24-hour dosing interval, the most judicious approach is to increase the dosage in 5- to 10-mg increments every 4 to 5 days. Following this conservative titration schedule, dosages of 60 to 80 mg/day can be achieved within 4 weeks of initiation.

Determining the Stable Dose of Methadone

The overall goals for the induction period and beyond are to attain a methadone dose that (1) suppresses opioid withdrawal symptoms throughout the 24-hour dosing interval, (2) eliminates craving or desire for other opioids, (3) creates sufficient tolerance to prevent euphoria caused by self-administration of illicit opioids, (4) eliminates the use of illicit opioids as evidenced by self-report and urine toxicology testing, and (5) minimizes side effects so that the patient is not experiencing intoxication and can function normally. Frequently, all these goals cannot be met by doses that are safely reached during the induction period. In that circumstance, ongoing methadone dose increases in increments of 5 to 10 mg every 5 to 7 days should be continued until these goals are achieved. Once the daily dose exceeds 40 mg, 10-mg increments generally are quite safe and appropriate. Finding the stable dose involves a clinical balancing act since doses needed to establish sufficient tolerance and eliminate illicit opioid use often result in some side effects. Clinical trial evidence demonstrates that methadone doses of 80 to 100 mg/day are superior to lower doses in reducing illicit opioid use and retaining patients in treatment (20). For most patients, the stable dose will reside in the range of 80 to 120 mg/day, though as a consequence of interindividual differences, some patients do well on lower doses and some require higher doses. Within 60 to 90 days of starting methadone, most patients will stabilize on a daily dose that remains constant indefinitely.

However, considering the variety of pharmacologic, environmental, and physiologic factors that can arise over time to influence methadone's activity, including its ability to induce its own metabolism, it is not unusual for patients to develop symptoms or signs of instability after a period on a stable dose. The instability may come to light via patient self-report of withdrawal symptoms, side effects, or illicit opioid use, or illicit opioid use might be detected on urine screening. In these situations the clinician should re-evaluate the patient, seek to address any contributing factors (such as newly diagnosed medical conditions or introduction of concomitant medications that could be interacting with methadone), and consider changes in the daily methadone dose. The dose can again be increased in 5- to 10-mg increments every 5 to 7 days until the criteria for stability are once more achieved.

Patients may also miss methadone doses because of failure to attend the clinic. If more than 1 consecutive day is missed, the patient should receive a medical evaluation, and the methadone dose may need to be temporarily reduced if a loss of tolerance is suspected. A common practice after 2 or 3 days is to restart the patient at 50% of his or her established maintenance dose; however, the reduction should not be less than the original initial dose. Providing that the patient tolerates the reduced amount of methadone, the dose can be increased by no more than 10 mg/day. Slower dose escalation is recommended for patients who are medically compromised or have problematic alcohol or benzodiazepine use. After missing 4 or more days of methadone, the most cautious course of action is to restart methadone at 30 mg or less, depending on the original initial dose. The methadone dose can then be retitrated upward in a fashion analogous to induction to return ultimately to the stable dose.

Methadone Serum Levels

In the majority of cases, stability on methadone can be achieved with close clinical monitoring and dose adjustments as clinically indicated. Some patients in contrast may fail to achieve stability as evidenced by ongoing illicit opioid use or by complaints of opioid craving or withdrawal symptoms. For a few select cases, obtaining serum methadone levels may help to illuminate the problem. No firm agreement exists on thresholds for an adequate serum concentration. Suggested minimally therapeutic trough levels range from 100 to 400 ng/mL (21). Peak serum levels also vary widely among stable patients in methadone treatment. The best available evidence indicates that the rate of decline from peak to trough, rather than absolute levels, optimally predicts the presence of withdrawal symptoms and instability (22), but determining the rate of decline requires multiple samples over a 24-hour period, a sampling regimen not possible outside of a research context. Although not perfect, the ratio of peak to trough may serve as a surrogate for the rate of decline. A peak-to-trough ratio of greater than 2:1 may be an indicator of inadequate coverage throughout the 24-hour dosing interval leading to clinical instability. Patients who exhibit such a pattern may be rapid metabolizers of methadone, who would respond best to a split-dosing regimen rather than to an increase in daily dose. Thus, to evaluate serum methadone levels, a trough level should be obtained 24 hours after the last dose and a peak level obtained about 3 hours after the last dose. Consideration of the absolute levels, the ratio between them, and the clinical context may guide rational methadone dosing.

Methadone Drug Interactions

Table 28.1 lists important potential drug–drug interactions involving methadone. Additive or synergistic effects can occur between methadone and other opioids or sedatives that also suppress respiratory drive leading to toxicity or overdose.

Given the numerous potential pathways for methadone metabolism, multiple drug–drug interactions are theoretically possible. Drugs that inhibit the enzymes involved in methadone metabolism could cause elevated methadone serum levels and increased opioid effects. For the most part, these types of expected interactions have not usually caused much in the way of clinically concerning effects. For example, a human laboratory study found that fluconazole (a CYP 3A4, 2C9, and 2C19 inhibitor) significantly increased methadone serum levels without causing any clinically observable effects (23). However, there is one case report of concomitant administration of fluconazole leading to methadone toxicity (24). Similarly, there is one case report of concomitant fluvoxamine (an inhibitor of CYP enzymes 3A4, 1A2, 2C9, and 2C19) administration leading to methadone toxicity (25).

TABLE 28.1 Common potential methadone drug–drug interactions

Class or specific drug	Interaction	Putative mechanism	Notes
Antiretrovirals			
Efavirenz, lopinavir, nevirapine	Reduction in serum methadone levels	Induction of CYP 450 enzymes	Clinically significant opioid withdrawal symptoms likely
Abacavir, etravirine, nelfinavir, ritonavir, squinavir, tipranavir	May reduce serum methadone levels	Induction of CYP 450 enzymes	Clinically pertinent opioid withdrawal symptoms usually not seen with these agents
Didanosine	Reduction in didanosine plasma concentration	Decreased bioavailability	Possible decreased efficacy of didanosine
Zidovudine	Increase in zidovudine plasma concentration	Unknown	Risk of zidovudine toxicity
Antidepressants			
Tricyclics: amitriptyline, clomipramine, desipramine, doxepin, imipramine, nortriptyline, protriptyline, trimipramine	Increases risk for constipation and sedation; increases risk for QT prolongation and arrhythmia	Anticholinergic effects; blockade of hERG channel	Clinical experience with combination indicates it is generally safe with careful clinical monitoring
Serotonin reuptake inhibitors: citalopram, escitalopram, fluvoxamine, fluoxetine, paroxetine, sertraline	May increase serum methadone levels; increased risk for serotonin syndrome	Inhibition of CYP enzymes; blockade of serotonin transporter	Clinical experience with combination indicates it is generally safe with careful clinical monitoring
Monoamine oxidase inhibitors: isocarboxazid, phenelzine, selegiline, tranylcypromine	Increased risk for serotonin syndrome	Inhibition of serotonin metabolism	Use with extreme caution and careful clinical monitoring
Serotonin/norepinephrine reuptake inhibitors: duloxetine, desvenlafaxine, venlafaxine	Increased risk for serotonin syndrome; increases risk for QT prolongation and arrhythmia (venlafaxine)	Blockade of serotonin transporter blockade of hERG channel (venlafaxine)	Clinical experience with combination indicates it is generally safe with careful clinical monitoring
Antibiotics			
Ciprofloxacin, clarithromycin, erythromycin, azithromycin	May increase methadone serum levels; increases risk for QT prolongation and arrhythmia	Inhibition of CYP enzymes; blockade of hERG channel	One case report of sedation (ciprofloxacin); clinical monitoring required
Rifampin	Reduction in serum methadone levels	Induction of CYP enzymes	Severe opioid withdrawal can occur; will need increased methadone dose

Antifungals		
Ketoconazole, fluconazole	May increase methadone serum levels	Inhibition of CYP enzymes	Little evidence for important clinical effects
Anticonvulsants		
Carbamazepine, phenytoin	Reduction in serum methadone levels	Induction of CYP enzymes	Severe opioid withdrawal can occur; will need increased methadone dose
Antiarrhythmics		
Procainamide, quinidine	Increases risk for QT prolongation and arrhythmia	Blockade of hERG channel	Careful clinical monitoring required
Amiodarone	May increase methadone serum levels; increases risk for QT prolongation and arrhythmia	Inhibition of CYP enzymes; blockade of hERG channel	Careful clinical monitoring required
Benzodiazepines	Additive CNS and respiratory depressant effects	Increased GABA activity	Careful clinical monitoring required
Barbiturates	Additive CNS and respiratory depressant effects	Increased GABA activity	Careful clinical monitoring required
Cimetidine	May increase methadone serum levels	Inhibition of CYP enzymes	No evidence of major clinical effect
Naltrexone	Precipitated opioid withdrawal	Displaces methadone from μ-opioid receptors	Contraindicated

Drug–drug interactions that are clinically significant induce the enzymes catalyzing the metabolism of methadone resulting in a decrease in the methadone serum level and emerging opioid withdrawal. Drugs known to cause this effect include the anticonvulsants, phenytoin, and carbamazepine; the antibiotic, rifampin; and antiretroviral medications, lopinavir, efavirenz, and nevirapine. These medications are best avoided in methadone-treated patients, but if their use is essential, often fairly substantial increases in the methadone dose are required to eliminate the emerging withdrawal symptoms. Other antiretroviral medications may alter methadone pharmacokinetics but do not appear to result in clinically observed withdrawal.

Finally, as described below, methadone can prolong the QT interval on the ECG. Numerous other drugs also have a similar effect. Although the issue has not been well studied, it seems probable that the combination of methadone with other drugs that prolong the QT interval could have additive effects increasing the risk for QT prolongation.

Managing Methadone Side Effects

Table 28.2 lists common methadone side effects. If troublesome side effects are present, and the patient has stopped illicit opioid use and does not have withdrawal symptoms, many side effects can be managed by incremental methadone dose reductions of 5 to 10 mg every 5 to 7 days until side effects are resolved, tolerable, or until withdrawal symptoms occur. If dose reductions are not reasonable because the patient has continued illicit opioid use or still has withdrawal symptoms, other interventions can be applied to manage some of the commonly occurring side effects.

Constipation is one of the most frequent and bothersome side effects in patients on methadone. Constipation can be managed by encouraging patients to drink more water, eating a diet higher in fiber content, and engaging in modest exercise. If these measures are ineffective, psyllium or other bulk-forming laxatives can be used but should be used with caution unless adequate fluid is maintained. Other patients respond to emollient laxatives such as docusate, or to stimulant laxatives (bisacodyl) or osmotic laxatives (lactulose). Although constipation is generally benign, it can obviously progress to impaction and small bowel obstruction, so early intervention to address it is warranted. Methylnaltrexone is an opioid-receptor antagonist that blocks the peripheral gastrointestinal opioid receptors, but does not cross the blood–brain barrier. It has been recently approved by the FDA as a subcutaneous preparation for the treatment of opioid-induced bowel dysfunction; the oral forms remain under investigation.

TABLE 28.2 Potential methadone side effects

Body system	Side effects
Body as a whole	Asthenia (weakness), edema, headache
Cardiovascular	Arrhythmias, bigeminal rhythms, bradycardia, cardiomyopathy, ECG abnormalities, extrasystoles, flushing, heart failure, hypotension, palpitations, phlebitis, QT interval prolongation, syncope, T-wave inversion, tachycardia, torsade de pointes, ventricular fibrillation, ventricular tachycardia
Digestive	Abdominal pain, anorexia, biliary tract spasm, constipation, dry mouth, glossitis
Metabolic and nutritional	Hypokalemia, hypomagnesemia, weight gain
Nervous	Agitation, confusion, disorientation, dysphoria, euphoria, insomnia, seizures
Respiratory	Pulmonary edema, respiratory depression, sleep apnea
Skin and appendages	Pruritis, urticaria, other skin rashes, and, rarely, hemorrhagic urticaria, diaphoresis
Special senses	Hallucinations, visual disturbances
Urogenital	Amenorrhea, antidiuretic effect, reduced libido, erectile dysfunction, urinary retention or hesitancy

Edema can also be an unpleasant side effect of methadone (26). How methadone causes edema remains unknown. Edema seldom responds to sodium restriction. It sometimes responds to a decrease in methadone dosage if the patient is sufficiently stable to undergo a decrease. If severe edema does not respond to these measures, diuretics, such as furosemide, often prove helpful. If a diuretic is prescribed, potassium levels should be checked periodically to assure that potassium depletion is not occurring.

Methadone can cause hormonal alterations related to sexual functioning. Methadone acts at the hypothalamus altering the release of gonadotropin-releasing hormone, leading to a reduction in follicle-stimulating hormone (FSH) and luteinizing hormone (LH) and subsequent suppression of testosterone levels. In men, reports of methadone side effects include orgasmic and erectile dysfunction, and decreased sexual desire. The reductions in FSH and LH normalize after several years of methadone treatment despite a persistent decrease in testosterone in some individuals (27). Sexual dysfunction may respond to a methadone dosage reduction. If that is not possible or does not help, erectile function often improves with use of phosphodiesterase type 5 inhibitors (presuming contraindications for this class of medications such as cardiac conditions are not present). Testosterone replacement can ameliorate sexual dysfunction among methadone treated men with low serum testosterone levels.

For women on methadone, depressed libido and oligomenorrhea or amenorrhea have been reported; however, some improvements are also noted after stabilizing in treatment. Irregular menses may lead some women to believe incorrectly that they cannot become pregnant or are pregnant when they are not. For symptomatic female patients, a medical workup is indicated that includes a discussion of the possibility of becoming pregnant without regular menses and about the use of birth control. Referral to an endocrinologist or gynecologist can identify or rule out other medical conditions that can cause amenorrhea or oligomenorrhea.

A hormonal effect of methadone that persists in some individuals after years of treatment is altered prolactin release. Rather than the normal diurnal variation, prolactin release becomes reactive to the peak level of methadone (27). The clinical symptoms associated with hyperprolactinemia include galactorrhea, menstrual disturbance, erectile dysfunction, or long-term loss of bone mineral density. A cross-sectional study found that three quarters of methadone-maintained patients had low bone mineral densities. Hormone levels were not measured in this study, but other modifiable factors contributing to low bone mineral density were lower body weight and heavy alcohol consumption (28).

Hyperhidrosis or excessive sweating (29) is another common complaint among patients on methadone. One potentially effective intervention is to lower the methadone dose if possible. In patients treated with additional drugs that induce hyperhidrosis such as cholinesterase inhibitors, selective serotonin reuptake inhibitors, or tricyclic antidepressants, using an alternative to one of these medications can decrease the severity of sweating. Methadone and other opioids induce release of histamine by degranulation of mast cells, which is implicated in the side effects of sweating and itching. Antihistamines are mast cell stabilizers, and two case reports suggest that antihistamines may alleviate sweating in methadone patients. The newer nonsedating antihistamines do not incur a risk of increase in the QT interval.

As noted above, methadone has a black box warning for QT interval prolongation. Some evidence suggests that a corrected QT interval longer than 500 msec increases the risk for torsades. At the present time, insufficient information on the cardiac effects of methadone is available to make definitive recommendations about how to handle this issue. It is reasonable to consider obtaining ECGs on methadone patients who have known structural heart disease or who have a history of syncope or a family history of sudden cardiac death, since there can be genetic predisposition to a prolonged QT interval. If patients on methadone have a corrected QT interval above 500 msec, consideration should be given to discontinuing other medications that also prolong the QT interval, to stopping illicit cocaine use, correcting electrolyte imbalances, and reducing the methadone dose if clinically feasible.

Methadone Medically Supervised Withdrawal and Tapering

Medically supervised withdrawal or tapering from methadone may be performed for several reasons. In the majority of cases, it should be avoided because relapse rates to dependence on illicit opioids tend to be high (30). If medically supervised withdrawal must be done, slower tapers lead to superior outcomes (31). Justifications for medically supervised withdrawal include patients who do not qualify for maintenance because they have had less than a 1-year history of opioid dependence, patients who must enter a controlled environment such as incarceration where methadone is not available, administrative tapers for patients who do not comply with program policies, and voluntary tapers for patients who evince a personal desire to be off methadone.

Patients who do not qualify for methadone maintenance because of less than a 1-year history of dependence may be appropriate for medically supervised withdrawal. One reasonable approach is to use a 180-day schedule to perform induction and stabilization, similar to what would be done for a maintenance patient and continue a stable dose to the 120-day mark. At that point, the dose can be tapered over 60 days with the understanding that the rate of taper should slow in the latter part of this interval. Shorter tapers can be conducted in analogous fashion.

For patients receiving an administrative discharge, the usual custom is to perform a taper over 21 days. Although this time frame almost universally militates against success, it does balance the patient having an opportunity to make alternative plans against the need to have the patient leave the program relatively quickly.

For patients requesting a voluntary taper, a number of signs of stability should be in place before considering a taper, including a substantial period without illicit drug use, a stable living situation, stable relationships, a stable source of income, and the absence of unstable medical or psychiatric conditions. The rate of taper should be adjusted to the patient's needs and expectations. It is not unusual for these types of tapers to require many months or even years depending on the starting dose. A typical rate would be a decrease of 5 to 10 mg from the daily dose every 1 to 2 weeks. It helps to inform the patient that a successful taper makes the patient feel better by reducing methadone side effects. If the patient starts to feel worse, the taper is going too rapidly. A good option is to allow the patient to halt the taper or regain the previous higher dose upon request if the patient experiences any instability. The taper should definitely be stopped if any obvious signs of instability such as a positive urine specimen or failure to comply with program rules occur. As the daily dosage drops below the 40 to 60 mg/day range, the rate of taper usually has to be decreased. Patients who successfully complete the taper should be encouraged to continue counseling and to make a decision to resume methadone if relapse seems imminent. Some patients may want to begin opioid antagonist therapy with naltrexone once they no longer have physiologic dependence, to protect themselves from relapse.

NONOPIOID SUBSTANCE USE

Patients who enter methadone-maintenance treatment for opioid dependence also have high rates of misusing other substances. Since methadone specifically targets only opioid dependence and since problematic use of other substances usually undermines stability in methadone maintenance, misuse of other substances oftentimes requires additional active interventions.

Alcohol

Among patients seeking treatment for opioid dependence, rates of alcohol dependence range from 24% for a current to 50% for a lifetime diagnosis (32,33). Excessive alcohol use causes serious medical and psychiatric morbidity, and particularly worsens the prognosis in chronic hepatitis C. Alcohol can act additively with methadone and other opioids to suppress CNS activity and respiratory drive, increasing the risk of overdose. Alcohol can also induce the activity of cytochrome P-450 enzymes (34), thereby enhancing the metabolism of methadone and destabilizing the patient. Patients who have indicators of alcohol problems tend to have poorer methadone treatment retention and more illicit drug use than patients without alcohol problems (35).

Monitoring for excessive or problematic alcohol use can prove challenging since alcohol is eliminated fairly rapidly via zero-order kinetics. Breathalyzers and routine urine tests for alcohol will only detect recent alcohol use but can and should be utilized. Tests for alcohol metabolites in urine such as ethyl glucuronide can screen for more remote alcohol use but are expensive and positive results can occur from the use of hand sanitizers, medications, and other products that contain even trace amounts of alcohol.

Active alcohol abuse or dependence when recognized in methadone maintenance should be treated aggressively. The mainstay of treatment involves one or more behavioral interventions including contingency management, motivational interviewing, relapse prevention, and 12-step facilitation with referral to Alcoholics Anonymous. Using the latter intervention would require some alterations for methadone patients who could experience stigmatization at 12-step meetings because of their methadone prescription. Pharmacologic interventions for alcohol dependence should also be considered, although naltrexone, as a μ-opioid antagonist, is contraindicated in methadone patients (as an acute dose of it will precipitate withdrawal in an opioid-dependent person). However, monitored disulfiram is used frequently. A study that compared monitored and required disulfiram to unmonitored disulfiram in methadone patients who were failing treatment because of severe alcohol dependence showed a dramatic and significant reduction in alcohol use in the monitored group (36), though a randomized-controlled trial found no difference in outcomes between disulfiram and placebo (37). Acamprosate has not been studied in methadone-maintenance patients.

Benzodiazepines

The prevalence of current benzodiazepine abuse in methadone-treated patients has been estimated between 24.9% and 50.6% (38). Patients use benzodiazepines for multiple reasons including to alleviate anxiety, to decrease restlessness or insomnia produced by stimulants, or to boost the effects of methadone, making it feel more like heroin. The respiratory depressant effects of methadone and benzodiazepines are synergistic. Use of benzodiazepines may require methadone dose reductions in the event of oversedation. If the benzodiazepines are prescribed for anxiety or insomnia, ideally the care can be coordinated and an alternative agent may be used. In the case of benzodiazepine dependence, it may not be realistic or safe to demand immediate abstinence from the benzodiazepine use. Abrupt cessation of benzodiazepines can cause a medically significant withdrawal syndrome. Options for treating benzodiazepine dependence among methadone patients include a slow outpatient taper, or admission to an inpatient unit for medically supervised withdrawal of benzodiazepines. Outpatient tapers often prove difficult because patients become symptomatic and continue use of illicit benzodiazepines. Experimental methods still undergoing study involve the substitution of anticonvulsants, which act through the gamma-aminobutyric acid (GABA) system, such as gabapentin, topiramate, or valproic acid for benzodiazepines. Use of sedatives other than benzodiazepines has become rare among methadone patients, but it should be addressed in a similar fashion to benzodiazepines.

Cocaine and Amphetamines

A diagnostic study of 716 patients who recently entered methadone treatment showed a lifetime rate of cocaine dependence of 64.7% and a current rate of 40.7% (32). In addition to the multitude of well-known toxic effects of cocaine, it can also exacerbate the risk for cardiac arrhythmia already potentially present during methadone treatment. Cocaine use during methadone treatment increases the likelihood of heroin use (39).

Behavioral treatments, particularly contingency management and cognitive–behavioral therapy, effectively reduce cocaine use among methadone patients (40). Several specific pharmacotherapy interventions for cocaine dependence among methadone patients have been tested with generally disappointing results with the exception of disulfiram, which shows considerable promise even among patients who do not have alcohol dependence (41). Disulfiram inhibits the enzyme dopamine-β-hydroxylase that catalyzes the transformation of dopamine into norepinephrine. This action potentially alters the balance between these two neurotransmitters in the brain, and thereby may mitigate the desire for and/or the effects of cocaine.

Because methamphetamine and other stimulant use among methadone patients seem to be infrequent, a paucity of data exists on this topic. Behavioral interventions would be similar to those used for cocaine.

Cannabis

Cannabis use among methadone patients is reported to range from 54% to 78.5% (42). In contrast to the very deleterious effects of alcohol, benzodiazepines, or cocaine use on methadone patients, cannabis use itself does not have a measurable negative effect on typical methadone treatment outcomes such as treatment retention, illicit opioid use, or employment. In fact, many methadone programs do not test for cannabis. Undoubtedly, some methadone patients with cannabis dependence suffer from the low motivation and cognitive disruption seen with that disorder and could benefit from cannabis abstinence. However, there is a growing body of experimental literature suggesting that stopping regular cannabis use may be difficult because of withdrawal symptoms including anxiety, depression, irritability, craving, decreased quantity and quality of sleep, and decreased appetite (43). As with other forms of substance dependence, patients with cannabis dependence usually respond to cognitive–behavioral therapy and contingency management (43). Methadone clinics can also approach the problem of cannabis use by giving positive rewards, such as take-home doses, preferential dosing, reduced fees, or counseling appointment times, for abstinence from cannabis.

Tobacco

The rate of tobacco smoking among methadone patients is about 80%, and many evince interest in quitting (44). Since methadone patients have a high prevalence of diseases caused or exacerbated by tobacco smoking, smoking cessation could have a substantial impact on health outcomes in this population. Also, heavy smoking strongly predicts cocaine and illicit opioid use among methadone patients (45). Long-term quit rates fall in the range of 5% when transdermal nicotine and intensive behavioral interventions are used. Other forms of smoking cessation pharmacotherapy such as bupropion, varenicline, or combination of transdermal nicotine with immediate release forms of nicotine replacement like gum or lozenge have not been investigated in methadone patients. Clearly, more research on both pharmacologic and behavioral interventions as well as more active application of clinical interventions known to work for tobacco dependence is needed among methadone patients.

CO-OCCURRING PSYCHIATRIC DISORDERS

Opioid-dependent patients on methadone maintenance exhibit high rates of co-occurring, non–substance-related, psychiatric disorders. Two large studies have used structured psychiatric interviews to assess psychiatric illness in opioid-dependent patients. Major depression ranged from a low of 8.7% for men in one study (32) to a high of 69% for women in the other study (33); rates of bipolar disorder ranged from 0% for women in one study to 10.8% in the other, with men falling in between; rates of anxiety disorders ranged from 6.1% to 25.4%. Rates of schizophrenia were similar to what is seen in the general population, about 1%. As for Axis II psychiatric disorders, overall rates of personality disorders range from 25.3% to 40.5% with antisocial personality being by far the most common. Neither of these studies assessed patients for posttraumatic stress disorder, but rates of posttraumatic stress disorder were determined to be 20% for women and 11% for men among methadone patients in a separate study of this specific disorder (46). Eating disorders and attention-deficit hyperactivity disorder have also been reported to occur not infrequently in methadone patients (47,48).

Assessment for co-occurring psychiatric disorders usually requires a thorough psychiatric interview. High rates of substance-induced psychiatric disorders obviously also occur among methadone patients. Ideally, observing a patient through a several week period of abstinence to see if symptoms remit may demonstrate that the disorder is not a primary psychiatric disorder and obviate the need for specific treatment. Particularly with depressive symptoms, many patients show improvement during their first week of methadone treatment (49).

It is generally believed that patients with substance dependence and co-occurring psychiatric disorders perform worse in treatment than do patients with only substance dependence, but few studies specifically examined this notion among methadone-maintenance patients. Nevertheless, active treatment directed at the non–substance-induced co-occurring disorders is recommended. In general, the treatment for these disorders should be identical to that provided to any psychiatric patient, including pharmacotherapy and psychotherapy.

Depression is one specific co-occurring disorder for which treatment among methadone patients has undergone rigorous investigation. Two double-blind, placebo-controlled trials of tricyclic antidepressants for depression among methadone patients showed that doxepin (50) in one study and imipramine (51) in the second study improved depressive symptoms significantly more than placebo, while having minimal effect on other treatment outcomes such as illicit drug use. Conversely, two placebo-controlled trials of serotonin reuptake inhibitors showed that neither fluoxetine (52) nor sertraline (53) was superior to placebo in treating depression in this population.

Aside from depression, a randomized-controlled trial of methylphenidate, bupropion, and placebo for attention-deficit hyperactivity disorder among methadone patients did not show differences on any outcomes for active medications compared to placebo (48).

Professional psychotherapy has not received rigorous investigation for specific disorders among methadone patients, but when psychiatric severity is assessed dimensionally rather than categorically, patients with low psychiatric severity derive no added benefit when psychotherapy is added to basic counseling, whereas patients with moderate or high psychiatric severity show significant improvements in outcome with the addition of psychotherapy to counseling (54).

CO-OCCURRING MEDICAL DISORDERS

Medical disorders are prevalent among opioid-addicted populations in part due to the route of drug administration. Injection drug users are at risk for infectious diseases such as pneumonia, tuberculosis, endocarditis, sexually transmitted diseases, soft tissue infections, bone and joint infections, CNS infections, and viral hepatitis. Clearly, HIV infection and acquired immunodeficiency syndrome pose a massive problem among injection drug users. Drug smoking also leads to medical complications, particularly pulmonary concerns. Cocaine and methamphetamine, taken by any route, can also cause myocardial ischemia and/or infarction as well as cardiac arrhythmias, cerebrovascular accidents, seizures, gastroduodenal ulceration, and acute renal failure. Excessive alcohol use has the potential to damage nearly every organ system. Methadone-maintenance patients need attention to these co-occurring medical disorders.

Both acute and chronic pain are not infrequent consequences of these co-occurring medical disorders or traumatic injury. A key principle in managing pain in methadone patients is that the daily methadone dose, which is intended to prevent withdrawal symptoms and opioid cravings, will not provide relief from either form of pain. When pain occurs, conservative measures such as nonsteroidal anti-inflammatory medications can be tried, but opioid analgesics should not be denied to patients on methadone if they have a painful condition for which a clinician would normally prescribe opioids. In fact, since patients on methadone may have opioid-induced hyperalgesia as well as a high level of opioid tolerance, higher doses of opioid analgesics may be required to control pain than would be used in an average, nonopioid-dependent individual with the same condition. Acute pain requiring opioids can be treated with any short-acting opioid to which the patient has a history of a good response. Chronic pain often responds well to additional amounts of methadone in pill form prescribed for pain and given in divided doses throughout the day, although other opioids can also be prescribed. If morphine is prescribed, it can conceivably confound interpretation of urine testing since heroin shows up on toxicology testing as morphine, one of heroin's major metabolites.

PSYCHOSOCIAL AND ANCILLARY SERVICES

Many patients with opioid dependence do not completely respond to methadone treatment alone. They may continue some degree of problematic substance use or struggle with core life issues such as relationships and employment. Some patients benefit from psychosocial interventions directed at the areas in which difficulties persist, although uncertainty remains as to the optimal intensity or modality of psychosocial treatments for these patients.

Studies of various intensities of psychosocial services in OTPs indicate that patients who receive minimal psychosocial services do not fare as well as those who receive moderate or high levels of services (55). However, the lower cost-effectiveness of more intensive services may nullify any slight advantage they hold over moderate services.

The accumulated general knowledge on modalities of psychotherapy indicates that individual therapist's skill at creating a therapeutic alliance has a stronger effect on outcomes in psychosocial interventions for substance dependence than the specific modality applied. Nevertheless, a variety of specific modalities have been applied to patients with opioid dependence such as individual drug counseling, cognitive–behavioral therapy, supportive–expressive psychotherapy, relapse prevention, contingency management, and medical management. A recent meta-analysis of psychosocial interventions for substance use disorders, that included interventions for opioid dependence, found that both cognitive–behavioral therapy and contingency management had positive moderate effects with contingency management holding a slight advantage (56). Psychotherapy performed better than drug counseling for patients with high psychiatric symptomatology (54).

Contingency management shapes behavior (e.g., illicit drug use) in a preferred direction (e.g., towards abstinence) by offering desired rewards contingent on behavior change, and numerous studies demonstrate its benefit in methadone maintenance (57). An approach that is already frequently applied in methadone programs, provision of methadone take-home doses contingent upon negative urine specimens, clearly increases abstinence rates (58). Another approach that shows tremendous promise grants vouchers that can be redeemed for goods or services contingent upon negative urine specimens but has not yet gained a strong foothold in clinical settings. This voucher-based contingency management approach leads to cocaine abstinence in 50% of methadone-maintained cocaine-abusing participants compared to none of the participants who receive vouchers that are not contingent upon a negative urine specimen (59). Reductions in opioid use also occur when vouchers are earned for cocaine abstinence. Using a technique in which patients who provide negative urine specimens draw vouchers from a bowl containing many vouchers of varying value significantly reduced stimulant use among methadone patients at an average cost for the awarded goods and services of $10 per week per participant (60). Ideally, in light of its efficacy, voucher-based contingency management will receive increasing use in methadone-maintenance programs.

As a consequence of long periods of opioid dependence, methadone-maintenance patients tend to have deficits in several life areas in addition to substance dependence and medical and psychiatric problems. They are likely to have legal difficulties, educational, vocational and financial problems, relationship and family issues, and an absence of healthy recreational activities. There is some evidence that targeting ancillary psychosocial services specifically to address these patient problem areas is beneficial (55). If such services are not available onsite, a referral network that facilitates connecting patients to needed services is desirable.

URINE TESTING

Drug testing identifies ongoing or sporadic drug use and potential safety issues. The results should be used as part of the treatment plan; a negative test should be used to discuss successful strategies, and a positive test to explore obstacles to abstinence and to identify additional recovery resources. Positive tests for illicit drugs may result in loss of take-home privileges. To avoid confusion between licit and illicit drugs, programs generally require the patient to report or bring in all prescriptions for controlled substances and to coordinate care with the prescriber. In the case of prescription opioids for pain, a confirmatory test can be obtained to distinguish the prescription opioid from heroin. The frequency of urine testing can be increased after a positive test result in order to clarify a lapse from a more extensive relapse.

Fear of sanction such as loss of take-home doses may lead a patient to avoid testing positive for drugs of abuse by tampering with the urine sample. Tampering methods include diluting the sample, adding substances designed to mask a positive test and substituting with a sample not containing drugs of abuse. To discourage tampering, programs are required to test on a random schedule. Reliance on urine observation to minimize falsification is not required, although at times it may be necessary. Temperature testing is less intrusive and can also identify altered specimens. A laboratory can check the validity of a urine sample by performing a urine creatinine analysis. The concentration of creatinine can be used to determine if the sample has been diluted by adulteration or by drinking an excessive amount of liquid.

Testing for methadone and methadone metabolite serves as an important diversion safeguard. Patients who are positive for methadone but negative for metabolite need to be evaluated. This result suggests that the methadone was put directly into the urine sample. Patients may legitimately provide a negative screen for methadone if they have a rapid metabolism or are on very low doses, or have missed doses. To avoid a false result, the commonly used less costly enzyme immunoassay can be confirmed with gas chromatography–mass spectrometry analysis.

TAKE-HOME STATUS

Regulations allow take-home doses of methadone for stable patients and, in fact, can ultimately be advanced to a maximum of a 1-month supply of take-home doses for patients in continuous treatment for 2 years or longer. Since patients highly value take-home doses, take-home privileges can be effectively used in a contingency management plan as described above. Patients who comply with program rules and responsibilities including abstinence from illicit drug use get rewarded with additional take-home doses. Patients who do not comply and/or supply positive urine specimens get punished by rapid removal of take-home doses. Such procedures actually reduce illicit drug use (58).

OTP physicians must consider the patient's ability to store, take, and transport take-home doses safely. Friends and family members other than the patient are susceptible to accidental overdose from take-home medication. Federal criteria for take-home privileges include: (1) absence of recent abuse of drugs (opioid or non-narcotic) including alcohol; (2) regularity of clinic attendance; (3) absence of serious behavioral problems at clinic; (4) absence of known recent criminal activity, for example, drug dealing; (5) stability of the patient's home environment and social relationships; (6) length of time in comprehensive maintenance treatment; (7) assurance that take-home medication can be safely stored within the patient's home; (8) determination that the rehabilitative benefit to the patient derived from decreasing frequency of clinic attendance outweighs the potential risk of diversion. Many programs are closed for dispensing on Sundays and holidays. Typically, it does not pose an undue risk to provide a take-home dose once per week on days the clinic is closed for patients who do not strictly meet all of these criteria. Occasionally, an individual patient may be so unstable that arrangements must be made to provide observed methadone dosing 7 days per week.

DIVERSION RISK REDUCTION PLAN

Physicians must weigh the risk of diversion against the benefits to the patient. For instance, when a urine drug test result is negative for methadone or metabolite, additional analysis is needed to determine if there is a logical explanation or indication of urine tampering or methadone diversion. Although diversion of take-home doses of methadone to individuals for whom it is not prescribed certainly occurs, few data exist to indicate the frequency of such events. A study of methadone medical maintenance (see below) in which subjects received either 5 or 6 days versus 27 days of take-home medication used random monthly medication callbacks by which subjects are notified to return to the clinic within 24 hours with all outstanding medication (61). In this scenario, if individuals do not have all expected medication in hand, diversion can be inferred. The study found that over a 12-month period of treatment 0.9% to 5.0% of subjects possessed an incorrect amount of medication at the time of callback, and 1.7% to 5.6% failed to return for the callback. In a survey in Australia of patients receiving methadone maintenance at community pharmacies, 12.6% admitted to ever having diverted or trying to divert their methadone, and 2.2% admitted to diverting or trying to divert methadone in the past 12 months (62). The number of take-home doses did not differ between diverters and nondiverters.

Thus, from the data available, methadone diversion is not an exceedingly common event, but some diversion of methadone will inevitably occur, so programs must develop and apply diversion reduction plans. Unfortunately, no data exist to guide programs toward the optimum approach. Diversion reduction plans must therefore rely on practicality and common sense. Careful application of criteria for take-home eligibility and removal of take-home privileges quickly with evidence of instability as enumerated above constitute the foundations of diversion reduction. Instituting a random callback system is also feasible and creates an additional safeguard. As conveyed by King et al. (61), programs can randomly phone a few patients each week and ask them to return within 24 hours with all methadone expected to be in their possession. Rare events of diversion will be detected by the callbacks, and all take-home privileges can be revoked from patients who fail the callbacks. Equally important, the callbacks may have a deterrent effect whereby patients who might be tempted to divert methadone refrain from doing so because of concern about failing a callback and losing their take-home privileges.

MANAGING PROBLEMATIC BEHAVIOR

Since methadone patients are by definition illicit drug users, since the prevalence of antisocial personality is high in this population, and since federal regulations stipulate certain requirements for the patients such as attendance at counseling, provision of urine specimens, and meeting specific criteria to obtain take-home doses, problematic behaviors by patients are bound to arise. Problematic behaviors include loss or misuse of take-home doses, loitering, drug possession or dealing on the premises, methadone diversion, theft, falsification of urine specimens, intoxication in the clinic, and, most seriously, verbal abuse, threats, or actual violence such as fighting.

Prevention of problematic behavior represents a necessary first step. Establishing a clear program structure and conveying to all patients a set of expectations and rules both orally and in writing at the outset and throughout treatment and then enforcing the expectations consistently and fairly will encourage patients to keep their behavior within appropriate boundaries. Reinforcing compliant behavior by provision of program privileges such as take-home doses and preferential dosing or appointment times will also support desired behavior. Regular counseling sessions provide patients an opportunity to adopt alternative, more functional coping strategies when they are faced with stressors that might lead them to engage in problematic behaviors.

When problematic behaviors do occur, the program has essentially two sanctions available as a consequence: (1) removal of take-home privileges or denial of take-homes for some specified time into the future and (2) program discharge. Oftentimes a dynamic tension exists between the direct interests of the patient and maintaining the integrity and safe milieu of the program necessitating difficult clinical and administrative decisions. Frequent discharge, even if it is not beneficial to the patient, becomes the only realistic option.

Occasionally patients return to the clinic to report theft, loss, or misuse of their take-home doses. Generally, unless the patient can provide a police report documenting that the take-homes were stolen, missing take-homes should not be replaced. If lost take-homes are replaced, diversion could be inadvertently encouraged. If the patient has admitted loss of take-home doses, there is clear evidence that the patient is not sufficiently responsible to manage take-home doses, and the patient should be placed on daily observed ingestion for some period of time. Similarly, if a patient reports running out of take-home doses because of taking a larger dose than prescribed, take-home privileges should be suspended, and the patient should be evaluated for a methadone dose increase.

Loitering can usually be handled through repeated warnings and removal of take-home privileges. Rarely would loitering require program discharge.

In contrast, drug possession or dealing on the premises, methadone diversion, and theft all involve criminal activity. Criminal activity seriously contaminates the milieu and interferes with the welfare of compliant patients. In most cases when such criminal activity is detected, program discharge is the most reasonable response. Falsification of urine specimens falls somewhere in between. A patient who attempts to falsify by, for example, bringing in someone else's urine or adulterating or diluting the specimen, presumably is motivated by a desire to obtain or maintain take-home doses that would be lost because of a drug-containing specimen. In that case, removal of take-home privileges for a specified time such as several months may be an adequate response to deter such behavior in the future. Repeated attempts at falsification may render discharge necessary.

A patient appearing intoxicated in the clinic poses both safety and liability concerns and requires several immediate actions. The patient should be evaluated by medical staff to determine if the methadone dose should be withheld or if is it safe to provide a partial dose such as 50% of the usual dose or less. If the intoxication appears serious, the patient should be transferred to an emergency room for monitoring and possible administration of naloxone if the intoxication is due to opioids or flumazenil if due to benzodiazepines. If the intoxication appears to be mild, the patient should be observed in the clinic until the intoxication resolves. If alcohol is involved, ideally a breathalyzer reading should be obtained, and the patient not released until below the legal limit. If the patient drove a vehicle to the clinic, the keys should be taken from the patient and not returned until the intoxication has resolved. Should the patient be noncompliant and attempt to drive while still intoxicated, the police should be called to protect public safety. Assuming the patient is cooperative, once the intoxication resolves, medical staff can determine if it is safe to give the patient methadone that day and initiate a plan to prevent further episodes of intoxication.

A repeated pattern of appearing intoxicated in the clinic raises the issue of whether the patient can be safely treated with methadone in an outpatient setting. If inpatient treatment is available, it should be strongly considered. If inpatient treatment is not available or is tried and fails to eliminate the episodes of intoxication, after ample warnings in writing with the patient as a signatory, discharge from methadone treatment may be the only option.

Verbal abuse, threats, or actual violence create a direct safety risk to other patients and staff, and, if permitted, make attending treatment or working at the program untenable. In these instances program, discharge is almost always the only reasonable course to pursue. Patients who incur an administrative discharge for any of these reasons would usually be given a 21-day methadone taper. In rare cases because of safety concerns, an immediate termination of methadone may be needed. Also, all clinics need to have an appeal or advocacy process whereby the patient can present any evidence that the purported infraction was not actually committed or that extenuating circumstances place the infraction in a different perspective. Even if a decision to remove take-home doses or discharge is not reversed, this process can be therapeutic for the patient by attempting to show that the program staff care about the patient as a person while not tolerating the behavior. Oftentimes, depending on the nature of the problematic behavior, transfer to another clinic can be facilitated or readmission at a later date can be planned contingent on resolution of the problematic behaviors.

METHADONE IN PREGNANCY

Methadone maintenance is the preferred treatment for opioid addiction during pregnancy. Because of its long duration of action, methadone provides reasonably constant opioid effects, thereby preventing the fetus from undergoing repeated cycles of excessive effect punctuated by periods of withdrawal that would occur in a pregnant woman using short-acting, illicit opioids (63). Case studies suggest that compared to no treatment, to treatment without medication, or to medically supervised withdrawal, methadone maintenance along with prenatal care reduces the risk of maternal and fetal complications (64). A recent study specifically examined outcomes for pregnant women receiving ongoing methadone maintenance compared to methadone withdrawal and found that those receiving maintenance stayed in treatment longer, attended more obstetrical visits, and more often delivered at the program hospital (63).

The basic approach to methadone treatment is similar for pregnant women as for other patients, but the physiology of pregnancy does demand careful attention to methadone dose adjustment. During the latter stages of pregnancy, particularly the third trimester, increasing blood volumes in pregnant women almost always creates the need for an increased dose of methadone. The need for this increase should be anticipated so that withdrawal symptoms and instability related to inadequate dose do not occur and create added stress on the fetus or lead to illicit opioid use. At times a single daily methadone dose does not fully prevent emergence of opioid withdrawal in a pregnant woman. In that case the patient should receive a split dose of methadone if it is logistically possible for the patient to attend the clinic twice daily or if the patient qualifies for take-home doses (64).

Methadone should be continued during and after delivery. For most women, the methadone dose needs to be reduced postpartum guided by careful clinical monitoring, generally either to a dose similar to the stable dose prior to pregnancy or, for women who began methadone maintenance during pregnancy, at approximately half the dosages they received in the third trimester (64).

Although methadone is excreted in breast milk, most mothers maintained on methadone should be encouraged to breast-feed because the health advantages of breast-feeding outweigh the risks of infant exposure to methadone. Exceptions occur for women who are HIV positive and/or who have ongoing use of illicit drugs or alcohol. Hepatitis C infection does not pose a contraindication to breast-feeding (64).

Methadone use during pregnancy predisposes the newborn to the neonatal abstinence syndrome (NAS), characterized by signs and symptoms of central and autonomic nervous system regulatory dysfunction (65). High variability occurs among infants in both incidence and severity of NAS, neither of which appear to be directly related to the maternal methadone dose level or duration of methadone exposure (65). Caretakers sometimes can treat infants with NAS solely with nonpharmacologic treatment, which generally involves reduction in external stimulation and physical soothing (66). Most, however, require pharmacologic treatment, which typically involves some form of opioid medication. Protocols vary from center to center, and no data currently support one strategy over another.

MEDICAL MAINTENANCE

Over the past 25 years, U.S. experimental models of methadone treatment for opioid dependence have been evaluated in which patients who have already stabilized in an OTP transfer their methadone care to a physician practicing in an office-based setting, otherwise known as medical maintenance. Typically, these patients come in to pick up their methadone once per week to once per month, see the physician, provide a urine specimen, and receive take-home doses until the next appointment. Both uncontrolled trials and randomized-controlled trials indicate that the majority of already stabilized patients succeed in medical-maintenance treatment and that patients randomly assigned to medical maintenance have equivalent outcomes to clinic-based patients (61). The studies also show that patients who do poorly in medical maintenance can readily return to routine clinic-based treatment (61). On a pragmatic level, while such medical-maintenance treatment of stabilized methadone patients is legally permissible in the United States via an exception to the methadone treatment regulations, the process to obtain such an exception is sufficiently cumbersome that very few medical-maintenance practices have been established outside the research setting.

INTERIM MAINTENANCE

In some areas of the United States, methadone treatment services are not readily and immediately available to all individuals seeking such treatment. Interim methadone maintenance is designed as a service that provides medication-only treatment as an alternative to having individuals who desire methadone treatment wait with no treatment until a slot in comprehensive treatment becomes available. As per federal regulations, interim methadone provides methadone induction and then a daily, stable observed dose of methadone with no take-home doses and no other services except emergency counseling. Although, as noted above, comprehensive methadone treatment shows superior outcomes to medication-only treatment, interim methadone compared to a wait-list control in at least three randomized-controlled trials demonstrated reduced illicit drug use and higher rates of subsequent entry into comprehensive methadone treatment (5).

CONCLUSION

Methadone maintenance has a long history of efficacy in the treatment of opioid dependence. Federal regulations provide specific requirements necessary to deliver methadone maintenance. Methadone has several pharmacologic characteristics, particularly its slow onset and long half-life, which make it ideal as a medication to treat opioid dependence but which also demand extensive knowledge and care for it to be prescribed safely. Medical personnel in OTPs must know proper procedures for methadone induction, how to determine an appropriate stable dose of methadone, how to manage side effects, and about methadone drug interactions.

Opioid-dependent patients treated with methadone often have complex presentations, with use of multiple substances in addition to opioids, and with a high prevalence of co-occurring medical and psychiatric disorders. Specific treatments directed toward these other disorders along with a moderate level of ongoing counseling can improve outcomes. Careful clinical monitoring including urine testing and a diversion risk reduction plan help to determine when take-home doses of methadone are indicated and can also help to prevent problematic behavior by patients which must be actively addressed when it occurs.

Methadone is a well-established treatment for pregnant women with opioid dependence and leads to improved fetal outcomes compared to no treatment. Increasing evidence shows that less restrictive forms of methadone maintenance, such as medical maintenance, and less intensive forms, such as interim maintenance, are safe and effective to treat the individual and address the public health and public safety aspects of opioid addiction. As the knowledge base about evidence-based practices in methadone maintenance continues to grow, this well-established modality should diversify and expand to treat an increasing number of opioid-dependent individuals throughout the 21st century.

REFERENCES

1. Barnett PG. The cost-effectiveness of methadone maintenance as a health care intervention. *Addiction*. 1999;94:479–488.
2. Darke S, Zador D. Fatal heroin 'overdose': a review. *Addiction*. 1996;91:1765–1772.
3. Mattick RP, Breen C, Kimber J, et al. Methadone maintenance therapy versus no opioid replacement therapy for opioid dependence. *Cochrane Database Syst Rev*. 2003:CD002209.
4. Marsch LA. The efficacy of methadone maintenance interventions in reducing illicit opiate use, HIV risk behavior and criminality: a meta-analysis. *Addiction*. 1998;93:515–532.
5. Schwartz RP, Highfield DA, Jaffe JH, et al. A randomized controlled trial of interim methadone maintenance. *Arch Gen Psychiatry*. 2006;63:102–109.
6. Gowing LR, Farrell M, Bornemann R, et al. Brief report: methadone treatment of injecting opioid users for prevention of HIV infection. *J Gen Intern Med*. 2006;21:193–195.
7. Gunne LM, Gronbladh L. The swedish methadone maintenance program: a controlled study. *Drug Alcohol Depend*. 1981;7:249–256.
8. Fugelstad A, Agren G, Romelsjo A. Changes in mortality, arrests, and hospitalizations in nonvoluntarily treated heroin addicts in relation to methadone treatment. *Subst Use Misuse*. 1998; 33: 2803–2817.
9. Leavitt SB, Shinderman M, Maxwell S, et al. When "enough" is not enough: new perspectives on optimal methadone maintenance dose. *Mt Sinai J Med*. 2000;67:404–411.
10. Ferrari A, Coccia CP, Bertolini A, et al. Methadone—metabolism, pharmacokinetics and interactions. *Pharmacol Res*. 2004;50: 551–559.
11. Inturrisi CE, Verebely K. The levels of methadone in the plasma in methadone maintenance. *Clin Pharmacol Ther*. 1972;13: 633–637.
12. Eap CB, Buclin T, et al. Interindividual variability of the clinical pharmacokinetics of methadone: implications for the treatment of opioid dependence. *Clin Pharmacokinet*. 2002;41:1153–1193.
13. Moody DE, Alburges ME, Parker RJ, et al. The involvement of cytochrome P450 3A4 in the N-demethylation of L-alpha-acetylmethadol (LAAM), nor LAAM, and methadone. *Drug Metab Dispos*. 1997;25:1347–1353.
14. Eap CB, Broly F, Mino A, et al. Cytochrome P450 2D6 genotype and methadone steady-state concentrations. *J Clin Psychopharmacol*. 2001;21:229–234.
15. Kharasch ED, Walker A, Whittington D, et al. Methadone metabolism and clearance are induced by nelfinavir despite inhibition of cytochrome P4503A (CYP3A) activity. *Drug Alcohol Depend*. 2009;101:158–168.
16. Inturrisi CE. The role of N-methyl-D-aspartate (NMDA) receptors in pain and morphine tolerance. *Minerva Anestesiol*. 2005;71:401–403.
17. Eap CB, Crettol S, Rougier JS, et al. Stereoselective block of hERG channel by (S)-methadone and QT interval prolongation in CYP2B6 slow metabolizers. *Clin Pharmacol Ther*. 2007;81: 719–728.

18. Corkery JM, Schifano F, Ghodse AH, et al. The effects of methadone and its role in fatalities. *Hum Psychopharmacol.* 2004;19:565–576.
19. Davis AM, Inturrisi CE. D-methadone blocks morphine tolerance and N-methyl-D-aspartate-induced hyperalgesia. *J Pharmacol Exp Ther.* 1999;289:1048–1053.
20. Strain EC, Bigelow GE, Liebson IA, et al. Moderate- vs high-dose methadone in the treatment of opioid dependence: a randomized trial. *JAMA.* 1999;281:1000–1005.
21. Eap CB, Bourquin M, Martin J, et al. Plasma concentrations of the enantiomers of methadone and therapeutic response in methadone maintenance treatment. *Drug Alcohol Depend.* 2000;61:47–54.
22. Dyer KR, Foster DJ, White JM, et al. Steady-state pharmacokinetics and pharmacodynamics in methadone maintenance patients: comparison of those who do and do not experience withdrawal and concentration–effect relationships. *Clin Pharmacol Ther.* 1999;65:685–694.
23. Cobb MN, Desai J, Brown LS Jr., et al. The effect of fluconazole on the clinical pharmacokinetics of methadone. *Clin Pharmacol Ther.* 1998;63:655–662.
24. Tarumi Y, Pereira J, Watanabe S. Methadone and fluconazole: respiratory depression by drug interaction. *J Pain Symptom Manage.* 2002;23:148–153.
25. Armstrong SC, Cozza KL. Med-psych drug–drug interactions update. *Psychosomatics.* 2001;42:435–437.
26. Mahe I, Chassany O, Grenard AS, et al. Methadone and edema: a case-report and literature review. *Eur J Clin Pharmacol.* 2004;59:923–924.
27. Kreek MJ, Hartman N. Chronic use of opioids and antipsychotic drugs: side effects, effects on endogenous opioids, and toxicity. *Ann NY Acad Sci.* 1982;398:151–172.
28. Kim TW, Alford DP, Malabanan A, et al. Low bone density in patients receiving methadone maintenance treatment. *Drug Alcohol Depend.* 2006;85:258–262.
29. Langrod J, Lowinson J, Ruiz P. Methadone treatment and physical complaints: a clinical analysis. *Int J Addict.* 1981;16:947–952.
30. Calsyn DA, Malcy JA, Saxon AJ. Slow tapering from methadone maintenance in a program encouraging indefinite maintenance. *J Subst Abuse Treat.* 2006;30:159–163.
31. Senay EC, Dorus W, Goldberg F, et al. Withdrawal from methadone maintenance. Rate of withdrawal and expectation. *Arch Gen Psychiatry.* 1977;34:361–367.
32. Brooner RK, King VL, Kidorf M, et al. Psychiatric and substance use comorbidity among treatment-seeking opioid abusers. *Arch Gen Psychiatry.* 1997;54:71–80.
33. Rounsaville BJ, Weissman MM, Kleber HD. The significance of alcoholism in treated opiate addicts. *J Nerv Ment Dis.* 1982;170:479–488.
34. Lieber CS. Microsomal ethanol-oxidizing system (MEOS): the first 30 years (1968–1998)—a review. *Alcohol Clin Exp Res.* 1999;23:991–1007.
35. Stenbacka M, Beck O, Leifman A, et al. Problem drinking in relation to treatment outcome among opiate addicts in methadone maintenance treatment. *Drug Alcohol Rev.* 2007;26:55–63.
36. Liebson IA, Tommasello A, Bigelow GE. A behavioral treatment of alcoholic methadone patients. *Ann Intern Med.* 1978;89:342–344.
37. Ling W, Weiss DG, Charuvastra VC, et al. Use of disulfiram for alcoholics in methadone maintenance programs. A veterans administration cooperative study. *Arch Gen Psychiatry.* 1983;40:851–854.
38. Gelkopf M, Bleich A, Hayward R, et al. Characteristics of benzodiazepine abuse in methadone maintenance treatment patients: a 1 year prospective study in an Israeli clinic. *Drug Alcohol Depend.* 1999;55:63–68.
39. Hartel DM, Schoenbaum EE, Selwyn PA, et al. Heroin use during methadone maintenance treatment: the importance of methadone dose and cocaine use. *Am J Public Health.* 1995;85:83–88.
40. Rawson RA, Huber A, McCann M, et al. A comparison of contingency management and cognitive-behavioral approaches during methadone maintenance treatment for cocaine dependence. *Arch Gen Psychiatry.* 2002;59:817–824.
41. Petrakis IL, Carroll KM, Nich C, et al. Disulfiram treatment for cocaine dependence in methadone-maintained opioid addicts. *Addiction.* 2000;95:219–228.
42. Saxon AJ, Calsyn DA, Greenberg D, et al. Urine screening for marijuana among methadone maintenance patients. *Am J Addict.* 1993;2:207–211.
43. Elkashef A, Vocci F, Huestis M, et al. Marijuana neurobiology and treatment. *Subst Abus.* 2008;29:17–29.
44. Nahvi S, Richter K, Li X, et al. Cigarette smoking and interest in quitting in methadone maintenance patients. *Addict Behav.* 2006;31:2127–2134.
45. Frosch DL, Shoptaw S, Nahom D, et al. Associations between tobacco smoking and illicit drug use among methadone-maintained opiate-dependent individuals. *Exp Clin Psychopharmacol.* 2000;8:97–103.
46. Villagomez RE, Meyer TJ, Lin MM, et al. Post-traumatic stress disorder among inner city methadone maintenance patients. *J Subst Abuse Treat.* 1995;12:253–257.
47. Mason BJ, Kocsis JH, Melia D, et al. Psychiatric comorbidity in methadone maintained patients. *J Addict Dis.* 1998;17:75–89.
48. Levin FR, Evans SM, Brooks DJ, et al. Treatment of methadone-maintained patients with adult ADHD: double-blind comparison of methylphenidate, bupropion and placebo. *Drug Alcohol Depend.* 2006;81:137–148.
49. Strain EC, Stitzer ML, Bigelow GE. Early treatment time course of depressive symptoms in opiate addicts. *J Nerv Ment Dis.* 1991;179:215–221.
50. Woody GE, O'Brien CP, Rickels K. Depression and anxiety in heroin addicts: a placebo-controlled study of doxepin in combination with methadone. *Am J Psychiatry.* 1975;132:447–450.
51. Nunes EV, Quitkin FM, Donovan SJ, et al. Imipramine treatment of opiate-dependent patients with depressive disorders. A placebo-controlled trial. *Arch Gen Psychiatry.* 1998;55:153–160.
52. Petrakis I, Carroll KM, Nich C, et al. Fluoxetine treatment of depressive disorders in methadone-maintained opioid addicts. *Drug Alcohol Depend.* 1998;50:221–226.
53. Carpenter KM, Brooks AC, Vosburg SK, et al. The effect of sertraline and environmental context on treating depression and illicit substance use among methadone maintained opiate dependent patients: a controlled clinical trial. *Drug Alcohol Depend.* 2004;74:123–134.
54. Woody GE, McLellan AT, Luborsky L, et al. Severity of psychiatric symptoms as a predictor of benefits from psychotherapy: the Veterans Administration-Penn study. *Am J Psychiatry.* 1984;141:1172–1177.
55. McLellan AT, Arndt IO, Metzger DS, et al. The effects of psychosocial services in substance abuse treatment. *JAMA.* 1993;269:1953–1959.

56. Dutra L, Stathopoulou G, Basden SL, et al. A meta-analytic review of psychosocial interventions for substance use disorders. *Am J Psychiatry*. 2008;165:179–187.
57. Griffith JD, Rowan-Szal GA, Roark RR, et al. Contingency management in outpatient methadone treatment: a meta-analysis. *Drug Alcohol Depend*. 2000;58:55–66.
58. Stitzer ML, Iguchi MY, Felch LJ. Contingent take-home incentive: effects on drug use of methadone maintenance patients. *J Consult Clin Psychol*. 1992;60:927–934.
59. Silverman K, Higgins ST, Brooner RK, et al. Sustained cocaine abstinence in methadone maintenance patients through voucher-based reinforcement therapy. *Arch Gen Psychiatry*. 1996;53:409–415.
60. Peirce JM, Petry NM, Stitzer ML, et al. Effects of lower-cost incentives on stimulant abstinence in methadone maintenance treatment: a national drug abuse treatment clinical trials network study. *Arch Gen Psychiatry*. 2006;63:201–208.
61. King VL, Kidorf MS, Stoller KB, et al. A 12-month controlled trial of methadone medical maintenance integrated into an adaptive treatment model. *J Subst Abuse Treat*. 2006;31:385–393.
62. Winstock AR, Lea T, Sheridan J. Prevalence of diversion and injection of methadone and buprenorphine among clients receiving opioid treatment at community pharmacies in New South Wales, Australia. *Int J Drug Policy*. 2008;19:450–458.
63. Jones HE, O'Grady KE, Malfi D, et al. Methadone maintenance vs. methadone taper during pregnancy: maternal and neonatal outcomes. *Am J Addict*. 2008;17:372–386.
64. Jones HE, Martin PR, Heil SH, et al. Treatment of opioid-dependent pregnant women: clinical and research issues. *J Subst Abuse Treat*. 2008;35:245–259.
65. Jansson LM, Choo R, Velez ML, et al. Methadone maintenance and breastfeeding in the neonatal period. *Pediatrics*. 2008;121:106–114.
66. Velez NM, Garcia IE, Garcia L, et al. The use of illicit drugs during pregnancy among mothers of premature infants. *PR Health Sci J*. 2008;27:209–212.

CHAPTER 29
Buprenorphine in the Treatment of Opioid Dependence

D. Andrew Tompkins ■ Eric C. Strain

INTRODUCTION

Opioid abuse and dependence remain substantial public health problems throughout much of the world. The United Nations estimates that between 15 and 21 million persons between the ages of 15 and 64 used illicit opioids in 2007, with the greatest use in Asia and Europe (1). In the United States, the 2008 National Survey on Drug Use and Health (NSDUH) estimated 1.7 million persons aged 12 and older were dependent or abusing prescription pain relievers and that 282,000 persons were dependent or abusing heroin (2). Prescription opioids have become widely available for the treatment of pain, and consequently have become more likely to be abused than heroin in the United States. Individual and societal costs of opioid dependence include incarceration, infectious diseases, increased health service utilization, loss of productivity, and death. Up until 1996, methadone, levomethadyl acetate, and naltrexone were the only pharmacologic agents approved to treat opioid dependence; in that year, France was the first country to approve the use of buprenorphine for this treatment. Since the late 1990s, buprenorphine has gained widespread use in the world. This chapter describes the history of buprenorphine, its associated pharmacokinetic and pharmacodynamic properties, the efficacy of this treatment, its optimal use in clinical practice, safety concerns, regulatory issues, and its use in special populations.

HISTORY

The chemical compound known as buprenorphine, 17-(cyclopropylmethyl)-alpha-(1,1-dimethylethyl)-4,5-epoxy-18,19-dihydro-3-hydroxy-6-methoxy-alpha-methyl-6,14-ethenomorphinan-7-methanol, hydrochloride, [5-alpha, 7-alpha (S)], was first synthesized in 1966 (Reckitt and Colman, Hull, UK) and quickly found use as a potent analgesic agent (3). Jasinski and colleagues learned about the unique partial agonist qualities of buprenorphine and hypothesized that this agent might also be used in the treatment of opioid dependence. In experiments they conducted at the Addiction Research Center, adult males with prior opioid dependence were maintained on 8 mg/day of subcutaneous (SC) buprenorphine; when these individuals were given acute doses of morphine, they experienced an attenuated euphoric response (4). When three of these same individuals were given acute doses of 4 mg SC naloxone, they had on average fewer withdrawal signs and symptoms than seven individuals maintained on morphine 30 mg SC four times daily, prompting the researchers to conclude buprenorphine had less risk of misuse and showed promise as a pharmacologic agent in the treatment of opioid dependence. These early results were substantiated when buprenorphine was shown to decrease heroin self-administration in heroin-dependent individuals (5). Buprenorphine was also shown to have a ceiling for euphoric effects, and it could almost completely block acute opioid effects for 24 hours with residual blockade of acute effects lasting for 98 hours after drug administration (6,7).

After these promising results, a sublingual (SL) version was developed for human clinical trials. Studies examining the efficacy of 8 mg SL buprenorphine as compared to low and high doses of methadone for maintenance therapy initially were conducted. One trial did not show a positive effect in terms of reducing relapse and improving retention in treatment over 52 weeks (8), whereas two other trials showed equivalence of buprenorphine with methadone (9,10) in terms of retention and opioid positive urine samples. Except for the flexible dosing strategy used in one study (10), these initial trials only tested a fixed 8 mg daily SL buprenorphine dose. Further trials showed superiority of 12 mg (11) and 16 mg doses of buprenorphine (12) to low dose methadone. In a major clinical trial (13), 220 opioid-dependent persons according to Diagnostic and Statistical Manual of Mental Disorders, 4th edition (DSM-IV) criteria (14) were randomized to low-dose methadone (20 mg), high-dose methadone (60 to 100 mg), buprenorphine (16 to 32 mg), or levomethadyl acetate (LAAM) (75 to 115 mg). Study retention rates were much greater and opioid use was much less in the high-dose methadone, LAAM, and buprenorphine treatment arms as compared to the low-dose methadone group. High-dose methadone had the highest retention rate (73%) followed by buprenorphine (58%) and LAAM (53%), although these results were not statistically different. LAAM had the lowest rate of opioid positive urinalysis per week (53%) followed by buprenorphine (62%) and methadone (62%). Given the preponderance of evidence, the U.S. Food and Drug Administration (FDA) gave approval for the use of buprenorphine (Subutex) and buprenorphine/naloxone (Suboxone) in the treatment of opioid dependence in the United States in October 2002, 6 years after approval in France.

As a partial agonist with a longer time to peak effect relative to morphine, buprenorphine has many useful features as a pharmaceutical treatment for opioid dependence. However, it is an opioid and has potential for abuse. Case reports of buprenorphine diversion and illicit use from New Zealand were published as early as 1983, where buprenorphine was marketed for analgesia as Temgesic (15). More reports came from other countries throughout the 1980s and early 1990s. Given a growing concern of diversion, a combination product with buprenorphine and naloxone was developed to decrease the risk of illicit use by injection. The abuse liability of the combination product was examined in a double-blind, randomized within subject study of persons maintained on low-dose methadone. The study showed that administration of SC buprenorphine 0.2 mg + naloxone 0.2 mg as well as buprenorphine 0.3 mg + naloxone 0.2 mg had similar subjective and objective effects as naloxone alone (16). These results suggested that the combination of the two medications had low abuse liability. However, the 1:1 ratio needed refinement, as there were many unpleasant opioid withdrawal effects in the sample.

To discover the optimal ratio of buprenorphine to naloxone, Mendelson and colleagues looked at ratios of buprenorphine to naloxone in morphine-maintained individuals (17). They found that ratios of 2:1 and 4:1 provided the maximum decrease in euphoric effects of morphine with the minimum amount of withdrawal effects. A further study confirmed that the optimal ratio was 4:1 buprenorphine to naloxone (18). Efficacy studies showed that the naloxone was not well absorbed when given in a SL formulation, and that the combination product (given in 16/4 mg daily doses for 4 weeks) produced similar reductions in illicit opioid use as buprenorphine 16 mg alone (19). An observational study demonstrated longer-term utility in 53 opioid-dependent persons treated in a primary care setting, but retention was still 38% at 2 years (20).

PHARMACOKINETICS

Buprenorphine has low oral bioavailability due to substantial first-pass metabolism in the small intestine and liver, so the medication has been administered intravenously (IV), intramuscularly (IM), sublingually, and transdermally (TD). Original efficacy studies in the treatment of opioid withdrawal and dependence used a SL buprenorphine solution dissolved in 30% ethanol, whereas buprenorphine is currently marketed as a SL tablet with and without the addition of naloxone. The most widely used buprenorphine formulations in the United States for opioid dependence are SL buprenorphine hydrochloride (Subutex) or buprenorphine hydrochloride combined with naloxone hydrochloride in a 4:1 ratio (Suboxone), both manufactured by Reckitt Benckiser Healthcare Ltd. (Hull, UK). A generic formulation of buprenorphine came onto the U.S. market in October 2009 and is manufactured by Roxane Laboratories (Columbus, OH).

Pharmacokinetic studies of the SL tablet (8 mg) compared to the SL buprenorphine solution (8 mg/mL) revealed a relative bioavailability of 49% (based on area under the curve [AUC]) in an acute dosing model of nondependent volunteers (21), but this could range between 60% and 70% (AUC) after 7 to 14 days of daily buprenorphine dosing (22,23). There is large intersubject variability in the SL absorption of buprenorphine, but there seems to be less intrasubject variability especially when examining the SL tablet formulation. SL absorption usually is dependent on saliva pH and length of time held under the tongue, but one study failed to find a clinically significant difference in buprenorphine absorption at differing saliva pHs and at times greater than 2.5 to 3 minutes held under the tongue (24). In clinical practice, patients are told to hold the tablet under their tongue until it dissolves, which occurs on average after 5 minutes. In some people, tablet particles can still remain after 10 minutes, but this does not affect bioavailability of buprenorphine.

Buprenorphine is highly lipophilic and therefore has a large volume of distribution. In plasma, it is usually protein bound but readily crosses the blood–brain barrier. Buprenorphine is metabolized by enzymatic transformation, mainly through the cytochrome P450 3A4 isozyme to the active metabolite norbuprenorphine (25). After glucuronidation, buprenorphine and its metabolites are excreted primarily through the fecal route (70%) as unconjugated buprenorphine or the metabolite norbuprenorphine. Around 30% is excreted in urine in the conjugated form, and dose adjustments usually do not need to be made in persons with severe renal impairment or who are on dialysis. Buprenorphine and its major metabolite are inhibitors of cytochrome P450 3A4 and 2D6 and could show significant drug–drug interactions if concomitant drugs that affect these enzymes are taken (26).

The addition of naloxone does not interfere with buprenorphine's pharmacokinetics but is mainly used as a deterrent against diversion and parenteral misuse of buprenorphine. There is very little absorption (≤10%) of SL administered naloxone. Naloxone is metabolized using similar enzymatic transformation and glucuronidation as buprenorphine, although its elimination half-life is much shorter (1 to 2 hours) when compared to buprenorphine. Naloxone can cause withdrawal effects if the tablet is crushed and injected in persons dependent on opioids (16,27). Likewise, as a partial agonist, buprenorphine itself can precipitate withdrawal if given to individuals maintained on other full mu-opioid receptor agonists, as buprenorphine has higher affinity to the receptor. This is a rare occurrence but has been seen, especially when transitioning high-dose methadone-maintained individuals to buprenorphine.

PHARMACODYNAMICS

Buprenorphine is a synthetic derivative of the morphine alkaloid thebaine and has approximately 25 to 40 times the analgesic potency of morphine when administered IV, and is 15 times more potent than intramuscular morphine when administered SL. Unlike morphine, buprenorphine displays both typical mu-opioid receptor agonist and antagonist properties, making it an ideal candidate for the treatment of opioid dependence. The agonist effects—miosis (clinically insignificant), respiratory depression, decreased gastrointestinal motility, euphoria, and sedation—occur at lower doses of the drug while antagonist effects occur only with increasing doses of buprenorphine given to persons maintained on another primary mu-opioid receptor agonist. These properties allow for a "ceiling effect" on respiratory depression, making for a better safety profile than pure mu-opioid receptor agonist (28).

The onset of buprenorphine's drug effect is slower than morphine, with mean peak effect seen between 40 and 60 minutes (producing a lower peak euphoric rush compared to other opioids), but the duration of action is longer, with a terminal half-life of 32 to 37 hours (4). Most likely this is a route of administration effect, as IV administered buprenorphine produces similar drug liking responses as IV morphine in persons with an opioid abuse history. The long terminal half-life allows for once daily or even less frequent dosing patterns (29). Buprenorphine's receptor binding properties help explain its partial agonist profile; it binds to mu-opioid receptors with greater affinity and can displace other agonists from these sites (30). Higher doses of an antagonist (3 and 10 mg/70kg IM naloxone or 3 mg/70 kg PO naltrexone) are required to displace buprenorphine from mu-opioid receptors as compared to methadone (31). Buprenorphine is also a weak kappa-opioid receptor antagonist, delta-opioid receptor antagonist, and opioid receptor-like 1 (ORL-1) agonist, but the full understanding of these actions is not yet known. It is currently hypothesized that one or more of these receptors could be involved in or mediate buprenorphine's bell-shaped dose–response curve. Buprenorphine's ORL-1 activity especially shows promise as the mechanism behind its ceiling effect for respiratory depression, as activation of this receptor antagonizes acute effects of morphine; however, more research into this area is needed.

EFFICACY IN THE TREATMENT OF OPIOID DEPENDENCE

This section examines the peer-reviewed papers reporting on results regarding the efficacy of buprenorphine and buprenorphine/naloxone in the treatment of opioid dependence (both maintenance and detoxification treatment). While the utility of detoxification as a treatment intervention has been called into question, detoxification followed by significant psychosocial rehabilitation does have proven benefit (32). It is with that overall treatment goal that opioid detoxification with buprenorphine is discussed.

Buprenorphine/naloxone and buprenorphine have been shown to provide greater suppression of opioid withdrawal symptoms in both inpatient and outpatient detoxification settings as compared to clonidine (33), dihydrocodeine (34), and lofexidine (35), and show similar results as methadone (36). Retention rates in these clinical trials have usually been higher in the inpatient as compared to outpatient setting, but one multisite trial conducted by the National Institute on Drug Abuse Clinical Trials Network did not find a significant difference between setting types (37). Drug abstinence at the end of outpatient detoxification is achieved at relatively low rates (17% to 29%) (38). Higher treatment success following opioid detoxification (as defined by study completion and drug-free urinalysis on the last day of study) is associated with better control of withdrawal symptoms during treatment, fewer comorbid substance use disorders (SUD) including nicotine dependence, and higher baseline anxiety levels (33). Long-term abstinence following detoxification, however, is rarely achieved or sustained unless significant ongoing rehabilitation and treatment is continued.

Consensus treatment guidelines advocate long-term maintenance therapy as a first-line strategy in adult opioid-dependent participants. In one of the first randomized controlled clinical trials of buprenorphine maintenance, daily SL buprenorphine (8 mg) was shown to be as effective as 60 mg methadone in terms of retention and opioid-negative urines, and superior to 20 mg methadone (9). Further double-blind clinical trials replicated these early results using a clinically relevant flexible dose schedule (10), although a Swiss multisite trial showed higher dose methadone (60 to 120 mg) had better retention rates than moderate dose buprenorphine (12 to 16 mg) (39). These early trials defined maintenance treatment as lasting between 8 and 16 weeks. Studies of longer duration (6 to 12 months) initially showed results favoring high-dose methadone compared to buprenorphine in terms of retention, opioid-free urine toxicology screens, and withdrawal symptoms (8,11). A recent meta-analysis by the *Cochrane Review* examined 24 randomized and controlled clinical trials and concluded that buprenorphine is less effective at retaining patients in treatment than methadone delivered at adequate doses (40). However, results for opioid-free urines showed no inferiority of buprenorphine and the authors concluded that buprenorphine is an effective intervention for the maintenance treatment of opioid dependence. Buprenorphine/naloxone combinations have also shown to be as effective as buprenorphine alone (19). Longer-term effectiveness trials in primary care clinics have shown buprenorphine to be a safe and successful treatment not only in the United States but also in over a dozen countries on six continents (41–45). These studies have shown that there is a large dropout rate in the first 3 months of treatment, but that this can be reduced somewhat by a quick induction phase to eliminate withdrawal symptoms. Given this large dropout rate, more research is needed into optimally choosing candidates for buprenorphine treatment. Patient variables such as gender, age, lifetime opioid use, and the particular opioid abused (heroin, methadone, or other prescription opioids) could be predictors of treatment outcomes as a few studies have shown.

OPTIMAL USE OF BUPRENORPHINE

The use of buprenorphine (most commonly buprenorphine/naloxone in the United States) in an outpatient medical practice for opioid dependence consists of three main phases: induction, stabilization/maintenance, and (if necessary) withdrawal. Induction onto buprenorphine, defined here as the first 24 to 72 hours of starting on buprenorphine, requires first a comprehensive medical evaluation to establish a diagnosis of opioid dependence, drug use history and any complicating medical, psychiatric disorders or SUD, concomitant medications, and drug allergies. There are no absolute contraindications to buprenorphine, except for documented previous allergic reactions to the medication or naloxone. The medication is not approved for children (<16 years of age) or pregnant women, but ongoing clinical trials are assessing safety and efficacy in these populations.

There are two separate induction strategies for persons previously on short-acting opioids (e.g., heroin or oxycodone) versus long-acting opioids (e.g., methadone). This discussion will first focus on buprenorphine induction for dependence on short-acting opioids. Patients should be told to come to the office in mild opioid withdrawal, usually 4 to 12 hours after their last dose of opioid. A clinician should verify the withdrawal syndrome with a standard rating scale such as the Clinical Opiate Withdrawal Scale (COWS) (46,47). Depending on the level of prior opioid use, the patient should be given 2/0.5 or 4/1 mg of SL buprenorphine/naloxone and monitored in the office for any side effects, including worsening opioid withdrawal or opioid toxicity. The patient should be instructed to place the tablet(s) under the tongue and keep them there for 3 to 5 minutes without talking or swallowing. If the mouth is dry, the patient should be instructed to drink water first before being administered the medication. If side effects occur, they should be treated with the appropriate medications. If withdrawal is not relieved by the initial buprenorphine dose, the patient can be redosed up to a recommended maximum total dose of 8/2 mg buprenorphine/naloxone on the first day. Previous research has shown that rapid induction of buprenorphine and buprenorphine/naloxone is safe and leads to better retention (42), so a patient should usually reach their maintenance dose (12 to 16 mg) on the second day. If the patient requires >16/4 mg per day, further titration can occur to a maximum dose of 32/8 mg on days 3 to 4.

There were some initial fears that giving persons already in mild opioid withdrawal SL naloxone in the form of buprenorphine/naloxone would worsen withdrawal, so the U.S. guidelines published in 2004 recommended using buprenorphine (without naloxone) during the initial induction and then switching to buprenorphine/naloxone (48). However, clinical experience and a recent clinical trial has shown that SL naloxone does not induce further withdrawal (49), and most practitioners start induction with buprenorphine/naloxone without sequelae. Buprenorphine/naloxone should be used for all phases of maintenance unless the subject has a documented allergy to naloxone; buprenorphine alone should be rarely used.

When the patient is dependent on long-acting opioids, the induction phase ideally requires an initial taper of the long-acting opioid. In the case of methadone, a person should be tapered to 30 to 40 mg daily dose if possible before buprenorphine induction (48). The patient should be instructed to present to the office 24 to 36 hours after the last methadone dose in order to show some mild opioid withdrawal. They should be told there is a small risk for worsening withdrawal symptoms after starting buprenorphine/naloxone. The rest of the induction phase is the same as with short-acting opioids. The patient should take no more methadone after the first dose of buprenorphine/naloxone. In case there are fears that a protracted methadone taper may trigger relapse before starting buprenorphine/naloxone, there is a study that has shown that there can be safe transition to buprenorphine/naloxone in some persons maintained on 100 mg of methadone (50). Results from that study suggest that small repeated doses of buprenorphine/naloxone (2/0.5 mg) spaced approximately 2 hours apart will decrease the risk of buprenorphine-precipitated withdrawal.

Although opioid dependence is typically required for buprenorphine maintenance, one exception requires more discussion. A physician may decide to prescribe buprenorphine to a person who is not currently opioid dependent but at high risk for relapse or developing opioid dependence; for example, a recently released prisoner with opioid dependence prior to incarceration or person using opioids after a recent detoxification attempt. This induction should start with a smaller buprenorphine/naloxone dose (2/0.5 mg) and should be titrated up to clinical effect more slowly (e.g., dose increases every 3 to 7 days).

Stabilization is the phase where the patient is maintained on the same dose of buprenorphine/naloxone and is referred/engaged in concurrent psychosocial counseling/rehabilitation. At this point, the patient may choose to take buprenorphine on alternate days, but this is not the general recommendation and is done rarely in clinical practice. Twice-daily dosing may also be required, especially in patients with comorbid pain.

Withdrawal from buprenorphine can be accomplished rapidly in an inpatient setting (≤3 days) or during a protracted outpatient taper. In the past, 0.3 mg IM buprenorphine was given two to three times daily for a rapid 3-day withdrawal. However, this treatment is no longer recommended and IM buprenorphine is not approved for opioid-dependent treatment. Instead, inpatient settings may use a SL buprenorphine taper. The superiority of moderate or long-term taper of buprenorphine has not yet been fully determined, although most studies show a substantial increase in opioid positive urines after any buprenorphine taper (33). Whether or not to stop buprenorphine treatment should be decided on a case-by-case basis by the physician and patient, weighing the risks of continued treatment against the risks of relapse following withdrawal.

LEGAL ISSUES

Office-based treatment of opioid dependence with buprenorphine did not come easily in the United States. Pharmacologic treatment of opioid dependence had been hindered by the Harrison Narcotic Act of 1914, which was interpreted by courts after 1917 to forbid physicians from prescribing opioids specifically for the treatment of opioid dependence. Prosecution of physicians violating this act and subsequent legislation continued until the American Medical Association and American Bar Association issued a joint report questioning these policies in 1958 (51). Methadone subsequently became available for the treatment of opioid dependence, and has proven to be a reliable and beneficial treatment. However, administrative fears of diversion, overdose, and physician prescribing practices led to very stringent and convoluted policies that governed its use, including an ability to dispense methadone only at approved clinics and hospital pharmacies. These policies, codified in the Narcotic Addict Treatment Act (NATA) of 1974, as well as a cadre of various state and local regulations, governed the medical treatment of opioid dependence up until 2001.

As stated earlier, buprenorphine showed early promise as a treatment for opioid dependence. However, it required an act of Congress in the United States to approve its use by individual physicians in an office-based setting. That bill was the 2000 Drug Addiction Treatment Act (DATA), which had taken 5 years of political maneuvering to become law (52). DATA allowed physicians to prescribe narcotics in an office-based setting and pharmacists to dispense certain narcotics (currently only buprenorphine) for the treatment of opioid dependence. The wording leaves open the possibility of "any approved narcotic drugs in schedule III, IV, or V ... for maintenance or detoxification treatment," so other medications may also be used in the future in office-based settings under DATA. DATA did specify requirements before physicians could legally prescribe buprenorphine for opioid dependence (Table 29.1). If a physician meets those requirements, he or she must apply for and receive a Department of Health and Human Services waiver (DHHS) waiver (http://www.buprenorphine.samhsa.gov) and be given a specific Drug Enforcement Agency (DEA) number before writing the first prescription.

Given concerns over diversion, DATA limited the number of buprenorphine-approved patients (initially 30 per physician group/institution) and prescribed a 3-year monitoring phase after buprenorphine was approved by the FDA for treatment of opioid dependence. In 2005, the effects of DATA on opioid dependence received a good review; thus DHHS expanded the number of potential buprenorphine patients per individual prescriber to the current levels (100 per year after the first year of approval) and removed the group practice restriction. Nevertheless, DHHS and DEA still have the authority to repeal the law without Congressional approval if those organizations are concerned about buprenorphine's effects on public health, making it easy to end office-based treatment of opioid dependence in the future.

In the United States, the rate of physicians applying for and receiving an DHHS waiver to prescribe buprenorphine has not been as quick as first predicted. As well, about half of all the physicians qualified to prescribe buprenorphine are addiction specialists (53). This indicates that primary care doctors are not expanding access to buprenorphine by becoming prescribers in the numbers that were originally projected. Reasons for this hesitation include lack of qualified counseling services, staff training, visit time required for in-

TABLE 29.1 Requirements for DATA Waiver

- Be a licensed physician (MD or DO)
- Possess a current DEA Number
- Have completed one of the following:
  1) Subspecialty Board Certification in Addiction Psychiatry from the American Board of Medical Specialties
  2) Addiction Certification from the American Society of Addiction Medicine
  3) Subspecialty Board Certification in Addiction Medicine from the American Osteopathic Association
  4) Not less than 8 hours of training on the treatment and management of opioid-addicted patients[a]
  5) Participated as an investigator in one or more clinical trials leading to the approval of a narcotic drug in Schedule III, IV, or V for maintenance or detoxification treatment
  6) Other training or experience as the State medical licensing board (of the State in which the physician will provide maintenance or detoxification treatment) considers to demonstrate the ability of the physician to treat and manage opioid-addicted patients
  7) Other training or experience as the Secretary of the Department of Health and Human Services (DHHS) considers to demonstrate the ability of the physician to treat and manage opioid-addicted patients (only a 3-year waiver)
- Have the capacity to refer patients to counseling and ancillary services
- Agree to have no more than 30 patients prescribed buprenorphine for opioid dependence in the first year after receiving a waiver and up to 100 patients after the first year
- Notify the Center for Substance Abuse Treatment in writing of the intent to begin dispensing or prescribing buprenorphine

[a]Sponsored by the American Society of Addiction Medicine, the American Academy of Addiction Psychiatry, the American Medical Association, the American Osteopathic Association, the American Psychiatric Association, or any other organization that the Secretary of DHHS determines is appropriate.

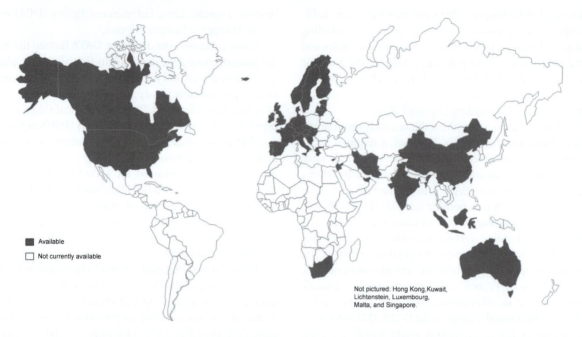

Figure 29.1. Countries where buprenorphine is prescribed for opioid dependence.

duction phase, lack of buprenorphine availability in local pharmacies, and pain medicine concerns (54). Future campaigns should address these needs in order to increase access to buprenorphine maintenance treatment.

Outside of the United States, countries have various legal restrictions on the prescribing and dispensing of buprenorphine and buprenorphine/naloxone. (See Fig. 29.1 for countries currently allowing the use of buprenorphine for the treatment of opioid dependence.) The following is not meant to be an exhaustive description of policies regulating buprenorphine in every country, as that would be beyond the scope of this chapter, but does illustrate the parameters of buprenorphine's use in non–U.S. countries. In France, the initial country to approve the use of buprenorphine for the treatment of opioid dependence, a national policy places physicians in primary care or specialized drug treatment facilities as the "gatekeepers" of patients' access to buprenorphine and allows community pharmacies to dispense it. Physicians can prescribe buprenorphine with up to a 28-day supply, but patients can only get up to 7 days of medication from the pharmacy unless the physician allows for longer periods (55). This system has led to buprenorphine being the primary medication used in opioid replacement therapy (ORT) throughout the country. Unlike France, Australia has both national and state laws that govern the use of buprenorphine for ORT (56). In this country, community pharmacists are the "gatekeepers" of patients' access to buprenorphine. Both physicians who prescribe buprenorphine and at least one pharmacist in the pharmacy that dispenses it must receive specialized buprenorphine training. States set up differing laws regarding take-home availability; but in general, all buprenorphine must be taken by the patient and witnessed by a staff member in a community pharmacy. National law does offer every other day or thrice-weekly dosing to stable patients who do not want to come daily for treatment. Finally, the "gatekeepers" in Italy (physicians) can only be found in specialized ORT facilities, and these prescribers must have received specialized training for buprenorphine (56). The medication is then dispensed daily in these facilities and must be witnessed, similar to methadone. In conclusion, eligibility criteria for buprenorphine, its prescribing and dispensing authority, or even the ability to offer ORT are governed by statutes that are essentially unique to each country where this medication is available.

SAFETY CONCERNS

The most common side effects from buprenorphine result from its opioid agonist properties and are seen when given to a nondependent person. These can include nausea, vomiting, sedation, and dizziness. Respiratory depression from buprenorphine, a serious and often fatal complication of other opioids, has been examined extensively in humans and animals. Studies concluded that there was a ceiling effect for respiratory depression unlike pure mu-opioid receptor agonist, and that this depression was not clinically significant (57,58). If severe respiratory depression does occur in the community, it is usually due to concurrent use of benzodiazepines and/or alcohol. This rare respiratory depression is difficult to treat with standard opioid antagonists; the best recommendation is to provide a continuous naloxone infusion until the buprenorphine has been cleared from the patient (59). However, case reports have also shown benefit from high-dose single injection of naloxone (4 to 6 mg IV bolus given within a correct dose window) (60) and doxapram, which stimulates respiratory drive via peripheral and central means (61).

There has also been particular interest on the cognitive and psychomotor effects of buprenorphine, especially as ORT is meant to help facilitate a person's return to employment, family involvement, and other important societal functions. However, many of the published studies examining acute and chronic dosing effects on cognition have methodologic problems that make conclusions difficult; for example, not matching groups on characteristics known to influence cognitive performance like premorbid IQ and allowing persons with active substance use to participate in studies. Nevertheless, some conclusions may be drawn that appear consistently throughout the literature. First, with a decrease in use of heroin or other illicit opioids while on buprenorphine maintenance, a person's executive function, selective attention, and concentration usually improve (42). Second, there appears to be relatively slower acute reaction time when comparing persons maintained on methadone to persons on buprenorphine (62). Third, buprenorphine seems to have less of an effect on decision-making skills than methadone (63). Finally, researchers have demonstrated that driving is not significantly impaired during buprenorphine maintenance; and, the addition of small amounts of alcohol (0.05% blood alcohol concentration) to chronic buprenorphine dosing does not show any worse performance than in non–drug abusing controls (64). Thus, the majority of the peer-reviewed studies indicate that buprenorphine may have less cognitive side effects than methadone; but like methadone, buprenorphine may help increase functioning to baseline by decreasing illicit substance use. However, better designed, prospective research is needed in this area to validate these conclusions.

In light of the growing concern over cardiac arrhythmias from QTc prolongation in methadone maintenance, studies have examined the risk for electrocardiogram abnormalities with buprenorphine and buprenorphine/naloxone. Researchers have concluded that buprenorphine does not significantly prolong the QTc at clinically indicated dosing ranges and may be safer than methadone (65). However, if patients are taking known inhibitors of cytochrome P450 3A4, such as certain medications to treat HIV, there is a slightly increased but not clinically significant risk of QTc prolongation (66).

Deaths associated with buprenorphine have received increased public scrutiny recently, especially as methadone-related overdoses have increased. The number of calls to U.S. Poison Control Centers after buprenorphine exposure has gone from 13 in 2000 to almost 6200 in 2008 (67) and a similar increase has been reported in France (68). In some countries, the number of reported deaths related to buprenorphine increased after its introduction, especially if combined with benzodiazepines. Whether this trend improves as physicians and patients become more knowledgeable about the medication remains to be seen. The experience in France, which approved buprenorphine in 1996, has shown that the death rate related to buprenorphine is lower than methadone (69), and there is early evidence for this same finding in Australia (70).

Diversion of buprenorphine was one of the original feared effects of office-based treatment. As the use of buprenorphine for opioid dependence has risen, diversion of supplies onto the black market has increased. In some locations outside of the United States where the heroin supply has been curtailed, this diversion is more frequent per capita than methadone (71). In the United States, a survey of 1000 patients seeking drug-abuse treatment at standard drug-abuse clinics showed that 35% of individuals self-reported misuse of buprenorphine to get high during the initial 2 years of treatment and this number fell to below 20% by the end of the survey period (72). In that same study, less than 3% of all persons presenting for ORT in 2007 gave buprenorphine as their drug of choice to get high. Vigilance should be maintained in the United States to prevent more diversion while not restricting this valuable pharmacotherapy from reaching patients in need.

Following diversion, illicit injection of buprenorphine (8 to 16 mg daily) has been associated with several cases of hepatitis, all in persons with underlying liver disease (i.e., hepatitis C and alcoholic hepatitis) (73). There is also evidence that hepatitis can occur in persons taking SL buprenorphine as prescribed (74,75), but these individuals also had underlying risk factors. Physicians should check liver function tests before induction and after maintenance has been achieved in those persons with known or at risk for liver dysfunction. Other side effects associated with the injection of SL buprenorphine are similar to most other illicit IV drugs, and include infectious endocarditis (76), myositis (77), acute limb ischemia sometimes requiring amputation (78), and embolic stroke (79).

Even with these risks of buprenorphine, two elegant studies have shown an overall decreased mortality in persons exposed to and compliant with ORT—including buprenorphine (43,80).

SPECIAL POPULATIONS

Although the FDA and most international governments have approved buprenorphine only for adults, recent research has shown promising results for buprenorphine's use in adolescents, pregnant women, and incarcerated populations. These populations are covered in depth elsewhere but deserve brief comment in this chapter. First, there is no FDA-approved treatment for opioid dependence in adolescents (<16 years old). However, one clinical trial showed promise for this medication's longer-term use in this population. Researchers randomized 152 persons aged 14 to 21 years with DSM-IV opioid dependence to either a 14-day buprenorphine detoxification and subsequent counseling or 12 weeks of buprenorphine maintenance along with counseling (81). Primary outcomes examined were opioid positive urine toxicology and treatment retention. At week 12, only 20.5% of adolescents randomized to detoxification remained in the study versus 70% in buprenorphine maintenance. There was no statistical difference in opioid positive urines between the groups at week 12, but there were significantly lower positive urines in the maintenance group at weeks 4 and 8. Maintenance participants had lower self-reported cocaine, marijuana, and injection drug use, and attended more counseling sessions than the detoxification group. During 12 month follow-up, the detoxification group was over twice as likely (OR 2.65) to have an opioid positive urine as the maintenance group. Overall, this trial pointed to the potential value of longer-term buprenorphine treatment for adolescents with opioid dependence. More research is needed on buprenorphine for this population, but it is likely to show value in including opioid agonist treatment for adolescents.

Buprenorphine (and buprenorphine/naloxone) is an FDA pregnancy category C medication, indicating not enough studies have been done to advise the use of this medication during pregnancy. The standard of care for opioid-dependent pregnant women has been methadone in a specialized treatment facility. There have been many peer-reviewed articles published on buprenorphine treatment of opioid dependence in pregnancy. In reviewing outcomes of these studies, authors examined birth weight, prematurity, neonatal abstinence syndrome (NAS), perinatal complications, and some long-term follow-up data on women and their offspring. In two studies comparing women without substitution therapy to buprenorphine and methadone, buprenorphine had less incidence of NAS compared to methadone (82,83), although other studies did not replicate this finding (84,85). When NAS was present, it had a later onset than methadone but seemed to be shorter in length. There was no difference in neonatal weight, length of hospitalization, or frequency of birth defects/neonatal demise in buprenorphine as compared to methadone-treated women (85–87). If women are to be prescribed buprenorphine currently, they should be informed that research is still ongoing into the neonatal and maternal outcomes. As well, induction onto buprenorphine may be complicated by precipitated withdrawal if the woman has been using long-acting opioids, but the maintenance phase typically has fewer dose adjustments (88). Finally, breastfeeding can usually continue if the mother remains on buprenorphine as there is low oral bioavailability of the medication. However, this recommendation is not yet backed by definitive studies.

The use of opioid agonist treatment in the prison system has been advocated by the Centers for Disease Control and Prevention (CDC) and the World Health Organization (WHO) due to the high incidence of substance use in the year prior to incarceration and obvious benefits to individual and public health (89,90). However, only 55% of facilities in the United States offer methadone currently, usually only for chronic pain and in pregnant women with opioid dependence; an even lower percentage of facilities offer buprenorphine (14%) (91). Internationally, 29 countries or territories offered ORT to prisoners in 2008, which was an increase over previous years (92). Most facilities prefer a drug-free detoxification environment to opioid agonist treatment. These facilities also do not always refer inmates to postrelease methadone or buprenorphine providers, doing so in less than half of all cases. Research is ongoing into the cost savings, decreased recidivism, decreased HIV transmission, and effects on substance relapse postrelease. This research is needed to help sway prisons and jails to treat opioid dependence just like any other disease during incarceration.

CONCLUSION

Buprenorphine provides patients and health care providers a new medication for the treatment of opioid dependence. It is often preferred over methadone by patients for its ease of use and safety/side effect profile. This chapter has shown the intense work done by researchers, lawmakers, physicians, advocates, and patients themselves to bring this treatment to the market. It does have unique risks and benefits, which should be weighed for every potential patient; it also appears to be roughly equivalent in many outcomes compared to methadone. Long-term data are still being collected, but the French experience shows the great benefits can occur with buprenorphine's widespread use. Hopefully, these results will be reproduced in the United States and worldwide for the benefit of all.

REFERENCES

1. United Nations Office on Drugs and Crime. *World Drug Report.* United Nations: New York; 2009.
2. Substance Abuse and Mental Health Services Administration. *Results of the 2008 National Survey on Drug Use and Health: National Findings.* (Office of Applied Studies, NSDUH Series H-36, HHS Publication No. SMA 09-4434). Rockvile, MD: Office of Applied Studies; 2009.
3. Cowan A, Doxey JC, Harry EJ. The animal pharmacology of buprenorphine, an oripavine analgesic agent. *Br J Pharmacol.* 1977;60:547–554.
4. Jasinski DR, Pevnick JS, Griffith JD. Human pharmacology and abuse potential of the analgesic buprenorphine: a potential agent for treating narcotic addiction. *Arch Gen Psychiatry.* 1978;35:501–516.
5. Mello NK, Mendelson JH. Buprenorphine suppresses heroin use by heroin addicts. *Science.* 1980;207:657–659.
6. Walsh SL, June HL, Schuh KJ, et al. Effects of buprenorphine and methadone in methadone-maintained subjects. *Psychopharmacology (Berl).* 1995;119:268–276.
7. Correia CJ, Walsh SL, Bigelow GE, et al. Effects associated with double-blind omission of buprenorphine/naloxone over a 98-h period. *Psychopharmacology (Berl).* 2006;189:297–306.
8. Ling W, Wesson DR, Charuvastra C, et al. A controlled trial comparing buprenorphine and methadone maintenance in opioid dependence. *Arch Gen Psychiatry.* 1996;53:401–407.
9. Johnson RE, Jaffe JH, Fudala PJ. A controlled trial of buprenorphine treatment for opioid dependence. *JAMA.* 1992;267:2750–2755.
10. Strain EC, Stitzer ML, Liebson IA, et al. Comparison of buprenorphine and methadone in the treatment of opioid dependence. *Am J Psychiatry.* 1994;151:1025–1030.
11. Schottenfeld RS, Pakes JR, Oliveto A, et al. Buprenorphine vs methadone maintenance treatment for concurrent opioid dependence and cocaine abuse. *Arch Gen Psychiatry.* 1997;54: 713–720.
12. Ling W, Charuvastra C, Collins JF, et al. Buprenorphine maintenance treatment of opiate dependence: a multicenter, randomized clinical trial. *Addiction.* 1998;93:475–486.
13. Johnson RE, Chutuape MA, Strain EC, et al. A comparison of levomethadyl acetate, buprenorphine, and methadone for opioid dependence. *N Engl J Med.* 2000;343:1290–1297.
14. American Psychiatric Association. *Diagnostic and Statistical Manual of Mental Disorders.* 4th ed. Text Revision. Washington, DC: American Psychiatric Association; 2000.
15. Harper I. Temgesic abuse. *N Z Med J.* 1983;96:777.
16. Bigelow GE, Preston KL, Liebson IA. Abuse liability assessment of buprenorphine–naloxone combinations. *NIDA Res Monogr.* 1987;76:145–149.

17. Mendelson J, Jones RT, Welm S, et al. Buprenorphine and naloxone combinations: the effects of three dose ratios in morphine-stabilized, opiate-dependent volunteers. *Psychopharmacology (Berl)*. 1999;141:37–46.
18. Fudala PJ, Yu E, Macfadden W, et al. Effects of buprenorphine and naloxone in morphine-stabilized opioid addicts. *Drug Alcohol Depend*. 1998;50:1–8.
19. Fudala PJ, Bridge TP, Herbert S, et al. Office-based treatment of opiate addiction with a sublingual-tablet formulation of buprenorphine and naloxone. *N Engl J Med*. 2003;349:949–958.
20. Fiellin DA, Moore BA, Sullivan LE, et al. Long-term treatment with buprenorphine/naloxone in primary care: results at 2–5 years. *Am J Addict*. 2008;17:116–120.
21. Nath RP, Upton RA, Everhart ET, et al. Buprenorphine pharmacokinetics: relative bioavailability of sublingual tablet and liquid formulations. *J Clin Pharmacol*. 1999;39:619–623.
22. Strain EC, Moody DE, Stoller KB, et al. Relative bioavailability of different buprenorphine formulations under chronic dosing conditions. *Drug Alcohol Depend*. 2004;74:37–43.
23. Compton P, Ling W, Moody D, et al. Pharmacokinetics, bioavailability and opioid effects of liquid versus tablet buprenorphine. *Drug Alcohol Depend*. 2006;82:25–31.
24. Mendelson J, Upton RA, Everhart ET, et al. Bioavailability of sublingual buprenorphine. *J Clin Pharmacol*. 1997;37:31–37.
25. Iribarne C, Picart D, Dreano Y, et al. Involvement of cytochrome P450 3A4 in N-dealkylation of buprenorphine in human liver microsomes. *Life Sci*. 1997;60:1953–1964.
26. Zhang W, Ramamoorthy Y, Tyndale RF, et al. Interaction of buprenorphine and its metabolite norbuprenorphine with cytochromes p450 in vitro. *Drug Metab Dispos*. 2003;31:768–772.
27. Stoller KB, Bigelow GE, Walsh SL, et al. Effects of buprenorphine/naloxone in opioid-dependent humans. *Psychopharmacology (Berl)*. 2001;154:230–242.
28. Walsh SL, Preston KL, Stitzer ML, et al. Clinical pharmacology of buprenorphine: ceiling effects at high doses. *Clin Pharmacol Ther*. 1994;55:569–580.
29. Petry NM, Bickel WK, Badger GJ. A comparison of four buprenorphine dosing regimens in the treatment of opioid dependence. *Clin Pharmacol Ther*. 1999;66:306–314.
30. Dum JE, Herz A. In vivo receptor binding of the opiate partial agonist, buprenorphine, correlated with its agonistic and antagonistic actions. *Br J Pharmacol*. 1981;74:627–633.
31. Eissenberg T, Greenwald MK, Johnson RE, et al. Buprenorphine's physical dependence potential: antagonist-precipitated withdrawal in humans. *J Pharmacol Exp Ther*. 1996;276:449–459.
32. Teesson M, Havard A, Ross J, et al. Outcomes after detoxification for heroin dependence: findings from the Australian Treatment Outcome Study (ATOS). *Drug Alcohol Rev*. 2006;25:241–247.
33. Ziedonis DM, Amass L, Steinberg M, et al. Predictors of outcome for short-term medically supervised opioid withdrawal during a randomized, multicenter trial of buprenorphine–naloxone and clonidine in the NIDA clinical trials network. *Drug Alcohol Depend*. 2009;99:28–36.
34. Wright NM, Sheard L, Tompkins CN, et al. Buprenorphine versus dihydrocodeine for opiate detoxification in primary care: a randomised controlled trial. *BMC Fam Pract*. 2007;8:3.
35. White R, Alcorn R, Feinmann C. Two methods of community detoxification from opiates: an open-label comparison of lofexidine and buprenorphine. *Drug Alcohol Depend*. 2001;65:77–83.
36. Gowing L, Ali R, White JM. Buprenorphine for the management of opioid withdrawal. *Cochrane Database Syst Rev*. 2009;(3):CD002025.
37. Ling W, Amass L, Shoptaw S, et al. A multi-center randomized trial of buprenorphine–naloxone versus clonidine for opioid detoxification: findings from the National Institute on Drug Abuse Clinical Trials Network. *Addiction*. 2005;100:1090–1100.
38. Horspool MJ, Seivewright N, Armitage CJ, et al. Post-treatment outcomes of buprenorphine detoxification in community settings: a systematic review. *Eur Addict Res*. 2008;14:179–185.
39. Uehlinger C, Deglon J, Livoti S, et al. Comparison of buprenorphine and methadone in the treatment of opioiddependence. Swiss multicentre study. *Eur Addict Res*. 1998;4 (suppl 1):13–18.
40. Mattick RP, Kimber J, Breen C, et al. Buprenorphine maintenance versus placebo or methadone maintenance for opioid dependence. *Cochrane Database Syst Rev*. 2008;(2):CD002207.
41. Gerra G, Leonardi C, D'Amore A, et al. Buprenorphine treatment outcome in dually diagnosed heroin dependent patients: a retrospective study. *Prog Neuropsychopharmacol Biol Psychiatry*. 2006;30:265–272.
42. Soyka M, Zingg C, Koller G, et al. Retention rate and substance use in methadone and buprenorphine maintenance therapy and predictors of outcome: results from a randomized study. *Int J Neuropsychopharmacol*. 2008;11:641–653.
43. Gibson A, Degenhardt L, Mattick RP, et al. Exposure to opioid maintenance treatment reduces long-term mortality. *Addiction*. 2008;103:462–468.
44. Leonardi C, Hanna N, Laurenzi P, et al. Multi-centre observational study of buprenorphine use in 32 Italian drug addiction centres. *Drug Alcohol Depend*. 2008;94:125–132.
45. Lawrinson P, Ali R, Buavirat A, et al. Key findings from the WHO collaborative study on substitution therapy for opioid dependence and HIV/AIDS. *Addiction*. 2008;103:1484–1492.
46. Wesson DR, Ling W. The Clinical Opiate Withdrawal Scale (COWS). *J Psychoactive Drugs*. 2003;35:253–259.
47. Tompkins DA, Bigelow GE, Harrison JA, et al. Concurrent validation of the Clinical Opiate Withdrawal Scale (COWS) and single-item indices against the Clinical Institute Narcotic Assessment (CINA) opioid withdrawal instrument. *Drug Alcohol Depend*. 2009;105:154–159.
48. Center for Substance Abuse Treatment. Clinical Guidelines for the Use of Buprenorphine in the Treatment of Opioid Addiction. *Treatment Improvement Protocol (TIP) U.S. Department of Health and Human Services, Rockville, MD. Series 40*. 2004.
49. Strain EC, Harrison JA, Bigelow JE. Induction of opioid-dependent individuals onto buprenorphine and buprenorphine/naloxone soluble film. Presented at the annual meeting, College on Problems of Drug Dependence, Reno, NV, June 24, 2009.
50. Rosado J, Walsh SL, Bigelow GE, et al. Sublingual buprenorphine/naloxone precipitated withdrawal in subjects maintained on 100 mg of daily methadone. *Drug Alcohol Depend*. 2007;90:261–269.
51. Musto D. The history of legislative controls over opium, cocaine, and their derivatives. In: Hamowy R, ed. *Dealing with Drugs: Consequences of Government Controls*. Lexington, MA: Lexington Books; 1987:37–71.
52. Jaffe JH, O'Keeffe C. From morphine clinics to buprenorphine: regulating opioid agonist treatment of addiction in the United States. *Drug Alcohol Depend*. 2003;70:S3–S11.
53. Fiellin DA. The first three years of buprenorphine in the United States: experience to date and future directions. *J Addict Med*. 2007;1:62–67.

54. Netherland J, Botsko M, Egan JE, et al. Factors affecting willingness to provide buprenorphine treatment. *J Subst Abuse Treat.* 2009;36:244–251.
55. Guichard A, Lert F, Brodeur JM, et al. Buprenorphine substitution treatment in France: drug users' views of the doctor–user relationship. *Soc Sci Med.* 2007;64:2578–2593.
56. Carrieri MP, Amass L, Lucas GM, et al. Buprenorphine use: the international experience. *Clin Infect Dis.* 2006;43(suppl 4): S197–S215.
57. Walsh SL, Preston KL, Bigelow GE, et al. Acute administration of buprenorphine in humans: partial agonist and blockade effects. *J Pharmacol Exp Ther.* 1995;274:361–372.
58. Dahan A, Yassen A, Romberg R, et al. Buprenorphine induces ceiling in respiratory depression but not in analgesia. *Br J Anaesth.* 2006;96:627–632.
59. Dahan A. Opioid-induced respiratory effects: new data on buprenorphine. *Palliat Med.* 2006;20(suppl 1):s3–s8.
60. van Dorp E, Yassen A, Sarton E, et al. Naloxone reversal of buprenorphine-induced respiratory depression. *Anesthesiology.* 2006;105:51–57.
61. Orwin JM. The effect of doxapram on buprenorphine induced respiratory depression. *Acta Anaesthesiol Belg.* 1977;28:93–106.
62. Soyka M, Hock B, Kagerer S, et al. Less impairment on one portion of a driving-relevant psychomotor battery in buprenorphine-maintained than in methadone-maintained patients: results of a randomized clinical trial. *J Clin Psychopharmacol.* 2005;25:490–493.
63. Pirastu R, Fais R, Messina M, et al. Impaired decision-making in opiate-dependent subjects: effect of pharmacological therapies. *Drug Alcohol Depend.* 2006;83:163–168.
64. Lenne MG, Dietze P, Rumbold GR, et al. The effects of the opioid pharmacotherapies methadone, LAAM and buprenorphine, alone and in combination with alcohol, on simulated driving. *Drug Alcohol Depend.* 2003;72:271–278.
65. Wedam EF, Bigelow GE, Johnson RE, et al. QT-interval effects of methadone, levomethadyl, and buprenorphine in a randomized trial. *Arch Intern Med.* 2007;167:2469–2475.
66. Baker JR, Best AM, Pade PA, et al. Effect of buprenorphine and antiretroviral agents on the QT interval in opioid-dependent patients. *Ann Pharmacother.* 2006;40:392–396.
67. Boyer EW, McCance-Katz EF, Marcus S. Methadone and buprenorphine toxicity in children. *Am J Addict.* 2009;19:89–95.
68. Kintz P. Deaths involving buprenorphine: a compendium of French cases. *Forensic Sci Int.* 2001;121:65–69.
69. Auriacombe M, Franques P, Tignol J. Deaths attributable to methadone vs buprenorphine in France. *JAMA.* 2001; 285:45.
70. Bell JR, Butler B, Lawrance A, et al. Comparing overdose mortality associated with methadone and buprenorphine treatment. *Drug Alcohol Depend.* 2009;104:73–77.
71. Winstock AR, Lea T, Sheridan J. Prevalence of diversion and injection of methadone and buprenorphine among clients receiving opioid treatment at community pharmacies in New South Wales, Australia. *Int J Drug Policy.* 2008;19:450–458.
72. Cicero TJ, Surratt HL, Inciardi J. Use and misuse of buprenorphine in the management of opioid addiction. *J Opioid Manag.* 2007;3: 302–308.
73. Berson A, Gervais A, Cazals D, et al. Hepatitis after intravenous buprenorphine misuse in heroin addicts. *J Hepatol.* 2001;34: 346–350.
74. Herve S, Riachi G, Noblet C, et al. Acute hepatitis due to buprenorphine administration. *Eur J Gastroenterol Hepatol.* 2004;16:1033–1037.
75. Zuin M, Giorgini A, Selmi C, et al. Acute liver and renal failure during treatment with buprenorphine at therapeutic dose. *Dig Liver Dis.* 2009;41:e8–e10.
76. Chong E, Poh KK, Shen L, et al. Infective endocarditis secondary to intravenous Subutex abuse. *Singapore Med J.* 2009;50:34–42.
77. Seet RC, Lim EC. Intravenous use of buprenorphine tablets associated with rhabdomyolysis and compressive sciatic neuropathy. *Ann Emerg Med.* 2006;47:396–397.
78. Partanen TA, Vikatmaa P, Tukiainen E, et al. Outcome after injections of crushed tablets in intravenous drug abusers in the Helsinki University Central Hospital. *Eur J Vasc Endovasc Surg.* 2009;37:704–711.
79. Joethy J, Yong FC, Puhaindran M. Another complication of subutex abuse. *Singapore Med J.* 2008;49:267–268.
80. Clausen T, Anchersen K, Waal H. Mortality prior to, during and after opioid maintenance treatment (OMT): a national prospective cross-registry study. *Drug Alcohol Depend.* 2008;94: 151–157.
81. Woody GE, Poole SA, Subramaniam G, et al. Extended vs short-term buprenorphine–naloxone for treatment of opioid-addicted youth: a randomized trial. *JAMA.* 2008;300: 2003–2011.
82. Binder T, Vavrinkova B. Prospective randomised comparative study of the effect of buprenorphine, methadone and heroin on the course of pregnancy, birthweight of newborns, early postpartum adaptation and course of the neonatal abstinence syndrome (NAS) in women followed up in the outpatient department. *Neuro Endocrinol Lett.* 2008;29:80–86.
83. Kakko J, Heilig M, Sarman I. Buprenorphine and methadone treatment of opiate dependence during pregnancy: comparison of fetal growth and neonatal outcomes in two consecutive case series. *Drug Alcohol Depend.* 2008;96:69–78.
84. Bakstad B, Sarfi M, Welle-Strand GK, et al. Opioid maintenance treatment during pregnancy: occurrence and severity of neonatal abstinence syndrome. A national prospective study. *Eur Addict Res.* 2009;15:128–134.
85. Fischer G, Ortner R, Rohrmeister K, et al. Methadone versus buprenorphine in pregnant addicts: a double-blind, double-dummy comparison study. *Addiction.* 2006;101:275–281.
86. Lejeune C, Simmat-Durand L, Gourarier L, et al. Prospective multicenter observational study of 260 infants born to 259 opiate-dependent mothers on methadone or high-dose buprenorphine substitution. *Drug Alcohol Depend.* 2006;82:250–257.
87. Jones HE, Johnson RE, Jasinski DR, et al. Buprenorphine versus methadone in the treatment of pregnant opioid-dependent patients: effects on the neonatal abstinence syndrome. *Drug Alcohol Depend.* 2005;79:1–10.
88. Jones HE, Martin PR, Heil SH, et al. Treatment of opioid-dependent pregnant women: clinical and research issues. *J Subst Abuse Treat.* 2008;35:245–259.
89. Centers for Disease Control and Prevention. *Substance Abuse Treatment for Injecting Drug Users: a Strategy with Many Benefits.* Atlanta, GA: CDC; 2002.
90. World Health Organization. *Interventions to Address HIV in Prison: Drug Dependence Treatment.* Geneva, Switzerland: WHO; 2007.
91. Nunn A, Zaller N, Dickman S, et al. Methadone and buprenorphine prescribing and referral practices in US prison systems: results from a nationwide survey. *Drug Alcohol Depend.* 2009;105:83–88.
92. Larney S, Dolan K. A literature review of international implementation of opioid substitution treatment in prisons: equivalence of care? *Eur Addict Res.* 2009;15:107–112.

CHAPTER 30: Naltrexone Pharmacotherapy

Emily Harrison ■ Ismene Petrakis

INTRODUCTION

Naltrexone hydrochloride is a nonselective, competitive opioid receptor antagonist which binds at the mu-, kappa-, and delta-opioid receptors and prevents opioids from binding at these receptors. Naltrexone is approved by the Food and Drug Administration (FDA) as a pharmacotherapy for the treatment of opioid dependence and for alcohol use disorders. While originally developed for use in opioid use disorders, its *clinical* effectiveness has been disappointing for opioid-dependent individuals. Instead, opioid *agonist* therapy with methadone or with the more recently approved mixed agonist/antagonist buprenorphine is usually the treatment of choice. Nevertheless, naltrexone continues to have a role in the treatment of opioid dependence, as an adjunctive medication during detoxification to shorten the course of detoxification or as maintenance therapy in highly motivated individuals. In contrast to the literature of naltrexone's efficacy in opioid dependence, a rich literature, including both clinical trials and laboratory studies, supports naltrexone's use in individuals with alcohol use disorders. Although not all patients benefit from its use, new research has suggested that certain patient characteristics such as family history of alcoholism and certain genetic polymorphisms are associated with the greatest efficacy. Naltrexone has also been evaluated as a potential treatment for other psychiatric disorders, such as pathological gambling and eating disorders, but its efficacy in these disorders has not been definitively established. This chapter reviews the clinical uses of naltrexone and the research evaluating its efficacy.

PHARMACOLOGY

The opioid receptor was first characterized in the 1970s and has subsequently been widely studied. Three types of opioid receptors have been identified and include the mu-, delta-, and kappa-opioid receptors. The opioid receptors are found primarily in the central nervous system and in the gastrointestinal tract, and mediate both the effects targeted by medications and the side effects of these agents. Opioids are chemicals that work by binding to the opioid receptors; they include medications (e.g., Percocet, oxycodone, OxyContin), drugs of abuse (notably heroin), and even occur endogenously (e.g., beta-endorphin). *Opiates* are those opioids which are either found in the resin of the opium poppy or are generated from its derivatives. Table 30.1 presents common opioids and opioid antagonists. Opioids when used medicinally are used primarily for their analgesic effects since they decrease the perception of pain, the reaction to pain, and pain tolerance (1). Other effects include sedation, constipation, and suppression of cough.

Extensive research has shown that substance use and abuse is mediated via the so-called reward circuit of the brain, which is a neurochemical pathway that connects mesolimbic and mesocortical structures. Dopaminergic neurons connect the midbrain ventral tegmental area via a mesolimbic dopaminergic pathway to cortical regions including the nucleus accumbens, amygdala, the hippocampus, and the prefrontal cortex. The reward potential of drugs of abuse is related to their ability to stimulate dopamine release in the mesolimbic pathway. Opiates are of particular interest in substance use disorders because activation of the opioid receptors results in dopamine release in the nucleus accumbens and is related to increased euphoria and feelings of well-being.

Naltrexone hydrochloride was first synthesized in the 1960s for use in the treatment of heroin dependence (2). Naltrexone has several routes of administration, including oral administration, implants, and suspended release injection. It is marketed under the trade names Revia and Depade; the extended release under the trade name Vivitrol. Naltrexone has a half-life of about 4 hours and the active metabolite 6-beta-naltrexol has a half-life of about 12 hours (3). Two related drugs include naloxone and methylnaltrexone bromide. Naloxone is shorter acting than naltrexone and not absorbed orally; it is the treatment of choice for opioid overdose and is part of the formulation of Suboxone, a combination treatment of buprenorphine and naloxone for opioid maintenance therapy. Methylnaltrexone bromide (Relistor) is marketed as a treatment for opioid-induced constipation.

Naltrexone and its active metabolite, 6-beta-naltrexol, are competitive antagonist at mu, kappa, and delta receptors. This competitive antagonism means naltrexone binds to the opioid receptor competing with opioid drugs (e.g., heroin and morphine). Naltrexone acts by reversibly blocking the physiological and subjective effects of opioids, thereby attenuating the euphoric effect of opioid drugs, rendering them less rewarding and less reinforcing. Naltrexone can also be used in opioid detoxification; however, it can precipitate opioid withdrawal and should be used with care in opioid-dependent populations. Although its mechanism of action suggests it would be an ideal medication for opioid dependence, its clinical utility is not supported by clinical studies.

TABLE 30.1	Opioids and opioid antagonists
Generic name	**Trade name(s)**[a]
Opioids	
Codeine	No trade names
Morphine	Astramorph, Avinza, Duramorph, Infumorph, Kadian, MS Contin, Oramorph, Roxanol
Diacetylmorphine (heroin)	No trade names
Hydrocodone	Vicodin, Lortab, Lorcet, Hycodan, Vicoprofen
Hydromorphone	Dilaudid
Oxycodone	Tylox, Percodan, Oxycontin
Oxymorphone	Opana, Numorphan, Numorphone
Fentanyl	Actiq, Fentora, Duragesic
Alphamethylfentanyl	No trade names
Sufentanil	Sufenta
Carfentanyl	Wildnil (animal use only)
Meperidine	Pethidine
Propoxyphene	Darvon-N, Darvon Pulvules
Methadone	Methadose, Dolophine
Levomethadyl acetate (LAAM)	Orlaam
Pentazocine	Talwin
Buprenorphine	Buprenex, Suboxone, Subutex
Tramadol	Ultram
Opioid antagonists	
Naltrexone	Revia, Depade
Nalmefene	Revex
Naloxone	Narcan

[a]All trade names are registered trademarks.

Naltrexone is also used in the treatment of alcohol dependence. Alcohol produces a wide variety of pharmacological effects on a number of different neurotransmitter systems including the dopamine, opioid, glutamate, serotonin, and GABA (gamma-aminobutyric acid) systems. Like all drugs of abuse, alcohol stimulates dopamine release in the mesolimbic pathway and dopaminergic release contributes to its reinforcing effects. However, dopamine release is not critical in promoting continued alcohol consumption. The rewarding effect of alcohol is also related to its ability to stimulate the opioid system. After preclinical evidence showed that naltrexone reduces alcohol euphoria and consumption in laboratory animals, naltrexone was examined as a possible treatment for alcohol use disorders in humans. Given the complexity of the reward circuitry and of alcohol's complex effects on multiple neurotransmitter systems, questions remain about the exact mechanism of action of naltrexone's effect on alcohol reward (4).

EFFICACY OF NALTREXONE

Opioid Dependence

Opioid dependence is a serious clinical problem leading to significant morbidity and mortality. It has been estimated that 0.1% to 0.4% of the population has opioid dependence; however, the number of individuals using opioids has increased dramatically with the availability of prescriptions such as Vicodin and OxyContin (1). Clinically, it is a syndrome manifested by continued use of opioids despite physical, social, or psychological consequences; usually individuals are physically dependent. The hallmarks of physical dependence include tolerance and withdrawal upon abrupt discontinuation of use. Abrupt cessation of opioids in an individual who is physically dependent leads to a well-characterized syndrome manifested by dysphoria, nausea, vomiting, rhinorrhea, watery eyes, mydriasis, and muscle aches, hence the term "kicking." Some of the symptoms are mediated by a hyperactivity of the noradrenergic system, particularly in the locus coeruleus. Detoxification from opioids can be accomplished by substitution and gradual tapering of a longer acting opioid (such as methadone). Alternatively, adrenergic agents, such as clonidine or lofexidine, are used to treat some of the symptoms of the opioid withdrawal syndrome by dampening the noradrenergic hyperactivity of the locus coeruleus. However, these agents do not alter its course (5). An alternative to detoxification is *agonist maintenance* therapy with methadone or the partial agonist buprenorphine, but that is beyond the scope of this chapter.

Naltrexone for Opioid Withdrawal/Detoxification

Since naltrexone binds to opioid receptors, administration of naltrexone in an opioid-dependent individual precipitates opioid withdrawal. Nevertheless, it has been used in the treatment of opioid withdrawal as an adjunct medication in order to accelerate the detoxification process. Naltrexone can be administered in combination with the α-adrenergic agent clonidine and other medications in an outpatient setting to produce rapid opioid withdrawal. In this application, naltrexone-assisted clonidine detoxification may reduce the time required for opioid detoxification from about 14 days down to 4 to 7 days (6). It should be noted that naltrexone can increase patient discomfort and reduce treatment compliance.

Naltrexone is also used in ultrarapid opioid withdrawal procedures. This accelerated withdrawal process occurs under general anesthesia in order to reduce the unpleasant effects of opioid withdrawal (7). As with rapid withdrawal, naltrexone is administered in combination with other medications (e.g., clonidine). The ultrarapid withdrawal process occurs over a 4- to 6-hour period, substantially shorter than the rapid withdrawal process. Ultrarapid opioid withdrawal is a significant medical procedure since it confers the risk of general anesthesia. Due to possible respiratory complications during and immediately postwithdrawal, an experienced anesthesiologist should be available (5). The opioid antagonist naloxone is used more commonly than naltrexone in ultrarapid opioid withdrawal (7).

Although patients are physiologically no longer dependent on opioids after withdrawal, craving for opioids occurs and could precipitate relapse. Following rapid and ultrarapid opioid withdrawal, maintenance with naltrexone (50 mg/day) is recommended to reduce levels of craving (5). However, following ultrarapid detoxification, rates of relapse are not substantially better than rates after more conventional methods of detoxification (8). Therefore, the risk/benefit ratio of ultrarapid detoxification seems to increase the risk without substantial benefit, when compared to more conventional methods.

Naltrexone for Maintenance Therapy

After abstinence is achieved, naltrexone can be used for maintenance therapy in order to prevent relapse. Due to the risk of precipitating withdrawal, abstinence from opioids is a prerequisite for the use of naltrexone as a maintenance pharmacotherapy. For patients who have not undergone documented detoxification, it is recommended that patients successfully complete a naloxone or naltrexone challenge to confirm abstinence prior to dosing. Naltrexone prevents relapse by blocking the effects of opioids, serving as a deterrent to further use.

Oral naltrexone was approved for use in opioid dependence in the United States by the FDA in 1984. Although in theory, naltrexone should be an ideal candidate for the treatment of opioid dependence, clinical data supporting naltrexone's efficacy in opioid dependence is not robust. Some reviews have suggested that naltrexone is not superior to placebo for retention or relapse rates. However, the studies are plagued by poor retention rates, which have been as low as 4% (1). Nevertheless, some evidence does suggest that naltrexone use is associated with lower heroin use and decreased criminal activity. When examining treatment studies with high retention rates, naltrexone decreased opioid use, craving, and even psychiatric symptoms compared to controls (1). Naltrexone seems to be particularly beneficial for patient populations who are highly motivated to remain opioid-free, such as health care professionals and legally mandated opioid-dependent individuals (1).

Doses and Routes of Administration

The standard prescribing dose of naltrexone is 50 mg/day, which is a dose that is sufficient to block the pharmacological effects of 25 mg of IV heroin for 24 hours (5). The frequency of naltrexone oral administration can vary from 50 mg/day to 100 mg/every other day to 150 mg/every third day: for every 50 mg dose, the duration of action extends by 24 hours. Therefore, a naltrexone dose of 100 mg is effective for 2 days and 150 mg for 3 days. Since higher doses can be taken less frequently, medication may be administered by others and this has the potential to improve compliance. Compliance is a major issue, as patients who want to resume opioid use can skip doses to resume drug use. Naltrexone use is not associated with tolerance or withdrawal.

While oral administration is currently the only approved route of administration for naltrexone, other routes under investigation include naltrexone implants and injectable sustained-release naltrexone. The advantage of the implants and sustained-release injections is the potential increase in compliance, compared to oral administration. Neither of these new routes of administration is currently approved by the FDA for the treatment of opioid dependence. Naltrexone implants typically last up to 4 to 6 weeks (however, some are formulated to last 4 to 6 months). Doses range from 1.1 to 2.2 to 3.3 g. The location of the implant is subcutaneous, in the abdomen or lateral chest wall (9). Individual variations in plasma naltrexone concentrations have been observed (10).

The first randomized clinical trial examining the safety and efficacy of naltrexone implants as maintenance treatment has recently been completed (11). In the study, 56 heroin-dependent patients received either a 6-month 2.2-g naltrexone implant or standard care. No placebo implant group was included. Opioid use was reduced in the naltrexone group, compared to the standard care control group. Although the majority of side effects were minimal, three patients experienced adverse events that necessitated the removal of the implant.

Injectable sustained-release naltrexone is another new development in naltrexone administration. A recent randomized clinical trial supports this route of administration as safe and well-tolerated (12). In the 8-week trial, 60 heroin-dependent participants were randomly assigned to receive sustained-release injections of 192 mg, 384 mg, or placebo naltrexone. These doses were selected because they are efficacious in the treatment of alcohol use disorders (13). Following detoxification, all participants successfully completed an oral naltrexone challenge test. Injections occurred at weeks 1 and 5. Although no significant reduction in heroin-positive urine samples was observed in the study, retention in treatment was dose dependent and participants were most likely to stay in treatment at the highest naltrexone dose. More research is needed to determine whether injectable sustained-release naltrexone should be considered a viable treatment for opioid dependence.

Opioid-Dependent Patients for Whom Naltrexone Is Optimal

As mentioned above, naltrexone is best for highly motivated patients who are interested in opioid abstinence. The addition of effective psychosocial treatments which address compliance can increase the effectiveness of naltrexone pharmacotherapy (14). For example, the inclusion of psychosocial treatments targeting compliance, involvement of the family, and family therapy all increase compliance (1). External motivation, such as risk of loss of license for health care professionals or those who are under legal mandate to remain abstinent, also increases compliance and therefore effectiveness of naltrexone.

Alcohol Use Disorders

Alcohol use disorders are one of the most common psychiatric disorders and are thought to affect 8% of the general population (15). Alcohol dependence is characterized by a pattern of continued drinking despite physical, psychological, or social consequences. Many, but not all individuals will have physical dependence, including tolerance to alcohol and withdrawal symptoms after abrupt cessation of alcohol use. Alcohol abuse is less serious, but characterized by a pattern of drinking that results in situations that are harmful: drinking in situations that are physically dangerous (i.e., driving while intoxicated), failure to fulfill work, school or home responsibilities, or continuing to drink despite relationship problems worsened by drinking. While alcohol dependence and abuse are the most serious of the alcohol use disorders, a far greater number of people exhibit hazardous drinking, or drinking that is associated with physical or psychological harm. While most treatments traditionally focus on alcohol abuse or dependence, emphasis on preventing hazardous drinking has become an increasingly important focus of treatment and research.

Pharmacologic management for alcohol use disorders can be characterized as treatment for detoxification from alcohol, treatment for the prevention of relapse, and treatment of comorbid psychiatric disorders. Medications for detoxification from alcohol and for comorbid psychiatric disorders are beyond the scope of this chapter. Naltrexone is one of the three medications approved by the FDA as a medication to prevent relapse alcoholism; the other two are disulfiram and acamprosate, and are reviewed elsewhere. Naltrexone is used to prevent relapse in abstinent individuals and to decrease heavy drinking in nonabstinent individuals. More recently it is being explored as a potential treatment for non–alcohol-dependent individuals who exhibit hazardous drinking.

Clinical Trials

In humans the efficacy of naltrexone treatment for alcohol use disorders was first demonstrated by Volpicelli and colleagues (16). In this landmark study, 70 alcohol-dependent male patients were randomized to receive 50 mg/day naltrexone or placebo for 12 weeks; all patients received outpatient psychotherapy. Patients receiving naltrexone reported less craving for alcohol and also reported fewer drinking days. In those individuals who drank alcohol, naltrexone slowed the rate of relapse to heavy drinking, defined as five or more alcoholic drinks in a day. These promising findings were replicated and extended by O'Malley and colleagues (17). In this study, 97 alcohol-dependent male and female patients were randomized to receive either 50 mg/day naltrexone or placebo for 12 weeks. They were also randomized to receive either cognitive behavioral therapy (emphasizing relapse prevention and coping skills) or supportive therapy. An interaction of naltrexone and therapy was observed, where abstinence from alcohol was more likely to occur in patients receiving active naltrexone and supportive therapy. However, in patients who drank alcohol, the combination of naltrexone and cognitive behavioral therapy was more efficacious. Together these two hallmark studies led to the FDAs approval of naltrexone for the treatment of alcohol use disorders in 1994. Since this approval, the majority of randomized clinical trials examining naltrexone have had positive results.

The first multisite study was conducted in the late 1990s (18). Patients ($N = 169$) received either 50 mg/day naltrexone or placebo for 12 weeks. All patients received psychosocial treatment and had been abstinent from alcohol for 5 to 30 days. The primary outcome of interest was the time to first heavy drinking day. No effect of naltrexone was observed when all patients were included in the analyses. However, when only compliant patients were included (defined by 80% medication consumption, and attendance at all follow-up appointments), naltrexone decreased the amount of alcohol consumed but did not change the time to the first heavy drinking day. The authors concluded that compliance is crucial in naltrexone treatment, indicating that naltrexone is best for highly motivated patients.

Several meta-analyses have examined the efficacy of naltrexone (19–21). Kranzler and Van Kirk (19) examined nine naltrexone studies. All studies were randomized clinical trials. The meta-analysis only considered data from intention-to-treat samples. The length of treatment varied across the included studies. They observed several indications that naltrexone is an efficacious treatment for alcohol use disorders. The effect size for naltrexone (12% to 19% better than placebo) was modest. Naltrexone decreased the percentage of drinking days, increased the likelihood of alcohol abstinence during study participation, and decreased the risk of relapse to heavy drinking. They concluded that naltrexone was a viable treatment for alcohol use disorders. Streeton and Whelan (20) examined seven naltrexone studies. All studies were randomized clinical trials that included 12 weeks of outpatient treatment, with varied psychosocial therapy. They concluded that naltrexone reduced relapse to heavy drinking and improves alcohol abstinence while on medication. At 6-month follow-up, no benefit of 12-week naltrexone, over placebo, was observed (21).

A more recent meta-analysis review of naltrexone as a treatment for alcohol use disorders was completed in 2005 by Srisurapanont and Jarusuraisin (22). Twenty-seven trials, spanning from 1992 to 2003, were included. All studies were randomized clinical trials. Eighteen studies compared naltrexone to placebo while others compared naltrexone to other medications such as acamprosate, disulfiram, nefazodone, and ondansetron. Five studies also included comparisons of psychosocial treatment length. The authors concluded that naltrexone reduced rates of relapse by 36% and reduced the rates of returning to alcohol drinking by 13% in short-term randomized clinical trials.

Some studies have reported negative findings with daily oral naltrexone. The largest negative study was the 52-week multisite VA Cooperative Study (23), which found no advantage of naltrexone over placebo. Participants were randomly assigned to one of three medication conditions: (a) 50 mg/day naltrexone for 12 months, (b) 50 mg/day naltrexone for 3 months, followed by placebo for 9 months, or (c) placebo for 12 months. Medication was offered as an adjunct treatment to individual counseling and programs, and attendance at Alcoholics Anonymous. Naltrexone, compared to placebo, did not delay or prevent relapse, decrease the percentage of drinking days, or decrease the number of drinks per drinking day in mostly male (98%) sample. In comparison with patients in other trials, patients in this study exhibited more severe and chronic alcohol dependence. This difference, among other characteristics, has been suggested as a rational for the negative results (24). A secondary analysis of the data suggests that naltrexone might have been beneficial for those alcohol-dependent patients with a consistent drinking pattern (25).

In the largest study to date, Project COMBINE examined the efficacy of naltrexone, in combination with combined behavioral intervention (CBI) and with another medication for alcohol use disorders (3 g/day acamprosate) in 1383 subjects (26). The study consisted of 16 weeks of treatment and the drinking outcomes of interest were the percentage of days abstinent and the time to first heavy drinking day. Participants were randomly assigned to naltrexone (100 mg), acamprosate (3 g), placebo, the combination or to no pill condition and to two psychosocial conditions that included medical management (MM), an intervention that could be modeled in a primary care or cognitive behavioral intervention (CBI). Randomization resulted in nine groups and the participants in groups 1 to 8 received MM, the ninth received CBI. The mean dose of naltrexone was 88 mg/day. The best outcomes were with those individuals who received MM and naltrexone or MM and CBI. Results supported the use of naltrexone in the treatment of alcohol dependence, but with a modest effect size.

An emergent use of oral naltrexone in young nondependent adults with hazardous drinking has been targeted administration of naltrexone, sometimes in combination with daily dosing. Patients are instructed to use the medication when they are expecting exposure to alcohol and alcohol-related cues. A recent study of early problem drinkers examined the efficacy of targeted naltrexone (27). In the study, 153 patients were randomly assigned to one of four groups: (a) 50 mg naltrexone daily, (b) placebo daily, (c) 50 mg naltrexone targeted, or (d) placebo targeted. The instruction for targeted naltrexone administration was to self-administer the medication in anticipation of a heavy drinking situation. Targeted naltrexone decreased both drinking and heavy drinking. This line of research continues in an ongoing randomized clinical trial (RCT00568958) in young adults, which is examining the efficacy of a low dose of targeted naltrexone (25 mg) in addition to daily naltrexone (25 mg) and counseling.

Concern about rates of compliance with oral naltrexone led to the development of 4-week extended-release injections. This formulation is marketed in the United States as Vivitrol. The FDA approved intramuscular naltrexone in 2006 for alcohol dependence. A 6-month randomized clinical trial examined the efficacy and tolerability of Vivitrol in 627 alcohol-dependent adults (13). Participants were randomly assigned to receive 380 mg naltrexone, 190 mg naltrexone, or placebo, and all received standardized psychosocial support. Both naltrexone doses were well tolerated. The 380 mg dose reduced heavy drinking more effectively than the 190 mg dose. Retrospective analyses of early treatment response indicated that Vivitrol was clinically effective within 2 days of injection (28) and was more efficacious if patients were already abstinent from alcohol (29). Gender effects were observed in this trial and a positive effect of naltrexone over placebo was observed in males, but not in women. The reasons for this gender difference are unclear and will be examined in future studies.

Laboratory Studies

Laboratory-based investigations have been conducted to further understand how naltrexone improves clinical outcomes for alcohol dependence. Several studies have suggested that naltrexone might reduce alcohol drinking by altering the subjective effects of alcohol. For example, Swift and colleagues (30) examined the effect of an acute dose of naltrexone on alcohol intoxication. Naltrexone decreased subjective ratings of alcohol-induced stimulation while increasing ratings of alcohol-induced sedation. In another study, chronic naltrexone (50 mg/day) administration led to decreased alcohol craving prior to drink consumption and decreased subjective alcohol-induced stimulation after consumption (31). Naltrexone has also been included in examinations of alcohol cue reactivity and is associated with decreased reactivity to alcohol cues compared to placebo (32).

Drinker characteristics such as family history of alcoholism have also been examined as possible predictors of response to naltrexone. A recent study explored the effect of chronic naltrexone administration and family history of alcoholism in a laboratory model of alcohol drinking (33). The study enrolled alcohol-dependent individuals and randomly assigned them to receive either 50 or 100 mg/day naltrexone or placebo. In the laboratory paradigm, participants consumed a priming dose of alcohol (equivalent to one alcoholic beverage) and then participated in an ad-lib drinking session for several hours. Naltrexone (100 mg/day) decreased the number of drinks consumed in family history positive males. These findings indicate that family history of alcoholism affects response to naltrexone and suggests that this effect might also be linked with gender.

Individuals with a family history of alcoholism can be about three times more likely to have a particular version (G allele vs. A allele) of the mu-opioid receptor gene (OPRM1) (34). A recent study investigated whether differences in this gene might influence the effect of naltrexone on response to alcohol. Forty participants received either 50 mg oral naltrexone or placebo. They then received intravenous alcohol to reach three targeted breath alcohol levels (0.02, 0.04, 0.06 g/dL). Under placebo, participants with the G allele variant reported greater subjective high from the alcohol. Under naltrexone, patients with the G allele reported greater blunting of alcohol-induced high, compared to patients with the A allele (35). These findings further strengthen the relationship between family history of alcoholism and response to naltrexone.

Doses and Routes of Administration

Oral naltrexone is marketed in the United States as Revia. The standard prescribing dose of naltrexone is 50 mg/day. This dose was first selected because it was efficacious in the treatment of opioid dependence. Some investigations have suggested that a higher dose (100 mg/day) results in better clinical outcomes. Naltrexone may be better tolerated if patients receiving oral naltrexone initiate treatment with 25 mg/day and then increase to 50 mg/day across 7 days. While the optimal length of treatment has not been determined, a typical length of treatment is 12 weeks. Oral administration is best for highly motivated patients, as the efficacy of naltrexone oral administration in the treatment of alcohol use disorders is enhanced in individuals who have high rates of medication compliance.

Another way to prescribe oral naltrexone, targeted administration in anticipation of exposure to alcohol, in combination with daily dosing is currently being evaluated.

Naltrexone is also available in a 4-week extended-release injection which is marketed in the United States as Vivitrol. Patients receive an intramuscular gluteal injection of serum that contains microspheres of encapsulated naltrexone (380 mg/injection). The microspheres degrade over time and naltrexone is continuously released. An advantage of this route of administration is that some side effects that some patients report with the rapid uptake of naltrexone when administered orally are minimized (13).

Naltrexone in Combination with Other Medications/Therapies

In most of the randomized clinical trials, naltrexone has been combined with some form of psychotherapy. Naltrexone has been evaluated with cognitive behavioral therapy, 12-step facilitation, supportive therapy, and medical management. It is recommended by the FDA that naltrexone be prescribed *in conjunction* with an adequate psychosocial intervention. In one of the landmark studies, naltrexone (vs. placebo) was paired with either cognitive behavioral therapy or supportive therapy (17). The interaction of naltrexone with therapy suggested that careful consideration of therapeutic styles should be considered when naltrexone is used as an adjunct pharmacotherapy.

Interest has grown, perhaps because of naltrexone's modest effect size, in combining naltrexone treatment with other medications to enhance alcohol use outcomes. Naltrexone has been given with other FDA-approved medications to treat alcoholism including acamprosate in the COMBINE trial (26), disulfiram in a multisite study in 254 dually diagnosed alcohol-dependent veterans (36) and with serotonin reuptake inhibitors as adjunctive medications (37). However, the addition of other medications does not seem to result in improved alcohol use outcomes compared to naltrexone alone. Studies evaluating naltrexone in combination with other medications, such as the anticonvulsant topiramate (NCT00769158) and the serotonergic agent ondansetron (NCT00027079), which have shown promise in treating alcoholism, are ongoing. Naltrexone has also been given safely to patients who are on psychiatric medications, including antipsychotics (38), antidepressants (23,39), and mood stabilizers (36,40).

Alcohol-Dependent Patients for Whom Naltrexone Is Optimal

Naltrexone is recommended for highly motivated patients, since efficacy rates seem to be highest among compliant patients (18). Recent studies have suggested that certain patient characteristics such as family history of alcoholism can also be a predictor of success with naltrexone (33). Some recent genetic research has indicated that a functional polymorphism of the OPRM1 (mu-opioid receptor) is associated with better naltrexone response (41). However, another study did not support this association (42). Differences in study sample characteristics have been suggested as a possible explanation for the mixed results.

SAFETY OF NALTREXONE

Side Effect Profile

Naltrexone is generally well tolerated. The most common side effects with 50 mg/day oral administration are nausea, headache, dizziness, fatigue, vomiting, anxiety, and sleeplessness; less common side effects include anxiety and sleepiness (20). Use of extended-release injections can reduce symptoms, such as nausea, that are associated with oral dosing. Some side effects specific to injections include pain, tenderness, induration, swelling, erythema, bruising, and pruritus at the injection site (13). Some side effects specific to naltrexone implants include infection of the implant site, pain at implant site, and allergic reactions (11).

Naltrexone is metabolized by the liver and can be associated with hepatotoxicity, although usually if given in much higher doses than the 50 mg currently recommended. Nevertheless, liver function tests should be evaluated before the use of naltrexone and periodically during treatment and it is generally recommended that individuals whose liver function tests are three to five times normal should not be prescribed naltrexone.

Questions have been raised about whether long-term therapy with naltrexone may be associated with dysphoria. Theoretically, dysphoria could occur because naltrexone, as an opioid receptor antagonist, competes with endogenous opioid peptides. A recent review, however, indicated that most studies have not found evidence of dysphoria with long-term naltrexone therapy (43).

Contraindications

It should be remembered that naltrexone is an opiate antagonist and as such is contraindicated in those patients with chronic pain who are being treated with opiates as it will precipitate withdrawal. In addition, worsening of pain has been reported with naltrexone (16). Before starting naltrexone, patients should discontinue narcotics for a minimum of 7 to 10 days. Patients taking naltrexone should be provided with a wallet card explaining that they are currently prescribed naltrexone. This safety measure will reduce complications for treatment in cases of emergency when opioid administration could be advisable. Naltrexone is contraindicated in pregnant and lactating women. As mentioned above, naltrexone should not be used in individuals who have seriously compromised liver function.

Use of Naltrexone in Other Populations

A growing body of literature is evaluating naltrexone's efficacy in dually diagnosed alcohol-dependent patients. This literature includes pilot studies, retrospective evaluations, secondary analyses, and a few randomized clinical trials. Naltrexone's efficacy is an important clinical issue since some evidence suggests that clinicians who treat patients with alcohol use disorders preferentially prescribe medications to individuals with comorbid psychiatric disorders. Utilization of naltrexone in the VA system nationally, despite a very low overall rate of prescribing (less than 2% of 194,001 patients with alcohol dependence were prescribed naltrexone), was higher in those patients with the presence of a comorbid mental disorder (44).

Several studies have suggested that naltrexone is both safe and effective for treating alcohol use disorders in individuals with comorbid psychiatric disorders. In a retrospective study on 72 psychiatric patients treated with naltrexone for their alcohol use disorder, 82% of patients significantly reduced their drinking (45). Naltrexone also decreased alcohol use and improved depressive symptoms in an open study with patients manifesting alcohol dependence (46). It has been hypothesized that patients with well-controlled psychiatric conditions might find naltrexone effective or that naltrexone might work synergistically with psychotropic medications in improving drinking outcomes (47). In a secondary analysis of the VA Cooperative Study of naltrexone, those subjects treated with antidepressants for depression and anxiety during the trial, naltrexone-treated individuals had better alcohol use outcomes than did individuals on placebo (48).

The first controlled, randomized clinical trial with naltrexone in patients with schizophrenia and comorbid alcohol dependence ($N = 31$) showed that naltrexone-treated individuals had fewer drinking days and heavy drinking days and reported less craving in comparison to individuals treated with placebo (38). All subjects were on stable doses of neuroleptic medication. Overall, naltrexone was well tolerated and did not cause a worsening of psychosis. A larger study evaluating naltrexone versus placebo in patients with comorbid schizophrenia has been recently completed (49,50), and results suggest that among patients who were compliant with medication, those on naltrexone had better outcomes than those who were on placebo (50). In patients with bipolar disorder ($N = 50$), naltrexone-treated patients had a trend toward better alcohol use outcomes than those on placebo (40).

A 12-week randomized clinical trial of naltrexone and disulfiram in individuals with Axis-I disorders and alcohol dependence, who were stable on psychiatric medications ($N = 254$), showed that individuals had better outcomes if treated with active medication compared to placebo. However, no difference in outcome in those treated by naltrexone compared to disulfiram and no advantage of the combination were observed (36). In evaluating outcome by diagnosis, individuals with posttraumatic stress disorder (PTSD) ($N = 93$) did particularly well on active medication, but again no differences between naltrexone or disulfiram and no advantage of the combination were observed (51). Individuals with psychotic spectrum disorders ($N = 61$) had worse overall alcohol outcomes than individuals with nonpsychotic spectrum disorders. They had better alcohol outcomes if treated with either naltrexone or disulfiram, compared to placebo, but again there was no clear advantage of the combination of disulfiram and naltrexone over either alone (52). Individuals with depression did not fare as well as those who had PTSD or psychosis (39).

Naltrexone has been evaluated for dually diagnosed patients with opioid dependence; however, opiate agonists such as methadone and buprenorphine have proven more effective for long-term treatment. Literature describing the use of agonist pharmacotherapies in opioid-dependent dual diagnosis patients is beyond the scope of this chapter.

Other Uses

Naltrexone has been evaluated for a number of other addictive and impulsive spectrum disorders, including cocaine dependence, tobacco dependence, problem gambling, kleptomania, and eating disorders. It has also been evaluated as an adjunctive medication in other psychiatric disorders and to treat opiate-induced adverse events.

Naltrexone has been evaluated for cocaine dependence, and given the high comorbidity with alcohol dependence, particular emphasis has been on treating those with both alcohol and cocaine dependence. In an early study, naltrexone was found to be less effective than disulfiram for cocaine- and alcohol-dependent individuals (53). For individuals with alcohol dependence who also use cocaine, doses higher than the standard 50 mg/day could be more effective than the standard dose. A recent study examining 50 mg/day naltrexone in 80 patients with cocaine and alcohol dependence did not observe a significant reduction in either cocaine or alcohol use (54).

Some randomized clinical trials have examined the effect of naltrexone on smoking cessation rates. In addition to examining naltrexone alone, the drug has also been used as an adjunct pharmacotherapy to other established treatments, such as nicotine replacement therapy (55). In general, findings have been inconsistent. The primary benefits of naltrexone for smoking cessation include that it might limit weight gain (56), and that it is useful in treating polydrug abuse (57).

Impulse Control Disorders: Problem Gambling and Kleptomania

Recent evidence suggests that chronic naltrexone administration reduces gambling urges and behaviors. An 18-week randomized clinical trial enrolled 77 problem gamblers who received either 50, 100, or 150 mg/day naltrexone, or placebo (58). Naltrexone improved clinical outcomes with no difference between doses. Family history of alcoholism has been identified as a clinical predictor of naltrexone response for problem gambling (59). However, naltrexone in the concurrent treatment of problem gambling and alcohol use disorder is not supported (60). In this 11-week randomized clinical trial, 52 participants received either naltrexone or placebo, and all received cognitive behavioral counseling. The dose of naltrexone started at 50 mg/day and was increased by 50 mg/day if patients reported no therapeutic effect; the actual mean dose for the naltrexone group was 100 mg/day. Naltrexone neither improved symptoms of problem gambling nor outcomes for the alcohol use disorder.

Naltrexone has also recently been used in the treatment of kleptomania. Doses have typically been higher than those used in the treatment of alcohol use disorders. An 8-week randomized clinical trials of naltrexone, compared to placebo, observed that naltrexone decreased stealing urges and behaviors (61). The naltrexone dose range was 50 to 150 mg/day, and the mean study dose was 116 mg/day. In another similar study, the mean effective dose was 135 mg/day (62).

Eating Disorders: Bulimia, Anorexia Nervosa, Binge Eating Disorder

Recent studies examining the efficacy of naltrexone in treating eating disorders have had mixed results. These studies used chronic naltrexone administration, with a standard 1-week medication lead-in period. Evidence for naltrexone's use in the treatment of eating disorders is limited. While there have been some indications that naltrexone improves clinical outcomes in the treatment of bulimia (63), other studies have had negative results (64). Limited evidence also suggests that naltrexone might be beneficial in the treatment of binge eating disorder (63). A report suggests that naltrexone can improve clinical outcome for anorexia nervosa in some patients (65).

MISCELLANEOUS

Naltrexone has been evaluated with limited success as an adjunctive treatment for schizophrenia (66) and depression (67) in individuals *without* comorbid substance use disorders. Naltrexone has also been used to alleviate opioid-induced adverse events. Low doses of naltrexone (6 mg/day) have been shown to reduce opioid-induced constipation and pruritus, without reversing analgesia (68).

CONCLUSIONS

Naltrexone is an oral opioid antagonist that competes with opioids to bind at opioid receptors. Although naltrexone was originally developed for the treatment of opioid dependence, research indicating that opioid receptors are involved in the effects of alcohol has led to the use of naltrexone for the treatment of alcohol use disorders as well. Naltrexone is safe and has clinical uses in both treatment of opioid dependence and alcohol dependence. Its role in opioid dependence is predominately as an adjunctive medication for opioid detoxification or for maintenance in highly motivated populations. In alcohol use disorders, naltrexone's efficacy is supported by most of the clinical trials, but it has a modest effect size. The standard starting dose of naltrexone is 50 mg/day for both opioid dependence and alcohol dependence. This dose is sufficient to block opioid receptors for 24 hours and has been found to be effective in treating alcohol use disorders. However, research evaluating the efficacy of different doses, particularly in alcohol use disorders, is underway. While oral administration is the most common route of administration, newer routes of administration include extended-release injections and implants. In opioid dependence, improving compliance is likely to improve its efficacy, and research into the use of extended-release injections is of high priority. In alcohol dependence, not all patients are sensitive to its therapeutic effects. Consideration should be given to patient characteristics that can increase positive outcomes, including family history of alcoholism. Further research on identifying characteristics, such as genotypes, of patients who most benefit from naltrexone therapy is also underway.

ACKNOWLEDGMENTS

This work was supported by a grant from NIAAA-T32-AA015496 (PI=Petrakis). We gratefully acknowledge the contributions of Erica Dean and Elizabeth Ralevski.

REFERENCES

1. Veilleux JC, Colvin PJ, Anderson J, et al. A review of opioid dependence treatment: pharmacological and psychosocial interventions to treat opioid addiction. *Clin Psychol Rev.* 2010;30:155–166.
2. Hollister LE. Clinical evaluation of naltrexone treatment of opiate-dependent individuals. *Arch Gen Psychiatry.* 1978;35:335–340.
3. Meyer MC, Straughn AB, Lo M-W, et al. Bioequivalence, dose-proportionality, pharmacokinetics of naltrexone after oral administration. *J Clin Psychiatry.* 1984;45:15–19.
4. Unterwald EM. Naltrexone in the treatment of alcohol dependence. *J Addict Med.* 2008;2(3):121–127.
5. Stotts AL, Dodrill CL, Kosten TR. Opioid dependence treatment: options in pharmacotherapy. *Exp Opin Invest Drugs.* 2009;10(11):1727–1740.
6. Vining E, Kosten TR, Kleber HD. Clinical utility of rapid clonidine–naltrexone detoxification for opioid abusers. *Br J Addict.* 1988;83:567–575.
7. Kaye AD, Gevirtz C, Bosscher HA, et al. Ultrarapid opiate detoxification: a review. *Can J Anesth.* 2003;50(7):663–671.
8. Lawental E. Ultra rapid opiate detoxification as compared to 30-day inpatient detoxification program—a retrospective follow-up study. *J Subst Abuse.* 2000;11(2):173–181.
9. Reece AS. Psychosocial and treatment correlates of opiate free success in a clinical review of a naltrexone implant program. *Subst Abuse Treat Prev Policy.* 2007;2:35–49.
10. Oslen L, Christophersen AS, Frogopsahl G, et al. Plasma concentrations during naltrexone implant treatment of opiate-dependent patients. *Br J Clin Pharmacol.* 2004;58(2):219–222.
11. Kunoe N, Lobmaier P, Vederhus JK, et al. Naltrexone implants after in-patient treatment for opioid dependence: randomized controlled trial. *Br J Psychiatry.* 2009;194:541–546.
12. Comer SD, Sullivan MA, Yu E, et al. Injectable, sustained-release naltrexone for the treatment of opioid dependence. *Arch Gen Psychiatry.* 2006;63:210–218.
13. Garbutt JC, Kranzler HR, O'Malley SS, et al. Efficacy and tolerability of long-acting injectable naltrexone for alcohol dependence. *JAMA.* 2005;293(13):1617–1625.
14. Tucker TK, Ritter AJ. Naltrexone in the treatment of heroin dependence: a literature review. *Drug Alcohol Rev.* 2000;19:73–82.
15. Grant BF, Dawson DA, Stinson FS, et al. The 12-month prevalence and trends in DSM–IV alcohol abuse and dependence: United States, 1991–1992 and 2001–2002. *Alcohol Res Health.* 2006;29(2):79–91.
16. Volpicelli JR, Alterman AI, Hayashida M, et al. Naltrexone in the treatment of alcohol dependence. *Arch Gen Psychiatry.* 1992;49(11):876–880.
17. O'Malley SS, Jaffe AJ, Chang G, et al. Naltrexone and coping skills therapy for alcohol dependence. A controlled study. *Arch Gen Psychiatry.* 1992;49(11):881–887.
18. Chick J, Anton R, Checinski K, et al. A multicentre, randomized, double-blind, placebo-controlled trial of naltrexone in the treatment of alcohol dependence or abuse. *Alcohol Alcohol.* 2000;35(6):587–593.
19. Kranzler HR, Van Kirk J. Efficacy of naltrexone and acamprosate for alcoholism treatment: a meta-analysis. *Alcohol Clin Exp Res.* 2001;29(5):1335–1341.
20. Streeton C, Whelan G. Naltrexone, a relapse prevention maintenance treatment of alcohol dependence: a meta-analysis of randomized controlled trials. *Alcohol Alcohol.* 2001;36(6):544–552.
21. O'Malley SS, Jaffe AJ, Chang G, et al. Six month follow-up of naltrexone and psychotherapy for alcohol dependence. *Arch Gen Psychiatry.* 1996;53(3):217–224.
22. Srisurapanont M, Jarusuraisin N. Opioid antagonists for alcohol dependence. *Cochrane Database System Rev.* 2005;1:1–45.
23. Krystal JH, Cramer JA, Krol WF, et al. Naltrexone in the treatment of alcohol dependence. *N Engl J Med.* 2001;345(24):1734–1739.
24. Fuller RK, Gordis E. Naltrexone treatment for alcohol dependence. *N Engl J Med.* 2001;345:1770–1771.
25. Gueorguieva R, Wu R, Pittman B, et al. New insights into the efficacy of naltrexone based on trajectory-based reanalyses of two negative clinical trials. *Biol Psychiatry.* 2007;61:1290–1295.
26. Anton RF, O'Malley SS, Ciraulo DA, et al. Combined pharmacotherapies and behavioral interventions for alcohol dependence. The COMBINE study: a randomized controlled trial. *JAMA.* 2006;295(17):2003–2017.
27. Kranzler HR, Armeli S, Tennen H, et al. Targeted naltrexone for early problem drinkers. *J Clin Psychopharmacol.* 2003;23(3):294–304.
28. Ciraulo DA, Dong Q, Silverman BL, et al. Early treatment response in alcohol dependence with extended-release naltrexone. *J Clin Psychiatry.* 2008;69(2):190–195.
29. O'Malley SS, Garbutt JC, Gastfriend DR, et al. Efficacy of extended-release naltrexone in alcohol-dependent patients who are abstinent before treatment. *J Clin Psychopharmacol.* 2007;27(5):507–512.
30. Swift RM, Whelihan W, Kuznetsov O, et al. Naltrexone-induced alterations in human ethanol intoxication. *Am J Psychiatry.* 1994;151(10):1463–1467.
31. Drobes DJ, Anton RF, Thomas SE, et al. Effects of naltrexone and nalmefene on subjective response to alcohol among non-treatment-seeking alcoholics and social drinkers. *Alcohol Clin Exp Res.* 2004;28(9):1362–1370.
32. Rohsenow DJ, Monti PM, Hutchison KE, et al. Naltrexone's effects on reactivity to alcohol cues among alcoholic men. *J Abnorm Psychology.* 2000;109(4):738–742.
33. Krishnan-Sarin S, Krystal JH, Shi J, et al. Family history of alcoholism influences naltrexone-induced reduction in alcohol drinking. *Biol Psychiatry.* 2007;62:694–697.
34. Ray LA, Hutchinson KE. A polymorphism of the mu-opioid receptor gene (OPRM1) and sensitivity to the effects of alcohol in humans. *Alcohol Clin Exp Res.* 2004;28(12):1789–1795.

35. Ray LA, Hutchison KE. Effects of naltrexone on alcohol sensitivity and genetic moderators of medication response: a double-blind placebo-controlled study. *Arch Gen Psychiatry.* 2007;64(9):1069–1077.
36. Petrakis IL, Poling J, Levinson C, et al. Naltrexone and disulfiram in patients with alcohol dependence and comorbid psychiatric disorders. *Biol Psychiatry.* 2005;57:1128–1137.
37. Farren CK, Scimeca M, Wu R, et al. A double-blind, placebo-controlled study of sertraline with naltrexone for alcohol dependence. *Drug Alcohol Depend.* 2009;99:317–321.
38. Petrakis IL, O'Malley SS, Rounsaville B, et al. Naltrexone augmentation of neuroleptic treatment in alcohol abusing patients with schizophrenia. *Psychopharmacology.* 2004;172:291–297.
39. Petrakis IL, Ralevski E, Nich C, et al. Naltrexone and disulfiram in patients with alcohol dependence and current depression. *J Clin Psychopharmacol.* 2007;27(2):160–165.
40. Brown ES, Beard L, Dobbs L, et al. Naltrexone in patients with bipolar disorder and alcohol dependence. *Depress Anxiety.* 2006;23:492–495.
41. Oslin DW, Berrettini W, Kranzler HR, et al. A functional polymorphism of the μ-opioid receptor gene is associated with naltrexone response in alcohol-dependent patients. *Neuropsychopharmacology.* 2003;28:1546–1552.
42. Gelernter J, Gueorguieva R, Kranzler HR, et al. Opioid receptor gene (OPRM1, OPRK1, and OPRD1) variants and response to naltrexone treatment for alcohol dependence: results from the VA Cooperative Study. *Alcohol Clin Exp Res.* 2007;31(4):555–563.
43. Pettinati HM, O'Brien CP, Rabinowitz AR, et al. The status of naltrexone in the treatment of alcohol dependence. *J Clin Psychopharmacol.* 2006;26(6):610–625.
44. Petrakis IL, Leslie D, Rosenheck R. Use of naltrexone in the treatment of alcoholism nationally in the Department of Veteran Affairs. *Alcohol Clin Exp Res.* 2003;27(11):1780–1784.
45. Maxwell S, Shinderman MS. Use of naltrexone in the treatment of alcohol use disorders in patients with concomitant major mental illness. *J Addict Dis.* 2000;19(3):61–69.
46. Salloum I, Cornelius J, Thase M, et al. Naltrexone utility in depressed alcoholics. *Psychopharmacology.* 1998;34(1):111–115.
47. Morris PL, Hopwood M, Whelan G, et al. Naltrexone for alcohol dependence: a randomized controlled trial.[comment]. *Addiction.* 2001;96(11):1565–1573.
48. Krystal JH, Gueorguieva R, Cramer J, et al. Naltrexone is associated with reduced drinking by alcohol dependent patients receiving antidepressants for mood and anxiety symptoms: results from VA Cooperative Study No. 425, "Naltrexone in the treatment of alcoholism". *Alcohol Clin Exp Res.* 2008;32(1):85–91.
49. Batki SL, Dimmock JA, Cornell M, et al. Directly observed naltrexone treatment of alcohol dependence in schizophrenia: preliminary analysis. *Alcohol Clin Exp Res.* 2002;26:83A.
50. Batki S, Dimmock J, Leontieva L, et al. Recruitment and characteristics of alcohol dependent patients with schizophrenia. *Alcohol Clin Exp Res.* 2005;29:78A.
51. Petrakis IL, Poling J, Levinson C, et al. Naltrexone and disulfiram in patients with alcohol dependence and comorbid post-traumatic stress disorder. *Biol Psychiatry.* 2006;60:777–783.
52. Petrakis IL, Nich C, Ralevski E. Psychotic spectrum disorders and alcohol abuse: a review of pharmacotherapeutic strategies and a report on the effectiveness of naltrexone and disulfiram. *Schizophr Bull.* 2006;32(4):644–654.
53. Carroll K, Ziedonis DM, O'Malley SS, et al. Pharmacologic interventions for abusers of alcohol and cocaine: a pilot study of disulfiram versus naltrexone. *J Drug Addict.* 1993;2:77–79.
54. Schmitz JM, Stotts AL, Sayre SL, et al. Treatment of cocaine–alcohol dependence with naltrexone and relapse prevention therapy. *Am J Addict.* 2004;13:333–341.
55. O'Malley SS, Cooney JL, Krishnan-Sarin S, et al. A controlled trial of naltrexone augmentation of nicotine replacement therapy for smoking cessation *Arch Intern Med.* 2006;166(6):667–674.
56. Toll BA, Leary V, Wu R, et al. A preliminary investigation of naltrexone augmentation of bupropion to stop smoking with less weight gain. *Addict Behav.* 2008;33:173–179.
57. Scholl RA, Lerman C. Current and emerging pharmacotherapies for treating tobacco dependence. *Exp Opin Emerg Drugs.* 2006;11(3):429–444.
58. Grant JE, Kim SW, Hartman BK. A double-blind, placebo-controlled study of the opiate antagonist naltrexone in the treatment of pathological gambling urges. *J Clin Psychiatry.* 2008;69(5):783–789.
59. Grant JE, Kim SW, Hollander E, et al. Predicting response to opiate antagonists and placebo in the treatment of pathological gambling. *Psychopharmacology.* 2008;200:521–527.
60. Toneatto T, Brands B, Selby P. A randomized, double-blind, placebo-controlled trial of naltrexone in the treatment of concurrent alcohol use disorder and pathological gambling. *Am J Addict.* 2009;18(3):219–225.
61. Grant JE, Kim SW, Odlaug BL. A double-blind, placebo-controlled study of the opiate antagonist, naltrexone, in the treatment of kleptomania. *Biol Psychiatry.* 2009;65:600–606.
62. Grant JE. Outcome study of kleptomania patients treated with naltrexone. A chart review. *Clin Neuropharmacol.* 2005;28(1):11–14.
63. Marrazzi MA, Markham KM, Kinzie J, et al. Binge eating disorder: response to naltrexone. *Int J Obes Relat Metab Disord.* 1995;19(2):143–145.
64. Mitchell JE, Christenson G, Jennings J, et al. A placebo-controlled, double-blind crossover study of naltrexone hydrochloride in outpatients with normal weight bulimia. *J Clin Psychopharmacol.* 1989;9(2):94–97.
65. Marrazzi MA, Bacon JP, Kinzie J, et al. Naltrexone use in the treatment of anorexia and bulimia nervosa. *Int Clin Psychopharmacol* 1995;10(3):163–172.
66. Sernyak M, Glazer WM, Heninger GR, et al. Naltrexone augmentation of neuroleptics in schizophrenia. *J Clin Psychopharmacol.* 1998;18(3):248–251.
67. Amiaz R, Stein O, Dannon PN, et al. Resolution of treatment-refractory depression with naltrexone augmentation of paroxetine—a case report. *Psychopharmacology.* 1999;143(4):433–434.
68. Friedman JD, Dello Buono FA. Opioid antagonists in the treatment of opioid-induced constipation and pruritus. *Ann Pharmacother.* 2001;35:85–91.

CHAPTER 31 — Vaccines for Substance Abuse

Frank M. Orson ■ Mark J. Biscone ■ Berma M. Kinsey ■ Thomas R. Kosten

INTRODUCTION

Vaccines for substance abuse offer a new and very different approach for treating for cocaine, nicotine, methamphetamine, heroin, and phencyclidine abuse. The socioeconomic problems of substance abuse are discussed in detail in other chapters; therefore, this chapter will discuss the influence of specific antibodies on drug pharmacodynamics and the experimental and clinical status for each of these abused substances. The basic concept for vaccine effects on the pharmacology of drugs is that antibodies can slow the rate of drug entry into the central nervous system (CNS), potentially reducing total drug concentrations. This is achieved through antibody binding of the substance in the bloodstream, since antibody molecules are too large to pass through the blood–brain barrier under normal conditions. This should result in a reduction in the reward sensations from drug ingestion, making the vaccinated-user less susceptible to psychological and physiologic reinforcement responses, so that the bonds of addiction might be more easily loosened.

Numerous issues remain to be fully investigated, but sufficient progress has been made in both experimental animal and human studies that more advanced clinical trials for the major abused substances will be conducted in the next few years. As will be discussed in detail, there are three distinct areas of limitation on vaccine effects relating to the influence on drug distribution and metabolism: the amount and persistence of antibody ordinarily elicited by vaccines, and the affinity of the antibody for the drug (1). The advantages of vaccines as a treatment for substance abuse, in contrast to conventional drug therapy approaches, are that if persistent, high levels of antibody can be elicited by a vaccine, compliance failures will be much less of a problem, and undesirable CNS side effects of the treatment itself would not be a concern, as they often are with small molecule agonists or antagonists. This chapter will discuss the effects of antidrug antibodies on drug pharmacodynamics in terms of both the quantitative and the qualitative properties of the antibodies, and will also review the current stages of vaccine development for nicotine, cocaine, methamphetamine, phencyclidine, and heroin. Vaccination resulting in long-term inhibition of the pharmacologic actions of abused drugs has great potential for assisting motivated addicts to begin and sustain abstinence from their specific abused substance.

CONCEPTUAL BASIS FOR DRUG VACCINES

Drugs associated with substance abuse enter the CNS following absorption or injection and occupy receptors that modulate neuron signaling, thus leading to the reward/reinforcement sensations associated with use of the specific drug. These sensations are dependent on the number of receptors occupied, as well as, in many cases, the rate at which receptor occupation occurs (2). Cocaine, for example, targets dopamine transporters and methamphetamine binds several different receptors (3), while morphine and heroin metabolites bind mu-opiate receptors. Preventing the rapid rise of receptor occupation in the brain will inhibit the maximal pleasurable and reinforcing effects of many abused drugs (4).

In order to influence drug pharmacodynamics, substance abuse vaccines must elicit high levels of specific IgG antibodies with good binding affinity, so that these antibodies can bind and hold most of the drug molecules within the circulation, reducing and delaying drug access to the brain. Antibody binding to target antigens has been extensively studied over the past several decades, and small molecule (hapten) binding in particular is quite well understood. The interactions between a small molecule (such as a drug of substance abuse) and an antibody can thus be accurately characterized as predominantly a function of antibody quantity and affinity, because antibody binding to a hapten does not result in significant changes in the structure or subsequent function of the antibody, in contrast to antibody binding to complex antigens. In the latter case, binding can create immune complexes, with alterations in the structure of the heavy chain portion of the antibody exposing complement binding sites, leading to activation of the complement cascade. Such changes in structure also result in attachment of the bound antibody to antibody receptors on cells of the reticuloendothelial system so that these complexes can be cleared from circulation. This clearance process can also cause activation of other immune functions that may lead to inflammatory responses in various tissues. Since binding of abused drugs, for example, cocaine, methamphetamine, or morphine, does not cause alterations in antibody structure, the half-life of the antibody is essentially unaffected. In fact, the half-life of the drug is often significantly prolonged as a result of binding to the antibody, except in the case of cocaine (discussed later).

To determine the initial, necessary goals for vaccine elicitation of antibody in terms of quantity and binding properties (affinity), the simple model of mass action equilibrium can be used, where K_a represents the association constant, [A] the free antibody concentration, [H] the concentration of free hapten, and [AH] the concentration of bound complex of drug and antibody at one combining site:

$$K_a = \frac{[AH]}{[A] \cdot [H]}$$

This equation is, for our purposes, sufficient to describe the basic interaction of a single drug molecule and a single antibody combining site, since the combining sites (two on IgG, for example) do not interact when bound with small molecules, either on the same antibody or between antibody molecules. At 50% occupancy of available antibody binding sites, the K_a predicted is accurate for IgG (5), the antibody isotype that dominates the antibody response with vaccines currently being studied. A more extensive discussion is provided elsewhere (1), detailing the alterations that occur at the extremes of antibody/drug concentration differences. In order to evaluate this equation, one must know the expected concentrations of free drug that are typically found in substance abusers depending on the drug of interest. Most of the drugs used achieve peak concentrations in the 0.5 to 1 μM range drug (6–8), although in heavy abusers, concentrations can sometimes be much higher (e.g., with morphine (9)).

From this information, and making reasonable assumptions about the expected binding affinity of the antibody responses, it is straightforward to determine the amounts of antibody required for binding a desired proportion of administered drug. Figure 31.1 shows a set of plots graphing the amount of antibody needed over a range of affinities for different doses to bind 75% of the peak concentration of the drug. As compared to the usual antibody responses needed for complete protection against toxins and microbes using standard vaccines, such as those against tetanus (1 to 2 μg/mL) or the *Haemophilus influenzae* b bacterium (0.15 μg/mL), the concentrations of antibody required for drug binding are quite high, up to 100 μg/mL or more for higher doses of drug. However, these levels are achievable in only a proportion of human patients using standard vaccine techniques (10). One interesting aspect of this plot is that it shows the relative independence of binding at affinities 30 μM^{-1} or higher (affinities that are typical of antibody in secondary (boosted) immune responses (11)). This is due to the fact that the specific concentrations of the target drug drive the response at a high proportion of binding. Each band in the figure flattens out beyond 30 and remains quite flat as the curve moves toward the right to higher affinities beyond that point. The binding at each higher dose then would require a step up in antibody concentration as can be appreciated on the right side of the figure. On the other hand, antibody affinities below 10 (typical of antibodies in primary immune responses (11)) are problematic for binding because much higher concentrations of antibody would be required with higher doses of drug (left side of figure). Although the actual requirements have not been precisely determined in clinical settings, the results from clinical trials for both nicotine (12) and cocaine vaccines (13) have shown that these estimates are clinically relevant. For both drugs, the higher 30% or so of high antibody responders showed significant reductions in drug use (cocaine) and quit rates (nicotine).

Simple binding to block uptake, however, is not the only consideration that affects drug pharmacodynamics. The speed with which the antibodies can bind to a drug will also influence its inhibition of drug entry into the CNS. As with many drugs of abuse, physiologic and subjective (the "rush") effects from smoked cocaine or methamphetamine are detectable within a few minutes of exposure (6). The antibody–antigen binding characteristics for haptens have been carefully studied over the years, and the initial attachment of an antibody combining site to its specific target molecule (the "on" rate) has been empirically determined in several model systems (14). Fortunately for substance abuse vaccine applications, these studies indicate that such initial antibody binding rates for small molecules are quite rapid and should not prove a hindrance to the effectiveness of vaccines, if they elicit a sufficiently high concentration of antibodies. IgG antibodies will bind the target molecules in a fully mixed sample essentially to equilibrium in less than 1 second (5), and consequently for ordinary administration routes and doses, the on rate of antibody binding is expected to be fast enough that maximal possible drug binding will occur in the bloodstream well before transfer of the drug to the brain is expected to take place. Achieving the high level responses necessary in vaccine recipients by optimizing vaccine design and administering with improved adjuvants should greatly reduce both the rate and the total drug accumulation in the brain from single doses.

Finally, although the above considerations do account for many of the clinical and experimental observations made

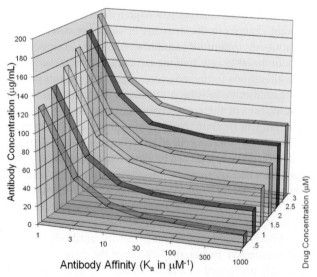

Figure 31.1. Affinity and dose effects on antibody requirements for 75% drug binding. The amount of antibody (Y axis, μg/mL) required to bind 75% of a specific peak drug concentration (Z axis, μM) is plotted for the specific antibody binding affinity, K_a (X axis, μM^{-1}).

with substance abuse drugs and vaccines thus far, some data from experimental animal studies suggest further effects of drug vaccines that are not fully understood. With nicotine vaccines in mice, for example, entry of a bolus dose of nicotine into the brain was blocked in vaccinated rats not previously treated with nicotine (15). Chronic nicotine treatment of such rats, however, which should result in some reduction of binding capacity of the antibody, showed lower levels of the nicotine bolus retained in the blood, but the mice still had a reduction in brain concentrations equivalent to the vaccinated mice without nicotine treatment. This might be explained in part by an increase in fat uptake (16), though the mechanisms for this observation remain obscure. Similarly, Owens' group has observed unexpected reductions in brain uptake of phencyclidine in experimental animals given a passive antibody infusion and then administered phencyclidine later at doses well above that expected to saturate the residual antibody (3). Thus some benefits of vaccination on drug pharmacodynamics may be operative, even at suboptimal antibody response levels.

ANTIBODY EFFECTS ON DRUG PHARMACODYNAMICS AND PHARMACOKINETICS

Most current ideas about reward from addictive substances combine aspects of "rate" and equilibrium binding pharmacologic theories to explain observations relating to drug action. The influence of both drug concentrations and pharmacodynamic features for cocaine, nicotine, methamphetamine, and opioids are important for their physiologic and subjective effects. Thus, a marked reduction in free-drug concentration in the blood by binding to specific antibodies would significantly inhibit drug action in the brain (e.g., if 75% to 90% of the drug is bound by high affinity antibody), since IgG-bound drug cannot readily cross the normal, noninflamed blood–brain barrier. In addition, it is well known experimentally that the rate of increase in receptor occupation in the CNS has a profound influence on the subjective effects of each of these drugs (17). Thus, less dramatic binding of the drug even by lower affinity antibody (e.g., resulting in 50% binding, perhaps) could still have a substantial influence on the rate of entry of free drug into the CNS. Even if the eventual total accumulation in the brain is similar to what would be achieved in the absence of antibody, the subjective CNS effects of the drug may be substantially or completely blunted, since the rate of receptor occupancy would be significantly reduced.

The pharmacokinetics of antibody-bound drug are thus related to the effects of antibody binding on a drug's metabolism, tissue distribution, and elimination pathways, as well as the antibody's intrinsic half-life and the effect of drug binding on antibody half-life through changes in the antibody structure, if any. Antibody binding to morphine, for example, prolongs morphine's terminal half-life in the bloodstream of experimental animals by two- to threefold (18), with essentially no effect on drug metabolism. In a vaccine study in rats, on the other hand, antibody binding of cocaine was shown to have little effect on cocaine half-life or metabolism, due in part to ongoing ester hydrolysis in the bloodstream, as well as no effect on clearance of the antibody (19).

Some antibodies can display catalytic properties, however. Selected monoclonal antibodies can enhance cocaine hydrolysis thus speeding the metabolic degradation of this drug in vivo (20). However, a vaccine that would elicit such catalytic antibodies from active immunization would be very difficult to design, given the broad variation in the structural features of the polyclonal antibodies elicited through immunization. Similar to morphine and in contrast to cocaine, antimethamphetamine antibodies have been shown to decrease methamphetamine clearance, prolong methamphetamine concentrations in serum, reduce conversion to amphetamine, and increase uptake in reticuloendothelial tissues like the liver (21). These features may well be related to the longer biologic half-life displayed by methamphetamine in comparison to cocaine, and especially to the fact that a substantial fraction of methamphetamine is not metabolized, but rather excreted unchanged in the urine. Nicotine also has a longer half-life in the body than cocaine, and the effects of antibodies on nicotine pharmacokinetics have been shown to resemble those on methamphetamine, with higher plasma concentrations after nicotine doses (22), and a half-life that is prolonged three- to sixfold.

A theoretical concern is that the potentially high affinity of the antidrug antibodies for drug metabolites, which, if present in high concentrations, may reduce the amount of antibody available for native drug binding. This is particularly a concern with cocaine. Benzoylecgonine is produced by hydrolysis of cocaine's methyl ester moiety, is structurally very similar to cocaine, and is essentially inactive pharmacologically. Heavy use of cocaine will result in substantial concentrations of benzoylecgonine in plasma, up to 10-fold higher than peak cocaine concentrations (23). Other metabolites, such as ecgonine methyl ester, and norcocaine are present in concentrations lower than cocaine itself. The half-life of benzoylecgonine is longer than that of cocaine, contributing to the high concentrations observed. Nicotine and its major metabolites, for example, cotinine, also present concerns regarding antibody binding competition. On the other hand, significant cross-reactivity of antimethamphetamine antibodies with amphetamine, a major methamphetamine metabolite, would be very desirable since amphetamine itself is pharmacologically active. Similarly, heroin is rapidly metabolized to 6-acetylmorphine and morphine in both the periphery and in the CNS. Both of these heroin metabolites are pharmacologically active. Fortunately, morphine conjugate vaccines can elicit antibodies capable of recognizing all three compounds (24).

NONTRADITIONAL VACCINE CONSTRUCTS

An alternative vaccine design is being developed at the University of Melbourne in David Jackson's laboratory in which a completely synthetic, self-adjuvanting epitope-based

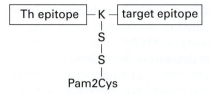

Figure 31.2. Self-adjuvanting vaccine structure. The helper T cell epitope and target epitope are attached to the lysine, and the internal adjuvant is the lipid moiety dipalmitoyl-S-glyceryl-cysteine (Pam2Cys) attached to the lysine through the serine residues.

vaccine is used to stimulate immune responses (25). The target epitope of the vaccine (in this case a substance abuse drug) is conjugated to a helper T cell (Th) epitope that also has the lipid moiety dipalmitoyl-S-glyceryl-cysteine (Pam2Cys) attached to it to function as the costimulatory signal for immune activation. The schematic design of this vaccine structure is shown in Figure 31.2.

A number of candidate antibody-inducing vaccines based on this design have been constructed, such as epitopes of either luteinizing hormone releasing hormone, gastrin, or a neutralizing epitope of group A streptococcus, and each has shown good responses in animal models (26). Epitopes from influenza virus, *Listeria monocytogenes* and tumor antigens that are recognized by cytotoxic T lymphocytes have been successful in demonstrating protection in various experimental animal systems. For antibody-inducing epitopes, the specific antibody levels elicited by the self-adjuvanting vaccine constructs in lab animals can be similar to that elicited by more traditional vaccines with standard adjuvants, such as complete Freund adjuvant (CFA), but without the toxicity associated with the latter agent. As a completely synthetic construct, the generic vaccine structure described here could have significant advantages in evaluation and development for rapid progression to human trials and clinical use. One such lipopeptide vaccine is expected to soon be in clinical trials in Australia.

Haptens like nicotine, cocaine, morphine, and methamphetamine are obvious potential immunogenic epitopes for such lipopeptide vaccine constructs using standard chemistries on a peptide synthesizer. Early experiments by Dr. Jackson in collaboration with our laboratory have shown that vaccines against amphetamine and cocaine elicited satisfactory levels of antidrug antibodies in mice. Once effectively formulated, a novel antidrug lipopeptide vaccine construct of this type would be inexpensive to produce with likely fewer side effect risks than the potentially toxic additional adjuvants traditionally required for most other vaccines. If so, it could be a real advance in vaccine design for clinical applications in substance abuse.

STATUS OF SPECIFIC DRUG VACCINES

Clinical trials with nicotine and cocaine vaccines have shown considerable promise, but still need improvement in the magnitude and consistency of the antibody responses to enhance clinical effectiveness. Antibody strategies for methamphetamine, morphine, and phencyclidine are still in preclinical development.

Nicotine

Cigarette smoking kills almost 5 million per year worldwide and further contributes to a worse clinical outcome in a variety of diseases. Successful escape from nicotine addiction in long-term smokers remains low despite the availability of several medications, counseling programs, and other treatments. Polls have shown that an overwhelming majority of tobacco users would like to quit the habit, which is fueled mainly by a strong physical dependence on nicotine. Given the widespread prevalence, adverse health consequences, motivated population of addicts, and failure of currently available treatments (27), nicotine is a critical therapeutic target for an effective vaccine.

Significant strides are being made in the area of nicotine vaccines, which will provide a new therapeutic option to help motivated individuals to finally break free of nicotine addiction. A number of these vaccines have successfully progressed to late Phase II and early Phase III clinical trials. Drug vaccines rely on the elicitation of specific antibodies that bind the drug in the bloodstream and thus prevent it from reaching specific receptors in the brain. This process effectively decouples the act of taking the drug and receiving the "reward" of the drug's effects. The antibodies must be present in sufficient quantities to deal with the majority of the drug amounts delivered. Whereas cocaine, heroin, and methamphetamine abuse is typically sporadic and taken in one bulk dose, nicotine is commonly delivered with frequent small doses. This can result in high plasma concentrations over a long duration. Furthermore, relapse to smoking after a period of abstinence frequently results from an ex-smoker being reacquainted with as little as a few puffs on a single cigarette, or even being in a smoky room occupied by current smokers. The presence of antibody at this precarious juncture could prevent any reward effect of the nicotine absorbed and thus help to prevent a relapse from occurring.

The effectiveness of eliciting antibodies targeting nicotine has been clearly demonstrated in animal models (12,15). In humans, three unique nicotine conjugate vaccines have completed Phase I clinical trials. All were well tolerated and able to elicit nicotine-specific antibodies, and cross-reactivity to human signaling molecules such as neurotransmitters was not observed. Following the NicVAX (Nabi Biopharmaceuticals) Phase I vaccine trial, a number of participants quit smoking for 30 days or more. This is particularly remarkable given that the trial was based around dosing and safety, not monitoring efficacy in smoking cessation. The majority of those individuals who quit were from the highest dose group, potentially linking dose/antibody response to successful smoking cessation. The NicVAX Phase IIB trial showed a 12-month continuous abstinence rate of 16% for the 400-μg schedule and 14% for the 200-μg schedule versus only 6% for the placebo group. Additionally, an improved immunization schedule was recently released based on the 400-μg dose, with an increase of subjects reaching the target antibody level from 50% to 80% at 14 weeks (12).

Substantial antinicotine antibody levels were also achieved utilizing the NicQb/NIC002 vaccine (Cytos Biotechnology AG). This was illustrated in the impressive quit rates attained for the upper third of antibody responders when compared to the placebo group (57% vs. 31%) (12). Data from the NIC002 Phase IIB trial was broken into three subgroups based on the antibody response to the vaccine: low, medium, and high responders. The 6-month continuous abstinence data showed 32% for the low, 32% for the medium, and 57% for the high responder groups compared to 31% for the placebo group, confirming the principle that only those with adequate antibody responses benefit significantly from immunization. After 12 months, the groups exhibited continuous abstinence rate of 26%, 21%, and 42%, respectively compared to the 21% of the placebo group. A second dose optimization trial, increasing the dose of conjugate from 100 to 300 μg, showed a 4.2-fold increase in specific antibody with up to 87% of patients achieving the antibody target level. Novartis purchased the rights to this vaccine, and the ongoing Phase IIB trial in smokers motivated to quit has been recently completed (28).

The trial involving the TA-NIC vaccine (Celtic Pharma, London) showed a similar positive response when the 12-month quit rate was compared between the highest dose group and the control group (38% vs. 8%) (29). A TA-NIC Phase IIB trial is currently planned. These studies show that vaccination against the nicotine molecule has immense potential to aid in the vast numbers of people seeking smoking cessation, especially if the quantity of specific antibodies induced can be optimized.

Cocaine

Cocaine continues to be a major problem in the United States and elsewhere in the world, resulting in both individual and family difficulties from the medical and legal perspectives, and economic and political disruptions from the local to the international level are pervasive (30). At least 14.5% of Americans (35.9 million) have tried cocaine at least once in their lifetimes as of 2007, and 2.3 million admitted to cocaine use in the past year, including 2.1 million in the prior month (31). The societal costs of this abuse are considerable as discussed in more detail elsewhere (see Chapter 14), but include the health care costs for up to 30% of drug-related emergency room (ER) visits that are up over 1% of all ER visits (32) as well as the direct health complications for individuals such as acute psychotic reactions, acute coronary syndromes, and strokes. Even though most individual abusers come to realize the dire consequences of their dependence, they often lack the ability to discontinue this highly addictive substance.

Medications to treat cocaine abuse have been sought for many years, but none has yet been sufficiently successful to achieve the status of approval. Behavioral therapies have been shown useful for a small percentage of cocaine addicts, but it is clear that new approaches are needed to complement those treatment programs. A therapeutic vaccine could be just an additional treatment, with or without new medications that are currently under study, since a vaccine would function via an entirely different and potentially complementary mechanism of action. Studies in experimental animals have shown that cocaine-specific antibody will significantly inhibit the accumulation of cocaine in the brain of rats and mice, demonstrating a reduction in locomotor activity induced by pharmacologic doses of cocaine, as well as an inhibition of the reinstatement of cocaine self-administration (19,33). This latter finding, as an accepted model of human cocaine addiction, may be the most pertinent for therapeutic applications of the clinical vaccine, since reinstatement of cocaine craving after a period of abstinence is one of the most difficult problems preventing the success of cocaine treatment programs (25). Complete avoidance of all exposure to the drug is certainly the best approach, but this is difficult to achieve, since even the most motivated individual may succumb to the temptation for cocaine use under a particularly stressful circumstance or in the context of social pressures for drug use. Thus, blocking the transient pleasure ordinarily felt from cocaine use may reduce or eliminate the craving response usually engendered in the previously abstinent individual.

A cholera toxin B conjugated COC preparation (TA-CD) has been developed and undergone preliminary clinical trials demonstrating safety and immunogenicity (34) and some clinical effectiveness (13). A 14-week Phase IIA trial, in which 18 cocaine-dependent subjects in early recovery were studied, the vaccine was well tolerated at two dose levels (100 μg × 4 injections or 400 μg × 5 injections). Cocaine-specific antibodies were detectable in immunized individuals for at least 6 months. Those subjects receiving the higher dose of vaccine developed significantly higher anticocaine antibody titers than those in the low dose group and were also more likely to maintain cocaine-free urines. In the Phase IIB double-blind placebo controlled trial, Martell et al. found that the TA-CD vaccine was able to stimulate specific antibody in almost all 57 immunized subjects (with none found in the 57 control subjects), but only about 30% of those immunized were able to produce levels of IgG antibody high enough to be expected to bind a major fraction of the cocaine that would enter the circulation after administration of a typical recreational dose of the drug. In addition, after booster dosing was completed at 12 weeks, antibody titers peaked at 16 weeks and then began an inexorable decline in virtually all subjects. Nonetheless, of those subjects who did achieve such antibody concentrations, a marked reduction in cocaine use was documented in thrice weekly urine tests for cocaine metabolites (13). For these subjects, more than 50% of their urine tests indicated no new use of the drug as determined by the Preston Rules during the period when their antibodies were present. In contrast, subjects who did not develop high levels of anticocaine antibody had no significant change in their cocaine use in the same period of the study.

One concern regarding cocaine vaccines, as well as other substance abuse vaccines, is that a vaccinated individual might be tempted to use increasing doses of drug to overwhelm the antibody block in order to achieve adequate concentrations in the brain to get the high sought from the substance. Theoretically, such increasing doses might result in higher risks of drug overdose toxicity, although higher doses in animal studies in our laboratory usually appear to overcome the block in a satisfactory pattern in relation to antibody. Interestingly, higher cocaine use did not appear to happen in most of the individuals with high antibody concentrations as documented by quantitative benzoylecgonine monitoring of urine samples in the Martell study. This may indicate that cocaine vaccines will be best applied clinically to those individuals who are motivated to quit their substance abuse. The implications of these preclinical and clinical studies are that cocaine conjugate vaccines may have a significant role to play in reducing cocaine abuse for those who wish to quit, especially with improvements in the vaccine design or administration methods that result in higher and more persistent cocaine-specific antibody levels.

A novel complementary therapy for vaccines that produce specific antibody to cocaine has been proposed as well. One of the two principal pathways for degradation of cocaine is through the enzyme butylcholinesterase, a nonspecific detoxifying hydrolase in circulation. This enzyme degrades cocaine by hydrolyzing the benzoyl ester of cocaine to produce benzoic acid and ecgonine methyl ester. Brimijoin et al. (35) and Zheng and Zhan (36) have markedly enhanced the hydrolytic function of this enzyme. Recent work on this enzyme has resulted in enhanced activity up to 50,000 times faster than the native enzyme. Although passive administration of the enzyme can be overcome by increasing doses of cocaine, combining a vaccine to produce antibody to bind the drug, and gene therapy to produce low to modest levels of the enzyme might be sufficient to block CNS entry by even very high doses of drug. Such an approach, while still relegated to the future clinically, is being actively developed in animal models.

Phencyclidine

Phencyclidine (PCP, "angel dust"), an N-methyl-D-aspartate (NMDA) receptor antagonist, is representative of a number of designer drugs that continue to be abused in some areas of the United States and around the world, despite the severe psychotic reactions that can occur with its use. Actual PCP dependence has been relatively uncommon, and as a result, vaccine development for PCP has been oriented primarily toward production of therapeutic antibodies, especially monoclonals, that can be used for passive, acute administration in emergency situations (37). The goal of eliciting monoclonal antibodies with a broad specificity for binding to a variety of PCP-related compounds has been challenging, although some progress has been made in that regard. Animal studies with PCP conjugate vaccines have shown that substantial quantities of induced antibodies can reduce the accumulation of PCP in the brain (38). Such antibodies can block the behavioral effects of PCP on locomotor activity and posturing, and passively administered polyclonal and monoclonal anti-PCP antibodies can also reverse the toxic effects of high PCP doses, suggesting that they may prove useful in treating patients who overdose on this drug (37). Unlike antibody blocking of other drugs thus far, infused monoclonal antibody against PCP has been found to block CNS effects of the drug much longer and at lower doses than would be expected based simply on predictions from drug pharmacokinetics and the antibody half-life (3). The mechanism by which this effect occurs remains unknown, although protection has been shown to persist in experimental animals for up to a month after administration, despite doses of PCP administered far in excess of the antibody binding capacity. Clinical application of this immunologic therapy to PCP overdose situations may be available in the near future.

Methamphetamine

Methamphetamine is a stimulant that is abused broadly in the United States, particularly in rural and suburban areas, with 1.3 million current year users in 2007 (39,40). The effects of methamphetamine to increase energy, a sense of well-being, and euphoria make this substance highly addictive, and once addiction is established it is very difficult to overcome (see Chapter 16 for more details). Unlike cocaine, which is rapidly hydrolyzed to inactive compounds, methamphetamine has a long half-life and is in part demethylated to amphetamine, which is itself an addictive stimulant. Much of the parent compound and its major metabolite are cleared by the kidney with a biologic half-life of 9 to 15 hours, depending on urinary pH. The effects of this stimulant are complex, because it affects multiple neurotransmitters in the nervous system, including dopamine, norepinephrine, serotonin, histamine, and gamma-aminobutyric acid, both blocking monoamine transporters and causing the release of monoamines from synaptic vesicles (3). As a result, it is likely to be less amenable to a specific drug antagonist, or even a substitute agonist agent, than cocaine, heroin/morphine, or nicotine.

Although a very small molecule near the lower limit of size for recognition of epitopes by the immune system (molecular weight of 149), antibodies can be made against it as a hapten when conjugated to a carrier protein like the other drugs discussed in this chapter. Owens et al. have characterized an extensive number of antibodies against methamphetamine (3). When a monoclonal antibody preparation is administered to rats, it is able to reverse the effects of 1 mg/kg methamphetamine given 30 minutes before the antibody, as might be useful in a drug overdose situation (41). Furthermore, methamphetamine self-administration in rats and locomotor activity in rats given high dose methamphetamine could also be inhibited by administration of monoclonal antibodies (3).

Active immunization with methamphetamine conjugate vaccines produces polyclonal antibodies, which will develop even with ongoing administration of methamphetamine (42), demonstrating that the immune responses to the conjugate vaccine were not inhibited by drug exposure during the vaccination process. This is particularly important considering the clinical application of the vaccines to active substance abusers. These experiments did not show inhibition of methamphetamine pharmacologic activity at the high doses administered; however, more recent studies have demonstrated that some blockade of methamphetamine activity by active immunization can be achieved (43). In these experiments, a phenyl ring linkage to the drug was used to conjugate to fused peptides (C5a, a complement component fragment that binds to dendritic cells, and a tetanus toxoid peptide sequence recognized by helper T cells). Rats were immunized with the conjugate vaccine weekly for 5 weeks, and in the absence of any other adjuvant, the resultant immune response showed modest antidrug IgG antibody by 6 weeks (1.7 µg/mL in sera). Nonetheless, vaccinated rats had to self-administer more methamphetamine than controls to overcome the presence of the antibody, which eventually became saturated with the drug, and the amount of measurable free antibody did not return to baseline until 34 days after administration of the drug was stopped. Conjugate vaccines constructed with more typical carrier proteins injected with conventional adjuvants in our laboratory, however, have been able to elicit much higher levels of specific antimethamphetamine IgG, up to 2 mg/mL, as measured by ELISA at 16 weeks after the original immunization and a booster dose at 3 weeks. As shown in Figure 31.3, the amount of specific antibody measured in the sera for each group of mice in the study is roughly proportional to the degree of inhibition of locomotor activity stimulated by single dose methamphetamine administration, similar to the observations cited above for passive monoclonal antibody administration. For the individual mice, 8/10 of vaccinated mice had a marked inhibition of methamphetamine-induced locomotor activation with a change in distance traveled of <500 cm. In contrast, 8/9 control mice had a difference in travel distance >1000 cm. These promising results suggest that a clinical vaccine that induced adequate levels of antidrug antibody would be expected to have a substantial impact on single doses of methamphetamine, and in combination with cognitive behavioral or other treatment regimens could provide an effective treatment tool to help prevent relapse to abuse of this highly addictive substance by motivated patients.

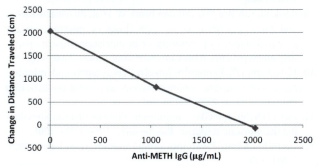

Figure 31.3. Specific IgG inhibits single dose methamphetamine increases in locomotor activity. Groups of mice were immunized with succinylmethamphetamine conjugated to ovalbumin using either alum or complete Freund's adjuvant (CFA) and boosted at 3 weeks. After 16 weeks, immunized and control groups were challenged with 5 µg/mL methamphetamine IP and locomotor activity was assessed as compared with saline injections. Mice immunized with CFA had over 2000 µg/mL anti-METH IgG and showed complete inhibition of locomotor activity. Partial inhibition was achieved with alum adjuvanted vaccinated mice as compared with controls having no antibody in circulation.

Heroin and Morphine

The concept of immunization against drugs of abuse was first realized in experimental animals more than 35 years ago with morphine (44,45). However, the discovery and development of synthetic narcotic derivatives such as methadone and buprenorphine shortly thereafter, and the successful implementation of these drugs in heroin abuse treatment programs, reduced the enthusiasm for narcotic vaccines, at least in developed countries. Unfortunately, the cost of these programs, and the resurgence of heroin/morphine abuse in recent years, especially in developing countries have illustrated clearly the limitations of this pharmacologic approach to the problem.

Narcotics abuse worldwide is dominated by heroin, especially, and morphine. In developed countries, however, there is an increasing problem with prescription drug abuse using synthetic narcotic derivatives (46), even including methadone which, as a partial mu-receptor agonist with a prolonged half-life, had not been considered initially to have a high abuse potential. The number of related compounds with narcotic abuse potential and the activity of heroin metabolites, as well as the extremely broad dose range of these drugs when actively abused pose special problems for a therapeutic immunization approach for these substances. Thus, the design of the conjugate vaccines in terms of linkage of the drug hapten to the carrier protein may be critical to their usefulness. Cross-reactivity with the major metabolites of heroin is crucial for antibody effects, since heroin is a prodrug that is rapidly converted to the pharmacologically active opiates 6-acetyl morphine and morphine by esterases present in both the periphery and the CNS (47). Early studies demonstrated that conjugate vaccines with a linkage through the 6-hydroxyl group elicited antibodies capable of binding heroin, 6-acetylmorphine, and morphine itself, the dominant compounds of interest, and similarly produced antibodies were later shown to bind glucuronide metabolites (48) that also have significant narcotic activity.

Early studies of morphine conjugate vaccines through a derivative of its 6-hydroxyl group elicited a polyclonal antibody response that bound heroin and 6-acetylmorphine, as well as morphine itself (49). The bound drug could be displaced from this binding by later addition of new morphine, indicating that bound molecules are eventually released for metabolism and elimination. In these studies, the authors also demonstrated that the antibodies were saturable, so that higher doses of drug could overcome the binding capacity of circulating antibodies. Of most clinical relevance, self-administration of heroin was reduced in actively immunized rhesus monkeys (45). Berkowitz et al. (24) showed that sequestration of the drug in the blood by antibody binding prolonged morphine half-life to explain at least a part of this effect. Anton et al. in recent studies (50) have shown that a conjugate vaccine using morphine linked through its 6-hydroxyl moiety to tetanus toxoid was capable of binding both morphine and heroin sufficiently so that rat reinstatement behavior for either morphine or heroin was inhibited. The antibodies could bind in vitro to heroin, morphine, and the active metabolites, similar to the findings in earlier studies, but they showed no binding to synthetic narcotics used in treatment, such as methadone and buprenorphine (50). Similar studies in our laboratory have demonstrated that conjugate vaccines to morphine through the 6-hydroxyl group are able to elicit high levels of antibody that are also able to inhibit the nociceptive action of morphine using hotplate assays in mice.

As discussed in the earlier section on antibody quantitation, the amount of antibody that may be expected from a very effective vaccine would be in the hundreds of micrograms/mL range, which, in molar concentration terms would be a few micromoles per liter. Due to tolerance in heavy users, heroin doses of up to 1600 to 1800 mg can be "safely" injected by some subjects, which would result in up to a 2 mM acute concentration (50). As a result the target population for vaccination in heroin/morphine abuse will have to be motivated addicts who have been withdrawn or are being withdrawn from opiates. Withdrawal leads to a reversal of tolerance so that the pharmacologically active drug dose will be within the range able to be inhibited by achievable antibody concentrations.

The well-known socioeconomic costs of narcotics abuse and especially the associated health complications of injected heroin abuse, including the spread of the human immunodeficiency virus (HIV), the hepatitis C virus, and other sexually transmitted diseases in many countries such as China, India, and Russia (1), has reestablished considerable enthusiasm for development of alternative therapeutic approaches for abuse of these substances, including active immunization. A successful vaccine against heroin abuse that could slow or even reverse the addiction would have profound effects on criminal behavior, social stability, and the transmission of HIV/AIDS and other blood borne or sexually transmitted diseases.

CONCLUSIONS

A number of addictive drugs have pharmacokinetic and pharmacodynamic characteristics that make them viable targets for vaccine development. On a theoretical basis, from the known properties of antibodies and the drug concentrations in blood expected for the abused drugs discussed, the quantity and quality of antibody elicited by an effective vaccine should be sufficient to reduce or block drug effects, often by both reducing and slowing the accumulation of drug in the brain. Animal studies with several conjugate drug vaccines and human studies with nicotine and cocaine vaccines have all shown promising results. Blocking immediate behavioral and toxic drug effects is valuable in itself, but even more promising from the addiction perspective is the inhibition of drug reinforcement, or craving, which is necessary to help prevent relapse to drug use by individuals motivated to quit. According to some animal experiments, the effects on reinforcement may not require levels of antibody blocking as high as would be expected for inhibition of the acute drug effects, a property that could dramatically extend the benefits of this approach to therapy. Drug vaccines should also effectively complement current counseling programs and potential future small molecule medications that may be developed to treat the growing worldwide problems posed by the addictions. Advances in vaccine conjugate design, carrier protein use, and especially adjuvant optimization will significantly enhance the quantity and quality of the antibodies produced, allowing drug vaccines to become useful clinical tools for the treatment of substance abuse.

ACKNOWLEDGMENTS

This study is supported by the Department of Veterans Affairs (VA) Merit Review Program and VISN 16 Mental Illness Research, Education and Clinical Center (MIRECC), the VA National Substance Use Disorders Quality Enhancement Research Initiative (QUERI), and the National Institute on Drug Abuse grants K05 DA 0454 (T.R.K.), P50-DA18197, R01 DA 026859 (F.M.O.), U01 DA 023898 (T.R.K., F.M.O.).

REFERENCES

1. Orson FM, Kinsey BM, Singh RAK, et al. Substance abuse vaccines. *Ann N Y Acad Sci.* 2008;1141:257–269.
2. Riviere GJ, Gentry WB, Owens SM. Disposition of methamphetamine and its metabolite amphetamine in brain and other tissues in rats after intravenous administration. *J Pharmacol Exp Ther.* 2000;292:1042–1047.
3. Gentry WB, Ruedi-Bettschen D, Owens SM. Development of active and passive human vaccines to treat methamphetamine addiction. *Hum Vaccin.* 2009;5:206–213.
4. Kosten T, Owens SM. Immunotherapy for the treatment of drug abuse. *Pharmacol Ther.* 2005;108:76–85.
5. Day ED. *Advanced Immunochemistry.* 2nd ed. New York, NY: Wiley-Liss; 1990.
6. Jenkins AJ, Keenan RM, Henningfield JE, et al. Correlation between pharmacological effects and plasma cocaine concentrations after smoked administration. *J Anal Toxicol.* 2002;26: 382–392.
7. Cook CE, Jeffcoat AR, Hill JM, et al. Pharmacokinetics of methamphetamine self-administered to human subjects by smoking S-(+)-methamphetamine hydrochloride. *Drug Metab Dispos.* 1993;21:717–723.
8. Russell MA, Feyerabend C, Cole PV. Plasma nicotine levels after cigarette smoking and chewing nicotine gum. *Br Med J.* 1976;1: 1043–1046.
9. Rook EJ, van Ree JM, van den Brink W, et al. Pharmacokinetics and pharmacodynamics of high doses of pharmaceutically prepared heroin, by intravenous or by inhalation route in opioid-dependent patients. *Basic Clin Pharmacol Toxicol.* 2006; 98:86–96.
10. Hatsukami DK, Rennard S, Jorenby D, et al. Safety and immunogenicity of a nicotine conjugate vaccine in current smokers. *Clin Pharmacol Ther.* 2005;78:456–467.
11. Eisen HN, Siskind GW. Variations in affinities of antibodies during the immune response. *Biochemistry.* 1964;3:996–1008.
12. Cerny EH, Cerny T. Vaccines against nicotine. *Hum Vaccin.* 2009; 5:200–205.
13. Martell BA, Orson FM, Poling J, et al. Cocaine vaccine for the treatment of cocaine dependence: a randomized double-blind placebo-controlled efficacy trial. *Arch Gen Psychiatry.* 2009;66: 1116–1123.
14. Barbet J, Rougon-Rapuzzi G, Cupo A, et al. Structural requirements for recognition of vasopressin by antibody; thermodynamic and kinetic characteristics of the interaction. *Mol Immunol.* 1981;18:439–446.
15. Hieda Y, Keyler DE, Ennifar S, et al. Vaccination against nicotine during continued nicotine administration in rats: immunogenicity of the vaccine and effects on nicotine distribution to brain. *Int J Immunopharmacol.* 2000;22:809–819.

16. Satoskar SD, Keyler DE, LeSage MG, et al. Tissue-dependent effects of immunization with a nicotine conjugate vaccine on the distribution of nicotine in rats. *Int Immunopharmacol.* 2003;3: 957–970.
17. Balster RL, Schuster CR. Fixed-interval schedule of cocaine reinforcement: effect of dose and infusion duration. *J Exp Anal Behav.* 1973;20:119–129.
18. Hill JH, Wainer BH, Fitch FW, et al. Delayed clearance of morphine from the circulation of rabbits immunized with morphine-6-hemisuccinate bovine serum albumin. *J Immunol.* 1975;114:1363–1368.
19. Fox BS, Kantak KM, Edwards MA, et al. Efficacy of a therapeutic cocaine vaccine in rodent models. *Nat Med.* 1996;2:1129–1132.
20. Matsushita M, Hoffman TZ, Ashley JA, et al. Cocaine catalytic antibodies: the primary importance of linker effects. *Bioorg Med Chem Lett.* 2001;11:87–90.
21. Laurenzana EM, Byrnes-Blake KA, Milesi-Halle A, et al. Use of anti-(+)-methamphetamine monoclonal antibody to significantly alter (+)-methamphetamine and (+)-amphetamine disposition in rats. *Drug Metab Dispos.* 2003;31:1320–1326.
22. Pentel PR, Dufek MB, Roiko SA, et al. Differential effects of passive immunization with nicotine-specific antibodies on the acute and chronic distribution of nicotine to brain in rats. *J Pharmacol Exp Ther.* 2006;317:660–666.
23. Williams RH, Maggiore JA, Shah SM, et al. Cocaine and its major metabolites in plasma and urine samples from patients in an urban emergency medicine setting. *J Anal Toxicol.* 2000;24:478–481.
24. Berkowitz BA, Ceretta KV, Spector S. Influence of active and passive immunity on the disposition of dihydromorphine-H3. *Life Sci.* 1974;15:1017–1028.
25. Simpson DD, Joe GW, Fletcher BW, et al. A national evaluation of treatment outcomes for cocaine dependence. *Arch Gen Psychiatry.* 1999;56:507–514.
26. Zeng W, Ghosh S, Macris M, et al. Assembly of synthetic peptide vaccines by chemoselective ligation of epitopes: influence of different chemical linkages and epitope orientations on biological activity. *Vaccine.* 2001;19:3843–3852.
27. Cerny EH, Cerny T. Vaccines against nicotine. *Human Vaccines* 2009;5:200-205.
28. Study to evaluate the efficacy, safety, tolerability and immunogenicity of 100 μg NIC002 vaccine in cigarette smokers who are motivated to quit smoking. In: U.S. Department of Health & Human Services, 2009. Available at: http://clinicaltrials.gov/ct2/show/NCT00736047
29. LeSage MG, Keyler DE, Pentel PR. Current status of immunologic approaches to treating tobacco dependence: vaccines and nicotine-specific antibodies. *AAPS J.* 2006;8:E65–E75.
30. Gootenberg P. *Andean Cocaine: The Making of a Global Drug.* Chapel Hill, NC: University of North Carolina Press; 2008.
31. Substance Abuse and Mental Health Services Administration. *Results from the 2008 National Survey on Drug Use and Health: National Findings* (Office of Applied Studies, NSDUH Series H-36, HHS Publication No. SMA 09-4434). Rockville, MD: Substance Abuse and Mental Health Services Administration;2009. Available at: http://oas.samhsa.gov/nsduh/2k8nsduh/2k8Results.pdf. Accessed August 9, 2010.
32. Substance Abuse and Mental Health Services Administration, Office of Applied Studies. *Drug Abuse Warning Network, 2006: National Estimates of Drug-Related Emergency Department Visits.* DAWN Series D-30, DHHS Publication No. (SMA) 08-4339. Rockville, MD: Substance Abuse and Mental Health Services Administration, Office of Applied Studies; 2008. Available at: http://dawninfo.samhsa.gov/files/ED2006/DAWN2k6ED.pdf. Accessed August 9, 2010.
33. Carrera MR, Ashley JA, Zhou B, et al. Cocaine vaccines: antibody protection against relapse in a rat model. *Proc Natl Acad Sci U S A.* 2000;97:6202–6206.
34. Orson FM, Kinsey BM, Singh RA, et al. Vaccines for cocaine abuse. *Hum Vaccin.* 2009;5:194–199.
35. Brimijoin S, Gao Y, Anker JJ, et al. A cocaine hydrolase engineered from human butyrylcholinesterase selectively blocks cocaine toxicity and reinstatement of drug seeking in rats. *Neuropsychopharmacology.* 2008;33:2715–2725.
36. Zheng F, Zhan CG. Rational design of an enzyme mutant for anti-cocaine therapeutics. *J Comput Aided Mol Des.* 2008;22: 661–671.
37. Laurenzana EM, Gunnell MG, Gentry WB, et al. Treatment of adverse effects of excessive phencyclidine exposure in rats with a minimal dose of monoclonal antibody. *J Pharmacol Exp Ther.* 2003;306:1092–1098.
38. Valentine JL, Owens SM. Antiphencyclidine monoclonal antibody therapy significantly changes phencyclidine concentrations in brain and other tissues in rats. *J Pharmacol Exp Ther.* 1996; 278:717–724.
39. Gao Y, LaFleur D, Shah R, et al. An albumin-butyrylcholinesterase for cocaine toxicity and addiction: catalytic and pharmacokinetic properties. *Chem Biol Interact.* 2008;175:83–87.
40. SAMHSA, Office of Applied Studies. *Results from the 2007 National Survey on Drug Use and Health: National Findings (NSDUH Series H-34, DHHS Publication No. SMA 08-4343).* Rockville, MD: SAMHSA, Office of Applied Studies; 2008. Available at: http://www.oas.samhsa.gov/nsduh/2k7nsduh/2k7results.cfm. Accessed August 9, 2010.
41. Gentry WB, Laurenzana EM, Williams DK, et al. Safety and efficacy of an anti-(+)-methamphetamine monoclonal antibody in the protection against cardiovascular and central nervous system effects of (+)-methamphetamine in rats. *Int Immunopharmacol.* 2006;6:968–977.
42. Byrnes-Blake KA, Carroll FI, Abraham P, et al. Generation of anti-(+)methamphetamine antibodies is not impeded by (+)methamphetamine administration during active immunization of rats. *Int Immunopharmacol.* 2001;1:329–338.
43. Duryee MJ, Bevins RA, Reichel CM, et al. Immune responses to methamphetamine by active immunization with peptide-based, molecular adjuvant-containing vaccines. *Vaccine.* 2009;27: 2981–2988.
44. Berkowitz B, Spector S. Evidence for active immunity to morphine in mice. *Science.* 1972;178:1290–1292.
45. Bonese KF, Wainer BH, Fitch FW, et al. Changes in heroin self-administration by a rhesus monkey after morphine immunisation. *Nature.* 1974;252:708–710.
46. Spiller H, Lorenz DJ, Bailey EJ, et al. Epidemiological trends in abuse and misuse of prescription opioids. *J Addict Dis.* 2009;28: 130–136.
47. Inturrisi CE, Schultz M, Shin S, et al. Evidence from opiate binding studies that heroin acts through its metabolites. *Life Sci.* 1983;33(suppl 1):773–776.
48. Beike J, Kohler H, Blaschke G. Antibody-mediated clean-up of blood for simultaneous HPLC determination of morphine and morphine glucuronides. *Int J Legal Med.* 1997;110:226–229.
49. Wainer BH, Fitch FW, Fried J, et al. A measurement of the specificities of antibodies to morphine-6-succinyl-BSA by competitive inhibition of 14 C-morphine binding. *J Immunol.* 1973;110: 667–673.
50. Anton B, Salazar A, Florez A, et al. Vaccines against morphine/heroin and its use as effective medication for preventing relapse to opiate addictive behaviors. *Hum Vaccin.* 2009;5:214–229.

CHAPTER 32 Acupuncture

Ji-Sheng Han ■ Cai-Lian Cui

INTRODUCTION AND HISTORY

Acupuncture (derived from the word *aces*, meaning a sharp point, and *puncture*, meaning to pierce) can be defined as a technique of inserting and manipulating fine filiform needles into specific points on the body to relieve pain and for various therapeutic purposes. The original acupuncture technique uses up-and-down and rotating maneuvers, termed as manual needling. In modern times, new methods of stimulating the acupuncture points (acupoints) include applications of electric current to needles inserted in the acupoints (electroacupuncture, EA), skin electrodes placed over the points (transcutaneous electrical acupoint stimulation, TEAS), injections into the points, or finger-pressure massage of selected points (acupressure), etc. In addition to the original 361 points, many new points have been described on specific body parts, leading to, for instance, scalp acupuncture, hand acupuncture, and (of particular interest for addiction treatment) ear acupuncture, also known as auricular acupuncture.

Although acupuncture and related acupoint therapies are most commonly known for their analgesic effects, it may be indicated for other medical applications such as nausea and vomiting of various etiologies (1). While a consensus on the clinical efficacy of acupuncture for the treatment of addictions has not yet been achieved unanimously, it has been amply demonstrated that acupuncture is an addiction treatment service now being sought by many potential patients.

Serendipitous Clinical Practice

The application of acupuncture in the treatment of opioid addiction originated from a serendipitous observation made by Dr. H. L. Wen in Hong Kong in 1972. A 50-year-old man was admitted to the Neurosurgical Unit of the Kwong Wah Hospital in Hong Kong, because of a brain concussion. He was a known opium addict of 5 years' duration. After the cerebral concussion had improved, the patient was asked whether he would agree to cingulotomy to relieve his drug-abuse problem. He agreed, and was then scheduled for surgery. During the operation for surgery, instead of local anesthesia being injected under the scalp (where the incision was to be made), acupuncture anesthesia (analgesia) was used. After stimulation for 15 to 30 minutes, the patient voluntarily stated that his withdrawal syndrome had completely cleared up. Physical examination revealed that he was free of withdrawal syndrome. The operation was canceled and the patient returned to the ward. The next day, two other patients, both of whom were opium abusers, appeared in the orthopedic wards. When they learnt of the experience of the previous patient, both agreed to the procedure. Both responded well to the half hour of acupuncture and electrical stimulation on the ear and body points and their withdrawal symptoms stopped. After the above observation, Dr. Wen and his colleague, Dr. Cheung subsequently reported that, in a study of 40 heroin and opium addicts, acupuncture combined with electrical stimulation (now being termed "electroacupuncture") was effective in relieving the symptoms of opioid withdrawal (2).

This method was later adopted in many clinical settings in Western countries, including the Lincoln Hospital in New York City. However, the body acupuncture points originally used by Wen and Cheung on the arm and hand were gradually omitted, retaining only the ear points for acupuncture and doing without additional electrical stimulation in drug-abuse treatment (3). The protocol developed at Lincoln Hospital by Dr. Michael Smith and his colleagues was subsequently promulgated by the National Acupuncture Detoxification Association (NADA) on a national basis, with formalized training and standards for the application of ear acupuncture in a group setting. This has been the predominant approach studied by clinical trials and practiced in the United States since then.

Translation from Basic Studies on Acupuncture Analgesia

The use of acupuncture as a method of anesthesia and/or analgesia for surgery in China in the late 1950s raised a great deal of interest among the public and the biomedical community. This led to exploration of the biologic mechanisms underlying the actions of acupuncture. Starting in 1965, the Department of Public Health of China sponsored extensive research in this area. The discovery of morphine-like substances (endorphins) in the mammalian brain in 1975 (4) had a great impact on modern concepts of pain and analgesia. It was soon clear that acupuncture (manual needling)-induced analgesia can be blocked by the opioid receptor antagonist naloxone, suggesting the involvement of endogenous opioid substances (5). Manual acupuncture or EA was shown to accelerate the production and release of endorphins which could then interact with various opioid receptors to relieve or prevent pain (6). Endorphins are a group of peptides possessing a variety of specific characteristics.

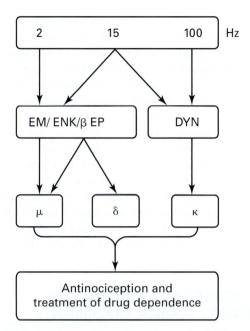

Figure 32.1. Frequency-dependent release of opioid peptides in the central nervous system. Four kinds of opioid peptides: EM, endomorphins; ENK, enkephalins; β EP, β-endorphin; DYN, dynorphins. Three kinds of opioid receptors: μ, δ, κ. Representative frequency of electroacupuncture: 2, 15, and 100 Hz.

Among those peptides, β-endorphin and enkephalin are primarily agonists of the μ- and δ-opioid receptors, whereas dynorphin is the agonist for the κ-opioid receptors. Interestingly, electrical stimulation of different frequencies can specifically induce the release of different endorphins. For example, low-frequency (2 to 4 Hz) EA stimulates release of the enkephalins that interact with μ- and δ-opioid receptors, whereas high-frequency (100 Hz) EA can stimulate the release of dynorphin to interact with κ-opioid receptors (7). These findings provided a biochemical explanation for the traditional acupuncture practice (see Fig. 32.1) and suggested that the usefulness of acupuncture might be much broader than pain control.

FROM PAIN MANAGEMENT TO OPIOID DEPENDENCE

China significantly suffered from problems of opiate addiction in the 1800s and early 1900s. This problem was minimized from 1949 to 1951 because of the complete closure of overseas trade involving opioids. However, concurrent with the implementation of the "open door policy" of the 1980s, large amounts of opiates began to be smuggled into border areas and increasing problems were seen with heroin addiction. It was natural to think that if acupuncture can release endogenous opioids in the brain to ease pain, why not make use of it to relieve opiate withdrawal symptoms? This idea was initially tested in rats made dependent on morphine. The withdrawal symptoms were significantly reduced by high-frequency (100 Hz) EA administered at the hind limbs. This effect was found to be much greater than that induced by low-frequency (2 Hz) stimulation (8). Encouraged by the experimental results, EA was applied clinically to previous heroin addicts to see if it suppressed withdrawal symptoms. Preliminary results were promising. However, it was soon found that it was not always feasible for patients to visit the clinic to obtain professional treatment one or more times a day, and, as a result, patients might drop out. Technology for self-administration (SA) of the stimulation was developed to see whether it would be possible for patients to treat themselves by using electrical acupoint stimulation without a needle, as part of the treatment program for their addiction problem.

Experimental findings obtained in the rat model showed that electrical stimulation applied to the surface of the skin overlaying the acupoint could produce analgesic effects similar to that produced by EA through the penetrating needles (9). Satisfactory results were also obtained for the treatment of heroin withdrawal in humans using the same method of electrical acupoint stimulation via skin electrodes (10). Later it was found that this device was also useful in suppressing the conditioned place preference (CPP) to morphine in the rat (11). This is an animal model mimicking craving for drugs of abuse. Subsequent human studies revealed that this form of stimulation could also inhibit the craving for heroin in addicted patients (see below).

ACUPUNCTURE AND VARIOUS KINDS OF MODIFICATIONS

Manual Needling

As discussed in the previous paragraphs, classical acupuncture involves the piercing of the skin by a sharp metallic needle and manipulation by up-and-down (plug-drag) and twisting (twirling) movements. The correct placement of the needle at the acupoint and the optimal manipulation are generally characterized by feedback from the patient concerning a subjective feeling called *de-qi*. This sensation, reported by patients to include heaviness, soreness, numbness, and sense of swelling, occasionally also involves the trembling of the local muscles. In the meantime, the operator of the needle (the acupuncturist) often has a feeling resembling that experienced during fishing when a fish is nibbling at or swallowing the bait. This is likely the result of the rhythmic contraction of muscle fibers surrounding the needle. According to the traditional acupuncturist, it takes years to really master the particular modes of manual stimulation, for example, to produce a feeling which is "warm" (like the whole mountain is burning), or, to produce a feeling which is "cold" (like the whole sky is freezing).

Electroacupuncture (EA)

It has been made clear that the analgesic effect induced by acupuncture can be completely blocked by local procaine injection deep into the acupoint, but not by its subcutaneous injection, suggesting that the signal of acupuncture originates mainly from nervous tissues (or tissues susceptible to procaine blockade) located in deep structures rather than in the superficial layer of the skin (12). Using single nerve fiber recording technique to record the afferent impulses of the nerve innervating the site of stimulation, it was found that the nerve fibers responsible for transmission of acupuncture signals belong to the group II (Aβ) fibers (13). Since the analgesic effect induced by manual needling can be totally abolished by local nerve blockade (12) or nerve transection, a neural mechanism is strongly implicated. It is thus rational to use electrical stimulation administered via the metallic needles in lieu of its mechanical movement. This has been called *EA*. The advantage of EA is that the frequency, amplitude, and pulse width of the electrical stimulation can be determined precisely and objectively, and therefore it can be replicated by other acupuncturists or experimenters without any difficulty. Moreover, the procedure of inserting the needle at a precise skin location, and changing the direction and the depth of the needle to an optimal status in order to achieve a maximal *de-qi*, is just the same as in manual needling. It is only at the end of the needle-placement procedure that the patient is connected to the electrical stimulator in place of further manual stimulation. This is exactly the procedure described by Dr. Wen in his first report, that is, "acupuncture and electrical stimulation" (2). Having said that, it should be mentioned that EA should optimally be given daily, or even several times per day during the period of detoxification, which may be difficult for outpatients who are at a distance away from the clinic. A procedure that can be operated by the patient at home under the supervision of the physician might be a desirable alternative to daily treatment in the clinic or inpatient care. In addition, because drug-addiction patients have a high incidence of bloodborne viral infections, it may be more convenient for invasive procedures to be replaced by noninvasive methods that do not produce sharp biohazardous waste.

Transcutaneous Electrical Acupoint Stimulation (TEAS)

An alternative to the use of EA is to take a transcutaneous route of electrical administration. However, since the skin has a very high impedance, which is more than 10 times that of the muscle tissue, it is necessary to use a constant current output device to assure a constant level of stimulation without being affected by the degree of moisture of the skin surface or the change of blood flow rate within the skin. Because the tip of the needle goes several millimeters or even centimeters below the skin, the placement of the skin electrodes should ensure the maximal stimulation of the deep structures underlying the acupoint. For example, to stimulate the Hegu point (coded as Large Intestine 4 [LI-4]) located in the thenar muscle of the hand, the correct placement of the skin electrodes should be one on the dorsal side and the other on the palm side of the point, so that the current is forced to pass through the thenar muscle with little deviation.

Regarding the frequency of stimulation, it is commonly accepted that conventional transcutaneous electric nerve stimulation (TENS) is based on the gate-control theory (14) that high-frequency (e.g., 100 to 200 Hz) low-intensity stimulation is preferable to activate the large-caliber nerve fibers in order to suppress the pain mediated by the unmyelinated small-caliber fibers. On the other hand, "acupuncture-like" stimulation is characterized by low-frequency (e.g., 2 to 4 Hz) high-intensity stimulation. The new approach of TEAS attempts to combine the TENS-like and the acupuncture-like stimulation to create what is hoped to be an optimal mode of stimulation to maximize the release of both classes of endorphins. A device that possesses these features was designed and named Han's Acupoint Nerve Stimulator (HANS), and used in a series of animal and clinical experiments, the details of which are given below.

NEUROBIOLOGY OF ACUPUNCTURE TREATMENT (ANIMAL EXPERIMENT)

Physical Dependence

Systemic studies reveal that the mechanism of acupuncture analgesia is attributed mainly to the increased release of endogenous opioid peptides in the central nervous system (CNS) (6,7). A rational extrapolation is that the activation of endogenous opioid systems by acupuncture should be useful to ease opiate withdrawal symptoms.

Early in the 1970s, it was reported that transauricular electrostimulation suppressed the naloxone-induced morphine withdrawal syndrome in mice and in rats. Auriacombe et al. (15) demonstrated that TENS with an intermittent high-frequency current effectively attenuated the abstinence syndrome in the rat after abrupt cessation of morphine administration. The mechanisms of action remained obscure. Based on our previous findings that low-frequency EA (e.g., 2 Hz) accelerated the release of β-endorphin and enkephalin in the CNS, whereas high-frequency EA (e.g., 100 Hz) accelerated the release of dynorphin (7,16) in the spinal cord, we tested the effect of EA in a naloxone-precipitated morphine withdrawal model of the rat. The results showed that 100-Hz EA was far more effective than 2-Hz in suppressing withdrawal syndrome (8). This outcome is hypothetically compatible with the previous reports that (a) 100-Hz EA accelerated the release of dynorphin in spinal cord (7) and (b) spinal dynorphin can suppress the withdrawal syndrome in heroin-dependent humans (17) and morphine-dependent rodents (18,19).

Recent study showed that chronic morphine treatment resulted in serious damage of the dopamine (DA) neurons in the ventral tegmental area (VTA) of the rats, manifested as shrinkage of the cell size, swelling of the rough endoplasmic reticulum, and blurring of the mitochondria. The electrophysiologic response of these DA neurons to morphine (1 mg/kg, i.v.) was also markedly reduced. When 100-Hz EA was given to these rats 24 hours after the last injection of morphine twice a day for 10 days, the morphine withdrawal syndrome were diminished, accompanied by a recovery of the VTA dopaminergic neurons, as compared to rats without EA treatment (20–22).

Psychic Dependence

There are several animal models (23) that can be used to study the psychic dependence on drugs of abuse, which is a central issue in addictive disorders. CPP is one of the frequently used models (24). In a two-chamber or three-chamber experimental apparatus, the drug (unconditioned stimulus) is injected in the animal in one of the chambers. Thus the drug effects become associated with the environmental stimuli unique to that chamber (e.g., color of the surroundings and texture of the floor). After repeated training, the rat will choose to stay longer on the drug-associated side than in a chamber associated with normal saline injection or no injection. The ratio between the time spent in the drug-associated side and the saline-associated side can be taken as an index for the degree of "craving." Using this model, experiments were conducted to test whether acupuncture suppresses the expression of the CPP.

Wang et al. (11) were among the first to explore the effect of EA on morphine CPP in the rat. CPP was significantly suppressed by a single session (30 minutes) of EA at 2 Hz and 2/100 Hz, but not 100 Hz. The results suggest that it is the low-frequency component of the EA that suppressed the morphine CPP. Since the effect of EA can be completely reversed by the opioid receptor antagonist naloxone at a dose of 1 mg/kg, which is sufficient to block the opioid μ and δ, but not the κ, receptors, it seems evident that the effect of EA is mediated by endogenously released μ- and δ-opioid agonists, most likely endorphins and enkephalins, to ease "craving" for exogenous opioids (in this case, the morphine).

In practical life, craving and relapse can be easily induced by stress or by a very small dose (priming dose) of opioids. This phenomenon can be reproduced in animals using the CPP model (25), and this reinstated CPP can also be suppressed by EA (26).

For simplicity and clarity of analysis, previous studies observed only the effects produced by a single session of EA. However, in clinical practice, acupuncture, or HANS is delivered daily in consecutive days or even several times a day. To mimic the clinical situation, animal experiments were designed using EA once a day for 3 or 5 consecutive days. In this case, not only 2-Hz, but also 100-Hz EA is effective in suppressing morphine CPP (27,28). The finding suggests that the efficacy of EA to suppress morphine-induced CPP depends not only on the frequency of EA (2 Hz better than 100 Hz), but also on the total number of sessions of EA being administered (5 times > 3 times > single session). This may be related to the degree of activation of the genes encoding opioid peptides. It was found that 2 and 100 Hz EA can selectively elevate preproenkephalin (PPE) and preprodynorphin (PPD) mNRA level, respectively (29,30), as well as an increase of the tissue content of DA in the nucleus accumbens (NAc) of morphine-induced CPP rats (31).

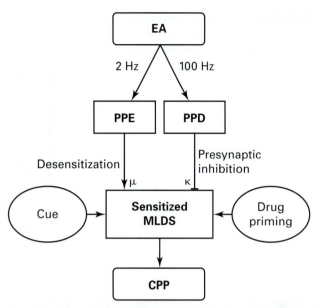

Figure 32.2. Diagram showing that the cue-induced CPP for morphine or drug priming-induced reinstatement of CPP can be suppressed by electroacupuncture of different frequencies. See details in the text. EA, electroacupuncture; PPE, preproenkephalin; PPD, preprodynorphin; MLDS, mesolimbic dopamine system.

The results mentioned above can be summarized in the diagram shown above. An environmental cue or small dose of drug can induce CPP or cause reinstatement of extinguished CPP by activation of the mesolimbic dopamine system (MLDS). The sensitized DA neurons can be suppressed by EA via different mechanisms: low-frequency EA activates the PPE neurons thereby desensitizing the DA neurons via μ-opioid receptors, whereas high-frequency EA activates the dynorphin system and causes the presynaptic inhibition of DA neurons via κ-opioid receptors (Fig. 32.2).

EFFICACY (HUMAN STUDIES)

Effect on Withdrawal Syndrome

For the treatment of the withdrawal syndromes in heroin addicts, HANS was used once a day for 30 minutes for a period of 10 days in a drug-addiction treatment center (32). Apart from the subjective answer to a standard questionnaire, two objective parameters were measured, that is, the heart rate and body weight of the patients.

Single Treatment

To observe the immediate effect of HANS on the heart rate of patients in withdrawal from heroin, the two pairs of output leads of the HANS were connected to four acupoints in the upper extremities. One pair at Hegu point (LI-4, at the dorsum of the hand on the thenar eminence) and Laogon (P-8, opposite to LI-4, on the palmar side), another pair on Neiguan (P-6, located at the palmar side of the forearm, 2 inches proximal to the palmar groove, between the tendons of the palmaris

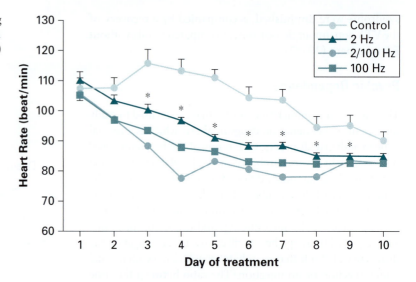

Figure 32.3. Heart rate of heroin addicts receiving HANS treatment once a day for 10 days. *$P < 0.01$ compared with the mock acupuncture ("control") group.

longus and flexor carpi radialis) and Waiguan (TE-5, on the dorsal surface of the forearm opposite the P-6). A "dense-and-disperse" mode of stimulation was administered, in which 2-Hz stimulation alternated automatically with 100-Hz, each lasting for 3 seconds. This mode of stimulation releases all four kinds of opioid peptides in the CNS (7). The control group received the same treatment, except that the electrodes were disconnected from the electronic circuitry. The average heart rate of the patients in opioid withdrawal was 109 beats per minute before treatment, significantly higher than the normal value of below 70. The dense-and-disperse mode stimulation for 30 minutes reduced the heart rate to 90 beats per minute. The full effect remained for only 20 minutes after the stimulation, and returned to its original level thereafter. So the effect was robust but short lasting.

Multiple Treatments

To observe the cumulative effect of multiple daily treatments with HANS, heroin-addiction patients were randomly divided into four groups, receiving HANS of 2, 100, or 2/100 Hz ("dense and disperse"). The control group received mock stimulation, with the electric circuitry disconnected. The treatment was delivered 30 minutes a day for 10 consecutive days.

In the control group receiving mock HANS, heart rate did not come down to a level of 100 beats per minute until 8 days after the treatment. Repeated daily EA treatment was effective in reducing the tachycardia of heroin withdrawal, with an effective order of dense-and-disperse > 100 Hz > 2 Hz (32) (Fig. 32.3). This result is compatible with the findings obtained in rats that the withdrawal syndrome is more effectively reduced by 100 Hz rather than 2 Hz stimulation, while the dense-and-disperse mode is always the best because of synergistic interaction between opioids.

In order to obtain a quantitative estimate of the effect of HANS in reducing withdrawal syndrome, the following protocol was established (33): HANS was used three times a day for the first 5 days and reduced to twice a day for the second 5 days and then once a day for a total of 14 days. Buprenorphine (Buprenex) i.m. was used as a supplement to HANS when the patient experienced withdrawal distress. To quantify the role of HANS in a combined HANS/buprenorphine treatment, 28 heroin-addiction patients were randomly divided into two groups, receiving buprenorphine only, or HANS plus buprenorphine. The results shown in Figure 32.4 indicate that the total amount of buprenorphine used in the HANS group was only 8.3% of that needed in the pure

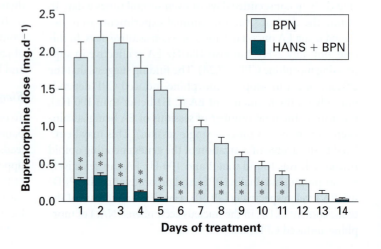

Figure 32.4. Influence of 2/100 Hz transcutaneous electric acupoint stimulation (with HANS device) on the requirement of buprenorphine (BPN) for heroin addicts during the period of detoxification. **$P < 0.01$ compared with the corresponding control group (BPN alone).

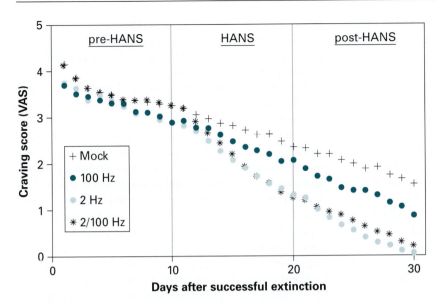

Figure 32.5. Effect of Han's Acupoint Nerve Stimulation (HANS) on craving scores in heroin addicts ($N = 29$ to 30 in each group). HANS of 2 and 2/100 Hz accelerated the decay of craving scores during the 10-day treatment period.

buprenorphine group. This can be taken as a quantitative estimate of the effect of HANS on opioid withdrawal symptoms. This is apparently a result of an accumulation of the therapeutic effect produced by repetitive treatments in the period of 14 days. Similar observations were made in another group of heroin-addicted subjects using a methadone reduction protocol as control group and HANS (2/100 Hz) plus methadone as the experimental group (34). The total dose of methadone used in the HANS group was only 25% of that in the control group.

Effect on Craving and Relapse

Drug addiction is a chronically relapsing disorder in the CNS. The cardinal behavioral feature of drug addiction is continued vulnerability to relapse after years of drug abstinence (35). Therefore, long-acting opioid (methadone, levo-alpha-acetylmethadol [LAAM], or buprenorphine) maintenance is the principal choice to prevent relapse to heroin. Alternately, for some patients, especially those with strong resources for social support, one may try to become drug free for the rest of their life. The following sections explore whether acupuncture helps to reduce craving and postpone or prevent the relapse.

Effect of HANS on Opiate Craving in Humans

To obtain a quantitative estimate of possible suppression of craving in response to acupuncture or related techniques, we used a visual analogue scale (VAS, 0 to 100 mm) to represent the degree of craving in a group of heroin-addicted patients who had completed the process of detoxification more than 1 month earlier. A total of 117 subjects with an initial VAS score higher than 20 were recruited, and were randomly assigned to four groups, receiving HANS treatment once a day for 10 days. This treatment period was preceded by a control pretreatment period for 10 days, and followed by another 10 days for the observation of after effects. Three groups were subjected to HANS treatment at frequency of 2, 100, or 2/100 Hz, respectively, and one group to mock HANS of minimal stimulation (using 5 mA threshold intensity at the beginning for 5 minutes and then switched off). There was a very slow decline of the VAS in the mock HANS control group. A dramatic decline of the degree of craving was observed in the groups receiving 2 or 2/100-Hz electric stimulation, but not in the group receiving 100-Hz stimulation. In summary, the results observed in humans coincided with the findings obtained in the rat that low-frequency HANS is more effective than high-frequency HANS in reducing the craving for opiates (26) (Fig. 32.5).

Drug Free for 1 Year as a Standard for Successful Prevention of Relapse

Heroin addiction is characterized by a high rate of relapse even after a long abstinence. Without taking special measures, the chance of complete drug abstinence for a period of 1 year is minimal. Consequently, we accept 1 year as a criterion of successful prevention of relapse. Based on the findings shown in the previous study concerning the effect of HANS on opiate craving, we encouraged detoxified addiction patients to take with them a unit of portable HANS when they were discharged from the detoxification center. It was strongly recommended to have at least one session (30 minutes) before going to bed to facilitate sleep. It was also suggested that they use the device anytime when there was a strong drug cue or a robust episode of craving. The anticraving effect was usually reported to appear within 20 minutes.

A follow-up study (2000 to 2001) was conducted on a group of 56 patients in Hainan island of south China, who used HANS at home with weekly consultation and a urine check twice a month. At the end of 12 months, only 9 were drug free based upon urine test results, so the 1 year relapse rate was 83.9% (16.1% success rate). A later study in Shanghai (2003) found a 1 year success rate of 26.8% (60 out of 224).

Compared with a 95% to 99% relapse rate at the end of 1 year in the majority of reports on heroin addiction in China (without methadone maintenance) (36), the above-mentioned results were encouraging.

SAFETY

Aversive Side Effects

Relatively few complications have been reported for acupuncture. Serious events including organ puncture and lung collapse are very rare, since most of the acupoints are located in the extremities. In fact, acupuncture is well known for its low rate of aversive side effects and high safety (1), compared with many standard pharmacologic treatments. The risk of acupuncture-mediated infection is minimized by strict adherence to the instructions for single use needle. For those still concerned, the use of skin electrodes rather than needles will reduce this risk from minimal to zero. The serendipitous electric shock is prevented by the design of the stimulation device such that once the modulatory keys are set, the whole device will be locked to avoid the incidental touch of the parameter keys.

Dependence Liability

Given the established finding that acupuncture and related techniques would increase the release of opioid peptides in the CNS (7), one may be concerned that acupuncture per se might produce dependence. While we have not heard of any report of this kind, this is a rational issue deserving careful exploration. In an experimental setting in the rat we tested the hypothesis that if EA produces pleasurable experience, repeated EA in a fixed experimental environment might cause CPP. This was verified by the finding in rats that EA of 2 Hz indeed cause significant, although mild, CPP (28,37). Translating into human behavior, one may expect that acupuncture or a related technique would be welcome by the patients, or at least to neutralize the possible inconvenience caused by needle punctures and to keep patients adhering to the acupuncture treatment schedule.

SPECIAL CONSIDERATIONS

Alcohol

Acupuncture was considered quite promising for the treatment of alcohol addiction in the 1980s (38). The same orthodox ear points suggested in the Lincoln Hospital/NADA protocol were used, and points 3 to 5 mm apart were used as nonspecific points for control. However, this result could not be replicated by Worner et al. (39) in the United States (56 cases) or by Sapir-Weise et al. (40) in Sweden (72 cases). In a recent randomized, placebo-controlled study of auricular acupuncture, Bullock et al. (41) conducted a large-scale clinical trial that included 503 cases. The outcome, however, was quite different from the original hypothesis. All four groups showed a significant improvement. These authors concluded that ear acupuncture did not make a significant contribution over and above that achieved by conventional treatment alone in the reduction of alcohol use.

Data show that the euphoric effect of alcohol is mediated by endogenous opioid peptides and the opioid antagonist naltrexone has been used to assist cognitive–behavioral therapy for alcoholics (42). Therefore, modulation of the endogenous opioid system should be considered as one of the approaches for the treatment of alcohol craving in alcoholic patients. Yoshimoto et al. (43) reported that rats subject to repeated restriction stress consume more alcohol than the control animals. EA at hind limb points zusanli (ST-36) significantly reduced the alcohol-seeking behavior, whereas the lumbar point Shenshu (BL-23) was not effective. The effect of EA stimulation at ST-36 was accompanied by an increase in DA level in the striatum, compared with that produced by EA at BL-23. These findings provide new information for understanding alcohol-drinking behavior and for treating human alcoholics. This was supported by a recent study of Overstreet et al. (44) who did an experiment in the P rats that showed special favor for alcohol consumption. EA applied at ST36 and SP6 of the rat with 2/100 Hz stimulation caused a significant reduction of alcohol consumption, which was reversed by naltrexone, a long-acting opioid receptor antagonist, suggesting that this effect is mediated by opioid receptors.

Smoking

A recent Cochrane review concluded that despite the relatively high number of studies, there was no consistent evidence that acupuncture was effective for smoking cessation. Lambert et al. (45) evaluated the efficacy of a standardized protocol of TEAS in alleviating the urge to smoke in nicotine-dependent individuals, during a 26-hour abstinence period. Electrical stimulation was applied on the Hegu (LI 4)/Laogon (PC 8) points of the hand, and Neiguan (PC 6)/Waiguan (TE 5) points of the upper arm, using 2/100 Hz alternating frequency and 10 mA intensity as the effective stimulation, and no stimulation or intermittent 5 mA minimal stimulation as the control. The results showed that 10 mA stimulation, but not the minimal stimulation, significantly reduced the craving for smoking. The results warrant further large-scale clinical trial.

Cocaine

Cocaine addiction is one of the most important challenges of substance abuse treatment for two reasons. First, according to the 2007 WHO report, cocaine has approached heroin in terms of drug users in the whole world (14 vs. 16 million persons), and surpassed heroin in terms of illicit drug market (71 vs. 65 billion dollars). Second, there is no effective pharmacologic treatment available for cocaine addiction.

Compared with heroin addiction, cocaine addiction shows a minimal withdrawal syndrome upon cessation of use, yet more prominent and longer-lasting craving, serving as one of the most important cues leading to its relapse. Therefore the most important issue is whether acupuncture can have an effect in suppressing and/or preventing cocaine craving. Data obtained from animal experiments with cocaine are discussed first, followed by a discussion of results from clinical trials.

Experimental Studies

In the last three decades, the SA technique has commonly been used to assess the degree of psychic dependence to cocaine in rats. In recent years, CPP has also been used for this purpose. Ren et al. (46) studied the expression of cocaine-induced CPP in rats, which was maintained for as long as 4 weeks at weekly checking, or for 13 days at a daily checking schedule. High-frequency (100 Hz) EA applied at hind leg points for 30 minutes was found to significantly reduce the CPP, whereas low-frequency (2 Hz) was without effect. This is in sharp contrast to opioid-induced CPP, where 2-Hz EA is much more effective than 100 Hz in suppressing its expression. The attenuation of cocaine CPP by 100-Hz EA may involve a κ-opioid mechanism. Indeed, the effect of 100 Hz EA can be blocked by the opioid antagonist naloxone only at a high dose (10 mg/kg). This dose is sufficient to antagonize all three subtypes of opioid receptors, including κ receptor. On the other hand, the lower doses (1 and 5 mg/kg) that are only able to inactivate μ- and δ-, but not κ-opioid receptors was not effective. These results may suggest a role for 100-Hz EA to reduce cocaine craving and to prevent relapse. Clinical trials of this approach are certainly warranted.

Clinical Trials

Ear acupuncture is often used for the treatment of cocaine addiction in the United States, using the same four to five ear points originally developed at Lincoln Hospital for use in the treatment of opioid addiction and promulgated by NADA for general use in addiction programs. Using this protocol, Smith et al. observed a series of 226 cases of users of cocaine or crack cocaine and found that 149 (65%) had more than 80% negative urine tests during the entire treatment period (47). While there was no control group, the success rate by itself was felt to be quite encouraging. This was supported by the work of Margolin (1993) and Avents (2000) with an observation population of 32 and 82, respectively.

Encouraged by the aforementioned results, a randomized, controlled, single-blind, multisite large-scale clinical trial was conducted from 1996 to 1999. The results were published in *JAMA* in 2002 (48). A total of 620 cocaine-dependent adults were randomly assigned to receive auricular acupuncture (four needles schedule), a needle-insertion control (four needles inserted into the helix of the ear), or a relaxation control. Treatments were offered five times weekly for 8 weeks. Main outcome measures were cocaine use during treatment and at the 3- and 6-month follow-up based on urine toxicology screening and retention in treatment. The conclusion was that within the clinical context of this study, acupuncture was not more effective than a needle-insertion or relaxation control in reducing cocaine use. The authors concluded that the results do not support the use of acupuncture as a stand-alone treatment for cocaine addiction, yet it may play an ancillary role for the treatment of cocaine addiction. This conclusion is apparently in contrast to that derived from the animal experiments, as well as results from the preceding pilot study. It seems that the psychosocial and rehabilitative services made available for patients during the second study were fairly minimal, while in the first, the services had been considerable (49).

Finally, in the planning of future large trials of acupoint therapy for cocaine addiction, attention should also be directed to the results obtained in rat experiments showing that the therapeutic effect of EA is frequency-dependent, that is, 100-Hz, rather than 2-Hz stimulation can suppress the cocaine-induced CPP. Therefore, it may be worthwhile to include 100-Hz EA (and possibly body EA) stimulation in future trials of acupuncture-related therapy for the treatment of cocaine addiction.

TECHNICAL COMMENTS ON USING ACUPUNCTURE IN THE TREATMENT OF ADDICTION

Ear Acupuncture versus Body Acupuncture

Although the ear concha is not included in the classical 14 meridians, there is no reason not to use ear points. On the other hand, there seems no reason to avoid the use of body points either. The original protocol of Dr. Wen in treating drug abuse in Hong Kong used four points in the hand and arm (connecting to electrical stimulator) and two points on the ear. Besides, while the sensation produced by piercing the ear is almost pure pain, pain is not a component of the typical experience of *de-qi* in the body acupuncture. In other words, ear acupuncture and body acupuncture should have equal chance to be used in the treatment of drug abuse.

Needle Staying versus Manual Needling

The results obtained in human studies (Fig. 32.6) suggest that manipulation of the needle produces a stronger physiologic effect than does needle staying (i.e., no manipulation) in the acupoint, at least when pain modulation is measured (50).

Acupuncture and Electroacupuncture versus Transcutaneous Electric Stimulation

A series of studies showed that the manipulation of the needle triggers a train of nerve impulses transmitted along the afferent nerve fibers to the CNS. The physiologic effects produced by acupuncture (e.g., the antinociceptive effect) can be readily blocked by the injection of local anesthetics deep into the acupoint (12), or along the afferent nerve. If nerve activation accounts for the transmission of the acupuncture signals, then similar effects should be induced whether nerve impulses are generated by manipulation of a needle (manual acupuncture, MA), or by electrical stimulation via the needles inserted into the point (EA), or even by electrodes placed

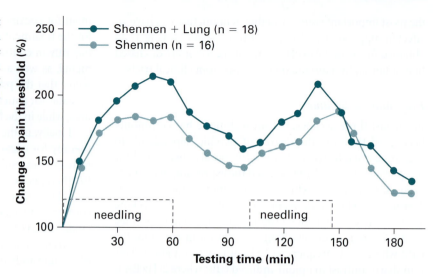

Figure 32.6. Influence of manual needling at ear acupoint Shenmen ($N = 16$) or Shenmen plus lung ($N = 18$) on pain threshold of the skin over the chest and abdomen in humans. The pain threshold increased during the period of needle manipulation and started to decrease when the needle stayed in situ.

on the surface of the skin over the point, forcing the current to pass through the underlying tissue (TEAS). In an experiment performed in the rat, the analgesic effects induced by EA (via needles) and by transcutaneous stimulation (via skin electrodes) were compared. No significant difference was found between the two approaches in the efficacy of inducing an antinociceptive effect (9). It is interesting to note that a similar mechanism seems to underlie the two analgesic effects. Thus, no matter whether the electrical stimulation is delivered via needles or skin electrodes, the opioid antagonist naloxone at a 2 mg/kg dose produced a complete reversal of 2-Hz stimulation-produced analgesia, a partial reversal of 15-Hz stimulation-induced analgesia, and no reversal on 100-Hz stimulation-produced analgesia (9), unless the dose of naloxone is increased to 10 to 20 mg/kg (7).

Opioid- versus Nonopioid-Mechanisms

The mechanism of acupuncture or EA relies, at least partly, on the frequency-dependent release of opioid peptides in the CNS (7). For example, high-frequency (100 Hz) stimulation is more efficacious in reducing opiate withdrawal syndrome, whereas low-frequency appears to be more effective in reducing opiate craving. In contrast to opiate addiction, effects on cocaine addiction may work through a slightly different mechanism, such that CPP for cocaine in the rat, a rodent model of cocaine craving, can be suppressed only by 100-Hz, but not 2-Hz, stimulation (46). These finding should be considered in the future study.

Design of Appropriate Control Group

Acupuncture, as a procedure (or group of related procedures), is far more difficult to subject to a double-blind clinical trial than is a drug. In this respect, clinical trials of acupuncture should be compared with trials for different types of psychotherapy or surgical procedures, rather than drug trials. In recent years, considerable methodologic progress has been made that will better answer many questions about acupuncture's efficacy. For example, the design of a mock needle that looks like it is penetrating the skin, but actually withdraws into a hollow space leaving a touch sensation on the skin mimics the *de-qi* experience (51). This is a single-blind design, because the acupuncturist knows the difference between the conventional needle and the mock needle.

To use EA at threshold intensity with intermittent trains is another option. For example, using a constant current device, the threshold intensity for a 4×4-cm skin pad is 5 mA for most subjects. A desirable intensity is two times the threshold, that is, 10 mA. On the other hand, one can use a minimal stimulation by (a) reducing the stimulation intensity to the threshold level (5 mA), and (b) reducing the time of stimulation by using an intermittent (on/off) schedule, that is, 10 seconds on and 20 seconds off, so that the stimulation time is cut by 2/3, yet the subject still feels the stimulations come and go (45).

SUMMARY

Acupuncture is an emerging treatment for drug abuse. This approach is different from that of pharmacologic treatments. For example, while methadone maintenance treatment is aiming at long-term replacement of methadone for heroin, acupuncture or TEAS attempts to strengthen the endogenous opioid system and eventually get rid of the drug. From a technical point of view, there is still considerable room for improvement, and more evidence of efficacy remains to be shown. For example, apart from the reduction of protracted withdrawal symptoms and craving, two further changes in body function help the patient to build confidence in maintaining abstinence. One is the disappearance of injection marks, and the other is the recovery of the depressed sexual function (52). The complicated network underlying drug abuse can be unraveled only through combined physiologic, neurobiologic, and psychological endeavors, and acupuncture may play a role at least as one of the tools in a comprehensive treatment approach.

REFERENCES

1. NIH Consensus Conference. Acupuncture. *J Am Med Assoc.* 1998;280:1518–1524.
2. Wen HL, Cheung SYC. Treatment of drug addiction by acupuncture and electrical stimulation. *Asian J Med.* 1973;9:138–141.
3. McLellan AT, Grossman DS, Blaine JD, et al. Acupuncture treatment for drug abuse: a technical review. *J Subst Abuse Treat.* 1993;10:569–576.
4. Hughes J, Smith TW, Kosteritz HW, et al. Identification of two related pentapeptides from the brain with potent opiate agonist activity. *Nature.* 1975;258:577–579.
5. Mayer DJ, Price DD, Rafii A. Antagonisms of acupuncture analgesia in man by the narcotic antagonist naloxone. *Brain Res.* 1977;121:368–372.
6. Han JS, Terenius L. Neurochemical basis of acupuncture analgesia. *Annu Rev Pharmacol Toxicol.* 1982;22:193–220.
7. Han JS. Acupuncture: neuropeptide release produced by electrical stimulation of different frequencies. *Trends Neurosci.* 2003;26:17–22.
8. Han JS, Zhang RL. Suppression of morphine abstinence syndrome by body electroacupuncture of different frequencies in rats. *Drug Alcohol Depend.* 1993;31:169–175.
9. Wang Q, Mao LM, Han JS. Comparison of the antinociceptive effects induced by electroacupuncture and transcutaneous electrical nerve stimulation in the rat. *Int J Neurosci.* 1992;65:117–129.
10. Wu LZ, Cui CL, Han JS. Han's acupoint nerve stimulator for the treatment of opiate withdrawal syndrome. *Chin J Pain Med.* 1995;1:30–35.
11. Wang B, Luo F, Xia YQ, et al. Peripheral electric stimulation inhibits morphine-induced place preference in rats. *Neuroreport.* 2000;11:1017–1020.
12. Research Group of Acupuncture Anesthesia, Peking Medical College. Effect of acupuncture on pain threshold of human skin. *Chin Med J.* 1973;(3):151–157.
13. Lu GW. Characteristics of afferent fiber innervations on acupuncture point Zusanli. *Am J Physiol.* 1983;245:R606–R612.
14. Melzack R, Wall PD. Pain mechanisms: a new theory. *Science.* 1965;130:971–979.
15. Auriacombe M, Tignol J, Moal ML, et al. Transcutaneous electrical stimulation with Limoge current potentiates morphine analgesia and attenuates opiate abstinence syndrome. *Biol Psychiatry.* 1990;28:650–656.
16. Han JS, Chen XH, Sun SL, et al. Effect of low- and high-frequency TENS on met-enkephalin-Arg-Phe and dynorphin A immunoreactivity in human lumbar CSF. *Pain.* 1991;47:295–298.
17. Wen HL, Ho WKK. Suppression of withdrawal symptoms by dynorphin in heroin addicts. *Eur J Pharmacol.* 1982;82:183–186.
18. Green PG, Lee NM. Dynorphin (1–13) attenuates withdrawal in morphine-dependent rats: effect of route of administration. *Eur J Pharmacol.* 1998;145:267–272.
19. Cui CL, Wu LZ, Han JS. Spinal kappa-opioid system plays an important role in suppressing morphine withdrawal syndrome in the rat. *Neurosci Lett.* 2000;295:42–48.
20. Chu NN, Zuo YF, Meng L, et al. Peripheral electrical stimulation reversed the cell size reduction and increased BDNF level in the ventral tegmental area in chronic morphine-treated rats. *Brain Res.* 2007;82:90–98.
21. Chu NN, Xia W, Yu P, et al. Chronic morphine-induced neuronal morphological changes in the ventral tegmental area in rats are reversed by electroacupuncture treatment. *Addict Biol.* 2008;13:47–51.
22. Hu L, Chu NN, Sun LL, et al. Electroacupuncture treatment reverses morphine-induced physiological changes in dopaminergic neurons within the ventral tegmental area. *Addict Biol.* 2009;14:431–437.
23. Markou A, Weiss F, Gold LH, et al. Animal models of drug craving. *Psychopharmacology (Berl).* 1993;112:163–182.
24. Bardo MT, Bevins RA. Conditioned place preference: what does it add to our preclinical understanding of drug reward? *Psychopharmacology (Berl).* 2000;153(1):31–43.
25. Wang B, Luo F, Zhang WT, et al. Stress or drug priming induces reinstatement of extinguished conditioned place preference. *Neuro Rep.* 2000;11(12):2781–2784.
26. Wang B, Zhang BG, Ge XC, et al. Inhibition by peripheral electric stimulation of the reinstatement of morphine-induced place preference in rats and drug-craving in heroin addicts. *J Peking University Health Sci.* 2003;85(3):241–247.
27. Shi XD, Ren W, Wang GB, et al. Brain opioid-receptors are involved in mediating peripheral electric stimulation-induced inhibition of morphine conditioned place preference in rats. *Brain Res.* 2003;981:23–29.
28. Chen JH, Liang J, Wang GB, et al. Repeated 2 Hz peripheral electrical stimulations suppress morphine-induced CPP and improve spatial memory ability in rats. *Exp Neurol.* 2005;194:550–556.
29. Shi XD, Wang GB, Ma YY, et al. Repeated peripheral electrical stimulations suppress both morphine-induced CPP and reinstatement of extinguished CPP in rats: accelerated expression of PPE and PPD mRNA in nucleus accumbens implicated. *Mol Brain Res.* 2004;130:124–133.
30. Liang J, Ping XJ, Li YJ, et al. Morphine-induced conditioned place preference in rats is inhibited by electroacupuncture at 2 Hz: role of enkephalin in the nucleus accumbens. *Neuropharmacology.* 2010;58:233–240.
31. Ma YY, Shi XD, Han JS, et al. Peripheral electrical stimulation-induced suppression of morphine-induced CCP in rats: a role for dopamine in the nucleus accumbens. *Brain Res.* 2008;1212:63–70.
32. Wu LZ, Cui CL, Han JS. Effect of Han's acupoint nerve stimulator (HANS) on the heart rate of 75 inpatients during heroin withdrawal. *Chin J Pain Med.* 1996;2:98–102.
33. Wu LZ, Cui CL, Han JS. Treatment on heroin addicts by 4-channel Han's Acupoint Nerve Stimulator (HANS). *J Beijing Med Univ.* 1999;31:239–242.
34. Wu LZ, Cui CL, Han JS. Reduction of methadone dosage and relief of depression and anxiety by 2/100 Hz TENS for heroin detoxification. *Chin J Drug Depend.* 2001;10:124–126.
35. Kalivas PW, Volkow ND. The neural basis of addiction: a pathology of motivation and choice. *Am J Psychiatry.* 2005;162:1403–1413.
36. Sun BQ, Ye YG, Qin LJ. A survey of the causes for relapse to drug in 615 cases of heroin abusers. *Chin J Drug Depend.* 2001;10:214–216.
37. Xia W, Chu NN, Liang J, et al. Electroacupuncture of 2 Hz has a rewarding effect: evidence from a conditioned place preference study in rats. *Evid Based Complement Alternat Med.* 2008; Doi:10.1093/ecam/nen043.
38. Bullock ML, Culliton PD, Olander RT. Controlled trial of acupuncture for severe recidivist alcoholism. *Lancet.* 1989;1:1435–1439.
39. Worner TM, Zeller B, Schwarz H, et al. Acupuncture fails to improve treatment outcome in alcoholics. *Drug Alcohol Depend.* 1992;30:169–173.

40. Sapir-Weise R, Berglund M, Frank A, et al. Acupuncture in alcoholism treatment: a randomized out-patient study. *Alcohol Alcohol*. 1999;34:629–635.
41. Bullock ML, Kiresuk TJ, Sherman RE, et al. A large randomized placebo-controlled study of auricular acupuncture for alcohol dependence. *J Subst Abuse Treat*. 2002;22:71–77.
42. Anton RF, Moak FH, Waid LR, et al. Natrexone and cognitive–behavioral therapy for the treatment of out patient alcoholics: results of a placebo-controlled trial. *Am J Psychiatry*. 1999;156:1758–1764.
43. Yoshimoto K, Kato B, Sakai K, et al. Electroacupuncture stimulation suppresses the increase in alcohol-drinking behavior in restricted rats. *Alcohol Clin Exp Res*. 2001;25:63S–68S.
44. Overstreet DH, Cui CL, Ma YY, et al. Electroacupuncture reduces voluntary alcohol intake in alcohol-preferring rats via an opiate-sensitive mechanism. *Neurochem Res*. 2008;33:2166–2170.
45. Lambert C, Berlin I, Lee TL, et al. A standardized transcutaneous electric acupoint stimulation for relieving tobacco urges in dependent smokers. *Evid Based Complement Alternat Med*. 2009; Doi:10.1093/ecam/nen074.
46. Ren YH, Wang B, Luo F, et al. Peripheral electric stimulation attenuates the expression of cocaine-induced place preference in rats. *Brain Res*. 2002;957:129–135.
47. Smith MO, Brewington V, Culliton PD, et al. Acupuncture. In: Lowinson JH, Ruiz P, Millman RB, et al., eds. *Substance Abuse, A Comprehensive Textbook*. 3rd ed. Baltimore, MD: Williams & Wilkins; 1997:484–492.
48. Margolin A, Kleber HD, Avants SK, et al. Acupuncture for the treatment of cocaine addiction: a randomized controlled trial. *J Am Med Assoc*. 2002;287:55–63.
49. Margolin A, Avants SK, Holford TR. Interpreting conflicting findings from clinical trials of auricular acupuncture for cocaine addiction: does treatment context influence outcome? *J Altern Complement Med*. 2002;8(2):111–121.
50. Research Group of Ear Acupuncture, Jiangsu College of New Medicine. The effect of ear acupuncture on the pain threshold of the skin at thoracic and abdominal region. In: *Theoretical Study on Acupuncture Anesthesia*. Shanghai, China: Shanghai People's Press; 1973:27–32.
51. Streitberger K, Kleinhenz J. Introducing a placebo needle into acupuncture research. *Lancet*. 1998;352:364–365.
52. Wu LZ, Cui CL, Han JS. Effect of 2/100 Hz transcutaneous electric nerve stimulation on sexual dysfunction and serum sex hormone of heroin addicts. *Chin J Integ Tradit Med West Med*. 2000; 20:15–18.

CHAPTER 33: Alcohol Abstinence Management

Richard N. Rosenthal

INTRODUCTION

For the most part, the treatment of alcohol dependence has been conceptualized by clinicians and the general public as a behavioral intervention, whether through involvement in mutual self-help groups such as Alcoholics Anonymous, or through intensive in- or outpatient rehabilitation, or through professional alcohol counseling. This reality is striking in that there have been effective medications available to assist in recovery from alcohol dependence since the early 1950s. Even with the fact that there at least five medications, four of which are currently FDA-approved, that contribute clinically useful impact in the treatment of alcohol dependence, the acceptance and implementation by the treatment community remains low (1,2). In general, medications for the treatment of alcohol dependence achieve their effect through either of two proposed mechanisms—stabilizing systems that have adapted to chronic alcohol exposure and which have become dysregulated with a reduction in alcohol intake, or interfering with the reinforcing effects of alcohol consumption.

HISTORY OF MEDICATION TREATMENT

Disulfiram

History of the Treatment

Disulfiram was a medication originally explored for use as an antiparasitic, and discovered to have aversive qualities in the context of alcohol drinking by Danish researchers Hald and Jacobsen in 1948 (3). In the United States, it was approved by the FDA for the treatment of alcohol dependence in 1951.

Pharmacology of the Medication/Treatment

Its mechanism of action is to block the oxidation of alcohol to acetate through the irreversible inhibition of the enzyme acetaldehyde dehydrogenase, which can increase plasma level of acetaldehyde 5 to 10 times than under normal circumstances of drinking. The buildup of acetaldehyde, which is the oxidation product of ingested alcohol via alcohol dehydrogenase, produces highly unpleasant symptoms in the patients, such as nausea, vomiting, throbbing headache, tachycardia, dysphoria, flushing, hypotension, vertigo, diaphoresis, and dyspnea (4). As such, the actual mechanism of disulfiram in the reduction of alcohol intake lies in its aversive qualities, and thus its ability to increase motivation for sobriety through potential or more rarely, actual punishment.

Efficacy of the Medication/Treatment

Although disulfiram has been in use for 60 years, there have not been a substantial number of well-controlled efficacy studies, and those that have been performed used various outcome measures with differing results (5). Some studies show an improvement in days drinking and reduction in quantities of alcohol consumed. In the largest ($N = 605$) clinical trial, a double-blind, placebo-controlled, 1-year, multicenter cooperative study by the Department of Veterans Affairs, there were no significant differences in the intention-to-treat analysis of abstinence rates among the three treatment groups receiving a daily dose of disulfiram 250 mg, disulfiram 1 mg (an inactive dose), or a vitamin (6). However, those in the disulfiram 250 mg group had significantly fewer drinking days than subjects in the other two groups. Only the groups who received disulfiram were told they might have an aversive reaction if they drank. Nonadherence was a confounding factor in this study, in that 80% of subjects did not take the study medication regularly. Interestingly, the small subset of patients across groups who were adherent with the protocol demonstrated reductions in their alcohol consumption.

A later randomized clinical trial took the adherence issues into consideration and put supervision of daily dosing of the study medication into the procedure, demonstrating significantly less drinking with 200 mg disulfiram compared to a vitamin C control (7). An open randomized 8-month clinical trial ($N = 100$) conducted a head-to-head comparison between disulfiram and acamprosate in subjects screened for good family support for adherence and follow-up (8). The disulfiram group had greater maintenance of abstinence (88% vs. 46%, $P = 0.0002$) and had increased time to relapse to heavy drinking (123 vs. 71 days, $P = 0.0001$), compared with the acamprosate group. Overall, disulfiram decreases drinking days, but there is not strong evidence that it supports maintenance of abstinence (10), and the lack of this stronger evidence is most likely due to patients' poor adherence with the study medication in the existing data sets.

Safety of the Medication/Treatment

Disulfiram is associated with rare but serious side effects such as hepatotoxicity, cholestatic and fulminant hepatitis, optic neuritis, peripheral neuritis, polyneuritis, and in high doses, psychotic symptoms (9). Contraindications to the use of disulfiram include ischemic heart disease and pregnancy. Disulfiram inhibits the induction of hepatic enzymes and thus may interfere with the metabolism of concomitantly administered medications. As such, disulfiram enhances the effects of the coumarin anticoagulants and the phenytoin anticonvulsants (4). In general, disulfiram is used safely in patients who clearly understand the need to avoid consumption or skin contact with all alcohol-containing materials, as even a small dose of alcohol can lead to a buildup of acetaldehyde. This means, in addition to abstaining from consumption of beverage alcohol, the patient must avoid contact or ingestion of alcohol found in foods, over-the-counter cold and other medications, mouthwashes, colognes, and lotions in order not to have an aversive reaction (10). Certain patients with poor control of impulses or poor judgment may be at higher risk for drinking when on disulfiram. Clearly, clinical judgment is a factor in choosing an optimal candidate, but diagnoses alone, while suggestive of potential problems in using disulfiram, are not sufficient as a contraindication against disulfiram use. For example, recent research has demonstrated that patients with co-occurring disorders that may impair cognition or judgment such as schizophrenia, depression, or post-traumatic stress disorder, can still make effective use of disulfiram therapy (11–13).

How the Medication/Treatment Is Optimally Used

Disulfiram is available in 250-mg tablets, and patients should start with an initial oral dose of 250 mg daily, and may be built up to 500 mg daily. Disulfiram should not be taken unless the blood alcohol concentration is zero or until the patient has not consumed any alcohol for at least 12 hours. In addition, as disulfiram is an irreversible aldehyde dehydrogenase inhibitor, the potential for a disulfiram reaction continues until new enzyme is synthesized, which may be up to 2 weeks after discontinuation of treatment. Typically, disulfiram is used for treating patients with prior failure of one or more courses of psychosocial treatment (10) and who are motivated to achieve complete abstinence (6). In patients newly diagnosed with alcohol dependence, disulfiram has not been recommended as a first-line medication, as there are other FDA-approved medications for the treatment of alcohol dependence with more benign side-effect profiles and ease of use. However, there are instances where it is imperative to demonstrate sobriety, such as in legal agreements and consent decrees, where the supervised use of disulfiram, combined with proper toxicologic evaluation, can increase the likelihood that a particular patient will be abstaining from alcohol over a given interval.

Adherence to the medication regimen is an important negative predictor of relapse since patients typically stop disulfiram if they are planning to start drinking again. As such, it is useful to investigate strategies that are likely to optimize exposure to the medication. Disulfiram in an implantable form has been investigated, but currently, the data are limited. As subject adherence with disulfiram dosing has been identified as an important factor in revealing its efficacy, several studies appear to support that supervised administration is an important strategy to optimize efficacy. In the 1986 VA study (6), across groups, those that demonstrated improvements in maintenance of abstinence were those who were adherent with the study medications. Since disulfiram works as an aversive contingency, rather than through neuromodulation, all subjects who took active or placebo medication were subject to the contingency. Supervision of disulfiram has been reported as a superior strategy for decades and even limited supervised administration appears to increase disulfiram's efficacy (14,15). In the open clinical trial comparing acamprosate to disulfiram described above, disulfiram generally had no specific effect unless its use was monitored and supervised by clinicians or significant others (8).

Special Considerations

A well-researched and effective behavioral strategy that optimizes the adherence to disulfiram is Behavioral Couples Therapy (BCT), which provides contingency for sobriety and increased social support for the patient's efforts to change. In BCT, a couple signs a contract stipulating that the partner will watch the patient taking a daily dose of disulfiram and record it on a calendar, then the patient and partner thank each other for their efforts, and will not argue or even discuss the patient's drinking behavior (16). A meta-analysis of randomized studies of BCT showed superior impact on frequency of alcohol use, consequences of use, and relationship satisfaction over individual interventions for alcohol and drug abuse (17).

Oral Naltrexone

History of the Treatment

Naltrexone is a μ-opioid antagonist that was approved in 1994 by the FDA for the prevention of relapse to heavy drinking in alcohol-dependent individuals (Table 33.1). As an opioid antagonist, it was originally approved and marketed as a treatment for opioid dependence. The use of oral naltrexone for opioid dependence, although pharmacologically active, has fallen into disuse due to high rates of medication nonadherence and treatment dropout (18).

Pharmacology of the Medication/Treatment

Endorphins and enkephalins, which are naturally occurring opiates, are released as a result of alcohol consumption (19). Dopamine (DA) is released from the nucleus accumbens (NAc) when these opiates bind to brain receptor sites, resulting in some of the pleasurable effects of alcohol. There may also be opioidergic but non-DA-mediated reward circuitry (20). Investigations of animal models of the role of opioids in alcohol-mediated reward have demonstrated that alcohol-preferring animals have reduced opioid peptides in their brains, and that alcohol is not self-administered by μ-opioid knockout mice (21). In research with humans, as compared to non-alcohol-dependent persons and their family members, a family history of alcoholism is associated with decreased baseline beta-endorphin levels and an exaggerated increase in beta-endorphin as a response to alcohol (22,23). This suggests that at least one component of the vulnerability to the development of alcohol dependence is based upon an increased sensitivity to alcohol-induced endorphine release and subsequent reinforcement. Naltrexone

TABLE 33.1 FDA-approved pharmacotherapies for alcohol dependence

Medication	Prescribing information		Mechanism of action	Common side effects	Contraindications	Drug interactions
	Dose	Comments				
Disulfiram (Antabuse) FDA approval: 1951	Oral: 250 mg daily (range: 125–500 mg)	■ No use ≤ 12 hours after drinking ■ Disulfiram reaction can occur up to 2 weeks after last dose ■ Avoid dietary alcohol intake ■ Periodic liver function tests recommended	Aldehyde dehydrogenase inhibitor	■ Optic neuritis ■ Peripheral neuritis ■ Hepatoxicity When taken with alcohol: ■ Nausea ■ Dizziness ■ Diaphoresis ■ Headache ■ Flushing	■ Concomitant use of alcohol or alcohol-containing products ■ Coronary artery disease ■ Severe myocardial disease	Warfarin, phenytoin, isoniazid, metronidazole, any alcohol-containing medication
Naltrexone (ReVia) FDA approval: 1994	Oral: 50 mg daily	■ No concurrent opioid use; screen for opioids ■ Avoid opioid analgesics ■ Periodic liver function tests recommended	Opioid antagonist	■ Nausea ■ Headache ■ Dizziness ■ Fatigue ■ Insomnia ■ Anxiety ■ Nervousness	■ Currently using opioids or in acute opioid withdrawal ■ Opioid analgesics ■ Acute hepatitis or liver failure	Opioid analgesics
Naltrexone (Vivitrol) FDA approval: 2006	Intramuscular injection: 380 mg monthly	■ No concurrent opioid use; screen for opioids ■ Avoid opioid analgesics ■ Patients should be warned for risk of allergic pneumonia	Opioid antagonist	■ Nausea ■ Headache ■ Vomiting ■ Insomnia ■ Decreased appetite ■ Diarrhea ■ Dizziness ■ Upper respiratory tract infections	■ Currently using opioids or in acute opioid withdrawal ■ Opioid analgesics ■ Acute hepatitis or liver failure	Opioid analgesics
Acamprosate (Campral) FDA approval: 2004	Oral: 1998 mg daily (666 mg t.i.d.)	■ With moderate renal impairment, reduce to 333 mg t.i.d. ■ Establish abstinence	NMDA/ glutamate receptor modulator	■ Diarrhea ■ Asthenia ■ Nausea ■ Pruritus ■ Flatulence	■ Severe renal impairment	No clinically relevant interactions

Adapted from Rosenthal RN. Current and future drug therapies for alcohol dependence. *J Clin Psychopharmacol.* 2006;26(suppl 1):S20–S29.

blocks the opioid-mediated release of DA in the NAc that is typically induced after alcohol consumption (24,25), thus diminishing alcohol's positive reinforcing effects. In addition, alcohol craving is reduced by naltrexone in both social drinkers (26) and alcohol-dependent patients (27), which may be another mechanism of action that is beneficial in recovery from alcohol dependence.

Efficacy of the Medication/Treatment

Two early trials demonstrated that when combined with psychosocial treatment, naltrexone was efficacious in treating alcohol dependence by reducing relapse to heavy drinking (Table 33.2). Volpicelli and colleagues (28) conducted a 12-week double-blind RCT in alcohol-dependent men ($N = 70$) who were postdetoxification and receiving outpatient psychosocial treatment, and compared naltrexone 50 mg/day versus placebo. Compared to 25% in the naltrexone-treated group, about 50% of the placebo-treated patients had relapsed to heavy drinking, defined as ≥5 drinks/day. The group treated with naltrexone also had significant reductions in alcohol craving over the 12-week period. O'Malley and colleagues (29) found similar results in an RCT of naltrexone 50 mg/day or placebo in male and female subjects with alcohol dependence ($N = 97$) who received either alcohol-targeted individual coping skills and relapse-prevention therapy or supportive therapy. Results of a later 12-week trial of naltrexone 50/mg a day compared to placebo in alcohol-dependent patients ($N = 97$) who were receiving psychosocial therapy, demonstrated that the rate of relapse to heavy drinking was significantly reduced only in naltrexone group patients who were adherent to the medication regimen (30).

Although most RCT of naltrexone demonstrate significant reductions in drinking behavior, a few have not (31,32). In a meta-analytic approach examining 14 RCTs of naltrexone and placebo, Bouza and colleagues found that administration of naltrexone over the short term (<12 weeks), significantly decreased the rate of relapse to heavy drinking (odds ratio, OR: 0.62 [0.52, 0.75], $P < 0.001$), but did not have a significant effect on the rate of abstinence (OR: 1.26 [0.97, 1.64], $P = 0.08$) (33) (Table 33.2). A Cochrane collaborative study performed a meta-analysis of 24 RCTs of naltrexone and placebo, finding that in short-term studies the rate of relapse to heavy drinking was reduced by 36% by naltrexone (relative risk, RR: 0.64, 95% CI 0.51 to 0.82). A smaller effect size was demonstrated for maintenance of abstinence (RR: 0.91, 95% CI 0.81 to 1.02) (34). There were too few studies ($N = 8$) to demonstrate benefits for prevention of relapse to heavy over the medium-term trials (>12 weeks), but some evidence for decreased craving over time and increased time to first drink were obtained. Project COMBINE, a 16-week multisite U.S. RCT ($N = 1383$), evaluated the effects of different combinations of acamprosate, naltrexone, and several behavioral

TABLE 33.2	Meta-analyses of randomized clinical trials of naltrexone and acamprosate[a]				
Study	Subject N	Study N	Relative benefit	Odds ratio [95% CI]	P-Value
Naltrexone					
Complete abstinence					
Bouza et al. (33)	1077	10	26%	1.26 [0.97, 1.64]	0.08
Srisurapanont et al. (34)	916	8	9%	0.91 [0.81, 1.02][a]	0.10
Relapse to heavy drinking					
Bouza et al. (33)	2072	14	38%	0.62 [0.52, 0.75]	<0.001
Srisurapanont et al. (34)	822	7	36%	0.64 [0.51, 0.82]	<0.001
Treatment retention					
Bouza et al. (33)	1892	11	6%	0.94 [0.80, 1.1]	0.5
Srisurapanont et al. (34)	1678	16	15%	0.85 [0.72, 1.01]	0.07
Acamprosate					
Complete abstinence					
Mann et al. (79)	4087	17	47%	1.47 [1.29–1.69]	<0.001
Bouza et al. (33)	3324	11	88%	1.88 [1.57, 2.25]	<0.001
Treatment retention					
Mann et al. (79)	4087	17	6%	[2.90–8.82]	0.01
Bouza et al. (33)	3959	12	29%	1.29 [1.13, 1.47][b]	<0.001

[a]Measures return to any drinking.
[b]Measures overall treatment adherence.
Adapted from Rosenthal RN. Current and future drug therapies for alcohol dependence. *Journal of Clinical Psychopharmacology.* 2006;26(suppl 1):S20–S29.

interventions in alcohol-dependent patients. The main result was that all treatment groups, including placebo, substantially reduced drinking (35). Secondary analyses demonstrated that relapse to heavy drinking was significantly reduced by naltrexone, but not acamprosate. This is an outcome that was present in most of the RCTs of naltrexone, and for which a significant effect was demonstrated in the meta-analyses described above.

Taken together, the evidence suggests that the main clinical effect of naltrexone, with respect to the treatment of alcohol dependence, is reduction in relapse to heavy drinking. This finding has implications based upon severity of symptoms, patient capacity and patient goals, as to how naltrexone should be included in treatment planning. There is a lesser effect on maintenance of complete abstinence.

Safety of the Medication/Treatment

Typical dosage for naltrexone is 50 mg once daily as an adjunct to psychosocial treatment of alcohol dependence. Naltrexone has a $t_{1/2}$ of only several hours in the plasma, but a major metabolite, 6-hydroxy-β-naltrexol, accumulates with regular dosing and demonstrates mild μ-opioid antagonism. Since naltrexone is an opiate antagonist, patients receiving naltrexone should be screened for opiate use so that administration does not precipitate acute withdrawal symptoms. Naltrexone-associated side effects are more frequent in the first days of therapy. The most common side effects are central nervous system symptoms (headache, dizziness, and fatigue) and gastrointestinal-related (nausea) symptoms (36). Naltrexone has few interactions with other medications as it is metabolized by a hepatic nonmicrosomal oxidase system. As μ-opioid receptors are blocked by naltrexone, naltrexone-treated patients will generally find opioids ineffective for analgesia. Therefore, patients taking naltrexone who are in acute pain, and who require an overriding dose of opioid medications for acute treatment should have this administered under the guidance of an anesthesiologist or a qualified clinician who can provide appropriate clinical support (37). A "black-box" warning exists for naltrexone in high doses, but at the recommended doses there is no evidence for hepatotoxicity. Reported hepatotoxicity in alcohol-dependent patients was attributable to elevations of liver enzymes that were reversible.

The optimal treatment duration with naltrexone has not been specified, but 3- to 6-month studies demonstrated low risk of treatment-emergent adverse events (AEs) or what is termed in systematic reviews a favorable harms profile (34,38). In addition, retention in treatment is not adversely impacted by naltrexone and may be improved (33,34).

How the Medication/Treatment Is Optimally Used

Pharmacogenetic considerations: The role of genetic markers in the clinical response to naltrexone for alcoholism has been examined. A particular single-nucleotide polymorphism (SNP) has been identified in exon 1 of the gene encoding for the μ-opioid receptor (*OPRM1*), which is a missense A-to-G (A118G) substitution coding for the amino acid aspartate instead of asparagine (Asn40Asp). This SNP is associated with altered μ-receptor response to endogenous opioids and to μ-opioid receptor antagonists, such that individuals carrying at least one copy of the Asp40 allele demonstrate increased alcohol-induced reward (39) and a greater decrease in the rewarding effects of alcohol in the context of naltrexone (40). Therefore, in certain cohorts of patients, naltrexone may be more efficacious, suggesting that better characterization of these higher responders is an appropriate venue for exploration. Several studies have examined in alcohol dependent subjects the effect of the Asn40Asp SNP on the clinical response to naltrexone (41–43) and have found that, compared to subjects homozygous for the Asn40 allele, carriers of the Asp40 allele in fact demonstrate superior response to naltrexone (41–44). In addition, Mitchell and colleagues conducted an RCT in heavy drinkers who were not seeking treatment for alcohol dependence (45). The studies by Oslin et al. (41) and Anton et al. (43) and a haplotype analysis by Oroszi et al. (44) on the Anton et al. (43) data set found that the μ-opioid receptor Asp40 allele predicted a positive clinical response to naltrexone, while the studies by Gelernter et al. (42) and Mitchell et al. (45) did not demonstrate that finding. In addition, a meta-analysis of 28 samples from 19 publications ($N = 8096$) of predominantly opioid- or alcohol-dependent subjects compared to controls showed no evidence for an association of the Asn40Asp polymorphism with alcohol dependence (46).

Ethnic and Racial Differences in Naltrexone Response

One factor in the varying results for the association of Asn40Asp SNP and clinical responsivity to naltrexone may be the ethnic differences in the tested subjects with regard to the frequency of the Asp40 SNP. The frequency of the Asn40Asp SNP is estimated to be less than 5% in individuals of African descent, whereas it is about four times greater in those of European descent, and up to 58% in Asians (47). If the OPRM1 Asp40 polymorphism renders increased response to μ-receptor antagonism, then those of African ancestry may be less likely to benefit from naltrexone. A secondary outcome analysis of the COMBINE study examined the effects of naltrexone among African Americans ($N = 100$) during the 16-week treatment and indeed found, when controlling for the behavioral interventions and acamprosate, that the beneficial effects attributed to naltrexone in the overall COMBINE sample, such as percent days abstinent and time to first heavy drinking, were not seen in the ethnic subsample (47). Whereas these data are initial and as yet unique, they offer a compelling hypothesis that a low frequency of a particular allele variant may have differential impact on responsivity to alcohol pharmacotherapy.

Special Considerations

It is reasonable to expect that due to adherence and judgment issues in patients with co-occurring disorders, treatment outcomes with naltrexone might be adversely affected. However, in an RCT, patients with schizophrenia treated with naltrexone for alcohol dependence had significantly fewer drinking days and heavy-drinking days (>5 drinks) and reported less craving (48). Petrakis and colleagues demonstrated in a second RCT that compared with placebo a replication in which naltrexone reduced heavy-drinking days as well as increased abstinent days in patients with schizophrenia (49). Therefore, the presence of co-occurring disorders should not be a barrier to use of naltrexone.

Injectable Naltrexone

History of the Treatment

Naltrexone was approved by the U.S. FDA in April 2006 in an injectable, extended-release formulation for the treatment of alcohol dependence (50,51).

Pharmacology of the Medication/Treatment

For the purposes of injection, 380 mg of naltrexone is encapsulated in biodegradable microspheres that slowly release naltrexone over a 30-day period after injection. The naltrexone released has the same μ-opioid antagonist properties as orally administered naltrexone. The microspheres are composed of a polylactide-co-glycolide polymer that is used extensively in other extended-release drugs, such as in absorbable sutures as well as in long-acting risperidone (Risperdal Consta). A pharmacokinetic analysis after injection of naltrexone 380 mg demonstrated sustained therapeutic plasma levels for 30 days, without significant drug accumulation (51). Plasma levels of naltrexone show peak concentrations 2 to 3 days after an intramuscular (IM) injection and demonstrate a slow decline for the next 30 days. Since oral naltrexone is dosed at 50 mg/day, over 30 days the monthly cumulative dose is 1500 mg, whereas an IM injection of naltrexone given every 30 days results in a lower monthly dose of 380 mg. IN addition, injectable long-acting naltrexone also does not demonstrate the typical daily fluctuations in plasma concentrations as associated with daily oral dosing of naltrexone (52).

Efficacy of the Medication/Treatment

In a multisite RCT in alcohol-dependent subjects ($N = 315$) of a depot formulation of naltrexone different from the one that is currently FDA-approved, treatment with depot naltrexone compared to placebo injection significantly increased the time to the first drink, decreased the number of drinking days during treatment, and supported a significantly greater rate of abstinence (18% vs. 10%) (53).

A 6-month, multisite, double-blind RCT evaluated the efficacy and safety of long-acting injectable naltrexone 190 or 380 mg (Vivitrol) in alcohol-dependent subjects ($N = 624$) over 24 weeks of treatment (50). Alcohol abstinence was not required of subjects at study entry and there was no lead-in with oral naltrexone prior to naltrexone injection. Patients received 12 sessions of psychosocial support. The primary outcome, targeted at the expected main effect of naltrexone in alcohol dependence, was the event rate (number of drinking days/total number of days at risk) of heavy drinking (≥5 standard drinks/day for men and ≥4 standard drinks/day for women). IM naltrexone reduced the rate of heavy drinking by 25% ($P = 0.03$) in the 380 mg group and by 17% ($P = 0.07$) in the 190 mg group, compared to placebo. Heavy-drinking days were reduced by 48% by long-acting injectable naltrexone including those actively drinking and patients who were abstinent at treatment entry. For subjects abstinent before injection, injectable naltrexone treatment effects were greater—compared to those actively drinking at injection who had a 21% decrease in the event rate of heavy drinking, those who had a period of 7-days abstinence prior to first injection had an 80% reduction ($P = 0.02$). Secondary outcomes included the event rates of risky drinking (>2 drinks/day for men and >1 drink/day for women) and of any drinking days. Injectable naltrexone was not associated with a significant reduction in risky drinking or rate of any drinking days (complete abstinence) compared to placebo.

In a subgroup of patients with at least 4 days of abstinence before injection ($N = 82$) IM naltrexone 380 mg prolonged abstinence (median time to first drink: 41 days vs. 12 days) and reduced the number of drinking days and heavy-drinking days. The rate of continuous abstinence at end of the study was 32% versus 11% ($P = 0.02$) (54). IM naltrexone 380 mg compared with placebo had beneficial effects on alcohol volumes and frequencies as well, with substantially increased time to first heavy-drinking event (>180 days vs. 20 days; $P = 0.04$), a 90% decrease in the median drinking days per month (0.7 vs. 7.2; $P = 0.005$), and a 93% decrease in heavy-drinking days per month (0.2 days vs. 2.9 days; $P = 0.007$). Taken together, IM naltrexone appears to have a positive effect even in actively drinking patients, but has stronger effects in abstinent individuals. However, there was no significant treatment outcome effect of subjects having abstinence as a treatment goal.

A 1-year open-label extension study was conducted with subjects consenting to continue after completing the initial 6-month study (55). Heavy drinking was significantly reduced in subjects receiving IM naltrexone. Compared to subjects who received naltrexone 380 mg IM during both the 6-month RCT and extension study, subjects who had been treated initially in the placebo arm of the study for 6 months who were switched to 380 mg IM naltrexone during extension study demonstrated the largest reduction in days of heavy drinking.

There appears to be a dose–response effect for IM naltrexone, with outcomes for 190 mg ($N = 26$) generally intermediate between that of the approved 380 mg IM dose and placebo (50,54).

In the intention-to-treat sample, an analysis of quality of life measures with the medical outcomes study 36-item short form demonstrated that compared with IM placebo, IM naltrexone 380 mg was associated with significant improvements in mental health ($P = 0.0496$), social functioning ($P = 0.010$), general health ($P = 0.048$), and physical functioning ($P = 0.028$) (56).

Overall, the clinical outcomes for long-acting injectable naltrexone in alcohol-dependent patients are consistent with the meta-analyses of RCTs of oral naltrexone in demonstrating reduction in relapse to heavy drinking. IM naltrexone has advantages over oral naltrexone in that it has less potential for hepatotoxicity, once-monthly administration is sufficient to sustain therapeutic plasma levels for a month, and the route of administration likely improves adherence in clinical populations.

Safety of the Medication/Treatment

Compared to the oral formulation of naltrexone, an advantageous pharmacokinetic property of IM naltrexone is its reduced first-pass elimination, which exposes the liver to less of the drug cumulatively and thus reduces the potential for hepatotoxicity. Pharmacokinetic studies comparing plasma concentrations after a single IM dose of naltrexone found similar levels of naltrexone and its primary metabolite 6β-naltrexol, and similar cumulative exposure over 63 days in subjects with mild (Child-Pugh grade A) and moderate (Child-Pugh grade B) hepatic impairment and in matched control subjects (57). Thus, this route of administration may be advantageous in using naltrexone with patients who have chemical or infectious hepatitis, or other liver impairment. Given the risk of hepatotoxicity with continued drinking, subjects treated with 380 mg IM naltrexone experience greater improvement in gamma-glutamyl transpeptidase levels compared to controls ($P = 0.03$) (54).

In the 6-month multisite RCT of treatment with long-acting injectable naltrexone, AEs occurring in at least 10% of subjects were nausea, headache, fatigue, decreased appetite, dizziness, and injection site pain. Discontinuation due to AEs occurred in 14% in the 380 mg and 6.7% in the 190 mg group and 6.7% in the placebo group (50).

How the Medication/Treatment Is Optimally Used

The greatest advantages of the long-acting IM formulation of naltrexone are the low dosing frequency, the more or less continuous exposure of μ-opioid receptors to naltrexone, and the high intrinsic medication adherence. The low dosing frequency can be helpful in supporting patients to return for the next dose. The nature of the formulation ensures that the patient will be exposed to the effects of the medicine for at least 30 days, until they return for the next dose administration. The fact that the medication can more easily be framed as a background for recovery can allow clinicians to focus upon delivering or providing for convergent (e.g., CBT to reduce acting on craving as the drug reduces craving) or complimentary (self-help groups to support abstinence) psychosocial interventions that work synergistically with naltrexone's main effects on drinking behavior (58).

Acamprosate

History of the Treatment

Acamprosate was approved for use by the U.S. FDA in July 2004 for the treatment of alcohol dependence in conjunction with psychosocial support. Its indication is for the maintenance of abstinence from alcohol in alcohol-dependent patients who are abstinent at treatment initiation (Table 33.1).

Pharmacology of the Medication/Treatment

Acamprosate is a taurine analogue that, similar to taurine, activates glycine receptors (GlyRs) in the NAc and also acts as a weak partial N-methyl-D-aspartate (NMDA) receptor antagonist. In animal models, strychnine-sensitive (competitive antagonist) GlyRs in the NAc and nicotinic acetylcholine receptors (nAChRs) in the ventral tegmental area are involved in regulating DA release and mediating alcohol-induced DA elevation in the mesolimbic DA system (59,60). In animal models of direct and systemic administration, acamprosate appears to decrease alcohol intake through primary interactions with GlyRs in the NAc and secondarily with the ventral tegmental nAChRs, both of which increase extracellular DA in the NAc (61,62).

In addition, acamprosate is believed to modulate glutamatergic hyperactivity associated with changes in the balance of excitatory and inhibitory neuroregulation in the context of chronic alcohol exposure. The normal balance between the neuronal excitation and inhibition that is regulated through gamma-aminobutyric acid (GABA), glutamate/NMDA, and other receptor systems is disrupted by acute alcohol exposure, leading to a net amplification of inhibitory process (63). However, chronic alcohol consumption elicits upregulation of excitatory NMDA receptors as a neuroadaptive mechanism to counterbalance the chronic inhibition. This resulting net excitation is a homeostatic mechanism compensatory to the chronic inhibitory action of alcohol, which restores the neuronal balance toward normal. When the chronic alcohol is precipitously removed in the chronically compensated state, such as when an alcohol-dependent person becomes acutely abstinent, the upregulated glutamate/NMDA receptor system functions unopposed, which results in a hyperexcitable state that is associated with acute withdrawal, as well as postwithdrawal phenomena (64,65). It has been proposed that acamprosate may modulate both ionotrophic and metabotrophic central NMDA receptors at regulatory sites, such as m-glu-R5 receptors, to normalize NMDA glutamatergic hyperexcitability and reestablish homeostasis in the absence of alcohol (66–70).

Efficacy of the Medication/Treatment

An analysis of outcomes in a clinical trial database consisting of data from double-blind RCTs—one short-term of 13 weeks (71) and two long-term of 48 weeks (72) and 52 weeks (73), were the basis of U.S. FDA approval of acamprosate in 2004 (Table 33.1). In all three RCTs, acamprosate (1332 and/or 1998 mg/day) was tested against placebo in the context of psychosocial support in abstinent subjects with a diagnosis of alcohol dependence who were detoxified. The short-term trial comparing placebo or acamprosate (1332 or 1998 mg/day) was a multisite study of French and Belgian subjects ($N = 188$). There was a significantly greater rate of complete abstinence in the acamprosate group at the end of the study (1998 mg/day acamprosate, 38%, vs. placebo, 13%, $P = 0.001$), as well as increased percent days abstinent (1998 mg/day acamprosate, 67%, vs. placebo, 29%, $P < 0.001$) and time to first drink (1998 mg/day acamprosate, 52.5 median days, vs. placebo, 17 median days, $P < 0.001$) (74). Similarly, in the long-term trials, complete abstinence rates were significantly greater in the acamprosate group in both the 48-week German study (72) ($N = 272$; pooled 1332/1998 mg/day acamprosate, 28%, vs. placebo, 13%, $P = 0.002$) and in the 52-week multisite French study (73) ($N = 538$; 1998 mg/day acamprosate, 16%, vs. placebo, 9%, $P = 0.044$). Both studies also demonstrated significant increases in percent days abstinent and time to first drink (74). In a 12-month medication-free follow-up evaluation of the German long-term RCT subjects, those previously randomized to receive acamprosate showed double the rate of abstinence at 1 year off of study medications (acamprosate, 39%, vs. placebo, 17%, $P = 0.003$) (72). The French 52-week RCT also showed that a significantly higher percentage of acamprosate-treated patients compared to placebo were able to regain abstinence after relapse to any drinking (acamprosate, 46.4%, vs. placebo, 34.6%, $P < 0.05$), demonstrating a relapse recovery effect (75).

Mason and colleagues compared against placebo the effects of acamprosate 1 g either twice daily or three times daily in a 6-month RCT in the United States ($N = 601$) and found no significant between groups difference in the percentage of abstinent days in the main analysis (54.3% for placebo, 56.1% for 2 g, 60.7% for 3 g) (76). However, there were differences in methodology and subject cohort between this study and the European trials described above. Unlike prior efficacy trials, the subjects in the U.S. trial were not required to be abstinent from alcohol prior to study entry, nor were they excluded by age limitation or elevated liver function tests. In addition, there was a higher percentage of polysubstance abuse among the subjects of the U.S. trial. Any of these factors may have contributed to the outcome differences between the U.S. and other studies. When the investigators performed a secondary analysis of the data from a subset of 241 subjects who initially had abstinence as a goal at study entry, controlling for baseline variables and treatment exposure, they found that compared to placebo, acamprosate was associated with a higher percentage of abstinent days (70.0% for 2 g, 58.1% for placebo; $P = 0.02$). These data suggest that for acamprosate treatment, motivation for abstinence may be an important factor in promoting a positive outcome.

A 26-week multisite RCT in Spain tested the efficacy of acamprosate that was administered at the beginning of medically supervised alcohol withdrawal rather than postdetoxification in patients with alcohol dependence ($N = 296$). Compared to the placebo-treated group, the acamprosate-treated group had a cumulative abstinence duration (CAD) 19 days longer at the study endpoint ($P = 0.0006$), and 16 days longer duration of abstinent days between the last episode of any drinking to the study endpoint (stable recovery duration) ($P = 0.021$) (77).

A secondary analysis of 15 European studies suggests a cumulative effect of acamprosate in reducing both the frequency of relapse and the amount of drinking during a relapse interval (78). The investigators evaluated relapse severity by defining it as the product of quantity and frequency of drinking by subjects at four intervals (30, 90, 180, and 360 days) across studies and found that compared to placebo, acamprosate was associated with less drinking among the subjects who relapsed ($P < 0.001$), and that the between-groups difference increased over time.

Two recent meta-analytic approaches support that acamprosate is efficacious in helping patients with alcohol dependence to maintain abstinence from alcohol (Table 33.2) (33,79). Pooled data from 17 placebo-controlled trials determined for acamprosate a significantly higher proportion of subjects maintaining complete abstinence and a relative benefit of 1.47 over placebo of attaining 6 months of complete abstinence, a moderate to strong effect (Mann et al. (79)). Similarly, in a different meta-analysis of 12 RCTs, acamprosate treatment was associated with a significant increase in the abstinence rate (OR: 1.88 [1.57, 2.25], $P < 0.001$) and the CAD (weighted mean difference, WMD: 26.55 [17.56, 36.54], $P < 0.001$) (33). Further, data from these systematic evaluations suggest that acamprosate has moderate benefits on overall treatment adherence and a small positive impact upon treatment retention (33,79).

Taken together, there is a good evidence base to conclude that acamprosate compared to placebo increases abstinence and decreases drinking days in patients with alcohol dependence. However, two large recent U.S. studies did not find similar results for the efficacy of acamprosate, and have dampened clinical enthusiasm for the medication (35,76). There may be differences in study methods and the characteristics of the populations being studied that may account for some of these striking and consistent differences in outcome. Nonetheless, there are strong data supporting acamprosate efficacy in long-term studies and its strongest effects have been demonstrated in subjects who have been recently detoxified.

Safety of the Medication/Treatment

Acamprosate, which does not undergo hepatic metabolism, is excreted entirely in the urine as unchanged drug (80), and does not interact significantly with other medications (81,82). When acamprosate is used with other medications such as disulfiram, diazepam, or even alcohol, there are no pharmacokinetic interactions (80). Acamprosate has a favorable safety and tolerability profile supported by the extant clinical trial data (83). Acamprosate was demonstrated to be safe, well tolerated, and compared to placebo, without significant discontinuation due to AEs in a meta-analysis of 10 RCTs (33). More recently, Rosenthal and colleagues (83) assessed the safety and tolerability of acamprosate by analyzing data from 13 short- and long-term RCTs ($N = 4234$). The incidence of treatment-emergent AEs was 61% for acamprosate and 56% for placebo ($P < 0.01$), the majority of which were reported across groups as transient, of mild or moderate severity, and were attributable to comparable discontinuation rates. For acamprosate compared to placebo, the highest frequency AEs were respectively, diarrhea (16% vs. 10%, $P < 0.01$) and flatulence (3% vs. 2%, $P < 0.01$), which occurred relatively infrequently. Transient diarrhea typically occurs in the first 4 weeks of treatment, with decreasing incidence over time, and is of mild to moderate severity (83). There were no increases in AEs among subjects taking additional medications frequently used to treat alcohol dependence.

How the Medication/Treatment Is Optimally Used

Acamprosate is formulated in a tablet containing 333 mg, which is recommended to be taken as two tablets three times a day. Given the strength of evidence for optimal response in already-abstinent patients, initiation of acamprosate treatment should begin as soon as possible after abstinence is achieved and the period of acute withdrawal has passed. Given recent research data demonstrating the benefit in study subjects who had lost abstinence, treatment should be continued even if a patient relapses (78).

Special Considerations

Patients with Impaired Renal Function Subjects with varying degrees of renal impairment were compared with healthy adult subjects in a pharmacokinetic study that measured total plasma clearance, renal clearance, C_{max}, and T_{max} after a single dose of acamprosate. Subjects with renal impairment differed significantly from healthy subjects on all measures, and a linear correlation between decreases in the clearance of creatinine and that of acamprosate was demonstrated (80). These data suggest that patients with impaired renal function could accumulate acamprosate with prolonged dosing. Therefore it is recommended that in patients with moderate renal impairment (creatinine clearance of 30 to 50 mL/min) the standard dose be halved to one 333 mg tablet three times a day. In patients with severe renal impairment (creatinine clearance <30 mL/min), acamprosate is not recommended (83).

Combination Treatment (Naltrexone and Acamprosate) Since the major effects of naltrexone and acamprosate determined in meta-analyses appear to be different and appear to work by different mechanisms, namely reduction in relapse to heavy drinking in the case of naltrexone, and maintenance of abstinence in the case of acamprosate, it is a reasonable strategy to test the efficacy in alcohol dependence by combining the two medications. Two studies have examined this approach, but demonstrating synergistic effects has been less than straightforward. The first study that demonstrated that a combination of medications might be superior to a single pharmacotherapeutic approach in treating alcohol dependence was conducted in Germany by Kiefer and colleagues (84). The investigators conducted a 12-week RCT of naltrexone 50 mg/day and acamprosate 1998 mg/day, singularly and in combination, in detoxified patients ($N = 160$) with alcohol dependence who also received weekly group therapy (84). The primary outcomes were the time to first drink, time to first relapse to heavy drinking (i.e., for men, ≥5 drinks/day and for women, ≥4 drinks/day), and CAD. Compared to placebo, all treatment groups, including each medicine alone and in combination, showed significant improvements in time to relapse. However, compared to acamprosate alone, the combination of acamprosate with naltrexone was significantly better in terms of time to relapse, but not better than naltrexone alone.

Feeney and colleagues (85) conducted a 12-week, single-location trial of acamprosate, naltrexone, or the combination in age-, sex-, and alcohol-severity-matched subjects with alcohol dependence ($N = 236$) who were recently detoxified, but not randomly assigned to groups. There were no significant between-groups differences with regard to CAD, total abstinence or days to relapse, but there were significantly more days to relapse in the combination group compared to the group receiving only acamprosate. In contrast to the findings of additive effects in combining naltrexone and acamprosate, superior to acamprosate alone (84,85), Project COMBINE, a multisite 16-week RCT did not find evidence with either low- or high-intensity behavioral interventions, of additive effects of combining naltrexone 100 mg/day and acamprosate 3 g/day compared to either drug alone (35). In this study, naltrexone was efficacious in reducing the risk of relapse to heavy drinking. However, this outcome was not improved in the group that received intensive, specialist-delivered behavioral therapy (combined behavioral intervention, itself efficacious) in addition to naltrexone. Surprisingly, neither the percent days abstinent, an expected evidence-based outcome for acamprosate, or relapse to heavy drinking were positively impacted by acamprosate as compared to placebo. Acamprosate's lack of efficacy was unexpected in this study and the result has been attributed to the overall level of improvement across treatment groups, the high placebo response rate, and methodological differences compared with the European studies (e.g., European subjects had required premedication abstinence, American subjects had more polysubstance abuse) in which the efficacy of acamprosate has been demonstrated (86).

Investigational or Off-Label Medications for Alcohol Dependence (Not Approved for Treatment of Alcohol Dependence by the U.S. Food and Drug Administration) Many classes of drugs are under active study for the treatment of alcohol dependence. This section focuses on a few of the more promising medications that are active on GABAergic, serotoninergic, and dopaminergic systems.

ANTICONVULSANTS AND OTHER GABAERGIC MEDICATIONS

Topiramate

History of the Treatment

As antiseizure medications tend to increase GABAergic activity or reduce glutamatergic activity, initial RCTs of several medications have been conducted in the treatment of alcohol dependence, including divalproex (87), and carbamazepine (88), with modest positive effects. However, topiramate has the most extensive evidence to date for efficacy in randomized, controlled trials.

Pharmacology of the Medication/Treatment

Topiramate's utility in the treatment of alcohol dependence is hypothesized to act to reduce alcohol's reinforcing effects in the central nervous system through binding a nonbenzodiazepine site on $GABA_A$ receptors so as to increase GABAergic activity (89) and also by inhibiting glutamatergic activity through binding and inhibiting activity of corticomesolimbic

AMPA/kainate glutamate receptors that have been upregulated due to chronic alcohol exposure (90).

Efficacy of the Medication/Treatment

Johnson et al. (91) conducted a double-blind 12-week RCT comparing topiramate (titrated up to 300 mg/day as tolerated) and placebo in alcohol-dependent subjects ($N = 150$) receiving outpatient psychosocial support (91). Drinks per day, drinks per drinking day, percentage of heavy-drinking days, and percentage of days abstinent were the primary outcome measures. Compared to those receiving placebo, the topiramate group had a 27.6% lower percentage of heavy-drinking days ($P = 0.0003$), and 26.2% more abstinent days ($P = 0.0003$). Continuing this line of efficacy research, a multisite 14-week double-blind U.S. RCT of topiramate (titrated up to 300 mg/day or maximum tolerated) and placebo was conducted by Johnson et al. in subjects with alcohol dependence ($N = 371$) who received a weekly treatment adherence enhancement therapy (92). Again, topiramate demonstrated a 16.2% mean reduction in the percentage of self-reported heavy-drinking days ($P < 0.001$) compared to placebo, and an 8.44% mean reduction in the rate of self-reported heavy-drinking days over the study interval ($P = 0.002$). Interestingly, there was also an improvement in the self-reported percentage of abstinent days ($P < 0.002$). As a corollary to the self-report measures, plasma gamma glutamyltransferase, a biomarker of alcohol consumption, was significantly reduced in the topiramate group as compared to placebo ($P < 0.001$). On data generated in the same study, another analysis was conducted to determine the effects of topiramate on physical health, obsessional thoughts and compulsions about using alcohol (a measure of craving), and psychosocial well-being (93). Topiramate compared with placebo had a significantly positive impact ($P < 05$) on alcohol-related obsessional thoughts and compulsions, psychosocial well-being, and aspects of quality of life, likely contributing to reducing the risk of relapse. Interestingly, a 12-week double-blind RCT compared topiramate (titrated to 300 mg/day), naltrexone (50 mg/day), and placebo in alcohol-dependent outpatients ($N = 155$) who were 1 week postdetoxification at study entry (94). Although there were no significant differences between naltrexone and topiramate, in time to first relapse, CAD and heavy-drinking weeks, topiramate was superior to placebo, and demonstrated trends toward superiority over naltrexone.

Safety of the Medication/Treatment

Over the approved therapeutic dose range of 200 to 800 mg/day, topiramate follows linear pharmacokinetics. The relative bioavailability is 80% and is not affected by food, with nearly complete oral absorption within 2 hours of administration (95). The drug is not widely metabolized in vivo and is mostly eliminated (70%) unchanged in the urine (95). Johnson et al. (91) reported no serious AEs in their initial RCT, but there were side effects that were reported in the topiramate group more commonly than in the placebo group, respectively, such as dizziness (28.0% vs. 10.7%, $P = 0.007$), paresthesia (57.3% vs. 18.7%, $P < 0.0001$), psychomotor slowing (26.7% vs. 12.0%, $P = 0.023$), memory/concentration impairment (18.7% vs. 5.3%, $P = 0.012$), and weight loss (54.7% vs. 26.7%, $P = 0.001$) (Table 33.3). In examining AEs occurring in greater than 10% of subjects, a similar profile was demonstrated in the multisite RCT as more common with topiramate versus placebo ($P < 0.05$), respectively, including: paresthesia (50.8% vs. 10.6%), altered taste perception (23.0% vs. 4.8%), anorexia (19.7% vs. 6.9%), difficulty concentrating (14.8% vs. 3.2%), dizziness (11.5% vs. 5.3%), and pruritis (10.4% vs. 1.1%) (92). In general, 85% of side effects occur during the period of titration and most of which tend to resolve with continued treatment, but about 20% of those treated in clinical trials drop out due to side effects (92,96). Individual genetic differences may modulate side effects of topiramate. A SNP of the GRIK1 gene coding for the kainate-selective GluR5 glutamate receptor subunit has been recently described in heavy drinkers, in which an allele variant was associated with greater severity of topiramate-induced side effects and also with serum levels of topiramate (97).

With respect to safety advantages of topiramate compared to placebo, measures of liver function (aspartate aminotransferase and alanine aminotranferase) and body mass index were reduced in a clinically small but significant way ($P < 0.001$). In addition compared to placebo, topiramate significantly reduced the mean plasma cholesterol level by 13.30 mg/dL ($P = 0.002$), mean systolic blood pressure by 9.70 mm Hg ($P < 0.001$) and mean diastolic blood pressure by 6.74 mm Hg ($P < .001$), returning blood pressure to the range of prehypertension levels (93).

How the Medication/Treatment Is Optimally Used

Topiramate should be titrated slowly starting at 25 mg/day and increasing at 25 mg/week until the patient reaches the 300 mg/day dose demonstrated effective in clinical trials. The slow titration decreases the frequency of neurocognitive side effects and discontinuation rates as compared to patients taking 50 mg/day and titrated at 50 mg/week, but takes 12 weeks to reach the target dose (98). It is unclear as to whether topiramate in doses less than 300 mg/day is effective in alcohol dependence. Given reports of seizures upon abrupt withdrawal of topiramate in patients without a prior seizure history, it is suggested that topiramate be tapered at the rate of 25% every 4 days for a period of 16 days (98).

Special Considerations

Patients with Impaired Renal Function The product packaging states that patients with moderately impaired kidney function (creatinine clearance 30 to 69 mL/min/1.73 m^2) had a 42% decrease in the clearance of topiramate. Since topiramate is mostly excreted unchanged in the urine, it is suggested that for patients with a creatinine clearance below 70 mL/min/1.73 m^2 and a resulting reduction in clearance of topiramate, 50% of the recommended dose should be given (95).

In postmarketing studies of topiramate, a normal anion gap hyperchloremic metabolic acidosis was a rare dose-related serious AE (95). Because topiramate is a weak carbonic anhydrase inhibitor, the kidneys may leach bicarbonate levels

TABLE 33.3 Non-FDA-approved pharmacotherapies for alcohol dependence

Medication	Prescribing information			Common side effects	Warnings/relative contraindications	Drug interactions
	Dose	Comments	Mechanism of action			
Topiramate (Topamax)	Oral: 300 mg daily (range: 200–800 mg)	1) Need slow titration to 300 mg 2) Typical increment of 25 mg/week ■ With moderate renal impairment, reduce dose 50% 3) Monitor patients for low serum bicarbonate	GABA$_A$ receptor activator; AMPA/kainate glutamate receptor inhibitor	■ Dizziness ■ Paresthesia ■ Psychomotor slowing ■ Memory impairment ■ Altered taste perception ■ Pruritis	■ Renal failure ■ Treatment with carbonic anhydrase inhibitors	■ Topiramate concentrations: ■ reduced by CYP2C9 inducers (e.g., valproic acid carbamazepine, phenytoin) ■ increased by 2C9 inhibitors (e.g., delavirdine)
Baclofen (Lioresal; Kemstro) FDA approval: 1994	Oral: 50 mg daily (range: 40–80 mg)	■ No concurrent opioid use; screen for opioids ■ Avoid opioid analgesics ■ Periodic liver function tests recommended	Stereoselective GABA$_B$ agonist	■ Drowsiness ■ Vertigo ■ Nausea ■ Abdominal pain	■ Use of CNS depressants ■ Renal failure	■ Potential synergy combined with any sedating medication
Serotonin reuptake inhibitors Fluoxetine (Prozac) Sertraline (Zoloft, Lustral)	Oral: 20 mg daily (range: 20–60 mg) Oral: 100 mg daily (range: 50–200 mg)	■ Beneficial effects may only be seen in those with late-onset alcohol dependence	Serotonin reuptake inhibition	■ Nausea ■ Insomnia ■ Dry mouth ■ Diarrhea ■ Decreased libido ■ Delayed ejaculation	■ Concomitant MAOI, pimozide, or thioridazine ■ Alcoholism onset <25 years old (may worsen alcoholism symptoms)	■ CYP2D6 inhibition ■ May increase levels of tightly protein bound drugs (e.g., warfarin, digitoxin)
Ondansetron (Zofran)	Oral: 4 µg/kg daily (range: 1–16 µg/kg)	■ Effect only demonstrated in early-onset alcoholics <25 years old	Serotonin-3 receptor antagonist	■ Constipation ■ Dizziness ■ Headache ■ Rash/pruritis	■ Long QT syndrome ■ Opioid Tx esp. Methadone	■ Potent inducers of CYP3A4 (e.g., phenytoin), may increase the clearance

such as can be seen with acetazolimide. Therefore during topiramate treatment, serum bicarbonate levels should be monitored at baseline and over the course of treatment. If a metabolic acidosis develops, of which parasthesias are a common sign, topiramate dose should probably be reduced or discontinued.

Baclofen

History of the Treatment

Baclofen is a potent and stereoselective $GABA_B$ agonist that has been used in clinical practice for the treatment of spasticity and is widely used as a muscle relaxant (99).

Pharmacology of the Medication/Treatment

In animal models, baclofen reduces the alcohol self-administration (100), suppresses acquisition and maintenance of alcohol drinking, relapse-like drinking, and the reinforcing, rewarding, stimulating, and motivational properties of alcohol in rodents (101).

Efficacy of the Medication/Treatment

In humans, 30 mg/day decreases alcohol withdrawal symptoms in alcohol-dependent patients in equivalence to that of diazepam (102). However, it is as yet unclear that baclofen when used in uncomplicated withdrawal has the same efficacy as benzodiazepines in reducing the incidence of seizures or delirium (103). In an open-label pilot study, Flannery and colleagues found significant reductions in drinks per drinking day and heavy-drinking days in alcohol-dependent subjects ($N = 13$) treated over 12 weeks with baclofen 10 mg three times daily with four sessions of motivational interviewing (104). In a 30-day double-blind RCT, Addolorato and colleagues compared 10 mg of baclofen three times daily with placebo in recently abstinent (12 to 24 hours) subjects ($N = 39$) with alcohol dependence and demonstrated significant increases in percentage total abstinence (70% vs. 21%; $P < 0.005$) and CAD (19.6 vs. 6.3 days; $P < 0.005$) (105). In addition, craving, as represented on the Obsessive Compulsive Drinking Scale, as well as on the individual obsessive and compulsive subscales, was significantly and increasingly reduced over the four weekly study timepoints by baclofen compared to placebo.

Safety of the Medication/Treatment

The common AEs associated with baclofen treatment were sleepiness, vertigo, nausea, and abdominal pain, all of which resolved in the first week of treatment. There were no serious AEs and baclofen did not appear to have abuse liability (105). No subjects in the baclofen group in the double-blind RCT discontinued medications as a result, none reported baclofen-induced euphoria, and none demonstrated withdrawal symptoms upon cessation of the study drug. So far, treatment with baclofen appears relatively safe, however, its abuse potential has not been well assessed and abrupt withdrawal has been linked to withdrawal-related delirium that appears not to be dose-related (106). The short-term efficacy of baclofen in the treatment of alcohol dependence is promising, but further controlled studies with larger numbers of subjects will be needed to make a compelling argument for its safety and appropriateness for general use.

Serotonergic Medications

Serotonin reuptake inhibitors (SRIs) have been demonstrated in animal studies to decrease the consumption of alcohol and enhance serotonergic function in the CNS, and they are used as antidepressants and anxiolytics in clinical treatment (37). Findings from RCTs of SRIs for the treatment of alcohol dependence are inconsistent and meta-analytic procedures on the data suggest that the best use of SRIs may be in treating major depression in patients with co-occurring alcohol dependence (107). One of the major issues with the efficacy of SRIs in the treatment of alcohol dependence appears to hinge on the discovery of a differential therapeutics based upon typology. Kranzler and colleagues found no significant reductions in drinking in an RCT comparing fluoxetine (up to 60 mg/day) to placebo in alcohol-dependent subjects receiving weekly cognitive behavioral therapy (CBT) ($N = 101$) who were not clinically depressed (108). However, discovery of true positive effects may be masked by the inclusion of non- or worse-responders in a clinical study. A secondary analysis of clinical trial data from the same study by alcohol subtype (Type A: earlier onset, more severity of dependence, and greater psychopathology or Type B: later onset, less severity of dependence, and less psychopathology) demonstrated that subjects with Type B alcohol dependence in the fluoxetine treatment group showed significantly worse drinking outcomes than those in the placebo group (109).

In another 14-week RCT of 200 mg sertraline in subjects with alcohol dependence stratified by Type A/B subtype ($N = 100$), the Type A subjects had fewer drinking days and had higher rates of complete abstinence when treated with sertraline compared to placebo (110). At 6 months follow-up after treatment with sertraline, the earlier results demonstrated by Kranzler and colleagues (109) of the negative impact of SRIs in Type B subjects, were extended: Type A alcoholic subjects maintained improved reductions in heavy drinking, whereas Type B alcoholic subjects demonstrated increased heavy drinking (111). In addition, the finding of adverse SRI effects in Type B alcoholics was also demonstrated by Chick and colleagues (112) in an RCT ($N = 493$) of fluvoxamine (up to 300 mg/day) that found in subjects with early onset alcohol problems, there was a higher relapse to heavy drinking than in placebo-treated subjects ($\leq$age 25). If early-onset, Type B alcoholics are demonstrated to have a higher ratio of impulsivity to cortical control than Type A alcoholics, then SRI's may work to worsen alcohol-related behaviors through reductions in harm-avoidance, which would push an already low balance between action and inhibition further toward action (113).

A different approach to modulating serotonergic function in the treatment of alcohol dependence was undertaken by

Johnson et al. (114) in comparing the efficacy of the 5-HT$_3$ receptor antagonist ondansetron (an antinausea medication) and placebo, in a 11-week, double-blind, RCT trial of subjects ($N = 271$) with either early- or late-onset alcohol dependence who also received adjunctive CBT. Although there was no significant effect in the overall subject cohort, subjects in the early-onset alcoholism group who received 1, 4, or 16 µg/kg ondansetron twice daily) showed significant reductions compared to placebo in self-reported drinking. Significant reductions in drinking compared with placebo were reported only in the early-onset alcoholism subset, findings that were corroborated by significant reductions in plasma carbohydrate-deficient transferrin. There were no significant differences in outcome with ondansetron or placebo in subjects with late-onset alcoholism. AE rates were similar for the both treatment groups, the most common for ondansetron and placebo, respectively, were headache (3.4% vs. 4.2%), constipation (5.0% vs. 1.4%), tachycardia (0.3% vs. 0%), and rash/pruritis (2.2% vs. 2.8%).

Taken together, these studies suggest that subtyping of patients with alcohol dependence may help resolve conflicting research findings on serotonergic treatment of alcohol dependence, and if validated, may support the use of SRIs and other serotonin-active agents in specially selected subpopulations of patients with alcohol dependence.

Directly Dopamine Active Medications

History of the Treatment

Data from preclinical research have illuminated the role of DA in the positively reinforcing and stimulant-like effects of alcohol, so a reasonable hypothesis is that by blocking DA, one may affect alcohol self-administration in animals, and perhaps drinking in humans. In rats, alcohol consumption induces release of DA from the NAc, the common reward system circuit implicated in the rewarding effects of all drugs of abuse (115). Mesostriatal DA activity is decreased in rodents by chronic alcohol administration (116). In persons with alcohol-dependence, DA and metabolites are decreased with chronic alcohol consumption, which is probably related to the dysphoria that they describe as a motivating factor in relapse (negative reinforcement) (117). As such, DA active medications might play a role in alcohol dependence by modulating hedonic tone.

When alcohol-dependent patients in human laboratory studies were pretreated with the antipsychotic medication haloperidol (a DA antagonist), it reduced craving and consumption of alcohol (118). Haloperidol also decreased the euphorigenic and stimulating effects of alcohol in social drinkers (119). Compared with heavy social drinkers given placebo before an alcohol challenge, those pretreated with 5 mg of the olanzapine (a DA antagonist) had a decreased urge to drink (120).

Whereas DA antagonists have held promise based upon reasonable, neurobiologically based hypotheses, preclinical research, and data from human laboratory studies, in randomized clinical trials for alcohol dependence the results have mostly been negative. In general, RCTs of both traditional and atypical antipsychotics have not demonstrated positive effects on craving or relapse in patients with alcohol dependence (120–123). However, one RCT of quetiapine 400 mg has demonstrated reductions in days of drinking and heavy drinking, but only in the subset of persons with Type B alcoholism (124).

CONCLUSIONS

Recently, the use of medications to treat alcohol dependence has received increased scrutiny due to its potential impact in improving drinking outcomes as well as enhancing the effectiveness of current behavioral treatment approaches. As our understanding of the underlying neurochemistry and neurobiology has progressed, medications have been developed that target specific neurotransmitter systems involved in the development and maintenance of alcohol dependence. Although there has been increasing progress in the differentiation of efficacious medicines for alcohol dependence, there are still many areas that need further development before we can claim to have constructed an appropriate differential therapeutics. As no pharmacologic intervention in alcohol dependence has yet been shown to have an effect on size warranting its use as a sole treatment, brief but well-rounded behavioral interventions, such as Medical Management (125,126) can add significant motivational support for adherence with pharmacologic treatment and engagement in other recovery-oriented activities (58). Alcohol-dependence medications given adjunctively with psychosocial treatment strategies improve drinking outcomes, yet adoption of these medical treatments in the broader addiction treatment community faces continuing obstacles such as lack of medical personnel, incompatible treatment philosophy, or clinical ignorance of efficacy (2). Pharmacologic interventions that target reductions in drinking without aiming for abstinence may have difficulty gaining clinical traction in the generally abstinence-oriented world of traditional alcoholism recovery programs.

Meta-analytic evidence from multiple clinical trials suggests that of the FDA-approved pharmacotherapies, acamprosate's strongest effects are in achieving and maintaining complete abstinence, while orally administered naltrexone's most robust effects are in decreasing heavy-drinking days. Given the recent finding of nonefficacy of acamprosate in US-based RCTs, and the subsequent analyses which have identified subgroups of responders even in those studies, further work is needed to better elucidate the best candidates for acamprosate treatment. Long-acting injectable naltrexone demonstrates a similar impact as oral naltrexone on heavy drinking, and offers further advantages over oral administration, including low dosing frequency, high intrinsic medication adherence, and reduced first-pass metabolism. These are the medications that should be used first-line. However, even though currently an off-label use of the medication in alcohol-dependent subjects, topiramate clearly fosters reductions in heavy-drinking days. Other medications have a less-robust evidence base, but there appears to be a signal based on age of onset for the effects of serotoninergic medications that warrants further study.

Whereas subacute and maintenance pharmacotherapeutic interventions have been a mainstay of treatment for chronic opioid dependence, it is as yet unclear whether medications are of benefit in the long-term treatment of chronic alcohol dependence. Similarly, other characteristics have yet to be clearly established, such as the optimal dosages and effectiveness of available pharmacotherapies in clinical settings, the optimal psychosocial interventions with each medication, and which subpopulations respond best to which medication.

It is hoped that pharmacotherapies for alcohol dependence may evolve into a more routine and widely used intervention as continuing evidence mounts demonstrating their effects in promoting abstinence and reducing in drinking behavior.

REFERENCES

1. McLellan AT, Carise D, Kleber HD. Can the national addiction treatment infrastructure support the public's demand for quality care? *J Subst Abuse Treat.* 2003;25(2):117–121.
2. Ducharme LJ, Knudsen HK, Roman PM. Trends in the adoption of medications for alcohol dependence. *J Clin Psychopharmacol.* 2006;26(suppl 1):S13–S19.
3. Hald J, Jacobsen E. A drug sensitizing the organism to ethyl alcohol. *Lancet.* 1948;2(6539):1001–1004.
4. Swift RM. Drug therapy for alcohol dependence. *N Engl J Med.* 1999;340:1482–1490.
5. Hughes JC, Cook CCH. The efficacy of disulfiram: a review of outcome studies. *Addiction.* 1997;92:381–395.
6. Fuller RK, Branchey L, Brightwell DR, et al. Disulfiram treatment of alcoholism. A veterans administration cooperative study. *J Am Med Assoc.* 1986;256:1449–1455.
7. Chick J, Gough K, Falkowski W, et al. Disulfiram treatment of alcoholism. *Br J Psychiatry.* 1992;161:84–89.
8. De Sousa A. An open randomized study comparing disulfiram and acamprosate in the treatment of alcohol dependence. *Alcohol Alcohol.* 2005;40:545–548.
9. Brewer C, Hardt F. Preventing disulfiram hepatitis in alcohol abusers: inappropriate guidelines and the significance of nickel allergy. *Addict Biol.* 1999;4:303–308.
10. Swift RM. Medications. In: Hester RK, Miller WR, eds. *Handbook of Alcoholism Treatment Approaches, Effective Alternatives.* Boston, MA: Pearson Education, Inc.; 2003:259–281.
11. Petrakis IL, Poling J, Levinson C, et al. VA New England VISN I MIRECC Study Group. Naltrexone and disulfiram in patients with alcohol dependence and comorbid psychiatric disorders. *Biol Psychiatry.* 2005;57:1128–1137.
12. Petrakis IL, Nich C, Ralevski E. Psychotic spectrum disorders and alcohol abuse: a review of pharmacotherapeutic strategies and a report on the effectiveness of naltrexone and disulfiram. *Schizophr Bull.* 2006;32:644–654. Epub 2006 Aug 3.
13. Petrakis IL, Poling J, Levinson C, et al. Naltrexone and disulfiram in patients with alcohol dependence and comorbid post-traumatic stress disorder. *Biol Psychiatry.* 2006;60:777–783.
14. Gerrein JR, Rosenberg CM, Manohar V. Disulfiram maintenance in outpatient treatment of alcoholism. *Arch Gen Psychiatry.* 1973; 28:798–802.
15. Brewer C, Streel E. Learning the language of abstinence in addiction treatment: some similarities between relapse-prevention with disulfiram, naltrexone, and other pharmacological antagonists and intensive "immersion" methods of foreign language teaching. *Subst Abus.* 2003;24:157–173.
16. O'Farrell TJ, Bayog RD. Antabuse contracts for married alcoholics and their spouses: a method to maintain antabuse ingestion and decrease conflict about drinking. *J Subst Abuse Treat.* 1986;3(1):1–8.
17. Powers MB, Vedel E, Emmelkamp PMG. Behavioral couples therapy (BCT) for alcohol and drug use disorders: a meta-analysis. *Clin Psychol Rev.* 2008;28:952–962.
18. Minozzi S, Amato L, Vecchi S, et al. Oral naltrexone maintenance treatment for opioid dependence. *Cochrane Database Syst Rev.* 2006;(1): Art. No.: CD001333. DOI: 10.1002/14651858. CD001333. pub2.
19. Gianoulakis C. Endogenous opioids and excessive alcohol consumption. *J Psychiatry Neurosci.* 1993;18:148–156.
20. Heimer L, Alheid GF. Piecing together the puzzle of basal forebrain anatomy. *Adv Exp Med Biol.* 1991;295:1–42.
21. Roberts AJ, McDonald JS, Heyser CJ, et al. mu-Opioid receptor knockout mice do not self-administer alcohol. *J Pharmacol Exp Ther.* 2000;293:1002–1008.
22. Gianoulakis C, Beliveau D, Angelogianni P, et al. Different pituitary beta-endorphin and adrenal cortisol response to ethanol in individuals with high and low risk for future development of alcoholism. *Life Sci.* 1989;45:1097–1099.
23. Gianoulakis C, Krishnan B, Thavundayil J. Enhanced sensitivity of pituitary beta-endorphin to ethanol in subjects at high risk of alcoholism. *Arch Gen Psychiatry.* 1996;53:250–257.
24. Gessa GL, Muntoni F, Collu M, et al. Low doses of ethanol activate dopaminergic neurons in the ventral tegmental area. *Brain Res.* 1985;348:201–203.
25. Benjamin D, Grant ER, Pohorecky LA. Naltrexone reverses ethanol-induced dopamine release in the nucleus accumbens in awake, freely moving rats. *Brain Res.* 1993;621:137–140.
26. Davidson D, Swift R, Fitz E. Naltrexone increases the latency to drink alcohol in social drinkers. *Alcohol Clin Exp Res.* 1996;20:732–739.
27. Monti PM, Rohsenow DJ, Hutchison KE, et al. Naltrexone's effect on cue-elicited craving among alcoholics in treatment. *Alcohol Clin Exp Res.* 1999;23:1386–1394.
28. Volpicelli JR, Alterman AI, Hayashida M, O'Brien CP. Naltrexone in the treatment of alcohol dependence. *Arch Gen Psychiatry.* 1992;49:876–880.
29. O'Malley SS, Jaffe AJ, Chang G, et al. Naltrexone and coping skills therapy for alcohol dependence. A controlled study. *Arch Gen Psychiatry.* 1992;49:881–887.
30. Volpicelli JR, Rhines KC, Rhines JS, et al. Naltrexone and alcohol dependence. Role of subject compliance. *Arch Gen Psychiatry.* 1997;54:737–742.
31. Kranzler HR, Modesto-Lowe V, Van Kirk J. Naltrexone vs. nefazodone for treatment of alcohol dependence. A placebo-controlled trial. *Neuropsychopharmacology.* 2000;22:493–503.
32. Krystal JH, Cramer JA, Krol WF, et al. Naltrexone in the treatment of alcohol dependence. *N Engl J Med.* 2001;345:1734–1739.
33. Bouza C, Angeles M, Munoz A, et al. Efficacy and safety of naltrexone and acamprosate in the treatment of alcohol dependence: a systematic review. *Addiction.* 2004;99:811–828.
34. Srisurapanont M, Jarusuraisin N. Naltrexone for the treatment of alcoholism: a meta-analysis of randomized controlled trials. *Int J Neuropsychopharmacol.* 2005;8:267–280.

35. Anton RF, O'Malley SS, Ciraulo DA, et al. Combined pharmacotherapies and behavioral interventions for alcohol dependence: the COMBINE study: a randomized controlled trial. *J Am Med Assoc.* 2006;295:2003–2017.
36. Croop RS, Faulkner EB, Labriola DF. The safety profile of naltrexone in the treatment of alcoholism. Results from a multicenter usage study. The Naltrexone Usage Study Group. *Arch Gen Psychiatry.* 1997;54:1130–1135.
37. Anton RF, Swift RM. Current pharmacotherapies of alcoholism: a U.S. perspective. *Am J Addict.* 2003;12(suppl 1):S53–S68.
38. Mason BJ. Rationale for combining acamprosate and naltrexone for treating alcohol dependence. *J Stud Alcohol Suppl.* 2005: Suppl 15:148–156; discussion 140.
39. Ray LA, Hutchison KE. A polymorphism of the mu-opioid receptor gene (OPRM1) and sensitivity to the effects of alcohol in humans. *Alcohol Clin Exp Res.* 2004;28:1789–1795.
40. Ray LA, Hutchison KE. Effects of naltrexone on alcohol sensitivity and genetic moderators of medication response: a double-blind placebo-controlled study. *Arch Gen Psychiatry.* 2007;64: 1069–1077.
41. Oslin DW, Berrettini W, Kranzler HR, et al. A functional polymorphism of the mu-opioid receptor gene is associated with naltrexone response in alcohol-dependent patients. *Neuropsychopharmacology.* 2003;28:1546–1552.
42. Gelernter J, Gueorguieva R, Kranzler HR, et al. Opioid receptor gene (OPRM1, OPRK1, and OPRD1) variants and response to naltrexone treatment for alcohol dependence: results from the VA Cooperative Study. *Alcohol Clin Exp Res.* 2007;31:555–563.
43. Anton RF, Oroszi G, O'Malley S, et al. An evaluation of mu-opioid receptor (OPRM1) as a predictor of naltrexone response in the treatment of alcohol dependence: results from the Combined Pharmacotherapies and Behavioral Interventions for Alcohol Dependence (COMBINE) study. *Arch Gen Psychiatry.* 2008;65:135–144.
44. Oroszi G, Anton RF, O'Malley S, et al. OPRM1 Asn40Asp predicts response to naltrexone treatment: a haplotype-based approach. *Alcohol Clin Exp Res.* 2009;33(3):383–393. Epub 2008 Nov 25.
45. Mitchell JM, Fields HL, White RL, et al. The Asp40 mu-opioid receptor allele does not predict naltrexone treatment efficacy in heavy drinkers. *J Clin Psychopharmacol.* 2007;27:112–115.
46. Arias A, Feinn R, Kranzler HR. Association of an Asn40Asp (A118G) polymorphism in the μ-opioid receptor gene with substance dependence: a meta-analysis. *Drug Alcohol Depend.* 2006; 83:262–268.
47. Ray LA, Oslin DW. Naltrexone for the treatment of alcohol dependence among African Americans: results from the COMBINE Study. *Drug Alcohol Depend.* 2009;105:256–258. Epub 2009 Aug 29.
48. Petrakis IL, O'Malley S, Rounsaville B, et al. Naltrexone augmentation of neuroleptic treatment in alcohol abusing patients with schizophrenia. [Published erratum in *Psychopharmacology (Berl).* 174(2):300.] *Psychopharmacology (Berl).* 2004;172:291–297.
49. Petrakis IL, Nich C, Ralevski E. Psychotic spectrum disorders and alcohol abuse: a review of pharmacotherapeutic strategies and a report on the effectiveness of naltrexone and disulfiram. *Schizophr Bull.* 2006;32:644–654.
50. Garbutt JC, Kranzler HR, O'Malley SS, et al. Efficacy and tolerability of long-acting injectable naltrexone for alcohol dependence: a randomized controlled trial. *J Am Med Assoc.* 2005;293: 1617–1625.
51. Johnson BA, Ait-Daoud N, Aubin HJ, et al. A pilot evaluation of the safety and tolerability of repeat dose administration of long-acting injectable naltrexone (Vivitrex) in patients with alcohol dependence. *Alcohol Clin Exp Res.* 2004;28:1356–1361.
52. Rosenthal RN. Out of the pipeline. Intramuscular naltrexone. Targeting adherence in alcohol dependency treatment. *Curr Psychiatry.* 2006;5:106–113.
53. Kranzler HR, Wesson DR, Billot L. Naltrexone depot for treatment of alcohol dependence: a multicenter, randomized, placebo-controlled clinical trial. *Alcohol Clin Exp Res.* 2004;28: 1051–1059.
54. O'Malley SS, Garbutt JC, Gastfriend DR, et al. Efficacy of extended-release naltrexone in alcohol-dependent patients who are abstinent before treatment. *J Clin Psychopharmacol.* 2007;27: 507–512.
55. Gastfriend DR, Dong Q, Loewy J, et al. *Durability of effect of long-acting injectable naltrexone.* Paper presented at: The American Psychiatric Association Institute; October 5–9, 2005; San Diego, CA.
56. Pettinati HM, Gastfriend DR, Dong Q, et al. Effect of extended-release naltrexone (XR-NTX) on quality of life in alcohol-dependent patients. *Alcohol Clin Exp Res.* 2009;33:350–356. Epub 2008 Nov 25.
57. Turncliff RZ, Dunbar JL, Dong Q, et al. Pharmacokinetics of long-acting naltrexone in subjects with mild to moderate hepatic impairment. *J Clin Pharmacol.* 2005;45:1259–1267.
58. Rosenthal RN, Ries RK. Medical Management techniques: integrating brief behavioral with pharmacological interventions in addiction treatment. In: Ries R, Fiellin D, Miller S, Saitz R, eds. *Principles of Addiction Medicine.* 4th ed. Philadelphia, PA: Lippincott, Williams & Wilkins, 2009:899–908.
59. Molander A, Söderpalm B. Glycine receptors regulate dopamine release in the rat nucleus accumbens. *Alcohol Clin Exp Res.* 2005a;29:17–26.
60. Molander A, Söderpalm B. Accumbal strychnine-sensitive glycine receptors: an access point for ethanol to the brain reward system. *Alcohol Clin Exp Res.* 2005b;29:27–37.
61. Chau P, Höifödt-Lidö H, Löf E, et al. Glycine receptors in the nucleus accumbens involved in the ethanol intake-reducing effect of acamprosate. *Alcohol Clin Exp Res.* 2010;34:39–45.
62. Chau P, Stomberg R, Fagerberg A, et al. Glycine receptors involved in acamprosate's modulation of accumbal dopamine levels: an in vivo microdialysis study. *Alcohol Clin Exp Res.* 2010;34:32–38.
63. De Witte P. Imbalance between neuroexcitatory and neuroinhibitory amino acids causes craving for ethanol. *Addict Behav.* 2004;29:1325–1339.
64. Kumari M, Ticku MK. Regulation of NMDA receptors by ethanol. *Prog Drug Res.* 2000;54:152–189.
65. Hoffman PL. NMDA receptors in alcoholism. *Int Rev Neurobiol.* 2003;56:35–82.
66. Naassila M, Hammoumi S, Legrand E, et al. Mechanism of action of acamprosate. Part, I characterization of spermidine-sensitive acamprosate binding site in rat brain. *Alcohol Clin Exp Res.* 1998;22:802–809.
67. al Qatari M, Bouchenafa O, Littleton J. Mechanism of action of acamprosate. Part II. Ethanol dependence modifies effects of acamprosate on NMDA receptor binding in membranes from rat cerebral cortex. *Alcohol Clin Exp Res.* 1998;22:810–814.
68. Harris BR, Prendergast MA, Gibson DA, et al. Acamprosate inhibits the binding and neurotoxic effects of trans-ACPD, suggesting a novel site of action at metabotropic glutamate receptors. *Alcohol Clin Exp Res.* 2002;26:1779–1793.
69. Harris BR, Gibson DA, Prendergast MA, et al. The neurotoxicity induced by ethanol withdrawal in mature organotypic hippocampal slices might involve cross-talk between metabotropic

glutamate type 5 receptors and *N*-methyl-D-aspartate receptors. *Alcohol Clin Exp Res.* 2003;27:1724–1735.

70. Heilig M, Egli M. Pharmacological treatment of alcohol dependence: target symptoms and target mechanisms. *Pharmacol Ther.* 2006;111:855–876.

71. Pelc I, Verbanck P, Le Bon O, et al. Efficacy and safety of acamprosate in the treatment of detoxified alcohol-dependent patients. A 90-day placebo-controlled dose-finding study. *Br J Psychiatry.* 1997;171:73–77.

72. Sass H, Soyka M, Mann K, et al. Relapse prevention by acamprosate. Results from a placebo-controlled study on alcohol dependence. *Arch Gen Psychiatry.* 1996;53:673–680.

73. Paille FM, Guelfi JD, Perkins AC, et al. . Double-blind randomized multicentre trial of acamprosate in maintaining abstinence from alcohol. *Alcohol Alcohol.* 1995;30:239–247.

74. Gage A, Chabac S, Goodman A. Acamprosate is effective for the treatment of alcohol dependence: reanalysis of three pivotal studies (abstract). *Alcohol Clin Exp Res.* 2005;29:161A.

75. Schneider E, Saikali K, Zhang D, et al. *Efficacy of acamprosate in regaining abstinence in alcohol-dependent patients who relapse (abstract).* Paper presented at: The Academy of Addiction Psychiatry 16th Annual Meeting and Symposium; 2005; Scottsdale, AZ.

76. Mason BJ, Goodman A, Chabac S, et al. Effect of oral acamprosate on abstinence in patients with alcohol dependence in a double-blind, placebo-controlled trial: the role of patient motivation. *J Psychiatric Res.* 2006;40:383–393.

77. Gual A, Lehert P. Acamprosate during and after acute alcohol withdrawal: a double-blind placebo-controlled study in Spain. *Alcohol Alcohol.* 2001;36:413–418.

78. Chick J, Lehert P, Landron F. Does acamprosate improve reduction of drinking as well as aiding abstinence? *J Psychopharmacol.* 2003;17:397–402.

79. Mann K, Lehert P, Morgan MY. The efficacy of acamprosate in the maintenance of abstinence in alcohol-dependent individuals: results of a meta-analysis. *Alcohol Clin Exp Res.* 2004;28:51–63.

80. Saivin S, Hulot T, Chabac S, et al. Clinical pharmacokinetics of acamprosate. *Clin Pharmacokinet.* 1998;35:331–345.

81. Wilde MI, Wagstaff AJ. Acamprosate. A review of its pharmacology and clinical potential in the management of alcohol dependence after detoxification. *Drugs.* 1997;53:1038–1053.

82. Acamprosate. *Drugs R D.* 2002;3:13–18.

83. Rosenthal RN, Gage A, Perhach JL, et al. Acamprosate: safety and tolerability in the treatment of alcohol dependence. *J Addict Med.* 2008;2:40–50.

84. Kiefer F, Jahn H, Tarnaske T, et al. Comparing and combining naltrexone and acamprosate in relapse prevention of alcoholism: a double-blind, placebo-controlled study. *Arch Gen Psychiatry.* 2003;60:92–99.

85. Feeney GF, Connor JP, Young RM, et al. Combined acamprosate and naltrexone, with cognitive behavioural therapy is superior to either medication alone for alcohol abstinence: a single centres' experience with pharmacotherapy. *Alcohol Alcohol.* 2006;41: 321–327.

86. Kranzler HR. Evidence-based treatments for alcohol dependence: new results and new questions. *J Am Med Assoc.* 2006;295: 2075–2076.

87. Brady KT, Myrick H, Henderson S, et al. The use of divalproex in alcohol relapse prevention: a pilot study. *Drug Alcohol Depend.* 2002;67:323–330.

88. Mueller TI, Stout RL, Rudden S, et al. A double-blind, placebo-controlled pilot study of carbamazepine for the treatment of alcohol dependence. *Alcohol Clin Exp Res.* 1997;21:86–92.

89. White HS, Brown SD, Woodhead JH, et al. Topiramate modulates GABA-evoked currents in murine cortical neurons by a nonbenzodiazepine mechanism. *Epilepsia.* 2000;41(suppl 1): S17–S20.

90. Johnson BA. Recent advances in the development of treatments for alcohol and cocaine dependence: focus on topiramate and other modulators of GABA or glutamate function. *CNS Drugs.* 2005;19(10):873–896.

91. Johnson BA, Ait-Daoud N, Bowden CL, et al. Oral topiramate for treatment of alcohol dependence: a randomised controlled trial. *Lancet.* 2003;361:1677–1685.

92. Johnson BA, Rosenthal N, Capece JA, et al. Topiramate for treating alcohol dependence. A randomized controlled trial. *J Am Med Assoc.* 2007;298:1641–1651.

93. Johnson BA, Rosenthal N, Capece JA, et al. Topiramate improves the physical health and quality of life of alcohol-dependent individuals: the US multi-site randomized controlled trial. *Arch Intern Med.* 2008;168(11):1188–1199.

94. Baltieri DA, Daró FR, Ribeiro PL, et al. Comparing topiramate with naltrexone in the treatment of alcohol dependence. *Addiction.* 2008;103(12):2035–2044. Epub 2008 Oct 8.

95. Topamax [package insert]. Raritan, NJ: Ortho-McNeil Pharmaceutical, Inc.; Revised April 2008.

96. Johnson BA, Ait-Daoud N, Akhtar FZ, et al. Oral topiramate reduces the consequences of drinking and improves the quality of life of alcohol-dependent individuals: a randomized controlled trial. *Arch Gen Psychiatry.* 2004;61:905–912.

97. Ray LA, Miranda R Jr, MacKillop J, et al. A preliminary pharmacogenetic investigation of adverse events from topiramate in heavy drinkers. *Exp Clin Psychopharmacol.* 2009;17(2):122–129.

98. Kenna GA, Lomastro TL, Schiesl A, et al. Review of topiramate: an antiepileptic for the treatment of alcohol dependence. *Curr Drug Abuse Rev.* 2009;2135–2142.

99. Davidoff RA. Antispasticity drugs: mechanisms of action. *Ann Neurol.* 1985;17(2):107–116.

100. Cousins MS, Roberts DC, de Wit H. GABA(B) receptor agonists for the treatment of drug addiction: a review of recent findings. *Drug Alcohol Depend.* 2002;65(3):209–220.

101. Maccioni P, Colombo G. Role of the GABA(B) receptor in alcohol-seeking and drinking behavior. *Alcohol.* 2009;43(7): 555–558.

102. Addolorato G, Leggio L, Abenavoli L, et al. Baclofen in the treatment of alcohol withdrawal syndrome: a comparative study vs diazepam, *Am J Med.* 2006;119(3):276.e13–276.e18.

103. Mayo-Smith MF. Pharmacological management of alcohol withdrawal: a meta-analysis and evidence-based practice guideline: American Society of Addiction Medicine Working Group on Pharmacological Management of Alcohol Withdrawal. *J Am Med Assoc.* 1997;278:144–151.

104. Flannery BA, Garbutt JC, Cody MW, et al. Baclofen for alcohol dependence: a preliminary open-label study. *Alcohol Clin Exp Res.* 2004;28(10):1517–1523.

105. Addolorato G, Caputo F, Capristo E, et al. Baclofen efficacy in reducing alcohol craving and intake: a preliminary double-blind randomized controlled study. *Alcohol Alcohol.* 2002;37(5): 504–508.

106. Leo RJ, Baer D. Delirium associated with baclofen withdrawal: a review of common presentations and management strategies. *Psychosomatics.* 2005;46:503–507.

107. Nunes EV, Levin FR. Treatment of depression in patients with alcohol or other drug dependence: a meta-analysis. *J Am Med Assoc.* 2004;291:1887–1896.

108. Kranzler HR, Burleson JA, Korner P, et al. Placebo-controlled trial of fluoxetine as an adjunct to relapse prevention in alcoholics. *Am J Psychiatry*. 1995;152:391–397.
109. Kranzler HR, Burleson JA, Brown J, et al. Fluoxetine treatment seems to reduce the beneficial effects of cognitive-behavioral therapy in type B alcoholics. *Alcohol Clin Exp Res*. 1996;20:1534–1541.
110. Pettinati HM, Volpicelli JR, Kranzler HR, et al. Sertraline treatment for alcohol dependence: interactive effects of medication and alcoholic subtype. *Alcohol Clin Exp Res*. 2000;24:1041–1049.
111. Dundon W, Lynch KG, Pettinati HM, et al. Treatment outcomes in type A and B alcohol dependence 6 months after serotonergic pharmacotherapy. *Alcohol Clin Exp Res*. 2004;28:1065–1073.
112. Chick J, Aschauer H, Hornik K. Efficacy of fluvoxamine in preventing relapse in alcohol dependence: a one-year, double-blind, placebo-controlled multicentre study with analysis by typology. *Drug Alcohol Depend*. 2004;74:61–70.
113. Hellerstein DJ, Kocsis JH, Chapman D, et al. Double-blind comparison of sertraline, imipramine, and placebo in the treatment of dysthymia: effects on personality. *Am J Psychiatry*. 2000;157(9):1436–1444.
114. Johnson BA, Roache JD, Javors MA, et al. Ondansetron for reduction of drinking among biologically predisposed alcoholic patients: a randomized controlled trial. *J Am Med Assoc*. 2000;284:963–971.
115. Di Chiara G, Imperato A. Ethanol preferentially stimulates dopamine release in the nucleus accumbens of freely moving rats. *Eur J Pharmacol*. 1985;115:131–132.
116. Diana M, Pistis M, Muntoni A, et al. Mesolimbic dopaminergic reduction outlasts ethanol withdrawal syndrome: evidence of protracted abstinence. *Neuroscience*. 1996;71:411–415.
117. Fulton MK, Kramer G, Moeller FG, et al. Low plasma homovanillic acid levels in recently abstinent alcoholic men. *Am J Psychiatry*. 1995;152:1819–1820.
118. Modell JG, Mountz JM, Glaser FB, et al. Effect of haloperidol on measures of craving and impaired control in alcoholic subjects. *Alcohol Clin Exp Res*. 1993;17:234–240.
119. Enggasser JL, de Wit H. Haloperidol reduces stimulant and reinforcing effects of ethanol in social drinkers. *Alcohol Clin Exp Res*. 2001;25:1448–1456.
120. Hutchison KE, Swift R, Rohsenow DJ, et al. Olanzapine reduces urge to drink after drinking cues and a priming dose of alcohol. *Psychopharmacology (Berl)*. 2001;155:27–34.
121. Guardia J, Segura L, Gonzalvo B, et al. A double-blind, placebo-controlled study of olanzapine in the treatment of alcohol-dependence disorder. *Alcohol Clin Exp Res*. 2004;28:736–745.
122. Marra D, Warot D, Berlin I, et al. Amisulpride does not prevent relapse in primary alcohol dependence: results of a pilot randomized, placebo controlled trial. *Alcohol Clin Exp Res*. 2002;26:1545–1552.
123. Wiesbeck GA, Weijers HG, Lesch OM, et al. Flupenthixol decanoate and relapse prevention in alcoholics: results from a placebo-controlled study. *Alcohol Alcohol*. 2001;36:329–334.
124. Kampman KM, Pettinati HM, Lynch KG, et al. A double-blind, placebo-controlled pilot trial of quetiapine for the treatment of Type A and Type B alcoholism. *J Clin Psychopharmacol*. 2007;27:344–351.
125. Pettinati HM, Weiss RD, Dundon W, et al. A structured approach to medical management: a psychosocial intervention to support pharmacotherapy in the treatment of alcohol dependence. *J Stud Alcohol Suppl*. 2005;(15):170–178; discussion 168–169.
126. Pettinati HM, Weiss RD, Dundon W, et al. *COMBINE Monograph Series, Volume 2. Medical Management Treatment Manual: A Clinical Research Guide for Medically Trained Clinicians Providing Pharmacotherapy as Part of the Treatment for Alcohol Dependence*. DHHS Publication No. (NIH) 04–5289. Bethesda, MD: NIAAA, 2004.
127. Rosenthal RN. Current and future drug therapies for alcohol dependence. *J Clin Psychopharmacol*. 2006;26(suppl 1):S20–S29.

CHAPTER 34

Alternative Pharmacotherapies for Opioid Addiction

Paul J. Fudala ■ Rolley E. Johnson

The development of methadone maintenance by Dole and Nyswander in the mid-1960s (1) ushered in the modern era of pharmacologic treatment for opioid dependence. Previously, except for a brief period of legalized opioid maintenance in several cities of the United States in the early 1900s, abrupt discontinuation of opioids or substitution of decreasing doses of methadone or shorter-acting legally prescribed opioids for patients' drugs of choice were used to "detoxify" opioid-dependent individuals. However, medically supervised withdrawal ("detox") alone is a generally unsuccessful treatment for opioid dependence because relapse typically occurs shortly after an individual completes a course of treatment. Medication-assisted therapy (i.e., opioid replacement therapy) in contrast, however, can enable patients to reduce or stop use of illicit opioids and to stabilize their lives. Still, many opioid-dependent individuals require recurrent or extended courses of treatment.

Since their introduction and approval, mu-opioid agonists such as methadone and the mu-opioid partial agonist buprenorphine have provided treatment options to millions of opioid-dependent individuals worldwide. The mu-opioid agonist methadyl acetate (LAAM) and the opioid antagonist naltrexone have provided for additional treatment options, though with much less of an impact than the former two medications. Efforts to develop new opioid-dependence treatment medications have focused on providing additional alternatives or formulations for those patients who cannot tolerate, do not respond to, or prefer not to take currently available medications. The development of treatment options with less abuse potential, abusability, likelihood for diversion, and risk for unintentional exposure has also been a strong consideration.

Interrupting the powerfully reinforcing effects of opioids and drug-seeking behavior requires a concerted effort by physicians, therapists, and other clinical personnel, as well as by the patients themselves and their families. This is particularly true once an addiction is established as a chronic condition, and will often require multiple interventions. Other chapters in this volume are specifically devoted to a discussion of methadone, buprenorphine, and naltrexone as opioid-dependence treatment agents. This chapter reviews the literature on additional pharmacotherapies which are or have been utilized, as well as some which are actively being investigated for opioid-dependence treatment. These include the opioid agonists LAAM, codeine, dihydrocodeine, morphine, and heroin, and also the nonopioid medications clonidine and lofexidine. Medications that have been assessed for opioid-dependence treatment but for which only very limited data are available (e.g., gabapentin, venlafaxine, topiramate, AV411) will not be considered here.

NONOPIOID TREATMENT ALTERNATIVES: CLONIDINE AND LOFEXIDINE

The acute opioid-withdrawal syndrome is a time-limited phenomenon, generally of brief duration. Following the abrupt termination of short-acting opioids such as heroin, morphine, or hydromorphone, withdrawal signs and symptoms usually subside by the second or third opioid-free day. Although the opioid-withdrawal syndrome can be extremely uncomfortable for the opioid-dependent individual, in contrast to the syndrome associated with the withdrawal of certain other drugs such as benzodiazepines and alcohol, it does not ordinarily pose a medical risk to the individual. The exception may be, however, in patients already severely compromised where dehydration secondary to vomiting, diarrhea, and sweating could be a significant factor in precipitating a medical crisis. Thus, there is a particular appeal for treating this syndrome symptomatically, especially with medications that do not themselves produce physical dependence. It must be recognized, however, that medically supervised withdrawal from opioids is only one of the initial steps in the treatment process of rehabilitating opioid-dependent individuals if complete and permanent abstinence is the treatment goal.

Clonidine is an α_2-adrenergic agonist that has been used for the treatment of various disorders including hypertension, autism, attention-deficit hyperactivity disorder, and various types of pain. Clonidine has been shown to be useful in the medically supervised withdrawal of patients from methadone, heroin, and other opioids, as well as preparing individuals for stabilization onto the opioid antagonist naltrexone.

The capacity of clonidine to ameliorate withdrawal-associated effects (e.g., lacrimation and rhinorrhea) is linked to its modulation of noradrenergic hyperactivity in the locus ceruleus (2,3). Additionally, clonidine may affect central serotonergic (4), cholinergic (5), and purinergic systems (6). It seems to be most effective in suppressing certain opioid-withdrawal signs and symptoms, such as restlessness and diaphoresis. However, clonidine is not well accepted by the addicted patient because it does not produce morphine-like subjective effects or relieve certain types of withdrawal distress, such as anxiety. Sedation and hypotension also limit its utility. No fixed-dosing guidelines are currently available and dosages are generally individualized to each patient based on therapeutic response and side-effect limitations.

Interestingly, clonidine abuse by users of illicit opioids and other drugs has been reported since the early 1980s (7). This abuse may be secondary to a desire to obtain various drug-related effects, such as sedation, euphoria, or hallucinations. Clonidine may also be used to prolong and enhance the effects of heroin or other opioids (8,9). One report described the intentional ingestion of clonidine patches by individuals on a chemical dependency unit who may have done so to obtain psychoactive effects or to alleviate opioid-withdrawal symptoms (10).

Secondary to an effort to identify an agent with less sedating and hypotensive effects than clonidine, a number of other α_2-adrenergic agonists (lofexidine, guanabenz, guanfacine) have been evaluated for their ability to moderate the opioid-withdrawal syndrome. Of these, lofexidine, a clonidine analogue licensed in the United Kingdom for opioid medical withdrawal treatment, has been the subject of much clinical evaluation. Lofexidine is being studied in the United States and enjoys widespread usage in the United Kingdom as the only α_2-adrenergic agonist approved there to relieve symptoms in patients undergoing withdrawal from opioids (11). Lofexidine is suggested to be used typically for a period of 7 to 10 days at maximal single doses of 0.8 mg, usually taken three times per day, in dosages ranging up to 2.4 mg/day (12).

Studies conducted in the early 1980s provided initial data indicating that lofexidine could be effective in suppressing some of the signs and symptoms of opioid withdrawal (13–15). More recent trials have provided further evidence for the efficacy of lofexidine. These trials included both open-label and double-blind evaluations, using both inpatient and outpatient populations.

When compared to methadone for the treatment of opioid-withdrawal signs and symptoms in polydrug-abusing opioid-dependent individuals, lofexidine treatment was associated with more severe symptomatology at various time points on and before the 10th (last) day of treatment, but both groups were observed to have a similar course of symptom decline thereafter (16). Both groups also showed similar rates of medical withdrawal treatment completion. In a subsequent open-label study by the same research group (17), the authors found that a 5-day lofexidine treatment regimen may attenuate opioid-withdrawal symptoms more rapidly than a 10-day lofexidine- or methadone-treatment schedule without exacerbating hypotensive side effects.

The combination of lofexidine and methadone has previously been associated with significant hypotension, sedation, and cognitive deficits compared to methadone alone (18). Most recently, the coadministration of lofexidine and methadone was found to induce QTc interval prolongation (19). Study subjects were stabilized on a targeted methadone maintenance dosage of 80 mg/day. After stabilization, subjects received lofexidine initially at a dose of 0.4 mg/day, eventually escalated to 1.6 mg/day. When maximal ECG responses were considered, statistically significant changes in heart rate (decrease), and PR, QRS, and QTc intervals (increase) were observed with the methadone/lofexidine combination compared to methadone alone. These results were secondary findings from a pilot dose-escalation study evaluating the safety of methadone and lofexidine coadministration referenced above (18).

When lofexidine was compared to clonidine, both treatments were generally found to produce similar therapeutic effects, but lofexidine typically was better tolerated. When lofexidine was compared to clonidine in an outpatient, double-blind trial, both medications produced positive treatment outcomes, but clonidine was associated with more hypotensive effects and required more home visits by medical staff (20). In a double-blind, inpatient study, lofexidine and clonidine were reported to be equally effective in treating the withdrawal syndrome. Clonidine, however, was associated with more hypotension and better treatment retention than was noted for lofexidine (21). In another double-blind, inpatient study using methadone-stabilized opioid-dependent individuals, both lofexidine and clonidine produced a similar suppression of withdrawal symptoms, but lofexidine was associated with less hypotension and fewer adverse events (22).

In an inpatient human laboratory study, oral pretreatment with placebo, lofexidine (0.4, 0.8, and 1.6 mg), and clonidine (0.1 and 0.2 mg) were compared in individuals maintained on 30 mg of methadone who received intramuscular naloxone doses of 0, 0.1, or 0.3 mg (a total of 18 separate experimental sessions). Both lofexidine and clonidine produced dose-related decreases in blood pressure and heart rate, but neither medication mitigated the subject-reported discomfort of precipitated opioid-withdrawal nor autonomic signs of withdrawal (23).

Additional studies using diverse paradigms have also supported the therapeutic effectiveness of lofexidine. For example, a naltrexone–lofexidine combination was associated with a more rapid resolution of the opioid-withdrawal syndrome than was a 7-day lofexidine-only treatment schedule, without substantial increases in withdrawal symptoms or hypotensive side-effects (24). When used in a 3-day opioid medical withdrawal procedure with adjunct medications (oxazepam, baclofen, ketoprofen, naloxone, and naltrexone), lofexidine-treated individuals showed significantly lower levels of withdrawal symptoms and fewer mood problems, as well as less sedation and hypotension (25).

When lofexidine was compared to buprenorphine in an open-label study, patients receiving buprenorphine reportedly had less-severe withdrawal symptoms and were more likely to complete medical withdrawal treatment (26). In another open-label evaluation, a noninferiority approach was utilized to compare buprenorphine to lofexidine in 210 randomized individuals undergoing medically supervised withdrawal from heroin. Sixty-five percent of those on buprenorphine and 46% of those on lofexidine completed medical withdrawal, with 46% in the buprenorphine and

36% in the lofexidine group reporting abstinence at 1 month. Interestingly, results from 271 individuals who declined randomization and chose their treatment instead were similar to those obtained from the randomized groups of individuals (27).

Twelve randomized controlled trials comparing buprenorphine to clonidine or lofexidine for modifying the signs and symptoms of opioid dependence in individuals who were primarily opioid dependent were reviewed (28). Findings indicated that buprenorphine was more effective than either clonidine or lofexidine in treating opioid withdrawal as evidenced by reduction in symptoms of opioid withdrawal, and by patients remaining in and completing medical withdrawal treatment.

LAAM: AN OPIOID AGONIST ALTERNATIVE TO METHADONE

LAAM is a derivative of methadone, and similar to methadone, is a synthetic mu-opioid agonist. LAAM was initially developed in the late 1940s by chemists in Germany seeking an analgesic substitute for morphine. The opioid effects produced by LAAM and its active metabolites, along with the potential for administering the parent drug on alternate days or on a three-times-weekly schedule (thus eliminating the need for "take-home" doses), fostered interest in its potential use as an alternative to methadone. For example, a single take-home dose of methadone can eliminate only one clinic visit per week, as methadone must be administered daily. However, a single take-home dose of LAAM could obviate the need for five clinic visits per week, as patients could receive in-clinic doses on Mondays and Wednesdays and a single take-home dose on Fridays.

While it was noted early in the development of LAAM that it could alleviate the signs and symptoms of opioid withdrawal following the termination of morphine administration, it was also observed that giving LAAM on a daily basis could lead to signs indicative of opioid toxicity, such as severe nausea and vomiting and respiratory depression. LAAM had also been shown to produce effects that were qualitatively similar to morphine and methadone. LAAM is converted to two pharmacologically active compounds by N-demethylation (*nor*-LAAM and *dinor*-LAAM) in addition to inactive compounds (29–31). The long half-lives of the *nor*-LAAM and *dinor*-LAAM metabolites, 48 and 96 hours, respectively, contribute to the extended duration of activity of LAAM (32).

Numerous studies (33,34) provided evidence for the effectiveness of LAAM as an opioid-dependence treatment agent, and LAAM was approved in the United States in 1993 for the management of opioid dependence. Most of these investigations, whether conducted prior to or following LAAM's approval in the United States, compared LAAM to methadone, since the latter is considered the standard for opioid-dependence treatment. Outcome measures most often assessed in these studies included the amount of time individuals remained in treatment, patients' illicit use of opioids and other drugs during the course of treatment, various elements related to individuals' social functioning (such as employment history and interactions with legal system), and general medical and psychiatric parameters, including adverse events potentially related to the treatment medication.

A number of factors limited the widespread use of LAAM, including regulatory issues, clinic-staff resistance, and the reluctance by practitioners to consider LAAM as a viable alternative to methadone (35). Most importantly, however, LAAM has been associated with serious cardiac adverse events, including *torsade de pointes* (36,37). Roxane Laboratories, which marketed LAAM, indicated in 2003 that it would no longer make LAAM available for clinical use. Although LAAM is still approved for use by the FDA, it is no longer approved for use in Europe.

OTHER OPIOID AGONISTS: MORPHINE, CODEINE, AND DIHYDROCODEINE

In addition to LAAM discussed above, other opioid agonists including codeine, dihydrocodeine, and morphine have been evaluated for the maintenance treatment of opioid dependence and medically supervised opioid withdrawal. Compared to methadone and buprenorphine, these medications have shorter durations of actions (although sustained-release formulations have been assessed and are used clinically), and may thus be less suitable as maintenance medications. Factors that need to be considered when assessing the viability of these potential treatment agents are cost; medical safety; abusability, abuse liability, and potential for diversion; ease of use; and patient acceptability, among others. None of these medications are approved for the treatment of opioid dependence in the United States. However, it has recently been reported that dihydrocodeine is the second most commonly prescribed opioid-dependence treatment medication (following methadone) by general practitioners in the United Kingdom (38).

In a retrospective investigation from Germany, medical withdrawal treatment outcome differences were assessed in codeine-substituted patients, methadone-substituted patients, and patients injecting heroin illicitly. The treatment regimen utilized methadone in a tapering dosage, and was independent of the opioid substance that patients were using (39). Methadone-substituted (50.4%) and codeine-substituted (45.5%) patients finished medical withdrawal treatment significantly more often than heroin-dependent patients (35.9%).

An open-label study of dihydrocodeine conducted in the United Kingdom assessed dihydrocodeine for the medical withdrawal of methadone-maintained patients (40). All patients initially had their methadone dosages reduced to 10 to 30 mg/day. Dihydrocodeine was then substituted for methadone, initially from 240 mg/day in four divided doses upwards to 600 mg/day over 7 days and then down to 60 mg/day over the next 7 days. Thirteen individuals successfully completed the program, with three of those beginning treatment with naltrexone. One individual relapsed to heroin use, and six dropped out of the program between days 3 and 11 during the dihydrocodeine treatment phase.

In a 3-year follow-up study in Germany, 199 individuals from a random sample of 297 individuals receiving codeine or dihydrocodeine maintenance treatment for opioid dependence were followed-up with regards to measures such as health, employment, criminal activity, and other outcome assessments (41). Out of the original sample of 297, 65% were still in treatment after 3 years. Over the 3-year period, 4% of the sample (12 patients) had died; 5 of the 12 were drug-related and 5 were AIDS-related. Generally, it was observed that there was improvement in their general physical condition, as well as medical and mental health. There was also a decreasing trend in criminal activity based on measures of conflicts with police, convictions, and imprisonment.

More recently, dihydrocodeine has been compared to buprenorphine and methadone with regards to addiction treatment efficacy (42). In what the authors described as the first likely randomized controlled trial of opioid dependence treatment involving dihydrocodeine, 235 patients were recruited for study participation, with 218 ultimately attending the initial treatment. In this open-label design, 110 patients were randomized to receive methadone and 108 to receive dihydrocodeine. There was no statistically significant difference between the groups for retention in treatment at follow-up, the primary outcome measure, when assessed at 6, 12, or 18 months. At 18 months, 88% of the dihydrocodeine patients remained in treatment compared to 77% on methadone. It was recommended, although not required, that patients remain with their assigned treatment for the duration of the study, or for as long as methadone or dihydrocodeine prescribing continued. Eighteen of the patients that had been randomized to receive dihydrocodeine changed to methadone; three changed from methadone to dihydrocodeine. The authors noted that the change from dihydrocodeine to methadone (which was the standard treatment) was achieved more easily than the converse since many clinicians were unwilling to prescribe dihydrocodeine unless the patient had been randomized to it. There was improvement over time compared to baseline on the various secondary outcome measures (including illicit opioid use, reported crime, and physical health), with no significant differences in these outcomes between groups.

In what was reported to be the first randomized controlled trial to compare buprenorphine and dihydrocodeine for opioid medical withdrawal, an open-label trial recruited 60 individuals who were using illicit opioids (43). Dose-reduction schedules for sublingual buprenorphine and oral dihydrocodeine were at the discretion of the treating physician but could not exceed 15 days. The primary outcome measure was abstinence from illicit opioids (as assessed by a urine sample) at the final study medication prescription. While a significantly higher proportion of individuals randomized to buprenorphine (21%) compared to dihydrocodeine (3%) provided an opioid-negative urine sample, only 23% of individuals overall completed the course of withdrawal medication and provided the required final urine sample.

Various studies have shown positive and encouraging results with regard to the use of slow-release oral morphine for the treatment of opioid dependence, and this medication has been used as an addiction pharmacotherapy in various countries. Formulations for once-daily administration have been developed, which could make the medication suitable for maintenance or medical withdrawal treatment.

Slow-release oral morphine has been evaluated in both comparative and noncomparative studies. In one of the former, 103 of 110 patients completed a 3-week study in Austria designed to assess treatment satisfaction (44). Patients reported significant reductions in somatic complaints, cravings for heroin and cocaine, and withdrawal symptoms compared to baseline. Cocaine consumption as assessed from urine drug screens was also significantly reduced; benzodiazepine consumption remained almost unchanged over the study period.

In another open-label study which assessed the safety and efficacy of slow-release oral morphine for the treatment of heroin dependence in Bulgaria, 19 of 20 patients completed the 6-month treatment protocol (45). Daily maintenance dosages averaged 760 mg, with a range of 440 to 1200 mg. No deaths or serious adverse events were reported. Psychosocial functioning and well-being improved, and a general improvement in patient health was observed. Concomitant use of methadone and other opioids was low, but this was based on self-report and was not verified with objective measures.

Slow-release oral morphine has also been compared to methadone. In an open-label crossover study, 18 methadone-maintenance patients were recruited to receive slow-release oral morphine once daily for approximately 6 weeks; methadone maintenance was resumed following this evaluation period (46). Patient outcomes were assessed during the transition between medications and also after at least 4 weeks on a stable dose of each medication. Three individuals dropped out of the study; two choosing to return to methadone maintenance. The mean initial methadone maintenance dosage was 78 mg (range 25 to 120 mg), while the mean final slow-release oral morphine dosage was 347 mg (range 120 to 570 mg). The transfer from methadone to slow-release oral morphine was not found to be associated with significant changes in the severity of opioid withdrawal across the first 5 days of treatment. The majority of the study patients preferred slow-release oral morphine to methadone.

The opioid agonist medications discussed above have the potential for being useful pharmacotherapies for addiction. However, as noted by Woody with regards to the use of long-acting morphine for opioid dependence treatment (and as can be extended to the development of codeine, dihydrocodeine, and other potential opioid agonist treatments), the medication development pathway would depend on a number of steps (47). These would include securing regulatory approval, getting the medication onto hospital and third-party payer formularies, developing reimbursement policies, and having clinicians use the medication.

HEROIN TREATMENT FOR OPIOID DEPENDENCE—A NEW APPROACH TO ADDRESSING ADDICTION

Following the first studies of heroin maintenance that were conducted in the United Kingdom in the 1970s (48) and the first trial of heroin-assisted treatment in Switzerland in 1994 (49), a number of studies conducted in North America and Europe have assessed the utility of using heroin to treat opioid-dependent individuals who typically were refractory to standard treatment such as methadone.

An excellent overview of some of the randomized controlled trials has recently been provided by Fischer and colleagues (50). Most of the studies involved the use of injected heroin, although utility of oral heroin (both immediate- and sustained-release) and inhaled heroin was also sometimes evaluated. Participants in the studies were typically individuals who did not respond adequately to methadone or other treatments; in some but not all cases, patients also received methadone. Main outcome measures often involved retention in treatment and assessments of illicit opioid and other drug use. Overall, the therapeutic outcomes of the various studies have been generally positive, although evidence of long-term benefit is generally lacking.

As noted by Lintzeris (51), results from randomized controlled trials have generally indicated that treatment with heroin, when compared to methadone treatment, is associated with comparable retention, improved health and functioning, and less self-reported illicit heroin use.

One of the most recently reported studies evaluated injectable heroin ($n = 115$) compared to oral methadone ($n = 111$) in study patients who had not benefited from at least two previous attempts at opioid dependence treatment, including methadone maintenance treatment at a dosage of 60 mg or more per day (52). This study was part of the North American Opiate Medication Initiative and was an open-label, randomized trial conducted in Canada (the cities of Montreal and Vancouver). Heroin was self-administered under supervision in the treatment clinics up to three times daily at a maximum dosage of 1000 mg/day; methadone was dispensed on a daily basis (no maximum dose indicated). The primary outcome measures were retention in addiction treatment at 12 months (or abstinence from opioids) and reduction in illicit drug use or other illegal activities. The results indicated that individuals assigned to heroin treatment were more likely to stay in treatment and reduce use of illegal drugs and engagement in illegal activities than those assigned to methadone. Sixteen of the 115 individuals in the heroin group had a life-threatening overdose or seizure during the study. One death occurred during the study, a methadone group individual who reportedly died from an opioid overdose.

Currently, heroin treatment for opioid dependence is a pharmacotherapeutic option in only a few countries, including the United Kingdom, the Netherlands, and Switzerland, and there are a limited number of individuals receiving such treatment. For example, it has been reported that in the United Kingdom in 2000, only 46 physicians had prescribed heroin and less than 450 patients were receiving it. In a retrospective review conducted to understand the basis for these low numbers, the criteria by which patients were determined to be eligible for heroin treatment and physicians' stated reasons for prescribing it were examined (53). The results indicated that generally, heroin was considered to be a treatment of last resort for those patients who already had a long history of injecting heroin, or for those who did not previously respond well to other treatments.

SUMMARY

Opioid dependence is a chronic, relapsing medical disorder, often described as a brain disease with behavioral components. It requires comprehensive, multimodal, long-term treatment, as many patients also abuse or are dependent upon other substances. Many also have other medical and psychiatric comorbidity. Various types of pharmacotherapies with different modes of action have been used and continue to be evaluated as treatments for opioid dependence. Because no single medication will be appropriate for every individual, it is important that clinicians have a variety of therapeutic agents available to them. Additionally, pharmacotherapy is not a treatment end in itself; other adjuncts to successful treatment may include psychotherapy, social rehabilitation, vocational training, and others. Intraindividual treatment may also change over time as patients cycle through periods of abstinence and drug use. Rational medication therapy begins with an understanding of not only the disease state generally, but also of the specific dynamics of the addiction process that affect the overall success of treatment.

REFERENCES

1. Dole VP, Nyswander M. A medical treatment for diacetylmorphine (heroin) addiction. A clinical trial with methadone hydrochloride. *J Am Med Assoc.* 1965;193:80–84.
2. Aghajanian GK. Tolerance of locus coeruleus neurones to morphine and suppression of withdrawal response by clonidine. *Nature.* 1978;276:186–188.
3. Crawley JN, Laverty R, Roth RH. Clonidine reversal of increased norepinephrine metabolite levels during morphine withdrawal. *Eur J Pharmacol.* 1979;57:247–250.
4. Redrobe JP, Bourin M. Clonidine potentiates the effects of 5-HT$_{1A}$, 5-HT$_{1B}$ and 5-HT$_{2A/2C}$ antagonists and 8-OH-DPAT in the mouse forced swimming test. *Eur Neuropsychopharmacol.* 1998;8:169–173.
5. Buccafusco JJ, Spector S. Influence of clonidine on experimental hypertension induced by cholinergic stimulation. *Experientia.* 1980;36:671–673.
6. Katsuragi T, Su C. Facilitation by clonidine of purine release induced by high KCl from the rabbit pulmonary artery. *Br J Pharmacol.* 1981;74:709–713.
7. Schaut J, Schnoll SH. Four cases of clonidine abuse. *Am J Psychiatry.* 1983;140:1625–1627.
8. Dennison SJ. Clonidine abuse among opiate addicts. *Psychiatr Q.* 2001;72:191–195.
9. Sharma A, Newton W. Clonidine as a drug of abuse. *J Am Bd Fam Pract.* 1995;8:136–138.

10. Rapko DA, Rastegar DA. Intentional clonidine patch ingestion by 3 adults in a detoxification unit. *Arch Intern Med.* 2003;163: 367–368.
11. Strang J, Bearn J, Gossop M. Lofexidine for opiate detoxification: review of recent randomised and open controlled trials. *Am J Addict.* 1999;8:337–348.
12. *Britlofex Summary of Product Characteristics.* Britannia Pharmaceuticals Limited. Available at: *http://www.lofexidine.co.uk/leaflets/bfl-spc-v3_07-2006.pdf*; accessed August 3, 2009.
13. Gold MS, Pottash AC, Sweeney DR, et al. Opiate detoxification with lofexidine. *Drug Alcohol Depend.* 1981;8:307–315.
14. Gold MS, Pottash AC, Sweeney DR, et al. Lofexidine blocks acute opiate withdrawal. *NIDA Res Monogr.* 1982;41:264–268.
15. Washton AM, Resnick RB, Geyer G. Opiate withdrawal using lofexidine, a clonidine analogue with fewer side effects. *J Clin Psychiatry.* 1983;44:335–337.
16. Bearn J, Gossop M, Strang J. Randomised double-blind comparison of lofexidine and methadone in the in-patient treatment of opiate withdrawal. *Drug Alcohol Depend.* 1996;43:87–91.
17. Bearn J, Gossop M, Strang J. Accelerated lofexidine treatment regimen compared with conventional lofexidine and methadone treatment for in-patient opiate detoxification. *Drug Alcohol Depend.* 1998;50:227–232.
18. Schroeder JR, Schmittner J, Bleiberg J, et al. Hemodynamic and cognitive effects of lofexidine and methadone coadministration: a pilot study. *Pharmacotherapy.* 2007;27:1111–1119.
19. Schmittner J, Schroeder JR, Epstein DH, et al. Electrocardiographic effects of lofexidine and methadone coadministration: secondary findings from a safety study. *Pharmacotherapy.* 2009; 29:495–502.
20. Carnwath T, Hardman J. Randomised double-blind comparison of lofexidine and clonidine in the out-patient treatment of opiate withdrawal. *Drug Alcohol Depend.* 1998;50:251–254.
21. Lin SK, Strang J, Su LW, et al. Double-blind randomised controlled trial of lofexidine versus clonidine in the treatment of heroin withdrawal. *Drug Alcohol Depend.* 1997;48:127–133.
22. Kahn A, Mumford JP, Rogers GA, et al. Double-blind study of lofexidine and clonidine in the detoxification of opiate addicts in hospital. *Drug Alcohol Depend.* 1997;44:57–61.
23. Walsh SL, Strain EC, Bigelow GE. Evaluation of the effects of lofexidine and clonidine on naloxone-precipitated withdrawal in opioid-dependent humans. *Addiction.* 2003;98:427–439.
24. Buntwal N, Bearn J, Gossop M, et al. Naltrexone and lofexidine combination treatment compared with conventional lofexidine treatment for in-patient opiate detoxification. *Drug Alcohol Depend.* 2000;59:183–188.
25. Gerra G, Zaimovic A, Giusti F, et al. Lofexidine versus clonidine in rapid opiate detoxification. *J Subst Abuse Treat.* 2001;21: 11–17.
26. White R, Alcorn R, Feinmann C. Two methods of community detoxification from opiates: an open-label comparison of lofexidine and buprenorphine. *Drug Alcohol Depend.* 2001;65:77–83.
27. Raistrick D, West D, Finnegan O, et al. A comparison of buprenorphine and lofexidine for community opiate detoxification: results from a randomized controlled trial. *Addiction.* 2005; 100:1860–1867.
28. Gowing L, Ali R, White JB. Buprenorphine for the management of opioid withdrawal. *Cochrane Database Syst Rev.* 2009;3: CD002025.
29. Leimbach DG, Eddy NB. Synthetic analgesics. III. Methadols, isomethadols and their acyl derivatives. *J Pharmacol Exp Ther.* 1954;110:135–147.
30. McMahon RE, Calp HW, Marshal FJ. The metabolism of alpha-dl-acetyl methadol in the rat: the identification of a probable active metabolite. *J Pharmacol Exp Ther.* 1965;149:436–445.
31. Moody DE, Alburges ME, Parker RJ, et al. The involvement of cytochrome P450 3A in the N-demethylation of 1-alpha-acetyl-methadol (LAAM), norLAAM and methadone. *Drug Metab Dispos.* 1997;25:1347–1353.
32. Walsh SL, Johnson RE, Cone EJ, et al. Intravenous and oral 1-alpha-acetylmethadol: pharmacodynamics and pharmacokinetics in humans. *J Pharmacol Exp Ther.* 1998;285:71–82.
33. Jaffe JH, Schuster CR, Smith BB, et al. Comparison of acetyl-methadol and methadone in the treatment of long-term heroin users. A pilot study. *J Am Med A.* 1970;211:1834–1836.
34. Anglin MD, Conner BT, Annon J, et al. Levo-alpha-acetyl-methadol (LAAM) versus methadone maintenance: 1-year treatment retention, outcomes and status. *Addiction.* 2007;102: 1432–1442.
35. Rawson RA, Hasson AL, Huber AM, et al. A 3-year progress report on the implementation of LAAM in the United States. *Addiction.* 1998;93:533–540.
36. Deamer RL, Wilson DR, Clark DS, et al. Torsades de pointes associated with high-dose levomethadyl acetate (ORLAAM). *J Addict Dis.* 2001;20:7–14.
37. Wedam EF, Bigelow GE, Johnson RE, et al. QT-interval effects of methadone, levomethadyl, and buprenorphine in a randomized trial. *Arch Intern Med.* 2007;167:2469–2475.
38. Strang J, Sheridan J, Hunt C, et al. The prescribing of methadone and other opioids to addicts: national survey of GPs in England and Wales. *Br J Gen Pract.* 2005;55:444–451.
39. Backmund M, Meyer K, Eichenlaub D, et al. Predictors for completing an inpatient detoxification program among intravenous heroin users, methadone substituted and codeine substituted patients. *Drug Alcohol Depend.* 2001;64:173–180.
40. Banbery J, Wolff K, Raistrick D. Dihydrocodeine—a useful tool in the detoxification of methadone-maintained patients. *J Subst Abuse Treat.* 2000;19:301–305.
41. Krausz M, Verthein W, Degkwitz P, et al. Maintenance treatment of opiate addicts in Germany with medications containing codeine—results of a follow-up study. *Addiction.* 1998;93: 1161–1167.
42. Robertson JR, Raab GM, Bruce M, et al. Addressing the efficacy of dihydrocodeine versus methadone as an alternative maintenance treatment for opiate dependence: a randomized controlled trial. *Addiction.* 2006;101:1752–1759.
43. Wright NMJ, Sheard L, Tompkins CNE, et al. Buprenorphine versus dihydrocodeine for opiate detoxification in primary care: a randomized controlled trial. *BMC Family Practice* 2007;8:3, accessed through http://www.biomedcentral.com/1471-2296/8/, on August 7, 2009.
44. Kraigher D, Jagsch R, Gombas W, et al. Use of slow-release oral morphine for the treatment of opioid dependence. *Eur Addict Res.* 2005;11:145–151.
45. Vasilev GN, Alexieva DZ, Pavlova RZ. Safety and efficacy of oral slow release morphine for maintenance treatment in heroin addicts: a 6-month open noncomparative study. *Eur Addict Res.* 2006;12:53–60.
46. Mitchell TB, White JM, Somogyi A, et al. Slow-release oral morphine versus methadone: a crossover comparison of patient outcomes and acceptability as maintenance pharmacotherapies for opioid dependence. *Addiction.* 2004;99:940–945.
47. Woody GE. New horizons: sustained release morphine as agonist treatment. *Addiction.* 2005;100:1758–1759.

48. Hartnoll RL, Micheson MC, Battersby A, et al. Evaluation of heroin maintenance in controlled trial. *Arch Gen Psychiatry*. 1980;37:877–884.
49. Fischer B, Rehm J, Kirst M, et al. Heroin-assisted treatment as a response to the public health problem of opiate dependence. *Eur J Public Health*. 2002;12:228–234.
50. Fischer B, Oviedo-Joekes E, Blanken P, et al. Heroin-assisted treatment (HAT) a decade later: a brief update on science and politics. *J Urban Health—Bull N Y Acad Med*. 2007;84:552–562.
51. Lintzeris N. Prescription of heroin for the management of heroin dependence: current status. *CNS Drugs*. 2009;23:463–476.
52. Oviedo-Joekes E, Brissette S, Marsh DC, et al. Diacetylmorphine versus methadone for the treatment of opioid addiction. *New Engl J Med*. 2009;361:777–786.
53. Metrebian N, Mott J, Carnwath Z, et al. Pathways into receiving a prescription for diamorphine (heroin) for the treatment of opiate dependence in the United Kingdom. *Eur Addict Res*. 2007;13:144–147.

CHAPTER 35 Sedative-Hypnotics Abstinence

R.C. Oude Voshaar

INTRODUCTION

Directly after their introduction in the 1960s, the potential of benzodiazepines to induce a state of physical dependence was described in chronic psychiatric patients who abruptly discontinued high-dose benzodiazepine treatment, that is, 300 to 600 mg per day of chlordiazepoxide (1). In the early 1970s, the first reports appeared in the scientific literature of patients who had escalated their benzodiazepine dosage beyond the upper limit of the recommended therapeutic range (2). These reports received little attention. Benzodiazepines were considered safe in clinical practice and only a small number of patients escalated their dosage beyond therapeutic levels. From large pharmacoepidemiologic studies it is estimated that only 1% to 2% of long-term benzodiazepine users escalate their dosage above 40 mg diazepam equivalents per day over the course of several years (3). The first study of physical dependence in normal-dose benzodiazepine usage was by Covi et al. (4), who described a withdrawal syndrome after the discontinuation of 20 weeks of chlordiazepoxide treatment (4). Subsequent studies proved that normal-dose dependence, as manifested by a physical withdrawal syndrome, was a real entity and occurred even if the dosage was tapered-off. About 15% to 25% of long-term (over 12 months) therapeutic dose users develop a definite withdrawal syndrome (5).

Research on the prevalence, characteristics, and treatment of sedative-hypnotic dependence largely relied on definitions of dependence that emphasized the physical aspect of dependence (6). Research in the late 1990s, however, showed that psychological aspects of dependence are important for sedative-hypnotic dependence (7). The first study using DSM-criteria for sedative-hypnotic dependence found past-year prevalence rates of 40% in primary care patients and 52% in psychiatric outpatients who used benzodiazepines at least 3 days a week (8). These figures may be falsely inflated by using DSM-III-R criteria, as the criteria for dependence have been changed in DSM-IV. A recent epidemiologic study reported a past-year prevalence rate of sedative-hypnotic dependence of 2.3% among community-dwelling elderly people, which corresponds to a prevalence rate of about 10% among past-year benzodiazepine users in the population (9).

The abuse and dependence potential of benzodiazepines have stimulated the development of nonbenzodiazepine hypnotics. These drugs, the so-called Z-drugs (zolpidem, zopiclon, zaleplon, and recently, eszopiclon), were supposed to be devoid of abuse and dependence by having chemical structures different from the benzodiazepines and by binding selectively to alpha1-subunit containing $GABA_A$-receptors. Although the abuse and dependence potential of these newer drugs are still considered remarkably lower than the classical benzodiazepines, evidence for significant abuse and their dependence potential is growing (10,11).

Today, it still remains controversial whether normal-dose dependence on sedative-hypnotic drugs should be regarded as a clinical problem or the best result for patients with treatment resistant (subthreshold) anxiety disorders and/or insomnia. Nonetheless, the reported prevalence rates of physical dependence associated with long-term benzodiazepine usage are high and vary between 2.2% and 17.6% in the community (12). Half of these long-term users meet DSM-IV criteria for specific disorders, for which the majority have never been treated according to current guidelines (13). Moreover, tapering-off their benzodiazepines does not worsen their psychopathologic symptoms (14,15).

HISTORY OF THE TREATMENT

Increasing knowledge on the dependence liability of sedative-hypnotic drugs as well as problems with stopping benzodiazepines in patients after long-term exposure prompted the development of treatment strategies to discontinue long-term benzodiazepine use. The first benzodiazepine discontinuation studies date from the early 1980s (16,17). Discontinuation strategies applied to long-term benzodiazepine users can be divided into two categories: minimal intervention programs, and systematic discontinuation programs. Minimal interventions are defined as simple intervention applicable to large groups of patients, for example, an advisory letter or a meeting in which long-term users are advised to stop their use. Systematic discontinuation programs are defined as tapering-off programs guided by a physician or psychologist. The main purpose of a systematic discontinuation program is to achieve a state of abstinence without experiencing significant withdrawal symptoms. These treatment programs can be further divided into systematic discontinuation alone or combined with either pharmacotherapy or psychotherapy. Psychotherapy has been added to these programs to achieve higher abstinence rates by either improving patients' coping skills with withdrawal symptoms or treating the underlying psychiatric symptoms. Pharmacotherapy has been added primarily to suppress withdrawal symptoms in order to achieve higher abstinence rates.

MINIMAL INTERVENTION PROGRAMS

Several minimal intervention strategies have been found to be successful in decreasing sedative-hypnotic drug usage in randomized controlled trials (18,19). Most evidence is found for the effect of sending a letter by the primary care physician to patients who have received benzodiazepine prescriptions for at least 3 months (most patients in these studies used benzodiazepines for years) (20). Other minimal intervention strategies that have proven successful include an advisory consultation by the primary care physician followed by either a self-help booklet or the opportunity to receive relaxation therapy and counseling by a nurse practitioner (18). Meta-analysis of these minimal intervention studies revealed that the odds of becoming fully abstinent is two to four times greater when compared to routine medical care or not raising the issue of discontinuation at all (18,19). These effects are robust and independent of the exact methodology of the individual studies, that is, randomization at patient level, randomization at the level of general practices (cluster-randomization), or comparison to a matched historical control group to correct for the hawthorne effect (i.e., less benzodiazepine prescribed by doctors due to increase in knowledge and awareness caused by participation in a benzodiazepine discontinuation program). Translated to clinical practice, approximately 25% of all long-term benzodiazepine users will completely quit their usage after a minimal intervention strategy and an even larger proportion reduce their daily dosage by more than 50% with such an approach. Over the following 2 years, half of the patients who had quit their usage completely will remain fully abstinent (50).

Minimal interventions have only been evaluated in primary care settings, thereby limiting their generalization to secondary care. Results apply to normal-dose, long-term benzodiazepine users with an average age around 60 years. Determinants of the success of a minimal intervention can be divided into three main categories, that is, usage characteristics including characteristics of the individual drugs, doctor variables, and patient variables. The most important and most consistently reported predictors of being able to discontinue long-term benzodiazepine use by a minimal intervention are a lower daily dosage at baseline and a shorter duration of use. Furthermore, the use of multiple different benzodiazepines is also a pharmacologic factor with a negative impact on outcome independent of dosage and duration of use (21,22). The use of multiple different benzodiazepines probably reflects a more severe or complicated condition, and discontinuation of more than one sedative-hypnotic drug may require closer monitoring and supervision of the patient. Particular pharmacologic differences such as half-life and potency are of little importance in predicting success (21–23).

Many papers note doctor characteristics and their attitudes as important determinants of high benzodiazepine consumption and subsequently disappointing success when applying dose reduction strategies. Several surveys indicate that physicians generally endorse benzodiazepines as an effective treatment for anxiety or insomnia, report quick action, and strong patient satisfaction (24). Furthermore, the risks associated with the use of benzodiazepines are minimized by doctors and monitoring or restricting renewal of benzodiazepine prescriptions is not regarded an important issue in clinical practice. Finally, many doctors are skeptic about the possibility of successful benzodiazepine discontinuation (24). Interestingly, a multilevel analysis of one of the largest benzodiazepine discontinuation studies showed that in primary care characteristics of physicians contributed marginally to a successful outcome, whereas patient characteristics were of major importance (23). However, little is known about which patient characteristics do influence the outcome of minimal intervention strategies. Age and gender only marginally influence outcome. The attitude about using benzodiazepines and coping strategies for dealing with dependence are probably the most important patient characteristics that influence outcome (25).

SYSTEMATIC DISCONTINUATION PROGRAMS

In contrast to minimal intervention, systematic discontinuation programs have been evaluated in different settings. Numerous discontinuation programs have been described, but the effectiveness of most programs is not substantiated by randomized controlled trials (26). Only two systematic discontinuation strategies have been compared with routine clinical care in a randomized controlled fashion (14,15,27). Both studies were conducted in primary care settings and yielded significantly higher success rates by a gradual dose reduction (GDR) approach compared to routine clinical care. The duration of both taper strategies, however, was quite different. Oude Voshaar et al. (14) evaluated a fixed discontinuation schedule of 25% per week, which resulted in an abstinence rate of 63%, whereas Vicens et al. (27) reduced the dosages with steps between 10% and 25% fortnightly resulting in an abstinence rate of 40%. The optimal duration of a tapering-off schedule remains speculative. A small pilot study with 42 patients found similar success rates when a fixed dosage reduction was compared to abrupt discontinuation (28), whereas extremely high abstinence rates up to 90% have been described in an uncontrolled study of "patient-tailored, symptom-guided benzodiazepine withdrawal" using a withdrawal schedule up to 15 months in a tertiary, specialized care centre (29). The rationale for a slow tapering-off program over months is the hypothesis that it takes time before brain systems regain control of the functions which have been damped down by benzodiazepine usage for years (http://www.benzo.org.uk/manual/index.htm). Supporters of "patient-tailored, symptom-guided benzodiazepine withdrawal" further state that "the rate of tapering should never be rigid but should be flexible and controlled by the patient, not the doctor, according to the patient's individual needs" (http://www.benzo.org.uk/manual/index.htm).

Most guidelines and researchers, however, advocate a fixed discontinuation schedule varying from 4 to 8 weeks in duration (14,26,30,31). Within this time period, withdrawal symptoms are generally acceptable for both low- and high-dose

TABLE 35.1	Conversion factors for benzodiazepine agonists in diazepam equivalents[a]	
Benzodiazepine agonist	Equivalent dosages	Conversion factor to diazepam equivalents
Alprazolam	0.5–1 mg	×10–20
Bromazepam	5–10 mg	×1–2
Brotizolam	0.25 mg	×40
Chlordiazepoxide	20–25 mg	×0.4–0.5
Clobazam	15–20 mg	×0.5–0.67
Clonazepam	0.5–8 mg	×1.25–20
Clorazepinezuur	10–15 mg	×0.67–10
Diazepam[a]	10 mg	×1
Flunitrazepam	1 mg	×10
Flurazepam	15–30 mg	×0.33–0.67
Ketazolam	15–60 mg	×0.16–0.67
Loprazolam	1–2 mg	×5–10
Lorazepam	1–2 mg	×5–10
Lormetazepam	1–2 mg	×5–10
Medazepam	10–20 mg	×0.5–1
Midazolam	7.5–10 mg	×1–1.33
Nitrazepam	10 mg	×1
Nordazepam	10 mg	×1
Oxazepam	20–50 mg	×0.2–0.5
Prazepam	10–20 mg	×0.5–1
Quazepam	20 mg	×0.5
Temazepam	20–30 mg	×0.5–0.67
Triazolam	0.125–0.5 mg	×20–80
Zaleplon[b]	20 mg	×0.5
Zolpidem[b]	5–20 mg	×0.5–2
Zopiclon[b]	7.5–15 mg	×0.66–1.33
Eszopiclon[b]	3 mg	×3.33

[a]An equivalent dosage of diazepam can be calculated by multiplying the dosage of the benzodiazepine with its conversion factor. This has to be done for each benzodiazepine-agonist separately, whereafter the equivalent dosages of diazepam can be summed up.

[b]Non-benzodiazepine agonist at the $GABA_A$-receptor.

benzodiazepine users. A feasible discontinuation schedule for clinical practice is the following (see also 14,30,31). Before tapering-off, benzodiazepine users should be transferred to an equivalent dosage of a long-acting benzodiazepine, for example, diazepam, and stabilized for 2 weeks. For patients taking more than one benzodiazepine, the dosages of the different benzodiazepines should be converted in diazepam equivalents and summed. By transferring all benzodiazepines into one long-acting benzodiazepine, fluctuations of blood levels are minimized, which results in higher discontinuation rates. Abstinence rates reported by published systematic discontinuation programs show that by transferring to a long-acting benzodiazepines an additional 5% to 10% of the patients will successfully quit (32).

Table 35.1 presents the equivalent dosages for all benzodiazepines. Due to the large pharmacokinetic differences between benzodiazepines, it is impossible to give exact equivalent dosages. This is reflected by the wide range of equivalent dosages reported by different researchers. For that reason, Table 35.1 is based upon different resources and shows the lower and upper limit of reported equivalents dosages (33; http://www.benzo.org.uk/manual/index.htm; 34). Although the preference for a specific long-acting agent is quite arbitrary, diazepam is often chosen due to the availability of 2 mg tablets that can be easily split in two halves of 1 mg each. Prescribing only diazepam 2 mg tablets has at least two advantages. First, the high number of diazepam 2 mg tablets that are often required to be taken before tapering begins confronts the patient with their "high dosage" and enhances their motivation to quit. A second, more pragmatic reason is the opportunity to gradually reduce the daily dosage without switching between tablets of different strengths. During the tapering-off phase, the daily dose of diazepam has to be reduced by 25% each week during weekly visits. Patients and clinicians have the opportunity to divide the last step into two steps of 12.5% for 4 days. The dose reduction period should be concluded 2 weeks after the last reduction step, because withdrawal symptoms rarely exceed a duration of more than 2 weeks.

Some issues need specific attention. First, it is important to collect all supplies of benzodiazepines kept by the patient at home before starting the discontinuation schedule. Benzodiazepine usage by partners or housemates must also be checked, and an agreement must be determined about how the patient and their partner will deal with these benzodiazepine stocks during the withdrawal period. Secondly, every dose reduction step should be accompanied by a consultation with the prescribing physician in order to evaluate withdrawal symptoms, exploring upcoming difficulties and last but not least, to be able to prescribe the exact number of 2 mg tablets of diazepam a patient needs till the next visit (rounding the number of tablets that have to be used each day to the upper whole digit). Patients can be given the opportunity to spread the prescribed daily dosage equally over the day. They do not have any limitations other than a maximum dosage that can be taken a day, but it may be wise to advise to take the largest number of tablets just before sleeping time. Hypnotic drug users should be warned about the possibility of some daytime sedation during the first 2 weeks. A next reduction step can always be postponed if the patient is not able to comply with it, but emphasize that the duration of their complaints (i.e., their withdrawal symptoms) will also be prolonged. In clinical practice, most withdrawal symptoms occur during the second half of the withdrawal phase (35). A complete resolution of withdrawal symptoms depends on the half-life of the agent that is withdrawn. For long-acting agents, all symptoms are generally resolved within 2 weeks, although anecdotal reports have been described of protracted withdrawal symptoms over years (36).

Different instruments can be used to measure benzodiazepine withdrawal symptoms during discontinuation. Two instruments are observer rated, the 34-item Physician Withdrawal Checklist (31) and the Clinical Institute Withdrawal Assessment—Benzodiazepine (CIWA-B) (37). For both instruments, however, data on validity and reliability are limited. The Benzodiazepine Withdrawal Symptom Questionnaire 1 & 2 (BWSQ1&2) have been developed for research purposes and are currently well validated (35,38). The BWSQ1 is a three-point scale, designed for single administration in epidemiologic research. It measures 20 symptoms (anxiety symptoms are not directly measured) retrospectively over the complete period of benzodiazepine use at times when the dosage was reduced or stopped. The BWSQ2 measures identical symptoms and is intended for repeated measurements during benzodiazepine withdrawal. Perceptual and sensory distortions, loss of appetite, as well as depressed mood play an important role in the BWSQ and a considerable overlap exists between the BWSQ and the CIWA-B questionnaires. A significant increase in scores during diazepam withdrawal differentiates patients who will be unsuccessful in stopping benzodiazepines and those who will be successful in the short term. Moreover, low scores on the BWSQ during the last taper phase predict a lower probability of using benzodiazepines in the following years (35). The BWSQ is therefore a suitable instrument to monitor withdrawal symptoms during treatment.

For interpretation of the scores as well as for motivating patients to continue withdrawal, it is important to acknowledge the difference between rebound symptoms, withdrawal symptoms, and the recurrence of a psychiatric disorder. Rebound is a recurrence of the original complaints of the patient before starting benzodiazepines but of a higher intensity. Withdrawal symptoms are purely related to the discontinuation of the drug and can partly overlap with the original disorder. A clear distinction remains difficult, but there are two specific differences between withdrawal and a relapse of anxiety. The first difference is the length of time between discontinuation of benzodiazepines and the appearance of symptoms, as well as the tendency of the symptoms to improve or worsen over time. True withdrawal symptoms usually develop within a few days after discontinuation, they are most severe directly after discontinuation but continue to lessen until they disappear within 2 weeks (varying on the half-life of the specific agents that was tapered). Relapse of anxiety generally manifests as anxious symptoms that return more than a week after benzodiazepine discontinuation and get progressively worse until treated. The second difference is the symptoms themselves. Several symptoms of withdrawal are not characteristic of anxiety, like sensitivity to light and sound, tinnitus, feelings of "electric shocks," tremors, myoclonic jerks, perceptual changes, and even seizures in case of high dosages. However, withdrawal symptoms also include many symptoms similar to anxiety, such as agitation, irritability, muscle cramps, fatigue, insomnia, headache, dizziness, and concentration difficulties. Therefore, rebound and withdrawal symptoms should never be a reason to stop tapering-off as a real recurrence of the disorder can only be established after rebound and withdrawal symptoms have been resolved. Withdrawal symptoms after low- and high-dose discontinuation are principally similar, but may differ in intensity. Epileptic seizures are extremely rare during discontinuation of benzodiazepines in therapeutic dosages, even in the case of abrupt discontinuation. In high-dose users, however, rapid discontinuation (within less than 1 week) may result in epileptic seizures especially in patients using benzodiazepine with a short half-life.

ADDITIONAL THERAPIES FOR SYSTEMATIC DISCONTINUATION PROGRAMS

Pharmacologic Interventions

Nonbenzodiazepine medications have also been examined in combination with systematic discontinuation programs to determine their efficacy and ability to increase success rates (18,19). These drugs have been selected based on their effect on peripheral or central receptors that are supposed to be involved in benzodiazepine withdrawal. Antidepressants and anxiolytic drugs have been examined for their anxiolytic effects. Anticonvulsants and sedative-hypnotic drugs have been examined based on their central GABAergic effects and/or sedative effects. Propranolol, a beta blocker, has been tested based upon the presence of adrenergically mediated withdrawal symptoms. Flumazenil, a benzodiazepine receptor antagonist, has been tested based upon the hypothesis that it would reset the $GABA_A$-receptor shift produced by prolonged benzodiazepine usage. Table 35.2 presents an overview of all randomized controlled trials to date.

Meta-analysis of all systematic discontinuation trials evaluating antidepressant drugs revealed a superior effect associated with the addition of an antidepressant. Subgroup analyses showed only significant effects for imipramine and trazodone. Although these results suggest differential effects between antidepressants, these differences are probably chance findings due to small sample sizes of the individual studies. In trials evaluating the addition of antidepressants, these agents are continued after having completed the benzodiazepine discontinuation. Several publications suggest that depressive patients have greater difficulty in stopping benzodiazepine use (39).

TABLE 35.2 Randomized clinical trial evaluating the additive effect of pharmacotherapy to systematic discontinuation alone

Pharmacotherapy	Studies (N)	Patients (N)	Pooled effect estimate odds ratio [95% CI]
Antidepressants			
■ Paroxetine	2	167	1.6 [0.8–3.0]
■ Imipramine	2	75	3.0 [1.2–7.8]
■ Dothiepin	1	87	0.6 [0.3–1.6]
■ Trazodone	2	108	2.6 [1.1–6.4]
Pooled analysis	7	437	1.6 [1.1–2.4]
Anticonvulsants			
■ Carbamazepine	3	99	1.0 [0.4–2.7]
■ Valproate	1	37	4.8 [1.1–20.3]
Pooled analysis	4	136	1.7 [0.8–3.8]
Anti-anxiety agents			
■ Buspirone	5	217	1.1 [0.7–1.9]
■ Progesterone	1	35	0.8 [0.2–3.2]
■ Alpidem	1	25	0.2 [0.0–0.9]
Pooled analysis	7	277	0.9 [0.6–1.4]
Sedatives-hypnotics			
■ Melatonin	2	72	2.5 [1.0–6.4]
■ Hydroxyzine	1	139	1.1 [0.4–2.9]
■ Cyamemazine	1	168	0.4 [0.2–0.8]
Pooled analysis	4	379	0.9 [0.6–1.5]
Other drugs			
■ Propranonol	2	71	0.8 [0.3–1.9]
■ Aspartate	1	144	0.9 [0.4–2.1]
■ Homeogene	1	41	2.0 [0.5–7.5]
■ Sedatif PC	1	46	1.5 [0.5–4.9]
■ Flumazenil	1	40	3.7 [1.0–14.0]

Note: Data from Oude Voshaar et al. (2006) (15,18,45).

This suggests that antidepressants may be successful due to positive effects on the underlying condition for which benzodiazepines were originally prescribed.

Anticonvulsants have not proven successful, with the exception of a large effect for valproate in a small trial. In contrast to what might be expected, non-benzodiazepine anti-anxiety drugs as well as sedative-hypnotic drugs do not have any beneficial effects. Based on stringent rules for evidence-based medicine, that is, meta-analysis of different trials from different research groups, only strong evidence exists for the lack of efficacy for buspirone. The same findings hold for trials of several individual drugs. Propranolol and carbamazepine, however, both attenuate the severity of withdrawal symptoms during a (gradual) dose reduction (16,40). This effect, however, does not translate into higher overall abstinence rates, with the exception for high-dose users (over 20 mg diazepam equivalents) and patients with panic disorder among which carbamazepine might have some effect (40,41).

In most studies, patients receive a maintenance dosage of the additive pharmacotherapy before the start of tapering. Three studies, however, evaluated abrupt substitution of the pharmacotherapy (19). It was found that acute substitution with propranolol or cyamemazine was actually less effective than GDR alone. Furthermore, acute substitution with Homéogène 46 and Sédatif PC was no more effective than abrupt cessation alone.

Psychological Interventions

Eight studies including a total of 499 patients have evaluated the efficacy of psychotherapy to facilitate systematic benzodiazepine discontinuation programs. As shown in Table 35.3, a pooled effect of these studies clearly shows the effectiveness of this strategy. Although all studies evaluated cognitive–behavioral therapy, the content of the psychotherapy largely varied between studies. This can be explained by differences in the specific patient populations under study. In three studies, patients with an underlying anxiety disorder (panic disorder or generalized anxiety disorder) were treated according to a CBT-protocol for these disorders. This resulted in significantly higher abstinence rates compared to tapering-off benzodiazepine without additive therapy. Similar results were found in studies including only patients with chronic insomnia. The two studies that included a mixed population selected only on the duration of long-term benzodiazepine use (14,15) or severity of benzodiazepine dependence (42) did not find any additional benefit associated with the use of CBT. The CBT in these studies was focused on benzodiazepine dependence and withdrawal, but only marginally on underlying symptoms of anxiety or insomnia.

Conclusion of Additive Therapy

The main conclusion of additive therapy is that pharmacotherapy or CBT is only effective during benzodiazepine tapering-off programs if focused on the underlying problem of the patient. The success rate in the control groups of these studies shows that in cases where an underlying psychiatric problem is present, the success of systematic discontinuation alone significantly decreases. If no depressive disorder, anxiety disorder of insomnia is present, as found in half of all long-term benzodiazepine users (13), systematic discontinuation alone is the preferred treatment.

TABLE 35.3 Gradual dose reduction (GDR) with and without additional cognitive–behavioral therapy

Comparisons	Patients (N)	Effect estimate odds ratio [95% CI]
CBT for anxiety disorders		
■ Baillargeon et al. (51)	33	9.8 [2.0–47.9]
■ Spiegel et al. (52)	21	1.1 [0.1–9.9]
■ Gosselin et al. (53)	61	5.0 [1.7–14.8]
Pooled analysis	115	4.7 [2.1–10.7]
CBT for insomnia		
■ Otto et al. (54)	52	6.2 [1.7–23.3]
■ Morin et al. (55)	65	5.0 [1.7–14.4]
Pooled analysis	117	5.5 [2.4–12.5]
CBT for substance use (BZD) disorders		
■ Vorma et al. (42)	76	0.4 [0.1–1.3]
■ Oude Voshaar et al. (50)	146	0.8 [0.4–1.5]
Pooled analysis	222	0.7 [0.4–1.2]
Overall pooled analysis	**499**	**1.8 [1.3–2.6]**

SPECIAL CONSIDERATIONS

Determinants of Successful Outcome

Numerous uncontrolled studies and studies evaluating additional therapies, shows that in general two out of three patients are able to discontinue their benzodiazepine usage successfully by systematic discontinuation (14,15,18,19). Long-term results show that approximately half of the successfully treated patients will remain fully abstinent over the following years. However, patients who were unable to quit completely as well as those patients who relapse, decrease their usage substantially. This is primarily explained by a change of their usage pattern (i.e., intermittent usage of benzodiazepine) and not by a reduction in the average daily dosage used. Psychiatric symptoms generally improve when patients stop using benzodiazepines (31,43). Even in a sample meeting criteria for DSM-IV sedative-hypnotic dependence, reduction of anxiety levels paralleled the reduction of the benzodiazepine dosage (44).

Several factors have been related to successful benzodiazepine discontinuation (for an overview to this topic, see Oude Voshaar et al. (45)). The most reliable predictor for discontinuation is a lower benzodiazepine dosage at the start of tapering-off. No differences have been reported between individual benzodiazepines during gradual discontinuation, although after *abrupt* cessation a shorter elimination half-life resulted in a lower abstinence rate. Demographic variables inconsistently influence taper outcomes. For example, both female and male sex as well as both younger and older ages have been related to successful taper outcome. The high success rates that can be achieved in elderly patients merits some attention, as many physicians are skeptical about the possibility of tapering-off benzodiazepines in elderly patients. A study among nursing home patients found a success rate of 80% (46). A high level of psychopathologic symptoms, especially anxiety and depressive symptoms, as well as the personality traits neuroticism, dependence and vulnerability, resulted in a lower abstinence rate (47). In addition, these personality traits led to the experience of a more severe benzodiazepine withdrawal syndrome upon discontinuation.

Examining all potential predictors together revealed that outcome depends more on nonspecific dependence characteristics, rather than the level of psychopathology, personality traits, or benzodiazepine type (45). Successful discontinuation is associated with a lower benzodiazepine dosage at the start of tapering, the ability of the patient to reduce their dosage already on their own prior to formal treatment, not using alcohol, and a higher degree of compliance with the prescribed benzodiazepine regime during their benzodiazepine treatment. Withdrawal symptoms, especially those experienced during the last half of the withdrawal period, also have an impact on the long-term abstinence (35). In contrast to many other substance use disorders, the treatment of benzodiazepine dependence has been poorly studied within the theoretical context of a psychological model of change. Available but preliminary evidence has yielded counterintuitive results. Patients in the more advanced stages of change in the transtheoretical model of behavioral change (i.e., preparation, action) were equally successful at achieving abstinence compared to patients in less-advanced stages (i.e., precontemplation, contemplation) (22).

Treatment Setting

The preferred treatment differs per setting. According to the principles of stepped care, minimal intervention should be considered the preferred treatment in primary care. In case a long-term benzodiazepine user is not able to discontinue his or her use with only minimal help, a systematic discontinuation program without any additive treatment should be offered. Patients suffering from a therapeutic dose dependency without clear evidence of an underlying psychiatric condition can be successfully treated in a primary care setting so long as the patient conforms to the guidelines discussed in Section 4.

If an underlying psychiatric condition is present, referral for second-line treatment is preferred. At this moment, it is important to acknowledge different natures of sedative-hypnotic dependence (48). First, there can be unintentional abuse by patients who begin using benzodiazepines to treat an affective disorder or insomnia but end up using them inappropriately. Most often, these patients use benzodiazepines for years while still suffering from underlying psychiatric conditions (13), whereas only a very small proportion will escalate their dosages over the years (3). The majority of evidence on systematic discontinuation of benzodiazepines (as described in Sections 4 and 5) is based on this population. Referral to both addiction and psychiatric clinics are realistic options, with a slight preference for the latter.

The second category is those patients who deliberately abuse benzodiazepines for their pleasant effects, in this paragraph referred to as intentional abusers of benzodiazepines. These patients usually take benzodiazepines in an attempt to get high and often abuse other substances for the same purpose. Multidrug users often take benzodiazepine simultaneously with other drugs to improve the euphoriant effects (especially of methadone), or use benzodiazepines to suppress the distress caused by withdrawal or adverse effects of other drugs like opiates, cocaine, or alcohol. Intentional abuse of benzodiazepines can results in both high-dose benzodiazepine dependence as well as benzodiazepine dependence complicated by a comorbid alcohol dependence and/or an other substance use disorders. A clinic specialized in (benzodiazepine) addiction should be preferred for this population as success rates drop to approximately 15% to 30% (42). Unfortunately, no specific guidelines are available for this important subgroup. Therefore, these patients should be treated according to the general principals of treating substance use disorders. Irrespective of the underlying problems, inpatient treatment seems superior for high-dose users, that is, patients using more than 30 mg diazepam equivalents a day. Other predictors of treatment success in patients with intentional abuse of benzodiazepines are a lower baseline dosage (within the high-dose range) and no previous withdrawal attempts (49). Among intentional abusers of benzodiazepines, patients with cluster B personality or borderline personality disorder are far less successful in achieving abstinence, suggesting the need of concomitant treatment for these disorders. In contrast, comorbid alcohol dependence and other psychiatric disorders did not influence treatment outcome in patients with intentional abuse of benzodiazepines (49). Despite low success rates in patients with intentional benzodiazepine abuse, those patients able to decrease their benzodiazepine levels significantly regained a much better quality of life at follow-up and experienced less psychopathologic symptoms.

CONCLUSIONS

Whether long-term benzodiazepine use must be discontinued should be considered in the context of diagnosis, current symptoms, side effects, treatment history, and alternative treatment modalities. If one decides to discontinue long-term benzodiazepine treatment, the following guidelines can be given. A first treatment should be started in primary care with a minimal intervention by providing general information to patients and encouraging them to stop the use of benzodiazepines by themselves through a taper. If patients are unable to stop their benzodiazepine use this way, a systematic discontinuation program should be offered to them, since half to two-thirds of the patients can be successfully discontinued. There is some evidence to suggest that patients must be transferred to a long-acting agent and tapered-off a by fixed discontinuation program. Additional treatment should only be given if there is evidence of an underlying psychiatric condition. In that case, patients should be referred to secondary care institutes. Although most evidence supports the use of cognitive–behavioral therapy focused on the underlying condition, available data suggest that antidepressants may also be an option. If these strategies fail, it remains unclear which treatment options should be used. We suggest the following options, depending on local circumstances and patient characteristics. Patients could be offered a symptom-guided taper-off scheme provided in a specialized care setting to prevent significant deterioration or relapse of the underlying disease during or after discontinuation. Patients using high dosages (>30 mg diazepam equivalent) as well as patients with comorbid substance use disorders other than benzodiazepines might be offered inpatient treatment.

REFERENCES

1. Hollister LE, Motzenbecker FP, Degan RO. Withdrawal reactions from chlordiazepoxide ("Librium"). *Psychopharmacologia.* 1961; 2:63–68.
2. Woody GE, O'Brien CP, Greenstein R. Misuse and abuse of diazepam: an increasingly common medical problem. *Int J Addict.* 1975;10:843–848.
3. Soumerai SB, Simoni-Wastila L, Singer C, et al. Lack of relationship between long-term use of benzodiazepines and escalation to high dosages. *Psychiatr Serv.* 2003;54:1006–1011.
4. Covi L, Lipman RS, Pattison JH, et al. Length of treatment with anxiolytic sedatives and response to their sudden withdrawal. *Acta Psychiatr Scand.* 1973;49:51–64.
5. Busto U, Sellers EM, Naranjo CA, et al. Withdrawal reaction after long-term therapeutic use of benzodiazepines. *New Engl J Med.* 1986;315:854–859.
6. Linssen SM, Breteler MHM, Zitman FG. Defining benzodiazepine dependence: the confusion persists. *Eur Psychiatry.* 1995;10:306–311.
7. Baillie AJ, Mattick RP. The benzodiazepine dependence questionnaire: development, reliability and validity. *Br J Psychiatry.* 1996;169:276–281.
8. Kan CC, Breteler MHM, Zitman FG. High prevalence of benzodiazepine dependence in outpatient users, based on DSM-III-R and ICD-10 criteria. *Acta Psychiatr Scand.* 1997;96: 85–93.
9. Préville M, Boyer R, Grenier S, et al. The epidemiology of psychiatric disorders in Quebec's older adult population. *Can J Psychiatry.* 2008;53:822–832.
10. Victorri-Vigneau C, Dailly E, Veyrac G, et al. Evidence of zolpidem abuse and dependence: results of the French Centre for Evaluation and Information on Pharmacodependence (CEIP) network survey. *Br J Clin Pharmacol.* 2007;64:198–209.
11. Licata SC, Rowlett JK. Abuse and dependence liability of benzodiazepine-type drugs: $GABA_A$ receptor modulation and beyond. *Pharmacol Biochem Behav.* 2008;90:74–89.
12. Zandstra SM, Führer JW, Van de Lisdonk EH, et al. Different study criteria affect the prevalence of benzodiazepine use. *Soc Psychiatry Psychiatr Epidemiol.* 2002;37:139–144.
13. Zandstra SM, van Rijswijk E, Rijnders CATh, et al. Long-term benzodiazepine users in family practice: differences from short-term users in mental health, coping behaviour and psychological characteristics. *Fam Pract.* 2004;21:266–269.
14. Oude Voshaar RC, Gorgels W, Mol AJJ, et al. Tapering off long-term benzodiazepine use with or without group cognitive-behavioural therapy: three condition, randomised controlled trial. *Br J Psychiatry.* 2003;182:489–504.
15. Oude Voshaar RC, Gorgels WJMJ, Mol AJJ, et al. Long-term outcome of two forms of randomised benzodiazepine discontinuation. *Br J Psychiatry.* 2006;188:188–189.
16. Tyrer P, Rutherford D, Huggett T, et al. Benzodiazepine withdrawal symptoms and propranolol. *Lancet.* 1981;1:520–522.
17. Tyrer P, Owen R, Dawling S, et al. Gradual withdrawal of diazepam after long-term therapy. *Lancet.* 1983;1:1402–1406.
18. Oude Voshaar RC, Couvée JE, Van Balkom AJLM, et al. Strategies to discontinue long-term benzodiazepine use: a meta-analysis. *Br J Psychiatry.* 2006;189:213–220.
19. Parr JM, Kavanagh DJ, Cahill L, et al. Effectiveness of current treatment approaches for benzodiazepine discontinuation: a meta-analysis. *Addiction.* 2009;104:13–24.
20. Gorgels WJ, Oude Voshaar RC, Mol AJ, et al. Discontinuation of long term benzodiazepine use by sending a letter to users in family practice: a prospective controlled intervention study. *Drug Alc Depend.* 2005;78:49–56.
21. Gorgels WJ, Oude Voshaar RC, Mol AJ, et al. Predictors of discontinuation of benzodiazepine prescription after sending a letter to long-term benzodiazepine users in family practice. *Fam Pract.* 2006;23:65–72.
22. Belleville G, Morin CM. Hypnotic discontinuation in chronic insomnia: impact of psychological distress, readiness to change, and self-efficacy. *Health Psychol.* 2008;27:239–248.
23. Stewart R, Niessen WJ, Broer J, et al. General practitioners reduced benzodiazepine prescriptions in an intervention study: a multilevel application. *J Clin Epidemiol.* 2007;60: 1076–1084.

24. Cook JM, Marshall R, Masci C, et al. Physicians' perspective on prescribing benzodiazepines for older adults: a qualitative study. *J Gen Intern Med.* 2007;22:303–307.
25. Bish A, Golombok S, Hallstrom C, et al. The role of coping strategies in protecting against long-term tranquillizer use. *Br J Med Psychol.* 1996;69:101–115.
26. Lader M, Tylee A, Donoghue J, et al. Withdrawing benzodiazepines in primary care. *CNS Drugs.* 2009;23:19–34.
27. Vicens C, Fiol F, Llobera J, et al. Withdrawal from long-term benzodiazepine use: randomised trial in family practice. *Br J Gen Practice.* 2006;56:958–963.
28. Sanchez-Craig M, Cappell H, Busto U, et al. Cognitive-behavioural treatment for benzodiazepine dependence: a comparison of gradual versus abrupt cessation of drug intake. *Br J Addict.* 1987;82:1317–1327.
29. Ashton H. Benzodiazepine withdrawal: outcome in 50 patients. *Br J Addict.* 1987;82:665–671.
30. Rickels K, Schweizer E, Case WG, et al. Long-term therapeutic use of benzodiazepines. I. Effects of abrupt discontinuation. *Arch Gen Psychiatry.* 1990;47:899–907.
31. Schweizer E, Rickels K, Case WG, et al. Long-term therapeutic use of benzodiazepines. II. Effects of gradual taper. *Arch Gen Psychiatry.* 1990;47:908–915.
32. Oude Voshaar RC. *Consecutive Treatment Strategies to Discontinue Long-Term Benzodiazepine Use. A Systematic Evaluation in General Practice.* Wageningen: Ponsen & Looijen BV; 2003.
33. WHO Collaborating Centre for Drugs Statistics Methodology. *Guidelines ATC Classification and DD Assignment.* Oslo: WHO/NCM; 1996.
34. Van den Broek WW, Moleman P. Benzodiazepine-agonsiten. In: Moleman P, ed. *Praktische Psychofarmacologie.* 5th ed. Houten: Prelum uitgevers; 2009:29–54.
35. Couvée JE, Zitman FG. The benzodiazepine withdrawal symptom questionnaire: psychometric evaluation during a discontinuation program in depressed chronic benzodiazepine users in general practice. *Addiction.* 2002;97:337–345.
36. Higgitt A, Fonagy P, Toone B, et al. The prolonged benzodiazepine withdrawal syndrome: anxiety or hysteria? *Acta Psychiatr Scand.* 1990;82:165–168.
37. Busto UE, Sykora K, Sellers EM. A clinical scale to assess benzodiazepine withdrawal. *J Clin Psychopharmacol.* 1989;9:412–416.
38. Tyrer P, Murphy S, Riley P. The benzodiazepine withdrawal symptom questionnaire. *J Aff Disord.* 1990;19:53–61.
39. Lader M. Anxiety or depression during withdrawal of hypnotic treatments. *J Psychosom Res.* 1994;38:113–123.
40. Schweizer E, Rickels K, Case WG, et al. Carbamazepine treatment in patients discontinuing long-term benzodiazepine therapy. Effects on withdrawal severity and outcome. *Arch Gen Psychiatry.* 1991;48:448–452.
41. Klein E, Colin V, Stolk J, et al. Alprazolam withdrawal in patients with panic disorder and generalized anxiety disorder: vulnerability and effect of carbamazepine. *Am J Psychiatry.* 1994;151:1760–1766.
42. Vorma H, Naukkarinen H, Sarna S, et al. Treatment of outpatient with complicated benzodiazepine dependence: comparison of two approaches. *Addiction.* 2002;97:851–859.
43. Rickels K, DeMartinis N, Garcia-Espana F, et al. Imipramine and buspirone in treatment of patients with generalized anxiety disorder who are discontinuing long-term benzodiazepine therapy. *Am J Psychiatry.* 2000;157:1973–1979.
44. Charney DA, Paraherakis AM, Gill KJ. The treatment of sedative-hypnotic dependence: evaluating clinical predictors of outcome. *J Clin Psychiatry.* 2000;61:190–195.
45. Oude Voshaar RC, Gorgels WJ, Mol AJ, et al. Predictors of long-term benzodiazepine abstinence in participants of a randomized controlled benzodiazepine withdrawal program. *Can J Psychiatry.* 2006;51:56–63.
46. Petrovic M, Pevernagie D, Van Den NN, et al. A programme for short-term withdrawal from benzodiazepines in geriatric hospital inpatients: success rate and effect on subjective sleep quality. *Int J Geriatr Psychiatry.* 1999;14:754–760.
47. Schweizer E, Rickels R, de Martinis N, et al. The effect of personality on withdrawal severity and taper outcome in benzodiazepine dependent patients. *Psychol Med.* 1998;28:713–720.
48. O'Brien CP. Benzodiazepine use, abuse, and dependence. *J Clin Psychiatry.* 2005;66[suppl 2]:28–33.
49. Vorma H, Naukkarinen HH, Sarna SJ, et al. Predictors of benzodiazepine discontinuation in subjects manifesting complicated dependence. *Subst Use Misuse.* 2005;40:499–510.
50. Oude Voshaar RC, Gorgels WJ, Mol AJ, et al. Predictors of relapse after discontinuation of long-term benzodiazepine use by minimal intervention: a 2-year follow-up study. *Fam Pract.* 2003;20:370–372.
51. Baillargeon L, Landreville P, Verreault R, et al. Discontinuation of benzodiazepine among older insomniac adults treated with cognitive-behavioural therapy combined with gradual tapering: a randomized trial. *Can Med Assoc J.* 2003;169:1015–1020.
52. Spiegel DA, Bruce TJ, Gregg SF, et al. Does cognitive behavior therapy assist slow-taper alprazolam discontinuation in panic disorder. *Am J Psychiatry.* 1994;151:876–881.
53. Gosselin P, Ladouceur R, Morin CM, et al. Benzodiazepine discontinuation among adults with GAD: A randomized trial of cognitive-behavioral therapy. *J Consult Clin Psychol.* 2006;74:908–917.
54. Otto MW, Pollack MH, Sachs GS, et al. Discontinuation of benzodiazepine treatment: efficacy of cognitive-behavioral therapy for patients with panic disorder. *Am J Psychiatry.* 1993;150:1485–1490.
55. Morin CM, Bastien C, Guay B, et al. Randomized clinical trial of supervised tapering and cognitive behavior therapy to facilitate benzodiazepine discontinuation in older adults with chronic insomnia. *Am J Psychiatry.* 2004;161:332–342.

CHAPTER 36: Nicotine Dependence Management

Douglas Ziedonis ■ David Kalman ■ Chris W. Johnson ■ Lisa A. Mistler

INTRODUCTION

Tobacco use is the leading preventable cause of illness and death in the United States and the second most common cause throughout the world (1–3). About 50% of all smokers are estimated to die from medical diseases worsened or caused by their smoking. This amounts to about 450,000 deaths per year in the United States and over 5 million deaths per year worldwide (4). As public awareness of the dangers associated with tobacco use has risen, the percentage of the US population classified as current smokers has declined, from nearly half the population in the mid-20th century to about 20% in 2008 (5). Compared to the general population, people with psychiatric disorders have much higher rates of nicotine dependence; at least 50% of people with posttraumatic stress disorder and depression and 60% of people with schizophrenia, bipolar disorder, and substance use disorders are dependent (6). These individuals also have more difficulty quitting tobacco use and may have other cofactors of poor outcome such as living with another smoker, lack of social support, higher severity of withdrawal symptoms, poor assertiveness skills, and depressed mood (7).

This chapter focuses on the clinical management of nicotine dependence, including ways to increase motivation for "lower motivated to quit" users as well as evidence-based pharmacological and behavioral therapy (BT) approaches for those ready to quit. Clinicians have a good range of evidence-based interventions that they can integrate into their clinical practice to help motivate patients to quit tobacco use (8).

There are many benefits to quitting tobacco use beyond reducing morbidity and mortality (9). One important strategy for motivating patients and their families to quit involves providing personalized feedback about the specific risks and benefits for them in addition to the general information on what they can expect to receive from quitting. For example, those who quit can expect quick improvement of cardiac functioning and reduced respiratory problems such as shortness of breath, cough, and infections such as influenza, pneumonia, and bronchitis. In the longer term, smoking cessation results in an increased life span and reduced morbidity due to decreased risk of coronary heart disease, stroke, dozens of different cancers including lung cancer, vision problems, wound healing, gum disease, peptic ulcers, and more generally, an improved health-related quality of life. Table 36.1 outlines some of the common health benefits over time. In addition there are many other advantages, including substantial financial savings, improved self-esteem, improved sense of taste and smell, and improved physical features such as whiter teeth, fresher breath, and less premature wrinkling of the skin.

HISTORY OF NICOTINE DEPENDENCE TREATMENT

Tobacco use had historically been seen as a habit or vice. The first tobacco-related Surgeon General's Report referred to tobacco smoking as a form of "habituation" (10). The first Diagnostic and Statistical Manual of Mental Disorders to classify nicotine dependence and nicotine withdrawal syndrome as disorders was in the DSM III (11). Nicotine is now recognized as the primary addictive ingredient in tobacco and nicotine dependence has many characteristics that are behaviorally and physiologically similar to other addictions (2,3). Specific evidence-based treatments, particularly pharmacological treatments, used by the medical profession for treating nicotine dependence are a relatively recent phenomenon. Community-based interventions developed earlier as the risks started to become apparent; the first formal psychosocial treatment method was developed in the early 1960s with support from the Seventh-day Adventist Church (12). The American Lung Association modeled its own group-treatment program on this early work. In the early 1980s, some smokers began to apply the 12-step principles of Alcoholics Anonymous to smoking cessation. This developed into Nicotine Anonymous (Nic-A), still a valuable resource for those attempting to quit. Evidence-based psychosocial approaches, including cognitive–behavioral treatments, have since been developed and will be reviewed later. The first tobacco cessation medication, nicotine gum, was approved by the Food and Drug Administration (FDA) in 1984, and the next medication to be approved in the United States was the nicotine patch in 1993. The off-label usage of the antidepressant bupropion for nicotine dependence therapy began in the mid 1980s; FDA approval was given in 1996. These initial forays into pharmacotherapy were followed by other nicotine-replacement medications, including the nicotine inhaler, nasal spray, and lozenge. Varenicline (a partial agonist at the nicotinic acetylcholine receptor [nAChR]) was approved for nicotine dependence treatment in 2006. There

TABLE 36.1	When smokers quit—the health benefits over time
20 minutes after quitting: Your heart rate and blood pressure drops. (Mahmud, A, Feely, J. Effect of smoking on arterial stiffness and pulse pressure amplification *Hypertension.* 2003;41:183.)	
12 hours after quitting: The carbon monoxide level in your blood drops to normal. (*US Surgeon General's Report*, 1988, p. 202)	
2 weeks to 3 months after quitting: Your circulation improves and your lung function increases. (*US Surgeon General's Report*, 1990, pp. 193, 194,196, 285, 323)	
1 to 9 months after quitting: Coughing and shortness of breath decrease; cilia (tiny hair-like structures that move mucus out of the lungs) regain normal function in the lungs, increasing the ability to handle mucus, clean the lungs, and reduce the risk of infection. (*US Surgeon General's Report*, 1990, pp. 285–287, 304)	
1 year after quitting: The excess risk of coronary heart disease is half that of a smoker's. (*US Surgeon General's Report*, 1990, p. vi)	
5 years after quitting: Your stroke risk is reduced to that of a nonsmoker 5 to 15 years after quitting. (*US Surgeon General's Report*, 1990, p. vi)	
10 years after quitting: The lung cancer death rate is about half that of a continuing smoker's. The risk of cancer of the mouth, throat, esophagus, bladder, cervix, and pancreas decrease. (*US Surgeon General's Report*, 1990, pp. vi, 131, 148, 152, 155, 164, 166)	
15 years after quitting: The risk of coronary heart disease is that of a non-smoker's. (*US Surgeon General's Report*, 1990, p. vi)	
Revised:10/26/2007 http://www.cancer.org/docroot/subsite/greatamericans/content/When_Smokers_Quit.asp	

are now seven FDA-approved medications, three of which are available over-the-counter (nicotine gum, patch, and lozenge). In addition to clinic-based interventions, internet quit programs and telephone quitlines have greatly enhanced access to psychosocial treatments in the past two decades.

NICOTINE DEPENDENCE PRACTICE GUIDELINES

There are several outstanding practice guidelines available that provide more extensive detail for the clinician and can be used as teaching tools. Each describes how they determined the level of evidence to support the recommendations in the guidelines. Table 36.2 outlines several prominent practice guidelines and relevant websites for them.

Nicotine dependence treatment begins by engaging the patient and assessing his or her readiness to change smoking behavior. Treatment should be tailored to the individual and his or her particular circumstances, motivational level, and other unique factors that influence him or her to use tobacco. This may include helping him or her increase motivation to quit and set a quit date, offering pharmacotherapy and psychosocial treatments, and helping him or her sustain abstinence and prevent relapse.

During the engagement phase, a careful assessment includes identifying the pattern of use and severity of dependence. The Fagerström Test for Nicotine Dependence, which assesses time to first cigarette of the day, the number of cigarettes smoked per day, and other smoking characteristics, can help to determine severity (13). Biochemical markers of tobacco use include cotinine levels in the blood and CO levels in expired air. Higher cotinine and CO levels are associated with an increased number of cigarettes per day and indicate the likely severity of nicotine withdrawal. For someone who regularly smokes 20 cigarettes per day, expired-air CO levels are typically in the 10 to 30 parts per million (ppm) range and cotinine levels in the 250 to 300 ng/mL range. The CO meter is easy to use and can be a useful motivational tool. The digital read out clearly demonstrates to a smoker the negative effect of smoking on blood oxygen saturation, an effect which is directly related to shortness-of-breath (a common symptom among smokers) and long-term risk of heart disease.

Assessment for history of prior quit attempts should include treatments used, if any, the length of abstinence, and the full context of relapse. If the patient used a medication, the clinician should review the dose and schedule of treatment, including effective use of medication, avoiding missed doses, and proper use, and also any side effects that developed (including determining whether any side effects may have been due to improper use). Prior psychosocial treatments might include group or individual treatment, American Lung Association and other community support groups, acupuncture, hypnosis, or Nic-A. An assessment should also be made of the person's current reasons for quitting, including his other motivation, commitment, and self-efficacy (perceived ability to quit). Another characteristic component of nicotine dependence treatment is helping the patient pick a "quit date" for when s/he will stop using tobacco products.

<table>
<tr><td colspan="2">**TABLE 36.2** National nicotine dependence treatment guideline</td></tr>
<tr><td colspan="2">Public Health Service/Treating Tobacco Use and Dependence: 2008 Update</td></tr>
<tr><td></td><td>Reference: Treating tobacco use and dependence: 2008 update. Rockville, MD: U.S. Department of Health and Human Services, Public Health Service; 2008 May:257pp.</td></tr>
<tr><td></td><td>Website: http://www.ahrq.gov/path/tobacco.htm</td></tr>
<tr><td></td><td>This is an update of the U.S. Department of Health and Human Services, Public Health Service. Fiore MC, Bailey WC, Cohen SJ, et al. Treating tobacco use and dependence. Clinical practice guideline. Rockville, MD: U.S. Depart of Health and Human Services, Public Health Service; 2000 June:197pp.</td></tr>
<tr><td colspan="2">American Psychiatric Association/Substance Use Disorder Practice Guideline</td></tr>
<tr><td></td><td>Reference: Work group on substance use disorders: treatment of patients with substance use disorders. 2nd ed. American Psychiatric Association. *Am J Psychiatry.* 2006;163(8 suppl):5–82.</td></tr>
<tr><td></td><td>Website: http://www.psychiatryonline.com/content.aspx?aID=141810&searchStr=nicotine+dependence</td></tr>
<tr><td></td><td>This is an update of the APA's 25. Hughes JR, Fiester S, Goldstein M, Resnick M, Rock N, and Ziedonis DM American Psychiatric Association's Practice Guidelines for the Treatment of Patients With Nicotine Dependence. *Am J Psychiatry.* 1996;153(10, entire supplement).</td></tr>
<tr><td colspan="2">US Preventive Services Task Force: Counseling and interventions to prevent tobacco use and tobacco-caused disease in adults and pregnant women</td></tr>
<tr><td></td><td>Reference: U.S. Preventive Services Task Force. Counseling and interventions to prevent tobacco use and tobacco-caused disease in adults and pregnant women: U.S. Preventive Services Task Force reaffirmation recommendation statement. *Ann Intern Med.* 2009;150(8):551–555.</td></tr>
<tr><td></td><td>Website: http://www.ahrq.gov/clinic/uspstf/uspstbac2.htm</td></tr>
<tr><td></td><td>This is an update of: U.S. Preventive Services Task Force (USPSTF). Counseling to prevent tobacco use and tobacco-caused disease: recommendation statement. Rockville, MD: Agency for Healthcare Research and Quality (AHRQ); 2003 Nov.:13pp.</td></tr>
</table>

PHARMACOLOGY OF SMOKED NICOTINE AND MEDICATIONS FOR NICOTINE DEPENDENCE

Pharmacological approaches are an important component of smoking cessation treatment (see Table 36.3), and a brief understanding of the pharmacology of smoked nicotine helps understand nicotine replacement and other medication strategies. The method by which nicotine is administered determines how quickly it crosses the blood–brain barrier and exerts psychoactive effects. Importantly, the strength of these effects is determined by how rapidly blood levels rise. Smoked tobacco is the most "efficient" method for delivering nicotine. Nicotine that is inhaled through a cigarette reaches the brain in less than 10 seconds and reaches peak arterial levels in 20 seconds (14). The half-life of nicotine is often given as 2 hours; however, it varies considerably from individual to

TABLE 36.3 Available pharmacologic therapies

Medication	Available doses (mg)	Minimum length of treatment	Increased odds of quitting versus placebo
Nasal spray	0.5 per spray	3–6 months	2×
Lozenge	2, 4	12 weeks	2×
Gum	2, 4	8–12 weeks	2×
Inhaler	4 per 80 inhalations	8–12 weeks	2×
Transdermal patch	21, 14, 7	8–12 weeks	2×
Bupropion XR	150	12 weeks	2×
Varenicline	0.5, 1	6 months	2× and 3×

individual, ranging from 1 to 4 hours (15). As a result of the short half-life, and because levels begin to fall only 15 to 20 minutes after a cigarette is smoked, nicotine plasma levels rise and fall rapidly many times throughout the day. As the blood levels fall, smokers experience withdrawal distress and an increased urge to smoke. As the levels rise, withdrawal distress is alleviated and the urge to smoke diminishes. Thus, among dependent smokers, the subjectively felt "need" for nicotine is driven, to a large extent, by negative reinforcement mechanisms which are especially potent due to the rapid rise in nicotine blood levels. Indeed, these considerations are central to understanding why dependence, itself, develops (16).

NICOTINE-BASED MEDICATIONS

There are currently five FDA-approved nicotine-based medications and two FDA-approved non-nicotine-based medications. Other nicotine-based approaches, including the electronic cigarette, or e-cigarette, are under consideration. The neurobiological targets of nicotine replacement therapy (NRT) are the same AChRs that tobacco products target. However, NRT works without exposing people to either the other harmful ingredients of tobacco products or to the extreme peaks and troughs in nicotine blood levels that contribute to and help maintain dependence. As a result, the abuse liability of NRTs is low. Among NRTs, the fastest peak plasma nicotine levels are achieved with the nasal spray (within 5 minutes), compared to the average cigarette in which peak arterial levels can reach 100 ng/mL within about 10 seconds. Therefore, smokers are able to titrate nicotine dose through smoking to keep within a certain peak/trough range that they prefer. Other nicotine replacement medications, including the lozenge, gum, and inhaler are far slower acting, with peak levels reached after about 45 minutes for the lozenge, around 30 minutes for the gum, and around 10 minutes for the inhaler. Peak levels with transdermal nicotine are reached much more slowly, after about 3 to 4 hours. Interestingly, despite the wide range of time-to-peak absorption of nicotine, these products appear to have similar abilities to alleviate withdrawal distress and urges and help individuals remain abstinent in the long term (17). Another important factor to consider is how much nicotine is available for delivery with different products and medications. Of note, a typical cigarette contains about 13 mg of nicotine and the average smoker absorbs about 1 to 2 mg into the body. This information can be helpful, along with cotinine or carbon monoxide levels, in determining doing titration of nicotine replacement medication. Other factors that are used as surrogates for level of nicotine dependence and dosing of medication include time to first cigarette and number of cigarettes per day which are two common measures that are used in studies to determine starting dosage of medications.

NON-NICOTINE-BASED MEDICATIONS

The FDA has approved two non-nicotine-based smoking cessation medications, bupropion and varenicline. The pharmacological actions of bupropion that mediate its efficacy in smoking cessation treatment remain to be clarified. However, there are several hypothesized connections between bupropion and smoking cessation. First, bupropion acts as an antagonist at nACh receptors, many of which are present throughout the mesolimbic system (18). The mesolimbic system mediates reinforcement and addictive liability across the spectrum of drugs of abuse. Second, depletion of dopamine is believed to contribute to symptoms of nicotine withdrawal; animal studies suggest that chronic administration of bupropion increases dopamine concentrations, perhaps through an effect on the dopamine transporter. Third, the effects of bupropion on noradrenergic pathways may also attenuate withdrawal symptoms. Bupropion inhibits firing of noradrenergic neurons in animals and decreases whole-body turnover of norepinephrine in humans. Thus, the efficacy of bupropion in smoking cessation treatment may be due, in part, to its effects on the mesolimbic dopaminergic and possibly noradrenergic systems involved in drug withdrawal (19).

The pharmacological actions of varenicline that mediate its efficacy in smoking cessation treatment are likely a function of its competitive nAChR antagonist properties. Varenicline is also an α4β2 nAChR partial agonist. As a partial agonist, the effect of varenicline on dopamine release is only about 35% to 60% compared to nicotine. Less dopamine activity reduces craving and withdrawal symptoms which also decreases the reinforcing aspects of nicotine (20).

EFFICACY OF THE MEDICATION

There is abundant support for the efficacy of the FDA-approved medications for nicotine dependence (7,21). This brief review draws from two comprehensive meta-analytic reviews of this body of work (21,22). Integrating the guidelines and findings of these reviews into clinical practice does take training and organizational change approaches (23) that will be discussed later in this chapter.

In clinical trials, about 14% of participants receiving placebo achieve long-term smoking abstinence of 6 months. The nicotine patch has been the most extensively investigated of the NRTs, and in meta-analyses, has been found to approximately double the odds that a smoker will achieve long-term abstinence. A similar odds ratio has been reported for the nicotine inhaler, lozenge, and nasal spray. Nicotine gum, used for up to 14 weeks, increased the odds of quitting by 50% compared to placebo. Interestingly, however, the odds of quitting doubled in trials of longer-term gum use.

Among the non-nicotine-based medications, bupropion has been the most extensively studied and meta-analyses show that this medication also approximately doubles the odds of quitting. The odds of quitting with varenicline appear to depend on dosage. The 1-mg dose approximately doubles and the 2-mg dose triples the odds of achieving long-term abstinence. When compared with the nicotine patch, varenicline improves the odds of quitting by 60%. By contrast, the efficacy of other medications is unchanged relative to the nicotine patch. However, it is worth noting that the efficacy of a new medication tends to erode somewhat over time. Finally, the two second-line medications for smoking cessation, nortriptyline and clonidine, also approximately double the odds of achieving long-term abstinence (21).

A small but growing number of clinical trials have also investigated the efficacy of combinations of smoking cessation medications. Studies of two combinations in particular—patch and gum, patch and nasal spray—have produced the best results. Participants who received one of these combinations were 3.6 times more likely to achieve abstinence compared to placebo (21). A recent study also found strong evidence for the efficacy of the nicotine patch plus the lozenge (24). Recognizing that tobacco dependence is a chronic relapsing disorder, researchers have also begun to investigate the efficacy of long-term medication treatment. As already noted, meta-analyses found greater efficacy of nicotine gum in studies in which the gum was used for more than 14 weeks compared to fewer than 14 weeks. In addition, one study has reported higher quit rates with long-term use of the nicotine patch (24), and the Cochrane analyses did not find a benefit of long-term patch use (22).

EFFICACY OF MEDICATION IN SMOKERS WITH PSYCHIATRIC DISORDERS

Researchers are increasingly turning their attention to investigating the efficacy of smoking cessation treatments in smokers with psychiatric disorders, where rates of smoking are two to four times higher than in the general population. Two randomized medication trials have been conducted with smokers with schizophrenia. George et al. (25) randomly assigned 32 smokers to bupropion or placebo. Quit rates were 47% and 15% at the end of treatment and 22% and 8% at 6-month follow-up in the bupropion and placebo conditions, respectively. Evins et al. (26) randomly assigned 53 smokers to bupropion or placebo. Quit rates were 16% and 0%, respectively, at the end of treatment. Evidence also suggests that smokers on atypical antipsychotics are more likely to achieve abstinence following a quit attempt than those taking typical antipsychotics. One speculation is that atypical antipsychotic-induced decreases in negative symptoms may improve quit rates by reducing the need to use nicotine to achieve these same effects. There is also little evidence that quitting smoking has an adverse effect on the symptoms of schizophrenia. Study samples have been too small in these studies to investigate differences according to smoking status, however.

Studies have also investigated the efficacy of smoking cessation treatments with alcoholics in early recovery. In a meta-analysis of eight clinical trials of concurrent smoking and alcohol treatment, the mean quit rate at follow-up for both intervention and control conditions was 7% (see Table 36.1 in Prochaska et al. (27) for a description of each study). In a more recent clinical trial, Kalman et al. (28) found no evidence for greater efficacy of a high dose (42-mg) versus standard dose of nicotine replacement, although these smokers tend to be highly nicotine dependent. However, in this study, the likelihood of achieving long-term nicotine abstinence was strongly moderated by length of abstinence from alcohol at time of enrollment in the trial. The smoking abstinence rate among participants with greater than 1 year of alcohol abstinence was 29%, 12% for participants with between 3 and 11 months of abstinence, and 0% among participants with only 2 months of abstinence (see Kalman et al. (29) for a review of this literature). Limited research has shown greater efficacy for combination pharmacotherapy (specifically patch plus gum) among smokers in early recovery.

Importantly, the preponderance of evidence does not indicate that smoking cessation compromises alcohol abstinence. In their meta-analysis, Prochaska et al. (27) found that participants in the concurrent intervention versus alcohol treatment only condition were significantly more likely to be abstinent from alcohol and other drugs. In addition, Kalman et al. (unpublished data) found that few (<10%) of these smokers report that quitting smoking has a negative effect on their ability to cope with urges to drink. Rohsenow et al. (30) found that smoking to cope with urges to drink does not predict relapse to alcohol following a quit attempt. However, in the largest study of tobacco treatment for smokers with comorbid alcohol dependence ($n = 499$), Joseph et al. (31) found that alcohol use outcomes for participants in the concurrent treatment condition were significantly poorer than for participants in the condition in which smoking cessation treatment was provided for 6 months following an alcohol treatment episode (the "delayed" condition). Accordingly, caution dictates that drinking status should be carefully monitored during a smoking quit attempt in this population.

Finally, Hughes (32) reviewed studies investigating the effect of a quit attempt on the emergence of major depression among smokers with a past history of depression. While rates varied widely (from 3% to 24%), within each study, these smokers were more likely to develop major depression following a quit attempt compared to smokers without a past history. Close monitoring of smokers with histories of depression is warranted during smoking cessation treatment. However, clinicians and patients should understand that depressed mood is not uncommon among smokers following a quit attempt and that it often resolves within 1 to 4 weeks. In other words, while careful monitoring of smokers with histories of major depression is advised, negative affect following cessation should not be considered an inevitable precursor to the emergence of a major depressive episode.

FUTURE DIRECTIONS IN PHARMACOTHERAPY

Several medications are currently undergoing evaluation for nicotine dependence. For example, tiagabine, a GABA agonist, diminished craving for cigarettes and increased cognitive performance compared to placebo (33). Preclinical research suggests that medications enhancing GABA decrease the rewarding effects of stimulants, including nicotine. Selegiline, an MAO-B inhibitor, has been shown to decrease craving (34) and there is preliminary evidence for its efficacy (35). PET studies suggest that MAO-B is reduced in the brains of smokers. After smoking cessation the enzyme activity returns to normal, leading to a drop in the level of dopamine and increases in craving. Selegiline is designed to prevent the effect of smoking cessation on dopamine levels and concomitant craving. Other future directions of medication development include vaccines and other immunologic strategies, including both passive and active immunization against nicotine. Using this model, antibodies would reduce the percentage of nicotine that is able to pass across the blood–brain barrier by binding to it, causing it to become a much larger molecule. As a consequence, less nicotine would reach central nervous system receptors and the rewarding and reinforcing effects of tobacco use would be reduced. The antibody-bound fraction of nicotine would also be protected against quick metabolism and excretion. Together, these effects would prolong the effects of nicotine and reduce the rate of required nicotine intake (36).

Stepped-care is a promising approach to treatment that, unfortunately, has been the subject of very limited investigation. In stepped-care, smokers are transitioned to more intensive treatments when smoking abstinence is not achieved with less intensive treatments. While more research needs to be done to determine the efficacy of stepped-care treatment, practitioners may want to consider such an approach with their patients. For example, a practitioner may advise a patient to use the nicotine patch and subsequently add the lozenge or gum if a lapse occurs. In considering this approach, it is important to note that the transition to the "higher" step should probably occur very quickly after a lapse since the great majority of smokers who lapse do not ultimately achieve abstinence. Finally, the practitioner may want to consider "switching" the patient from a nicotine-based to a non-nicotine-based medication. Again, however, the efficacy of this approach awaits further research.

OPTIMAL USE OF THE MEDICATION, INCLUDING SAFETY CONCERNS

Medications are optimally used by individualizing a prescribed regimen to fit each patient's unique needs, including the amount of daily tobacco use and severity of nicotine dependence, comorbid psychiatric and medical conditions, concurrently-taken medications, and patient values and preferences. It is particularly important to educate patients about the appropriate use of medications. For example, "chewing" nicotine gum is a "bite and park" technique. A second example is that patients must understand the effect of acidic beverages on the buccal absorption of nicotine from the gum, lozenge, and inhaler. Two common ways to optimize the medications include the concurrent use of two medications for nicotine dependence (such as patch and a short-acting NRT; bupropion and NRT; etc.) and integrating behavioral and/or other psychosocial treatments with medications. The most recent nicotine dependence treatment practice guidelines (7,21, see Table 36.2) recommend the integration of nicotine dependence treatment medications with behavioral and supportive psychosocial approaches. The chapter will now discuss each of the seven FDA approved medications in more detail, including available dose strengths, indications for particular doses, suggested amount of treatment time, practical considerations, and safety concerns. Of note, serious side effects from nicotine replacement medications overall are rare. There is a range of opinion as to whether these medications should be used by the pregnant smoker; however it is clear that ongoing smoking is a serious concern for the mother and child.

Nicotine Gum

Nicotine gum is available in doses of 2 and 4 mg. Although the 2-mg gum is recommended for people who smoke fewer than 25 cigarettes per day and the 4-mg gum is recommended for people who smoke 25 or more cigarettes per day, many clinicians will just recommend the 4-mg dose during smoking cessation or forced abstinence situations (such as on an airplane or in a locked medical unit). Smokers should use at least one piece every 1 to 2 hours for the first 6 weeks but not exceed 24 pieces in any 24-hour period. The gum is typically used for 8 to 12 weeks, although as noted earlier, some research has shown that longer duration of use is associated with greater efficacy. As with other NRTs, the gum is effective when it is used to maintain a steady plasma nicotine level. Therefore, while it can also be used to cope with urges as they occur, it is unlikely to be effective when only used ad libitum.

Nicotine gum releases nicotine from an ion-exchange resin. The gum should be chewed slowly until a peppery taste is achieved (usually after two or three "chews") and then placed between the teeth and cheek for a few minutes. The process is then repeated until the taste dissipates (after about 30 minutes). The nicotine released has a medicinal effect only when it is absorbed through the oral mucous membranes. It should not be swallowed because absorption depends on the pH of the medium and nicotine cannot be absorbed in a highly acidic medium. For this same reason, acidic beverages (e.g., coffee, soft drinks) should not be used for 30 minutes before or 30 minutes after gum use. Finally, nicotine gum is not recommended for patients with temporomandibular joint problems, dental problems, and dentures.

Side effects and adverse effects of nicotine gum can include local irritation in the mouth, tongue, and throat, mouth ulcers, hiccups, jaw ache, gastrointestinal symptoms (flatulence, indigestion, and nausea), anorexia, and palpitations. Chewing the gum too fast can cause lightheadedness, dizziness, hiccups, nausea, vomiting, or insomnia. Another frequently occurring side effect of chewing nicotine gum is the apparent constriction of the muscles of the throat. As nicotine constricts the blood vessels in the gums, use of nicotine gum for a longer period of time can lead to gum diseases, owing to inadequate blood flow. Heartburn can occur as a side effect of nicotine gum use if the nicotine containing saliva is swallowed rather than absorbed bucally.

Nicotine Toxicity

Nicotine toxicity, while rare, can occur if the individual continues the usual smoking patterns while also using NRT. Although concurrent use can occur with any type of NRT product with tobacco products, clinicians have been most careful when prescribing the NRT patch since this is a long-acting product. In most cases, individuals who start NRT patch might slip and also use a few cigarettes while trying to quit. This does not mean that the NRT should be discontinued; however, the clinician should work with the patient in an attempt to determine the ongoing triggers and whether some short-acting NRT (gum, lozenge, spray, or inhaler) might be added to the NRT patch or if there are some BT strategies that could be helpful to manage ongoing cravings. Tobacco users try to avoid nicotine intoxication symptoms when smoking or using other forms of tobacco. Symptoms of nicotine overdose include chest pain, irregular heartbeat, nausea, vomiting, along with severe dizziness, blurring of vision, and seizures.

Nicotine Lozenge

The nicotine lozenge is available in 2 and 4-mg dosages. The 2-mg lozenge is recommended for tobacco users who are less heavily addicted (e.g., smoke their first cigarette of the day more than 30 minutes after waking in the morning). The 4-mg dose is recommended for more heavily addicted users. Suggested dosing is at least nine lozenges per day during the first 6 weeks of treatment, with one lozenge every 1 to 2 hours. The lozenges should be used for up to 12 weeks with a dose taper to one lozenge every 2 to 4 hours starting in week 7 and further tapering to one lozenge every 4 to 8 hours in weeks 10 to 12. Usage should not exceed 20 lozenges per day. As with the gum and inhaler, nicotine absorption occurs through the oral mucous membranes and users should be instructed to avoid acidic food and drink for 30 minutes before and after use.

Side effects and adverse effects of the nicotine lozenge can include irritation of the teeth, gums and throat, indigestion, diarrhea or constipation, flatulence, insomnia, hiccups, headache, and coughing. The lozenges should be sucked slowly and gently, and not chewed or swallowed, as this may cause heartburn or indigestion. Nicotine toxicity may occur if not used as directed.

Nicotine Patch

Nicotine patches are available in 21, 14, and 7-mg dosages. A typical nicotine dependence treatment regimen can be 8 to 12 weeks, and one method starts the patient on a 21-mg patch for 1 month, followed by 2 weeks of the 14-mg dose and 2 weeks with a 7-mg dose. Some clinicians just prescribe the 21-mg dose for the full 8 to 12 weeks and do not taper to lower mg dose patches. The nicotine patch allows nicotine to be slowly absorbed through the skin. At the start of each day, the patient should place the patch on a relatively hairless, clean location (typically between the neck and waist), rotating the location every day to avoid local skin irritation. The patch may be removed at night if the patient experiences disruption of normal sleep. The nicotine patch provides continuous release of nicotine. Peak nicotine levels are reached after 4 to 6 hours and then gradually decline over the course of the rest of the day, dropping to very low but detectable levels during the night. The 21-mg patch provides the user with about 16-mg of nicotine over a 24-hour period. The transdermal patch does not allow for self-titration of dose, like the other NRT products (gum, spray, inhaler, and lozenge) which can be taken to help quell momentary craving or withdrawal distress.

Side effects and adverse effects of the nicotine patch can include local skin reactions or erythema (25%), itching, burning, or tingling when the patch is applied. This usually goes away within an hour, and is a result of nicotine coming in contact with the skin. Some patients complain of vivid and sometimes unpleasant dreams and/or insomnia with overnight patch use; this is more frequent with the 24-hour patch and one remedy is to remove the patch while sleeping.

Nicotine Nasal Spray

The nicotine nasal spray contains aerosolized nicotine that is delivered to the nostril. Each spray contains 0.5 mg of nicotine. One dose consists of two sprays of 0.5 mg each, one to each nostril (1-mg of nicotine total). Each bottle contains enough nicotine for roughly 50 doses. Initial treatment should be 1 to 2 doses every hour, increasing as needed for relief of withdrawal symptoms. Minimum recommended dosage is eight doses per day. Usage should not exceed 40 doses per day. Recommended duration of therapy with the nasal spray is 3 to 6 months. Nicotine from the nasal spray is absorbed through nasal mucous membranes, resulting in more rapid absorption than NRTs absorbed through oral mucous membranes or transdermally. Therefore, the nasal spray may be appropriate for smokers who respond strongly to the "hit" of nicotine that cigarettes provide. Patients should avoid sniffing, swallowing, or inhaling through the nose while administering doses, as this may increase irritation. The spray is best administered with the head tilted backwards slightly.

Side effects and adverse effects of the nicotine nasal spray can include local airway irritation (i.e., coughing, rhinorrhea, lacrimation, nasal irritation), though tolerance to these appears to develop relatively quickly. Systemic effects include nausea, headache, dizziness, tachycardia, and sweating (37). The spray replicates the repeated administration of nicotine seen in smokers, potentially resulting in reinforcing peaks. As such, an initial concern regarding the spray was the potential for abuse due to the relatively rapid time course to peak blood level, although cases of abuse have been rare.

Nicotine Inhaler

The nicotine inhaler consists of a perforated cartridge filled with 10-mg of nicotine and an additive to reduce irritation from inhaled nicotine. A draw from the inhaler is similar to the average draw from a cigarette and produces about 0.1 μmol of nicotine at room temperature, with nicotine delivery decreasing sharply below 40°F. Similar to other NRTs, the recommended time on the medication is about 12 weeks and this might be extended based on individual situation and need for tapering off. The inhaler must be "puffed" and, therefore, imitates the upper airway stimulation experienced while smoking, though absorption is in fact primarily through the oropharyngeal mucosa. As such, acidic foods such as coffee and soft drinks should be avoided for half an hour before and after use. Efficacy of the inhaler is optimized by frequent use. Users should consume at least six cartridges per day. Each cartridge delivers a 4-mg dose of nicotine over 80 inhalations.

Side effects and adverse effects of the nicotine inhaler are similar to those of the spray and can include local irritation, cough, headache, nausea, dyspepsia. Local irritation in mouth and throat was reported by 40% of patients using the inhaler as compared to 18% of patients on placebo. Coughing (32% active vs. 12% placebo) and rhinitis (23% active vs. 16% placebo) were also higher for those using the inhaler.

Bupropion SR (Zyban, Wellbutrin)

This is a heterocyclic, atypical antidepressant that blocks the reuptake of both dopamine and norepinephrine. It is a strong antagonist to the $\alpha_3\beta_2$ nicotinic receptor and weaker antagonist to the $\alpha_4\beta_2$ and α_7 nicotinic receptors (38). Treatment for nicotine dependence with bupropion SR should begin about 1 to 2 weeks before the patient's quit date. The PDR recommends a dose of 150-mg should be taken each morning for 3 days, followed by a dose of 150-mg twice daily for the remainder of the treatment. From clinical experience, some patients benefit from a longer time period (1 week) before the dose is increased to 300 mg per day. Dosage should not exceed 300 mg daily. Similar to other nicotine dependence treatments, the PDR recommends 12 weeks for treatment; however, individual situations may suggest using the medication for a longer time period.

Bupropion SR's efficacy in nicotine dependence treatment is not due to its antidepressant properties, although it has been found helpful in patients with a prior history of depression. Of note, NRT has also been shown to be effective in helping people with a prior history of depression. If insomnia occurs with bupropion SR, taking the second daily dose earlier in the evening may be helpful. Alcohol should be used moderately while taking bupropion SR, and patients should be evaluated for alcohol dependence or any other substance use disorders. Bupropion SR is contraindicated in patients with a history of seizures or eating disorders, and patients who have used an MAO inhibitor in the past 14 days.

Side effects and adverse effects of bupropion are more limited with this medication in smoking cessation studies compared to studies of depressed patients, although the reason for this is not understood. Some of the common side effects include dry mouth, insomnia, nausea, and skin rashes. Less frequently, use of bupropion is also associated with hostility, agitation, depressed mood, suicidal thoughts and behavior, and attempted suicide. As a result of these concerns, the FDA requires a black-box warning about these possible adverse effects and recommends that the provider monitor any changes in patient mood or behavior while the patient is taking bupropion. This warning about neuropsychiatric problems is also present for varenicline. Finally, as noted, bupropion should not be used for patients who have an eating disorder or who have a history of seizures.

Varenicline (Chantix)

This is a partial agonist of the $\alpha_4\beta_2$ subtype of the nAChR and a full agonist at α_7 neuronal nicotinic receptors (39). Typical nicotine dependence treatment with varenicline involves an initial upward titration of dose. The patient should be instructed to take varenicline on a full stomach, starting at 0.5 mg once daily for the first 3 days followed by 0.5 mg twice daily for 4 days. The patient then takes 1 mg twice daily for 3 months. The patient should be instructed to cease smoking on day 8 of the treatment, when the dosage increases to 1 mg twice daily. Varenicline is approved for up to 6 months. If insomnia becomes an issue, the second pill of the day should be taken at supper instead of bedtime. Dosage of varenicline in patients with significant kidney disease (creatinine clearance ≤30 mL/min) or who are currently on dialysis should be reduced.

Side effects and adverse effects of varenicline can include constipation, flatulence, headache, increased appetite, nausea, vomiting, vivid, strange or unusual dreams, insomnia, taste changes (20). These were the most common adverse events, occurring at twice the rate as with placebo or in more than 5% of subjects. Less frequently, use of varenicline is also associated with hostility, agitation, depressed mood, suicidal thoughts and behavior, and attempted suicide. As a result of these concerns, the FDA requires a black-box warning about these possible adverse effects and recommends that the provider monitor any changes in patient mood or behavior while the patient is taking varenicline.

PSYCHOSOCIAL TREATMENT

Psychosocial treatments are an important component of nicotine dependence treatment. Unfortunately, psychosocial treatments are underutilized and most often not a component of treatment. Treatment is most likely to be medication only. There are many reasons for this, including poor reimbursement, lack of provider training in the techniques, and emphasis on medications due to direct to consumer advertising. All the treatment guidelines recommend the use of psychosocial treatment, and some individuals do not want a medication, preferring to use BT or some other type of psychosocial treatment.

The core psychosocial treatments for nicotine dependence are similar to other substance use disorders, including Cognitive Behavioral Therapy (CBT) (relapse prevention), Motivational Enhancement Therapy/Motivational Interviewing (MET/MI), and 12-step facilitation (7). CBT and MET have been adapted and evaluated specifically for nicotine dependence, both as brief interventions in primary care and more intensive interventions in smoking cessation clinics. Internet- and telephone-based interventions are also broadly available and effective. In general, psychosocial treatments aid in smoking cessation by increasing patient awareness of the risks of tobacco use and the benefits of quitting; increasing motivation to quit, and engage in treatment; providing support for changes in behaviors and activities that will help sustain abstinence over time; encouraging use of medications. Of note, there is a need for more research on treatment that is tailored to specific risk factors such as different psychiatric disorders, motivational levels, and severity of dependence. A comprehensive evaluation and reevaluation if treatment is not working can help with improving treatment outcomes and delivering patient-centered care (40).

Assessing motivation to quit smoking is important. The transtheoretical model describes five stages of motivational readiness to change a behavior: precontemplation, contemplation, preparation, action, and maintenance stages (41). Patients not interested in quitting or who are not willing to readily engage in a discussion about quitting are in the precontemplation stage. Patients willing to discuss the pros and cons of quitting, however, who are not willing to quit for many months are in the contemplation stage. Those who are planning to quit in the next month are in the preparation stage. Those ready to make a quit attempt are in the action stage, and those successfully abstinent for at least 3 to 6 months are in the maintenance stage (41). There are outstanding resources available that provide detail on specific approaches for these different motivational levels. For this chapter, the focus will be on two broad categories into which clinical programs often divide their treatments: those for lower motivated patients (patients in the precontemplation or contemplation stages of change) and those for more highly motivated patients (patients in the preparation or action stages of change).

Lower Motivated Patients

Many patients are lower motivated and do not initially want to stop using tobacco products. Different strategies can be used to help motivate these individuals, including MET, brief personalized feedback interventions, reducing barriers to accessing treatment, connecting to support groups or Healthy Living/Wellness oriented groups, educating their family members, and recommending they speak to others who have quit. Some strategies to help patients prepare for quitting include suggesting they monitor their own tobacco use, which may lead to recognition of how much and in what situations patients are smoking, discussion about the benefits of quitting and risks of continued use, and assessing who could provide support and who or what might be the barriers to change.

MET strategies try to help the individual increase their motivation and commitment to quit. The approach gives the clinician a framework of maintaining empathy, optimism, and a nonconfrontational style in the context of lower motivation and lack of agreement on a goal of abstinence. MET works very well with Prochaska and DiClemente's stages of change model which recommends modifying the strategies based on the patient's readiness for change (42). When patients appear to have no internal motivation to quit, a confrontational style predictably elicits patient resistance and nonengagement in treatment. By "joining up" with patients and meeting them at their stage of change, clinicians are more likely to be able to develop realistic goals with the patient. These might be limited to increasing awareness about risks and benefits, providing knowledge about treatment options, and understanding the particular motivators for and barriers to change. As motivation increases patients may feel more comfortable setting a goal to reduce or eliminate cigarette use only in a specific place (like in the car or home) versus complete abstinence. Brief personal feedback interventions by a physician or other medical staff can increase the likelihood of treatment success two- to tenfold (43,44). Personalized feedback that has been shown to help increase motivation includes giving feedback on the patient's cost of cigarettes for 1 year (cost per day = packs × costs per pack × 365 days), carbon monoxide score (if you have a CO meter), and information on the relationship of the patient's own specific health concerns (cardiac, pulmonary, impotence, wrinkles, wound healing, etc). Other helpful feedback includes discussing the interaction of a patient's medications with tobacco metabolism, and the negative effect on low-density lipids from smoking.

Higher Motivated Patients

The general approach to the motivated client is to initially engage with them by doing a comprehensive assessment, give them information on treatment options, confirm the motivation to quit, learn about potential barriers and strengths, and set a quit date. Helping them quit includes preparing for the quit date, selecting the medication option that they prefer, enlisting supportive friends or family, and engaging in some type of psychosocial treatment (individual, group, internet, Quitline). This phase includes learning about cues and triggers and anticipatory guidance on how to manage these, learning about nicotine withdrawal and the appropriate use of medications to manage the symptoms, and psychosocial strategies to help manage cravings, withdrawal symptoms, and triggers to use. CBT and BT in general are appropriate treatment options for most dependence issues including nicotine dependence. BT involves the identification of affective, cognitive, and environmental cues that trigger tobacco use behavior. Awareness of these trigger cues is helpful in planning intervention strategies to prevent relapse upon their presentation. BT strategies often normalize the role of abstinence lapses during the progress of treatment ("slips") such that "falling off the wagon" is not viewed as an irreparable failure. Discussion of management techniques for withdrawal symptoms, such as sleep disturbance and irritability, can be useful and can allow individuals to learn techniques from others when performed in a group setting. This can also occur as part of a separate relapse prevention coping skills training. Stress management and relaxation training are often used as secondary interventions to buttress behavioral methods. Stimulus control strategies involve the removal or alteration of cues that have been strongly associated with tobacco use, for example, avoiding certain situations that are likely to increase craving. Problems with the group format include low compliance, lack of availability of groups, and a general reluctance to participate on the part of some patients. Problems with the individual format include higher cost and the need for more counselors per population (45).

Despite little controlled research examining psychosocial intervention with spouses and significant others or families, social support for individuals who are attempting to quit using tobacco appears to enhance treatment success. Immediate family and social circles can be involved in treatment via education about supportive roles and behaviors. Concerned others can be engaged as well, providing assessment information or helping to enhance patient motivation. Conjoint sessions with family members may help with motivation, education, and sustaining changes. This may also address a barrier if a family member is a tobacco user.

Hypnosis, acupuncture, and laser therapy are approaches that some individuals believe have been beneficial in their efforts to stop using tobacco. The empirical evidence does not support use of these therapies, though poor study methodology makes a definite conclusion impossible to make (40,46,47). Hypnosis claims to reduce or even ameliorate the desire to use tobacco or to help solidify a commitment to quit. Acupuncture is a traditional Chinese therapy that aims to reduce the withdrawal symptoms associated with tobacco cessation through the insertion of needles into specific areas of the body. Laser therapy purports to operate under the same mechanisms of action as acupuncture using low-level lasers instead of traditional needles.

Many areas now have meetings of Nic-A groups that are structured similarly to Alcoholics Anonymous groups. These groups are based on the 12-step approach to recovery. Nic-A is a relatively new organization and does not therefore have the extensive network that other 12-step programs have developed over time. No formal controlled studies looking at the benefits obtained by attending Nic-A have been conducted. Written self-help materials such as those distributed within Nic-A can play a vital role in patient education, especially regarding the negative health effects of tobacco, the benefits of quitting, and the nature of the addiction. Self-help literature, internet resources, and Nic-A can be efficiently incorporated into formal treatments as well as brief interventions, individual and group treatments.

SPECIAL CONSIDERATIONS

There is no one ideal treatment method for nicotine dependence. Special management issues exist for a number of populations and individual circumstances. Treatment of nicotine dependence in psychiatric populations requires particular attention. Individuals presenting as nicotine dependent with a co-occurring mental illness, another addiction, or all three are more likely to require modifications to traditional nicotine dependence treatment. One critical issue in treatment planning is the actual timing of treatment. There is literature supporting concurrent treatment and also supporting the delay of nicotine dependence treatment until the other issues are stabilized. Successful nicotine cessation in persons with active alcohol dependence is less likely than in individuals recovering from alcohol dependence, though some treatment programs have addressed both simultaneously with success. NRT appears to be especially helpful among smokers with co-occurring mental illness and addiction. Appropriate treatment of the mental illness or other addiction is integral to successful co-treatment, including appropriate medication and therapy methodologies. Individuals presenting with a co-occurring disorder often benefit from an initial motivational enhancement approach that bolsters their sense of self-efficacy and readiness to change (43). Adding BT may help to confront the social and other skill deficits that are often at hand among persons suffering from these co-occurring problems (48). Successful treatment for nicotine dependence has been shown in several studies to be positively associated with recovery from alcohol dependence (48–50). However one notable study, inconsistent with the majority of related literature, suggested that despite reaching a greater number of patients by offering tobacco and alcohol dependence treatment at the same time, concurrent treatment may have an adverse effect on alcohol abstinence when compared to the delay of nicotine dependence treatment (31).

ADDRESSING TOBACCO THROUGH ORGANIZATIONAL CHANGE

The better integration of nicotine dependence treatment into routine clinical practice requires system changes as well as training and education of staff and physicians. All the evidence-based practice guidelines also include information on doing system change. The Addressing Tobacco Through Organizational Change (ATTOC) model has been

TABLE 36.4	Internet resources
NIDA website: http://smoking.drugabuse.gov/
NIDA for Teens: The Science behind Drug Abuse: http://teens.drugabuse.gov/
Surgeon General website: http://www.surgeongeneral.gov/tobacco/
Smoke Free: www.smokefree.gov/
Clearing the Air (2008)—for all smokers interested in quitting
Medication Guide: www.smokefree.gov/medication-guide.aspx
National Cancer Institute
Talk to an Expert By Instant Messaging—LiveHelp—https://cissecure.nci.nih.gov/livehelp/welcome.asp
■ Receive information and advice about quitting smoking through real time text messaging with a National Cancer Institute smoking cessation counselor. Support is offered in English only during specified hours of operation.
By Telephone call from anywhere: 1-877-44U-QUIT (1-877-448-7848)
■ Smoking cessation counselors from the National Cancer Institute are available to answer smoking-related questions in English or Spanish, Monday through Friday, 9:00 AM to 4:30 PM local time.
Any State Quitline: 1-800-QUITNOW (1-800-784-8669 / TTY 1-800-332-8615)
■ This toll-free telephone number connects you to counseling and information about quitting smoking in your state
American Cancer Society (ACS) 1-800-ACS-2345
American Lung Association 1-800-LUNG-USA
For Military Personnel—Quit Tobacco. Make Everyone Proud: www.ucanquit2.org/
■ This site provides tobacco cessation information to members of the U.S. military and is sponsored by the Department of Defense
American Heart Association: http://www.americanheart.org/presenter.jhtml?identifier=4731
Cochrane Reports: http://www.cochrane.org/reviews/en/ab006219.html

used in all types of clinical settings, including inpatient, outpatient, community-based outreach, mental health, addiction, general medical, emergency room settings, etc. (23). The ATTOC model helps an agency/practice to develop specific patient, staff, and environmental goals that will help assure improved patient care, staff recovery, staff training, new policy development, communication, and environmental restrictions or campus tobacco-free initiatives. Staff training is not enough for changing the culture of clinical practice to integrate nicotine dependence treatment. Table 36.4 provides a list of internet sites that can be helpful for patients and staff education.

CONCLUSIONS

Nicotine dependence treatment is efficacious and cost-effective. Blending medications and psychosocial treatments improves clinical outcomes, as does the use of multiple medications for the more severely dependent. There are specific strategies for patients with different levels of motivation; using motivation-based treatment approaches may help patients create more realistic goals in which they are more invested. In addition to individual and group counseling approaches, the use of internet sites and telephone quitlines allow for greater access to help for many. Nic-A is another free resource; however this network is much smaller than that of Alcoholics Anonymous or other 12-step Fellowship groups.

REFERENCES

1. Centers for Disease Control and Prevention. Annual smoking-attributable mortality, years of potential life lost, and economic costs—United States, 1995–1999. *Morb Mortal Wkly Rep.* 2002; 51:300–303.
2. Surgeon General. *The Health Consequences of Smoking: Nicotine Addiction.* Washington DC: U.S. Govt. Print; 1988.
3. American Psychiatric Association. *Diagnostic and Statistical Manual of Mental Disorders (DSM IV).* 4th ed. Washington DC: APA; 1994.
4. World Health Organization. WHO Report on the Global Tobacco Epidemic. The MPOWER package. Geneva: World Health Organization; 2008.
5. Heyman KM, Barnes PM, Schiller JS. *Early Release of Selected Estimates Based on Data From the 2008 National Health Interview Survey.* Hyattsville, MD: National Center for Health Statistics; 2009.
6. Kalman DA, Morissette SB, George TP. Co-morbidity of smoking in patients with psychiatric and substance use disorders. *Am J Addict.* 14:106–123.

7. Kleber HD, Weiss RD, Anton Jr. RF, et al. *Practice Guideline for the Treatment of Patients with Substance use Disorders*. 2nd ed. Washington DC: American Psychiatric Press; 2006.
8. World Health Organization. *World Health Report 2002: Reducing Risks, Promoting Healthy Life*. Geneva: World Health Organization; 2002.
9. Surgeon General. *The Health Benefits of Smoking Cessation*. Washington DC: U.S. Govt. Print; 1990.
10. Surgeon General. *Smoking and Health. Report of the Advisory Committee to the Surgeon General of the Public Health Service*. Washington DC: U.S. Govt. Print; 1964.
11. American Psychiatric Association. *Diagnostic and Statistical Manual of Mental disorders (DSM-III)*. 3rd ed. Washington DC: APA; 1980.
12. McFarland JW, Gimbel HW, Donald WAJ, et al. The 5-day programme to help individuals stop smoking. *Conn Med*. 1964;28: 885–890.
13. Heatherton TF, Kozlowski LT, Frecker RC, et al. The Fagerstrom Test for Nicotine Dependence: a revision of the Fagerstrom Tolerance Questionnaire. *Br J Addict*. 1991;86:1119–1127.
14. Rose JE, Behm FM, Westman EC, et al. Arterial nicotine kinetics during cigarette smoking and intravenous nicotine administration: implications for addiction. *Drug Alcohol Depend*. 1999; 56:99–107.
15. Benowitz NL, Jacob P III, Jones RT, et al. Interindividual variability in the metabolism and cardiovascular effects of nicotine in man. *J Pharmacol Exp Ther*. 1982;221:368–367.
16. Henningfield JE, Keenan RM. Nicotine delivery kinetics and abuse liability. *J Consult Clin Psychol*. 1993;61:743–750.
17. Etter JF, Stapleton JA. Nicotine replacement-therapy for long-term smoking cessation: a meta-analysis. *Tob Control*. 2006;15: 280–285.
18. Watkins SS, Koob GF, Markou A. Neural mechanisms underlying nicotine addiction: acute positive reinforcement and withdrawal. *Nicotine Tob Re*s. 2000;2(1):19–37.
19. Hurt RD, Sachs DPL, Glover ED, et al. A comparison of sustained-release bupropion and placebo for smoking cessation. *N Engl J Med*. 1997;337:1195–1202.
20. Keating GM, Siddiqui AA. Varenicline: a review of its use as an aid to smoking cessation therapy. *CNS Drugs*. 2006;20(1): 945–960.
21. Fiore MC, Jaen CR, Baker TB, et al. *Treating Tobacco Use and Dependence, 2008 Update. Clinical Practice Guideline*. Rockville, MD: U.S. Department of Health and Human Services. Public Health Service; 2008.
22. Stead LF, Perera R, Bullen C, et al. Nicotine replacement for smoking cessation. *Cochrane Database Syst Rev*. 2008;(1): CD000146 pub3.
23. Ziedonis DM, Zammarelli L, Seward G, et al. Addressing tobacco use through organizational change: a case study of an addiction treatment organization. *J Psychoactive Drugs*. 2007;39(4): 451–459.
24. Piper M, Smith S, Schlam T, et al. A randomized placebo-controlled clinical trial of 5 smoking cessation pharmacotherapies. *Arch Gen Psychiatry*. 2009;66(11):1253–1262.
25. George TP, Vessicchio JC, Termine A, et al. A placebo-controlled trial of bupropion for smoking cessation in schizophrenia. *Biol Psychiatry*. 2002;52:53–61.
26. Evins AE, Cather C, Deckersbach T, et al. A double-blind placebo-controlled trial of bupropion sustained-release for smoking cessation in schizophrenia. *J Clin Psychopharmacol*. 2005;25(3):218–225.
27. Prochaska JJ, Delucchi K, Hall SM. A meta-analysis of smoking cessation interventions with individuals in substance abuse treatment or recovery. *J Consult Clin Psychol*. 2004;72: 1144–1156.
28. Kalman D, Kahler CW, Garvey AJ, et al. High-dose nicotine patch therapy for smokers with a history of alcohol dependence: 36-week outcomes. *J Subst Abuse Treat*. 2006;30:213–217.
29. Kalman D, Kim S, DiGirolamo G, et al. Addressing tobacco use disorder in smokers in early remission from alcohol dependence: the case for integrating smoking cessation services in substance use disorder treatment programs. *Clin Psychol Rev*. 2010;30:12–24.
30. Rohsenow DJ, Colby SM, Martin RA, et al. Nicotine and other substance interaction expectancies questionnaire: relationship of expectancies to substance use. *Addict Behav*. 2005;30(4): 629–641.
31. Joseph AM, Willenbring ML, Nugent SM, et al. A randomized trial of concurrent versus delayed smoking intervention for patients in alcohol dependence treatment. *J Stud Alcohol*. 2004; 65:681–691.
32. Hughes JR. Depression during tobacco abstinence. *Nicotine Tob Res*. 2007;9:443–446.
33. Sofuoglu M, Mouratidis M, Yoo S, et al. Effects of Tiagabine in combination with intravenous nicotine in overnight abstinent smokers. *Psychopharmacology*. 2005;2994(181):504–510.
34. Biberman R, Neumann R, Katzir I, et al. A randomized controlled trial of oral selegiline plus nicotine skin patch compared with placebo plus nicotine skin patch for smoking cessation. *Addiction*. 1998;98(10):1403–1407.
35. George TP, Vessicchio JC, Termine A, et al. A preliminary placebo-controlled trial of selegiline hydrochloride for smoking cessation. *Biol Psychiatry*. 2003;53:136–143.
36. LeSage MG, Keyler DE, Pentel PR. Current status of immunologic approaches to treating tobacco dependence: vaccines and nicotine-specific antibodies. *AAPS J*. 2006;8(1):65–75.
37. Sutherland G, Stapleton JA, Russell MAH, et al. Randomised controlled trial of nasal nicotine spray in smoking cessation. *Lancet*. 1992;340:324–329.
38. Slemmer JE, Martin BR, Damaj MI. Bupropion is a nicotinic antagonist. *J Pharmacol Exp Ther* 295:321–327.
39. Mihalak KB, Carroll FI, Luetje CW. Varenicline is a partial agonist at α4β2 and a full agonist at α7 neuronal nicotinic receptors. *Mol Pharmacol*. 2006;70:801–805.
40. Hajek P, Stead LF, West R, et al. Relapse prevention interventions for smoking cessation. *Cochrane Database Syst Rev*. 2005;(1). Art. No.: CD003999. DOI: 10.1002/14651858. CD003999.pub2.
41. Prochaska JO. Stages and process of self-change of smoking: toward an integrative model of change. *J Consult Clin Psychol*. 1983;51:390–395.
42. Prochaska JO, Di Clemente CC, Norcross J. In search of how people change: applications to addictive behavior. *Am Psychol*. 1992;47:1102–1114.
43. Klesges RC, Klesges LM, Myers AW, et al. The effects of phenylpropanolamine on dietary intake, physical activity, and body weight after smoking cessation. *Clin Pharmacol Ther*. 1990;47: 747–754.
44. Steinberg ML, Ziedonis DM, Krejci JA, et al. Motivational interviewing with personalized feedback: a brief intervention for motivating smokers with schizophrenia to seek treatment for tobacco dependence. *J Consult Clin Psychol*. 2004;72(4): 723–728.

45. Hajek P, Belcher M, Stapleton J. Enhancing the impact of groups: an evaluation of two group formats for smokers. *Br J Clin Psychol.* 1985;24:289–294.
46. Abbot NC, Stead LF, White AR, et al. Hypnotherapy for smoking cessation. *Cochrane Database Syst Rev.* 1998;(2): Art. No.: CD001008. DOI: 10.1002/14651858.CD001008.
47. White AR, Rampes H, Campbell JL. Acupuncture and related interventions for smoking cessation. *Cochrane Database Syst Rev.* 2006;(1): Art. No.: CD000009. DOI: 10.1002/14651858. CD000009.pub2.
48. Hughes JR. Possible effects of smoke-free inpatient units on psychiatric diagnosis and treatment. *J Clin Psychiatr.* 1993;54: 109–114.
49. Friend KB, Pagano ME. Smoking cessation and alcohol consumption in individuals in treatment for alcohol use disorders. *J Addict Dis.* 2005;24:61–75.
50. Hughes JR. Treatment of smoking cessation in smokers with past alcohol/drug problems. *J Subst Abuse Treat.* 1993;10: 181–187.

PART 2 ■ Psychosocial and Other Treatments

CHAPTER 37

Self-Help Programs Focused on Substance Use: Active Ingredients and Outcomes

Rudolf H. Moos ■ Christine Timko

Self-help groups (SHGs), often called mutual help or support groups, are an important component of the system of care for individuals with substance use disorders (SUDs). SHGs are composed of individuals who share a common problem, such as a SUD, and who meet regularly to exchange support and information about how to manage and overcome that problem and lead more meaningful lives; in general, these groups do not have professionally trained leaders. SUD patients have high rates of posttreatment relapse and additional episodes of specialized care; participation in SHGs tends to improve the likelihood of achieving and maintaining remission and to reduce the need for further professional care. SHGs offer a safe, structured setting in which members can express their feelings, improve their communication and interpersonal skills, clarify the reasons for their substance abuse, learn self-control, and identify new activities and life goals. Thus, several professional organizations, including the American Psychiatric Association and the American Society of Addiction Medicine, recommend referrals to SHGs as an adjunct to the treatment of patients with SUDS.

SUBSTANCE USE FOCUSED SELF-HELP PROGRAMS

Twelve-Step Self-Help Programs

The most prevalent substance use focused self-help programs, including Alcoholics Anonymous (AA), Narcotics Anonymous (NA), and Cocaine Anonymous (CA), follow traditional 12-step principles. AA is a fellowship whose primary purpose is to help individuals with alcohol-related problems maintain sobriety. It is structured around the 12 steps (e.g., admission of powerlessness over alcohol, belief in a higher power) and 12 traditions (e.g., an emphasis on common welfare and recognition that personal recovery depends on AA unity). Other key aspects of AA involve open and closed-group meetings, sponsorship, and literature that describes AA, shares AA tenets, and provides guidance to recovering individuals. AA estimates that there are about 1.2 million members and 52,000 groups in the United States and more than 2 million members and 105,000 groups worldwide (see www.aa.org).

NA is a fellowship of recovering individuals with drug use problems. NA grew out of AA and is similar to AA in that it provides a structured support network in which members share information about overcoming addiction and living productive, drug-free lives through adherence to the 12 steps and 12 traditions. NA encourages complete abstinence from all drugs, including alcohol, but, consistent with AA, accepts the use of prescribed medications for psychiatric and medical disorders. NA has about 44,000 weekly meetings in more than 120 countries worldwide (see www.na.org).

CA is a fellowship open to individuals who want to stop using cocaine, including "crack" cocaine and other mind-altering substances. CA's program of recovery was adapted from AA and, like AA, uses the 12-step recovery method. There are an estimated 30,000 members and more than 2,000 groups (see www.ca.org).

Traditional 12-step SHGs may have some limitations for individuals who have both substance use and psychiatric disorders, in part because they may be less able to bond with other members who do not share experiences associated with psychiatric problems. Double Trouble in Recovery (DTR) is a 12-step fellowship adapted from the 12-step method of AA; it is designed to meet the unique needs of dually diagnosed individuals. It has amended step 1 and step 12 of the 12-steps to include mental disorders so that, for example, step 1 is "We admitted we were powerless over mental disorders and substance abuse—that our lives had become unmanageable." In addition, it specifically addresses the problems and benefits associated with psychiatric medications (see www.doubletroubleinrecovery.org).

Alternative Self-Help Programs

Many individuals do not believe in 12-step principles or traditions and find it hard to accept the idea of submitting themselves to a Higher Power. This fact has led to the growth of several self-help programs that are not based on the 12 steps, including SMART Recovery, Secular Organizations for Sobriety (SOS), LifeRing, and Women for Sobriety (WFS). (see Chapter 38 for further details on these alternative self-help programs.)

Self-Management and Recovery Training (SMART Recovery) espouses a rational treatment orientation and focuses on teaching individuals new coping skills and more logical ways of thinking and acting. It emphasizes practical methods of changing maladaptive behavior rather than a 12-step or spiritual approach. SMART's four-point program includes: (1) building and maintaining motivation to abstain, (2) learning how to cope with urges, (3) managing thoughts, feelings, and behavior, and (4) balancing momentary and enduring satisfactions (see www.smartrecovery.org).

SOS provides support for individuals who seek to achieve and maintain sobriety, a forum to express thoughts and feelings about recovery, and a nonreligious or secular approach that does not depend on the 12 steps or traditions. Members are expected to acknowledge their addiction and take personal responsibility for achieving and maintaining sobriety. Members tend to be well-educated individuals who have been in professional treatment; many members also attend AA (see www.secularsobriety.org).

LifeRing is another secular alternative to AA and NA. It is similar to AA/NA in that it is oriented toward abstinence; however, it is based on the belief that the positive social reinforcement of the group, rather than a Higher Power, can support individuals in their quest to lead a clean and sober life. Members are encouraged to rely on the group process to guide them toward the development of an individualized path to recovery. In addition to regular in-person group meetings, LifeRing sponsors internet-based chat rooms, a recovery focused message board, and specialized email forums (see www.unhooked.com).

Many women attend and benefit from AA or NA, but some women are alienated by the emphasis on powerlessness, humility, and surrender and/or express discomfort with face-to-face self-disclosure in group meetings populated mostly by men. These issues led to the development of WFS, which shares AA's focus on meditation and spirituality, but espouses the idea that sobriety depends on taking personal responsibility for one's behavior rather than on a Higher Power. WFS provides an alternative for women who prefer an emphasis on improving self-esteem, independence, and personal responsibility, and who wish to explore personal issues in groups with other women (see www.womenforsobriety.org).

SELF-HELP GROUPS AND SUBSTANCE USE AND QUALITY OF LIFE OUTCOMES

The majority of research on substance use focused SHGs has been conducted on 12-step groups. In general, the findings show that individuals with SUDs who regularly attend and become involved in 12-step groups tend to experience better substance use and quality of life outcomes than individuals who do not participate in these groups.

Self-Help Groups and Substance Use Outcomes

Project MATCH (Matching Alcoholism Treatments to Client Heterogeneity) was a large clinical trial that compared the outcome of 12-step facilitation, cognitive–behavioral, and motivational enhancement treatment for patients with alcohol use disorders. Patients who attended AA more often in each 3-month interval after treatment were more likely to maintain abstinence from alcohol in that interval. In addition, more frequent AA attendance in the first 3 months after treatment was related to a higher likelihood of abstinence and fewer alcohol-related consequences in the subsequent 3 months; these findings held for patients in each of the three types of treatment (1).

Comparable findings have been obtained in several other studies. For example, alcohol-dependent individuals who participated in SHGs in the first and second years after intensive outpatient treatment were more likely to be abstinent in the second and third years, respectively; attendance at two or more meetings per week was associated with less severe relapses (2). Outpatients with SUDs who attended more 12-step SHG meetings in the prior 6 months were more likely to be abstinent at both 6-month and 5-year follow-ups (3).

Individuals who attend SHGs over a longer interval are more likely to maintain abstinence than are individuals who stop attending. Patients who participated in a minimum of six meetings in the prior 6 months had better substance use outcomes at 6- and 30-month follow-ups; in addition, this level of attendance prior to the 6-month follow-up was associated with better 30-month outcomes. Individuals who discontinued attendance or attended intermittently had substance use levels that were similar to those of individuals who reported no regular attendance (4).

In a prospective study of individuals with alcohol use disorders, a longer duration of attendance in AA in the first year after help-seeking was associated with a higher likelihood of 1-, 8-, and 16-year abstinence and freedom from drinking problems (Fig. 37.1). Moreover, after controlling for the duration of AA attendance in year 1, the duration of attendance in years 2 to 3 and 4 to 8 was related to a higher likelihood of 16-year abstinence (5).

These findings hold for participation in NA and for SUD patients with different diagnoses. According to Witbrodt and Kaskutas (6), individuals who attended more 12-step group meetings in the first 6 months after seeking treatment were more likely to be abstinent at a 6-month follow-up; those who

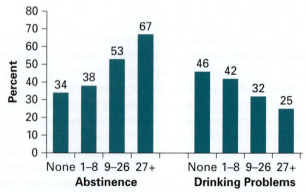

Figure 37.1. Alcohol-related outcomes at 16 years by duration of participation (number of weeks) in AA in the first year ($N = 461$).

attended more meetings in the subsequent 6 months were more likely to be abstinent at a 12-month follow-up. Comparable findings were obtained for patients with alcohol use disorder diagnoses only, patients with drug use disorder diagnoses only, and patients with both drug and alcohol use disorder diagnoses.

Attendance is an important indicator of participation, but it may not adequately reflect the depth of an individual's involvement in a SHG, as shown by such indices as number of steps completed, acceptance of 12-step ideology, and self-identification as a group member. In this respect, patients with cocaine use disorders who regularly engaged in 12-step activities but attended meetings inconsistently had better drug use outcomes than patients who attended consistently but did not regularly engage in 12-step activities (7). Moreover, independent from their level of 12-step group attendance, patients who believed more strongly in 12-step ideology were more likely to be abstinent independent of their level of 12-step group attendance (8).

Maintaining attendance without significant involvement may indicate reluctance to fully accept 12-step group ideology and the goal of abstinence. Individuals who attend SHGs but are unable to embrace key aspects of the program are less likely to benefit from it. Thus, optional SHG attendance may be more closely associated with better substance use outcomes than is SHG attendance that is expected as part of a treatment program, perhaps because voluntary participation reflects more motivation for change than does expected or coerced participation (9).

Self-Help Groups and Quality of Life Outcomes

SHGs also appear to promote positive quality of life outcomes, as indicated by more personal and social resources and better social functioning. With respect to personal resources, participation in SHGs has been associated with increases in self-efficacy for abstinence, and decreases in distress, depression, and psychiatric symptoms. According to Suire and Bothwell (10), individuals who worked all 12 steps had more self-esteem and social confidence and were more optimistic and trusting than were individuals who had not worked all 12 steps. In addition, some studies have shown an association between participation in SHGs and higher levels of spirituality and perceived meaning of life.

Affiliation with 12-step SHGs tends to promote more reliance on approach coping and less on avoidance coping. In this vein, compared to patients who had no continuing care after residential treatment, at a 1-year follow-up patients who attended 12-step SHGs tended to rely more on coping responses aimed toward reducing substance use, such as stimulus control (e.g., removing reminders of drinking from home), counterconditioning (e.g., engaging in physical activity instead of drinking), self-reevaluation (noting that dependency on substances reduces self-esteem), and reinforcement management (rewarding themselves for trying to stop drinking) (11). In addition, a longer duration of AA attendance has been linked to more reliance on approach and less on avoidance coping at both 1-year and 8-year follow-ups (12).

There also is a relatively robust relationship between SHG involvement and better social support and functioning. For example, individuals with alcohol use disorders who attend more AA meetings, and those who attend AA longer, tend to report more support from friends (12). Similarly, individuals with drug use disorders who attended NA once a week or more had more friends and social resources than their peers who did not attend NA or attended infrequently (13).

In a review of this area, Groh and colleagues (14) concluded that more involvement in AA was associated with larger friendship networks, primarily due to acquiring an AA sponsor and the development of new 12-step friends. Involvement in AA was also linked to more support for abstinence from friends and to higher quality friendships and more general support. The strength of affiliation among AA members may be comparable to or even stronger than that for close friends and family members.

LINKAGES BETWEEN SELF-HELP GROUPS AND TREATMENT

Many individuals participate in both SUD treatment and SHGs; in general, these two sources of help tend to bolster involvement in each other and contribute to better substance use outcomes.

PARTICIPATION IN SELF-HELP GROUPS AND TREATMENT

Compared with individuals who initially entered only AA, individuals who entered both treatment and AA participated in AA as much or more in the subsequent 15 years. Individuals who stayed in treatment longer in the first year after initiating help-seeking subsequently showed more sustained participation in AA. More extended treatment later in individuals' help-seeking careers was not associated with later participation in AA, which suggests that treatment providers' referrals to AA have more influence in the context of an initial treatment episode (15).

There also is a more specific link in that, compared to patients who participate in treatment not oriented toward 12-step principles, patients who participate in 12-step facilitation treatment, which introduces patients to 12-step philosophy and encourages them to join a group and get a sponsor, are more likely to affiliate with 12-step SHGs. These patients are more likely to attend meetings, talk to a sponsor, read 12-step literature, incorporate the steps into their daily life, and talk to friends in 12-step groups (1,16). Similarly, patients with cocaine use disorders who receive individual drug counseling based on 12-step philosophy are more likely to attend and participate in SHGs than are comparable patients who receive supportive-expressive or cognitive treatment.

In Project MATCH, patients who developed a stronger alliance in treatment were more likely to attend AA during and after treatment (1). More generally, a supportive and spiritually oriented treatment environment can enhance participation in 12-step activities. In this vein, patients in more supportive treatment environments increased 12-step involvement during treatment; that is, they were more likely to acquire a sponsor and 12-step friends and to read 12-step literature. Moreover, when patients who had a high risk of dropping out of SHGs after treatment were treated in a more supportive environment, their risk of dropout declined (17).

These findings suggest that participation in treatment tends to strengthen SHG affiliation, which may bolster the effects of treatment. A supportive treatment milieu and strong treatment alliance may enhance patients' motivation for recovery and strengthen the impact of counselors' recommendations to maintain affiliation with SHGs. Moreover, treatment that emphasizes the value of SHGs in recovery encourages more SHG involvement than treatment that does not have this emphasis.

TREATMENT, SELF-HELP GROUPS, AND SUBSTANCE USE OUTCOMES

Participation in treatment and participation in SHGs have independent effects on substance use outcomes that tend to augment each other. In the long-term study of individuals with alcohol use disorders described earlier, individuals who participated in both treatment and AA were more likely to be remitted at both 1- and 16-year follow-ups than were individuals who received only treatment in the first year (15). Similarly, among clients with drug use disorders, longer episodes of treatment and weekly or more frequent SHG attendance have been independently associated with 6-month abstinence. Moreover, in a nationwide sample, alcohol-dependent individuals who participated in 12-step SHGs in addition to treatment were more than twice as likely to achieve an abstinent recovery as were individuals who obtained formal treatment alone (18).

The orientation of treatment can also influence the outcome of SHG participation: According to Humphreys and colleagues (16), as the treatment emphasis on 12-step approaches increased, the positive relationship of SHG participation to better substance use outcomes became stronger. More specifically, there was a stronger relationship between 12-step SHG participation and better substance use outcomes among patients from 12-step treatment programs than among patients from cognitive–behavioral or eclectic programs.

Essentially comparable findings were obtained in the NIDA Collaborative Cocaine Treatment study. Patients in individual drug counseling that emphasized 12-step principles changed more in 12-step beliefs and behaviors than did patients in supportive-expressive therapy and cognitive therapy, which placed less emphasis on 12-step ideology. These patients also experienced better substance use outcomes; changes in patients' 12-step beliefs and behaviors explained or mediated part of this effect (19).

Participation in SHGs may even compensate for the lack of services provided in treatment. In a study of dually diagnosed patients in residential programs, more attendance at 12-step SHGs was associated with better discharge and 1-year substance use and psychiatric outcomes. The benefits of 12-step SHG attendance depended on the intensity of services provided during treatment. More 12-step SHG attendance during treatment was associated with better alcohol and drug outcomes at discharge only among patients treated in low-service-intensity programs; more attendance after treatment was associated with better psychiatric and family/social functioning at 1 year only among patients receiving low-service-intensity care (20).

SELF-HELP GROUPS AND HEALTH CARE UTILIZATION AND COSTS

Involvement in SHGs can reduce the use and costs of health care. Compared to individuals who initially obtained professional outpatient care, individuals who entered AA had less income and education and experienced more adverse consequences of drinking at baseline, suggesting somewhat worse prognoses. Nevertheless, individuals who initially sought help from AA had alcohol-related and psychosocial outcomes comparable to those who initially obtained outpatient treatment, and they had 45% lower alcohol-related health care costs over a 3-year period.

By increasing their patients' reliance on SHGs, professional treatment programs that emphasize 12-step approaches may lower subsequent health care costs. In this vein, compared with patients treated in cognitive–behavioral programs, patients treated in 12-step programs were more involved in SHGs at both 1- and 2-year follow-ups after discharge from acute treatment. In contrast, patients treated in cognitive–behavioral programs received more inpatient and outpatient care after discharge, resulting in 64% higher 1-year and 30% higher 2-year annual health care costs. Patients treated in 12-step programs also had higher rates of abstinence at both 1-year and 2-year follow-ups (21).

PERSONAL FACTORS, PARTICIPATION, AND SELF-HELP GROUP OUTCOMES

In a search to identify individuals who may be especially well-suited for participation in SHGs, researchers have examined a range of personal factors, including severity and impairment related to substance use, and disease model beliefs and religious/spiritual orientation. In addition, some studies have considered the suitability of SHGs for individuals with substance use and psychiatric disorders, women, youth, and members of racial and ethnic minority groups.

SEVERITY AND IMPAIRMENT

Individuals who are heavier substance users, have more substance-related problems, and are more dependent on substances are more likely to affiliate with SHGs. More impaired clients also are more likely to continue SHG attendance and less likely to drop out after treatment than less impaired clients are.

Compared to individuals with less severe substance use problems, those with more severe problems may benefit more from SHG involvement. Morgenstern and colleagues (22) found that patients with more severe substance use and psychosocial problems who had high levels of SHG affiliation had better 6-month substance use outcomes; outcomes were poor when group affiliation was low. For patients who had less severe problems, levels of SHG affiliation were not related to outcomes. Individuals with more severe problems may benefit more from the support and structure of SHGs because it helps to alleviate their distress and increase their self-control and interpersonal and coping skills.

Consistent with these ideas, 12-step SHG attendance appears to be more effective for individuals who have relapsed than for those who have maintained interim recovery status. In this regard, for patients who resumed drinking at a 1-year follow-up after residential treatment, those who attended 12-step SHGs after relapse were more likely to be abstinent at 4- to 5-year follow-ups than were those who did not attend these groups. However, among patients who were abstinent at the 1-year follow-up, those who attended SHGs were no more likely to remain abstinent at 4- to 5-year follow-ups than were those who did not attend these groups (23). These findings suggest that 12-step SHGs may be more effective at initiating than maintaining abstinence.

DISEASE MODEL BELIEFS AND RELIGIOUS/SPIRITUAL ORIENTATION

Individuals whose beliefs are more consonant with a 12-step orientation are more likely to affiliate with 12-step SHGs. More specifically, patients who believe in the disease model of substance use, and have an abstinence goal and an alcoholic or addict identity tend to become more involved in SHGs and are less likely to drop out (17). Patients with both SUDs and posttraumatic stress disorders (PTSD) whose beliefs matched 12-step philosophy participated more in SHG activities; more participation was associated with less distress for these patients but with more distress for patients whose beliefs did not match 12-step principles as well (24).

Because of the emphasis on spirituality in 12-step SHGs, there has been speculation that less religious or spiritually inclined individuals may participate and benefit less from these groups. In fact, individuals with stronger religious beliefs are more likely to attend and become involved in 12-step SHGs and are less likely to drop out. In a 3-year study that examined the role of religiosity in AA, more spiritually oriented individuals attended more meetings than secular individuals did; in addition, secular and religiously uncommitted individuals had a sharper decline in AA involvement than spiritual and religious individuals did. These findings suggest that 12-step SHGs are somewhat less engaging for more secular individuals (25). Nevertheless, when they become involved in SHGs, less religious individuals appear to derive as much or more benefit from them as more religious individuals do.

Acceptance-based responding, or awareness of internal experiences that enable an individual to respond adaptively to stressors such as craving, may explain part of the effect of spirituality/religiosity on enhanced 12-step SHG involvement. In this vein, individuals who are higher on spirituality/religiosity tend to increase more in acceptance-based responding. In turn, acceptance-based responding has been linked to increased 12-step SHG involvement (26).

INDIVIDUALS WITH SUBSTANCE USE AND PSYCHIATRIC DISORDERS

A high proportion of patients with SUDs have co-occurring psychiatric disorders. In general, except for individuals with psychotic disorders, dually diagnosed individuals appear to attend and benefit from substance-use-focused 12-step SHGs as much as do individuals with only SUDs. A study of patients discharged from hospital-based residential treatment showed that dually diagnosed patients attended a comparable number of 12-step SHG meetings in the 3 months before 1-, 2-, and 5-year follow-ups as did patients with only SUDs. SHG attendance was similarly associated with a higher likelihood of 5-year remission for both groups of patients (27).

A few studies have focused on individuals with specific psychiatric disorders. Patients with SUDs and PTSD participated as much in 12-step SHGs after treatment as did patients with only SUDs. The dually diagnosed patients who participated more in SHGs were more likely to be abstinent and experienced less distress; they also were more likely to maintain stable remission (28). Some aspects of 12-step SHGs, such as their spiritual emphasis and provision of support, may be especially helpful to trauma survivors by lessening their sense of shame and hopelessness and providing an enhanced sense of purpose in life.

The situation may be different for individuals who have SUDs and co-occurring major depression. Compared to patients with only SUDs, those who also had major depression were less likely to become involved in 12-step SHGs after treatment. At a 2-year follow-up, the association between SHG involvement and abstinence was stronger for patients who had only SUDs than for patients who also had major depression. Depressed individuals may have interpersonal problems that make it harder to develop friendships and to acquire and relate to a sponsor; thus, they may need more support and guidance to become involved in and benefit from 12-step SHGs (29).

Some dually diagnosed individuals may do especially well in dual-focused 12-step SHGs, such as DTR. In fact, individuals who experience more severe consequences of drug use and more psychiatric symptoms are more likely to maintain attendance in DTR, which is associated with better adherence to medication regimens. With respect to outcomes, individuals who affiliate more strongly with DTR are less likely to continue to use substances and tend to improve more in self-efficacy for recovery, leisure time activities, feelings of well-being, and social relationships (30).

Women

Women with alcohol or drug use disorders are at least as likely as are men to attend SHGs and continue to participate in them. Participation in SHGs is also associated with as good or better outcomes for women as for men. In a comparison of women and men with alcohol use disorders, women were more likely than men to attend AA and went to more AA meetings in the first year after initiating help-seeking. More extended participation in AA was associated with a higher likelihood of remission for both women and men; however, the positive association between a longer duration of AA attendance and stable remission was stronger for women (31).

Compared to men, women may be more in tune with 12-step philosophy, which involves acceptance of powerlessness over the abused substance and dependence on a higher power to attain sobriety. Women with SUDs often report low self-esteem, an external locus of control, stable attributions for failure, and frequent substance use when feeling powerless or inadequate. These personal characteristics are congruent with 12-step ideology, which expects individuals with substance use problems to admit past wrongdoing, acknowledge inability to control substance use, and trust a higher power to achieve recovery.

Youth

Many adolescents attend SHGs after treatment and those who do tend to experience better substance use outcomes. In a study that followed adolescents for 8 years, Kelly and colleagues (32) found that AA/NA attendance in the first 6 months and 12 months posttreatment was associated with a higher likelihood of abstinence at each subsequent follow-up. Attendance at just one meeting per week was associated with better outcomes and attendance at three or more meetings per week was associated with complete abstinence.

More broadly, adolescents who have more severe alcohol and drug problems and are more motivated for abstinence are more likely to attend 12-step SHGs. Adolescents often attribute their relapses to social situations and the pressure to use substances. Therefore, they may benefit from contact with a sponsor who can be a role model, structure that helps them avoid high-risk situations, participation in substance-free social events, and the opportunity to try out a new lifestyle (33).

However, adolescents' attendance tends to decline over time, in part due to boredom and lack of perceived fit with the group. There also are important barriers to SHG participation for adolescents, including less severe substance use problems and less motivation for abstinence, practical problems arranging transportation to and from meetings, discomfort with the emphasis on spirituality, and issues that are quite different than those of older members, many of whom are concerned with marital and employment problems that are less relevant to adolescents.

MEMBERS OF RACIAL AND ETHNIC MINORITY GROUPS

Compared to Caucasians, African Americans may be more likely to attend SHGs, increase their affiliation during treatment, identify as AA members, experience a spiritual awakening in AA, and do service at AA meetings; in addition, they appear to be less likely to drop out of SHGs after treatment. Certain characteristics of 12-step SHGs may especially appeal to African American patients, including the fact that meetings are widely available and open to anyone, are free of charge, and have a strong social and spiritual component.

In order to meet their unique recovery needs, African Americans appear to integrate cultural factors and a unique language and perspective in the process of affiliation with AA. According to Durant (34), African Americans are more likely to associate their problems with racism and economic disadvantage than with alcohol abuse; they are less likely to accept the disease concept of alcoholism. Nevertheless, they respond to modeling and support from mentors and sponsors, modify the moral aspects of AA to meet their spiritual needs, and adapt the AA world view to better fit their racial and cultural background.

Compared to non-Hispanic white individuals, Hispanic individuals may be less likely to attend AA after treatment, perhaps because they tend to turn to their existing family and community support system. For example, In Project MATCH, Hispanic individuals attended AA less often after 12-step treatment than non-Hispanic white patients did. Nevertheless, as judged by self-identification as an AA member, having an AA sponsor, experiencing a spiritual awakening, and celebrating an AA birthday, they were as committed to AA as were non-Hispanic whites. Moreover, attendance at AA tends to be associated with decreased alcohol consumption among Hispanic individuals, just as it is among non-Hispanic whites (35).

Twelve-step SHGs have been criticized as less well-suited for American Indian groups because they entail the disclosure of personal problems, emphasize Western religious beliefs, and have a philosophy of powerlessness over alcohol that runs counter to the mores of many tribes on self-reliance and stoicism. Although self-help cannot be universally appropriate for all American Indian tribes, due to the tribes' cultural diversity, it can be appropriate for some. Native American modifications of SHGs incorporate elements of the medicine wheel, purification sweat, and sacred pipe as healing devices. The 12 steps have been blended with the medicine wheel in the Wellbriety Movement, a culture-specific recovery approach for Native Americans.

ACTIVE INGREDIENTS OF SELF-HELP GROUPS

The effectiveness of SHGs in curtailing substance use is based largely on four key ingredients: (1) abstinence-specific and general support that emphasizes the value of identification with abstinence-oriented role models and strong bonds with family, friends, work, and religion; (2) the goal direction and structure of a consistent belief system that espouses a substance-free lifestyle; (3) involvement in rewarding activities that do not involve substance use, including helping others overcome substance use problems; and (4) an emphasis on bolstering members' self-efficacy and coping skills (36).

These critical factors appear to be common change factors that underlie long-term recovery from substance abuse. In support of this idea, a survey of SHGs, including traditional 12-step groups, SMART Recovery, SOS, and WFS, showed that active involvement in a support group was associated with a higher likelihood of long-term remission irrespective of the particular group to which the individual belonged (37).

ABSTINENCE-SPECIFIC AND GENERAL SUPPORT

SHGs are an important source of abstinence-specific and general support, and may be especially effective in counteracting the influence of substance users in a social network. SHGs provide modeling of substance use refusal skills, ideas about how to avoid relapse-inducing situations, practical advice for staying sober, and helpful hints about how to address everyday life problems. Individuals who continue to attend AA more regularly after treatment are more likely to have social network members who support cutting down or quitting substance use than are individuals who attend AA less regularly. In fact, the increase in friends' abstinence-oriented and general support explains part of the positive influence of SHG involvement on remission (3,38).

Individuals who have fewer heavy drinkers in their social network, more people who encourage reduction in drinking, and more AA-based support for reducing drinking, are more likely to initiate and maintain abstinence. In addition, the number of AA-based social network members who support reduced drinking tends to explain part of AA's effect on abstinence. Involvement in AA also may protect individuals from the potential negative influence of a "wet" social network.

GOAL DIRECTION AND STRUCTURE

SHGs provide a context of goal direction and structure in the form of a shared ideology that enhances individuals' immersion into the group. The shared ideology, which is reinforced by explaining group beliefs in understandable terms, specifying changes needed to maintain sobriety, and providing the 12 steps as a guide for change, helps members negotiate the recovery process. AA norms appear to result in more personal and intimate self-disclosures, and less conflict, in AA groups than in non-AA support groups.

There also is a system of taking turns in AA that exemplifies its egalitarian nature and low levels of conflict. In this vein, members acknowledge and identify with previous speakers' contributions and do not openly confront or challenge them, thereby communicating acceptance, maintaining solidarity, and reducing the potential for disagreement. AA members tell life stories aligned with AA principles, which supports the development of shared identities characterized by dependence on AA and relevance to the 12 steps (39).

The emphasis on spirituality is a key aspect of the goal direction in 12-step SHGs. In this sense, AA can be seen as a spiritual recovery movement that rewards compliance with its norms by engaging individuals in a social system that promotes new meaning in their lives. According to Zemore (40), increases in patients' 12-step involvement from baseline to a 1-year follow-up predicted a higher likelihood of abstinence at follow-up. This relationship was partially explained by an increase in religious practices and spirituality, indicating that spiritual change may contribute to recovery within the context of SHG involvement.

REWARDING ACTIVITIES

Another active ingredient of SHGs involves their role in engaging members in rewarding substance-free social pursuits. Members who are more involved in group meetings and related activities, such as doing service and becoming a sponsor, are more likely to achieve and maintain abstinence. Involvement in community groups predicted 1-year abstinence among drug-dependent individuals independent of attendance at AA/NA and being a sponsor. Adolescents may also benefit from the substance-free and sober social events and activities and avoidance of high-risk social situations associated with SHGs. By helping their members become more socially integrated, SHGs increase the likelihood of sustained abstinence.

SHGs also provide members an opportunity to help other individuals in need through service at meetings and other pro-social and altruistic behaviors. Recovering individuals who become sponsors or are otherwise engaged in helping other alcoholic individuals are less likely to relapse and tend to experience fewer depressive symptoms. Similarly, compared to DTR members who were less involved in sharing at meetings and helping other members, those who were more involved in these activities were more likely to remain abstinent (30). The type of helping that occurs in SHGs, which includes personal contact with peers who have similar problems, may be especially beneficial in that it enhances the helper's social status, social bonding, and sense of purpose (41).

SELF-EFFICACY AND COPING SKILLS

Affiliation with AA tends to be associated with increases in members' motivation for abstinence and self-efficacy to avoid drinking. Findings from Project MATCH showed that self-efficacy predicted a higher likelihood of abstinence and explained part of the association between participation in AA and abstinence. In addition, AA attendance at 6 months posttreatment predicted self-efficacy at 9 months, which predicted abstinence at 15 months. Self-efficacy to avoid drinking explained part of the effect of AA attendance on abstinence for both less severe (Type A) and more severe (Type B) alcoholic individuals (42).

A study that assessed patients in 12-step treatment during treatment and at 1- and 6-month follow-ups focused on several common change factors, including commitment to abstinence, self-efficacy, and active cognitive and behavioral coping. More affiliation with AA in the month after treatment was associated with increases in these change factors and with better 1- and 6-month substance use outcomes. These common change factors appeared to explain all of the effect of AA affiliation on 6-month substance use outcomes (43).

As noted earlier, individuals who are more involved in 12-step groups tend to rely more on approach and less on avoidance coping. According to Humphreys and coworkers (38), approach coping responses explained part of the effect of involvement in SHGs on the reduction of substance use. Affiliation with SHGs also promotes more reliance on coping skills directed toward reducing substance use. The active ingredients of SHGs that foster improvement in coping skills likely include modeling of substance use refusal skills, ideas about how to manage relapse-inducing situations, and practical advice for coping with craving.

These effective ingredients of SHGs reflect four critical factors that aid long-term recovery of SUDs: (1) forming bonds and obtaining social support from new relationships and role models, such as a new spouse/partner, friend, or sponsor; (2) supervision or monitoring, such as by a sponsor or spouse/partner, and the provision of positive consequences for continued remission; (3) involvement in rewarding activities that do not involve substance use, such as a program of exercise, spiritual or religious pursuits, or social and service activities that include helping other people; and (4) affiliation with a group that provides a sustained source of hope and self-confidence.

FACILITATING PARTICIPATION IN SELF-HELP GROUPS

In general, individuals participate much longer and more intensively in SHGs than they do in treatment. Many individuals with SUDs depend more on SHGs than on treatment as their dominant resource, probably because SHG meetings are accessible and free, entry is easy, and rewarding long-term social networks are likely to develop. However, there are many obstacles to participation, including lack of motivation and perceived need for help, and dropout rates may approach 75% in 12 months. Accordingly, treatment providers need to strengthen their efforts to help patients engage in these groups.

Relatively few patients begin SHG attendance after treatment; thus, participation should be initiated during treatment to maximize the likelihood that it will persist after treatment. Some useful ways for treatment staff to strengthen the SHG referral process include providing an introduction to a sponsor or recovery guide, addressing potential barriers such as lack of transportation and child care services, and maintaining contact to enhance continuing attendance. For example, when counselors educate patients about 12-step concepts during treatment and provide access to meetings and well-functioning role models who are in recovery, patients tend to find 12-step SHGs more palatable and to increase their involvement in 12-step activities.

12-STEP AND SOCIAL NETWORK TREATMENT

Treatment oriented toward 12-step principles increases the likelihood that an individual will participate and affiliate with 12-step SHGs. More specifically, 12-step facilitation treatment effectively promotes participation in 12-step SHGs among both alcohol- and drug-dependent clients (44). Adaptations of 12-step treatment have been developed for patients with substance use problems seen in nonspecialty care settings (45) and for patients with substance use and other psychiatric disorders. An adaptation for dual diagnosis patients that includes medication compliance and social skills, on-site DTR groups, and case managers who help patients find and attend meetings, appears to be successful in increasing 12-step SHG participation (46).

A socially focused treatment that tries to shape a patient's social network to reinforce sobriety in part by emphasizing the importance of AA can also increase participation in AA. According to Litt and colleagues (47), network support treatment successfully enhanced patients' involvement in AA, increased the proportion of abstinent individuals in patients' social networks, and strengthened the extent to which the social network encouraged abstinence. For individuals who are disinclined to engage fully in treatment, intensive case management may be another way to enhance participation in treatment and in SHGs.

BRIEFER INTERVENTIONS

There also are brief interventions, such as motivational interviews, that appear to help get patients engaged in SHGs. Clients who receive motivational enhancement interventions are more likely to participate in 12-step SHG meetings than do clients in usual care. However, Kahler and colleagues (48) found that a 1-hour motivational enhancement intervention was more effective than a 5-minute brief advice condition, but only for patients with relatively little prior self-help participation. Motivational enhancement involves discussing both the perceived costs and benefits of 12-step SHG involvement and, in so doing, may engender an increase in ambivalence for some patients who are strongly committed to attending AA/NA.

Timko and DeBenedetti (49) designed a three-session intensive referral condition for patients entering outpatient SUD treatment. Counselors gave patients a schedule of SHG meetings, encouraged patients to join a group, work the first steps, and obtain a sponsor; arranged AA/NA members to escort patients to meetings, made contracts with patients to attend meetings, and followed-up by checking with patients about whether they had attended meetings and obtained a sponsor. Compared to patients in a standard referral condition, patients in the intensive referral condition were more likely to attend 12-step SHG meetings, read 12-step literature, provide service during a meeting, consider themselves to be a 12-step group member, celebrate a 12-step birthday, and have a sponsor.

Similarly, in a study of adolescent SUD programs, clinicians from sites at which clients had high SHG attendance rates were more likely to have used active strategies to connect youth with SHGs. These clinicians monitored clients' meeting attendance, prescreened sponsors, and taught clients how to find an appropriate sponsor. They also often worked with local members of AA or NA to conduct meetings at the treatment site; members helped clients find sponsors, arranged transportation to meetings, and linked adolescents to sober social activities within the recovery community (50).

CONCLUSIONS

A high priority for future research is to specify the characteristics of individuals who are most likely to benefit from SHGs and to consider the benefits and barriers to joining SHGs and beliefs associated with participation. We also need more information about the optimal duration and frequency of participation for individuals who vary in the severity of their disorder and level of personal and social resources. Other issues to address include identifying personal and contextual predictors of dropout and of the duration of participation, and developing an integrative model of the role of SHGs and other life context factors as joint influences in the course of relapse and remission.

Most generally, the finding that a longer duration of participation in SHGs predicts better substance use outcomes indicates that SHGs are most beneficial when they become an ongoing supportive aspect of individuals' lives. Extended 12-step group engagement may initiate and maintain the personal and social changes needed to solidify stable remission, especially abstinence-specific and general support, goal direction and structure, involvement in rewarding substance-free activities, and enhanced self-efficacy and coping skills. SHGs represent an important part of the array of effective interventions that can change the enduring aspects of individuals' life contexts and increase the likelihood of a long-term course of recovery.

Key Points
1. Sustained attendance at SHGs is associated with a higher likelihood of abstinence and better substance use outcomes.
2. Involvement in SHGs may accrue benefits over and above those of attendance itself.
3. Delay in participation and dropout from SHGs foreshadows poorer substance use outcomes.
4. Participation in SHGs can substitute for, bolster, and help to explain the benefits of treatment; it can also reduce health care utilization and costs.
5. Less religious individuals appear to benefit from SHGs as much as do individuals who are more religious.
6. In general, expect for individuals with psychotic disorders, individuals with both substance use and psychiatric disorders appear to attend and benefit from substance-use-focused 12-step SHGs as much as do individuals with only SUDs.
7. Women with alcohol or drug use disorders are at least as likely as are men to attend SHGs and to benefit from them.
8. Many adolescents with SUDs attend SHGs after treatment and those who do tend to experience better substance use outcomes.
9. SHGs contribute to better substance use outcomes by providing support, goal direction and structure; exposure to abstinent role models, rewarding substance-free activities, and a focus for building self-confidence and coping skills.

ACKNOWLEDGMENTS

Department of Veterans Affairs Health Services Research and Development Service funds and NIAAA grant AA15685 supported preparation of the manuscript. We thank Bernice Moos for help in reviewing the literature. Due to space limitations, only selected references are provided. The views expressed here are the authors' and do not necessarily reflect the views of the Department of Veterans Affairs.

REFERENCES

1. Tonigan JS, Connors GJ, Miller WR. Participation and involvement in alcoholics anonymous. In: Babor TF, Del Boca FK, eds. *Matching Alcoholism Treatments to Client Heterogeneity: The Results of Project MATCH*. New York, NY: Cambridge University Press; 2003:184–204.
2. Kelly JF, Stout R, Zywiak W, et al. A 3-year study of addiction mutual-help group participation following intensive outpatient treatment. *Alcohol Clin Exp Res*. 2006;30:1381–1392.
3. Weisner C, DeLucchi K, Matzger H, et al. The role of community services and informal support on five-year drinking trajectories of alcohol dependent and problem drinkers. *J Stud Alcohol*. 2003;64:862–873.
4. Kissin W, McLeod C, McKay J. The longitudinal relationship between self-help group attendance and course of recovery. *Eval Program Plan*. 2003;26:311–323.
5. Moos R, Moos B. Participation in treatment and Alcoholics Anonymous: a 16-year follow-up of initially untreated individuals. *J Clin Psychol*. 2006;62:735–750.
6. Witbrodt J, Kaskutas LA. Does diagnosis matter? Differential effects of 12-step participation and social networks on abstinence. *Am J Drug Alcohol Abuse*. 2005;31:685–707.
7. Weiss RD, Griffin ML, Gallop RJ, et al. The effect of 12-step self-help group attendance and participation on drug use outcomes among cocaine-dependent patients. *Drug Alcohol Depend*. 2005;77:177–184.
8. Fiorentine R, Hillhouse MP. Exploring the additive effects of drug misuse treatment and twelve-step involvement: does twelve-step ideology matter? *Subst Use Misuse*. 2005;35:367–397.
9. Zemore SE, Kaskutas LA. Services received and treatment outcomes in day hospital and residential programs. *J Subst Abuse Treat*. 2008;35:232–244.
10. Suire JG, Bothwell RK. The psychosocial benefits of alcoholics anonymous. *Am J Addict*. 2006;15:252–255.
11. Johnson J, Finney J, Moos R. End-of-treatment outcomes in cognitive–behavioral and 12-step substance use treatment programs: do they differ and do they predict 1-year outcomes? *J Subst Abuse Treat*. 2006;31:41–50.
12. Timko C, Finney J, Moos R. The 8-year course of alcohol abuse: gender differences in social context and coping. *Alcohol Clin Exp Res*. 2005;29:612–621.
13. Davey-Rothwell MA, Kuramoto SJ, Latkin CA. Social networks, norms, and 12-step group participation. *Am J Drug Alcohol Abuse*. 2008;34:185–193.
14. Groh DR, Jason LA, Keys CB. Social network variables in alcoholics anonymous: a literature review. *Clin Psychol Rev*. 2008;28:430–450.
15. Moos R, Moos B. Paths of entry into alcoholics anonymous: effects on participation, perceived benefit, and outcome. *Alcohol Clin Exp Res*. 2005;29:1858–1868.
16. Humphreys K, Huebsch P, Finney J, et al. A comparative evaluation of substance abuse treatment: V. Substance abuse treatment can enhance the effectiveness of self-help groups. *Alcohol Clin Exp Res*. 1999;23:558–563.
17. Kelly J, Moos R. Dropout from 12-step self-help groups: Prevalence, predictors, and counteracting treatment-related effects. *J Subst Abuse Treat*. 2003;24:241–250.
18. Dawson DA, Grant BF, Stinson FS, et al. Estimating the effect of help-seeking on achieving recovery from alcohol dependence. *Addiction*. 2006;101:824–834.

19. Crits-Christoph P, Gibbons MBC, Barber JP, et al. Mediators of outcome of psychosocial treatments for cocaine dependence. *J Consult Clin Psychol*. 2003;71:918–925.
20. Timko C, Sempel JM. Intensity of acute services, self-help attendance, and one-year outcomes among dual diagnosis patients. *J Stud Alcohol*. 2004;65:274–282.
21. Humphreys K, Moos R. Encouraging post-treatment self-help group involvement to reduce demand for continuing care services: two-year clinical and utilization outcomes. *Alcohol Clin Exp Res*. 2007;31:64–68.
22. Morgenstern J, Bux DA, Labouvie E, et al. Examining mechanisms of action in 12-step community outpatient treatment. *Drug Alcohol Depend*. 2003;72:237–247.
23. McKellar JD, Harris AH, Moos R. Patients' abstinence status affects the benefits of 12-step self-help group participation on substance use disorder outcomes. *Drug Alcohol Depend*. 2009;99:115–122.
24. Ouimette PC, Humphreys K, Moos R, et al. Self-help participation and functioning among substance use disorder patients with posttraumatic stress disorder. *J Subst Abuse Treat*. 2001;20:25–32.
25. Kaskutas LA, Turk N, Bond J, et al. The role of religion, spirituality, and alcoholics anonymous in sustained sobriety. *Alcohol Treat Q*. 2003;21:1–16.
26. Carrico AW, Gifford EV, Moos R. Spirituality/religiosity promotes acceptance-based responding and twelve-step involvement. *Drug Alcohol Depend*. 2007;89:66–73.
27. Ritsher JB, McKellar JD, Finney JW, et al. Psychiatric comorbidity, continuing care, and mutual-help as predictors of five-year remission from substance use disorders. *J Stud Alcohol*. 2002;63:709–715.
28. Ouimette PC, Moos R, Finney J. Two-year mental health service use and course of remission in patients with substance use and posttraumatic stress disorders. *J Stud Alcohol*. 2000;61:247–253.
29. Kelly J, McKellar JD, Moos R. Major depression in patients with substance use disorders: relationships to 12-step self-help involvement and substance use outcomes. *Addiction*. 2003;98:499–508.
30. Magura S. Effectiveness of dual focus mutual aid for co-occurring substance use and mental health disorders: a review and synthesis of the "double trouble" in recovery evaluation. *Subst Use Misuse*. 2008;43:1904–1926.
31. Moos R, Moos B, Timko C. Gender, treatment, and self-help in remission from alcohol use disorders. *Clin Med Res*. 2006;4:163–174.
32. Kelly JF, Brown SA, Abrantes A, et al. Social recovery model: an 8-year investigation of adolescent 12-step group involvement following inpatient treatment. *Alcohol Clin Exp Res*. 2008;32:1468–1478.
33. Kelly JF, Myers MG. Adolescents' participation in alcoholics anonymous and narcotics anonymous: review, implications, and future directions. *J Psychoact Drugs*. 2007;39:259–269.
34. Durant A. African-American alcoholics: an interpretive/constructivist model of affiliation with alcoholics (AA). *J Ethnicity Subst Abuse*. 2005;4:5–21.
35. Arroyo JA, Miller WR, Tonigan JS. The influence of Hispanic ethnicity on long-term outcome in three alcohol treatment modalities. *J Stud Alcohol*. 2003;64:98–104.
36. Moos R. Active ingredients of substance use focused self-help groups. *Addiction*. 2008;103:387–396.
37. Atkins RG, Hawdon JE. Religiosity and participation in mutual aid support groups for addiction. *J Subst Abuse Treat*. 2007;33:321–331.
38. Humphreys K, Mankowski E, Moos R, et al. Enhanced friendship networks and active coping mediate the effect of self-help groups on substance abuse. *Ann Behav Med*. 1999;21:54–60.
39. O'Halloran S. Symmetry in interaction in meetings of Alcoholics Anonymous: the management of conflict. *Discourse Soc*. 2005;16:535–560.
40. Zemore SE. A role for spiritual change in the benefits of 12-step involvement. *Alcohol Clin Exp Res*. 2007;31:76S–79S.
41. Zemore SE, Pagano ME. Kickbacks from helping others: health and recovery. In: Galanter M, Kaskutas LA, eds. *Recent Developments in Alcoholism*. Vol. 18. New York, NY: Springer; 2008:141–166.
42. Bogenschutz MP, Tonigan JS, Miller WR. Examining the effects of alcoholism typology and AA attendance on self-efficacy as a mechanism of change. *J Stud Alcohol*. 2006;67:562–567.
43. Morgenstern J, Labouvie E, McCrady BS, et al. Affiliation with Alcoholics Anonymous after treatment: a study of its therapeutic effects and mechanisms of action. *J Consult Clin Psychol*. 1997;65:768–777.
44. Walitzer KS, Dermen KH, Barrick C. Facilitating involvement in Alcoholics Anonymous during out-patient treatment: a randomized clinical trial. *Addiction*. 2009;104:391–401.
45. Kelly J, McCrady BS. Twelve-step facilitation in on-specialty settings. In: Galanter M, Kaskutas LA, eds. *Recent Developments in Alcoholism*. Vol. 18. New York, NY: Springer; 2008:321–346.
46. Laudet A, Stanick V, Sands B. An exploration of the effect of on-site 12-step meetings on post-treatment outcomes among polysubstance-dependent outpatient clients. *Eval Rev*. 2007;31:613–646.
47. Litt MD, Kadden RM, Kabela-Cormier E, et al. Changing network support for drinking: initial findings from the network support project. *J Consult Clin Psychol*. 2007;75:542–555.
48. Kahler CW, Read JP, Stuart GL, et al. Motivational enhancement for 12-step involvement among patients undergoing alcohol detoxification. *J Consult Clin Psychol*. 2004;72:736–741.
49. Timko C, DeBenedetti A. A randomized controlled trial of intensive referral to 12-step self-help groups: one-year outcomes. *Drug Alcohol Depend*. 2007;90:270–279.
50. Passetti LL, Godley SH. Adolescent substance abuse treatment clinicians' self-help meeting referral practices and adolescent attendance rates. *J Psychoact Drugs*. 2008;40:29–40.

CHAPTER 38 Alternative Support Groups

Arthur T. Horvath

INTRODUCTION

This chapter overviews five support groups for addictive behavior. These groups are in many aspects fundamentally different from and hence alternatives to 12-step groups such as Alcoholics Anonymous (AA; which is discussed in Chapter 37). In order of longevity these groups are Women for Sobriety (WFS), Secular Organizations for Sobriety/Save Our Selves (SOS), Moderation Management (MM), SMART Recovery (SMART), and LifeRing Secular Recovery (LifeRing). They appear to comprise, as of 2009, the complete list of widely available non-12-step and nonreligious addiction support groups. This chapter is oriented toward providing information that would help professionals and their patients identify whether alternatives in general, and which alternatives in particular, might be helpful for a particular patient.

Groups not covered in this chapter are those with a religious orientation (e.g., Overcomers Outreach; Overcomers in Christ; the Calix Society; Jewish Alcoholics, Chemically Dependent Persons, and Significant Others), those which offer only a small number of meetings (e.g., Men for Sobriety), and Rational Recovery (RR), which as of January 2000, no longer offers support groups.

HISTORY OF ALTERNATIVE SUPPORT GROUPS

The modern alternatives to 12-step groups are relatively young and unknown. AA, the original 12-step group, began in 1935. The oldest of the alternatives, WFS, began in 1976. Despite the continued predominance of 12-step groups in the United States, the alternatives appear slowly to be gaining recognition. Where available, they have become valuable options for professionals and their patients to consider in treatment planning.

Although these alternatives arose in response to the perceived mismatch between some individuals and 12-step groups, the alternatives nevertheless have significant similarities with 12-step groups. All 12-step and alternative groups are without substantial empirical support of effectiveness. All offer 60- to 90-minute meetings at no charge but request donations. All are essentially self-supporting, primarily through member donations and the sale of recovery materials (including newsletters, books, workbooks, audio- and videotapes, and software, some of which may be produced by lay individuals or professionals not directly affiliated with the organization). All have recommended reading lists. All have an extensive official and/or unofficial Internet presence. This presence evolves as Internet communication evolves, and currently includes online meetings (text and/or voice), listserves, message boards, blogs, and chat rooms. All (except MM) are abstinence-oriented. All (except SMART and LifeRing) were founded by an individual who had a new perspective about recovery from addictive behavior. All are nonprofit corporations.

Nevertheless, the programmatic and organizational differences between these alternatives and 12-step groups are substantial and numerous. None emphasize reliance on a "higher power" for recovery. On the other hand, none are opposed to religious or spiritual beliefs in their members. None offer formal sponsorship of new members by experienced members. All are supportive, both in principle and in practice, of appropriate professional treatment for addictive behavior. None expect members to attend for life, but rather to attend for as long as (or whenever) it is helpful. Typical attendance during the period of active involvement is one to three meetings per week, but there are few guidelines about frequency of attendance (vs. AA's "90 meetings in 90 days"). All apparently appeal primarily to higher-functioning individuals (although this may be an artifact of the effort often required to locate these alternatives). All are accepting, both in principle and in practice, of individuals with neurotic (but not necessarily psychotic) comorbidity, and all encourage professional treatment of these conditions. All are flexible in the application of their program principles to the individual case. All are supportive of 12-step groups for individuals who benefit from them. All suggest that some individuals may be impeded in their recovery by 12-step groups, or benefit more from alternative groups, or both. All are very small (in comparison to AA's more than approximately 100,000 meetings worldwide). All operate on very limited budgets. All appear to be evolving more rapidly than 12-step groups.

The differences between 12-step groups and alternatives with respect to meetings and meeting leaders are also substantial and numerous. All groups typically devote major portions of their meetings to discussion ("cross talk"). None have speaker meetings (although their leaders may give separate public presentations). All have, or prefer to have, small meetings (approximately 6 to 12 members), to allow ample opportunity for individual participation. All have meeting formats, but tolerate (or even encourage) significant variation based on local custom or preference. None have extensive meeting rituals. All are led by a facilitator who guides the discussion. The facilitator is typically a peer, and a member of the group's

> **Box 38.1   Contact information for alternative support groups**
>
> **Women for Sobriety (WFS)**
> PO Box 618
> Quakertown, PA 18951–0618
> 215-536-8026 (voice)
> 215-538-9026 (fax)
> www.womenforsobriety.org
>
> **Secular Organizations for Sobriety/Save Our Selves (SOS)**
> 4773 Hollywood Blvd
> Hollywood, CA 90027
> 323-666-4295 (voice)
> 323-666-4271 (fax)
> www.sossobriety.org
>
> **Moderation Management (MM)**
> 22 W 27th Street, 5th Floor
> New York, NY 10001
> www.moderation.org
>
> **SMART Recovery (SMART)**
> 7304 Mentor Avenue, Suite F
> Mentor, OH 44060
> 866-951-5357 (toll free)
> 440-951-5357 (voice)
> 440-951-5358 (fax)
> www.smartrecovery.org
>
> **LifeRing Secular Recovery (LifeRing)**
> 1440 Broadway, Suite 312
> Oakland, CA 94612-2023
> 800-811-4142 (toll free)
> 510-763-0779 (voice)
> 510-763-1513 (fax)
> www.lifering.org
>
> **American Self-Help Clearinghouse**
> www.selfhelpgroups.org

recovery program (but a significant minority of facilitators in some alternatives are behavioral health professionals). Because of the responsibility involved in being a facilitator, all appear to experience difficulty finding facilitators. Because of the lack of a lifetime membership requirement, all experience difficulty retaining facilitators. All aspire to international availability, as qualified facilitators can be identified.

The five alternatives differ from one another primarily on their view of addiction as a disease. WFS takes a disease approach. SOS and LifeRing leave this issue up to the individual, but emphasize physiologic aspects of addiction more than psychological ones. MM views addictive behavior as a learned maladaptive behavior, not a disease. SMART originally also viewed addiction as a learned maladaptive behavior, but in 2008 changed to accepting belief in addiction as a disease (or not) as a personal belief of the participant.

Contact information for each organization is included in Box 38.1, which also includes the American Self-Help Clearinghouse. This clearinghouse maintains a searchable database of over 1100 national, international, model, and online support groups, some of them for addictive behavior, and a database of local support group clearinghouses. These databases can be used to locate specialized support groups for various faiths, occupations, and addictive behaviors.

DESCRIPTION OF EACH ALTERNATIVE SUPPORT GROUP

Women for Sobriety

History

WFS was founded in 1976 by Jean Kirkpatrick, PhD, to address the unique problems of women alcoholics. She suggested that these problems include self-value, self-worth, guilt, and humiliation. Kirkpatrick's own experience was that AA was only partially helpful to her as a woman alcoholic.

Despite professional treatment and AA attendance, Kirkpatrick had a 30-year drinking history, including hospital and mental hospital admissions, hit-and-run accidents (during blackouts), and jail time. She had recurring episodes of depression and attempted suicide several times. She nevertheless earned a doctorate in sociology from the University of Pennsylvania by age 50. She died in June 2000, at the age of 77.

Kirkpatrick's AA experience was one that she believes is typical for women. The recounting of the harm caused by drinking seemed to be good for men in AA and reminded them of their reasons not to relapse. For her, however, recounting painful and often humiliating past drinking experiences seemed to make even more difficult the task of accepting herself and gaining mastery of her life. Additionally, AA did not address how societal views of women (vs. men) alcoholics posed additional challenges for recovering women.

Program

WFS has two primary publications (1,2). The WFS newsletter is *Sobering Thoughts*. WFS is intended for women alcoholics (including those who also have prescription medication problems). Kirkpatrick suggested that for some women AA may be more effective at achieving initial sobriety, because initially a woman may be overwhelmed by the complexity of the WFS program. After several months of abstinence, however, most women are believed to be ready to appreciate the idea that women need a different approach to recovery.

Kirkpatrick was ultimately able to stop drinking in her early 50s by relying on the philosophies of the Unity Church,

> **Box 38.2 The WFS "New Life" acceptance program**
>
> Level I: Accepting alcoholism as a physical disease.
>   "I have a life-threatening (drinking) problem that once had me."
>
> Level II: Discarding negative thoughts, putting guilt behind, and practicing new ways of viewing and solving problems.
>   "Negative thoughts destroy only myself."
>   "Problems bother me only to the degree I permit them to."
>   "The past is gone forever."
>
> Level III: Creating and practicing a new self-image.
>   "I am what I think."
>   "I am a competent woman and have much to give life."
>
> Level IV: Using new attitudes to enforce new behavior patterns.
>   "Happiness is a habit I will develop."
>   "Life can be ordinary or it can be great."
>   "Enthusiasm is my daily exercise."
>
> Level V: Improving relationships as a result of our feelings about self.
>   "Love can change the course of my world."
>   "All love given returns."
>
> Level VI: Recognizing life's priorities: emotional and spiritual growth, self-responsibility.
>   "The fundamental object of life is emotional and spiritual growth."
>   "I am responsible for myself and my actions."
>
> From Kirkpatrick J. *WFS "New Life" Acceptance Program* [brochure]. Quakertown, PA: Women for Sobriety, 1993, with permission. Copyright Jean Kirkpatrick, 1993.

Emerson, and Thoreau. Several years after achieving sobriety, she formulated the principles of WFS, based in part on these philosophies. She also included in WFS cognitive–behavioral change techniques, and an emphasis on health promotion and peer support.

WFS views alcoholism as a physical disease that a woman can grow beyond by learning new self-enhancing behavior via:

1. Positive reinforcement (approval and encouragement)
2. Cognitive strategies (positive thinking)
3. Letting the body help (relaxation techniques, meditation, diet, and physical exercise)
4. Dynamic group involvement.

Box 38.2 presents the WFS "New Life" Acceptance Program.

Meeting Format

WFS meetings are led by a Certified Moderator. Certification is based on having at least 1 year of continuous sobriety, reading *Turnabout* (1), subscribing to the WFS newsletter, and passing a written test about WFS principles and their application in meetings. WFS instituted certification to assure that moderators with a history of AA attendance understood the differences between WFS and AA principles and meeting formats.

Meetings are open to all women alcoholics. Newcomers are given a packet of introductory information. Meetings begin with a reading of the Statement of Purpose, followed by introductions ("Hello, my name is Jean, and I'm a competent woman"). Most of the meeting is devoted to discussion of member's concerns, and how the "New Life" Acceptance Program (see Box 38.2) can be applied to them. Following discussion each member is asked to describe something positive she has accomplished in the past week.

The meeting closes with the members standing, holding hands, and saying: "We are capable and competent, caring and compassionate, always willing to help another, bonded together in overcoming our addictions."

Secular Organizations for Sobriety/Save Our Selves

History

Secular Organizations for Sobriety/Save Our Selves (SOS) was established in 1985 by Jim Christopher, in Hollywood, CA. Christopher had been sober since 1978, initially using AA. He separated from AA early in his recovery, because he wanted an approach that was based on personal responsibility rather than reliance on a higher power. In 1985, he wrote "Sobriety without Superstition" for *Free Inquiry*, a leading U.S. secular humanist journal. Because of the strong positive response to the article he founded SOS.

Program

SOS has two primary publications (3,4), and publishes the *SOS International Newsletter*. Originally intended for alcoholics, SOS has been extended to the full range of addictive behavior (both substance and activity addictions), and in some cases to family members as well. SOS is for individuals who desire recovery but are uncomfortable with the spiritual content of 12-step groups and would prefer a personal responsibility approach. Specialized groups for family members, youth, or youth in dysfunctional families are also allowed. The only requirements of an SOS meeting are that it be secular and promote total abstinence.

SOS views the cycle of addiction as having three elements: physiologic need for the substance, the learned habit of using and all the associations to using, and the denial of both the need and the habit. Over time the addiction becomes the highest priority, and it begins to destroy the rest of life. However, the cycle of addiction can be replaced by the cycle of

> **Box 38.3 Suggested guidelines for sobriety of SOS**
>
> 1. To break the cycle of denial and achieve sobriety, we first acknowledge that we are alcoholics or addicts.
> 2. We reaffirm this truth daily and accept without reservation the fact that, as clean and sober individuals, we cannot and do not drink or use, no matter what.
> 3. Since drinking or using is not an option for us, we take whatever steps are necessary to continue our Sobriety Priority lifelong.
> 4. A quality of life—"the good life"—can be achieved. However, life is also filled with uncertainties. Therefore, we do not drink or use regardless of feelings, circumstances, or conflicts.
> 5. We share in confidence with each other our thoughts and feelings as sober, clean individuals.
> 6. Sobriety is our priority, and we are each responsible for our lives and our sobriety.

sobriety: acknowledgement of the addiction, acceptance of the disease or habit, and making sobriety the highest priority in life (the "Sobriety Priority"). The Sobriety Priority is a cognitive strategy to be applied daily, to weaken associations to using, and to allow new associations to develop. SOS accepts that participants may use a wide variety of techniques or approaches in recovery. SOS emphasizes that it concerns itself only with helping participants accomplish the Sobriety Priority, and not with transforming the rest of life. With sobriety secured, participants are in a much better position to grow as individuals, but this remains a personal matter. Box 38.3 reproduces the Suggested Guidelines for Sobriety.

Meeting Format

The suggested meeting format includes an opening statement summarizing the purpose of the meeting, announcements (e.g., the availability of new literature), anniversaries (of sobriety), the reading of the Suggested Guidelines for Sobriety, and introductions of all present. The meeting proper is next ("This meeting is now open. We ask that you try to keep your sharing to a reasonable length of time so that everyone can participate."). The closing includes passing the hat, and a ritual ("Let's close by giving ourselves a hand for being here to support and celebrate each other's sobriety.")

The members of each SOS group are allowed to create a meeting structure that meets their needs. Most SOS meetings have an active exchange of information, experiences, and ideas.

Moderation Management

History

MM was founded in 1993 by Audrey Kishline to support individuals who desire to moderate their alcohol consumption. Her own experience had been that it was difficult to obtain support for this goal.

During her 20s, Kishline's drinking increased to the level of a moderate problem. She eventually sought treatment. Ultimately, this treatment included two inpatient stays, an aftercare program, and consultation with at least 30 alcoholism treatment professionals, all of whom diagnosed her as "alcoholic." She also attended AA regularly for several years, attending hundreds of meetings. Her initial reaction to treatment was that her drinking became more severe. She suggested that at least in part this increase was a self-fulfilling prophecy based on what she had learned about alcoholism as a disease over which she was powerless. She also suggested that over several years she gradually matured out of her drinking problem, as she became more involved in the responsibilities and activities of life (e.g., marriage, children, homemaking, college courses, hobbies, and friends). As this maturing occurred, her beliefs about herself also evolved. Rather than believing herself to have a disease, she chose to abstain because of the kind of life she wanted to lead.

Several years prior to writing her 1994 book (5), Kishline chose to return to moderate drinking. She asserted that she was misdiagnosed initially, and that moderation of her alcohol consumption had been overlooked as an option for her. She founded MM in the hope that the moderation option would not be overlooked for others in similar situations.

Kishline had a drunk driving crash on March 25, 2000, in which she killed two passengers in an oncoming car. A fact left out of many media reports was that at the time of the crash Kishline had stopped attending MM and had been attending AA for about 2 months. It would not appear to be reasonable to blame either AA or MM for her behavior.

Program

MM originally had one primary publication (5), but switched to another (6). MM is intended for individuals who fit the description "problem drinker" rather than "alcoholic." There are two fundamental requirements for membership: a willingness to accept responsibility for one's own behavior and a desire to moderate (or stop) drinking. MM is not aimed at individuals who have experienced significant withdrawal symptoms from alcohol, who have medical conditions exacerbated by alcohol (e.g., heart disease, diabetes, gastrointestinal problems, and so on), or who are experiencing other relevant conditions including pregnancy or desired pregnancy, a behavioral health disorder, being on medications that interact negatively with alcohol, or being in personal crisis. Lastly, MM is not designed for individuals who are already abstaining successfully after a history of severe dependence.

MM recommends that as early as possible in their MM involvement members abstain for 30 days, during which time they examine how drinking has affected their lives, write down their life priorities, consider the quantity, frequency, and circumstances of their past drinking, and learn the moderation guidelines MM suggests. Members might also complete the Drinker's Checkup, a free interactive program available on the MM website, or the Short Alcohol Dependence Data Questionnaire (SADD) (7), also available on the MM website. On the SADD scores from 1 to 9 suggest low dependence on alcohol, 10 to 19 medium dependence, and 20 or higher (maximum score 45) high dependence. Individuals who score below 16 are considered good candidates for MM. Those who score between 16 and 19 are encouraged to obtain professional assessment before attending a moderation program. Individuals who score 20 and above are encouraged to pursue abstinence. Even individuals with low scores are not discouraged from pursuing abstinence, but are offered the alternative of MM as a means to abstain.

MM hopes to reach problem drinkers early in their problem drinking career by offering an approach that appeals to common sense and does not require excessive effort (relative to the intensity of the problem). MM is therefore partly a prevention program (see Section 8). If an individual is not successful following MM's moderation guidelines, the individual is encouraged to pursue abstinence.

MM views drinking problems as arising from bad habits, rather than being the manifestations of a disease. MM is based on empirically supported cognitive–behavioral moderation training (see Chapter 44). Box 38.4 reprints the nine steps of MM. MM suggests that 6 to 18 months of once-weekly attendance is usually needed for successful completion of its program.

MM understands moderate drinking to be (for men) no more than 4 standard drinks per day, no more than 4 drinking days per week, and no more than 14 standard drinks per week. A standard drink is the amount of alcohol in a 12-ounce bottle of beer, a 5-ounce glass of wine, or a 1.5-ounce shot of liquor, all of which, because of differing concentrations, have approximately equal amounts of pure alcohol. For women, moderate drinking is understood to be no more than 3 standard drinks per day, no more than 4 drinking days per week, and no more than 9 standard drinks per week. Both sexes are encouraged not to drink and drive, or to drink in situations where the drinker or others might be endangered.

Meeting Format

Meetings are led by a moderator, and begin with the reading of an opening statement describing the purpose of MM, followed by a reading of the nine steps (see Box 38.4) and ground rules for members. Visitors (the meetings are open) and newcomers are invited to introduce themselves. Anyone who recently completed the recommended initial 30 days of abstinence is acknowledged.

The first working section of the meeting is devoted to giving every member the opportunity to update the group on the member's activities since the member's last meeting. Feedback by others may be offered. The next working section is general discussion. If no one has a topic to discuss, the moderator suggests one, which would typically be one of the ideas or techniques covered in the MM book. The meeting ends with the reading of a closing statement.

Smart Recovery

History

SMART (Self-Management and Recovery Training) incorporated as a nonprofit organization in 1992 under the name Rational Recovery Self-Help Network. The organization entered into an agreement with Jack Trimpey, the founder and owner of Rational Recovery Systems, to use the name Rational Recovery and to operate Rational Recovery support groups. The board of directors, of which Trimpey was a member, had evolved from an informal group of advisors, mostly mental health professionals, that Trimpey had assembled for an initial meeting in 1991. Trimpey took the leading role in establishing and incorporating the organization.

Beginning about 1993 there was increasing disagreement between Trimpey and the organization about how the organization would be managed, and the nature of its program. These developments culminated in 1994 with the mutual agreement between Trimpey and the organization to separate. This separation was accomplished by changing the organization's name. Individual support groups made their own decisions about which affiliation to maintain. As of 2000, RR groups have ceased altogether.

Box 38.4 The nine steps of MM

1. Attend meetings and learn about the program of MM.
2. Abstain from alcoholic beverages for 30 days and complete steps three through six at this time.
3. Examine how drinking has affected your life.
4. Write down your priorities.
5. Take a look at how much, how often, and under what circumstances you used to drink.
6. Learn the MM guidelines and limits for moderate drinking.
7. Set moderate drinking limits and start weekly "small steps" toward positive lifestyle changes.
8. Review your progress at meetings and update your goals.
9. After achieving your goal of moderation, attend MM meetings any time you feel the need for support, or would like to help newcomers.

From Kishline A. *Moderate Drinking: The Moderation Management Guide for People Who Want to Reduce Their Drinking.* New York, NY: Crown;1995, with permission. Copyright Audrey Kishline, 1994.

> **Box 38.5 SMART Recovery purposes and methods**
>
> 1. We help individuals gain independence from addictive behavior.
> 2. We teach how to:
>   - Enhance and maintain motivation to abstain
>   - Cope with urges
>   - Manage thoughts, feelings, and behavior
>   - Balance momentary and enduring satisfactions.
> 3. Our efforts are based on scientific knowledge, and evolve as scientific knowledge evolves.
> 4. Individuals who have gained independence from addictive behavior are invited to stay involved with us, enhance their gains, and help others.
>
> Reprinted with permission of SMART Recovery. Copyright SMART Recovery, 1996.

Program

SMART has two primary publications (8,9) and extensive training materials for meeting facilitators. The SMART newsletter is *SMART Recovery: News and View*. There is a specialized application for SMART in correctional facilities, the InsideOut program (10), which was developed on a grant from the National Institute on Drug Abuse. The InsideOut program includes a facilitator manual and videotape, participant workbook, and male and female participant videotapes. SMART is intended for individuals who desire to abstain from any addictive behavior (substance or activity), or who are considering abstinence. SMART assumes that there are degrees of addictive behavior, and that all individuals to some degree experience it. Individuals for whom the negative consequences of addictive behavior have become substantial are the ones likely to be considering or desiring abstinence.

The SMART program is consistent with a cognitive–behavioral perspective, which does not require a belief in addiction as a disease. However, just as participants are free to have any conception (or not) of a higher power, they are similarly free to have any understanding of addiction as a disease. Box 38.5 reprints the SMART purposes and methods statement.

There are four primary goals for an individual in the SMART program: motivational maintenance and enhancement, effective urge coping, rational thinking (leading to effective emotional and behavioral management), and lifestyle balance. In service of these goals, many cognitive–behavioral and other psychological techniques are taught. With respect to changing addictive behavior itself, the program draws from established references of the cognitive–behavioral approach (11). Self-help literature on addictive behavior (12–14), as well as cognitive–behavioral self-help literature on a broad range of topics, including mood management, assertiveness training, relationships, effective communication, and stress management, is also recommended (15), and techniques derived from this literature are incorporated into the SMART program. Consistent with SMART's previous affiliation with RR, as well as its cognitive–behavioral orientation, Rational Emotive Behavior Therapy (REBT) techniques and terms (16) are a prominent but not an essential aspect of the SMART program.

Meeting Format

Meetings are open unless closed by local custom. Meetings begin with an opening statement by the facilitator. The statement describes the four primary goals of the SMART program, and outlines the meeting to follow. Participants check in and establish an agenda for who will be the primary focuses of the discussion. The major portion of the meeting follows, consisting of discussion guided by the facilitator on the four primary goals of the SMART program, and the Tools SMART continues to evolve to accomplish these goals, as they apply to the individual situations discussed. One of the principal approaches is to consider "activating events" volunteered by the members. Activating events can include urges, life circumstance changes, thoughts, social interactions, or other experiences that lead or potentially lead to undesired emotions or behavior, including addictive behavior. Activating events are typically analyzed using Ellis' ABCDE method (16). The Disputation step, in which irrational ideas are disputed, can draw upon the entire range of scientific knowledge about addictive behavior. After passing the hat for donations, the formal meeting concludes with a check out, possibly to include each participant proposing a personal homework project, which would put into action the ideas or techniques from the meeting that have been significant for that participant.

LifeRing Secular Recovery

History

LifeRing Secular Recovery (LifeRing) began as the Northern California set of SOS meetings. In 1999, a federal court ruling prohibited SOS from using that name in Northern California. Representatives of the Northern California meetings, on May 23, 1999, adopted the name LifeRing Secular Recovery. During 2000, LifeRing emerged as an organization independent of SOS. A constitutional congress ratified bylaws on February 17, 2001. Some former SOS meetings from outside of Northern California are now affiliated with LifeRing.

Program

LifeRing has two primary publications (17,18). One LifeRing motto is "empower your sober self." LifeRing views the addicted individual as a person in conflict between an "addict self" and "sober selves." Recovery is the process of reinforcing and building connections between the sober selves until they merge into a resilient and predominating sober self. Each participant is encouraged to develop a Personal Recovery Program.

LifeRing uses the "Three-S" philosophy of Sobriety, Secularity, and Self-Help. Sobriety is understood as complete abstinence from alcohol and other drugs. Another LifeRing motto is "we do not drink or use, no matter what." LifeRing welcomes participants of any religious belief or none. Religious or spiritual beliefs are not part of the LifeRing program (Secularity), which focuses on enhancing human effort to overcome addiction. LifeRing meetings focus on reinforcing the participant's striving to maintain sobriety. Individual motivation and effort are understood as the foundations of change of change (Self-Help).

The LifeRing program suggests that there are as many ways to get sober as there are individuals. No one approach will work for all. A successful recovery plan probably involves some learning by experimentation. Therefore, the LifeRing publications emphasize a wide range of tools, including changing one's self-image, understanding the effects of substances, eating well, exercising, and recalling the bad effects of one's use, etc.

Meeting Format

Box 38.6 reprints the suggested opening statement for meetings. Meeting facilitators are termed convenors. Convenors are normally required to have 6 months of recovery. Meetings typically focus on answering the question "how was your week?" Convenors aim to foster a discussion that is informal, supportive, and conversational. The discussion focuses on the challenges to recovery the participants have faced in the previous week, and the ones they expect to face in the upcoming week.

EVIDENCE OF EFFICACY

With respect to experimental evidence of efficacy, alternatives and 12-step groups are similar. Although the 12-step literature is substantially larger, neither has definitive evidence of efficacy. However, the ultimate justification of a support group will not be established by an efficacy study. Millions have attended 12-step groups despite their lack of evidence of efficacy. Although alternatives have lower attendance, they continue to exist, in one instance for more than 30 years. Support groups exist because recovering individuals choose to attend them.

An unfortunate aspect of alternatives is the failure of many professionals to educate patients about their existence. Evidence is emerging about how many professionals exhibit this failing (19), despite numerous calls for both professionals and nonprofessionals to adopt a broader perspective on recovery (20–22).

The majority of the evidence about alternatives addresses the issues of who might differentially benefit from one support group versus another, and who attends these groups. Penn (23) found comparable outcomes for participants in a 12-step or SMART-oriented day-treatment program for the addicted mentally ill. The investigators needed to make the 12-step arm of the study more client-centered (as SMART already is), in order to reduce the subject dropout rate. Atkins (24) found that although participation in any support group is related to good recovery outcomes, subjects whose individual beliefs better matched the support group had greater levels of participation and better outcomes. Nonreligious subjects were less likely to participate in 12-step groups. Religious respondents were less likely to participate in SOS. Religiosity had little impact on SMART Recovery participation.

Box 38.6　LifeRing opening statement for meetings

Opening statement

This is a regular open meeting of LifeRing Secular Recovery. LifeRing is a self-help support group for all people who want to get and stay clean and sober. We feel that in order to remain in recovery, we have to make sobriety the top priority in our lives. By sobriety, we mean complete abstinence from alcohol and other addictive drugs. Out of respect for people of all faiths and none, we conduct our meetings in a secular way, which means that, during this hour we do not use prayer or talk about religion. We rely in our recovery on our own efforts and on the help of the group members and other friends. Everything that we share at this meeting is completely confidential and stays in this room. If you are under the influence of alcohol or drugs now, we ask that you maintain silence at this meeting. You may speak with members afterward.

The meeting format is flexible. We generally begin by checking in and talking about the highlights and heartaches of our past week in recovery, and what we plan to do to stay clean and sober in the coming week. We encourage cross talk throughout the meeting. By cross talk we mean questions and positive, supportive feedback. Positive experiences from your own recovery are welcome. Please allow enough time for everyone to participate by limiting your speaking time if necessary. If this is your first time at this meeting of LifeRing—Welcome. Please introduce yourself by your first name. If you would like, tell us how long you have been in recovery and then tell us about your past week and your coming week in recovery. If you would like to know more about the LifeRing approach, we have LifeRing books and handouts available here. Thank you.

Reprinted with permission of LifeRing Secular Recovery.

As to who is attending WFS and why, Kaskutas (25–28) studied women who attended WFS only, or both WFS and AA. Their responses support the suggestion that women may need a different approach to recovery. Women who attended only WFS reported that they did not feel that they fit in at AA, that AA was too negative, that they disliked the "drunkalogues" and the focus on the past, and that AA is better suited to men's needs than to women's needs. Women attended WFS for support and nurturance, for a safe environment, for discussion about women's issues, and for the emphasis on positives and self-esteem. Attending WFS for 1 year was associated with an increase in self-esteem. For women who attended both WFS and AA, insurance against relapse and AA's availability were frequently cited reasons to attend AA. Respondents were primarily white, educated, middle aged, and middle or upper class. Most had also participated in individual psychotherapy. Kaskutas and colleagues (29,30) have begun to consider how recoveries in both WFS and 12-step groups can be understood from the broader perspectives of world views and spiritual activities. It seems likely that studying WFS participants—and eventually participants in the entire range of alternative support groups—will greatly expand our understanding of the diversity of recovery.

SOS participants are predominantly white, educated, and nontheistic (31). Most have had negative experiences with AA. Connors and Derman (32) found similar demographics, but less negative experience with AA. Both surveys found that SOS involvement was associated with sobriety.

MM participants are white, middle-class, and well-educated. They appreciate the nondisease approach to recovery, and find the emphasis on choice and self-control a better match for their values (33). MM tends to attract more women and younger participants (34). There are mixed findings about level of physical dependence on alcohol (34–36). Individuals who inquire about MM then actually attend MM have more serious alcohol problems than those who simply inquire (35). Perhaps as MM has become better known it has attracted more women and individuals with higher levels of alcohol problems (36).

SMART Recovery participants have a significantly higher level of internal locus of control than do AA members (37). LifeRing presents the results of a membership survey on its website. The membership is comparable to the other alternatives.

HOW ALTERNATIVE SUPPORT GROUPS ARE OPTIMALLY USED?

If an individual has no experience with addictive behavior support groups, sampling all that are available would seem most sensible. Further research may provide guidance regarding the initial matching of individuals to addictive behavior support groups. However, given the general paucity of *treatment* matching findings, we might expect to discover that it is difficult to predict which individuals will do better in which support groups. The wisest course of action in practice, until clear findings suggest otherwise, would appear to be encouraging patients to sample the available support groups and make their own choices.

If an individual has no strong preferences, 12-step groups would seem more desirable than the alternatives simply because of their availability and size (which increase the likelihood that suitable models of success would be identified). If alternatives are preferred, and more than one is reasonably proximate and not inappropriate for one's gender (WFS) or goal (MM), on what basis might one be selected over another? Although the information provided here may be helpful, probably the best test of compatibility is the individual's reaction to each available meeting. Because the quality of these meetings is quite dependent on the style and ability of the facilitator, it seems likely that the group environment the facilitator engenders may be a larger factor in the desirability of an individual meeting than the organization's official program or meeting format. Consequently, where more than one alternative is available, an individual might attend selected meetings of each. Just as there is presumably a high degree of variability in the helpfulness of 12-step sponsors, there is presumably a high degree of variability in the helpfulness of the individual meetings of alternative support groups.

Excellent advice has been offered on how to integrate mental health treatment with 12-step attendance (20). This advice is needed because of the apparent contradictions between these two perspectives. There appear to be far fewer of such contradictions for the individual attending an alternative. Similarly, because alternatives, like mental health treatment, tend to emphasize self-empowerment, and 12-step groups tend to emphasize powerlessness, contradictions are also likely to arise if the individual attends both alternative and 12-step groups and/or treatment. However, many individuals are able to look past these contradictions and experience benefits from both approaches. Some, for instance, appreciate the social support of 12-step groups (which are also more available), but rely on alternatives for their primary orientation to recovery.

If no suitable group is available, an option for the motivated individual, depending on the desired affiliation, would be to start one's own group. Given that teaching a subject is often the best way to learn it, this option has much to recommend it. The objection that those in early recovery should be guided by those in long-term recovery overlooks the fact that recoveries without this guidance occur routinely (38,39). If attending or starting a group is not an option, the literature of one or more of these alternatives may by itself be helpful. As previously noted, all the alternatives have extensive Internet presences, which may be of benefit to those who can access them.

SPECIAL CONSIDERATIONS

Not included in this chapter are estimates of the number of groups each organization offers. None of these organizations has a substantial administrative staff. The careful monitoring of currently active meetings is necessarily a low priority, given the challenges faced in disseminating information about the existence of these organizations. The order of magnitude for the number of each organization's meetings is "hundreds," whereas for AA the order of magnitude is "tens of thousands." Of more significance to the provider or patient is whether there are meetings in the patient's locality.

However, all of these organizations are making increasing use of the communication options the Internet continues to develop. Therefore, the absence of local meetings appears to be a decreasing impediment to active involvement in these organizations for individuals willing to go online. Although meetings-per-week is an obvious metric in the face-to-face world, we need to await the development of widely recognized metrics in the virtual world in order to assess the relative sizes of the online communities each of these organizations is sponsoring. A noteworthy aspect of these virtual communities is that, with the use of screen names, the anonymity in recovery that AA suggested as valuable is now a realistic option.

Serious ethical and legal issues may arise when an individual, for considered and responsible reasons, chooses to pursue an alternative approach to recovery, but a treatment provider or third party insists on 12-step group attendance and/or 12-step-oriented treatment. It would appear to be unethical to insist that an individual use a 12-step approach to recovery if the individual wishes to pursue another approach. However, insistence on a 12-step recovery approach continues to be widespread (19).

If the third party is the government, then a series of U.S. Federal Circuit Court decisions that began in 1996 is relevant. These five decisions (2nd, 3rd, 7th, 8th, and 9th Circuit) have held that government-required 12-step attendance violates the establishment clause of the U.S. Constitution's First Amendment (40). Although the distinction between a religious and spiritual approach is widely made in the 12-step community (with 12-step groups being considered of the latter type), these decisions have held that 12-step groups are religious enough that a citizen cannot be ordered by the government to attend one. The U.S. Supreme Court has already declined to hear an appeal of the decision in the 2nd Circuit. It appears likely that further decisions around this precedent will be in lower courts, perhaps for the purpose of awarding damages. Given the frequency with which judges, probation, and parole officers order individuals in the criminal justice system to "attend AA," the ramifications of these decisions, for alternative support groups in particular and the addiction treatment community in general, are just beginning to be recognized.

CONCLUSIONS

A fundamental conclusion about alternative support groups is that they could be highly valuable resources for many individuals, but awareness of their existence is slight and growing very slowly. This conclusion gives rise to a number of questions. Will enough individuals attend alternatives so that one or more may come to exist as equal members of the recovery community, and not merely as "alternatives?" Will widespread awareness of the existence of alternatives increase the number of individuals involved in support groups (or recovery or treatment) or will they draw their participants only from those who otherwise would have attended 12-step groups? How much time will be needed before there is widespread awareness of these recovery resources? What are the root causes of the slow growth of awareness about alternatives, and what can be done to address these causes? If awareness continues to grow too slowly, would some form of affirmative action be appropriate, and who would sponsor this affirmative action?

ACKNOWLEDGMENTS

The author gratefully acknowledges the assistance of the organizations described in this chapter. Nevertheless, all opinions and any errors are attributable solely to the author.

REFERENCES

1. Kirkpatrick J. *Turnabout. New Help for the Woman Alcoholic.* New York, NY: Bantam Books; 1990.
2. Kirkpatrick J. *Goodbye Hangovers, Hello Life: Self-Help for Women.* New York, NY: Ballantine Books; 1986.
3. Christopher J. *How to Stay Sober. Recovery without Religion.* Buffalo, NY: Prometheus Books; 1988.
4. Christopher J. *Unhooked. Staying Sober and Drug Free.* Buffalo, NY: Prometheus Books; 1989.
5. Kishline A. *Moderate Drinking: The Moderation Management Guide for People Who Want to Reduce Their Drinking.* New York, NY: Crown; 1996.
6. Rotgers F, Kern MF, Hoeltzel R. *Responsible Drinking: A Moderation Management Approach for Problem Drinkers.* Oakland, CA: New Harbinger; 2002.
7. Raistrick D, Dunbar G, Davidson R. Development of a questionnaire to measure alcohol dependence. *Br J Addict.* 1983;78:89–95.
8. SMART Recovery. *SMART Recovery Handbook.* Mentor, OH: Author; 2004.
9. SMART Recovery. *Facilitator Manual.* Mentor, OH: Author; 2006.
10. Inflexxion. *InsideOut: A SMART Recovery Correctional Program.* Newton, MA: Author; 2002.
11. Hester RK, Miller WR, eds. *Handbook of Alcoholism Treatment Approaches: Effective Alternatives.* Boston, MA: Allyn & Bacon; 2002.
12. Ellis A, Velten E. *When AA Doesn't Work for you: Rational Steps to Quitting Alcohol.* Fort Lee, NJ: Barricade; 1992.
13. Prochaska JO, Norcross JC, DiClemente CC. *Changing for Good: The Revolutionary Program that Explains the Six Stages of Change and Teaches You How to Free Yourself from Bad Habits.* New York: William Morrow; 1994.
14. Horvath AT. *Sex, Drugs, Gambling and Chocolate: A Workbook for Overcoming Addictions.* San Luis Obispo, CA: Impact; 1999.
15. Norcross JC, Santrock JW, Campbell LF, et al. *Authoritative Guide to Self-Help Resources in Mental Health, Revised Edition.* New York, NY: Guilford Press; 2003.
16. Ellis A, Harper RA. *A New Guide to Rational Living.* Englewood Cliffs, NJ: Prentice-Hall; 1975.
17. Nicolaus M. *Recovery by Choice: Living and Enjoying Life Free of Alcohol and Drugs.* Oakland, CA: LifeRing; 2001.
18. Nicolaus M. *Empowering Your Sober Self.* Hoboken, NJ: Jossey-Bass; 2009.

19. Fenster J. Characteristics of clinicians likely to refer clients to 12-step programs versus a diversity of post-treatment options. *Drug Alcohol Depend.* 2006;83(3):238–246.
20. McCrady B, Horvath AT, Delaney SI. Self-help groups. In: Hester RK, Miller WR, eds. *Handbook of Alcoholism Treatment Approaches: Effective Alternatives.* 3rd ed. Boston, MA: Allyn & Bacon; 2002:165–187.
21. Buddie AM. Alternatives to twelve-step programs. *J Forensic Psychol Pract.* 2004;4(3):61–70.
22. Saladin ME, Ana EJS. Controlled drinking: more than just a controversy. *Curr Opin Psychiatry.* 2004;17(3):175–187.
23. Penn PE, Brooks AJ. Five years, Twelve Steps, and REBT in the treatment of dual diagnosis. *J Ration Emot Cogn Behav Ther.* 2000;18(4):197–208.
24. Atkins RG, Hawdon J. Religiosity and participation in mutual-aid support groups for addiction. *J Subst Abuse Treat.* 2007;33(3):321–331.
25. Kaskutas LA. What do women get out of self-help? Their reasons for attending Women for Sobriety and Alcoholics Anonymous. *J Subst Abuse Treat.* 1994;11:185–195.
26. Kaskutas LA. Predictors of self esteem among members of Women for Sobriety. *Addict Res.* 1996;4(3):273–281.
27. Kaskutas LA. Pathways to self-help among Women for Sobriety. *Am J Drug Alcohol Abuse.* 1996;22(2):259–280.
28. Kaskutas LA. A road less traveled: choosing the "Women for Sobriety" program. *J Drug Issues.* 1996;26(1):77–94.
29. Humphries K, Kaskutas LA. World views of Alcoholics Anonymous, Women for Sobriety, and Adult Children of Alcoholics/Al-Anon mutual help groups. *Addict Res.* 1995;3(3):231–243.
30. Zemore SE, Kaskutas, LA. Helping, spirituality and Alcoholics Anonymous in recovery. *J Stud Alcohol.* 2004;65(3):383–391.
31. London WM, Courchaine KE, Yoho DL. Recovery experiences of SOS members. Preliminary findings. In: Christopher J, ed. *SOS Sobriety: The Proven Alternative to 12-step Programs.* Buffalo, NY: Prometheus Books; 1992:45–59.
32. Connors G, Derman K. Characteristics of participants in Secular Organizations for Sobriety (SOS). *Am J Drug Alcohol Abuse.* 1996;22(2):281–295.
33. Klaw E, Humphreys K. Life stories of Moderation Management mutual help group members. *Contemp Drug Probl.* 2000:27(4):779–803.
34. Humphreys K, Klaw E. Can targeting nondependent problem drinkers and providing internet-based services expand access to assistance for alcohol problems? A study of the Moderation Management self-help/mutual aid organization. *J Stud Alcohol.* 2001;62(4):528–532.
35. Klaw E, Horst D, Humphreys K. Inquirers, triers, and buyers of an alcohol harm reduction self-help organization. *Addict Res Theory.* 2006;14(5):527–535.
36. Kosok A. The Moderation Management programme in 2004: what type of drinker seeks controlled drinking? *Int J Drug Policy.* 2006;17(4):295–303.
37. Li EC, Feifer C, Strohm M. A pilot study: locus of control and spiritual beliefs in Alcoholics Anonymous and SMART Recovery. *Addict Behav.* 2000;25(4):633–640.
38. Sobell LC, Cunningham JA, Sobell MB. Recovery from alcohol problems with and without treatment: prevalence in two population surveys. *Am J Public Health.* 1996;86:966–972.
39. American Psychiatric Association. *Diagnostic and Statistical Manual of Mental Disorders.* 4th ed. Washington, DC: Author; 2000.
40. Apanovitch DP. Religion and rehabilitation: the requisition of God by the state. *Duke Law J.* 1998;47:785–852.

CHAPTER 39: The Therapeutic Community

William B. O'Brien ■ J. Gabriel Piedrahita ■ Francisco (Sebastian) P. Bacatan, Jr.

In the presence of fellow therapeutic community residents and guests, a beautiful and confident young lady, a proud Daytop graduate, stood at the podium and related her tragic life journey. Her name was Sheila. This is her story (1):

Sheila's mother was 22 years old, attractive, and naïve. She met a dashing foreign importer from Germany in an eastside restaurant in New York City where she worked as a waitress. They struck up a friendship immediately, which soon developed into a serious relationship. She soon found herself pregnant, the information which she revealed to him on the eve of his return to his homeland. He explained that he had a wife and family back home, that he cared for her and that he would be back to the U.S.

Sheila's mother, now deserted, experienced the loneliness and abandonment that all women in like situations feel, but in addition, she feared her parents' reaction. As the pregnancy progressed, she stayed closer to her apartment in the east Bronx, NY, and away from her parents. The baby (Sheila) was born at New York Lincoln Hospital. No one else was there with this young mother; no one was to know of the birth. Once discharged with her baby, Sheila's mother moved among her Bronx neighbors, all strangers, in her quest to find someone who wanted a baby. Sheila's mother gave her baby away. She, then, returned to her work at the restaurant. The crisis had passed. So did Sheila, into the hands of strangers.

After a few weeks, the grandparents, worried sick over the sudden absence of their daughter, Sheila's mom, traveled from their upstate home in Utica, NY, to her Bronx apartment to ease their fears. They did not find Sheila's mom. She was at work at the restaurant. However, before they left the apartment building, the superintendent's wife informed them of the baby and their daughter's successful efforts to give the child away. Though struggling with the good feelings of a grandchild against the backdrop of a daughter-in-panic giving her child away, they decided to go to the restaurant and confront their daughter. That resulted in an hysterical scene, from which they drew bits and pieces of information: yes, she had a baby girl; not sure of the father; the baby is with an unknown couple not far from her apartment; she cannot recall the street and apartment.

It took the grandparents six weeks to find the couple and their granddaughter, which they swiftly claimed, bringing her with them on their return to Utica, NY. The grandfather, however, had somewhat of a drinking problem, creating not a few heated arguments, leaving Sheila a very uncertain, emotionally damaged girl. Very soon, Sheila became frightened by the grandparents' constant fighting and grandpa's drinking.

At age 9, Sheila's mother reappeared for the first time at the grandparents' home to claim her daughter since she learned that her welfare allotment could be increased. Sheila was, at first, reluctant to go but eventually was assured by her mother that she loved and wanted her.

Sheila returned to live with her mother from her 9th to 15th year. When she arrived on Daytop's doorstep, Sheila was a devastated young girl using drugs to block out her mom's drinking, her mother's many boyfriends' abuse and sexual advances. By age 15, she had 4 pregnancies, 3 abortions, and a baby boy, all by her mother's boyfriends.

She soon found the Daytop therapeutic community much more than a port in the storm. She grew to trust, to give and receive true love, to respect herself and no longer to feel worthless and cheap. Even her appearance changed from a disheveled young girl to an attractive, sparkling young lady. In Daytop's long journey, few found in Daytop a truer home more than tragic Sheila.

This is one of the sad tales of young people who come to the therapeutic community, wounded, experiencing loneliness and helplessness; who receive assistance in redirecting their lives; and who go through the experience of brokenness, witnessing the death of a loved one, a separation or divorce of one's parents, neglect and companion difficulties, failure in school, domestic violence, sexual abuse, unwanted pregnancies, and abortion. This catalogue of crises and problems seems endless. They speak of poverty, boredom, and broken homes. They describe excitement and comradeship provided by their gangs. One common denominator ran through all these unfortunate stories: drugs.

WHAT IS A THERAPEUTIC COMMUNITY?

The therapeutic community is a drug-free, self-help program, a highly structured, family-like environment where positive peer interaction assumes center stage (2–8). The therapeutic community is different from other drug treatment approaches, mainly in its use of the community as the key agent of change (3,6,9). This approach is referred to as "the community method" (2). The therapeutic community believes that drug abuse is not in itself a disease but merely a manifestation of underlying problems that the addicted need to overcome with the encouraging support of a caring community. The therapeutic community impresses upon the drug abusers that "only you can do it, but you cannot do it alone" (6).

RELIGIOUS ROOTS OF THE THERAPEUTIC COMMUNITY

The root of the term "religion" is the Latin term "ligare," from which our terms "ligament" and "ligature" arise. Thus, re-ligion means, literally, a reconnection, reunion, reconciliation" (10).

The concept and dynamics of the modern-day therapeutic community can be traced deeply into the past, even as far back as the early intertestamentary communities (11–13). Glaser (11) established the connection between the modern-day therapeutic communities with the early biblical communities and concluded that the therapeutic community has strong religious roots. In the 1947 discovery of the Dead Sea Scrolls, there is a description of Qumran, a community that flourished roughly around 200 BC to AD 50 (14). Some scholars observed that the problems experienced by the members of the Qumran community are somewhat akin to those experienced by the residents of today's therapeutic communities (11; see also 12,13,15).

Glaser (11) indicated one can readily recognize that the problems reflected in the "Rule of the Community" of Qumran were dealt with in a similar way as they are in the modern-day therapeutic community: conforming one's spirit and actions to the dictates of the community. This was accomplished in the Qumran community through mutual criticism, while in the therapeutic community it is achieved through the process of the encounter group. The resemblance between these two (mutual criticism and group encounter) is reflected in this brief excerpt found in the Dead Sea Scrolls:

> They shall rebuke one another in truth, humility, and charity. Let no man [sic] address his companion in anger, or ill-temper, or obduracy, or envy prompted by the spirit of wickedness. Let him not hate him (because of the wickedness of his uncircumcised heart), but let him rebuke him on the very same day lest he incur guilt because of him. Furthermore, let no man [sic] accuse his companion before the congregation without having first admonished him in the presence of witnesses (11).

According to De Leon (2), Glaser (11), and Rom-Rymer (15), another similarity between the Qumran community and the present-day therapeutic community is their strong adherence to the rules and norms of the community. The Dead Sea Scrolls' "Manual of Discipline" has a rule that reads: "You shall reprove your neighbor, lest you bear sin because of him" (16). The Qumran community had a deep awareness of the close involvement they had with each other. If one saw another commit sin and did nothing about it, that person is as guilty of that sin as the person who had committed it (16). In the therapeutic community, members, likewise, have this same awareness of co-responsibility and involvement through the practice of responsible concern by being one's "brother's/sister's keeper."

Roots in Early Christian Church

Although the link between the Qumran community and Jesus's early community is yet to be established, it is widely assumed that the "beliefs of the inter-testamentary community and those of the Synoptic Gospels stemmed from the same historical period and, perhaps, the same sources" (11). Both communities were intent upon the task of reconnecting themselves to God and neighbor through "full, unreserved, open confession of fault followed by appropriate restitution or penance" (13). These are central features of the present-day therapeutic community. O. Hobart Mowrer, a noted research psychologist at the University of Illinois, had done extensive research into the linkages between the present-day therapeutic community and the early Christian formulation (11,15,17). He pointed out that early Christianity was essentially a small group movement that celebrated fellowship or "koinonia." Koinonia is the anglicization of a Greek word ($\kappa o\iota\nu\omega\nu\iota\alpha$) that connotes fellowship, sharing in common, communion, a People of God, and rooted and grounded in love (18). The first mention of koinonia in scriptures is Acts 2:42: "They devoted themselves to the apostles' teaching and to fellowship, to the breaking of bread and to prayer." Fellowship is a central ingredient of Christian life. Believers in Christ are to come together in love, faith, mutual support, and encouragement. There were no churches or cathedrals, but rather small groups of people meeting in homes (13), most likely in the homes of prominent members of the community (19). It is this element of koinonia that maintains the sense of unity and communion among the diverse Christian groups and their leaders (19,20).

Mowrer (10) explained that it is here, in these small communities, that we find the ancient practice of "exomologesis." Exomologesis is a Greek word meaning "confession," joined with publicly manifested repentance (21). The practice of exomologesis perdures in the present-day therapeutic community (17). It demands complete openness about one's life, both past and present, followed by crucial behavioral change, with the avowed support and encouragement from other members of the community (17). Central to the process was the demonstration of public contrition before the entire congregation. Further, "spiritual reinstatement" was achieved by the imposition of a public penance commensurate with the offense (22), pleas for forgiveness along with plans for restitution. The closing phase is celebrated with warm fellowship (koinonia). Mowrer (10) described this process in the early Christian community as a healing experience.

> A small-groups movement in which alienated, sinful, "neurotic persons" confessed before their peers while accepting the penance imposed under the guidance of the particular "congregation" (or house church) to which they belonged. From all indications, this ... experience was [found to be] "highly therapeutic" while this early version of Christianity survived and prospered ... because it was redemptive and rehabilitative in an intensely practical [as well as in] psychologically and socially important ways (10).

Scholarly research into the primitive Christian Church of the first four centuries indicates that many of the practices of the first Christian community were conducted with similar intent as that of the present-day therapeutic community (15). It was with the arrival of Constantine the Great (AD 325), ruler of the Roman Empire (12), that the practice of exomologesis began to gradually disappear in favor of a private, "auricular" confession solely to a priest (10), until it was completely abandoned in the 13th century at the Lateran Council in 1215 (23).

The Protestant Reformation in the 16th century (12,20) decided to eliminate the "middle man," that is, the priest confessor, but as Mowrer (12) argues, the move failed to reestablish exomologesis, the practice of openness, mutual support, and admonition in a small group as practiced in the early church.

However, centuries later, the original healing practice of exomologesis found its way back into self-help groups, namely, the Oxford Group, People of the Way, and Alcoholics Anonymous (11; see also 3,12,13,15), but, most particularly, into the modern therapeutic communities. Exomologesis becomes, then, a characteristic of the therapeutic community to build a "common unity" of purpose and interests toward self-knowledge and growth (koinonia). The healing dimension of this koinonia comes from an aligned relationship that overrides each person's distorted perception of self and its interactions and fulfills the human yearning for belonging and relevance. Koinonia connotes not only being together but also doing together in a frank, close relationship that overcomes brokenness and divisiveness and so promoting wholeness with self, others, and the environment. Koinonia empowers and renews its members to interact in a beneficial multilevel relationship.

MULTIDIMENSIONAL APPROACH TO HEALING

The basic premise of the therapeutic community is that the person (substance abuse client) "enjoys" a disorder that affects all aspects of his or her life (3). It is a disorder of the whole person (3,4,6,7,24–26). Individual attitudes and behaviors, emotional management, and one's personal values, all these are slated for change. Such a multidimensional goal can be negotiated in a communal setting. Throughout the years, the therapeutic community has enhanced substance abuse treatment, intervention, prevention, and educational services for both adolescents and adults. It has emphasized a holistic approach to healing, using interdisciplinary staff, proven paraprofessionals, as well as family members to provide a wide variety of services to accommodate the need portfolios of adolescents as well as of adults (29). It utilizes multiple approaches in responding to the changing needs of its clients.

"The distinctive feature of the therapeutic community is … that the community itself … is the primary teacher and is the primary healer," proclaims De Leon (24). He notes further that as teacher, the community is capable of transmitting skills; as healer, the community is capable of mediating the variety of life experiences, which become healing experiences. Since the disorder in question involves the whole person, the multidimensional goal of changing the individual can be managed in a 24-hour, 7-day a week context for purposes of lasting learning and healing. Individual change moves forward through the intervention of peer challenge and role modeling across the therapeutic environment. In the therapeutic community, one discovers an interesting composite made up of the environment, the systems, and the structure, which, taken together, are capable of achieving healing along with educational dividends (2). In the therapeutic community, "the disorder of the whole person means that change is multidimensional." "Individual change is viewed along several dimensions of behavior, perceptions, and experiences" (2), and, for purposes of facilitating change, multiple interventions are open to the community.

The therapeutic community also recognizes the need to engage other agencies, utilizing a cross-reference system, embracing different approaches in an effort to provide a holistic, healthy structure for substance abuse clients in recovery. The Daytop therapeutic community, for example, invites speakers from other agencies to facilitate educational seminars, such as Planned Parenthood, Teen Challenge, and others. It encourages residents to attend weekly Alcoholics Anonymous meetings. The Daytop therapeutic community participates in the Youth Assistance Program (YAP), where young residents visit the local correctional facilities. This is a program where the inmates of the facility provide their own insights into the problems of youth today as seen through the prism of their personal experiences (1). It is vital that in addressing the problems, substance abuse clients must utilize multilevel approaches while building partnerships with sister agencies in the community. In dealing with the substance abuse clients, one needs to consider an approach that is centered upon the partnership of family, school, and community forces. There is a strong need to address the interrelatedness of the differing systems of the larger community in order to have an effective treatment program. According to the African saying that "it takes a whole village to raise a child," correspondingly "it takes a whole community to raise an integrated person." In the therapeutic community, there is strong emphasis upon the need for rebuilding a sense of community, or village, in which everyone reasserts his or her shared responsibility in the process of nurturing the substance abuse clients.

HEALING THROUGH A CARING FAMILY ENVIRONMENT

Family is vital in the life of substance abuse clients. It is the setting where the valuable aspects of self-esteem, self-acceptance, and sense of responsibility are nurtured. Although ideally the family is where these should be in play, the fact is that there are many substance abuse clients who do not enjoy stable and healthy families. These clients are numbered "among the damaged" because their families have been severely wounded and stand clearly in need of healing. It is impossible to learn these tasks when one lacks a healthy, functioning family setting (27). It is true that "the therapeutic community can never [fully] replace the functional family, [but] it is a temporary place enjoying the support with the natural family" (28). In this case, the therapeutic community is a place where the family can also relearn and refashion itself.

The therapeutic community recognizes the importance of healing not only for the wounded clients in treatment but for the families as well (27). Here the community provides a safe harbor of care, nurture, and emotional support for troubled clients and their families. In the Daytop therapeutic community, there is a special focus on the family through its Family Association Programs for purposes of identifying imbalances while empowering parents to recalibrate their lives by embracing new values. In Daytop there is a saying: "We try to heal the soul of the family!" (27) By "soul," Daytop does not refer to one's inner force or beliefs, but rather one's entire self. The therapeutic community has given evidence of some success due to its efforts in soul-caring by providing the quintessential nourishing family environment, which, more often than not, has been found wanting in the original familiar situation. The English word "care" comes from the Latin word "cura," which connotes, among other things, attention and healing. This consideration stands at the portals of the therapeutic community, a formula for living that encourages individuals and families to embrace one's soul-life as the inner core of their being (27). The process of healing (care of self and one's soul) is not accomplished in isolation but, rather, in the collective journey traveled through family with each member supporting the other.

Herein lies the root of the therapeutic community outreach to families of substance abuse clients, which serves to heal relationships between members within the family unit. It aspires to increase the solidarity of the family while promoting its own well-being. The therapeutic community family outreach opens up avenues for confronting tensions, conflicts, and consequent maladjustments in the vast sea of family tensions through efforts of reorganization and reintegration. The therapeutic community offers innovative approaches for understanding the soul-life of the family unit as well as the blueprints for organizing families in support of each other. This approach in promoting the well-being of the family is an example of family systems theory. It represents a holistic approach, which positions every part of family life in terms of the "family as a whole." The dynamics of family system theory in the therapeutic community is reflected in this story (1):

> A 14-year-old boy from Long Island, NY came to Daytop because of his alcohol and drug problems. The Daytop director evaluated the family situation and discovered that the father had a serious drinking problem. He confronted the parents with the challenge that, if they seriously desired to help their son, the father needed to deal with his problem immediately. There was a special urgency, as the director advised, for both parents to join the Family Association. The director later reported that the father had stopped drinking, joined AA, and both parents became active members in the association. The entire family now is engaged in weekly family therapy as part of the son's treatment program.

HEALING THROUGH CARING PEERS

On the occasion of her visits to one of the therapeutic communities, Brieland (29) recorded the experience of a young resident: "I went on drugs because I wanted to belong. I wanted to have friends. However, they weren't friends, were they? A friend wouldn't give you something that he knew would harm you? However, I have true friends here, real friends" (29).

True friendships and positive peer role models serve as primary agents of change in the therapeutic community. De Leon (2) asserts that the strength of the community in the context of healing and change (psychological and social learning) "relates to the number and quality of its peers serving as role models." The therapeutic community requires a multiplicity of role models (roommates, older and younger residents, as well as senior and junior staff) to maintain the integrity of the community while ensuring the promotion of individual growth and healthy relationships.

William Glasser, who is recognized as "the father of reality therapy," contends that human beings have some basic needs that must be satisfied in order to exist in a reasonably satisfying life (30). The first is the need for a relationship of mutual respect and affection with at least one other person. Bassin (30) further asserts that Glasser's concept of love goes beyond any romantic and sexual connotation. Essentially, it relates to the vital ingredients of concern, acceptance, and respect. A second universal need indicated by Glasser is the feeling of self-worth, which is produced to a greater degree by the love of a responsible person and the return of that love (30). Glasser argues that when one is unable to fulfill the needs for love and worth, one experiences pain, loneliness, and discomfort. The therapeutic community fulfills these two basic needs, particularly by providing a caring setting where residents feel nurtured and supported, physically and psychologically safe, as well as understood and accepted by others. It is a place that fulfills the essential need to be connected and to belong. The therapeutic community is set apart from other approaches due to the strategic use of healthy peer relationships to facilitate change and growth (2,3).

HEALING THROUGH CARING MENTORS

In the therapeutic community, members are expected to serve as role models for purposes of "maintaining the integrity of the community as well as of ensuring the wide acceptance of social learning" (2). A greater investment of responsibility is expected from staff and senior members of the community who serve as "caring mentors" for newer members. Staff and senior residents act as guides in assisting others in their recovery (3). The credentials of therapeutic community mentors are their own experiences in self-help recovery. When new members walk through the doors of a therapeutic community residence, they are not met by doctors, professors, or priests. Someone equally wounded greets them. That someone has been where the new members now find themselves at entry, and that someone has successfully traveled the path toward recovery. These therapeutic community mentors serve as caring guides for new members through the processes of self-discovery and change. They ensure that new members of the community receive exposure to a range of growth experiences through positive interactions with others. To serve as caring mentors in the lives of younger residents is a paramount responsibility of staff and senior residents.

St. Thomas Aquinas stressed: *Nemo dat quod non habet*, "You cannot give what you do not have." In the therapeutic community, every staff and senior members must model the expected behaviors and values demanded by this idealistic community. Each member is reminded of the significance of the axiom "talk the talk and walk the walk," in the process of effectively guiding other members of the community toward growth and change. Palmer (31) argues, "we teach who we are." According to him, "selfhood" of the significant adult remains a key factor in the formation of the young. To make a difference in their lives, one needs to bear the identity and authenticity of an integrated person. Such integrity springs from the inner persona of the adult. He argues further that the courage to teach reveals a primordial demand to first probe the "heart's longing to be connected with the largeness of life, a longing that animates both love and work" (31). Likewise, these are the underlying tenets of the therapeutic community: in changing oneself, we change others; in helping others, we help ourselves. The common struggles in life are the backdrop for one's connectedness with others as well as one's commitment to help.

HEALING THROUGH HONESTY AND RESPONSIBLE CONCERN

O. Hobart Mowrer maintains that the practice of honesty, responsible love, and concern is intrinsically therapeutic (29). The therapeutic community provides honesty with a new dimension: radical self-disclosure and transparency. It is here where one discovers healing and wholeness. When a resident feels "nurtured, supported, and safe as well as accepted by others," he or she is more likely to participate in the community and risk the challenge to change (2). The "tough love and rugged honesty" of the therapeutic community is always within the context of a caring and nurturing setting, which Winnicot refers to as a "holding environment" (32). Carl Rogers, the "father of client-centered therapy," explained that the healing outcome from the environment of the therapeutic community springs from the encounter process that is at the heart of that caring environment (29). "Shame, fear, anger, guilt, confusion, despair, and aloneness" (2) are some of the early pains experienced by members of the community, and these are "associated with circumstantial stress, pressures, and psychological injuries" of the past, as well as from isolation. However, the therapeutic community offers an environment that fosters nurturing and caring, along with physical and psychological safety as well as social relatedness. As Abraham Maslow (33) indicated in his commentary on his visit in 1965 to Daytop Staten Island, "in order to be open and trusting, one must first create a safe environment where the participant is able to experience a true sense of belonging and of being respected as a person." Even though within and without the therapeutic community–setting, past traumas have a way of resurfacing and haunting, in a safe setting, such as the caring family of the therapeutic community, confronting these traumas and resolving them constitute a liberating experience.

When there is genuine dialogue between people, each person is seen, understood, and acknowledged by the other (34). What emerges from this is a meeting between people at a deeper level. When someone speaks candidly to another person, with defenses discarded, they are placing a call upon that person to respond to them at a profound level. They are calling out for that person to recognize them at their particular stage of struggling to exist in their everyday lives. When someone calls out in this way, it is impossible not to respond. Tucker (34) claims: "a meeting between you and that person suddenly takes place. . . . Once one has responded, one has taken responsibility for another."

HEALING THROUGH RESPONSIBILITY

In exploring the meaning of responsibility, Bratter (35) argues that the English word "response" appears to be less proactive than the French term "repondre," or the German "antworten." He explains that the German term "verantwortung" appears more comprehensive. It suggests answering for one's actions. "Ability" connotes being able to accomplish a task that coincides with the therapeutic community's overall definition of "responsibility" (35). He defines the word "responsibility" where the emphasis is placed on the person's ability to respond to external challenges with reasonable judgment. Bratter (35) cited Patterson to emphasize this point:

> The meaning of life is not found in questioning the purpose of existence. It arises from the response which man [sic] makes to life, to situations, and to tasks with which life confronts him. Although there are biological, psychological, and sociological factors influencing man's [sic] response, there remains the element of choice. He cannot always control the conditions by which he is confronted, but he can control his responses to them. Man [sic] is thus responsible for his responses, his choices, [and] his actions.

In the therapeutic community, the residents and staff are immersed in dialogue on how to be responsible through the continual, candid feedback of the group. This is the goal of psychotherapy, according to Bratter (35), to help the individual assume responsibility for self, in the sense of recognizing the active, responsible force in one's life; being capable of making decisions; and assuming consequences. Along with this acceptance, the recognition of responsibility toward others follows upon a readiness to discover the obligations arising from the values one holds, whether they relate to one's children, parents, friends, employees, colleagues, the community, or one's country (35). Each person is responsible for the other. Daytop's Millbrook Center in Upstate New York has become a mecca for visitors. In the *Capsule Anecdotes–Daytop Stories*, it shares the memorable visit of one of the recent guests to that center:

> Very young adolescents with youthful enthusiasm and ever-present smiles greet the visitor. Following swiftly behind is the offer to provide a guided tour of the premises and the program content. Guests become intrigued by this lovely, smiling youngster and wonder whether s/he actually had been an addict. "Just as sweet as my own children," the guests are overheard to say. However, something unique tends to distinguish this youngster from most kids. A youthful but clear sense of responsibility. They reach out to assist the visitors up the steps.

They hold the door. They offer them a glass of water and so on. Actually, in the course of these visitor tours, in which this particular visitor was fortunate to participate, one was so impressed with this incident. "An incident suddenly drew our young tour guide away from us to the side of a young girl crying. She had just received word that her mother was rushed to the hospital after an auto accident. Begging our forbearance for a few minutes, our guide sat down with the trembling, sobbing "sister," holding her hand and sharing her tears. Once he saw that another resident arrived on the scene to continue concern for the grieving "sister," he apologized to us and continued his tour as if nothing happened. So much gentle responsibility wrapped in a 15-year-old boy. "We were so impressed!" the guest declared (1).

In the therapeutic community, responsibility is regarded as an essential part of a mutually dependent relationship between the individual and the society. Being part of the community means taking on the full responsibilities of membership while accepting the consequences when these responsibilities do not bear fruit. One cannot be satisfied with a passive, noncontributing membership style. On the contrary, one must be aware of his or her role in accepting full responsibility in the larger community. "Accountability and responsibility are integral tools for interrupting self-defeating lifestyles" (36) while facilitating the recovery process in the community.

The therapeutic community encourages its members to care for and support each other. "I am my brother's/sister's keeper," the Christian principle holds, while in the therapeutic community, it reaches further, "in helping my brothers/sisters, I, also, help myself!" Helping each other includes helping peers to struggle (37). Helping others becomes a key component in the process of helping oneself. It echoes what Mowrer frequently insisted upon: "The best way to help yourself is to help others" (29).

HEALING THROUGH ONE'S WOUNDENESS

The dynamics of the therapeutic community encourages and empowers individuals to embark upon a journey into self-knowledge and personal growth. Recognizing the difficulties on the path to gathering a candid picture of oneself, just as the eye cannot reflect upon itself, the therapeutic community itself serves as a complete reflection of a member's potential. At the same time, it surfaces patterns of denial, hypocrisy, manipulation, and self-deception where they exist. Harris (18) states, "we do not have a sense of our own [selves] unless other people mirror it back to us." Such a process opens up an avenue to accept in oneself uncertainties, inadequacies, helplessness, as well as instances of lack of control. This is what Kurtz and Ketcham (38), in *The Spirituality of Imperfection*, describe as the discovery that "something is awry; that there is, after all, something 'wrong' with us." Entering the therapeutic community in itself is a cry for help. The experience becomes a form of grasping at one's limitations, maladaptive behaviors, fears, and negative attitudes. In another sense, the community becomes a holding environment that provides the individual with a safe place to accept imperfection, to develop a vision of life, and to implement a curative way of living in which those imperfections can be constructively addressed (38).

In this journey of declaring ownership for one's limitations and wounds, the recognition of one's own weaknesses fosters the development of compassion. The member gradually discovers that both the weaknesses and the destructive behavior of others are not really far from one's own behavioral performance. One can also be convinced early on that the craving for love expressed by others resides also deep in one's own heart. Such a glimpse of compassion serves to support the caring environment that permeates all activities in the community. A Daytop staff member shared a glimpse of his early experience as a staff member, working with the adolescents at Daytop Millbrook (1). He approached the director one day with this observation, "I cannot understand why these kids were on drugs!" The director, an ex-addict, looked at him and said, "If you cannot understand why these kids are here, you will never be able to move them. You will never be able to touch their lives and you will never be able to help them." He refers to this episode as the beginning of his personal journey. It was the beginning of an inventory of his own imperfections or "woundedness" to be better equipped to compassionately accompany the young people in Daytop. He concluded: "Even professional people working in the therapeutic community cannot position themselves to assist the young people at Daytop unless they first recognize in themselves a certain 'woundedness'. This recognition stands at the gates of the therapeutic community!" (1).

There is a general assumption that the more perfect one appears, the more one will be loved (35). Actually, the reverse is more often true. The more willing one is to admit human weakness, the more lovable he or she becomes (35). Kurtz and Ketcham (38) likewise claim that one's woundedness, helplessness, and powerlessness are essential to the fabric of being human. They moreover declare: "To deny our errors is to deny ourselves." In the therapeutic community, the more willing we are to admit human weakness and failure, the more effective we become in guiding and healing others. The more willing we are to be in touch with our limitations, the more understanding we become with others. The more we are in touch with our woundedness, the more we are able to express compassion (1). "Acknowledging the solidarity of shared humanness remains a fundamental requirement for effectively helping and counseling the wounded," Albers (36) further points out. The struggle to be oneself and to acknowledge one's humanity among others is, indeed, a struggle, but "when there is a real commitment, there is community" (34).

THERAPEUTIC COMMUNITY: THE WOUNDED HEALER

The therapeutic community was born out of the crying need of a suffering and an anguished group of social outcasts "who forged an instrument for change that came to be known as the 'therapeutic community'" (39). The therapeutic community founders soon discovered that peer group influence was extremely effective in bringing on change and in learning how to live again. Through peers, wounded people were able to relate deeply and emotionally on the basis of shared experience, a common ground of woundedness, and on this premise they moved forward in an historic effort to assist each other to reclaim their lives via mutual support and peer modeling.

The therapeutic community actualizes the paradox of the wounded healer. Its members can be described as the "twice-born" mentioned in *The Varieties of Religious Experience* of William James (40): "The "twice-born" have known tragedy, failure, and defeat and they have named them as such; but they also have a new sense of possibility of somehow rising above such experience … It is only in the embracing of our torn self, only in the acceptance that there is nothing "wrong" with feeling "torn," that we can hope for whatever healing is available and can, thus, become as "whole" as possible. Our own brokenness allows us to become whole" (38).

The community represents a living paradox that embraces the human condition as "both/and" (both a wounded warrior and a healer; both a saint and a sinner) rather than "either/or" (either a wounded warrior or a healer; either a saint or a sinner). The healing experience of the therapeutic community transcends its own boundaries. Nouwen (41) points out that to a "wounded healer," a compassionate person, nothing human is alien: "compassion breaks through the boundaries of language and national boundaries, rich and poor, educated and illiterate … this compassion pulls people into the larger sphere where they can see that every human face is the face of a neighbor. There is the necessity to recognize the suffering of his time in his own heart and make that recognition the starting point of his service." He claims that the "willingness to see one's own limitations and 'woundedness' as rising from the depth of the human condition" remains a potent source of healing (41). The therapeutic community staffs and facilitators need to recognize their own woundedness to be able to heal the wounds of others.

CONCLUSION: THE THERAPEUTIC COMMUNITY, A HEALING KOINONIA

The central inquiry of this chapter is to discuss the healing components of the therapeutic community as a koinonia (community). It proposes that the therapeutic community, as koinonia, offers an effective healing approach in dealing with wounded substance abuse clients. For people who do not fall into this labeled "wounded" category, it serves to confirm and strengthen positive traits of character. The therapeutic community rebuilds a person's self-esteem, self-image, self-respect, and self-dignity. It restores a sense of hospitality to self and to others. The therapeutic community assumes a certain maturity through responsible concern for peers.

The therapeutic community affirms the fundamental values common to all religions, but particularly to the Christian faith. It stands as a model for the holistic and multidimensional treatment approach in addressing the needs of the substance abuse client as a whole person. The therapeutic community is a paradigm for comprehensive treatment programs that incorporates partnership with families, schools, and other community forces in a common effort to promote a healthy and caring environment for their clients. It offers other helping agencies a pattern for building small communities through caring peer relationships, which facilitate change and growth through honesty, responsible concern, and responsibility. The therapeutic community recognizes the necessity of being in touch with one's vulnerability, one's "woundedness," and this provides helping professionals and educators with a framework for ministering more effectively to wounded substance abuse people. The journey of fashioning and refashioning peoples' lives remains the crowning moment of the community effort. The therapeutic community is in many ways a *koinonia* where the "wounded" are healed through the embrace of an *agape* and caring community. As a young Daytop graduate declared, "The therapeutic community is truly an Easter place!"

REFERENCES

1. Bacatan F. *An Analysis of the Daytop Therapeutic Community Using Maria Harris's Koinonia Curriculum: Implications for the Religious Education of Youth* [doctoral dissertation]. Bronx, NY: Fordham University. Available at: www.il.proquest.com.
2. De Leon G, ed. *Community as Method: Therapeutic Communities Special Populations and Settings*. Westport, CT: Praeger Publishers; 1997.
3. De Leon G. *The Therapeutic Community: Theory, Model and Method*. New York, NY: Springer Publishing Company; 2000.
4. Kooyman M. *The Therapeutic Community for Addicts: Intimacy, Parent Involvement Treatment Outcome*. Amsterdam, the Netherlands: Swets & Zeitlinger; 1992.
5. Kooyman M. The history of therapeutic communities: a view from Europe. In: Rawlings B, Yates R, eds. *Therapeutic Communities for the Treatment of Drug Users*. Philadelphia, PA: Jessica Kingsley Publishers Ltd; 2001:59–78.
6. O'Brien, WB. *You Can't Do It Alone: The Daytop Way to Make Your Child Drug Free*. New York, NY: Simon & Schuster; 1993.
7. Perfas F. *Therapeutic Community: A Practice Guide*. Lincoln, NE: iUniverse Inc; 2003.
8. Perfas F. *Therapeutic Community: Social Systems Perspective*. Lincoln, NE: iUniverse Inc; 2004.
9. National Institute on Drug Abuse. *Therapeutic Community. Report Series*, August 2002; NIH Publication No. 02-4877.
10. Mowrer OH. *Abnormal Reactions or Actions: An Autobiographical Answer*. Dubuque, IA: WM. C. Brown Company Publishers; 1966.
11. Glaser FB. The origin of the drug-free therapeutic community: a retrospective history. *Addict Ther*. 1978;2(special issues 3 & 4):3–15.
12. Mowrer OH. Therapeutic community groups and communities in retrospect and prospect. In: Vamos P, Devlin J, eds. *The Proceedings of the First World Conference on Therapeutic Communities*. Montreal, Que.: Portage Press; 1977.
13. O'Brien WB. Therapeutic communities around the world. In: Angelini F, ed. *Proceedings of the Sixth International Conference: Drugs and Alcoholism against Life*. Vatican City: Vatican Press; 1991.

14. Baigent M, Leigh R. *The Dead Sea Scrolls Deception*. New York, NY: Summit Books; 1991.
15. Rom-Rymer J. *An Empirical Assessment of Mowrer's Theory of Psychopathology Applied to a Therapeutic Community* [doctoral dissertation]. Tallahassee, FL: The Florida State University; 1981.
16. Emerson J. *The Dynamics of Forgiveness*. Philadelphia, PA: The Westminster Press; 1966.
17. O'Brien WB. The therapeutic community in retrospect and prospect. *The International Congress on Drugs and Alcohol, Jerusalem*; September 13–18, 1981.
18. Harris M. *Fashion Me a People: Curriculum in the Church*. Louisville, KY: John Knox Press; 1989.
19. Cwiekowski F. *The Beginnings of the Church*. Mahwah, NJ: Paulist Press; 1988.
20. Sanks H. *Salt, Leaven and Light: The Community Called Church*. New York, NY: The Crossroad Publishing Company; 1997.
21. Forest J. *Confession: Doorway to Forgiveness*. Maryknoll, NY: Orbis Books; 2002.
22. Clebsch W, Jaekle C. *Pastoral Care in Historical Perspective*. Englewood Cliffs, NJ: Prentice-Hall; 1964.
23. Tentler TN. *Sin and Confession on the Eve of Reformation*. Princeton, NJ: Princeton University Press; 1977.
24. De Leon G. Therapeutic community treatment research fact: what we know. *"Know Thy Self" Evolutionary Course of the Therapeutic Communities: The Third Generation. Proceedings of the 13th World Conference of Therapeutic Communities*. Athens, Greece: Lithographic Establishment of ΚΕΘΕΑ; 1990:245–248.
25. Sugarman B. *Daytop Village: A Therapeutic Community*. New York, NY: Holt, Rinehart & Winston Inc; 1974.
26. O'Brien WB, Devlin CJ. The therapeutic community. In: Lowinson J, Ruiz P, Millman R, et al., eds. *Substance Abuse: A Comprehensive Textbook*. 3rd ed. New York, NY: William & Wilkins; 1997:400–405.
27. O'Brien WB. Natural family & TC family. In: Avanzini F, ed. *The Family in the Society: Which Future? Volume I: Proceedings of the XV World Conference of Therapeutic Communities*. Verona, Italia: Centro Studi; 1992:391–394.
28. Donati P. Family and modernization today: redefining identities and relationships. In: Avanzini F, ed. *The Family in the Society: Which Future? Volume I: Proceedings of the XV World Conference of Therapeutic Communities*. Verona, Italia: Centro Studi; 1992:29–48.
29. Brieland C. *Triumph over Tragedy: The Story of the Therapeutic Community*. Milford, PA: Promethean Institute and Division of Daytop Village; 1993.
30. Bassin A. Go help your brother! Triad theory and reality therapy for drug addicts, part 1: some theoretical tidbits. *Addict Ther*. 1975;1(3):34–41.
31. Palmer P. *The Courage to Teach: Exploring the Inner Landscape of a Teacher's Life*. San Francisco, CA: Jossey-Bass; 1998.
32. Abram J. *The Language of Winnicott: A Dictionary and Guide to Understanding His Works*. Northvale, NJ: Jason Aronson Inc; 1997.
33. Maslow A. *The Farther Reaches of Human Nature*. New York, NY: Viking Press; 1993.
34. Tucker S, ed. *A Therapeutic Community Approach to Care in the Community: Dialogue and Dwelling*. Philadelphia, PA: Jessica Kingsley Publishers Ltd; 2000.
35. Bratter TE. Rebirth, responsibility, reality, and respect: the four R's of the American self-help therapeutic community. *Addict Ther*. 1978;3(1):51–66.
36. Albers R. Families and substance abuse. In: Anderson H, Browning D, Evison I, et al., eds. *The Family Handbook*. Louisville, KY: Westminster John Knox Press; 1998:187–191.
37. Sugarman B. Structure, variations and context: a sociological view of the therapeutic community. In: De Leon G, Zeingefuss JT, eds. *Therapeutic Communities for Addictions: Readings in Theory, Research, and Practice*. Springfield, IL: Charles C. Thomas; 1986:65–82.
38. Kurtz E, Ketcham K. *The Spirituality of Imperfection: Storytelling and the Search for Meaning*. New York, NY: Bantam Books; 1992.
39. Rangell M. Daytop village: treatment by peers. *Addict Ther*. 1975;1(2):57–59.
40. James W. *The Varieties of Religious Experience*. New York, NY: Simon & Schuster Inc; 1997.
41. Nouwen H. *The Wounded Healer*. New York, NY: Image Books, Doubleday; 1990.

CHAPTER 40 Network Therapy

Marc Galanter ■ Helen Dermatis

Psychotherapy for people dependent on alcohol and other drugs presents unique problems for the office-based practitioner. Among these are the ever-present vulnerability to relapse to substance use and high dropout rates. In order to address this problem, we can consider how engaging the input of people close to an addicted person can help in achieving a stable abstinence and deal with the vulnerability to dropout from treatment. To understand this option, it is first important to understand that certain conditioned drug-seeking behaviors may be extinguished if appropriate aversive stimuli are interposed after triggers to drug use are presented.

A drug user can become entangled in an interlocking web of self-perpetuating reinforcers that contribute to the persistence of drug abuse, despite compromising consequences, and the user's imperviousness to a traditional, psychodynamic psychotherapeutic approach does not necessarily take such conditioning factors into account. This is because neither the user nor the therapist is typically aware of their existence due to the unconscious nature of the conditioned response of drug seeking. The therapist's attempt to alter the course of the stimulus–response sequence is therefore often not viable, even with the aid of a willing patient, as neither party is necessarily aware that a conditioned sequence is taking place.

Sufficient exploration, however, can reveal the relevant stimuli and their effect through conditioned sequences of drug-seeking behavior. I initially described a technique for guided recall of relevant conditioned stimuli in a psychotherapeutic context, whereby the alcoholic or addict may become aware of the sequence of circumstances that can precipitate relapse (1). Once this is done, the patient's own distress at the course of the addictive process, generated by the patient's own motivation for escaping the addictive pattern, may be mobilized. This motivational distress then serves as an aversive stimulus. The implicit assumption behind this therapeutic approach is that the patient in question wants to alter his or her pattern of drug use and that the recognition of a particular stimulus as a conditioned component of addiction will then allow the patient, in effect, to initiate the extinction process. If a patient is committed to achieving abstinence from an addictive drug such as alcohol or cocaine but is in jeopardy of occasional slips, this cognitive labeling can facilitate consolidation of an abstinent adaptation.

As we shall see, the input of people close to the patient can help to reveal triggers to drugs use that may not have been apparent to the patient. Such an approach is less valuable in the context of (a) a lack of motivation for abstinence, (b) fragile social supports, or (c) compulsive substance abuse unmanageable by the patient in the patient's usual social settings. Hospitalization or replacement therapy (e.g., methadone or buprenorphine) may be necessary in such cases, because ambulatory stabilization through psychotherapeutic support is often not feasible, even with the support of family and close peers. On the other hand, for willing patients, or ones whom family and friends have convinced to cooperate, the network approach can be most valuable.

THE NETWORK THERAPY TECHNIQUE

This approach can be useful in addressing a broad range of addicted patients characterized by the following clinical hallmarks of addictive illness. When they initiate consumption of their addictive agent, be it alcohol, cocaine, opiates, or depressant drugs, they frequently cannot limit that consumption to a reasonable and predictable level; this phenomenon has been termed *loss of control* by clinicians who treat persons dependent on alcohol or drugs (2). Second, they have consistently demonstrated relapse to the agent of abuse; that is, they have attempted to stop using the drug for varying periods of time but have returned to it, despite a specific intent to avoid it.

This treatment approach is not necessary for those abusers who can learn to set limits on their use of alcohol or drugs; their abuse may be treated as a behavioral symptom in a more traditional psychotherapeutic fashion. Nor is it directed at those patients for whom the addictive pattern is most unmanageable, such as addicted people with unusual destabilizing circumstances such as homelessness, severe character pathology, or psychosis. These patients may need special supportive care such as inpatient detoxification or long-term residential treatment.

Key Elements

Three key elements are introduced into the Network Therapy technique. The first is a cognitive–behavioral approach to relapse prevention, which has been considered valuable in addiction treatment (3,4). Emphasis in this approach is placed on triggers to relapse and behavioral techniques for avoiding them, in preference to exploring underlying psychodynamic issues.

Second, support of the patient's natural social network is engaged in treatment. Peer support in Alcoholics Anonymous (AA) has long been shown to be an effective vehicle for promoting abstinence, and the idea of the therapist's intervening with family and friends in starting treatment was employed in one of the early ambulatory techniques specific to addiction (5). The involvement of spouses (6) has since been shown to be effective in enhancing the outcome of professional therapy.

Third, the orchestration of resources to provide community reinforcement suggests a more robust treatment intervention by providing a support for drug-free rehabilitation (7). In this relation, Khantzian pointed to the "primary care therapist" as one who functions in direct coordinating and monitoring roles in order to combine psychotherapeutic and self-help elements (8). It is this overall management role over circumstances outside as well as inside the office session that is presented to trainees, in order to maximize the effectiveness of the intervention.

CBT and Social Support

Cognitive–Behavioral Therapy This format for treatment has been shown to be effective for a wide variety of substance use disorders, including alcohol (9), marijuana (10), and cocaine dependence (11). It is premised on the original findings by Wikler (12) on conditioning models of drug seeking in heroin-addicted subjects.

The CBT approach is goal oriented and focuses on current circumstances in the patient's life. In Network Therapy, reference in both individual and conjoint sessions can be made to salient past experiences. CBT sessions are typically structured, so, for example, patients begin each network session with a recounting of recent events directly relevant to their addiction and recovery. This is followed by active participation and interaction of therapist, patient, and network members in response to the patient's report. CBT emphasizes psychoeducation in the context of relapse prevention, so that circumstances, thoughts, and interpersonal situations that have historically precipitated substance use are identified and the patient (and network members as well) are taught to anticipate where such triggers can precipitate substance use.

The process of guided recall, noted previously, is particularly important because it allows the therapist both individual sessions with the patient alone and network sessions—in conjunction with network members along with the patient—to guide the patient to recognize a sequence of conditioned stimuli (triggers) that play a role in drug seeking. Such triggers may not initially be apparent to the patient or network members, but with encouragement and prompting, they can emerge over the course of an exploration of the circumstances that have led, either in the past or in a recent "slip," to substance use.

Social Support This issue has been studied in a variety of data sets in relation to the recovery from substance use disorders. For example, in the federal Project MATCH, three modalities—twelve-step facilitation, motivational enhancement, and cognitive–behavioral approaches—were compared. In a secondary analysis of findings from this multisite study, it was found (13) that certain aspects of social support were most predictive of abstinence outcomes. Two social network characteristics that had a positive effect on outcome were the size of the supportive social network in the person's life and the number of members who were abstainers (or recovering alcoholics). I have found that nonproblem drinking participants are important to a long-term clinical outcome. As a matter of fact, a large number of network members, when their participation is effectively maintained over time, can counter a variety of circumstances that may undermine a patient's abstinence. Additionally, they can provide varied aspects of support relative to the patient's experience in recovery. And indeed, they should be free of substance-related problems. Of interest in this context, it has been reported that men are more typically encouraged by their wives to seek help, whereas women are more often encouraged by mothers, siblings, and children (14).

Community Reinforcement Family involvement in substance abuse treatment has long been shown to be effective in improving outcome, and there are numerous approaches that make use of social network involvement in treatment, including Behavioral Couples Therapy (15), Marital Therapy (16), and the Community Reinforcement Approach (17,18).

More specifically, a Community Reinforcement and Family Training (CRAFT) program includes many aspects of treatment that were employed in Network Therapy. The CRAFT approach was developed to encourage drinkers to enter therapy and reduce drinking, in part by eliciting support of concerned others, as well as to enhance satisfaction with life among members of the patient's social network who were concerned about his or her drinking. As in Network Therapy, the CRAFT program includes a functional analysis of the patient's substance use, that is to say, understanding the substance use with respect to its antecedents and consequences. Like Network Therapy, it also serves to minimize reciprocal blaming and defensiveness among the concerned significant others and to promote a patient's sobriety-oriented activities.

In one large trial in which concerned significant others were randomized to one of three conditions, a comparison was made between Al-Anon-facilitated therapy, an approach similar to the Johnson Institute interventions, and the CRAFT model (25). In that study, the CRAFT intervention was found to be more effective in engaging treatment-refusing, alcoholic subjects. Similar positive findings were obtained in studies on CRAFT with illicit drug users (19,20). On the other hand, in another study, concerned significant others were successfully trained to apply a modified Johnson Intervention technique in the absence of a therapist, and this approach was found to be successful in itself (21).

Initial Encounter: Starting a Social Network

So how does one go about developing Network Therapy? The patient should be asked to bring his or her spouse or a close friend to the first session. Alcoholic patients often dislike certain things they hear when they first come for treatment and may deny or rationalize, even if they have voluntarily sought help. Because of their denial of the problem, a significant other is essential to both history taking and implementing a viable treatment plan. A close relative or spouse can often cut through the denial in a way that an unfamiliar therapist cannot and can therefore be invaluable in setting a standard of realism in dealing with the addiction.

Some patients make clear that they wish to come to the initial session on their own. This is often associated with their desire to preserve the option of continued substance abuse and is born out of the fear that an alliance will be established independent of them to prevent this. Although a delay may be tolerated for a session or two, it should be stated unambiguously at the outset that effective treatment can be undertaken only on the basis of a therapeutic alliance built around the addiction issue that includes the support of significant others and that it is expected that a network of close friends and/or relatives will be brought in within a session or two at the most.

The weight of clinical experience supports the view that abstinence is the most practical goal to propose to the addicted person for his or her rehabilitation (22,23). For abstinence to be expected, however, the therapist should assure the provision of necessary social supports for the patient. Let us consider how a long-term support network is initiated for this purpose, beginning with availability of the therapist, significant others, and a self-help group.

In the first place, the therapist should be available for consultation on the phone and should indicate to the patient that he or she wants to be called if problems arise. This makes the therapist's commitment clear and sets the tone for a "team effort." It begins to undercut one reason for relapse, the patient's sense of being on his or her own if unable to manage the situation. The astute therapist, however, will assure that he or she does not spend excessive time on the telephone or in emergency sessions. The patient will therefore develop a support network that can handle the majority of problems involved in day-to-day assistance. This generally will leave the therapist to respond only to occasional questions of interpreting the terms of the understanding among himself or herself, the patient, and support network members. If there is a question about the ability of the patient and network to manage the period between the initial sessions, the first few scheduled sessions may be arranged at intervals of only 1 to 3 days. In any case, frequent appointments should be scheduled at the outset if a pharmacologic detoxification with benzodiazepines is indicated, so that the patient need never manage more than a few days' medication at a time.

What is most essential, however, is that the network be forged into a working group to provide necessary support for the patient between the initial sessions. Membership ranges from one to several persons close to the patient. Larger networks have been used by Speck (24) in treating schizophrenic patients. Contacts between network members at this stage typically include telephone calls (at the therapist's or patient's initiative), dinner arrangements, and social encounters and should be preplanned to a fair extent during the joint session. These encounters are most often undertaken at the time when alcohol or drug use is likely to occur. In planning together, however, it should be made clear to network members that relatively little unusual effort will be required for the long term and that after the patient is stabilized, their participation will amount to little more than attendance at infrequent meetings with the patient and therapist. This is reassuring to those network members who are unable to make a major time commitment to the patient as well as to those patients who do not want to be placed in a dependent position.

Defining the Network's Membership

Once the patient has come for an appointment, establishing a network is a task undertaken with active collaboration of patient and therapist. The two, aided by those parties who join the network initially, must search for the right balance of members. The therapist must carefully promote the choice of appropriate network members, however, just as the platoon leader selects those who will go into combat. The network will be crucial in determining the balance of the therapy. This process is not without problems, and the therapist must think in a strategic fashion of the interactions that may take place among network members. The following case illustrates the nature of their task.

A 25-year-old graduate student had been abusing cocaine since high school, in part drawing from funds from his affluent family, who lived in a remote city. At two points in the process of establishing his support network, the reactions of his live-in girlfriend, who worked with us from the outset, were particularly important. Both he and she agreed to bring in his 19-year-old sister, a freshman at a nearby college. He then mentioned a "friend" of his, apparently a woman whom he had found attractive, even though there was no history of an overt romantic involvement. The expression on his girlfriend's face suggested that she did not like this idea, although she offered no rationale for excluding this potential rival. However, the idea of having to rely for assistance solely on two women who might see each other as competitors was unappealing. The therapist therefore finessed the idea of the "friend," and both she and the patient moved on to evaluating the patient's uncle, whom he initially preferred to exclude, despite the fact that his girlfriend thought him appropriate. It later turned out (as expected) that the uncle was perceived as a potentially disapproving representative of the parental generation. The therapist encouraged the patient to accept the uncle as a network member nonetheless, so as to round out the range of relationships within the group, and did spell out my rationale for his inclusion. The uncle did turn out to be caring and supportive, particularly after he was helped to understand the nature of the addictive process.

Defining the Network's Task

As conceived here, the therapist's relationship to the network is like that of a task-oriented team leader, rather than that of a family therapist oriented toward insight. The network is established to implement a straightforward task, that of aiding the therapist in sustaining the patient's abstinence. It must be directed with the same clarity of purpose that a task force is directed in any effective organization. Competing and alternative goals must be suppressed, or at least prevented from interfering with the primary task.

Unlike family members involved in traditional family therapy, network members are not led to expect symptom relief for themselves or self-realization. This prevents the development of competing goals for the network's meetings. It also assures the members protection from having their own motives scrutinized and thereby supports their continuing involvement without the threat of an assault on their psychological defenses. Because network members have—kindly—volunteered to participate, their motives must not be impugned. Their constructive behavior should be commended. It is useful to acknowledge appreciation for the contribution they are making to the therapy. There is always a counterproductive tendency on their part to minimize the value of their contribution. The network must, therefore, be structured as an effective working group with high morale. This is not always easy.

A 45-year-old single woman served as an executive in a large family-held business—except when her alcohol problem led her into protracted binges. Her father, brother, and sister were prepared to banish her from the business but decided first to seek consultation. Because they had initiated the contact, they were included in the initial network and indeed were very helpful in stabilizing the patient. Unfortunately, however, the father was a domineering figure who intruded in all aspects of the business, evoking angry outbursts from his children. The children typically reacted with petulance, provoking him in return. The situation came to a head when both of the patient's siblings angrily petitioned me to exclude the father from the network, 2 months into the treatment. This presented a problem because the father's control over the business made his involvement important to securing the patient's compliance. The patient's relapse was still a real possibility. This potentially coercive role, however, was an issue that the group could not easily deal with. The therapist decided to support the father's membership in the group, pointing out the constructive role he had played in getting the therapy started. It seemed necessary to support the earnestness of his concern for his daughter, rather than the children's dismay at their father's (very real) obstinacy. It was clear to the therapist that the father could not deal with a situation in which he was not accorded sufficient respect and that there was no real place in this network for addressing the father's character pathology directly. The hubbub did, in fact, quiet down with time. The children became less provocative themselves, as the group responded to my pleas for civil behavior.

The Use of Alcoholics Anonymous

Use of self-help modalities is desirable whenever possible. For the alcoholic, certainly, participation in AA is strongly encouraged. Groups such as Narcotics Anonymous, Pills Anonymous, and Cocaine Anonymous are modeled after AA and play a similarly useful role for drug abusers. One approach is to tell the patient that he or she is expected to attend at least two AA meetings a week for at least 1 month, so as to become familiar with the program. If after a month the patient is quite reluctant to continue, and other aspects of the treatment are going well, the patient's nonparticipation may have to be accepted.

Some patients are more easily convinced to attend AA meetings; others may be less compliant. The therapist should mobilize the support network as appropriate, so as to continue pressure for the patient's involvement with AA for a reasonable trial. It may take a considerable period of time, but ultimately a patient may experience something of a conversion, wherein the patient adopts the group ethos and expresses a deep commitment to abstinence, a measure of commitment rarely observed in patients who undergo psychotherapy alone. When this occurs, the therapist may assume a more passive role in monitoring the patient's abstinence and keep an eye on the patient's ongoing involvement in AA.

Use of Pharmacotherapy in the Network Format

For the alcoholic, disulfiram may be of marginal use in assuring abstinence when used in a traditional counseling context (25), but becomes much more valuable when carefully integrated into work with the patient and network, particularly when the drug is taken under observation. A similar circumstance applies to the use of oral naltrexone for stabilizing abstinence in an opioid-dependent person. In the case of alcohol, it is a good idea to use the initial telephone contact to engage the patient's agreement to abstain from alcohol for the day immediately prior to the first session. The therapist then has the option of prescribing or administering disulfiram at that time. For a patient who is earnest about seeking assistance for alcoholism, this is often not difficult, if some time is spent on the phone making plans to avoid a drinking context during that period. If it is not feasible to undertake this on the phone, it may be addressed in the first session. Such planning with the patient almost always involves organizing time with significant others and therefore serves as a basis for developing the patient's support network.

The administration of disulfiram under observation is a treatment option that is easily adapted to work with social networks. A patient who takes disulfiram cannot drink; a patient who agrees to be observed by a responsible party while taking disulfiram will not miss his or her dose without the observer's knowledge. This may take a measure of persuasion and, above all, the therapist's commitment that such an approach can be reasonable and helpful.

Disulfiram typically is initiated with a dose of 500 mg, and then reduced to 250 mg daily. It is taken every morning, when the urge to drink is generally least. Particulars of administration in the context of treatment has been described (26).

As noted previously, individual therapists traditionally have seen the addicted person as a patient with poor prognosis. This is largely because in the context of traditional psychotherapy, there are no behavioral controls to prevent the recurrence of drug use, and resources are not available for behavioral intervention if a recurrence takes place—which may occur. A system of impediments to the emergence of relapse, resting heavily on the actual or symbolic role of the network, must therefore be established. The therapist must have assistance in addressing any minor episode of drinking so that this ever-present problem does not lead to an unmanageable relapse or an unsuccessful termination of therapy.

How can the support network be used to deal with recurrences of alcohol use, when in fact, the patient's prior association with these same persons did not prevent him or her from drinking? The following example illustrates how this may be done when social resources are limited. In this case, a specific format was defined with the network to monitor a patient's compliance with a disulfiram regimen.

A 33-year-old public relations executive had moved to New York from a remote city 3 years before coming to treatment. She had no long-standing close relationships in the city, a circumstance not uncommon for a single alcoholic in a setting removed from her origins. She presented with a 10-year history of heavy drinking that had increased in severity since her arrival, no doubt associated with her social isolation. Although she consumed a bottle of wine each night and additional hard liquor, she was able to get to work regularly. Six months before the outset of treatment, she attended AA meetings for 2 weeks and had been abstinent during that time. She had then relapsed, though, and became disillusioned about the possibility of maintaining abstinence. At the outset of treatment, it was necessary to reassure her that prior relapse was in large part a function of not having established sufficient outside supports (including more sound relationships within AA) and of having seen herself as failed after only one slip. However, there was basis for real concern as to whether she would do any better now, if the same formula was reinstituted in the absence of sufficient, reliable supports, which she did not seem to have. Together the therapist and she came up with the idea of bringing in an old friend whom she saw occasionally and whom she felt she could trust. They made the following arrangement with her friend. The patient came to sessions twice a week. She would see her friend once each weekend. On each of these thrice-weekly occasions, she would be observed taking disulfiram, so that even if she missed a daily dose in between, it would not be possible for her to resume drinking on a regular basis, undetected. The interpersonal support inherent in this arrangement, bolstered by conjoint meetings with her and her friend, also allowed her to return to AA with a sense of confidence in her ability to maintain abstinence.

Format for Medication Observation by the Network

1. Take the medication every morning in front of a network member.
2. Take the pill so that that person can observe you swallowing them.
3. The observer writes down the time of day the pills were taken on a list prepared by the therapist.
4. The observer brings the list in to the therapist's office at each network session.
5. The observer leaves a message on the therapist's answering machine on any day in which the patient had not taken the pills in a way that ingestion was not clearly observed.

Meeting Arrangements

At the outset of therapy, it is important to see the patient with the group on a weekly basis for at least the first month. Unstable circumstances demand more frequent contacts with the network. Sessions can be tapered off to biweekly and then to monthly intervals after a time.

To sustain the continuing commitment of the group, particularly that between the therapist and the network members, network sessions should be held every 3 months or so for the duration of the individual therapy. Once the patient has stabilized, the meetings tend less to address day-to-day issues. They may begin with the patient's recounting of the drug situation. Reflections on the patient's progress and goals, or sometimes on relations among the network members, then may be discussed. In any case, it is essential that network members contact the therapist if they are concerned about the patient's possible use of alcohol or drugs and that the therapist contact the network members if the therapist becomes concerned about a potential relapse.

Adapting Individual Therapy to the Network Treatment

As noted previously, network sessions are scheduled on a weekly basis at the outset of treatment. This is likely to compromise the number of individual contacts. Indeed, if sessions are held once a week, the patient may not be seen individually for a period of time. The patient may perceive this as a deprivation unless the individual therapy is presented as an opportunity for further growth predicated on achieving stable abstinence assured through work with the network.

When the individual therapy does begin, the traditional objectives of therapy must be arranged so as to accommodate the goals of the substance abuse treatment. For insight-oriented therapy, clarification of unconscious motivations is a primary objective; for supportive therapy, the bolstering of established constructive defenses is primary. In the therapeutic context that is described here, however, the following objectives are given precedence.

Of primary importance is the need to address exposure to substances of abuse or to cues that might precipitate alcohol or drug use (27). Both patient and therapist should be sensitive to this matter and explore these situations as they arise. Second, a stable social context in an appropriate social environment—one conducive to abstinence with minimal disruption of life circumstances—should be supported. Considerations of minor disruptions in place of residence, friends, or job need not be a primary issue for the patient with character disorder or neurosis, but they cannot go untended here. For a considerable period of time, the substance abuser is highly vulnerable to exacerbations of the addictive illness and in some respects must be viewed with the considerable caution with which one treats the recently compensated psychotic.

Finally, after these priorities have been attended to, psychological conflicts that the patient must resolve, relative to his or her own growth, are considered. As the therapy continues, these come to assume a more prominent role. In the earlier phases, they are likely to reflect directly issues associated with previous drug use. Later, however, as the issue of addiction becomes less compelling from day to day, the context of the treatment increasingly will come to resemble the traditional psychotherapeutic context. Given the optimism generated by an initial victory over the addictive process, the patient will be in an excellent position to move forward in therapy with a positive view of his or her future.

A LONGER COURSE

The following case description illustrates how a network was engaged in treating a patient in long-term care for his addictive problem.

A 22-year-old man left a message on the therapist's answering machine asking if he could make an appointment. When called back, he said he wanted help to address his heroin habit. He said, "I gotta get clean." In response to a few questions, he described himself as a 30-year-old, single artist who clearly had aspirations to achieve wider recognition. He had been using heroin intranasally on and off for 3 years, but for the past 6 months was "sniffing" large doses at least twice a day.

At the initial encounter, given concern about his reliability, the therapist asked to engage collateral support for the patient. He asked if they could both speak on the phone with a friend or a close family member of his who could be a resource for him until the next session. Although he was somewhat wary, he agreed to their calling a cousin with whom he had a close relationship and who had repeatedly expressed concern over his drug use. The three agreed that the cousin would meet him for dinner right before the next scheduled session, and come with him to that appointment.

The patient appeared with his cousin 4 days later. He was somewhat tremulous, and reported that he and a friend, also addicted to heroin, had decided to detoxify themselves abruptly with some naltrexone that his friend had acquired. They supported each other, suffering miserably over the intervening days.

This patient was a good candidate for Network Therapy: his continuous dependence on heroin had been less than a year in duration, and this was less than appropriate for maintenance on buprenorphine or methadone. It would be desirable to avoid his dependency for the long term on an opioid if that could be avoided—and he did not want that option anyway. His network was constituted of three people: his cousin, a close friend, and an uncle 20 years his senior, whom he viewed as a mentor and friend. For the first 3 weeks, individual and network sessions were alternated each week. Over the subsequent weeks, the frequency of network meetings was decreased relative to the therapist's sense of the patient's stability in treatment. After 6 months the network members came to a session only once every month or two.

A second component of the treatment was to provide protection from relapse by having the patient take oral naltrexone, an opioid antagonist, which blocks the effect of an agonist, heroin or otherwise, such as hydrocodone. It was arranged that he would take two 50-mg pills twice weekly (Monday and Wednesday), and three on a third occasion (Friday). He would do this in front of his cousin, who lived only one block away from him. This naltrexone regimen was continued over the course of the ensuing 10 months, and after that on the patient's own recognizance.

At the outset of treatment, the therapist had stipulated that the patient was not to use marijuana, alcohol, or other drugs, explaining to him and the network how any of these could lead to a relapse. He was also expected to give a urine sample for toxicology at random times in order to assure abstinence from drugs. The patient did indeed say at one point in the treatment that he felt supported in avoiding marijuana by virtue of the fact that he did not want to have a positive urine toxicology.

The therapist had often discussed with the patient his vulnerability to alcoholism given his family history. Alcohol was a blight on his family, as his father always drank heavily every evening, making him very uncomfortable during his occasional visits to home. After 3 months in treatment, however, the patient said that he had "never bargained for not drinking at all" and that he didn't quite see himself as abstinent from alcohol for the long term. As the therapist and he discussed this, they agreed that it was best that he stay abstinent for at least a year, and toward the end of that time his options could be discussed. The issue was also discussed with the network members, who were wary of the patient embarking on something other than total abstinence, but the therapist pointed out that a test of drinking was "better during treatment than afterwards." This was discussed at some length, and the patient implemented a diary of his drinking, limited to no more than two beers a day and no wine or hard liquor.

At one point during the subsequent treatment, tragedy befell the family, as the patient's younger brother, who also drank abusively, had an auto accident while drunk and was gravely injured. After this, the patient had continued to keep his drinking diary, but a month after his brother's accident, he decided that he was better off remaining abstinent, and decided to do so. He did indeed maintain abstinence over a year of subsequent ongoing psychotherapy for general adaptive issues, and reported being abstinent 3 years after that.

RESEARCH ON NETWORK THERAPY

Network Therapy is included under the American Psychiatric Association (APA) Practice Guidelines (28) for substance use disorders as an approach to facilitating adherence to a treatment plan. The Substance Abuse and Mental Health Services Administration (SAMHSA) includes a description of Network Therapy in its National Registry of Evidence-Based Program and Practices (29), and Network Therapy is listed in one of its Treatment Improvement Protocols (TIP) as Substance Abuse Treatment and Family Therapy (30). To date, five studies have demonstrated its effectiveness in treatment and training. Each addressed the technique's validation from a different perspective: a trial in office management, studies of its effectiveness in the training of psychiatric residents and of counselors who work with cocaine-addicted persons, an evaluation of acceptance of the network approach in an Internet technology transfer course, and a trial evaluating the impact of Network Therapy relative to medication management in heroin-addicted persons inducted on to buprenorphine. In addition, Network Therapy components that have been adapted and combined with other psychosocial treatments to treat patients with opioid or alcohol dependence are described below.

An Office-Based Clinical Trial

A chart review was conducted on a series of 60 substance-dependent patients, with follow-up appointments scheduled through the period of treatment and up to 1 year thereafter (31). For 27 patients, the primary drug of dependence was alcohol; for 23, it was cocaine; for 6, it was opiates; for 3, it was marijuana; and for 1, it was nicotine. In all but eight of the patients, networks were fully established. Of the 60 patients, 46 experienced full improvement (i.e., abstinence for at least 6 months) or major improvement (i.e., a marked decline in drug use to nonproblematic levels). The study demonstrated the viability of establishing networks and applying them in the practitioner's treatment setting. It also served as a basis for the ensuing developmental research supported by the National Institute on Drug Abuse.

Treatment by Psychiatry Residents

We developed and implemented a Network Therapy training sequence in the New York University Psychiatric Residency Program and then evaluated the clinical outcome of a group of cocaine-dependent patients treated by the residents. The psychiatric residency was chosen because of the growing importance of clinical training in the management of addiction in outpatient care in residency programs, in line with the standards set for specialty certification.

A training manual was prepared on the network technique, defining the specifics of the treatment in a manner allowing for uniformity in practice. It was developed for use as a training tool and then as a guide for the residents during the treatment phase. Network Therapy tape segments drawn from a library of 130 videotaped sessions were used to illustrate typical therapy situations. A Network Therapy rating scale was developed to assess the technique's application, with items emphasizing key aspects of treatment (32). The scale was evaluated for its reliability in distinguishing between two contrasting addiction therapies, Network Therapy and systemic family therapy, both presented to faculty and residents on videotape. The internal consistency of responses for each of the techniques was high for both the faculty and the resident samples, and both groups consistently distinguished the two modalities. The scale was then used by clinical supervisors as a didactic aid for training and to monitor therapist adherence to the study treatment manual.

We trained third-year psychiatry residents to apply the Network Therapy approach, with an emphasis placed on distinctions in technique between the treatment of addiction and of other major mental illness or personality disorder. The residents then worked with a sample of 47 cocaine-addicted patients. Once treatment was initiated, 77% of the subjects did establish a network, that is, bring in at least one member for a network session. In fact, 1.47 collaterals on average attended any given network session, across all the subjects and sessions. This is notable, because compliance after initial screening was not necessarily assured. Almost all of those who completed a 24-week regimen (15 of 17) produced urines negative for cocaine in their last three toxicologies. On the other hand, only a minority of those who attended the first week but who did not complete the sequence (4 of 18) met this outcome criterion (33). The residents, inexperienced in drug treatment, achieved results similar to those reported for experienced professionals (34,35). These comparisons supported the feasibility of successful training of psychiatry residents naive to addiction treatment and the efficacy of the treatment in their hands.

To better understand the role of therapeutic alliance in Network Therapy, Glazer et al. (36) reviewed videotaped network sessions on 21 out of the 47 cocaine-addicted patients and rated them on level of patient–therapist alliance using the PENN Helping Alliance Rating Scale and the Working Alliance Inventory. The tapes that were selected to be rated were those that represented the participants' first videotaped Network Therapy session. Results showed a significant positive correlation between therapeutic alliance and outcomes as measured by the percentage of cocaine-free urine toxicology screens and by eight consecutive cocaine-free urines.

Treatment by Addiction Counselors

This study was conducted in a community-based addictions treatment clinic, and the Network Therapy training sequence was essentially the same as the one applied to the psychiatry residents (37). A cohort of 10 cocaine-dependent patients received treatment at the community program with a format that included Network Therapy, along with the clinic's usual package of modalities, and an additional 20 cocaine-dependent patients received treatment as usual and served as control subjects. The Network Therapy was found to enhance the outcome of the experimental patients. Of 107 urinalyses conducted on the Network Therapy patients, 88% were negative, but only 66% of the 82 urine samples from the control subjects were negative, a significantly lower proportion. The mean retention in treatment was 13.9 weeks for the network patients, reflecting a trend toward greater retention than the 10.7 weeks for control subjects.

The results of this study supported the feasibility of transferring the network technology into community-based settings with the potential for enhancing outcomes. Addiction counselors working in a typical outpatient rehabilitation setting were able to learn and then incorporate Network Therapy into their largely twelve-step-oriented treatment regimens without undue difficulty and with improved outcome.

Use of the Internet

We studied ways in which psychiatrists and other professionals could be offered training by a distance-learning method using the Internet, a medium that offers the advantage of not being fixed in either time or location. An advertisement was placed in *Psychiatric News*, the newspaper of the APA, offering an Internet course combining Network Therapy with the use of naltrexone for the treatment of alcoholism.

The sequence of material presented on the Internet was divided into three didactic "sessions," followed by a set of questions, with a hypertext link to download relevant references and a certificate of completion. The course took about 2 hours for the student to complete. Our assessment was based on 679 sequential counts, representing 240 unique respondents who went beyond the introductory web page (38). Of these respondents, 154 were psychiatrists, who responded positively to the course. A majority responded "a good deal" or "very much" (a score of 3 or 4 on a four-point scale) to the following statements: "It helped me understand the management of alcoholism treatment" (56%), "It helped me learn to use family or friends in network treatment for alcoholism" (75%), and "It improved my ability to use naltrexone in treating alcoholism" (64%). The four studies described in this section support the use of Network Therapy as an effective treatment for addictive disorders. They are especially encouraging given the relative ease with which different types of clinicians were engaged and trained in the network approach. Because the approach combines a number of well-established clinical techniques that can be adapted to delivery in typical clinical settings, it is apparently suitable for use by general clinicians and addiction specialists.

Network Therapy in Buprenorphine Maintenance

Galanter et al. (39) evaluated the impact of Network Therapy relative to a control condition (medical management, MM) among 66 patients who were inducted on to buprenorphine for 16 weeks and then tapered to zero dose. Network Therapy resulted in a greater percentage of opioid-free urines than did MM (65% vs. 45%). By the end of treatment, Network Therapy patients were more likely to experience a positive outcome relative to secondary heroin use (50% vs. 23%). The use of Network Therapy in office practice may enhance the effectiveness of eliminating secondary heroin use during buprenorphine maintenance.

ADAPTATIONS OF NETWORK THERAPY TREATMENT

Rothenberg et al. (40) adapted Network Therapy and combined it with relapse prevention and a voucher reinforcement system in the treatment of opioid-dependent patients who were enrolled in a 6-month course of treatment with naltrexone referred to as behavioral naltrexone therapy (BNT). The Network Therapy component involved one significant other who could monitor adherence to naltrexone. In addition to the patient receiving vouchers for each day of abstinence and each pill taken, the network member was reinforced with a voucher for each pill recorded as monitored. The primary treatment outcome was retention in treatment. Patients who used methadone at baseline did more poorly than those using only heroin, as demonstrated in the retention rates: 39% vs. 65% and 0% vs. 31%, respectively, at 1 month and 6 months.

Copello et al. (41) combined elements of Network Therapy with social aspects of the community reinforcement approach and relapse prevention referred to as social behavior and network therapy (SBNT) in the treatment of persons with alcohol drinking problems. A number of social skills training strategies are incorporated into the treatment, especially those involving social competence in relation to the development of positive social support for change in alcohol use. Every individual involved in treatment is considered a client in his or her own right, and the person with alcohol problems is referred to as the focal client. The core element of the approach is mobilizing the support of the network even though this may involve network sessions that are conducted in the absence of the focal client. In their initial feasibility study with 33 clients, there were two cases in which sessions were held with network members in the absence of the focal client, and in both cases re-engagement of the focal client in treatment was achieved. Out of the 33 clients enrolled in the study, 23 formed a network with the mean number of network members equal to 1.82 and the mean number of network sessions equal to 5.24. In a multisite, randomized controlled trial of 742 clients with alcohol problems, the UKATT research team (42) compared SBNT to motivational enhancement therapy (MET). Both treatment groups exhibited similar reductions in alcohol consumption and alcohol-related problems and improvement in mental functioning over a 12-month period.

Additional studies involving the UKATT study sample were conducted assessing (a) cost-effectiveness (43), (b) client-treatment matching effects (44), and (c) clients' perceptions of change in alcohol drinking behaviors (45). The UKATT team evaluated the cost-effectiveness of SBNT relative to MET. SBNT resulted in a fivefold cost savings in health, social, and criminal justice service expenditures and was similar to cost-effectiveness estimates obtained for MET. The UKATT research team (44) tested a priori hypotheses concerning client-treatment matching effects similar to those tested in Project MATCH. The findings were consistent with Project MATCH in that no hypothesized matching effects were significant. Orford et al. (45) interviewed a subset of clients ($n = 397$) who participated in this trial to assess their views concerning whether any positive changes in drinking behavior had occurred and to what they attributed those changes. At 3 months after randomization to treatment, SBNT clients made more social attributions (e.g., involvement of others in supporting behavior change) and MET clients made more motivational attributions (e.g., awareness of the consequences of drinking).

Copello et al. (46) adapted SBNT for persons presenting with drug problems. Of 31 clients enrolled in the study, 23 received SBNT and had outcomes data available at 3-month follow-up. Reductions in the amount of heroin used per day and increases in family cohesion and family satisfaction were documented. Open-ended interviews with clients, network members, and therapists were conducted in a qualitative investigation of respondents' perceptions of SBNT (47). Major themes that emerged from the analysis of interview responses included the value of SBNT in (a) increasing network support for reducing drug use, (b) promoting open and honest communication between clients and network members about drug use, and (c) increasing network members' understanding of drugs and the focal person's behavior. Williamson et al. (47) suggest that these features of SBNT may be more prominent when the problem is one of illicit drug use than when the problem involves alcohol use.

PRINCIPLES OF NETWORK TREATMENT

Start a Network as Soon as Possible

1. It is important to see the alcohol or drug abuser promptly, because the window of opportunity for openness to treatment is generally brief. A week's delay can result in a person's reverting back to drunkenness or losing motivation.
2. If the person is married, engage the spouse early on, preferably at the time of the first phone call. Point out that addiction is a family problem. For most drugs, you can enlist the spouse in assuring that the patient arrives at your office with a day's sobriety.
3. In the initial interview, frame the exchange so that a good case is built for the grave consequences of the patient's addiction, and do this before the patient can introduce his or her system of denial. That way you are not putting the spouse or other network members in the awkward position of having to contradict a close relation.
4. Then make clear that the patient needs to be abstinent, starting now. (A tapered detoxification may be necessary sometimes, as with depressant pills.)
5. When seeing an alcoholic patient for the first time, start the patient on disulfiram treatment as soon as possible, in the office if you can. Have the patient continue taking disulfiram under observation of a network member.
6. Start arranging for a network to be assembled at the first session, generally involving one of the patient's family or close friends.
7. From the very first meeting you should consider how to ensure sobriety till the next meeting, and plan that with the network. Initially, their immediate company, a plan for daily AA attendance, and planned activities may all be necessary.

Manage the Network with Care

1. Include people who are close to the patient, have a long-standing relationship with the patient, and are trusted. Avoid members with substance problems, because they will let you down when you need their unbiased support. Avoid superiors and subordinates at work, because they have an overriding relationship with the patient independent of friendship.
2. Get a balanced group. Avoid a network composed solely of the parental generation, or of younger people, or of people of the opposite sex. Sometimes a nascent network selects itself for a consultation if the patient is reluctant to address his or her own problem. Such a group will later supportively engage the patient in the network, with your careful guidance.
3. Make sure that the mood of meetings is trusting and free of recrimination. Avoid letting the patient or the network members feel guilty or angry in meetings. Explain issues of conflict in terms of the problems presented by addiction; do not get into personality conflicts.
4. The tone should be directive. That is to say, give explicit instructions to support and ensure abstinence. A feeling of teamwork should be promoted, with no psychologizing or impugning members' motives.
5. Meet as frequently as necessary to ensure abstinence, perhaps once a week for a month, every other week for the next few months, and every month or two by the end of a year.
6. The network should have no agenda other than to support the patient's abstinence. But as abstinence is stabilized, the network can help the patient plan for a new drug-free adaptation. It is not there to work on family relations or help other members with their problems, although it may do this indirectly.

Keep the Network's Agenda Focused

1. *Maintaining abstinence.* The patient and the network members should report at the outset of each session any exposure of the patient to alcohol and drugs. The patient and network members should be instructed on the nature of relapse and plan with the therapist how to sustain abstinence. Cues to conditioned drug seeking should be examined.
2. *Supporting the network's integrity.* Everyone has a role in this. The patient is expected to make sure that network members keep their meeting appointments and stay involved with the treatment. The therapist sets meeting times and summons the network for any emergency, such as relapse; the therapist does whatever is necessary to secure stability of the membership if the patient is having trouble doing so. Network members' responsibility is to attend network sessions, although they may be asked to undertake other supportive activity with the patient.

3. *Securing future behavior.* The therapist should combine any and all modalities necessary to ensure the patient's stability, such as a stable, drug-free residence; the avoidance of substance-abusing friends; attendance at twelve-step meetings; medications such as disulfiram or blocking agents; observed urinalysis; and ancillary psychiatric care. Written agreements may be handy, such as a mutually acceptable contingency contract with penalties for violation of understandings.

Make Use of Alcoholics Anonymous and Other Self-Help Groups

1. Patients should be expected to go to meetings of AA or related groups at least two to three times, with follow-up discussion in therapy.
2. If patients have reservations about these meetings, try to help them understand how to deal with those reservations. Issues such as social anxiety should be explored if they make a patient reluctant to participate. Generally, resistance to AA can be related to other areas of inhibition in a person's life, as well as to the denial of addiction.
3. As with other spiritual involvements, do not probe the patients' motivation or commitment to AA once engaged. Allow them to work out things on their own, but be prepared to listen.

REFERENCES

1. Galanter M. Cognitive labeling: psychotherapy for alcohol and drug abuse: an approach based on learning theory. *J Psychiatr Treat Eval.* 1983;5:551–556.
2. Jellinek EM. *The Disease Concept of Alcoholism.* New Haven, CT: Hillhouse; 1963.
3. Marlatt GA, Gordon J. *Relapse Prevention: Maintenance Strategies in the Treatment of Addictive Behaviors.* New York: Guilford Press; 1985.
4. Beck AT, Wright FD, Newman CF, et al. *Cognitive Therapy of Substance Abuse.* New York: Guilford Press; 1993.
5. Johnson VE. *Intervention: How to Help Someone Who Doesn't Want Help.* Minneapolis: Johnson Institute; 1986.
6. McCrady BS, Stout R, Noel N, et al. Effectiveness of three types of spouse-involved behavioral alcoholism treatment. *Br J Addict.* 1991;86:1415–1424.
7. Azrin NH, Sisson RW, Meyers R. Alcoholism treatment by disulfiram and community reinforcement therapy. *J Behav Ther Psychiatry.* 1982;13:105–112.
8. Khantzian EJ. The primary care therapist and patient needs in substance abuse treatment. *Am J Drug Alcohol Abuse.* 1988;14:159–167.
9. Morgenstern J, Longabaugh R. Cognitive-behavioral treatment for alcohol dependence: a review of the evidence for its hypothesized mechanisms of action. *Addiction.* 2000;95:1475–1490.
10. Stephens RS, Babor TF, Kadden R, et al. The marijuana treatment project: rationale, design, and participant characteristics. *Addiction.* 2002;94:109–124.
11. Carroll KM. *A Cognitive-Behavioral Approach: Treating Cocaine Addiction.* Rockville, MD: National Institute on Drug Abuse; 1998.
12. Wikler A. Dynamics of drug dependence: implications of a conditioning theory for research and treatment. *Arch Gen Psychiatry.* 1973;28:611–616.
13. Zywiak WH, Wirtz PW. Decomposing the relationships between pretreatment social network characteristics and alcohol treatment outcome. *J Stud Alcohol.* 2002;63(1):114–121.
14. Beckman LJ, Amaro H. Personal and social difficulties faced by women and men entering alcoholism treatment. *J Stud Alcohol.* 1986;47:135–145.
15. Fals-Stewart W, O'Farrell TJ, Feehan M, et al. Behavioral couples therapy versus individual-based treatment for male substance-abusing patients. *JSAT.* 2000;18:249–254.
16. O'Farrell TJ. Marital therapy in the treatment of alcoholism. In: Jacobson NS, Gurman AS, eds. *Clinical Handbook of Marital Therapy.* New York, NY: Guilford Press; 1986:513–535.
17. Azrin NH, Sisson RW, Meyers R, et al. Alcoholism treatment by disulfiram and community reinforcement therapy. *J Behav Ther Exp Psychiatry.* 1982;13:105–112.
18. Meyers RJ, Smith JE, Lash DN. The community reinforcement approach. *Recent Dev Alcohol.* 2003;16:183–195.
19. Kirby KC, Marlowe DB, Festinger DS, et al. Community reinforcement training for family and significant others of drug abusers: a unilateral intervention to increase treatment entry of drug users. *Drug Alcohol Depend.* 1999;56:85–96.
20. Meyers RJ, Miller WR, Smith JE, et al. A randomized trial of two methods for engaging treatment-refusing drug users through concerned significant others. *J Consult Clin Psychol.* 2002;70:1182–1185.
21. Landau J, Stanton DM, Brinkman-Sull D, et al. Outcomes with the ARISE approach to engaging reluctant drug- and alcohol-dependent individuals in treatment. *Am J Drug Alcohol Abuse.* 2004;30(4):711–748.
22. Helzer JE, Robins LN, Taylor JR, et al. The extent of long-term drinking among alcoholics discharged from medical and psychiatric facilities. *N Engl J Med.* 1985;312:1678–1682.
23. Gitlow SE, Peyser HS, eds. *Alcoholism: A Practical Treatment Guide.* New York: Grune & Stratton; 1980.
24. Speck R. Psychotherapy of the social network of a schizophrenic family. *Fam Process.* 1967;6:208.
25. Fuller R, Branchey L, Brightwell DR, et al. Disulfiram treatment of alcoholism. A veterans administration cooperative study. *JAMA.* 1986;256:1449–1455.
26. Gallant DM. *Alcoholism: A Guide to Programs, Intervention and Treatment.* New York: Norton; 1987.
27. Galanter M. Network therapy for addiction: a model for office practice. *Am J Psychiatry.* 1993;150:28–36.
28. American Psychiatric Association. Practice guidelines for the treatment of patients with substance use disorders: alcohol, cocaine, opioids. *Am J Psychiatry.* 1995;152(11):1–59.
29. SAMHSA's National Registry of Evidence-Based Programs and Practices. *Network Therapy Review.* Available at: http://www.nrepp.samhsa.gov/porgramfulldetails.asp?PROGRAM_ID=61. [Review conducted February 2007.]
30. Center for Substance Abuse Treatment. *Substance Abuse Treatment and Family Therapy. Treatment Improvement Protocol (TIP) Series, No. 39.* DHHS Publication No. (SMA) 05-4006. Rockville, MD: Substance Abuse and Mental Health Services Administration; 2004.
31. Galanter M. Network therapy for substance abuse: a clinical trial. *Psychotherapy.* 1993;30:251–258.
32. Keller D, Galanter M, Weinberg S. Validation of a scale for network therapy: a technique for systematic use of peer and family

support in addiction treatment. *Am J Drug Alcohol Abuse.* 1997; 23:115–127.
33. Galanter M, Dermatis H, Keller D, et al. Network therapy for cocaine abuse: use of family and peer supports. *Am J Addict.* 2002;11:161–166.
34. Carroll KM, Rounsaville BJ, Gordon LT, et al. Psychotherapy and pharmacotherapy for ambulatory cocaine abusers. *Arch Gen Psychiatry.* 1994;51:177–187.
35. Higgins ST, Budney AJ, Bickel WK, et al. Achieving cocaine abstinence with a behavioral approach. *Am J Psychiatry.* 1993;150:763–769.
36. Glazer SS, Galanter M, Megwinoff O, et al. The role of therapeutic alliance in network therapy: a family and peer support-based treatment for cocaine abuse. *Subst Abuse.* 2003;24(2): 93–100.
37. Keller D, Galanter M, Dermatis H. Technology transfer of network therapy to community-based addiction counselors. *J Subst Abuse Treat.* 1999;16:183–189.
38. Galanter M, Keller DS, Dermatis H. Using the internet for clinical training: a course on network therapy. *Psychiatr Serv.* 1997;48:999. Available at: http://mednyu/substanceabuse/course.
39. Galanter M, Dermatis H, Glickman L, et al. Network therapy: decreased secondary opioid use during buprenorphine maintenance. *J Subst Abuse Treat.* 2004;26:313–318.
40. Rothenberg JL, Sullivan MA, Church SH, et al. Behavioral naltrexone therapy: an integrated treatment for opiate dependence. *J Subst Abuse Treat.* 2002;23:351–360.
41. Copello A, Orford J, Hodgson R, et al. Social behaviour and network therapy: basic principles and early experiences. *Addic Behav.* 2002;27:345–366.
42. UKATT Research Team. Effectiveness of treatment for alcohol problems: findings of the randomised UK alcohol treatment trial (UKATT). *BMJ.* 2005;331:541–543.
43. UKATT Research Team. Cost effectiveness of treatment for alcohol problems: findings of the randomised UK alcohol treatment trial (UKATT). *BMJ.* 2005;331:544–549.
44. UKATT Research Team. UK alcohol treatment trial: client-treatment matching effects. *Addiction.* 2008;103:228–238.
45. Orford J, Hodgson R, Copello A, et al. To what factors do clients attribute change? Content analysis of follow-up interview with clients of the UK alcohol trial. *J Subst Abuse Treat.* 2009;36:49–58.
46. Copello A, Williamson E, Orford J, et al. Implementing and evaluating social behaviour and network therapy in drug treatment practice in the UK: a feasibility study. *Addict Behav.* 2006;31: 802–810.
47. Williamson E, Smith M, Orford J, et al. Social behavior and network therapy for drug problems: evidence of benefits and challenges. *Addict Disord Treat.* 2007;6:167–179.

CHAPTER 41 Individual Psychotherapy

Joan E. Zweben

INTRODUCTION

This chapter describes the elements of individual therapy from the perspective of therapists working in the community as well as those working in addiction treatment programs. It gives an overview of the treatment tasks for therapists who are not specialists in the addiction field but are aware of the roles of alcohol and other drug use in undermining their patients' progress in other areas. It also reviews the tasks of the therapist or counselor who works within a structured addiction treatment program.

A great deal of addiction treatment is conducted in groups, and the relative expense of individual sessions can lead to downplaying their value. However, such sessions can play a key role in promoting the engagement and retention that is associated with positive substance abuse treatment outcomes. It is imperative that the therapists have familiarity with the stages and tasks of recovery and have the ability to tailor interventions accordingly. Individual therapy with a clinician familiar with addiction and recovery can make a significant contribution to the patient's quality of life at all stages.

No single definition allows us to distinguish between therapists and counselors, but historically the terms have been used to indicate level of training and scope of practice. Therapists, by custom and by law in many states, have advanced degrees in psychiatry, psychology, or social work and corresponding state licenses to practice autonomously. Counselors working in substance abuse treatment programs may or may not have credentials, and usually have circumscribed roles that include case management, exploring current obstacles to recovery efforts and teaching of early recovery skills. They may conduct individual sessions, depending upon particular organizational licenses and state laws.

Noncredentialed counselors were integrated into treatment teams on inpatient units in the 1950s, when the Minnesota model was developed at Hazelden (1), and when it became apparent that the mental health model that defined alcohol problems as a symptom of an underlying disorder was not producing good results. Counselors in 12-step recovery were brought in to create a new model that treated alcoholism as an independent disorder that must be addressed as such. Therapeutic communities (TCs), developed and expanded in the 1960s, also relied predominantly on noncredentialed staff in recovery (2–4). Some of these clinicians and managers were hired into the private sector programs and brought important perspectives on the importance of affiliating with a culture that supports recovery.

Some of these counselors have little training, except what they receive onsite, but many states require some form of credentialing, usually certification, and such programs can be quite demanding. Some require 200 to 300 hours of course work, plus supervised field placement experience. Many of the counselors are quite gifted and their street skills have made them keen observers of human behavior. In the last decade, the U.S. federal Center for Substance Abuse Treatment (CSAT) put extensive efforts into defining the competencies required for counselors in addiction treatment settings (5). They address the following issues:

- What professional standards should guide substance abuse treatment counselors?
- What is an appropriate scope of practice for the field?
- Which competencies are associated with positive outcomes?
- What knowledge, skills, and attitudes (KSAs) should all substance abuse treatment professionals have in common?

This effort by CSAT has provided a framework for curriculum development to the credentialing bodies, and also a structure for the selection, onsite training, and evaluation of counselors in the workplace.

CSAT also offers a *Directory of Addiction Study Programs (DASP)* (http://nattc.org/dasp/main.asp), a comprehensive list of institutions offering a certificate, associate, bachelor, master, and/or doctoral program in substance use disorders treatment. Included in this directory are institutions offering a concentration, specialty or minor in the addiction field.

THERAPISTS AND COUNSELORS WITHIN A SPECIALTY TREATMENT PROGRAM

Individual therapists and counselors have a variety of roles, depending on whether they are in specialty programs or private practice, and whether they are licensed or not. Both counselors and therapists in specialty programs may be utilized to do a comprehensive assessment, but whether this includes a precise evaluation of a mental disorder that coexists with the addictive disorder depends on whether the clinician has the training and appropriate license to do so. Although it can be difficult to get an accurate diagnosis, uncontaminated by substance-induced symptoms, it is nonetheless important to make a provisional diagnosis or a sufficiently clear description of symptoms to allow for treatment planning. This diagnosis can be revised as further information emerges.

Entry into a specialty program is often precipitated by a crisis and this is often best managed in individual sessions. It is tempting for family members and outside therapists to breathe a sigh of relief once the patient is admitted to a residential or inpatient program, but engaging family members and outpatient therapists at this stage gives an excellent opportunity to promote their involvement in the treatment episode (6,7) and in the patient's long-term recovery. Even a single meeting with family members permits the therapist to work more effectively with the patient toward good resolution of the current crisis. Some desirable outcomes of the crisis intervention are relief from stress and fear, enhancing the patient's confidence in the utility of professional help, harnessing the opportunities in the crisis, and increasing awareness that the alcohol and other drug use is only one element that needs to be addressed.

Structured programs rely heavily on group interventions, and these have some distinct advantages (8). Indeed, some staff may take the position that individual sessions undermine group participation. However, individual sessions have strategic value in promoting engagement, particularly for patients who are not yet comfortable disclosing important issues in a group format. It is important that therapists repeatedly encourage patients to bring important issues to the group as soon as they surface, and fears of further disclosure can be addressed.

Licensed therapists usually have strong clinical skills to bring to this effort. Individual sessions offer more time to explore issues related to motivation, work on ambivalence about abstinence, discuss incidents where behavioral strategies appeared to break down, and focus on the interplay between alcohol and other drug use and other psychiatric disorders that may be present. Although all of this can be done in the group setting, time constraints can preclude the kind of thorough discussion that improves results.

Therapists in Independent Practice

Finding a Therapist with Adequate Proficiency

The task of finding a therapist who is competent to assess and treat substance abuse issues is more complicated than one might assume. Unfortunately, academic degrees and professional licenses may not accurately represent specific skills to address substance abuse. Graduate or medical schools do not necessarily integrate thorough training in the assessment and treatment of addictive disorders into their core curricula, nor are their supervisors always prepared to address these issues in clinical training settings. Indeed, the older and more "seasoned" the clinical supervisor, the less the likelihood that he or she has had formal training in addressing substance abuse. Some seek it out, but many assume their basic training will serve them with only modest modifications and underestimate the importance of specialized knowledge. Licensed professionals have been known to be too wedded to their theoretical models, or their temperament may hamper their ability to revise their practices in the light of emerging evidence.

The claim that "I have been seeing alcohol and drug users for many years" does not settle questions of competence. Therapists become comfortable with the practices they have developed over time and are not usually in a position to study their dropouts. Many patients report minimizing or concealing their alcohol and other drug use for years, whereas their therapists focus on psychodynamic issues. When such issues become apparent, some therapists assume that a referral to 12-step programs or other forms of self-help is adequate to address the addiction. In the absence of specific knowledge about conducting a drug and alcohol assessment, they are ill equipped to determine if this will be enough.

The issue of the therapist or counselor's recovery status has been debated for decades. Many patients indicate that having a therapist in recovery increases their confidence that they will be understood and be given helpful guidance. However, some recovering people, like some licensed professionals, can be quite rigid and may find sophisticated ways to blame the patient if the treatment is not working. Although this issue has not been extensively studied, there are currently no data that support the notion that recovery status leads to greater or lesser effectiveness. The same is true for licenses and credentials. It is likely that in the end, therapist variables will be shown to have a major influence on substance abuse treatment outcome, as it has in psychotherapy itself (9). In the psychotherapy literature, therapist variables (the quality of the relationship, therapist effects such as positive regard) account for 18% of the variance, and the specific treatment method accounts for 5% to 8% (9).

In selecting good therapists for referral, it is helpful to consider

- Evidence of basic knowledge, through course work or continuing education activities
- Recent updates in training
- Good relationship skills, as reflected in patient and colleague feedback and patient satisfaction surveys.

Finding a Specialty Program

Therapists in the community are in a prime position to intervene early on developing problems with alcohol and other drugs, and if they are proficient, they may save the patient decades of self-destructive behavior. However, the patient may reach a point where more structure is needed than a private practitioner can provide and referral to a specialty program is in order. Patients rarely welcome such a recommendation. Indeed, it can take months or even years to prepare a psychotherapy patient to enter a specialty program, as these patients often do not recognize the significance of their alcohol and other drug use in their distress. A rapidly changing landscape in which programs open, close, or are acquired by different corporate entities makes it difficult to know which programs are sound. General considerations when choosing a program should include

- Whether the program has a current license from the Commission on Accreditation of Rehabilitation Facilities (CARF) or the Joint Commission (aka the Joint Commission on the

Accreditation of Health Care Organizations) or another certifying entity recognized by the state where the program is located.
- If not part of a local medical center, whether the program has a close relationship or current referral agreement with local primary and specialty care, including detoxification if needed.
- If the program involves family members in therapy and recovery planning. This means that geographical considerations should usually take precedence over prestige, unless financial resources permit participation no matter what the location.
- If the program uses evidence-based practices and explains them clearly to family members.
- If the program either provides or has access to medications, including psychotropic medications and medications used to treat addiction (such as buprenorphine or methadone). The program should not discriminate against patients needing specific types of medications. It is especially important that programs do not discourage patients needing opioid agonists or partial agonists from utilizing such medication as part of a comprehensive program of recovery.
- If the program is willing to maintain a collaborative relationship with the therapist in the community and include the therapist when possible in recovery planning meetings.

It is very important to assess financial resources and plan for a long-term recovery process. In private sector programs, what is offered as data on outcomes often originates from the marketing department and the average patient or family member is not equipped to evaluate the data they are shown. Interestingly, public sector programs are under more pressure to utilize evidence-based practices and document outcomes, and are often subject to third-party scrutiny. High prestige programs are often touted as the most desirable and some families mortgage their retirement in order to send their loved one for a month or more. The key question is what resources will be needed for the long term? What services will need to be continuous? For example, a patient with complex medical and psychiatric problems will possibly need a team that includes several physician specialists and a therapist, one of whom must agree to coordinate the care over the long term. The choice of inpatient or residential treatment should rest on whether the patient will get the needed services there, and what is offered in the brochure may not correspond to what is readily available once the patient enters the program. Inpatient/residential treatment may be an excellent way to sort out the patient's different problems, but the long-term structure and treatment plan will determine success. Unfortunately, the patient who has regular crises can elevate the anxiety of family members and even the therapist, resulting in magical expectations for specialty treatment. Not all essential activities need to be provided by professionals. There is a growing emphasis on a recovery-management approach that provides long-term supports and recognizes multiple pathways to healing (10). This paradigm shift requires relinquishing a crisis-oriented, acute care model that focuses on isolated treatment episodes in favor of a broader perspective in which professional treatment plays an important but not exclusive role.

Possible Conflicts between Therapists and Addiction Specialists

Smooth working relationships take time to develop, and many exist between addiction specialists and therapists in the community. It is helpful for the addiction specialist to recognize that time spent educating other professionals about treating addictive disorders has a multiplier effect, in that many other patients will benefit. Stigma is alive and potent; many therapists still have a stereotyped view of individuals with alcohol and other drug problems, especially about their prognosis. However, with training, therapists can become quite proficient at handling mild to moderate substance abuse problems and in preparing patients for specialty treatment if it will be needed. This puts them in a prime position to do prevention and early intervention, a valuable service to their patients.

Although it is increasingly common to find graduate programs providing education and supervision about the treatment of addictive disorders, older, seasoned therapists are the least likely to have received such training except for brief intensive workshops, often required for initial licensure or license renewal. Therapists who have been in practice for several decades may enjoy excellent reputations as clinicians, but may not appreciate their own limitations in addressing alcohol- and drug-using behavior. Since therapists do not systematically follow their dropouts, they can become comfortable with their way of handling these issues without knowing true outcomes.

Conflicts are also possible between some traditional models of psychotherapy and principles of addiction treatment. For example, insight-oriented psychodynamic therapy places great value on insight into root causes as a primary source of behavior change, whereas addiction treatment stresses the importance of structure and systematic transmission of specific skills to change drug-using behavior. Addiction specialists are more likely to be directive, particularly in early recovery, whereas psychodynamic therapists have more varied styles. These differences can be managed with good communication. Community therapists have an enormous contribution to make in early identification and intervention and to improve quality of life for the recovering patient.

Another major source of tension between psychotherapists and addiction specialists can also be the failure to understand the importance of self-help group participation. This is addressed later in this chapter.

Strengths and Limits of Office-based Therapy

There are distinct advantages to office-based therapy, and challenging disadvantages. Social stigma and the possibility of severe negative consequences to admitting substance use cause many individuals to avoid or delay seeking help for extended periods of time, especially in group settings. An office setting affords far greater reassurance of privacy and confidentiality. It is a far less threatening point of entry into treatment, and for those already in psychotherapy, there is an excellent opportunity to avoid the full-blown consequences of a substance use disorder through identification and early intervention by a therapist who is already trusted. There is greater possibility of flexible, individualized care. Most addiction treatment programs rely heavily on group interventions, for very good reasons. They often do a comprehensive assessment but are limited in their ability to offer individualized treatment. They also may be rigid in their rules, making it difficult to deal with patients who are ambivalent about their goals, or promote premature discharge of patients who are unable to achieve abstinence quickly or who relapse after doing well. Patients may also resist self-help group participation, the cornerstone of most addiction treatment programs. This resistance may often be more effectively dealt with in an individual therapy modality. A more complete discussion of patients who can benefit from office-based treatment can be found elsewhere (8).

Office-based treatment may have significant limitations, especially for the practitioner who does not have strong connections to other resources, including specialty addiction treatment programs. It is important for the therapist to identify an addiction medicine specialist to identify, evaluate, and treat addiction-related medical conditions. Early psychosocial treatment typically requires multiple visits each week, and patients may not be able to afford this, or their insurance may not cover anything but licensed addiction treatment programs. Individuals whose alcohol or other drug use is severely out of control usually require the firm structure of an inpatient, residential, or intensive outpatient specialty program to be launched into a successful recovery process. This is especially true if the patient is a suicide risk, or at risk of harming others. Therapists may be unwilling or unable to provide drug and alcohol testing in the office, and unable to find a monitoring program in the community. This undercuts his or her ability to have an objective marker of progress. It is highly desirable for therapists working with individuals to have an addiction recovery group available, either in his or her practice or in the community. This may be difficult to achieve. In short, the solo practitioner must assemble a variety of the resources normally found within structured programs to be prepared to meet the needs of the addicted patient.

In summary, the therapist in the community is in an ideal position to do early intervention, provide assistance to those with mild-to-moderate problems, and prepare patients to enter a specialty treatment program if that becomes appropriate. They can make an invaluable contribution to the quality of recovery, particularly if they develop an understanding of what it takes and are sensitive to relapse warning signs.

History of the Treatment

Individual psychotherapists have long attempted to address alcohol and other drug use within their preferred models. Leon Wurmser (11,12) represented a classic psychoanalytic view and recommended that the therapist provide and maintain an attitude of warmth, kindness, and flexibility in contrast to a more authoritarian approach adopted by many addiction treatment programs. He described substance abusers as having severe pathology due to childhood trauma, which must be addressed for treatment to be effective.

Edward Khantzian emphasized the user's vulnerabilities in self-regulation and self. He viewed drug use as self-medication in which individuals seek the specific actions or effects of each class of drugs in order to relieve or change a range of painful affect states (13–15). He thought that modified dynamic group therapy was an excellent way to address patients' difficulties in understanding and regulating feelings, self-esteem, relationships, and self-care. Henry Krystal introduced the concept of alexithymia, describing substance abusers' difficulty with recognizing, naming, tolerating, and verbalizing emotions (16). He viewed this as emanating from early failure to individuate from the mother and was not optimistic about the potential of psychotherapy to remedy these deficits. The early theorists relied on resolution of the underlying problems to address the substance abuse.

Stephanie Brown is perhaps the first person to write comprehensively about addressing alcoholism in the context of psychodynamic psychotherapy, from a perspective more focused on the addictive behavior itself (17–19). Her first book was published at a time when it was very unlikely that the patient's alcoholism would be recognized and appropriately addressed by physicians, psychologists, and other helping professionals. At that time, many recovering individuals felt mistrust of professionals, feeling they had been discouraged from pursuing abstinence and their entry into recovery had been delayed, sometimes by decades, by a well-meaning professional. Alcoholics Anonymous (AA) was viewed with condescension by many professionals. Her book, rich with clinical examples, described the recovery process in developmental stages: drinking, transition, early and ongoing recovery, and described the therapist's tasks at each stage. Recovery was more than the absence of drinking; it was a complex developmental process with many permutations. Her discussion of the potential partnership between AA and psychotherapy went beyond encouraging a positive attitude on the part of professionals and outlined a model for how the therapist could enhance the synergy. Because she skillfully integrated the perspective of a psychodynamic therapist with that of a recovering person, this book was greatly appreciated by psychotherapists in the community. Since her methodology was qualitative and observational, her work has not been widely recognized by researchers. Evidence from controlled trials is discussed later in this chapter.

Unique Features of the Treatment Approach

Setting Goals: Harm Reduction versus Abstinence

The issue of harm reduction versus abstinence as a treatment goal can be a significant aspect of the therapeutic encounter in individual psychotherapy for a patient with a substance use disorder, and the therapist should be familiar with these concepts and their own stance on this feature of treatment. Harm reduction is a public health strategy intended to reduce the impact of particular behaviors on individuals, families, and communities. Abstinence is on one end of the continuum of harm reduction and controversy exists about the merits of intermediate goals.

The controversy over harm reduction versus abstinence goals has existed for at least a decade, with some polarization still evident but also a blending of practices over time. There is a research literature supporting a variety of benefits from both interventions, but to date there is no controlled trial comparing the results of random assignment to programs with each goal. We know that abstinence-oriented treatment produces a small percentage (possibly 20%) of continuous, unbroken abstinence over a period of many years. Nonetheless, it yields significant benefits of reduction of alcohol and other drug use, reduction of drug-associated crime, improvement in family, medical (including psychiatric) status, and family functioning. We do not know if harm reduction treatment programs (as opposed to specific harm reduction interventions) produce comparable benefits. They may well do so, but they have not been rigorously studied in the same way. A more extensive discussion of harm reduction approaches by some of its main proponents can be found elsewhere (20,21).

In this author's view, harm reduction can be seen as a continuum on which total abstinence produces the most extensive and stable gains, but behavior changes short of that still produce meaningful benefits. Many, perhaps most, patients enter treatment with a deep desire to practice controlled use, but those who seek treatment in specialty settings have typically spent much of their lives trying to do so, with serious negative consequences. Those who achieve abstinence for extended periods of time, with occasional slips or short relapses, can often maintain their gains. We know that abstinence-oriented programs, despite their imperfections, produce substantial harm reduction. We do not know if harm reduction programs produce equivalent harm reduction. These important studies still need to be conducted.

Patients seen in private practice may be possible candidates to choose their own harm reduction goals. These should be consistent with health guidelines on consumption, for example, limits on alcohol (www.niaaa.nih.gov/FAQs). There are no sure methods for selecting who will do well with a harm reduction approach, but a short personal history of substance use, no family history of problematic substance use, and no physical dependence on the substance are commonly used criteria. Disqualifiers include pregnancy, medical and psychiatric conditions exacerbated by use, and hazardous interactions with prescribed medications. In the case of illicit drugs, the risks of procuring, possessing, and using the substances are a consideration. Therapist neutrality should be carefully communicated so that the therapist is not seen as endorsing these behaviors.

Therapists who are not substance abuse specialists need to familiarize themselves with immediate and delayed negative effects of alcohol and other drugs (covered in detail in this book) the patient is taking in order to be able to identify and discuss negative consequences. The majority of addiction specialists are convinced by their observations that once a person has crossed the boundary into uncontrolled use, he or she is unlikely to be able to return to controlled use of their primary drug of abuse *and* all other intoxicants. The clinician can acknowledge that the patient will select his or her own goals despite our recommendations, but we can avoid suggesting that one goal is as good as another and can emphasize that abstinence offers the widest margin of safety and the best foundation for progress.

Therapists can use harm reduction as an engagement strategy, collaborating with the patient on a treatment contract that acknowledges that if the patient cannot stay within limits, abstinence becomes the goal. This provides a structure for the patient to discover time-worn principles for himself or herself if these are relevant. It allows the therapist to keep the alliance with the patient in focus while giving forthright feedback on the patient's decision making. It is important to avoid a power struggle over abstinence goals, but it is equally important to give clear recommendations. Patients can be asked to make specific commitments to a goal, and then keep notes of their experiences. Many patients decide the struggle to maintain controlled use is exhausting and total abstinence is actually a relief.

Careful documentation is especially important when the therapist supports harm reduction goals, as liability issues can be significant if the patient causes harm to others in the course of active alcohol and other drug use.

Engagement

Motivational Enhancement

Counselors trained in substance abuse treatment settings are more likely to have been exposed to systematic motivational interviewing and enhancement techniques, due to extensive training efforts over the last 15 years. These techniques, described in detail in Treatment Improvement Protocol #35 (22) (available at no charge from the National Clearinghouse for Alcohol and Drug Information, http://ncadi.samhsa.gov/), are reviewed in Chapter 46 of this book. It is a set of principles geared to the individual's stage of change. These stages include

- Precontemplation, in which the patient is unaware or underaware that alcohol and other drug use is a problem.
- Contemplation, in which the patient is aware that there is a problem, but highly ambivalent and not yet committed to action.
- Preparation, in which the patient is feeling more positive about taking action, or making small steps.
- Action, in which the patient is taking visible steps toward quitting.
- Maintenance, in which the patient is focusing on maintaining gains, including mastering relapse prevention strategies.

Clinicians within specialty programs may assume that the patient who has been admitted is in the Action stage and may underestimate the ambivalence that is still lurking. Patients themselves downplay it for fear of disappointing their caregivers and peers. Others, under coercion, may be biding their time until they are once again free to drink and use. Individual sessions can provide a place where there is adequate time to elicit ambivalence and perhaps actual plans to use, and address them more thoroughly.

There are a number of psychodynamic reasons for continued substance use that may be useful to address. Fear of failure can increase resistance to making an abstinence commitment. The patient, wishing to avoid another discouraging experience, does not commit wholeheartedly to the effort. Closely related to this is a feeling of hopelessness or fear of the unknown. If the patient has a significant other who drinks and/or uses, the thought of abstinence and recovery can bring appropriate fears that the relationship might not survive. If domestic violence has been part of the relationship, vulnerability may be further enhanced. An addiction pattern in the family of origin can be another psychological obstacle. Despite the pain caused by the addiction, patients may feel on some level that drinking and using are how one belongs in this family, and abstinence will effectively make them an orphan. Patient may feel survival guilt in relation to family members or other significant persons. This self-reproach for leaving others behind may be another contributor to fears, particularly if the patient has previously had some successful time in recovery. Many of these feelings and beliefs may not be conscious, or may only be partially conscious, and can benefit from careful exploration that usually does not occur in groups because of time constraints. In the early abstinence stage, the goal of this exploration is to identify specific obstacles that often mystify the patient. Most arrive in treatment when they are suffering significant negative consequences and often do not understand their own resistance in the face of overwhelming evidence that alcohol and other drugs are having a destructive influence in their lives. The therapist should make clear that it is not necessary to resolve complex emotional issues in order to change drug-using behavior. Labeling the key issues can allow them to move on. Work on resolution takes place later on a foundation of abstinence.

The conviction that drinking and using are a form of self-medication is another prevalent reason to resist an abstinence commitment. Patients often have plausible reasons for their beliefs and it is unwise to discount their position. An educational posture is likely to be the most productive. Most patients focus on the initial effect of the drug, and do not adequately weigh the longer-term effects, even when they know what these are. For example, many cite the euphoria and feelings of relaxation that accompany the first drink of the day as a reason why they are sure that it helps them manage stress. Even though they usually "know" that alcohol is a central nervous system depressant, they do not connect drinking with their worsening depression over time. The therapist can alert them to the difficulties of focusing on a drug's immediate reward and ask them to notice and discuss the unfolding consequences. Journal-keeping is an excellent way to do this, but careful inquiry can also bring insight about the longer-term consequences. The therapist should be prepared to identify specifics related to the patient's drug(s) of choice:

Susan had begun using methamphetamine in her 20s when she began feeling overwhelmed caring for her three children and noticed she was becoming more and more depressed. Methamphetamine energized her and made her feel able to manage her increasingly complicated life. Over time, however, her depression and desperation worsened and she began using more and more of the drug just to get through her day. She sought psychiatric help, but she went through a series of antidepressants and reported that "they didn't work." Upon inquiry, she was able to identify turning points in the escalation of her use, and consider the possibility that her self-medication strategy was in fact resulting in longer and deeper episodes of depression, and counteracting any benefits of the medications.

Preparing the Patient for Specialty Treatment if Needed

Patients do not greet the recommendation to specialty treatment with enthusiasm for a variety of reasons. Many resent the pressure to give up their drugs and do not yet have strong enough incentives to undertake the task. Many communities do not have an appropriate program. For example, working patients often seek an intensive outpatient program with evening sessions, but residential treatment is the only option. The patient may lack insurance coverage or other financial resources for payment. Some large public sector programs offer specific programs for higher functioning patients who can pay and these are typically less expensive than other high-profile programs that advertise extensively. However, they may provide excellent treatment, particularly since their funding requires attention to evidence-based practices.

It must be acknowledged that addiction treatment programs vary widely in quality and patient resistance may be justified in terms of local lore or professional reputation. The clinician must assess whether the potential benefits of the program outweigh its shortcomings. A safe environment with a firm structure alone is an enormous benefit that may outweigh other objections. Patients may insist that they can only benefit from a program tailored to their preferences (e.g., no 12-step elements), which either does not exist or is otherwise unavailable. The clinician can adopt a "take what you need and leave the rest" stance when encouraging a more realistic approach. It may also be useful to take the position that "it is necessary that you want a better life for yourself so badly that you are willing to do a lot of things you do not like." In any case, the therapeutic alliance is the clinician's strongest asset and if the patient needs specialty treatment, it is likely that a crisis will eventually present itself as the catalyst for action.

It should be noted that recovery is a long-term process that may or may not require continuing professional treatment, so families must manage their resources with this long-term view. It is common for therapists and family members to be anxious and exhausted coping with the alcoholic or drug user, and reach for residential/inpatient treatment as the only acceptable solution. Skillful advertising promotes the idea that high-end treatment can be the "cure" for addiction and families can spend hard earned savings to provide this level of service. It is important that an addiction specialist makes a careful assessment to determine which actual services will meet the needs of the patient.

Connecting Presenting Problems with Alcohol and Other Drug Use

Many patients do not connect their alcohol and other drug use with the troubles that propel them to seek therapy, so the therapist must help them make that link. This requires familiarity with the different drugs of abuse, not only their short-term effects but also the longer-term consequences that unfold days or weeks after the episode of use, or after the patient has gone from occasional to regular use. The therapist should not attempt to "prove" that the patient's problems are the result of drinking and/or using, but should make the connection and encourage the patient to think about it, including keeping a journal to promote closer observation. For example, the woman described above (Susan) who used methamphetamine to energize her to cope with her three children may not connect her worsening depression with her stimulant use. The husband whose wife is frustrated over his "not being there" may not acknowledge the role of marijuana in their marital difficulties. In addition to the detailed descriptions of drug effects contained in this volume, clinicians should keep a recent reference book at hand, such as the well-known guide by Marc Schuckit (23) to confirm the links between alcohol and other drug use and specific psychiatric symptoms. Alcohol and other drugs are great imitators of or contributors to conditions that therapists see regularly. These include low self-esteem, interpersonal conflict, sexual problems, difficulties in following through at home or work, "boredom" in relationships or at work, and a host of other complaints.

Setting Goals

Patients entering a specialty addiction treatment program usually do so with the expectation that they accept abstinence as a goal. However, it is important to make room for an ongoing discussion of ambivalence, which is always present to some degree. For some patients, a wavering commitment to abstinence surfaces once they feel better and begin to convince themselves that they "can handle it now." Others harbor fantasies of controlled use from the outset. Some treatment programs convey the impression that ambivalence is somehow a sign of failure or lack of commitment to recovery and thus discourage disclosure. It is important to convey that ambivalence is normal and open discussion can provide insight and encouragement. This is an excellent opportunity to reinforce the idea that cravings or feelings do not have to be acted upon.

A variety of programs, especially those designed for the severely mentally ill and those addressing HIV/AIDS, provide low-threshold admission in which the goal is to engage the patient and focus on whatever goals are acceptable to reduce harm to self and others. In these programs, setting specific goals that are realistic, incremental, and achievable is important. Early successes increase motivation and engagement, and some patients eventually find themselves committing to total abstinence even when they had no intention of doing so when they entered the program.

Regardless of program orientation, some risk factors require immediate attention. Imminent danger to self and/or others must be addressed immediately. Vigorous intervention is required for patients who are suicidal, homicidal, psychotic, or at risk for serious violence at home or elsewhere. Other dangers include driving while intoxicated, having unprotected sex with strangers, or patterns of self-mutilation. Patients may also need a medically managed withdrawal. Drugs such as cocaine, methamphetamine, or marijuana can be discontinued immediately without medical consequences. Alcohol may require a medicated withdrawal; this should be assessed by a physician before stopping abruptly. Benzodiazepines and other sedative–hypnotics require physician assessment and management for withdrawal. Withdrawal from opiates is not in itself life-threatening, but the stress of withdrawal can be dangerous to patients with other medical conditions, such as heart disease. A full discussion of management of withdrawal can be found in relevant chapters in this book.

Patients may also enter treatment at risk for serious and possibly irreversible psychosocial consequences if substance use continues. These include the loss of a job, breakup of an important relationship, loss of professional licensure, loss of child custody and/or visitation, and incarceration. Patients with these kinds of dilemmas may cooperate with recommendations for early treatment goals or they may refuse to accept recommendations. In the latter case, it is possible that skilled motivational enhancement interventions that maximize the patient's legitimate choices at each point may prove successful in enlisting cooperation. It is important for the therapist to take an appropriately active stance while avoiding fruitless overcontrolling behavior that reflects a power struggle rather than firm guidance.

Establishing Abstinence: Stabilization Phase

Mastering the Behaviors of Abstinence

Cognitive–behavioral and contingency management strategies have been extensively researched and can be employed as a component of psychotherapy to assist patients to establish and maintain abstinence (see Chapters 44, 45, and 47). Early recovery skills include the ability to anticipate and manage cravings and urges. As stated in the popular video series, *Beat the Street*, "Avoid if you can; cope if you must." Assertiveness is often a problem, and a variety of approaches teach patients how to assert themselves without being apologetic, how to refuse alcohol and other drugs, how to extract themselves from compelling but dangerous situations, and how to establish a protective structure that will facilitate progress. It is important to identify family members and others who can be relied upon to provide support in the recovery process. Often, it takes effort to reconnect with such people, or develop new relationships, and the therapist can provide an arena to discuss difficulties and make a plan to address them.

It is useful to distinguish between alcohol and other drug use that occurs in the early stages of recovery from that which occurs after abstinence has been relatively stable for an extended period of time. The first reflects a failure to establish stable abstinence, whereas a relapse after a sustained period of time often requires a different approach. In both cases, it is useful to start with an examination of ambivalence about recovery, as a shift in motivation must be addressed first. It is common to find counselors or therapists turning toward their array of techniques, offering them, looking for new ones, and becoming frustrated when the patient does not follow through or comes back with a report that "it didn't work." Return of ambivalence is often the basis for lapses or relapses on the part of the patient. A lapse is a relatively circumscribed episode of use that does not involve a major deterioration in functioning. A relapse is a continuation of use over a period of time and often involves a regression to patterns characteristic of the worse period of active use. In the latter, recovery is no longer a priority, behavior reverts to old survival skills (such as lying to avoid accountability), and the patient returns to old people, places, and things. To the extent that the relapse involves such serious regression, the therapist must in effect start over to help the patient re-establish abstinence. However, it is also important to "do the detective work" on how and when decisions were made that made alcohol and other drug use inevitable. Unresolved grief over the loss of an important relationship may be a factor, or job problems or family illness may precipitate or contribute to the relapse. It is very common for patients to describe feeling bored or overconfident at time abstinent progresses, or feeling they do not need to continue activities such as 12-step program attendance that were important to recovery.

Identifying and Addressing Co-occurring Disorders

Although there is general consensus that psychotherapy should focus on discontinuing drug use before addressing other issues (24), in practice this may not work. Patients may insist that their traumatic experiences haunt them and they cannot be expected to give up their alcohol and other drug use until they make some progress toward putting their feelings to rest. Women in domestic violence situations who seek treatment in substance abuse settings may not be able to focus on their substance abuse until they receive some help for the threats from their relationship. Brown and colleagues (25) offer a Steps of Change Model that proposes that substance-abusing women seeking help may have a hierarchy of readiness, based on the urgency of their issues. Those in battering relationships may be ready to make changes in their exposure to violence before they are fully receptive to substance abuse treatment. The clinician who offers meaningful help is in a good position to engage the patient about the substance use. Treatment priorities should not be determined by rigid formulas, but the therapist can work within a recovery-oriented framework and address topics consistent with where the patient is in the recovery process. Thus, specific content can be discussed at any time, but the goals can shift from engagement, to stabilization (symptom management), to mastery.

Trauma issues are frequently cited as a reason why patients cannot make an abstinence commitment. They express fear that their symptoms will become unmanageable and refuse to proceed further until these issues are "resolved." They can be reminded that establishing safety is the first step to resolving trauma issues and they cannot be safe if they continue to drink and use. The therapist must give adequate attention to preparing the patient for the possibility of an upsurge of symptoms by making a careful assessment of the patient's resources and enhancing coping skills for that troubled time. Seeking Safety (26) is an empirically validated, manualized treatment for stabilization of such patients in early recovery. It offers a wealth of strategies to strengthen patient-coping skills and is well regarded by clinicians and patients alike.

Family and Social Issues

Couples and family issues are addressed elsewhere in this volume. Suffice it to say that the patient will benefit from family interventions designed to coach others about how to support the recovery process. Dislocations in family functioning are also best dealt with in a coordinated fashion, with goals related to what the patient can handle at each stage of recovery. Although Alanon can be invaluable to family members, its emphasis on disengagement may conflict with the need to develop and strengthen the social supports that are needed in recovery. The therapist's goal is to address inappropriate forms of enmeshment and facilitate health and social connections.

Facilitating the Use of Self-Help Programs

One of the most important tasks of the therapist is to facilitate the use of the self-help system. These programs fill a variety of needs that cannot be met by professional treatment alone: a community that supports the recovery process, a wide range of role models, structured activities to fill the gaps left by the absence of alcohol and other drug use, and a process for personal development that has no financial barriers. It is not interchangeable with professional therapy or substance abuse treatment, but complements and augments its effects.

There are now a variety of self-help groups (e.g., LifeRing, SMART Recovery; see Chapter 38), but the 12-step system is the largest in the world, with a great variety of groups in most urban environments and some resources in rural communities (see Chapter 37). At high risk times, such as holidays, there are often meetings at all hours of the day and night, providing a safety structure unmatched by anything except residential treatment. High-profile celebrities have made the public aware that meetings are attended by members of all social classes. A patient who is truly working the steps is often an excellent therapy participant, in that he or she is "open, honest, and willing," that is, committed to the kind of self-examination that therapy requires.

A variety of studies support the view that 12-step participation (usually AA) is beneficial and promotes long-term sobriety (27–31). Supportive interventions such as arranging for someone to take a newcomer to a meeting facilitate attendance (32), but attendance in itself is not enough. Recent research indicates that an intensive intervention to promote participation did increase involvement and was in turn associated with improved outcomes for both alcohol and other drug use (33). This finding held even for patients with considerable previous 12-step program experience and formal treatment. There is only a moderate correlation between attendance and involvement, the latter being more related to positive outcomes (34). Earlier studies distinguished between attendance and involvement, the latter being measured by such things as finding and working with a sponsor, chairing meetings, working the steps, and doing service (35–37). These studies also supported the view that involvement was related to positive outcomes.

Opinions about the value of particular research methods can skew the debate on AA effectiveness. The prestigious *Cochrane Reviews* analyzed eight experimental trials involving 3417 people and concluded that none of the studies unequivocally demonstrated the effectiveness of AA or 12-step facilitation (TSF) approaches for reducing alcohol dependence or associated problems (38). On July 25, 2006, the *New York Times* reported "review sees no advantage in 12-step programs." Unfortunately, this type of headline fails to acknowledge the limitations of the *Cochrane Reviews*. In general, their exclusive focus on experimental studies dismisses a large body of relevant research, particularly important with respect to 12-step programs because patients cannot be randomized to AA or no AA. It is not possible to control whether they attend or not. The randomized studies that do exist are based on more indirect methods. Kaskutas, principal investigator in some of the studies, has offered critiques of this specific review (39), citing serious errors in how the studies are described and classified. For example, she notes the conflating of the manualized TSF intervention, used in professional treatment settings, with the 12-step self-help group. She also notes that experimental evidence is only one of six criteria for establishing causation, and the evidence from other types of studies is compelling (39).

On a more clinical note, it is important for the therapist to facilitate engagement in a self-help program, particularly in the early stages of recovery. If the patient is in a structured program, this task is made easier in that participation to attend self-help meetings is usually encouraged or required, and attending with peers who feel just as anxious reduces some obstacles. The therapist in private practice or in a nonspecialty organizational setting may have a more difficult task. Some therapists "require" attendance at meetings as a way to address addictive behavior. For the patient, this approach underestimates the complexity of acknowledging that drinking and/or using is a problem and that behavior needs to change. Just attending a meeting can be very charged and there are many reasons for patients to resist. In addition, self-help meetings do not address all aspects of the problem; hence, therapists need to develop proficiency at handling some of the clinical issues.

Common resistances to participation in 12-step meetings includes a generalized discomfort with strangers, or about being the outsider in a group where everyone knows one another; fears of being swallowed up by a "cult"; distaste for the rituals, especially the opening statement "I am an alcoholic/addict"; and awkwardness about "that religious stuff." The therapist can encourage examination of these issues, while conveying the expectation that at some point the patient will give meetings a fair try. Eliciting the patient's picture about what meetings are like can provide an opportunity to correct misconceptions or to encourage the patient to compare what they fear or imagine with what meetings are actually like. It is productive to explore the charged issues, as these are usually reflective of broader problem areas. It is very important to give the patient permission to be ambivalent and to air negative feelings with the therapist. It may be useful to ask the patient to report first on what they disliked and then on what they learned. Negative feelings about meetings in no way preclude reaping benefits. "Take what you need and leave the rest" is an AA slogan that allows many to continue to attend. However, the therapist should monitor engagement and ask regularly about what would foster greater involvement. It is enormously useful for the therapist to provide a place for patients to talk about what is happening on a regular basis. A more extensive discussion on the intersection between self-help groups and psychotherapy can be found elsewhere (8,17).

One of the best ways to become more effective in facilitating the use of the self-help system is for the therapist to attend a variety of meetings that might be appropriate to his or her patient population. Since the 12-step system is the largest in the world, it is important to familiarize oneself with those meetings in the community. Alternative groups are also available, but they are typically fewer in number and hence less able to offer a firm support system. If the therapist is not in recovery, it is important to look for an "open meeting" in the 12-step system. It is particularly useful to note: (a) what you think, feel, and do prior to attending the meeting, while there, and afterwards; (b) what you observe about the group process; and (c) what are the strengths and limits of this group process compared to a therapy group. The self-help system and psychotherapy complement each other and it is important to understand the similarities and differences. Some therapists are uncomfortable with the "no–cross talk" rule, because they think the person sharing needs support they do not get. However, speakers are usually approached by others immediately after the meeting, and it has been proposed that social support is one of the main effective elements offered by the 12-step system (40,41).

Patients on psychotropic medication and those with severe mental illness should be coached and supported in meeting selection and attendance. Some meetings are more tolerant of medication and/or eccentric behavior, and it is helpful to have some starting suggestions. The AA literature (42) states very clearly that medication prescribed by a physician familiar with addiction is compatible with recovery and not the business of other AA members. Nonetheless, some meeting participants express their opinions freely and may bring pressure to bear on the patient to discontinue medication. This is particularly problematic when coming from a sponsor. Therapists should familiarize themselves with the AA pamphlet on medication and provide copies in the office. Role-plays on the handling of intrusive peers can be beneficial. Those with cognitive impairments can benefit from coaching about how to behave in meetings. The therapist can review the opening rituals, go over what happens in the meetings, and remind the patient that meetings are not a place to share delusions. The 12-step structure at its best is welcoming and stable but not overly intrusive. This will vary among meetings, but those working with mental health patients can identify appropriate meetings from the recommendations of other patients.

Difficulties with a sponsor are more complicated and the therapist must remain respectful of the sponsor relationship while challenging a sponsor's inappropriate positions. Patients often cite their relationship to their sponsor as one of the most important elements in their recovery. However, patients may select sponsors who are very rigid and controlling, often re-enacting unhealthy relationship themes from childhood. The therapist can point out that a sponsor is not given a permanent appointment. People have different sponsors at different times in recovery, depending on what they need at the time. Here again, the patient may need specific help to extricate himself or herself from a negative situation.

Ongoing Recovery Issues

While individual psychotherapy can be useful in the early stages of substance abuse treatment, it also has great potential to improve the quality of recovery by addressing issues that remain after a period of extended abstinence. Patients usually need to improve their ability to identify, modulate, tolerate, and appropriately express their feelings. They need to learn to manage their feelings without being self-destructive. In collaboration with a skilled therapist, they need to learn to distinguish between strong but appropriate feelings, feelings that represent a pathologic condition such as major depression (that may need medication), and ones that may be detrimental to their psychological health. Recovering people may be intolerant of affects, but they may also be too reluctant to seek psychotropic medications, as "using a pill to feel better" is understandably a charged issue. The appropriate use of medications is not only important for a satisfying recovery, but also it can play a key role in preventing relapse as well.

Interpersonal issues are usually an important focus in ongoing recovery, as key relationships have usually been distorted by alcohol and other drug use. The selection of a mate while drinking and using usually raises issues about the durability of the relationship once abstinence is stable. During the using phase, the more intact partner or spouse often takes over key functions, such as parenting and management of finances. Recovery often brings dissatisfactions with power imbalances in relationships, which need to be carefully renegotiated on a realistic timetable. Even changes for the better raised anxiety levels and the therapist can be an important anchor as well as guide through the turmoil. Other common issues include separation and individuation, self-esteem, and issues related to childhood trauma or other sources of post-traumatic stress disorder (PTSD).

A wide range of psychotherapies can be beneficial during extended abstinence, but it is crucial that the therapist have an appreciation of relapse potential once the patient begins to explore anxiety-provoking material. It is particularly easy to underestimate vulnerability in patients who are articulate and high functioning. Patients typically do not want to disappoint their therapists by announcing that relapse has occurred. Therapists should work with the patient to make a list of relapse warning signs for that individual and should inquire periodically about fantasies or cravings about drugs, or "exceptions" such as a drink here and there. Carelessness about attire, getting inadequate sleep, and loss of a previously regular exercise schedule can also be indications of a relapse state of mind or an actual relapse.

Research-based Principles and Interventions

The last decade has seen increasing emphasis on integrating evidence-based practices into addiction treatment programs. Private practitioners may be insulated from these expectations, unless their managed care payers impose requirements. In this case, there may be a "pick from this list" approach that constrains the ability to do individualized treatment planning or an arduous appeals process that discourages initiative. In the course of this discussion, it is important to keep in mind that evidence-based *principles* are as important as specific interventions found that showed efficacy in clinical trials (43). Examples of key elements of principles that guide funders include

- There is a strong correlation between retention in treatment and positive outcomes. Thus, we need to engage and retain patients, not discharge them for manifesting their substance-using behaviors.
- Services that are sufficiently comprehensive and continuous over time produce better outcomes. This includes attending to practical issues such as housing and transportation.
- Medications are compatible with recovery and improve outcomes when appropriately used.
- Addictive disorders behave like other chronic disorders and need to be addressed in a chronic care model, not an acute care model.
- Harm reduction approaches yield benefits in terms of public health and safety.

Controlled Trials

The first systematic investigations of psychotherapy in the treatment of addiction were conducted by George Woody and colleagues (44,45) who examined the role of psychotherapy for a male veteran population in a methadone maintenance program. Patients received individual drug counseling, supportive–expressive therapy, or cognitive–behavioral therapy plus drug counseling. The patients receiving psychotherapy improved considerably more than those who received drug counseling alone, with no differences found between types of therapy. The addition of psychotherapy was most important for patients with a high level of psychiatric symptoms.

This random assignment controlled trial legitimated the use of psychotherapy in addiction treatment, although financial constraints have always limited its use.

More recently, Project MATCH (46) demonstrated that individual therapy sessions of cognitive–behavioral coping skills therapy, motivational enhancement therapy, or TSF therapy all produced reductions in drinking outcomes from baseline to 1 year after treatment. These psychosocial treatments were well defined and manuals have been made available by both the National Institute on Alcohol Abuse and Alcoholism (NIAAA) (47,48) and the CSAT (49). It is important to remember that this study was conducted under highly controlled conditions, with far more resources than community-based programs enjoy. Fidelity checks are required in treatment trials to assure that the treatment is conducted with consistency across settings. It is in effect a form of clinical supervision, using a trained professional to review and rate audio or videotapes. Many funders of community treatment will not pay for clinical supervision. Nonetheless, it is possible that the manuals will be helpful to practitioners and training supervisors in community settings.

Specific evidence-based interventions that have been widely disseminated include motivational enhancement therapy, cognitive–behavioral therapy, contingency management (50), community reinforcement approaches, Seeking Safety (for PTSD and substance abuse), and certain family therapies. These have shown positive results in efficacy trials and vary in the extent to which effectiveness trials, which demonstrate that they work in the community, have been conducted. In any case, it is widely acknowledged that they may need to be adapted to be responsive to cultural variations. However, not enough is known about what critical elements must be maintained to preserve their potency. Practitioners are advised to familiarize themselves with these approaches, as they offer valuable tools to assist patients at different points in the recovery process. A more extensive review of research-based interventions can be found in Rounsaville et al. (51).

Meta-analysis

Unfortunately, there are no meta-analyses of psychotherapy for the treatment of substance use disorders. This reflects the relative lack of well-controlled studies of psychotherapy for substance abuse treatment. Inasmuch as the majority of patients seen in specialty settings for substance use disorders have at least one other co-occurring mental disorder, it is important to integrate effective treatments for those disorders when possible. While insufficient work has been done on the main combinations of substance use disorders and other disorders, a variety of interventions have been studied and found beneficial (52).

A recent meta-analysis (53) notes that short-term treatments are insufficient for many patients with complex disorders and examines the effectiveness of long-term psychodynamic psychotherapy (LTPP) on this challenging group of patients. The analysis included studies of patients with personality disorders, eating disorders, depressive and anxiety disorders, and combinations of these disorders (but did not include patients with substance use disorders). For many of the patients, the disorders were chronic, that is, lasting more than 1 year. There were 23 studies, involving 1053 patients (none on psychotropic medication), in this meta-analysis. Both RCTs ($n = 11$) and carefully designed observational studies ($n = 12$) were included. The comparative analyses showed significantly better outcomes in overall effectiveness, target problems, and personality functioning than shorter forms of therapy. Within-group effect sizes were large (0.78–1.98) and stable, even across complex mental disorders. It is important to note that substance use disorders were not a part of this meta-analysis, and it is likely that a good working knowledge of addiction and recovery is essential for producing good outcomes in LTPP.

Therapeutic Alliance

Perhaps the earliest recognition of the importance of the therapeutic alliance was documented in a classic study of the usefulness of psychotherapy for opiate-dependent patients, which influenced subsequent psychosocial studies (54). Researchers and clinicians have since confirmed that some counselors or therapists achieve better outcomes (55–57) and emphasis is shifting to include examination of common factors in addition to specific interventions. Therapeutic alliance is also related to treatment dropout (58,59). Unfortunately, there has not been sufficient in-depth examination of this variable. How can programs select for clinicians with greater capability of forming an alliance? To what extent can this be taught? How can therapists be trained to deal with conflicts or ruptures in the alliance? What teaching or supervision methods are most effective? Is it better to focus on the clinician's ability to form and maintain an alliance, or on methods of obtaining fidelity to a manual? Although these are not mutually exclusive, the current emphasis on implementing specific evidence-based interventions will likely require hard choices in an era of diminishing resources.

CONCLUSIONS

Individual therapy has been studied because it allows for better control in trials on specific interventions, such as motivational enhancement or cognitive–behavioral therapy, but far too little is known about its optimal use in addiction treatment and recovery. Since it is relatively expensive to provide, it is important to understand when it is essential, desirable, unnecessary, or even contraindicated in a specialty program. Patients often report that having individual attention allows them to settle into treatment and make a sustained commitment, but it is not possible at this time to disentangle the relative contributions of different activities. For therapists working in private practice in the community, it is crucial to appreciate what must be done to effectively address alcohol and other drug use within the ongoing therapeutic relationship. It is also important to know how to prepare a patient for specialty treatment if needed. Interventions have been developed that show efficacy in controlled trials, but these are rarely used by private practitioners in the community.

Manuals exist for treatments with a strong evidence base, but little work has been done on how to disseminate them among private practitioners and train such clinicians in their use. Inasmuch as most patients with alcohol and other drug problems do not seek help in specialty settings, it is important to understand how best to strengthen the ability of community practitioners to address this issue.

ACKNOWLEDGMENTS

Thanks to Beth Manning, PhD, and Suzanne Gelber, PhD, for contributing insights to this chapter. NIDA Grant #U10 DA015815.

REFERENCES

1. McElrath D. The Minnesota Model. *J Psychoactive Drugs*. 1997;29(2):141–144.
2. Deitch DA. The treatment of drug abuse in the therapeutic community: historical influences, current considerations, future outlook. *Drug Abuse in America: Problem in Perspective.* 1973;4: 158–175. Rockville, MD: National Commission on Marijuana and Drug Abuse.
3. DeLeon G. Residential therapeutic communities in the mainstream: diversity and issues. *J Psychoactive Drugs*. 1995;27(1): 3–15.
4. DeLeon G. *The Therapeutic Community: Theory, Model, and Method*. New York: Springer; 2000.
5. Center for Substance Abuse Treatment. *Addiction Counseling Competencies: The Knowledge, Skills, and Attitudes of Professional Practice*. (Vol. DHHS Publication No. (SMA) 06-4171.). Rockville, MD: Substance Abuse and Mental Health Services Administration; 2006: TAP 21.
6. Conner KR, Shea RR, McDermott MP, et al. The role of multifamily therapy in promoting retention in treatment of alcohol and cocaine dependence. *Am J Addict*. 1998;7(1):61–73.
7. Zweben A, Pearlman S, Li S. Reducing attrition from conjoint therapy with alcoholic couples. *Drug Alcohol Depend*. 1983;11: 239–245.
8. Washton AM, Zweben JE. *Treating Alcohol and Drug Problems in Psychotherapy Practice: Doing What Works*. New York: Guilford Press; 2006.
9. Norcross JC, Lambert MJ. The therapy relationship. In: Norcross JC, Beutler LE, Levant RF, eds. *Evidence-Based Practices in Mental Health*. Washington DC: American Psychological Association; 2006:208–217.
10. White WL. *Recovery Management and Recovery-Oriented Systems of Care: Scientific Rationale and Promising Practices*. Northeast Addiction Technology Transfer Center, Great Lakes Addiction Technology Transfer Center, Philadelphia Department of Behavioral Health/Mental Retardation; 2008.
11. Wurmser L. Psychoanalytic considerations of the etiology of compulsive drug use. *J Am Psychoanal Assoc*. 1974;22: 820–843.
12. Wurmser L. *The Hidden Dimension: Psychodynamics in Compulsive Drug Use*. New York: J. Aronson; 1978.
13. Khantzian EJ. Some treatment implications of the ego and self disturbances in alcoholism. In: Bean MH, Zinberg NE., eds. *Dynamic Approaches to the Understanding and Treatment of Alcoholism*. New York: Macmillan; 1981:163–193.
14. Khantzian EJ. The self-medication hypothesis of substance use disorders: a reconsideration and recent applications. *Harv Rev Psychiatry*. 1997;4:231–244.
15. Khantzian EJ, Halliday KS, McAuliffe WE. *Addiction and the Vulnerable Self: Modified Dynamic Group Therapy for Substance Abusers*. New York: The Guilford Press; 1990.
16. Krystal H. *Integration and Self Healing: Affect, Trauma, Alexithymia*. Hillsdale, NJ: The Analytic Press; 1988.
17. Brown S. *Treating the Alcoholic: A Developmental Model of Recovery*. New York, NY: Wiley Inter-Science; 1985.
18. Brown S. *Treating Adult Children of Alcoholics: A Developmental Perspective*. New York, NY: Wiley; 1988.
19. Brown S, Lewis V. *The Alcoholic Family in Recovery: A Developmental Model*. New York, NY: The Guilford Press; 1999.
20. Denning P. *Practicing Harm Reduction Psychotherapy*. New York, NY: The Guilford Press; 2000.
21. Denning P, Little J, Glickman A. *Over the Influence: The Harm Reduction Guide for Managing Drugs and Alcohol*. New York, NY: Guilford Press; 2004.
22. Miller WR. *Enhancing Motivation for Change in Substance Abuse Treatment* (Vol. 35). Rockville, MD: U.S. Department of Health and Human Services; 1999.
23. Schuckit MA. *Drug and Alcohol Abuse*. New York, NY: Springer-Verlag; 2005.
24. Rounsaville B, Carroll KM, Back S. Individual Psychotherapy. In: Lowinson JH, Ruiz P, Millman RD, et al., eds. *Substance Abuse: A Comprehensive Textbook*. New York, NY: Williams & Wilkins; 2005.
25. Brown VB, Melchior LA, Panter AT, et al. Women's steps of change and entry into drug abuse treatment. A multidimensional stages of change model. *J Subst Abuse Treat*. 2000;18(3): 231–240.
26. Najavits LM. *Seeking Safety: A Treatment Manual for PTSD and Substance Abuse*. New York, NY: Guilford; 2002.
27. Bond J, Kaskutas LA, Weisner C. The persistent influence of social networks and alcoholics anonymous on abstinence. *J Stud Alcohol*. 2003;64(4):579–588.
28. Donovan DM, Wells EA. Tweaking 12-step: the potential role of 12-Step self-help group involvement in methamphetamine recovery. *Addiction*. 2007;102(suppl 1):121–129.
29. Moos RH, Moos BS. Participation in treatment and Alcoholics Anonymous: a 16-year follow-up of initially untreated individuals. *J Clin Psychol*. 2006;62(6):735–750.
30. Ouimette PC, Moos RH, Finney JW. Influence of outpatient treatment and 12-step group involvement on one-year substance abuse treatment outcomes. *J Stud Alcohol*. 1998;59(5): 513–522.
31. Timko C, Moos RH, Finney JW, et al. Long-term outcomes of alcohol use disorders: comparing untreated individuals with those in alcoholics anonymous and formal treatment. *J Stud Alcohol*. 2000;61(4):529–540.
32. Sisson RW, Mallams JH. The use of systematic encouragement and community access procedures to increase attendance at Alcoholics Anonymous and Al-Anon meetings. *Am J Drug Alcohol Abuse*. 1981;8(3):371–376.
33. Timko C, Debenedetti A, Billow R. Intensive referral to 12-step self-help groups and 6-month substance use disorder outcomes. *Addiction*. 2006;101(5):678–688.
34. Owen PL, Slaymaker V, Tonigan JS, et al. Participation in alcoholics anonymous: intended and unintended change mechanisms. *Alcohol Clin Exp Res*. 2003;27(3):524–532.
35. Emrick CD, Tonigan JS, Montgomery H, et al. Alcoholics Anonymous: What is currently known? In: McCrady B, Miller WR, eds.

Research on Alcoholics Anonymous: Opportunities and Alternatives. New Brunswick, NJ: Rutgers University Press; 1993.

36. Johnson JE, Finney JW, Moos RH. End-of-treatment outcomes in cognitive–behavioral treatment and 12-step substance use treatment programs: do they differ and do they predict 1-year outcomes? *J Subst Abuse Treat.* 2006;21:41–50.
37. Toumbourou JW, Hamilton M, U'Ren A, et al. Narcotics Anonymous participation and changes in substance use and social support. *J Subst Abuse Treat.* 2002;23(1):61–66.
38. Ferri M, Amato L, Davoli M. Alcoholics Anonymous and other 12-step programmes for alcohol dependence. *Cochrane Database Syst Rev.* 2006;(3) Art. No.: CD005032. DOI: 10.1002/14651858.CD005032.
39. Kaskutas LA. Comments on the Cochrane Review on Alcoholics Anonymous effectiveness. *Addiction.* 2008;103:1402–1405.
40. Kaskutas LA, Ammon L, Delucchi K, et al. Alcoholics Anonymous careers: patterns of AA involvement five years after treatment entry. *Alcohol Clin Exp Res.* 2005;29(11):1983–1990.
41. Kaskutas LA, Bond J, Humphreys K. Social networks as mediators of the effect of alcoholics anonymous. *Addiction.* 2002;97(7): 891–900.
42. Alcoholics Anonymous. *The AA member—medications and other drugs. Report from a group of physicians in AA.* New York, NY: Alcoholics Anonymous World Services; 1984.
43. Miller WR, Zweben JE, Johnson W. Evidence-Based Treatment: Why, What, Where, When and How? *J Subst Abuse Treat.* 2005;29: 267–276.
44. Woody GE, Luborsky L, McLellan AT, et al. Psychotherapy for opiate addicts: Does it help? *Arch Gen Psychiatry.* 1983;40: 639–645.
45. Woody GE, McLellan AT, Luborsky L, et al. Psychotherapy for substance abuse. *Psychiat Clin North Am.* 1986;9(3):547–562.
46. Project Match Research Group. Matching alcoholism treatments to client heterogeneity: Project Match posttreatment drinking outcomes. *J Stud Alcohol.* 1997;58:7–29.
47. Kadden R, Carroll K, Donovan D, et al., eds. *Cognitive–Behavioral Coping Skills Therapy Manual.* Rockville, MD: U.S. Department of Health and Human Services; 1995.
48. Nowinski J, Baker S, Carroll K. *Twelve Step Facilitation Therapy Manual* (Vol. 1). Rockville, MD: U.S. Department of Health and Human Services; 1994.
49. Miller WR, Zweben A, DiClemente CC, et al. *Motivational Enhancement Therapy Manual.* Rockville, MD: U.S. Department of Health and Human Services; 1994.
50. Dutra L, Stathopoulou G, BAsden SL, et al. A meta-analytic review of psychosocial interventions for substance use disorders. *Am J Psychiatry.* 2008;165(2):179–187.
51. Rounsaville BJ, Carroll KM, Beck SE. Individual psychotherapy. In: Ries RK, Fiellin DA, Miller SC, et al., eds. *Principles of Addiction Medicine.* Philadelphia, PA: Lippincott Williams & Wilkins; 2009:769–785.
52. Ries RK, Miller SC, Fiellin DA, et al., eds. *Principles of Addiction Medicine.* Philadelphia, PA: Lippincott Williams & Wilkins; 2009.
53. Leichsenring F, Rabung S. Effectiveness of long-term psychodynamic psychotherapy: a meta-analysis. *JAMA.* 2009;300(13): 1551–1565.
54. Luborsky L, Barber JP, Siqueland L, et al. Establishing a therapeutic alliance with substance abusers. *NIDA Res Monogr.* 1997;165:233–244.
55. Carroll KM, Nich C, Rounsaville BJ. Contribution of the therapeutic alliance to outcome in active versus control psychotherapies. *J Consult Clin Psychol.* 1997;65(3):510–514.
56. McLellan AT, Woody GE, Luborsky L, et al. Is the counselor an "active ingredient" in substance abuse rehabilitation? An examination of treatment success among four counselors. *J Nerv Ment Dis.* 1988;176:423–430.
57. Petry NM, Bickel WK. Therapeutic alliance and psychiatric severity as predictors of completion of treatment for opioid dependence. *Psychiatr Serv.* 1999;50(2):219–227.
58. Cournoyer LG, Brochu S, Landry M, et al. Therapeutic alliance, patient behaviour and dropout in a drug rehabilitation programme: the moderating effect of clinical subpopulations. *Addiction.* 2007;102(12):1960–1970.
59. Meier PS, Donmall MC, McElduff P, et al. The role of the early therapeutic alliance in predicting drug treatment dropout. *Drug Alcohol Depend.* 2006;83(1):57–64.

CHAPTER 42 Group Therapy

Arnold M. Washton

INTRODUCTION

The history of group therapy adapted specifically for treating substance use disorders (SUDs) is not easily traced, but over the past several decades group therapy has evolved into the most prevalent form of substance abuse treatment in the United States. Group therapies are used for treating all types of SUDs (including those involving the use of alcohol, cocaine, opioids, sedatives, marijuana, and various combinations of these and other substances) and for individuals suffering from co-occurring psychiatric and addictive disorders. A broad spectrum of group therapy models (e.g., cognitive/behavioral, psychoeducational, motivational, interpersonal, 12-step, psychodynamic) are utilized by substance abuse treatment programs and practitioners operating from differing theoretical orientations. Most group-based interventions for SUDs incorporate a variety of therapeutic strategies and techniques consistent with recent trends toward integrative rather than monolithic approaches (1).

For purposes of this chapter, group therapy is defined as treatment delivered to a preselected cohort of addicted individuals in the context of regularly scheduled group therapy sessions led by a professionally trained group leader—typically an addition therapist, counselor, or other mental health professional with relevant training and experience. Considering that this is only one chapter in a comprehensive textbook, the present discussion of group-based interventions for addiction is unavoidably limited. More extensive coverage of this topic can be found in other publications (2–5).

The topics addressed in this chapter are (a) efficacy of group therapy for addiction, (b) advantages and limitations of group approaches, (c) differences between group therapy and self-help groups, (d) patient selection factors, (e) groups designed for different stages of recovery, and (f) group management considerations.

EFFICACY

Although group therapy has emerged as the most popular treatment modality for SUDs, empirical evidence of its clinical efficacy is sparse. Most studies have compared the effectiveness of different models of group therapy, but only a handful have compared group to individual therapy and results are inconsistent.

Bowers and al-Redha (6) found that alcohol-dependent patients who received couples therapy in a group format showed greater reductions in alcohol consumption at 6-month follow-up than patients who received couples therapy individually. In addition, there was some indication that couples treated in the group format reported more improved marital adjustment and higher ratings of relationship satisfaction than couples treated individually.

Schmitz et al. (7) compared outpatient delivery of the same 12-session cocaine relapse prevention (RP) program in group versus individual therapy formats. Although the proportion of patients producing cocaine-free urine samples at the end of treatment did not differ between formats, group RP patients reported using cocaine on significantly fewer days during treatment and experienced fewer cocaine-related problems than did individual RP patients. Follow-up data collected at 12 and 24 weeks posttreatment revealed no significant differences between formats regarding cocaine use or any other outcome measures, leading the authors to conclude that the efficacy of RP interventions is not strongly influenced by delivery format. Similarly, Graham et al. (8) found no significant differences in outcome regarding substance use between individual and group delivery of a structured RP approach. Only one psychosocial outcome measure (social support from friends at 12-month follow-up) showed a significant difference that favored the group format.

Weiss et al. (9) found that in patients struggling with concurrent bipolar and SUDs, integrated group therapy designed to address both disorders was more effective than group drug counseling alone in reducing both drug use and psychiatric symptoms. Rosenblum et al. (10) reported that substance abusers in a soup kitchen who received motivationally enhanced group counseling were significantly more likely than others who received concrete services only (i.e., information, referral, advocacy) to show reduced drinking and increased participation in some type of substance abuse intervention (e.g., formal treatment and/or 12-step groups) during the follow-up period. A study by Crits-Christoph et al. (11) comparing the effectiveness of four psychosocial treatments for cocaine-dependent outpatients indicated that patients receiving a combination of group drug counseling plus individual drug counseling were more likely to show decreased drug use over time than patients who received group drug counseling only or group drug counseling plus individual psychotherapy.

An extensive study by Panas et al. (12) involving 7815 patients from 63 publicly funded outpatient substance abuse treatment programs has provided perhaps the strongest empirical evidence to date of the efficacy of group approaches. This study found that type of treatment, defined as proportion of group to individual therapy, was strongly and positively associated with various treatment performance measures including completion of treatment and achievement of treatment goals.

Although the above studies provide some empirical support for the effectiveness of group-based treatment interventions, more extensive research in this area is sorely needed. Acknowledging this pressing need, Morgan-Lopez and Fals-Stewart (13) describe various methodologic and other obstacles that have tended to stifle substance abuse group therapy research. In addition to problems inherent in evaluating and measuring group process, these obstacles include data analytic complexities caused by group member interactions, changing group membership over time, and limited control over treatment delivery ingredients.

Despite the absence of a solid empirical base for utilizing group therapy as the treatment of first choice for addiction, the current popularity of group interventions appears to be based largely on its historically long-standing use as the mainstay of addiction treatment programs in the United States, its cost-effectiveness, and on the apparent goodness of fit between certain clinical needs/characteristics of addicted individuals and the combination of therapeutic forces that group therapy uniquely provides.

ADVANTAGES OF GROUP THERAPY

From an economic standpoint, group therapy is more cost-effective to deliver than individual therapy, making it increasingly attractive in current efforts to reduce health care costs. Due to limited resources, most treatment programs, especially those supported by public funds, are unable to make individual therapy routinely available to their patients. As compared to individual therapy, group therapy allows a larger number of patients to be treated by fewer clinicians on a given workday. Importantly, group therapy enjoys a high rate of patient acceptance and desirability among individuals seeking treatment for SUDs. In fact, patients seeking addiction treatment often prefer group to individual treatment.

One of the most striking therapeutic benefits of group-based interventions for SUDs is readily apparent to clinicians who routinely provide this type of treatment. Namely, that groups often have a unique ability to empower clients to change even after individual therapy and/or other interventions have failed. When people struggling with a common adversity join together in pursuit of a common goal, a variety of potent forces are mobilized that motivate and inspire them to overcome the adversity. This same phenomenon is evident, for example, in how people cope with the aftermath of natural disasters and other severely traumatic or life-threatening situations.

Group therapy incorporates a unique combination of therapeutic forces not available in other forms of treatment (3,5). Groups provide therapeutic opportunities for (a) mutual identification and reduced feelings of isolation and shame; (b) peer acceptance, support, and role modeling; (c) confrontation and realistic feedback; (d) peer pressure, social support, structure, and accountability for making positive changes; (e) acquisition of new coping skills; (f) exchange of factual information; and (g) instillation of optimism and hope. The gathering together of people who share a common problem often creates a bond between them, stemming from a sense of mutual identification and an expectation of being intuitively understood. This is critically important in counteracting the intense feelings of isolation, shame, and guilt that addicted individuals often experience. The social stigma of addiction and profound humiliation of having lost control over one's behavior makes rapid acceptance into a peer group all the more important for newcomers. The group instills optimism and hope by giving newcomers a chance to make contact with others who are succeeding in making positive changes and by instantly supplying newcomers with a positive support network committed to the pursuit of common goals. Groups often enhance treatment retention as a by-product of the bonding that develops between group members. Groups provide a forum for developing better coping abilities and avoiding common pitfalls in recovery. Because groups typically place high value on self-disclosure, active participation, compliance with group norms (e.g., abstinence, punctuality, attendance, honesty), a spirit of cooperation among group members, and facing rather than avoiding problems, it is difficult for resistant or noninteractive patients to "hide out" in small groups because all members are expected to routinely participate in group discussions.

LIMITATIONS OF GROUP THERAPY

Given the numerous advantages of group therapy, what might be some of its limitations and when might individual therapy be preferable? First, unlike individual therapy where patients enjoy total privacy and confidentiality, group therapy inevitably requires patients to disclose their identity and personal problems to strangers. This can be a problem especially for patients who live in small communities where the chances of encountering people who might know them can be substantial. While maintaining strict confidentiality regarding group members' identities and the content of sessions is a cardinal rule of group therapy, there is no way to control what group members might say or do outside of group sessions. Despite increasing public enlightenment about addiction as a widespread disorder affecting people from all walks of life, unwanted disclosure of information about an individual's alcohol or drug problem still holds the potential to damage careers, reputations, and relationships.

A second limitation of group therapy is that the content and pace of the treatment is determined by the group as a whole and not by the needs of any one individual. Inevitably there are times when group therapy is out of step with the needs of some members while appropriately addressing the needs of others. This limitation is most evident in open membership groups where new members are admitted throughout the life of the group as others leave. Each time newcomers enter an ongoing group, the continuity of treatment is interrupted as attention shifts back to newcomer issues. By contrast, individual therapy allows the therapist to address patient's issues as they arise and to spend as much time within a session or as many sessions as necessary to deal with these issues.

A third limitation of groups is that typically only a small portion of the therapy time is devoted to the needs of any one individual. This is offset to some extent by the benefits that group members may derive indirectly from participating in discussions that focus on the issues of other members. Nonetheless, individual therapy devotes 100% of the therapy time to the needs of one person, which may be more likely to engender change or perhaps do so more rapidly.

A fourth limitation is that group therapy may not be suitable or appropriate for all addicted individuals. While many, if not most, can benefit from group therapy and prefer it to other forms of treatment, others are simply not good candidates for group treatment. Patients with severe borderline personality disorders often find the intense interpersonal interaction and scrutiny in group sessions intolerably stressful. Similarly, patients who are avoidant, shy, or schizoid may be unable to participate actively in group discussions or form meaningful connections with other group members. Apart from psychiatric impairment, some patients simply do not want to be in group therapy for whatever reasons and flatly refuse to participate, preferring individual therapy instead. Although further exploration of this unreceptive stance may help to allay certain commonly held fears and misconceptions about group therapy (e.g., expectations of harsh confrontation by peers), some patients remain adamant about not wanting group therapy and it is important for clinicians to respect these patients' wishes.

GROUP THERAPY VERSUS SELF-HELP GROUPS

Group therapy and self-help groups such as Alcoholics Anonymous (AA) are not good substitutes for one another. Each forum provides a unique form of help and, ideally, they should be seen as synergistic rather than competing activities. Self-help groups have many advantages, but the in-depth attention given to psychological and personal issues that take place in professionally led recovery groups is simply not available in self-help meetings. Many individuals are not comfortable revealing personal details of their lives in the public forum of a self-help meeting and are more inclined to do so in the smaller, more intimate setting of a group therapy session. In group sessions, members are strongly encouraged to give objective feedback to one another, whereas in self-help meetings giving feedback (known as "cross talk") is not permitted. These are not criticisms of self-help groups, which contain their own unique blend of therapeutic forces, but fundamental differences between these two very different forms of help for people struggling with the problem of addiction. Unlike group therapy, self-help meetings are characterized by peer rather than professional leadership, an absence of screening or exclusion criteria, unlimited size of membership, widespread availability, and an absence of time limits on the length of participation which may extend over a participant's lifetime.

PATIENT SELECTION FACTORS

A formal selection process is required to ensure that patients are placed in groups best suited to meet their needs. Ideally, screening of potential group members should be conducted by the clinician who leads the group. No matter how rigorous the selection process may be, it is sometimes impossible to ensure that the composition of patients placed in a group is ideal for conducting the group's therapeutic work. The goal of patient selection should be to achieve a reasonable degree of homogeneity and heterogeneity among group members (3). It is important that all group members find a basis for identifying with one or more of the other members because admitting a newcomer into the group who shares few characteristics with other members may create problems for that individual and for the group as a whole. At the same time, diversity enhances the richness of the group experience. Group members can differ in age, gender, race, socioeconomic status, educational level, and other variables as long as one member is not the lone "outlier" (3). Generally, newcomers will fare better when there are at least one or two other group members with whom they can readily identify. Individuals who are different from all other group members in one or more important respects (e.g., one woman among a group of men, one gay person among heterosexuals, one seriously impaired person among highly functional people) are likely to feel out of place in the group, not participate actively in group discussions, and/or drop out prematurely.

Group membership should not be limited only to patients who have the same primary drug of choice, considering that the addictive disorder, not the drug use itself, is the focus of treatment. Heterogeneity in this regard can help group members realize that different substances often lead to the same constellation of problems and that changes required to deal effectively with these problems are very similar, regardless of a person's substance(s) of choice. When a newcomer happens to be the only person in a group with a particular drug of choice, identification and bonding with other group members can be compromised. For example, a lone cocaine user may feel out of place in a group where alcohol is the substance of choice of all other members. It is important to help such patients identify as soon as possible the similarities between addictions to different types of substances and encourage them to identify with these similarities rather than the differences in order to feel part of the group and derive maximum therapeutic benefit from being there. Despite similarities, however, the group should not ignore some of the unique problems associated with the use of different types of substances such as residual cognitive impairments following chronic alcohol use, lingering withdrawal symptoms of depression and insomnia following cessation of opioid use, and sexual acting-out behaviors often associated with cocaine and methamphetamine use. Addressing substance-specific issues straightforwardly, proactively, and whenever they arise can help to promote group cohesiveness and induct patients with different substances of choice into the group.

In addition to the above, other important patient selection factors include the patient's desired treatment goals, motivation or reasons for entering the group, and stage of readiness for change. Individuals committed to the goal of total abstinence from all psychoactive substances usually do not mix well in groups with those who choose nonabstinence goals such as harm reduction, moderation, or partial abstinence (i.e., abstinence from the most problematic substance, but not others). Those pursuing a goal of total abstinence from all psychoactive substances often feel irritated and unsafe in groups where others are not committed to the same goal and may feel that the presence of these group members not only adversely affects their own motivation to refrain from all substance use, but also distracts the group from its primary mission of supporting abstinence. Similarly, those not choosing total abstinence are likely to feel criticized and out of place in a group where all other members are committed to abstinence. Thus, patients with incompatible or opposing goals are not likely to work well together in groups and their seemingly irreconcilable differences can consume too much of the group's time and thwart the therapeutic work. Traditionally, substance abuse treatment groups have restricted membership to patients who are committed to total abstinence or at least willing to comply with an abstinence requirement during their tenure in the group. Recognizing that many patients who seek help for SUDs are not ready or willing to accept total abstinence as their goal, harm reduction and moderation groups have emerged as alternatives for these patients, whether or not abstinence is their ultimate goal (14,15).

Similarly, mixing mandated and nonmandated patients can be problematic. Group members mandated into treatment under threat of serious consequences (e.g., loss of personal freedom, job, driver's license, professional licensure) are frequently mistrustful and reticent to participate openly and actively in group discussions. Their presence in a group frequently disrupts group cohesiveness and inhibits the participation of voluntary members who may respond negatively to others who are perceived as being in the group only to avoid severe consequences. This is not necessarily an insurmountable problem, if properly addressed, but doing so can consume an inordinate amount of group time and requires a great deal of intervention by the group leader to manage this difficult and often contentious issue. Nonetheless, even with the group leader's best efforts, there is no guarantee that this issue will be resolved to the satisfaction of all group members and some of the nonmandated patients may end up leaving the group prematurely, feeling that it is simply not the best place for them to get the help they need.

GROUPS FOR DIFFERENT STAGES OF RECOVERY

Phase-Specific Groups

Work on the application of the stages of change model (16) to group therapy indicates that substance abuse treatment groups function best when all members are in a similar stage of change (15,17). Ideally, groups should be composed of individuals either in the early stages of precontemplation, contemplation, and preparation or those in the latter stages of action and maintenance. The types of therapeutic interventions that work best in the treatment of addiction often depend on what phase of recovery or stage of change the person is in. Individuals grappling with addiction typically progress through a series of phases as they move from active use toward sustained abstinence and recovery. Accordingly, many treatment programs offer phase-specific groups that focus on the tasks and goals most relevant to each stage. This may include motivation enhancement or pretreatment induction groups for those who need preparatory work before making an abstinence commitment or participating in a formal treatment program, early abstinence groups for those in the process of breaking free of alcohol/drug use, and RP or continuing care groups for those in the middle and later stages of recovery. This stratification of groups offers a number of clinical advantages: (a) it focuses the group work on the specific problems, tasks, and goals relevant to each phase; (b) it provides predefined progress markers that give group members a sense of personal accomplishment as they complete one phase and move on to the next; (c) it makes it easier for individuals to identify and relate to stage-specific issues being addressed in the group and to bond with other group members who are dealing with similar issues; and (d) it facilitates patient placement into a group best suited to meet his or her needs at each stage of the recovery process. The rationale for stratification is based on the assumption that matching treatment interventions to meet the specific needs of patients as they progress through different stages of recovery is likely to enhance clinical outcomes. There is a natural progression from an initial focus on breaking free of substance use, to securing abstinence, to preventing relapse, and eventually to addressing a variety of psychological issues. The dividing lines between different stages are somewhat arbitrary and the rate of progression through each stage varies from person to person.

Mixed-Phase Groups

Despite the numerous advantages of phase-specific groups, there are also drawbacks. One significant disadvantage is that the group composition may change too frequently and become disruptive as members move from one phase to the next. Another limitation is that private practitioners or small treatment programs may not have sufficient caseloads or manpower to reliably maintain different groups for patients in each phase of treatment and thus mixed-phase groups may be the only feasible alternative. In a mixed-phase model, participants stay in a group as long as needed to achieve their treatment goals and/or as long as their participation in the group remains productive. Individuals struggling with addiction move through the change process at such different rates that it is not possible to specify in advance how long it will take for a given group member to achieve his or her treatment goals. As compared to phase-specific groups, mixed groups contain a broader array of patients at different phases of recovery: some in the early phases, others farther along in the process, and still others somewhere in between. All have an opportunity to interact with one another in a group setting and derive mutual benefits from doing so. A potential drawback, however, is that inevitably there will be times when the group membership becomes skewed as, for example, when a majority of members is in the early phases of recovery. When this happens the smaller number of more advanced members may become disenchanted or bored with the types of issues that consume the group's time.

Early Recovery Groups

Early recovery groups focus on issues most relevant to the beginning stages of treatment: helping members to establish initial abstinence, stabilize their overall functioning, acknowledge and accept their addiction problem, work through initial ambivalence and reluctance about giving up alcohol/drug use, establish a social support network, become bonded to other members and integrated into the group, overcome early relapses and other setbacks without dropping out, deal effectively with both immediate and delayed consequences of their addiction, and begin the process of identifying and changing some of the dysfunctional self-defeating cognitions, emotions, and behaviors intertwined with their addiction. This is an ideal wish list and certainly not every group member will achieve all of these goals during their tenure in the group. In the absence of financial constraints that limit length of stay, tenure in a group varies according to how quickly patients progress toward achieving their goals, ranging usually from several months to as much as a year, if circumstances permit.

Newcomers struggling to establish or maintain initial abstinence usually need specific guidance and support from other group members on early recovery issues such as (a) discarding all drug supplies and paraphernalia, (b) avoiding contact with dealers, users, parties, bars, and other high-risk situations, (c) learning how to recognize self-sabotaging behaviors and other "setups" for drug/alcohol use, and (d) learning how to manage urges and cravings. Once initial abstinence is established, the focus predictably shifts to stabilization of the individual's functioning. Often, a profound sense of disappointment emerges in the newly abstinent patient soon after the patient realizes that life is still fraught with problems despite having given up alcohol/drugs. This realization may lead the patient to seriously question whether the struggle of staying abstinent is really worthwhile, especially if and when delayed consequences of prior substance use such as financial, legal, and relationship problems begin to surface while the patient is actually doing well. Support and advice from established group members who have "been there" can be extremely helpful at this point to counteract the newcomer's tendency to impulsively self-medicate their resentment, anxiety, and fear.

The issues discussed in early recovery groups are largely patient-driven so that members' problems, crises, and issues can be effectively dealt with as they arise. The leader often plays a very active, and at times directive, role in guiding the group discussion by keeping it focused on relevant issues, encouraging participation of all members and ensuring that members provide helpful therapeutic feedback to one another without lecturing, advice-giving, hostile confrontation, and other unhelpful behaviors. At times, the group leader may suggest that a certain topic or issue be addressed in the group based on important themes that have emerged in recent group sessions. Where appropriate, the leader may take a portion of the session to review group rules or guidelines such as those regarding how group members can give good feedback to one another, especially when there is an influx of new members. In early recovery groups, members are actively encouraged to maintain contact with one another outside the group. This stands in marked contrast to traditional (psychodynamic) group psychotherapy where outside contact between group members is viewed as undesirable "contamination" that must be avoided.

Relapse Prevention and Continuing Care Groups

The essential tasks and goals of RP and continuing care groups are to help patients' strengthen their commitment to abstinence, work through residual ambivalence about giving up alcohol and drugs, and both learn and practice RP strategies. Although RP is the primary focus of this phase, the group should not focus exclusively on substance use but on a wider range of issues in greater depth. These issues may include the recovery tasks of repairing damaged relationships, forming new ones, working toward resolving the lingering impact of developmental and trauma issues, enhancing self-esteem, and creating a reasonably satisfying lifestyle that is free of alcohol and other drugs. Relapses that occur after abstinence has been firmly established and practiced for at least several months are frequently caused not so much by environmental triggers (which is more typical during the early phases) as by failure of the patient to cope adequately with negative emotions generated by interpersonal conflicts and other types of life problems and stressors. Research on the relapse process indicates that the most common precipitants of relapse are negative mood states, interpersonal conflict, and social pressures to use alcohol/drugs (18). Among the many topics addressed in this phase of treatment are how to identify negative feelings; how to manage anger; how to avoid impulsive decision-making; how to relax and have fun without drugs; how to give and receive constructive criticism; how to be assertive without being aggressive; and how to deal with problems in interpersonal relationships.

In addition to providing coping skills training, it is equally important to sensitize patients to relapse warning signs so that appropriate measures can be taken to "short-circuit" what is often a progressive backsliding in attitudes and behaviors. Explaining the relapse dynamic (1,19) as a progressive identifiable process that is set in motion long before returning to substance use empowers group members to interrupt what otherwise might be an insidious slide toward relapse, which they are unable to recognize while it is happening. Moreover, group members must be alerted to the possibility that flare-ups can occur many months (or even years) after stopping alcohol and drug use.

RP groups should also address psychological issues that go beyond the basic cognitive and behavioral factors that promote a return to substance use. This involves exploring in detail the inner emotional life of each group member and interpersonal problems that repeatedly give rise to the compulsive desire to "self-medicate" (20). Patients with long, destructive histories of substance use often lack the ability to identify, manage, tolerate, and appropriately express feelings. The ultimate goal here is not merely the acquisition of self-knowledge and insight but fundamental change in the individual's characteristically maladaptive patterns of thinking, feeling, behaving, and interacting. For example, learning how to tolerate unpleasant feelings instead of impulsively obliterating them with chemicals is an essential part of group treatment at this stage. At an appropriate time the group should also address members' long-standing, deep-seated problems that may stem from parental alcoholism, physical/sexual abuse, or other developmental and life traumas. Coordination between individual and group therapy is especially vital here. Moreover, whenever such sensitive highly charged issues are being discussed, the group leader must be especially mindful of the possibility that group members may be at increased risk of relapse. Even when in-depth exploration of difficult issues appears to be well-tolerated, patients should always be alerted to the possibility of relapse as an attempt to avoid painful issues.

GROUP MANAGEMENT CONSIDERATIONS

Leadership Roles and Responsibilities

The group leader serves a variety of essential functions. These include (a) establishing and enforcing group rules in a caring, consistent, nonpunitive manner to protect the group's integrity and progress; (b) screening, preparing, and orienting potential newcomers to ensure suitability and proper placement in the group; (c) keeping group discussions on track and focused on important issues to maximize the therapeutic benefit for all group members; (d) emphasizing, promoting, and maintaining a caring, nonjudgmental, therapeutic climate in the group that both counteracts self-defeating attitudes and promotes self-awareness, expression of feelings, honest self-disclosure, and adaptive alternatives to drug use; (e) managing problem members who are disruptive to the group in a timely and consistent manner to protect the membership and integrity of the group; and (f) educating patients about selected aspects of alcohol/drug use, addiction, recovery, and related issues.

Effective leadership of an addiction recovery group demands that the leader adopt a certain posture in the group that differs significantly from that of traditional psychodynamically oriented psychotherapy groups, particularly in the early stages of recovery. In traditional groups, the therapist gently guides and focuses the attention of group members on matters pertaining to group process, group dynamics, and the complicated interpersonal interaction among group members. With the exception of carefully timed comments, the therapist may remain quiet and nondirective in the customary mode of psychodynamic psychotherapy. By contrast, in early abstinence groups the therapist must work actively to keep the group focused on concrete here-and-now issues that pertain directly to addiction-related issues. The therapist plays a very active and directive leadership role that includes questioning, confronting, advising, and educating group members on relevant issues. The therapist keeps the group task-oriented and reality-based, and serves as the major catalyst for group discussion. Addressing substance-related issues is always the number one priority of the group, and the therapist must be sure always to keep the group focused on this task.

It is not the group leader's role to direct or control the group discussion, but rather to facilitate a process whereby members learn how to interact with one another in an increasingly open, honest, empathetic manner that promotes positive change. When a group is working properly, the leader functions as a coach or guide, staying in the background while the group takes responsibility for the therapeutic work. When the group is not working properly, the leader is doing a lot of talking and/or spending a lot of time exhorting members to participate more actively in group discussions. Well-functioning groups require deliberate and persistent intervention by the group leader to return maximum responsibility for what goes on in sessions to the group's members, consistent with the psychotherapeutic principle of analyzing resistance before dealing with content (3,19). It is much more important to help group members recognize their passivity than it is to try to drag them into doing the therapeutic work. As compared to early recovery groups, where the group leader plays a much more active role, later stage groups should be helped to focus increasingly on group process and become reliably self-correcting when the discussion strays offtrack or becomes unproductive.

Preparing New Members for Group Entry

Preparing new patients for group entry involves not only orienting them to basic group ground rules, but also establishing realistic goals and expectations. Before admitting new patients to a group, the group leader should ideally meet individually with each prospective newcomer for at least one or two sessions to assess motivation, clarify myths and misconceptions about group therapy, and address resistances to group participation. Prospective members should also be informed about how the group works, how to give useful feedback, and how to refrain from unhelpful group behaviors (3,19). Before newcomers attend a first group meeting they should agree in writing to adhere to the group ground rules.

Managing Peer Confrontation and Feedback

Peer confrontation can be extremely effective in helping group members achieve a more realistic assessment of their maladaptive attitudes and behaviors. But heavy-handed, excessive, and poorly timed confrontation can be countertherapeutic and damaging. Some patients enter groups with the mistaken idea that humiliation and aggressive confrontation are the ways to force resistant group members to face reality. Sometimes harsh confrontations are rationalized as attempts to be "truly honest" with members who are seen as "resistant" or not conforming to group expectations and norms. Group members typically have less tolerance for negative attitudes and obfuscations than do group leaders, especially when these attitudes are reminiscent of their own problems. Likely targets for attack are members who repeatedly relapse, those who are experienced as defiant, superficial, or insincere, and those who minimize their problem and make little attempt to bond with other members. The group leader should not allow unpopular, frustrating, resistant, or severely troubled group members to be verbally scapegoated and bludgeoned by their peers, even when the content of what is being said is entirely accurate. Harsh or excessive confrontation must not be used as a means to push unpopular or troubled members out of the group and discourage them from coming back. It is often the style rather than content of peer confrontation that determines its impact on the recipient. The main goal of confrontation is to make the person more receptive to change without eliciting defensiveness or destructive acting-out behavior.

Managing Common Problems

Among the most common problems that arise in group therapy are the following: chronic lateness and absenteeism, hostility and other disruptive behaviors, lack of active participation, superficial presentations, proselytizing and hiding behind AA, and playing cotherapist. Because of space limitations, these problems are touched on only briefly here. More in-depth discussion of these issues can be found elsewhere (3,19).

Lateness and Absenteeism

An atmosphere of consistency and predictability is essential for group therapy to be effective. Because most patients have histories of irresponsible behavior during active addiction, when this type of behavior arises in the group it should not be ignored. A pattern of repeated lateness and/or absenteeism adversely affects group morale and cohesion. It is almost always a sign of ambivalence about being in the group and should be addressed as such.

Hostility and Other Disruptive Behaviors

Sometimes the content of what a member says in a group session is less important than the way he or she says it. The group leader must attend the session continuously to affect body language, voice intonation, and overall communication style of group members. Some members are chronically antagonistic, argumentative, and sarcastic. They repeatedly devalue the group, complain about how poorly it is run, point out minor inconsistencies, and reject advice or suggestions offered by other group members or the group leader. The group leader should not ignore these types of negative behaviors. An appropriate intervention by the group leader might be to say, "I wonder if anyone else is experiencing Tom's remarks as hostile and devaluing? Can someone offer him feedback about how he's coming across and how it is affecting the atmosphere in the group?" The group leader should guide the ensuing discussion to make sure that group members do not use this as an opportunity to assault and demean the problem group member for "bad" behavior, but rather help him to see the self-defeating nature of his actions as well as the negative impact of his behavior on the entire group.

Silence and Lack of Participation

Some group members sit quietly on the sidelines as observers of the group discussion, glad to have the focus of attention not be on them. Silent members may secretly harbor feelings of ambivalence, resentment, and annoyance about being in treatment, and doubt whether they need to be in the group at all. Some members are just shy and need gentle coaxing and encouragement from the group to open up. An example of how to address a silent group member might be as follows: "I've noticed that Dale has not participated at all during the past two or three group sessions. Maybe the group can try to find out what's holding her back and perhaps encourage or make it easier for her to join in the discussion?"

Superficial Presentations

Terse or superficial presentations that focus on facts rather than feelings and reveal little or nothing about the presenter are another forms of patient resistance to the group's therapeutic work. In these situations, the group leader can intervene by saying something like, "I've noticed that when Jason talks about himself his statements are very brief and factual. They tell us very little about what's on his mind or what he is actually feeling. I'm wondering if others share my observations and concerns." Similarly, some group members present lengthy stories recounting external events and circumstances full of irrelevant details and devoid of emotional content. This is often indicative of a member who is just going through the emotions of being in treatment to satisfy a spouse, employer, or mandate. The group leader might intervene by saying, "Jeff, you've just given the group a very long and detailed account of the events of last week, but we heard very little about how you were feeling these past few days on the heels of your recent relapse. I'm wondering if other group members are getting the type of information from you that they would need to give you meaningful feedback. I notice that some group members look bored and uninterested. How are you all feeling right now?"

Proselytizing and Hiding Behind AA

This is one of the most difficult problems to address in group therapy for addiction (13,20). In almost every recovery group there are likely to be some members solidly linked into AA or other 12-step programs who insist with unwavering conviction that AA is the one and only pathway to successful recovery. They may be openly intolerant of other members who do not embrace AA and take it as their mission to proselytize the benefits of AA in the hopes of converting nonbelievers. Additionally, they may complain that there is not enough "recovery talk" in the group and that the format of group sessions does not sufficiently parallel that of an AA meeting. These individuals will often polarize the group into opposing factions: those who embrace AA enthusiastically and wholeheartedly versus those who are more tempered in their posture toward AA or reject it completely. If this polarization is not addressed, it will ultimately destroy group cohesion, create an unsafe climate in the group, divert valuable attention from other important issues, and stall the group's therapeutic work. (It is important for group leaders to acknowledge that although AA can be extremely helpful to people struggling with addiction, many are not receptive at first to the 12-step program and should be coaxed rather than coerced into giving AA a try. Moreover, there is a general consensus among addiction treatment professionals that no single method of recovery is best for everyone with an addiction problem.) A potentially helpful intervention may include saying something like, "Well group, we could probably debate the pros and cons of AA here for many sessions and still not reach agreement among everyone in the room. I think it would be more useful to talk about how group members feel that there is a serious split among you on this issue and how it is affecting what we do here in the group."

Playing Cotherapist

Some group members play the role of therapist's helper that serves (unconsciously) as a diversion or smokescreen for dealing with their own issues. They often try to perform certain of the group leader's functions such as keeping the group discussion on track, confronting other members on inappropriate behaviors, and reinforcing group norms. Because their input is often very helpful to the group it is easy for other members and sometimes the group leader to overlook the fact that the self-appointed "cotherapist" spends so much time being a helper that his or her own issues are rarely, if ever, addressed. An appropriate intervention might include saying something like, "Robert, you've been extremely helpful to other group members and it's very clear that everyone here values your input. But I'm wondering if the group can take some time to get to know you a little better and try to help you identify what you want to work on here."

Responding to a Group Member's Substance Use

When a group member reports that he or she has used alcohol/drugs since the last group session, the group must give first priority to addressing this issue. In doing so, the group leader should role model a direct, compassionate, nonpunitive response. The group leader's task is to help the group utilize the discussion of a member's use as an opportunity to learn something useful. Suggested guidelines for dealing with a group member's recent alcohol/drug use are as follows: (a) Ask the individual to give the group a detailed account of the sequence of feelings, events, and circumstances that led up to the use. (b) Invite others to ask the patient about early warning signs, self-sabotage, and other factors that may have preceded the actual substance use. (c) Ask others to share any suggestions or feedback they can offer the patient about the use and how to prevent it from happening again. Also ask them to share their feelings about the episode, reminding them to avoid any tendency they may have to scapegoat the patient or to act out feelings of anger and frustration with negative comments. (d) With the patient's active participation, ask the group to develop a list of suggested strategies and behavioral changes to guard against the possibility of further substance use.

Although most group members respond supportively to a fellow member's substance use, there is an unspecified limit as to how many times this will happen. When a group member shows little evidence of using previous suggestions about how to prevent further use, other members may start to become intolerant and feel that this individual may be jeopardizing the integrity of the group. Peer confrontation can become very intense when dealing with relapse issues and the group leader must guard vigilantly against the group's tendency to scapegoat or ostracize the struggling member.

SUMMARY

This chapter discusses the efficacy, advantages, and limitations of group therapy as well as various practical considerations involved in group formation and leadership. Group therapy has evolved over several decades into the treatment of choice for addiction. Stage-specific groups that address the changing needs of patients as they move through different phases of recovery help to enhance patient-treatment matching and clinical outcomes. Although clinically effective, group therapy is not the best or only treatment option for every individual with an addiction problem. Group therapy should not be used as a stand-alone treatment but ideally as just one component of a more comprehensive multimodality treatment approach. Group leaders serve many important and complex functions including deciding which patients to bring together in a group, keeping group discussions focused on relevant topics, and handling various types of problems that arise during group sessions. In addition to its therapeutic benefits for patients, groups provide a valuable source of personal and professional growth, even for the most seasoned clinician.

REFERENCES

1. Washton AM, Zweben JE. *Treating Alcohol and Drug Problems in Psychotherapy Practice: Doing What Works.* New York, NY: Guilford Press; 2006.
2. Flores PJ, Georgi JM, eds. *Substance Abuse Treatment: Group Therapy.* Treatment Improvement Protocol (TIP) No. 41. Substance Abuse and Mental Health Services Administration, DHHS Publication No. (SMA) 05-3991. Rockville, MD; 2005.
3. Vannicelli M. *Removing the Roadblocks: Group Psychotherapy with Substance Abusers and Family Members.* New York, NY: Guilford Press; 1992.

4. Spitz HI, Brook DW. *The Group Therapy of Substance Abuse*. New York, NY: Haworth Medical Press; 2002.
5. Yalom I. *The Theory and Practice of Group Psychotherapy*. New York, NY: Basic Books; 1995.
6. Bowers TG, al-Redha MR. A comparison of outcome with group marital and standard individual therapies with alcoholics. *J Stud Alcohol*. 1990;51:301–309.
7. Schmitz JM, Oswald LM, Jacks SM, et al. Relapse prevention treatment for cocaine dependence: group vs. individual format. *Addict Behav*. 1997;22(3):405–418.
8. Graham K, Annis HM, Brett PJ, et al. A controlled field trial of group versus individual cognitive–behavioral training for relapse prevention. *Addiction*. 2002;91(8):1127–1140.
9. Weiss RD, Griffin ML, Kolodziei ME, et al. A randomized trial of integrated group therapy versus group drug counseling for patients with bipolar disorder and substance dependence. *Am J Psychiatry*. 2007;164(1):100–107.
10. Rosenblum A, Magura S, Kayman DJ, et al. Motivationally-enhanced group counseling for substances users in a soup kitchen: a randomized clinical trial. *Drug Alcohol Depend*. 2005;80:81–103.
11. Crits-Christoph P, Siqueland L, Blaine J, et al. Psychosocial treatment of cocaine dependence: results of National Institute on Drug Abuse Collaborative Cocaine Treatment Study. *Arch Gen Psychiatry*. 1999;56:493–502.
12. Panas L, Caspi Y, Fournier E, et al. Performance measures for outpatient substance abuse services: group versus individual counseling. *J Subst Abuse Treat*. 2003;25:271–278.
13. Morgan-Lopez AA, Fals-Stewart W. Analytic complexities associated with group therapy in substance abuse treatment research: problems, recommendations, and future directions. *Exp Clin Psychopharmacol*. 2006;14(2):265–273.
14. Little J. Harm reduction group therapy. In: Tatarsky A, ed. *Harm Reduction Psychotherapy: A New Treatment for Alcohol and Drug Problems*. Northvale, NJ: Jason Aronson; 2002:310–346.
15. Velasquez MM, Maurcr GG, Crouch C, et al. *Group Treatment for Substance Abuse: A Stages-of-Change Therapy Manual*. New York, NY: Guilford Press; 2001.
16. Prochaska JO, DiClemente CC, Norcross JC. In search of how people change: applications to addictive behaviors. *Am Psychol*. 1992;47:1102–1114.
17. Washton AM. Outpatient groups at different stages of substance abuse treatment: preparation, initial abstinence, and relapse prevention. In: Brook DW, Spitz HI, eds. *The Group Therapy of Substance Abuse*. New York, NY: Haworth Medical Press; 2002:99–119.
18. Marlatt GA, Gordon J. *Relapse Prevention: Preparing People to Change Addictive Behaviors*. New York, NY: Guilford Press; 1985.
19. Washton AM. Group therapy: a clinician's guide to doing what works. In: Coombs RH, ed. *Addiction Recovery Tools: a Practical Handbook*. Thousand Oaks, CA: Sage Publications; 2001: 239–256.
20. Khantzian EJ, Halliday KS, McAuliffe WE. *Addiction and the Vulnerable Self: Modified Dynamic Group Therapy for Substance Abusers*. New York, NY: Guilford Press; 1990.

CHAPTER 43
Family/Couples Approaches to Treatment Engagement and Therapy

William Fals-Stewart ■ Wendy K. K. Lam

INTRODUCTION

Historically, alcoholism and drug addiction have been viewed by the majority of treatment providers and researchers, as well as by the public at large, as problems of the "individual." In turn, intervention approaches focused largely or exclusively on the diagnosed individual. During the last four decades, this conceptualization has slowly given way to a greater awareness of family members' crucial roles in the etiology and maintenance of, not to mention the long-term recovery from, various kinds of addictive behaviors. Consequently, treatment providers and researchers alike have placed greater emphasis on understanding drinking and drug use from a family systemic perspective and, in turn, on exploring how consideration of partner and family dynamics may be understood and used to address individuals' substance abuse.

As it turns out, the preponderance of available evidence reveals that marital and family therapy approaches are among the most efficacious in terms of prevention, change initiation, and treatment of substance use disorders. Indeed, some have argued that these intervention approaches are the most effective methods for treating alcoholism and drug abuse, principally because of the substantial improvements seen across a very broad range of outcomes (e.g., substance use reduction, improved child functioning, reduced domestic violence).

In this chapter, we will (a) present a brief history of couple- and family-based perspectives and treatment approaches; (b) describe the unique features of these treatment approaches that differentiate them from other models; (c) discuss the various partner- and family-involved approaches for substance use that focus on treatment engagement and active therapeutic models, and review the available evidence of efficacy for these approaches; (d) present optimal implementation techniques used by the most efficacious couple- and family-based approaches; and (e) identify special considerations that clinicians and researchers alike may be likely to encounter when conducting couples- and family-based treatment with substance-abusing couples. Lastly, the chapter will conclude with an exploration of possible future directions with respect to partner- and family-involved therapies with substance-abusing patients.

HISTORY OF FAMILY- AND COUPLES-BASED APPROACHES FOR SUBSTANCE ABUSE TREATMENT

The traditional framework from which substance use disorders are viewed is succinctly captured in the commonly stated axiom among treatment providers, "Alcoholism and drug abuse are individual problems best treated on an individual basis." It is a long-standing clinical philosophy that had held sway in the substance abuse treatment community for much of the last half century and had a very powerful influence on the treatment of alcoholism and other drug use disorders (1). By the early 1970s, there was an acknowledgement among many providers that the focus on the individual was necessary, but not sufficient, since it did not adequately consider the contextual factors that served to support patients' continued use or relapse. Despite the very dominant individual-focused paradigm, the family and home environments were simply too important to ignore. This shift toward consideration of the family when treating addictive behavior was legitimized in a special report given to the U.S. Congress in the early 1970s by the National Institute on Alcohol Abuse and Alcoholism; that body described couple and family therapy as "one of the most outstanding current advances in the area of psychotherapy of alcoholism" and recommended funding of controlled studies to test the effectiveness of these promising methods (2).

Since that time, the call to examine family-based treatment approaches for substance abuse has been answered by many different research groups, initially with small-scale studies and, as evidence of effectiveness accumulated, followed by large-scale randomized clinical trials. Results of this programmatic line of research yielded findings that were both consistent and highly positive; compared to individual-based therapies, partner- and family-involved interventions were more efficacious in terms of substance use reductions, improvements in patients' psychosocial adjustment, and amelioration of serious family problems, such as domestic violence and children's maladjustment (3,4). As a result, an increasing number of treatment providers and the programs in which they work began intervening with the family as a way to reduce or eliminate abusive drinking or drug use by one or more of its members. In the last decade, the Joint Commission on Accreditation of Health Care Organizations standards for accrediting substance abuse treatment programs in the United States required that an adult family member who lives with an identified substance-abusing patient be included at least in the initial assessment (5). Thus, in the last 50 years, some involvement of the family in the treatment of substance abuse moved from being viewed in most circles as inappropriate all the way to a component of competent standard practice.

FAMILY TREATMENT FOR SUBSTANCE MISUSE: UNIQUE AND DEFINING FEATURES

Definitions: Marriage and Family

When considering what makes partner- or family-focused interventions for alcoholism and drug abuse unique, a deceptively simple answer is that these treatments focus on or otherwise involve intimate partners or other family members. Although certainly true, how does one define terms like "marriage" and "family"? In many important respects, what defines these terms has been and very much remains in a state of flux. To gain appreciation of this, one needs to only reference headlines or watch the news about the heated debates among those who favor or are opposed to same-sex marriage. How our society and our culture, as well as other societies and cultures, define and operationalize these terms is among the great sociopolitical debates of our generation. Simply stated, there is no encompassing definition of *family* or *marriage*; this has always been the case. Different societal norms and attitudes influence definitions of such cultural constructions, and because cultures and beliefs change over time, the definition of what is meant by marriage and family changes in concert.

However, at least for the purpose of operationalizing these terms to identify an "intervention unit," it nonetheless seems possible to distill certain qualities and characterizations of these institutions that are somewhat consistent under a variety of circumstances and conditions. In the most inclusive sense, family or marriage (or at least an intimate relationship—marriage carries legal elements as well as sociocultural ones) implies an enduring involvement on an emotional level with other people. For practical purposes, family can be defined according to the individual's closest emotional connections, of which marriage is a subset. In other words, the individual constructs who is his or her family or his or her partner(s), which is not to be confused, of course, with those persons the individual "likes." Thus, our definition moves beyond the pure genetic, biologic, or legal definitions, but also encompasses emotional and behavioral connections defined by the individual who identifies "partner" and "family." As a practical consideration, it is common for providers to identify a romantic partner as one with whom the patient has married or lived with for at least a year. For individuals who work with broader family systems, such systems are often partially defined by those with whom the patient currently lives (e.g., married partner and children) or lived with while growing up (e.g., family of origin members, such as parents and siblings). From this perspective, we see the family can take many different forms, including, but not limited to,
(a) a traditional nuclear family in which members are cohabiting in household (where either one or both parents are working); (b) a household or family headed by a single parent; (c) a "blended" family resulting from divorce, separation, and remarriage; (d) a same-sex couple with or without custodial children; (e) a multigenerational household including grandparents, parents, and children; and even (f) long-term cohabiting partners who are not romantically linked but define themselves as a family (6). Depending on the need of the patient, any of these can ultimately become the familial unit of intervention.

The Interplay between Substance Use and Marital/Family Maladjustment

Compared to traditional individual-focused interventions for alcoholism and drug abuse, family-based approaches try to understand these disorders from a systems perspective. People are not islands. They interact with others in their social and environmental network; they influence those networks and those networks influence them. Although there are certainly many social networks (e.g., work, school, and church), the family is very often the most proximal, influential, and powerful. Proponents of family-based intervention approaches universally hold that the power of the family can be used to help bring about healthful behavioral change.

The interconnection between substance use and familial distress appears to be marked by what can be best described as "reciprocal causality." Certain commonly observed characteristics and behaviors of alcoholics and drug abusers (e.g., denial of problems, checking out of interactions and general cognitive distortion of information) are not conducive to positive family environments. In turn, these characteristics contribute high relationship and family distress, which makes for an environment that serves to promote (inadvertently or otherwise) continued use or relapse (7). Thus, as shown in Figure 43.1, the link between substance use and

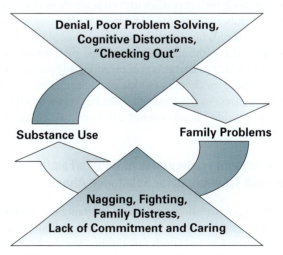

Figure 43.1. "Vicious cycle" between substance abuse and family problems.

relationship problems is not unidirectional, with one consistently causing the other, but rather each can serve as a precursor to the other, creating a "vicious cycle" from which couples that include a partner who abuses drugs or alcohol often have difficulty escaping (8).

There are several family environment antecedent conditions and reinforcing consequences of substance use. Couples, marital, and family problems (e.g., poor communication and problem-solving, arguing, and financial stressors) often serve as precursors to excessive drinking or drug use, and unfortunately, resulting family interactions can inadvertently help to facilitate continued drinking or drug use once these behaviors have developed. For example, substance abuse often provides more subtle adaptive consequences for the family members, such as facilitating the expression of emotion and affection (e.g., caretaking when a parent or partner is suffering from a hangover). Finally, even when recovery from the alcohol or drug problem has begun, marital and family conflicts can, and very often do, precipitate relapses.

Lastly, the family is an extremely important molding influence for children, with deleterious effects on children's emotional and behavioral functioning well-established in both the scientific and the lay press. As part of the family of the substance-abusing patient, children in the home become caught in the dynamics of the "vicious cycle" created by substance abuse within the family (8,9). Distress within the couple spills over into their parenting and the family environment to impact children (10); sometimes, in turn, children's distress may feed back into the family's functioning. For example, alcoholic parents are less likely than nonalcoholic parents to monitor what their children are doing, which can lead to affiliation of their adolescent children with drug-using peers (11), creating another source of family conflict. Parental substance abuse thus often has direct and serious physical, emotional, behavioral, and economic consequences on parenting and children. Moreover, the ancillary short- and long-term negative influences created within the family are often no less destructive. Exposure to violence, interparental conflict, and stress, which are comparatively high in families with an alcoholic or drug-using family member, compromises children's functioning, and may increase their likelihood of becoming substance users in adolescence (12). Although researchers and providers tend to think of the deleterious effects of parenting and parental substance misuse on children (which are indisputable), it is also clear that stress in the family that can be created by children helps to provide a family context conducive to continued use or relapse.

Foundational Frameworks of Couple/Family-Focused Treatments for Substance Abuse

The strong interrelationship between substance use and family interaction supports the use of interventions that address both substance misuse and family functioning. Approaches to relationship- and family-focused treatments for substance abuse take many different forms, but most are founded largely or exclusively on one of three foundational frameworks (13,14).

The best known of these and the most widely used is the *family disease approach*, which views alcoholism and other drug abuse as an illness experienced by the family, suffered not only by the substance user but also by family members.

Interventions founded on this perspective, such as Al-Anon and related approaches, focus on the patient and his or her detachment from family members during the recovery process. Family members are taught there is nothing they can do to stop the substance user besides stop enabling behaviors, and instead are encouraged to focus on their own recovery. As such, any family member involvement in treatment, if it occurs, is conducted in parallel to that of the substance-abusing individual, rather than as an integrated part of the patients' treatment. In many ways, although interactions are considered, this framework remains most closely tied to individual-based conceptualizations of substance use, which place the primary responsibility of change within the individual patient.

The *family systems approach* applies the principles of general systems theory to families, with particular attention paid to ways in which families maintain a dynamic balance between substance use and family functioning and whose interactional behavior is organized around alcohol or drug use. From this perspective, the family system provides a context that enables excessive drinking and/or drug use. Alcoholism and other addictive disorders are diseases that flourish in and are enabled by family systems. Family members react to the identified patient with particular behavioral patterns. They may enable the substance misuse to continue by shielding the patient from the negative consequences of his or her actions. Such behaviors are referred to as *codependence*. In this way, the person with the drug or alcohol use problem is said to suffer from the *disease of addiction*, whereas the family members suffer from the *disease of codependence*.

In a general sense, treatment evolving from a family systems perspective aims at identifying the function that substance use within the family serves, and then restructuring interaction patterns associated with drinking or drug use to make that maladaptive behavior unnecessary in the maintenance of the family system functioning. Structural (15) and strategic (16) theory and therapy methods fall within this broader systems framework.

The *behavioral model* assumes that family interactions serve to reinforce alcohol- and drug-using behavior. The goal of couple and family therapy from this perspective is to eliminate reinforcement for substance use by the family, which is often unintentional, and to promote reinforcement of behavior conducive to abstinence.

Family-based behavioral models are the foundation for the most commonly used interventions with alcoholic and drug-abusing couples. From this perspective, three general reinforcement patterns are typically observed in couples with a substance-abusing partner: (a) reinforcement for substance-using behavior in the form of attention or caretaking, (b) shielding the substance user from experiencing negative consequences related to his or her drinking or drug use, and (c) punishing substance use behavior. Behaviorally oriented treatment focuses on changing spousal and other family members' interactions that serve as stimuli for abusive substance use or that trigger relapse. More adaptive and reinforcing interaction antecedents, such as improving communication and problem-solving abilities and strengthening coping skills, are developed in ways that reinforce sobriety.

EFFICACY OF COUPLES- AND FAMILY-INVOLVED APPROACHES

During the last several decades, many different couples-based and family therapy approaches have been developed (or at least modified) to engage and treat substance-abusing patients; a large and growing body of research evidence supports their effectiveness. Because of the multiple forms of family-based approaches that have been used to address substance abuse, and the wide array of outcomes explored by both treatment providers and investigators, it is well beyond the scope of this chapter to discuss them all. Among the most frequently referenced in the research and clinical literatures include (a) community reinforcement and family training, (b) behavioral couple therapy (BCT), (c) solution-focused couple therapy (SFCT), (d) brief strategic family therapy, (e) multisystemic family therapy, and (f) multidimensional family therapy. In some cases, some of these are minor variations of each other, although many would argue that some of the nuanced differences may have a great influence on treatment response and outcomes for a given patient and his or her family.

For reasons that are more pragmatic than conceptual or theoretic, family-involved therapeutic interventions for alcoholism and substance abuse have been categorized as either *partner-focused approaches* (that include intimate partners as part of the intervention) or *family approaches* (that address larger family systems that may or may not include the dyadic system). Of course, in practice and research, this distinction often becomes blurry; for example, some partner-involved therapies for substance abuse have also incorporated substantial elements of parent training to improve children's adjustment (17,18). Nonetheless, such distinctions between couples- and family-involved therapies offer some organizational structure to any discussion of such treatment methods and how they may be used to engage or treat substance-abusing individuals within these families.

Partner- and Family-Involved Approaches to Engagement

Treatments developed to help substance-using individuals to recognize problem behavior and seek help to change have involved both partners and other family members. The Community Reinforcement Approach (CRA) is based on an assumption that by shifting patterns of reinforcement and contingencies across environmental influences and events, an individual substance abuser's behavior can change. Within this broad community framework, the family is one of many critical environmental influences of interest (19). Given the importance of family, CRA was modified to focus on the family. The resulting *Community Reinforcement and Family Training* [CRAFT; (20)] aims to teach family members (most often spouses of substance abusers) how to (a) encourage the substance abuser to evaluate whether or not drinking or drug use is problematic, (b) support sobriety, (c) seek out and encourage treatment for substance abuse, and (d) participate in that treatment in a way that is most beneficial.

A more coercive approach, the *Johnson Institute Intervention*, commonly referred to as an "Intervention," involves training family and significant others to confront an alcohol or drug abuser, request that he or she seek treatment, and impose consequences for not seeking help (21). The goal of this program is treatment engagement by the substance abuser. The approach is controversial (on practical and ethical bases), and there is limited evidence of effectiveness with the widely diverse population of individuals with alcohol use disorders (22).

Unilateral family therapy (UFT) is used to help family members develop or strengthen coping skills, to enhance healthful family functioning, and to help create a family environment that is conducive to sobriety or at least reduced drinking and drug use. UFT outlines a series of graded steps that families can use prior to initiating any sort of confrontation with the substance abuser to recognize his or her problem and seek formal treatment. Although research is limited, in a small-scale trial, participation in UFT was associated with significantly greater likelihood that individuals with drinking problems would enter treatment or reduce their drinking (23).

It is also important to mention certain related approaches that, rather than focus on initiating change, emphasize self-healing. For example, Dittrich (24) has developed a *group program for wives of treatment-resistant substance abusers*. Following the family disease framework, this treatment is designed to help partners cope with their own emotional distress rather than trying to motivate the substance-abusing partner to seek help or otherwise change. This particular approach borrows heavily from Al-Anon, the most commonly used source of support for family members of substance abusers, which advocates family members detach from the substance abusers in a loving way, accept they are powerless to control the substance abuser, and seek support from other Al-Anon members.

Results of randomized clinical trials have compared some of these approaches in terms of their efficacy in engaging patients in treatment. One investigation compared the CRAFT, Al-Anon, and Johnson Institute Intervention approaches for effectiveness in getting individuals with drinking problems into formal treatment. The highest overall treatment rate for the alcoholic family members was associated with the CRAFT therapy (64%). The majority of families in the Johnson Institute condition chose not to complete the intervention; in fact, 70% failed to follow up with the critical confrontation session. Because Al-Anon is not designed to facilitate entry into treatment, it is not surprising that this was not a common outcome (25).

Couple-Based Approaches to Treatment

The majority of couple- and family-involved approaches to substance abuse have focused on efforts to treat the substance abuser to attain and adjust to sobriety, and to maintain these gains. Two commonly referenced couple approaches, BCT and SFCT, dominate the research and practice areas of couple therapy, respectively.

BCT (3) has, to date, the strongest empirical support for its effectiveness (26). When using BCT with a married or cohabiting alcoholic or drug-abusing patient, a therapist treats the partners together and works to build support from within the dyadic system for abstinence. In a global sense, emphasis is placed on increasing reinforcement with the dyadic system for abstinence. To accomplish that goal, BCT seeks to strengthen the relationship by improving partners' communication and having partners participate in relationship enhancement exercises (e.g., participating in mutually shared rewarding activities, and observing and recognizing caring behaviors). As the relationship strengthens, partners are taught skills and engage in exercises to positively reinforce aspects of sober living.

Empirical support for the effectiveness of BCT with alcoholic and drug-abusing couples is extensive. Multiple studies have compared drinking and relationship outcomes for alcoholic patients and their partners treated with BCT to various forms of therapy that involve only the individual patient (e.g., individual counseling sessions and group therapy). Results of these investigations have been very consistent, revealing a pattern of less frequent drinking, fewer alcohol-related problems, happier relationships, and lower risk of marital separation for alcoholic patients who received BCT than for patients who receive only individual-based treatment (27).

Although the research on the effects of BCT for married or cohabiting patients that abuse drugs other than alcohol is more recent, the outcomes have been no less impressive than those obtained for alcoholic couples. Compared to individual treatment for the substance-abusing partner only, BCT for drug-abusing men and their non-substance-abusing female partners resulted in fewer days of drug use, fewer drug-related arrests and hospitalizations, a longer time to relapse after treatment completion, and more positive relationship adjustment (28). Although BCT studies with alcoholic and drug-abusing patients have recruited samples that consisted largely or exclusively of married or cohabiting male patients and their non-substance-abusing female partners, preliminary investigations with married or cohabiting female patients and their non-substance-abusing male partners have yielded positive results similar to those for substance-abusing men (29,30). Interestingly, the use of BCT with alcohol- and drug-abusing couples also has important effects on other aspects of family functioning that are not primary targets of the intervention, including improvements in custodial children's emotional and behavioral adjustment (even though the children did not participate in BCT nor was parenting an emphasis of the intervention) (31) and reductions in domestic violence (32).

SFCT (33) primarily emphasizes solutions to the presenting issue or concern, rather than the origins of the problem. Simply stated, SFCT is a strengths-based, solution-focused brief therapy approach to couple distress and substance use. The basic conceptualization of relationship problems in SFCT is that distressed couples (a) are locked into a negative mindset, (b) are stuck in problem talk, (c) have inherent strengths but are not seeing or utilizing them, and (d) are not noticing the exceptions to when the problem occurs. In SFCT, problem talk is completely discouraged; the goal of the therapist is to help the couple identify and coconstruct active solutions to the problem, often found in the exceptions (i.e., those times when the problem does not occur), and identify small achievable goals that may enhance optimism for further behavioral change. The therapy is brief, sometimes lasting only one to two sessions, and rarely more than ten. Few empirical outcome evaluations of the use of solution-focused therapies with substance-abusing populations have been conducted, although it appears that treatment providers believe it to be effective and commonly use this approach with these patients (34). Empirical evaluations, however, are needed to determine the accuracy of the provider beliefs.

Family Approaches to Treatment

As noted, no one family-involved intervention has come to dominate family therapy for alcoholism and drug addiction. Upon reflection, this is not a surprise; as opposed to partner-involved therapy (which inherently narrows the intervention unit to intimate partners), family therapy has a much larger field of family types and, relatedly, family issues that it is called upon to address. The bulk of the controlled clinical research trials that include a family component in substance abuse treatment examine adults with partners in couple-based approaches. However, it is also important to consider the role of family and significant others in the treatment of adolescents who struggle with alcohol problems. Thus, in addition to the models listed above, three other approaches that have been developed for use primarily with substance-abusing adolescents and their families are reviewed: (a) brief strategic family therapy (BSFT), (b) multidimensional family therapy (MDFT), and (c) multisystemic family therapy (MST). Each of these approaches integrates structural (13) and strategic (14) theory and principles within a family systems perspective, and although highly intensive, has developed a strong base of empirical support.

In BSFT (35), substance-abusing behavior is seen to develop in response to unsuccessful attempts at dealing with developmental challenges. Rigid family structures are also believed to contribute to the development of adolescent substance abuse. The therapist attempts to intervene in the system through the parents by changing parenting practices, improving the parent–adolescent relationship, and teaching conflict resolution skills. A series of randomized trials has demonstrated empirical support for BSFT at engaging and treating substance-using adolescents and their families, including Hispanic youth and families; a multisite effectiveness trial is currently under way (36).

MDFT (37) views adolescent substance abuse as a result of multiple interacting factors, which may include failure to meet developmental challenges as well as other forms of abuse or trauma. The primary goals of treatment are to improve adolescent, parental, and overall family functioning, which in turn will impact the substance-abusing and other problematic behaviors. MDFT is a very flexible approach; the treatment length is determined by the treatment provider, setting, and family and may include a combination of individual and family sessions. MDFT begins with a thorough multisystem assessment of both developmental ecologic risk and protective factors. This information is then used to create an MDFT case conceptualization, which identifies the strengths and weaknesses in the adolescent's multiple systems and becomes the basis of treatment. MDFT has demonstrated strong efficacy in reducing substance use and delinquency with juvenile justice–involved adolescents (38).

MST (39) is based on Bronfenbrenner's social ecologic model of behavior, seeking to understand the substance-abusing behavior within a broader, real-world context. MST assumes that substance abuse is influenced by variables from multiple systems, targeting change in other areas (e.g., arrests, out-of-home placements, and mental health) as well as substance use. Thus, one of the goals of treatment is to assess the strengths and needs of each system and their relationship to the presenting problem. Family members play a large role in determining treatments goals. MST focuses on the present and targets a broad set of specific and well-defined problems through the use of daily and weekly assignments. The MST therapist is responsible for addressing and overcoming any barriers that may result during the course of treatment.

With its broad, ecologic, and family focus, MST was not originally designed to target substance use specifically. As such, initial studies examining substance-related outcomes of MST among violent and chronic juvenile offenders showed long-term effects on substance use–related outcomes through adulthood (e.g., drug-related arrests or convictions) (40), though less consistently valid substance use reductions (41). Recent pilot and larger trials that integrate MST with other contingency management strategies aimed specifically at reducing substance use suggest promising effects on both self-report and biologic substance use reductions (42).

OPTIMAL IMPLEMENTATION OF FAMILY-BASED TREATMENT

There is considerable debate among providers about how to implement family-based treatments as part of an overall package to address alcoholism and substance abuse. It is sometimes asserted among some providers that participation in family treatment should not occur until the identified patient has been sober for at least a year. There are at least three problems with that recommendation: (a) given that so many patients who received treatment in substance abuse treatment settings relapse during the year after leaving treatment, only a limited number of patients would actually be sober for a year and be eligible for family-involved treatment; (b) if patients remains sober for a year, they often will not meet the necessary diagnostic criteria for a substance abuse treatment program to be able to provide services (in many states, a current diagnosis of a substance use disorder is required for admission); and (c) there is no empirical support that delaying family treatment enhances efficacy.

Optimally, it is important to include a family member or members in the intervention package as early as possible. In our experience, family members often bring a different perspective than the patient on the family and its role in the etiology and maintenance of the patient's drinking and drug use behavior. They can also give providers a sense of whether or not the family will be functionally supportive of the patient's efforts to maintain a sober lifestyle, as well as how much focus will need to be placed on the family as treatment unfolds. As a general rule of thumb, the best time to implement family-focused treatment for substance abuse is as soon as possible. An early assessment can inform providers about the possible role of the family in the patient's treatment.

Lastly, in an ideal situation, there should be family therapy providers who do "family work" with patients, which is provided as a complement to individual-focused treatments by yet another provider. Such staffing allows for certain therapeutic boundaries to exist between partner- and family-focused therapy sessions and individual-focused sessions. In reality, many programs do not have the resources to enjoy the luxury of having separate providers for family therapy. Nonetheless, it is often out of necessity that a single provider serves as the individual counselor and the family counselor. In our experience, one person can effectively serve as the individual counselor and the family counselor. When that is the only way that family therapy can be provided, it is important to establish confidentiality boundaries between what is discussed in family therapy versus what is discussed in individual therapy. Typically, the contents of the individual sessions are kept confidential from the family therapy sessions (3).

SPECIAL CONSIDERATIONS

There are several clinically significant considerations in implementing effective family intervention with substance abusers that may challenge its use. One that is commonly encountered among couples and families with a substance-abusing member is violence. In situations where the risk of types of violence that are severe (i.e., aggression that has the potential to result in serious injury or is life threatening), the immediate intervention goal is safety; in these situations, partner and family therapy is contraindicated (43). For some families, there may, in fact, be legal restrictions (i.e., restraining orders or no contact orders) that preclude conjoint family sessions.

Another factor to consider is whether more than one actively substance abusing family member is present—particularly if these individuals have formed a drinking or drug use partnership of some type. Sometimes referred to as "double-trouble couples," these family systems may support continued use versus abstinence (44). Research on family-based approaches for these situations is lacking, and it is often recommended that individual therapy be used prior to engaging family members in these circumstances.

Another critical consideration is the existence of high levels of blame and rumination from family members (usually the partner) toward the substance-abusing individual. There may also exist important practical barriers to partner or family intervention; these include (a) geographic distances among family members or among family members and the treatment provider; (b) family members who are divorced, incarcerated, or otherwise separated; (c) coordination of family members' and treatment providers' schedules; and (d) securing reimbursement for services delivered to multiple individuals in the context of formal treatment.

FUTURE DIRECTIONS AND CONCLUSIONS

Although there is an increasing awareness of the efficacy of partner- and family-involved approaches to alcoholism and drug abuse, there are several important gaps in the research literature and in general practice that reflect the next generation of research in this area. More specifically, the following five areas seem most pressing: (a) disseminating evidence-based marital and family treatments to community-based treatment programs, (b) applying these approaches with specific populations, (c) examining mechanism of action, (d) exploring the use of partner- and family-involved approaches as part of a stepped care model, and (e) addressing the behavioral and emotional needs of non-substance-abusing partners.

Dissemination

Although marital and family approaches for substance abuse have very strong research support, they are not widely used in community-based alcoholism and drug abuse treatment settings. For example, Fals-Stewart and Birchler (45) conducted a national survey of 398 randomly selected U.S. substance abuse treatment programs and found fewer than 10% of the programs used any form of partner-involved therapy. Despite its proven efficacy, BCT in particular was viewed as too costly to deliver and requiring too many sessions. Investigators and treatment providers will need to work in concert to identify barriers and ways to overcome them, so these very powerful methods can reach patients in need of them.

Specific Populations

Although the body of empirical literature supporting the use of marital and family therapy for substance abuse is substantial, it is critical to also recognize its limitations. Among these are the types of families that are typically the subject of such studies, which usually include largely white, male substance-abusing patients. Studies on the efficacy of marital and family therapy approaches for women with substance use disorders are far less common, although available evidence does suggest that they are efficacious (30). Even fewer studies have examined partner- and family-involved interventions with same-sex couples, although a very recent trial yielded encouraging results (46).

Relatedly, it is also important to recognize that BCT trials have focused on couples in which only one partner has a drug or alcohol problem. Dual-using partners, or "double-trouble" couples, represent a very unique challenge. In our experience, women who are married to or are in relationships with substance-abusing men have particularly bad outcomes compared to women in relationships with men who do not use alcohol or other drugs. This comes as no surprise, given that women in double-trouble couples fail to get support for abstinence in their homes. Methods to engage both partners and promote mutual abstinence (e.g., contingency management for both partners and motivational interviewing) are worthy next steps to address the needs of these patients.

A great deal of research has been conducted related to both family therapy and culture and ethnicity, but very little of this has appeared in the family therapy literature on substance abuse. This represents what is likely the most important gap in the extant empirical literature to date. Observations with over 1500 substance-abusing couples in randomized clinical trials suggest that BCT may have benefits across some, but not all, racial/ethnic groups. Understanding the degree to which the "vicious cycle" of substance use affects families in universal ways and can thus be treated similarly, as well as the degree to which other cultural and ethnic factors must be considered to achieve benefits for diverse families, will be critical for the research and practice fields to address.

Lastly, despite all efforts to engage partners and families, there are patients whose partners or family members will simply not be involved in treatment. There can be any number of reasons for this; a patient may simply refuse, the family members may refuse, or scheduling between participants and providers becomes impossible. These patients represent a clearly definable population in their own right. An intriguing option is to engage in family therapy by working only with the patient to promote family change. Such an approach eschews the multiple barriers that clinicians often face when trying to engage and treat larger family systems. As paradoxical as they may first appear, one-person couple therapy and one-person family therapy have shown promise in preliminary pilot-sized trials (47,48). However, more comprehensive efficacy trials are needed to explore observed positive effects in these one-person family interventions compared to standard individual and partner- and family-involved treatments.

Mechanisms of Action

We now have confidence that many treatments are effective, some more than others, but despite the successful efforts of substance abuse treatment researchers to conduct rigorous clinical trials and spell out in treatment manuals what the treatments consist of, little research has formally investigated what the active ingredients of these treatments are. In other words, what are the mechanisms of action that make certain partner- and family-involved approaches curative? If these factors can be identified, then these approaches can be modified to maximize efficiency and effectiveness of treatment.

Partner- and Family-Involved Treatment in the Context of Stepped Care

Since partner- and family-involved therapies have been shown to be efficacious across a number of different formats [e.g., abbreviated formats (49), multifamily, and one-person couples treatment], some of these interventions may be good candidates for a stepped care approach (50), moving from least to most intensive as treatment response dictates. As an example, married or cohabiting patients entering treatment can enter a therapy group, without the participation of their partners, which focuses on relationship issues. Patients for whom it is clinically indicated can then move to a multicouple group format that would include their partners. Couples who require more conjoint treatment can participate in a planned abbreviated couple therapy; if that is insufficient, then patients and their partners can participate in the standard form of couple therapy, which is the most intensive, requiring the most time and greatest commitment by both providers and partners.

Partners as Patients

In our experience, partners of substance-abusing patients have a host of emotional and behavioral problems. These range from increased risk for infection from sexually transmitted diseases, victimization from intimate partner violence, and increased levels of psychological depression. Intervention models, such as BCT, lean heavily on the non-substance-abusing partners to support and promote abstinence. It is quite plausible that if the emotional and behavioral needs of these partners are not adequately addressed, they will have fewer resources to bring to partner-involved intervention approaches, leading to overall poorer treatment response and outcomes for the substance-abusing patient and the couples more broadly. An important next step in this overall programmatic line of research is to examine the moderating effects of the psychological adjustment of non-substance-abusing partners on treatment response and outcome and, if such factors moderate effects, design interventions that address the unique needs of these partners.

CONCLUSION

As has been well documented in the scientific and lay press, the emotional, economic, and societal toll of alcoholism and drug abuse is incalculable. The effects of substance use disorders affect not only the patients but also those around them; in fact, those emotionally closest to the substance-abusing patient often suffer the most. Partner- and family-involved approaches have had such well-documented success because such methods view outcomes across multiple dimensions of functioning that go well beyond the frequency of substance use toward outcomes like child and family adjustment, family violence, relationship quality, and so forth. By seeking to foster family environments conducive to abstinence, marital and family approaches have great potential to help maintain long-term and even multigenerational healthful change.

ACKNOWLEDGMENTS

This chapter was supported, in part, by grants from the National Institute on Drug Abuse (R01DA12189, R01DA014402, R01DA014402-SUPL, R01DA015937, and R01DA016236) and the National Institute on Alcohol Abuse and Alcoholism (R21AA013690).

REFERENCES

1. Jellinek EM. *The Disease Concept of Alcoholism.* New Haven, CT: Hillhouse; 1960.
2. Keller, M. Trends in treatment of alcoholism. In: *Second Special Report to the U.S. Congress on Alcohol and Health.* Washington, DC: Department of Health, Education, and Welfare; 1974: 145–167.
3. O'Farrell TJ, Fals-Stewart W. Alcohol abuse. *J Marital Fam Ther.* 2003;29:97–120.
4. Stanton MD, Shadish WR. Outcome, attrition, and family-couples treatment for drug abuse: a meta-analysis and review of the controlled, comparative studies. *Psychol Bull.* 1997;122:170–191.
5. Brown ED, O'Farrell TJ, Maisto SA, et al., eds. *Accreditation Guide for Substance Abuse Treatment Programs.* Newbury Park, CA: Sage Publications; 1997.
6. McCrady BS. Family and other close relationships. In: Miller WR, Carroll KM, eds. *Rethinking Substance Abuse: What the Science Shows and What We Should Do about It.* New York: Guilford Press; 2006.
7. Birchler GR, Fals-Stewart W, O'Farrell TJ. Couple therapy for alcoholism and drug abuse. In: Gurman AS, ed. *Clinical Handbook of Couple Therapy.* 4th ed. New York: Guilford; 2008: 523–544.
8. Fals-Stewart W, O'Farrell TJ, Birchler GR. Behavioral couples therapy for substance abuse: rationale, methods, and findings. *Sci Pract Perspect.* 2004;2:30–41.
9. Lam WK, Fals-Stewart W, O'Farrell TJ. Dynamics in substance-abusing families and treatment implications. In: Straussner SLA, Fewell CH, eds. *Children of Alcohol and Other Drug Abusing Parents: Treatment Issues and Interventions.* NY: Springer; in press.
10. Fals-Stewart W, Kelley ML, Fincham FD, et al. Emotional and behavioral problems of children living with drug-abusing fathers: comparisons with children living with alcohol-abusing and non-substance-abusing fathers. *J Fam Psychol.* 2004;18: 319–330.
11. Chassin L, Pillow DR, Curran PJ, et al. The relation of parent alcoholism to adolescent substance use: a test of three mediating mechanisms. *J Abnorm Psychol.* 1993;102:3–19.
12. Chassin L, Curran PJ, Hussong AM, et al. The relation of parent alcoholism to adolescent substance use: a longitudinal follow-up study. *J Abnorm Psychol.* 1996;10:70–80.
13. Gondoli DM, Jacob T. Family treatment of alcoholism. In: Watson R, ed. *Drug and Alcohol Abuse Reviews: Vol. 1. Prevention and Treatment of Drug and Alcohol Abuse.* New York: Humana Press; 1990:245–262.

14. Fals-Stewart W, O'Farrell TJ, Birchler GR. Family therapy techniques. In: Rotgers F, Morgenstern J, Walters ST, eds. *Treating Substance Abuse: Theory and Technique*. New York: Guilford; 2003:140–165.
15. Minuchin S, Fishman HC. *Family Therapy Techniques*. Cambridge, MA: Harvard University Press; 1981.
16. Haley J. *Problem-Solving Therapy*. San Francisco: Jossey-Bass; 1976.
17. Lam WK, Fals-Stewart W, Kelley ML. Effects of parent skills training with Behavioral Couples Therapy for alcoholism: a randomized clinical pilot trial. *Addict Behav*. 2008;33:1076–1080.
18. Lam WK, Fals-Stewart W, Kelley ML. Parent training with behavioral couples therapy for paternal substance abuse: effects on substance abuse, parental relationship, parenting, and CPS involvement. *Child Maltreat*. 2009;14:243–254.
19. Roozen HG, Boulogne JJ, van Tulder MW, et al. A systematic review of the effectiveness of the community reinforcement approach in alcohol, cocaine and opioid addiction. *Drug Alcohol Depend*. 2004;74:1–13.
20. Smith JE, Meyers RJ. Community reinforcement and family training. In: Fisher GL, Roget's NA, eds. *Encyclopedia of Substance Abuse Prevention, Treatment, and Recovery*. Thousand Oaks, CA: Sage Publications; 2008:219–221.
21. Johnson VE. *Intervention: How to Help Someone Who Doesn't Want Help*. Center City, MN: Hazelden; 1986.
22. Connors GJ, Donovan DM, DiClemente CC. *Substance Abuse Treatment and the Stages of Change: Selecting and Planning Interventions*. New York: Guilford; 2001.
23. Thomas EJ, Santa C, Bronson D, et al. Unilateral family therapy with spouses of alcoholics. *J Soc Serv Res*. 1987;10:145–162.
24. Dittrich JE. A group program for wives of treatment resistant alcoholics. In: O'Farrell TJ, ed. *Treating Alcohol Problems: Marital and Family Intervention*. New York: Guilford; 1993:78–114.
25. Miller WR, Meyers RJ, Tonigan JS. Engaging the unmotivated in treatment for alcohol problems: a comparison of three strategies for intervention through family members. *J Consult Clin Psychol*. 1999;67:688–697.
26. Powers M, Vedel E, Emmelkamp P. Behavioral couples therapy (BCT) for alcohol and drug use disorders: a meta-analysis. *Clin Psychol Rev*. 2008;28:952–962.
27. Fals-Stewart W, O'Farrell TG, Birchler GR, et al. Behavioral couples therapy for alcoholism and drug abuse: where we've been, where we are, and where we're going. *J Cogn Psychother*. 2005;19:231–249.
28. Fals-Stewart W, Birchler GR, O'Farell TJ. Behavioral couples therapy for male substance-abusing patients: effects on relationship adjustment and drug-using behavior. *J Consult Clin Psychol*. 1996;64:959–972.
29. Winters J, Fals-Stewart W, O'Farrell TJ, et al. Behavioral couples therapy for female substance-abusing patients: effects on substance use and relationship adjustment. *J Consult Clin Psychol*. 2002;70:344–355.
30. Fals-Stewart W, Birchler GR, Kelley ML. Learning sobriety together: a randomized clinical trial examining behavioral couples therapy with alcoholic female patients. *J Consult Clin Psychol*. 2006;74:579–591.
31. Kelley ML, Fals-Stewart W. Couples- versus individual-based therapy for alcoholism and drug abuse: effects on children's psychosocial functioning. *J Consult Clin Psychol*. 2002;70:417–427.
32. Fals-Stewart W, Clinton-Sherrod M. Treating intimate partner violence among substance abusing dyads: the effect of couples therapy. *Prof Psychol Res Pract*. 2009;40:257–263.
33. Lipchik E. *Beyond Technique in Solution-Focused Therapy*. New York: Guilford Press; 2002.
34. Herbeck DM, Hser Y, Teruya C. Empirically supported substance abuse treatment approaches: a survey of treatment providers' perspectives and practices. *Addict Behav*. 2008;33:699–712.
35. Szapocznik J, Hervis O, Schwartz S. *Therapy Manuals for Drug Addiction: Brief Strategic Family Therapy for Adolescent Drug Abuse*. Bethesda, MD: National Institute on Drug Abuse; 2003.
36. Robbins MS, Szapocznik J, Horigian VE, et al. Brief strategic family therapy for adolescent drug abusers: a multi-site effectiveness study. *Contemp Clin Trials*. 2009;30:269–278.
37. Liddle HA. Treating adolescent abuse using multidimensional family therapy. In: Weisz J, Kazdin A, eds. *Evidence-Based Psychotherapies for Children and Adolescents*. 2nd ed. New York: Guilford Press; 2009.
38. Liddle HA. Family-based therapies for adolescent alcohol and drug use: research contributions and future research needs. *Addiction*. 2004;99:76–92.
39. Cunningham PB, Henggeler SW. Engaging multiproblem families in treatment: lessons learned throughout the development of multisystemic therapy. *Fam Process*. 1999;38:265–281.
40. Schaeffer CM, Borduin CM. Long-term follow-up to a randomized clinical trial of multisystemic therapy with serious and violent juvenile offenders. *J Consult Clin Psychol*. 2005;73:445–453.
41. Henggeler SW, Rowland MD, Randall J, et al. Home-based multisystemic therapy as an alternative to hospitalization of youths in psychiatric crisis: clinical outcomes. *J Am Acad Child Adolesc Psychiatry*. 1999;38:1331–1339.
42. Randall J, Cunningham PB. Multisystemic therapy: a treatment for violent substance-abusing and substance-dependent juvenile offenders. *Addict Behav*. 2003;28:1731–1739.
43. Fals-Stewart W, Kennedy C. Addressing intimate partner violence in substance abuse treatment. *J Subst Abuse Treat*. 2005;5:5–17.
44. Fals-Stewart W, Birchler GR, O'Farrell TJ. Drug-abusing patients and their intimate partners: dyadic adjustment, relationship stability, and substance use. *J Abnorm Psychol*. 1999;108:11–23.
45. Fals-Stewart W, Birchler GR. A national survey of the use of couples therapy in substance abuse treatment. *J Subst Abuse Treat*. 2001;20:277–283.
46. Fals-Stewart W, O'Farrell TJ, Lam WK. Behavioral couple therapy with gay and lesbian couples. *J Subst Abuse Treat*. 2009;37:379–387.
47. Morgan-Lopez A, Fals-Stewart W. Analytic methods for modeling longitudinal data from rolling therapy: groups with membership turnover. *J Consult Clin Psychol*. 2007;75:580–593.
48. Szapocznik J, Kurtines WM, Foote FH, et al. Conjoint versus one-person family therapy: some evidence for the effectiveness of conducting family therapy through one person. *J Consult Clin Psychol*. 1983;51:889–899.
49. Fals-Stewart W, Lam WK. Brief behavioral couples therapy for drug abuse: a randomized clinical trial examining clinical efficacy and cost effectiveness. *Fam Syst Health*. 2008;26:377–392.
50. Sobell MB, Sobell LC. Stepped care as a heuristic approach to the treatment of alcohol problems. *J Consult Clin Psychol*. 2000;68:573–579.

CHAPTER 44

Cognitive Behavioral Therapy

Kathleen M. Carroll

INTRODUCTION AND OVERVIEW

Cognitive behavioral treatments are among the most well-defined and rigorously studied psychotherapeutic interventions for substance use disorders. While this chapter focuses almost primarily on cognitive behavioral therapy (CBT), it should be noted that CBT shares several features with several other empirically supported behavioral approaches reviewed in this volume. First, cognitive, behavioral, and motivational therapies are applicable across a broad range of substance use disorders. That is, well-controlled trials have supported their efficacy across alcohol, stimulant, marijuana, and opioid-dependent populations. Second, these approaches were developed from well-founded theoretical traditions with established theories and principles of human behavior. Third, these approaches are highly flexible and can be implemented in a wide range of clinical modalities and settings. Moreover, they are compatible with a variety of pharmacotherapies and, in many cases, foster compliance and enhance the effects of pharmacotherapies including methadone, naltrexone, and disulfiram. Finally, these approaches are relatively brief/short-term and highly focused approaches that emphasize rapid, targeted change in substance use and related problems. In this manner, they are very compatible in a health care environment that is increasingly influenced by managed care, best clinical practice models, and professional accountability.

At the most simple level, CBT attempts to help individual patients recognize, avoid, and cope. That is, recognize the situations in which they are most likely to use drugs or alcohol, avoid those situations when possible or appropriate, and learn to cope more effectively with a range of problems and problematic behaviors associated with substance use. CBT has two critical components and defining features: First, a thorough functional analysis of the role alcohol and illicit drugs play in the individual's life. For each instance of substance use the patient experiences during treatment, the therapist and patient will identify the patient's thoughts, feelings, and circumstances before the substance use, as well as the patient's thoughts, feelings, and circumstances after the episode of substance use. Early in treatment, the functional analysis plays a critical role in helping the patient and therapist assess the determinants, or high-risk situations, that are likely to lead to substance use, as well as shed light on some of the reasons the individual may be using drugs or alcohol. The second critical component of CBT is skills training. In CBT, this consists of a highly individualized training program that helps substance users change old habits associated with their drug use and learn or relearn more adaptive skills and responses.

HISTORY

Cognitive behavioral treatments have their roots in classical behavioral theory and the pioneering work of Pavlov, Watson, Skinner, and Bandura (1,2). Pavlov's work on classical conditioning demonstrated that a previously neutral stimulus could elicit a conditioned response after being paired repeatedly with an unconditioned stimulus. Furthermore, repeated exposure to the conditioned stimulus without the unconditioned stimulus would eventually lead to extinction of the conditioned response. The power of classical conditioning was demonstrated in drug abuse by Wikler (3) who confirmed that opioid addicts exhibited conditioned withdrawal symptoms upon exposure to drug paraphernalia. Today, classical conditioning theory is the basis of several behavioral approaches to substance use treatment, such as cue exposure and stimulus avoidance as an early component of many addiction counseling approaches.

Second, Skinner's work on operant conditioning demonstrated that behaviors that are positively reinforced are likely to be exhibited more frequently. The field of behavioral pharmacology, which has convincingly demonstrated the reinforcing properties of abused substances in both humans and animals, is grounded in operant conditioning theory and principles. Behavior therapies assume that drug use and related behaviors are learned through their association with the positively reinforcing properties of the drugs themselves as well as their secondary association with other environmental stimuli. CBT attempts to disrupt this learned association between drug-related cues or stimuli and drug craving or use by understanding and changing these behavior patterns. A wide range of behavioral interventions, including those that seek to provide alternate reinforcers to drugs use or reduce reinforcing aspects of abused substances, also are based on operant conditioning theory.

CBTs conceive substance use disorders as complex, multidetermined problems, with a number of influences playing a role in the development or perpetuation of the disorder. These may include family history and genetic factors; the presence of comorbid psychopathology; personality traits such as sensation seeking or impulsivity; and a host of environmental factors, including substance drug availability and lack of countervailing influences and rewards. Though CBTs primarily emphasize the reinforcing properties of substances as central to the acquisition and maintenance of substance abuse and dependence, these etiologic influences are seen as heightening risk or vulnerability to the development of substance use problems. For example, some individuals may find substances unusually highly rewarding secondary to genetic vulnerability, comorbid depression, a high need for sensation seeking, the modeling of family and friends who use substances, or environments devoid of alternative reinforcers.

CBTs also reflect the pioneering work of Ellis and Beck that emphasizes the importance of the person's thoughts and feelings as determinants of behavior. CBT evolved in part from dissatisfaction with the extreme positions of radical behaviorism (e.g., emphasis on overt behaviors) and classical psychoanalysis (emphasis on unconscious conflicts or representations). CBT emphasizes how the individual perceives and interprets life events as important determinants of behavior (4). A person's conscious thoughts, feelings, and expectancies mediate an individual's response to the environment. CBT also seeks to help patients become aware of maladaptive cognitions and then learn to challenge and change them.

Just as CBT assumes that many individuals essentially "learn" to become substance users over time, through complex interplays of modeling, classical conditioning, or operant conditioning, each of these principles is invoked in CBT to help the patient stop using drugs and alcohol. For example, modeling is used to help the patient learn new behaviors (e.g., how to refuse an offer of drugs, how to break off or limit a relationship with a drug-using associate) by having the patient participate in role plays with the therapist during the treatment. That is, the patient learns to respond in new, unfamiliar ways by first watching the therapist model those new strategies and then practicing those strategies within the supportive context of the therapy hour.

Operant conditioning concepts are used several ways in CBT. First, through a detailed examination of the antecedents and consequences of substance use, the therapist attempts to develop an understanding of the reasons the patient may be more likely to use in a given situation and to understand the role that drugs or alcohol play in their life. This "functional analysis" of substance use is used to identify the high-risk situations in which the patient is likely to use drugs and thus to provide the basis for learning more effective coping behaviors in those situations. Second, the therapist attempts to help the patient develop meaningful alternate reinforcers to drug use; that is, other activities and involvements (relationships, work, hobbies) that serve as viable alternatives to drugs and alcohol use and help the patient remain abstinent. Finally, a detailed examination of the consequences, both long- and short-term, of their substance use, is used as a strategy to build or reinforce the patient's resolve to reduce or eliminate their substance use.

Classical conditioning concepts also play an important role in CBT, and particularly in interventions directed at reducing some forms of craving for drugs. Just as Pavlov demonstrated that repeated pairings of a conditioned stimulus with an unconditioned stimulus could elicit a conditioned response, he also demonstrated that repeated exposure to the conditioned stimulus without the unconditioned stimulus would, over time, result in extinction of the conditioned response. Thus, the therapist attempts to help the patient understand and recognize conditioned craving, identify his/her own idiosyncratic array of conditioned cues for craving, avoid exposure to those cues, and cope effectively with craving when it does occur without using the drug so that conditioned craving is reduced and eliminated over time.

Learning serves as an important metaphor for treatment process throughout. CBT therapists tell patients that a goal of the treatment is to help them "unlearn" old, ineffective behaviors and "learn" new ones. Patients, particularly those who are demoralized by their failure to change their substance use, or for whom the consequences of addiction have been severe, are frequently surprised to think about substance use as a type of skill, as something they have learned to do over time: In effect they have learned a complex set of skills that enabled them to acquire the money needed to buy drugs and alcohol (which often led to another set of licit or illicit skills), avoid detection, and so on. Patients who can reframe their self-appraisals in terms of being "skilled" in this way can often see that they also have the capacity to learn a new set of skills, this time, though, skills that will help them remain abstinent (5).

UNIQUE FEATURES

Durability

While CBT is not necessarily more effective than other evidence-based therapies for substance use disorders, where it appears to stand out is in its durability. An important development in our conception of substance use disorders is that they are chronic relapsing disorders and thus treatment should be conceived of as producing behavior change and maintaining it over the lifespan, rather than brief, disjointed, acute episodes of care (6). Thus, a major disadvantage of many addiction pharmacotherapies in this context is that they can be very effective while the patient is taking them, but relapse is common once the medication stops.

CBT, however, is associated with particularly durable effects. Several studies have documented a "sleeper effect," in which patients exposed to CBT continue to improve even after they leave treatment (7–9). This is illustrated in Figure 44.1, which shows patterns of drug use within treatment and during the follow-up period for CBT versus supportive clinical management among cocaine-dependent individuals. The durability of effects from CBT is found in its applications to other areas (10) as well, and may be associated with its emphasis on conveying effective, generalizability skills that may benefit the individual long after they leave treatment.

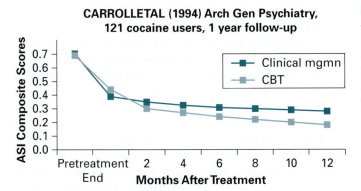

Figure 44.1. "Sleeper effect" of CBT. Severity of cocaine use within treatment (pretreatment end) and through follow-up (end-12 months) by treatment condition (CBT vs. supportive clinical management). (Data from Carroll KM, Rounsaville BJ, Nich C, et al. One year follow-up of psychotherapy and pharmacotherapy for cocaine dependence: delayed emergence of psychotherapy effects. *Arch Gen Psychiatry*. 1994;51:989–997.)

Unique and Common Factors of CBT

All behavioral or psychosocial treatments include both common factors as well as unique factors or active ingredients (11). Common factors refer to dimensions of treatment that are shared across most therapies. These common factors include the provision of education, a convincing rationale for the treatment, enhancing expectations of improvement, the provision of support and encouragement, and in particular the quality of the therapeutic relationship. A positive therapeutic relationship, or alliance, has repeatedly been associated with better outcome in a range of psychotherapies (12), including those for substance use disorders. A positive working relationship is an essential component of virtually all therapies, but, by itself, is not necessarily sufficient to produce change.

Unique factors refer to a treatment's "active ingredients" or those techniques and interventions that distinguish or characterize particular psychotherapies. While common factors are shared, unique factors are those that are not shared across different therapies. CBT, like most therapies, consists of a complex combination of common and unique factors. For example, in CBT mere delivery of skills trainings without grounding in a positive therapeutic relationship leads to a dry, overly didactic approach that alienates or bores most patients and ultimately has the opposite effect of that intended. It is important to recognize that CBT is thought to exert its effects through this intricate interplay of common and unique factors and a major task of the therapist is to achieve appropriate levels of balance between attending to the relationship and delivering skills training. For example, without a solid therapeutic alliance, it is unlikely that a patient will either stay in treatment, be sufficiently engaged to learn new skills, or to share successes and failures in trying new approaches to old problems. Conversely, empathic delivery of skills training as tools to help the patient manage his/her life more effectively, with the therapist giving the message of "I see you really struggling with your craving for cocaine [for example], I think we can come up with some effective ways to help you understand what is happening better and help you deal with it," may form the basis of a strong working alliance (5).

To specify CBT in terms of its common and unique factors and to clarify the range of therapist interventions that are consistent and inconsistent with this approach, CBT interventions will be described in terms of the system recommended by Waltz and colleagues (13): First, CBT's essential and unique interventions, that is, active ingredients that are specific or unique to CBT. Second, CBT's recommended interventions, those that are thought to be "active" and important, but which are not necessarily unique to CBT. Third, interventions, behaviors, or processes that are acceptable within the therapy but are not essential or unique. Finally, interventions, behaviors, or processes that are proscribed, or not consistent with this approach. Each of these has been explicated in a detailed process rating system (14) and validated in several randomized clinical trials of CBT.

Essential and Unique Interventions of CBT

In CBT, the key active ingredients that distinguish it from other therapies and the elements that must be delivered in order for the patient to be considered as being "adequately exposed" to CBT include

- Conducting functional analyses of substance use
- Providing individualized skills training in strategies such as recognizing and coping with craving, monitoring, challenging, and changing thoughts about substance use, problem-solving skills, planning for emergencies, recognizing seemingly irrelevant decisions, and refusal skills.
- Examining the patient's cognitive processes related to substance use
- Identifying and debriefing the past and future high-risk situations
- Encouraging and reviewing extrasession implementation of skills (homework)
- Practicing skills within sessions

Recommended Interventions

Interventions that are essential, but not necessarily unique to CBT include the following:

- Discussing, reviewing, reformulating the patient's goals for treatment
- Monitoring substance use and craving
- Monitoring general functioning
- Exploring positive and negative consequences of substance use

- Exploring the relationship between affect states and substance use
- Providing feedback on urinalysis results
- Setting a clear agenda for each session
- Making process comments as indicated
- Discussing the advantages of an abstinence goal and exploration of the patient's ambivalence
- Meeting resistance with exploration and a problem-solving approach
- Supporting patient efforts to institute behavior change, assessing the level of family support

Acceptable Interventions

Interventions that are not required or strongly recommended as part of CBT but are not incompatible with this approach include

- Being involved in self-help activities as a coping skill
- Identifying means of self-reinforcement for abstinence
- Exploring discrepancies between patient's stated goals and actions
- Eliciting concerns about substance use and consequences (e.g., decision balance)

Proscribed Interventions

Interventions that are proscribed because they are distinctive of other forms of empirically validated approaches to treatment include the following (note, however, that CBT can be combined effectively with other approaches):

- Extensive self-disclosure by the therapist
- Use of a confrontational style or a confrontation-of-denial approach
- Requiring the patient attend self-help groups (as in Twelve-Step Facilitation)
- Use of disease model language or slogans (as in Twelve-Step Facilitation)
- Extensive exploration of interpersonal aspects of substance use (as in interpersonal or supportive-dynamic approaches)
- Extensive discussion or interpretation of underlying conflicts or motives (as in supportive-dynamic approaches)
- Provision of direct reinforcement for abstinence (e.g., vouchers, tokens, as in contingency management [CM] approaches)

EVIDENCE OF EFFICACY

CBT has been shown to be effective across a wide range of substance use disorders (15–18), including alcohol dependence (19,20), marijuana dependence (21,22), cocaine dependence (23–26), and nicotine dependence (27–29). CBT has also been shown to be compatible with a number of other treatment approaches, including pharmacotherapy (30,31) and traditional counseling approaches (32) and thus can be implemented in a wide range of settings. These findings are consistent with evidence supporting the effectiveness of CBT across a number of other psychiatric disorders as well, including depression, anxiety disorders, and eating disorders.

CBT has been used with a range of substance use disorders for over 30 years. As our understanding of CBT has deepened over time, this series of studies has been marked by progressively larger effect sizes for CBT over comparison or control conditions. This is illustrated in our series of randomized controlled trials on CBT at Yale. In our first randomized trial, we conducted a direct comparison of CBT with another active therapy, Interpersonal Psychotherapy (IPT), adapted for cocaine users. In that trial, CBT was not found to have a main effect over IPT, but was found to be significantly more effective among the more severely dependent cocaine abusers (33), suggesting that the higher levels of structure and emphasis on skills may have been particularly helpful for the more severely impaired cocaine users.

Severity of cocaine dependence as a moderator of CBT effects was also replicated in our next study (23). This study used a 2 × 2 factorial design, where desipramine was compared with placebo and CBT compared to supportive Clinical Management, a supportive psychotherapy control condition. This study was also the first to describe that after the study treatments were terminated, those that had been assigned to CBT continued to reduce the frequency of their cocaine use throughout the 1-year follow-up (the "sleeper effect") (8). Evidence of continued improvement associated with CBT in turn led to increasing interest in mechanisms that might underlie this effect, with skill training and behavioral practice through homework assignments as prime candidates, as described in more detail in the sections below.

Thus, in our next study, which was the first to report a significant main effect for CBT over supportive Clinical Management and which replicated the "sleeper effect" for CBT over a 1-year follow-up (34), we also evaluated the acquisition of coping skills in CBT and their relationship to outcome in this population. We developed and validated a role-play task for assessing the acquisition of coping skills in CBT (35); the task involved the patient listening to a series of audiotaped high-risk situations (e.g., "what would you do if you found yourself at a party where you didn't think cocaine would be available, and then noticed a lot of people going in and out of a back room?" "What would you do if you started feeling really intense craving?"). The patient's responses were audiotaped and then rated for quality of response, type of coping response, and number of responses generated using a rating method demonstrated to be highly reliable. In this study, evaluation of the role play task demonstrated the following: (1) coping skills increased significantly after CBT, (2) patients demonstrated increases in coping skills that were parallel to those taught in the treatment they had been assigned (i.e., differential acquisition of specific behavioral and cognitive coping strategies in CBT with respect to alternate behavioral therapies), and finally, (3) greater acquisition of CBT-specific behavioral and cognitive coping skills was associated with significantly less cocaine use over the 1-year follow-up (34).

In our most recently completed trial (36), 121 cocaine-dependent individuals were randomized to one of four conditions in a 2 × 2 factorial design: disulfiram (250 mg/day) plus CBT, disulfiram plus IPT, placebo plus CBT, and placebo plus IPT. Across outcome measures and for the full intention-to-treat sample (as well as across all subsamples including treatment initiators and treatment completers), patients assigned to CBT reduced their cocaine use significantly more than those assigned to IPT, and patients assigned to disulfiram reduced their cocaine use significantly more than those assigned to placebo. Effects of CBT plus placebo were comparable to those of the CBT–disulfiram combination. This was our first trial to identify a significant main effect for CBT over another active behavioral therapy (IPT). Furthermore, although retention was a significant predictor of better drug use outcomes, the CBT by time effect remained statistically significant after controlling for retention. Thus, this series of trials has demonstrated increasingly strong effects for CBT over time and our follow-up studies have consistently indicated high durability of CBT compared to other approaches.

Another particularly exciting development in the field of drug dependence treatment has been the very strong empirical support for CM approaches, where participants receive incentives (i.e., vouchers redeemable for goods and services, chances to draw prizes from a bowl) contingent on demonstrating acquisition of treatment goals (e.g., submitting drug-free urine specimens, attending treatment sessions) (37). Given that CM has strong immediate effects but those effects tend to weaken after the contingencies are terminated, while CBT tends to have more modest effects initially but is comparatively durable, several investigators have begun to evaluate various combinations of CBT and CM, reasoning that the relative strengths and weaknesses of these may be offset by combining them. For example, Rawson and colleagues (9) recently compared group CBT, voucher CM, and a CBT/CM combination in conjunction with standard methadone maintenance treatment for cocaine-using methadone maintenance patients. During the acute phase of treatment, the groups assigned to CM had significantly better cocaine use outcomes than the group assigned to CBT. However, during the follow-up period, a CBT "sleeper" effect emerged again, where the group assigned to CBT essentially caught up to the CM groups by the 52-week follow-up (9). Similar results were found for a parallel study conducted among a large sample ($N = 171$) of stimulant-dependent individuals treated as outpatients (38), where CM was associated with better retention and substance use outcomes during treatment but outcomes for CBT and CM were comparable at 1 year.

Epstein and colleagues (39), conducted a similar study, again in the context of intensive methadone maintenance, where participants were offered CM, group CBT, or a combination of CM plus CBT, in addition to standard individual counseling. Results largely paralleled those found in the Rawson study, in that the investigators reported large initial effects for CM, with drop off after the termination of the contingencies, and the best 1-year outcomes for the CM + CBT combination.

OPTIMAL USE, CBT TECHNIQUES, AND STRATEGIES

At the most simple level, most CBT approaches attempt to help individual patients recognize the situations in which they are most likely to use, avoid those situations when appropriate, and cope more effectively with a range of problems and problematic behaviors associated with substance use by implementing a range of cognitive and behavioral coping strategies. Specific techniques vary widely with the type of cognitive behavioral treatment used, and there are a variety of manuals, protocols, and training programs available that describe the techniques associated with each approach (5,40–43).

As noted earlier, two key defining features of most cognitive behavioral approaches for substance use disorders are (a) an emphasis on a functional analysis of drug use, that is, understanding drug use with respect to its antecedents and consequences, and (b) an emphasis on skills training. Cognitive behavioral approaches include a range of skills to foster or maintain abstinence. These typically include strategies for (a) Understanding the patterns that maintain drug use and developing strategies for changing these patterns. This often involves self-monitoring of thoughts and behaviors that take place before, during, and after high-risk situations or episodes of drug use. (b) Fostering the resolution to stop substance use through exploring positive and negative consequences of continued use (also known as the decisional balance technique). (c) Understanding craving, craving cues, and the development of skills for coping with craving when it occurs. These include a variety of affect regulation strategies (distraction, talking through a craving, "urge surfing," and so on). (d) Recognizing and challenging the cognitions that accompany and maintain patterns of substance use. (e) Increasing awareness of the consequences of even small decisions (e.g., which route to take home from work), and the identification of "seemingly irrelevant" decisions that can culminate in high-risk situations. (f) Developing problem-solving skills, and practicing application of those skills to substance-related and more general problems. (g) Planning for emergencies and unexpected problems and situations that can lead to high-risk situations. (h) Developing skills for assertively refusing offers of drugs, as well as reducing exposure to drugs and drug-related cues.

These basic skills are useful in their application to helping patients control and stop substance use, but it is essential that therapists also point out how these same skills can be applied to a range of other problems. For example, use of a functional analysis can be used to understand the determinants of a wide range of behavior patterns, skills used to cope with craving can easily be applied to other aspects of affect control, the principles used in the sessions on seemingly irrelevant decisions can easily be adapted to understanding a wide range of behavior chains, and substance use refusal skills can easily be transferred to more effective and assertive responding in a number of situations. We think it is essential that, when therapists teach coping skills, they emphasize and demonstrate that the skills can be applied immediately to control substance use, but can also be used as general strategies that can be used across a wide range of situations and problems the patient may encounter in the future.

Broad-spectrum cognitive behavioral approaches, such as those described by Monti and colleagues (41) and adapted for use in Project MATCH (40), expand to include interventions directed to other problems in the individual's life that are seen as functionally related to substance use. These interventions may include general problem-solving skills, assertiveness training, strategies for coping with negative effect, awareness of anger and anger management, coping with criticism, increasing pleasant activities, enhancing social support networks, and job-seeking skills, among others.

In comparison to many other behavioral approaches, CBT is typically highly structured. That is, CBT is generally brief (12 to 24 weeks) and organized closely around well-specified treatment goals. Usually an articulated agenda exists for each session and the clinical discussion remains focused around issues directly related to substance use. Progress toward treatment goals is monitored closely and frequently, with frequent monitoring of substance use through urine toxicology screens, and the therapist takes an active stance throughout treatment. Generally, sessions take place within a weekly scheduled therapy "hour." In broad-spectrum cognitive behavioral approaches, sessions often are organized roughly in thirds (the 20/20/20 rule) (5), with the first third of the session devoted to the assessment of the patient's substance use and general functioning in the past week and report of current concerns and problems; the second third is more didactic and devoted to skills training and practice; and the final third allows time for therapist and patient to plan for the week ahead and discuss how new skills will be implemented (5). The therapeutic relationship is seen as principally collaborative. Thus, the role of the therapist is one of consultant, educator, and guide who can lead the patient through a functional analysis of his/her substance use, aid in identifying and prioritizing target behaviors, and consult in selecting and implementing strategies to foster the desired behavior changes.

While structured and didactic, CBT is a highly individualized and flexible treatment. That is, rather than viewing CBT treatment as cookbook "psychoeducation," the therapist carefully matches the content, timing, and nature of presentation of the material to the individual patient. The therapist attempts to provide skills training at the moments the patient is most in need of them. That is, the therapist does not belabor topics such as breaking ties with cocaine suppliers with a patient who is highly motivated and has been abstinent for several weeks. Similarly, the therapist does not race through material in an attempt to "cover" all of it in a few weeks; for some patients, it may take several weeks to master a basic skill.

Extrasession Practice as a Possible Mediator of CBT

In CBT, therapists encourage patients to practice new skills; such practice is a central and essential component of treatment. The degree to which the treatment is a "skills training" over merely a "skills exposure" approach has to do with the degree to which there is opportunity to practice and implement coping skills, making extrasession practice and homework all the more important. It is critical that patients have the opportunity to try out new skills within the supportive context of treatment. Through first-hand experience, patients can learn what new approaches work or do not work for them, where they have difficulty or problems, and so on. There are many opportunities for practice within CBT, both within sessions and outside of them. Within each session, there are opportunities for patients to rehearse and review ideas, raise concerns, and get feedback from the therapist.

As noted earlier, there has been growing interest in understanding not only what treatments work, but how they work. Understanding the mechanisms of action of CBT and other empirically validated therapies has heretofore received very little attention in the literature, but is an area of great importance. Understanding treatment mechanisms can not only advance the development of more effective treatment strategies, but also result in more powerful, efficient, and ultimately less-expensive treatments.

The converging evidence suggesting that CBT is a particularly durable approach has led to increased focus on unique or distinctive aspects of CBT that might account for its durability. Encouraging clients to implement and practice skills outside of sessions via homework assignments is one possible mechanism for this effect. Homework encourages practice of skills outside sessions and possibly generalization of skills to other problems, and emphasis on extrasession practice assignments is a unique feature of CBT (44). Moreover, investigators evaluating CBT in nonsubstance use psychiatric disorders have noted the importance of homework in CBT's effectiveness.

The relationship of homework compliance, skills acquisition, and outcome in CBT has received comparatively little attention in the substance abuse literature. Thus, in a recent trial for cocaine dependence treatment (45), we evaluated homework completion in detail, collecting data on the specific type of homework assigned and how well it was done (e.g., fully, partially, no attempt made) at every session. We found strong relationships between homework compliance and outcome. Compared with the participants assigned to CBT who did not do homework or who did it only rarely, the participants who did homework consistently *stayed in treatment significantly longer, had more consecutive days of cocaine abstinence* (a strong predictor of long-term outcome), and *fewer cocaine-positive urines during treatment*. Similar effects were found for the subset of participants who completed treatment in this study, suggesting that the effects of homework compliance on better substance use outcomes were not completely accounted for by differential retention. In addition, we found strong relationships between homework compliance and acquisition of coping skills, as well as between homework completion and participants' ratings of their confidence in avoiding use in a variety of high-risk situations. Participants who completed homework had significant increases over time in their self-reported confidence in handling a variety of high-risk situations, while scores for the subgroup that did not do homework did not change over time.

Farabee and colleagues (46) evaluated the extent to which cocaine users reported engaging in a series of specific drug-avoidance activities (e.g., avoiding drug-using friends and places where cocaine would be available, exercising, using thought-stopping) after CBT versus alternate treatments (e.g., CM and a control condition). They found that, by the end of treatment, participants assigned to CBT reported more frequent engagement in drug-avoidance activities than participants in the comparison treatments. Furthermore, the frequency of drug-avoidance activities was strongly related to better cocaine use outcomes over the 1-year follow-up. Taken together, these studies suggest that CBT interventions that foster the patients' engagement in active behavior change may play a key role in CBT's comparative durability.

SPECIAL CONSIDERATIONS

Training and Competence in CBT

The growing evidence base for CBT and the increased emphasis on incorporating empirically supported therapies into clinical practice has also led to greater focus on training and dissemination. Although standard methods used to train clinicians to use CBT in clinical efficacy trials have generally been associated with high levels of treatment fidelity and comparatively small levels of variation in treatment delivery, these methods (intensive didactic workshop training plus structured feedback on supervised training cases) had not been empirically evaluated, nor are they commonly used in training clinicians to use novel approaches (47).

A comparatively new development in dissemination and technology transfer is the application of rigorous clinical trials methodology to evaluate different methods of training clinicians to implement empirically validated therapies such as motivational interviewing and CBT. In one study (48), 78 clinicians were assigned to one of three training conditions: (1) review of the NIDA CBT manual only ("Manual Only") (5), (2) access to a web-based training site, which included additional frequently asked questions, role plays and practice exercises, plus the manual ("Web"), or (3) a 3-day didactic seminar plus up to three sessions of supervision from a CBT expert trainer based on actual session tapes submitted by the participants ("Seminars + Supervision"). Outcomes focused on clinician behavior and included (a) between-group comparisons of the clinicians' ability to demonstrate key CBT techniques based on structured role plays administered before and after training, and (b) scores on a CBT knowledge quiz. The videotaped role plays were scored by independent raters, blind to the participants' training condition as well as time (e.g., pre- vs. post training) and on an adherence/competence ratings of specific CBT techniques from the Yale Adherence and Competence Scale (YACs) (14).

Although all groups demonstrated improved adherence and competence scores over time, the only training condition that reached levels of skill consistent with those required of clinicians participating in our CBT efficacy trials was the Seminar + Supervision condition, with intermediate ratings for the Web condition. The mean effect size for the Seminar + Supervision versus Manual only condition comparisons was consistent with a large effect (0.69), while the average effect size for the Web versus Manual only condition contrasts was consistent with a medium size effect (0.30). In addition, the Seminar + Supervision condition was associated with significantly more clinicians reaching criterion levels for adequate fidelity than those assigned to the Manual only condition (54% vs. 15%).

These findings underscore that merely making manuals available to clinicians has little enduring effect on clinicians' ability to implement new treatments. This has important implications for current efforts to disseminate new treatments. These findings also suggest that face-to-face training followed by direct supervision and credentialing may be essential for effective technology transfer and raise questions regarding whether practitioners should feel competent (from an ethical perspective) to administer an empirically supported treatment on the basis of reading a manual alone. Finally, the findings suggest that standard strategies used to train clinicians in clinical trials can be effective for community-based clinicians and may be pursued as a strategy for future dissemination trials and bridging the gap between research and practice.

Addressing Limitations of CBT

Despite CBT's emerging empirical support, future research is needed to address its limitations. CBT is a relatively complex approach, in that it is comparatively complicated to train clinicians to use this approach or to implement it effectively in clinical practice. As a result, competent delivery of CBT has been shown to be very rare in clinical practice. Independent review of clinician audiotapes from the "treatment as usual" condition in a multisite trial supported by the NIDA Clinical Trials Network indicated that, although the clinicians professed using a high level of CBT in their clinical work, interventions associated with CBT (e.g., skill training, focus on cognitions) were extremely rare (49).

Another relative weakness of CBT may be the cognitive demands it places on patients, in that they are asked to learn a range of new concepts and skills, including to monitor and remember cognitions and inner states, implement new skills while in stressful situations, and so on. Recent data suggests that substance users with higher levels of cognitive impairment may have poorer outcome in CBT than those who are less impaired (50). This suggests that clinicians using CBT strategies should monitor the cognitive skills of their patients, and in cases where the patients may have memory, attention, or impulse control problems, to adapt the implementation of CBT accordingly, with slower progression through concepts, frequent repetition of material and checking back with the patient to assess understanding, and providing more structure on extrasession assignments.

Potential strategies for addressing these issues include greater emphasis on understanding CBT's mechanisms of action, so that ineffective components of CBT can be removed and treatment delivery simplified. A more novel strategy is to harness the ability and breadth of technology to standardize CBT and make it more widely available to those that may benefit from it. We have developed a computer-assisted version of CBT, called CBT4CBT (computer-based training in cognitive behavioral therapy). The content of CBT4CBT is based closely on our NIDA CBT manual (5), but it is delivered in six sessions, or modules, and makes extensive use of the multimedia capabilities of computers to convey CBT principles and illustrate implementation of new cognitive and behavioral strategies (51). That is, key CBT concepts are taught through short movies, or vignettes, which feature engaging characters in realistic settings confronting a number of challenging situations as well as a number of interactive games and exercises to teach CBT strategies. Thus, users are able to see multiple examples of how CBT principles can be implemented, rather than hear sometimes too abstract or incomplete presentations from their therapists.

In a clinical trial where CBT4CBT was delivered in addition to standard outpatient treatment, exposure to the program was associated with significantly fewer drug-positive urine specimens submitted and longer durations of abstinence during treatment (51). In addition, data from a 6-month follow-up indicated the durability of these effects in that the "sleeper effect" of CBT appeared to extend to its computer-based version (52), which appeared to have been mediated by significantly higher levels of skill acquisition among those who used the CBT4CBT program (53). Finally, participants' level of neuropsychological functioning did not appear to be associated with outcome in the CBT4CBT program, perhaps because little or no reading of text was required, users can control the rate of speed of material presented, can repeat material as often as they wish, and they can select the types of exercises and issues they would like to address, thereby reducing the "cognitive load" of CBT. Although CBT4CBT and other computer-assisted programs have great potential to make empirically supported therapies more widely available and to broaden the base of substance abuse treatment, and some of the early data on their effectiveness is very encouraging, substantially more testing and evaluation is needed before they can be widely distributed.

SUMMARY

CBT is a behavioral approach that has strong theoretical and empirical support with a variety of substance abusing populations, as well as a broad range of disorders that tend to co-occur with addiction, including depressive and anxiety disorders. Moreover, these approaches can be combined and integrated effectively with a range of other empirically supported behavioral therapies as well as pharmacotherapies. CBT also appears to be particularly durable, an important feature among the addictions, which are characterized by frequent relapse. In recent years, clinical researchers have recently emphasized moving these approaches more broadly into the clinical community, and thus a range of practical resources (e.g., books, videotapes, manuals, training resources, and programs) for implementing them effectively in clinical practice are available, and data from recent trials evaluating computer-assisted version of CBT have been promising. Thus, due to its comparatively strong evidence base, flexibility, broad applicability across a range of patient types and settings, and durability, CBT should be a component of all substance abuse clinicians' repertoire.

ACKNOWLEDGMENT

Support was provided by NIDA grants P50 DA09241, U10 DA13038, R37 DA15969, and K05-DA00457.

REFERENCES

1. Craighead WE, Craighead LW, Ilardi SS. Behavioral therapies in historical perspective. In: Bongar BM, Beutler LE, eds. *Comprehensive Textbook of Psychotherapy: Theory and Practice.* New York, NY: Oxford University Press; 1995:64–83.
2. Rotgers F. Behavioral theory of substance abuse treatment: bringing science to bear on practice. In: Rotgers F, Keller DS, Morgenstern J, eds. *Treating Substance Abusers: Theory and Technique.* New York, NY: Guilford Press; 1996:174–201.
3. Wikler A. Dynamics of drug dependence: implications of a conditioning theory for research and treatment. *Arch Gen Psychiatry.* 1973;28:611–616.
4. Meichenbaum DH. Cognitive-behavioral therapy in historical perspective. In: Bongar BM, Beutler LE, eds. *Comprehensive Textbook of Psychotherapy: Theory and Practice.* New York, NY: Oxford University Press; 1995:140–158.
5. Carroll KM. *A Cognitive-Behavioral Approach: Treating Cocaine Addiction.* Rockville, MD: NIDA; 1998.
6. McLellan AT, Lewis DC, O'Brien CP, et al. Drug dependence, a chronic medical illness: implications for treatment, insurance, and outcomes evaluation. *JAMA.* 2000;284:1689–1695.
7. Donovan DM, Anton RF, Miller WR, et al. Combined pharmacotherapies and behavioral interventions for alcohol dependence (The COMBINE Study): examination of posttreatment drinking outcomes. *J Studies Alcohol Drugs.* 2008;69:5–13.
8. Carroll KM, Rounsaville BJ, Nich C, et al. One year follow-up of psychotherapy and pharmacotherapy for cocaine dependence: delayed emergence of psychotherapy effects. *Arch Gen Psychiatry.* 1994;51:989–997.
9. Rawson RA, Huber A, McCann MJ, et al. A comparison of contingency management and cognitive-behavioral approaches during methadone maintenance for cocaine dependence. *Arch Gen Psychiatry.* 2002;59:817–824.
10. Hollon SD. Does cognitive therapy have an enduring effect? *Cognit Ther Res.* 2003;27:71–75.

11. Castonguay LG, Goldfried MR, Wiser S, et al. Predicting the effect of cognitive therapy for depression: a study of unique and common factors. *J Consult Clin Psychol.* 1996;64:497–504.
12. Horvath AO, Symonds BD. Relation between working alliance and outcome in psychotherapy: a meta-analysis. *J Couns Psychol.* 1991;38:139–149.
13. Waltz J, Addis ME, Koerner K, et al. Testing the integrity of a psychotherapy protocol: assessment of adherence and competence. *J Consult Clin Psychol.* 1993;61:620–630.
14. Carroll KM, Nich C, Sifry R, et al. A general system for evaluating therapist adherence and competence in psychotherapy research in the addictions. *Drug Alcohol Depend.* 2000;57:225–238.
15. Dutra L, Stathopoulou G, Basden SL, et al. A meta-analytic review of psychosocial interventions for substance use disorders. *Am J Psychiatry.* 2008;165:179–187.
16. Carroll KM. Relapse prevention as a psychosocial treatment approach: a review of controlled clinical trials. *Exp Clin Psychopharmacol.* 1996;4:46–54.
17. Irvin JE, Bowers CA, Dunn ME, et al. Efficacy of relapse prevention: a meta-analytic review. *J Consult Clin Psychol.* 1999;67:563–570.
18. Magill M, Ray LA. Cognitive-behavioral treatment with adult alcohol and illicit drug users: a meta-analysis of randomized controlled trials. *J Stud Alcohol Drugs.* 2009;70:516–527.
19. Morgenstern J, Longabaugh R. Cognitive-behavioral treatment for alcohol dependence: a review of the evidence for its hypothesized mechanisms of action. *Addiction.* 2000;95:1475–1490.
20. Miller WR, Wilbourne PL. Mesa Grande: a methodological analysis of clinical trials of treatments for alcohol use disorders. *Addiction.* 2002;97:265–277.
21. MTP Research Group. Treating cannabis dependence: findings from a multisite study. *J Consult Clin Psychol.* 2004;72:455–466.
22. Stephens RS, Roffman RA, Curtin L. Comparison of extended versus brief treatments for marijuana use. *J Consult Clin Psychol.* 2000;68:898–908.
23. Carroll KM, Rounsaville BJ, Gordon LT, et al. Psychotherapy and pharmacotherapy for ambulatory cocaine abusers. *Arch Gen Psychiatry.* 1994;51:177–197.
24. Carroll KM, Nich C, Ball SA, et al. Treatment of cocaine and alcohol dependence with psychotherapy and disulfiram. *Addiction.* 1998;93:713–728.
25. McKay JR, Alterman AI, Cacciola JS, et al. Group counseling versus individualized relapse prevention aftercare following intensive outpatient treatment for cocaine dependence. *J Consult Clin Psychol.* 1997;65:778–788.
26. Rohsenow DJ, Monti PM, Martin RA, et al. Brief coping skills treatment for cocaine abuse: 12-month substance use outcomes. *J Consult Clin Psychol.* 2000;68:515–520.
27. Fiore MC, Smith SS, Jorenberg DE, et al. The effectiveness of the nicotine patch for smoking cessation: a meta-analysis. *JAMA.* 1994;271:1940–1947.
28. Hall SM, Reus VI, Munoz RF, et al. Nortripyline and cognitive-behavioral therapy in the treatment of cigarette smoking. *Arch Gen Psychiatry.* 1998;55:683–690.
29. Patten CA, Martin JE, Myers MG, et al. Effectiveness of cognitive-behavioral therapy for smokers with histories of alcohol dependence and depression. *J Stud Alcohol.* 1998;59:327–335.
30. Anton RF, Moak DH, Waid LR, et al. Naltrexone and cognitive-behavioral therapy for the treatment of outpatient alcoholics: results of a placebo-controlled trial. *Am J Psychiatry.* 1999;156:1758–1764.
31. O'Malley SS, Jaffe AJ, Chang G, et al. Naltrexone and coping skills therapy for alcohol dependence: a controlled study. *Arch Gen Psychiatry.* 1992;49:881–887.
32. Morgenstern J, Morgan TJ, McCrady BS, et al. Manual-guided cognitive behavioral therapy training: a promising method for disseminating empirically supported substance abuse treatments to the practice community. *Psychol Addict Behav.* 2001;15:83–88.
33. Carroll KM, Rounsaville BJ, Gawin FH. A comparative trial of psychotherapies for ambulatory cocaine abusers: relapse prevention and interpersonal psychotherapy. *Am J Drug Alcohol Abuse.* 1991;17:229–247.
34. Carroll KM, Nich C, Ball SA, et al. One year follow-up of disulfiram and psychotherapy for cocaine-alcohol abusers: sustained effects of treatment. *Addiction.* 2000;95:1335–1349.
35. Carroll KM, Nich C, Frankforter TL, et al. Do patients change in the way we intend? Treatment-specific skill acquisition in cocaine-dependent patients using the Cocaine Risk Response Test. *Psychol Assess.* 1999;11:77–85.
36. Carroll KM, Fenton LR, Ball SA, et al. Efficacy of disulfiram and cognitive-behavioral therapy in cocaine-dependent outpatients: a randomized placebo controlled trial. *Arch Gen Psychiatry.* 2004;64:264–272.
37. Higgins ST, Silverman K. *Motivating Behavior Change Among Illicit-Drug Abusers.* Washington, D.C.: American Psychological Association; 1999.
38. Rawson RA, McCann MJ, Flammino F, et al. A comparison of contingency management and cognitive-behavioral approaches for stimulant-dependent individuals. *Addiction.* 2006;101:267–274.
39. Epstein DE, Hawkins WE, Covi L, et al. Cognitive behavioral therapy plus contingency management for cocaine use: findings during treatment and across 12-month follow-up. *Psychol Addict Behav.* 2003;17:73–82.
40. Kadden R, Carroll KM, Donovan D, et al. *Cognitive-Behavioral Coping Skills Therapy Manual: A Clinical Research Guide for Therapists Treating Individuals with Alcohol Abuse and Dependence.* Rockville, MD: NIAAA; 1992.
41. Monti PM, Rohsenow DJ, Abrams DB, et al. *Treating Alcohol Dependence: A Coping Skills Training Guide in the Treatment of Alcoholism.* New York, NY: Guilford Press; 1989.
42. Marlatt GA, Gordon JR. *Relapse Prevention: Maintenance Strategies in the Treatment of Addictive Behaviors.* New York, NY: Guilford; 1985.
43. Annis HM, Davis CS. Relapse prevention. In: Hester RK, Miller WR, eds. *Handbook of Alcoholism Treatment Approaches.* New York, NY: Pergamon Press; 1989;170–182.
44. Kazantzis N, Deane FP, Ronan KR. Homework assignments in cognitive and behavioral therapy: a meta-analysis. *Clin Psychol Sci Pract.* 2000;7:189–202.
45. Carroll KM, Nich C, Ball SA. Practice makes progress: homework assignments and outcome in the treatment of cocaine dependence. *J Consult Clin Psychol.* 2005;73:749–755. PMCID: PMC2365906.
46. Farabee D, Rawson RA, McCann MJ. Adoption of drug avoidance strategies among patients in contingency management and cognitive-behavioral treatments. *J Subst Abuse Treat.* 2002;23:343–350.
47. Weissman MM, Verdeli H, Gameroff MJ, et al. National survey of psychotherapy training in psychiatry, psychology, and social work. *Arch Gen Psychiatry.* 2006;63:925–934.

48. Sholomskas D, Syracuse G, Ball SA, et al. We don't train in vain: a dissemination trial of three strategies for training clinicians in cognitive behavioral therapy. *J Consult Clin. Psychol.* 2005;73:106–115. PMCID: PMC2367057.
49. Santa Ana E, Martino S, Ball SA, et al. What is usual about 'treatment as usual': audiotaped ratings of standard treatment in the Clinical Trials Network. *J Subst Abuse Treat.* 2008;35:369–379. PMCID: PMC2712113.
50. Aharonovich E, Hasin DS, Brooks AC, et al. Cognitive deficits predict low treatment retention in cocaine dependent patients. *Drug Alcohol Depend.* 2006;81:313–322.
51. Carroll KM, Ball SA, Martino S, et al. Computer-assisted cognitive-behavioral therapy for addiction. A randomized clinical trial of 'CBT4CBT'. *Am J Psychiatry.* 2008;165:881–888. PMCID: PMC2562873.
52. Carroll KM, Ball SA, Martino S, et al. Enduring effects of a computer-assisted training program for cognitive-behavioral therapy: a six-month follow-up of CBT4CBT. *Drug Alcohol Depend.* 2009;100:178–181. PMCID: PMC2742309.
53. Kiluk BD, Nich C, Babuscio TA, et al. Quantity versus quality: acquisition of coping skills in computer-assisted cognitive behavioral therapy for substance abuse. *Addiction*, in press.

CHAPTER 45

Contingency Management in the Treatment of Substance Use Disorders: Trends in the Literature

Stephen T. Higgins ■ Stacey C. Sigmon ■ Sarah H. Heil

Substance use disorders (SUDs) are highly prevalent in the United States, as they are in virtually all other developed countries, and tremendously costly both economically as well as in terms of personal loss. While there has been a great deal of progress in developing evidence-based treatments for SUDs, there is no question that new and more effective interventions are needed. One widely recognized need is for interventions that are explicitly designed to increase the likelihood of initiating and sustaining behavior change over time, that is, interventions to combat the waxing and waning of commitment or motivation over time that is a hallmark of SUDs. The focus of this chapter is on contingency management (CM), a treatment approach that is particularly well suited to that task.

CM interventions involve the systematic application of reinforcing or punishing consequences to promote and sustain behavior change (1). When used in the treatment of SUDs, CM interventions are usually focused on increasing abstinence from drug use, but also can address areas such as increasing clinic attendance, adherence to medication, and other therapeutic regimens. Investigators have been exploring the use of CM interventions for treatment of SUDs since the 1960s, but there has been tremendous growth in this area of investigation in the past two decades. That growth is illustrated in Figure 45.1, which shows the cumulative number of yearly citations on the topic of SUDs identified through a PubMed search of the term contingency management. The level of growth is striking and as will be characterized below associated with a high degree of efficacy across different types of SUDs, special populations, and therapeutic targets.

There are sound scientific rationales for the use of CM in treating SUDs. CM is based on the principles of operant conditioning, that is, the study of how environmental consequences alter the future probability of voluntary behavior. Behavior that is followed by reinforcing consequences increases in future probability while behavior that is followed by punishing consequences decreases. There is overwhelming scientific evidence that drug use, including drug use by those with SUDs, conforms to the principles of operant conditioning (2). Additionally, an emerging area of behavioral economic research on delay discounting documents that individuals with SUDs exhibit a greater discounting of the value of temporally delayed reinforcement than do matched controls without SUDs (3). Considering that most of the naturalistic reinforcement for discontinuing drug use (improved physical health, family life, employment) are delayed in time while those derived from drug use are relatively immediate, it makes sense that systematically providing substitute reinforcement contingent on therapeutic progress as is done in CM might be helpful in bridging the temporal gap between discontinuing drug use and reaping naturalistic rewards for doing so (2). Moreover, chronic drug use can directly diminish frontal lobe cortical functions (executive functions) that underpin effective goal-directed behavior across time and one's ability to focus on longer-term outcomes. Such diminished frontal lobe functioning quite plausibly leaves individuals with SUDs more vulnerable to the mesolimbic-based, relatively immediate reinforcement that drug use represents (3). CM appeals to that same mesolimbic brain reward system to promote recovery from SUDs—that is, CM uses the same processes that drive addiction, but to promote recovery. A final rationale is that in addition to increasing activity in mesolimbic brain areas, response-contingent incentives increase activity in brain regions associated with top-down cortical functions underpinning attention, error monitoring, and other executive functions that are important to successful long-term goal seeking (4,5) and are often diminished among those with SUDs (6).

VOUCHER-BASED CONTINGENCY MANAGEMENT

This chapter is focused on voucher-based CM, which is the most thoroughly researched form of CM used in the treatment of SUDs (1). With this approach, patients earn vouchers exchangeable for retail items, or a comparable monetary-based consequence, contingent on meeting therapeutic goals—usually abstinence from drug use, but sometimes attendance at therapy sessions or compliance with medication regimens. Interventions involving vouchers exchangeable for backup prizes (7) or where cash payments were used (8) are included as part of the voucher-based literature in this chapter.

Basic Elements of Voucher-Based CM

Behavioral Principles and Core Procedures

In this section, we review some basic elements of implementing an effective CM intervention. All CM interventions involve the systematic use of the basic behavioral science

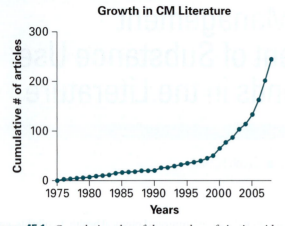

Figure 45.1. Cumulative plot of the number of citations identified in a PubMed search of the term "contingency management" involving substance use disorders (SUDs). The search included all citations through October of 2009.

principles of positive or negative reinforcement and positive or negative punishment. Voucher-based CM emphasizes positive reinforcement involving the delivery of a reinforcing stimulus (e.g., voucher) contingent on the occurrence of a therapeutic goal. The other principle used in voucher-based CM is negative punishment, which involves the removal of a reinforcing stimulus (e.g., special privileges) contingent on the occurrence of an undesirable response. As is outlined further below, this punishment component of voucher-based CM is in the form of a reset contingency wherein the value of vouchers that can be earned is reduced contingent upon evidence of recent drug use or failure to attend a scheduled test to confirm compliance with the contingency. In summary, then, voucher-based CM relies largely on systematic and frequent use of positive reinforcement and a modest use of negative punishment to increase abstinence, deter relapse, and to encourage compliance with scheduled assessments and other therapeutic targets.

Effective voucher-based CM interventions usually include the following features: (1) a well-articulated contract, in writing when possible, to stipulate what behavior change is expected of the patient, what the consequences will be when the behavior change does and does not occur, and the start and stop dates of the intervention; (2) an operationally defined therapeutic target that allows for independent observer agreement on the occurrence or nonoccurrence of the target; (3) use an objective means of verifying occurrence of the target behavior whenever possible; (4) a well-specified schedule for monitoring compliance with the contract; (5) a schedule that includes frequent opportunities for the patient to interact with and learn from the reinforcement contingencies; (6) a minimal number of behaviors that are simultaneously being targeted for change; (7) short temporal delays between verifying compliance with the therapeutic target and delivering the programmed consequences; (8) a consequence of sufficient magnitude, intensity, or value to function as an effective reinforcer. Importantly, the last two points (delay in delivering consequences and magnitude/intensity/value of the consequence) are fundamental to effective use of reinforcement and were demonstrated to be statistically significant moderators of treatment effect size in our prior meta-analysis on voucher-based CM (9).

An Exemplar of Voucher-Based CM: Smoking Cessation in Pregnant Women

To provide a concrete example of an effective voucher-based CM program, in this section we describe the intervention and related results from a study on smoking cessation among pregnant women (10). This study was selected to serve as the exemplar because the voucher program used is relatively prototypical and the results achieved provide an excellent example of the substantial improvements in outcomes that can be achieved through effective use of the voucher-based CM approach.

Participants in this study were 82 women who were still smoking upon entering prenatal care. They were randomly assigned to an abstinence-contingent voucher condition wherein vouchers exchangeable for retail items were earned contingent on biochemically verified abstinence from recent smoking or to a noncontingent control condition wherein vouchers were delivered independent of smoking status. The details of the voucher conditions were described in the written consent form, which was supplemented by discussion with staff upon treatment assignment, and all study participants had to pass a brief written quiz designed to document understanding of the voucher contingencies before commencing with treatment. In addition to the vouchers, women received whatever was usual care for smoking cessation through their obstetric providers.

Women began their cessation effort on a Monday and reported to the clinic daily for 5 consecutive days for abstinence monitoring. The frequency of abstinence monitoring decreased to twice weekly in week 2 where it remained for the next 7 weeks, then decreased to once weekly for 4 weeks, and then to every other week until delivery. This schedule provided ample opportunity for frequent reinforcement of abstinence. During the postpartum period, abstinence monitoring was increased to once weekly again for 4 weeks related to the increased risk of relapse postpartum, and then decreased to every other week through 12 weeks postpartum at which point the voucher program was discontinued. Voucher values in the abstinence-contingent condition began at $6.25 for a negative test on the first day of the cessation effort and escalated by $1.25 for each consecutive negative specimen up to a maximum of $45.00 where it remained through the remainder of the intervention save for positive results or a missed visit. These values were tested in an earlier pilot trial and shown to be effective (11). Positive test results or failure to provide a scheduled specimen reset the value of vouchers back to their initial low level, but two consecutive negative tests restored the voucher value to the pre-reset level consistent with the punishment component noted above. If a woman abstained completely throughout the antepartum and postpartum periods, she could earn approximately $1150 in purchasing power; mean voucher earnings in this condition was $461 ± 456. Women in the noncontingent-voucher condition received vouchers independent of smoking status and at values of $15.00 per visit antepartum and $20.00 per visit postpartum, which were estimated based on our earlier pilot study to be comparable to average earnings in the contingent condition. Mean voucher amount provided to women in the noncontingent condition was $413 ± 163, which did not differ significantly from earnings in the contingent condition. Smoking status was biochemically verified based on breath CO specimens ≤6 ppm during the initial 5 days of the intervention and urine cotinine (≤80 ng/mL) from week 2 through the remainder of the study. Because of cotinine's relatively long half-life, it cannot be used to verify smoking status in the initial days of the quit attempt. Two ultrasound examinations were performed at approximately 30- and 34-weeks gestation for the purpose of estimating fetal growth.

Biochemically verified 7-day point-prevalence abstinence was significantly greater among women in the contingent- compared to the noncontingent-voucher conditions at the end-of-pregnancy assessment (41% vs. 10%) and 12-week postpartum assessments (24% vs. 3%) (Fig. 45.2). Mean weeks of continuous abstinence during the antepartum period was also significantly greater in the contingent- than the noncontingent-voucher conditions, with those in the former achieving 9.7 ± 1.9 weeks compared to 2.0 ± 0.8 weeks among those in the latter. Additionally, a significantly greater percentage of women assigned to the contingent- than the noncontingent-voucher conditions sustained abstinence through the third trimester (27% vs. 3%), which is the trimester where fetal growth appears to be especially impacted by maternal smoking. Treatment effects were no longer significant at the 24-week assessment (8% vs. 3%) in this trial whereas they had been in the prior trial (27% vs. 0%). Collapsing across trials, a treatment effect is discernible at the 24-week assessment (16% vs. 2%), but that should be confirmed in future trials that are better powered to estimate treatment effects after the intervention is discontinued.

Ultrasound assessments of treatment effects on fetal growth showed there was a significantly greater increase in estimated fetal weight in the contingent compared to the noncontingent treatment conditions (Fig. 45.3, top panel). In addition, estimated growth rates for two of the three individual parameters used to compute fetal weight (fetal femur length, fetal abdominal circumference) were significantly greater in the contingent than the noncontingent conditions (Fig. 45.2, bottom panels). We consider these fetal-growth effects to provide important physical evidence of the substantive contributions that CM can make to improving treatment outcomes among pregnant women with SUDs.

Overall, the increases in abstinence and fetal growth observed in this trial are quite promising. This work is being followed-up with further scientific efforts to improve outcomes with pregnant smokers and with plans to extend the approach into community practice.

Reviewing the Literature

Our group previously published a meta-analysis on voucher-based CM (9). That review covered the years 1991 to 2004, with March 2004 representing the last publication month from which studies were included. In this section, we provide a review of the voucher-based CM literature picking up where the earlier review left off, while omitting the one published report from 2004 that was included in the prior review (12). The review for the present chapter ends in October 2009, related to meeting the chapter submission deadline for this edited volume.

We included studies that met the following criteria: (a) involved contingent vouchers or a related monetary-based CM intervention, (b) published in a peer-reviewed journal, (c) included an experimental comparison condition, (d) used a research design wherein treatment effects attributable to CM could be dissociated from other aspects of treatment, and (e) was an original prospective, experimental study that reported previously unpublished data (i.e., not retrospective or a subset of a previously published study). There are three differences between these inclusion criteria and those used in the prior review that merit mention. First, in the prior review studies were excluded if they were not conducted with individuals seeking or enrolled in treatment for SUDs. We have elected not to use that inclusion criterion in the present study as excluding individuals who are not in treatment excludes the vast majority of individuals with SUDs and because CM interventions can be used effectively to alter drug use in nonclinical settings. Second, we previously excluded studies involving fewer than

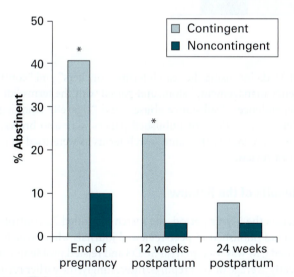

Figure 45.2. Point-prevalence abstinence at the end of pregnancy, 12, and 24 weeks postpartum. Women in the contingent condition ($n = 37$) received voucher-based CM contingent on biochemically verified smoking abstinence, and those in the noncontingent condition ($n = 40$) received vouchers independent of smoking status. *Indicates a significant difference between conditions ($p < 0.05$). (Reprinted with permission from Heil SH, Higgins ST, Bernstein IM, et al. Effects of voucher-based incentives on abstinence from cigarette smoking and fetal growth among pregnant women. *Addiction.* 2008;103:1009–1018.)

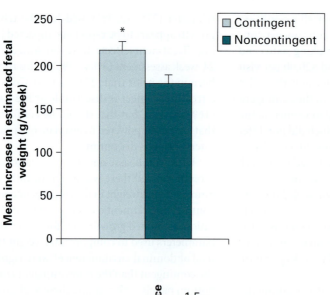
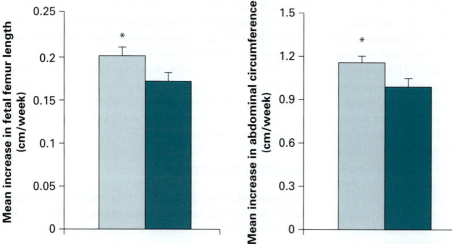

Figure 45.3. Mean (±SEM) rates of growth in estimated fetal weight (**top panel**), fetal femur length (**bottom left panel**), and fetal abdominal circumference (**bottom right panel**) between ultrasound assessments conducted during the third trimester. See Figure 45.1 for description of conditions. *Indicates a significant difference between conditions ($p < 0.05$). (Reprinted with permission from Heil SH, Higgins ST, Bernstein IM, et al. Effects of voucher-based incentives on abstinence from cigarette smoking and fetal growth among pregnant women. *Addiction*. 2008;103:1009–1018.)

10 subjects. While studies involving small sample sizes can be misleading when estimating effect size, which was the main purpose of the prior review, specifying a minimal number of subjects is arbitrary. Instead, we now include studies that met the other inclusion criteria independent of sample size as long as they included inferential statistics so that all studies had a common criterion for supporting inferences about treatment efficacy. Third, the present review does not attempt a quantitative review as was done in the meta-analysis, although descriptive summaries of the proportion of trials reporting statistically significant treatment effects of the voucher intervention are reported. Time and other resource limitations precluded us from conducting another meta-analysis. We required use of a no-voucher or noncontingent-voucher control condition for inclusion in the meta-analysis related to our goal of accurately estimating effect size of the contingent voucher condition, but that criterion was omitted for the present review. We still required inclusion of an experimental comparison condition, but it could be in the form of an alternative type or intensity of treatment.

The literature search for the present review was conducted using PubMed, the search engine of the U.S. National Library of Medicine, using the search terms "vouchers" and "contingency management," alone and paired with the terms "drug dependence," "substance abuse," and "cigarette smoking." Reference sections of published papers were also browsed. These are largely the same search terms as were used in our prior review.

Results of the Review

Across the 5-year period, the search identified 72 controlled studies published in peer-reviewed journals where voucher-based CM was used to treat SUDS and related problems for a yearly average of 14.4 reports. Interestingly, the earlier review covering 13.25 years identified 55 controlled studies or 4.2 reports/year. This more than threefold increase in reports/year on voucher-based CM is consistent with the striking growth in this area of treatment outcome research noted above and illustrated in Figure 45.1. Five of these reports were excluded from further consideration due to failure to meet inclusion criteria, leaving 67 reports that satisfied inclusion criteria.

Consistent with the prior review, the vast majority of studies (50 reports or 75%) focused on increasing abstinence from drug use. The remaining studies fall into two categories, (1) those examining either the efficacy of a contingency requiring abstinence from drug use and other therapeutic goals or comparing contingencies on abstinence to those on other therapeutic goals (10 reports or 15%) and (2) another set of reports examining the efficacy of contingencies on other therapeutic goals including adherence to medication regimens, retention in community SUDs treatment, and attendance at work therapy (7 reports or 10%). Also consistent with our prior review is the overwhelming degree of support for efficacy. Statistically significant treatment effects of CM were reported in 88% (59/67) of the reports reviewed, with that breaking down further to 90% (45/50) among studies focused on abstinence only, 70% (7/10) among studies targeting abstinence and other behaviors or comparing those two approaches, and 100% (7/7) among studies targeting medication compliance, treatment retention, and attendance at work therapy. The somewhat lower level of success in studies targeting behavior change for multiple targets simultaneously compared to more focused targets is also consistent with prior CM reviews (9).

Trends in the Recent Literature

In this section, we have organized the studies into what we deem to be seven trends discernible in approximately 5 years of the voucher-based CM literature covered by this review. While studies are often of relevance to more than one trend, we assigned each report to a primary trend. The trends identified were (a) extending the intervention to additional SUDs, (b) treatment of special populations, (c) extending use into community settings, (d) improving longer-term outcomes, (e) combining the intervention with pharmacotherapies, (f) investigating various parametric questions, and (g) using the intervention as a research tool rather than treatment intervention per se. Each of the 67 studies included in the review was assigned to one of those seven trends, with each of the trends including a specific table (Tables 45.1 to 45.7) listing key characteristics from each of the studies included under that trend. We comment briefly on each of the trends below. It merits mention that additional studies are cited in the text and reference section below because of their relevance to a point of discussion, but unless they are also listed in one of the tables they were not among the 67 studies included in the review.

Extending the Intervention to Additional Substance Use Disorders

While once the major trend in this area of investigation, extension of voucher-based CM to new types of SUDs is only a small part of current research efforts (see Table 45.1). In the present review only two examples of this type of research were identified. One involved trials further establishing the efficacy of voucher-based CM in the treatment of marijuana dependence and the other extending its efficacy to treatment of methamphetamine dependence. Three excellent controlled trials added support to other trials already in the literature on the efficacy of voucher-based CM for increasing abstinence in marijuana-dependent individuals (13–15). Evidence on the efficacy of voucher-based CM in treating methamphetamine dependence surfaced initially in trials among mixed samples of cocaine- and methamphetamine-dependent patients. A controlled trial by Rawson et al. (16) showing the efficacy of

TABLE 45.1 Extending the intervention to additional SUDs

Study	n	Setting	Voucher duration (weeks)	Maximum voucher earnings	Voucher delivery	Statistically significant treatment effect?	Voucher target(s)
Budney et al. (13)	90	DF	12	$570.00	I	Y	Marijuana use
Carroll et al. (14)	136	DF	8	$540.00	I	Y	Marijuana use
				$340.00	I	Y	Counseling attendance
Kadden et al. (15)	240	DF	7	$385.00	I	Y	Marijuana use
Rawson et al. (16)	171	DF	16	$988.75	I	Y	Cocaine + methamphetamine use

Note: Numbers next to each citation refer to its position in the reference section; *n*, sample size, all groups combined; setting, setting in which study occurred; DF, drug-free clinic; M, medication clinic; MM, methadone maintenance; NTS, not a treatment setting; voucher duration (weeks), number of weeks that voucher intervention was in place; maximum voucher earnings, total possible voucher earning across duration of the intervention; statistically significant treatment effect, presence or absence of significant treatment effect at $p < 0.05$; voucher target, the target of the voucher intervention. Voucher delivery: I, immediate (at the same visit the reinforcement was earned); D, delayed (at a visit after the reinforcement was earned).

CM alone and in combination with cognitive–behavior therapy for increasing abstinence and retention in these "stimulant-dependent" samples among patients enrolled in methadone therapy is an excellent example. Included in the section below on extending voucher-based CM to community clinic settings are two multisite trials that also support the efficacy of CM in treating these mixed samples of cocaine- and methamphetamine-dependent patients (17,18).

Extending the Intervention to Special Populations

The use of voucher-based CM to treat SUDs in special populations is a trend that was discernible in the prior review and that continues to gain momentum in the period covered by the present review (Table 45.2). For example, nine reports in the present review described results from studies testing the efficacy of voucher-based CM for smoking cessation in special populations, including adolescents (19), college students (20–22), pregnant women (10,11), and individuals enrolled in treatment for other SUDs (23,24), and one with individuals residing in rural areas isolated from usual smoking-cessation services (25). All reported significant treatment effects although all but the Heil et al. (10) trial in pregnant women were relatively preliminary investigations.

Another special population with whom voucher-based CM has promise is the dually diagnosed, with four studies on that topic identified in this review and all reporting significant treatment effects (26–29). Two of the studies supported the feasibility of using contingent vouchers to promote abstinence from cocaine and alcohol (26) and marijuana (29) in the dually diagnosed population while the two other studies (27,28) represented a more thorough investigation of the efficacy of contingent vouchers for promoting abstinence and job seeking among veterans enrolled in compensated work therapy. Considering that compensated work therapy programs operate in Veterans Hospitals located throughout the United States, they service large numbers of veterans suffering with SUDs and other psychiatric disorders, and improvements in the program are needed, this appears to be a promising area where voucher-based CM could make a substantive contribution.

Other studies in special populations identified in the review further supported a well-established application of contingent vouchers to increase participation in vocational training among chronically unemployed, intravenous drug abusers (30,31). Two randomized clinical trials were identified supporting the efficacy of contingent vouchers for increasing adherence with antiretroviral medications in HIV-positive illicit drug-dependent individuals while the incentives were in place, although effects dissipated following termination of the intervention (32,33). The studies on vocational training are part of the programmatic research effort by Silverman and colleagues on the use of abstinence-contingent work therapy as a form of maintenance therapy discussed above. The studies on adherence with antiretroviral medications suggest that some form of contingent-vouchers maintenance therapy may be an important future direction to investigate with that population as well. Lastly, the present review identified one study supporting the efficacy of voucher-based CM for improving outpatient retention of pregnant illicit drug abusers (34), but this is an area of investigation ripe for further development.

Extending the Intervention into Community Clinics

An important research effort has been on moving voucher-based CM from university-based research clinics into community clinics. That effort is succeeding on multiple fronts that were discernible in the present literature review (Table 45.3). One direction in this effort has been led by Petry and colleagues using an adaptation of the original voucher-based CM intervention that amounts to using lower-value incentives. In at least six controlled studies that were identified in the present review, the intervention was shown to increase abstinence and/or clinic attendance/treatment retention among illicit drug abusers enrolled in community clinics, including the two multisite trials noted above (7,17,18,35–37). This research effort is important because with lower-value incentives community clinics operating on limited budgets are likely to be more open to adopting this evidence-based intervention. Important to keep in mind, though, and often misunderstood, is that there is overwhelming evidence that the size of the treatment effect obtained with voucher-based CM decreases as the value of the incentives decreases, and there is no evidence that Petry and colleagues have surmounted that obstacle. They have shown that one can use lower-value incentives than are typically used in conventional voucher arrangements and still improve outcomes in community clinics, which is important. What they have not shown empirically is that their adaptation of the original schedule arrangement has any influence on outcome or that they can obtain larger treatment effects at lower costs compared to prototypical voucher programs. Indeed, in two trials conducted by Petry and colleagues (37,44) where their arrangement was compared to a prototypical voucher arrangement using comparable incentive values, there were no significant differences between the two arrangements in treatment outcomes.

Sometimes overlooked but quite impressive are successful efforts by other investigators to use lower value CM programs in community clinics (38,39). Again, there is no evidence to suggest that these investigators have devised a method for producing treatment effect sizes comparable to those achieved at higher voucher values but at a more affordable cost, but, rather, they are showing that costs can be lowered to more affordable levels and still retain significant benefit in terms of improving treatment outcomes.

Another research development relevant to the successful dissemination of voucher-based CM into community clinics in the United States and abroad is a project conducted in Spain wherein vouchers exchangeable for goods donated by community businesses were efficacious in treatment of cocaine dependence (40). Lastly, but very importantly, Volpp and colleagues (8) reported a successful controlled trial using monetary reinforcement of abstinence from cigarette smoking among employees of a large corporation. Moving the voucher-based CM into work settings offers tremendous opportunity for successful dissemination of this approach, especially if employers are willing to cover intervention costs.

TABLE 45.2 Extending the intervention to special populations

Study	n	Setting	Voucher duration (weeks)	Maximum voucher earnings	Voucher delivery	Statistically significant treatment effect?	Voucher target(s)
Heil et al. (10)	77	DF	42[b]	$1180.00[b]	—	Y	Smoking (CO → cotinine)
Higgins et al. (11)	58	DF	38[b]	$1090.60[b]	—	Y	Smoking (CO → cotinine)
Krishnan-Sarin et al. (19)	28	DF	4	$313.75	—	Y	Smoking (CO + cotinine)
Correia and Benson (20)	88	NTS	1	$40.00 (low), $80.00 (high)	—	Y	Smoking (CO)
Irons and Correia (21)	12	NTS	1	$65.00	—	Y	Smoking (CO + cotinine)
Tevyaw et al. (22)	110	NTS	3	$283.50	—	Y	Smoking (CO reduction → abstinence)
Dunn et al. (23)	20	MM	2	$362.50	—	Y	Smoking (CO → cotinine)
Robles et al. (24)	16	DF	4	$598.00	—	Y	Smoking (CO + cotinine)
Stoops et al. (25)	68	DF	6	$793.00	—	Y	Smoking (CO reduction → abstinence)
Tracy et al. (26)	30	DF	4	$81.60[a]	Could not be determined	Y	Cocaine + alcohol use
Drebing et al. (27)	19	NTS (VA hospital)	16	$736.00	—	Y	Cocaine + opioids + alcohol use
			32	$270.00	—	Y	Employment and related tasks
Drebing et al. (28)	100	NTS (VA hospital)	16	$560.00	—	Y	Cocaine + opioids + alcohol use
			32	$610.00	—	Y	Employment and related tasks
Sigmon and Higgins (29)	7	NTS	12	$930.00	—	Y	Marijuana use
Wong et al. (30)	4	MM	10	Could not be determined	—	Y	Employment behavior (% on-time arrival)

Continued

TABLE 45.2 Extending the intervention to special populations (*Continued*)

Study	n	Setting	Voucher duration (weeks)	Maximum voucher earnings	Voucher delivery	Statistically significant treatment effect?	Voucher target(s)
Wong et al. (31)	5	MM	14.4	Could not be determined	I	Y	Employment behavior (% completed work shifts)
Rosen et al. (32)	56	HIV clinic	16	$800.00[a]	I	Y	HIV medication adherence
Sorenson et al. (33)	66	MM	12	$1172.40	I	Y	HIV medication adherence
Svikis et al. (34)	91	DF	2	$525.00	I	Y	Treatment attendance

Note: Numbers next to each citation refer to its position in the reference section; *n*, sample size, all groups combined; setting, setting in which study occurred; DF, drug-free clinic; M, medication clinic; MM, methadone maintenance; NTS, not a treatment setting; voucher duration (weeks), number of weeks that voucher intervention was in place; maximum voucher earnings, total possible voucher earning across duration of the intervention; statistically significant treatment effect, presence or absence of significant treatment effect at $p < 0.05$; voucher target, the target of the voucher intervention. Voucher delivery: I, immediate (at the same visit the reinforcement was earned); D, delayed (at a visit after the reinforcement was earned).

[a]Calculated based on expected average max earnings stated in text.
[b]Calculated based on average antepartum weeks + 12 postpartum weeks in study.

TABLE 45.3 Extending the intervention to community clinics

Study	n	Setting	Voucher duration (weeks)	Maximum voucher earnings	Voucher delivery	Statistically significant treatment effect?	Voucher target(s)
Petry et al. (7)	77	MM	12	Could not be determined (prize)	I	Y	Cocaine use
						Y	Group counseling attendance
Volpp et al. (8)	878	NTS (GE)	52	$650.00	D	Y	Smoking (cotinine)
				$100.00	Could not be determined	Y	Completion of smoking-cessation program
Peirce et al. (17)	338	MM	12	$400.00[a]	I	Y	Stimulants + alcohol use
Petry et al. (18)	415	DF	12	$400.00[a]	I	Y	Stimulants + alcohol use
Alessi et al. (35)	103	DF	12	Could not be determined (prize)	I	Y	Cocaine + opioids + alcohol use
				Could not be determined (prize)	I	N	Group counseling attendance
Ledgerwood et al. (36)	75	DF	16	Could not be determined (prize)	I	Y	Group counseling attendance
Petry et al. (37)	142	DF	12	$456.00	I	Y	Cocaine + opioids + alcohol use
				$426.00	I	Could not be determined	Treatment goal completion
				Could not be determined (prize)	I	Y	Cocaine + opioids + alcohol use
				Could not be determined (prize)	I	Could not be determined	Treatment goal completion
Brooner et al. (38)	236	MM	24	$3201.00	I	Y	Cocaine + opioids + barbiturates + benzodiazepines + alcohol
Rowan-Szal et al. (39)	61	MM	8	$8.00	I	Y	Cocaine use

Continued

TABLE 45.3 Extending the intervention to community clinics (*Continued*)

Study	n	Setting	Voucher duration (weeks)	Maximum voucher earnings	Voucher delivery	Statistically significant treatment effect?	Voucher target(s)
Garcia-Rodriguez et al. (40)	96	DF		$8.00	I	Could not be determined	Counseling attendance
				Could not be determined (stars)	Could not be determined	Could not be determined	Treatment goal completion
Marlowe et al. (41)	269	NTS (Drug Court)	12	$1134.00 (low), $2268.00 (high)	I	Y	Cocaine use
			52	$390.00	I	N	Drug court program compliance
Henggler et al. (42)	161	NTS (Juvenile Drug Court)	52	Could not be determined	I	Y	Cocaine + amphetamines + marijuana use
Prendergast et al. (43)	163	NTS (Drug Court)	26	$520.00	I	N	Cocaine + opioids + methamphetamine + benzodiazepines + marijuana + alcohol
				$520.00	I	N	Treatment task completion
				$1040.00	I	N	Both

Note: Numbers next to each citation refer to its position in the reference section; *n*, sample size, all groups combined; setting, setting in which study occurred; DF, drug-free clinic; M, medication clinic; MM, methadone maintenance; NTS, not a treatment setting; voucher duration (weeks), number of weeks that voucher intervention was in place; maximum voucher earnings, total possible voucher earning across duration of the intervention; statistically significant treatment effect, presence or absence of significant treatment effect at $p < 0.05$; voucher target, the target of the voucher intervention. Voucher delivery: I, immediate (at the same visit the reinforcement was earned); D, delayed (at a visit after the reinforcement was earned).

[a]Calculated based on expected average max earnings stated in text.

Important to mention in this section are three additional international examples relevant to the goal of integrating CM into community practices. First, a project is currently under way in the United Kingdom (UK) examining the feasibility of nationwide adoption of voucher-based CM for treatment of SUDs following a recommendation in that direction from the National Institute on Clinical Excellence, an independent body in the UK responsible for providing national guidance on health promotion (45). Second, voucher-based CM specifically for smoking cessation among pregnant women has been implemented into routine clinical practice in certain locations in the UK. For example, a program entitled "Give it up for Baby" in Tayside, Scotland uses vouchers exchangeable for grocery items to promote smoking cessation with economically disadvantaged mothers, the group most at risk for smoking during pregnancy (46). Third, while not targeting SUDs, some mention of conditional cash transfer (CCT) programs warrants mention in any discussion on dissemination of CM into community practices. CCT programs are aimed at eliminating chronic poverty and are operating in many low- and middle-income countries worldwide (47). In these programs, mothers earn cash supplements contingent on adherence with infant inoculations, supplemental feeding, and school enrollment and attendance, among other health-related goals. Tens of millions of families are participating in these programs, which, without question, represent the largest CM effort ever undertaken.

Combining the Intervention with Pharmacotherapies

A clear trend involving studies with voucher-based CM and medications is evident in the present literature review (Table 45.4), with some studies examining the relative efficacy of voucher-based CM and medications, others investigating combined effects, and still others looking at whether CM can enhance compliance with medications known to be efficacious but where adherence is problematic (48–57). Eight of the 10 trials report results supporting the efficacy of the CM intervention, but beyond that the results from this emerging and potentially very important area of investigation are quite mixed. Perhaps the clearest finding is one by Oliveto and colleagues (52) showing that the efficacy of voucher-based CM for cocaine abstinence among opioid-dependent patients enrolled in substitution therapy was conditional on an adequate dose of the medication. That study provided important experimental confirmation of what was long part of voucher-based CM for treating opioid-dependent populations. Results from a trial by Poling et al. (53) offer a suggestion that combining bupropion therapy with CM for treatment of cocaine dependence facilitates the efficacy of the medication. The Poling et al. trial is a novel and interesting finding that while less intuitive than the Oliveto et al. (52) finding is logically comparable, and if replicable suggests great promise for combining CM and pharmacotherapy.

This area of investigation is currently lacking any programmatic direction that is readily discernible, but certainly appears to have great potential. Worth mentioning is that the community CM program for smoking cessation among pregnant smokers described above combines the intervention with free nicotine replacement therapy for mothers who are interested in both and where a pharmacist or provider agrees that pharmacotherapy is indicated (46).

Investigating Longer-Term Outcomes

From early in the development of the voucher-based CM approach to treatment of cocaine dependence there has been interest in its longer-term outcomes. Research on how to directly improve longer-term outcomes has taken two complementary directions that are discernible in the results of the present review (Table 45.5). The first seeks to build on correlational data suggesting that key to fostering longer-term abstinence is increasing during-treatment abstinence. In an experimental test of this notion conducted with cocaine-dependent outpatients, Higgins et al. (58) demonstrated that increasing during-treatment abstinence by using vouchers with greater monetary value also improves longer-term abstinence levels during a 2-year period of posttreatment follow-up.

The second direction of research on this topic of improving longer-term outcomes is focused on voucher-based maintenance therapy. This important effort is being led by Silverman and colleagues who are systematically investigating whether integrating voucher-based CM for abstinence from drug use with vocational training initially and then paid employment thereafter may be a means for developing a self-sustaining intervention that can remain in place long-term (59–62). As would be expected in such an ambitious undertaking, some revisions in the protocol have been necessary (59), but the two most recent trials have resulted in positive outcomes that are quite promising in terms of supporting the feasibility of establishing an efficacious maintenance intervention of voucher-based CM for treatment of chronically unemployed, urban, intravenous cocaine- and opioid-dependent outpatients (60,61).

Conducting Parametric Studies

As is appropriate and necessary in treatment development, many studies in the CM literature address various parametric questions about this treatment approach. We identified 13 reports of that nature in the present literature review (Table 45.6). The focus of these studies ranges broadly, but includes a wealth of potentially important, creative, and essential investigations about how to optimize and further expand this efficacious treatment approach. Examples include experiments on prototypical voucher-based CM combined with computer delivered therapy (63), Internet-based CM delivered alone and without regular in-person interaction (64), different scheduling arrangements to optimize outcomes (65,66), and the possibility of using group rather than individual reinforcement contingencies (67). Some of these studies offer important but clearly incremental advances, while others offer novel advances. All are important and underscore the health of this area of research.

Using the Intervention as a Research Tool

An application of substantial scientific value but rarely discussed is the use of voucher-based CM as a research tool. A recent trial by Mueller et al. (75) provides another interesting

TABLE 45.4 Combining the intervention with pharmacotherapies

Study	n	Setting	Voucher duration (weeks)	Maximum voucher earnings	Voucher delivery	Statistically significant treatment effect?	Voucher target(s)
Glenn and Dallery (48)	14	M: Nic patch	5 days	$56.25	I	Y	Smoking (CO)
Gross et al. (49)	60	M: Buprenorphine	12	$269.00	I	N	Cocaine + opioids use
Jones et al. (50)	199	M: l-Tryptophan	12	$1155.00	I	Y	Cocaine use
Mooney et al. (51)	97	M: Nic gum	15 days	$100.00	Could not be determined	Y	Self-reported nicotine gum use
Oliveto et al. (52)	140	M: LAAM	12	$738.00	D	Y	Cocaine + opioids use
Poling et al. (53)	106	M: Methadone, bupropion	12	$462.00	I	Y	Cocaine + opioids use
			25	$472.00	I	Could not be determined	Treatment task completion
Schmitz et al. (54)	87	M: Naltrexone	12	$997.50	I	N	Cocaine use
Schottenfeld et al. (55)	162	M: Methadone or buprenorphine	12	$997.50	I	Y	Cocaine + opioids use
Shoptaw et al. (56)	229	M: Sertraline	12	$997.50	I	Y	Methamphetamine use
Wiseman et al. (57)	20	M: Nic patch	2	$100.00	I	Y	Smoking (CO)

Note: Numbers next to each citation refer to its position in the reference section; *n*, sample size, all groups combined; setting, setting in which study occurred; DF, drug-free clinic; M, medication clinic; MM, methadone maintenance; NTS, not a treatment setting; voucher duration (weeks), number of weeks that voucher intervention was in place; maximum voucher earnings, total possible voucher earning across duration of the intervention; statistically significant treatment effect, presence or absence of significant treatment effect at $p < 0.05$; voucher target, the target of the voucher intervention. Voucher delivery: I, immediate (at the same visit the reinforcement was earned); D, delayed (at a visit after the reinforcement was earned).

TABLE 45.5	Investigating longer-term outcomes						
Study	n	Setting	Voucher duration (weeks)	Maximum voucher earnings	Voucher delivery	Statistically significant treatment effect?	Voucher target(s)
Higgins et al. (58)	100	DF	12	$499.00 (low), $1995.00 (high)	I	Y	Cocaine use
Knealing et al. (59)	47	MM	36	$5718.00	I	N	Cocaine + opioids use
DeFulio et al. (60)	51	MM	52	Not provided	I	Y	Cocaine use
Silverman et al. (61)	56	MM	26	Not provided	I	Y	Cocaine use
Silverman et al. (62)	78	MM	52	$5800.00	I	Y	Cocaine use

Note: Numbers next to each citation refer to its position in the reference section; n, sample size, all groups combined; setting, setting in which study occurred; DF, drug-free clinic; M, medication clinic; MM, methadone maintenance; NTS, not a treatment setting; voucher duration (weeks), number of weeks that voucher intervention was in place; maximum voucher earnings, total possible voucher earning across duration of the intervention; statistically significant treatment effect, presence or absence of significant treatment effect at $p < 0.05$; voucher target, the target of the voucher intervention. Voucher delivery: I, immediate (at the same visit the reinforcement was earned); D, delayed (at a visit after the reinforcement was earned).

example (Table 45.7). In this instance, CM was used as a research tool in examining the potential contribution of individual differences in executive function to relapse vulnerability in a laboratory model of smoking abstinence. Our group has effectively used CM in a series of experimental studies focused on examining how an initial period of smoking abstinence alters relapse risk (76–79).

The potential utility of voucher-based CM as a research tool seems to have tremendous unrealized potential. The technology gives researchers the potential to experimentally alter drug use practices in severely addicted individuals for sustained periods of time while they reside in their usual drug-using environments. The questions that can follow from that are enormous, including, for example, changes in brain function and structure as well as behavioral and lifestyle outcomes.

SUMMARY/CONCLUSIONS

Voucher-based CM is an efficacious approach to the treatment of SUDs that is based on a clear and compelling set of scientific principles and evidence-based rationales. The approach also has a set of reasonably well-articulated recommended practices for effective CM treatment that we reviewed above. By coupling our review of those core principles and recommended practices with a detailed example of how they can be put into action in the form of a voucher-based CM treatment for pregnant smokers, we hope that readers interested in adopting this approach may be able to gain helpful practical insights from this chapter on how to do so.

Rather than focus the review on the entire almost 20 years of voucher-based CM research, we elected to examine the 5 most recent years. The results from that review show a field that is growing at a very healthy pace, with a total of 72 controlled studies published in peer-reviewed journals over 5 years at a rate of 14.4 articles/year. Importantly, this pace of growth does not appear to have compromised efficacy. Overall, 88% of the articles reviewed in this chapter reported statistically significant treatment effects, which is consistent with the high levels of efficacy that were noted in our earlier review (9).

In trying to organize this rapidly growing literature, we identified seven trends. The practice of extending the approach to new SUDs appears to be leveling off as it would have to. The developments noted in the present review with marijuana and methamphetamine use disorders are important, especially considering the prevalence of the former and the high toxicity and individual and community disruption associated with the latter. The one relatively glaring hole in an otherwise impressive record of extending CM to all major SUDs is alcohol use disorders. No studies on that topic were identified in the present review, which is in keeping with earlier reviews. The major obstacle to extending CM to alcohol use disorders has been technical. That is, reliable methods for biochemically verifying recent abstinence have been associated with detection windows that are too short (e.g., breath alcohol levels) or too long (e.g., gamma-glutamyltransferase) for effective use in CM interventions. Whether recent technological developments such as continuous transdermal alcohol-monitoring devices will permit a break in this logjam remains to be seen, but this is an area with great potential for growth and where voucher-based CM may be able to make important contributions.

TABLE 45.6 Conducting parametric studies

Study	n	Setting	Voucher duration (weeks)	Maximum voucher earnings	Voucher delivery	Statistically significant treatment effect?	Voucher target(s)
Petry et al. (44)	74	MM	12	$585.00 in vouchers	—	Y	Cocaine use
				$300.00[a] in prizes	—	Y	
Bickel et al. (63)	135	Buprenorphine maintenance	23	$1316.75	—	Y	Cocaine + opioids use
Dallery et al. (64)	20	DF	18 days	$171.50	—	Y	Smoking (CO reduction → abstinence)
Roll and Shoptaw (65)	18	Could not be determined	12	$1035.00	Could not be determined	Y	Methamphetamine use
Roll and Howard (66)	19	NTS	5 days	$147.50	—	Y	Smoking (CO)
Kirby et al. (67)	22	MM	Could not be determined	Could not be determined (prize)	—	N	Cocaine + group counseling attendance + medication adherence
Correia et al. (68)	47	MM	2	$300.00	—	Y	Cocaine use
Katz et al. (69)	211	Opioid detox	5 days	$100.00	—	Y	Cocaine + opioids use
Lamb et al. (70)	37	NTS	12	$1320.00	—	Y	Smoking (CO reduction)
Petry et al. (71)	131	DF	12	Could not be determined	—	Y	Cocaine + opioids + alcohol use
					—	Could not be determined	Treatment task completion

Preston et al. (72)	67	MM	12	Could not be determined (prize)	I	N	Cocaine use
						Cocaine + opioids use
Sigmon et al. (73)	46	MM	12 days[b]	$1200.00	I	Y	Cocaine (abstinence vs. reduction)
Vandrey et al. (74)	12	MM	40 days	$350.00 in cash	D	Y	Cocaine use
				$350.00 in vouchers	D	Y	

Note: Numbers next to each citation refer to its position in the reference section; *n*, sample size, all groups combined; setting, setting in which study occurred; DF, drug-free clinic; M, medication clinic; MM, methadone maintenance; NTS, not a treatment setting; voucher duration (weeks), number of weeks that voucher intervention was in place; maximum voucher earnings, total possible voucher earning across duration of the intervention; statistically significant treatment effect, presence or absence of significant treatment effect at $p < 0.05$; voucher target, the target of the voucher intervention. Voucher delivery: I, immediate (at the same visit the reinforcement was earned); D, delayed (at a visit after the reinforcement was earned).

[a]Calculated based on expected average max earnings stated in text.

[b]12 days randomly reinforced during a 24-week period.

TABLE 45.7 Using the intervention as a research tool

Study	n	Setting	Voucher duration (weeks)	Maximum voucher earnings	Voucher delivery	Statistically significant treatment effect?	Voucher target(s)
Mueller et al. (75)	19	NTS	6 days[a]	$404.00	I	Y	Smoking (CO)
Alessi et al. (76)	34	NTS	12 days	$427.50	I	Y	Smoking (CO)
Chivers et al. (77)	58	NTS	2	$507.50	I	Y	Smoking (CO)
Lussier et al. (78)	63	NTS	2	$507.50	I	Y	Smoking (CO)
Yoon et al. (79)	34	NTS	2	$507.50	I	Y	Smoking (CO → cotinine)

Note: Numbers next to each citation refer to its position in the reference section; *n*, sample size, all groups combined; setting, setting in which study occurred; DF, drug-free clinic; M, medication clinic; MM, methadone maintenance; NTS, not a treatment setting; voucher duration (weeks), number of weeks that voucher intervention was in place; maximum voucher earnings, total possible voucher earning across duration of the intervention; statistically significant treatment effect, presence or absence of significant treatment effect at $p < 0.05$; voucher target, the target of the voucher intervention. Voucher delivery: I, immediate (at the same visit the reinforcement was earned); D, delayed (at a visit after the reinforcement was earned).

[a]Six lab visits.

The use of voucher-based CM with special populations is an exciting and growing area with potentially important contributions being made with pregnant women, adolescents, and those with other psychiatric disorders, among other groups. Recent developments with pregnant cigarette smokers and in vocational training with dually diagnosed veterans appears to hold particular promise in terms of this treatment approach becoming widely used in clinical practice. An area where we see unrealized potential is in the use of voucher-based CM in treating pregnant women dependent on illicit drugs. There is no programmatic body of CM research focused specifically on this population.

Efforts to move voucher-based CM into community clinics have been tremendously successful in terms of demonstrating efficacy in those settings. Where progress has been slower is in adoption of the practices into routine clinical care, especially in the United States. As was noted above, efforts are under way exploring broad implementation in the UK where they have a single-payor health care system, but in the US system how to pay for incentive-based interventions remains a major obstacle to broad dissemination into community SUDs clinics. Important to recognize, though, is that there are other important community venues for intervening on SUDs besides treatment clinics. Indeed, employment settings, drug courts, other criminal justice settings, community agencies such as Women, Infants, and Children (WIC) offices and community health centers may eventually prove to be a better match with the voucher-based CM approach than community SUDs treatment clinics.

Progress is being made toward using voucher-based CM to improve longer-term outcomes. There is strong evidence that voucher-based CM interventions produce effects that carry over into the posttreatment period and progress is being made in how to improve upon that situation by increasing during-treatment success. The development of longer-term or maintenance CM interventions is a parallel and essential effort that is also progressing well. Indeed, when one considers the broad agreement that SUDs are chronic relapsing disorders, the need for maintenance interventions is obvious. Again, it may be the case that the venues for implementing such longer-term interventions ends up being something other than or at least in addition to conventional community SUDs treatment clinics.

Also rather clear is the importance of effectively combining voucher-based CM with pharmacotherapies. This review revealed numerous efforts in that direction, but as yet nothing that is particularly promising other than the use of voucher-based CM in methadone and other opioid-substitution clinics.

Attention to various parametric questions about effective CM treatment is an ongoing theme in this literature that all signs indicate will and should continue. Despite the striking growth in the number of studies appearing in the voucher-based CM literature and high rates of success in terms of significant findings, there is a daunting amount more to be learned about how to optimize the use of financial incentives for behavior change around SUDs as well as other health-related behavior. We anticipate that this is an area that will see growing attention as government and private enterprises attempt to curb the spiraling health care costs associated with SUDs and other health-related behaviors.

Last, but by no means least, we see promising growth in the use of voucher-based CM as a research tool. That was evident in trials on neuropsychological factors (75) as well as the effects of initial abstinence on relapse risk (76–79). This remains a highly underutilized strength of voucher-based CM, but the trend from the present review shows growth in this area that is likely to continue as evidence accumulates on the scientific advantages of doing so.

ACKNOWLEDGMENTS

Preparation of this chapter was supported in part by research grants DA009378, DA008076, DA07242, and DA019550 from the National Institute on Drug Abuse.

REFERENCES

1. Higgins ST, Silverman K, Heil SH, eds. *Contingency Management in Substance Abuse Treatment*. New York, NY: The Guilford Press; 2008.
2. Higgins ST, Heil SH, Lussier JP. Clinical implications of reinforcement as a determinant of substance use disorders. *Annu Rev Psychol*. 2004;55:431–461.
3. Bickel WK, Miller ML, Kowal BP, et al. Behavioral and neuroeconomics of drug addiction: competing neural systems and temporal discounting processes. *Drug Alcohol Depend*. 2007;90(suppl 1):S85–S91.
4. Aston-Jones G, Cohen JD. Adaptive gain and the role of the locus coeruleus-norepinephrine system in optimal performance. *J Comp Neurol*. 2005;493:99–110.
5. Muller J, Dreisbach G, Goschke T, et al. Dopamine and cognitive control: the prospect of monetary gains influences the balance between flexibility and stability in a set-shifting paradigm. *Eur J Neurosci*. 2007;26:3661–3668.
6. Garavan H, Hester R. The role of cognitive control in cocaine dependence. *Neuropsychol Rev*. 2007;17:337–345.
7. Petry NM, Martin B, Simcic F. Prize reinforcement contingency management for cocaine dependence: integration with group therapy in a methadone clinic. *J Consult Clin Psychol*. 2005;73:354–359.
8. Volpp KG, Troxel AB, Pauly MV, et al. A randomized, controlled trial of financial incentives for smoking cessation. *N Engl J Med*. 2009;360:699–709.
9. Lussier JP, Heil SH, Mongeon JA, et al. A meta-analysis of voucher-based reinforcement therapy for substance use disorders. *Addiction*. 2006;101:192–203.
10. Heil SH, Higgins ST, Bernstein IM, et al. Effects of voucher-based incentives on abstinence from cigarette smoking and fetal growth among pregnant women. *Addiction*. 2008;103:1009–1018.
11. Higgins ST, Heil SH, Solomon LJ, et al. A pilot study on voucher-based incentives to promote abstinence from cigarette smoking during pregnancy and postpartum. *Nicotine Tob Res*. 2004;6:1015–1020.
12. Petry NM, Tedford J, Austin M, et al. Prize reinforcement contingency management for treating cocaine users: how low can we go, and with whom? *Addiction*. 2004;99:349–360.
13. Budney AJ, Moore BA, Rocha HL, et al. Clinical trial of abstinence-based vouchers and cognitive-behavioral therapy for cannabis dependence. *J Consult Clin Psychol*. 2006;74:307–316.
14. Carroll KM, Easton CJ, Nich C, et al. The use of contingency management and motivational/skills-building therapy to treat young adults with marijuana dependence. *J Consult Clin Psychol*. 2006;74:955–966.
15. Kaddem RM, Litt MD, Kabela-Cormier E, et al. Abstinence rates following behavioral treatments for marijuana dependence. *Addict Behav*. 2007;32:1220–1236.
16. Rawson RA, McCann MJ, Flammino F, et al. A comparison of contingency management and cognitive behavioral approaches for stimulant-dependent individuals. *Addiction*. 2006;101:267–274.
17. Peirce JM, Petry NM, Stitzer ML, et al. Effects of lower-cost incentives on stimulant abstinence in methadone maintenance treatment: a national drug abuse treatment clinical trials network study. *Arch Gen Psychiatry*. 2006;63:201–208.
18. Petry NM, Peirce JM, Stitzer ML, et al. Effect of prize-based incentives on outcomes in stimulant abusers in out patient psychosocial treatment programs: a national drug abuse treatment clinical trials network study. *Arch Gen Psychiatry*. 2005;62:1148–1156.
19. Krishnan-Sarin S, Duhig AM, McKee SA, et al. Contingency management for smoking cessation in adolescent smokers. *Exp Clin Psychopharmacol*. 2006;14:306–310.
20. Correia CJ, Benson TA. The use of contingency management to reduce cigarette smoking among college students. *Exp Clin Psychopharmacol*. 2006;14:171–179.
21. Irons J.G, Correia CJ. A brief abstinence test for college student smokers: a feasibility study. *Exp Clin Psychopharmacol*. 2008;16:223–229.
22. Tevyaw TO, Colby SM, Tidey JW, et al. Contingency management and motivational enhancement: a randomized clinical trial for college student smokers. *Nicotine Tob Res*. 2009;11:739–749.
23. Dunn KE, Sigmon SC, Thomas GS, et al. Voucher-based contingent reinforcement of smoking abstinence among methadone-maintained patients: a pilot study. *J Appl Behav Anal*. 2008;41: 527–538.
24. Robles E, Crone CC, Whiteside-Mansell L, et al. Voucher-based incentives for cigarette smoking reduction in a women's residential treatment program. *Nicotine Tob Res*. 2005;7:111–117.
25. Stoops WW, Dallery J, Fields NM, et al. An internet-based abstinence reinforcement smoking cessation intervention in rural smokers. *Drug Alcohol Depend*. 2009;105:56–62.
26. Tracy K, Babuscio T, Nich C, et al. Contingency Management to reduce substance use in individuals who are homeless with co-occurring psychiatric disorders. *Am J Drug Alcohol Abuse*. 2007;33:253–258.
27. Drebing CE, Van Ormer EA, Krebs C, et al. The impact of enhanced incentives on vocational rehabilitation outcomes for dually diagnosed veterans. *J Appl Behav Anal*. 2005;38:359–372.
28. Drebing CE, Van Ormer EA, Mueller L, et al. Adding contingency management intervention to vocational rehabilitation: outcomes for dually diagnosed veterans. *J Rehabil Res Dev*. 2007;44:851–865.
29. Sigmon SC, Higgins ST. Voucher-based contingent reinforcement of marijuana abstinence among individuals with serious mental illness. *J Subst Abuse Treat*. 2006;30:291–295.
30. Wong CJ, Dillon EM, Sylvest CE, et al. Contingency management of reliable attendance of chronically unemployed substance abusers in a therapeutic workplace. *Exp Clin Psychopharmacol*. 2004;12:39–46.
31. Wong CJ, Dillon EM, Sylvest C, et al. Evaluation of a modified contingency management intervention for consistent attendance in therapeutic workplace participants. *Drug Alcohol Depend*. 2004;74:319–323.
32. Rosen MI, Dieckhaus K, McMahon TJ, et al. Improved adherence with contingency management. *AIDS Patient Care STDS*. 2007;21:30–40.
33. Sorensen JL, Haug NA, Delucchi KL, et al. Voucher reinforcement improves medication adherence in HIV-positive methadone patients: a randomized trial. *Drug Alcohol Depend*. 2007;88:54–63.

34. Svikis DS, Silverman K, Haug NA, et al. Behavioral strategies to improve treatment participation and retention by pregnant drug-dependent women. *Subst Use Misuse.* 2007;42:1527–1535.
35. Alessi SM, Hanson T, Wieners M, et al. Low-cost contingency management in community clinics: delivering incentives partially in group therapy. *Exp Clin Psychopharmacol.* 2007;15:293–300.
36. Ledgerwood DM, Alessi SM, Hanson T, et al. Contingency management for attendance to group substance abuse treatment administered by clinicians in community clinics. *J Appl Behav Anal.* 2008;41:517–526.
37. Petry NM, Alessi SM, Marx J, et al. Vouchers versus prizes: contingency management treatment of substance abusers in community settings. *J Consult Clin Psychol.* 2005;73:1005–1014.
38. Brooner RK, Kidorf MS, King VL, et al. Comparing adaptive stepped care and monetary-based voucher interventions for opioid dependence. *Drug Alcohol Depend.* 2007;88(suppl 2):S14–S23.
39. Rowan-Szal GA, Bartholomew NG, Chatham LR, et al. A combined cognitive and behavioral intervention for cocaine-using methadone clients. *J Psychoactive Drugs.* 2005;37:75–84.
40. Garcia-Rodriguez O, Secades-Villa R, Higgins ST, et al. Effects of voucher-based intervention on abstinence and retention in an outpatient treatment for cocaine addiction: a randomized controlled trial. *Exp Clin Psychopharmacol.* 2009;17:131–138.
41. Marlowe DB, Festinger DS, Dugosh KL, et al. An effectiveness trial of contingency management in a felony preadjudication drug court. *J Appl Behav Anal.* 2008;41:565–577.
42. Henggeler SW, Halliday-Boykins CA, Cunningham PB, et al. Juvenile drug court: enhancing outcomes by integrating evidence-based treatments. *J Consult Clin Psychol.* 2006;74:42–54.
43. Prendergast ML, Hall EA, Roll J, et al. Use of vouchers to reinforce abstinence and positive behaviors among clients in a drug court treatment program. *J Subst Abuse Treat.* 2008;35: 125–135.
44. Petry NM, Alessi SM, Hanson T, et al. Randomized trial of contingent prizes versus vouchers in cocaine-using methadone patients. *J Consult Clin Psychol.* 2007;75:983–991.
45. Pilling S, Strang J, Gerada C. Psychosocial interventions and opioid detoxification for drug misuse: summary of NICE guidance. *Br Med J.* 2007;335:203–205.
46. Ballard P, Radley A. Give it up for baby: a smoking cessation intervention for pregnant women in Scotland. *Public Health Commun Mark.* 2009;III:147–160 (www.gwumc.edu/sphhs/departments/pch/phcm/.../cases_3_09.pdf).
47. Lagarde M, Haines A, Palmer N. Conditional cash transfers for improving uptake of health interventions in low- and middle-income countries: a systematic review. *J Am Med Assoc.* 2007;298:1900–1910.
48. Glenn IM, Dallery J. Effects of internet-based voucher reinforcement and a transdermal nicotine patch on cigarette smoking. *J Appl Behav Anal.* 2007;40:1–13.
49. Gross A, Marsch LA, Badger GJ, et al. A comparison between low-magnitude voucher and buprenorphine medication contingencies in promoting abstinence from opioids and cocaine. *Exp Clin Psychopharmacol.* 2006;14:148–156.
50. Jones HE, Johnson RE, Bigelow GE, et al. Safety and efficacy of L-tryptophan and behavioral incentives for treatment of cocaine dependence: a randomized clinical trial. *Am J Addict.* 2004;13:421–437.
51. Mooney M, Babb D, Jensen J, et al. Interventions to increase use of nicotine gum: a randomized, controlled, single-blind trial. *Nicotine Tob Res.* 2005;7:565–579.
52. Oliveto A, Poling J, Sevarino KA, et al. Efficacy of dose and contingency management procedures in LAAM-maintained cocaine-dependent patients. *Drug Alcohol Depend.* 2005;79:157–165.
53. Poling J, Oliveto A, Petry N, et al. Six-month trial of bupropion with contingency management for cocaine dependence in a methadone-maintained population. *Arch Gen Psychiatry.* 2006;63:219–228.
54. Schmitz JM, Lindsay JA, Green CE, et al. High-dose naltrexone therapy for cocaine-alcohol dependence. *Am J Addict.* 2009;18:356–362.
55. Schottenfeld RS, Chawarski MC, Pakes JR, et al. Methadone versus buprenorphine with contingency management or performance feedback for cocaine and opioid dependence. *Am J Psychiatry.* 2005;162:340–349.
56. Shoptaw S, Huber A, Peck J, et al. Randomized, placebo-controlled trial of sertraline and contingency management for the treatment of methamphetamine dependence. *Drug Alcohol Depend.* 2006;85:12–18.
57. Wiseman EJ, Williams DK, McMillan DE. Effectiveness of payment for reduced carbon monoxide levels and noncontingent payments on smoking behaviors in cocaine-abusing outpatients wearing nicotine or placebo patches. *Exp Clin Psychopharmacol.* 2005;13:102–110.
58. Higgins ST, Heil SH, Dantona R, et al. Effects of varying the monetary value of voucher-based incentives on abstinence achieved during and following treatment among cocaine-dependent outpatients. *Addiction.* 2007;102:271–281.
59. Knealing TW, Wong CJ, Diemer KN, et al. A randomized controlled trial of the therapeutic workplace for community methadone patients: a partial failure to engage. *Exp Clin Psychopharmacol.* 2006;14:350–360.
60. DeFulio A, Donlin WD, Wong CJ, et al. Employment-based abstinence reinforcement as a maintenance intervention for the treatment of cocaine dependence: a randomized controlled trial. *Addiction.* 2009;104:1530–1538.
61. Silverman K, Wong CJ, Needham M, et al. A randomized trial of employment-based reinforcement of cocaine abstinence in injection drug users. *J Appl Behav Anal.* 2007;40:387–410.
62. Silverman K, Robles E, Mudric T, et al. A randomized trial of long-term reinforcement of cocaine abstinence in methadone-maintained patients who inject drugs. *J Consult Clin Psychol.* 2004;72:839–854.
63. Bickel WK, Marsch LA, Buchhalter AR, et al. Computerized behavior therapy for opioid-dependent outpatients: a randomized controlled trial. *Exp Clin Psychopharmacol.* 2008;16:132–143.
64. Dallery J, Glenn IM, Raiff BR. An internet-based abstinence reinforcement treatment for cigarette smoking. *Drug Alcohol Depend.* 2007;86:230–238.
65. Roll JM, Shoptaw S. Contingency management: schedule effects. *Psychiatry Res.* 2006;144:91–93.
66. Roll JM, Howard JT. The relative contribution of economic valence to contingency management efficacy: a pilot study. *J Appl Behav Anal.* 2008;41:629–633.
67. Kirby KC, Kerwin ME, Carpenedo CM, et al. Interdependent group contingency management for cocaine dependent methadone maintenance patients. *J Appl Behav Anal.* 2008;41:579–595.
68. Correia CJ, Sigmon SC, Silverman K, et al. A comparison of voucher-delivery schedules for the initiation of cocaine abstinence. *Exp Clin Psychopharmacol.* 2005;13:253–258.

69. Katz EC, Chutuape MA, Jones H, et al. Abstinence incentive effects in a short-term outpatient detoxification program. *Exp Clin Psychopharmacol.* 2004;12:262–268.
70. Lamb RJ, Morral AR, Kirby KC, et al. Contingencies for change in complacent smokers. *Exp Clin Psychopharmacol.* 2007;15: 245–255.
71. Petry NM, Alessi SM, Carroll KM, et al. Contingency management treatments: Reinforcing abstinence versus adherence with goal-related activities. *J Consult Clin Psychol.* 2006;74:592–601.
72. Preston KL, Ghitza UE, Schmittner JP, et al. Randomized trial comparing two treatment strategies using prize-based reinforcement of abstinence in cocaine and opiate users. *J Appl Behav Anal.* 2008;41:551–563.
73. Sigmon SC, Correia CJ, Stitzer ML. Cocaine abstinence during methadone maintenance: effects of repeated brief exposure to voucher-based reinforcement. *Exp Clin Psychopharmacol.* 2004; 12:269–275.
74. Vandrey R, Bigelow GE, Stitzer ML. Contingency management in cocaine abusers: a dose-effect comparison of goods-based versus cash-based incentives. *Exp Clin Psychopharmacol.* 2007; 15:338–343.
75. Mueller ET, Landes RD, Kowal BP, et al. Delay of smoking gratification as a laboratory model of relapse: effects of incentives for not smoking, and relationship with measures of executive function. *Behav Pharmacol.* 2009;20:461–473.
76. Alessi SM, Badger GJ, Higgins ST. An experimental examination of the initial weeks of abstinence in cigarette smokers. *Exp Clin Psychopharmacol.* 2004;12:276–287.
77. Chivers LL, Higgins ST, Heil SH, et al. Effects of initial abstinence and programmed lapses on the relative reinforcing effects of cigarette smoking. *J Appl Behav Anal.* 2008;41:481–497.
78. Lussier JP, Higgins ST, Badger GJ. Influence of the duration of abstinence on the relative reinforcing effects of cigarette smoking. *Psychopharmacology.* 2005;181:486–495.
79. Yoon JH, Higgins ST, Bradstreet MP, et al. Changes in the relative reinforcing effects of cigarette smoking as a function of initial abstinence. *Psychopharmacology.* 2009;205:305–318.

CHAPTER 46
Motivational Interviewing and Enhancement

Carlo C. DiClemente ■ Onna R. Van Orden ■ Katherine S. Wright

INTRODUCTION

One of the true innovations in the field of substance abuse treatment in the past 15 years has been the adoption of sophisticated motivational interventions. Lack of motivation to change is common in substance abuse stemming from the capacity of substances to create habitual addictive patterns of behavior that include physiologic and psychological dependence. This has led some to call addictions "diseases of denial" and to suggest that confrontation, experiencing severe consequences, and "hitting bottom" are the most effective methods for breaking through the addicted individual's denial. For the most part, this perspective has changed dramatically over the past 15 years. There is growing recognition that lack of motivation is not simply a problem of addiction but is a part of all human intentional behavior change (1–3). Motivation is multidimensional involving a series of tasks that include creating concern, decision making, firm intentions, commitment, planning, and sustained implementation (4). These tasks are not new and are critical for understanding individual behavior change whether it happens through self-change or with the assistance of treatment or mutual help programs (5).

Motivational interviewing (MI) was developed as an intervention style and a set of strategies based on motivational principles to address the typical motivational conundrum faced by treatment providers: most treatments are action-oriented, but most patients are ambivalent, unmotivated, and not ready for change. MI is best thought of as an intervention that attempts to empower the individual and evoke change rather than an intensive treatment. This chapter will describe the MI approach, offer some evidence for efficacy of this treatment, and describe how it can be used in substance abuse treatment.

HISTORY OF MOTIVATIONAL INTERVIEWING

MI was born out of two converging lines of research that emerged at the end of the 1970s and the beginning of the 1980s. The seminal work by Edwards and colleagues indicated that brief interventions of advice and information were as effective as more extensive formal treatments when used with a broad range of individuals with alcohol problems (6). These findings spurred Miller to begin developing and evaluating brief interventions for excessive drinking. Such interventions, like the Drinker Check-Up, were designed to influence problem drinkers to change their drinking behavior using an assessment format that included objectively and empathically delivered feedback. Early on, minimal interventions were viewed as more relevant for problem drinkers rather than heavier or dependent drinkers. This was influenced by the belief that "true alcoholics" would not be able to benefit from these interventions because dependence compromised and crippled motivation. In fact, inability to change despite trying to do so became one of the symptoms that supported a dependence diagnosis adopted by the DSM-III-R. Nevertheless, evaluations of the Drinker Check-Up program indicated that many individuals with serious alcohol problems were able to moderate, if not quit, drinking (7). Interest grew among providers in using minimal, motivational interventions for substance abuse, primarily for alcohol abuse and dependence.

At the same time, Prochaska and DiClemente were developing the Transtheoretical Model, which described intentional behavior change in a series of stages that individuals negotiated by use of a number of behavior change principles or processes (8). This model was proposed as an integrative, eclectic framework that could make sense of the puzzling outcomes of many treatment comparison trials indicating that different types of therapies seemed to produce equivalent outcomes when evaluated in clinical trials (9). This model delineated preaction stages (Precontemplation, Contemplation, and Preparation/Decision Making) indicating that there were tasks and steps that were necessary to get individuals ready for action. Their early research also indicated that there may be separate sets of strategies that could be used to influence early-stage transitions, which might differ from action-oriented strategies that would be more important in the later action stages (Action and Maintenance) (10). It should be noted that many researchers were focusing on decision-making as well as beliefs and intentions contributing to the zeitgeist that led to the creation of cognitive-behavioral treatments that focused both on cognitive variables as well as behavioral learning principles as critical ingredients for change (11).

Miller began to concentrate on motivation and brought together these two lines of research in his review of motivation in substance abuse (12). He also co-sponsored with Nick Heather the third International Conference on the Treatment of Addictions Behaviors held in Berwyck, Scotland in 1984, the theme of which was self-regulation and the stages of change (13). On a sabbatical in Australia, Bill Miller teamed up with Welsh researcher, Stephen Rollnick, and together they developed what is now known as MI (2). Their work made explicit critical elements of successful brief interventions and focused on early-stage motivational challenges that individuals must resolve for successful modification of their problematic substance use. Although originally focused on addictions, this approach came to be used for a variety of health behavior problems (1,14). MI also became an integral intervention component for developing Screening, Brief Intervention, Referral, and Treatment (SBIRT) approaches for early intervention in drug abuse and other problematic health behaviors (15). In addition, MI interventions were developed into an independent, brief treatment called Motivational Enhancement Treatment (MET) (16). Both the first and second editions of the MI book became widely used as a training manual that described the basic principles and strategies as well as how the approach has been adapted for a variety of problems and integrated into many different intervention settings. Today MI is being used in pretreatment interventions as a component of a larger integrated approach, as a free-standing treatment (MET), and as a basic brief intervention used by a multidisciplinary and heterogeneous group of providers. Most importantly, the emergence of MI has reflected and promoted a dramatic change in perspective about how to approach and interact with individuals with substance abuse and how to engage motivational considerations in a constructive, respectful, and empowering manner.

UNIQUE FEATURES OF MOTIVATIONAL INTERVIEWING

MI is not a complete therapy intended to provide support, coping skills, and problem solving over a long period of time. As its name indicates, it is a way of talking and interacting with an individual that is designed to activate the person's concern, considerations, and intentions to change and to support the individual's sense of confidence and efficaciousness in making the change. It is specifically intended to help resolve ambivalence, to promote consideration of values, to reevaluate the current status quo and the potential for change, and to support realistic self-efficacy and planning to make a change. It consists of a *style* of interacting that can be used throughout the provider's encounter with a substance abuser as well as a series of *strategies* that can be used to address various obstacles and considerations that hinder the flow of motivation and change for specific clients. Table 46.1 provides an overview of these features of MI. In addition, specific skills are needed for practitioners to be able to implement these strategies.

The style or spirit of MI is marked by critical attitudes and values that underlie the entire approach. The key dimensions of the MI-style are Collaboration, Evocation, and Autonomy. Important elements that characterize an MI encounter between the provider and the client are empathy, respect, a collaborative relationship, belief in the capacity for change, and elicitation of motivational considerations, commitment, and change language from the client. Spirit and style are core elements that distinguish MI from other approaches that are more expert-oriented, openly directive, confrontational, and therapist-dominated. Many of the core MI elements are similar to those described in a good therapeutic or working relationship between therapist and client. However, MI-style is a unique combination of elements from Carl Rogers' nondirective approach, from humanistic/existential therapy, and from emerging scientific principles of communication, interpersonal interaction, engagement, and motivation.

The core MI strategies include expressing empathy, using open-ended questions, reflective listening, summarizing and clarifying client thoughts and experiences, affirming client strengths and capacity, eliciting change talk, rolling with resistance, asking permission before giving advice, and presenting a menu of options. There are also more specific techniques that can be used in each of these areas that are outlined in Table 46.1. The objective of the use of these strategies and techniques is to elicit and promote "change language" from the client. Change language consists of any client statements and expressions that reflect a Desire, Ability, Reasons or Need to change or a Commitment to take some action to change (DARN-C language). On hearing any DARN-C language, providers are expected to emphasize them and encourage exploration by reflecting on these client expressions using reflective listening techniques or highlighting them in various types of summaries (collecting, linking, and transitional).

Implementing MI requires practitioners to have or develop both the style of communication and the basic skills to enable them to use the strategies and techniques outlined in Table 46.1. The style, strategies, and skills that comprise MI may come more naturally to some health practitioners than to others. The style requires a respectful, empowering attitude toward the client and the intervention process. MI is neither intended to undermine the role of the provider as a professional, who has important knowledge and specific skills and aids, nor to blur the boundary between client and professional. However, an MI practitioner would need to have attitudes and communication skills that are consonant with collaboration, empathy, listening before speaking, tolerance of client ambivalence and lack of motivation, and the ability to collect, understand, reflect, and summarize what is being said in the encounter. The ability to listen and pay attention not only to clients' words, but also to their demeanor, emotions, and language is at the heart of being able to engage in reflective listening and to offer accurate and provocative reflections. Minimizing assumptions and prejudgments of client capacity, motivation, and ability to change is also critical to eliciting change talk and being affirming. Although many practitioners indicate that they are using MI in their practice, fewer seem to be using the entire scope of style, strategies, techniques, and skills that are outlined and

TABLE 46.1 Key elements of a motivational style of counseling

Style	Strategies	Techniques

Collaboration
  Even power distribution
  Client involved in decisions
Evocation
  Communicate belief in the capacity for change
  Understand client experience
Autonomy
  Respect
  Acknowledge client's freedom
A Motivational _Style_ of Counseling: "a skillful clinical style for eliciting from patients their own good motivations for making behavior changes."[b]
Motivational Counseling _Strategies_: methods to enhance client engagement in the change process, supported by the use of several motivational counseling techniques.
Motivational Counseling _Techniques_: specific behaviors that will enable a counselor to perform effective motivational counseling strategies.
	Open-ended questions
	  Elicit longer responses
	Affirm the client
	  Provide tailored support
	Reflective listening
	  Clarify client's meaning
	Summarizing statements
	  Reflect deeper understanding
	Rolling with resistance
	  Come alongside client
	Eliciting change talk
	  Highlight and resolve ambivalence
	Empathy
	  Acceptance supports change
		Open-ended questions
		  Begin with words such as "how", phrases such as "tell me about…" or statements that implicitly ask for a response
		Affirm the client
		  Notice strengths
		  Acknowledge efforts
		  Be appropriate to setting and culture
		Reflective listening
		  Simple reflection
		  Amplified reflection
		  Understatements
		  Double-sided reflection
		Summarizing statements
		  Collect
		  Link
		  Transition
		Rolling with resistance
		  Reframe
		  Shift focus
		  Enhance discrepancy
		Additional skills
		  Avoid blurting out responses
		  Ask permission to give advice
		  Present a menu of options
		  Attend to DARN-C language[a]

[a]DARN-C is an acronym for the client's Desires, Abilities, Reasons, and Needs for change, and their use of Commitment language to enhance self-efficacy for change.
[b]Rollnick S, Miller WR, Butler CC. *Motivational Interviewing in Health Care: Helping Patients Change Behavior.* New York, NY: Guilford Press; 2008:6.

demonstrated by the developers of the MI approach. Simply using open-ended questions and reflections do not encompass the broad scope of knowledge, skills, and behaviors needed to fully implement MI. Because of its popularity, there are many adaptations of MI (AMI) that do not include all of the elements and are not executed with the rigorous skill development, feedback and supervision, and detailed analyses of taped sessions that reflect a more comprehensive and faithful application of MI (17).

EFFICACY OF MI WITH DIFFERENT POPULATIONS

A large number of studies have evaluated MI and AMI across a wide range of behaviors. The following review will describe findings in this literature highlighting the efficacy of MI with various types of addictive behaviors and populations and update the reviews of its application to various substances and in a variety of settings (3). In their review on AMI interventions prepared for the second edition of the MI book, Burke, Arkowitz, and Dunn concluded that "in general, AMIs are more effective than no treatment … are not significantly different from credible alternative treatments … and are efficacious, both as stand-alone treatments and as preludes to other treatments" (pp. 241–242).

In a later meta-analysis of randomized controlled trials (RCT) testing the efficacy of AMI across health behaviors, Burke, Arkowitz, and Manchola used strict criteria for inclusion as an AMI RCT, including random assignment, control group, and adequate measures. In addition, they included only studies of individual therapy with interventions that used MI techniques separate from other treatments. They found 15 studies focused on alcohol, 5 with drug addictions, and just 2 for smoking cessation that met these criteria. These authors concluded that "AMIs were equivalent to other active treatments and yielded moderate effects (from 0.25 to 0.57 [Cohen's d]) compared with no treatment and/or placebo for problems involving alcohol, drugs, and diet and exercise"

(p. 843) (18). These reviews indicate that AMI interventions are efficacious but not necessarily better than other credible interventions.

Techniques of MI, however, may be more efficacious when addressing preaction motivational tasks and engagement with the intervention. One multisite drug-abuse treatment study found that MI strategies integrated into the initial intake and evaluation sessions of outpatient treatment were associated with significantly better treatment retention at 28-day follow-up. However, the intervention did not impact self-reported overall substance use at either 28-day or 84-day follow-up (19). Miller, Yahne, and Tonigan also found a single session of MI early in either inpatient or outpatient substance abuse treatments did not produce an increase in self-reported percent days abstinent from substances at either 3, 6, 9, and 12 months posttreatment as validated by urine toxicology and collateral reports (20). Limited exposure to MI especially when joined with a more extensive treatment does not appear to be effective to produce differential changes in substance use behavior compared to active controls among a heterogeneous group of treatment-seeking substance abusers. However, AMIs did demonstrate some positive effects on treatment engagement and retention in inpatient or outpatient substance abuse programs. Studies focused on specific substances of abuse may provide a better test of potential efficacy of MI approaches. These are reviewed below, with the caveat that additional research is needed on the efficacy of MI for the treatment of specific substances of abuse, particularly illicit substances.

Alcohol

MI interventions for alcohol abuse and dependence have been studied more extensively than for any other addictive behavior. A large number of studies examined MI and AMI types of interventions for alcohol use, abuse, and dependence and found that AMI interventions had a moderate advantage compared either with other interventions or no intervention at all. Vasilaki, Hosier, and Cox, updating three previous reviews, concluded that brief interventions using MI were particularly effective in reducing alcohol consumption (21). The review included only RCTs that examined MI as a treatment to reduce alcohol consumption in comparison to no treatment or a comparison treatment. They reviewed 22 RCTs, published between 1983 and 2003, that satisfied Miller and Rollnick's definition of MI as "a client-centered, directive method for enhancing intrinsic motivation to change by exploring and resolving ambivalence," (p. 328) among other criteria. Only 15 studies were included in the final meta-analysis, as 7 did not meet the methodologic quality criteria for inclusion. Nine compared brief MI with no treatment and nine compared it to other treatments with three studies falling into both categories. Mean duration of the MI intervention across these studies was 87 minutes.

The strongest conclusion of this review was that MI was significantly more effective in reducing alcohol consumption at a 3-month follow-up among nondependent drinkers when compared with no-treatment controls. When compared to other treatments, results were mixed. MI had greater efficacy than a standard care or treatment-as-usual (TAU) control in four studies. In five studies, MI was more effective than a comparison treatment (CBT, skills-based counseling, and directive-confrontational counseling), but in three other studies MI was equivalent to an alternative treatment. One of these was the large-scale, multisite alcohol treatment study, Project MATCH, in which researchers utilized, with high fidelity, a treatment condition comprised of four comprehensive MET sessions and found it produced comparable results to two other more extensive 12-session treatments (22). The review concluded that MI was useful as a brief intervention and more successful when the client was a young adult who was a heavy drinker rather than an older adult with more severe dependence. It is notable, however, that in none of these studies was MI found to be less effective than other treatments or a no-treatment control (21).

Group differences in efficacy tended to be greater at 3-month compared to 6-month follow-ups, perhaps suggesting that its effects may fade with time. This does not always seem to be the case, however, since other studies have found support for sustained reductions in alcohol-related problems as well as reductions in the quantity and frequency of drinking at 12-month follow-up interviews (23). Studies of reduction in drinking with AMI interventions have also shown support for its use in screening and brief interventions across a number of settings (24,25).

In alcohol studies examining MI as a treatment option compared to no treatment, MI fared well. Heavy-drinking participants receiving one individual sessions of MI reduced their drinking throughout the 6-week follow-up period (26). Another study showed both MI and control groups reducing their drinking over a 2-month follow-up period, with subjects in the MI condition significantly reducing their binge-drinking above and beyond the comparison group (27). McCambridge and Strang also found significant reductions in alcohol use 3 months after a single MI session, although this may have been a subclinical sample (28). However, in other RCTs, no differences were found between MI and no-treatment or TAU control groups on drinking outcomes (29,30). In one such study, both MI and control groups reduced their alcohol consumption at the 6-month postintervention follow-up point but did not differ from one another (30). In another, the significant difference between MI and the control group found at the third month had disappeared by the sixth month of follow-up (29).

In summary, MI has demonstrated efficacy compared to no treatment, TAU, and some comparison treatments for alcohol abuse and dependence. Results appear to be strongest with younger and less-dependent drinkers. There are also some indications that these brief interventions may produce effects that fade in some groups of drinkers. The research supports use of MI for brief interventions and for outpatient treatment for individuals with a range of excessive drinking problems.

However, the exact parameters of who can most benefit from these types of interventions and in which settings they are most effective have not yet been definitively determined.

Opiates

RCTs involving AMI with opiate abusers, either as brief interventions or strategies included throughout treatment, demonstrate inconsistent evidence of treatment efficacy. Out-of-treatment heroin users who received a single, brief motivational intervention during a routine medical visit showed higher rates of abstinence from heroin 6 months later (24). However, in another RCT examining methadone maintenance treatment retention street-recruited injection drug users who received four sessions of MI aimed at entering drug treatment and reducing drug use did not stay in treatment longer than those receiving a four-session risk reduction intervention aimed at safer injection and sex behaviors (31). Earlier studies of MET have also found little support for efficacy in the treatment of opiate users in terms of outcomes and mixed effects on treatment engagement (18).

Amphetamines or Stimulants

There are few studies of MI with amphetamine or stimulant users that were RCTs. However in one RCT, Baker and colleagues compared the effectiveness of two treatment conditions containing one initial MI session followed by either two or four cognitive-behavior therapy sessions with a control group receiving only a self-help booklet to reduce amphetamine use (32). Participants in both treatment groups were significantly more likely than those in the control group to report abstinence from amphetamines, although not confirmed with urinalyses. Abstaining participants also reported less benzodiazepine use, tobacco smoking, polydrug use, injecting risk-taking behavior, criminal activity level, psychiatric distress, and depression.

Cocaine and Crack

Few RCTs have evaluated MI with cocaine users. However, in the same RCT examining heroin use, Bernstein and colleagues found that out-of-treatment cocaine users who received a single, brief MI session during a routine medical visit showed higher rates of abstinence from cocaine at 6-month follow-up, findings consistent with prior reviewed studies of motivational interventions for cocaine use with low-motivated participants (24).

Tobacco

In their meta-analysis of controlled trials examining efficacy of AMIs, Burke, Arkowitz, and Manchola concluded that there was not yet enough evidence to support MI for smoking cessation (18). Few studies met their criteria for an AMI controlled trial. Since that review, however, McCambridge and Strang found a moderate effect size for the reduction of self-reported tobacco use at 3-month follow-up compared to an education-only group for a single MI session with over 200 young persons (ages 16 to 20) using alcohol, cannabis, and/or tobacco (28). Conversely, another study compared abstinence rates across four treatment groups of African American light smokers (<10 cigarettes per day) and found that receiving more directive, advice-oriented health education counseling combined with either nicotine gum or placebo gum was associated with higher cotinine-verified abstinence rates at 6 months compared to a treatment that included an MI component (33).

For older adult patients in the CARES program, there was some support for MET tailored for smoking cessation and delivered by nurses during homecare visits to patients who smoke. A sample of these patients showed more than twice the abstinence rates and significantly more quit attempts and fewer cigarettes smoked per day than those who received only the AHCPR guideline smoking cessation treatment (34). Although there are not many RCTs in this area, MI strategies are often incorporated into smoking cessation interventions in primary care, quitlines, and group formats.

Cannabis

The evidence is mixed for efficacy of MI or MET use in treatment of cannabis abuse or dependence. Few RCTs focus on cannabis use alone and studies vary widely with regard to number of sessions (1 to 12), length of posttreatment follow-up periods (3 to 15 months), and populations (adolescents and young adults, with or without nonacute psychotic disorders or other substance dependencies). Two multisite RCTs involved in the Cannabis Youth Treatment (CYT) used MET in combination with Cognitive Behavioral Therapy (CBT) as part of three of the five treatment options studied. MET was delivered in 2 individual sessions, followed by either 3 CBT group sessions in the first condition (MET/CBT5) or 10 CBT group sessions in the second (MET/CBT12). A third treatment option, called the Family Support Network, added parent education meetings, home visits, and case management. The fourth and fifth treatment options involved case management, 10 to 14 sessions with a therapist, and additional skills training. All five CYT interventions showed significant, positive posttreatment clinical outcomes, measured as rates of abstinence and community functioning up to 12 months later. Minimal differences were found between the conditions, and the MET/CBT5 and MET/CBT12 were found to be among the most cost-effective interventions (35).

McCambridge and Strang found reductions in substance use after 3 months following the single MI session that was greater for heavy alcohol and cannabis users than for heavy cigarette smokers (28). In addition, cannabis use was reduced more in youth considered "high-risk." Another study found greater reductions in cannabis use after a nine-session treatment combining MET with CBT compared with a two-session treatment of MET alone (36). Baker and colleagues reported less promising results in patients with nonacute psychotic disorders; after 10 sessions of MI combined with CBT compared to TAU, short-term improvements were found for reduction of cannabis use but differences disappeared at the 12-month posttreatment rating (37). The populations involved in these studies of MI interventions for cannabis treatment differ from traditional substance treatment studies: psychiatric populations, adolescents, and pregnant women.

EFFICACY OF MOTIVATIONAL INTERVIEWING WITH SPECIAL POPULATIONS

MI has also been used and evaluated with special populations with a variety of substance abuse problems. Special populations, as the title suggests, bring to treatment special considerations that can influence the efficacy of MI-style interventions. In the context of substance use, these populations often experience unique psychosocial, developmental, or contextual factors that can impact change in a variety of ways. Such factors can influence the dose and strategies of motivational interventions that are needed as well as evaluations of efficacy. Empirical studies of these populations warrant separate discussion.

Psychiatric Populations

Two RCTs involving larger doses of MI incorporated throughout treatment for drug abuse showed positive effects of MI on substance use outcomes in dual diagnosis or psychiatric treatment settings. One study of 129 stabilized outpatients meeting DSM criteria for drug dependence (cocaine, heroin, or cannabis) and serious mental illness (schizophrenia, schizoaffective disorder, or major affective disorders), evaluated the efficacy of Behavioral Treatment for Substance Abuse in Severe and Persistent Mental Illness (BTSAS), a multicomponent intervention that included a session MI at baseline, 3 months, and 6 months during treatment, social skills training, and urinalysis evaluation with monetary contingency management for abstinence (38). Compared to a sample of patients receiving supportive discussion treatment, BTSAS participants showed significantly higher percentage of clean urine samples throughout the intervention, longer time to dropout, and higher ratings on self-reported community functioning and quality of life. Utilizing a tailored MI and CBT combined intervention, Baker and colleagues conducted an RCT with a sample of persons with nonacute psychotic disorders. Compared to those receiving TAU, participants receiving one-to-four sessions of MI followed by five-to-ten CBT sessions showed reductions in amphetamine use at 12-month follow-up, although not significantly different from those receiving TAU (37). Reductions in self-reported depression found at 6-month follow-up were also noted for the MI group.

Although general effectiveness for smoking cessation is not established, brief MI interventions may be effective for promoting smoking cessation among patients with serious mental illness. A single MI session with a sample of tobacco smokers with schizophrenia or schizoaffective disorder produced higher rates of contacting tobacco treatment providers and attending a first counseling session for smoking cessation, as compared to educational interventions or advice alone (39). Such findings are promising considering the exceptionally high rates of smoking among adults with SMI.

Adolescents

In addition to the positive findings of studies using MI with cannabis using adolescents, recent studies have demonstrated effectiveness in promoting modification of smoking behavior among adolescents. In a multisite RCT conducted in 37 high schools, specially trained school nurses delivered four one-on-one MI, style smoking cessation interventions to students who smoked in the past month *and* were interested in quitting. Students in the MI condition reported significantly greater abstinence rates and likelihood of quitting at both 6-week and 3-month follow-up compared to a TAU group (40). One MI session in a medical setting given to nontreatment-seeking adolescent smokers demonstrated greater reductions in smoking at 3-month follow-up, biochemically confirmed, as compared to those who received only standardized brief advice to quit smoking (41). Finally, MI used with adolescent problem drinkers demonstrated a sustained decrease in the average number of drinking days per month and frequency of high-volume drinking over a 12-month period compared to controls (42). There is solid support for using MI approaches with adolescents for harm reduction, prevention, and intervention.

Pregnant Women

MI-style interventions have shown promise in helping pregnant smokers to quit or reduce smoking and move along the stages of change, using brief interventions as well as more extensive and manualized interventions (43). However, recent RCTs have produced nonsupportive findings when examining substance use outcomes. MI added to standard health care information researchers provided at home by specially trained midwives did not produce reduction or cessation compared to the standard care (44). Four sessions of individually delivered MET provided to pregnant smokers in methadone maintenance in a hospital-based prenatal program were not more effective than standard care for smoking cessation. Another study of drug abusing pregnant women (cocaine, marijuana, amphetamine or methamphetamine, alcohol, or PCP), compared substance use outcomes between two groups of women referred for treatment (45). Both groups received TAU and either three sessions of MI or an educational control treatment. Treatment condition had no effect on retention or substance use outcomes in this trial. In contrast, cost-effectiveness research comparing MI to usual care has demonstrated an estimated savings in maternal medical costs, quality-adjusted life-years and life-years by selecting MI interventions for relapse prevention among low-income pregnant smokers over other special clinical interventions (46).

SUMMARY

The evidence for the efficacy of MI across substances of abuse and special populations is supportive overall. However, a number of studies have results that are equivocal or fail to support the superiority of this approach. In areas where it has been evaluated more extensively (alcohol, cannabis, and some health behaviors), there is evidence that it is a viable brief intervention, is more efficacious than some comparison treatments, and is usually better than standard care at least for shorter-term outcomes. With other substances, like opiates and cocaine, evidence is less available and what exists is partially supportive. There also seem to be important problem and population dimensions that impact efficacy and effectiveness. Greater severity seems to decrease efficacy of brief interventions, as would be understandable. Some problem areas, like smoking, have yet to demonstrate superiority of MI approaches for cessation, but there is promising evidence for reduction with younger populations. AMIs also seem useful with special populations and can be used with psychiatric and adolescent populations, but the evidence for use with pregnant women is mixed and may depend on the outcome desired and the multiple problems faced by this population.

Overall, MI has received empirical support as an intervention for (a) brief interventions, (b) as an adjunct to other treatments, and (c) sometimes as a free-standing treatment depending on the type of substance, severity of the problem, and the multiplicity of client problems. It has also been successfully used with various special populations including those with psychiatric problems and with adolescents. Its utility with pregnant women seems more problematic in stringent tests of the intervention. Evidence for the superiority of MI to other credible and viable interventions and treatments, however, has yet to be established in many areas. The utility of AMI approaches for treatment engagement and retention is promising but also needs additional controlled research.

HOW THE TREATMENT IS OPTIMALLY USED

Since MI is predominantly a style of interacting that includes a number of strategies and techniques, it can take many different forms and be adapted for use in many different settings. It seems to have been used most successfully as an intervention to address ambivalence and defuse resistance to change in brief interventions. However, this approach has been adapted for use in a more extensive, though still rather brief formats, including MET and also incorporated as a component in combination treatments with cognitive-behavioral approaches (47). As noted in the review above, there is evidence for effectiveness for each type of use with one or another of the substances of abuse. Optimal use of MI would depend on the type of problem and population, the objective of the intervention, the skill and training of the providers, and the nature of the intervention setting. We will describe and reference applications that have been used in various studies.

Burke, Arkowitz, and Dunn concluded that the state of the current research was such that very little is known about precisely how MI works to elicit various treatment outcomes (3). Some research indicates that the impact may be mediated by the motivational style of warmth and empathy communicated by the counselor, or the effect of offering tailored assessment feedback, or by promoting treatment participation which then affects behavioral outcomes. Nonetheless, it appears that both brief and more extensive MI-style treatments show efficacy. Following are descriptions of the unique features of each MI treatment that has shown significant effects in at least one of the following outcomes: substance use, substance-related problems, treatment engagement, retention or compliance, quality of life, and general functioning. Developers of these various MI-style interventions have been working to better understand the optimal combination of MI dose and strategy for promoting change in substance abuse.

Brief Interventions

Brief motivational interventions tend to take place in one-to-four sessions either as a substitute for treatment, a brief motivational intervention in an opportunistic setting or moment, or as a part of a screening brief intervention, referral, and treatment protocol. Brief interventions are administered instead of, or early in, treatment and sometimes as a pretreatment intervention to engage a client in treatment. These interventions focus on applying the styles, strategies, and select techniques of MI in order to help the client resolve ambivalence about change and move toward reducing or abstaining from substance use. Brief MI interventions also can be used to promote engaging in treatment creating a supportive environment for the client through empathy and active listening. Variations depend upon the setting and client goals.

Primary Care/Medical/Health Care Settings

Although patient-centered communication is becoming a standard element of medical student education, MI offers a very specific way to interview and negotiate change with patients particularly about chronic disease risk behaviors including smoking, diet, cancer screening, physical activity, and alcohol and drug use (1). Brief health behavior change interventions (from 5 to 20 minutes) by general and specialty medical practitioners or other health care providers (nurses, physician assistants, or behavior change specialists) often have incorporated MI strategies in their design (18). These interventions can be structured and well-defined like the Five A's for smoking cessation: Ask about current substance use, Advise clients to consider reducing or quitting their substance use, Assess their readiness to quit, Assist client in finding options for treatment or change plan, and Arrange for a follow-up (48). These interventions can also consist of a semiscripted individual interview during a routine medical visit and have also been incorporated in home health care visits for elderly and for pregnant women (24,44).

Screening and brief interventions for alcohol and drug abuse that often incorporate an MI-style and one or more of the strategies and techniques (open-ended questions, reflective listening, summarizing, and choice) are being used in many different opportunistic as well as substance abuse treatment settings. The amount of time allocated to these types of interventions ranges from 20 minutes to roughly an hour in a single session; settings range from emergency rooms or trauma centers to rural health care centers; and treatment can be focused on alcohol or drug use behaviors with patients including college students, young adult, and heavy or hazardous drinkers (21,23,25–28). Slightly longer brief MI-based interventions consisting of a couple of sessions or with additional feedback and/or contact by phone or mail have also been used with various populations in health care settings (36).

Pretreatment and Addictions Treatment

MI strategies have also been incorporated into one, 2-hour assessment and evaluation session or in pretreatment sessions at the beginning of substance abuse treatment programs (18,19). MI has also been extended into a stand-alone treatment that has been manualized for use in alcoholism treatment in the form of MET (16) that consists of four one and a half hour sessions spread over 12 weeks. This treatment has been used in other treatment trials (UK alcoholism treatment trial, UKATT) and has been adapted for use with various types of substances (49). However, more frequently, AMI have combined it with other forms of treatment either by making MI-style and strategies part of the entire program or by combining MI sessions with additional CBT sessions or combining the two types of treatment into an eclectic mix (50). MI has also been combined with other treatments for managing substance abuse problems in individuals with mental illness (38).

SPECIAL CONSIDERATIONS

There are a number of important considerations and concerns about MI that affect evaluations and recommendations for use. We will describe these in the following categories: fidelity and training, evaluations challenges, and barriers to effective use of MI.

Fidelity and Training

Many practitioners have been exposed to MI in presentations, workshops, and trainings. Some of the assumptions, principles, and techniques are familiar and similar to what practitioners believe are basic skills already learned in their formation as clinicians (empathy, listening, and respect for clients). However, the familiarity is deceptive and the ease of implementation is overestimated by many. What individuals mean when they assert that they are using MI varies greatly. The developers have been very cognizant of the need for screening and extensive training of practitioners (51,52). They have also used detailed evaluations of taped interactions to assess fidelity to the MI approach in various research studies (17). Evaluating MI-consistent and -inconsistent behaviors of practitioners seem to be critical for fidelity and effectiveness with the inconsistent behaviors predictive of worse outcomes (53). Although style and strategies/techniques have been taught, the essential skills needed to execute MI approaches with fidelity have not been clearly delineated. It does seem that clinicians who have difficulty being or appearing empathic or being nonjudgmental about the specific behavior being discussed, have difficulty sitting back and listening, cannot tolerate ambivalence, or get hooked by resistance behaviors will have a difficult time using MI (54). Adequate training and selection of practitioners is a critical consideration for implementing MI with fidelity.

In professional communications and evaluations it is also important to be clear when using or assessing MI approaches. Practitioners and programs should clearly identify how they are using MI in their program. Are they incorporating only the style and spirit, only some strategies, or are they trying to adopt the entire approach? MI is primarily motivational. What are they doing to assist and support other dimensions of behavior change for their clients? When combining MI with other approaches, how are practitioners making sure these treatments are compatible and what is the explicit strategy for integration or combination of MI with the other approaches? These are critical questions for implementation and especially for evaluation of MI as a brief or more extensive interventions technique.

Evaluation Challenges

In addition to fidelity of implementation and the skill and practices of the individual practitioners who are using MI in the various settings described above, there are a number of other challenges for accurate evaluation of MI. Caution should be used in reading studies and evaluations in the literature. It is not clear what are the appropriate outcomes for evaluating MI interventions. Behavior change is often the intervention goal, yet MI is focused on the motivational dimensions of change and empowerment of the individual to choose to change. Goals of clients and goals of interventions vary greatly. An abstinence-based alcoholism treatment program could have a client with a personal goal of moderation, and successful MI would be marked by reduction in use and not necessarily abstinence. A variety of other outcomes would be appropriate beyond drinking or drug use: stage movement, harm reduction, treatment engagement and retention, general functioning, quality of life, and reduction of substance-related consequences. In fact, some studies have shown that results may include some of these outcomes, like reduction in consequences, without necessarily seeing differences in drinking levels (42).

Another important dimension to be considered in the evaluation of MI is the heterogeneity of the individuals included in the intervention. Dramatic differences were observed in the ages, gender, problem severity, consequences, and sociodemographic characteristics of participants in the previously reviewed studies. Results often indicate that sometimes individuals with less severe problems and sometimes those with more consequences benefit most from MI. Studies with adolescents, who might be considered good candidates for this approach because of adolescent oppositionality, have had positive but mixed findings. Initial indications are that MI works equally well for men and women but there are a number of smoking cessation studies with pregnant women where these women have not responded to this approach. When treatment goals include behavior changes needed to address multiple problems or health behaviors, most interventions find this challenging, and MI is no exception. Motivation for each problem area may be distinct, and brief interventions are more problematic with reciprocally complicating conditions. In terms of populations and settings, the critical dimensions of with whom and how MI works have not yet been resolved.

A final consideration about the evaluation of MI pertains to researchers conducting the studies. Burke and colleagues noted in their review that studies conducted by proponents of MI produced higher effect sizes, on average, than other studies. This could be due to investigator allegiance effects and/or execution of MI in terms of training and supervision, or the intense monitoring involved in these studies. However a practical implication of this observation is that well-implemented and supervised MI has greater efficacy.

Barriers to Implementing MI

There are a number of barriers that practitioners and trainers of MI approaches should address in their work and the following seem to be among the most important:

- Most clinics use closed-ended questions during intake procedures to establish diagnosis and treatment options. Although often necessary for efficient triaging of patients, this type of interaction is contrary to the spirit and strategies of MI. Shifting between intake mode and MI mode presents a challenge since interactions with the client have been established in the intake that are difficult to change. Efforts must be made to distinguish intake mode from MI intervention to reduce confusion.
- MI promotes client talk and provider listening. During brief interventions providers are often fearful that promoting client talk will extend the session beyond what is feasible, allowable, reimbursable, and practical. Providers who have only limited time need to be taught not only how to promote client conversation but also how to direct and manage client conversations to meet the demands of the setting and the time allocated for this intervention. Using transitional and closing summaries, skillful messaging about having heard the client's concerns, and effective management of boundaries imposed by limits of time are critical to health care providers implementing and keeping brief interventions brief.
- Standardizing MI interventions is difficult and creating manuals that overdetermine provider behaviors and responses are problematic. Programs that want to include MI have to provide for some structure as well as some flexibility in implementation.
- MI is not nondirective. Individuals beginning to learn MI often mistake reflective listening as never giving advice or setting limits. Nothing could be further from the truth. Miller and Rollnick describe MI as a directive but nonconfrontational approach that does not eliminate the role and expertise of the provider (3).

CONCLUSION

MI is an innovative style of interacting with individuals who have substance abuse problems that includes a set of strategies and techniques and also demands a specific skill set. Although not a complete therapy designed to intervene intensively during the entire scope of the change process from lack of interest and ambivalence to sustained change, its style and principles can be used to engage, motivate, and guide individuals throughout the change process. MI can be used as a brief intervention or combined with multiple other types of treatments either as a backdrop or a companion treatment. There is a growing body of research that indicates efficacy for a variety of populations and problems. However, supporting evidence is not unequivocal and there is a need for additional research on the scope of its effectiveness. Practitioners can incorporate MI-style and strategies with benefit especially in addressing the needs of less motivated clients. Careful implementation while paying attention both to the limitations and the multiple potential ways of integrating MI into both prevention and treatment of substance abuse is recommended.

REFERENCES

1. Rollnick S, Miller WR, Butler CC. *Motivational Interviewing in Health Care: Helping Patients Change Behavior*. New York, NY: Guilford Press; 2008.
2. Miller WR, Rollnick S. *Motivational Interviewing: Preparing People to Change Addictive Behavior*. New York, NY: Guilford; 1991.
3. Miller WR, Rollnick S. *Motivational Interviewing: Preparing People for Change*. 2nd ed. New York, NY: Guilford Press; 2002.
4. DiClemente CC. Mechanisms, determinants and processes of change in the modification of drinking behavior. *Alcohol Clin Exp Res*. 2007;31:13s–20s.
5. DiClemente CC. *Addiction and Change: How Addictions Develop and Addicted People Recover*. New York, NY: Guilford Press; 2003.
6. Edwards G. Alcoholism: a controlled trial of treatment and advice. *J Stud Alcohol Drugs*. 1977;38:1004–1031.
7. Miller WR, Sovereign RG, Krege B. Motivational interviewing with problem drinkers II: the Drinker's Check-up as a preventive intervention. *Behav Psychother*. 1988;16:251–268.
8. Prochaska JO, DiClemente CC. *The Transtheoretical Approach: Crossing the Traditional Boundaries of Therapy*. Homewood, IL: Dow Jones-Irwin; 1984.
9. Prochaska JO, DiClemente CC, Norcross JC. In search of how people change: applications to addictive behaviors. *Am Psychol*. 1992;47:1102–1114.

10. Prochaska JO, DiClemente CC. Toward a comprehensive model of change. In: Miller WR, Heather N, eds. *Treating Addictive Behaviors: Processes of Change.* New York, NY: Plenum Press; 1986:3–28.
11. Janis IL, Janis IL, Mann L. *Decision Making: A Psychological Analysis of Conflict, Choice, and Commitment.* New York, NY: Free Press; 1977.
12. Miller WR. Motivation for treatment: a review with special emphasis on alcoholism. *Psychol Bull.* 1985;98:84–107.
13. Miller WR, Hester RK. The effectiveness of alcoholism treatment: what research reveals. In: Miller WR, Heather N, eds. *Treating Addictive Behaviors: Processes of Change.* New York, NY: Plenum Press; 1986:121–174.
14. Rollnick S, Mason P, Butler C, eds. *Health Behavior Change: A Guide for Practitioners.* Edinburgh, UK: Churchill Livingstone; 1999.
15. Barry KL. Consensus panel chair. *Treatment Improvement Protocol (TIP) Series 34: Brief Interventions and Brief Therapies for Substance Abuse.* SAMHSA Publication No (SMA) 99-3353. Rockville, MD: U.S. Department of Health and Human Services; 1999.
16. Miller WR, Zweben A, DiClemente CC, et al. *Motivational Enhancement Therapy Manual: A Clinical Research Guide for Therapists Treating Individuals with Alcohol Abuse and Dependence.* Rockville, MD: U.S. Department of Health and Human Services; 1992.
17. Moyers TB, Martin T, Manuel JK, et al. Assessing competence in motivational interviewing. *J Subst Abuse Treat.* 2005;28:19–26.
18. Burke BL, Arkowitz H, Menchola M. The efficacy of motivational interviewing: a meta-analysis of controlled clinical trials. *J Cons Clin Psychol.* 2003;71:843–861.
19. Carroll KM, Ball SA, Nich C, et al. Motivational interviewing to improve treatment engagement and outcome in individuals seeking treatment for substance abuse: a multisite effectiveness study. *Drug Alcohol Depend.* 2006;81:301–312.
20. Miller WR, Yahne CE, Tonigan JS. Motivational interviewing in drug abuse services: a randomized trial. *J Cons Clin Psychol.* 2003; 71:754–763.
21. Vasilaki EI, Hosier SG, Cox WM. The efficacy of motivational interviewing as a brief intervention for excessive drinking: a meta-analytic review. *Alcohol Alcsm.* 2006;41:328–335.
22. Project MATCH Research Group: Matching alcoholism treatments to client heterogeneity: Project MATCH posttreatment drinking outcomes. *J Stud Alc Drugs.* 1997;58:7–29.
23. Hester RK, Squires DD, Delaney HD. The Drinker's Check-up: 12-month outcomes of a controlled clinical trial of a stand-alone software program for problem drinkers. *J Subst Abuse Treat.* 2005;28:159–169.
24. Bernstein J, Bernstein E, Tassiopoulos K, et al. Brief motivational intervention at a clinic visit reduces cocaine and heroin use. *Drug Alcohol Depend.* 2005;77:49–59.
25. Gentilello LM, Rivara FP, Donovan DM, et al. Alcohol interventions in a trauma center as a means of reducing the risk of injury recurrence. *Ann Surg.* 1999;230:473–484.
26. Beckham N. Motivational interviewing with hazardous drinkers. *J Am Acad Nurse Pract.* 2007;19:103–110.
27. Feldstein SW, Forcehimes AA. Motivational interviewing with underage college drinkers: a preliminary look at the role of empathy and alliance. *Am J Drug Alc Abuse.* 2007;33:737–746.
28. McCambridge J, Strang J. The efficacy of single-session motivational interviewing in reducing drug consumption and perceptions of drug-related risk and harm among young people: results from a multi-site cluster randomized trial. *Addiction.* 2004; 99:39–52.
29. Connors GJ, Walitzer KS, Dermen KH. Preparing clients for alcoholism treatment: effects on treatment participation and outcomes. *J Cons Clin Psychol.* 2002;70:1161–1169.
30. Emmen MJ, Schippers GM, Wollersheim H, et al. Adding psychologist's intervention to physician's advice to problem drinkers in the outpatient clinic. *Alcohol Alcsm.* 2005;40:219–226.
31. Booth RE, Corsi KF, Mikulich-Gilbertson SK. Factors associated with methadone maintenance treatment retention among street-recruited injection drug users. *Drug Alcohol Depend.* 2004;74: 177–185.
32. Baker A, Lee NK, Claire M, et al. Brief cognitive behavioural interventions for regular amphetamine users: a step in the right direction. *Addiction.* 2005;100:367–378.
33. Nollen NL, Mayo MS, Cox LS, et al. Predictors of quitting among African American light smokers enrolled in a randomized, placebo-controlled trial. *J Gen Intern Med.* 2006;21: 590–595.
34. Borrelli B, Novak S, Hecht J, et al. Home health care nurses as a new channel for smoking cessation treatment: outcomes from project CARES (Community-nurse Assisted Research and Education on Smoking). *Prev Med.* 2005;41:815–821.
35. Dennis M, Godley SH, Diamond G, et al. The Cannabis Youth Treatment (CYT) study: main findings from two randomized trials. *J Subst Abuse Treat.* 2004;27:197–213.
36. Babor TF. Brief treatments for cannabis dependence: findings from a randomized multisite trial. *J Cons Clin Psychol.* 2004;72: 455–466.
37. Baker A, Bucci S, Lewin TJ, et al. Cognitive-behavioural therapy for substance use disorders in people with psychotic disorders: randomised controlled trial. *Br J Psychiatry.* 2006;188: 439–448.
38. Bellack AS, Bennett ME, Gearon JS, et al. A randomized clinical trial of a new behavioral treatment for drug abuse in people with severe and persistent mental illness. *Arch Gen Psychiatry.* 2006; 63:426–432.
39. Steinberg ML, Ziedonis DM, Krejci JA, et al. Motivational interviewing with personalized feedback: a brief intervention for motivating smokers with schizophrenia to seek treatment for tobacco dependence. *J Cons Clin Psychol.* 2004;72:723–728.
40. Pbert L, Osganian SK, Gorak D, et al. A school nurse-delivered adolescent smoking cessation intervention: a randomized controlled trial. *Prev Med.* 2006;43:312–320.
41. Colby SM, Monti PM, Tevyaw TOL, et al. Brief motivational intervention for adolescent smokers in medical settings. *Addict Behav.* 2005;30:865–874.
42. Spirito A, Monti PM, Barnett NP, et al. A randomized clinical trial of a brief motivational intervention for alcohol-positive adolescents treated in an emergency department. *J Pediatr.* 2004; 145:396–402.
43. Velasquez MM, Hecht J, Quinn V, et al. Application of motivational interviewing to prenatal smoking cessation: training and implementation issues. *Tob Control.* 2000;9:iii36–iii40.
44. Tappin DM, Lumsden MA, Gilmour WH, et al. Randomised controlled trial of home based motivational interviewing by midwives to help pregnant smokers quit or cut down. (Cover story). *Br Med J.* 2005;331:373–375.
45. Mullins SM, Suarez M, Ondersma SJ, et al. The impact of motivational interviewing on substance abuse treatment retention: a randomized control trial of women involved with child welfare. *J Subst Abuse Treat.* 2004;27:51–58.

46. Ruger JP, Weinstein MC, Hammond SK, et al. Cost-effectiveness of motivational interviewing for smoking cessation and relapse prevention among low-income pregnant women: a randomized controlled trial. *Value Health*. 2008;11:191–198.
47. Anton RF, O'Malley SS, Ciraulo DA, et al. Combined pharmacotherapies and behavioral interventions for alcohol dependence: the COMBINE study: a randomized controlled trial. *J Am Med Assoc*. 2006;295:2003–2017.
48. Fiore MC, Jaen CR, Baker TB, et al. *Treating Tobacco Use and Dependence 2008 Update: Clinical Practice Guideline*. Rockville, MD: U.S. Department of Health and Human Services; 2008.
49. UKATT: Effectiveness of treatment for alcohol problems: findings of the randomised UK alcohol treatment trial (UKATT). *Br Med J*. 2005;331.
50. Velasquez MM, Maurer GG, Crouch C, et al. *Group Treatment for Substance Abuse: A Stages-of-Change Therapy Manual*. New York, NY: Guilford Press; 2001.
51. Miller WR, Yahne CE, Moyers TB, et al. A randomized, controlled trial of methods to help clinicians learn MI. *J Cons Clin Psychol*. 2006;72:1050–1062.
52. Rosengren DB. *Building Motivational Interviewing Skills: A Practitioner Workbook*. New York, NY: Guilford Press; 2009.
53. Moyers TB, Martin T, Houck JM, et al. From in-session behaviors to drinking outcomes: a causal chain for motivational interviewing. *J Cons Clin Psychol*. 2009;77:1113–1124.
54. Moyers TB, Manuel JK, Wilson P, et al. A randomized trial investigating training in motivational interviewing for behavioral health providers. *Behav Cogn Psychother*. 2008;36:149–162.

CHAPTER 47: Relapse Prevention

Dennis C. Daley ■ G. Alan Marlatt ■ Antoine Douaihy

Substance use disorders (SUDs) represent a serious public health problem in the United States. They are associated with many serious medical, psychiatric, family, occupational, legal, financial, and spiritual problems. SUDs not only cause impairment and suffering on the part of the affected individual, but they also create a significant burden for the family and society (1). The conceptual model of addiction as a chronic disorder requiring long-term management has been widely accepted within the substance abuse treatment field (2). Despite the fact that longitudinal studies have repeatedly demonstrated that substance abuse treatment is associated with major reductions in substance use, other studies showed that the majority of individuals relapse at some point following a treatment episode and many of them subsequently reenter treatment (3). To better understand addiction, it is useful to take a "life course perspective," in which substance use, treatment, relapse, and recovery are not viewed as discrete and single events but rather as stages in a chronic and cyclical process where drug use patterns and treatment episodes influence later experiences (4,5). Relapse prevention (RP) is a cognitive–behavioral approach with the goal of identifying and addressing high-risk situations for relapse, and assisting individuals in maintaining desired behavioral changes. RP strategies are often incorporated into individual and group treatment manuals. RP techniques may be supplemented by other treatments for SUDs such as pharmacotherapy or mindfulness meditation (6,7).

This chapter provides an overview of relapse and RP. We define lapse, relapse, and recovery, and review treatment outcome studies, empirical studies of RP approaches, relapse precipitants, models of RP, and the recent conceptualization of relapse as a dynamic process. We then integrate the RP literature by discussing cognitive and behavioral strategies that clinicians can implement with patients with any type of SUD to reduce lapse and relapse risk. Finally we briefly discuss future research directions and their relevance to clinical care.

OVERVIEW OF LAPSE, RELAPSE, AND RECOVERY

Lapse and Relapse

The term *lapse* refers to the initial episode of alcohol or other drug use following a period of abstinence, whereas the term *relapse* refers to failure to maintain behavior change over time: "a breakdown or setback in the person's attempt to change or modify a target behavior" (8). Other conceptualization of relapse includes complex multidimensional composite indices of outcome/relapse, taking into account the different aspects of return to problematic behavior and the presence or absence of related consequences that go beyond the simple concept of abstinence–lapse–relapse and fit more into the concept of a harm-reduction approach (9). So relapse can be viewed not only as the event of resumption of a pattern of substance abuse or dependence, but also as a process in which indicators or warning signs appear prior to the individual's actual substance use (2).

A lapse may end quickly or lead to a relapse of varying proportions. Shiffman (10), for example, reported that 63% of smoking lapsers who called his Stay-Quit line were smoking 2 weeks later; only 37% were able to stop their lapses. Other studies had shown that a lapse does not necessarily lead to a full-blown relapse in users of opiates (11) and tobacco (12). Based on different conceptualization and methodologic approaches to understanding relapse, relapse is better understood as both a dichotomous outcome and a process involving a series of prior related events and the predictors of these events interfering with behavior change (13). A dynamic conceptual and clinical assessment model would better capture all the variables of relapse as it unfolds across time (14). The effects of the initial lapse are mediated by the person's affective and cognitive reactions. A full-blown relapse is more likely with the individual who has a strong perception of violating the abstinence rule (self-blame and loss of perceived control that individuals experience after the violations of self-imposed rules) (15). Although some individuals experience a full-blown relapse and return to pretreatment levels of substance abuse, others use alcohol and drugs problematically, but do not return to previous levels of abuse or dependence and suffer less-harmful effects as a result. Relapsers vary in the quantity and frequency of substance use as well as in the medical and psychosocial sequelae that accompany a relapse.

Recovery

Most researchers implicitly define "recovery" in terms of substance use only and most often as abstinence, either total abstinence or from the specific substance under study (4). Several terms have been used such as remission, resolution, abstinence, and recovery. Some authors use DSM-IV Criteria (16) to define recovery. The emphasis on abstinence and equating it with recovery has been connected with the influence of abstinence-based 12-step recovery principles and it has been also embraced by the American Society of Addiction Medicine definition of recovery as "overcoming both physical and psychological dependence to the psychoactive drug while making a commitment to sobriety" (17). Recovery was generally described as a process rather than an end point, and even among participants who did not define recovery in terms of substance use, abstaining from all mood-altering substances was perceived as a prerequisite to the other benefits of recovery (18). McLellan and colleagues have pointed out that "Typically the immediate goal of reducing alcohol and drug use is necessary but rarely sufficient for the achievement of the longer-term goals of improved personal health and social function and reduced threats to public health and safety—that is, recovery," (2: p. 448). Therefore recovery from SUDs is the process of initiating abstinence from alcohol or other drug use, as well as making intrapersonal and interpersonal changes to maintain this change over time. Specific changes and improvements vary among people with SUDs and can occur in any of the following areas of functioning: physical, psychological, behavioral, interpersonal, family, social, spiritual, and financial (13). It is generally accepted that recovery tasks are contingent on the stage or phase of recovery the individual is in (19). Recovery is mediated by the severity and degree of damage caused by the SUD, the presence of a comorbid psychiatric or medical illness, and the individual's perception, motivation, gender, ethnic background, and support system. Gender similarities and differences have been more recently explored in the treatment, relapse and recovery cycle. Women are one third less likely to transition form one status to another (recovery, treatment, incarceration, and using) and predictors of transitioning to different statuses vary by gender (20). Numerous longitudinal studies have shown that on average, people reached sustained abstinence only after three to four episodes of different kinds of treatments over a number of years (4,21). Scott and colleagues (4) showed that over a 2-year period, 82% of drug users transitioned one or more times between use, incarceration, treatment, and recovery. An average of 32% changed over 90 days, with movement in every direction, and treatment increased the likelihood of getting to recovery (6). The risk of relapse is particularly problematic in the first 3 years of abstinence and never completely goes away (22). Although some individuals may achieve full recovery, others achieve a partial recovery. The latter may experience multiple relapses over time.

Recovering from a SUD involves psychoeducation, increasing self-awareness, developing coping skills for sober living, and following a program of change (13). The program of change may involve professional treatment, participation in self-help programs (Alcoholics Anonymous [AA], Narcotics Anonymous [NA], Cocaine Anonymous [CA], Crystal Meth Anonymous [CMA], Rational Recovery, SMART Recovery, Men or Women for Sobriety, or Dual Recovery Anonymous [DRA]), psychotherapy, pharmacotherapy, case management, and self-management approaches. The information and skills learned as part of RP offer an excellent mechanism to prepare for the maintenance phase of recovery. In the earlier phases of recovery, the individual typically relies more on external support and help from professionals, sponsors, or other members of support groups. As recovery progresses, more reliance is placed on oneself to handle problems and the challenges of living a sober lifestyle. Flynn and colleagues (23) followed a group of opioid users 5 years after treatment and compared those who were in recovery and those who were not. The subjects in recovery were more likely to benefit from family and friends as a support group. In addition, those subjects were nearly four times more likely to perceive themselves as improving their quality of life.

TREATMENT OUTCOME STUDIES

Numerous reviews of the treatment outcome literature, as well as studies of specific clinical populations receiving treatment, document variable rates of relapse among alcoholics, smokers, and drug abusers. Despite the high relapse rates reported in some studies, treatment has a positive effect on multiple domains of functioning for treated alcoholics and drug-dependent individuals. Outcome is best viewed by considering multiple domains: substance use, as well as social, familial, and psychological functioning. SUDs are not unlike other chronic or recurrent medical or psychiatric conditions in that recovery is not a linear process and relapses do occur, yet significant improvements are often made.

Miller and Hester reviewed more than 500 alcoholism outcome studies and reported that more than 75% of subjects relapsed within 1 year of treatment (24). In another analysis of the alcohol treatment outcome literature, Miller and colleagues reported that there was a "significant" treatment effect on at least one alcohol measure for at least one follow-up point for 146 of 211 studies (25, p. 17).

McLellan and colleagues reviewed more than 100 clinical trials of drug abuse treatment and found that most patients show favorable outcomes at the 1-year follow-up period: 40% to 60% are continuously abstinent and 15% to 30% are not using drugs addictively (26). Catalano and colleagues reviewed studies of relapse rates and found relapse rates ranging from 25% to 97% for opioid addiction and from 75% to 80% for tobacco dependence within 1 year of treatment (27). Relapse rates were lowest among opiate addicts who graduated from a therapeutic community in which they resided for a minimum of 18 to 24 months. Hoffmann and Harrison (28) followed 1957 adult patients with alcohol and/or drug problems who were treated in five different treatment centers in the St. Paul, Minnesota, area. They reported that approximately 50% of patients were abstinent for the entire 2-year period. The Comprehensive Assessment and Treatment Outcome Research (CATOR) group, an independent evaluation service for the substance abuse field, followed 8087 patients from 38 inpatient programs and 1663 patients from 19 different outpatient programs for 1 year (29). Sobriety rates at 1 year were 60% for inpatient and 68% for outpatient subjects successfully contacted at 6 and 12 months. Even when these rates are adjusted and assume a 70% relapse rate for missing cases, sobriety rates at 1 year are 44%

and 52% for the inpatient and outpatient cohorts. Numerous reports by the National Institute on Drug Abuse, and the Center for Substance Abuse Treatments document the following positive outcomes for treatment of alcohol and drug abuse: cessation or reduction of substance use; decreases in posttreatment medical care and medical costs; decreases in work problems including absenteeism and working under the influence; decreases in traffic violations and other arrests; and improvement in psychological, social, and family functioning (30).

Individuals who relapse do not always return to pretreatment levels of substance use. The actual quantity and frequency of use may vary dramatically. A cocaine or heroin addict who injected large quantities of drugs on a daily basis for years may return to substance use after treatment. Yet this individual may not return to daily use, and the quantity of drugs used may be significantly less than the pretreatment level. Because drug and alcohol use is only one outcome measure, an individual may show improvement in other areas of life functioning despite an actual lapse or relapse to substance use. Patients who remain in treatment the longest have the best outcomes (30). A recent review exploring gender differences in alcohol and substance abuse relapse showed that for women, marriage and marital stress were risk factors for alcohol relapse and among men, marriage lowered the relapse risk (31). Recent research is attempting to identify predictors of treatment performance and outcome (32).

Empirical Studies of RP

A growing number of studies have evaluated the effectiveness and efficacy of RP approaches for SUDs. Carroll (33) reviewed 24 randomized controlled trials on the effectiveness of RP among smokers (12 studies), alcohol abusers (6 studies), marijuana abusers (1 study), cocaine abusers (3 studies), the opiate addicted (1 study), and other drug abusers (1 study). Carroll reported that the strongest evidence for efficacy of RP is with smokers and concluded that "there is good evidence for RP approaches compared with no-treatment controls … [and that] outcomes where RP may hold greater promise include reducing severity of relapses when they occur, durability of effects after cessation, and patient-treatment matching" (33: p. 53). Patients with higher levels of impairment along dimensions such as psychiatric severity and addiction severity appear to benefit most from RP when compared to those with less-severe levels of impairment. Thus, RP may be especially helpful for patients with co-occurring psychiatric disorders.

A meta-analysis of 26 clinical trials by Irvin and colleagues involving 9504 participants supports the efficacy of Marlatt and Gordon's RP model (34). This analysis found the strongest treatment effects for RP with participants who had problems with alcohol and polysubstance use, the effects were weaker for smoking and cocaine. Randomized trials of RP for smoking showed that additional support elements such as stress management and abstinence "resource renewal" may be needed in a smoking intervention (35).

Carroll and colleagues (36) conducted a study of outpatient cocaine abusers in which they compared RP to interpersonal psychotherapy (IPT). RP was more effective than IPT for patients with more severe cocaine problems and, to some extent, for those with higher psychiatric severity. In another study of outpatient cocaine abusers, Carroll and colleagues (37) compared the outcomes of 12 weeks of treatment in which patients were randomized to psychotherapy (cognitive–behavioral RP or an operationalized clinical management condition) and pharmacotherapy (desipramine hydrochloride or placebo). Patients were followed for 1 year and the research team found a significant psychotherapy-by-time effect, indicating a delayed improved response to treatment for patients who received RP. A study by Wells and colleagues (38) of outpatient cocaine abusers comparing RP and 12-step counseling found that subjects in both treatment conditions reduced their use of cocaine, marijuana, and alcohol use at 6 months posttreatment. However, subjects in the 12-step counseling condition showed greater improvement in alcohol use when compared to those receiving RP at the 6-month follow-up period. Another study followed 121 patients with cocaine dependence that were randomized to one of four conditions in a 2×2 factorial design: disulfiram plus CBT, disulfiram plus IPT that did not include RP components, placebo plus CBT, and placebo plus IPT. The patients assigned to CBT reduced their cocaine use more significantly than those assigned to IPT, and patients assigned to disulfiram reduced their cocaine significantly more than those assigned to placebo. In addition, the CBT × time effect remained statistically significant after controlling for retention, which was a significant predictor of better drug use outcomes (39).

A study of inpatient alcoholic veterans found that results consistently favored veterans receiving RP over those receiving a discussion group (40). Subjects in the RP group drank less, had fewer episodes of intoxication, experienced less severe lapses for shorter periods of time, and stopped drinking significantly sooner after a relapse compared to subjects in the discussion group. Another study of alcoholics receiving inpatient treatment found that there was greater treatment adherence and satisfaction, reduced lengths of inpatient treatment, and fewer alcohol-related arrests among patients receiving RP compared to patients receiving other treatment modalities (41). A study of hospitalized male alcoholics found that patients treated with RP compared to interpersonal process therapy drank on fewer days, drank less alcohol, completed more aftercare, and had a slightly higher rate of continuous abstinence at 6-month follow-up (42).

Two large studies comparing the effectiveness of CBT to other active treatments that emphasize the use of 12-step fellowship have demonstrated no difference between conditions at follow-up. Results of Project MATCH (Matching Alcoholism Treatments to Client Heterogeneity), a large-scale multisite, randomized clinical trial of three manual-driven treatments (cognitive–behavioral therapy: CBT; motivational enhancement therapy: MET; twelve-step facilitation therapy: TSF), showed significant reductions in days of alcohol use and drinks per day at both the 1- and 3-year follow-up periods (43). The second study was naturalistic, involved veterans, and showed that patients in all three conditions (CBT, TSF, or a combination of both) performed equally well at 1-year follow-up (44).

Recent randomized controlled trials support the reported efficacy of combined CBT-like therapies and naltrexone for alcohol-dependent individuals (45). The COMBINE (Combined Pharmacotherapies and Behavioral Intervention) study suggested that medical management of an alcohol-dependent patient with a physician providing treatment with naltrexone and basic advice and information is as effective as CBT. That trial enrolled 1383 alcohol-dependent subjects and randomly assigned them to one of eight groups that could include naltrexone, acamprosate, or both of the drugs, with or without what was identified as a cognitive–behavioral intervention (CBI). One group received the CBI alone without the placebo. The patients who received a medication also received medical management that was fairly rigorous (9 appointments over 16 weeks), during which a physician or a nurse discussed the patient's diagnosis and progress and suggested attendance to AA. Those who got the CBI received up to 20 sessions, which was comparable with a streamlined version of outpatient alcoholism treatment. Subjects receiving medical management with naltrexone, CBI or both, fared better on drinking outcomes, whereas acamprosate showed no evidence of efficacy, with or without CBI. Putting it more into clinical implications, the percentage of subjects with a good clinical outcome were 58% for those who received only medical management and placebo, 74% for those who received medical management with naltrexone only, 74% for those who received medical management with naltrexone and CBI, and 71% for those who received medical management with placebo and CBI. The subjects were followed for a year after the 16-week treatment, and although the patterns of efficacy remained much the same, there were appreciable falloff for all groups (46–48).

Some data support the view that the response to RP treatment is quite comparable between cocaine-dependent individuals and those dependent on methamphetamine (49). Rawson and colleagues conducted a study with methamphetamine-dependent individuals assessing the effectiveness of the Matrix treatment protocol which is based on cognitive–behavioral principles of Marlatt and Gordon, 1985 (8) and used in an intensive outpatient treatment setting (50), versus "treatment as usual" in eight community treatment organizations. The in-treatment gains made by participants in the Matrix suggest that this treatment approach has positive effects.

The empirical literature on evaluating RP strategies for cannabis dependence has incorporated other strategies. A multisite study involving 450 marijuana-dependent individuals demonstrated that an integrated CBT and Motivational Interviewing (MI) was more effective than MI alone, which in turn was more effective than a delayed treatment control condition (51). There are no efficacy studies evaluating RP specifically for abuse of club drugs, hallucinogens, inhalants, and steroids (52).

The most recent meta-analysis that focused solely on smoking and included 42 studies of controlled trials with at least 6 months follow-up, most of which used skills training approaches, showed small and no significant effects for the behavioral interventions (53). These findings are in contrast with the strong meta-analytic evidence for the efficacy of interventions consistent with RP for smoking cessation reported in the U.S. Public Health Services Clinical Practice Guideline (54).

Two trials have compared the delivery of RP in individual versus group format and found no difference in group versus individually delivered RP (55).

Several studies have included spouses in the RP intervention (56). A study of the first relapse episodes and reasons for terminating relapses for men with alcoholism who were treated with their spouses found that the relapses of patients receiving RP in addition to behavioral marital therapy were shorter than those of patients not receiving the RP (56). In a study of married alcoholics, O'Farrell and colleagues (57) found that in couples assessed to be "high distress," abstinence rates were highest for those who received behavioral marital therapy in combination with RP. Alcoholics who received RP after completing behavioral marital therapy had more days of abstinence, fewer days drinking, and improved marriages than did those who received only behavioral marital therapy (58). A more recent study (59) evaluated conjoint treatments in 90 men with alcohol problems and their female partners. Couples were followed for 18 months after treatment. Across the three outpatient treatments (alcohol behavioral couples therapy: ABCT; ABCT/RP; ABCT with interventions encouraging AA involvement: AA/ABCT), drinkers who provided follow-up data maintained abstinence on almost 80% of days during follow-up with no differences in drinking or marital happiness outcomes between groups.

There are limitations to studies on RP. First, some studies have used RP as the single treatment intervention for cessation of drinking rather than for maintenance of change once drinking was stopped. Second, studies usually do not differentiate between subjects who are motivated to change substance use behavior and those who have little or no motivation to change. Third, in some studies, sample sizes are small and there is not enough power to detect statistical differences between experimental and control conditions. Fourth, studies do not always use random assignment or operationalize the therapy being compared against RP, making it difficult to determine what factors contribute to treatment effects. And last, the follow-up period is often short-term (6 months or less). Despite these limitations, however, there is empirical evidence that RP strategies enhance the recovery of individuals with SUDs. Furthermore, RP is now listed on SAMHSA's National Registry of Evidence-based Programs and Practices (NREPP) website (www.nrepp.samsha.gov) as an "Evidence-based Practice."

RELAPSE DETERMINANTS

Research by Marlatt and colleagues led to classifying relapse for alcoholics, smokers, heroin addicts, gamblers, and overeaters in two broad categories, intrapersonal and interpersonal determinants (8). Intrapersonal determinants contributing to relapse include: emotional states, coping, outcome expectancies, self-efficacy, craving, and motivation. According to this research, the category that most frequently affected relapse of alcoholics, smokers, and heroin addicts was negative emotional states. Thirty-eight percent of alcoholics, 37% of smokers, and 19% of heroin addicts relapsed in response to a negative affective state that they were unable to manage effectively.

Intrapersonal Determinants

1. *Emotional States*: In the original relapse taxonomy (8) and in the replication of the taxonomy (60), negative affect was the best predictor of outcomes. Baker and colleagues have recently identified negative affect as the primary motive for drug use. According to this model, excessive substance use is motivated by positive and negative affective regulation such that substances provide negative reinforcement when they provide relief from negative affective states (61). Thus, clinicians should incorporate interventions to help patients regulate their emotions and decrease negative emotional states.
2. *Coping*: Coping has been shown to be a critical predictor of substance use treatment outcomes and is often the strongest predictor of behavioral lapses in the moment (62,63). Several types of coping have been identified such as stress, temptation, cognitive and behavioral coping, as well as approach and avoidance coping. Active cognitive and behavioral coping strategies have been shown to be significantly related to abstinence outcomes, whereas the use of avoidance coping tends to be associated with negative outcomes (63).
3. *Outcome Expectancies*: Outcome expectancies are typically described as an individual's anticipation of the effects of a future experience. Anticipation of the effects of a substance has been identified as one of the primary cognitions related to substance use and relapse (64). Outcome expectancies may be affecting substance use behavior via the relationship between negative emotional states and beliefs about substances relieving negative affect (65). Both negative and positive expectancies are related to relapse, with negative expectancies being protective against relapse and positive expectancies being a risk factor for relapse (12). Individuals endorsing positive expectancies at the beginning of treatment may benefit from an intervention challenging them (66).
4. *Self-efficacy*: Self-efficacy is defined as the degree to which an individual feels confident and capable of performing a certain behavior in a specific situational context (67). Self-efficacy is a predictor of outcomes across all types of addictive behaviors, including gambling, smoking, and drug use (68). Increased self-efficacy following RP intervention was related to improved outcomes (69). Most likely the relationship between self-efficacy and outcomes is bidirectional, meaning that individuals who are more successful report greater self-efficacy and individuals who have lapsed report lower self-efficacy. The mechanism by which self-efficacy influences outcome is not clear (69). Thorough assessment of self-efficacy during treatment and interventions designed to strengthen it are major components of any RP intervention.
5. *Motivation*: Motivation may be related to the relapse process in two distinct ways: the motivation for behavior change and the motivation to engage in the problematic behavior. This illustrates the issue of ambivalence experienced by many patients attempting to change an addictive behavior (70). The ambivalence is related to both self-efficacy and outcome expectancies. The transtheoretical model of change incorporates five stages of readiness to change: precontemplation, contemplation (ambivalence), preparation, action, and maintenance. Each stage characterizes a different level of readiness for change, with precontemplation indicating the lowest level of change (71). Motivation to change is transactional, reflected in and affected by interpersonal interaction. The transtheoretical model of change provides a framework for understanding the change process and MI provides a means of facilitating the change process. Thus, assessment of motivation and commitment to change during treatment and interventions such as MI designed to resolve ambivalence and strengthen motivation are critical components of any RP intervention.
6. *Craving*: Craving is possibly the most studied and poorly understood construct in the field of SUD research. Addiction research did not show any significant association between subjective craving and objective measures of relapse (72). For example, Sayette and colleagues (73) demonstrated that cue exposure was predictive of nicotine craving, but only for smokers who are deprived of nicotine. Craving has been described as a cognitive experience focused on the desire to use a substance and is often related to the expectancies for the desired effect of the drug, whereas urge has been defined as the behavioral intention to use a substance. Studies on the role of cue reactivity in addiction showed that drug-related stimuli elicit craving but cue reactivity is not a consistent predictor of relapse. Cue reactivity could have an impact on the treatment of addictive behaviors (74).

Interpersonal Determinants

Interpersonal precipitants of relapse include relationship conflict, social pressure to use substances, and positive emotional states associated with some type of interaction with others (8,75). Functional social support or the level of emotional support is highly predictive of long-term abstinence rates across several addictions (76). The quality of social support or the level of support from nonsubstance abusers has also been related to relapse (76). Stanton provided an overview of interpersonal dynamics as a high-risk situation for relapse. However, the relationship between interpersonal factors and relapse is not entirely clear (77). Clearly, the role of social support is a critical component of RP. An extension of RP that involves including spouses or significant others in conjoint therapy, such as behavioral marital therapy (78), has strong empirical support (59).

OVERVIEW OF MODELS OF RP

A variety of models of RP are described in the literature. The more common approaches include (a) Marlatt and Gordon's cognitive–behavioral approach, which has been adapted for other clinical populations such as sex offenders, overeaters, and individuals with problems controlling sexual behaviors; (b) Annis' cognitive–behavioral approach, which incorporates concepts of Marlatt's model with Bandura's self-efficacy theory; (c) Daley's psychoeducational approach; (d) Gorski's neurologic impairment model; (e) Zackon, McAuliffe, and Chien's addict aftercare model; (f) the Matrix neurobehavioral model of treatment of Rawson et al., which includes RP as a central component of treatment; (g) Washton's intensive outpatient model; (h) the coping/social skills training model of Monti et al.; and (i) the Cue Extinction (CE) model developed by Childress et al. (79).

Many inpatient, partial hospital, and outpatient treatment programs have incorporated various aspects of these RP approaches. Some programs offer specific "relapse tracks" that are geared specifically for patients who have relapsed following a period of sustained recovery. The focus of these programs is primarily on problems and issues associated with relapse (79). Despite their differences, these RP approaches have many components in common. They focus on the need for individuals with a SUD to develop new coping skills for handling high-risk situations and relapse warning signs; to make lifestyle changes to decrease the need for alcohol, drugs, or tobacco; to increase healthy activities; to prepare for interrupting lapses so that they do not end in a full-blown relapse; and to prepare for managing relapses so that adverse consequences may be minimized. All RP approaches emphasize the need to have a broad repertoire of behavioral, cognitive, and interpersonal coping strategies to help prevent a relapse. Most are time-limited or brief, making them more feasible in the current climate of managed care.

The Cognitive–Behavioral Model of Relapse

Marlatt (8) proposed a cognitive–behavioral model of the relapse process shown in Figure 47.1, which centers on identifying high-risk situations and the individual's response to the situations. A high-risk situation is defined as a circumstance in which an individual's attempt to refrain from a particular behavior (ranging from any use of a substance to heavy use) is threatened. The high-risk situation is defined as any experience, emotion, setting, thought, or context, and varies from person to person and within each individual. High-risk situations often arise without warning (80). If the individual lacks an effective coping strategy and/or confidence to deal with the situation (low self-efficacy), the tendency is to give in to temptation. The decision to use or not use is then mediated by the individual's outcome expectancies for the initial effects

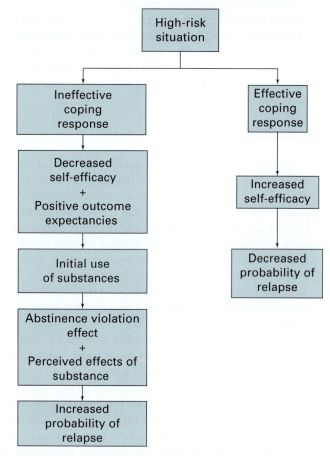

Figure 47.1. Cognitive–behavioral model of relapse.

of using the substance. Individuals who decide to use the substance may be vulnerable to the "abstinence violation effect," which is the self-blame and loss of perceived control that individuals experience after the violation of self-imposed rules, which undermines their commitment to abstinence goals. The lapse is more likely to lead to a full-blown relapse if the individual perceives it as an irreparable failure.

The Cognitive–Behavioral Model of Relapse, Revised

This reconceptualized cognitive–behavioral model of relapse focuses on the dynamic interactions between multiple risk factors and situational determinants. Seemingly insignificant changes in levels of risk (e.g., slight decrease in mood ratings) may kindle a downward spiral of increased craving leading to a lapse episode often initiated by a minor cue (14). For example, increased level of stress may trigger a high-risk situation in which a decrease in coping ability considerably increases the likelihood of the person's using an ineffective coping response, thereby leading to an increased probability of a lapse (81). As shown in Figure 47.2, the reconceptualized dynamic model of relapse allows for several configurations of distal (e.g., years of dependence,

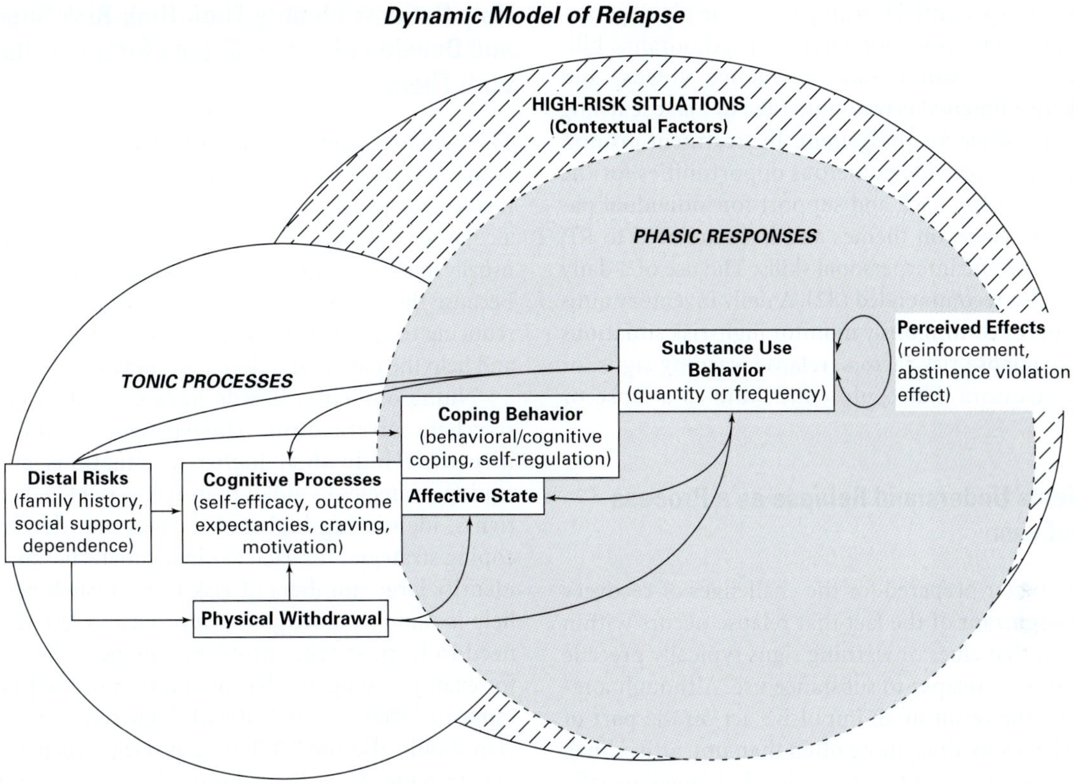

Dynamic Model of Relapse

Figure 47.2. Dynamic model of relapse.

family history, social support, and comorbid psychiatric disorders) and proximal (e.g., emotional states, craving, cognitive vigilance, and situational response efficacy) relapse risks (14). Distal risks (solid lines) are defined as stable predispositions that increase an individual's vulnerability to lapse, whereas proximal risks (dotted lines) are immediate precipitants that actualize the statistical probability of a lapse. Connected boxes are hypothesized to be nonrecursive —that is there is a reciprocal causation between them (e.g., coping skills influencing drinking behaviors and in turn drinking influences coping (11). These feedback loops (indicated by double-headed arrows) allow for the interaction between coping skills, cognitions, craving, affective state, and substance use behavior. The role of contextual factors is indicated by the large stripped circle in Figure 47.2, with situational cues (e.g., walking by the liquor store) playing an important role in the relationship between risk factors and substance use behavior. The white and gray circles represent tonic and phasic processes (the phasic one is contained within the high-risk situation circle). The circle on the far left (solid border) represent tonic processes which indicate the individual's vulnerability to relapse. Tonic processes provide the foundation for the possibility of a lapse. The phasic response (dotted border) incorporates situational, cognitive, affective, physical states, and coping skills. The phasic response is conceptualized as the turning point of the system where behavior response may lead to a sudden change in substance use behavior. On the other hand, an individual can de-escalate the risk of relapse by utilizing effective coping strategies. Recent empirical studies demonstrate that responding in a high-risk situation is related to both distal and proximal risk factors operating within the two phasic and tonic processes. Understanding the complexity of the relapse process alerts the clinicians about the importance of a comprehensive assessment about the individual's background, coping skills, substance use history, self-efficacy, and emotional states. The consideration of how these factors are intertwined within a high-risk situation allows the clinicians to help patients continually assess their own vulnerability to relapse.

CLINICAL RP INTERVENTIONS

This section discusses practical RP interventions that can be used in multiple treatment contexts. These interventions reflect the approaches of numerous clinicians and researchers who have developed specific models of RP and/or written patient-oriented RP recovery materials and the authors' experience working with patients with alcohol dependence and drug addictions, including patients with comorbid psychiatric conditions. The interventions reflect the models of RP discussed earlier. Whereas some of these interventions can be used by the patient as part of a self-management recovery program, other interventions involve eliciting support or help from family members or significant others. The literature emphasizes individualizing RP strategies, taking into account the patient's level of motivation, severity of substance use, gender, ego functioning, and sociocultural environment.

The use of experiential learning (e.g., role playing, fantasy, behavioral rehearsal, monodramas, psychodrama, bibliotherapy, use of workbooks, interactive videos, and homework assignments) is recommended to make learning an active experience for the patient. In treatment groups, action techniques provide numerous opportunities for the clinician to elicit feedback and support for individual patients, identify common themes and issues related to RP, and practice specific interpersonal skills. The use of a daily inventory is also recommended (82). A daily inventory aims to get patients to continuously monitor high-risk situations and identify relapse risk factors, relapse warning signs, or significant stressors that could contribute to a lapse or relapse.

Help Patients Understand Relapse as a Process and as an Event

Patients are better prepared for the challenges of recovery if they are cognizant of the fact that relapse occurs within a context and that clues or warning signs typically precede an actual lapse or relapse to substance use. Although a relapse may be the result of an impulsive act on the part of the recovering individual, more often than not, attitudinal, emotional, cognitive, and/or behavioral changes usually manifest themselves prior to the actual ingestion of substances. An individual's clues or warning signs can be conceptualized as links in a relapse chain (8,13). Many relapsers reported to the authors that their warning signs appeared days, weeks, or even longer before they used substances (Fig. 47.3). Patients under treatment for the first time can benefit from reviewing common relapse warning signs identified by others in recovery. The authors have found it helpful to have relapsers review their experiences in great detail so that they can learn the connections among thoughts, feelings, events or situations, and relapse to substance use. An evaluation of one of the authors' psychoeducational model of RP and a workbook used in conjunction with this program by 511 patients found that "Understanding the Relapse Process" was rated as the most useful topic (83).

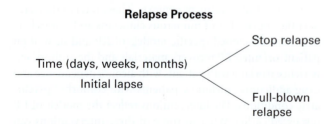

Figure 47.3. Relapse process.

Help Patients Identify Their High-Risk Situations and Develop Effective Coping Strategies to Deal with Them

The need to recognize the risk of relapse and high-risk factors is an essential component of RP. High-risk factors, or critical incidents, typically are those situations in which patients used alcohol or other drugs prior to treatment. High-risk factors usually involve intrapersonal and interpersonal situations (84). Because the availability of coping skills is a protective factor reducing relapse risk, the clinician should assess coping skills and help the patient develop new ones as needed (13).

Numerous clinical aids have been developed by researchers and clinicians to help patients identify and prioritize their individual high-risk situations and develop coping strategies to aid in their recovery (13). For some patients, identifying high-risk factors and developing new coping strategies for each are inadequate, because they may identify large numbers of risk factors. Such patients need help in taking a more global approach to recovery and may need to learn specific problem-solving skills. Marlatt (8), for example, suggests that in addition to teaching patients "specific" RP skills to deal with high-risk factors, the clinician should also use "global" approaches such as skill training strategies (e.g., behavioral rehearsal, covert modeling, and assertiveness training), cognitive reframing (e.g., coping imagery and reframing reactions to lapse or relapse), and lifestyle interventions (e.g., meditation, exercise, and relaxation). Figure 47.4 summarizes one paradigm for conceptualizing high-risk factors.

Help Patients Identify and Manage Alcohol or Drug Cues as well as Cravings

There is a growing body of research suggesting that patients' desire or craving for alcohol or other drugs can be triggered by exposure to environmental cues associated with prior use (72). Cues such as the sight or smell of the substance of abuse may trigger cravings that become evident in cognitive (e.g., increased thoughts of using) and physiologic (e.g., anxiety) changes. The advice given in AA, NA, CA, and CMA: "avoid people, places, and things" associated with substance abuse, was developed as a way of minimizing exposure to cues that trigger cravings that can be so overwhelming that they contribute to a relapse. A practical suggestion is to encourage patients to remove from their homes substances as well as paraphernalia (pipes, mirrors, needles, etc.) used for taking drugs. Cue exposure treatment is one method used to help reduce the intensity of the patient's reactions to cues (85). This treatment involves exposing the patient to specific cues associated with substance use. Cue exposure also involves teaching or enhancing coping skills (e.g., systematic relaxation, behavioral alternatives, visual imagery, and cognitive interventions) to improve the patient's confidence in his or her ability to resist the desire to use.

Because it is impossible for patients to avoid all cues that are associated with substance use, the clinician can

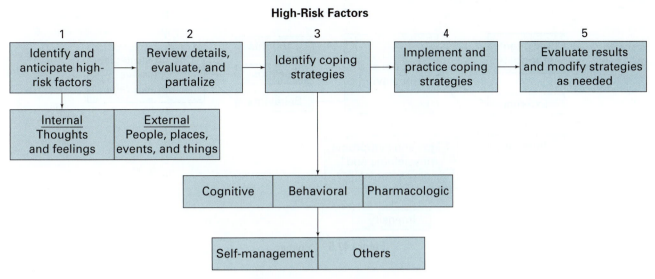

Figure 47.4. High-risk factors.

teach the patient a variety of practical techniques to manage cravings (13). Patients should learn information about cues and how they trigger cravings for alcohol or other drugs. Monitoring and recording cravings, associated thoughts, and outcomes can help patients become more vigilant and prepared to cope with them. Helpful cognitive interventions for managing cravings include changing thoughts about the craving or desire to use, challenging euphoric recall, talking oneself through the craving, thinking beyond the high by identifying negative consequences of using (immediate and delayed) and positive benefits of not using, using AA/NA/CA/CMA recovery slogans and delaying the decision to use. Behavioral interventions include avoiding, leaving, or changing situations that trigger or worsen a craving, redirecting activities or getting involved in pleasant activities, getting help or support from others by admitting and talking about cravings and hearing how others have survived them, attending self-help support group meetings, or taking anticraving medications such as naltrexone or acamprosate. Shiffman and colleagues (10) recommend that ex-smokers carry a menu card that lists various ways to cope with a craving to smoke, a strategy that can also address alcohol or other drug cravings. Another effective way to cope with urges to use substances is a meditation imagery technique known as "urge surfing" (8,86). To help patients deal with the urge to use without giving in, they are taught to visualize the urge as a rising ocean wave that they will learn to "surf" without getting "wiped out" by the craving. Figure 47.5 represents a paradigm that the authors have found useful when helping patients understand and manage cravings.

Help Patients Understand and Deal with Social Pressures to Use Substances

Direct and indirect social pressures often lead to increased thoughts and desires to use substances, as well as anxiety regarding one's ability to refuse offers to drink alcohol or use other drugs. Figure 47.6 outlines one method of helping patients understand and deal with social pressures. The first step is to identify high-risk relationships (e.g., living with or dating an active drug abuser or alcoholic) and situations or events in which the patient may be exposed to or offered substances (e.g., social gatherings where people smoke cigarettes or drink alcohol). The next step is to assess the effects of these social pressures on the thoughts, feelings, and behaviors of the patient. Planning, practicing, and implementing coping strategies is the next step. These coping strategies include avoidance and the use of verbal, cognitive, or behavioral skills. Using role playing to rehearse ways to refuse offers of drug or alcohol is one very practical and easy-to-use intervention. The final step of this process involves teaching the patient to evaluate the results of a given coping strategy and to modify it as needed. Pressures to use alcohol or other drugs may result from relationships with active drug users or alcoholics. The patient needs to assess his or her social network and learn ways to limit or end relationships that represent a high risk for relapse.

Help Patients Develop and Strengthen a Supportive Recovery Social Network

Several authors have addressed RP from a broader perspective that involves the family or significant others (78). O'Farrell and colleagues (57,58) developed a RP protocol for use in combination with behavioral marital therapy. Involvement of immediate families or significant others in the recovery process provides them with an opportunity to deal with the impact of substance use on their lives as well as their own issues (e.g., enabling behaviors, preoccupation, feelings of anger, shame, and guilt). Families are then in a much better position to support the recovering member. The authors have seen family members sabotage the recovery of the addicted member in a multiplicity of overt and covert ways. Such behavior is usually an indication that they have not had an opportunity to deal with their own issues or heal from their emotional pain.

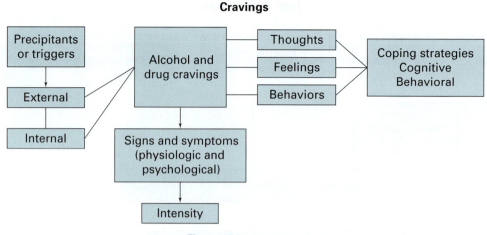

Figure 47.5. Cravings.

Patients can be encouraged to get involved in AA, NA, CA, CMA, or other support groups. Sponsors, other recovery and personal friends, and employers may become part of an individual's RP network (87). Patients generally should not try to recover in isolation, particularly during the early stages of recovery. Following are some suggested steps for helping patients develop a RP network. First, the patient needs to identify whom to involve in or exclude from this network. Others who abuse substances, harbor extremely strong negative feelings toward the recovering person, or generally are not supportive of recovery usually should be excluded. The patient should then determine how and when to ask for support or help. Behavioral rehearsal can help the patient practice ways to make specific requests for support. Rehearsal also helps increase confidence as well as clarifies thoughts and feelings regarding reaching out for help. Many patients, for example, feel guilty or shameful and question whether or not they deserve support from others. Yet others have such strong pride that the thought of asking others for support is very difficult to accept. Rehearsal may also clarify the patient's ambivalence regarding ongoing recovery, and it helps better understand how the person being asked for support may respond. This prepares the patient for dealing with potential negative responses from others. Patients should be advised to emphasize that recovery is ultimately their responsibility. An action plan can then be devised, practiced, implemented, and modified as needed. Some patients find it helpful to put their action plan in writing so that all of those involved have a specific document to refer to. The action plan can address the following issues: how to communicate about and deal with relapse warning signs and high-risk situations; how to interrupt a lapse; how to intervene if a relapse occurs; and the importance of exploring all the details of a lapse or relapse after the patient is stable so that it can be used as a learning experience. Having a plan can make both the recovering person and family feel more in control even if faced with the possibility of an actual relapse. Additionally, it helps everyone take a proactive approach to recovery rather than sit back passively and wait for problems to occur. The authors' clinical experience has been that patients and families who are involved in such discussions are much more likely to intervene earlier in the relapse process than those not involved in these discussions.

Help Patients Identify and Develop Effective Coping Strategies to Manage Negative Emotional States

Negative affective states are associated with relapse across a range of addictions (8). Several investigators reported that depression and anxiety were major factors in a substantial

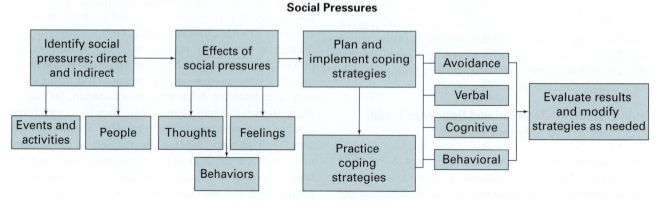

Figure 47.6. Social pressures.

number of relapses (88). Shiffman and colleagues (10) found that coping responses for high-risk situations were less effective for smokers who were depressed. Other negative affective states associated with relapse include anger, anxiety, and boredom. The acronym HALT used in 12-step Programs (which stands for, "don't get too hungry, angry, lonely, or tired") speaks to the importance of the recovering alcoholic's or drug addict's not allowing himself or herself to get too angry or lonely. These two emotional states are seen as high-risk factors for many.

Helping patients improve their ability to identify and manage their emotions is a helpful treatment strategy (13). Interventions for helping patients develop appropriate coping skills for managing negative emotional states vary, depending on the sources, manifestation, and consequences of these emotions. For example, strategies for dealing with depression that accompanies the realization that addiction caused havoc in one's life may vary from those for dealing with depression that is part of a bipolar or major depressive illness that becomes manifest after the patient is substance-free and creates significant personal distress.

Help Patients Identify and Learn Strategies to Cope with Cognitive Distortions

Cognitive distortions or errors in thinking are associated with a wide range of mental health and SUDs (89). These distortions have also been implicated in relapse to substance use as well. Twelve-step programs refer to cognitive distortions as "stinking thinking" and suggest that recovering individuals need to alter their thinking if they are to remain alcohol- and drug-free. Teaching patients to identify their cognitive errors (e.g., black-and-white thinking, "awfulizing," overgeneralizing, selective abstraction, catastrophizing, or jumping to conclusions) and evaluate how these affect the relapse process is often very helpful. Patients can then be taught to use counter thoughts to challenge their faulty beliefs or specific negative thoughts. The authors provide patients with a sample worksheet to help them learn to change and challenge relapse thoughts. This worksheet has three directives: (a) list the relapse-related thought; (b) state what is wrong with it; and (c) create new statements. A list of seven specific thoughts commonly associated with relapse is used to prompt patients in completing this therapeutic task. These examples include, "relapse can't happen to me"; "I'll never use alcohol or drugs again"; "I can control my use of alcohol or other drugs"; "a few drinks, tokes, pills, lines won't hurt"; "recovery isn't happening fast enough"; "I need alcohol or other drugs to have fun"; and "my problem is cured." Patients seldom have difficulty coming up with additional examples of specific thoughts that can contribute to a relapse. Many of the AA, CMA, and NA slogans were devised to help alcoholics and drug addicts alter their thinking and survive desires to use substances. Slogans such as "this, too, will pass," "let go and let God," and "one day at a time" often help the individual work through thoughts of using.

Help Patients Work Toward a Balanced Lifestyle

In addition to identifying and managing high-risk relapse factors, recovering individuals often need to make more global changes to restore or achieve a balance in their lifestyle (8,13). Development of a healthy lifestyle is seen as important in reducing stress that makes one more vulnerable to relapse. The patient's lifestyle can be assessed by evaluating patterns of daily activities, sources of stress, stressful life events, daily hassles and uplifts, balance between wants (activities engaged in for pleasure or self-fulfillment) and shoulds (external demands), health and exercise patterns, relaxation patterns, interpersonal activities, and religious beliefs. Helping patients develop positive habits or substitute indulgences (e.g., jogging, meditation, relaxation, exercise, hobbies, or creative tasks) for substance abuse can help to balance their lifestyle (13,90).

Help Patients Develop a Relapse Management Plan

Since addiction has been clearly identified as a chronic relapsing illness, it is highly recommended that patients have an emergency plan to follow if they lapse, so that a full-blown relapse can be avoided. If a full-blown relapse occurs, however, the patient needs to have strategies to stop it. The specific intervention strategies should be based on the severity of the patient's lapse or relapse, coping mechanisms, and prior history of relapse. Helpful interventions include getting patients to use self-talk or behavioral procedures to stop a lapse or relapse, asking family, 12-step sponsors, friends, or professionals for help, carrying an emergency card with names and phone numbers of others who can be called on for support, or carrying a reminder card that gives specific instructions on what to do if a lapse or relapse occurs (13). Marlatt recommends developing a relapse contract with patients that outlines specific steps to take in the event of a future relapse. The aim of this contract is to formalize or reinforce the patient's commitment to change. Analyzing lapses or relapses is a valuable process that can aid ongoing recovery. This helps to reframe a "failure" as a "learning" experience and can help the individual prepare for future high-risk situations.

Consider the Use of Pharmacologic Intervention as an Adjunct to Psychosocial Treatment

Because some patients benefit from pharmacologic interventions to attenuate or reduce cravings for alcohol or other drugs, enhance motivation to stay sober, and increase confidence in their ability to resist relapse, a therapist should consider using a pharmacologic intervention as an adjunct to psychosocial treatment (91). None of the medications approved for the treatment of alcohol dependence has proven effective without some form of concurrent behavioral intervention. In addition, research shows that the combined effects of the pharmacologic and behavioral treatment are additive for smoking cessation (92). Medications can also be very helpful in preventing relapse to opioid dependence. Unfortunately, despite a significant number of clinical trials with good outcomes, medications are still underutilized by physicians treating patients with addictions.

Assess Patients for Co-occurring Psychiatric Disorders and Facilitate Specialized Treatment if Needed

Numerous studies of community samples, psychiatric treatment populations, and substance abuse treatment populations evidence high rates of dual diagnoses (SUD co-occurring with a psychiatric disorder) (93). Dual-diagnosis patients are at higher risk for substance use relapse than those with only a substance use diagnosis resulting from the effect of psychiatric symptomatology on motivation, judgment, and functioning. In addition, dual-diagnosis patients who resume substance use frequently fail to adhere to psychiatric treatment and comply poorly with pharmacotherapy, psychotherapy, and/or self-help program attendance (94). In a quality assurance/improvement study conducted by one of the authors of 25 substance abusers with mood disorders and 25 substance abusers with schizophrenia who were rehospitalized as a result of significant worsening of psychiatric condition, it was found that alcohol and drug abuse relapse played a significant role in 60% of these psychiatric relapses. In a study comparing psychiatric patients with ($n = 127$) and without ($n = 102$) substance abuse comorbidity, one of the authors found that the patients with co-occurring disorders were significantly more likely to relapse and be hospitalized (95). RP strategies can be adapted and tailored to the specific problems and symptoms of the patient's psychiatric disorder. Monitoring target moods or behaviors, participating in pleasant activities, developing routine and structure in daily life, learning to cope with persistent psychiatric symptoms associated with chronic or recurrent forms of psychiatric illness, and identifying early warning signs of psychiatric relapse and developing appropriate coping strategies are helpful interventions for dual diagnosis patients (13).

Negative mood states that are part of an affective disorder (major depression, bipolar disease, etc.) or anxiety disorder (phobia, panic disorder, etc.) may require pharmacotherapy in addition to psychotherapy and involvement in self-help programs. Patients on medications for these or other psychiatric disorders may also benefit from developing strategies for dealing with well-meaning members of self-help programs who encourage them to stop their medications because it is perceived as detrimental to recovery from their SUD.

Facilitate the Transition to Follow-up Outpatient Treatment For Patients Completing Residential or Hospital-Based Treatment

Many patients make significant gains in structured, hospital-based or residential substance abuse treatment programs only to have these negated as a consequence of failure to adhere to ongoing outpatient or aftercare treatment (96). Interventions used to enhance treatment entry and adherence that lower the risk of relapse include the provision of a single session of motivational therapy prior to discharge from inpatient treatment, the use of telephone or mail reminders of initial treatment appointments, integrating motivational interventions in early recovery, and providing reinforcers for appropriate participation in treatment activities or for providing drug-free urines. Studies of patients with schizophrenia and a SUD (97) or patients with mood and SUDs (98) show that providing a single motivational therapy session prior to hospital discharge leads to a nearly twofold increase in the show rate for the initial outpatient appointment. Patients who show for their initial appointment and successfully "enter" outpatient treatment have a reduced risk of treatment dropout and subsequent psychiatric and/or substance use relapse.

CONCLUSION

Relapse is complex, dynamic, and unpredictable. A variety of RP clinical treatment models have been developed for patients with alcohol, tobacco, or other addictions. Many of the cognitive and behavioral interventions described in these RP approaches can be adapted for use with patients who have additional problems, such as other compulsive disorders, impulse control disorders, or comorbid psychiatric illnesses. RP interventions aim to help patients maintain change over time and address the most common issues and problems raising vulnerability to relapse. Studies indicate that RP has efficacy in reducing both relapse rates and the severity of lapses or relapses. RP strategies can be used throughout the continuum of care in primary rehabilitation programs, dual-diagnosis hospital programs, residential programs, halfway houses, or therapeutic community programs, as well as in partial hospital, outpatient, and aftercare programs integrated with other treatments such as pharmacotherapy. In addition, family members can be included in educational and therapy sessions and involved in the development of RP plans for members with SUDs. Many of the RP approaches described in the literature could play an important role in the development of short-term or brief interventions such as MI. Incorporating the RP techniques within the brief intervention will be beneficial for patients attempting to abstain or reduce their substance use after treatment and they can be provided in individual or group sessions, making them attractive and cost effective. RP techniques need to be studied more rigorously in diverse samples of populations including ethnic minority groups and adolescents. Future research should focus on refining the understanding of the dynamic reconceptualization of the relapse process and developing better data analytic methods for assessing behavior change. Clinical researchers should focus their efforts on better dissemination of RP strategies to community-based providers of drug and alcohol services. Neuroimaging studies are needed to better understand the underlying neuronal substrates of craving, decision-making, and the implications for RP.

REFERENCES

1. Center for Substance Abuse Treatment (CSAT). Treatment cuts medical costs. In: SAMSHA CSAT. *Substance Abuse in Brief.* Rockville, MD: Substance Abuse and Mental Health Services Administration; 2000.
2. McLellan AT, McKay JR, Forman R, et al. Reconsidering the evaluation of addiction treatment: from retrospective follow-up to concurrent recovery monitoring. *Addiction.* 2005;100(4):447–458.
3. Grella CE, Hser YI, Hsieh SC. Predictors of drug treatment reentry following relapse to cocaine use in DATOS. *J Subst Abuse Treat.* 2003;25(3):145–154.
4. Scott CK, Foss MA, Dennis ML. Pathways in the relapse-treatment-recovery cycle over 3 years. *J Subst Abuse Treat.* 2005;28(suppl 1):S63–S72.
5. Hser Yi, Longshore D, Anglin MD. The life course perspective on drug use: a conceptual framework for understanding drug use trajectories. *Eval Rev.* 2007;31(6):515–547.
6. Marlatt GA, Donovan DM, eds. *Relapse Prevention.* 2nd ed. New York, NY: Guilford Press; 2005.
7. Marlatt GA. Buddhist psychology and the treatment of addictive behavior. *Cogn Behav Pract.* 2002;9:44–49.
8. Marlatt GA, Gordon J, eds. *RP: A Self-Control Strategy for the Maintenance of Behavior Change.* New York, NY: Guilford Press; 1985.
9. Marlatt GA, Witkiewitz K. Harm reduction approaches to alcohol use: health promotion, prevention, treatment. *Addict Behav.* 2002;27:867–886.
10. Shiffman S. Relapse following smoking cessation: a situational analysis. *J Consult Clin Psychol.* 1982;50:71–86.
11. Gossop M, Stewart D, Browne N, et al. Factors associated with abstinence, lapse, or relapse to heroin use after residential treatment: protective effects of coping responses. *Addiction.* 2002;97:1259–1267.
12. Gwantley CJ, Shiffman S, Balabanis B, et al. Dynamic self-efficacy and outcome expectancies: prediction of smoking lapse and relapse. *J Abnorm Psychol.* 2005;114(4):661–675.
13. Daley DC, Marlatt GA. *Overcoming Alcohol and Drug Problem: Effective Recovery Strategies. Therapist Guide.* 2nd ed. New York, NY: Oxford University Press; 2006.
14. Witkiewtiz K, Marlatt GA. Realpse prevention for alcohol and drug problems: that was Zen, this is Tao. *Am Psychol.* 2004;59(4):224–235.
15. Marlatt GA. Situational determinants of relapse and skill-training interventions. In: Marlatt GA, Gordon J, eds. *RP: A Self-Control Strategy for the Maintenance of Behavior Change.* New York, NY: Guilford Press; 1985:71–127.
16. American Psychiatric Association. *Diagnostic and Statistical Manual of Mental Disorders.* American Psychiatric Press 4th ed. (DSM-IV). Washington, DC; 1994.
17. American Society of Addiction Medicine. *Patient Placement Criteria for the Treatment of Substance Use Disorders.* Chevy Chase, MD: American Society of Addiction Medicine; 2001.
18. Laudet AB. What does recovery mean to you? Lessons form the recovery experience for research and practice. *J Subst Abuse Treat.* 2007;33(3):243–256.
19. Brown S. *Treating the Alcoholic: A Developmental Model of Recovery.* 2nd ed. New York, NY: Wiley; 1995.
20. Grella CE, Scott CK, Foss MA, et al. Gender similarities and differences in the treatment, relapse, and recovery cycle. *Eval Rev.* 2008;32(1):113–137.
21. Dennis ML, Scott CK, Funk R, et al. The duration and correlates of addiction treatment careers. *J Subst Abuse Treat.* 2005;28:S51–S62.
22. Dennis ML, Scott CK. Managing addiction as a chronic condition. *Addict Sci Clin Pract.* 2007;4(1):45–55.
23. Flynn PM, Joe GW, Broome KM, et al. Recovery from opioid addiction in DATOS. *J Subst Abuse Treat.* 2003;25:177–186.
24. Miller W, Hester R. Treating the problem drinker: modern approaches. In: Miller WR, ed. *The Addictive Behaviors: Treatment of Alcoholism, Drug Abuse, Smoking and Obesity.* New York, NY: Pergamon Press; 1980.
25. Miller WR, Brown JM, Simpson TL, et al. What works? A methodological analysis of the alcohol treatment outcome literature. In: Hester R, Miller WR, eds. *Handbook of Alcoholism Treatment Approaches.* 2nd ed. Boston, MA: Allyn & Bac; 1995:12–44.
26. McLellan A, Lewis DC, O'Brien CP, et al. Drug dependence, a chronic mental illness: implications for treatment, insurance, and outcomes evaluation. *J Am Med Assoc.* 2000;284(13):1689–1695.
27. Catalano R, Howard M, Hawkins J, et al. Relapse in the addictions rates, determinants, and promising prevention strategies. In: *1988 Surgeon General's Report on Health Consequences of Smoking.* Washington, DC: U.S. Government Printing Office; 1988.
28. Hoffmann N, Harrison P. *CATOR 1986 Report: Findings Two Years After Treatment.* St Paul, MN: CATOR; 1986.
29. Hoffman NG, Miller NS. Treatment outcomes for abstinence-based programs. *Psychiatr Ann.* 1992;22(8):402–408.
30. National Institute on Drug Abuse (NIDA). Principles of drug addiction treatment: a research based guide. *NIDA Notes.* 1997;12(5):1–8.
31. Walitzer KS, Dearing R. Gender differences in alcohol and substance use relapse. *Clin Psychol Rev.* 2006;26:128–148.
32. Hillhouse MP, Marinelli P, Gonzales R, et al.; the Methamphetamine Treatment Project Corporate Authors. Predicting intreatment performance and post-treatment outcomes in methamphetamine users. *Addiction.* 2007;102(s1):84–95.
33. Carroll KM. RP as a psychosocial treatment: a review of controlled clinical trials. *Exp Clin Psychopharmacol.* 1996;4(1):46–54.
34. Irvin JE, Bowers CA, Dunn ME, et al. Efficacy of RP: a meta-analytic review. *J Consult Clin Psychol.* 1999;67(4):563–570.
35. Hajek P, Stead LF, West R, et al. Relapse prevention interventions for smoking cessation. *Cochrane Database Syst Rev.* 2005(1):CD003999.
36. Carroll KM, Rounsaville BJ, Gawin FH. A comparative trial of psychotherapies for ambulatory cocaine abusers: RP and interpersonal psychotherapy. *Am J Drug Alcohol Abuse.* 1991;17(3):229–247.
37. Carroll KM, Rounsaville BJ, Nich C, et al. One-year follow-up of psychotherapy and pharmacotherapy for cocaine dependence. Delayed emergence of psychotherapy effects. *Arch Gen Psychiatry.* 1994;51(12):989–997.
38. Wells EA, Peterson PL, Gainey RR, et al. Outpatient treatment for cocaine abuse: a controlled comparison of RP and twelve-step approaches. *Am J Drug Alcohol Abuse.* 1994;20(1):1–17.
39. Carroll KM, Fenton L, Ball S, et al. efficacy of disulfiram and cognitive behavioral therapy for cocaine dependent outpatients. *Arch Gen Psychiatry.* 2004;64:264–272.
40. Chaney E, O'Leary M. Skill training with alcoholics. *J Consult Clin Psychol.* 1978;46(5):1092–1104.
41. Koski-Jannes A. *Alcohol Addiction & Self-Regulation: A Controlled Trial of Relapse Prevention Program for Finnish Inpatient Alcoholics.* Finland: Finnish Foundation for Alcohol Studies: Helsinki; 1992.
42. Ito JR, Donovan DM, Hall JJ. RP and alcohol aftercare: effects on drinking outcome, change process, and aftercare attendance. *Br J Addict.* 1988;83:171–181.

43. Project MATCH. Matching alcoholism treatments to patient heterogeneity: Project MATCH three-year drinking outcomes. *Alcoholism Clin Exp Res*. 1998;22(6):1300–1311.
44. Ouimette PC, Finney JW, Moos RH. 12-Step and cognitive behavioral treatment for substance abuse: a comparison of treatment effectiveness. *J Consult Clin Psychol*. 1997;65:230–240.
45. Anton RF, Moak DH, Latham P, et al. Naltrexone combined with either cognitive behavioral or motivational enhancement therapy for alcohol dependence. *J Clin Psychopharmacol*. 2005;25: 349–357.
46. Anton RF, O'Malley SS, Ciraulo DA, et al. Combined pharmacotherapy and behavioral interventions for alcohol dependence. *J Am Med Assoc*. 2006;295:2003–2017.
47. The COMBINE Study Group. Testing combined pharmacotherapies and behavioral interventions for alcohol dependence (The COMBINE Study): rationale and methods. *Alcohol Clin Exp Res*. 2003;27:1107–1122.
48. The COMBINE Study Group. Testing combined pharmacotherapies and behavioral interventions for alcohol dependence (The COMBINE Study): a pilot feasibility study. *Alcohol Clin Exp Res*. 2003;27:1123–1131.
49. Rawson RA, Huber A, Brethen PB, et al. Methamphetamine and cocaine users: differences and treatment retention. *J Psychoactive Drugs*. 2000;32:233–238.
50. Rawson RA, McCann M, Flammino F, et al. A comparison of contingency management and cognitive behavioral approaches for cocaine and methamphetamine dependent individuals. *Arch Gen Psychiatry*. 2002;59:817–824.
51. MTP Research Group. Brief treatments for cannabis dependence: findings from a randomized multi-site trial. *J Consult Clin Psychol*. 2004;72:455–466.
52. Kilmer JR, Cronce JM, Paler PS. Relapse prevention for abuse of club drugs, hallucinogens, inhalants, and steroids. In: Marlatt GA, Donovan D, eds. *Relapse Prevention*. 2nd ed. New York, NY: Guilford Press; 2005:208–247.
53. Lancaster T, Hajeck P, Stead L, et al. Prevention of relapse after quitting smoking: a systematic review of trials. *Arch Intern Med*. 2006;166:828–835.
54. Fiore MC, Bailey WC, Cohen SJ, et al. *Treating Tobacco Use and Dependence: Clinical Practice Guideline*. Rockville, MD: U.S. Department of Health and Human Services, Public Health Service; 2000.
55. Marques AC, Formigoni ML. Comparison of individual and group cognitive behavioral therapy for alcohol and/or drug dependent patients. *Addiction*. 2001;96:832–837.
56. Maisto SA, McKay JR, O'Farrell TJ. Relapse precipitants and behavioral marital therapy. *Addict Behav*. 1995;20(3):383–393.
57. O'Farrell TJ. Couples RP sessions after a behavioral marital therapy couples group program. In: O Farrell TJ, ed. *Treating Alcohol Problems: Marital and Family Interventions*. New York, NY: Guilford Press; 1993:305–326.
58. O'Farrell TJ, Choquette KA, Cutter HS, et al. Behavioral martial therapy with and without additional couples RP sessions for alcoholics and their wives. *J Stud Alcohol*. 1993;54(6):652–666.
59. McCrady BS, Epstein EE, Kahler CW. Alcoholics Anonymous and relapse prevention as maintenance strategies after conjoint behavioral alcohol treatment for men: 18-months outcomes. *J Consult Clin Psychol*. 2004;72:870–878.
60. Lowman C, Allen J, Stout RL, et al. Replication and extension of Marlatt's taxonomy of relapse precipitants: overview of procedures and results. *Addiction*. 1996;91(suppl):51–71.
61. Tennen H, AffleckG, Armelie S, et al. A daily process approach to coping: linking theory, research and practice. *Am Psychol*. 2000;55:626–636.
62. Carels RA, Douglass OM, Cacciapaglia HM, et al. An ecological momentary assessment of relapse crises in dieting. *J Consult Clin Psychol*. 2004:72(2):341–348.
63. Maisto SA, Zywiak WH, Connors GJ. Course of functioning one year following admission for treatment of alcohol use disorders. *Addict Behav*. 2006;31(1):69–79.
64. Juliano LM, Brandon TH. Effects of nicotine dose, instructional set, and outcome expectancies on the subjective effects of smoking in the presence of a stressor. *J Abnorm Psychol*. 2002;111:88–97.
65. Demmel R, Nicolai J, Gregorzik S. Alcohol expectancies and current mood states in social drinkers. *Addict Behav*. 2006;31(5): 859–867.
66. Corbin WR, McNair LD, Carter JA. Evaluation of a treatment appropriate cognitive intervention for challenging alcohol outcome expectancies. *Addict Behav*. 2001;26(4):475–488.
67. Bandura A. *Self-Efficacy: The Exercise of Control*. New York, NY: Freeman; 1977.
68. Sklar SM, Annis HM, Turner NE. Group comparisons of coping self-efficacy between cocaine and alcohol abusers seeking treatment. *Psychol Addict Behav*. 1999;13:123–133.
69. Brown TG, Seraganian P, Tremblay J, et al. Process and outcome changes with relapse prevention versus 12-step aftercare programs for substance abusers. *Addiction*. 2002;97(6): 677–689.
70. Miller WR, Rollnick S. *Motivational Interviewing: Preparing People for Change*. 2nd ed. New York, NY: Guilford Press; 2002.
71. Prochaska JO, DiClemente CC. *The Transtheoretical Approach: Crossing the Traditional Boundaries of Therapy*. Malabar, FL: Krieger; 1984.
72. Drummond DC, Litten RZ, Lowman C, et al. Craving research: future directions. *Addiction*. 2000;95(suppl 2):247–255.
73. Sayette MA, Martin CS, Hall JG, et al. The effects of nicotine deprivation on craving response covariation in smokers. *J Abnorm Psychol*. 2003;112:110–118.
74. Carter BL, Tiffany ST. Meta-analysis of cue reactivity in addiction research. *Addiction*. 1999;94:327–340.
75. Marlatt GA. Cognitive assessment and intervention procedures for RP. In: Marlatt GA, Gordon J, eds. *RP: A Self-Control Strategy for the Maintenance of Behavior Change*. New York, NY: Guilford Press; 1985:201–279.
76. Dobkin PL, Civita M, Paraherakis A, et al. The role of functional social support in treatment retention and outcomes among outpatient adult substance abusers. *Addiction*. 2002;97: 347–356.
77. Armeli S, Todd M, Mohr C. A daily process approach to individual differences in stress-related alcohol use. *J Pers*. 2005; 73(6):1–30.
78. Winters J, Fals-Stewart W, O'Farrell TJ, et al. Behavioral couples therapy for female substance-abusing patients: effects on substance use and relationship adjustment. *J Consult Clin Psychol*. 2002;70:344–355.
79. Daley DC, Marlatt GA, Spotts CE. Relapse prevention: clinical models and intervention strategies. In: Graham AW, et al., eds. *Principles of Addiction Medicine*. 3rd ed. Chevy Chase, MD: American Society of Addiction Medicine; 2003:467–485.
80. Hawkins RC, Hawkins CA. Dynamics of substance abuse: implications for chaos theory for clinical research. In: Chamberlain L, Butz MR, eds. *Clinical Chaos: A Therapist's Guide to Nonlinear Dynamics and Therapeutic Change*. Philadelphia, PA: Brunner/Mazel; 1998.
81. Rabois D, Hagga DA. The influence of cognitive coping and mood on smoker's self efficacy and temptation. *Addict Behav*. 2003;28:561–573.

82. Gorski T, Miller M. *Staying Sober Workbook*. Independence, MO: Independence Press; 1988.
83. Daley DC. Five perspectives on relapse in chemical dependency. *J Chem Depend Treat*. 1989;2:3–26.
84. Connors GJ, Longabaugh R, Miller WR. Looking forward and back to relapse: implications for research and practice. *Addiction*. 1996;91, Suppl: S191–196.
85. National Institute on Drug Abuse (NIDA). *Cue Extinction Techniques: NIDA Technology Transfer Package*. Rockville, MD: National Institutes of Health; 1993.
86. Ostafin BD, Marlatt GA. Surfing the urge: experiential acceptance moderates the relationship between automatic alcohol motivation and hazardous drinking. *J Soc Clin Psychol*. 2008;27:426–440.
87. Peters RH, Witty TE, O'Brien JK. The importance of the work family with structured work and RP. *J Appl Rehabil Counsel*. 1993;24(3):3–5.
88. Pickens R, Hatsukami D, Spicer J, et al. Relapse by alcohol abusers. *Alcohol Clin Exp Res*. 1985;9(3):244–247.
89. Beck A, Wright F, Liese B. *Cognitive Therapy of Substance Abuse*. New York, NY: Guilford Press; 1994.
90. Marlatt GA, Chawla N. Meditation and alcohol use. *South Med J*. 2007;100:451–453.
91. Douaihy A, Daley D, Stowell KR, et al. Relapse prevention: clinical strategies for substance use disorders. In: Witkiewtiz K, Marlatt GA, eds. *Therapist's Guide to Evidence-Based Relapse Prevention*. Burlington MA, USA: Academic Press Publications, Elsevier; 2007:37–71.
92. Hughes JR. Combined behavioral therapy and pharmacotherapy for smoking cessation: an update. *NIDA Res Monogr*. 1995;150: 92–109.
93. Daley D, Moss HB. *Dual Disorders: Counseling Patients with Chemical Dependency and Mental Illness*. 3rd ed. Center City, MN: Hazelden; 2002.
94. Daley D, Zuckoff A. *Improving Treatment Compliance: Counseling and System Strategies for Substance Use and Dual Disorders*. Center City, MN: Hazelden; 1999.
95. Zuckoff A, Daley DC. Engagement and adherence issues in treating persons with non-psychosis dual disorders. *Psychiatr Rehabil Skills*. 2001;5(1):131–162.
96. deLeon G. Aftercare in therapeutic communities. RP in substance misuse [Special Issue]. *Int J Addict*. 1990–1991;25(9A–10A): 1225–1237.
97. Swanson AJ, Pantalon MV, Cohen KR. Motivational interviewing and treatment adherence among psychiatric and dually diagnoses patients. *J Nerv Ment Dis*. 1999;187(9):630–635.
98. Daley D, Zuckoff A. Improving compliance with the initial outpatient session among discharged inpatient dual diagnosis patients. *Soc Work*. 1998;43(5):470–473.

SECTION 7 ■ MANAGEMENT OF ASSOCIATED MEDICAL CONDITIONS

CHAPTER 48: Maternal and Neonatal Complications of Alcohol and Other Drugs

Karol Kaltenbach ■ Hendrée Jones

INTRODUCTION

Attention given to the concerns over the use of licit and illicit substances by pregnant women by both researchers and members of the public has varied considerably over the past several decades. The approaches to this public health problem have included a spectrum of punitive and treatment-oriented approaches with both extremes alternating as the principal or primary approach.

The public's concern and the subsequent behavioral and medical research on the effects of prenatal exposure to substances is grounded in the theory that disturbances during development in utero are a direct result of these substances altering the physical and/or nervous system of the child. Considerable research conducted in the area has approached the issue using a behavioral teratology frame of reference. Behavioral teratology investigates how substances that may or may not be inconsequential to the mother may harm the developing embryo and fetus. The type, duration, and severity of the harm are dependent upon multiple factors including the exposure dosage and the time during gestation when the exposure occurs. Moreover, harm to the central nervous system (CNS) during development may not manifest itself until later in development (1). As will be illustrated in this chapter, preclinical or animal model studies provide data to elucidate the biologic mechanisms that relate to both the negative effects of prenatal exposure to substances as well as protective effects of interventions to ameliorate or reverse the effects of this exposure. Both animal and clinical data also emphasize that the mechanisms associated with effects of prenatal exposure to substances on the fetus or child are multifactorial and encompass physiology, biology, genetics, epigenetics, dynamic relations between child and caregiver, and the environmental contexts in which the child develops.

This chapter summarizes the literature regarding the maternal and neonatal complications of licit (alcohol, nicotine, benzodiazepines, prescription opioids, and inhalants) and illicit (heroin, cocaine, amphetamines, hallucinogens, and marijuana) substances. Unfortunately, the political and regulatory distinction between legal and illegal substances has led the public to erroneously assume that there is a relationship between the legality of a substances and its ability to negatively impact fetal development and growth. As will be illustrated in this chapter, if substances were ranked in terms of the severity of their devastating consequences to fetal and maternal health, the two legal substances of alcohol and tobacco would likely decidedly trump the negative consequences associated with illicit substances such as cocaine, heroin, and marijuana. While the public and scientific communities have paid an enormous amount of attention to in utero cocaine effects, the effects associated with prenatal cocaine exposure appear more subtle than the prenatal effects of tobacco (2) and tobacco is used by the vast majority of women who use cocaine during pregnancy. Thus, it should be recognized that although the information in this chapter is ordered by classes of substances, these classes simply serve as organizing principles rather than representing the typical pattern of the ways drugs are used by women who become pregnant. In reality, pregnant women frequently use multiple substances that may have additive or even synergistic effects on the health and well being of the mother, fetus, and neonate.

This chapter is divided into 11 sections. The first section provides a summary of the prevalence of substance use by pregnant women. The second section summarizes the social characteristics and historical overview of the use of licit and illicit substances by pregnant women. The remaining sections summarize the information known about the maternal and neonatal consequences of prenatal exposure to alcohol, opioids, cocaine, amphetamine, inhalants, marijuana, nicotine, benzodiazepines, and hallucinogens, together with information relevant for the health care provider in regard to the use of these drugs by pregnant women.

Prevalence

According to U.S. national survey data from pregnant women of childbearing age (between 15 and 44 years of age, inclusive), 5.1% reported using illicit drugs in the past month. This

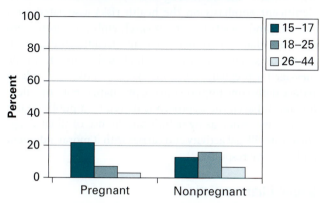

Figure 48.1. Illicit drug use in the past month by age of females of childbearing age. (From National Survey of Drug Use and Health Data, 2007–2008.)

used opioids (including heroin, OxyContin, and pain relievers), 0.4% used cocaine, and 0.2% used inhalants (3). Alcohol use in the past month was reported by 10.6% of pregnant women, while 4.5% reported binge drinking, and 0.8% reported heavy alcohol use. Similar to illicit drug use, these rates were significantly lower than the rates reported for their same-age nonpregnant counterparts, 54.0%, 24.2%, and 5.5%, respectively (3).

Among childbearing-age women, past month cigarette use was lower among pregnant (16.4%) than nonpregnant (27.3%) women (Fig. 48.2). Similar to the patterns seen with past month illicit drug use, the pattern of fewer pregnant than nonpregnant women reporting use was seen in each age subgroup with the exception of 15- to 17-year-old girls, for whom the rate of cigarette smoking appeared somewhat higher for pregnant than nonpregnant girls (20.6% vs. 14.7%). Moreover, the same pattern of decreasing numbers of women reporting cigarette use over the trimesters was also evident (3).

HISTORICAL OVERVIEW

Drug use by women and pregnant women in particular is certainly not a contemporary phenomenon. Stephan Kandall (4) provides an excellent discussion of the history of drug use among women in the United States from the mid-1800s, but it has only been since the end of the 20th century that significant attention has been directed at the use of licit and illicit substances by women with concern regarding use during pregnancy. The confluence of changes include the experience gained from the thalidomide tragedy (that drugs taken during pregnancy may be a teratogen); the strong stance by the Surgeon General in 1965 that smoking may be hazardous to your health; changes in federal drug policy during the 1960s that included treatment as an important approach; and the scientific report of the association between maternal drinking and infant abnormalities in 1971 that led to a new concern regarding the effects of drug use during pregnancy.

rate is similar to the rates reported since 2003 among pregnant women. However, this rate was significantly lower than the rate (9.8%) for nonpregnant women in the same childbearing age group (3). When this age group is categorized into subgroups, the same pattern of less reported use among pregnant than nonpregnant women was observed, except among girls 15 to 17 years of age (Fig. 48.1). In this latter subgroup, those girls who were pregnant had a higher rate of reported substance use in the past month relative to those girls who were not pregnant, that is 21.6% versus 12.9% (3). There is evidence to suggest that illicit drug use decreases over the course of pregnancy with 7.2%, 5.0%, and 2.8% of pregnant women reporting past month use of illicit drugs in the first, second, and third trimester, respectively (Fig. 48.2).

Examining the classes of substances used by pregnant women in the last month, 3.8% reported marijuana use, 0.8%

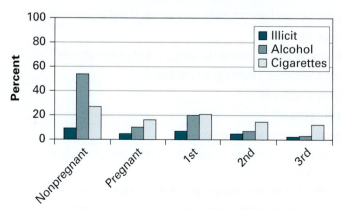

Figure 48.2. Drug use in the past month by females of childbearing age: pregnancy and trimester status. (From National Survey of Drug Use and Health Data, 2007–2008.)

However, this focus has not necessarily led to a strong cumulative body of scientific evidence, as both public and scientific interest is often driven by the politics of the day. For example, there has been a steady focus on delineating the effects of prenatal alcohol and nicotine exposure, in concert with consistent public health education to reduce/eliminate the use of these substances during pregnancy, including advisories from the Office of the Surgeon General on Alcohol Use in Pregnancy in 2005, and Treating Tobacco Use and Dependence in 2008. Yet, the trajectory of attention on illicit drugs is more restricted in that studies investigating the effects of illicit prenatal drug exposure are usually conducted primarily during the time periods in which societal concern is the greatest. For example, the majority of studies investigating opioid exposure were conducted in the late 1970s and early 1980s corresponding to the aftermath of the widespread heroin addiction of the 1960s; as the crack/cocaine epidemic spread throughout the country in the late 1980s and early 1990s attention shifted to prenatal cocaine exposure; and with the recent upsurge in the illegal manufacture of methamphetamines, we are just now beginning to accrue data on methamphetamine exposure. This dichotomy reflects some of the issues between use of licit and illicit drugs. Alcohol use in moderation is socially acceptable and has deep-seated cultural and religious roots; for pregnant women, the message is simply abstinence during pregnancy. (However, for pregnant women who are alcohol dependent, the problems are very complex and are often intertwined with tobacco and illicit drug abuse.) While there has been significant emphasis on the health risks associated with smoking and society has progressively embraced group zero tolerance, that is, no smoking in public facilities, the decision to smoke is viewed as an individual choice, and again the message for pregnant women is to cease smoking or at least reduce daily consumption during pregnancy. For both alcohol and tobacco the approach is driven by a public health perspective; whereas by definition, the use of illicit drugs constitutes illegal activity and carries with it moral judgment and punitive responses.

Social Characteristics

When addressing the complications of maternal drug abuse or dependence during pregnancy, it is important to understand the overall context in which maternal drug abuse usually occurs. In the early 1980s, notable work by Beth Reed and others (5) was some of the first to recognize that the issues of maternal drug dependence must be addressed within the context of the fundamental role gender plays in defining identity; coping skills; psychological social and cultural realties; and

TABLE 48.1 Needs of pregnant women with substance abuse problems and the services they require

Presenting issues	Services
Medical comorbidities	Obstetrical services
	Nutritional counseling
	HIV, sexually transmitted infections and hepatitis B and C testing and counseling
	Smoking cessation intervention
	Appropriate sub-specialty referrals, for example, cardiology, pulmonology, hepatology, dental
Psychiatric comorbidities	Psychiatric services
	Pharmacologic and behavioral treatment
Childhood and/or current exposure to physical, sexual, and psychological abuse	Trauma specific services
	Referral to Rape Crisis Centers, Help lines for court and legal information
Family relationship problems	Family therapy services
	Referral of partner/family member to substance abuse treatment
Lack of education and vocational training	GED or other employment training or services
Involvement with criminal justice	Community legal services
	Referral to drug court
Involvement with child protective services	Child assessment and referral services
	Parenting intervention services, especially for the care of newborns and young children
	Child care within substance abuse treatment program

available resources. Drug-dependent women most often suffer from low self-esteem, depression, and anxiety; are usually the primary caregivers for their children; have a high incidence of victimization; and are involved in relationships with men who are also drug dependent (6). This early work of Reed is supported by work of Comfort and Kaltenbach (7) and others in the nineties and by Jones et al. (8) and others in the subsequent decade. Although the actual prevalence varies across studies, the consistency in the data allows for a general characterization. Overall, substance abusing pregnant women tend to have completed approximately 11 years of education, are most likely to be unmarried, have a history of substance abuse in their families, have a history of physical and sexual victimization, have significant health and/or mental health problems, have current problems with criminal justice, have current and/or past involvement with Child Protective Services, lack stable housing, and are unemployed with poor vocational training. As such they are a very vulnerable population with little support and few if any resources (7). Yet they are often the targets of prejudicial and judgmental treatment by health care providers and coercive policies implemented by child welfare systems, juvenile/family court, and the criminal justice system. Although no state statute makes it a crime for pregnant women to become pregnant or give birth, in extreme cases, "fetal abuse" statutes have been used to prosecute pregnant women. "Fetal abuse" statutes are those statues in which existing child abuse statutes were applied to include maternal prenatal conduct, have been used to prosecute pregnant women for drug use (9). In these cases, where the fetus was determined to be a "child," pregnant women have been arrested for possession of a controlled substance, delivering drugs to a minor or charged with child abuse. By 2000, some 200 pregnant women in 30 states had been prosecuted on such interpretations of fetal abuse (10).

These actions frequently deter women from seeking prenatal care and treatment for their substance use disorders. Their chaotic lifestyle and lack of prenatal care results in an array of medical and obstetrical complications, reducing the chances of a healthy pregnancy outcome regardless of the effects of the drug(s) they are abusing. Table 48.1 delineates the complex needs of pregnant women with substance use disorders and the services that should be provided in addition to substance abuse treatment.

ALCOHOL

Effects of Prenatal Exposure to Alcohol on the Neonate

Considerable research has consistently shown the adverse physical and behavioral effects on children whose mothers consumed alcohol during pregnancy. The early literature on this topic described a fetal alcohol syndrome (FAS) that included three defining aspects. The first aspect consists of facial malformations that can include small eyes, inner epicanthal folds, a thin upper lip, a long smooth philtrum, and midfacial hypoplasia. The second aspect is notable delays in growth and growth restriction (in head size and physical height). These delays are evident prenatally and there is typically failure to catch up at any point in life postnatally. The third aspect is CNS/neurodevelopmental abnormalities (e.g., neurologic hard or soft signs, behavioral problems, learning disabilities as appropriate for age) (11,12). Because there are some individuals who were prenatally exposed to alcohol who exhibit some but not all FAS aspects, newer terms have been developed to refine the characterization of their problems. These terms include alcohol-related neurodevelopmental disorder (ARND), alcohol-related birth defects (ARBD), and the largest umbrella term, fetal alcohol spectrum disorder (FASD). FASD encompasses all adverse effects demonstrated in individuals prenatally exposed to alcohol (12). FASDs are estimated to occur in 2% to –4% of all live births and are associated with severe cognitive, behavioral, adaptive, social, and emotional regulatory outcomes. These primary problems can set the occasion for vulnerabilities in childhood- or adult-onset secondary problems, particularly in the domains of psychiatric illnesses, including substance use disorders, social relations, school performance, and legal issues (see Paley & O'Connor (13) for a review).

An important question in both the clinical and research domains is whether there is a "safe" amount of alcohol to consume during pregnancy. Heavy (three or more drinks per week or one or more drink per day) alcohol consumption during pregnancy is associated with low birth weight and preterm birth and these outcomes are proximate causes of neonatal morbidity and death and predictors of long-term developmental outcomes (14). A summary of FASDs would be incomplete without the acknowledgment of the importance of the animal models that have confirmed the exact nature and extent of the effects of prenatal alcohol exposure on the fetus by demonstrating the linkage between in utero alcohol exposure and compromised physical attributes and behavior (see Kelly et al. (15) for a review).

Information for Clinicians Regarding Alcohol Exposure During Pregnancy

Ideally, the use of alcohol during pregnancy should be avoided as no "safe" amount of alcohol has been identified. While some women are able to spontaneously quit their use of alcohol before or upon pregnancy awareness, other women are not in a life position to accomplish this behavior change. Thus, it is important to identify as early as reasonably possible pregnant women who are drinking in order to provide them with opportunities for intervention to change their drinking behavior.

In the absence of reliable biomarkers to detect alcohol consumption over many days or weeks, screening methods have by necessity relied on self-report. Although denial and stigma are always concerns for inaccurate reporting, there are alcohol use screening tools designed for pregnant women. The T-ACE is one tool that has been validated for screening pregnant women for at-risk alcohol consumption. The T-ACE is recommended by the American College of Obstetricians and Gynecologists (ACOG) and the National Institute on

Alcohol Abuse and Alcoholism for screening and can reliably detect alcohol use across all ethnic/racial minority groups. It asks four questions about a woman's *tolerance* for alcohol, if she has ever been *annoyed* by other people criticizing her drinking, if she has ever felt she needs to *cut down* her drinking and if she ever has an *eye-opener* drink first thing in the morning (16).

Following a positive screen for at-risk drinking, pregnant women need to be assessed for current dependence on alcohol. Those women who are determined to be dependent need treatment in specialty centers. For those women who are not dependent, research shows the benefits of brief interventions, administered by health professionals in the context of care visits, for reducing at-risk drinking (14). ACOG also offers a FASD tool kit for assisting health care providers in screening, intervention, and assistance for pregnant patients with at-risk drinking (14).

While there is continually growing evidence to document the associated negative effects of prenatal exposure to alcohol on the fetus, neonate, and child, the research agenda has recently expanded to include a focus on understanding the complex interactions that exist between caregivers and the child prenatally exposed to alcohol. How these dynamics can alter the subsequent behavior of the child in his/her maturity is also of interest. Animal models have proven to be instrumental in providing guidance for how environmental enrichment and exercise are related to improvements in alcohol's developmental effects (15).

Alcohol exposure may produce epigenetic (gene expression is changed in absence of changing the organism's actual DNA) effects as a result of the direct actions of alcohol on the DNA of the in-utero exposed child or from changes which result from compromised caregiver–infant behaviors early in postnatal life (15).

Although much is known about the adverse effects associated with prenatal exposure to alcohol, the effects of this substance in combination with other substances, including, particularly, cigarette smoking, has received less scientific attention. There is some evidence to suggest a synergistic effect of prenatal exposure to both alcohol and cigarette smoking on low birth weight, premature birth, and prenatal growth restriction (17).

OPIOIDS

Effects of Prenatal Exposure to Opioids on the Neonate

Although there are a number of drugs classified as opioids, including buprenorphine, codeine, fentanyl, heroin, hydrocodone, methadone, meperidine, morphine, and oxycodone, the primary opioids used/abused by pregnant women are heroin, oxycodone, methadone, and buprenorphine (3). Opioids are not categorized as a teratogen (18), but they do easily cross the placenta. Infants exposed to opioids in utero are born passively dependent and neonatal abstinence occurs in 55% to 94% of newborns (19).

Neonatal abstinence is characterized by signs and symptoms of CNS hyperirritability; gastrointestinal (GI) dysfunction; respiratory distress; and vague autonomic symptoms that include yawning, sneezing, mottling, and fever. Infants generally develop tremors, which may progress to the point where they occur spontaneously without any stimulation. A high-pitched cry, hyperactive Moro reflex, increased muscle tone, sleep disturbances, and irritability are also present. Respiratory dysregulation is indicated by nasal stuffiness and rapid respiration. The rooting reflex is increased and infants often suck frantically on their fists or thumbs, yet have difficulty feeding because of an uncoordinated sucking reflex. Additional GI dysfunction is characterized by regurgitation and diarrhea (20).

Infants undergoing withdrawal must be assessed to determine the severity of the withdrawal and whether to initiate pharmacotherapy to treat it. The most widely used assessment instrument used in U.S. hospitals is the Neonatal Abstinence Score (20) commonly referred to as the Finnegan score (21). There are several other scoring instruments, for example, Green and Suffet (22), Lipsitz (23), and a number of hospitals use a "modified" Finnegan (8). Whatever scoring system is utilized, the purpose is to objectively assess the onset, progression, and diminution of abstinence symptoms. It provides a mechanism for determining if pharmacotherapy is indicated, monitoring the infant's response to treatment, and initiating a taper when control is achieved. For example, using the Finnegan score, infants are assessed 2 hours after birth and then every 4 hours at a minimum. Pharmacotherapy is indicated when the total abstinence score is 8 or greater for three consecutive scores, or 12 or greater for two consecutive scores. Once abstinence is controlled using the prescribed dosage schedule, the dose administered to achieve control is maintained for 72 hours and then a dosage reduction schedule is initiated (20).

The American Academy of Pediatrics (19) recommends opioid therapy for the treatment of opioid abstinence. Short-acting opioids administered orally are well tolerated by neonates, can be easily titrated to control abstinence, and offer a wide margin of safety between therapeutic and toxic doses (24). There are limited data evaluating the efficacy of different drug regimes in the treatment of neonatal abstinence (see American Academy of Pediatrics (19) for a review); however, there appears to be clinical consensus that use of diluted tincture of opium or morphine sulfate is indicated, as they have been reported as the most commonly used agents in hospitals throughout the United States (21). Buprenorphine has recently been investigated as a treatment option. Kraft et al. (25) conducted a randomized open-label study of the use of buprenorphine in comparison to standard of care neonatal opium solution in the treatment of 26 neonates in opioid withdrawal, and reported the mean length of treatment for infants receiving neonatal opium solution was 32 days compared with 22 days for infants receiving buprenorphine. While these findings were not significant ($p < 0.077$), there is a suggestion of improved efficacy that requires further investigation. Clonidine for neonatal opioid withdrawal has also been recently evaluated in a randomized, double blind clinical trial by Agthe et al. (26). They found the addition of oral clonidine with the use of diluted tincture of opium reduced the length of treatment by 27% compared to infants receiving diluted tincture of opium and placebo. Both of these studies reflect renewed interest in empirically determining the efficacy of treatment medications for neonatal abstinence.

There is significant variability in the onset and duration of neonatal abstinence. The time of onset of withdrawal ranges from shortly after birth to 2 weeks of age but on average, occurs within 72 hours after birth (20). In addition to individual variability, abstinence due to methadone exposure is more prolonged and more severe than for heroin exposure (27). Although the data to date are quite limited, there is also some suggestion that abstinence due to buprenorphine exposure requires less medication and a shorter hospital stay than for methadone-exposed infants (8). There are relatively no data to date on the characterization of neonatal abstinence from oxycodone exposure. Variability in neonatal abstinence can also be due to concomitant drug use. Benzodiazepine use among methadone maintained pregnant women has been found to increase the length of treatment for neonatal abstinence by an average of 14.4 days (28). Nicotine has also been reported to increase the duration of neonatal abstinence in infants born to methadone maintained women (29).

The type of opioid used may also have an effect on perinatal outcomes, including prematurity and birth weight. Infants exposed to heroin have high rates of intrauterine growth restriction and prematurity (30) and infants exposed to both heroin and methadone have lower birth weights than infants born to women enrolled in a methadone maintenance program (31). In a study by Kandall et al., infants born to women receiving methadone maintenance had a mean birth weight of 2961 g, which has been an exceptionally consistent finding across studies for the past 30 years (31). There are few data comparing infants born to women maintained on methadone and those born to women maintained on buprenorphine but available data suggest that birth weight does not differ (8).

Although neurodevelopmental outcomes assessed by the NICU Network Neurobehavioral Scale (NNNS) have found infants exposed to opioids differ from nondrug exposed comparison infants on orientation scores and stress abstinence scores at 1 month of age, with adjustment for covariates of socio-economic status (SES), birth weight and polydrug use, there were no significant effects (32). The Maternal Life Style Study (discussed in more detail under section "Cocaine" in this chapter) examined cognitive, motor, and behavioral outcomes at 1, 2, and 3 years of age in a cohort of 1227 children (cocaine exposed $n = 474$; opioid exposed $n = 50$; cocaine and opioid $n = 48$; and nondrug exposed $n = 655$). After controlling for covariates, including frequency and quantity of substance use per trimester, maternal education, SES, home environment, maternal/caregiver IQ, and maternal psychological symptoms, there were no significant differences on the Bayley Scales of Infant Development between the opioid exposed infants and other groups (33).

Information for Clinicians Regarding Opioid Exposure During Pregnancy

Different opioids manifest different clinical issues for opioid-dependent pregnant women. Heroin use is illegal and is characterized by a chaotic lifestyle; medical complications associated with parenteral opioid use can include hepatitis, HIV, septicemia, and cellulitis. Obstetrical complications are related to a lack of prenatal care. Moreover, the effects of heroin last only 3 to 5 hours, so the fetus is subjected to repeated episodes of opioid withdrawal, increasing the risk of morbidity and mortality (34). It is essential that efforts be made to engage pregnant heroin-dependent women in treatment.

Methadone is a synthetic opioid medication that is used in the treatment of opioid dependence and methadone maintenance is recommended as the standard of care in the management of opioid dependence during pregnancy (35). Effective methadone maintenance prevents the onset of withdrawal for 24 hours, reduces or eliminates craving, and blocks the euphoric effects of other opioids. In pregnancy, methadone prevents erratic maternal opioid drug levels, and protects the fetus from repeated episodes of withdrawal (34). Additionally, through regulation, it ensures that prenatal care will be available. In the United States, methadone may only be prescribed for maintenance within a licensed opioid treatment program (OTP). Under federal methadone regulations, 42CFR8.12, pregnant women must be given priority for admittance to an OTP and the program must, at a minimum, coordinate prenatal care with a medical provider if they do not have the capacity to provide obstetrical services. When effective methadone maintenance is provided with a comprehensive program that includes prenatal care, the incidence of obstetric and fetal complications and neonatal morbidity and mortality can be reduced (34).

One of the most contentious clinical issues in providing methadone maintenance to pregnant women is the question of dose. A prevailing concern has centered on whether there is a dose response to the severity of neonatal abstinence. Recommendations have often proposed low methadone doses in an attempt to reduce or eliminate neonatal abstinence. Although there have been well over 30 studies that have investigated the relationship between dose and severity of withdrawal, the findings are contradictory. While a number of studies have reported significant relationships, the majority found no relationship. As such there is not compelling evidence to reduce maternal dose to avoid neonatal abstinence. Conversely, there is evidence that higher doses are associated with less illicit drug use (36) and reducing methadone dose may lead to illicit substance use, and hence increase risk to both mother and fetuses (34).

Although methadone has been used for the treatment of opioid dependence for over 40 years, recent concerns have emerged regarding an association between methadone and

QTc interval prolongation, with torsade de pointes associated with very high dose methadone. There have been a number of publications with recommendations such as obtaining a pretreatment ECG, a follow-up ECG within 30 days, and annually. For patients with QTc interval greater than 500 msec it has been recommended that consideration be given to discontinuing or reducing methadone dose (37). To date, there are no data on QTc intervals in pregnant opioid-dependent women maintained on methadone so this presents a unique challenge for clinical care in this population.

Buprenorphine, a partial mu-opioid agonist, was approved for use in the treatment of opioid dependency in the United States in 2002; however, it was not approved for use in pregnancy. Nevertheless, there are many instances in which a woman has been successfully maintained on buprenorphine when she becomes pregnant. In such cases, the prescribing physician and patient may decide that the benefits of remaining on the current medication outweigh any risk. To date, there are only published data from two small, randomized clinical trials on the safety and efficacy of buprenorphine compared to methadone in the treatment of pregnant women (8,38). However, there are a large number of studies, primarily case reports and prospective studies from Europe, in which buprenorphine has been used with pregnant women. The reports indicate that buprenorphine during pregnancy provides the same benefits as other opioid agonist medications (39). Moreover, there is limited evidence to suggest that infants born to women maintained on buprenorphine may have less severe neonatal abstinence and require less treatment compared to methadone (8).

The presence of methadone or buprenorphine in breast milk has been an important question in the clinical management of opioid dependence during pregnancy. There are limited data regarding buprenorphine, but the evidence indicates that only small amounts of buprenorphine pass into breast milk and the well-established poor oral bioavailability of buprenorphine suggests that absorption via breast milk may be low (40). From as early as 1974, there have been a number of studies that have reported low concentrations of methadone in breast milk (see Jansson et al. (41) for a review) and in 2001, the American Academy of Pediatrics (42) recommendation on drugs and breast-feeding eliminated the dose restriction on methadone, making methadone maintenance treatment compatible with breast-feeding regardless of maternal dose. The general recommendation is that opioid maintained mothers can breast-feed if they are not HIV positive, not using illicit drugs, and do not have a disease or infection is which breast-feeding is contraindicated.

COCAINE

Effects of Prenatal Exposure to Cocaine on the Fetus and Neonate

Cocaine is an alkaloid prepared from the leaves of the Erythroxylon coca plant. It blocks the presynaptic reuptake of the neurotransmitters norepinephrine and dopamine, producing an excess of transmitter at the postsynaptic sites. Activation of the sympathetic nervous system by this mechanism produces vasoconstriction, an acute rise in arterial pressure, tachycardia, and a predisposition to ventricular arrhythmias and seizures (43). Cocaine use rose dramatically in the 1980s and was accompanied by ubiquitous media coverage due to numerous high-profile deaths and the shift from expensive cocaine powder to the far cheaper crack/cocaine. The minimal cost and potent euphoria that crack/cocaine provided gave rise to the "cocaine epidemic" including significant use among pregnant women. This led to major concerns on the effects on the fetus and neonate as cocaine easily crosses the placenta. The animal and adult literature on the effects of cocaine on the cardiovascular system provided support for such concern as did the potential for the potent vasoconstrictive properties of cocaine to cause congenital malformations.

The first studies on the effects of prenatal cocaine exposure published in the mid-1980s reported alarming outcomes with increased incidence of spontaneous abortion, abruptio placentae, premature labor and delivery, intrauterine growth restriction, risk of congenital malformation of the genitourinary tract, neurobehavioral effects, and risk of perinatal cerebral infarction (see Volpe (44) for a review). However, subsequent studies in the late 1980s and early 1990s have failed to replicate the early findings. In response to such disparities Lutiger et al. (45) conducted a meta-analysis to evaluate the reproductive risks of cocaine. The reproductive effects assessed included rates of small for gestational age (SGA) births, low birth weight, prematurity, abruptio placentae, malformation, spontaneous abortion, fetal demise, and Sudden Infant Death Syndrome (SIDS). They reviewed 45 scientific papers reporting on the effects of cocaine used during pregnancy and identified 20 eligible for meta-analysis. They included comparisons of four groups; no drug use, cocaine alone, polydrug users who did not use cocaine, and polydrug users who used cocaine. None of the comparisons found an increased risk of abruptio placentae, cardiac malformations, or sudden infant death associated with cocaine use. They found very few adverse reproductive effects were associated with cocaine when the polydrug cocaine use group was compared to the nonocaine polydrug use group. When the comparison groups consisted of no drug use, the polydrug cocaine group had a higher risk of spontaneous abortions; similarly they found in comparisons of the cocaine alone and no drug use groups, there was a higher risk for in utero death in addition to genitourinary tract malformations for the cocaine alone group. They concluded that the discrepancies suggest that a variety of adverse reproductive effects commonly associated with prenatal cocaine exposures may be caused by confounding factors clustering in cocaine users.

In addition to contradictory reproductive risk data, there were also inconsistent findings regarding adverse neurobehavioral effects and developmental outcomes. In an effort to provide a critical synthesis of existing studies, Frank et al. (46) conducted a review of all articles published between 1984 and

2000 that included the words cocaine, crack/cocaine, pregnancy, prenatal exposure, delayed effects, children, and related disorders. Seventy-four published articles were identified. Studies were then excluded if they failed to mask children's exposure status; had no control group; subjects were not prospectively recruited; samples were largely confounded with exposure to opioids, methamphetamines or phencyclidine; and/or samples were predominately comprised of HIV positive mothers. Thirty-six studies met the inclusion criteria for this analysis. These studies were comprised of 17 independent cohorts from 14 cities; some cohorts were the subjects reported in multiple articles, either at different ages or with analyses of different variables. In summary, their review found that after controlling for tobacco and alcohol exposure, cocaine did not effect physical growth and that for children up to age 6, there is little impact of prenatal cocaine exposure on children's scores on nationally normed cognitive assessments (see Frank et al. (46) for a full review).

To address the many methodologic issues in the cocaine literature prospectively, the Maternal Lifestyle Study (MLS), a multisite longitudinal study was implemented through the NICHD Neonatal Research Network. This study included a cohort of 522 cocaine exposed and 655 comparison mother/child dyads. In addition to a large cohort, this study included extensive assessment on the multiple domains of child, mother, and environment and was designed to address the multiple associated factors that impact our understanding of the effects of prenatal cocaine exposure including polydrug use, the caregiving environment, sample size, and medical conditions (47). The MLS study has confirmed that cocaine exposure is not associated with mental, motor or behavioral deficits through 3 years of age after controlling for birth weight and environmental risks (33), but has also demonstrated that cocaine may effect areas of the brain that are not manifested until later in development. Specifically, the neural systems most likely to be affected by cocaine exposure are involved in discrete neurobehavioral functions such as attention, arousal, and motivation.

Two studies from the same longitudinal cohort examined the effect of prenatal cocaine exposure on attention and response inhibition as measured by continuous performance tests (CPTs) at ages 5 and 7 in a sample of 219 cocaine exposed and 196 comparison children and found cocaine associated increases in omission errors at ages 5 and 7, slower reaction times, and decreased consistency in performance at age 7 (48). They also investigated the risk for developing a learning disability by age 7 (cocaine exposed $n = 212$, comparison $n = 197$), and found that the cocaine exposed children had a 2.8 times greater risk of developing a learning disability by age 7 than the nonexposed children (49).

Several other studies have focused on a specific function. Singer et al. (50) examined their cohort at 9 years of age and found that the cocaine exposed group ($n = 192$) had poorer perceptual reasoning IQ than a noncocaine exposed group ($n = 179$). Mays et al. (51) examined performance on a spatial working memory task in 75 cocaine exposed and 55 nondrug exposed 8- to 10-year-old children. In this study, cocaine exposed children had significantly slower correct moves per second and number of errors per trial. The clinical significance of these studies remains unclear. Much more research is needed to both definitely establish the presence of subtle impairments in attentional states and executive functions and what may be meditating factors in children of mothers who used cocaine during their pregnancy.

Information for Clinicians Regarding Cocaine Exposure During Pregnancy

Women who use cocaine during pregnancy have a complex array of obstetrical/medical risks, including a high incidence of alcohol, tobacco and marijuana use, syphilis, gonorrhea, and hospitalizations related to violence (32), making their obstetrical management difficult. To date, there are no specific medical treatments for cocaine use in pregnancy; referrals should be made to either outpatient or residential treatment programs.

Unlike opioids, cocaine does not produce an abstinence syndrome but infants may initially exhibit signs of irritability, tremulousness, and liability after birth. While these are transient, they may both exacerbate and be exacerbated by the caregiving environment. Mothers may benefit from individualized direction and support on how to structure the caretaking environment to provide an optimal environment for her newborn.

Breast-feeding is contraindicated for mothers who are using cocaine because cocaine is present in breast milk and may produce an acute neurotoxic disorder including irritability, hypertonia, tremors, and seizures (42).

AMPHETAMINES

Effects of Prenatal Exposure to Amphetamines on the Fetus and the Neonate

Amphetamine and methamphetamine are commonly known stimulants. They have a somewhat different mechanism of action from cocaine. Amphetamine and methamphetamine reverse the action of the monoamine transporters. They also stimulate dopamine, norepinephrine, and serotonin release and increase the availability of these neurochemicals at the postsynaptic receptor. Methamphetamine is a known potent drug with neurotoxic effects. A review of the effects of prenatal exposure to amphetamines and methamphetamines concluded that cleft palates, cardiac anomalies, and deficits in fetal growth are evident in both animal studies and documented human exposure cases (52).

There are very limited data regarding the long-term outcomes following prenatal exposure to amphetamine and/or methamphetamine. The largest study to date, the Infant Development, Environment, and Lifestyle (IDEAL) Study, demonstrated that in general, both the prevalence and frequency of methamphetamine use decreased from the first to the third trimester of pregnancy (84.3% vs. 56.0% vs. 42.4%, and 3.1 vs. 2.4 vs. 1.5 days/week). Among this group of methamphetamine-using pregnant women, one third were deemed as consistently high users throughout pregnancy and had fewer prenatal care visits than those groups who were able to reduce their use during pregnancy (53). Prenatal exposure to amphetamines has been associated with low birth weight, with infants being 3.5 times more likely to be small for gestational age, and showing decreased arousal, movement disorders, and increased stress in the neonatal period (54). The cognitive function in children ages 3 to 4 years showed that compared to non-methamphetamine-exposed children, methamphetamine-exposed children had poorer performance on a visual motor integration task as well as evidence of abnormal acceleration of neuronal and glial development in these brain regions (55).

Information for Clinicians Regarding Amphetamine Exposure During Pregnancy

The identification of amphetamine use during pregnancy can be challenging and no self-report tools exist that are specific for pregnant women. There are biologic tests available that can detect the recent use of amphetamines and methamphetamine. At delivery, biologic matrices such as umbilical cord, meconium, urine, and hair have been used to determine the presence of these drugs at birth. While it is possible to identify a pregnant woman and her in-utero exposed neonate and to characterize the detrimental effects of this substance exposure on her and her child, treatment interventions to reduce or eliminate such use are needed. To the best of our knowledge, there are no specific behavioral or medication treatments that have been designed and/or have evidence to support their use in pregnant women who use amphetamine or methamphetamine. Specific to pregnant women, ensuring prenatal care attendance, regular assessment for fetal growth, and intervention with other substance use (e.g., concurrent alcohol use is prevalent in these stimulant users) seem especially important for these pregnant women.

INHALANTS

A diverse group of chemicals are known as organic solvents (frequently known as inhalants). These chemicals have multiple household and industrial uses. Most people encounter solvents in their daily life with the use of items such as cleaning fluids and glues (containing aromatic hydrocarbons like toluene or benzene), paint stripper or correction fluid (containing alkyl halides like 1,1,1-trichloroethane [TCE]), fuels or lighter fluids (aliphatic hydrocarbons like propane, gasoline, butane), air fresheners (aliphatic nitrites like isoamyl), nail polish remover (like ketones), and nitrous oxide which was used in pressurized whip cream dispensers and is still used in medical and dental settings. With awareness and proper use, most individuals experience only low-level exposure to these chemicals. There are infrequent occasions when industrial accidents have exposed individuals to acute, high levels of these chemicals. There are also individuals who voluntarily expose themselves to repeated high-levels of organic solvents. The voluntary exposure or abuse of organic solvents is typically performed by inhaling vapors to become intoxicated. The various inhalation routes include "bagging" (inhaling fumes after spraying into a bag), "huffing" (inhaling solvent fumes from a cloth placed over nose and mouth), "sniffing" or "snorting" (see Jones and Balster (56) for a review).

Associated Effects of Prenatal Exposure to Abused Inhalants on the Neonate

While there are numerous types of organic solvents that have been reported to be abused, there are few data about abuse of these inhalants during pregnancy. As such, only those organic solvents with the most human prenatal exposure data are discussed below. While little is known about the specifics of abused inhalants during pregnancy, it is known that these types of substances are quite toxic and can be fatal if misused.

Toluene

The initial report concluding an association between inhalant abuse during pregnancy and negative birth outcome was published in 1979. It was in this report that the term "fetal solvent syndrome" was used to describe the constellation of physical effects including low birth weight, small head size, and facial dysmorphology that was present in children born to mothers with known abuse of toluene during pregnancy (57). Since that time, there have been numerous other case reports describing the effects of prenatal exposure to abused inhalants on the child. The largest report provided a summary of 35 deliveries from 15 solvent-abusing women. These cases were compared to a control group of infants and showed that, on average, toluene-exposed neonates were at increased risk for being premature, of lower birth weight, smaller birth length, smaller head circumference, and to have intrauterine growth restriction. Developmental follow-up of the toluene-exposed children showed that compared to a control group, on average, there was growth restriction in terms of height and weight as well as developmental delays in cognitive, speech, and motor skills (58).

Given the similarities between toluene and alcohol, a direct comparison of the teratologic effects of prenatal toluene and alcohol exposure has been undertaken. There were both overlapping and unique anomalies associated with prenatal exposure to either substance. Similar features included a thin upper lip, midfacial hypoplasia, and small palpebral fissures. Head and facial features that appeared unique to toluene were micrognathia, ear anomalies, a narrow bifrontal diameter, abnormal scalp hair patterns, down turned corners of the mouth, and a large fontanelle (59). Craniofacial features unique to fetal alcohol exposure included a more pronounced hypoplasia of the philtrum and nose (59). The reasons underling the similar physical alterations may be either similar mechanisms of action of the two drugs, the restricted range of craniofacial abnormalities that can occur at birth, and/or the fact that the toluene-exposed children may have also been prenatally exposed to alcohol during gestation.

Gasoline

There is at least one report of two infants born to a mother who repeatedly sniffed gasoline during pregnancy. Both neonates had low birth weight, and were small in length and head circumference for their gestational age. Following delivery, they exhibited hypotonia followed by hypertonia. At later follow-up they were observed to have minor facial and physical abnormalities (60).

It is important to remember the complexities of the lives of women who abuse substances while pregnant and the inhalant literature, like other in utero literature, often minimizes the possible contribution of multiple factors such as nutrition, licit substance use (nicotine and alcohol), stress, and psychiatric comorbidities that may play important yet undefined roles in exacerbating or mitigating the effects on maternal and neonatal outcomes.

Information for Clinicians Regarding Inhalant Abuse During Pregnancy

Signs and symptoms of toluene or other solvent abuse can include: stains (e.g., paint) on the body or clothing, a noticeable chemical odor, sores around the mouth and/or nose, irritated eyes and/or nose, drunken appearance, nausea, anorexia, irritability, or excitability (see Jones and Balster (56) for review). More recently, solvent withdrawal signs have been discussed in the literature and may include fatigue and difficulty concentrating, fast heart beat, depressed mood, trembling, or twitching (61). Given the short duration of action, it is unlikely that tests of bodily fluids will be able to detect the use of inhalants or their metabolites. Thus, asking questions to women suspected of abusing inhalants during pregnancy about the amount and frequency of their inhalant use in a nonjudgmental and neutral manner may be the most effective method for determining abuse.

Renal tubular acidosis is one of the most frequent signs of solvent abuse. The effects of acidosis on pregnancy outcome are concerning. Maternal acidemia has been shown to decrease blood flow and oxygenation, which can compromise fetal development. While a reversible complication, renal tubular acidosis can result in hypokalemia, hypophosphatemia, hypomagnesemia, hypocalcemia, and rhabdomyolysis. Chronic use can result in neurotoxic damage with cerebellar degeneration and cortical atrophy. Hypokalemia and hypophosphatemia can result in debilitating muscle weakness. Further, hypokalemia may also result in cardiac arrhythmias. Hypomagnesemia can result in severe hypocalcemia and a related parathyroid hormone suppression (62).

While it is possible to identify a pregnant woman who abuses inhalants and to characterize the detrimental effects of the abuse on her and her child, treatment interventions to reduce or eliminate such abuse are needed. To the best of our knowledge, there are no specific treatments for pregnant women who abuse inhalants. Specific to pregnant women, ensuring prenatal care attendance and regular assessment for preterm labor, fetal growth, and renal tubular acidosis seems especially important for these pregnant women. Currently, there are no medications or treatments that reverse acute solvent intoxication.

In terms of the neonate, there have been reports of a neonatal withdrawal following prenatal exposure to abused solvents (63). However, standardized measures to evaluate such withdrawal are lacking. It might be expected that mothers showing signs of intoxication at delivery should have neonates monitored for alcohol-like withdrawal signs, so that appropriate intervention can be provided to the neonate.

MARIJUANA

Effects of Prenatal Exposure to Marijuana on the Fetus and Neonate

Reports and studies of the effects of in utero exposure to marijuana have shown modest and inconsistent effects. For example, of five reports that include prospective and retrospective studies using a combination of methods to determine marijuana exposure, only one showed a significant effect on birth outcomes (64). A prospective study characterizing prenatal marijuana exposure showed significant effects on birth weight adjusted for gestational age and length at birth (65). In contrast, the IDEAL study demonstrated that marijuana use was not significantly related to the examined fetal growth parameters of gestational-age adjusted birth weight and being SGA (66).

Interestingly, several studies have reported a mixture of negative and beneficial effects of in utero exposure to marijuana even in those studies that controlled for maternal weight gain due to marijuana's appetite stimulant effects. For example, a prospective study of prenatal marijuana exposure during gestation showed a modest but significantly negative effect of marijuana use during the first trimester of pregnancy on birth length, yet an average increase of 139 g in birth weight in women reporting one or more marijuana joints per day in the third trimester (67).

Information for Clinicians Regarding Marijuana Exposure During Pregnancy

While the majority of the evidence supports minimal to no effects associated with prenatal exposure to marijuana on birth outcomes, the literature is limited by methodologic challenges such as reliance on self-report, few prospective studies assessing exposure over the entire pregnancy, and controlling for multiple environmental and individual factors that could relate to the outcomes observed (64).

Although the current literature does not support a consistent negative pattern of effects on birth outcomes following prenatal exposure to marijuana, this absence of evidence should not be taken as reassurance that prenatal exposure to marijuana is without risks. There is accumulating evidence showing that the endocannabinoid system plays a major role in CNS patterning. This patterning occurs in areas that are relevant for mood, memory, and reward. A recent review suggested a possible association with in utero marijuana exposure and genetic changes of neural systems that are relevant to endocannabinoid function (68).

There are also data to support the conclusion that prenatal marijuana exposure has a negative relationship with executive functioning which is largely mediated by the prefrontal region of the brain which develops somewhat later in childhood maturation (69).

Like other substances that have been discussed in this chapter, there are tools to detect the presence of marijuana in multiple biologic matrices. The window of detection of the presence of marijuana in the mother during pregnancy and/or the neonate at birth may be somewhat longer compared to the other substances that are abused. As of yet, treatment interventions (behavioral, medication, or a combination of the two) to reduce or eliminate marijuana use during gestation are lacking. To the best of our knowledge, there are no specific behavioral or medication treatments that have been designed and/or have evidence to support their use in pregnant women.

NICOTINE/TOBACCO PRODUCTS

Effects of Prenatal Exposure to Tobacco Products on the Fetus and Neonate

Like alcohol, considerable attention has focused on characterizing and understanding the adverse effects on children born to mothers who smoke cigarettes or use other nicotine-containing products during pregnancy. The rates of cigarette smoking women who continue to smoke cigarettes after finding out that they are pregnant decreased in the United States for several decades and have now plateaued. Women who smoke cigarettes during pregnancy are more likely to be younger, single, have less academic success and/or employment stability, and depend on governmental medical assistance compared to their nonsmoking counterparts (70). Women who continue to smoke cigarettes and/or tobacco products during pregnancy are more likely to have spontaneous abortions, ectopic pregnancies, premature rupture of membranes, placenta previa, placenta abruption, fetal growth restriction, preterm birth, and SIDS relative to women who do not smoke during pregnancy (71,72). The adverse effects of secondhand smoke are also evident with increases in the risk for SIDS and infant respiratory distress (see Pauly & Slotkin (70) for a review).

While the exact mechanisms underlying the negative prenatal and neonatal effects of smoking have yet to be elucidated, it is known that nicotine binds to nicotinic acetylcholine receptors (nAChRs). These receptors are ligand-gated ion channels that are present throughout the fetal nervous system. Preclinical studies have shown that nicotine and its activation of nAChRs results in alterations in neuronal activity and life. However, the presence of other chemicals in addition to nicotine makes it difficult to disentangle the in utero effects of nicotine relative to the other chemicals in human exposures (73).

The negative effects associated with prenatal tobacco exposure during pregnancy have been reported to extend from the neonatal period into adolescence. A recent review on this topic concluded that prenatal tobacco exposure is associated with negative effects in infancy (e.g., attention levels, self-regulation ability), childhood (e.g., inattention and externalizing behaviors), and adolescence (attention deficit hyperactivity disorder and nicotine dependence (74)).

Information for Clinicians Regarding Tobacco Exposure During Pregnancy

Given the negative effects on both mother and fetus associated with prenatal exposure to tobacco products, there is a need to examine the current treatments for tobacco cessation in pregnant women.

The cessation of cigarette use during pregnancy can result in beneficial effects, with quitting smoking as late as the last trimester resulting in a near normal–birth weight infant (75). Currently, uncertainty exists about the use of nicotine replacement therapy during pregnancy given the modest ability of these medications to achieve smoking cessation in pregnant women while also minimizing harm to the fetus and children exposed to these type of medication (70). Other medications such as bupropion, which acts to inhibit the presynaptic reuptake of dopamine and norepinephrine, may hold promise for reducing both smoking and depression, which is a frequent comorbid disorder found in pregnant smokers.

Given that any medication has some associated risk, and definitive efficacy and safety data are lacking for medication treatments, behavioral interventions should be the first line of treatment for smoking cessation during pregnancy. One of the most promising interventions for reducing tobacco use in pregnant women is voucher-based reinforcement therapy that is delivered contingent upon smoking abstinence. This intervention has been shown to effectively reduce cigarette smoking and improve fetal growth (76). However, the optimal choice of treatment for cigarette smoking during pregnancy depends on multiple factors including the patient's desire for a particular treatment, her previous treatment response, and any patient-specific medical precautions/contraindications (77).

BENZODIAZEPINES

Benzodiazepines are among the most frequently prescribed medications to pregnant women. Commonly prescribed benzodiazepines are diazepam (Valium); alprazolam (Xanax); lorazepam (Ativan); clonazepam (Klonopin); and chlordiazepoxide (Librium). Benzodiazepines affect the inhibitory neurotransmitter gamma-aminobutyric acid (GABA) and appear to act on the limbic, thalamic, and hypothalamic levels of the CNS to produce sedative and hypnotic effects, reduction of anxiety, anticonvulsant effects, and skeletal muscle relaxation (78).

Effects of Prenatal Exposure to Benzodiazepine on the Fetus and Neonate

The only benzodiazepine that has been systematically studied among pregnant women is diazepam. Initial reports found an increased incidence of cleft lip and cleft palate with exposure to diazepam during pregnancy, but prospective studies do not support these findings and most reviewers have concluded that diazepam is not teratogenic (78).

Neonatal abstinence syndrome has been reported for infants with prolonged interuterine exposure to diazepam with symptoms closely resembling opioid withdrawal (79). Symptoms include hypertonia, irritability, abnormal sleep patterns, inconsolable crying, tremors, bradycardia, cyanosis, poor sucking, apnea, diarrhea, vomiting, and risk of aspiration of feeds (78). If treatment is indicated, phenobarbital is the recommended medication (24).

Information for Clinicians Regarding Benzodiazepine Exposure During Pregnancy

While benzodiazepine use during pregnancy may be indicated for treatment of specific medical problems, they have a high potential for abuse when used with other depressants such as alcohol and opioids. Benzodiazepine dependence is one of the major challenges faced by clinicians providing methadone maintenance for opioid dependence and it is especially problematic in the treatment of pregnant women. The abuse of benzodiazepines in methadone maintained patients has the potential to increase the CNS depressant effects of methadone and as such is considered a risk factor for fatal overdose. Exacerbating this risk is that abuse of benzodiazepines is associated with poor psychological functioning and less reduction in illicit drug use (80). Management of benzodiazepine use is further complicated both by the potential for seizures in rapid withdrawal and by patient resistance to a benzodiazepine taper due to fear of seizures. Withdrawal from benzodiazepines should be conducted by a prolonged gradual taper accompanied with extensive psychological support.

Infants born to women maintained on methadone who use/abuse benzodiazepines require significantly longer treatment for neonatal abstinence than infants born to methadone maintained women who do not use benzodiazepines (28). Effective management of the abstinence is made more difficult because of possible delayed onset of benzodiazepine withdrawal, which can occur as late as 12 to 21 days after birth. In addition, opioids used in the treatment of neonatal abstinence have no effect on withdrawal from a nonopioid. While phenobarbital is recommended as a drug of choice for nonopioid related withdrawal (19,24), the optimal treatment for infants with concomitant opioid and benzodiazepine withdrawal is not know (28).

Breast-feeding is contraindicated for mothers using diazepam as diazepam has the potential to cause lethargy, sedation, and weight loss in infants. There is little data on breast-feeding while taking alprazolam but based on available evidence of a case report and a cohort study of five cases, caution is indicated. No adverse effects have been reported with the use of lorazepam or chlordiazepoxide during breast-feeding (78). However, as previously discussed, breast-feeding is contraindicated with any illicit drug use, and in the case of misuse of prescription drugs it would be prudent to follow this same guideline.

HALLUCINOGENS

Hallucinogens, including LSD, Peyote, and PCP/Phencyclidine, all cause serious negative psychological effects and because of their erratic nature their use can be dangerous (e.g., "bad trips" and flashbacks associated with LSD use, and seizures and coma associated with high doses of PCP). Despite severe adverse outcomes related to these drugs, there is very little data on their effect in pregnant women. The limited data that exist include a few small retrospective studies, case reports, and one prospective study examining perinatal outcome associated with maternal PCP use.

Effects of Prenatal Exposure to PCP on the Fetus and Neonate

In a study that screened over 2000 pregnant women for PCP use early in pregnancy, a verbal history of use was reported by 149 pregnant women and current use documented by urine drug screens was identified in 23 pregnant women. Data collection was completed for 94 study patients, including 14 with confirmed current use, and 94 matched controls. The control group was unique from most studies in that they differed from the study group only in PCP use and the mean number of other drugs used; both groups frequently abused marijuana, cocaine, barbiturates, alcohol, and glue. Significantly more abnormal neurobehavioral findings, that is, decreased attention and depressed neonatal reflexes, were associated with maternal phencyclidine use, both in the sample which included all users and the subsample of confirmed users. Moreover, multiple regression analyses showed the number of abnormalities was related to PCP use and not other drugs. No significant relationships were found between abnormal anatomic findings and maternal PCP use. The authors qualify their results with the caution that while this study suggests PCP is not an anatomic teratogen, it does not confirm it (81). The abnormal neurobehavioral findings are consistent with a case study that reported two infants whose mothers used PCP during pregnancy to have symptoms similar to opioid withdrawal, that is, jitteriness, hypertonia, and hyperreflexia (82).

Information for Clinicians Regarding PCP Exposure During Pregnancy

As with most of the drugs discussed in this chapter, there are no specific treatment interventions to reduce or eliminate PCP use during pregnancy. As reported by Golden et al. (81), pregnant PCP users were characterized as using multiple drugs so general behavioral drug treatment interventions should be utilized.

For infants who exhibit moderate to severe CNS hyperirritability, treatment with phenobarbital is suggested (24). Breast-feeding is contraindicated as PCP has been found in breast milk (42).

SUMMARY

As previously discussed, information for each class of drug was presented independently for purposes of organization but most pregnant women with a substance use disorder use/abuse multiple drugs. There are numerous iterations of combinations, for example, opioid-dependent women may use and/or be dependent on cocaine, alcohol, marijuana, and/or benzodiazepines, cocaine users typically use and/or are dependent on alcohol and/or marijuana and opioids, methamphetamine users may also use alcohol and marijuana, and a large majority who use illicit drugs smoke cigarettes. The use of multiple drugs may have additive or synergistic effects on both the mother and neonate.

It is also important to understand that while the focus of this chapter is on the use of alcohol and other drugs during pregnancy, the substance use almost always precedes the pregnancy. All too frequently, the situation reflects a woman with a chronic substance use disorder who becomes pregnant, and thus brings to the pregnancy multiple bio-psycho-social problems that may impact on the health and well being of both her and her child.

As such, the effect of drug use during pregnancy is often confounded by numerous factors including multiple drug use, psychiatric comorbidities, exposure to violence and victimization, lack of prenatal care, poor nutrition, and living in an impoverished community. Attention to the use of drugs during pregnancy should be viewed within the context of multiple risks, the need to eliminate vulnerabilities, stigma and prejudice, and to the need to provide comprehensive care to promote a healthy outcome for both mother and child.

REFERENCES

1. Vorhees CV. Concepts in teratology and development toxicology derived from animal research. *Ann NY Acad Sci*. 1989;562:31–41.
2. Slotkin TA. Fetal nicotine or cocaine exposure: which one is worse? *J Pharmacol Exp Ther*. 1998;285(3):931–45.
3. SAMHSA. *Office of Applied Studies*. National Survey on Drug and Health; 2007 and 2008.
4. Kandall SR. *Substance and Shadow: Women and Addiction in the United States*. Cambridge, MA: Harvard University Press; 1996.
5. Beschner GM, Reed BG, Mondanaro J, eds. *Treatment Services for Drug Dependent Women*. Vol. 1. Rockville, MD: NIDA Res Monogr DHHS Pub. No (ADM); 1981.
6. Reed BG. Intervention strategies for drug dependent women: an introduction. In: Beschner GM, Reed BG, Mondanaro J. eds. *Treatment Services for Drug Dependent Women*. Vol. 1. Rockville MD: NIDA Res Monogr DHHS Pub. No (ADM); 1981:1–25.
7. Comfort M, Kaltenbach K. Biopsychosocial characteristics and treatment outcomes of pregnant cocaine-dependent women in residential and outpatient substance abuse treatment. *J Psychoactive Drugs*. 1999;31(3):279–289.
8. Jones HE, Johnson RE, Jasinski DR, et al. Buprenorphine versus methadone in the treatment of pregnant opioid-dependent patients: effects on the neonatal abstinence syndrome. *Drug Alcohol Depend*. 2005;79(1):1–10.
9. Scott T. Repercussions of the crack baby epidemic: why a message of care rather than punishment is needed for pregnant drug-users. 19 *Natl Black Law J*. 2006;203–221.
10. Paltrow L, Cohen D, Carey C. *Year 2000 Overview: governmental responses to pregnant women who use alcohol and other drugs*. Joint document produced by the Women's Law Project, Philadelphia, PA and National Advocates for Pregnant Women, New York, NY; 2000.
11. Jones KL, Smith DW, Ulleland CN, et al. Pattern of malformation of chronic alcoholic mothers. *Lancet*. 1973;1(7815):1267–1271.
12. Warren K, Floyd L, Calhoun F, et al. *Consensus Statement on FASD*. Washington DC: National Organization on Fetal Alcohol Syndrome; 2004.
13. Paley B, O'Connor MJ. Intervention for individuals with fetal alcohol spectrum disorders: treatment approaches and case management. *Dev Disabil Res Rev*. 2009;15(3):258–267.
14. Bailey BA, Sokol RJ. Pregnancy and alcohol use: evidence and recommendation for prenatal care. *Clin Obstet Gynecol*. 2008; 51(2): 436–444.
15. Kelly SJ, Goodlett CR, Hannigan JH. Animal models of fetal alcohol spectrum disorders: impact of the social environment. *Dev Disabil Res Rev*. 2009;15(3):200–208.
16. Sokol RJ, Martier SS, Ager JW. The T-ACE questions: practical prenatal detection of risky drinking. *Am J Obstet Gynecol*. 1989; 160(3):853–868.
17. Odendaal HJ, Steyn DW, Elliott A, et al. Combined effects of cigarette smoking and alcohol consumption on perinatal outcome. *Gynecol Obstet Invest*. 2009;67(1):1–8.
18. Scalli AR. Identifying teratogens: the tyranny of lists. *Reprod Toxicol*. 1997;11(4):555–559.
19. American Academy of Pediatrics Committee on Drugs. Neonatal drug withdrawal. *Pediatrics*. 1998;101(6):1079–1088.
20. Finnegan LP, Kaltenbach K. Neonatal abstinence syndrome. In: Hoekelman RA, Friedman SB, Nelson NM, et al., eds. *Primary Pediatric Care*. 2nd ed. St Louis, MO: Mosby Yearbook; 1992; 1367–1378.
21. Sarkar S, Donn SM. Management of neonatal abstinence syndrome in neonatal intensive care units: a national survey. *J Perinatol*. 2006;26(1):15–17.
22. Green M, Suffet F. The neonatal narcotic index: a device for the improvement of care in the abstinence syndrome. *Am J Drug Alcohol Abuse*. 1981;8(2):203–213.
23. Lipsitz PJ. A proposed narcotic withdrawal score for use with newborn infants. *Clin Pediatr*. 1975;14(6):592–594.
24. Finnegan LP, Kandall SR. Neonatal abstinence syndromes. In: Aranda J, Jaffe SJ, eds. *Neonatal and Pediatric Pharmacology: Therapeutic Principles in Practice*. 3rd ed. Philadelphia, PA: Lippincott, Williams & Wilkins; 2004:848–857.
25. Kraft WK, Gibson E, Dysart K, et al. Sublingual buprenorphine for treatment of neonatal abstinence syndrome: a randomized trial. *Pediatrics*. 2008;122(3):e601–e607.
26. Agthe AG, Kim GR, Mathias KB, et al. Clonidine as an adjunct therapy to opioids for neonatal abstinence syndrome: a randomized controlled trial. *Pediatrics*. 2009;123(5):e849–e856.
27. Rajegowda BK, Glass L, Evans HE, et al. Methadone withdrawal in newborn infants. *J Pediatr*. 1972;81(3):532–534.
28. Seligman NS, Salva N, Hayes EJ, et al. Predicting length of treatment for neonatal abstinence syndrome in methadone-exposed neonates. *Am J Obstet Gynecol*. 2008;199(4):396.e1–396.e7.
29. Choo RE, Huestis MA, Schroeder JR, et al. Neonatal abstinence syndrome in methadone exposed infants is altered by level of prenatal tobacco exposure. *Drug Alcohol Depend*. 2004;75(3): 253–260.

30. Naeye RL, Blanc W, Leblanc W. Fetal complications of maternal heroin addiction: abnormal growth infections and episodes of stress. *J Pediatr.* 1973;83(6):1055–1061.
31. Kandall SR, Albino S, Lowinson J, et al. Differential effects of maternal heroin and methadone use on birthweight. *Pediatrics.* 1976;58:681–685.
32. Bauer CR, Shankaran S, Bada HS, et al. The maternal lifestyle study: drug exposure during pregnancy and short-term maternal outcomes. *Am J Obstet Gynecol.* 2002;186(3):487–495.
33. Messinger DS, Bauer CR, Das A, et al. The maternal lifestyle study: cognitive motor and behavioral outcomes of cocaine-exposed and opiate-exposed infants through three years of life. *Pediatrics.* 2004;113(6):1677–1685.
34. Kaltenbach K, Berghella V, Finnegan L. Opioid dependence during pregnancy: effects and management. In: Wood JR, ed. *Obstetrics and Gynecology Clinics of North America*. Philadelphia, PA: WB Saunders; 1998:139–152.
35. National Institutes of Health Consensus Development Panel. Effective medical treatment of opiate addiction. *J Am Med Assoc.* 1998;280(22):1936–1943.
36. McCarthy JJ, Leamon MH, Parr MS, et al. High-dose methadone maintenance in pregnancy: maternal and neonatal outcomes. *Am J Obstet Gynecol.* 2005;193(3 Pt 1):606–610.
37. Krantz MJ, Martin J, Stimmel B, et al. QTc interval screening in methadone treatment. *Ann Intern Med.* 2009;150(6):1–26.
38. Fisher G, Ortner R, Rohrmeister K, et al. Methadone versus buprenorphine in pregnant addicts: a double blind, double-dummy comparison study. *Addiction.* 2006;101(2):275–281.
39. Johnson RE, Jones HE, Fischer G. Use of buprenorphine in pregnancy: patient management and effects on the neonate. *Drug Alcohol Depend.* 2003;70(2 Suppl):S87–S101.
40. Johnson RE, Jones HE, Jasinski DR, et al. Buprenorphine treatment of pregnant opioid-dependent women: maternal and neonatal outcomes. *Drug Alcohol Depend.* 2001;63(1):97–103.
41. Jansson LM, Velez M, Harrow C. Methadone maintenance and lactation: a review of the literature and current management. *J Hum Lact.* 2004;20(1):62–71.
42. American Academy of Pediatrics Committee on Drugs. The transfer of drugs and other chemicals into human milk. *Pediatrics.* 2001;108(3):776–789.
43. Cregler LL. Medical complications of cocaine abuse. *N Engl J Med.* 1986;315(23):1495–1500.
44. Volpe JJ. Effects of cocaine use on the fetus. *N Engl J Med.* 1992;327(6):399–407.
45. Lutiger B, Graham K, Einarson TR, et al. Relationship between gestational cocaine use and pregnancy outcome; a meta-analysis. *Teratology.* 1991;44(4):405–414.
46. Frank DA, Augustyn M, Knight WG, et al. Growth, development, and behavior in early childhood following prenatal cocaine exposure. *J Am Med Assoc.* 2001;285(12):1613–1625.
47. Lester BM, Tronick EZ, LaGasse L, et al. The maternal lifestyle study: effects of substance exposure during pregnancy on neurodevelopmental outcome in 1-month old infants. *Pediatrics.* 2002;110(6):1182–1192.
48. Accornero VH, Amado AJ, Morrow CE, et al. Impact of prenatal cocaine exposure on attention and response inhibition as assessed by continuous performance tests. *J Dev Behav Pediatr.* 2007;28(3):195–205.
49. Morrow CE, Culberston JL, Accornero VH, et al. Learning disabilities and intellectual functioning in school-aged children with prenatal cocaine exposure. *Dev Neuropsychol.* 2006;30(3):905–931.
50. Singer LT, Nelson S, Short E, et al. Prenatal cocaine exposure: drug and environmental effects at 9 years. *J Pediatr.* 2008;153(1):105–111.
51. Mays L, Snyder PJ, Langlois E, et al. Visuospatial working memory in school-aged children exposed in utero to cocaine. *Child Neuropsychol.* 2007;13(3):205–218.
52. Plessinger MA. Prenatal exposure to amphetamines: risks and adverse outcomes in pregnancy. *Obstet Gynecol Clin North Am.* 1998;25(1):119–138.
53. Della Grotta S, Lagasse LL, Arria AM, et al. Patterns of methamphetamine use during pregnancy: results from the infant development, environment, and lifestyle (IDEAL) study. *Matern Child Health J.* 2010 Jul;14(4):519–527.
54. Smith LM, Lagasse LL, Derauf C, et al. Prenatal methamphetamine use and neonatal neurobehavioral outcome. *Neurotoxicol Teratol.* 2008;30(1):20–28.
55. Chang L, Cloak C, Jiang CS, et al. Altered neurometabolites and motor integration in children exposed to methamphetamine in utero. *Neuroimage.* 2009;48(2):391–397.
56. Jones HE, Balster RL. Inhalant abuse in pregnancy. *Obstet Gynecol Clin North Am.* 1998;25(1):153–167.
57. Toutant C, Lippmann S. Fetal solvents syndrome. *Lancet.* 1979;1(8130):1356.
58. Arnold GL, Kirby RS, Langendoerfer S, et al. Toluene embryopathy: clinical delineation and developmental follow-up. *Pediatrics.* 1994;93(2):216–220.
59. Pearson MA, Hoyme HE, Seaver LH, et al. Toluene embryopathy: delineation of the phenotype and comparison with fetal alcohol syndrome. *Pediatrics.* 1994;93(2):211–215.
60. Hunter AG, Thompson D, Evans JA. Is there a fetal gasoline syndrome? *Teratology.* 1979;20(1):75–79.
61. Ridenour TA, Bray BC, Cottler LB. Reliability of use, abuse, and dependence of four types of inhalants in adolescents and young adults. *Drug Alcohol Depend.* 2007;91(1):40–49.
62. Wilkins-Haug L, Gabow PA. Toluene abuse during pregnancy: obstetric complications and perinatal outcomes. *Obstet Gynecol.* 1991;77(4):504–509.
63. Tenenbein M, Casiro OG, Seshia MM, et al. Neonatal withdrawal from maternal volatile substance abuse. *Arch Dis Child Fetal Neonatal Ed.* 1996;74(3):F204–F207.
64. Schempf AH. Illicit drug use and neonatal outcomes: a critical review. *Obstet Gynecol Surv.* 2007;62(11):749–757.
65. Zuckerman B, Frank DA, Hingson R, et al. Effects of maternal marijuana and cocaine use on fetal growth. *N Engl J Med.* 1989;320(12):762–768.
66. Smith LM, LaGasse LL, Derauf C, et al. The infant development, environment, and lifestyle study: effects of prenatal methamphetamine exposure, polydrug exposure, and poverty on intrauterine growth. *Pediatrics.* 2006;118(3):1149–1156.
67. Day N, Sambamoorthi U, Taylor P, et al. Prenatal marijuana use and neonatal outcome. *Neurotoxicol Teratol.* 1991;13(3):329–334.
68. Jutras-Aswad D, DiNieri JA, Harkany T, et al. Neurobiological consequences of maternal cannabis on human fetal development and its neuropsychiatric outcome. *Eur Arch Psychiatry Clin Neurosci.* 2009;259(7):395–412.
69. Fried PA, Smith AM. A literature review of the consequences of prenatal marihuana exposure: an emerging theme of a deficiency in aspects of executive function. *Neurotoxicol Teratol.* 2001;23(1):1–11.
70. Pauly JR, Slotkin TA. Maternal tobacco smoking, nicotine replacement and neurobehavioural development. *Acta Paediatr.* 2008;97(10):1331–1337.

71. Ernst M, Moolchan ET, Robinson M. Behavioral and neural consequences of prenatal exposure to nicotine. *J Am Acad Child Adolesc Psychiatry*. 2001;40(6):630–641.
72. Haustein KO. Cigarette smoking, nicotine and pregnancy. *Int J Clin Pharmacol Ther*. 1999;37(9):417–427.
73. Thompson BL, Levitt P, Stanwood GD. Prenatal exposure to drugs: effects on brain development and implications for policy and education. *Nat Rev Neurosci*. 2009;10(4):303–312.
74. Cornelius MD, Day NL. Developmental consequences of prenatal tobacco exposure. *Curr Opin Neurol*. 2009;22(2):121–125.
75. Ahlsten G, Cnattingius S, Lindmark G. Cessation of smoking during pregnancy improves foetal growth and reduces infant morbidity in the neonatal period: a population-based prospective study. *Acta Paediatr*. 1993;82(2):177–181.
76. Heil SH, Higgins ST, Bernstein IM, et al. Effects of voucher-based incentives on abstinence from cigarette smoking and fetal growth among pregnant women. *Addiction*. 2008;103(6):1009–1018.
77. Oncken CA, Kranzler HR. What do we know about the role of pharmacotherapy for smoking cessation before or during pregnancy? *Nicotine Tob Res*. 2009;(11):1265–1273.
78. Iqbal MM, Sobhan T, Ryals T. Effects of commonly used benzodiazepines on the fetus, the neonate and the nursing infant. *Psychiatr Serv*. 2002;53(1):39–49.
79. Rementeria JL, Bhatt K. Withdrawal symptoms in neonates from intrauterine exposure to diazepam. *J Pediatr*. 1977;90(1):123–126.
80. Brands B, Blake J, Marsh DC, et al. The impact of benzodiazepine use on methadone maintenance treatment outcomes. *J Addict Dis*. 2008;27(3):37–48.
81. Golden NL, Kuhnert BR, Sokol RJ, et al. Neonatal manifestations of maternal phencyclidine exposure. *J Perinat Med*. 1987;15(2):185–191.
82. Strauss AA, Modaniou HD, Bosu SK. Neonatal manifestations of maternal phencyclidine (PCP) abuse. *Pediatrics*. 1981;68(4):550–552.

CHAPTER 49: Medical Complications of Drug Use/Dependence

Joshua D. Lee ■ Jennifer McNeely ■ Marc N. Gourevitch

Medical illness takes a heavy toll among drug users. Four principal factors contribute to drug users' higher risk for many medical conditions. Direct toxicities of illicit drugs are responsible for a wide variety of medical sequelae (e.g., cocaine-related cardiotoxicity). Behaviors associated with drug use (injection, exchanging sex for money or drugs) place drug users at elevated risk for specific conditions (such as endocarditis and sexually transmitted diseases [STDs]). Socioeconomic disadvantage and poverty engender life circumstances (e.g., congregate housing) that confer increased environmental risk for infections such as tuberculosis. Finally, diminished access to and effective use of care, and disruption of daily routines by active drug use (impeding self-care behaviors such as adherence with medication or appointments) adversely affect clinical outcomes.

This chapter begins by reviewing general principles of care for drug users with medical conditions, with additional attention to issues of overlapping syndromes, medication adherence, and prevention of common complications. We then review a range of specific illnesses associated with injection drug use (IDU) and with noninjection use of heroin and cocaine. Medical syndromes associated with acute use of specific drugs (e.g., intoxication, overdose, and withdrawal) are covered elsewhere in this volume.

CARE OF DRUG USERS WITH MEDICAL CONDITIONS

The Doctor–Patient Relationship and Principles of Care

To gather from patients the information needed to provide effective care, the relationship between patient and clinician must be grounded in trust. This may take time to establish, and is fostered by the physician's adoption of a nonjudgmental, engaged stance. Shame and diminished self-esteem are prevalent traits among drug users. Physicians should avoid critical remarks regarding ongoing drug use, as patients often respond by withholding clinically important information they think might provoke such reactions in the future.

Like other chronic illnesses, substance use is a persistent condition typically characterized by exacerbations and remissions. Clinicians are generally comfortable managing exacerbations of other chronic diseases and familiar with strategies to induce remission or to slow progression of diseases they cannot cure. When a drug user resumes drug use after a period of abstinence, however, clinicians often become discouraged or angry. Clinicians who accept relapse as a common clinical presentation of drug use, and who are aware of available treatment options, are likely to remain more successfully engaged with the drug-using patient, enhancing the quality and continuity of care provided.

The issue of confidentiality frequently arises when caring for the drug-using patient. A direct approach is most effective here as well. When the physician is part of a larger treatment team with the common expectation that patient data will be shared among team members, such an arrangement is best made clear to the patient toward the beginning of the relationship. Splitting and perceived betrayal can thereby be minimized. The physician must be familiar with the laws governing confidentiality of patients' substance abuse behaviors and treatment. Appreciation of this issue by the treating clinician will enhance development of trust in the clinician by the patient.

To engage the patient most effectively, the provider must determine and address the patient's agenda. While the clinician may be eager to bring a patient's hypertension under control, the patient may be more concerned about his insomnia. By inquiring about and addressing the primary concerns of the patient, the clinician reveals interest in helping the patient, who may in turn be more open to working with the physician to address medical conditions that are of less immediate concern to the patient.

Inquiring in a nonjudgmental fashion about concurrent drug use should be routinely performed at most, if not all, visits. Type of substance, frequency of use, and route of administration are particularly important to ascertain. When examining the drug-using patient, attention should be focused on the systems directly affected by the substances the patient is known to use, while not neglecting evidence of use of other drugs. Special attention should be paid to the presence of a variety of signs. Injection ("track") marks may be recent (appearing as fresh punctate marks, often with mild surrounding erythema) or old (linear scars representing the confluence of multiple past injection sites). They are found wherever veins are accessible, most often in the antecubital fossae, on the forearms, hands, and legs, and less commonly in the neck and groin. Lymphedema of the hands, fresh or old healed abscesses, and cellulitis are common among current or former injectors. A cardiac murmur consistent with mitral or tricuspid regurgitation may suggest a past or current history of endocarditis. The nasal septum should always be examined for erosion or infection, suggesting intranasal drug use.

Drug users, often heavy users of the health care system, typically receive fragmented care. For example, a patient's substance abuse treatment, human immunodeficiency virus (HIV)-related care, general primary care, and psychiatric care may each be delivered by distinct providers at distinct sites. Integrating care improves health care outcomes, and should be a goal of service delivery (1,2). The more information the physician has on hand regarding the components of a patient's care, the greater the chances that medication interactions or complications from overlapping medical and psychiatric comorbidities will be averted. It is incumbent on the clinician to inquire about concurrent drug use and related treatment, new medications, and new diagnoses when patients receive care in more than one location. Effective integration of drug use–related and general medical care can be achieved through a variety of models (3,4).

Overlapping Symptoms and Syndromes

A clinical challenge that arises when assessing and caring for the drug-using patient is distinguishing symptoms and signs related to drug use itself from those of comorbid medical and psychiatric conditions.

Constitutional symptoms, while frequently related to drug use and withdrawal, may also reflect systemic illness. Thus, fever after drug injection may reflect use of an impure drug mixture or the first sign of endocarditis. Myalgias, chills, nausea, vomiting, and diarrhea—all hallmarks of withdrawal from narcotics and alcohol—may likewise reflect gastroenteritis or another infectious process, or the side effects of interferon treatment for hepatitis C infection. Weight loss, commonly associated with heavy cocaine use, must also prompt consideration of systemic infection (e.g., tuberculosis), malignancy, or HIV infection. Dyspnea in the crack smoker may be caused by chronic pulmonary dysfunction related to drug inhalation, or to asthma, or to community-acquired or HIV-related pneumonia. Seizures may occur in the context of drug withdrawal (e.g., alcohol or benzodiazepines) or as a result of prior trauma or intercurrent infection. The same principles apply to the overlap between many psychiatric syndromes and syndromes of intoxication or withdrawal.

Adherence

Studies of adherence among drug users have focused largely on adherence to antiretroviral therapy among HIV-infected drug users. Though lack of adherence to treatment recommendations is widespread in the general population, particular emphasis has been given to defining correlates of adherence among substance users, reflecting a general sense that substance users may have difficulty adhering to medical treatments, and concern that poor adherence among persons with HIV infection will foster development and transmission of resistant virus (5,6).

Active drug or alcohol use has been identified as one of the few relatively consistent predictors of poor adherence, and this is particularly true for cocaine users (7). However, past history of drug or alcohol abuse has not been consistently associated with poor adherence, and a number of studies have found that persons no longer actively using drugs, as well as some active users, are able to adhere to antiretroviral therapy with success comparable to that of nonusers. For both active and former substance users, engagement in substance use treatment, particularly if on-site primary care is available, seems to facilitate access and adherence to HAART (highly active antiretroviral therapy) and other medical therapies (4). Untreated depression is strongly associated with poor adherence (8).

Interactions between medications and methadone can pose a unique barrier to adherence among drug users receiving methadone treatment. It is critical that such interactions be identified in clinical practice, as precipitation of opioid withdrawal by an antiretroviral agent that induces methadone metabolism may result in resumption of heroin use or nonadherence with the medication that is causing (or perceived to be causing) the interaction (9). Salient examples of medications that precipitate clinically significant increases in cytochrome P450-mediated methadone metabolism include the nonnucleoside reverse transcriptase inhibitors efavirenz and nevirapine, the tuberculosis antibiotic rifampin, and the anticonvulsant phenytoin. Though much less common, medications such as fluoxetine that inhibit methadone metabolism can precipitate oversedation and, theoretically at least, overdose. As a rule, it is important to remain alert to possible interactions between methadone and antiretrovirals or other medications; this is reviewed extensively elsewhere (see Chapter 53 in this volume) (10).

Assessing adherence in clinical settings can be challenging. Despite its tendency to overestimate adherence, self-report remains the most practical measure, and is most likely to facilitate discussion between patients and providers about the reasons for nonadherence. Self-report appears most valid when patients are asked about the number of missed doses within a short time frame (1 to 7 days), and when assessments are gathered on more than one occasion and responses are averaged over time. Clinicians' estimates of patient adherence have been repeatedly shown to be inaccurate and should not be substituted for a thorough adherence assessment.

Prevention of Complications

Disproportionate emphasis is often placed on drug treatment over prevention of the potential adverse consequences of use. Harm reduction takes a different approach, placing priority on minimizing the negative sequelae of drug use and promoting healthy behaviors, and acknowledging that abstinence may not be an immediate goal for all patients. This is similar to the way that physicians treat other chronic diseases, such as diabetes, hypertension, and HIV. The goal is to minimize adverse consequences associated with the condition—in this case, illicit drug use. Despite the fact that a "cure" (i.e., sustained abstinence) may not be a realistic near-term solution for many drug users, much can still be done to minimize the impact of drug use on the patient's health. In creating the opportunity for patient and provider to work together toward meaningful and achievable behavioral change, this approach can be more effective and engaging for patient and provider alike.

Harm reduction interventions can encompass a wide range of activities, from basic medical care, to social work and mental health services, to instruction in safer injection techniques. Cornerstones of the harm reduction approach are interventions that address major causes of morbidity and mortality among drug users, namely IDU, overdose, and sexual risk behavior.

Injection Drug Use

Injection drug use (IDU), through the use of shared injection equipment, remains an important driver of the HIV/AIDS and hepatitis C virus (HCV) epidemics. Over one third (36%) of AIDS cases in the United States, and the majority of cases among women, can be attributed directly or indirectly to IDU (11). HCV is the most common blood-borne infection in the United States, and IDU is the leading risk factor for transmission (12). The majority of these infections can be prevented through the once-only use of syringes and other injection equipment, as recommended by the U.S. Department of Health and Human Services (13). Though rates of new HIV infections have decreased among IDUs, largely as a result of increased access to sterile syringes, education, and resultant changes in injection behaviors, access to clean injecting equipment remains a challenge for many users (14). For health care and other treatment providers, providing counseling on the importance of once-only use of syringes and assisting clients with access to sterile syringes are essential components of preventive care for IDUs, and present opportunities for improved communication and establishment of trust between patient and provider.

While there is state-by-state variation in laws, syringes may be legally obtained by three methods: over-the-counter purchase, prescription, and through syringe exchange programs (SEPs) or authorized agencies (15). Each of these options has advantages and disadvantages, and different methods may be preferred by different groups of IDUs. Syringe exchange is the most widely studied, with effectiveness in reducing the spread of HIV demonstrated in multiple studies and federal government reviews (16). Syringe exchange is legal in many states, and there are now about 200 programs operating in 38 states and territories of the United States (17). Despite a 21-year ban on U.S. federal funding, (finally lifted at the end of 2009), many SEPs have been supported by state and local government funds, as well as private charity. Yet the effectiveness of the SEP approach is limited by lack of accessibility, with limited locations and hours of operation. Providing sterile injection equipment in pharmacies, either over the counter or by prescription, offers a potential solution, but may also be limited by cost, availability, and an individual's reluctance to disclose that they are engaged in IDU.

Overdose

Drug overdose is a leading cause of death among young adults, second only to motor vehicle accidents in deaths due to unintentional injury (18). In 2005, the latest year for which data are available, there were over 22,000 drug overdose deaths, far exceeding the number of deaths due to homicide in the United States (19). In recent years drug overdose deaths have risen dramatically, increasing by 68% between 1999 and 2004 (18). This increase is primarily attributed to deaths caused by use of potent prescription opioid analgesics, while deaths due to heroin and other illicit drugs have remained essentially stable.

Nonetheless, drug overdose remains common among illicit drug users. The overall mortality rate among out-of-treatment drug users is exceedingly high; six times that of an age-matched sample in a recent British study, which found that the majority (68%) of these deaths were attributable to overdose (20). A New York City study found that over 57% of users interviewed had witnessed at least one drug overdose, and over half knew someone who had died of an overdose (21).

While rates are increasing among adolescents and young adults, the 25- to 44-year age group is at greatest risk for fatal drug overdose. While less is known about overdose among prescription drug users, among heroin users it appears that long-term injectors are at greatest risk, particularly when using opioids in combination with benzodiazepines or alcohol (22). Returning to use after a period of opioid abstinence (and subsequent decreased tolerance), such as following an episode of drug treatment or incarceration, is associated with a significantly increased risk of overdose. Older users, and particularly those with other medical problems, are also at high risk for fatal overdose (22).

Overdose deaths can be prevented, and health care and other service providers working with substance users, particularly opioid users, have important contributions to make toward this goal. Persons leaving substance abuse treatment or incarceration should be educated about overdose risk, particularly that associated with potent or long-acting prescription opioids and using opioids in combination with alcohol, sedatives, and cocaine. In many U.S. cities (e.g., New York City, San Francisco, Baltimore, Chicago, Pittsburgh), and some rural areas (e.g., Wilkes County, North Carolina), service providers are distributing naloxone to drug users and teaching them how to administer it in case of opioid overdose. Naloxone ("Narcan") is a potent opioid antagonist commonly used medically to reverse opioid overdose. It can be administered as an intramuscular injection or intranasally, and has a favorable safety profile with essentially no abuse potential. Evaluation of the New York City program showed that distribution and administration to IDUs is feasible and safe, and indicated that such programs may be able to reduce overdose deaths on a larger scale (23).

Sexual Risk Behavior

Because of the disinhibiting effects of many drugs, the stimulant effects of others, and the relationship of drug procurement to risky sexual behavior, substance users are also at higher risk for sexually transmitted diseases (STDs), including HIV. Substance users are more likely to encounter circumstances where they have less authority over their sexual activity, because of engagement in commercial sex work, exchange of sex for drugs, and intimate partner violence (24).

Stimulant use is associated with increased sexual risk behavior among heterosexuals as well as men who have sex with men (MSM) (25). It is strongly correlated with HIV incidence among MSM, with users of methamphetamine and crack cocaine reporting higher numbers of sexual partners and exchanging sex for drugs or money, and those who use drugs during sex being more likely to engage in unprotected intercourse and other high-risk sexual behaviors (26,27). Binge alcohol use is also an important, but sometimes overlooked, factor in high-risk sexual behavior (28). Injection drug users also remain at high risk for sexual spread of HIV, with the majority (63%) reporting unprotected vaginal sex and almost half (47%) having more than one sexual partner (29).

Providers working with active substance users should always ask about high-risk sexual activity and screen for past or current intimate partner violence. Substance users should be counseled on the importance of condom use and other safe sex practices for prevention of HIV and other STDs, and engaged in discussion of the risks of sexual activity under the influence of alcohol and other drugs. Screening for intimate partner violence and regular testing for HIV and STDs is recommended for all substance users (further discussed below).

Immunization

Active substance users are at high risk for a number of vaccine-preventable infections. Substance users should receive annual vaccination against influenza. Tetanus booster vaccination every 10 years is recommended for the general population, and should be strictly observed for IDUs given the association of tetanus with IDU. Pneumococcal vaccination is recommended for individuals with unhealthy alcohol use, HIV, and other chronic conditions (including heart, lung or liver disease, diabetes, sickle cell disease), and thus is indicated for many substance users. All illicit drug users who lack immunity to hepatitis A should be vaccinated. Hepatitis B vaccination is explicitly recommended for IDUs, and the Centers for Disease Control and Prevention (CDC) guidelines recommend universal vaccination of adults attending drug treatment, STD clinics, correctional facilities, and other settings serving populations at high risk for infection. HAV and HBV vaccines are further discussed in the section "Viral Hepatitis" below.

CARDIOVASCULAR DISEASE AND CANCER: CONFLUENT RISKS AND ASSOCIATED OUTCOMES

Leading Health Indicators

The leading causes of mortality in the United States are heart disease and cancer, which together account for nearly half of all deaths annually (30). Stroke (cerebrovascular diseases, 6%), chronic lower respiratory diseases including COPD (5%), and accidents (5%) complete the top five causes of death. Each of these conditions are strongly associated with addictive disorders, with tobacco and alcohol making the greatest contribution overall but drugs such as opioids, cocaine, and amphetamine taking a heavy toll as well. A recent study estimated that tobacco smoking was the leading modifiable risk factor for mortality, outstripping hypertension, diet, exercise, and being overweight, and accounting for approximately 467,000 (or 1 of every 5 to 6) deaths, while alcohol resulted in a net 64,000 excess deaths annually (31). Globally, disease burdens linked to tobacco are projected to increase (32).

Cardiovascular Disease

Tobacco and Cardiovascular Disease

Tobacco control efforts are based on well-understood causal associations between smoking and both heart disease as well as malignancy. For the most part, tobacco addiction prevention and treatment takes place largely outside of the domain of the traditional addiction treatment delivery system. The importance of addressing smoking cessation among patients presenting with other substance use disorders cannot be overstated, as the comorbidity of tobacco dependence with alcohol, opioids, and stimulant abuse and dependence is exceptionally high (33).

Nicotine, the principal addictive component of both inhaled and smokeless tobacco, is a CNS stimulant and associated with increases in blood pressure and heart rate. Nicotine itself, however, has not been clearly implicated as a cause of atherosclerosis, lipid abnormalities, sudden cardiac death, or stroke in humans (34–36). Consistent with this finding is the fact that nicotine replacement therapy (NRT) has not been linked to increased CVD events or death. Rather, NRT is a mainstay of secondary CVD prevention among smokers following myocardial infarction or other cardiac events (37,38). Nicotine, then, is the compound within tobacco products that by virtue of its addictive properties drives repeated exposure to the over 4000 known components in cigarette smoke including carbon monoxide and free-radical-promoting volatile chemicals (34,39). The cumulative effect of cigarette smoke compounds on the chronic user is an intravascular environment of hypoxia, inflammation and decreased immune function, abnormal lipid metabolism, and platelet, thrombotic, and vasomotor dysfunction, all of which act synergistically to initiate and promote atherothrombotic disease progression.

Smoking cessation and sustained abstinence are thus critical CVD risk reduction goals. Nurses' Health Study data indicate that women who quit smoking may reduce CVD mortality risk to that of never-smokers within 10 to 14 years of quitting, and all-cause mortality to normal levels within roughly 20 years (40,41). The impact on individuals' risk profiles of reducing the quantity of cigarettes smoked but continuing to smoke is less clear (42,43).

Alcohol and Cardiovascular Disease

Unique among addictive substances, alcohol relates to CVD risk and mortality in a "J"- or "U"-shaped fashion. Multiple large epidemiologic studies have observed a similar relationship: moderate alcohol use is protective against cardiac events including myocardial infarction and stroke compared to no use, while excessive, chronic use is clearly harmful. Among the general population, moderate alcohol use, defined as ≤2 drinks/day (men)/≤1 drink/day (women), when previously established and in the absence of alcohol or other addictive disorders, may be considered a component of a healthful "lifestyle." Persons coping with alcohol and other drug use disorders, however, can be unequivocally counseled toward abstinence, as failure to control daily drinking promotes precursors, particularly hypertension, and eventual CVD and death. On balance, roughly 90,000 deaths in the United States (2005) can be attributed to alcohol including those due to CVD, compared to 26,000 deaths from CVD, stroke, and diabetes averted due to moderate alcohol use (31).

The cardioprotective effects of moderate alcohol use appears to reflect increased high density lipoproteins (HDLs), vasodilation and lowered blood pressure, enhanced insulin sensitivity and with it lowered risk for hyperglycemia and diabetes, and reduced risk of inflammation, thrombosis, and arrhythmias. In contrast, chronic, heavy alcohol use fosters a maladaptive hyperautonomic state marked by catecholamine up-regulation and hypertension, promotion of thrombosis and arrhythmias, lipid dysregulation, insulin resistance and diabetes, and direct myocardial toxicity that can result in alcoholic cardiomyopathy and heart failure. Risks extend to binge drinking as well, a risk factor (as is daily heavy drinking) for atrial fibrillation.

Cocaine, Stimulants, MDMA, and Cardiovascular Disease

Cocaine is a clear cardiotoxin and proarrhythmic agent, and any level of use is associated with increased risk of CVD, sudden cardiac death, and stroke. Among persons 18 to 45 years of age in the United States, cocaine accounts for up to 25% of acute myocardial infarctions (44). Despite this high population-attributable risk, cocaine-associated myocardial infarctions occur in only 1% to 6% of patients who present to emergency departments with cocaine-associated chest pain (45,46). Although all cocaine users are at risk, most patients with cocaine-associated myocardial infarction are young, nonwhite, male, cigarette smokers, without other risk factors for atherosclerosis, and with a history of repeated cocaine use. Only half of such patients have evidence of atherosclerotic coronary artery disease on subsequent angiography (47).

The most common medical symptom associated with cocaine use is chest pain, which may reflect myocardial ischemia or infarction. Cocaine use increases the risk of acute myocardial infarction by several mechanisms, including coronary vasoconstriction or vasospasm, increased adrenergic activity (which intensifies myocardial oxygen demand by increasing blood pressure, ventricular contractility, and heart rate), and increased platelet adhesion, aggregation, and intravascular thrombosis (48,49). In one recent study, users of cocaine had a transient 24-fold increase in the risk of myocardial infarction in the hour immediately following cocaine use (50). The occurrence of myocardial infarction after cocaine use is unrelated to the quantity ingested, route of administration, or blood levels of cocaine or its metabolites (49,51). In addition to acute myocardial ischemia and infarction, cocaine use is linked to dissection of the thoracic aorta and coronary arteries, cardiac rhythm and conduction abnormalities, left ventricular dysfunction, dilated cardiomyopathy, hypertension, and tachycardia. Cocaine use may be a stronger independent risk factor than other drugs for endocarditis, particularly involving left-sided valves (52).

Cocaine, amphetamine, methamphetamine, and MDMA intoxication can all be marked by tachycardia, hypertension, chest pain, arrhythmias, myocardial ischemia, infarction, and sudden death. Though longitudinal observational data linking stimulant abuse or dependence to CVD is lacking, it is likely that chronic stimulant dependence heightens the risk of atherosclerotic heart disease, cardiomyopathies, and sudden death from arrhythmias and infarction (53).

Opioids, Cannabis, and Cardiovascular Disease

Opioid- and cannabis-dependent populations are at higher risk for ischemic heart disease, largely reflecting comorbid tobacco and alcohol dependence. Injection use of opioids, and resulting embolic and infectious complications, including endocarditis, also poses obvious cardiac risks. Methadone, the opiate agonist used in the pharmacotherapy of opioid dependence, has been associated in some patients with prolongation of the QTc interval on the electrocardiogram and uncommonly with ventricular arrhythmia (torsade de pointes). Other data hint at a potential cardioprotective effect of long-term exposure to opiates (54). Isolated cannabis use and dependence have not been clearly linked to excess mortality or CVD, and most longitudinal cohort studies linking cannabis smoking to heart disease are confounded by tobacco use (55).

Management of Ischemic Heart Disease in Persons with Substance Abuse

In persons with substance abuse or dependence, care for hypertension, lipid disorders, diabetes, and heart disease is best addressed in concert with individuals' addiction treatment. Lack of engagement in substance abuse treatment should not, however, preclude careful attention to and care of these comorbid medical conditions.

Regarding modifiable risk factors, all adults should be screened for hypertension, high cholesterol (men age ≥35, women age ≥45 with no other risk factors), and excess weight, with diabetes screening recommended for adults with blood pressure of ≥135/80 mm Hg (56). A low-salt, high-fiber diet and regular exercise are beneficial both as primary and secondary CVD prevention. Men ≥40 years, postmenopausal women, and those with CVD risk factors including smoking should consider daily aspirin therapy. Smoking cessation, elimination of unhealthful alcohol use, and avoidance of cocaine and other stimulants are clearly of particular importance among patients with drug abuse or dependence.

Hypertension control should be focused on reaching and maintaining a "goal blood pressure" of below 140/90 mm Hg, or lower (<130/80 mm Hg) in the setting of diabetes, proteinuric chronic kidney disease, or known CVD. Treatment should follow national guidelines (57). Of note, clonidine, a central alpha-2-agonist and oft-encountered antihypertensive medication among addicted persons, is not appropriate as monotherapy for hypertension due to lack of efficacy, the need for twice daily dosing, reports of its abuse as a sedative, and the risk of potentially fatal rebound hypertension.

While primary CVD prevention in the form of cholesterol lowering is of modest benefit to those with this single modifiable risk factor, the benefit to those with known CVD or multiple risk factors can be quite substantial. Statin therapy, the cornerstone of lipid management, has consistently reduced CVD events and total mortality in large randomized control trials. Fibrate and nicotinic acid therapies are generally less well tolerated but are also effective. Antiplatelet and antithrombic therapy is recommended both as primary prevention (aspirin) and following an ischemic event (aspirin, clopidogrel). The increased risks of major bleeding must be taken into account among those with platelet dysfunction, bleeding disorders, liver failure, or other predisposing conditions, such as gastric ulcers, all of which are more common in alcohol-dependent patients.

Cancer

Tobacco and Lung Cancer

Unlike cardiovascular disease or other common cancers (e.g., breast or colon cancer), in which a constellation of modifiable factors such as weight, blood pressure, and diet combine with tobacco dependence to heighten disease and mortality risk, lung cancer has cigarette smoking as by far its most important cause. This is true of both non-small-cell (85% of all lung cancers; includes squamous cell and adenocarcinoma) and small-cell (15%) tumors (58). Lung cancer is the leading cause of cancer death in the United States (158,664 deaths in 2006) and globally, and lung cancer incidence and death rates closely follow geographic variations in smoking rates (59). This reflects a lack of effective lung cancer screening mechanisms, as well as persistently poor rates of remission and survival following diagnosis. The importance of primary prevention, centering on tobacco control efforts, cannot be overstated. Unlike CVD, in which smoking cessation is an important component of treatment and secondary prevention, there are few second chances following a lung cancer diagnosis. Five-year survival in the United States following a diagnosis of any lung cancer remains quite low (around 15%), with little improvement over the last 40 years.

Generally, lung and other cancers evolve as cumulative environmental exposures interact with genetic susceptibility. Over time, direct tissue injury from tobacco smoke promotes premalignant genetic mutations and tissue changes including dysplasia, clonal patches, and angiogenesis, which progress to malignant cell invasion, early-stage cancer, and eventual metastasis (58). Returning to baseline levels of lung cancer risk comparable to that of never-smokers occurs slowly following successful cessation. In women, while a significant (21%) reduction in risk appears within the first 5 years of quitting, excess risk compared to never-smokers may take up to 30 years to disappear (40). From a perspective of lung cancer risk reduction, then, current smokers should be encouraged to quit as soon as possible and should be supported in abstinence for as long as possible.

Tobacco and Other Cancers

Smoking, smokeless tobacco use, and second-hand smoke are causative factors in most nonlung malignancies, including leukemias, head and neck and esophageal cancers, and cancers of the pancreas, liver, stomach, cervix, kidney, large bowel, and bladder (60). In addition, chronic tobacco use mediates the majority of lung and nonlung cancers in persons dependent on other substances, including alcohol, stimulants, cannabis, and opioids. Of note, smoking is not clearly linked to increased risk for colorectal or breast cancers, both of which are more common in heavy drinkers.

Alcohol and Cancer

Alcohol consumption is a risk factor for the second and third most common causes of cancer mortality in 2006, colorectal cancer (55,170 deaths United States) and breast cancer (41,430 deaths), though a dose-dependent association between alcohol intake and colorectal cancer risk is not firmly established (61). Alcohol may increase estrogen and androgen levels in women, among other plausible mechanisms for alcohol's promotion of breast cancer (62). Alcohol is linked to most cancers of the digestive tract, particularly squamous cell carcinomas, including those of the oral cavity, head and neck, esophagus, and liver (hepatocellular carcinoma [HCC]), though it is not associated with stomach cancers. HCC arises in the setting of cirrhosis, the most common cause of which is heavy alcohol consumption, and the risk of alcohol-induced HCC is heightened in the setting of viral hepatitis. The effectiveness of screening for breast and colorectal cancers is well established in the general population, though guidelines do not vary by level of alcohol use (56). Colorectal cancer screening in all adults consists of fecal occult blood testing, sigmoidoscopy, or colonoscopy beginning at age 50 to age 75 years. Screening mammography every 1 to 2 years is recommended for women age ≥40 years.

Viral Causes of Cancer among Drug Users

HIV, human papilloma virus (HPV), hepatitis B virus (HBV), and HCV are each prevalent among drug users and associated with increased risk of malignancy. Cervical cancer screening is recommended for all women who have been sexually active and have a cervix (56).

ALCOHOLIC PANCREATITIS, LIVER DISEASE, AND VIRAL HEPATITIS

Addiction and Gastrointestinal Disease

Disorders of the intestinal tract and liver among addicted persons are primarily mediated by chronic heavy alcohol use and viral hepatitis. As noted above, alcohol and tobacco use are strongly associated with head and neck and esophageal cancers, particularly squamous cell carcinomas, and tobacco is a strong risk factor in gastric cancers. Excessive alcohol use in the setting of viral hepatitis (often contracted through high-risk sexual behavior or IDU) confers particularly high risk of hepatocellular injury, development of cirrhosis, and HCC.

Alcoholic Pancreatitis

Pancreatitis and alcoholic liver disease are well-known consequences of chronic alcohol misuse. The incidence of acute pancreatitis in developed countries correlates with rates of alcohol consumption as well as with gallbladder disease, the two chief causes of pancreatitis (63). Mortality varies by center, with rates of 5% to 30%. Death from pancreatitis usually follows multiorgan failure (0 to 2 weeks from onset) and sepsis (>2 weeks). Overconsumption of ethanol results in toxic levels of its metabolites, including acetaldehyde and fatty acid ethyl esters, which are thought to increase production of digestive and lysosomal enzymes by pancreatic acinar cells and thereby initiate the cascade of inflammatory and autodigestive pancreatic injury.

The management of acute pancreatitis consists largely of supportive measures, including pain control, intravenous fluids, fasting, electrolyte corrections, and insulin-based control of hyperglycemia. Alcohol abstinence is of course mandatory. Risk factors for disease severity include older age (>55 years), obesity, organ failure at admission, and pleural effusion or pulmonary infiltrates. Single or multiple episodes of acute pancreatitis may result in chronic pancreatitis, marked by fibrosis and mononuclear infiltrate (vs. neutrophilic in acute pancreatitis), chronic abdominal pain often following meals, and pancreatic insufficiency with fat malabsorption and glucose intolerance.

Alcoholic Liver Disease

Alcoholic liver disease ranges across a spectrum from asymptomatic fatty liver to alcoholic hepatitis, cirrhosis, and end-stage liver failure. Alcohol is primarily metabolized by the liver by way of the alcohol dehydrogenase pathway. Chronic, heavy alcohol use may also induce secondary microsomal enzyme oxidation pathways. Both pathways generate toxic metabolites including acetaldehyde and free radical oxygen intermediates. Hypoxia associated with alcohol metabolism, increased levels of cytokines, neutrophil migration, and liver macrophagic Kupffer cell activation all contribute to hepatocellular injury, chronic inflammation, and eventual fibrosis.

The incidence of alcoholic liver disease is quite variable, with cirrhosis developing in approximately 50% of persons who consume at least 1 pint of spirits (roughly 210 g of ethanol) daily for >20 years (64). Most persons consuming eight or more standard drinks per day, however, will develop precursor conditions such as alcoholic fatty liver. Physical signs that often accompany the presence of alcohol-related liver disease include right upper quadrant pain, enlarged or reduced liver edge, general muscular atrophy, bleeding disorders, and peripheral neuropathies. Elevated serum transaminase levels, particularly a ratio of elevated AST to ALT of >2 in the setting of chronic heavy alcohol use, is highly suggestive of alcoholic liver disease. Imaging (including ultrasound, CT, or MRI) can detect fatty changes, cirrhosis, or liver tumors. Liver biopsy is not required for the diagnosis of alcoholic liver disease, but is often used to exclude other causes of liver disease and to establish disease severity.

Alcoholic fatty liver is a direct, reversible effect of ethanol ingestion, and usually does not progress to alcoholic hepatitis or cirrhosis. It is often asymptomatic or characterized by mild abdominal pain; laboratory tests are often normal. Alcoholic fatty liver is characterized by macrovesicular steatosis and mitochondrial distortion, and is usually indistinguishable from other causes of fatty liver including obesity, pregnancy, drug toxicity, or viral hepatitis. Alcoholic hepatitis is characterized by fever, hepatomegaly, jaundice and anorexia, and elevated serum transaminase levels, and can be accompanied by ascites in fulminant cases. Neutrophil infiltration and Mallory bodies on biopsy are highly suggestive of alcoholic injury as opposed to viral hepatitis. Cirrhosis may coexist with alcoholic hepatitis, and both usually begin in the pericentral liver with progression to panlobular regions. Cirrhotic fibrosis is the accumulation of scar or extracellular matrix. Progression of cirrhosis is marked by portal hypertension, varices, ascites, and lower body edema, jaundice, coagulopathies, and eventual fulminant hepatic failure with encephalopathy.

Abstinence from alcohol use is a critical goal among persons with alcohol-related hepatitis and cirrhosis, while the presence of alcoholic fatty liver indicates a person should clearly reduce if not cease drinking. Early alcoholic cirrhosis may be partially reversible with abstinence, and 5-year transplant-free survival among persons with cirrhosis and clinical decompensation is approximately twice as high among persons able to abstain (60%) compared to those who continue to drink (30%) (65). Liver transplant is highly effective in end-stage alcoholic liver disease, though this has traditionally been offered only to highly selected patients agreeing to abstinence and with good social support and functioning. A period of ≥6 months of abstinence, though somewhat arbitrary, has become a standard pretransplant criteria, and usually involves a pledge of abstinence as well as enrollment in a comprehensive treatment program (66).

Viral Hepatitis

Hepatitis A

Hepatitis A virus (HAV) is the leading cause of acute viral hepatitis in the United States, and results in significant morbidity and health care costs (67). Hepatitis A is a nonenveloped ribonucleic acid (RNA) virus that is excreted in stool and usually transmitted by fecal–oral contact, although transmission through blood is also possible. Most cases of HAV occur during community-wide outbreaks, but a high proportion of these cases occur in persons who report using drugs (68). The prevalence of anti-HAV antibodies is particularly high among drug users; in one study, the prevalence among injection drug users was twice that in the general population (69).

Transmission between drug users is hypothesized to occur primarily by the fecal–oral route when people gather together to smoke, snort or swallow drugs, and secondarily by percutaneous transmission through sharing needles and other injection supplies. Drug use (including injection and noninjection use) is now recognized as a significant risk factor for transmission of hepatitis A, and drug users are among the groups recommended for HAV vaccination.

Hepatitis A is generally an acute, localized disease, with uncommon cases involving relapse or extrahepatic manifestations. Unlike hepatitis B, a carrier state does not exist for HAV. The usual incubation period for HAV is 28 days (range: 15 to 40 days), and most adults are asymptomatic during acute infection. When symptoms occur, they typically include a mild prodromal illness of fever, headache, malaise, and nonspecific gastrointestinal symptoms, followed by dark urine, jaundice, tender hepatosplenomegaly, and postcervical lymphadenopathy. This classic presentation occurs in more than 80% of symptomatic patients and is self-limited, lasting less than 8 weeks. Most patients are treated supportively and experience complete resolution by 3 to 6 months. Importantly, a rarer and more severe form of HAV has been described in patients with hepatitis C or other chronic liver disease, and is associated with fulminant liver failure and a high mortality rate (up to 35%) (70).

The diagnosis of acute HAV is made by detecting anti-HAV antibodies in patients with symptoms consistent with hepatitis. Abnormal liver enzyme tests are not specific for hepatitis A. IgM anti-HAV antibodies can be detected 1 to 2 weeks after exposure and persist for 3 to 6 months. IgG anti-HAV antibodies can be detected 5 to 6 weeks after exposure and persist for decades, conferring lifelong protection against HAV reinfection. The high prevalence of HAV exposure among drug users suggests that this population is at particularly high risk for HAV infection. In addition, chronic hepatitis caused by hepatitis B or C is extremely common among injection drug users, making them more susceptible to developing severe fulminant hepatitis with acute HAV suprainfection. HAV as well as HBV vaccination of drug users is therefore indicated to both protect the individual from a potentially fatal condition, and to reduce HAV transmission to others. HAV vaccine is administered intramuscularly as two injections given 6 months apart. In addition to the HAV vaccine, a combined HAV/HBV vaccine (Twinrix) has been shown to be effective in IDUs (69). While IDU may reduce vaccine immunogenicity, HAV vaccination has been shown to be effective in IDU populations, though they are more likely than the general population to require both vaccinations of the scheduled 2-vaccine series to obtain full immunity (69). Because of the high prevalence of prior infection and anti-HAV antibodies among drug users, HAV serology should be checked in adults and experienced IDUs, though providers may choose to give the first dose of vaccine prior to receiving these results.

Hepatitis B

As many as 1.4 million people in the United States are living with chronic hepatitis B (HBV) infection, with new infections occurring at a rate of over 40,000 annually despite the availability of an effective vaccine (71). The prevalence of HBV infection among IDUs is particularly high (40% to 80%), accounting for an estimated 4% to 12% of all chronic HBV infections in the U.S. population (72). Hepatitis B is a deoxyribonucleic acid (DNA) virus that is predominantly acquired through sexual contact (homosexual and heterosexual), but also by IDU and occupational exposure. Among drug users, HBV is transmitted parenterally through the sharing of needles and other contaminated injection equipment, or high-risk sexual behavior (73). HBV acquisition is a relatively early event for most injection drug users, with 50% to 70% of injectors seroconverting within the first 5 years of initiating injection (74). In one study, HBV incidence ranged from 12% to 31% per year among young (age 18 to 30 years) injection drug users (75). Young IDUs thus manifest the highest incidence of new HBV infections in the United States, with transmission linked to injection practices (sharing needles and other injecting equipment) and high-risk sexual behavior (not using a condom and/or having multiple sexual partners) (76). It is now recommended that injection drug users be routinely screened for hepatitis B infection (serologic testing for HBsAg) if they are not known to be immune (73).

The outcome of acute HBV infection is variable. Approximately 40% of patients develop clinical symptoms of acute hepatitis, though fulminant hepatic failure is a rare complication, affecting just 1 in 1000 patients (71). The incubation period, defined by the appearance of clinical symptoms, ranges from 1 to 6 months. Early in infection, circulating HBV surface antigen (HBsAg) can be detected prior to the development of either clinical symptoms or elevated hepatic transaminases. This is followed by the production of hepatitis B e antigen (HBeAg), and then by elevations in transaminases. The first evident immune response is the production of antibodies to HBV core antigens (anti-HBc), which appear shortly after HBsAg. Anti-HBc plays no role in host defense, but is a reliable marker of past HBV infection. HBV surface antibody (anti-HBs) confers immunity to hepatitis B and may be present in those who have been successfully vaccinated against HBV as well as in those with a history of HBV infection.

Among all patients with acute hepatitis B, 5% to 10% develop chronic infection with persistent HBsAg positivity. Chronic HBV is associated with cirrhosis and hepatocellular cancer, and leads to 4000 deaths from cirrhosis and 800 deaths from HCC annually in the United States (77). While all those with active infection should be evaluated for treatment, not all will require immediate therapy. Treatment has the potential to reduce the risk of progressive chronic liver disease and its longer-term complications such as HCC, while also reducing the individual's infectivity to others. There are multiple treatment options for chronic HBV, including interferon-alfa and nucleoside reverse transcriptase inhibitors (lamivudine, adefovir, entecavir, telbivudine, tenofovir). All patients should be evaluated for HIV infection prior to starting HBV therapy, since coinfection rates are high, response to HBV treatment can be blunted in HIV-infected persons, and HBV monotherapy can engender HIV resistance to antiretroviral treatment.

The hepatitis B vaccine is immunogenic, effective, and safe. Though vaccination has been recommended for injection drug users by the CDC since 1982, uptake in this population has remained consistently low (less than 30%) (69). Multiple barriers to successful vaccination among IDUs include generally poor access to health care services, lack of awareness of the need for vaccination among drug users and health care workers alike, and the relative complexity of the vaccine schedule (75). The recommended vaccine consists of three intramuscular injections at 0, 3, and 6 months. The full sequence results in protective levels of anti-HBs in more than 90% of young (≤40 years old) healthy adults, though its effectiveness is somewhat diminished in persons who are older, smoke, are overweight, or are immunocompromised (by HIV-infection, diabetes mellitus, renal failure, or chronic liver disease). Though completion of all three doses is recommended, protective antibodies develop in 30% to 55% of adults after a single dose, and in up to 75% after two doses, so a significant proportion of those who do not receive the full series may still be protected (75). An alternative schedule with just two doses, administered 6 months apart, may result in anti-HBs levels similar to those obtained with the three-dose schedule (78).

Drug treatment programs as well as syringe exchange and targeted street outreach programs have been successful in achieving high rates of vaccination completion (70% to 85%) among injection drug users. Vaccination of the entire population during infancy or early adolescence, as has been recommended by the CDC since 1991, will eventually reduce the incidence of HBV infection, but this guideline has yet to be fully implemented, with the result that many adults remain susceptible to HBV infection. Greater efforts are necessary to vaccinate drug users against HBV, and should involve all potential settings in which drug users have contact with health care providers. These include drug treatment programs, health departments, jails and prisons, needle exchange programs, ambulatory clinics, and hospital emergency rooms. Drug users should be screened with HBV serologies (HBsAg and either anti-HBc or anti-HBs) but (as with HAV vaccination) the first dose of vaccine may be given at the same visit after blood is drawn for testing (73).

Hepatitis C

Approximately 4 million people have evidence of exposure to HCV in the United States, of whom 78% have chronic infection (12). HCV is the most common chronic liver disease in the United States, and accounts for the majority of liver transplants. Hepatitis C is a retrovirus with six major genotypes, genotype 1 being most common in the United States and Europe. It is very efficiently transmitted by contact with infected blood, and more rarely through sexual exposure. In the United States, up to 8% of HCV-infected persons are HIV coinfected (79).

IDU is the primary route of transmission of HCV infection (12). Among injectors, there is considerable geographic variation in HCV seroprevalence but rates are consistently high, ranging from 14% to 51% in major U.S. cities (80). Acquisition of HCV infection is often rapid following initiation of drug injection, with greater than one in three IDUs becoming infected within the first 5 years after initiating injecting (81). Transmission risk increases with injection frequency and with injecting a mixture of cocaine and heroin ("speedball") (81). Sharing of drug preparation equipment, including cookers and the filtration cotton, is also clearly associated with incident infection. Although sharing of intranasal cocaine sniffing equipment (e.g., straws) has also been considered a possible route of HCV transmission, these data are inconclusive (81). Sexual transmission of HCV, although much less efficient than injection-related transmission, can also be a route of infection among drug users. Multiple sex partners and comorbid STDs increase the risk of sexual acquisition of HCV (82), and noninjection drug users trading sex for money or drugs may be at particularly high risk.

Most patients do not seek medical attention during acute infection with hepatitis C because clinical manifestations are often mild, though 20% to 30% may experience fatigue, abdominal pain, poor appetite, or jaundice during the acute phase (82). Following initial infection with HCV, approximately 15% to 20% of persons appear to permanently clear the virus, and 80% to 85% of persons develop chronic infection. HCV-induced cirrhosis develops in an estimated 15% to 20% of those with chronic infection, and HCV-related end-stage liver disease (ESLD) now constitutes the most common indication for liver transplantation in the United States (83). Factors associated with accelerated progression of HCV-related liver disease include coinfection with HIV, older age at time of infection, and alcohol consumption. HCC develops almost exclusively in HCV-infected individuals who have developed cirrhosis, at a rate of 1% to 4% per year (83).

Among those who naturally ward off chronic infection, there is no evidence that protective immunity develops against future reinfection with HCV. Nevertheless, reinfection of injectors appears to be a relatively uncommon occurrence (84). This is of particular relevance to injection drug users and others who may be repeatedly exposed to the virus over time.

Serologic determination of HCV infection is generally accomplished by testing for the presence of anti-HCV antibodies. Serum levels of HCV RNA are assessed in antibody-positive persons. If HCV RNA is absent in the presence of anti-HCV antibodies, the patient is assumed to have cleared the infection. Those with detectable HCV RNA should undergo genotype determination, as this will influence subsequent treatment. Because of the substantial overlap in risk factors and implications for treatment, HIV testing should be offered concurrently with testing for HCV. HCV treatment eligibility is determined primarily by considering the extent of plasma viremia, hepatic fibrosis, and inflammation. The National Institutes of Health's *2002 Consensus Development Conference Statement on Management of Hepatitis C* explicitly states that persons should not be excluded from receiving HCV treatment solely on the basis of active drug or alcohol use, and methadone treatment is also not considered a contraindication to treatment (85). This position was reiterated in the more recent American Association for the Study of Liver Disease (AASLD) practice guidelines (12). As with all patients with chronic medical conditions, the decision to embark on a sustained course of treatment, during which side effects are likely and a successful response uncertain, must be made on a case-by-case basis. Factors to consider include the patient's motivation, past adherence with chronic therapies, HCV genotype, medical and psychiatric comorbidities, likelihood of success, and engagement in medical care.

Currently, best HCV treatment results are obtained with a combination of pegylated interferon alpha, administered by subcutaneous injection, and ribavirin, taken orally. Response to treatment is typically evaluated after 12 weeks: if an insufficient drop in HCV viral load is observed, treatment is discontinued. Of the three HCV genotypes most prevalent in the United States, genotypes 2 and 3 are most responsive to treatment, which is typically continued for 6 months in such patients. Twelve months of treatment is considered standard for persons with genotype 1 infection. A patient is deemed to have a successful end-of-treatment response (ETR) when HCV viremia is undetectable after treatment completion. A sustained viral response (SVR) is defined as persistence of viral eradication (as measured by nondetectable viremia) 6 months following completion of treatment, and is the best predictor of long-term treatment response. Rates of SVR in clinical trials approximate 45% following 48 weeks of treatment of patients with genotype 1 infection, and 80% following 24 weeks of treatment of patients with genotypes 2 and 3 infections. Treatment duration is longer and rates of SVR lower in those coinfected with HIV and HCV, but given the opportunity for HCV treatment to alleviate the rapid progression of liver disease in these patients, treatment is recommended except in those cases where its adverse effects outweigh potential benefits (12).

Although it remains uncertain whether a SVR to treatment signifies a true "cure" of the patient's HCV infection, prevention of long-term sequelae of HCV infection is clearly associated with successful treatment (86). Repeat treatment of nonresponders (those unable to clear virus) and relapsers may be considered based on the initial therapy received and patient characteristics. Treatment of nonresponders with maintenance pegylated interferon is an area of active investigation but is not currently recommended, based on initial results indicating that while HCV viremia and markers of inflammation are reduced, there is no significant difference in progression to cirrhosis (12). Newer therapies, including protease inhibitors and derivatives of current treatment agents (interferons and ribavirin) are currently under investigation, and some have shown promising results in clinical trials.

Side effects from treatment with peglyated interferon and ribavirin are significant. Major complications of interferon are constitutional symptoms and psychiatric manifestations. Depression, prevalent to begin with among HCV-infected drug users, is often precipitated or worsened by treatment of HCV with interferon (86). Screening for depression and other psychiatric disorders at baseline and periodically during treatment is an important component of care. The major complications of ribavirin are hematologic, with significant anemia, neutropenia, or both often complicating treatment.

Configuring services to optimize delivery of hepatitis C treatment to eligible drug users is challenging. Several of the stages of care (e.g., screening, evaluation of eligibility for treatment, which typically involves liver biopsy, and treatment itself) are often conducted by distinct health care providers. To the extent possible, integration of the several aspects of the patient's care is an important goal (87). For patients engaged in substance abuse treatment, providing hepatitis C related care on-site at the treatment program is an attractive option, facilitating interdisciplinary management of the medical, psychiatric, and substance abuse treatment aspects of care (88). For example, patients receiving methadone maintenance treatment often request an increase in their methadone dose during combination treatment of their HCV infection, presumably because of the similarity between interferon-related side effects and the symptoms of opioid withdrawal. Other patients, learning that they are infected with HCV decades after they stopped injecting, may be profoundly discouraged by this unwanted "blast from the past," to the point that it jeopardizes their recovery. Such complex clinical issues are ideally addressed in an interdisciplinary setting. Patients' access to the various members of the treatment team can be facilitated when they are colocated in a common site. SEPs provide another promising setting into which HCV-related services can effectively be integrated for active drug users (89).

In several studies, only a small proportion of eligible HCV-infected drug users enroll in HCV treatment, and even fewer complete the treatment course (90,91). Improved strategies for provider and patient education, defining surrogate markers for fibrosis that could spare the step of liver biopsy, developing less-toxic therapies, and successfully treating comorbid psychiatric and substance abuse disorders, are urgently needed in view of the very heavy burden of HCV infection among persons with a history of substance abuse.

Efforts to prevent HCV transmission and acquisition, often given less attention than diagnosing and treating existing infection, are vitally important. HCV antibody testing should be widely offered to all persons with current or former drug or alcohol misuse. Persons testing negative should receive tailored counseling. If they are injecting drugs, use of sterile syringes and not sharing any injecting related equipment should be discussed and encouraged. IDUs should receive sterile injecting equipment and/or referral to SEPs or pharmacies that dispense syringes, and safer routes of use (e.g., intranasal) suggested, while simultaneously working with the patient to reduce or eliminate their drug use. Safer sex practices, particularly for persons with multiple partners, should be supported as well. Persons testing positive for HCV, if injecting drugs, should be counseled not to share needles and syringes or other injecting equipment such as cookers, cotton, and other implements that could come into contact with blood.

Secondary prevention efforts include routine vaccination against hepatitis A and hepatitis B for all HCV-infected persons. Evidence suggests that hepatitis A can be particularly fulminant in some HCV-infected persons (71), and some data implicate hepatitis B as a factor associated with accelerated progression of HCV-related liver disease. Increasingly it is recommended that HIV treatment be initiated earlier in patients who are coinfected with HCV, even among those with higher CD4 counts, based on some evidence that HAART may decrease liver damage in this population (92). Alcohol consumption is associated with more rapid progression of HCV-related liver disease and with diminished response to treatment (93). There is uncertainty as to whether a modest degree of alcohol consumption is detrimental, because most studies have found this effect to be associated with moderate to heavy levels of drinking. Counseling HCV-infected persons to eliminate or at least minimize alcohol consumption is strongly encouraged.

Hepatitis D

Hepatitis D (delta) virus (HDV), an incomplete RNA virus that requires coinfection with active HBV to become active, is transmitted in the same manner as HBV and is prevented by HBV vaccination. It is endemic in the Mediterranean region and in parts of Asia, Africa, and South America and appears to have been spread to nonendemic areas such as the United States and Northern Europe by IDU. Outbreaks of severe and fulminant hepatitis, primarily as a result of coinfection with HDV and HBV, have been reported in injection drug users and their sexual contacts (94).

There are two mechanisms of HDV infection: coinfection with HBV, and superinfection of HBsAg carriers. In coinfection, HBV and HDV are acquired together, and there is a higher incidence of fulminant hepatic failure (up to 20%) than with HBV infection alone. Thirty percent of patients with acute fulminant hepatitis B have coinfection with HDV, and the case fatality rate is almost 5%. Similarly, when a chronic HBV carrier is superinfected with HDV, subsequent liver disease is more severe and more rapidly progressive than with HBV infection alone (95). HDV superinfection should be strongly considered when a stable chronically infected HBV carrier has an exacerbation of chronic liver disease or an episode resembling acute hepatitis B. Treatment for chronic HDV in patient with evidence of liver disease may be beneficial, but optimal treatment regimens are not clearly defined and are best undertaken as part of a clinical trial.

Other Viral Causes of Hepatitis

Other viruses have the potential to cause hepatic disease among drug users as well, including Epstein–Barr virus, herpes simplex virus, and cytomegalovirus, each of which may bring about hepatitis-associated illnesses. Most often these viruses are spread through direct contact, but they can be spread parentally as well. Although relatively rare in comparison to HAV, HBV, HCV, and HDV, it is important to consider these pathogens in the differential diagnosis of hepatitis among drug users.

SEXUALLY TRANSMITTED DISEASES

Sexually transmitted diseases (STDs) are common among substance users, often associated with sexual risk incurred in the setting of intoxication (particularly among users of stimulants such as cocaine and amphetamines) as well as with exchange of sex for money or drugs. Crack use is particularly strongly associated with sex in exchange for money or directly for drugs, and crack-smoking sex workers report very-high-risk sexual practices, as well as low rates of condom use. STDs that present commonly among drug users include syphilis, gonorrhea, chlamydia, genital herpes simplex virus, HPV, and trichomoniasis. In addition, HIV is transmitted among drug users both sexually and parentally; a full discussion of HIV infection is found elsewhere in this volume.

Syphilis

Syphilis is a readily curable, bacterial genital ulcer disease caused by *Treponema pallidum*. After declining throughout the 1990s, the number of reported cases of syphilis in the United States began increasing in 2001, with current rates of 3.8 cases per 100,000 being almost double those of a decade ago (96). This increase has been largely driven by outbreaks in some cities among men who have sex with men (MSM), with drug and alcohol use playing a significant role in transmission. Among drug users, rates of incident syphilis are very high, with lifetime prevalence ranging from 2% to 19% (97). Risk behaviors consistently associated with syphilis incidence among drug users include crack cocaine use, multiple sex partners, and the exchange of sex for money or drugs (98).

Patients who have syphilis may seek treatment for clinical signs of primary infection (usually a painless chancre), secondary infection (manifestations that include but are not limited to skin or mucocutaneous lesions), or tertiary infection (typically neurologic or cardiac complications). Latent infections, or those lacking clinical manifestations, are detected by serologic testing. Latent syphilis acquired within the preceding year is referred to as early latent syphilis; all other cases of latent syphilis are either late latent syphilis or latent syphilis of unknown duration (98).

Because of their high risk for syphilis exposure, drug users should be screened annually with RPR (rapid plasma reagin) or VDRL (Venereal Disease Research Laboratory) nontreponemal tests. Given the high rate of false–positive nontreponemal tests, positive results should be confirmed with a treponemal antibody test (e.g., FTA-ABS, TP-PA). Nontreponemal titers usually correlate with disease activity; a fourfold change in titer, equivalent to a change of two dilutions (e.g., from 1:16 to 1:4 or from 1:8 to 1:32), indicates a clinically significant difference between two nontreponemal test results obtained using the same serologic test. Nontreponemal tests usually become nonreactive with time after treatment; however, in some patients, nontreponemal antibodies can persist at a low titer for a long period of time, sometimes for the life of the patient. Most patients who have reactive treponemal tests will have reactive tests for the remainder of their lives, regardless of treatment or disease activity. However, 15% to 25% of patients treated during the primary stage revert to being serologically nonreactive after 2 to 3 years. Treponemal antibody titers correlate poorly with disease activity and should not be used to assess treatment response. HIV serology should be checked in all patients with serologic evidence of syphilis.

Like all other patients, drug users with STDs should be treated with single-dose regimens, if possible. Benzathine penicillin (2.4 million units) is the preferred single-dose regimen for early syphilis (primary, secondary, or early latent), and has been used effectively for more than 50 years to achieve clinical resolution and to prevent sexual transmission and late sequelae. Treatment of late latent or tertiary syphilis, which requires a series of three weekly injections of benzathine penicillin (total of 7.2 million units), usually does not affect transmission and is intended to prevent occurrence or progression of late complications (99). All treatment requires follow-up quantitative nontreponemal tests to assess treatment response. High rates of compliance with screening and treatment for syphilis among drug users have been achieved when these services are offered on-site in substance-abuse treatment programs (99).

Gonorrhea and Chlamydia

Gonorrhea (*Neisseria gonorrhoeae*) and chlamydia (*Chlamydia trachomatis*) are the most common bacterial STDs in the United States, with an estimated 600,000 cases of gonorrhea and close to 3 million cases of chlamydia each year (97). As with syphilis, rates of gonorrhea and chlamydia are much higher among drug users than among the general population. In cross-sectional studies of drug-using populations, close to half reported having had gonorrhea, and rates of current gonorrhea or chlamydia infection exceeded 5% (100).

These bacterial infections are a major cause of urethritis and proctitis in men, and cervicitis and pelvic inflammatory disease (PID) in women. However, because they are often asymptomatic, particularly in women, gonococcal and chlamydial infections are often detected only by screening tests. Screening is essential to prevent complications, including ascending infection, infertility, ectopic pregnancy, and chronic pelvic pain. In recent years, screening of women has been facilitated by highly sensitive new tests that do not require a pelvic exam or urethral swab, but instead amplify nucleic acid obtained from urine using a ligase chain reaction for *C. trachomatis* and *N. gonorrhoeae* (NAAT testing). Regular screening for gonorrhea and chlamydia is now recommended for sexually active women by the United States Preventive Services Task Force (56). Annual screening of substance-using women and of substance-using MSM should be performed.

Several antibiotics are effective in the single-dose treatment of gonorrhea, with cephalosporins including cefixime (Suprax) and ceftriaxone (Cefizox) being preferred. With increasing rates of quinolone resistance, ciprofloxacin (Cipro), ofloxacin (Floxin), and levofloxacin (Levaquin) are not recommended for the treatment of gonorrhea among MSM or in areas with high rates of resistance (99). Treatment of gonorrhea and chlamydia is generally offered simultaneously, because of the frequency of dual infection. Efficacious regimens for the treatment of chlamydia include azithromycin (Zithromax) or doxycycline (Vibramycin), but azithromycin is preferred because it can be given in a single, directly observed dose. As with other STDs, patients should be instructed to notify and refer their sex partners for testing and treatment.

Genital Herpes

Genital herpes simplex virus type 2 (HSV-2) infection is the most common infectious cause of genital ulcer disease, with at least 50 million persons infected in the United States (99). Although most cases of genital herpes are caused by HSV-2, genital infections with herpes simplex virus type 1 (HSV-1) are increasingly recognized. Serologic evidence of HSV-2 infection increases with age and number of sexual partners, and is more common among drug users. In recent studies, the prevalence of antibodies to HSV-2 among drug users has ranged from 44% to 58% (101).

The classic presentation of HSV-2 is with multiple vesicular or ulcerative genital lesions, but many infections may be asymptomatic. Shedding of virus occurs even in the absence of lesions, and HSV-2 transmission usually occurs at times of subclinical or asymptomatic shedding.

Optimal management of genital herpes includes antiviral therapy (with acyclovir [Zovirax], famciclovir [Famvir], or valacyclovir [Valtrex]), along with appropriate counseling on the natural history of infection, risk for sexual and perinatal transmission, and methods to prevent further transmission (99). Systemic antiviral drugs partially control symptoms when used to treat recurrent episodes, and may be used as daily suppressive therapy in those with frequent recurrences (≥6 per year). However, these drugs neither eradicate latent virus nor affect the risk for, frequency of, or severity of recurrences after the drug is discontinued. Recognizing the symptoms and signs of clinical episodes of HSV infection and promptly seeking treatment are key factors in reducing transmission rates.

Human Papilloma Virus

HPV infections are the causative agents for genital wart disease and cervical carcinoma, and are transmitted primarily through sexual contact. The prevalence of HPV is as high as 50% among sexually active adolescent and young adult women, and risk factors for HPV include number of sexual partners, early age of first sexual intercourse, drinking and drug use related to sexual behavior, and partner's number of sexual partners.

The two major manifestations of genital HPV infection are external genital warts, usually caused by HPV-6 and HPV-11, and squamous intraepithelial lesions of the cervix that are detected by cytologic screening. The major types of HPV associated with squamous intraepithelial lesions are HPV-16, -18, -31, -33, and -45. These HPV types also cause squamous cell cancer of the vagina, vulva, anus, and penis. A vaccine against HPV types 6, 11, 16, and 18 (Gardisil) has recently become available, and is recommended for girls and women age 9 to 26. It is best administered prior to onset of sexual activity, but does have utility in women who have been exposed to HPV if they have not been infected with all four types covered by the vaccine. Vaccination does not preclude the need for routine cervical cancer screening. Women who use drugs should be screened with Papaniculou (Pap) smears according to standard guidelines. Testing for HPV is often used to determine which women with low-grade cervical abnormalities on Pap require additional evaluation, but its utility as a primary screening test is still under review. At present, no therapy has been identified that effectively eradicates persistent subclinical HPV infection.

Trichomoniasis

Trichomonas vaginalis is a protozoan that causes vaginitis in women, and is highly prevalent among drug-using women. Recent availability of self-administered vaginal swab tests has obviated the need for pelvic exams followed by wet mount microscopy or vaginal culture in screening for trichomonas, making routine testing more feasible for a larger number of women. Because it is frequently asymptomatic, screening for trichomoniasis should be routine among drug-using women. Recommended treatment is with metronidazole or tinidazole, both of which can be given as a single dose (99). Patients should be counseled to abstain from alcohol during treatment and for 24 hours following completion of metronidazole and 72 hours after tinidazole. As with other STDs, sexual partners should also be treated.

SKIN AND SOFT-TISSUE INFECTIONS

Skin and soft-tissue infections are more common both among injection and noninjection drug users compared to general populations. Methicillin-resistant *Staphylococcus aureus* (MRSA) has become the most common causative agent of community-acquired soft-tissue infections. Isolates are usually not susceptible to beta-lactam antibiotics previously used most widely, including first-generation cephalosporins (i.e., cephalexin) and extended-spectrum penicillins (i.e., amoxicillin-clavulanate) (102,103).

Frequent, recurrent abscesses and cellulitis are prevalent among injection drug users, developing at a rate of roughly one episode every 3 years (104). Risk of abscess has been associated with route of injection, with intramuscular ("muscling") or subcutaneous ("skin popping") injection conveying greater risk for abscess than intravenous injection. Other risk factors identified include higher injection frequency (105) and injecting a mixture of cocaine and heroin (speedball) (105). Common sites of abscess are, in order of descending frequency, arm, leg, buttocks, deltoid, and head/neck (106).

The bacteriology of injection-associated abscess has been better defined than that of cellulitis, reflecting the greater likelihood of isolating an organism. *Staphylococcus aureus* is the most common pathogen in these infections, followed by *Streptococcus* species. The majority of *S. aureus* isolates in both the community and hospital settings now demonstrate resistance to beta-lactam antimicrobials (methicillin, oxacillin, dicloxacillin, cefazolin, cephalexin), while susceptibility to vancomycin, clindamycin, rifampin, trimethoprim-sulfamethoxazole, and tetracycline is generally high (107). Mixed aerobic/anaerobic infections are more common among injection-associated abscesses than abscesses identified in other clinical settings. Studies of the microbiologic flora in heroin and on injection equipment have also been conducted. While a variety of organisms were identified in this manner, *S. aureus* was not, suggesting that the injection drug user's skin, not the drug or equipment used, is the likely source for staphylococcus-related abscesses (108). Indeed, strains of *S. aureus* isolated from drug users presenting to the hospital with serious *S. aureus*-related infections are similar to the strains colonizing the same population of drug users in the community (109).

Prevention of skin and soft-tissue infections among noninjectors consists of good general and hand hygiene, avoidance of skin–skin contact, and treatment and decolonization of MRSA case clusters and household contacts. Among injectors, attention to sterile injection equipment and techniques is vital, including routinely cleansing the injection site with alcohol or soapy water prior to injection and sterilization of drug being injected by heating prior to injection ("cooking"—a step taken to help dissolve the drug), which may inactivate harmful bacteria (110).

Treatment of abscess typically requires incision and drainage, and small (≤5 cm) wounds may not require adjunctive antibiotics (111). Larger lesions or those with surrounding cellulitis or systemic symptoms require antibiotics for 1 to 2 weeks, depending on response. In the emerging era of MRSA, evidence-based guidelines for the presumptive treatment of soft-tissue infections are not yet established. Reasonable choices for empiric MRSA coverage include clindamycin, trimethoprim-sulfamethoxazole, and tetracyclines, and therapy designed to cover both MRSA and group A *streptococci* would include a beta-lactam and one of these older MRSA-active agents. Rifampin as an element of combination therapy is also supported by susceptibility data, though it is important not to use it alone to avoid rapid development of resistance. Floroquinolones, including ciprofloxacin, should not be used alone for the same reason, and because floroquinolone resistance is prevalent among MRSA isolates (112). Parenteral therapy including vancomycin should be considered for patients with extensive tissue involvement and diabetes or other immunodeficiencies.

INFECTIVE ENDOCARDITIS

In the pre-HIV era, endocarditis was the infection most classically associated with IDU, and it remains common among injectors today. An estimated 2% to 5% of active IDUs per year will develop infective endocarditis (IE), and the risk is even higher among those who are HIV-infected (113). IE remains a highly morbid condition among IDUs, with estimates of mortality ranging from 7% to 37%, although rates may be lower (approximately 10%) among those with right-sided endocarditis (114).

IE among drug users can affect any heart valve. Although native valve endocarditis in the general population is most often left-sided, IE is more commonly right-sided (tricuspid valve) when associated with IDU. This is thought to be due to a variety of factors, including direct valvular endothelial damage from impurities of the drug injected into the venous system (rendering right-sided valves most susceptible to bacterial infection), predilections of certain skin flora for right-sided valve surfaces, and direct effects on the valvular endothelium of specific drugs (which may present in higher concentrations to right-sided than to left-sided valves) (52).

Many organisms are reported to cause endocarditis among injecting drug users. Although both the skin and the injected drug are implicated as the source of the pathogen causing endocarditis, the skin is thought to be the prime source in most cases (115). Reports of the prevalence of specific pathogens vary by location and over time, likely reflecting diverse rates of colonization with specific pathogens, and variations in injection practices and source of drug. Overall, *Staphylococcus aureus* is most frequently reported, accounting for more than 50% of IE cases among IDUs, among whom methicillin-resistant infections are common (116). Other prevalent IE pathogens include streptococci and enterococci, and a variety of gram-negative and fungal infections can be seen as well. Polymicrobial presentations are more common among injection drug users than among others with endocarditis (116).

Persistent bacteremia is a hallmark of IE. The revised Duke criteria provide a consistent standard for diagnosis. Several authors have developed clinical prediction rules to determine the likelihood that a given febrile injector presenting to the emergency department has endocarditis. Such algorithms remain relatively inexact, however, leading many to conclude that most febrile injection drug users should be admitted to the hospital for observation or empiric treatment until the diagnosis of endocarditis can be excluded (116,117).

An extended course of parenteral antibiotics remains the mainstay of treatment of IE. Advances in treatment in the past decade include oral therapy for selected patients and shorter (2 weeks) duration of treatment for patients with uncomplicated right-sided methicillin-sensitive *S. aureus* endocarditis. Though use of such regimens is appropriately limited to cases meeting specific criteria, these advances are important for injecting drug users, as venous access is often problematic in those with a substantial injection history, and prolonged hospital stays are generally difficult for injectors and noninjectors alike. The presence of HIV infection does not diminish the efficacy of treatment for endocarditis. Significant HIV-related immunosuppression, however, is associated with increased endocarditis-associated mortality (118). Access to sterile injection equipment and adherence to sterile injection technique are the practices most likely to reduce injectors' risk of endocarditis. The principles of prevention discussed above in the context of skin and soft-tissue infections apply to endocarditis as well.

TUBERCULOSIS

Drug users are at increased risk for tuberculosis infection and disease. The prevalence of latent tuberculosis infection (LTBI) among drug users varies by locale and population studied, but rates of approximately 15% to 25% are typical (119,120). Drug users are heterogeneous with respect to their risk for LTBI, and research suggests that smokers of crack cocaine are at particularly high risk for tuberculosis infection (121).

It is uncertain whether drug use is associated with an increased risk of developing tuberculosis disease among persons with LTBI, though the presence of HIV infection clearly does increase this risk (121). Chemoprophylaxis is effective in reducing the likelihood of later developing active disease. Regular screening for and, when detected, treatment of LTBI should thus be offered to all drug users (122). The prevalence of tuberculin reactivity among HIV-seropositive drug users is generally lower than among HIV-uninfected persons, reflecting the diminished delayed-type hypersensitivity response associated with more advanced immunosuppression (123). Two-step ("booster") tuberculin skin testing may increase the sensitivity of this testing method. Interferon gamma release assays (QuantiFERON-TB Gold In-Tube and T-SPOT) are blood tests for TB that are now approved for use in place of the tuberculin skin test and may have increased sensitivity among substance-using populations, and also eliminates the need for patients to make a return visit to a health care provider for interpretation of skin test results (124).

Treatment of tuberculosis in drug users should follow standard guidelines (125). Because fragmented medical care is common in this population, it is particularly important to remain attentive to the possibility of multidrug resistant TB in those who are not appropriately responsive to treatment. Rifampin (Rifadin), one of the most effective antituberculosis medications, is a potent inducer of methadone metabolism, often precipitating opioid withdrawal symptoms in methadone-maintained persons. Carefully managed methadone dose increases, or even splitting of the methadone dose so it is administered twice daily, can resolve this complication. Alternatively, rifabutin (Mycobutin), which has similar activity to rifampin but far less impact on methadone metabolism, can sometimes substitute for rifampin. Such changes should generally be made in consultation with an expert in tuberculosis treatment. Directly observed therapy (DOT) can be a highly effective means to optimize adherence with treatment for LTBI or of active tuberculosis, particularly for patients engaged in opioid-agonist treatment with methadone, or who live in a congregate setting (e.g., shelter, residential drug treatment) (126).

PNEUMONIA AND CHRONIC LUNG DISEASE

Community-acquired pneumonia is common among drug users, particularly those with HIV infection. Recent studies have determined that the incidence of pneumonia ranges from 4.4 to 14.2 per 1000 person-years among HIV-negative drug users, and from 47.8 to 90.5 per 1000 person-years among HIV-positive drug users (127,128). Pneumonia is also the most common reason for hospitalizations among drug users, accounting for 27% of hospital admissions in one study (129).

Many factors contribute to drug users' increased susceptibility to pneumonia, including depression of the gag reflex by alcohol and drugs, leading to aspiration of oropharyngeal and gastric secretions; impaired pulmonary function as a consequence of cigarette smoking; and weakened immunity as a consequence of malnutrition and continuous antigenic stimulation. In addition, HIV-infection is associated with a markedly increased risk of bacterial pneumonia, and recurrent bacterial pneumonia has been included as an AIDS-defining illness since 1993. The risk for pneumonia among HIV-infected drug users is approximately five times that of non–HIV-infected drug users.

Encapsulated bacteria, most commonly *Streptococcus pneumoniae*, followed by *Haemophilus influenzae*, are the most frequent causes of pneumonia in both HIV-positive and HIV-negative drug users, and are highly associated with classic symptoms of sputum production, chest pain, and fever (130). Atypical bacteria, including *Mycoplasma pneumoniae*, *Chlamydia pneumoniae*, and *Legionella* species are also common among drug users, and are more likely to cause dry cough and headache than classic pneumonia symptoms. *Pneumocystis carinii*, *Mycobacterium tuberculosis*, and *Mycobacterium avium* are common among HIV-infected drug users, as discussed further elsewhere in this volume. Pulmonary tuberculosis should always be included in the differential diagnosis of drug users with pneumonia, and annual tuberculin skin testing of drug users is recommended. In addition, pneumococcal vaccine and annual influenza vaccines should be offered to all drug users.

Chronic lower respiratory diseases including chronic obstructive pulmonary disease (COPD) are the fourth leading cause of death in the United States. Tobacco smoking is by far the most important environmental risk factor for COPD. Cannabis use, while associated with COPD-like symptoms including airflow obstruction, chronic cough, bronchitis, and decreased exercise tolerance, is not a clear cause of COPD in studies that control for tobacco use (131).

Pulmonary Complications of Crack Cocaine Use

Crack cocaine and to a lesser extent intranasal cocaine use are associated with pulmonary complications. Intranasal cocaine may cause nonspecific bronchial irritation that results in wheezing in persons with a history of obstructive lung disease. Crack cocaine, on the other hand, can precipitate a broad spectrum of pulmonary complications, including asthma exacerbations (fatal and near-fatal asthma); barotrauma (pneumomediastinum and pneumothorax); noncardiogenic pulmonary edema; diffuse alveolar hemorrhage; recurrent pulmonary infiltrates with eosinophilia; nonspecific interstitial pneumonitis; bronchiolitis obliterans with organizing pneumonia; pulmonary vascular abnormalities; and "crack lung" (acute pulmonary infiltrates associated with chest pain, hemoptysis, and a spectrum of clinical and histologic findings) (132). Among crack smokers, the prevalence of respiratory symptoms (cough, black sputum production, wheezing, dyspnea, or hemoptysis) is greater than 50% (133).

DRUG USE AND NEUROLOGIC DISEASE

Tobacco, alcohol, and stimulant use are all clear risk factors for cerebrovascular events, including ischemic strokes and hemorrhage, which together comprise the third leading cause of mortality in the United States (137,119 deaths in 2006). As with CVD, smoking promotes atherosclerotic cerebrovascular disease progression and hypertension. Alcohol, as with cardiac events, relates to ischemic stroke risk in a J-shaped fashion, with moderate use being protective and heavy use increasing risk. Any alcohol use, however, appears associated with a greater risk of hemorrhagic stroke. Cerebral vasoconstriction has been implicated as the mechanism of acute cocaine-associated neurologic complications, including ischemic and hemorrhagic stroke, in several case reports and case-control studies (134). In addition, long-term cocaine and amphetamine use appears to predispose patients with incidental neurovascular anomalies, such as aneurysms and arteriovenous malformations, to present with intracranial or subarachnoid hemorrhages at an earlier point than nonusers.

Cocaine- or amphetamine-induced seizures are a relatively rare but severe manifestation of stimulant toxicity. These are usually single, tonic–clonic, resolve without intervention, and are more likely to occur in patients with a history of prior seizures. Altered mental status, delirium, and seizure are well-described symptoms of severe alcohol and sedative-hypnotic withdrawal.

Injection drug users are at increased risk for systemic infections that may affect the central nervous system, including endocarditis, viral hepatitis, and HIV. Endocarditis is associated with neurologic complications in 20% to 40% of patients, including cerebral embolism and infarction, hemorrhage from ruptured mycotic aneurysms, meningitis, encephalopathy, and parenchymal, subdural, or epidural abscesses (135). HIV infection may cause neurologic complications either directly or through opportunistic infections that attack the central nervous system.

Focal central nervous system infections occur commonly among drug users, although most focal infections result from embolization of infected vegetations among patients with endocarditis. The most frequent focal infections are brain abscesses, which may also result from local spread of an ear or sinus infection, hematogenous dissemination from a distant focus, such as infection in the lung, skin, bone, or pelvis, or trauma with an open fracture or foreign body injury. Spinal epidural abscesses are also common, and are caused by direct local extension of vertebral osteomyelitis, hematogenous spread from distant infection, or blunt spinal trauma.

Toxin-mediated diseases, including tetanus and botulism, comprise an additional important category of central nervous system infections among injection drug users. These infections usually result from intramuscular or subcutaneous injection of drugs, which predisposes to the inoculation of *Clostridium* species and the release of disease-producing toxin. Tetanus is caused by *Clostridium tetani*, and causes intense, sustained muscular spasms that may be localized or generalized. Localized tetanus causes muscle rigidity, pain, and enhanced deep tendon reflexes, while generalized tetanus causes respiratory failure and requires treatment in an intensive care unit. Wound botulism is caused by *C. botulinum*, and has been associated in particular with the injection of black tar heroin (136). Wound botulism initially causes blurred vision, dysarthria, and dysphagia, but may lead to descending muscle paralysis and respiratory failure. A high index of suspicion is necessary to diagnose these uncommon but rapidly progressive toxin-mediated diseases among drug users who present with neurologic symptoms. All injection drug users should be immunized against tetanus.

OTHER MEDICAL COMPLICATIONS

While other medical sequelae of drug use cannot be properly reviewed here because of space limitations, the reader is directed to recent reviews of pulmonary (137) and renal (138) complications.

REFERENCES

1. Laine C, Hauck WW, Gourevitch MN, et al. Regular outpatient medical and drug abuse care and subsequent hospitalization of persons who use illicit drugs. *J Am Med Assoc*. 2001;285(18):2355–2362.
2. Weisner C, Mertens J, Parthasarathy S, et al. Integrating primary medical care with addiction treatment: a randomized controlled trial. *J Am Med Assoc*. 2001;286(14):1715–1723.
3. O'Connor PG, Selwyn PA, Schottenfeld RS. Medical care for injection-drug users with human immunodeficiency virus infection. *N Engl J Med*. 1994;331(7):450–459.
4. Samet JH, Friedmann P, Saitz R. Benefits of linking primary medical care and substance abuse services: patient, provider, and societal perspectives. *Arch Intern Med*. 2001;161(1):85–91.
5. Osterberg L, Blaschke T. Adherence to medication. *N Engl J Med*. 2005;353:487–497.
6. Blower SM, Gershengorn HB, Grant RM. A tale of two futures: HIV and antiretroviral therapy in San Francisco. *Science*. 2000;287:650–654.
7. Arnsten JH, Demas PA, Grant RW, et al. Impact of active drug use on antiretroviral therapy adherence and viral suppression in HIV-infected drug users. *J Gen Intern Med*. 2002;17:377–381.
8. Malta M, Strathdee SA, Magnanini MM, et al. Adherence to antiretroviral therapy for human immunodeficiency virus/acquired immune deficiency syndrome among drug users: a systematic review. *Addiction*. 2008;103(8):1242–1257.
9. Gourevitch MN, Friedland GH. Interactions between methadone and medications used to treat HIV infection. *Mt. Sinai J Med*. 2000;67(5–6):429–436.
10. Bruce RD, Altice FL, Gourevitch MN, et al. Pharmacokinetic drug interactions between opioid agonist therapy and antiretroviral medications: implications and management for clinical practice. *J Acquir Immune Defic Syndr*. 2006;41(5):563–572.
11. Centers for Disease Control and Prevention. Fact Sheet: Drug-associated HIV transmission continues in the United States. Available at: http://www.cdc.gov/hiv/resources/Factsheets/idu.htm. Accessed August 12, 2009.
12. Armstrong GL, Wasley A, Simard EP, et al. The prevalence of hepatitis C virus infection in the United States, 1999 through 2002. *Ann Intern Med*. 2006;144(10):705–714.
13. U.S. Department of Health and Human Services, Public Health Service. HIV Prevention Bulletin: Medical advice for persons who inject illicit drugs. Available at: http://www.cdcnpin.org/Reports/MedAdv.pdf. Accessed August 12, 2009.
14. Hall HI, Song R, Rhodes P, et al. Estimation of HIV incidence in the United States. *J Am Med Assoc*. 2008;300(5):520–529.
15. Stancliff S, Agins B, Rich JD, et al. Syringe access for the prevention of blood borne infections among injection drug users. *BMC Public Health*. 2003;3:37.
16. Normand J, Vlahov D, Moses LE, eds. *Preventing HIV Transmission: The Role of Sterile Needles and Bleach*. Washington, DC: National Academy Press; 1995.
17. Harm Reduction Coalition. Syringe Access. Available at: http://www.harmreduction.org/article.php?list=type&type=49. Accessed August 12, 2009.
18. Centers for Disease Control and Prevention. Unintentional poisoning deaths—United States, 1999–2004. *MMWR Morb Mortal Wkly Rep*. 2007;56(05):93–96.
19. Centers for Disease Control (CDC) Congressional Testimony. United States Senate subcommittee on Crime and Drugs Committee on the Judiciary and the Caucus on International Narcotics Control. Trends in unintentional drug overdose deaths. March 12, 2008. Available at: http://www.cdc.gov/Washington/testimony/2008/t20080312a.htm. Accessed August 12, 2009.
20. Gossop M, Stewart D, Treacy S, et al. A prospective study of mortality among drug misusers during a 4-year period after seeking treatment. *Addiction*. 2002;97(1):39–47.
21. Tracy M, Piper TM, Ompad D, et al. Circumstances of witnessed drug overdose in New York City: implications for intervention. *Drug Alcohol Depend*. 2005;79(2):181–190.
22. Sporer KA, Kral AH. Prescription naloxone: a novel approach to heroin overdose prevention. *Ann Emerg Med*. 2007;49(2):172–177.
23. Piper TM, Stancliff S, Rudenstine S, et al. Evaluation of a naloxone distribution and administration program in New York City. *Subst Use Misuse*. 2008;43(7):858–870.

24. Moore M, Stuart GL, Meehan JC, et al. Drug abuse and aggression between intimate partners: a meta-analytic review. *Clin Psychol Rev*. 2008;28:247–274.
25. Centers for Disease Control and Prevention. Methamphetamine use and HIV risk behaviors among heterosexual men—preliminary results from five northern California counties, December 2001–November 2003. *MMWR Morb Mortal Wkly Rep*. 2006;55(10):273–277.
26. Colfax G, Vittinghoff E, Husnik MJ, et al. Substance use and sexual risk: a participant- and episode-level analysis among a cohort of men who have sex with men. *Am J Epidemiol*. 2004;159(10):1002–1012.
27. Ober A, Shoptaw S, Wang P, et al. Factors associated with event-level stimulant use during sex in a sample of older, low-income men who have sex with men in Los Angeles. *Drug Alcohol Depend*. 2009;102:123–129.
28. Raj A, Reed E, Santana MC, et al. The associations of binge alcohol use with HIV/STI risk and diagnosis among heterosexual African American men. *Drug Alcohol Depend*. 2009;101:101–106.
29. Centers for Disease Control and Prevention. HIV-associated behaviors among injecting-drug users—23 cities, United States, May 2005–February 2006. *MMWR Morb Mortal Wkly Rep*. 2009;58(13):329–332.
30. Heron MP, Hoyert DL, Murphy SL, et al. Deaths: Final data for 2006. National vital statistics reports. Vol. 57, no. 14. Hyattsville, MD: National Center for Health Statistics; 2009.
31. Danaei G, Ding EL, Mozaffarian D, et al. The preventable causes of death in the United States: comparative risk assessment of dietary, lifestyle, and metabolic risk factors. *PLoS Med*. 2009;6(4):e1000058.
32. Murray CJ, Lopez AD. Alternative projections of mortality and disability by cause 1990–2020: global burden of disease study. *Lancet*. 1997;349(9064):1498–1450.
33. Kalman D, Morissette SB, George TP. Co-morbidity of smoking in patients with psychiatric and substance use disorders. *Am J Addict*. 2005;14(2):106–123.
34. Ambrose JA, Barua RS. The pathophysiology of cigarette smoking and cardiovascular disease: an update. *J Am Coll Cardiol*. 2004;43(10):1731–1737.
35. Hansson J, Pedersen NL, Galanti MR, et al. Use of snus and risk for cardiovascular disease: results from the Swedish Twin Registry. *J Intern Med*. 2009;265(6):717–724.
36. Arabi Z. Metabolic and cardiovascular effects of smokeless tobacco (Review). *J Cardiometab Syndr*. 2006;1(5):345–350.
37. Stead LF, Perera R, Bullen C, et al. Nicotine replacement therapy for smoking cessation. *Cochrane Database Syst Rev*. 2007(4):CD000146.
38. Rigotti NA, Munafo MR, Stead LF. Interventions for smoking cessation in hospitalised patients. *Cochrane Database Syst Rev*. 2007;(3):CD001837.
39. Chelland Campbell S, Moffatt RJ, Stamford BA. Smoking and smoking cessation—the relationship between cardiovascular disease and lipoprotein metabolism: a review. *Atherosclerosis*. 2008;201(2):225–235.
40. Kenfield SA, Stampfer MJ, Rosner BA, et al. Smoking and smoking cessation in relation to mortality in women. *J Am Med Assoc*. 2008;299(17):2037–2047.
41. Kawachi I, Colditz GA, Stampfer MJ, et al. Smoking cessation in relation to total mortality rates in women: a prospective cohort study. *Ann Intern Med*. 1993;119(10):992–1000.
42. Bjartveit K, Tverdal A. Health consequences of sustained smoking cessation. *Tob Control*. 2009;18(3):197–205.
43. Tverdal A, Bjartveit K. Health consequences of reduced daily cigarette consumption. *Tob Control*. 2006;15(6):472–480.
44. Qureshi AI, Suri MF, Guterman LR, et al. Cocaine use and the likelihood of nonfatal myocardial infarction and stroke: data from the Third National Health and Nutrition Examination Survey. *Circulation*. 2001;103(4):502–506.
45. Feldman JA, Fish SS, Beshansky JR, et al. Acute cardiac ischemia in patients with cocaine-associated complaints: results of a multicenter trial. *Ann Emerg Med*. 2000;36(5):469–476.
46. Weber JE, Chudnofsky CR, Boczar M, et al. Cocaine-associated chest pain: how common is myocardial infarction? *Acad Emerg Med*. 2000;7(8):873–877.
47. Lange RA, Hillis LD. Cardiovascular complications of cocaine use. *N Engl J Med*. 2001;345(5):351–358.
48. Siegel AJ, Mendelson JH, Sholar MB, et al. Effect of cocaine usage on C-reactive protein, von Willebrand factor, and fibrinogen. *Am J Cardiol*. 2002;89(9):1133–1135.
49. Kloner RA, Rezkalla SH. Cocaine and the heart. *N Engl J Med*. 2003;348(6):487–488.
50. Mittleman MA, Mintzer D, Maclure M, et al. Triggering of myocardial infarction by cocaine. *Circulation*. 1999;99(21):2737–2741.
51. Blaho K, Logan B, Winbery S, et al. Blood cocaine and metabolite concentrations, clinical findings, and outcome of patients presenting to an ED. *Am J Emerg Med*. 2000;18(5):593–598.
52. Frontera JA, Gradon JD. Right-side endocarditis in injection drug users: review of proposed mechanisms of pathogenesis. *Clin Infect Dis*. 2000;30(2):374–379.
53. Yeo KK, Wijetunga M, Ito H, et al. The association of methamphetamine use and cardiomyopathy in young patients. *Am J Med*. 2007;120(2):165–171.
54. Marmor M, Penn A, Widmer K, et al. Coronary artery disease and opioid use. *Am J Cardiol*. 2004;93:1295–1297.
55. Sidney S. Comparing cannabis with tobacco—again. *Br Med J*. 2003;327(7416):635–636.
56. US Preventive Services Task Force. *Guide to Clinical Preventive Services, 2008: Recommendations of the U.S. Preventive Services Task Force*. AHRQ Publication No. 08–05122, September 2008. Agency for Healthcare Research and Quality, Rockville, MD. Available at: http://www.ahrq.gov/clinic/pocketgd08/. Accessed August 8, 2009.
57. Chobanian AV, Bakris GL, Black HR, et al. The seventh report of the Joint National Committee on Prevention, Detection, Evaluation, and Treatment of High Blood Pressure: The JNC 7 Report. *J Am Med Assoc*. 2003;289:2560.
58. Herbst RS, Heymach JV, Lippman SM. Lung cancer. *N Engl J Med*. 200825;359(13):1367–1380.
59. Jemal A, Thun MJ, Ries LA, et al. Annual report to the nation on the status of cancer, 1975–2005, featuring trends in lung cancer, tobacco use, and tobacco control. *J Natl Cancer Inst*. 2008;100(23):1672–1694.
60. Sasco AJ, Secretan MB, Straif K. Tobacco smoking and cancer: a brief review of recent epidemiological evidence. *Lung Cancer*. 2004;45(suppl 2):S3–S9.
61. Thun MJ, Peto R, Lopez AD, et al. Alcohol consumption and mortality among middle-aged and elderly U.S. adults. *N Engl J Med*. 1997;337(24):1705–1714.
62. Singletary KW, Gapstur SM. Alcohol and breast cancer: review of epidemiologic and experimental evidence and potential mechanisms. *J Am Med Assoc*. 2001;286(17):2143–2151.
63. Vege SS, Yadav D, Chari ST. Pancreatitis. In: Talley NJ, Locke GR, Saito YA, eds. *GI Epidemiology*. 1st ed. Malden MA: Blackwell Publishing; 2007.

64. Lelbach WK. Organic pathology related to volume and pattern of alcohol use. In: Gibbins RJ, Israel Y, Kolant H, et al., eds. *Research Advances in Alcohol and Drug Problems*. New York, NY: Wiley; 1974:93–198.
65. Adachi M, B renner DA. Clinical syndromes of alcoholic liver disease. *Dig Dis*. 2005;23(3–4):255–63.
66. Weinrieb RM, Van Horn DH, McLellan AT, et al. Interpreting the significance of drinking by alcohol-dependent liver transplant patients: fostering candor is the key to recovery. *Liver Transpl*. 2000;6(6):769–776.
67. Kemmer NM, Miskovsky EP. Infections of the liver. *Infect Dis Clin North Am*. 2002;14(3):605–615.
68. Baral S, Sherman SG, Millson P, et al. Vaccine immunogenicity in injecting drug users: a systematic review. *Lancet Infect Dis*. 2007;7:667–674.
69. Villano SA, Nelson K, Vlahov D, et al. Hepatitis A among homosexual men and injection drug users: more evidence for vaccination. *Clin Infect Dis*. 1997;25(3):726–728.
70. Vento S, Garofano TRC, Cainelli F, et al. Fulminant hepatitis associated with hepatitis A virus superinfection inpatients with chronic hepatitis C. *N Engl J Med*. 1998;338(5):286–290.
71. Centers for Disease Control and Prevention. Disease burden from viral hepatitis A, B, and C in the United States. Available at: http://www.cdc.gov/hepatitis/PDFs/disease_burden.pdf. Accessed August 12, 2009.
72. Centers for Disease Control and Prevention. Recommendations for identification and public health management of persons with chronic hepatitis B virus infection. *MMWR Morb Mortal Wkly Rep*. 2008;57(RR08):1–20.
73. Neaigus A, Gyarmathy VA, Miller M, et al. Injecting and sexual risk correlates of HBV and HCV seroprevalence among new drug injectors. *Drug Alcohol Depend*. 2007;89:234–243.
74. Quaglio G, Lugoboni F, Mezzelani P, et al. Hepatitis vaccination among drug users. *Vaccine*. 2006;24:2702–2709.
75. Des Jarlais DC, Diaz T, Perlis T, et al. Variability in the incidence of humanimmunodeficiency virus, hepatitis B virus, and hepatitis C virus infection among young injecting drug users in New York City. *Am J Epidemiol*. 2003;157:467–471.
76. Seal KH, Edlin BR. Risk of hepatitis B infection among young injection drug users in San Francisco: opportunities for intervention. *West J Med*. 2000;172:16–20.
77. Hoofnagle JH, Di Bisceglie AM. The treatment of chronic viral hepatitis. *N Engl J Med*. 1997;336(5):347–356.
78. Koff RS. Hepatitis Vaccines. *Infect Dis Clin North Am*. 2001;15(1):83–95.
79. Ghany MC, Strader DB, Thomas DL, et al. Diagnosis, management, and treatment of hepatitis C: an update. *Hepatology*. 2009;49(4):1335–1374.
80. Amon JJ, Garfein RS, Ahdieh-Grant L, et al. Prevalence of hepatitis C virus infection among injection drug users in the United States, 1994–2004. *Clin Infect Dis*. 2008;46:1852–1858.
81. Yen T, Keeffe EB, Ahmed A. The epidemiology of hepatitis C virus infection. *J Clin Gastroenterol*. 2003;36(1):47–53.
82. Lauer GM, Walker BD. Hepatitis C virus infection. *N Engl J Med*. 2001;345(1):41–52.
83. El-Serag HB. Hepatocellular carcinoma and hepatitis C in the United States. *Hepatology*. 2002;36(5 suppl 1):S74–S83.
84. Backmund M, Meyer K, Edlin BR. Infrequent reinfection after successful treatment for hepatitis C virus infection in injection drug users. *Clin Infect Dis*. 2004;39(10):1540–1543.
85. National Institutes of Health consensus development conference statement. Management of hepatitis C. 2002 June 10–12, 2002. *HIV Clin Trials*. 2003;4(1):55–75.
86. Castera L, Zigante F, Bastie A, et al. Incidence of interferon alfa-induced depression in patients with chronic hepatitis C. *Hepatology*. 2002;35(4):978–979.
87. Edlin BR, Kresina TF, Ramond DB, et al. Overcoming barriers to prevention, care, and treatment of hepatitis C in illicit drug users. *Clin Infect Dis*. 2005;40(suppl 5):S276–S285.
88. Litwin AH, Harris KA, Nahvi S, et al. Successful treatment of chronic hepatitis C with pegylated interferon in combination with ribavirin in a methadone maintenance treatment program. *J Subst Abuse Treat*. 2009;37(1):32–40.
89. Pratt CC, Paone D, Carter RJ, et al. Hepatitis C screening and management practices: a survey of drug treatment and syringe exchange programs in New York City. *Am J Public Health*. 2002;92(8):1254–1256.
90. Reed C, Stuver SO, Tumilty S, et al. Predictors of treatment for hepatitis C virus (HCV) infection in drug users. *Subst Abuse*. 2008;29(1):5–15.
91. Broers B, Helbling B, Francois A, et al. Barriers to interferon-alpha therapy are higher in intravenous drug users than in other patients with acute hepatitis C. *J Hepatol*. 2005;42(3):323–328.
92. Hammer SM, Eron JJ, Reiss P, et al. Antiretroviral treatment of adult HIV infection: 2008 recommendations of the international AIDS Society—USA Panel. *JAMA*. 2008;300(5):555–570.
93. Mochida S, Ohnishi K, Matsuo S. Effect of alcohol intake on the efficacy of interferon therapy in patients with chronic hepatitis C as evaluated by multivariate logistic regression analysis. *Alcohol Clin Exp Res*. 1996;20(9 suppl):371A–377A.
94. Lettau LA, McCarthy JG, Smith MH, et al. Outbreak of severe hepatitis due to delta and hepatitis B viruses in parenteral drug abusers and their contacts. *N Engl J Med*. 1987;317(20):1256–1262.
95. Saracco G, Rosina F, Brunetto MR, et al. Rapidly progressive HBsAg-positive hepatitis in Italy: the role of hepatitis delta virus infection. *J Hepatol*. 1987;5(3):274–281.
96. Centers for Disease Control and Prevention. Sexually Transmitted Disease Surveillance, 2007. Atlanta, GA: U.S. Department of Health and Human Services; December 2008. Available at: http://www.cdc.gov/std/stats07/Surv2007FINAL.pdf. Accessed August 12, 2009.
97. Tyndall MW, Patrick D, Spittal P, et al. Risky sexual behaviours among injection drugs users with high HIV prevalence: implications for STD control. *Sex Transm Infect*. 2002;78(suppl 1):i170–i175.
98. Centers for Disease Control and Prevention. Sexually transmitted diseases treatment guidelines, 2006. *MMWR Morb Mortal Wkly Rep*. 2006;55(RR-11):1–94.
99. O'Connor PG, Molde S, Henry S, et al. Human immunodeficiency virus infection in intravenous drug users: a model for primary care. *Am J Med*. 1992;93(4):382–386.
100. Hwang LY, Ross MW, Zack C, et al. Prevalence of sexually transmitted infections and associated risk factors among populations of drug abusers. *Clin Infect Dis*. 2000;31(4):920–926.
101. Kanno MB, Zenilman J. Sexually transmitted diseases in injection drug users. *Infect Dis Clin North Am*. 2002;16(3):771–780.
102. Daum RS. Clinical practice. Skin and soft-tissue infections caused by methicillin-resistant *Staphylococcus aureus*. *N Engl J Med*. 2007;357(4):380–390.

103. King MD, Humphrey BJ, Wang YF, et al. Emergence of community-acquired methicillin-resistant *Staphylococcus aureus* USA 300 clone as the predominant cause of skin and soft-tissue infections. *Ann Intern Med*. 2006;144(5):309–317.
104. Spijkerman IJ, van Ameijden EJ, Mientjes GH, et al. Human immunodeficiency virus infection and other risk factors for skin abscesses and endocarditis among injection drug users. *J Clin Epidemiol*. 1996;49(10):1149–1154.
105. Murphy EL, DeVita D, Liu H, et al. Risk factors for skin and soft-tissue abscesses among injection drug users: a case-control study. *Clin Infect Dis*. 2001;33(1):35–40.
106. Takahashi TA, Merrill JO, Boyko EJ, et al. Type and location of injection drug use-related soft tissue infections predict hospitalization. *J Urban Health*. 2003;80(1):127–136.
107. Naimi TS, LeDell KH, Como-Sabetti K, et al. Comparison of community- and health care-associated methicillin-resistant *Staphylococcus aureus* infection. *J Am Med Assoc*. 2003;290(22): 2976–2984.
108. Tuazon CU, Hill R, Sheagren JN. Microbiologic study of street heroin and injection paraphernalia. *J Infect Dis*. 1974;129(3): 327–329.
109. Holbrook KA, Klein RS, Hartel D, et al. *Staphylococcus aureus* nasal colonization in HIV-seropositive and HIV-seronegative drug users. *J Acquir Immune Defic Syndr Hum Retrovirol*. 1997; 16(4):301–306.
110. Vlahov D, Sullivan M, Astemborski J, et al. Bacterial infections and skin cleaning prior to injection among intravenous drug users. *Public Health Rep*. 1992;107(5):595–598.
111. Rajendran PM, Young D, Maurer T, et al. Randomized, double-blind, placebo-controlled trial of cephalexin for treatment of uncomplicated skin abscesses in a population at risk for community-acquired methicillin-resistant S*taphylococcus aureus* infection. *Antimicrob Agents Chemother*. 2007;51(11): 4044–4048.
112. Moran GJ, Krishnadasan A, Gorwitz RJ, et al. Methicillin-resistant *S. aureus* infections among patients in the emergency department. *N Engl J Med*. 2006;355(7):666–674.
113. Sande MA, Lee BL, Mills J, et al. Endocarditis in intravenous drug users. In: Kaye D, ed. *Infective Endocarditis*. New York, NY: Raven Press; 1992.
114. Hecht SR, Berger M. Right-sided endocarditis in intravenous drug users: prognostic features in 102 episodes. *Ann Intern Med*. 1992;117(7):560–566.
115. Brown PD, Levine DP. Infective endocarditis in the injection drug user. *Infect Dis Clin North Am*. 2002;16(3):645–665.
116. Samet JH, Shevitz A, Fowle J, et al. Hospitalization decision in febrile intravenous drug users. *Am J Med*. 1990;89(1):53–57.
117. Marantz PR, Linzer M, Feiner CJ, et al. Inability to predict diagnosis in febrile intravenous drug abusers. *Ann Intern Med*. 1987;106:823–828.
118. Ribera E, Miró JM, Cortes E, et al. Influence of human immunodeficiency virus 1 infection and degree of immunosuppression in the clinical characteristics and outcome of infective endocarditis in intravenous drug users. *Arch Intern Med*. 1998; 158(18):2043–2050.
119. Salomon N, Perlman DC, Friedmann P, et al. Prevalence and risk factors for positive tuberculin skin tests among active drug users at a syringe exchange program. *Int J Tuberc Lung Dis*. 2000;4(1):47–54.
120. Howard AA, Klein RS, Schoenbaum EE, et al. Crack cocaine use and other risk factors for tuberculin positivity in drug users. *Clin Infect Dis*. 2002;35(10):1183–1190.
121. Markowitz N, Hansen NI, Hopewell PC, et al. Incidence of tuberculosis in the United States among HIV-infected persons. The Pulmonary Complications of HIV Infection Study Group. *Ann Intern Med*. 1997;126(2):123–132.
122. Jasmer RM, Nahid P, Hopewell PC. Clinical practice. Latent tuberculosis infection. *N Engl J Med*. 2002;347(23):1860–1866.
123. Graham NM, Nelson KE, Solomon L, et al. Prevalence of tuberculin positivity and skin test anergy in HIV-1-seropositive and -seronegative intravenous drug users. *J Am Med Assoc*. 1992;267(3):369–373.
124. Grimes CZ, Hwang LY, Williams ML, et al. Tuberculosis infection in drug users: interferon-gamma release assay performance. *Int J Tuberc Lung Dis*. 2007;11(11):1183–1189.
125. Centers for Disease Control and Prevention. Treatment of tuberculosis. *MMWR Morb Mortal Wkly Rep*. 2003;52(RR-11):1–77.
126. Gourevitch MN, Hartel D, Schoenbaum EE, et al. Lack of association of induration size with HIV infection among drug users reacting to tuberculin. *Am J Respir Crit Care Med*. 1996;154 (4 pt 1):1029–1033.
127. Safaeian M, Wilson LE, Taylor E, et al. HTLV-II and bacterial infections among injection drug users. *J Acquir Immune Defic Syndr*. 2000;24(5):483–487.
128. Scheidegger C, Zimmerli W. Incidence and spectrum of severe medical complications among hospitalized HIV-seronegative and HIV-seropositive narcotic drug users [Comment]. *AIDS*. 1996;10(12):1407–1414.
129. Palepu A, Tyndall MW, Leon H, et al. Hospital utilization and costs in a cohort of injection drug users [Comment]. *Can Med Assoc J*. 2001;165(4):415–420.
130. Park DR, Sherbin VL, Goodman MS, et al. The etiology of community-acquired pneumonia at an urban public hospital: influence of human immunodeficiency virus infection and initial severity of illness. *J Infect Dis*. 2001;184(3):268–277.
131. Tetrault JM, Crothers K, Moore BA, et al. Effects of marijuana smoking on pulmonary function and respiratory complications: a systematic review. *Arch Intern Med*. 2007;167(3):221–228.
132. Tashkin DP. Airway effects of marijuana, cocaine, and other inhaled illicit agents [Review] [139 refs]. *Curr Opin Pulm Med*. 2001;7(2):43–61.
133. Haim DY, Lippmann ML, Goldberg SK, et al. The pulmonary complications of crack cocaine: a comprehensive review. *Chest*. 1995;107(1):233–240.
134. McEvoy AW, Kitchen ND, Thomas DG. Intracerebral haemorrhage and drug abuse in young adults. *Br J Neurosurg*. 2000; 14(5):449–454.
135. Tunkel AR, Pradhan SK. Central nervous system infections in injection drug users. *Infect Dis Clin North Am*. 2002;16(3): 589–605.
136. Shapiro RL, Hatheway C, Swerdlow DL. Botulism in the United States: a clinical and epidemiologic review. *Ann Intern Med*. 1998;129(3):221–228.
137. Pruett BD, Baddour LM. Sinopulmonary complications of illicit drug use. *Infect Dis Clin North Am*. 2002;16(3):623–643, viii.
138. Crowe AV, Howse M, Bell GM, et al. Substance abuse and the kidney. *Q J Med*. 2000;93(3):147–152.

CHAPTER 50

Psychiatric Complications of HIV-1 Infection and Drug Abuse

Harold W. Goforth ■ L. Brett Caram ■ Jorge Maldonado ■ Pedro Ruiz ■ Francisco Fernandez

The human immunodeficiency virus type 1 (HIV-1) has infected 60 million individuals worldwide, of which 42 million are still living with the infection. The spread of the virus continues at a rate of 14,000 newly infected individuals per day, and 5 million persons contracted the virus in 2003 (1). According to the Centers for Disease Control and Prevention (CDC), the number of persons living with HIV in the United States is estimated to have been 384,906 as of December 2002, and a total of 501,669 have died from the disease (2). Progress has been made since the introduction of zidovudine (AZT) as the first antiretroviral agent, and the advent of highly active antiretroviral therapy (HAART) in 1996 decreased both the mortality and the incidence of AIDS. Unprotected sexual intercourse, injection drug use (IDU), and contaminated blood and blood product transfusions are well-known mechanisms of HIV-1 transmission. Other risk factors include crack cocaine use in women (3) and use of marijuana or volatile nitrites ("poppers") in the male homosexual population (4).

Concurrent substance abuse and psychiatric disorders in patients who are infected with the HIV are common. Prevalence rates vary significantly across reported studies and range from 10% to nearly 70% depending on the study (5,6). As many as half of patients have at least one psychiatric disorder, and nearly 40% abuse drugs other than marijuana. Twelve percent met criteria for drug dependence during the previous 12 months (5). In addition, bipolar II disorder, cyclothymic, and hyperthymic temperaments have been linked with up to 70% of the HIV population (6) and are associated with increased novelty seeking and risk-taking behavior in this population, which is suggestive of increased rates of unsafe sexual practices and needle.

In an attempt to make clinicians more aware and more capable of managing these complex and challenging patients, we review the psychiatric complications associated with HIV infection, neurobehavioral aspects, neuropathology, and treatment options for psychiatric disorders associated with the HIV-1 infection.

SCOPE OF THE PROBLEM

The highest rates of HIV infection are in patients with dual diagnosis of severe mental illness and substance use disorder. In one study of HIV-positive participants with comorbid substance use and psychiatric problems ($n = 1848$), HIV prevalence was 4.7% in patients having a diagnosis of both substance abuse and mental illness, whereas HIV prevalence was only 2.4% in patients diagnosed with a substance abuse disorder alone. Psychiatric illness appeared to almost double the risk of HIV—especially in those with concurrent poor psychosocial supports (7). These findings were confirmed by a cross-sectional survey of 3806 adults living with HIV across four major metropolitan areas in the United States, which showed that 72% of respondents reported at least occasional use of various drugs, and 40% of respondents reported frequent use of various drugs—only 28% declared abstinence from all drugs (8). In the group reporting frequent use of drugs, more were likely to be identified as heterosexual, had public health insurance, and endorsed increased symptoms of depression (7,8), which illustrates the complexities of the relationship between the triply diagnosed of mental health-substance abuse and HIV infection.

DRUG ABUSE DISORDERS

Alcohol use alone has been linked to multiple risk factors associated with HIV, including STD histories, condom nonuse, multiple sex partners, and lower HIV-related knowledge. These risks appear to increase substantially with increasing amounts of alcohol use and those demonstrating abstinence from alcohol appear to have the lowest risk profile. The impact of alcohol upon these risk factors remains present even in the absence of other drug abuse (9).

Intravenous drug use (IVDU) has long been associated with an increased prevalence of comorbid psychiatric diagnosis—especially dysthymia and depression. Depressive syndromes in IVDU populations have also been linked to increased willingness to share needles, syringes, and other paraphernalia, which further increases the risk of HIV transmission (10,11). Even after controlling for multiple confounding variables including age, race, gender, number of days on which injection drugs were used, and the average number of injections per injection day, a diagnosis of depression is significantly associated with injection risk behavior (12). Other data confirm that depressed patients are more likely to engage in sex with IVDU populations, heightening an already substantial risk of transmission (13). Being physically abused as an adult and Latino race appears to be a significant predictor of depression among HIV-seropositive intravenous drug users of both genders. However, data show that women appear to experience increased depressive symptoms as compared to men, and correlates of depression in both men and women include perceived functional limitation, greater negative feelings regarding condom use, lower social support, and a lower sense of empowerment/external locus of control (14).

Methamphetamine-dependent men who have sex with men (MSM) also demonstrate high lifetime rates of psychiatric disorders including major depression and anxiety disorders. Generalized anxiety disorder, specific phobia, bipolar disorder, and major depressive disorder have all been linked to higher rates of sexually transmitted infections including gonorrhea and HIV (15). Naturalistic interview studies have demonstrated the wide prevalence of a cycle of severe depression and anxiety in the context of methamphetamine use as well as persistent anhedonia. Almost all respondents in such studies reported that crystal methamphetamine was severely damaging to social relationships with a resultant increase in self-isolation, random sexual encounters, and increased numbers of sexual partners with a decreased likelihood of condom use (16).

PSYCHIATRIC DISORDERS IN HIV INFECTION

Common mental disorders among individuals with HIV and substance abuse include adjustment disorders, sleep disorders, depressive disorders, mania, dementia, delirium, pain, psychosis, and sleep disorders. A careful psychiatric assessment is necessary in order to engage in differential diagnostic considerations and differential therapeutics.

Mania and Bipolar Disease

Bipolar disease in the context of HIV is especially problematic in that it involves cyclical moods that not only predispose its sufferer's to the risk factors of depression, but also heightened risks of contracting HIV due to features of mania that include impulsivity, hypersexuality, and increased goal-directed behavior. Patients with comorbid HCV/HIV are at increased risk for comorbid psychiatric disorders including bipolar type (6). Severity of bipolar illness has also been associated with HIV risk profile including high rates of unprotected intercourse (69%), multiple partners (39%), sex with prostitutes (24%, men only), and sex trading (10%) (17).

Schizophrenia

Patients with serious and persistent mental illness (SPMI) have been noted to have approximately twice the incidence of HIV as compared to patients without SPMI, and there is also a greater incidence of infection with HCV (18). However, the source of this increased risk has been debated and some data suggest that in the absence of comorbid substance abuse, these patients do not share an elevated risk for acquiring HIV compared to other non-SPMI populations (19). Identification of comorbid SPMI is important in an HIV population given that comorbidity incurs a worse prognosis for both the schizophrenia as well as the HIV due to factors such as psychosocial instability and adherence (18).

Depression

Depression is the most common co-occurring mood disorder with HIV, with rates increasing in the context of advancing age. Depression has been closely linked to apathy in HIV-seropositive populations, and both apathy and depression are linked to combination antiretroviral therapy (CART) nonadherence (20), and a greater frequency of injection drug risk behavior among depressed injection drug users (12).

HIV-seropositive women are a special risk group with regard to depression and intravenous drug use, and they present with both increased severity of depression as well as an elevated incidence of depression (21). Women also report the poorest quality of life scores in the context of HIV infection, in spite of showing some protection against cognitive decline with respect to male counterparts (22). Drug use, violence, and depression have been deemed a "tripartite HIV risk" among African-American women and are underexplored areas of research—again highlighting the need for effective psychiatric services in this at-risk group.

PSYCHOSOCIAL ISSUES

Sexual Abuse

Childhood sexual experiences have been linked as a strong predictor to psychological distress as well as risk of substance abuse and HIV transmission risk (23,24). Among MSM, those with a history of childhood sexual abuse were more likely to engage in high-risk sexual behavior including unprotected receptive anal intercourse, engage in trading sex for money or drugs, report being HIV seropositive, and experience nonsexual relationship violence (24). Individuals who experienced forced sexual contact as a child have a higher risk for showing increased rates of substance abuse and HIV transmission risk as compared to a no exposure to sexual abuse group (23). An assessment of these groups should include a discussion of patterns of risk exposure and childhood sexual experience to better tailor interventions to the specific individual. The role of past trauma in placing individuals at risk of HIV has also been found in large populations of HIV-seropositive women, with posttraumatic stress disorder (PTSD) being associated with the practice of receptive anal sex and prostitution (25). Importantly, both childhood trauma and depression appear to predispose to ineffective coping, which may predispose this group to additional burdens of depression and disease.

Risk Taking Behavior

Previous cross-sectional data has illustrated a close relationship between substance abuse, depression, and behavior, but it is difficult to infer causal relationships from this data. Longitudinal data can better support causal associations, and one such study examining the relationship between depression and sexual risk behaviors in a community sample of 332 inner-city drug abusers found that increasing severity of depression predicted sexual encounters with multiple partners as well as sexual encounters with known injection drug users (26). Other studies have confirmed a link between mental health and risk-taking behavior, even when controlling for substance abuse patterns, across a variety of populations. One study examining a subset analysis of STD clinic patients meeting criteria for major depressive disorder (13) found that depressed patients were more likely to have sex for money or drugs, have a greater number of lifetime sexual partners, and a higher likelihood of abusing alcohol or other substances. The HIV behaviors associated with depression persisted even when controlling for substance abuse.

Similarly, another longitudinal study examining HIV risk behaviors and drug use among Latino heroin and cocaine injectors not in treatment demonstrate a close association between both mental health and substance abuse. Intravenous drug users in this study reported high rates of both depression (52%) as well as severe anxiety (37%) and high rates of alcohol intoxication in the last 30 days (18%). Those showing polysubstance abuse (alcohol and IVDU) were more likely to share needles and paraphernalia, as well as engage in casual sex, prostitution, and unprotected sex (27). Similar patterns among comorbid mental health disorders, substance abuse, and increased sexual risk taking have also been identified in young age populations. One study examining a cohort of newly homeless youth who were followed longitudinally for up to 24 months demonstrated that drug use was a significant predictor of having multiple sexual partners as well as decreased condom use. Similarly, living in a nonfamily setting also was a significant predictor of sexual risk-taking behavior and condom use (28).

A large analysis of 736 enrolled MSM participants in the EXPLORE study described patterns of use with methamphetamines, poppers, and cocaine as well as sexual risk behavior. Younger participants were more likely to increase their use of drugs over time, and high-risk sexual behavior was more common during periods characterized by increased methamphetamine, popper, or sniffed cocaine use. Importantly, a within-person analysis found that both light drug use (less than weekly use) and heavy drug use periods were significantly associated with engaging in unprotected anal sex with HIV-seropositive or unknown status partners as compared to periods of no drug use (29). Importantly, these data suggest that a risk-reduction model of addressing substance abuse in this population is likely to be ineffective in reducing HIV transmission, while engagement in an abstinence model appears safer and more effective. Similar data regarding the risk of moderate alcohol use upon nonadherence also support an abstinence model over a risk-reduction one (30).

Adherence to CART

Previous studies examining the relationship between depression and HIV transmission have shown mixed results, but the role of depression upon adherence to CART has been confirmed in multiple studies on the subject. A recent longitudinal study on adherence rates from 2001 to 2004 of HIV-seropositive patients with concurrent mental illness and substance abuse demonstrated several concerning patterns. Almost 73% of participants met criteria for major depressive disorder, and depression was linked to nonadherence (31). Given that mental health diagnosis and substance abuse problems are common among patients infected with HIV, a great deal of attention has been devoted to the study of these factors and their impact upon adherence. Large cross-sectional studies demonstrated that mental health diagnoses including depression, generalized anxiety disorder, or panic disorder predicted nonadherence to CART therapy over the previous week compared to non-psychiatrically ill counterparts. Nonadherence was also associated with cocaine, amphetamines, or sedative use in the previous month, but cocaine demonstrated the largest effect size in the drug abuse group, while generalized anxiety disorder showed the largest odds of nonadherence among the mental health diagnoses. However, alcohol abuse showed the largest odds ratio of nonadherence among all diagnoses combined (30). Based upon available data, a history of substance abuse in the absence of current abuse does not predict nonadherence, which illustrates the importance of active interventions designed to curb substance abuse and dependence.

The presence of depression has also been linked as an independent risk factor in not only nonadherence but also HIV disease progression, viral load, and CD8 activation. This pattern has been documented in a study of CART-treated HIV-infected drug users. Clinical predictors of disease progression included nonadherence to CART as well as a higher score of depressive symptoms following CART initiation that remained significant even after controlling for nonadherence behavior (32). Other affective syndromes including complicated bereavement and chronic grief have also been linked to disease progression in HIV-infected populations (33).

However, encouragingly, depressed HIV patients who receive psychiatric treatment with antidepressants are more likely than untreated patients to receive appropriate care for their HIV disease and increase adherence to HIV interventions. Antidepressant therapy for treatment of depression in this population has also been demonstrated to be associated with a lower monthly cost of medical care services based on at least one study examining merged Medicaid and surveillance data (34).

CENTRAL NERVOUS SYSTEM

When HIV was initially discovered, it was though to affect only CD4 lymphocytes; however, it was recovered from brain, spinal fluid, and peripheral nerves in 1985, which showed its potential for direct central nervous system (CNS) infection. Since that time, HIV-1 has been shown to penetrate the blood–brain barrier (BBB) early in the course of the infection, is replicated in brain tissue using monocytes and multinucleated macrophages as hosts, and becomes an anatomic reservoir for the disease. The mechanisms whereby HIV-1 penetrates the nervous system remain inadequately understood, but the virus appears to enter the brain through endothelial gaps in brain capillaries, via the choroid plexus, or as a proviral form contained in a latently infected cell (monocyte), which differentiates into a macrophage once inside the CNS to become a productively infected cell. The virus is known to invade and destroy subcortical areas such as the basal ganglia and temporolimbic structures, as well as support cells such as astrocytes, which share similar CD4 receptors with their well-known lymphocyte host (35). This effect may be exaggerated in substance-abusing populations (36).

Clinically, patients suffer from a wide spectrum of cognitive impairments related to CNS HIV disease including personality changes, and motor dysfunctions that range from subclinical symptoms without impairment of work or daily activities to severe dementia with paraplegia and incontinence. The prevalence of HIV-associated dementia (HAD) was approximately 30% in the 1990s, but has decreased to approximately 11% with the advent of HAART therapy (35). Its severity appears related in part to the degree of inflammatory response in the brain (33). In patients with moderate to severe dementia, multinucleated giant cells (MNGC) are found in 25% to 50% of patients (37). Microglial and glial changes, along with MNGC, can be found in any part of the CNS but are more common in deep white matter of the cerebral hemispheres, basal ganglia, and brainstem (37). White matter pallor with astrogliosis, diffuse or focal vacuolation associated with axonal or myelin loss, and cortical atrophy are other changes that are less commonly observed (38). Rather than a true demyelination process of the oligodendritic myelin sheath, the pallor is a result of an increase in interstitial water content, most likely caused by a leaky BBB.

Peripheral Nervous System Pathology and Myopathy in HIV-1 Infection

Patients with HIV-1 infection may also present with a wide variety of symptoms involving the peripheral nervous system (PNS). Distal symmetric peripheral neuropathy (DSPN) is the most common presentation among patients with generalized neuropathies (39). Initial symptoms include trophic changes in the lower extremities, paresthesias, sensory loss, edema, and weakness. Medication-induced neuropathies have a clinical presentation that is similar to DSPN except that they present concurrent with the use of antiretrovirals. Inflammatory demyelinating polyradiculoneuropathy may be acute (AIDP), presenting at the time of seroconversion and the initial manifestation of HIV-1 infection, or chronic (CIDP), presenting as subacute or chronic weakness in upper and lower extremities, diminished deep tendon reflexes, and mild sensory abnormalities. Cranial nerves may also be involved, and mononeuritis multiplex can present as an abrupt-onset mononeuropathy with periodic additional abrupt mononeuropathies in other distributions and may involve the cranial nerves as well. Pain may accompany any of the neuropathies and may be both severe and incapacitating. Less common presentations of PNS dysfunction include progressive polyneuroradiculopathy with early impairment of bladder and rectal sphincter control, and autonomic neuropathy with postural hypotension, diarrhea, and sudden arrhythmias with the risk of death (40).

Myopathy associated with HIV-1 infection has three different histologic findings: (a) polymyositis; (b) necrotizing myopathy without inflammatory infiltrates; or (c) nemaline rod myopathy. Clinically, myositis presents as painless progressive weakness involving the shoulder and pelvic girdle muscles, elevated creatinine kinase, and electromyographic abnormalities. Treatment with prednisone alone or in combination with plasmapheresis is generally effective. Historically, one of the more important causes of myopathy among HIV-1–infected patients was related to AZT, which usually developed after 9 months to 1 year of treatment and manifest as leg weakness and wasting of the buttock muscles (40). However, AZT myopathy is more unusual now given that high doses of AZT are rarely used in favor of other available CART regimens.

Diagnosis and Management of HIV-1 Secondary Neurologic Complications

HIV-1 CNS involvement may occur at any time, but opportunistic infections and HIV-1–related malignancies affecting the nervous system are usually a late manifestation of the HIV-1 infection, occurring most often in patients with a CD4 count less than 50 cells/mm^3. Table 50.1 indicates potential CNS pathologies secondary to HIV-1 infection. No significant differences in the incidence of neurologic disease between IVDUs and non-IVDUs have been reported (41).

Toxoplasma gondii infection is a common cause of focal intracerebral lesions in patients with AIDS. However, primary infection is usually asymptomatic. Focal encephalitis with headache, fever, confusion, and motor weakness is the most common clinical presentation. Individuals with toxoplasmosis encephalitis are almost uniformly seropositive for antitoxoplasma immunoglobulin G antibodies. Computed

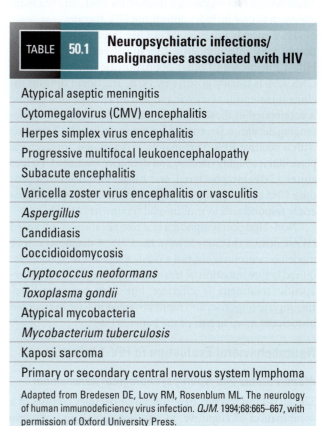

TABLE 50.1 Neuropsychiatric infections/malignancies associated with HIV

Atypical aseptic meningitis
Cytomegalovirus (CMV) encephalitis
Herpes simplex virus encephalitis
Progressive multifocal leukoencephalopathy
Subacute encephalitis
Varicella zoster virus encephalitis or vasculitis
Aspergillus
Candidiasis
Coccidioidomycosis
Cryptococcus neoformans
Toxoplasma gondii
Atypical mycobacteria
Mycobacterium tuberculosis
Kaposi sarcoma
Primary or secondary central nervous system lymphoma

Adapted from Bredesen DE, Lovy RM, Rosenblum ML. The neurology of human immunodeficiency virus infection. *QJM*. 1994;68:665–667, with permission of Oxford University Press.

tomography (CT) scan or magnetic resonance imaging (MRI) often shows multiple contrast enhancing lesions with associated edema. The majority of clinicians rely on empiric diagnosis, since definitive diagnosis requires a brain biopsy. Detection of *T. gondii* by PCR in cerebrospinal fluid (CSF), although highly specific, has low sensitivity and is usually negative once therapy has started. At times, individuals who are severely immune deficient may not mount an antibody response. Primary prophylaxis with daily DS TMP-SMX is recommended in toxoplasma-seropositive individuals with a CD4 count less than 100 cells/mm^3. This can be discontinued when the CD4 count is >200 for 3 or more months. The initial choice of therapy for toxoplasmosis encephalitis includes pyrimethamine, sulfadiazine, and leucovorin (42,43).

Cryptococcus neoformans is a common cause of meningitis and the prevalent CNS fungal infection in patients with AIDS. The typical clinical presentation includes subacute meningitis with fever, malaise, and headache in a patient with a CD4 count of less than 50 cells/mm^3. Cryptococcal antigen is invariably detected in CSF. Treatment usually includes amphotericin B deoxycholate combined with flucytosine for at least 2 weeks followed by fluconazole (44).

Other secondary neurologic infections associated with HIV-1 include progressive multifocal leukoencephalopathy (PML) secondary to polyoma virus JC virus, cytomegalovirus (CMV) infection encephalitis and polyradiculopathy, herpes simplex virus (HSV) encephalitis, neurosyphilis, mycobacterial infection, and other fungal infections. The incidence of PML after widespread use of HAART has significantly declined (45). There remains no established therapy for PML, and the main approach to care includes optimizing HIV therapy.

HSV encephalitis is a rare but life-threatening complication of HSV infection, especially in patients with advanced HIV-1 infection and other opportunistic infections of the CNS. CSF is usually positive by PCR. Treatment options include intravenous acyclovir and foscarnet. Syphilitic disease is accelerated in those infected with HIV, and there is wide-ranging debate on screening for neurosyphilis in HIV patients with a positive RPR. Fortunately, if diagnosed, intravenous penicillin is a highly effective and definitive treatment. Herpes zoster, CMV, mycobacterial, and fungal infections that produce CNS complications in HIV-1–infected individuals generally respond well to multimodal treatment (42,43).

Non–Hodgkin lymphoma is a complication of advanced HIV-1 disease that may involve the CNS. A diagnosis can be made via neuroimaging, but a tissue diagnosis is typically required before initiation of treatment. Multiagent chemotherapeutic treatment is effective but may be short-lived. Incomplete responses and rapid progression have been noted historically in up to half of the patients (46).

Neurobehavioral Evaluation in HIV-1 Infection

Mental Status and Neuropsychological Assessment

The HIV-1–associated cognitive/motor complex consists of a combination of cognitive, motor, behavioral, and affective disturbances that may be severe and sufficient for the diagnosis of AIDS. It may be the presenting manifestation of HIV-1 infection or it may cause mild symptoms and may not be associated with significant impairment in the social or occupational functioning levels of these patients. Data support that asymptomatic HIV-1–positive patients have an elevated rate of cognitive dysfunction as compared to HIV-1–negative controls, but these are usually subtle impairments that are unrelated to the level of immunosuppression or to depression and are most evident in individuals with lower cognitive reserve. It is generally accepted by clinicians that HIV-1–related cognitive impairment can occur at any time during the course of the disease, but cognitive abnormalities in asymptomatic patients are associated with an increased risk of morbidity and mortality (47).

Although varying psychological tests have been used to determine or evaluate the earlier signs of HIV-1 effects on mental function, no definitive test can be used, either alone or in combination with others, to establish a diagnosis of HIV-1–associated cognitive/motor complex. A careful cognitive history can be an extremely useful adjunct in the differential diagnosis of the etiologies of cognitive dysfunction in HIV-1–infected patients with cognitive complaints.

The most significant signs of cognitive impairment related to HIV-1 infection include early, mild problems with abstraction, learning, language, verbal memory, and psychomotor speed that progress to more serious difficulties with attention and concentration, slowing of information processing, slowed psychomotor speed, impaired cognitive flexibility, impairment in nonverbal abilities of problem solving, visuospatial integration and construction, and nonverbal memory in the late phases of the infection. The early stages of cognitive impairment associated with HIV-1 affect psychomotor tasks (such as the Wechsler Adult Intelligence Scale digit symbol and block design, and the trail making test part B from the Halstead–Reitan Neuropsychological Test Battery), memory tasks (such as the delayed visual reproduction subtest from the Wechsler Memory Scale); and the delayed recall of the Rey–Osterrieth Complex Figure. Psychomotor and neuromotor tasks may reveal HIV-1–related cognitive dysfunction and are sensitive measures for the early detection of HIV-1–related cognitive impairment (48).

The neuropsychological tests used for assessment of dementia generally appraise complex language-associated functions (such as aphasia and apraxia), higher level cognitive functions of verbal and nonverbal abstract reasoning and problem solving, and perceptual functioning of the different sensory modalities. However, as more has been learned about the HIV-1–associated cognitive/motor complex, it has become apparent that these neuropsychological assessments are not reliably sensitive or useful for detecting the often subtle impairments of the early stages of HIV-1's effects on the CNS or function (48).

CSF Studies

CSF reflects changes consistent with HIV-1 infection, including the presence of HIV-1 virions, abnormally elevated IgG levels, HIV-1–specific antibodies, mononuclear cells, and oligoclonal bands. HIV-1 replicates in the brain with independent dynamics from other organs, making the CSF viral load more representative for the assessment of CNS infection (49). It correlates with the degree of neurocognitive dysfunction and has a role in monitoring the response to antiretroviral medications in the CNS (48). Although other CSF studies have been used in the assessment of CNS compromise in HIV-1 infection, their use is now limited because serum viral load measurements have replaced them in clinical practice. CSF β_2-microglobulin has shown a high correlation between its concentration and both the severity of the dementia and the level of systemic disease. Although elevation in the myelin basic protein and its degradation was found in patients with HIV-1–associated cognitive/motor complex and with PML, this was not seen in patients with other opportunistic infections. An abnormally low CSF CD4:CD8 ratio may have importance for treatment considerations and prognostic value for HIV dementia (49,50).

Neuroimaging

MRI and to a lesser extent CT and are useful tools in the diagnosis of secondary infections and brain tumors. Primary CNS HIV-1 infection can be associated with characteristic imaging features including cortical atrophy, ventricular enlargement, diffuse or patchy periventricular white matter abnormalities, and, in children, calcification of the basal ganglia and delayed myelination. MRI is more sensitive than CT, and is now considered the neuroimaging criterion standard. Both, however, are useful as diagnostic tools and have utility in assessing the prognosis of these patients (51).

Magnetic resonance spectroscopy (MRS) measures levels of metabolites in brain tissue. MRS in HIV disease, particularly HIV dementia, shows increases in choline and reductions in N-acetylaspartate suggestive of neuroinflammation and neuronal injury. In some studies, these findings correlate with the severity of the HIV dementia along with CD4 counts and viral load (52).

Electrophysiology

There is currently relatively little role for electrophysiology in the diagnosis and management of uncomplicated HIV patients outside of that subset in whom one is assessing for the presence of epilepsy or other CNS lesions. However, research data using electrophysiologic techniques has provided some interesting findings. The percentage of patients with abnormal electroencephalograms appears to increase as the systemic disease progresses, and a low amplitude pattern may be found in advanced dementia and atrophy on neuroimaging. In asymptomatic patients, studies have found conflicting results, but the best available data support a very limited role, if any, of CNS dysfunction in nonimmunocompromised HIV patients. Evoked potential studies have also been useful in detecting preclinical abnormalities in neurologically and physically asymptomatic HIV-1–seropositive patients by showing significant delays in latency of response to the brainstem auditory-evoked potential, somatosensory-evoked potentials from tibial nerve stimulation, and visual-evoked potentials. However, these are rarely used clinically at this point in time (53).

Treatment of Neuropsychiatric Disorders

Mental disorders secondary to medical conditions such as delirium, dementia, mood disorders, psychosis, and anxiety disorders are the most common neuropsychiatric conditions associated with HIV-1 infection (54). One of the most perplexing aspects of these presentations is that HIV-1–related neuropsychiatric manifestations very closely resemble other primary psychiatric (functional) disorders. Like syphilis, HIV-1 infection often confounds precise diagnostic criteria because of its characteristic as a "great imitator."

Delirium

It is estimated that as many as 30% of hospitalized medical/surgical patients may have an undetected delirium process. Delirium is a predictor of outcome in hospitalized AIDS patients, and delirious patients have higher mortality rates, longer lengths of inpatient hospitalizations, and a greater need for long-term care as compared to a group of nondelirious AIDS patients with similar demographics and markers of medical morbidity (55). Standardized and validated instruments exist for delirium screening and should be used routinely (56).

There are diverse suggestions for the etiology of HIV-1–related delirium. However, it is important to attempt to determine the particular etiology for each individual patient because certain causes are life-threatening or may lead to permanent brain damage. These conditions include Wernicke encephalopathy, hypoglycemia, hyperglycemia, hypoxemia, hemodynamic instability with cerebral hypoperfusion, infections, metabolic disturbances, and electrolyte imbalances. Herpes and *T. gondii* encephalitis, cryptococcal meningitis, space-occupying lesions from cerebral tumors, PML, and neurotoxicities from antiviral agents should also be included in the differential diagnosis of delirium in HIV-1 patients. In a substance-abusing population, the detection of intoxication or withdrawal is important in the differential diagnostic considerations (57).

Prompt pharmacologic interventions may help remediate the various behavioral abnormalities associated with the delirium process. High-potency neuroleptics remain the standard of care for delirious patients, although their use in HIV-infected patients brings an increased risk of significant treatment-emergent side effects. At low doses, haloperidol and chlorpromazine (a low-potency neuroleptic) in both oral and intravenous formulations have been used effectively and with few adverse events in the treatment of delirium in hospitalized AIDS patients. Atypical antipsychotics are used now as first-line agents, and are both effective and better tolerated as compared to traditional neuroleptics. The experience, however, is still limited, especially in HIV-1–infected individuals, and they must be used with caution (58).

Lorazepam is useful in the management of severely agitated delirious HIV-1–infected patients when used in combination with a neuroleptic. Lorazepam alone, however, appears to be ineffective and is associated with worsening delirium (59). The notable exception to this is when treating delirium associated with GABAergic withdrawal such as delirium tremens, benzodiazepine withdrawal, or barbiturate withdrawal. Benzodiazepines are the treatment of choice in these scenarios.

Dementia

It is beyond the scope of this chapter to review the different classes of antiretroviral drugs and their use in clinical practice in the context of HIV-cognitive impairment and dementia. The use of antiretroviral agents are generally recommended when CD4 count is below 350 cells/mm^3 or plasma HIV RNA is above 100,000 copies/mL. There are no established guidelines for HIV-associated cognitive and dementing illness. Like that of systemic therapy, the use of antiretroviral therapy (ART) in HIV-cognitive impairment and dementia is to produce complete virologic suppression in both plasma and the CNS.

Various drugs that are effective against HIV-1 are approved by the Food and Drug Administration (FDA) for clinical use. Initial therapy for HIV has either a PI backbone or a nonnucleoside reverse transcriptase inhibitors (NNRTI) backbone, and then includes a dual NRTI component. It is recommended, currently, that therapy begin if a patient has HIV symptoms regardless of CD4 count, or in any asymptomatic individual with a CD4 count <350 cells/mm^3. However, there is ongoing research regarding the exact optimal point at which to initiate HAART. With regard to CNS symptoms, studies show that CART improves cognitive functioning among patients with minor cognitive changes who are otherwise asymptomatic and reduces the neurocognitive deficits when used long-term, therefore reducing the risk of HAD (60).

CNS distribution of the NRTIs is best characterized of anti-HIV agents. AZT and stavudine are significantly better in terms of CNS penetration than didanosine, although the data regarding CNS penetrance with stavudine in clinically used doses are conflicting. Early data regarding abacavir are also promising with at least one study showing that it penetrates into CNS at levels high enough to inhibit local HIV populations. A recent review covering this data also notes that NRTIs are able to prevent infection of resting CD4 lymphocytes and macrophages to varying degrees depending on the specific agent (60).

NNRTIs including nevirapine, efavirenz, and delavirdine are increasingly important components of CART regimens and are highly active against HIV-1. In addition, they are detectable in the CNS even though they are highly protein bound, which may limit CNS access—especially for delavirdine. Efavirenz has been shown to reach effective CNS levels to inhibit local HIV replication and can be given once daily due to its long half-life. Nevirapine shows the least protein binding (60%) and is also quite lipophilic. It has shown an approximate 10 times greater propensity to cross the BBB than other NNRTIs, so it is likely the NNRTI of choice when targeting CNS symptoms (60).

Protease inhibitors are large-molecular-weight agents and are relatively highly protein bound, but they also show high lipophilicity. Unfortunately, they are actively removed from the CSF due to acting as substrates of P glycoprotein efflux transporter that pumps PIs across the BBB. Some reports have suggested that nelfinavir, ritonavir, and lopinavir doe not reach effective CSF concentrations. It has also been noted that available studies that evaluated the benefit of PI-based regimens also contained multiple NRTIs as part of the CART regimen. Indinavir may be the best penetrator into the CSF, but its dosing is inconvenient and difficult, so it is rarely used in favor of simpler regimens designed to promote adherence. Lopinavir has been shown to reach effective CSF concentrations to inhibit HIV replication as well. Saquinavir, nelfinavir, amprenavir, and ritonavir all appear to be weakly and insufficiently CNS penetrant to prevent the replication of local RNA populations (60). The optimal CART regimen for the treatment of cognitive impairment is not known (61). However, in future, optimizing CNS penetration of CART therapy by utilizing more CNS penetrant agents may be useful in further treating HIV associated cognitive disorders (62).

The psychostimulants such as methylphenidate and dextroamphetamine have been used effectively to manage symptoms of decreased concentration, or memory deficits among patients with HIV-related cognitive impairment and HAD. Case reports and uncontrolled clinical trials treating patients with methylphenidate (30 to 90 mg/day) or dextroamphetamine (30 to 60 mg/day) all showed significant improvement (63,64).

Mood Disorders

While mood disorders associated with HIV-1 infection are most frequently depressive, manic and hypomanic disturbances have also been described. The diagnostic process for evaluating mood disorders is complex, requiring careful consideration of the interaction of medical conditions, substances, and behavioral factors. Depressive spectrum disorders are commonly observed in patients with HIV-1–related disorders ranging from normal sadness to major affective disorders, as well as mood disorders that may be substance induced or a consequence of a general medical condition. Although it has been suggested that clinicians rely on psychological rather than somatic symptoms of depression to fulfill diagnostic criteria for depression in the medically ill, an all-inclusive approach is often the simplest and most clinically effective. Depression in medically ill patients is underdiagnosed and undertreated, and this is particularly true of HIV-1–infected persons who suffer an increased incidence of depression when compared with other medically ill patients or the general population (58).

Suicidal thoughts are frequently a symptom of depression, and patients need to be assessed carefully. Risk factors include social isolation, perceived lack of social support, adjustment disorder, personality disorder, alcohol abuse, HIV-1–related interpersonal or occupational problems, and a past history of depression. Other risk factors include current major depression, previous suicide attempt, and history of alcohol abuse. One should never blithely consider the notion of "rational suicide" as an understandable reaction to this devastating and socially stigmatized disease. Because of impaired decision-making capacities and cognitive inefficiencies associated with HIV-1 disease, it is vital that clinicians respond promptly to any and all reports of suicidal ideation. A thorough assessment of the patient includes a realistic appraisal of the psychosocial situation and of the motivation for completing the suicide, along with any appropriate neurodiagnostic assessment to rule out a potentially reversible organic mental disorder (65).

Antidepressants with greater affinity for the central muscarinic receptor should be avoided for symptomatic HIV-1–infected patients, which can mask or aggravate HIV-1–related cognitive impairment or precipitate delirium. Another adverse side effect of these agents is the possibility of excessive drying of the mucous membranes, which introduces the possibility of oral candidiasis that is often refractory to treatment in HIV-1–infected patients. Antidepressants that are preferable for HIV-1–infected individuals include selective serotonin reuptake inhibitors (SSRIs), and other second-generation antidepressants such as bupropion, venlafaxine, mirtazapine, and psychostimulants (58).

Fluoxetine has been shown to be safe in HIV populations, but inhibition of the CYP450 2D6 and 3A4 isozymes is problematic in patients with HIV. Similarly, paroxetine is not recommended in this population for the same reasons. Sertraline and citalopram have also been shown to be effective and well tolerated. Venlafaxine is also a reasonable choice because of its low interactions with other drugs (58).

Patients being treated with lithium carbonate or monoamine oxidase inhibitors before their diagnosis with HIV-1 disease should usually continue to take that medication. Increased vigilance in toxicity monitoring with a concomitant dosage alteration may be necessary as HIV-1 disease progresses, especially when infectious complications cause severe diarrhea or any other form of fluid loss due to the emergence of nephrotoxicity and neurotoxicity from lithium toxicity (66). Psychostimulants such as methylphenidate and dextroamphetamine may be tried in depressed patients who are symptomatic of HIV-1 infection, in those depressed patients in whom rapid improvement in symptoms is needed or who are cognitively impaired or who suffer from both depression and dementia. Methylphenidate is a safe and effective treatment for these syndromes. Response usually occurs within hours of the first administration and includes psychomotor activation, appetite stimulation, and qualitative as well as quantitative improvement in higher cortical functions. The initial administration of methylphenidate is usually 5 to 10 mg orally, and an adequate therapeutic response usually requires less than 30 mg daily. Methylphenidate can be continued safely for several months after the patient's symptoms remit. Special care should be taken in using dextroamphetamine, which has been noted to unmask or aggravate abnormal involuntary movements in AIDS dementia patients. The use of psychostimulants in managing depressive or cognitive symptomatology in drug-abusing patients is questionable, so they should be used cautiously if at all (64).

Sleep Disorders

Insomnia is one of the most prevalent neuropsychiatric disorders in HIV-seropositive populations. Estimates as high as 70% have been noted in some studies, if one looks at the incidence of insomnia across the HIV disease process. Insomnia has been linked to reduced quality of life as well as treatment nonadherence. However, there has been very limited research on the treatment of insomnia in this setting. Readers are referred to a comprehensive review of HIV-associated insomnia by Omonuwa and colleagues (67). Essentially, there appear to be four primary factors that impact the assessment and treatment of insomnia in individuals with HIV: (a) medications used to treat HIV, (b) antibiotics used to treat opportunistic infections, (c) the HIV infection itself, and (d) conditions frequently associated with HIV infection.

Insomnia is defined as persistent difficulty falling asleep, staying asleep, or nonrestorative sleep which is associated with impaired daytime function. Insomnia is common in the general population, but the prevalence of insomnia in HIV-positive individuals appears to be higher. It is easy to assume that HIV-associated insomnia is due to the stress of a highly stigmatized and potentially life-threatening physical illness, but this view is contradicted somewhat by a study of asymptomatic HIV-positive men, which showed that even prior to experiencing HIV/AIDS symptoms, there were more shifts to stage 1, increased awakenings, and lower sleep efficiency. The sleep changes that occur in HIV infection have been quantified in several studies employing polysomnography; however, the data are conflicting. There are reports of an increase in slow wave sleep that occurs primarily during later sleep cycles, but this finding has failed to be replicated in other studies. Similarly, increased sleep latency, a reduction in the percentage of stage 2 sleep, and an increase in the number of nocturnal awakenings have been reported but have not been confirmed by subsequent studies. The pathophysiology of insomnia in HIV is equally unclear. It is agreed that insomnia becomes highly prevalent in the later stages of HIV infection, and this may be due to disruption of sleep centers via HIV-mediated neurotoxic effects, medication effects, opportunistic infections, HAD, and chronic depression (67).

The NNRTI efavirenz has the distinction of being the antiviral medication best documented to be associated with sleep disturbances. Nervous system adverse events including dizziness, insomnia, and fatigue are among the most common associated with this medication. Sleep effects of efavirenz include difficulty with sleep initiation and maintenance, as well as vivid nightmares. An ambulatory polysomnographic study found that all patients on efavirenz had longer sleep latencies, reduced sleep efficiency, and reduced REM sleep. Efavirenz serum levels appear to correlate with changes in sleep. However, the sleep disruption associated with efavirenz appears to self-extinguish in the majority of patients over time, and every effort should be made to support the infectious disease team during this time so that patients can remain on this agent if needed (67).

A large number of different prescription medications are used to treat insomnia. These medications can be broadly categorized as benzodiazepines, nonbenzodiazepine hypnotics, antidepressants, and antipsychotics. The benzodiazepines are a relatively old group of compounds that exert a therapeutic effect on sleep via allosteric modulation of the γ-aminobutyric acid (GABA) receptor complex and enhance the inhibition that occurs when GABA. Commonly used benzodiazepines include triazolam, temazepam, flurazepam, quazepam, lorazepam, oxazepam, and alprazolam. Major alterations in half-life and effect have been noted with the agents that require oxidation in the presence of protease inhibitors, so if a benzodiazepine is to be used, then we recommend that it either be temazepam, lorazepam, or oxazepam in this patient population. Other alternatives include the typical benzodiazepine-like agents such as zolpidem, zaleplon, and eszopiclone. The reader is referred to a comprehensive review of these agents for up to date concerns over drug–drug interactions (67). All these agents are Schedule IV under the Drug Enforcement Administration, which is reflective of the fact that they do have some potential to be habit forming over time in susceptible individuals.

Antidepressants are frequently used in the treatment of insomnia, but none are FDA approved for this indication. The most commonly used agents include sedating tricyclic antidepressants, mirtazapine, and trazodone. However, in contrast to the benzodiazepines, they have less abuse potential in vulnerable patient populations. Tricyclics must be used with caution as they can cause sedation, orthostasis, weight gain, dry mouth, constipation, and cardiac dysrhythmia; although some data exist to suggest that very low dose doxepin can avoid these side effects while improving both sleep onset insomnia and sleep maintenance insomnia. Other alternative antidepressants include mirtazapine and trazodone. Among the antipsychotics that are frequently used off-label for sleep, quetiapine and olanzapine appear to be common choices. Care must be taken in the selection of these choices, as atypical antipsychotics can exacerbate and cause a metabolic syndrome. No atypical antipsychotic has placebo-controlled data to support their use in treating primary insomnia. However, for those patients who are refractory to other measures and who understand the associated risks, they can clinically be useful per our experience (67,68).

Psychosis

Nearly 10% of patients with HIV infection have a diagnosed psychosis of one type or another (68). There are several potential causes for psychosis and the initial evaluation for psychosis includes the same medical workup as that for delirium and dementia (69). Some are preexisting conditions unrelated to the HIV infection, whereas others are thought to result from delirium and CNS involvement of the HIV infection. Others may result from drug use inclusive of rare iatrogenic causes such as that which occurs with efavirenz (70). Many patients with HIV-associated psychosis also manifest symptoms of cognitive decline, such as HMCMD or HAD. In fact, psychotic symptoms may precede the onset of dementing illness (71). There is also a high association between psychosis and HIV-related mood disorders.

Treatment of psychosis in the context of HIV-disease, whether or not there is concurrent CNS involvement, requires timely intervention. This is best accomplished with neuroleptics. However, patients with HIV infection are more sensitive to side effects such as extrapyramidal reactions and neuroleptic malignant syndrome. This is particularly true with high-potency typical neuroleptics, whereas confusion and seizures are more frequent with low-potency neuroleptics. The atypical antipsychotics (risperidone, paliperidone, olanzapine, quetiapine, aripiprazole, and ziprasidone) have also been shown to control HIV-related psychosis without having the same treatment emergent side effects (72). Quetiapine has been shown to have the least antiparkinsonian effects (73), and should be considered for patients with symptomatic HIV-related CNS disease given the associated subcortical damage related to HIV infection. Risperidone is an effective alternative and has been reported to be well tolerated in low doses (74). Low doses should be used in any regimen involving protease inhibitors because of potentially heightened risk of extrapyramidal reactions (75) and alterations in consciousness that have been reported with such combinations (76,77).

One major area of concern for the use of atypical antipsychotic agents in patients with HIV infection receiving HAART is in the development or exacerbation of metabolic syndrome (72). In such instances where there is a major concern for potentially exacerbating metabolic syndrome, the practitioner can choose to prescribe those with a lower incidence of metabolic effects, such as aripiprazole or ziprasidone. Another concern with the use of atypical antipsychotics is the possibility of cytochrome P450 interactions, especially with protease inhibitors. Although not well studied, the possible use of paliperidone, which has the lowest affinity, should be considered in this patient population (78).

Anxiety

Anxiety disorders affect some 17% to 36% of patients with HIV infection with adjustment disorder with anxious mood, generalized anxiety disorder, and panic disorder (79). Persistent and chronic anxiety following notification of seropositive status affects about 20% of patients and, in time, may evolve into a fully developed PTSD. This may be problematic as avoidant behaviors secondary to untreated HIV-related anxiety may diminish treatment compliance and interfere with medical management of HIV disease.

In the differential diagnoses of anxiety, one should always be concerned about the common association with depression, and a careful assessment to rule out depressive illness is critical. Anxiety may also arise from multiple medical conditions, especially in patients with pain, respiratory compromise due to pneumonia, and delirium as well as substance-induced anxiety. As with other HIV-related psychiatric disorders, a comprehensive medical evaluation is essential (69), including an extensive review of medications. Antiretroviral medications, like efavirenz, have been associated with anxiety, irritability, restlessness, agitation, and insomnia (68).

Treatment with psychotherapy, self-hypnosis, and biofeedback is very effective in anxiety disorders (68). Moreover, all psychotherapies are useful for the development of adaptive behaviors that allow the individual to reduce anxiety while improving coping capacity. Combining pharmacotherapy with a benzodiazepine during psychotherapy may be necessary for acute reduction of symptoms. This is best accomplished with the use of intermediate-acting benzodiazepines without active metabolites such oxazepam or lorazepam. Similarly, with chronic refractory anxiety, lorazepam is a better choice because of its ease of use and low neurotoxicity (68,76).

In the management of anxiety in individuals with co-occurring substance abuse, antidepressants and antiepileptic agents are preferred to benzodiazepines (68). All SSRIs and venlafaxine have been reported to be effective and should be considered initial first-line therapies. Also, the combination of a benzodiazepine with an antidepressant or with buspirone can be helpful, but the risk of addiction remains a concern. Use of gabapentin, tiagabine, or pregabalin either alone or in combination with antidepressants has been reported to be safe and effective (72). In cases where painful neuropathy is causing or exacerbating anxiety, the antiepileptic agents should be tried initially with the hopes of improving both disease states.

In cognitively impaired and patients with HAD, benzodiazepines should be avoided as it may further compromise cognitive function and may uncover or exacerbate disinhibition, frontal lobe dysfunction, confusion, and delirium. While the use of antihistamines is sometimes recommended in managing anxiety, our clinical experience suggests otherwise. Anxious patients, especially those with cognitive compromise, do not do well with antihistamines. The use of trazodone in low doses (25 to 50 mg t.i.d.) is preferable (68).

Pain in HIV Patients

HIV patients experience pain commonly, and prevalence of pain within 2 weeks has been estimated to be greater than 60% based on one outpatient survey. Patients answering this survey were noted to have multiple sources of pain and on average experienced 2.5 different pains in the preceding 2 weeks. Average pain scores were rated as 5.4 out of 10, and worst mean pain rated as 7.4 out of 10 indicative of moderately severe pain. The pain levels were noted to interfere with functional status across a variety of measures. Other factors influencing pain included the number of current HIV-related symptoms, treatment for HIV-related infections, and the absence of antiretroviral medications. Female gender, non-Caucasian race, and number of HIV-related physical symptoms were significantly associated with pain intensity, indicating perhaps a different pain experience in these vulnerable groups (80).

The most common source of HIV-linked pain is HIV-associated painful neuropathy, which appears to affect up to 30% of patients with HIV over the course of their disease (39). The causes of this painful neuropathy appear myriad and manyfold, but typically involves both direct neurotoxic effects of HIV as well as potential effects from antiretroviral medications—especially the NRTIs (e.g., stavudine). In addition to these causes, patients may have additive neuropathy from such reasons as diabetes mellitus, nutritional deficiencies, or the late results of syphilis. Hyperalgesia and paresthesias are common manifestations of HIV-associated neuropathy, and diminished ankle-jerk reflexes are also frequently noted. Electromyographic data show abnormal sensory and motor conduction supportive of a dying-back axonopathy. Neuropathy is virtually always progressive (39).

Tricyclic antidepressants have the most data with regards to non-HIV neuropathic pain management, but they must be used cautiously in HIV-seropositive patients due to anticholinergic effects and decreased tolerance. There is also data to suggest that tricyclics may be ineffective for HIV-related painful neuropathy (81). Alternative agents for treating HIV-related neuropathic pain include anticonvulsants (gabapentin or pregabalin), newer generation antidepressants (venlafaxine or duloxetine), or lidocaine topical applications (patches). Unfortunately, none of these agents has been subjected to rigorous testing in a double-blind, placebo-controlled trial in HIV-seropositive patients or in those whose pain is due to HIV-associated painful neuropathy (82).

Even though HIV-seropositive patients are at increased risk of adverse drug reactions, use of opiates can be safe and effective if comorbidities and potential drug–drug interactions are considered at the time of prescribing. There has historically been concern over chronic use of opiates in persistent nonmalignant cancer pain, but multiple evidence-based trials and position statements by pain societies including the American Academy of Pain Medicine support the chronic use of opiates in managing persistent pain due to a variety of etiologies. Multiple randomized high-quality trials of opiates have demonstrated efficacy for diverse pain conditions including musculoskeletal pain, osteoarthritis, low-back pain, painful diabetic neuropathy, and postherpetic neuralgia. To date, no adequate trial has been conducted using opiates to control the pain of HIV-associated neuropathy, but clinical experience supports their judicious use. Long-term data remains suboptimal, and further studies are needed to better understand the role of opiates in long-term management of pain, regardless of etiology.

Tolerance to the respiratory depressant effect of opiates develops quickly in patients, so this can generally be avoided by slow and careful titration. Chronic opiate therapy may also suppress endocrine function in hypothalamic, pituitary, gonadal, and adrenal hormones that leads to fatigue, depression, and diminished libido (83). When evaluating depression in patients using chronic opiates and HIV, attention to endocrine markers becomes more important in the differential diagnosis. Addiction to opiates when used for established medical indications is rare. Opioid abuse may become a concern, however, especially among those with earlier addiction histories. Published guidelines and statements from state medical boards and pain organizations are available to assist physicians in the assessment of responsible opioid use.

Substance Use/Abuse and Treatment

Injection drug users are less likely to receive ART than any other population. Factors associated with poor access to treatment include active drug use, younger age, and female gender, suboptimal health care, not being in a drug treatment program, recent incarceration, and lack of health care provider expertise. Yet these individuals should be considered and can be treated effectively. Nursing outreach interventions over

3 months including home visits have demonstrated improvements in making and keeping appointments, integration of care among HIV, substance abuse and mental health providers and improved access, adherence, and retention of patients in CART (84).

Another study examining the effects of an intensive outpatient cocaine treatment program over 9 months found that risky behavior among participants was correlated with high-intake problem severity and psychological symptomatology. Over the course of treatment, the amount of risky behavior was found to decrease significantly among those participating actively in the treatment program. The decrease in risky behavior was linked to decreased substance abuse, but it did not appear affected by demographic variables or type or duration of treatment in this study (85).

Other potential data-driven intervention models include brief peer-delivered educational interventions, which have demonstrated effectiveness in reducing crack cocaine use, IDU, and the number of IDU sex partners. Methadone maintenance treatment (MMT) programs remain an essential part of the treatment of dually diagnosed patients. Increased numbers of patients in MMT show IVDU abstinence. MMT has been demonstrated to dramatically reduce both illicit opiate use as well as criminal activity. More recent data support that MMT also reduces incarceration rates, which would likely diminish the risk factor of sharing needles while incarcerated and lower exposure to high-risk practices (86). In addition, opiate treatment–resistant dually diagnosed patients show better long-term survivability in MMT programs than their nondually diagnosed counterparts (87).

Non-MMT programs centering around group activity and support also demonstrate significant roles for the treatment of this complex population, and involvement in either MMT or non-MMT programs is associated with improved ART adherence (88). Buprenorphine programs are likewise associated with improved CART adherence, although they are widely underused in HIV-seropositive populations in the United States. France appears to be most experienced with buprenorphine programs in HIV-positive populations, and data support their effectiveness in this population (89) even though both methadone and buprenorphine have significant drug–drug interactions with HAART medications.

Methadone is primarily metabolized via cytochrome P450 3A4 and this cytochrome is also responsible for the metabolism of multiple HAART medications—most notably, the protease inhibitors. Consequently, drug–drug interactions and potential complications involving methadone/buprenorphine prescribed concurrently with HAART include changes in pharmacokinetics as well as other effects such as a prolonged QTc interval. Ritonavir produces strong 3A4 inhibition initially but has also been documented to induce 3A4 when administered chronically. Therefore, it is clear that drug–drug interactions are difficult to predict over time and require careful monitoring. For instance, initiation of a ritonavir or other protease-containing ART regimen in a patient on stable MMT may result in opiate toxicity and overdose due to early cytochrome inhibition. Conversely, lopinavir is a potent inducer of methadone metabolism with one study finds that the combined effects of lopinavir/ritonavir administered to MMT patients include significant reductions in the methadone area under the concentration–time curve and reductions in the maximum serum concentration in the setting of increased methadone oral clearance (90). Consequently, the authors also noted increased rates of opiate withdrawal in this population, highlighting the need for careful monitoring of patients during either MMT initiation or HAART initiation. Buprenorphine is also metabolized by 3A4, and concurrent ritonavir acutely inhibits its metabolism producing higher levels as with methadone. However, conflicting data also demonstrate relative safety in using buprenorphine in the setting of protease inhibitors and nonnucleoside reverse transcriptase inhibitors (NNRTIs) as well (91).

SUMMARY

HIV-1 infection is a major health and social issue of our time, with drug abuse, unprotected sexual intercourse, and transfusion of contaminated products being well-determined risk factors. As the prevalence of HIV-1 infection continues to increase, advances in treatments permit the prognosis to improve. Neuropsychiatric complications are now accurately diagnosed more often and our understanding of their etiologies and effective treatment regimens continues to improve. Signs of neuropsychiatric disorders are now detected earlier, allowing prompt and aggressive management of these potentially devastating complications of the HIV-1 infection. The overall prognosis for these patients at the moment of seroconversion continues to improve, along with the quality of their lives. The contribution of neuropsychiatry is of great importance as we pay attention to the neurobehavioral aspects of HIV-1 disease in these individuals.

REFERENCES

1. UNAIDS. *Report on Global HIV/AIDS Epidemic: "the Bangkok Report."* Barcelona: XV International conference on AIDS; 2004.
2. Centers for Disease Control and Prevention. HIV/AIDS surveillance report. *MMWR Morb Mortal Wkly Rep.* 2002;14(2):1–48.
3. Buehler JW, Petersen, LR, Jaffe HW. Current trends in the epidemiology of HIV/AIDS. In: Volberding PA, Sande MA, eds. *The Medical Management of AIDS.* Philadelphia: WB Saunders; 1995:3–21.
4. Ostrow AG. Substance abuse and HIV infection. *Psychiatr Clin North Am.* 1994;17:69–89.
5. Rabkin JG, Ferrando S, Jocobsberg L, et al. Prevalence of axis I disorders in an AIDS cohort: a cross-sectional, controlled study. *Compr Psychiatry.* 1994;38:146–154.
6. Perretta P, Akiskal H, Nisita C, et al. The high prevalence of bipolar II and associated cyclothymic and hyperthymic temperments in HIV patients. *J Affect Disord.* 1998;50:215–224.
7. Bing EG, Burnam M, Longshore D, et al. Psychiatric disorders and drug use among human immunodeficiency virus infected adults in the United States. *Arch Gen Psychiatry.* 2001;58:721–728.
8. Lightfoot M, Rogers T, Goldstein R, et al. Predictors of substance use frequency and reductions in seriousness of use among persons living with HIV. *Drug Alcohol Depend.* 2005;77:129–138.

9. Morrison TC, DiClemente R, Wingood G, et al. Frequency of alcohol use and its association with STD/HIV-related risk practices, attitudes, and knowledge among an African-American community recruited sample. *Int J STD AIDS.* 1998;9:608–612.
10. Abbott PJ, Weller SB, Walker SR. Psychiatric disorders of opioid addicts entering treatment. *J Addict Dis.* 1994;13:1–11.
11. Braine N, Des Jarlais D, Goldblatt C, et al. HIV risk behavior among amphetamine injectors at US syringe exchange program. *AIDS Educ Prev.* 2005;17:515–524.
12. Stein MD, Solomon D, Herman D, et al. Depression severity and drug injection HIV risk behaviors. *Am J Psychiatry.* 2003;160: 1659–1662.
13. Hutton HE, Lyketsos C, Zenilman J, et al. Depression and HIV risk behaviors among patients in a sexually transmitted disease clinic. *Am J Psychiatry.* 2004;161:912–914.
14. Valverde EE, Purcell D, Waldrop-Valverde D, et al. Correlates of depression among HIV positive women and men who inject drugs. *J Acquir Immune Defic Syndr.* 2007;46:S96–S100.
15. Shoptaw S, Peck J, Reback C, et al. Psychiatric and substance dependence comorbidities, sexually transmitted diseases, and risk behaviors among methamphetamine dependent gay and bisexual men seeking outpatient drug abuse treatment. *J Psychoactive Drugs.* 2003;35:S161–S168.
16. Mimiaga MJ, Fair A, Mayer K, et al. Experiences and sexual behaviors of HIV infected MSM who acquired HIV in the context of crystal methamphetamine use. *AIDS Educ Prev.* 2008;20:30–41.
17. Meade CS, Graff F, Griffin M, et al. HIV risk behavior among patietns with co-occuring bipolar and substance use disorders: associations with mania and drug abuse. *Drug Alcohol Depend.* 2008;92:296–300.
18. Cournos F, McKinnon K, Sullivan G. Schizophrenia and comorbid human immunodeficiency virus or hepatitis C virus. *J Clin Psychiatry.* 2005;66:S27–S33.
19. Himelhoch S, McCarthy J, Ganoczy D, et al. Understanding associations between serious mental illness and HIV among patients in the VA Health System. *Psychiatr Serv.* 2007;58: 1165–1172.
20. Rabkin JG, Ferrando S, van Gorp W, et al. Relationships among apathy, depression, and cognitive impairment in HIV/AIDS. *J Neuropsychiatry Clin Neurosci.* 2000;12:451–457.
21. Morrison MF, Petitto J, Ten-Have T, et al. Depressive and anxiety disorders in women with HIV infection. *Am J Psychiatry.* 2002; 159:789–796.
22. Wisniewski AB, Apel S, Selnes O, et al. Depressive symptoms, quality of life, and neuropsychological performance in HIV/AIDS: the impact of gender and injection drug use. *J Neurovirol.* 2005;11:138–143.
23. Arreola S, Neilands T, Pollack L, et al. Childhood sexual experiences and adult health sequelae among gay and bisexual men: defining childhood sexual abuse. *J Sex Res.* 2008;45:246–252.
24. Kalichman SC, Gore-Felton C, Benotsch E, et al. Trauma symptoms, sexual behaviors, and substance abuse: correlates of childhood sexual abuse and HIV risks among men who have sex with men. *J Child Sex Abus.* 2004;13:1–15.
25. Hutton HE, Treisman G, Hunt W, et al. HIV risk behaviors and their relationship to posttraumatic stress disorder among women prisoners. *Psychiatr Serv.* 2001;52:508–513.
26. Williams CT, Latkin CA. The role of depressive symptoms in predicting sex with multiple and high risk partners. *J Acquir Immune Defic Syndr.* 2005;38:69–73.
27. Matos TD, Robles R, Sahai H, et al. HIV risk behaviors and alcohol intoxication among injection drug users in Puerto Rico. *Drug Alcohol Depend.* 2004;76:229–234.
28. Quach LA, Wanke C, Schmid C, et al. Drug use and other risk factors related to lower body mass index among HIV-infected individuals. *Drug Alcohol Depend.* 2008;95:30–36.
29. Colfax G, Coates T, Husnik M, et al. The EXPLORE Study Team: Longitudendal patterns of methamphetamine, popper (amyl nitrite), and cocaine use and high-risk sexual behavior among a cohort of San Francisco men who have sex with men. *J Urban Health.* 2005;82:S62–S70.
30. Tucker JS, Burnam M, Sherbourne C, et al. Substance use and mental health correlates of nonadherence to antiretroviral medications in a sample of patients with human immunodeficiency virus infection. *Am J Med.* 2003;114:573–580.
31. Berger-Greenstein JA, Cuevas C, Brady S, et al. Major depression in patients with HIV/AIDS and substance abuse. *AIDS Patient Care STDS.* 2007;21:942–955.
32. Bouhnik AD, Preau M, Vincent E, et al. MANIF 2000 Study Group: Depression and clinical progression in HIV infected drug users treated with highly active antiretroviral therapy. *Antivir Ther.* 2005;10:53–61.
33. Goforth HW, Lowery J, Cutson T, et al. Impact of bereavement on progression of AIDS and HIV infection: a review. *Psychosomatics.* 2009;50:433–439.
34. Sambamoorthi U, Walkup J, Olfson M, et al. Antidepressant treatment and health services utilization among HIV infected Medicaid patients diagnosed with depression. *J Gen Intern Med.* 2000;15:311–320.
35. Sharma D, Bhattacharya J. Cellular and molecular basis of HIV-associated neuropathogenesis. *Indian J Med Res.* 2009;129:637–651.
36. Kenedi CA, Joynt KE, Goforth HW. Comorbid HIV encephalopathy and cocaine use as a risk factor for new-onset seizure disorders. *CNS Spectr.* 2008;13:230–234.
37. Sharer LR. Pathology of HIV1 infection of the central nervous system. A review. *J Neuropathol Exp Neurol.* 1992;51:3–11.
38. Smith TW, DeGirolami U, Henin D. Human Immunodeficiency virus leukoencephalopathy and the microcirculation. *J Neuropathol Exp Neurol.* 1990;49:357–370.
39. Cornblath DR, McArthur J. Predominantly sensory neuropathy in patients with AIDS and AIDS-related complex. *Neurology.* 1988;38:794–796.
40. Miller RG. Neuropathies and myopathies complicating HIV infection. *J Clin Apheresis.* 1991;6:110–121.
41. Malouf R, Jacquette G, Dobkin J. Neurologic disease in human immunodeficiency virus-infected drug abusers. *Arch Neurol.* 1990;47:1002–1007.
42. Cunha BA. Central nervous system infections in the compromised host: a diagnostic approach. *Infect Dis Clin North Am.* 2001;15:567–590.
43. Pruitt AA. Nervous system infections in patients with cancer. *Neurol Clin.* 2003;21:193–219.
44. Furrer H, Fux C. Opportunistic infections: an update. *J HIV Ther.* 2002;7:2–7.
45. Khanna N, Elzi L, Mueller N, et al. Incidence and outcome of progressive multifocal leukoencephalopathy over 20 years of the Swiss HIV cohort study. *Clini Infect Dis.* 2009;48:1459–1466.
46. Kaplan LD, Northfelt DW. Malignancies associated with AIDS. In: Sande MA, Volberding PA, eds. *The Medical Management of AIDS.* Philadelpia: WB Saunders; 1995:555–590.
47. Ellis RJ, Calero P, Stockin M. HIV infection and the central nervous system: a primer. *Neuropsychol Rev.* 2009;19:144–151.
48. Woods SP, Moore D, Weber E, et al. Cognitive neuropsychology of HIV-associated neurocognitive disorders. *Neuropsychol Rev.* 2009;19:152–168.

49. Lambotte O, Deiva K, Tardieu M. HIV-1 persistence, viral reservoir, and the central nervous sytem in the HAART era. *Brain Pathol.* 2003;13:95–103.
50. Brew BJ, Letendre S. Biomarkers of HIV related central nervous system disease. *Int Rev Psychiatry.* 2008;20:73–88.
51. Bakshi R. Neuroimaging of HIV and AIDS related illnesses: a review. *Front Biosci.* 2004;9:632–646.
52. Chang L, Ernst T, Leonido-Yee M, et al. Cerebral metabolic abnormalities correlate with clinical severity of HIV-1 cognitive motor complex. *Neurology.* 1999;52:100–108.
53. Harrison MJ, Newman S, Hall-Craggs M, et al. Evidence of CNS impairment in HIV infection: clinical, neuropsychological, EEG, and MRI/MRS study. *J Neurol Neurosurg Psychiatry.* 1998;65: 301–307.
54. Owe-Larsson B, Saell L, Salamon E, et al. HIV infection and psychiatric illness. *Afr J Psychiatry.* 2009;12:115–128.
55. Fernando SJ, Freyburg Z. Neuropsychiatric aspects of infectious disease. *Crit Care Clin.* 2008;24:889–919.
56. Morandi A, Jackson J, Ely E. Delirium in the intensive care unit. *Int Rev Psychiatry.* 2009;21:43–58.
57. Fernandez F, Holmes VF, Levy JK. Consultation liaison psychiatry and HIV-related disorders. *Hosp Commun Psychiatry.* 1989; 40:146–153.
58. Brogan K, Lux J. Management of common psychiatric conditions in the HIV-positive population. *Curr HIV/AIDS Rep.* 2009;6:108–115.
59. Breitbart W, Marotta R, Platt M, et al. A double-blind trial of haloperidol, chlorpromazine, and lorazepam in the treatment of delirium in hospitalized AIDS patients. *Am J Psychiatry.* 1996; 153:231–237.
60. McGee B, Smith N, Aweeka F. HIV pharmacology: barriers to the eradication of HIV from the CNS. *HIV Clin Trials.* 2006; 7:142–153.
61. Cysique LA, Brew BJ. Neuropsychological function and antiretroviral treatment in HIV/AIDS: a review. *Neuropsychol Rev.* 2009;19:169–185.
62. Letendre S, Marquie-Beck J, Capparelli E, et al. Validation of the CNS penetration effectiveness rank for quantifying antiretroviral penetration into the central nervous system. *Arch Neurol.* 2008;65:65–70.
63. Fernandez F, Levy J, Galizzi H. Response of HIV-related depression to psychostimulants: case reports. *Hosp Commun Psychiatry.* 1988;39:628–631.
64. Fernandez F, Levy JK, Sampley HR. Effects of methylphenidate in HIV-related depression: a comparative trial with desipramine. *Int J Psychiatry Med.* 1995;25:53–67.
65. Komiti A, Judd F, Grech P, et al. Suicidal behaviour in people with HIV/AIDS: a review. *Aust N Z J Psychiatry.* 2001;35: 747–757.
66. Fernandez F, Levy JK. Psychopharmacology in HIV spectrum disorders. *Psychiatr Clin North Am.* 1994;17:135–148.
67. Omonuwa TS, Goforth HW, Preud'homme X, et al. The pharmacologic management of insomnia in patients with HIV. *J Clin Sleep Med.* 2009;5:251–262.
68. Fernandez F. Ten myths about HIV infection and AIDS. *Focus.* 2005;3:184–193.
69. Bradley M, Muskin P. 5-step workup of HIV patients. *Current Psychiatry.* 2007;6(12):11–17.
70. Lowenhaupt E, Matson K, Qureishi B, et al. Psychosis in a 12-year-old HIV positive girl with an increased serum concentration of efavirenz. *Clin Infect Dis.* 2007;45:e128–e130.
71. Lyketsos CG, Schwartz J, Fishman M, et al. AIDS mania. *J Neuropsychiatry Clin Neurosci.* 1997;9:277–279.
72. Goodkin K. Psychiatric aspects of HIV spectrum disease. *Focus.* 2009;7:303–310.
73. Parsa MA, Bijan B. Quetiapine (Seroquel) in the treatment of psychosis in patients with Parkinson's disease. *J Neuropsychiatry Clin Neurosci.* 1998;10:216–219.
74. Singh AN, Golledge H, Catalan J. Treatment of HIV related psychotic disorders with risperidone: a case series of 21 cases. *J Psychosom Res.* 1997;42:489–493.
75. Kelly DV, Beique LC, Bowmer MI. Extrapyramidal symptoms with ritonavir/indinavir plus risperidone. *Ann Pharmacother.* 2002;36:827–830.
76. Fernandez F. Psychopharmacological interventions in HIV infections. *New Dir Ment Health Serv.* 1990;48:43–53.
77. Jover F, Cuadrado J, Andreu L, et al. Reversible coma caused by risperidone-ritonavir interaction. *Clin Neuropharmacol.* 2002;25: 251–253.
78. Dolder C, Nelson M, Deyo Z. Paliperidone for schizophrenia. *Am J Health-System Pharm.* 2008;65:403–413.
79. Fernandez F. Anxiety and neuropsychiatry of AIDS. *J Clin Psychiatry.* 1989;50:S9–S14.
80. Breitbart W, McDonald M, Rosenfeld B, et al. Pain in ambulatory AIDS patients. I: Pain characteristics and medical correlates. *Pain.* 1996;68:315–321.
81. Saarto T, Wiffen P. Antidepressants for neuropathic pain. *Cochrane Database Syst Rev.* 2007;17:CD005454.
82. Verma S, Estanislao L, Mintz L, et al. Controlling neuropathic pain in HIV. *Curr HIV/AIDS Rep.* 2004;1:136–141.
83. Daniell HW. Hypogonadism in men consuming sustained-action oral opioids. *J Pain.* 2002;3:377–384.
84. Andersen M, Tinsley J, Milfort D, et al. HIV health care access issues for women living with HIV, mental illness, and substance abuse. *AIDS Patient Care STDS.* 2005;19:449–459.
85. Gottheil E, Lundy A, Weinstein S, et al. Does intensive outpatient cocaine treatment reduce AIDS risky behaviors? *J Addict Dis.* 1998;17:61–69.
86. Werb D, Kerr T, Marsh D, et al. Effect of methadone treatment on incarceration rates among injection drug users. *Eur Addict Res.* 2008;14:143–149.
87. Maremmani I, Pani P, Mellini A, et al. Alcohol and cocaine use and abuse among opioid addicts engaged in a methadone maintenance treatment program. *J Addict Dis.* 2007;26:61–70.
88. Kapadia F, Vlahov D, Wu Y, et al. Impact of drug abuse treatment modalities on adherence to ART/HAART among a cohort of HIV seropositive women. *Am J Drug Alcohol Abuse.* 2008;34:161–167.
89. Carrieri MP, Amass L, Lucas G, et al. Buprenorphine use: the international experience. *Clin Infect Dis.* 2006;43:S197–S215.
90. McCance-Katz EF, Rainey P, Friedland G, et al. The protease inhibitor lopinavir-ritonavir may produce opiate withdrawal in methadone-maintained patients. *Clin Infect Dis.* 2003;37:476–482.
91. McCance-Katz EF, Moody D, Smith P, et al. Interactions between buprenorphine and antiretrovirals. II. The protease inhibitors nelfinavir, lopinavir/ritonavir, and ritonavir. *Clin Infect Dis.* 2006;43:S235–S246.

CHAPTER 51 Acute and Chronic Pain

Russell K. Portenoy

When acute, tolerable and appropriate to injury, pain is biologically essential, signaling the need to identify the source of injury, seek help, and rest while healing occurs. When the severity of acute pain is high enough to initiate maladaptive stress responses, however, or its signaling imperatives have passed, treatment to relieve the pain or mitigate its effects is necessary to promote healing, well-being, and functional restoration.

When pain persists, it is never biologically adaptive. Indeed, chronic pain should be recognized as a heterogeneous and complex entity that should be considered a potentially serious illness in its own right (1). Chronic pain is associated with mood disturbance, sleep disorder, loss of function and impaired quality of life, and caregiver burden. It also is a public health problem of immense magnitude. In the United States, a recent evaluation by an expert committee noted that the estimated prevalence of chronic pain—at least 30% of adults and 20% of children in the United States—creates a societal burden that is greater than that of diabetes, heart disease and cancer combined, including direct costs of at least $100 billion per year attributed to pain-related health care utilization and lost productivity (1).

The assessment and management of acute and chronic pain are within the purview of all clinicians. The ability to apply basic principles of pain management, and to refer appropriately, should represent skills that are broadly acquired and kept up to date. Pain medicine also is a subspecialty, and although the numbers of specialists are relatively small—just a few thousand in the United States—patients with complex chronic pain problems should ideally have access to professionals with specialist competencies, if needed.

There is a complex relationship between pain management and the clinical issues surrounding the problems of drug abuse, addiction, and diversion. The key role played by opioid drugs, which are both essential medical treatments and a major source of abuse, has justified exploration of this relationship. The interface between pain and drug abuse is broad in scope, potentially including issues that extend from basic science to public policy. For clinicians, the focus is on the role of potentially abusable drugs, especially the opioids, and on the challenges in providing effective pain management to patient populations with the comorbidity of a substance use disorder.

Historically, there has been an unfortunate lack of communication between specialists in pain management and specialists in addiction medicine. In recent years, this has been recognized as a problem in need of redress and a new level of discourse has begun. This discourse broadly promotes *balance* for both the clinical and public health perspectives. A balanced approach to the clinical use of abusable substances applies to all the relevant communities—health professionals, regulators, law enforcers, policymakers, and the public. It acknowledges that all patients must have access to prescription drugs to treat legitimate medical needs, and strongly affirms that those who are charged with protecting the public health through regulation or law enforcement must pursue their agendas in a way that does not obstruct appropriate medical care. It also emphasizes, however, that there is a clear obligation on the part of both health professionals and patients to understand the need to assess, minimize, and manage all known risks, including the potential for abuse, addiction, and diversion.

The goals of this chapter are (a) to provide an overview of the principles of pain assessment and pain management, with a focus on opioid pharmacotherapy and (b) to explore some of the specific issues that arise when treating patients for pain in the context of a substance use disorder.

PRINCIPLES OF PAIN ASSESSMENT

Assessment is the essential prerequisite to the safe and effective treatment of acute or chronic pain. Although it is often straightforward in the setting of an acute traumatic event, a comprehensive assessment should be entertained even in this setting to ensure that the plan of care is safe, likely to provide benefit, and capable of addressing the impact of the pain and comorbid conditions. When pain becomes chronic and the plan of care anticipates a longer, and perhaps indefinite, time frame, the need for a more detailed pain assessment is clear and all the elements of this assessment become more challenging.

The information obtained through pain assessment derives from an appropriate history, physical examination, review of records, and often confirmatory laboratory and radiographic procedures. The most important part of the history is to provide sufficient information to characterize the pain complaint and determine the impact of the pain on multiple functional domains (Table 51.1).

The rest of the history also is important, particularly exploration of medical and psychiatric pathology. The chronic pain patient with a serious medical disorder may have pain attributable to the disease, related to its treatment, or unrelated to either. The patient should be asked about the severity and extent of

TABLE 51.1	Key pain-related information obtained in a routine pain assessment
■ *Nature of the pain complaint, including*
■ Temporal features, including onset (abrupt or gradual), course (improving, progressing, stable), and daily pattern (diurnal variation, episodes of severe pain)
■ Location, including primary site or sites, referral, and whether it is deep or superficial
■ Severity, usually queried in terms of a score on a "0" to "10" numeric scale for pain "on average" and pain "at its worst"
■ Quality, often prompted by cues such as "aching," "burning," or "throbbing"; and factors that provoke or relieve the pain
■ *Prior and current evaluation of the pain, including*
■ Where it has been treated and by whom;
■ What laboratory, radiographic, or electrodiagnostic studies have been carried out; and whether prior records are available
■ *Prior and current treatments for the pain and their outcomes*
■ *Current impact of the pain, including effects on*
■ Physical function, such as the ability to perform activities of daily living and instrumental activities of daily living (e.g., shopping, cleaning), engage in exercise or other physical activities, enjoy restorative sleep
■ Psychological function, such as the effect on mood, coping, and adaptation
■ Social and familial functioning, including the impact on relationships with significant others (including marital and family relationships, and, if appropriate, sexual functioning) and other social interactions
■ Financial status and health system aspects, including financial resources, need for disability payments, and medical insurance status

disease, past and current treatments, and the goals of care going forward. Comorbid medical problems also must be recorded.

All chronic pain patients should be queried about other symptoms, including chronic fatigue, insomnia, and appetite changes. Psychological symptoms, such as anxiety or depressed mood, also should be ascertained.

Past and present psychiatric history is extremely relevant and requires focused questioning. Questions should explore the lifetime history of anxiety or depressive disorders, and a question about the occurrence of preadolescent abuse should be considered, particularly in the case of chronic pain associated with disability and other psychological or psychiatric concerns.

The comorbidity of substance use should be explored in all patients with chronic pain, including those with medical illness. Specific questions about the current and earlier use of tobacco and alcohol, illicit drugs, and the nonmedical use of prescription drugs should be asked. If an opioid or another potentially abusable drug has been given for a medical purpose, it is appropriate to ask whether there have been any concerns, either on the part of the patient or family, or on the part of the prescriber, concerning the way in which these drugs have been used by the patient. If a history of substance abuse is elicited, the interview should clarify the specific behaviors, both at the present time and in the past, in an effort to clarify the diagnosis or determine the need for further evaluation or referral.

Information about medical disorders in the family typically is elicited as part of the routine history. With the chronic pain patient, however, this history should be expanded and include questions about chronic pain and psychiatric disorders, including problematic use of alcohol or drugs.

The physical examination of patients with pain attempts to characterize the factors that contribute to the pain diagnosis and ascertain the status of comorbidities. A review of the existing medical records, and often additional laboratory or imaging procedures, is necessary to confirm and expand the understanding.

Framework for Interpreting the Nature of the Pain

A useful framework that may assist in the interpretation of information obtained about the nature of the pain focuses on a set of key considerations. These include the distinction between acute and chronic pain and the utility of syndromic, etiologic, and pathophysiologic diagnosis.

Acute Pain versus Chronic Pain

Acute pain may be defined as pain that has been, or is anticipated to be, experienced for a relatively short period, typically no more than days to weeks. The most common types of acute pains are linked to recognizable tissue injury following trauma, including surgical trauma. Less common types are related to medical conditions or to primary pain diagnoses such as headache. Acute pains can be monophasic (e.g., following surgery) or recurrent. They may be recognized as a syndrome even in the absence of tissue injury (e.g., migraine), or be expected as part of an underlying pathology producing cumulative damage (e.g., sickle cell disease).

Chronic pain (also called persistent pain) may be defined by a temporal criterion alone, which is conventionally either 3 months or 6 months. Alternatively, chronic pain may be defined using other clinical criteria, specifically: *pain that persists beyond the healing of the inciting lesion, occurs in the context of a lesion that is not likely to heal, or is transitory but frequently recurrent.*

The phenomenology of acute and chronic pain differs in many ways beyond duration. Acute pain usually is caused by an event or disorder with a known anticipated time course. It is usually well localized and has a familiar aching, throbbing, or stabbing quality. These qualities are not absolute, however, and pain related to some visceral processes (e.g., bowel obstruction) and some neuropathic processes (e.g., painful polyneuropathy) typically have other characteristics (see Etiology and Pathophysiology). Irrespective of the underlying cause, acute pain may be associated with sympathetic responses, such as tachycardia, hypertension, tachypnea, and sweating, and the emotional response of anxiety. These emotional and autonomic concomitants of acute pain may be absent, however, especially if the pain is expected or the intensity is not intense.

In contrast to acute pain, chronic pain usually is less well localized, has both intensity and qualities that vary, and typically is not associated with any type of sympathetic response. If a mood change occurs, it typically is in the spectrum of depression.

Acute pain related to some type of tissue injury or damage usually is perceived to be reflective of a "normal" response to a noxious stimulus, a response that is the human output of the neural process of "nociception" investigated in the laboratory. From this perspective, pain is a perception of the sensation of a noxious stimulus, which itself is subserved by the biologic processes of nociception; as a perception, pain is always subject to influence by both thoughts and emotions linked to past experience and current psychosocial status.

Chronic pain is not biologically adaptive and presumably requires some type of pathologic change in nociception. It is assumed that chronic pain, like other illnesses, always is subject to powerful influence by cognitive and psychological processes that can either promote pain relief, coping, and function or contribute to distress and impairment.

The experience of chronic pain does not eliminate the risk of concurrent acute pain. Indeed, episodes of acute severe pain are common among those with persistent pain. When this occurs in the context of long-term opioid treatment, the term *breakthrough pain* is applied. Breakthrough pain occurs in populations with cancer and noncancer pains; its prevalence among opioid-treated chronic pain patients in community settings is at least one third (2,3). The association of breakthrough pain with adverse physical and psychosocial outcomes, and the recent advent of opioid drugs specifically indicated for cancer-related breakthrough, justifies the effort to separately assess these episodes and consider treatment that targets them specifically.

Etiology and Pathophysiology

One of the goals of the pain assessment is to identify the etiology of the pain—the lesion or the disorder that is responsible for activating or sustaining nociception. In many situations, such as acute postoperative pain, the etiology is obvious. In some chronic pain disorders, such as pain related to osteoarthritis or osteoporosis, the etiology also seems clear in relation to a specific site of chronic tissue injury. Etiology is uncertain in many other disorders, such as chronic headache, fibromyalgia, chronic back pain, and many types of neuropathic pain.

The potential value in an etiologic diagnosis lies in the ability to offer disease-modifying therapy to some patients. If an etiology can be identified and is treatable, and treatment has both a favorable therapeutic index and consistency with the goals of care, primary disease-modifying therapy should be entertained as a part of a pain management strategy. For example, joint replacement therapy, if feasible and appropriate, is a highly effective intervention for chronic pain related to advanced osteoarthritis. An etiologic diagnosis also may allow primary therapy for other aims (e.g., prevention of a complication, such as pathologic fracture) and may help clarify prognosis in some cases.

The term *pathophysiology* refers to the mechanisms that sustain the pain. These mechanisms cannot be determined in humans with clinical pain, and the information provided by the pain assessment can only be used to infer the existence of a category of mechanisms. Although this is undoubtedly a gross simplification of extremely complex processes underlying pain perception, labeling by inferred pathophysiology has become clinically accepted for pain syndromes other than headache because it suggests assessment and treatment strategies that have proved clinically useful.

In general, most pain syndromes are believed to be sustained by tissue injury and/or changes in sensory processing. Pains other than common types of headache are described as *nociceptive*, *neuropathic*, or *mixed*. Occasionally, pain syndromes are believed to have a predominating psychological pathogenesis, and rarely, pain syndromes occur that are unclassifiable (best termed *idiopathic pain*).

Nociceptive pain, which is subdivided into *somatic* and *visceral* subtypes, is defined as pain that appears to be commensurate with the degree of ongoing activation of nerves by tissue injury and related processes. Nociceptive pain typically is inferred to exist when tissue damage is identified and appears to be a sufficient explanation for the pain. If the damage occurs in somatic structures, such as joint, muscle, or soft tissue, it results in somatic pain; if the damage occurs in viscera, it results in visceral pain. Pains classified as nociceptive are believed to be responsive to peripherally directed interventions that reduce the source of injury.

In terms of phenomenology, somatic pain usually has a familiar quality, such as aching or throbbing. It is well-localized, worsened with movement, and may be associated with signs of inflammation. Visceral pain varies with the organ involved. When due to obstruction of hollow viscus, the pain usually is poorly localized, referred to specific cutaneous sites, gnawing or aching in quality, and often associated with nausea. Visceral pain related to involvement of connective tissue, such as the liver capsule or muscle, is more well localized and typically sharp and aching in quality.

Neuropathic pain may be defined as pain related to disease or dysfunction of the nervous system, or as pain that is inferred to be sustained by aberrant sensory processes induced in either the peripheral nervous system, the central nervous system, or both. There are important subtypes, including pain related to compression or entrapment of nerve (e.g., median neuropathy from carpal tunnel syndrome or radiculopathy from a herniated nucleus pulposis), pain related to neuroma formation after transaction of a peripheral nerve (e.g., stump pain), pain related to toxic or metabolic injury to all nerves (e.g., painful peripheral neuropathy), and pain related to central nervous system processes (such as pain due to spinal cord injury or poststroke central pain). The diagnosis may be suggested by the associated neurologic disorder, the phenomenology of the pain itself, or associated features that define a discrete syndrome.

The phenomenology of neuropathic pain is heterogeneous. Some patients describe the pain as a familiar aching, but others describe dysesthesias (abnormal uncomfortable sensations, which are perceived as unfamiliar), which may include pain descriptors such as burning, tingling, squeezing, or electrical. There may or may not be specific abnormalities on examination, such as allodynia (pain with light touch), hyperalgesia (relatively increased pain to a noxious stimulus), and hyperpathia (exaggerated pain response, often with spread, after-sensation, and emotional overreaction). Patients with neuropathic pain also may have coexisting sources of nociceptive pain, the phenomenology of which may further complicate the patient's description of the pain.

The diagnosis of neuropathic pain may suggest the use of selected types of analgesics, including numerous drugs used primarily as antidepressants or anticonvulsants (4). Numerous studies also have established that opioids are efficacious (4), and for this reason, inferences about pain pathophysiology (nociceptive vs. neuropathic) should not be the deciding factor whether or not to try an opioid for chronic pain.

Pain Syndromes

Syndrome identification is extremely useful in pain assessment because it may provide information about underlying organic processes, suggest an efficient evaluation, guide the selection of treatments, and indicate prognosis. The International Association for the Study of Pain has developed a taxonomy of pain, the goal of which is to establish criteria for the diagnosis of specific pain syndromes (5).

Although the term *chronic pain syndrome* does not appear in a taxonomy of pain, the literature may apply it to patients with chronic pain associated with a high level of disability and psychiatric comorbidity. These associated manifestations have long suggested the potential value of a multidisciplinary approach to management that emphasizes both comfort and functional restoration. Indeed, the clinical challenge posed by the management of the patient with pain and disability was a prime driver of the development of pain medicine as a subspecialty. Although most patients with acute pain and, presumably, most with chronic pain do not have the type of overriding disability that is implied by the label, it is important to acknowledge the needs of this subgroup. Whereas most patients with pain can be managed adequately by a single clinician who expertly administers one or more treatments, patients with a complex chronic pain illness may benefit most from the involvement of specialists in various disciplines, who together implement a multimodality approach intended to address pain and its consequences, and comorbid conditions. A specialist in addiction medicine may be an appropriate member of a multidisciplinary pain management team.

PAIN AND SUBSTANCE ABUSE

The clinical interface between pain and substance abuse can be best illuminated by a focus on the use of potentially abusable drugs used in the management of acute and chronic pain. The most important of these drugs are the opioids. Opioid therapy is the mainstay approach for the treatment of severe acute pain and chronic pain related to active cancer or another advanced medical illness. Although yet controversial, opioid therapy for the treatment of chronic noncancer pain is well established in some countries and rapidly growing in the United States and others. The safe and effective use of opioid drugs requires competencies in pain assessment and management in all patient populations, and these skills must be most highly refined when these drugs are used to manage pain in populations with substance abuse histories.

Terminology and Characteristics of Relevant Phenomena

Many of the terms used to describe opioid-related phenomena, such as tolerance, are difficult to translate to the clinical setting. An understanding of terminology is a foundation to the development of clinical strategies that promote safe and appropriate prescribing. The effort to bring together the perspectives of specialists in pain management and addiction medicine to refine the meanings of key terms has been a notable advance (6).

Tolerance

Tolerance is a pharmacologic property of opioid drugs defined by the need for increasing doses to maintain effects (7). Tolerance can be induced reliably in animal models with little exposure to a drug and occurs to different opioid effects at varied rates and extents. Although there are subtypes based on the impact of learning and pharmacokinetic changes, it is the occurrence of the so-called analgesic pharmacodynamic tolerance—loss of analgesic effects associated with biologic processes induced in cells by the binding of the drug to its receptors—that characterizes opioid tolerance and raises clinical concerns.

If pharmacodynamic tolerance to analgesic effects were to occur regularly, it would be a major impediment to the clinical effectiveness. Alternatively, if the development of tolerance to the positive psychic effects of opioids, and the consequent need to increase doses to regain these effects, routinely drove aberrant use, this too would compromise the long-term utility of these drugs. The latter process has been perceived as a key step in the pathogenesis of addiction (8).

There is no question that tolerance can occur to diverse opioid effects, including analgesia, and that tolerance can be induced with little drug exposure. Clinical observation suggests that tolerance to some effects, such as somnolence and nausea, develops quickly. This is widely perceived to be a clinically favorable outcome, increasing the safety of the drugs and allowing the dose escalation necessary to attain analgesia. In contrast, tolerance to analgesic effects seems to be an uncommon driver of dose escalation to maintain analgesia. Although some patients with pain do report diminishing analgesic effects in the absence of any other reason for changes in pain—the scenario that suggests the occurrence of analgesic tolerance—most patients demonstrate relatively stable dose requirements for prolonged periods. In the cancer population, for example, the need for dose escalation typically occurs only in the setting of a progressive lesion; for example, patients who self-administer morphine for several weeks to control pain from chemotherapy-induced mucositis do not increase the dose after an initial rapid titration (9). Surveys of patients with nonmalignant pain treated with systemic or neuraxial opioids for prolonged periods also demonstrate variable dose requirements over time, with stability in most patients who have no obvious disease progression (10). These observations suggest that analgesic pharmacodynamic tolerance is a pharmacologic phenomenon that can be reliably demonstrated in animal models, presumably occurs to some degree during opioid administration for pain, but has a variable presentation and relatively little impact in the routine management of most patients receiving long-term opioid therapy (7).

The importance of tolerance in the context of abuse and addiction also is uncertain. Although traditionally included in the definition of addiction (11), a newer conceptualization no longer makes reference to it (6). The phenomenon of tolerance may be important for some patients in the development of an addictive pattern of drug use, but overall it appears to be neither necessary nor sufficient for the appearance of addiction.

Physical Dependence

Like tolerance, *physical dependence* is a pharmacologic property of opioid drugs. It is defined solely by the occurrence of an abstinence syndrome (withdrawal) following abrupt dose reduction or administration of an antagonist. Because some degree of physical dependence can be produced with very little opioid exposure, and neither the dose nor duration of administration required to produce clinically significant physical dependence in humans is known, most practitioners assume that the potential for an abstinence syndrome exists after an opioid has been administered repeatedly for only a few days.

Physical dependence has been perceived as an impediment to the discontinuation of an ineffective or problematic therapy, suggesting to some clinicians that the decision to try an opioid for more than a short time means that therapy will be difficult or impossible to stop. The belief that a trial of long-term opioid therapy is something of a "life sentence" presumably leads some clinicians to consider an opioid trial as a last resort.

Physical dependence also has been considered another key element in the pathogenesis of addiction (8). In this view, the need to reduce the adverse effects of withdrawal drives drug-seeking behavior. Like tolerance, physical dependence traditionally has been included in the definition of addiction (11).

Paradoxically, extensive clinical experience suggests that physical dependence actually is a rare concern in practice. Abstinence phenomena seldom present significant challenges to the safe discontinuation of an ineffective or problematic therapy, as long as dose reduction and concurrent therapies are well managed. This has been amply demonstrated by the success of opioid detoxification by multidisciplinary pain programs and the routine cessation of opioid therapy in cancer patients who become fully analgesic following a pain-relieving procedure.

Similarly, physical dependence may or may not be apparent among those who abuse opioid drugs. As a result, it is best to define addiction in a way that fully distinguishes it from physical dependence (6). In short, physical dependence presumably occurs in all opioid-treated patients after a short time, but very few become addicted, and the occurrence of physical dependence, as determined by abstinence phenomena, may or may not be prominent among those who become addicted. Just like tolerance, the capacity to experience uncomfortable withdrawal may be a factor in the development of an addictive pattern of drug use in some cases, but it appears to be neither necessary nor sufficient for the development of the disease of addiction.

Use of the term *addiction* as a synonym for physical dependence appears to be entrenched in the U.S. medical culture. This unfortunate practice reinforces the stigma associated with opioid therapy and should be rejected. The term addiction should only be applied to a specific syndrome characterized by a highly maladaptive pattern of drug use. If the clinician wishes to characterize the potential for withdrawal, the term *physical dependence* must be used. Labeling the patient as *dependent* also should be discouraged, because its imprecision fosters confusion between physical dependence and addiction. For the same reason, use of the term habituation should be eschewed; in the clinical setting, this term is often used indiscriminately to refer to tolerance, physical dependence, or the development of craving.

Addiction

The development of a definition for addiction jointly endorsed by professional societies for pain and addiction in the United States represents an important piece of the effort to improve communication across disciplines (6). According to the statement endorsed by the American Pain Society (APS),

American Academy of Pain Medicine (AAPM), and American Society of Addiction Medicine:

> [a]ddiction is a primary, chronic, neurobiologic disease, with genetic, psychosocial, and environmental factors influencing its development and manifestations. It is characterized by behaviors that include one or more of the following: impaired control over drug use, compulsive use, continued use despite harm, and craving.

This definition reinforces the conclusion that a diagnosis of addiction requires an assessment of drug-related behaviors to establish the existence of a seriously maladaptive pattern of drug use. Craving may involve rumination about the drug and an intense desire to secure its supply. Compulsive use may be indicated by escalating consumption of the drug without medical justification or sanction by a clinician. Continued use despite harm could involve outcomes that are problematic for physical or psychosocial well-being, work or other role functioning, or relationships with health professionals. Although an addictive pattern of opioid use may involve phenomena recognized as likely tolerance or physical dependence, neither of these biologic processes is necessary for a diagnosis.

Abuse, Misuse, and Other Terms

Other terms commonly used in the setting of opioid treatment also have challenged precise definition. *Drug abuse* may be considered any type of drug use that is outside accepted societal and cultural norms. This definition is practical, but nonetheless implies that there is broad consensus about the nature of normative behavior. This is not always true, particularly during periods of changing perceptions (e.g., with respect to marijuana use) or when clinicians and patients do not share cultural backgrounds. Nonetheless, it is generally accepted that drug abuse includes any use of an illicit drug and any use of a legal drug in a manner that is contrary to clinician instructions, or to regulations or laws. Importantly, patients with the disease of addiction may or may not be actively abusing drugs, and most drug abuse is undertaken by individuals who do not otherwise meet criteria for a diagnosis of addiction.

Drug diversion should be considered apart from abuse or addiction. Diversion or the transfer of a licit drug into an illegal marketplace is considered a criminal act and the individuals responsible may or may not be personally using the drug in question. Indeed, physicians in the United States who have been prosecuted for drug trafficking typically have not been accused of abusing the drugs they prescribed.

In the clinical setting, drug-related behaviors that are egregious enough to be labeled drug abuse may be positioned on a continuum of problematic *nonadherence behaviors*. Nonadherence behaviors, which also have been called *aberrant drug-related behaviors* and sometimes *red-flag behaviors*, are varied and may be difficult to interpret (Table 51.2). Although it is widely agreed that a very serious nonadherence behavior, such as forging prescriptions, represents both drug abuse and a probable sign of addiction, a less severe behavior, such as repeated requests for early prescription refills, is more challenging to characterize. Many clinicians use the term *misuse* as a way to distinguish these less egregious nonadherence behaviors.

To date, there has been no standardization of this language into a more precise diagnostic terminology that is broadly applicable across both non-medical and medical settings. The labeling of drug abuse and addiction (substance abuse disorder and substance dependence disorder in the psychiatric parlance adopted in the American Psychiatric Association's *Diagnostic and Statistical Manual of Mental Disorders* [DSM] (11)) clearly is simpler when drug use does not involve a drug that has been prescribed for a legitimate medical purpose.

Interpreting Nonadherence Behaviors in the Medical Context

All patients who are given an opioid or other controlled prescription drug for medical purposes must be routinely evaluated for drug-related behaviors throughout the course of treatment. In the ambulatory setting, nonadherence is particularly challenging. In some cases, it takes the form of undertreatment. This problem is seldom discussed but may be a significant issue, particularly when treating pain associated with a serious medical illness. The decision to take less medication than prescribed may be related to cost, fear of side effects or addiction, family concerns, or other factors. Education and support of the patient and family may require specific targeting of these concerns.

When nonadherence takes the form of excessive opioid use, the behaviors can be labeled as misuse or abuse, or perhaps addiction, depending on the nature of the problem. The type of assessment necessary to assess these drug-related behaviors is a core clinical competency for addiction specialists, essential for establishing a diagnosis and evaluating a treatment plan, but is relatively novel for pain specialists and other clinicians. This is an area of practice that must be improved. There is a broad consensus in the United States that clinicians who prescribe opioids or other controlled prescription drugs to manage medical disorders must possess basic skills in assessing drug-related behaviors in terms of the risks associated with abuse, addiction, and diversion. Those who do not, or who encounter patients who pose a high level of challenge in assuring adherence, should not prescribe without help.

The complexity inherent in evaluating nonadherence behaviors may be lessened by applying a "differential diagnosis." In some cases, the behaviors are sufficiently extreme (e.g., injection of an oral formulation) to immediately suggest the diagnosis of addiction (Table 51.2). In other cases, the behaviors are less egregious and could reflect other diagnoses, such as impulsive behavior driven by unrelieved pain (a phenomenon broadly labeled "*pseudoaddiction*"), a psychiatric disorder other than addiction, or a mild encephalopathy with confusion about drug intake. Occasionally, aberrant behaviors indicate criminal intent (i.e., intent to divert).

The phenomenon of *pseudoaddiction* illustrates the complexity of this differential diagnosis. Pseudoaddiction was originally described anecdotally in a cancer patient who demonstrated behaviors consistent with drug craving that

TABLE 51.2 Aberrant drug-related behaviors

Behaviors Probably More Suggestive of Addiction
- Selling prescription drugs
- Prescription forgery
- Stealing or "borrowing" drugs from others
- Injecting oral formulations
- Obtaining prescription drugs from nonmedical sources
- Concurrent abuse of alcohol or illicit drugs
- Multiple dose escalations or other noncompliance with therapy despite warnings
- Multiple episodes of prescription "loss"
- Repeatedly seeking prescriptions from other clinicians or from emergency rooms without informing prescriber or after warnings to desist
- Evidence of deterioration in the ability to function at work, in the family, or in society that appear to be related to drug use
- Repeated resistance to changes in therapy despite clear evidence of adverse physical or psychological effects from the drug

Behaviors Probably Less Suggestive of Addiction
- Aggressive complaining about the need for more drug
- Drug hoarding during periods of reduced symptoms
- Requesting specific drugs
- Openly acquiring similar drugs from other medical sources
- Unsanctioned dose escalation or other noncompliance with therapy on one or two occasions
- Unapproved use of the drug to treat another symptom
- Reporting psychic effects not intended by the clinician
- Mildly impaired cognition or subtle signs of impaired function

disappeared when the opioid regimen was increased (12). The term became accepted because of broad clinical experience affirming that aberrant behavior can be driven by desperation caused by uncontrolled pain. The degree of "aberrancy" is relevant, however, and it is essential to recognize that pseudoaddiction can coexist with other drivers of aberrant use, including addiction itself. Indeed, it is a common observation that the stress associated with pain may drive relapse among those with the known diagnosis of addiction. The diagnosis of pseudoaddiction should not be used to explain illicit acts or a clearly maladaptive pattern of compulsive drug use.

Given the differential diagnosis of aberrant drug-related behavior and the extraordinary heterogeneity of the population with painful disorders, the clinician who discerns an episode of nonadherence must determine if the problem is likely to be transitory—perhaps an impulsive action related to a pain flare, to worsening of a comorbid psychiatric disorder, or to some severe situational stressor—or is likely to be more serious and abiding. This may require more time and observation after additional structure has been introduced into the planned therapy (e.g., urine drug screening, frequent visits, or other strategies; see Structuring Therapy to Reduce Risk).

The diagnostic challenges are most significant in the ambulatory setting during long-term treatment of chronic pain, particularly when the severity of the nonadherence behavior is limited. For example, the patient with unrelieved pain who deliberately takes extra doses of an opioid and fails to contact the physician until an early refill is needed has engaged in aberrant drug-related behavior. The diagnosis is uncertain initially, and the future plan of care would clearly be different if the behavior reflected incipient addiction, pseudoaddiction, or, possibly, both phenomena. Interpretation of the behavior also may not be possible the first time that it occurs. A decision to continue the therapy usually would be justified and closer monitoring of drug-related behaviors would hopefully ensue. Other data, such as the results of urine drug screening, may be obtained and strongly influence the interpretation of the initial event and future behaviors. A diagnosis of the aberrant behavior should be withheld until observations are sufficient to provide a rationale.

The potential for mislabeling nonadherence behaviors as addiction is particularly great in the patient with a remote or current history of substance abuse. Although opioids may be clearly indicated, any evidence of aberrant drug-related behavior may generate great concern that relapse has occurred. This concern is well placed if the aberrant behaviors are egregious (e.g., prescription forgery), but the more common scenario involves less serious behaviors that are far more difficult to interpret. Pain complaints may be voluble and disproportionate to the degree of evident pathology. The patient may appear to require unusually high doses or may request specific drugs. Interactions with the medical staff may be perceived to have a manipulative quality in which the patient appears to be unusually knowledgeable about opioid treatment or presents a posture of negotiation about therapy. It is extremely important that the clinicians caring for these patients recognize that these behaviors may or may not reflect abuse or addiction. Pseudoaddiction may be common, set in motion by both a lack of trust that limits the aggressiveness with which pain is approached and the appropriate concerns raised by an analysis of risk and benefit during treatment with a potentially abusable drug. The challenge is to understand that risk management is part of the therapeutic plan of care; avoid assumptions while continuing to assess behaviors appropriately; and if worrisome drug-related behaviors occur, clarify the differential diagnosis in a manner that is justified by the data available. In the absence of data, both clinicians and patients are best served by clear documentation that information is not sufficient to interpret the behavior.

PRINCIPLES OF OPIOID THERAPY

The safe and effective prescribing of opioid drugs for acute or chronic pain requires skills in optimizing favorable pharmacologic outcomes (reducing pain and minimizing side effects) and reducing the risks associated with misuse, abuse, addiction, and diversion. These skills must be translated into a set of pragmatic decisions: Who should be selected for opioid therapy, how should the drug be selected and administered, and how should the treatment be structured to minimize the risks of abuse?

Selection of Patients for Opioid Therapy

There is a long-standing international consensus that opioid therapy is the mainstay treatment for patients with acute severe pain and patients with chronic pain related to active cancer or another type of advanced medical illness. Selection of an opioid to treat pain in these settings should be viewed as the "default" position; the decision to do otherwise should have a clear rationale.

In contrast to this view, there is no consensus about the role of opioid therapy to treat other types of chronic pain. The populations with chronic pain are very heterogeneous, represent many types of disorders and very diverse comorbidities, and largely encompass patients receiving care in community settings by clinicians who are not pain specialists. These populations include the increasing number of patients with pain caused by stable or indolent medical illness (including those who are cancer survivors with chronic pain) or a primary pain-related diagnosis (e.g., chronic headache and fibromyalgia).

The decision to select a patient with chronic noncancer pain cannot be based on the existing evidence of effectiveness. Although there have been many clinical trials of opioid therapy for noncancer pain, and these trials have been collated into systematic reviews (13), the existing evidence can provide little insight other than generally supporting the conclusion that opioids are efficacious for all types of pain and that some patients appear to benefit during long-term therapy (and a substantial minority stop treatment over time). There is no evidence of long-term effectiveness and no evaluation of comparative effectiveness, either comparing opioid regimens or comparing opioids with other treatment approaches for pain (14).

Given the lack of evidence, an expert panel charged to create evidence-based guidelines for opioid treatment by the APS and the AAPM were forced to rely mostly on expert opinion (15). Although most of the recommendations offered in this guideline were strong, they were almost all based on low-quality evidence.

The APS–AAPM panel endorsed the view that a trial of opioid therapy with the intent to continue it long-term if beneficial can be considered for any patient with chronic noncancer pain but the decision to offer this therapy requires a detailed assessment designed to determine whether the benefits would be likely to outweigh the risks. It is reasonable to consider four questions in reaching this conclusion:

- *What is conventional practice for this type of patient and this type of pain?*
- *Are there other therapies that have equivalent or better therapeutic indices and might be considered instead?*
- *Are there relatively high risks of adverse pharmacologic effects as a result of medical comorbidities or concurrent treatments?*
- *Is the patient likely to be a responsible drug user, or is the risk of problematic drug-related behavior high?*

The answers to these questions do not exclude any patient from treatment but should help position the treatment against other options and, equally important, help the clinician decide whether treatment might be undertaken only with the help of a consultant or perhaps only through referral to a clinician with more experience or more resources.

Importantly, the initiation of an opioid therapy with the intention to continue it indefinitely if the outcomes be favorable should be conceptualized as a *trial*, even if it is taking place after the patient has been receiving an opioid for some time but without commitment to long-term therapy. Patients should understand that this therapeutic trial will attempt to optimize outcomes and monitor the effectiveness of treatment and drug-related behavior. Like all trials, the outcomes may support the conclusion to continue treatment, change treatment, or stop treatment.

Optimizing the Outcomes of Opioid Pharmacotherapy

Based on receptor interactions, opioid analgesics can be classified as pure agonists or agonist–antagonists (Table 51.3).

TABLE 51.3 Characteristics of Commonly Used Opioid Analgesics

	Equianalgesic doses[a] (mgs)	Half-life (hours)	Peak effect (hours)	Duration (hours)	Toxicity	Comments
Morphine-like Agonists						
Morphine	10 IM 20–60 PO[b]	2–3 2–3	0.5–1 1.5–2	3–6 4–7	Constipation, nausea, sedation, hypogonadism most common; respiratory depression rare in practice	Standard comparison for opioids; available in rectal formulation
Modified-release morphine	20–60 PO[b]	—	3–4	8–24	—	Several formulations, including an abuse deterrent form
Hydromorphone	1.5 IM 7.5 PO	2–3 2–3	0.5–1 1–2	3–4 3–6	Same as morphine	Available in rectal formulation
Modified-release hydromorphone	7.5 PO	—	3–4	24	Same as hydromorphone	—
Oxycodone	20 PO	2–3	1–2	3–6	Same as morphine	Combined with aspirin or acetaminophen, for moderate pain; available orally without coanalgesic for severe pain
Modified-release oxycodone	20 PO	2–3	3–4	8–12	Same as oxycodone	Available in an abuse deterrent form
Fentanyl	100 μg	7–14	Minutes	Minutes with acute and 4–6 hours with chronic dosing	Same as morphine	IV sometimes used for acute pain; commonly used as an anesthetic
Fentanyl transdermal system	See package insert	—	—	48–72	Same as morphine	Transdermal system commonly used to treat chronic pain; possibly less constipation than oral morphine; not widely abused by those with a history of substance abuse

(*Continued*)

TABLE 51.3 Opioid analgesics (*Continued*)

	Equianalgesic doses[a]	Half-life (hours)	Peak effect (hours)	Duration (hours)	Toxicity	Comments
Fentanyl-containing rapid-onset formulations	Start with lowest doses	—	Varies by product; all within 30 minutes	1	—	Formulations available in the United States and Europe include an oral transmucosal lozenge, an effervescent tablet, a buccal patch, a sublingual tablet, and a nasal spray
Oxymorphone	1 IM 15 PO	3–6 3–6	0.5–1 1–2	3–6 3–6	Same as morphine	Available in rectal formulation
Modified-release oxymorphone	15 PR	2–3	3–4	8–12	Same as oxymorphone	—
Meperidine	75 IM 300 PO	2–3 2–3	0.5–1 1–2	3–4 3–6	Same as morphine + central nervous system (CNS) excitation; contraindicated in those on monoamine oxidase (MAO) inhibitors	Not preferred because of potential toxicity Not preferred because of potential toxicity
Heroin	5 IM	0.5	0.5–1	4–5	Same as morphine	Analgesic action because of metabolite, predominantly morphine; not available in the United States
Levorphanol	2 IM 4 PO	11–16	0.5–1 1–2	3–6 3–6	Same as morphine	With long half-life, accumulation could occur after beginning or increasing dose, but seldom a problem
Methadone	10 IM 20 PO	12–>150	0.5–1.5 1–2	4–8	Same as morphine plus QTc prolongation	Risk of delayed toxicity as a result of accumulation; concern about cardiac effects and unanticipated high potency in some settings; requires knowledge for safe use as an analgesic
Codeine	130 IM 200 PO	2–3	1.5–2	3–6	Same as morphine	Usually combined with nonopioid

Propoxyphene napsylate	—	12	1.5–2	3–6	Same as morphine plus seizures and cardiac toxicity with overdose	Not preferred because of toxic metabolite; often combined with nonopioid
Propoxyphene hydrochloride	—	12	1.5–2	3–6	Same as napsylate	Same as napsylate
Hydrocodone	—	2–4	0.5–1	3–4	Same as morphine	Available only as acetaminophen and ibuprofen combination
Dihydrocodeine	—	2–4	1–2	3–4	Same as morphine	Only available combined with acetaminophen or aspirin

Partial Agonists

Buprenorphine	0.4 IM 0.8 SL	20–73	0.5–1 2–3	4–6 6–12	Same as morphine, except less risk of respiratory depression or endocrine effects	Can produce withdrawal in opioid-dependent patients; has ceiling for analgesia but the clinical relevance of this is uncertain; sublingual tablet (with and without naloxone) are available in the United States and indicated for office-based agonist therapy of addiction, but, are used for pain infrequently; low-dose transdermal patch is available in some countries and is widely used for chronic pain

Mixed Agonist–Antagonists

Pentazocine	60 IM 180 PO	2–3 2–3	0.5–1 1–2	3–6 3–6	Same profile of effects as buprenorphine, except for greater risk of psychotomimetic effects	Produces withdrawal in opioid-dependent patients; oral formulation combined with naloxone or nonopioid available in the United States; ceiling doses and side-effect profile limit role in chronic pain
Nalbuphine	10 IM	4–6	0.5–1	3–6	Same as buprenorphine	Produces withdrawal in opioid-dependent patients
Butorphanol	2 IM 2 intranasal	2–3	0.5–1	3–4	Same profile of effects as nalbuphine	Produces withdrawal in opioid-dependent patients; no oral formulation

(*Continued*)

TABLE 51.3 Opioid analgesics (*Continued*)

	Equianalgesic doses[a]	Half-life (hours)	Peak effect (hours)	Duration (hours)	Toxicity	Comments
Dezocine	10 IM[c]	1.2–7.4	0.5–1	3–4	Same profile of effects as nalbuphine	Produces withdrawal in opioid-dependent patients; no oral formulation
Centrally Acting Drugs with Opioid Actions						
Tramadol	—	6–7	1–2	4–6	Similar to morphine	Analgesic action related to monoamine (norepinephrine and serotonin) reuptake blockade and opioid effect; maximum dose is usually 600 mg/day because of concern about toxicity, including seizures and serotonin syndrome
Tapentadol	—	4	1–2	4–6	Similar to morphine but may have fewer adverse GI effects	Analgesic action related to monoamine (norepinephrine) reuptake blockade and opioid effect; maximum dose is usually 400 mg/day because of concern about toxicity, including seizures and serotonin syndrome

[a]Dose that provides analgesia equivalent to 10 mg IM morphine. These ratios are useful guides when switching drugs or routes of administration. When switching drugs, reduce the equianalgesic dose of the new drug by 25% to 50% to account for incomplete cross-tolerance. The only exception to this is methadone, which appears to manifest a greater degree of incomplete cross-tolerance than other opioids; when switching to methadone, reduce the equianalgesic dose by 90%.

[b]Extensive survey data suggest that the relative potency of IM:PO morphine of 1:6 changes to 1:2–3 with chronic dosing.

[c]Approximate equianalgesic dose suggested from meta-analysis of available comparative studies.

The agonist–antagonist drugs include a mixed agonist–antagonist subclass (including butorphanol, nalbuphine, pentazocine, and dezocine) and a partial agonist subclass (including buprenorphine). The agonist–antagonists have a ceiling effect for analgesia and for respiratory depression, can reverse the effects of pure agonists in patients who are physically dependent, and are less preferred by individuals who abuse opioid drugs. Two other centrally acting analgesics, tramadol and tapentadol, have opioid activity mediated by the mu-receptor and often are categorized with the opioid agonists. These drugs have a mixed analgesic mechanism involving both mu-agonism and monoaminergic reuptake blockade.

Opioid Selection

The treatment of acute pain may be accomplished with any of the opioid drugs. In the ambulatory setting, the most common approach to the treatment of moderate or severe pain in the patient with very limited or no prior opioid exposure involves the administration of a short-acting oral opioid, which may be combined with either acetaminophen or aspirin. In the United States, these drugs include hydrocodone, codeine, dihydrocodeine, oxycodone, tramadol, and tapentadol. Oral meperidine and propoxyphene also are used but are not preferred because of the potential for adverse effects. Although meperidine has lesser contractile effects on smooth muscle in preclinical models, this characteristic has no established benefits in the clinical setting; the drug is not preferred for either acute or chronic pain because of the potential for toxicity due to accumulation of an active metabolite, normeperidine, which may produce dysphoria, tremulousness, hyperreflexia, and seizures. Propoxyphene also has a toxic metabolite and produces a similar spectrum of potential toxicities, as well as serious cardiac toxicity with overdose.

In the inpatient setting, acute pain is usually managed with a pure mu-agonist such as morphine or hydromorphone, which is usually administered intravenously. The only certain advantage of this route is a faster onset of effect, the advantages of which often are worth pursuing as long as drug administration is in a monitored environment.

The agonist–antagonist opioids also can be used to treat acute pain. These drugs have less abuse potential than the pure agonist drugs, but the lack of oral formulations and the pharmacologic profile (e.g., ceiling effect) has limited their utility. Intranasal butorphanol has gained some acceptance in headache management, and the parenteral mix agonist–antagonists are sometimes used in monitored settings, such as emergency departments.

The partial agonist buprenorphine is available as a transdermal patch in some countries and has gained wide acceptance in the management of pain in the opioid-naive patient. In the United States, the sublingual tablets of buprenorphine that are approved for the treatment of addiction have been used off-label for pain, but experience is very limited. Some clinicians believe that buprenorphine may be especially useful for pain when the patient has a past or current history of drug abuse, but this potential advantage has yet to be established empirically.

In the most common scenario for the treatment of acute pain in the opioid-naive ambulatory patient, a combination product containing an opioid, for example, hydrocodone, and a nonopioid, for example, acetaminophen, is used. The dose may be increased as needed until the maximum safe dose of the nonopioid coanalgesic is reached. For acetaminophen, this is usually considered to be 2.7 to 4 g/day, and even lower (e.g., <2 g/day) in patients with known liver disease or heavy alcohol use.

Patients who have chronic pain and who are opioid-naive also usually receive a short-acting opioid as a first trial. Experienced clinicians do offer some of these patients a long-acting drug from the start, but this strategy does not appear to be common. Usually, the decision to continue opioid treatment for the long term is accompanied by a switch to a drug with a long duration of effect. The opioids conventionally used in the United States in this situation include morphine, hydromorphone, fentanyl, oxycodone (used as a single entity), oxymorphone, levorphanol, and methadone.

All of the long-acting pure mu-agonist drugs should be viewed as alternatives in practice. Although morphine is the most commonly used drug for severe pain on a global level, there is now a large clinical experience that establishes very substantial individual variation in the response to different opioids. A patient may experience markedly different side effects when changed from one opioid to another and the balance between analgesia and side effects cannot be predicted based on the experience with a different drug. This variation is the basis for the so-called *opioid rotation*, the practice of switching opioids when side effects interfere with effective therapy (16).

There are a few drug-specific characteristics that may influence the decision to try one or another of the pure mu-agonist opioids. The specific role of morphine, for example, has evolved with recognition of its active metabolites. Morphine 6-glucuronide (M-6-G) binds to the mu-receptor and presumably contributes to both analgesia and side effects observed during morphine therapy; morphine 3-glucuronide (M-3-G), which is produced at higher concentrations than M-6-G and is not an opioid, may cause toxicity such as myoclonus and agitation. Both these metabolites accumulate in patients with renal insufficiency. Patients with renal insufficiency should be administered morphine cautiously, and those with unstable renal function might be better served by an opioid without active metabolites, such as fentanyl (17).

Fentanyl is available in a transdermal formulation and transmucosal formulations (indicated for cancer-related breakthrough pain; see Route of Opioid Administration). Transdermal fentanyl is very well accepted and may be preferred due to the ability to avoid additional pills, a dosing frequency of every 2 to 3 days, or the possibility of a lower rate of constipation than observed with oral drugs (18).

Most of the long-acting pure mu-agonist drugs used for chronic pain have relatively short elimination half-lives but have prolonged effects because of a delivery system that slowly releases the drug in the gut. The time required to approach steady state with these drugs is determined largely by the half-life of release and absorption, rather than elimination. The modified release oral opioids containing morphine, oxycodone, hydromorphone, or oxymorphone, for example, usually require 2 to 3 days to be at steady state, far longer than would be explained by the elimination half-life of the specific drugs delivered.

The potential benefits associated with the long-acting, modified release formulations—more convenience and better adherence to therapy—also may be accomplished by using a drug with a long half-life. Two drugs currently available in the United States, namely levorphanol and methadone, have considerably longer half-lives and may be used as long-acting drugs for chronic pain management. Five to six half-lives must pass before steady state is approached after dosing is begun or altered. With levorphanol, which has a half-life of 11 to 16 hours, this period extends to several days; if the treatment is carefully monitored for this period, further accumulation is unlikely. The long and variable half-life of methadone does complicate therapy, however, and is one of the characteristics of this drug that must be understood to ensure its safe use as an analgesic.

The use of methadone in the treatment of pain has been growing steadily during the past decade, driven by its low cost, high efficacy in some clinical situations, and perceived value in reducing the risk of abuse in patients predisposed to addiction. This increasing use, which was initially welcomed by pain specialists as a means to improve access to effective pain therapy, has been associated with reports of negative outcomes—including mortality—in some populations (19). Recognition that the use of methadone may be associated with a relatively high level of risk has led to re-examination of its pharmacology in relation to analgesia and other effects.

Methadone has a half-life that typically is about 24 hours but ranges from less than 15 hours to more than 150 hours (20); there is no way to predict the outliers from clinical presentation. The time required to approach steady state is 5 days or less in most patients but can extend to a few weeks in some. Without knowing for certain how much time is required after dosing is initiated or the dose is increased before the plasma concentration stops rising, a relatively long period of monitoring is required following each dose adjustment to avoid unanticipated delayed toxicity. This need for monitoring is most critical in patients predisposed to opioid side effects, including those with advanced age or major organ dysfunction.

This potential for prolonged accumulation of drug due to half-life is not the only source of risk associated with methadone. When administered to a patient already receiving a pure mu-agonist opioid, the potency of the methadone is related to the dose of the prior drug and can be much higher than expected. The potency almost always is more than would be anticipated from review of the classic equianalgesic dose tables used to guide opioid switching (16). This unanticipated high potency is believed to be related to the *d*-isomer, which represents 50% of the commercially available racemic mixture in the United States. This isomer blocks the *N*-methyl-D-aspartate receptor, and as a result, may yield independent analgesic effects and partially reverse opioid tolerance. Thus, when methadone racemate is given to patients receiving another opioid, the opioid-mediated analgesic effects produced by the *l*-isomer are augmented by the *d*-isomer's effects on tolerance. Because there is presumably more tolerance at higher doses, methadone becomes more potent with higher doses of the prior opioid. To accommodate the potential for increased potency, a switch to methadone from another opioid is most safely accomplished by reducing the calculated equianalgesic dose by 75% to 90% (16). Failure to take this potential potency into account will lead to early overdoses.

It is now appreciated that methadone is among a large group of drugs that can prolong the QTc interval (21,22), presumably placing patients at risk for the development of a life-threatening cardiac arrhythmia, torsades de pointe. Although the risk of severe prolongation (above 500 msec) appears very low and there is no consensus concerning ECG monitoring, it is reasonable to obtain a baseline ECG in patients who may be predisposed to a prolonged QTc interval, such as those with heart disease or concurrent treatment with cardioactive drugs. An ECG also is prudent when the dose reaches an arbitrary levels, for example, above 100 mg/day, and periodically thereafter if the dose continues to be escalated.

Clinicians who prescribe methadone as an analgesic must be clear about the differences between this use and its administration for opioid addiction. In the United States, any clinician may prescribe methadone for pain, but a special license is required to use the drug in maintenance therapy for addiction. In contrast to the once-daily administration that is adequate for treating addiction, the use of methadone as an analgesic requires multiple daily doses—typically three or four—in most patients. Patients who are receiving methadone maintenance for the treatment of addiction can receive methadone as an analgesic as well, but this requires a separate prescription.

Route of Opioid Administration

For chronic therapy, the oral and transdermal routes for opioid delivery are well accepted. The advent of oral modified release formulations allowed more convenient dosing, either once daily or twice daily, and the transdermal route offered 48- to 72-hour dosing interval. These formulations also may improve treatment adherence, with theoretical benefits on pain control. They are not preferred when rapid dose titration is needed for severe pain. The transdermal route may be favored by some patients to reduce the pill burden or gain from the potential for lesser constipatory effects; it is relatively contraindicated when the patient is likely to experience spikes of fever, which may alter the delivery characteristics of the patch and lead to periods of increased drug absorption. The use of the transdermal system also is limited by the difficulties involved in delivering high doses and the need for an alternative route to provide supplemental doses for breakthrough pain.

The rectal route occasionally is used for prolonged therapy, particularly at the end of life. Rectal administration of modified release oral formulations has proved useful anecdotally.

The parenteral route typically is used for the treatment of acute severe pain in a monitored setting. The rationale for intravenous bolus therapy, including intravenous patient-controlled analgesia, is the ability to provide pain relief quickly following a dose and titrate more effectively, unencumbered by the delay associated with oral absorption. Subcutaneous bolus injection also is widely used, particularly in the setting of pain related to advanced illness. In contrast, intramuscular injection is rarely appropriate, given the pain it causes, the risk of hematoma, and the occurrence of variable absorption from different muscles.

Several parenteral drug delivery options exist for the patient in need of long-term treatment but lacking in the ability to swallow or absorb opioid drugs. The usual context is pain related to medical illness. Although repeated subcutaneous injection can be used, continuous infusion techniques are generally preferred because they reduce the need for nursing support, eliminate the potential for bolus effects (side effects at peak concentration or pain breakthrough at the end of the dosing interval), and can be implemented in the home with relative ease. Any opioid available in an injectable formulation can be used for continuous infusion. Long-term intravenous administration is possible if the patient has an indwelling venous access device; long-term subcutaneous infusion can be accomplished using a 25-gauge butterfly needle that can be placed at any convenient site and left under the skin for a week before changing.

A variety of techniques for intraspinal opioid delivery (known as neuraxial analgesia) have been adapted to long-term treatment, and there is emerging evidence that properly selected patients can benefit greatly from this approach (23). The clearest indication is intolerable somnolence or confusion in a patient who is not experiencing adequate analgesia during systemic opioid treatment of a pain syndrome located below the level of mid chest. Continuous epidural infusion, which can be accomplished through either a percutaneous or implanted epidural catheter, is usually preferred if the patient has advanced medical illness and a life expectancy measured in just a few months. Otherwise, subarachnoid infusion using a totally implanted system should be considered. In a population with cancer pain, a controlled trial comparing neuraxial infusion and comprehensive medical management demonstrated that the spinal opioid treatment improved pain, side effects, quality of life, and even survival (24).

The potential for intraspinal infusion has increased further with the use of drug combinations. An opioid, such as morphine or hydromorphone, is usually combined with a local anesthetic, such as bupivacaine. Clonidine is often added, and other drugs may be considered for refractory pain, including other opioids, baclofen, midazolam, and ziconotide. Ziconotide is a unique calcium-channel blocker available only for neuraxial infusion and has been shown to be effective for cancer pain in controlled trials (25). As new drugs are tested for intraspinal therapy, the indications for the approach are likely to increase.

The decision to pursue a trial of neuraxial infusion is occasionally influenced by a history of substance abuse. Patients with severe pain problems, who pose a challenge in risk management, might be considered for a technique capable of providing an effective opioid regimen without patient access to the drug. Based on clinical experience, this strategy may be beneficial for the patient in recovery, but demonstrably prone to relapse. Given the need for close monitoring and follow-up after pump implantation, a patient with active addiction, or a serious comorbid psychiatric disorder, generally would not be considered appropriate.

During the past decade, there has been extensive effort applied to the development of transmucosal opioid delivery systems. This effort has been driven by the recognition that breakthrough pain may be a serious problem for a substantial proportion of opioid-treated chronic pain patients (2,3) and that conventional management with a short-acting oral opioid fails to address the problem adequately. The transmucosal formulations incorporate a lipophilic drug, such as fentanyl, into a delivery system that can yield more rapid absorption than oral dosing, and thereby produces an onset of analgesia that more closely matches the time course of a typical breakthrough pain (26). The first system available, oral transmucosal fentanyl citrate (OTFC) placed the drug into a candy matrix that is sucked, allowing partial absorption through the buccal mucosa. An effervescent fentanyl buccal tablet and a fentanyl impregnated film also are available in the United States, and other systems available in Europe, including intranasal and sublingual formulations, are undergoing development for the U.S. market. There have been no comparative trials among the rapid-onset formulations and very little evaluation of any of these formulations relative to the conventional oral formulations used for breakthrough pain. Nonetheless, all are efficacious for breakthrough pain, and all yield analgesia more promptly than oral drugs. Given the demonstrated time–action relationship of these drugs, it is reasonable to consider a trial of one or another if breakthrough pain has a very quick time course or if a conventional oral agent fails to provide adequate relief.

Although the development of the rapid-onset opioid formulations may address an unmet clinical need for a more effective treatment for breakthrough pain, they have also raised concerns about potential adverse effects, including the risk of abuse, precipitation or relapse of addiction, and unintentional overdose. In the United States, these concerns have been highlighted by the degree to which the available formulations, which are indicated for cancer-related breakthrough pain, are being used off-label for noncancer pain. Although there are yet no empirical data supporting the view that these drugs are especially problematic in terms of abuse, addiction or diversion, the U.S. government has taken a proactive course and required the so-called "risk evaluation and mitigation strategies" (REMS) for each agent. The REMS programs are intended to improve safety and enhance monitoring of adverse outcomes. Although it is still too early to determine the impact of these or other REMS programs, the mandate demonstrates both the growing level of concern about prescription drug abuse and a strong regulatory response to this concern.

Dosing Guidelines

The success of opioid therapy derives less from the selection of the drug and route than from the clinical strategies used in initiating and altering the dose. In the setting of acute pain, dosing usually involves a conventional starting dose provided on an "as needed" basis, irrespective of the specifics of the drug, route, or treatment setting. Although side effects such as nausea or somnolence are common during the initial period of drug administration, the overall balance between analgesia and side effects usually is favorable from the start. If not, the treatment should be changed promptly. If the problem is a side effect that typically can be easily managed, such as nausea, the change may involve coadministration of a drug to treat this. If the problematic side effect is difficult to manage, the opioid should be changed. If the problem is not a side effect, but rather a lack of efficacy after several doses, consideration should be given to an increase in the dose, conventionally by an amount in the range of 33% to 100%.

The management of acute severe pain in the relatively opioid-naive patient using either an oral or parenteral agent is highly successful. The simplicity and effectiveness of the strategy explains its widespread acceptance by health professionals. In contrast, the effort to optimize the outcomes during long-term therapy requires a far greater set of competencies, including skills in pharmacotherapy and risk management (15). Guidelines intended to optimize the pharmacologic outcomes have been developed for chronic cancer-related pain (27,28) and represent the starting point for long-term therapy in all populations and settings.

Dose "By the Clock" For continuous or frequently recurring pain, "fixed schedule" (around-the-clock) dosing is usually preferred and long-acting drugs are used conventionally. Coadministration of a short-acting opioid, offered on an "as-needed" basis (known as a "rescue" dose or "escape" dose), may be used to manage breakthrough pains. Rescue dosing is widely considered to be a standard of care during management of pain related to active cancer but should not be considered routine in other populations. Like the decision to initiate a therapeutic trial of an opioid regimen with the intention to continue it long-term if outcomes are favorable, the decision to coadminister a short-acting drug for breakthrough pain should be taken only after an analysis of potential risks and benefits.

Although there is no evidence that the around-the-clock administration of a long-acting opioid confers any benefit over the use of short-acting opioids during the treatment of chronic pain (29), it is nonetheless taken as axiomatic that regular dosing with long-acting drugs is better because of the potential for improved convenience and adherence, and reduced pain fluctuation associated with bolus effects. On theoretical grounds, it also might be beneficial to use a long-acting drug (without access to a short-acting drug for breakthrough pain) in the effort to reduce the likelihood that the patient predisposed to addiction would experience a flare of the latter disorder induced by rapid changes in drug concentration.

For all of these putative benefits, experienced clinicians generally endorse the use of around-the-clock administration of a long-acting drug for chronic pain. The message provided to patients is that it is better in terms of both relief and side effects to prevent pain than to treat it after it occurs.

Given this widespread perception, it is a remarkable observation that a large proportion of opioid-treated patients receive prescriptions for short-acting medication for prolonged periods of time. These drugs are usually prescribed on an as-needed basis. The reasons for this are unknown but presumably include the failure on the part of some clinicians to properly conceptualize long-term treatment as grounded in a commitment to continue indefinitely. To the extent that this is so, it represents an unmet need for clinician education and support. As noted, current guidelines indicate that the clinician should, at some point, proceed from short-term therapy to a trial of long-term therapy, during which outcomes are evaluated to decide explicitly whether the patient is a candidate for ongoing opioid management of a chronic pain problem (15).

It also is likely, however, that some proportion of long-term as-needed therapy actually follows from the clinical observation that the benefits exceed any problems. Some patients prefer long-term access to a short-acting drug as needed because they value the sense of control over the therapy and the ability to adjust the dose on a daily basis. Other perceive benefit in better control of side effects. For example, the elderly patient with chronic pain from osteoarthritis who benefits from opioid therapy but struggles with constipation may learn that a reduction in dose for 1 or 2 days favorably influences bowel function; this outcome may have more value than the potential improvements in pain control associated with regular dosing of a long-acting drug. The use of a short-acting drug also may be useful in those with widely fluctuating pains, for whom the ability to rapidly titrate the dose higher, and reduce the dose quickly, overrides other concerns. Although the around-the-clock administration of a long-acting drug should be strongly considered whenever the transition to long-term therapy is made, flexibility based on a good assessment is appropriate.

Individualize the Dose In the setting of acute pain management, the dose may need to be adjusted promptly to optimize effects. The typical patient has little or no opioid exposure, and the overall outcomes associated with a conventional dose can quickly be determined. For example, the ambulatory patient might be treated with an opioid–nonopioid combination product, or with tramadol or tapentadol, at the lowest dose available. The inpatient might be treated with intravenous patient-controlled analgesia using a standard protocol (e.g., morphine 1 mg every 6 minutes as needed, or equivalent) or with intravenous injection (e.g., morphine 5 mg intravenously every two hours as needed). If the starting dose is not effective, it should be increased.

If the patient with acute pain has substantial prior opioid exposure, either as a result of long-term opioid therapy for pain or methadone maintenance, the initial dose of the drug for acute pain typically needs adjustment. Based on clinical experience, there are strategies to identify the proper dose quickly. One approach involves the calculation of the dose delivered over 3 to 4 hours (i.e., one eighth to one sixth the total daily dose), which is then converted to a dose of the drug used for acute pain based on standard equianalgesic data; this dose is then reduced by 25% to 50% to account for variation and incomplete cross-tolerance (16). The result of the first dose is monitored and the dose is adjusted upward with the subsequent permitted dose, usually 3 or 4 hours later. An alternative approach is to give a conventional starting dose for an opioid-naive patient, with a plan to repeat it (with or without a 50% increase) after a long enough period to observe the peak effect of the first dose (e.g., 20 to 30 minutes if using morphine). Additional dose escalations may be needed if the dose remains ineffective. These repeated doses can be given at short intervals until the patient reports that a dose has yielded effect. The subsequent regimen uses this dose, administered every three hours as needed.

Individualization of the dose during long-term opioid therapy is far more challenging and, again, is the key to the overall success of the therapy. The goal is to identify a dose through repeated titration that is associated with a favorable balance between analgesia and side effects. Once a pure mu-opioid agonist drug and route of administration are selected, the dose should be incremented until adequate analgesia occurs or intolerable and unmanageable side effects supervene. If a favorable dose is found, it should be continued, but should pain reappear during the course of therapy, retitration should be considered in an effort to recapture the favorable balance between analgesia and side effects.

There are several approaches to dose escalation at the start of therapy, or later should pain worsen after a period of stability. The size of the increase is usually selected as either the total quantity of rescue drug consumed during the previous day (or if this is changing, the average of the past 2 to 3 days), or as 33% to 50% of the current total daily dose. The increment can be larger (75% to 100% of the total daily dose) if pain is severe and the patient is medically stable, or smaller if the patient is already experiencing opioid toxicity or is predisposed to adverse effects because of advanced age or coexisting major organ dysfunction. Caution is also reasonable if the patient has a limited prior opioid exposure.

Dose titration typically identifies a dose that yields a favorable balance between analgesia and side effects for a stable period. Many patients appear to find the same dose effective for many months or years. This phenomenon belies the inevitability of tolerance as a problem in the long-term administration of opioid drugs.

Although doses typically stabilize for prolonged periods during long-term management, dose escalation is usually required at intervals to maintain analgesia. Patients who ultimately require relatively high opioid doses typically evolve through a series of "retitrations" driven by reappearance of moderate or severe pain after a period of stable, effective therapy. In the patient with pain as a consequence of medical illness, the need for a dose increase can usually be explained by some overt change in clinical status, such as worsening of a pain-producing structural lesion. This implies that the reappearance of pain after a period of stability may call for reevaluation of the underlying pain-producing disease. Pain may worsen in the absence of a progressive lesion, however, and the assessment at this time also should address the potential of other biomedical factors (e.g., change in the underlying pathophysiology of the pain) or factors related to an emerging psychosocial or psychiatric problem.

Although dose escalation after a period of stability to regain benefit that has been lost should always be considered, this action should not be viewed as automatic. Depending on the assessment, it may be appropriately combined with other interventions (a treatment that targets a factor assessed as driving the pain, a treatment that is independently coanalgesic, or both) or eschewed all together in lieu of an alternative strategy.

During the steady increase in the use of opioid therapy to manage persistent pain, it has been commonly accepted that the pure mu-agonists do not have a ceiling effect for analgesia and the maximal dose is immaterial as long as the patient attains a favorable balance between analgesia and side effects. Although this is true from a pharmacologic perspective, the guideline to titrate the dose without regard to the total dose must be qualified. Few patients with any type of chronic pain require relatively high doses of an opioid. Although the dose that is considered "high" is entirely arbitrary, data from the pharmaceutical industry in the United States indicate that a large majority of patients receive a total daily dose less than the equivalent of 200 mg of morphine, and it is reasonable on this basis to consider doses that exceed this level to be high. The need for a high dose is not, in itself, a problem—indeed, pain specialists commonly treat patients with doses above this and some patients ultimately stabilize on doses equivalent to several grams of morphine daily while demonstrating good pain control, minimal side effects, and responsible drug use. Nonetheless, the reality that high doses escalation by itself should never be made in isolation to judge the effectiveness and safety of an opioid regimen. Nonetheless, the reality that high doses are seldom needed obligates the clinician to be particularly careful when the dose requires escalation to high levels. The clinician should reassess the nature of the pain and comorbidities (including the potential for substance use disorder), the rationale for therapy, the availability of alternative treatments, and the outcomes associated with dose escalation (15). This reassessment should be well documented and repeated as necessary.

The concerns raised about the use of relatively high opioid doses have increased with elucidation of the physiology of *opioid-induced hyperalgesia* (30). This term refers to a neurophysiologic phenomenon characterized by an opioid-induced lowering of pain threshold and increase in pain response to noxious stimuli. Clearly demonstrated in preclinical models, the empirical data in patients are very limited. Case reports suggest that opioid treatment can result in the so-called "paradoxical pain" but that the phenomenon is rare and heterogeneous. One subtype is characterized by generalized pain and allodynia associated with tremulousness, confusion, and myoclonus, which occur in the setting of escalating doses of systemic or neuraxial opioid; this subtype is not naloxone reversible and appears to be fundamentally different than the opioid-induced hyperalgesia that is observed in animal models. Other patients may have a type of opioid-induced hyperalgesia that is mediated by the opioid receptor, but at this time, the extent to which this type of phenomenon influences outcomes during opioid therapy is entirely unknown. There are insufficient data to conclude that opioid-induced hyperalgesia represent anything more than a rare adverse event. In the absence of relevant symptoms and signs, such as escalating pain as the dose is increased, or signs of delirium, it is not appropriate to limit or withhold opioid treatment in an effort to prevent or reverse opioid-induced hyperalgesia.

Be Aware of Relative Potencies Potency refers to the dose required to produce a given effect. It is entirely distinct from efficacy, which may be defined as the anticipated effect produced by a given dose, or effectiveness, which is the extent to which the drug has a favorable therapeutic index in the clinical setting. Potency is an issue in opioid prescribing only when there is a planned switch from one drug to another—opioid rotation. The dose of the second drug must be selected based on its potency relative to the drug it is replacing; the dose should be high enough to ensure no flare of pain or abstinence phenomena, but low enough to minimize the risk of toxicity.

Studies of relative potency began five decades ago with the development of a scientific methodology. Using morphine as a standard, relative potencies have been determined for most pure agonist drugs. This information was used to construct an equianalgesic dose table (Table 51.3), which summarizes the results of relative potency studies and provides a guide for the practice of opioid rotation. A recent evidence-based guideline for opioid rotation emphasize that the equianalgesic table is only a starting point for a guideline (16). The first step in this guideline involves calculation of the equianalgesic dose using the values in the standard table. This calculated equianalgesic dose typically is reduced by 25% to 50% in recognition of individual variation and incomplete cross-tolerance between drugs. There are, however, two important exceptions to this: First, a switch to methadone should be accompanied by a 75% to 90% reduction in the calculated equianalgesic dose as a result of the potential for an unanticipated high potency as discussed previously, and second, a switch to the transdermal fentanyl patch should have no immediate dose reduction because the equianalgesic dose ratios that were built into the initial commercialization of this product were conservative.

The evidence-based guideline further suggests a second step in opioid rotation (16). After calculation of the equianalgesic dose and immediate dose reduction in most cases, a second decision is needed about an additional change, specifically either an increase or a decrease by 15% to 25%. An increase should be considered if pain is severe, and a decrease should be considered if the patient is medically frail, the doses are relatively high, or significant opioid toxicity is present. Although there are no empirical data demonstrating the safety and effectiveness of this two-step strategy, the approach is proposed as a flexible method that is likely to transition a patient from one opioid drug to another with relatively low risk of adverse consequences associated with either overdosing or underdosing.

If a so-called rescue medication is coadministered for breakthrough pain, the conventional dose selected is 5% to 15% of the total daily dose, and the dosing interval in the ambulatory population is usually 1 to 2 hours, as needed. If the rescue drug is changed to another, the same calculations using relative potency estimates can be done to select an appropriate starting dose. As noted, the key exception to this guideline is posed by the rapid-onset fentanyl formulations. Controlled studies have not confirmed that the dose administered on a scheduled basis predicts the effective size of the rescue (31) and guidelines for the use of these formulations should include a low starting dose in all cases (e.g. 200 to 400 μg of the OTFC), followed by dose titration.

Treat Side Effects Treatment of opioid-induced side effects is an integral part of opioid therapy (27,32). Management of side effects enhances comfort and allows continued upward dose titration of the opioid drug, if necessary. Although respiratory depression fosters the greatest concern, tolerance to this adverse effect develops quickly and it is rarely a problem. The most common and persistent side effect during long-term treatment is constipation. Although less prevalent, persistent sedation or mental clouding also may occur and limit dose escalation.

Although the evidence is very limited (33), there is a large experience supporting the use of laxative therapy for opioid-induced constipation. Treatment is needed by a high proportion of those who receive opioids in the context of serious medical illness, most of whom have other factors contributing to constipation; a smaller proportion of patients without these factors require ongoing treatment. The conventional approach involves either the administration of a stool softener, docusate, in combination with a contact cathartic, such as bisacodyl or senna, or the administration of an osmotically active agent. The latter products include poorly absorbed sugars, specifically lactulose or sorbitol, or propylene glycol. The treatment of opioid-induced constipation that is refractory to these therapies may involve trials of drugs that have been used anecdotally, such as a prokinetic agent (metaclopramide), an acetylcholinesterase inhibitor (e.g., donepezil), lubiprostone, misoprostol or colchicine. More specifically, refractory constipation can be treated with an opioid antagonist. Methylnaltrexone is now approved in the United States as a parenteral opioid antagonist specifically indicated for refractory constipation; the studies suggest that more than one half of treated patients respond with a bowel movement, most within an hour of dosing (34). There also is limited experience with oral naloxone for severe opioid-induced constipation.

Patients who experience persistent somnolence or mental clouding during opioid therapy may improve with elimination of nonessential centrally acting drugs or opioid rotation. Another strategy is to treat the symptom using a psychostimulant, such as methylphenidate or modafinil.

There have been very few studies of this approach but extensive clinical experience has been favorable (32). The potential side effects of the psychostimulants, including anxiety, tremulousness, anorexia, and insomnia, must be considered, however, particularly if dose escalation is required to gain benefit. Equally important, the psychostimulants are potentially abusable drugs and the decision to implement a trial, and the approach to monitoring treatment over time, requires consideration of the potential for abuse and diversion, similar to the opioid itself.

Other side effects are common with short-term administration but seldom compromise long-term therapy. These include nausea, itch, dry mouth, and urinary retention. Like other side effects, the management may consider opioid rotation or specific treatment of the symptom.

In recent years, there has been increasing concern about side effects related to the neuroendocrine effects of opioid drugs, specifically drug-induced hypogonadism. Most opioid-treated men have hypothalamic hypogonadism, and although the prevalence of this complication in women is uncertain, the levels of sex hormones in women receiving opioid drugs are relatively low compared to those who are not (35,36). Hypogonadism may be associated with sexual dysfunction and infertility, mood disturbance, fatigue, and osteoporosis. Although the impact of these potential outcomes in the diverse populations with chronic pain is unknown, pain specialists now generally advocate for measurement of testosterone and free testosterone in opioid-treated men with symptoms that may suggest hypogonadism. There is no consensus about the approach to take with opioid-treated women, but it is reasonable to consider hormonal therapy in premenopausal women who become symptomatically hypogonadal during opioid treatment.

Recently, concern also has focused on the potential for opioids to cause sleep-disordered breathing (37). The data are limited but a form of central sleep apnea associated with changes in sleep architecture should be considered a potential risk during long-term therapy. A survey of chronic pain patients suggested that the prevalence of this adverse effect is very high when assessed with polysomnograhy and that the risk of serious sleep apnea is highest among those patients treated with methadone and those who are receiving concurrent treatment with a benzodiazepine (38). Given concerns about the increase in mortality among opioid-treated pain patients (39), the potential for this effect should be taken seriously. Patients with untreated sleep apnea syndrome, and those at risk by virtue of obesity, short neck, snoring, or daytime somnolence that predates treatment, should be treated cautiously. It is best to avoid benzodiazepines in these at-risk patients and to consider referral for a sleep study and treatment of a sleep disorder, if present.

Monitoring Outcomes

Regardless of the pain syndrome or setting of care, opioid therapy must be monitored in terms of analgesic effects, side effects, impact on functioning, and drug-related behaviors. In the setting of chronic pain management, changes in therapy should be considered if an initial favorable balance between analgesia or side effects change for the worse, physical or psychosocial functioning decline, or nonadherence behaviors occur. A simple framework for monitoring has been summarized using the mnemonic, the "Four A's" (Table 51.4). Documentation of outcomes in the medical record should periodically describe the assessment of each element. This may be facilitated by use of a chart tool, such as the Pain Assessment and Documentation Tool (40).

Risk Assessment and Management

Monitoring for aberrant drug-related behavior should be considered a best practice during treatment with any potentially abusable drug in any clinical situation. Opioid therapy in all treatment contexts always carries a risk associated with its abuse liability. In some situations, such as acute pain management in monitored settings or the treatment of chronic pain in those with advanced medical illness, the risks may be very low or the management of these risks may be relatively simple. In other situations, such as the treatment of a chronic pain problem in the patient with a recent history of polysubstance abuse, the risks are very high. Irrespective of the level of risk, the most efficient and appropriate framework is a *universal precautions* approach. This approach, which has been emphasized in the setting of chronic pain management (41), should be broadly generalized. It empowers clinicians to act in patients' best interests by putting the emphasis on assessment and encouraging rational clinical decisions and appropriate documentation.

Laws and Regulations Governing Controlled Prescription Drugs

In the United States, there are three levels to the regulations and laws that govern the use of controlled prescription drugs: (a) international laws and treaties, (b) federal laws and regulations, and (c) state laws and regulations. A basic knowledge of the framework provides the background for clinical risk management; a more detailed understanding of specific regulations and laws is necessary to practice.

The International Narcotics Control Board was established in 1968 as an independent body charged with the implementation of the United Nations drug conventions. It attempts to ensure that adequate supplies of controlled drugs are available for medical and scientific uses while minimizing diversion to illicit purposes. The board monitors international trade in drugs and government control systems. It has no direct interaction with clinicians.

In the United States, the Drug Enforcement Administration (DEA) and the Food and Drug Administration (FDA) work together to regulate drugs. The DEA was created in 1970 as part of the Controlled Substances Act (CSA), which embodies so-called Title II and Title III of the Comprehensive Drug Abuse Prevention and Control Act. The goal of this legislation was to create a closed system for monitoring and providing access to abusable drugs with legitimate medical purpose. The CSA created different "schedules" of drugs

TABLE 51.4	The four A's approach to monitoring long-term opioid therapy
Analgesia	
■ Assess pain intensity over time, preferably in terms of a documented measurement, using either of the following scales:	
■ A 0–10 numeric scale, one for average pain during the past week and one for worst pain during the past week	
■ Percent relief scale, using the period prior to long-term opioid treatment as a baseline	
Adverse Effects	
■ Document symptoms that are side effects, e.g., constipation, mental clouding, or sedation	
■ Document monitoring for other side effects, such as hypogonadism and sleep-disordered breathing	
Activities	
■ Document impact of treatment on at least several functional domains, potentially including	
■ Physical activities	
■ Role functioning	
■ Mood	
■ Coping	
■ Social interactions and family interactions	
■ Sexual functioning	
■ Impact of other symptoms such as insomnia and fatigue	
Aberrant Drug-Related Behavior	
■ Document assessment of drug-related behavior, with the scope and specific elements defined by the level of structure applied to the therapy; potential assessments include	
■ Global assessment	
■ Adherence to instruction, including prescription, required consultations, and acquisition of medical reports	
■ Results of urine drug screening	
■ Reports of drug-related impairment at work or other activities	

based on the risk of abuse and diversion, medical use, and safety. Schedule I drugs, such as heroin and marijuana, are believed to have a high potential for abuse, a lack of accepted safety, and no current federally accepted medical use. Schedule II drugs such as morphine, fentanyl, hydromorphone, levorphanol, methadone, oxycodone, oxymorphone, methylphenidate, dextroamphetamine, and dronabinol are believed to have a high potential for abuse but have currently accepted for medical uses. Drugs classified into schedules III through V, such as hydrocodone and codeine, are medically useful and have progressively less abuse potential.

The DEA is a law enforcement agency and relies on the criminal justice system to enforce the CSA. Although most of its activity is focused on reducing the flow of illicit drugs, it is responsible for investigating and stopping the trafficking of controlled prescription drugs. The filter through which it evaluates clinician behavior is framed by two key elements that must characterize every prescription for a controlled drug: (a) it must be provided in *the usual course of professional practice* and (b) it must be *for a legitimate medical purpose*.

The two key elements of a legal prescription under the CSA are similar to the criteria used by medical boards, which are charged with ensuring that medical practice is appropriate to the standard of care. Although this commonality between criteria used to judge physician prescribing behavior under criminal statute and criteria used to judge physician behavior under civil medical practice laws raises concern about fairness (similar behaviors can be addressed as a criminal or a civil violation without clear criteria for distinguishing them), it does simplify understanding of the legal and regulatory framework for prescribing. It is essential that the documentation in the medical record demonstrates that the person who receives a prescription for a controlled drug is a patient in a doctor–patient relationship and has a medical indication for the drug, and that the prescription is given and monitored in a manner consistent with medical care.

In contrast to the DEA, the FDA is not primarily a law enforcement agency. It is a regulatory body that determines whether a drug is legal for prescribing and dispensing. Historically, the FDA has limited its purview to the assessment of safety and efficacy. With the passage of the 2007 FDA Amendments Act, however, the agency has been required to improve the safety of controlled prescription drugs through proactive approaches that reduce the risk of unintentional overdose, drug abuse, and addiction. These approaches, known collectively as REMS, are presently evolving. Newly approved opioid drugs now have individual REMS, all of which focus on education of physicians, pharmacists, and patients, and some of which include enhanced monitoring through registries or the use of specialty pharmacies. In the near future, it is likely that REMS will be applied uniformly to some classes of controlled prescription drugs, such as modified release opioids and rapid-onset formulations for breakthrough pain. The FDA has indicated its commitment to maintain access to these drugs for the patients who need them, but there is concern that REMS may increase the reluctance of prescribers to offer Schedule II opioids. This remains to be determined.

In the United States, each state works with the federal government to oversee the movement of controlled prescription drugs and minimize abuse and diversion. Each state also has sole responsibility for maintaining standards of health care practice through licensure of professionals. Law enforcement is conducted through numerous agencies, and medical practice and licensure are governed through state medical boards. Both the existence of medically inappropriate language in state laws and regulations and the empirical demonstration of knowledge gaps among the members of state boards have been recognized as potential barriers to appropriate medical use of opioid drugs (42). In an effort to improve this situation, the Federation of State Medical Boards, a national organization, has drafted a model policy for the medical use of controlled substances ("Model Policy for the Use of Controlled Substances for the Treatment of Pain"), which has now been adopted, at least in part, by most states (43).

Structuring Therapy to Reduce Risk

From the perspective of universal precautions, all patients who are prescribed an opioid should undergo an assessment designed to stratify the risk of abuse, addiction, and diversion. If prescribing is initiated, the plan of care should include strategies for adherence monitoring appropriate for the level of risk.

Risk stratification relies on clinical assessment, potentially supplemented by one of the present numerous questionnaires. Clinical assessment alone typically is used in the setting of acute pain management. Prescribing may be occurring in a monitored environment and is planned for a short time. The most important concern is whether the patient has a personal history of alcohol or drug abuse, and if so, whether the nature of this history is likely to increase the risk that that patient will engage in aberrant behaviors during the relatively brief period of prescribing.

When a decision about potential long-term therapy is being entertained, the challenge of the assessment and its implications is greater. From the clinical perspective, it is widely accepted that the risk of abuse or addiction is increased in those with (a) a personal history of drug abuse, (b) a family history of drug abuse, or (c) a history of major psychiatric pathology. Although it is obvious that each factor may be complex, positive findings in any of these three domains should raise concerns, particularly if supported by ancillary information. This information may include a past experience of physical or sexual abuse, regular contact with high-risk individuals or environments, prior criminal behavior, or heavy smoking.

During the past decade, multiple tools have been developed to assist the clinician in predicting which patients are at higher risk for developing abuse behaviors during long-term therapy. None of these tools has been adequately validated (44). The tool that has been best validated is the Screener and Opioid Assessment for Patients with Pain (44,45); less well validated, but briefer instruments—the Opioid Risk Tool, the Diagnosis, Intractability, Risk and Efficacy Inventory, and the Cut Down, Annoyed, Guilty, Eye-Opener Tool, Adjusted to Include Drugs—also are in use. Numerous other questionnaires vary in length, validation, specific outcomes assessed, and clinical utility (46). At present, the decision to incorporate a tool in practice is a matter of clinical judgment.

Based on the clinical assessment or information obtained using a questionnaire, each patient who is prescribed a controlled drug can be categorized in terms of the risk for nonadherence behavior. Patients with no past or current history of alcohol or drug abuse, no family history of these disorders, and no major psychopathology may be considered low risk; others may be considered to be at higher risk. As described previously, the assessed level of risk is one element that must be considered in the initial decision to initiate a trial of opioid therapy with the intention of long-term treatment if outcomes are favorable. If the patient is perceived to be a candidate, the level of risk also should be considered in the decision to obtain consultation for assistance in therapy, or possibly referring the patient to a more experienced clinician or structured program.

If the decision is made to prescribe, treatment must be structured in a manner that allows monitoring and control commensurate with the assessed risk. If the patient has acute pain and is treated in a monitored environment, there may be few additional elements of monitoring necessary. In the ambulatory setting, however, even short-term therapy for acute pain must consider risk and structure therapy appropriately.

If the patient has chronic pain, the decision to undertake opioid treatment with the intention to continue treatment indefinitely should begin with a trial, during which nonadherence behavior and other outcomes can be assessed. This overall approach to chronic therapy—risk stratification followed by the structuring of therapy during an initial treatment trial, after which the plan of care for longer-term management can be defined—is appropriate for all types of patients with persistent pain, including those with pain related to serious illness.

There are no guidelines for the initial structuring of therapy in a manner that matches risk with an appropriate degree of monitoring and control. Many of the strategies are well known by those who work with patients who have the disease of addiction, but their adaptation to the context of opioid prescribing for pain is a matter of clinical judgment. Some approaches are straightforward, such as the requirement for all medical records before prescribing is begun; requirement that contact be maintained with other physicians, counselors or sponsors, or drug treatment program; requirement for consultation with a mental health professional with expertise in the addictions; prescription of small quantities; and frequent visits to the office.

Urine drug screening is a widely accepted approach for adherence monitoring (47,48), but there is debate about the most appropriate method for implementing this strategy in practice. Although there is agreement that high-risk patients should be screened at the start of treatment, and periodically thereafter, some experienced clinicians advocate universal testing repeatedly during therapy. All clinicians who treat patients with long-term opioid therapy should develop a system for urine drug screening, decide proactively on an approach, and learn how to interpret the findings.

The so-called "opioid agreement" is another controversial tool in the structuring of treatment (49). Although a document that is reviewed by the patient and the clinician at the start of opioid therapy may be used effectively as an educational device, it also could contribute to the stigmatization of opioid therapy, undermine goals by stating requirements (e.g., no driving) that are inconsistent with common practice, or encourage the patient to dissemble by threatening negative consequences that may be out of proportion to the behaviors that occur. If the document gives a clinician a false sense of security, it could unintentionally reduce the vigilance necessary in monitoring treatment. Finally, an agreement that includes specific promises theoretically could be used adversely in a medicolegal dispute.

Given the controversy, each clinician must decide whether the use of an agreement is appropriate and likely to be beneficial. If one is selected, it is best to conceptualize it as a tool to enhance patient understanding and expectations about the therapy and provide very specific instructions. A model for this type of agreement has been created by the American Academy of Pain Medicine (50).

Monitoring Therapy and Addressing Nonadherence

Monitoring outcomes using the framework of the "Four A's" (Table 51.4) will ensure that drug-related behaviors are included among the key outcomes evaluated. The intensity and type of monitoring will determine the information available. For the patient who is assessed as low risk, monitoring of drug-related behaviors may take the form of simple questions about adherence, the answers to which may be documented. For patients at higher levels of assessed risk, these questions may be complemented by the results of urine drug screening, which evaluates for the presence of the prescribed drug and the absence of nonprescribed drugs; pill counts; information from the pharmacy; or reports from other clinicians, sponsors, or programs.

The occurrence of nonadherence behavior of any type should be documented and initiate a thoughtful response. The following elements should be considered:

1. Clarify the nature and severity of the behavior with all existing information; plan to acquire additional information if needed.
2. Evaluate the *differential diagnosis* of the behavior. The following diagnoses are not mutually exclusive: (a) addiction, either de novo (iatrogenic addiction) or relapse; (b) pseudoaddiction; (c) other psychiatric disorder associated with impulsive drug-related behavior, such as an anxiety disorder or a personality disorder; (d) encephalopathy (e.g., an early dementia or a confusional state) associated with disinhibition, automatic behavior, or memory disturbance; (e) family issues driving aberrant drug-related behavior; and (f) criminal intent.
3. Decide whether the plan of care must address a new concern, regardless of the next steps for pain. For example, if a de novo diagnosis of addiction is suspected, the plan of care should include proposed management of this newly diagnosed and serious disorder. The patient should be told of the suspected diagnosis, and, if necessary, referred for further assessment and treatment. Any other new medical or psychiatric diagnosis, or suspected diagnosis, should be documented and addressed, again irrespective of the parallel plan for pain management.
4. Decide whether the behavioral problems warrant an end to the therapeutic relationship. The ethical foundation of medicine requires that the decision to continue or discontinue any specific therapy be separated from the decision to continue the therapeutic relationship. Discharge of the patient from the medical practice should only occur if the patient's behavior, such as a criminal act or repeated lying, so undermines the therapeutic relationship that ongoing care is not possible. If this is the case, the patient should be informed in writing, given the names and locations of other sources of medical care, and told that emergency care is still available (this can be delegated to a local hospital-based emergency department). If the patient is taking medications that would be unsafe to stop abruptly, he or she should either be referred to a program that provides detoxification or be given a prescription for a tapering dose of the drug. The tapering of an opioid usually can be accomplished quickly by reducing the dose by 50% every 3 days, with an end when the dose reaches that equivalent to about 30 to 60 mg of oral morphine per day.
5. Whether or not the decision is to promptly discharge the patient from the medical practice, a strong suspicion of diversion should lead to a prompt discontinuation of prescribing. Prescription of a controlled substance to someone who is likely to be diverting the drug is prohibited in the United States under the federal CSA. A high index of suspicion that diversion is occurring should be followed by no further prescribing, or if this would place the patient in imminent risk of serious medical compromise, prescribing for no more than a few days with instructions to taper the dose.
6. With the exception of the patient who is likely to be engaged in criminal activity, the clinician is not legally obligated to discontinue prescribing if aberrant drug-related behavior

occurs. Nonetheless, continued prescribing despite clear evidence that serious nonadherence is occurring would not be consistent with good clinical practice. If aberrant drug-related behavior is encountered, the clinician must decide if the type of behavior or its underlying diagnosis (e.g., relapse of an addictive disorder) creates so much risk or burden that the treatment must be discontinued, even as the offer of continued management of pain or other medical problems is made. This has been called an *exit strategy*. If, however, the clinician perceives a high likelihood that the nonadherence behavior will stop and monitoring can be improved, then opioid treatment should be continued.

7. If the decision is made to continue prescribing, the treatment should be promptly re-structured to accomplish three goals: First, prescriber control over the therapy must be regained and the new structure should help the patient maintain control over impulsive use. Second, the new structure for prescribing should enhance the ability to monitor the therapy. Third, the goals of good pain control and maintenance or improvement of function should be retained. The restructuring of the therapy to regain control and enhance monitoring should consider all of the strategies that are used when long-term treatment is initiated for the first time (see Structuring Therapy to Reduce Risk). This may include a written agreement, frequent visits, small quantities prescribed, urine drug screening, and required consultations, perhaps with a specialist in addiction medicine or pain medicine.

8. The documentation surrounding the response to aberrant drug-related behavior should be comprehensive and demonstrate both the rationale for clinical actions and the actions themselves.

Other Issues in the Treatment of the Substance Abuser with Pain

Based on clinical experience, some of the salient differences among subsets of those with substance use disorders can be explored in terms of their impact on the principles discussed above.

Patients with a Remote History of Substance Abuse

Patients with a remote history of alcohol or drug abuse should be stratified as relatively high risk irrespective of the context and setting of opioid prescribing. These patients require more intensive monitoring because of both a presumed increased risk of abuse and addiction and the potential for undertreatment pain. Undertreatment may be related to clinician or patient factors, or both. The stigma associated with a substance abuse history may lead medical or nursing staff to assume that pain reports reflect drug-seeking and should be addressed by the withholding of treatment. Conversely, patients may fear that treatment with an opioid or other abusable drug may lead to relapse, and for this reason, they withhold complaints or underdose. The optimal management of the patient with pain and remote history of addiction must incorporate careful, ongoing assessment and education of the staff and the patient.

Patients in Methadone Maintenance Programs

Patients enrolled in methadone maintenance programs vary in the extent to which craving is controlled and drug abuse behaviors are occurring. Chronic pain is highly prevalent in this population but access to pain therapy is limited (51). Should a patient receiving methadone for addiction seek pain care, the assessment should clarify the nature and effectiveness of the program (the patient should specifically consent in writing to information sharing with the program, and the clinician who manages the pain should determine the results of recent urine drug screening and related information maintained by the program); this assessment should judge the strength of the recovery and the extent to which the patient has access to supports that may help to sustain it. Opioid therapy should be considered for long-term therapy only if there is evidence that the patient's recovery has been established sufficiently to justify a trial and other pain management strategies are unavailable or have proven to be ineffective.

Generally, patients who are considered for opioid therapy should be continued on their daily dose of methadone. This applies to all treatment settings. Occasionally, the patient undergoing methadone treatment for addiction responds so well to long-term opioid therapy for pain that the specific treatment for addiction can be withdrawn (52). This decision should be taken only if there is evidence over time to support it, and only after careful discussion with the patient and clinicians at the methadone treatment program.

If acute or chronic pain is considered for opioid therapy, the methadone-treated population is likely to be at high risk of undertreatment. Negative stereotyping by medical staff may increase the reluctance to prescribe, and the opioid dose selected may be less likely to work because of opioid tolerance related to the concurrent methadone administration. If persistent pain reports are interpreted as a manipulative attempt to obtain opioids for purposes other than analgesia, the therapeutic relationship may become conflicted and the clinician's goals for analgesia may be superseded by the desire to prevent drug abuse. This concern is legitimate if the patient develops a return of aberrant drug-taking behaviors, but if "drug seeking" reflects only the need for pain relief, undertreatment will result from the failure to respond.

The methadone-treated patient can be treated with methadone or another opioid for pain. If methadone is used, dosing for pain usually requires drug administration every 6 to 8 hours, and like other opioids, this regimen can be coadministered with a once-daily dose of methadone given by the program. As described previously, documentation in the medical record must be meticulous in the United States, describing the opioid treatment (including methadone, if given) as treatment for pain and not addiction. The specific dose of the opioid used for pain may be substantially higher than anticipated, although this does not occur in all cases (53). When initiating treatment with opioid, it is best to begin with standard doses and titrate these doses rapidly should the outcomes be unhelpful.

Patients Receiving Opioid-Agonist Therapy with Buprenorphine

Buprenorphine offers another option for opioid agonist therapy of addiction and is increasing in use. It is now being used as an analgesic in many countries. The assessment, assumption of high risk, careful selection of patients for consideration of opioid therapy, need to structure therapy in a manner to mitigate risk, and requirement for careful documentation during pain therapy all parallel the approach taken with methadone-maintained patients.

The pharmacology of buprenorphine is characterized by high-affinity binding to the mu-receptor, a half-life longer than a day, and partial agonism. The high affinity raises concern that the buprenorphine-treated patient may not respond to administration of a pure mu-agonist drug, at least at typical doses. There is very little experience with the coadministration of another pure mu-agonist drug to the buprenorphine-treated patient, either for acute pain or for chronic pain (54). Although it is possible that the patient who experiences severe pain during buprenorphine treatment for addiction could be managed by increasing and dividing the dose of buprenorphine, there also is very little experience with this approach. Based on anecdotal experience, acute pain should be treated initially with mu-agonist opioid doses that are conventional for the setting, but if the response is poor, the dose should be rapidly titrated. In most cases, the buprenorphine should be continued at the prior dose while this is carried out. For chronic pain, the same principles would apply, with the expectation that there is a dose of a pure mu-agonist that may provide added pain relief. Research is needed to clarify the outcomes associated with the management of acute and chronic pain in buprenorphine-treated patients.

Active Drug Abusers

Patients with active alcohol or drug abuse are presumed to be at high risk for nonadherence. In the monitored setting, acute pain can be managed using conventional means, such as intravenous patient-controlled analgesia, but staff must be prepared to manage the type of problems that may be associated with drug abuse, including the development of withdrawal phenomena, comorbid psychiatric disease, and responses to opioid drugs for pain that may be difficult to interpret.

In the ambulatory setting, the use of a controlled prescription drug in the context of current abuse is very challenging. Prescribing is not acceptable if diversion is expected, and even if it is not the case, the abusing patient may be perceived as incapable of honest reporting and this, too, would contraindicate therapy.

All cases deserve careful assessment, however, and there may be scenarios in which a trial of opioid treatment might be considered. For example, the patient who is actively abusing alcohol or marijuana and is entering a treatment program with close monitoring may be assessed as more likely to proceed into recovery if pain is controlled. Given the heterogeneity of the population abusing drugs, the question that must be addressed is whether the specifics of the situation warrant the risk of an appropriately structured treatment trial.

CONCLUSION

Although an exploration of the issues at the interface between pain and substance abuse focuses on the opioid drugs, decision making in the clinical setting must be informed by a broader knowledge of the varied modalities used to manage acute and chronic pain. Recent texts describe the breadth of therapies—pharmacologic and nonpharmacologic—that can be employed in the management of pain (55) and the influence of a patient's substance use history on the selection and implementation of these therapies (56). The optimal treatment of acute or chronic pain, irrespective of the pain diagnosis and the unique characteristics of the patient, always must consider the risks and benefits of an opioid-based treatment trial against the risks and benefits of other potential strategies. This analysis requires familiarity with other analgesic approaches, an understanding of conventional practice, and good judgment that takes into account the feasibility and goals that surround the plan of care.

The relatively straightforward decision to use a conventional intravenous opioid regimen for any patient who is opioid-naive and experiencing acute severe pain in the inpatient setting has little in common with the complexity of the decisions involved in the treatment of other populations. This complexity is most apparent in the development of a plan for the patient with opioid addiction who has developed a serious chronic pain disorder. Clinicians who assume responsibility for the management of pain often must coordinate consultations and cotreatment by a group of professionals who can provide insight into the options for pain management, the nature of the associated medical and psychiatric disorders, and the strategies that can be used to reduce the risk of therapeutic nonadherence, undertreatment, or drug abuse. The principles that underlie the safe and effective use of opioid drugs provide the foundation for the development of broader strategies for pain management that promise compassionate and competent care for every patient with pain.

REFERENCES

1. The Mayday Fund Special Committee. Available at: http://www.maydaypainreport.org. Accessed on September 7, 2010.
2. Portenoy RK, Bruns D, Shoemaker B, et al. Breakthrough pain in community-dwelling patients with cancer pain and noncancer pain: part 1—prevalence and characteristics. *J Opioid Manage.* 2010, in press.
3. Portenoy RK, Bruns D, Shoemaker B, et al. Breakthrough pain in community-dwelling patients with cancer pain and noncancer pain: part 2—impact on function, mood, and quality of life. *J Opioid Manage.* 2010, in press.
4. Dworkin RH, O'Connor AB, Audette J, et al. Recommendations for the pharmacological management of neuropathic pain: an overview and literature update. *Mayo Clin Proc.* 2010;85(3 suppl):S3–S14.
5. Merskey H, Bogduk N. *Classification of Chronic Pain*, 2nd ed. Seattle: IASP Press; 1994.

6. Savage SR, Joranson DE, Covington EC, et al. Definitions related to the medical use of opioids: evolution towards universal agreement. *J Pain Symptom Manage.* 2003;26(1):655–657.
7. Rosenblum A, Marsch L, Joseph H, et al. Opioids and the treatment of chronic pain: controversies, current status and future directions. *Exp Clin Psychopharm.* 2008:16:405–416.
8. Wikler A. *Opioid Dependence: Mechanisms and Treatment.* New York, NY: Plenum Press; 1980.
9. Chapman CR, Hill HF. Prolonged morphine self-administration and addiction liability: evaluation of two theories in a bone marrow transplant unit. *Cancer.* 1989;63:1636–1644.
10. Adriaensen H, Vissers K, Noorduin H, et al. Opioid tolerance and dependence: an *inevitable* consequence of chronic treatment? *Acta Anaesthesiol Belg.* 2003;54(1):37–47.
11. American Psychiatric Association. *Diagnostic and Statistical Manual of Mental Disorders.* 4th ed., Text Rev. Washington, DC: American Psychiatric Association; 2000.
12. Weissman DE, Haddox JD. Opioid pseudoaddiction—an iatrogenic syndrome. *Pain.* 1989;36:363–366.
13. Noble M, Treadwell JR, Tregear SJ, et al. Long-term opioid management for chronic noncancer pain. *Cochrane Database Syst Rev.* 2010 Jan 20;(1):CD006605.
14. Chou R, Ballantyne JC, Fanciullo GJ, et al. Research gaps on use of opioids for chronic noncancer pain: findings from a review of the evidence for an American Pain Society and American Academy of Pain Medicine clinical practice guideline. *J Pain.* 2009;10(2):147–159.
15. Chou R, Fanciullo GJ, Fine PG, et al. American Pain Society-American Academy of Pain Medicine Opioids Guidelines Panel: Clinical guidelines for the use of chronic opioid therapy in chronic noncancer pain. *J Pain.* 2009;10(11):3–30.
16. Fine PG, Portenoy RK, and the Ad Hoc Expert Panel on Evidence Review and Guidelines for Opioid Rotation. Establishing "best practices" for opioid rotation: conclusions of an expert panel. *J Pain Symptom Manage.* 2009;38:418–425.
17. Dean M. Opioids in renal failure and dialysis patients. *J Pain Symptom Manage.* 2004;28:497–504.
18. Ahmedzai S, Brooks D. Transdermal fentanyl versus sustained-release oral morphine in cancer pain: preference, efficacy, and quality of life. The TTS-Fentanyl Comparative Trial Group. *J Pain Symptom Manage.* 1997;13:254–261.
19. Modesto-Lowe V, Brooks D, Petry N. Methadone deaths. Risk factors in pain and addicted populations. *J Gen Intern Med.* 2010;25(4):305–309.
20. Plummer JL, Cherry DA, Cousins MJ, et al. Long-term spinal administration of morphine in cancer and non-cancer pain: a retrospective study. *Pain.* 1991;44:215–220.
21. Kornick CA, Kilborn MJ, Santiago-Palma J, et al. QTc interval prolongation associated with intravenous methadone. *Pain.* 2003;105:499–506.
22. Cruciani RA, Homel P, Yap Y, et al. QTc measurements in patients on methadone. *J Pain Symptom Manage.* 2005;29:385–391.
23. Patel VB, Manchikanti L, Singh V, et al. Systematic review of intrathecal infusion systems for long-term management of chronic non-cancer pain. *Pain Physician.* 2009;12(2):345–360.
24. Smith TJ, Staats PS, Deer T, et al. Implantable Drug Delivery Systems Study Group. Randomized clinical trial of an implantable drug delivery system compared with comprehensive medical management for refractory cancer pain: impact on pain, drug-related toxicity, and survival. *J Clin Oncol.* 2002;20:4040–4049.
25. Staats PS, Yearwood T, Charapata SG, et al. Intrathecal ziconotide in the treatment of refractory pain in patients with cancer or AIDS: a randomized controlled trial. *J Amer Med Assoc.* 2004; 291:63–70.
26. Zeppetella G, Ribeiro MD. Opioids for the management of breakthrough (episodic) pain in cancer patients. *Cochrane Database Syst Rev.* 2006:CD004311.
27. American Pain Society. *Principles of Analgesic Use in the Treatment of Acute Pain and Cancer Pain.* 5th ed. Skokie, IL: American Pain Society; 2003.
28. Ripamonti CI, Bareggi C. Pharmacology of opioid analgesia: clinical principles. In: Bruera EB, Portenoy RK, eds. *Cancer Pain: Assessment and Management.* New York: Cambridge University Press; 2010:195–229.
29. Chou R, Clark E, Helfand M. Comparative efficacy and safety of long-acting oral opioids for chronic non-cancer pain: a systematic review. *J Pain Symptom Manage.* 2003;26(5):1026–1048.
30. Bannister K, Dickenson AH. Opioid hyperalgesia. *Curr Opin Support Palliat Care.* 2010;4(1):1–5.
31. Portenoy R, Taylor D, Messina J, et al. A randomized, placebo-controlled study of fentanyl effervescent buccal tablets for breakthrough pain in opioid-treated patients with cancer. *Clin J Pain.* 2006;22:805–811.
32. Benyamin R, Trescot AM, Datta S, et al. Opioid complications and side effects. *Pain Physician.* 2008;11(2 suppl):S105–S120.
33. Ahmedzai SH, Boland J. Constipation in people prescribed opioids. *Clin Evid. (Online)* 2007;Jun 1:pii:2407.
34. McNicol E, Boyce DB, Schumann R, et al. Efficacy and safety of mu-opioid antagonists in the treatment of opioid-induced bowel dysfunction: systematic review and meta-analysis of randomized controlled trials. *Pain Med.* 2008;9:634–659.
35. Daniell HW. Opioid endocrinopathy in women consuming prescribed sustained-action opioids for control of non-malignant pain. *J Pain.* 2008;9:28–36.
36. Daniell HW. Hypogonadism in men consuming sustained-action oral opioids. *J Pain.* 2002;3:377–384.
37. Walker JM, Farney RJ. Are opioids associated with sleep apnea? A review of the evidence. *Curr Pain Headache Rep.* 2009;13: 120–126.
38. Webster L, Choi Y, Desai H, et al. Sleep-disordered breathing and chronic opioid therapy. *Pain Med.* 2008;9:425–432.
39. Paulozzi LJ, Budnitz DS, Yongli X. Increasing deaths from opioid analgesics in the United States. *Pharmacoepidemiol Drug Saf.* 2006;15:618–627.
40. Passik SD, Kirsh KL, Whitcomb LA, et al. A new tool to assess and document pain outcomes in chronic pain patients receiving opioid therapy. *Clin Ther.* 2004;26:552–561.
41. Gourlay DL, Heit HA, Almahrezi A. Universal precautions in pain medicine: a rational approach to the treatment of chronic pain. *Pain Med.* 2005;6(2):107–112.
42. Gilson AM, Ryan KM, Joranson DE, et al. A reassessment of trends in the medical use and abuse of opioid analgesics and implications for diversion control: 1997–2002. *J Pain Symptom Manage.* 2004;28:176–188.
43. Federation of State Medical Boards of the United States, Inc. Model Policy for the Use of Controlled Substances for the Treatment of Pain. Available at: http://www.fsmb.org/pdf/ 2004_grpol_Controlled_Substances.pdf. Accessed on September 7, 2010.
44. Chou R, Fanciullo GJ, Fine PG, et al. Opioids for chronic non-cancer pain: prediction and identification of aberrant drug-related behaviors: a review of the evidence for an American Pain Society and American Academy of Pain Medicine clinical practice guideline. *J Pain.* 2009;10(2):131–146.

45. Moore TM, Jones T, Browder JH, et al. A comparison of common screening methods for predicting aberrant drug-related behavior among patients receiving opioids for chronic pain management. *Pain Med.* 2009;10(8):1426–1433.
46. Passik SD, Kirsh KL, Casper D. Addiction-related assessment tools and pain management: instruments for screening, treatment-planning, and monitoring compliance. *Pain Med.* 2008;9(suppl 2):S145–S166.
47. Cone EJ, Caplan YH. Urine toxicology testing in chronic pain management. *Postgrad Med.* 2009;121(4):91–102.
48. Manchikanti L, Manchukonda R, Pampati V, et al. Does random urine drug testing reduce illicit drug use in chronic pain patients receiving opioids? *Pain Physician.* 2006;9(2):123–129.
49. Fishman SM, Kreis PG. The opioid contract. *Clin J Pain.* 2002;18:S70–S75.
50. The American Academy of Pain Medicine. Available at: http://www.painmed.org/pdf/controlled_substances_sample_agrmt.pdf. Accessed on September 7, 2010.
51. Rosenblum A, Joseph H, Fong C, et al. Prevalence and characteristics of chronic pain among chemically dependent patients in methadone maintenance and residential treatment facilities. *JAMA.* 2003;289:2370–2378.
52. Cruciani R, Estaban S, Seewald RM, et al. MMTP patients with chronic pain switching to pain management clinics. A problem or an acceptable practice? *Pain Med.* 2008;9(3):359–364.
53. Kantor TG, Cantor R, Tom E. A study of hospitalized surgical patients on methadone maintenance. *Drug Alcohol Depend.* 1980;6:163173.
54. Heit HA, Gourlay DL. Buprenorphine: new tricks with an old molecule for pain management. *Clin J Pain.* 2008;24(2):93–97. [Erratum in: *Clin J Pain.* 2008;24(4):370].
55. Fishman SM, Ballantyne JC, Rathmell P, eds. *Bonica's Management of Pain.* Philadelphia, PA: Lippincott Williams & Wilkins; 2009.
56. Smith HS, Passik SD, eds. *Pain and Chemical Dependency.* New York: Oxford University Press; 2008.

CHAPTER 52

Substance Use Disorders in Individuals with Co-occurring Psychiatric Disorders

Sylvia J. Dennison

INTRODUCTION

Use of, and withdrawal from, alcohol and other substances of abuse can cause, mimic, or mask psychiatric symptoms. The overlap of signs and symptoms makes it difficult to accurately diagnose all conditions present. However, failing to diagnose any co-occurring disorders (COD) increases the likelihood that the individual's treatment needs will not be met, worsening the patient's prognosis.

For some time, individuals with both psychiatric and substance problems have been called "dually diagnosed." This term is now felt to be confusing, appearing to imply, as it does, that only two conditions exist. Currently, individuals who concomitantly suffer from one or more psychiatric and one or more substance-related problems are said to have COD. The population of individuals with COD poses a particular challenge to the treating professional. A working understanding of psychiatric conditions and the motivation for substance use are important, as is the impact various substances of abuse have on psychiatric conditions. It is not enough for the treatment provider to deal with only one problem. If the treating professional is not proficient in the approach to one or the other problems, it is incumbent upon him to see to it that the COD client gets the additional care he needs.

HISTORY

That psychiatric and substance use disorders commonly co-occur is now well recognized, as are the facts that such co-occurrence is predictive of high utilization of services and poor treatment adherence. Prior to this recognition, fractionation of care was the norm, with mental health providers refusing to treat substance abusers, substance abuse treatment providers refusing to work with those with mental illnesses, and both camps often missing the presence of one or the other disorders.

Once it became clear there was a population for whom addiction alone was not the problem, the issue of cause and effect became a subject of debate. Arguments arose regarding which came first. Was the person depressed because he was drinking heavily, or did he drink heavily because he was depressed? Was she psychotic because she was a daily marijuana user, or did she choose to smoke the drug because, as she claimed, it calmed her nerves and helped her rest? Was he anxious because he chronically abused benzodiazepines and felt the rebound effect, or did he use the benzodiazepines because of his chronic state of anxiety?

Traditional providers of addiction treatment saw the problem as substance abuse and any other unacceptable behaviors as simply excuses to justify continued drug use. The more psychologically minded developed the theory that the addicted individual used his drug(s) of choice as a means of treating uncomfortable or unacceptable impulses (1), the so-called self-medication hypothesis of addictive disorders (2).

Regardless of the cause(s) of ongoing substance use, many mental health treatment providers refused to treat any other psychopathology until the substance use disorder had been addressed and the individual abstinent, sometimes for many months. Unfortunately, such an approach condemned the individual with an untreated mental illness to a high likelihood of early relapse and an overall poorer outcome (1,3).

This fragmented approach to treatment left many, if not most, COD patients without treatment of any sort. For those who did seek treatment, early dropout was common. By the late 1980s, it was increasingly recognized that a new, coordinated approach to care was essential for meeting the needs of persons with COD. In response, the concept of "No wrong door" was introduced (4). No matter where the COD patient presented, providers were admonished to be ready to intervene on his behalf to make treatment immediately available. This approach meant that the alcohol-dependent client with depression must be given access to mental health care at the earliest possible time just as the bipolar client with cocaine dependence must receive immediate help for his stimulant habit.

The cost, morbidity, and mortality of COD prompted the U.S. government, in 2003, to create the Co-Occurring Center for Excellence (COCE) through the Substance Abuse and Mental Health Services Administration (SAMHSA). Its purpose was to function as a resource for the dissemination of information regarding evidence-based approaches to this population as well as to foster the adoption of such practices (5). Over its 5-year course, the COCE served as a clearinghouse for information, data collection, and grants for research on COD. Though its mission is over, this is still a valuable resource. COCE can be accessed at http://coce.samhsa.gov.

A consensus panel, also convened by SAMSHA, provided a definition of COD, a definition that will be used throughout this review. That is, that people with COD are

> ... individuals who have at least one psychiatric disorder as well as an alcohol or drug disorder. While these disorders may interact differently in any person (e.g., an episode of depression may trigger a relapse into alcohol abuse, or cocaine use may exacerbate schizophrenic symptoms) at least one disorder of each type can be diagnosed independently of the other. (6)

EPIDEMIOLOGY

Simply suffering from a mental illness greatly increases the likelihood that the individual will have a comorbid substance use disorder. According to the SAMHSA (7), in 2002 there were over 17.5 million American adults with serious mental illnesses, of whom nearly a quarter had a comorbid substance use disorder. Despite the numbers involved, more than half of those with COD received no treatment for either disorder and only 11.8% received treatment for both.

Further reports from SAMSHA (8) suggest that the cost of treatment of mental health and substance abuse will top $239 billion by 2014. This is a fivefold increase over costs from 1986 ($42 billion) and double that of 2003 ($121 billion). Importantly, these data reflect only the direct costs of treatment, not the additional costs of substance-related illnesses, decreased productivity, police intervention, and incarceration (Table 52.1).

Recognizing that preventing the emergence of COD is preferable to treating established illness, research has focused on the issue of which disorder came first. Unfortunately, the data are often contradictory. Some studies showed early onset of substance misuse in adolescence predicts the later development of some types of psychiatric disorders (9). Others found that childhood or other early psychiatric symptoms predict the later emergence of substance use disorders (10,11). Yet another (12) suggested either could precede or follow the other depending on the exact psychiatric diagnosis and the specific substance of abuse, all of which make the development of prevention strategies very difficult.

Just as there may be a difference in the timing of onset of symptoms of substance use problems and of psychiatric symptoms, there is a difference in the frequency with which the various psychiatric disorders are associated with substance use problems. For example, any affective disorder appears to be frequently associated with substance use disorders with slightly more than 40% of cases of unipolar depression associated with alcohol problems (13). Bipolar disorder is associated with any substance use disorder in more than 40% of cases (14) and an additional 17% of unipolar respondents associated with a nonalcohol substance use disorder (13). Further, the presence of a substance use disorder increases the frequency of depressive episodes in individuals with either type of disorder (15) as well as that of suicide in depressed individuals (16).

According to the Surgeon General's Report (17), as many as 65% of persons with at least one mental disorder " ... also have a lifetime history of a least one substance use disorder." A major source of data for that declaration comes from the Epidemiological Catchment Area study (18), considered one of the most comprehensive studies of COD and a rich source of information for nearly 20 years. A replication study is under way to update the information, and analysis of those data is now under way. It is likely that replication data will provide the same invaluable service as provided by its predecessor. However, for now the original study is the source of much of the data shown here. In this study, Regier et al. (18) found that among individuals with schizophrenia, from 25% in community samples to 66% of individuals in specialized samples such as Veterans Affairs, community mental health, and inpatient samples are estimated to have comorbid substance use disorders. The anxiety disorders, on the other hand, have a much more variable rate of comorbidity, depending on the specific diagnosis. Nevertheless, substance use disorders co-occur at a much higher rate among individuals with anxiety disorders than among the general population (19), with the possible exception of social phobia (20).

The co-occurrence of psychiatric and substance use disorders has social, economic, and prognostic implications. When substance misuse and mental illness co-occur, the risk is great that, in general, the individual will not do as well as if he had not developed such a comorbid problem. Poverty and homelessness (21) are more frequent, as are the risks of being both victim and perpetrator of violent assault (22–24). It is important to note that while most violent crimes are not committed by the mentally ill, those that are perpetrated by members of this population are more likely to be committed by those with COD. Furthermore, among the mentally ill, substance use also increases the risk of both accidental and homicide deaths (25). Yet another issue that has taken on extreme importance is that of greater risk taking among COD clients in terms of sexual behaviors and needle sharing. Such behaviors have resulted in an increased risk for HIV and similar medical conditions in this population (26,27) (Table 52.2).

Comorbidity, in short, is associated with a greater number of social and health consequences than either disorder alone. Thus, although substance misuse per se is a source of significant social and medical morbidity and mortality, in the case of the mentally ill, the problems become magnified many times over.

TABLE 52.1	Direct cost of treating COD (in billions of dollars)
1986	42
2003	121
2014 (projected)	239

TABLE 52.2	Consequences of co-occurring disorders
Increased likelihood of poverty	
Increased likelihood of homelessness	
Increased likelihood of being the victim of abuse	
Increased likelihood of being a perpetrator of violence	
Increased likelihood of engaging in high-risk behaviors	
Increased risk of death via homicide, suicide, and accidental means	

EVALUATION OF THE PATIENT WITH CO-OCCURRING DISORDERS

That it is extremely important to detect the presence of co-occurring conditions early in the evaluation process cannot be overstated. Identification of such conditions subsequent to initial hospitalization for psychiatric disorders results in more hospitalizations and poorer long-term outcome (28).

Having said this, it is also clear assessing the COD client is more complicated than assessing patients with either condition as, again, substance use and psychiatric disorders can mimic, mask, or exacerbate the symptoms of each other. It is obvious that a psychiatric workup is necessary if such has not already been done. Helpful information includes the patient's past diagnoses, if the patient is aware of what they may have been, past hospitalizations for psychiatric reasons, what prompted the psychiatric admission, response to treatment, family history of psychiatric problems, what medications he has had in the past and how he reacted to each. Furthermore, the interviewer should ask about suicidal ideation, both current and past, as well as attempts.

It is also useful to determine if the psychiatric symptoms predated the onset of the individual's substance misuse. Note should be made as to whether or not the patient's psychiatric condition improves, disappears, or worsens when the patient isn't using the substance(s). Unfortunately, it is often impossible to determine either of the above. If the patient uses substances daily and has no substantial periods of clean time, it will not be possible to know if his symptoms improve with abstinence. Likewise, if the patient has been using substances for many years, memory may not prove accurate as to whether the substance misuse or the psychiatric symptoms came first.

Although assuring the safety of the patient must always be a consideration in dealing with the chemically dependent, it is of paramount importance when dealing with the COD individual who poses a greater risk for dangerous behaviors. Patients in the immediate poststimulant dysphoric state or who are acutely under the influence of depressants such as alcohol are at an increased risk of self-harm, regardless of whether or not they have a comorbid psychiatric condition. Both acute and chronic use of substances of abuse, however, vastly magnify the risk of suicide in individuals with depression and other chronic, severe mental illnesses, including schizophrenia and bipolar illness. Thus, at intake and at frequent intervals throughout the treatment process, the patient's risk of suicide must be assessed.

The treatment provider must be prepared to make judgments about the safety of using medications in patients who may be acutely under the influence of a substance in order to adequately treat this complicated population. For this reason, a brief review of some common medication–street substance interactions follows in the next section. An excellent and much more comprehensive review of drug–drug interactions can be found in Ciraulo et al. (29).

Typical assessment questions must be asked of the COD patient—age at onset of use, what is used, quantity, and how the substance is administered, that is, orally, intranasally, intravenously, rectally, etc. The method called a time line followback may be helpful to jog the patient's memory as to episodes of use. In this technique the patient uses a calendar to remind himself of specific dates or events during which he was actively using. In addition, just as in a non-COD population, collateral information should be obtained if at all available. Oral screening tools used to assess for alcohol and other substance abuse may be less helpful in the COD population, though there is still a place for the Michigan Alcohol Screening Test (MAST) and Drug Abuse Screening Test (DAST) with this population. Use of these tools is described elsewhere and will not be discussed here. It must be borne in mind, though, that the COD population is more likely to experience social isolation, and be unemployed and homeless, rendering some typical questions moot.

While the user may identify himself as having a problem with a specific substance, it is important to ask about substances used with the drug of choice. For example, while readily admitting that he is addicted to cocaine, the same patient may neglect to mention, as feeling it is irrelevant, that he is also ingesting a fifth of hard liquor during cocaine binges. This knowledge is necessary in order to avoid missing such needs as safe withdrawal from alcohol and to screen for further physical damage that may result from such concomitant use.

Understanding the user's motivation for substance use can also be helpful in developing an overall treatment plan. The individual suffering from panic disorder and agoraphobia in middle school, for example, may find that alcohol, at least temporarily, will help relieve her anxiety symptoms (30). Fear of the return or worsening of anxiety symptoms in abstinence may impede her progress toward abstinence. Likewise, nicotine has been shown to lessen the cognitive problems associated with schizophrenia (31), a fact that the psychotic user may be exploiting, either consciously or unconsciously.

As noted previously, it has been postulated that the person with COD is self-medicating with his drug of choice, something argued for a couple of decades. Regardless of the motivation for use, the facts above citing the potential benefits of the substances abused make it important to ask the user what it is he wants to feel as a result of use of his drug(s) of choice. It is possible that the only answer will be "to get high." However, it is also possible that there is truly a benefit

TABLE 52.3	Psychiatric evaluation of the COD patient		
Psychiatric symptoms			
	Age of onset	Pre/postsubstance use disorder	
	Hospitalizations for psychiatric reasons?	Substance related?	
	Diagnose(s)? (list all)	Effect of substance (ab)use on symptoms	
Family history of SUD			
	Who?		
	Their diagnoses		
	Also with substance use disorders?		
Past treatment episodes (nonmedication)			
	Types (e.g., hospitalization, day hospital, etc.)	Number of times	
	Response to treatment		
History of suicide attempts			
	By what means?	Number of times	
	Substance related? (under the influence, in withdrawal, etc.)	If so, what substance?	
Nicotine/caffeine use			
	Amount/frequency		
	Effect		
History of prescription use			
	Name	Compliant with treatment?	
	Abusing substances concomitantly?	What?	
	Effect of medication		
History of abuse of prescriptions			
	Own medications? Others' medications?	Why?	
	What (list all)		
	Frequency		
	Response		
	Effect on psychiatric symptoms		
History of over-the-counter drug abuse			
	What (list all)		
	Frequency		
	Response	Was this the desired response? If not, what was the desired response?	
	Using prescription medications at times?		

that the user is seeking. Such information can be invaluable in establishing treatment goals.

Use and abuse of common substances such as caffeine and tobacco should be explored in any addicted population. However, it takes on even greater importance with COD clients. Caffeine may significantly worsen symptoms of anxiety and panic (32). Nicotine, on the other hand, may increase the metabolism of a variety of psychoactive medications, resulting in a need for ever greater doses in order to treat psychiatric symptoms (29). The latter is particularly important in hospitals and other facilities that forbid smoking, as the abrupt withdrawal of nicotine can result in a rapid rise in psychiatric medications and the emergence of uncomfortable side effects.

Prescription and over-the-counter drug abuse should also be asked about. If the individual is getting early refills on any prescription, even those not typically thought of as intoxicants, efforts should be made to determine the reason. Clonidine, for example, may be abused to help mitigate the effects of opiate withdrawal. However, at high enough doses, this alpha-adrenergic antihypertensive can result in a "drug store high," a mild sedation in its own right (33). Likewise, highly anticholinergic agents such as benztropine, used, among other things, to counter the side effects of some antipsychotic medications, are well recognized for their significant abuse potential (34). Further, readily available over-the-counter medications containing dextromethorphan can induce a common, and potentially lethal, high, especially in alcohol abusers.

As with any substance-dependent individual, the COD patient should have intake and random drug screens performed. It is also essential, though, that the clinician be familiar with what the toxicologic tests available in his facility are actually testing for. For example, some emergency rooms and laboratories do not include PCP or LSD in their routine screens, yet these substances are often around (8). Further, buprenorphine is surfacing as a recreational drug and also may not be on routine tests. Thus, it is helpful to be familiar with what one is really asking for in a "routine screen."

Medical screening is highly important in this population. As noted earlier, COD patients, especially those with psychotic disorders, are more likely to engage in high-risk behaviors than the non-COD population. Thus, the incidence of HIV, hepatitis C, and other health problems is quite high (35) (Table 52.3).

TREATMENT

Historically, three basic approaches to treatment of COD patients were used: sequential, parallel, and integrated models. In the sequential model, first one and then the other condition was treated. The idea was that one condition had to be under control before the second could be adequately addressed. Of course, determining which condition to treat first presented a significant problem. In addition, addiction-treatment programs have not typically been designed to meet the needs of the mentally ill, while mental health providers were reticent to treat intoxicated patients and ill-equipped to handle them (36).

In the parallel model, both conditions were addressed simultaneously, but in different programs with different staff. Poor communication between staff and the potential for the patient to receive mixed messages posed substantial risk, however. Further, treatment philosophies often clashed and goals were often markedly different between addiction and mental health treatment programs.

Finally, in the integrated model, both conditions are treated simultaneously by providers knowledgeable about both conditions. This is the approach most strongly supported by providers and by evidence-based studies (37).

To address some of the deficiencies inherent in existing programs, there has been a major initiative at the national level to educate mental health and addiction-treatment providers in each other's specialties. Cross-training is promoted at national, state, and local levels. Special certification programs have been developed to standardize and measure necessary levels of knowledge and skills, and to promote quality programming for treating individuals with COD. Where once treatment programs consisted, in many respects, of promoting the principles of Alcoholics Anonymous and other 12-step, self-help programs, it is now accepted that working with the dually disordered is a much more complex task than this. The treatment provider must help the patient gain an understanding of the patient's substance use disorder, of the patient's mental illness, and of the impact one has on the other. Further, research suggests that family, legal, and vocational services be included in "integrated treatment."

A way of conceptualizing the severity of the needs of any given patient has been developed, the four quadrants of COD. Most states use this model for assessing which patients have the greatest needs. The practitioner working with patients with COD should be familiar with this concept. However, it is not as meaningful for the individual or small group of practitioners as it is for larger systems of care. Thus, a great deal of time will not be spent reviewing this beyond the brief description below.

In the quadrant model, the mental illness and the substance use disorder are viewed individually in terms of severity of symptoms, and then grouped together to determine the level of care the individual needs. Less severe mental disorder and substance use disorder are quadrant I, severe mental illness and less severe substance use disorder quadrant II, less severe mental disorder with more severe substance use disorder quadrant III, and severe levels of both substance and psychiatric disorders quadrant IV. Clearly, the latter is viewed as requiring the highest level of care and may include housing, legal intervention, treatment for each disorder, and coordination among a number of entities in order to meet the individual's needs. The reader is referred to the Center for Substance Abuse Treatment (CSAT) publication *Treatment Improvement Protocol* (TIP) number 42 (37) for a comprehensive review of how this is used in dealing with COD (Fig. 52.1).

Comprehensive treatment for COD individuals demands that programming provide integrated mental health and addiction treatment and includes flexibility, repetition, long-term support, and medication where necessary (38). Increasing

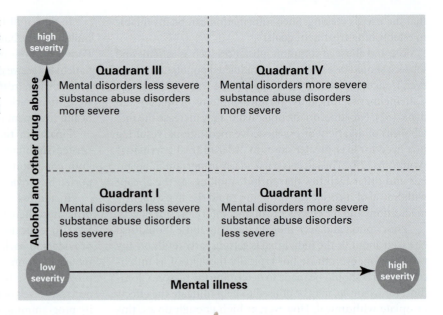

Figure 52.1. Quadrant model for patient care. Adapted from Center for Substance Abuse Treatment. *Substance Abuse Treatment for Persons with Co-occurring Disorders. Treatment Improvement Protocol (TIP) Series 42.* DHHS Publication No. (SMA) 05-3922. Rockville, MD: Substance Abuse and Mental Health Services Administration; 2005.

evidence suggests that individuals with COD are more likely to seek treatment in mental health programs with addiction-treatment components (39) and less likely to receive the breadth of treatment recommended for treating COD clients in addiction treatment–based programs (40). Further, provision of on-site mental health care results in better psychological functioning and decreased substance use (41).

Medication(s) When Necessary

There is no question that some psychiatric conditions can be treated with psychotherapy, behavioral interventions, and other psychotherapeutic techniques. There has been considerable concern among addiction-treatment providers that jumping in quickly with a pill to treat a patient's discomfort sends a wrong message. That is, it signals that only a substance, not personal learned strengths and skills, can help the individual through hard times. The problem with the latter reasoning, though, is that the addicted person with a co-occurring psychiatric condition who presents for treatment typically hasn't learned the alternate means of dealing with his hallucinations or depression, or he wouldn't be there in the first place. Furthermore, psychotherapeutic interventions take time to be learned and rehearsed and, while effective for some psychiatric conditions, are not as beneficial for others. In addition, the dually disordered are at a high risk of dropout and relapse. Waiting for lengthy interventions to take effect may ensure the patient's early withdrawal from treatment long before a positive response can occur. Finally, at least for the severely mentally ill, medication is typically a first, not a last, choice. Early and vigorous intervention with medication, where indicated, using nonaddictive agents may help the patient stay in treatment and gain confidence that he can learn the techniques he needs for dealing with his substance use and psychiatric disorders.

That having been said, when dealing with the COD individual, as with any other person with a substance use disorder, when medication is deemed necessary, every effort should be made to use medications that (a) do not induce euphoria, (b) do not cause dependence, (c) are effective in the individual who is actively using substance(s) of abuse, and (d) are safe when used by the active user (Table 52.4).

Psychiatric Conditions, Medications, and Substances of Abuse

The following is not an exhaustive review of all possible medications to treat the various psychiatric conditions, but an effort to give the reader an overview of the types of information available regarding medications that have proven safe and effective in relieving psychiatric symptoms in patients with psychiatric disorders who continue to actively use substances of abuse. It cannot be overstated that the clinician must be vigilant about the possibility that a problem will arise with the medicated individual who is also abusing other substances. It is always possible the individual is using more substances than the treatment provider is aware of, increasing the possibility of a negative consequence.

Depression, Antidepressants, and Mood Stabilizers

Depression and mania can be improved by active treatment with medication even when the patient continues to abuse alcohol, opiates, nicotine, and perhaps marijuana. To date, no

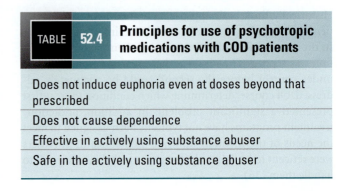

TABLE 52.4 Principles for use of psychotropic medications with COD patients

Does not induce euphoria even at doses beyond that prescribed
Does not cause dependence
Effective in actively using substance abuser
Safe in the actively using substance abuser

medication has been shown to be unequivocally superior in improving such symptoms among individuals abusing psychostimulants.

Tricyclic antidepressants (TCAs) and selective serotonin reuptake inhibitors (SSRIs) decrease depressive symptoms in unipolar depression in actively drinking alcoholics (42,43). The clinician is advised to make TCAs available in very limited supplies, however, to a member of this population, because of the potential for a lethal interaction with alcohol. Concomitant abuse of benzodiazepines, alcohol, cocaine, and marijuana is common among opiate-dependent individuals. This fact, and that much of the research available regarding opiate addicts, comes from methadone-maintenance patients, making it necessary to view data on this population with caution. Nevertheless, there is evidence that simply stabilizing opiate-dependent individuals on methadone improves depressive symptoms. Tricyclics and SSRIs also improve depression in individuals actively using opiates. It should be noted, however, that abuse of TCAs by methadone-maintenance patients is a well-known phenomenon in clinics; thus, such drugs should be used only with close supervision and with only small quantities available. Sertraline may cause an initial rise in methadone levels, which will normalize after a brief interval. There is some evidence that SSRI medication may cause a slight improvement in depressive symptoms in individuals actively abusing marijuana. Thus, erring on the side of the patient and offering to treat these symptoms with medication may be reasonable.

Lithium is relatively ineffective in treating substance-dependent individuals with mania. Furthermore, there is an increased risk of toxicity with this medication if the individual is using alcohol or marijuana. Thus, this mood stabilizer should be avoided in COD clients with bipolar disorder or cyclothymia (29). Divalproex improves manic symptoms in actively drinking alcoholics with this disorder, although close observation of liver functions is essential. In one study, gabapentin decreased alcohol abuse in bipolar patients with alcohol problems (44). However, abuse of this medication is becoming increasingly recognized (45). Quetiapine appears to decrease both manic symptoms and cocaine cravings in dually disordered patients with bipolar disorder and substance use problems. It too appears to be abused by individuals in some populations, however (46). Carbamazepine must be introduced and used with caution among individuals on methadone, because it lowers this opiate's levels, leading to withdrawal (29). Tiagabine may decrease cocaine use in some individuals and has been effectively used for the treatment of bipolar disorder (47). Topiramate is sometimes used as a mood stabilizer and appears to decrease alcohol consumption in some alcohol-dependent individuals, producing interesting possibilities for the use of this agent in COD patients (48).

Psychoses and Antipsychotic Medications

Actively treating psychosis improves retention in both addiction and mental health treatment. Despite concern about the possible interaction between antipsychotics and alcohol, there is little in the literature to support this worry. This may, of course, reflect the long-held habit of withholding antipsychotic medications when individuals with psychoses began to imbibe. Thus, it is reasonable to use this medication with caution in the COD patient. High doses of typical antipsychotic medications in conjunction with cocaine appear to increase the risk of dystonic reactions and perhaps neuroleptic malignant syndrome. Whether or not this applies to other psychostimulants is not known. Risperidone, olanzapine, and clozapine improve symptoms and retention among schizophrenic psychostimulant abusers. Clozaril also appears to decrease substance use in general in COD populations (49). Nicotine acts in competition with some antipsychotic medications (such drugs as haloperidol, fluphenazine, olanzapine, and clozapine), effectively lowering the levels of these agents. It is important for the treatment provider to keep this in mind in the event that a patient is abruptly forced to discontinue his routine dose of nicotine or to have it drastically reduced. The patient's level of neuroleptic medication may become suddenly far greater than it had been, resulting in greatly increased side effects and discomfort.

Anxiety Disorders

Treating anxiety symptoms in individuals actively using alcohol, psychostimulants, and opiates improves retention in treatment and provides some degree of symptom relief. Benzodiazepines are among the top three most-abused prescription drugs in the United States and may be abused by nearly half of individuals seeking treatment for substance misuse. These facts, and that there is some evidence of a disinhibiting effect of some benzodiazepines when used by alcohol-dependent individuals, serve as relative, not absolute, contraindications to their use in this population. Alprazolam, in particular, has been suggested as having this effect. If this class of medication is used, it is advisable to use such agents with caution, in acute situation rather than as a maintenance strategy, under close supervision, and briefly, if at all possible. Furthermore, longer-acting agents should be used. TCAs, SSRIs, and venlafaxine are helpful in relieving anxiety symptoms in individuals with coexisting alcohol and anxiety problems. The existence of so many non-dependence-inducing, effective medications begs the question of necessity of using potentially addictive agents for the treatment of anxiety disorders for any but very short-term problems. Venlafaxine undergoes extensive hepatic metabolism, and close observation of liver functions is advised in individuals abusing alcohol. Many cases of fatal reactions have been reported of opiate-dependent individuals using and abusing benzodiazepines. Consequently, use of this class of agents for individuals with this problem is not advised. Rather, a trial of an SSRI, as in depression, is preferable. Buspirone appears to be effective in reducing symptoms of generalized anxiety disorders in actively drinking alcoholics (50). However, it is also extensively metabolized in the liver, making close monitoring essential.

Use of Disulfiram and Anti-Craving Medications in COD Populations

The use of disulfiram in any population is sometimes controversial, but among those with severe mental illnesses, much more so. Manufacturers themselves warn about the possible emergence of psychosis as a result of the use of this drug. However, with close monitoring for a worsening of psychiatric symptoms, this medication has proven beneficial in reducing alcohol consumption in some populations (51). It appears that acamprosate may be safe and effective for helping reduce alcohol consumption in individuals with mental illnesses, though definitive studies are lacking. Naltrexone may also be safe and effective in reducing alcohol consumption in this population (52). If there is any suspicion of covert use of opiates, however, this medication should be avoided.

SPECIAL CONSIDERATIONS: TOBACCO USE IN CO-OCCURRING DISORDERS

That ongoing tobacco use is associated with increased risk of relapse in substance abusers has become increasingly accepted over the last two decades. However, it also appears that ongoing tobacco use is associated with increased likelihood of early dropout from treatment (53). Historically, individuals with COD, especially those with psychotic disorders, were not expected, or even encouraged, to stop smoking. Infamously, cigarettes were used to bribe inpatients for good behaviors. For example, compliance with rules could result in the individual being rewarded with a cigarette at hourly intervals. There was a popularly held, and fully discredited, belief that there was something about schizophrenia that somehow protected against the development of cancer, so there was no need to treat nicotine dependence.

It is now quite clear that smoking cessation in COD patients is something that should be strongly promoted. However, it must be borne in mind that nicotine has some very positive effects on symptoms of psychiatric disorders, making it an even more attractive drug than it would otherwise be. The COD patient may require a great deal more support, repetition, and help with motivation than might otherwise be the case. Treatment of individuals with co-occurring disorders should include nicotine cessation training as an integral part of any programming, both to aid in retention and to improve overall patient health.

CONCLUSION

Individuals with both substance use and psychiatric disorders constitute a substantial and difficult-to-treat subsection of the addiction population. Addressing only the substance use predicts a lack of improvement in the psychiatric condition and early relapse to alcohol and other drug use. Addressing only the psychiatric condition likewise is unlikely to result in a decrease in substance use. Early and vigorous treatment for each condition should be initiated, including use of medications where indicated. In the latter case, care must be taken that medications used should be proved safe in the individual actively abusing alcohol and other substances, effective in treating the psychiatric condition when the individual is actively using, and nonaddictive where at all possible.

Much remains to be done to demonstrate that one therapeutic modality is clearly superior to another for the treatment-specific comorbid conditions, though studies are under way. It is clear, however, that concomitant treatment of all conditions present—medical, psychiatric, and substance related—must occur if there is any likelihood of improvement in any condition. It is also clear that this complicated and diverse population will present challenges for the treatment community for some time to come.

REFERENCES

1. Brower KJ, Aldrich MS, Robinson EA. Insomnia, self-medication and relapse to alcoholism. *Am J Psychiatry*. 2001;158(3):399–404.
2. Khantzian EJ. The self-medication hypothesis of addictive disorders: focus on heroin and cocaine dependence. *Am J Psychiatry*. 1985;142(11):1259–1264.
3. Xie H, McHugo GJ, Fox MB, et al. Substance abuse relapse in a ten-year prospective follow-up of clients with mental and substance use disorders. *Psychiatr Serv*. 2005;56(10):1282–1287.
4. Department of Health and Human Services. *Improving Substance Abuse Treatment: The National Treatment Plan Initiative. Changing the Conversation*. Rockville, MD: Center for Substance Abuse Treatment; 2000:12.
5. Center for Substance Abuse Treatment, Division of Systems Improvement. *Co-occurring Center for Excellence (COCE)*. Rockville, MD: Substance Abuse and Mental Health Services Administration; 2009.
6. Center for Substance Abuse Treatment. *Substance Abuse Treatment for Persons with Co-occurring Disorders*. Rockville, MD: Substance Abuse and Mental Health Services Administration; 2005.
7. National Survey on Drug Use and Health. *Adults with Co-occurring Serious Mental Illness and a Substance Use Disorder*. Rockville, MD: Office of Applied Studies, Substance Abuse and Mental Health Services Administration; 2004.
8. Substance Abuse and Mental Health Services Administration, Office of Applied Studies. *Drug Abuse Warning Network, 2006: National Estimates of Drug-Related Emergency Department Visits*, SAaMHS Administration, ed. Rockville, MD: Department of Health and Human Services; 2008.
9. Johnson RJ, Kaplan HB. Stability of psychological symptoms: drug use consequences and intervening processes. *J Health Soc Behav*. 1990;31(3):277–291.
10. Kessler RC, McGonagle KA, Zhao S, et al. Lifetime and 12-month prevalence of DSM-III-R psychiatric disorders in the United States: results from the National Comorbidity Survey. *Arch Gen Psychiatry*. 1994;51:8–19.
11. Wilens T, Biederman J, Kwon A, et al. Risk of substance use disorders in adolescents with bipolar disorder. *J Am Acad Child Adolesc Psychiatry*. 2004;43(11):1380–1386.
12. Falk DE, Yi HY, Hilton ME. Age of onset and temporal sequencing of lifetime DSM-IV alcohol use disorders relative to comorbid mood and anxiety disorders. *Drug Alcohol Depend*. 2008;94(1):234–245.
13. Hasin DS, Stinson FS, Hasin DS, et al. Epidemiology of major depressive disorder: results from the National Epidemiologic Survey on Alcoholism and Related Conditions. *Arch Gen Psychiatry*. 2005;62(10):1097–1106.
14. Merikangas KR, Akiskal HS, Angst J, et al. Lifetime and 12-month prevalence of bipolar spectrum disorder in the National Comorbidity Survey Replication. *Arch Gen Psychiatry*. 2007;64(5):543–552.

15. Jaffee WB, Griffin ML, Gallop R, et al. Does alcohol use precipitate depression among patients with co-occurring bipolar and substance use disorders. *J Clin Psychiatry.* 2009;70(2):171–176.
16. Angst J, Angst F, Stassen HH. Suicide risk in patients with major depressive disorder. *J Clin Psychiatry.* 1999;60(suppl 2):57–62.
17. Department of Health and Human Services. *Mental Health: A Report of the Surgeon General.* Rockville, MD: Substance Abuse and Mental Health Services Administration; 1999.
18. Regier DA, Farmer ME, Rae DS. Comorbidity of mental disorders with alcohol and other drug abuse: results from the Epidemiological Catchment Area Study. *J Am Med Assoc.* 1990;264(19):2511–2518.
19. Walfish S, Massey R, Krone A. Anxiety and anger among abusers of different substances. *Drug Alcohol Depend.* 1990;25(3):253–256.
20. Merikangas KR, Angst J. Comorbidity and social phobia: evidence from clinical, epidemiologic and genetic studies. *Eur Arch Psychiatry Clin Neurosci.* 1995;244(6):297–303.
21. McNiel DE, Binder RL, Robinson JC. Incarceration associated wtih homelessness, mental disorder, and co-occurring substance abuse. *Psychiatr Serv.* 2005;56:840–846.
22. Goodman LA, Dutton MA, Harris M. The relationship between violence dimensions and symptom severity among homeless mentally ill women. *J Trauma Stress.* 1997;10(1):51–70.
23. Holt RL, Montesinos S, Christensen RC. Physical and sexual abuse history in women seeking treatment at a psychiatric clinic for the homeless. *J Psychiatr Pract.* 2007;13(1):58–60.
24. Elbogen EB, Johnson SC. The intricate link between violence and mental disorder: results from the National Epidemiological Survey on Alcohol and Related Conditions. *Arch Gen Psychiatry.* 2009;66(2):152–161.
25. Rasanen P, Tihonen J, Isohanni M. Schizophrenia, alcohol abuse, and violent behavior: a 26 year follow up study of an unselected birth cohort. *Schizophr Bull.* 1998;24(3):437–441.
26. Dausey DJ, Desai RA. Psychiatric comorbidity and the prevalence of HIV infection in a sample of patients in treatment for substance abuse. *J Nerv Ment Dis.* 2003;191(1):10–17.
27. Walkup J, Blank MB, Gonzalez JS, et al. The impact of mental health and substance abuse factors on HIV prevention and treatment. *J Acquir Immune Defic Syndr.* 2008;47(suppl 1):S15–S19.
28. Irmiter C, Barry KL, Cohen K, et al. Sixteen year predictors of substance use disorder diagnoses for patients with mental health disorders. *Subst Abuse.* 2009;30(1):40–46.
29. Ciraulo DA, Shader RI, Greenblatt DJ, et al., eds. *Drug Interactions in Psychiatry.* 3rd ed. Philadelphia PA: Lippincott Williams and Wilkins; 2006.
30. Wilson GT, Abrams D. Effects of alcohol on social anxiety and physiological arousal: cognitive versus phenomenological processes. *Cogn Theory Res.* 1977;1(3):195–210.
31. Levin ED, Wilson W, Rose JE, et al. Nicotine-haloperidol interaction and cognitive performance in schizophrenics. *Neuropsychopharmacology.* 1966;15(5):429–436.
32. Bruce M, Scott N. Shine P. Anxiogenic effects of caffeine in patients with anxiety disorders. *Arch Gen Psychiatry.* 1992;49:867–869.
33. Dennison SJ. Clonidine abuse among opiate addicts. *Psychiatr Q.* 2001;72(2):191–195.
34. Buhrich N, Weller A, Kevans P. Misuse of anticholinergic drugs by people with serious mental illnesses. *Psychiatr Serv.* 2000;51:928–929.
35. Rosenberg SD, Drake RE, Brunette MF, et al. Hepatitis C virus and HIV co-infection in people with severe mental illness and substance use disorders. *AIDS.* 2005;19(suppl 3):526–533.
36. Brooks AJ, Penn PE. Comparing treatments for dual diagnosis: twelve-step and self-management and recovery management. *Am J Drug Alcohol Abuse.* 2003;29(2):359–383.
37. Center for Substance Abuse Treatment. Substance abuse treatment for persons with co-occurring disorders. In: *Treatment Improvement Protocol (TIP) Series 42.* Rockville, MD: Substance Abuse and Mental Health Services Administration; 2005.
38. Ries RK. Co-occurring alcohol use and mental disorders. *J Clin Psychopharmacol.* 2006;26(suppl):S30–S36.
39. Drug and Alcohol Services Administration. *The DAIS Report: Facilities Offering Special Programs or Groups for Clients with Co-occurring Disorders, 2004,* Office of Applied Studies, ed. Arlington, VA: Substance Abuse and Mental Health Services Administration; 2006.
40. Havassy BE, Alvidrez J, Mericle AA. Disparities in use of mental health and substance abuse services by persons with co-occurring disorders. *Psychiatr Serv.* 2009;60(2):217–223.
41. Grella C, Stein JA. Impact of program services on treatment outcomes of patients with comorbid mental and substance use disorders. *Psychiatr Serv.* 2006;57(7):1007–1015.
42. McGrath PJ, Nunes EV, Stewart JW. Imipramine treatment of alcoholics with primary depression: a placebo-controlled clinical trial. *Arch Gen Psychiatry.* 1996;53(3):232–240.
43. Cornelius JR, Sallou IM, Ehler JG. Fluoxetine in depressed alcoholics: a double-blind, placebo-controlled trial. *Arch Gen Psychiatry.* 1997;54(8):700–705.
44. Perugi G, Frare F. Effectiveness of adjunctive gabapentin in resistant bipolar diosrder: is it due to anxious alcohol abuse comorbidity? *J Clin Psychopharmacol.* 2002;22(6):584–591.
45. Pittenger C, Desan PH. Gabapentin abuse and delirium tremens upon gabapentin withdrawal. *J Clin Psychiatry.* 2007; 68(3):483–484.
46. Pierre JM, Shnayder I, Wirshing DA, et al. Intranasal quetiapine abuse. *Am J Psychiatry.* 2004;161:1718.
47. Gonzalez G, Sevarino K, Sofuoglu M, et al. Tiagabine increases cocaine-free urines in cocaine-dependent methadone treated patients: results of a randomized pilot study. *Addiction.* 2003;98(11):1625–1632
48. Johnson BA, Ait-Daoud N, Akhtar FZ, et al. Oral topiramate reduces the consequences of drinking and improves quality of life of alcohol-dependent individuals. *Arch Gen Psychiatry.* 2004;61(9):905–912.
49. Brunette MF, Drake RE, Xie H, et al. Clozapine use and relapses of substance use disorder among patients with co-occurring schizophrenia and substance use disorders. *Schizophr Bull.* 2006;32:637–643.
50. Tollefson GD, Montague-Clouse J, Tollefson SL. Treatment of comorbid generalized anxiety in a recently detoxified alcoholic population with a selective serotonergic drug (buspirone). *J Clin Psychopharmacol.* 1992;12(1):19–26.
51. Mueser KT, Noordsy DL, Fox L, et al. Disulfiram treatment for alcoholism in severe mental illness. *Am J Addict.* 2003;12(3):242–252.
52. Maxwell S, Shinderman MS. Use of naltrexone in the treatment of alcohol use disorders in patients with concomitant major mental illness. *J Addict Dis.* 2000;19(3):61–69.
53. Graff F, Griffin ML, Weiss RD. Predictors of dropout from group therapy among patients with bipolar and substance use disorders. *Drug Alcohol Depend.* 2008;94(1–3):272–275.

CHAPTER 53 Medication Interactions

Carolina L. Haass-Koffler ■ Elinore F. McCance-Katz

INTRODUCTION

The World Health Organization reports that drug interactions are a major source of morbidity and mortality. Drug interactions can occur with the coadministration of therapeutic medications with alcohol, with other prescriptions drugs, with an illegal or illicit substance, or with other pharmacologic interventions that are used in the treatment of substance use disorders (SUDs). Unfortunately, *in vitro* findings regarding effects of medications and other substances on enzyme function and/or cell-based assays are sometimes not predictive of the clinical manifestation(s) that may be observed when substances are simultaneously consumed in humans. This lack of predictive value underscores the fact that there is a need to conduct drug interaction studies in humans whenever possible. This chapter will summarize many clinically significant drug interactions and underscore the need for clinical staff to consider possible drug interactions depending on the clinical presentation in order to improve clinical outcomes.

Mortality data published by the Drug Abuse Warning Network (DAWN) have shown that the majority of nonsuicidal deaths occur in multidrug users. Those data contributed to the idea that accidental deaths are more likely to occur when drug interactions alter pharmacokinetic (PK) and/or pharmacodynamic (PD) properties of coadministered drugs to produce detrimental effects. The sections in this chapter will describe the current knowledge of the many critical and common drug interactions as they occur in humans. First, we will review drug interactions between opioid therapies used to treat opioid dependence and other medications with a focus on viral therapeutics, since human immunodeficiency virus (HIV) and other co-occurring infectious diseases have a disproportionate effect on drug users. Interactions between opioids, prescription analgesics, and other medications will also be reviewed since there has been, in recent years, a steady increase in emergency department visits involving prescription medications, according to the DAWN surveys. The limited literature on the use of stimulants with other drugs and alcohol will be reviewed. Finally, interactions between tobacco products and other medications will be briefly reviewed, particularly as they relate to those who suffer from other SUDs or concurrent mental illness.

BRIEF OVERVIEW OF MECHANISMS FOR DRUG INTERACTIONS

Drug interactions can occur through several mechanisms, and one or more of these mechanisms may be responsible for observed clinical manifestations. The mechanisms for drug interactions include effects of drugs on hepatic metabolism by cytochrome P450 (CYP) enzymes; on glucuronidation; on the function of the efflux transporter, P-glycoprotein (P-gp); and on absorption of drugs. PD interactions are also important. Some drugs, when taken in combination, can exhibit synergism that might increase drug effects resulting in toxicity.

Drugs can exert effects on hepatic metabolism by the alteration of CYP enzyme functioning. For example, the U.S. Food and Drug Administration (FDA) has classified CYP 3A4 inhibitors as strong, moderate, or weak, based on their effects on CYP 3A4 substrate metabolism (Table 53.1). Increased systemic exposure to buprenorphine, a CYP 3A4 substrate, is noted following concomitant administration with ketoconazole, a strong CYP 3A4 inhibitor. While *in vitro* assays can demonstrate inhibition of CYP 450 enzymes, we often learn of inducing properties of a drug through clinical observation. For instance, the HIV antiretroviral (ARV) medication, nelfinavir, is known to inhibit CYP 3A4; however, it has been associated with reductions in the plasma concentrations of methadone, possibly due to induction of other CYP 450 enzymes involved in its clearance (1).

Glucuronidation is a mechanism by which many drugs are eliminated by rendering metabolites water soluble so that they can then be excreted. For example, methadone can inhibit zidovudine (AZT) glucuronidation, resulting in increased concentrations of that drug, which may, in turn, be associated with AZT toxicity (2). Drug interactions can also be associated with specific drug effects on the P-gp efflux transporter. For example, cocaine has been shown to induce the efflux pump, P-gp (3), which could potentially result in lower concentrations of drugs that are substrates of P-gp.

Other mechanisms of drug interactions include production of active metabolites resulting from coconsumed drugs and degradation of drugs in the gastrointestinal (GI) tract as a result of decreased GI mobility induced by another drug taken concomitantly. It has been shown that simultaneous cocaine and alcohol consumption results in the formation of

TABLE 53.1	Classification of CYP3A4 inhibitors		
	Strong CYP3A inhibitors	**Moderate CYP3A inhibitors**	**Weak CYP3A inhibitors**
	Cause ≥5-fold increase in AUC[a] of sensitive CYP3A substrate	Cause ≥2 but <5-fold increase in AUC of sensitive CYP3A substrate	Cause ≥1.25 but <2-fold increase in AUC of sensitive CYP3A substrate
	Atazanavir, clarithromycin, indinavir, itraconazole, ketoconazole, nefazodone, nelfinavir, ritonavir, darunavir/ritonavir, lopinavir/ritonavir, saquinavir/ritonavir, telithromycin	Aprepitant, diltiazem, erythromycin, fluconazole, fosamprenavir, grapefruit juice, verapamil	Cimetidine

[a]AUC, area under the curve.

cocaethylene, a cocaine-like compound that can contribute to toxicities associated with the abuse of these substances (4). Altered absorption can also be associated with clinically significant drug interactions, as in the case of methadone slowing GI mobility, which in turn can expose pH-sensitive drugs to an environment that can result in their degradation. For example, if stavudine, a pH-sensitive drug, is exposed for a longer period to the acidic environment of the stomach, increased degradation and subsequent subtherapeutic stavudine concentrations occur. This renders stavudine less beneficial in patients with co-occurring opioid dependence and HIV disease who receive methadone maintenance and stavudine as part of their HIV treatment regimen (5).

PD interactions can result when two or more drugs with similar pharmacologic effects are coadministered. For example, when buprenorphine and benzodiazepines (e.g., alprazolam) have been injected together, deaths have resulted that are thought to be related to depression of the central nervous system (CNS) with a resulting decrease in respiration (6). When given alone, buprenorphine has been shown to have a ceiling effect at which higher doses do not produce further opioid agonist effects (7); however, its injection with benzodiazepines may result in a potentially life-threatening drug interaction (8).

It can be difficult to determine what mechanism(s) are responsible for adverse drug interactions. Controlled studies in humans that include simultaneous administration of medications and measurement of plasma drug concentrations are important for understanding PK and PD drug interactions; these interactions are important in the treatment of medical and mental disorders.

DRUG INTERACTIONS BETWEEN OPIOIDS USED FOR TREATMENT OF OPIOID DEPENDENCE AND OTHER MEDICATIONS

Currently approved medications for the treatment of opioid dependence include methadone, buprenorphine, and L-acetyl-methadol (LAAM). However, LAAM is not currently available, and methadone is the most widely used medication for the treatment of opioid addiction. Buprenorphine is increasingly being used to treat opioid dependence, and its availability by prescription should result in more widespread use for treatment of opioid addiction.

Each of these opioids is metabolized by CYP 3A4 (9), although methadone metabolism is contributed to by CYP 2B6 and 2D6 (10) and a small fraction of buprenorphine metabolism occurs via CYP 2C8 (11). CYP 3A4 is responsible for the metabolism of a wide variety of drugs. Some drugs (which may or may not be substrates of CYP 3A4) may alter the function of CYP 3A4 either by inducing the enzyme and thereby increasing the metabolism of drugs that are substrates of this enzyme or by inhibiting the enzyme, resulting in increased exposure to a drug that would normally be metabolized by CYP 3A4. Those with opioid dependence often have co-occurring illnesses—both medical and psychiatric—which require medication therapy. Some of these medications may alter the function of CYP 3A4, resulting in adverse drug interactions.

The potential for adverse drug interactions in methadone-maintained patients has been recognized for many years when opiate withdrawal symptoms were observed in those prescribed rifampin for the treatment of tuberculosis (11), and similarly, phenytoin (12) and/or carbamazepine were prescribed for the treatment of seizure disorders. This interaction of carbamazepine and methadone was noted when carbamazepine was studied as a pharmacotherapy for the treatment of cocaine dependence in methadone-maintained individuals and was found to be associated with opiate withdrawal and decreased the methadone trough (13). In the ensuing years, other adverse drug interactions, mainly between opioid therapies and medications prescribed for illnesses that occur at high frequency in opioid-dependent patients, have been observed (e.g., ARV therapies such as zidovudine [AZT], whose metabolism may be inhibited by methadone inhibition of glucuronidation, leading to AZT toxicity; or induction of methadone metabolism by efavirenz, leading to opiate withdrawal; or increased buprenorphine and norbuprenorphine concentrations in those receiving the protease inhibitor (PI) combination of atazanavir/ritonavir, which has been associated with cognitive dysfunction in some; or opioid toxicity observed in methadone-treated patients receiving the antibiotic ciprofloxacin). However, the availability of other medications to treat opioid dependence, albeit with little known of potential drug interactions with those therapeutics, led to a question of whether it might be possible to "match" patients with opioid dependence to medication regimens that would be associated with fewer drug interactions, thus improving clinical outcomes in those with co-occurring conditions.

DRUG INTERACTIONS BETWEEN OPIOIDS AND ANTIRETROVIRAL MEDICATIONS

Opioid-dependent patients frequently engage in high-risk behaviors that make them more susceptible to some infectious diseases. This possibility is conferred through engaging in high-risk behaviors such as sharing of injection equipment (syringes, needles, cotton, etc.) that may be contaminated with infectious agents and/or by high-risk sexual behaviors.

The treatment of choice for opioid dependence in the individual who is opioid addicted and who also has HIV disease is opioid therapy; methadone has been the most frequently utilized medication for the treatment of opioid addiction in this population. To a far lesser extent, LAAM was utilized in this population until it became unavailable, and more recently, buprenorphine is being utilized in opioid-dependence treatment in those with HIV/AIDS. Drug interactions between methadone or buprenorphine and HIV medications are summarized in Table 53.2.

The first medication to be FDA approved as a treatment for HIV/AIDS was zidovudine (AZT). This nucleoside reverse transcriptase inhibitor (NRTI) was used as a single agent to treat HIV disease prior to the use of multidrug therapy (highly active antiretroviral therapy [HAART] in those with HIV/AIDS). When methadone-maintained patients with HIV were prescribed AZT, some developed symptoms that appeared to be consistent with opioid withdrawal including muscle/joint pain, insomnia, anxiety, and depression. Examination of the methadone trough in these patients showed therapeutic concentrations. This led to a PK study in which both methadone and AZT concentrations

TABLE 53.2 Drug interactions between methadone or buprenorphine and HIV medications

NRTIs	Methadone	Buprenorphine
AZT	↑ AZT concentrations; possible AZT toxicity	No clinically significant interaction
Didanosine (ddI) (buffered tablets)	Significant ↓ ddI concentrations	Not studied
ddI (enteric-coated), lamivudine, tenofovir	No clinically significant interaction	No clinically significant interaction
Stavudine	Significant ↓ stavudine concentrations	Not studied
Abacavir	Withdrawal noted in some receiving amprenavir plus abacavir	Not studied
NNRTIs		
Nevirapine, efavirenz	Opioid withdrawal may occur	No clinically significant effect
Etravirine	No clinically significant interaction	Not studied
Delavirdine	↑ Methadone (and LAAM) concentrations; no cognitive impairment	↑ Buprenorphine concentrations; no cognitive impairment
PI		
Saquinavir	No clinically significant interaction	Not studied
Nelfinavir	↓ Methadone concentrations; few adverse events reported	No interaction
Amprenavir	↓ Methadone concentrations and withdrawal in some receiving abacavir and amprenavir	Under study
Lopinavir/ritonavir	↓ Methadone concentrations and withdrawal in some	No clinically significant interaction
Atazanavir/ritonavir	No clinically significant interaction	Significant ↑ in buprenorphine and norbuprenophine; cognitive impairment possible
Ritonavir	No clinically significant interaction	No interaction

LAAM, L-acetyl-methadol.

were examined in those with heroin addiction and AIDS. Methadone treatment was associated with a 41% increase in AZT exposure. In some patients, this was sufficient to result in AZT toxicity, which can resemble opiate withdrawal (2). The possible explanations for these findings included that of slowed GI transit associated with methadone treatment resulting in increased absorption of AZT and/or the possibility that methadone inhibited glucuronidation (the principal means of AZT metabolism). A second study examined the effect of other opioid-dependence pharmacotherapies on AZT metabolism. This study showed that, unlike methadone, both LAAM and buprenorphine nonsignificantly lowered AZT concentrations over an 8-hour dosing interval, while naltrexone, an opioid antagonist medication, had no effect on AZT concentrations (14). The results from this study indicated that methadone interactions with specific medications might not be reflective of interactions that could occur with other opioids. This led to further investigations to determine the presence of drug interactions between HIV medications and opioids used in opioid-dependence treatment (methadone, LAAM, and buprenorphine).

Current pharmacotherapy treatment of HIV disease includes a combination of medications from at least two classes. The backbone of HAART consists of either a PI, often boosted by low-dose ritonavir—a PI that inhibits CYP 3A4 enzyme activity and therefore can delay metabolism of PIs that are substrates of CYP 3A4—or a nonnucleoside reverse transcriptase inhibitor (NNRTI). In addition, two NNRTIs are added to complete the regimen. Some of these medications have significant effects on CYP 3A4 including induction by some drugs and inhibition by others.

Further investigation of drug interactions between methadone and ARV medications revealed that other medications with CYP 3A4-inducing properties were also associated with opiate withdrawal when administered concomitantly with methadone. For example, one of the first medications in a line of potent ARV therapeutics, nevirapine, was associated with significant opiate withdrawal in methadone-maintained patients (15). Similarly, another NNRTI, efavirenz, was also associated with significant opiate withdrawal in patients with HIV disease who were also receiving methadone-maintenance therapy (16). The first combination PI, lopinavir/ritonavir, was also associated with onset of opiate withdrawal in methadone-maintained patients, particularly in those with the methadone trough levels that were in the lower end of the therapeutic range (17).

Should medications used to treat HIV alter methadone metabolism, there are two principal adverse events of concern. The first is that of the onset of opiate withdrawal symptoms. If opioid-maintained individuals with HIV disease experience opiate withdrawal with HAART, they may not adhere to the prescribed HIV treatment regimen. Poor adherence to HIV therapeutics has been linked to ongoing drug abuse (18). Poor adherence can also result in development of viral resistance and failure of the HIV therapeutic regimen, underscoring the need for those providing methadone-maintenance therapies to be aware of the potential for adverse drug interactions in their patients with HIV/AIDS who are receiving HAART. Another possibility is that of opioid toxicity, which can potentially result in cognitive impairment or respiratory depression. While there have been clinical episodes of opioid toxicity thought to be precipitated by the use of methadone with an ARV medication that inhibits methadone metabolism, to date, only one drug interaction study has been conducted in human volunteers that shows significant increases in methadone concentrations and LAAM concentrations when administered with an ARV (again, an NNRTI drug) known to inhibit CYP 3A4, delavirdine (19). No significant opioid toxicity was observed in this study, but delavirdine was dosed only for 7 days in this drug-interaction study. With ongoing treatment as in clinical care, the potential for developing opioid toxicity should be considered. Results from drug interaction studies in humans showing significant interactions with methadone have resulted in the U.S. FDA decision that full approval of any HIV medication would require a drug interaction study to be conducted between methadone and the drug under FDA consideration.

One of the significant findings from drug interaction studies that have been conducted thus far between opioids and HIV medications is the lack of clinically significant effects of PK drug interactions detected between buprenorphine and ARV medications. Unlike what has been reported for methadone, buprenorphine/naloxone-treated individuals have not reported withdrawal symptoms or symptoms of opioid intoxication, even when a significant shift in buprenorphine exposure occurs. For example, when methadone-maintained patients with HIV disease are administered HAART containing efavirenz, a potent inducer of CYP 450 enzymes including 3A4 and 2B6, significant opiate withdrawal has been observed (20); rapid methadone dose increases are often required to relieve these withdrawal symptoms. Despite the fact that concentrations of buprenorphine and of norbuprenorphine, its active metabolite formed as a result of metabolism by CYP 3A4, are substantially reduced following efavirenz administration, withdrawal symptoms were not observed in a clinical study (21). One possible explanation for the lack of opiate withdrawal associated with declines in buprenorphine exposure is that the combined effect of buprenorphine and norbuprenorphine is sufficient to prevent opiate withdrawal; methadone, conversely, has no active metabolites. When methadone metabolism is induced, no active metabolites are formed, opioid blood levels drop, and the patient then experiences withdrawal. Another possible explanation is that the high affinity of buprenorphine for the μ-opioid receptor (7) might prevent opiate withdrawal even in the presence of low plasma concentrations. Two other ARV medications shown to be associated with opiate withdrawal symptoms in methadone-maintained patients, nevirapine and lopinavir/ritonavir, have both been shown not to produce opiate withdrawal in buprenorphine-treated patients (21,22).

One caveat to the otherwise benign profile of drug interactions between buprenorphine and ARV medications thus far is the effect of atazanavir and atazanavir/ritonavir, a frequently utilized PI combination in those with HIV/AIDS (23). Atazanavir is an inhibitor of CYP 3A4 and an inhibitor of glucuronidation, both pathways for buprenorphine clearance. Concomitant administration of atazanavir and buprenorphine produces significant increases in buprenorphine and norbuprenorphine plasma concentrations. While a drug interaction study with buprenorphine and atazanavir showed no evidence of cognitive impairment, several participants did experience increased sedation (23). There is a report in the literature of cognitive impairment having developed in several patients with HIV/AIDS being treated with atazanavir/ritonavir who began buprenorphine/naloxone treatment for opioid dependence (24). These findings indicate that patients receiving these medications in combination should be monitored clinically for symptoms of opioid excess. This interaction has not been observed with methadone; therefore, methadone might be a better treatment for opioid dependence in those who will be treated with atazanavir/ritonavir. However, the preponderance of drug interaction study data indicates that buprenorphine offers advantages over methadone in the treatment of opioid dependence in those with HIV/AIDS due to a relative lack of adverse drug interactions and the ability to dose both buprenorphine and ARV medications at standard clinical dosages without concern for subtherapeutic concentrations or toxicities.

DRUG INTERACTIONS BETWEEN OPIOIDS AND MEDICATIONS USED TO TREAT OTHER INFECTIOUS DISEASES

Hepatitis C Medications: Interferon

Hepatitis C virus infection (HCV) is a common co-occurring infection in opioid-dependent individuals; at particularly high risk are those who are injection drug users and who have engaged in high-risk injection practices (25). Many of those with co-occurring HCV will require treatment for this infection. The current standard of care for treatment of HCV is a combination of interferon and ribavirin. Thus far, two drug interaction studies have been conducted exploring the potential for adverse drug interactions between opioid therapies and HCV medications.

Methadone has been studied in combination with interferon and no significant drug interaction was identified (26). The impetus for this study was complaints of adverse symptoms in methadone-maintained patients receiving treatment for HCV. However, the administration of interferon and ribavirin is itself known to be associated with a variety of adverse events (e.g., nausea, anorexia, myalgias, depression, and insomnia), some of which may be mistaken for opiate withdrawal symptoms. There is no additional contribution to the medication side effects that can occur with medications used in the treatment of HCV due to drug interactions with methadone. Buprenorphine has yet to be studied in this population.

Tuberculosis Medications: Rifampin

The adverse drug interaction between methadone and rifampin, a mainstay of tuberculosis treatment, has long been known. Rifampin is an inducer of CYP 3A4, which has been associated with opiate withdrawal in methadone-maintained patients. Rifabutin appears not to produce this adverse drug interaction to the same degree as rifampin (27) and is recommended as a substitute for rifampin in this population. The interaction between buprenorphine and rifampin is currently under study. Several study participants to date have experienced opiate withdrawal requiring early study termination underscoring the potency of rifampin as a CYP 3A4 inducer (28). A second study to determine whether the alternative medication, rifabutin, is associated with adverse drug interactions in buprenorphine-treated patients is currently under way. Isoniazid is an inhibitor of CYP 3A4 (29) and has not been reported to produce significant adverse drug interactions in combination with methadone.

TABLE 53.3 Interactions between methadone or buprenorphine and other antivirals or antibiotics

Hepatitis C Antivirals	Methadone	Buprenorphine
Interferon	No clinically significant interaction	Not studied
Ribavirin	Not studied	Not studied
Tuberculosis Antibiotics		
Rifampin	Opioid withdrawal may occur	Opioid withdrawal may occur
Rifabutin	No clinically significant interaction	Not studied
Other Antibiotics		
Fluconazole, Variconizole, Ciprofloxacin, Clarithromycin	↑methadone plasma concentrations	Not studied

Antibiotics

Opioid dependence, particularly that associated with injection drug use, is associated with a variety of infectious processes that often require antibiotic treatment. Frequent complications of injection drug use include skin infections such as abscesses, cellulitis, endocarditis, and sepsis. There are limited reports of adverse drug interactions between methadone and antibiotic medications. However, ciprofloxacin, a widely used antibiotic effective for a large number of infections, has been associated with opioid toxicity when administered to methadone-maintained patients (30). Some antifungal medications including fluconazole and voriconazole are potent inhibitors of CYP 3A4 and may also be associated with increases in opioid exposure. Increases in opioid exposure may be better tolerated in those receiving treatment with buprenorphine as compared to methadone or LAAM. The reason for this is that buprenorphine is a partial agonist associated with a ceiling effect in terms of its opioid agonist effects (7). Increasing doses of buprenorphine do not produce proportional opioid agonist effects, meaning that respiratory depression, a common cause of morbidity and mortality with toxic doses of full µ-opioid agonists, is less likely to occur in those treated with buprenorphine. Interactions between methadone and buprenorphine with HCV or tuberculosis medications and other antibiotics are listed in Table 53.3.

DRUG INTERACTIONS BETWEEN OPIOIDS AND BENZODIAZEPINES

Benzodiazepine (BZD) use is prevalent in the population of those with SUDs and, specifically, in those with opioid dependence. Epidemiologic studies have suggested that co-occurring psychiatric disorders such as depression, anxiety, sleep disorders, and polysubstance abuse contribute to the high rate of BZD use among opioid-dependent individuals.

Methadone and buprenorphine could have PK interactions with BZDs since they share CYP enzyme metabolic pathways. Many BZDs are weak competitors for CYP 3A4; methadone is metabolized by a variety of CYP isoforms (31). Buprenorphine is metabolized by CYP 3A4, but is also a weak inhibitor of this enzyme (32). There are few clinical studies that have investigated PK interactions between BZDs administered concomitantly with methadone (33,34), but none have directly studied PK interactions between BZDs and buprenorphine. Human clinical studies are needed to investigate the simultaneous use of opioids and BZDs at therapeutic doses in order to determine the possible clinical consequences resulting from PK interactions between these medications.

Currently, PD interactions are the major concern in those who ingest both methadone or buprenorphine and BZDs. It is of clinical importance to note that methadone and BZDs are administered orally when used therapeutically, while buprenorphine tablets are administered sublingually. Buprenorphine, an opioid partial agonist, has been shown to have a ceiling effect at which higher doses do not produce further opioid agonist effects (7); however, when abused in combination with BZDs intravenously, significant morbidity and mortality has been reported (6,8). A synergism between opioids and BZDs to produce respiratory depression may result from common intracellular transduction pathways between opioids and the $GABA_A$ receptor system, resulting in increased chloride ion conduction and decreased membrane excitability (35). Methadone alone has been shown to produce respiratory depression in humans; this effect may be potentiated by coadministration of BZDs. The degree of respiratory depression observed with methadone and BZD administration has been reported to be greater than that observed when BZDs are simultaneously administered with buprenorphine (36,37). In contrast, buprenorphine and BZDs when administered by the injected route may produce severe adverse events as a result of rapid attainment of high (toxic) plasma concentrations of the drugs. This may result in a synergism between the two medications and consequent depression of the CNS as well as a potentially lethal decrease in respiration (6).

ADVERSE EFFECTS RELATED TO DRUG INTERACTIONS

Adverse effects related to drug interactions can be quite harmful to patients requiring opioid therapy for treatment of opioid dependence. For those who experience opiate withdrawal symptoms related to induction of opioid metabolism, it is quite possible that nonadherence to prescribed regimens will occur, which could result in poor clinical outcomes, worsening of disease, and increased substance abuse. In situations in which a drug interaction results in inhibition of opioid metabolism, it is possible that adverse events could include cognitive impairment, decreased respiration, and possible adverse effects on cardiac conduction.

In recent years, increasing attention has focused on the effect of LAAM and methadone on cardiac QT interval. LAAM was removed from the market in Europe and was black-box-labeled in the United States following a series of deaths linked to the occurrence of cardiac dysrhythmias including Torsades de Pointes. Both LAAM and methadone have been shown to block hERG (human ether-a-go-go) potassium channels, which can be associated with slowed electrical conduction in the heart, in some cases producing arrhythmia. In some, this has been observed to be correlated with the use of higher doses of methadone (>100 mg daily).

Another potential manifestation of this adverse event can occur when patients who are opioid maintained are treated with medications that induce metabolism of the opioid. For example, some patients being treated with methadone will require an increase in methadone dose to prevent withdrawal when treated with medications that induce its metabolism. A case report of such a patient discussed the onset of Torsades de Pointes in the patient receiving treatment with lopinavir/ritonavir who had their methadone dose increased due to the onset of opiate withdrawal. When the lopinavir/ritonavir was stopped, the methadone dose was not decreased, leading to the development of excessive methadone plasma concentrations and cardiac arrhythmia (38). It is important to consider this potential sequence of events that can lead to a serious adverse drug interaction in patients with co-occurring conditions requiring treatment with medications that may induce methadone metabolism. In contrast to these findings, buprenorphine has not, to date, been associated with cardiac QT interval prolongation (39).

DRUG INTERACTIONS BETWEEN PRESCRIPTION OPIOID ANALGESICS AND OTHER MEDICATIONS

Morphine exerts its analgesic effects through agonism at μ-opioid receptors. It is metabolized chiefly through glucuronidation by two enzymes: UDP-glucuronosyltransferase (UGT) 2B7, which produces the 6-conjugate (M6G), and UGT 1A3, which produces the 3-conjugate (M3G) (40). The M3G metabolite possesses neuroexcitatory effects, while M6G is responsible for the analgesic effects (41). Both genetic variability of the UGT enzymes 2B7 and 1A3 and drugs that inhibit or induce UGT enzymes could affect the M3G–M6G ratio. However, patient response to morphine analgesia is not well understood because the UGT enzyme system is not as well studied as the CYP 450 enzyme system (42). Inhibitors of UGT enzymes that might decrease the formation of both metabolites include tricyclic antidepressants such as amitriptyline, nortriptyline, and clomipramine (43). Morphine's glucuronidation may be competitively inhibited by morphine itself (44) as well as by the coadministration of chloramphenicol or diazepam (45). Some *in vitro* studies have shown that morphine might be a P-gp substrate (46). Therefore, the inhibition of P-gp would be permissive of morphine entrance through the blood–brain barrier, potentially enhancing its CNS effects including analgesia. Whether this potentiation occurs is still unclear; however, drugs that are P-gp inhibitors that could theoretically enhance CNS morphine effects would include the immunosuppressant, cyclosporine; the calcium channel blocker, diltiazem; and the antifungal medication, itraconazole (47).

Hydromorphone and oxymorphone are morphine analogues that are both metabolized by UGT enzymes (48). Hydromorphone is the CYP 2D6–produced metabolite of hydrocodone, and like morphine, it is minimally metabolized by CYP enzymes. To date, there is no published literature regarding PK alteration and changes in clinical efficacy of hydromorphone when UGT enzymes are inhibited or induced (44).

Opioid analgesics such as methadone, oxycodone, and hydrocodone share the same CYP 2D6 pathway for metabolism with numerous other drugs. When multiple substrates of CYP 2D6 are ingested concurrently, altered drug levels may occur, but are difficult to predict. In one known example, methadone has been reported to inhibit CYP 2D6 and may alter the PK of the antidepressant desipramine, a substrate of CYP 2D6 (49). Methadone has been reported to be associated with increased desipramine levels (50). Other tricyclic antidepressants (imipramine), antipsychotics (risperidone and other phenothiazines), analgesics (codeine), antiarrhythmics (flecainide), and some beta-blockers are also substrates of CYP 2D6 and may have the potential for adverse drug interactions based on increased plasma concentrations if given with methadone (49). Dextromethorphan, a substrate of CYP 2D6, has been associated with delirium in a patient receiving methadone (51). This adverse event abated with cessation of dextromethorphan and was attributed to the effect of methadone on dextromethorphan clearance.

Buprenorphine is chiefly metabolized by CYP 3A4. Opioid toxicity or opioid withdrawal is expected as a consequence of drug–drug interactions with 3A4 inhibitors (azole antifungals, macrolide antibiotics, and nefazodone) and inducers (rifampin and some antiepileptics). However, the ability to predict those interactions is difficult (52), and thus far few drug–drug PK interactions have been associated with adverse events in those receiving buprenorphine and other medications concurrently.

DRUG INTERACTIONS BETWEEN STIMULANTS AND OTHER MEDICATIONS

Psychostimulants produce euphoria, mood elevation, sharpened sensory perception, increased energy, and in some, extraversion. Adverse effects typically predominate when high doses are ingested or as a result of drug interactions when stimulants are ingested with other medications. As sympathomimetic agents, psychostimulants produce cardiovascular effects, including hypertension and increased cardiac output. Interactions may occur with the coadministration of psychotropic and cardiovascular medications. The increase in CNS and cardiovascular stimulation that might occur could be related to serotonergic syndrome, which is a constellation of symptoms that includes neuromuscular hyperactivity, autonomic hyperactivity, and altered mental status (53). Psychostimulants might interact adversely with antidepressants as a result of excess serotonin activity, particularly monoamine oxidase inhibitors (MAOI) or selective serotonin reuptake inhibitors (SSRI), and produce symptoms of serotonin toxicity. Fatal case reports have confirmed evidence of the relationship between serotonin syndrome and coadministration of MAOIs, SSRIs, and illegal stimulants (54).

Amphetamines and MDMA (3,4-methylenedioxymethamphetamine, also known by the street name, Ecstasy) are metabolized primarily by CYP 2D6, showing nonlinear kinetics with unpredictable effects. Drugs that inhibit CYP 2D6 may increase the serum concentration of amphetamine and MDMA, leading to risk of toxicity (55). Inhibitors of CYP 2D6 include several SSRIs (e.g., paroxetine and fluoxetine), ARV medications (e.g., ritonavir), and antiarrhythmics (e.g., quinidine).

Cocaine- and methamphetamine-addicted individuals are usually multidrug users, and their conditions are often complicated by co-occurring mental disorders. The opioid-dependent population has been shown to use cocaine at high rates. Among opioid-dependent individuals, up to 50% use cocaine while being treated for opioid dependence (56). Those patients may require multidrug therapy and close monitoring for drug interactions since opioid-cocaine dependence has been associated with poor clinical outcomes in opioid-dependence treatment (57).

Cocaine has recently been shown to diminish buprenorphine concentrations (58). The underlying PK interaction between those drugs is not obvious since each had been reported to be metabolized by different pathways. Lower buprenorphine plasma concentrations may result from induction of buprenorphine metabolism through an effect of cocaine on CYP 3A4 (59) or through an ability of cocaine to induce the efflux pump, P-gp (3). Another possible explanation is that cocaine metabolites are known to be vasoconstrictors, which might reduce buprenorphine absorption sublingually (60). Cocaine use appears to have a similar, but less dramatic, effect on methadone concentrations. This reduced effect may be related to the fact that methadone is metabolized by several CYP 450 enzymes; therefore, the effect of cocaine on CYP 3A4 function regarding methadone metabolism is diminished in the presence of otherwise normal metabolic processing by the liver relative to effects observed for buprenorphine, which is primarily metabolized by CYP 3A4. Methamphetamine has not been associated with adverse drug interactions in combination with either methadone or buprenorphine to date.

A randomized trial of buprenorphine for the treatment of concurrent opiate and cocaine dependence showed that buprenorphine was well tolerated at dose ranges between 2 and 16 mg. Most adverse events appeared to be related to concurrent illnesses common in this population or to opiate withdrawal rather than to direct side effects of the pharmacologic interventions (61).

Disulfiram (also known by the trade name Antabuse) is an FDA-approved treatment for alcohol dependence and has shown promise as a treatment for cocaine dependence as well. Initially, disulfiram was evaluated in patients with co-occurring cocaine and alcohol dependence (62). Study participants in the disulfiram arm of the study used less cocaine; however, it was not clear if the reduction of stimulant use was due to the reduction in alcohol intake or a direct action of disulfiram to reduce cocaine use. A more recent study evaluated disulfiram as treatment for cocaine dependence in a population of primary cocaine users without alcohol dependence. This randomized, placebo-controlled study that included cognitive–behavioral therapy or interpersonal psychotherapy showed that disulfiram exerted a direct effect in reducing cocaine use rather than a secondary effect in reducing concurrent alcohol use (63). The observed effect of disulfiram was postulated to be associated with reduced cocaine consumption resulting from its ability to inhibit the function of aldehyde dehydrogenases. Aldehyde dehydrogenase inhibition is responsible for the disulfiram–alcohol interaction as well as the inhibition of dopamine beta-hydroxylase and of the aldehyde dehydrogenase–mediated metabolism of serotonin to 5-hydroxyindoleacetic acid; the latter two may be associated with reduction in positive effects of cocaine use. When receiving disulfiram treatment, study participants have reported reduction in cocaine-associated subjective effects such as "high" and "rush"; cardiovascular toxicity was not observed (64). Furthermore, the safety of disulfiram for the treatment of alcohol and cocaine dependence was studied in randomized clinical trials that showed that disulfiram generally has an acceptable side-effect and drug-interaction profile (65).

DRUG INTERACTIONS BETWEEN ALCOHOL AND OTHER MEDICATIONS

Alcohol is a potent CNS depressant that may interact with many drugs; it affects multiple systems within the brain, but mainly it acts as an agonist at GABA receptors. When used concurrently with other depressants such as benzodiazepines (BZDs) and opioids, increased sedation and serious depression of respiratory and/or cardiac function can result.

Alcohol is primarily absorbed through the stomach and the small intestine and largely metabolized by the liver. Hepatic alcohol metabolism occurs via alcohol dehydrogenase, catalase, and the microsomal CYP 450 pathway, which leads to the oxidation of alcohol to acetaldehyde. Drugs that share the same CYP P450 metabolic pathway as alcohol may interact in several ways, including reduction in hepatic metabolism of other drugs resulting from acute alcohol ingestion, increased drug clearance in the presence of chronic alcohol intake, and reduced elimination of drugs resulting from alcoholic liver disease.

Benzodiazepines

Alcohol may have significant interactions with BZDs, medications that are commonly prescribed for anxiety and insomnia. BZDs (e.g., diazepam, lorazepam, alprazolam, clonazepam, and temazepam) are generally considered safe when used alone; however, they can be dangerous if taken with alcohol. BZDs and alcohol can act synergistically in that these drugs facilitate inhibition at GABA receptors and alcohol decreases the excitatory effect of glutamate at N-methyl D-aspartate (NMDA) receptors. This mechanism may help to explain fatal overdose in the presence of opioids and/or BZD and alcohol (66). BZDs may enhance the adverse psychomotor effect of ethanol since it has been reported that BZD concentrations are elevated following a single dose of alcohol and BZD (67). PK changes are expected with both acute and chronic drinkers; however, clinical studies have shown that following a 10 mg (intravenous) dose of diazepam or 1 mg (oral) dose of alprazolam, chronic alcoholics had significantly lower concentrations of the BZDs than healthy nonalcoholics, suggesting that PK alterations may be more prominent in alcoholics with chronic consumption of large amounts of alcohol and who may be more likely to have impaired liver function (68).

All BZDs are expected to result in additive CNS depression with alcohol; however, not all BZDs have similar clinical effects when ingested with alcohol. The concurrent use of BZDs and alcohol is an important issue in patient care, since alcohol and BZDs show cross-tolerance, and abuse of BZDs is frequently observed among alcohol abusers (69). Abuse of BZDs should be monitored, and substance-related disorders resulting from BZD abuse should be treated in these patients. In general, alcohol-abusing patients are not good candidates for BZD therapy and are at higher risk for adverse drug interactions if these drugs are co-abused.

Bupropion

The antidepressant and smoking cessation medication bupropion is metabolized to hydroxybupropion, which is an inhibitor of and substrate for CYP 2D6. Patients with a history of alcohol use metabolize bupropion faster with consequent production of active metabolites; therefore, the use of bupropion and alcohol may increase the risk of lowering the seizure threshold (especially during alcohol withdrawal), which is a known adverse event associated with bupropion use in persons with alcohol dependence. Bupropion treatment of depression or nicotine dependence should be carefully considered in a patient with an alcohol use disorder or known misuse of alcohol.

Methadone

A PD interaction has been reported to occur between alcohol and methadone. Although a direct effect on PK of methadone has not been found, severe adverse events including deaths have occurred in patients who co-ingest these substances (70). Interestingly, no drug interaction of clinical significance has been detected between methadone and disulfiram (71). These findings underline the need to treat co-occurring alcohol disorders in opioid-addicted patients receiving opioid agonist therapy. Clinical reports of adverse events related to alcohol ingestion in buprenorphine-treated patients have not been published to date.

Cocaine

Cocaine metabolism is mainly accomplished through hydrolysis by esterases in the serum and liver. In the presence of alcohol, cocaine undergoes transesterification, resulting in production of cocaethylene, an active metabolite that is structurally similar to cocaine. Cocaethylene is less potent than an equivalent cocaine dose with respect to neurochemical, pharmacologic, and behavioral properties (4); however, when cocaine and alcohol are used together, some studies have suggested that cocaethylene may have the potential to increase cocaine-associated toxicities (72,73). A placebo-controlled, double-blinded study reported that the behavioral and physiologic effects of intranasal cocaethylene in humans are similar to those of cocaine (74). Like cocaine, cocaethylene produces euphoria and increases both heart rate and systolic blood pressure; the slower elimination of cocaethylene could result in its accumulation, with increased potential for toxicity with binge use of cocaine and alcohol. Data from some human studies have shown much higher concentrations of cocaethylene, even exceeding those of cocaine following fatal overdose (72,73).

Methylphenidate

Methylphenidate (MPH) is normally metabolized to an inactive substance, ritalinic acid (75). Coadministration with ethanol produces an active metabolite, ethylphenidate, obtained via metabolism by carboxylesterases in the liver. Coadministration of MPH with ethanol is also believed to elevate MPH plasma concentrations, decrease clearance, and increase half-life of the drug (75,76), underscoring a potential for toxicity with co-abuse of these drugs.

DRUG INTERACTIONS BETWEEN CIGARETTE SMOKE OR NICOTINE AND OTHER MEDICATIONS

Cigarette smoke is known to contain, in addition to nicotine, thousands of different ingredients (e.g., polycyclic aromatic hydrocarbons, N-nitrosamines, and aromatic amines) (77). Those compounds, especially aromatic hydrocarbons, through tobacco combustion may induce CYP 1A1, 1A2, and 2E1 with consequent change of metabolism and elimination of other drugs that are taken at the same time (78).

Induction of CYP 1A2 by cigarette smoking is responsible for many clinically relevant drug interactions, making therapeutic outcomes unpredictable and possibly leading to toxicities. Several classes of drugs that are metabolized by CYP 1A2 include atypical antipsychotics, SSRIs, BZDs, and beta-blockers (78,79). In addition to toxicity related to PK interactions, smoking may also be associated with other adverse events such as increased risk of cardiovascular and cerebrovascular disease. Some of these risks could potentially be exacerbated by drug interactions (78).

A major concern with cigarette smoking with regard to drug interactions is that those affected by other comorbid conditions, for example, schizophrenia and/or alcohol use disorders, have higher rates of cigarette smoking than the general population (80). Smoking is the most prevalent of the SUDs in patients suffering from schizophrenia (81). Between 72% and 90% of those with schizophrenia are smokers compared with 24% of the general population (82). In the alcohol-dependent population, over 80% are tobacco smokers (83), and an epidemiologic study has revealed that smokers have a 4% to 10% increased risk of developing an alcohol use disorder (84). As a result of cigarette smoking with its associated induction of CYP 1A2, increased metabolism and/or decreased plasma concentrations may be observed for many antipsychotics (olanzapine, clozapine, fluphenazine, haloperidol, and chlorpromazine) and other adjunctive therapies for schizophrenia including antidepressants (imipramine, clomipramine, and fluvoxamine), and BZDs (alprazolam, lorazepam, oxazepam, and diazepam) (85). The possibility of alcohol abuse in those with co-occurring mental illness and those who smoke cigarettes may place these individuals at risk for adverse drug–drug interactions as their clinical condition is likely to require that they be treated with several medications.

The potential drug interactions that might occur in cigarette smokers are numerous. Patients who smoke and require other concomitant medications may need higher medication doses than nonsmokers. Clinicians should monitor medication responses and dose accordingly being aware of the potential for drug–drug interactions. If an individual on medications is able to quit smoking, additional monitoring of medication responses and adverse events should be undertaken, given the possible changes associated with the cessation of chronic nicotine exposure. It is also possible that doses of some medications may need to be reduced following smoking cessation.

CONCLUSION

Drug interactions between presently ingested substances, both licit and/or illicit, are a leading cause of morbidity and mortality. This chapter gives a broad overview of drug interactions among illicit substances (i.e., cocaine), legal drugs (i.e., alcohol and tobacco), prescription medications (i.e., ARV and analgesics), and other pharmacotherapies to treat SUDs (e.g., methadone, buprenorphine, and disulfiram). Patients requiring medications to treat SUDs often have co-occurring medical (e.g., HIV/AIDS) and mental (e.g., schizophrenia) illnesses that will require additional medication treatment. These clinical realities place patients with SUDs at greater risk for potentially toxic drug interactions. Furthermore, the clinical management of patients with polysubstance (i.e., opioid/cocaine/alcohol) abuse is common and complex, and can have unpredictable outcomes.

Much remains to be learned about medication interactions between drugs ingested by those with SUDs. Most medications in combination with illicit substances have not been directly studied in humans. *In vitro* studies and preclinical findings indicating the likelihood of drug interactions are not always predictive of what will occur in humans. The ongoing study of frequently prescribed medications and illicit substances alone and in combination will help to inform clinical care and to increase safety of medication treatments in this vulnerable and high-risk population.

REFERENCES

1. Kharasch ED, Walker A, Whittington D, et al. Methadone metabolism and clearance are induced by nelfinavir despite inhibition of cytochrome P4503A (CYP3A) activity. *Drug Alcohol Depend.* 2009;101:158–168.
2. McCance-Katz EF, Jatlow P, Rainey P, et al. Methadone effects on zidovudine (AZT) disposition (ACTG 262). *J Acquir Immune Defic Syndr Hum Retrovirol.* 1998;18:435–443.
3. Lopez P, Velez R, Rivera V. Characteristics of P-glycoprotein (Pgp) upregulated in chronic cocaine users and HIV infected persons. *Retrovirology.* 2005;2(suppl 1):142.
4. McCance-Katz EF, Price LH, Kosten TR, et al. Cocaethylene: pharmacology, physiology, and behavioral effects in humans. *J Pharmacol Exp Ther.* 1995;274:215–223.
5. Rainey PM, Friedland G, McCance-Katz EF, et al. Interaction of methadone with didanosine (ddI) and stavudine (d4T). *J Acquir Immune Defic Syndr Hum Retrovirol.* 2000;24:241–248.
6. Obadia Y, Perrin V, Feroni I, et al. Injecting misuse of buprenorphine among French drug users. *Addiction.* 2001;96:267–272.
7. Walsh SL, Preston KL, Stitzer ML, et al. Clinical pharmacology of buprenorphine: ceiling effects at high doses. *Clin Pharmacol Ther.* 1994;55:569–580.
8. Reynaud M, Petit G, Potard D, et al. Six deaths linked to concomitant use of buprenorphine and benzodiazepines. *Addiction.* 1998;93:1385–1392.
9. Iribarne C, Berthou F, Baird S, et al. Involvement of cytochrome P450 3A4 enzyme in the n-demethylation of methadone in human liver microsomes. *Chem Res Toxicol.* 1996; 9:365–373.
10. Kharasch ED, Hoffer C, Whittington D, et al. Role of hepatic and intestinal cytochrome P450 3A and 2B6 in the metabolism, disposition, and miotic effects of methadone. *Clin Pharmacol Ther.* 2004;76:250–269.
11. Picard N, Cresteil T, Djebli N, et al. In vitro metabolism study of buprenorphine: evidence for new metabolic pathways. *Drug Metab Dispos.* 2005;33(5):689–695.
12. Tong TG, Pond SM, Kreek MJ, et al. Phenytoin-induced methadone withdrawal. *Ann Intern Med.* 1981;94:349–351.
13. Kuhn KL, Halikas JA, Kemp KD. Carbamazepine treatment of cocaine dependence in methadone maintenance patients with dual opiate-cocaine addiction. *NIDA Res Monogr.* 1989;95: 316–317.
14. McCance-Katz EF, Rainey PM, Friedland G, et al. Effect of opioid dependence pharmacotherapies on AZT disposition. *Am J Addict.* 2001;10:296–307.
15. Altice FL, Friedland GH, Cooney EL. Nevirapine induced opiate withdrawal among injection drug users with HIV infection receiving methadone. *AIDS.* 1999;13:957–962.
16. Boffito M, Rossati A, Reynolds HE, et al. Undefined duration of opiate withdrawal induced by efavirenz in drug users with HIV infection and undergoing chronic methadone treatment. *AIDS Res Hum Retroviruses.* 2002;18:341–342.
17. McCance-Katz EF, Rainey P, Friedland G, et al. The protease inhibitor lopinavir/ritonavir may produce opiate withdrawal in methadone-maintained patients. *Clin Infect Dis.* 2003;37: 476–482.
18. Arnsten JH, Demas PA, Grant RW, et al. Impact of active drug use on antiretroviral therapy adherence and viral suppression in HIV-infected drug users. *J Gen Intern Med.* 2002;17:377–381.
19. McCance-Katz EF, Rainey P, Smith P, et al. Drug interactions between opioids and antiretroviral medications: interaction between methadone, LAAM, and delavirdine. *Am J Addict.* 2006;15: 23–34.
20. McCance-Katz EF, Gourevitch MN, Arnsten J, et al. Modified Directly Observed Therapy (MDOT) for injection drug users with HIV disease. *Am J Addict.* 2002;11: 271–278.
21. McCance-Katz EF, Moody DE, Morse G, et al. Interactions between buprenorphine and antiretrovirals I: non-nucleoside reverse transcriptase inhibitors I: efavirenz and delavirdine, *Clin Infect Dis.* 2006;43(suppl 4):S224–S234.
22. McCance-Katz EF, Moody DE, Morse G, et al. Interactions between buprenorphine and antiretrovirals II: protease inhibitors, nelfinavir, lopinavir/ritonavir, or ritonavir. *Clin Infect Dis.* 2006;43(suppl 4):S235–S246.
23. McCance-Katz EF, Moody DE, Morse GD, et al. Interaction between buprenorphine and atazanavir or atazanavir/ritonavir. *Drug Alcohol Depend.* 2007;91:269–278.
24. Bruce RD, Altice FL. Three case reports of a clinical pharmacokinetic interaction with buprenorphine and atazanavir plus ritonavir. *AIDS.* 2006;20:783–784.
25. Sulkowski MS, Mast EE, Seeff LB, et al. Hepatitis C virus infection as an opportunistic disease in persons infected with human immunodeficiency virus. *Clin Infect Dis.* 2000;(suppl 1): S77–S84.
26. Berk SI, Litwin AH, Arnsten JH, et al. Effects of pegylated interferon alfa-2b on the pharmacokinetic and pharmacodynamic properties of methadone: a prospective, nonrandomized, crossover study in patients coinfected with hepatitis C and HIV

receiving methadone maintenance treatment. *Clin Ther.* 2007;29: 131–138.
27. Brown LS, Sawyer RC, Li R, et al. Lack of a pharmacologic interaction between rifabutin and methadone in HIV-infected former injecting drug users. *Drug Alcohol Depend.* 1996;43: 71–77.
28. McCance-Katz EF. Drug interactions between opioids and antiretroviral medications: why should we care? Unique models for comprehensive substance abuse treatment: joint session with the international society of addiction medicine. ASAM Annual Meeting, New Orleans, LA, May 2009.
29. Desta Z, Soukhova NV, Flockhart DA. Inhibition of cytochrome P450 (CYP450) isoforms by isoniazid: potent inhibition of CYP2C19 and CYP3A. *Antimicrob Agents Chemother.* 2001;45: 382–392.
30. Karin H, Segerdahi M, Gustafsson LL, et al. Methadone, ciprofloxacin and adverse drug reactions. *Lancet.* 2000;356: 2069–2070.
31. Erber JG, Rhodes RJ, Gal J. Stereoselective metabolism of methadone N-demethylation by cytochrome P4502B6 and 2C19. *Chirality.* 2004;16:36–44.
32. Chang Y, Moody DE. Effect of benzodiazepines on the metabolism of buprenorphine in human liver microsomes. *Eur J Clin Pharmacol.* 2005;60:875–881.
33. Preston KL, Griffiths RR, Cone EJ, et al. Diazepam and methadone blood levels following concurrent administration of diazepam and methadone. *Drug Alcohol Depend.* 1986; 18: 195–202.
34. Kobayashi K, Yamamoto T, Chiba K, et al. Human buprenorphine N-dealkylation is catalyzed by cytochrome P450 3A4. *Drug Metab Dispos.* 1998;26:818–821.
35. Nutt DJ, Malizia AL. New insights into the role of the GABAA–benzodiazepine receptor in psychiatric disorder. *Br J Psychiatry.* 2001;179:390–396.
36. Lintzeris N, Mitchell TB, Bond A, et al. Interactions on mixing diazepam with methadone or buprenorphine in maintenance patients. *J Clin Psychopharmacol.* 2006;26:274–283.
37. Lintzeris N, Mitchell TB, Bond A, et al. Pharmacodynamics of diazepam co-administered with methadone or buprenorphine under high dose conditions in opioid dependent patients. *Drug Alcohol Depend.* 2007;91:187–194.
38. Lüthi B, Huttner A, Speck RF, et al. Methadone-induced Torsade de Pointes after stopping lopinavir-ritonavir. *Eur J Clin Microbiol Infect Dis.* 2007;26:367–369.
39. Wedam EF, Bigelow GE, Johnson RE, et al. QT-interval effects of methadone, levomethadyl, and buprenorphine in a randomized trial. *Arch Intern Med.* 2007;167:2469–2475.
40. Coffman BL, Rios GR, King CD, et al. Human UGT2B7 catalyzes morphine glucuronidation. *Drug Metab Dispos.* 1997;25: 1–4.
41. Smith MT. Neuroexcitatory effects of morphine and hydromorphone: evidence implicating the 3-glucuronide metabolites. *Clin Exp Pharmacol Physiol.* 2000;27:524–528.
42. Armstrong SC, Cozza KL, Benedek DM. Med-psych drug-drug interactions update. *Psychosomatics.* 2002;43:245–247.
43. Wahlström A, Lenhammar L, Ask B, et al. Tricyclic antidepressants inhibit opioid receptor binding in human brain and hepatic morphine glucuronidation. *Pharmacol Toxicol.* 1994;75: 23–27.
44. Armstrong SC, Cozza KL. Pharmacokinetic drug interactions of morphine, codeine, and their derivatives: theory and clinical reality, part I. *Psychosomatics.* 2003;44:167–171.
45. Grancharov K, Naydenova Z, Lozeva S, et al. Natural and synthetic inhibitors of UDP-glucuronosyltransferase. *Pharmacol Ther.* 2001;89:171–186
46. Crowe A. The influence of P-glycoprotein on morphine transport in Caco-2 cells. Comparison with paclitaxel. *Eur J Pharmacol.* 2002;440:7–16.
47. Yu DK. The contribution of P-glycoprotein to pharmacokinetic drug-drug interactions. *J Clin Pharmacol.* 1999;39:1203–1211.
48. Radominska-Pandya A, Czernik PJ, Little JM, et al. Structural and functional studies of UDP-glucuronosyltransferases. *Drug Metab Rev.* 1999;31:817–899.
49. Ereshefsky L, Riesenman C, Lam YW. Antidepressant drug interactions and the cytochrome P450 system. The role of cytochrome P450 2D6. *Clin Pharmacokinet.* 1995;29(suppl 1): 10–18.
50. Maany I, Dhopesh V, Arndt IO, et al. Increase in desipramine serum levels associated with methadone treatment. *Am J Psychiatry.* 1989;146:1611–1613.
51. Lotrich FE, Rosen J, Pollock BG. Dextromethorphan-induced delirium and possible methadone interaction. *Am J Geriatr Pharmacother.* 2005;3:17–20.
52. Armstrong SC, Cozza KL. Pharmacokinetic drug interactions of morphine, codeine, and their derivatives: theory and clinical reality, Part II. *Psychosomatics.* 2003;44:515–520.
53. Dvir Y, Smallwood P. Serotonin syndrome: a complex but easily avoidable condition. *Gen Hosp Psychiatry.* 2008;30:284–287.
54. Kłys M, Kowalski P, Rojek S, et al. Death of a female cocaine user due to the serotonin syndrome following moclobemide-venlafaxine overdose. *Forensic Sci Int.* 2009;184:e16–e20.
55. Oesterheld JR, Armstrong SC, Cozza KL. Ecstasy: pharmacodynamic and pharmacokinetic interactions. *Psychosomatics.* 2004; 45:84–87.
56. Disney ER, Kidorf M, King VL, et al. Prevalence and correlates of cocaine physical dependence subtypes using the DSM-IV in outpatients receiving opioid agonist medication. *Drug Alcohol Depend.* 2005;79:23–32.
57. Fiellin DA, Sullivan L, Moore BC, et al. The impact of cocaine use on outcomes in office-based buprenorphine treatment [Abstract]. College on Problems of Drug Dependence, San Juan, PR; 2008.
58. McCance EF, Rainey PM, Moody DE. Effect of cocaine use on buprenorphine pharmacokinetics in humans. *Am J Addict.* 2010;19:38–46.
59. Pellinen P, Stenbäck F, Kojo A, et al. Regenerative changes in hepatic morphology and enhanced expression of CYP2B10 and CYP3A during daily administration of cocaine. *Hepatology.* 1996;23:515–523.
60. Madden JA, Konkol RJ, Keller PA, et al. Cocaine and benzoylecgonine constrict cerebral arteries by different mechanisms. *Life Sci.* 1995;56:679–686.
61. Montoya ID, Gorelick DA, Preston KL, et al. Randomized trial of buprenorphine for treatment of concurrent opiate and cocaine dependence. *Clin Pharmacol Ther.* 2004;75:34–48.
62. Carroll KM, Nich C, Ball SA, et al. Treatment of cocaine and alcohol dependence with psychotherapy and disulfiram. *Addiction.* 1998;93:713–728.
63. Carroll KM, Fenton LR, Ball SA, et al. Efficacy of disulfiram and cognitive behavior therapy in cocaine-dependent outpatients: a randomized placebo-controlled trial. *Arch Gen Psychiatry.* 2004; 61:264–272.
64. Baker JR, Jatlow P, McCance-Katz EF. Disulfiram effects on responses to intravenous cocaine administration. *Drug Alcohol Depend.* 2007;87:202–209.

65. Malcolm R, Olive MF, Lechner W. The safety of disulfiram for the treatment of alcohol and cocaine dependence in randomized clinical trials: guidance for clinical practice. *Expert Opin Drug Saf.* 2008;7:459–472.
66. White JM, Irvine RJ. Mechanisms of fatal opioid overdose. *Addiction.* 1999;94:961–972.
67. Sellers EM, Busto U. Benzodiazepines and ethanol: assessment of the effects and consequences of psychotropic drug interactions. *J Clin Psychopharmacol.* 1982;2:249–262.
68. Sellman R, Pekkarinen A, Kangas L, et al. Reduced concentrations of plasma diazepam in chronic alcoholic patients following an oral administration of diazepam. *Acta Pharmacol Toxicol (Copenh).* 1975;36:25–32.
69. Hollister LE. Interactions between alcohol and benzodiazepines. *Recent Dev Alcohol.* 1990;8:233–239.
70. Kreek MJ. Opioid interactions with alcohol. *Adv Alcohol Subst Abuse.* 1984;3:35–46.
71. Kreek MJ. Metabolic interactions between opiates and alcohol. *Ann N Y Acad Sci.* 1981;362:36–49.
72. Hearn WL, Rose S, Wagner J, et al. Cocaethylene is more potent than cocaine in mediating lethality. *Pharmacol Biochem Behav.* 1991;39:531–533.
73. Jatlow P, Elsworth JD, Bradberry CW, et al. Cocaethylene: a neuropharmacologically active metabolite associated with concurrent cocaine-ethanol ingestion. *Life Sci.* 1991;48:1787–1794.
74. McCance-Katz EF, Price LH, McDougle CJ, et al. Concurrent cocaine-ethanol ingestion in humans: pharmacology, physiology, behavior, and the role of cocaethylene. *Psychopharmacology (Berl).* 1993;111:39–46.
75. Patrick KS, Straughn AB, Minhinnett RR, et al. Influence of ethanol and gender on methylphenidate pharmacokinetics and pharmacodynamics. *Clin Pharmacol Ther.* 2007;81:346–353.
76. Markowitz JS, DeVane CL, Boulton DW, et al. Ethylphenidate formation in human subjects after the administration of a single dose of methylphenidate and ethanol. *Drug Metab Dispos.* 2000;28:620–624.
77. Schein JR. Cigarette smoking and clinically significant drug interactions. *Ann Pharmacother.* 1995;29:1139–1148.
78. Zevin S, Benowitz NL. Drug interactions with tobacco smoking. An update. *Clin Pharmacokinet.* 1999;36:425–438.
79. Kroon LA. Drug interactions and smoking: raising awareness for acute and critical care providers. *Crit Care Nurs Clin North Am.* 2006;18:53–62.
80. Littleton J, Barron S, Prendergast M, et al. Smoking kills (alcoholics)! Shouldn't we do something about it? *Alcohol Alcohol.* 2007;42:167–173.
81. Cuffel BJ. Comorbid substance use disorder: prevalence, patterns of use, and course. In: Drake RE, Mueser KT, eds. *Dual Diagnosis of Major Mental Illness and Substance Disorder: Recent Research and Clinical Implications.* San Francisco: Jossey-Bass; 1996:93–105.
82. Hughes JR, Hatsukami DK, Mitchell JE, et al. Prevalence of smoking among psychiatric outpatients. *Am J Psychiatry.* 1986;143:993–997.
83. Miller NS, Gold MS. Comorbid cigarette and alcohol addiction: epidemiology and treatment. *J Addict Dis.* 1998;17:55–66.
84. Grant BF, Hasin DS, Chou SP, et al. Nicotine dependence and psychiatric disorders in the United States: results from the national epidemiologic survey on alcohol and related conditions. *Arch Gen Psychiatry.* 2004;61:1107–1115.
85. Evins AE, Cather C, Deckersbach T, et al. A double-blind placebo-controlled trial of bupropion sustained-release for smoking cessation in schizophrenia. *J Clin Psychopharmacol.* 2005;25:218–225.

SECTION 8 ■ MODELS OF PREVENTION

CHAPTER 54 School-Based Programs

Gilbert J. Botvin ■ Kenneth W. Griffin

INTRODUCTION

The problem of substance abuse has been a source of concern to health professionals, community leaders, and law enforcement agencies over the past several decades. Considerable effort and resources have been spent attempting to understand the etiology of substance use and abuse and to identify effective prevention and treatment strategies. Research concerning the onset and developmental progression of substance abuse indicates that most youth initiate substance use by experimenting with alcohol and cigarette smoking during adolescence. For a subset of these youth, experimentation escalates to frequent and regular use, and for some, the use and abuse of more serious illicit drugs can ultimately lead to drug dependence and substance abuse disorder. Furthermore, substance abuse can lead to a variety of negative health, legal, social, and pharmacologic outcomes in young adulthood (1).

Preventive interventions and related initiatives to reduce substance abuse have been the focus of a great deal of research. A wide variety of activities have been used to achieve the goal of reduced drug abuse, particularly among adolescents. These prevention activities range from educational and skills training activities that take place within schools, families, and communities to mass media public service announcements (PSAs), policy initiatives such as requiring health warning labels on cigarettes and alcohol, changes in school rules (i.e., "zero-tolerance" policies), and laws and regulations including increased cigarette taxes and minimum purchasing age requirements (2). However, the bulk of the drug abuse prevention research in the United States in the past 25 to 30 years has concentrated on school-based prevention programs. Because the general pattern of substance use initiation and escalation is well documented, many prevention programs aim to prevent early-stage substance use or delay the onset of use among adolescents. Typically, these programs are provided to middle school or junior high school students and target the use of tobacco, alcohol, and marijuana because these are the most widely used substances in the United States and because preventing them may reduce the risk for the abuse of other illicit drugs and their associated negative outcomes. Research shows that the most effective approaches to the prevention of adolescent drug abuse are derived from psychosocial theories (3) and focus primarily on the psychosocial risk and protective factors that promote the initiation and early stages of substance use (4).

PREVALENCE AND CURRENT TRENDS

National survey data show that prevalence rates of alcohol, tobacco, and illicit drug use among adolescents peaked in the late 1970s and early 1980s. More recently, we have seen a gradual decline in prevalence rates for several substances among adolescents, although there have been increases observed in others. Data from the 2008 Monitoring the Future Study (5) found that among high school seniors, almost half (45%) report ever using cigarettes, and one out of five high school seniors reported being current smokers. This represents a large improvement from the late 1970s, when twice as many high school seniors (two of every five) were current smokers. Rates of alcohol and marijuana use have also decreased since the late 1970s although not as much as cigarette smoking. In the past 10 years, prevalence rates for alcohol and marijuana use have gradually declined for high school seniors; however, both substances are still widely used. Alcohol use is the most prevalent substance use behavior among teens, and marijuana is the most prevalent illicit drug used. In 2008, more than half (55%) of 12th graders reported having been drunk at least once in their life, and one in four reported binge drinking (five or more drinks in a row) in the past 2 weeks. About 47% of high school seniors reported ever using marijuana in 2008, and 32% reported use in the past year. After marijuana, the most commonly abused drugs among high school seniors were amphetamines (11%), inhalants (10%), sedatives and tranquilizers (9% each), hallucinogens (9%), and Ecstacy (MDMA) at 6% lifetime prevalence. The misuse of over-the-counter (OTC) medications is also a growing problem among young people. The active ingredient in many cough suppressants, dextromethorphan (DXM), can produce hallucinations or dissociative, "out-of-body" experiences when taken in very large doses. Approximately 6% of 12th graders reported ever using an OTC cough and cold medication to get high in the past year (6).

THE IMPORTANCE OF PREVENTION

Although there have been significant advances in the effectiveness of drug abuse treatment in recent years, many treatment modalities are expensive, labor intensive, and plagued by high rates of recidivism. Clinicians are confronted by a disorder that often proves to be refractory to change. Patients frequently remain in pathogenic environments in which social networks continue to support substance abuse and the availability of drugs is ubiquitous. Prevention is important because it offers a logical alternative to treatment. Many experts believe it is easier and less expensive to prevent substance abuse than it is to treat such an insidious disorder once it has developed. However, from a historical perspective, most initial efforts to develop effective substance abuse prevention programs achieved only a limited degree of success. Many failed completely because they were based on erroneous assumptions about the causes of drug abuse. The first major breakthrough came at the end of the 1970s in the area of school-based smoking prevention. That work stimulated a great deal of prevention research and led to the development of several promising prevention approaches. Since the 1980s, empiric evidence from a growing number of carefully designed and methodologically sophisticated research studies indicates that prevention works, and recent research suggests that substance use prevention is also cost-effective (7).

THE SCHOOL AS THE SITE OF PREVENTION EFFORTS

The development and testing of approaches for preventing adolescent substance abuse have largely focused on middle/junior high school students. Schools have served as the primary setting for prevention efforts in large part because they offer the most efficient access to large numbers of adolescents. Furthermore, in addition to their traditional educational mission, schools often take steps to address a variety of social and health problems among students, particularly those that present a significant barrier to the achievement of educational objectives. The U.S. Department of Education, for example, has included "drug-free schools" as one of its goals for improving the quality of education in this country. Many states mandate schools to provide their students with programs in health education and/or tobacco, alcohol, and drug education as well as teenage pregnancy and AIDS education.

CHAPTER OVERVIEW

This chapter provides a summary of developments in school-based substance abuse prevention over the past three decades. It begins with a discussion of what is currently known about the etiology and developmental progression of substance use and the implications for prevention. Traditional and contemporary prevention approaches are described and the evidence for their effectiveness is summarized. A major focus of this chapter is on the current generation of theory-based substance abuse prevention approaches and the results of research testing their short- and long-term effectiveness. The final section summarizes conclusions to be drawn from this body of research, directions for future research, and implications for public health policy.

ETIOLOGY AND IMPLICATIONS FOR PREVENTION

To provide a context for understanding existing substance abuse prevention efforts and for developing a prescription for the most effective preventive interventions possible, it is necessary to be familiar with the factors associated with the initiation and maintenance of tobacco, alcohol, and drug abuse. Furthermore, it is important to identify when the onset and escalation of substance use typically occur to determine the most appropriate point of intervention. An understanding of the developmental course of substance abuse is also central, in terms of both the progression from nonuse to experimentation to abuse and the general sequence of using specific psychoactive substances or classes of substances.

Etiologic Determinants

A variety of risk factors for early-stage substance use have been identified, as well as several protective factors that offset the effects of risk (4). Furthermore, a number of theoretical models have been developed or applied to phenomenon of alcohol and drug use among youth (3). A large body of literature demonstrates that substance abuse results from the complex interaction of a number of different factors, including cognitive, attitudinal, social, personality, pharmacologic, biologic, and developmental factors (8,9).

Social Factors

Social factors are the most powerful influences promoting the initiation of tobacco, alcohol, and drug abuse. These include the behavior and attitudes regarding substance use among significant others such as parents, older siblings, and friends (10). Studies reveal that parents' use of alcohol, tobacco, marijuana, and other illicit drugs, and parental attitudes that are not explicitly against use, often translate into higher levels of use among children and adolescents. Poor family relationships and inadequate parenting practices (i.e., lack of parental monitoring) have been identified as risk factors for youth substance use. Other social influences include popular media portrayals showing substance use as an important part of popularity, sophistication, success, sex appeal, and good times (11). Both the modeling of substance use behavior by media personalities and the positive messages about substance use in popular music, movies, and other media are powerful sources of influence that promote and support substance use (12).

Cognitive and Attitudinal Factors

Individuals who are unaware of the adverse consequences of tobacco, alcohol, and drug use, as well as those who have positive attitudes toward substance use, are more likely to become substance users than those with either more knowledge or more negative attitudes toward substance use (13). In addition, individuals who believe that substance use is "normal" and that most people smoke, drink, or use drugs are more likely to be substance users. Positive expectations about the effects of substance use are also predictive of substance use behavior (14).

Personality Factors

Substance use is associated with a number of psychological characteristics. Substance users have lower mood, self-esteem, assertiveness, personal control, and self-efficacy than nonusers, and are more anxious, impulsive, and rebellious than nonusers (7). The clinical literature also suggests that individuals with a specific psychiatric condition or symptoms (e.g., anxiety and depression) may use particular substances as a way of alleviating these feelings. For example, through experimentation with different substances, highly anxious individuals may find that alcohol or other depressants help them to feel less anxious, and they might use those substances as a way of regulating their feelings of anxiety. This has been referred to in the literature as the self-medication hypothesis (15).

Pharmacologic Factors

The pharmacology of commonly abused substances varies, although animal research has shown that several drugs of abuse (cocaine, amphetamine, morphine, nicotine, and alcohol), each with different molecular mechanisms of action, affect the brain in the same way by increasing strength at excitatory synapses on midbrain dopamine neurons (16). Furthermore, virtually all of these substances produce effects that are highly reinforcing and dependency producing. For tobacco, alcohol, and most illicit drugs, tolerance develops quickly, leading to increased dosages and an increased frequency of use. Once a pattern of dependent use has been established, termination of use produces dysphoric feelings and physical withdrawal symptoms.

Behavioral Factors

Substance use is highly associated with a variety of health-compromising or problem behaviors. Individuals who use one substance are more likely to use others. Indeed, substance abuse among young people is often considered to be part of a general syndrome reflecting a particular value orientation (17). Youth who smoke, drink, or use drugs tend to get lower grades in school, are not generally involved in adult-sanctioned activities such as sports and clubs, and are more likely than nonusers to become involved in antisocial or delinquent behavior, aggressiveness, and premature sexual activity (18,19). Furthermore, it is believed that these problem behaviors have the same or highly similar causes, which have significant implications for prevention. Notably, it may be possible to develop a single preventive intervention capable of having an impact on several associated behaviors at the same time.

Initiation and Developmental Course

Since the 1960s, some degree of experimentation with substance use has become commonplace in contemporary American society. This is particularly true with respect to alcohol, tobacco, and marijuana, which are the most widely used and abused substances in society. For most individuals, experimentation with tobacco, alcohol, and marijuana typically takes place during the adolescent years. First use and intermittent experimentation generally occur almost exclusively within the context of social situations. After a period of experimentation and regular use, some individuals develop patterns of use characterized by both psychological and physiologic dependence. The initial social and psychological motivations for using drugs eventually yield to one driven increasingly by pharmacologic factors.

Substance Use Progression

Research indicates that experimentation with one substance frequently leads to experimentation with others in a logical and generally predictable progression (20). Most individuals begin by using alcohol and tobacco, progressing later to the use of marijuana. This developmental progression corresponds closely to the prevalence of these substances in our society, with alcohol being the most widely used, followed by tobacco and then marijuana. Some individuals may also use inhalants early in this sequence because of the wide availability. For some individuals this progression may eventuate in the use of depressants, stimulants, hallucinogens, and other drugs. However, many individuals either may discontinue use after a short period of experimentation or may not progress from the use of one substance to the use of others. The likelihood of progressing from one point in the developmental sequence to another can best be understood in probabilistic terms, with an individual's risk of moving to greater involvement with drugs increasing at each additional step in the developmental progression.

Knowledge of the developmental progression of substance use is important because it has implications for the focus and timing of preventive interventions. Interventions targeted at the use of substances occurring toward the beginning of this progression have the potential of not only preventing the use of those substances, but also of reducing or eliminating the risk of using other more serious substances further along the progression.

Adolescence and Substance Abuse Risk

Adolescence is frequently characterized as a period of great physical and psychological change (21). During adolescence, individuals typically experiment with a wide range of behaviors and lifestyle patterns. This occurs as part of the natural process of separating from parents, developing a sense of autonomy and independence, establishing a personal identity, and acquiring the skills necessary for functioning effectively in an adult world. However, many of the developmental changes that are necessary prerequisites for becoming healthy adults increase an adolescent's risk of smoking, drinking, or using drugs. Adolescents who are impatient to assume adult roles may smoke, drink, or use drugs as a way of appearing more grown-up and laying claim to adult status. Adolescents may also engage in substance use because it provides them with a means of establishing solidarity with a particular peer group, rebelling against parental authority, or establishing their own individual identity.

As the result of normal cognitive development, adolescents shift from a "concrete operational" mode of thinking, which is characteristically rigid, literal, and grounded in the "here and now," to a "formal operational" mode of thinking, which is more relative, abstract, and hypothetical (22). It has been suggested that these changes in the manner in which adolescents think may serve to undermine previously acquired knowledge relating to the potential risks of smoking, drinking, or using drugs. For example, the "formal operational" thinking of the adolescent facilitates the discovery of inconsistencies or logical flaws in arguments being advanced by adults concerning the health risks associated with substance use. Similarly, cognitive development during early adolescence may enable young people to formulate counterarguments to antidrug messages, which may, in turn, permit rationalizations for ignoring potential risks, particularly if substance use is perceived to have social or personal benefits.

Conformity needs and conformity behavior increase rapidly during preadolescence and early adolescence, and decline steadily from middle to late adolescence. However, an individual's susceptibility to conformity pressure may vary greatly, depending on values and a variety of psychological factors, as well as the relative importance of peer acceptance. Finally, because adolescents characteristically have a sense of immortality and invulnerability, they tend to minimize the risks associated with substance use and overestimate their ability to avoid personally destructive patterns of use.

PREVENTION STRATEGIES

In view of the adverse health, social, and legal consequences of substance abuse and the difficulty of achieving sustained abstinence once addictive patterns of use have developed, it is apparent that the most promising approach to the problem of substance abuse is prevention. Prevention efforts have taken place on several different levels and have taken many forms. Prevention has been conceptualized in terms of supply and demand reduction models and as primary, secondary, and tertiary prevention. Each encompasses a different aspect of prevention, and has substantially different operational implications.

Supply and Demand Reduction

Supply reduction efforts are based on the fundamental assumption that substance use can be controlled by simply controlling the supply or availability of drugs. This has been the driving force behind the activities of law enforcement agencies, particularly with respect to the interdiction of drugs by governmental agencies such as the Drug Enforcement Administration (DEA), the Federal Bureau of Investigation (FBI), and local police departments. Demand reduction efforts, on the other hand, are conceptualized as those that attempt to dissuade, discourage, or deter individuals from using drugs or reducing the desire to use drugs. Demand reduction includes prevention, education, and treatment programs.

Types of Prevention

Consistent with usage in the field of public health, primary prevention interventions are designed to reach individuals before they have developed a specific disorder or disease. As such, they target a general population of individuals who, for the most part, have not yet begun using tobacco, alcohol, or other drugs. The goal of these approaches is to prevent substance use and abuse by intervening upon individual and/or environmental factors viewed as promoting or supporting this type of health-compromising behavior. Secondary prevention involves screening and early intervention. Tertiary prevention involves preventing the progression of a well-established disorder to the point of disability. However, one criticism of this classification system is that it is difficult to distinguish between tertiary prevention and treatment in that both involve care for persons with an established disorder.

In a 1994 report on preventive intervention research, the Institute of Medicine (23) proposed a new framework for classifying intervention programs as part of a continuum of care that includes prevention, treatment, and maintenance (Fig. 54.1). While originally proposed as a system to classify interventions for mental disorders, the framework has been widely adopted and the terminology is now applied to other types of interventions. In this framework, prevention is reserved only for interventions that occur prior to the initial onset of a disorder. Prevention is further divided into three types: universal, selective, and indicated preventive interventions. These categories define prevention according to the groups to whom the interventions are directed, rather than the stage of illness progression.

Universal prevention programs focus on the general population and aim to deter or delay the onset of a condition or risk behavior. While the level of risk for developing the condition may vary among individuals, universal programs recognize that all members of a population share some level of risk and can benefit from prevention programs that provide information and skills to help individuals avoid the outcome or condition. Selective prevention programs target selected high-risk groups or subsets of the general population believed to be at high risk because of membership in a particular group. Risk groups for selective interventions may be based on biologic, social, psychological, or other risk factors. Selective interventions for drug abuse prevention, for example, might recruit groups such

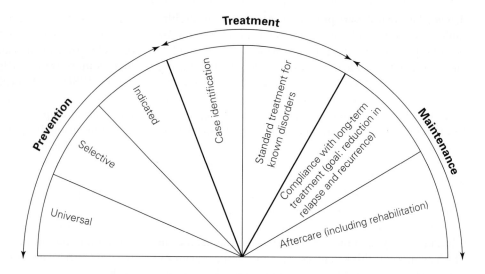

Figure 54.1. Institute of Medicine continuum of care model. (Reprinted with permission from Institute of Medicine. *Reducing Risks for Mental Disorders: Frontiers for Preventive Intervention Research.* Washington, DC: National Academy Press; 1994.)

as children of drug users, pregnant women, or residents of high-risk neighborhoods. An individual's level of risk is presumed to be higher than average because of their membership in the selected group. Indicated prevention programs are designed for those already engaging in the behavior, or showing early danger signs, or engaging in related high-risk behaviors. Indicated programs for drug abuse prevention, for example, would be appropriate for individuals that recently initiated substance use, with the goal of reducing their chances of a further escalation in use that can develop into a drug abuse problem. Thus, while recruitment and participation in a selective intervention is based on subgroup membership, recruitment and participation in an indicated intervention is based on early warning signs demonstrated by an individual.

Substance abuse prevention efforts can be divided into five general strategies:

- Information dissemination approaches
- Affective education approaches
- Alternatives approaches
- Social resistance skills approaches
- Broader competence enhancement approaches, which emphasize personal and social skills training

Table 54.1 summarizes these prevention strategies, which are discussed in the following sections.

Information Dissemination

Ubiquitous on the prevention landscape are programs that rely on the dissemination of factual information. The hallmark of these programs is the primary focus on providing factual information such as the pharmacology and the adverse consequences of use. Information dissemination approaches to substance abuse prevention are based on a rational model of human behavior. Substance abuse is seen as being the result of insufficient knowledge of the adverse consequences of using psychoactive drugs. Thus, the prescription for preventing substance abuse is to educate adolescents about the dangers of smoking, drinking, or using drugs. It is assumed that exposure to factual information about the dangers of using drugs will lead to changes in attitudes, which, in turn, will lead to nonsubstance use behavior. Within the context of the information dissemination approach, individuals are seen as being essentially rationale individuals that are likely to avoid the harms of substance use once they become aware of factual information about these harms.

Information dissemination programs have taken the form of public information campaigns and school-based tobacco, alcohol, and drug education programs. Public information campaigns have involved the use of pamphlets, leaflets, posters, and PSAs to increase public awareness of the problem of tobacco, alcohol, or drug abuse and alter societal norms concerning use. School programs have involved classroom curricula, assembly programs featuring guest speakers (frequently policemen or health professionals), and educational films.

Many informational approaches have been designed to deter substance use by emphasizing, even dramatizing, the risks associated with substance use. The underlying assumption of fear-arousal approaches is that evoking fear is more effective than a simple exposition of the facts. These approaches go beyond a dispassionate presentation of information by providing a clear and unambiguous message that substance use is dangerous. In addition, traditional prevention programs have sometimes focused on the immorality of substance use. Program providers not only teach the objective facts, but also "preach" to students about the evils of smoking, drinking, or using drugs, and exhort them not to engage in those behaviors.

Examination of the empiric evidence concerning the effectiveness of the different approaches to tobacco, alcohol, and drug abuse prevention indicates quite clearly that while informational approaches may in some cases increase knowledge and change attitudes regarding substance use, these approaches fail when it comes to the most important outcome: reducing or preventing alcohol, tobacco, and other drug use. Increasing knowledge has little or no impact on substance

TABLE 54.1 Overview of major school-based prevention approaches

Approach	Focus	Methods
Information dissemination	Increase knowledge of drugs, their effects, and the consequences of use; promote antidrug use attitudes	Didactic instruction, discussion, audio/video presentations, displays of substances, posters, pamphlets, school assembly programs
Affective education	Increase self-esteem, responsible decision making, interpersonal growth; generally include little or no information about drugs	Didactic instruction, discussion, experiential activities, group problem-solving exercises
Alternatives	Increase self-esteem, self-reliance; provide variable alternatives to drug use; reduce boredom and sense of alienation	Organization of youth centers, recreational activities; participation in community service projects; vocational training
Resistance skills	Increase awareness of social influence to smoke, drink, or use drugs; develop skills for resisting substance use influences; increase knowledge of immediate negative consequences; establish nonsubstance use norms	Class discussion; resistance skills training; behavioral rehearsal; extended practice via behavioral "homework"; use of same-age or older peer leaders
Competence enhancement	Increase decision making, personal behavior change, anxiety reduction, and communication, social, and assertive skills; apply generic skills to resist substance use influences	Class discussion; cognitive–behavioral skills training (instruction, demonstration, practice, feedback, reinforcement)

use or on intentions to engage in tobacco, alcohol, or drug use in the near future (24). As such, the evaluation studies refute the basic assumption of the information dissemination model: that increased knowledge alone is sufficient for behavior change. Furthermore, research in health communications has found that fear appeals used as part of informational approaches are generally not effective in changing behavior, although these approaches as well may contribute to change in attitudes about drug use. It is also clear that appeals to the immorality of substance use are unlikely to be persuasive to students at highest risk for substance use.

Considering the complex etiology of substance abuse, it is not surprising that approaches that rely on the provision of factual information are ineffective. Information dissemination approaches are inadequate because they are too narrow in their focus and are based on an incomplete understanding of the factors promoting substance use and abuse. Although knowledge about the negative consequences of substance use is important, it is only one of many factors considered to play a role in the initiation of substance use among adolescents.

Affective Education

Substance abuse prevention efforts have also used affective education approaches, which are based on a different set of assumptions than information dissemination approaches. Less emphasis is placed on factual information about the adverse consequences of substance abuse, and more emphasis is placed on students' personal and social development. Affective education approaches focus on increasing self-understanding and acceptance through activities such as values clarifications and responsible decision making; improving interpersonal relations by fostering effective communication, peer counseling, and assertiveness; and increasing students' abilities to fulfill their basic needs through existing social institutions. A common component of many affective education programs is the inclusion of norm-setting messages concerning responsible substance use.

The results of evaluation studies testing the effectiveness of affective education approaches have been as discouraging as evaluations of informational approaches. Although affective education approaches have, in some instances, been able to demonstrate an impact on one or more of the correlates of substance use, they have not produced an impact on substance use behavior (25). While some of the components of affective education that focus on personal skills (e.g., communication and assertiveness) may be helpful as part of a larger prevention strategy, they are not effective in changing drug use behavior when emphasized on their own.

Alternatives

One method of preventing substance abuse that has been a part of both community-based and school-based interventions has been to restructure part of the adolescent's environment to provide them with alternatives to substance use and activities associated with substance use. Several different alternatives approaches have been developed. The original model for alternatives typically involved the establishment of youth centers providing a particular activity or set of activities in the community (e.g., hobbies, team sports, and community service). It was assumed that if adolescents could be provided with real-life experiences that would be as appealing as substance use, their involvement in these activities would actually take the place of involvement with substance use. Another type of alternatives approach is Outward Bound and similar programs. These activities are organized in the hope that they would alter the affective-cognitive state of an individual and that they would change the way individuals felt about themselves and others and how they saw the world. This approach focuses on healthy activities frequently designed to promote teamwork, self-confidence, and self-esteem.

While these approaches may seem worthwhile, few alternatives approaches have been evaluated properly, and those that have been evaluated are ineffective in preventing substance use behavior. Most alternative activities have limited theoretical or conceptual connection to substance abuse prevention. Although some activities related to academics, religion, or physical fitness training may be associated with nonsubstance use (26), these are unlikely to be attractive activities for high-risk young people. Furthermore, certain alternative activities may expose young people to environments or settings where substance use is normative, such as some social, entertainment, and vocational activities, and therefore may increase the risk for substance use. Like affective education, some components of alternative activities that help young people develop specific skills may be helpful as part of a larger prevention strategy, but by themselves these approaches are not effective in changing drug use behavior.

Toward Theory-Based Interventions: Psychological Inoculation

The pioneering prevention research of Evans and his colleagues at the University of Houston toward the end of the 1970s triggered a major departure from traditional approaches to tobacco, alcohol, and drug abuse prevention. Unlike previous approaches that focused on information dissemination and/or fear arousal, the strategy developed initially by Evans and his colleagues (27) focused on the social and psychological factors believed to be involved in the initiation of cigarette smoking.

Evans's work was strongly influenced by persuasive communications theory as formulated by McGuire (28) and a concept called "psychological inoculation." Psychological inoculation is analogous to that of inoculation used in infectious disease prevention. Persuasive communications designed to alter attitudes, beliefs, and behavior are conceptualized as the psychosocial analogue of "germs." To prevent "infection" it is necessary to expose the individual to a weak dose of those "germs" in a way that facilitates the development of "antibodies" and thereby increases resistance to any future exposure to persuasive messages in their more virulent form.

The application of the concept of psychological inoculation as a smoking prevention strategy is fairly straightforward. Smoking is conceptualized as being the result of social influences (persuasive messages) to smoke from peers and the media that are either direct (offers to smoke from other adolescents or cigarette advertising) or indirect (exposure to high-status role models who smoke). If adolescents are faced with peer pressure to try cigarettes, for example, they can be forewarned and prepared by providing them with the necessary skills for countering such pressure. They can be trained on what to say in specific situations to diffuse or negate attempts at peer pressure, and they can be taught to form counterarguments in situations when they see older youth posturing and acting "tough" by smoking.

The intervention initially developed by Evans consisted of a series of films designed to increase students' awareness of the various social pressures to smoke that they would be likely to encounter as they progressed through the critical junior high school period. Also included in these films were demonstrations of specific techniques that could be used to effectively resist various pressures to smoke. The prevention strategy developed by Evans also included two other important components: periodic assessment of smoking with feedback to students and information about the immediate physiologic effects of smoking. Smoking was assessed by questionnaire on a biweekly basis, and saliva samples were collected as an objective measure of smoking status. The rate of smoking in each classroom (which was considerably lower than most adolescents thought) was publicly announced to correct the misperception that cigarette smoking is a highly normative behavior (i.e., that everybody is doing it).

In the first major test of this prevention strategy, Evans compared students receiving assessment/feedback with those receiving monitoring/feedback plus inoculation against a control group (29). The students in the two treatment conditions exhibited smoking onset rates that were about 50% lower than that observed in the control group. The overall reduction in smoking onset was dramatic in view of the history of failed prevention efforts that preceded this study. The success of the study conducted by Evans triggered an explosion of prevention research and offered the first real evidence that preventive interventions could produce effects on substance use behavior.

Resistance Skills Training

Several variations in the prevention model originally developed by Evans have been tested over the years. Similar to Evans's model, these interventions were designed to increase students' awareness of the various social influences to engage in substance use. A distinctive feature of these prevention models is that they place more emphasis on teaching students specific skills for effectively resisting both peer and media pressures to smoke, drink, or use drugs. These resistance skills training programs (also referred to as "social influence" or "refusal skills training" approaches) are based on a conceptual model stressing the fundamental importance of social factors in promoting the initiation of substance use among adolescents. These influences come from the family (parents and older siblings), peers, and the mass media. Adolescents may be predisposed toward substance use because substance use behavior is modeled by parents or older siblings, or because of the transmission of positive messages and attitudes concerning substance use. Similarly, individuals who have friends who smoke, drink, or use drugs are more likely to become substance users themselves as a result of issues relating to modeling and the need for peer acceptance (as well as the greater availability of substances). Finally, on the larger societal level, high-status role models in the mass media may promote substance use by increasing perceived positive norms and expectations with respect to substance use. As Bandura (30) indicated, all social influences are themselves a product of the interaction between individual learning histories and forces in both the community and the larger society. Through social learning processes, a young person may expect various positive outcomes from substance use, such as increased alertness, relief from anxiety, or enhanced social status. While expectations of reward can be learned from direct experience with substance use, positive expectancies are initially typically learned by observing the expectations, attitudes, and behaviors regarding substance use of significant others like parents, siblings, peers, and media personalities.

Research on resistance skills training approaches initially focused primarily on preventing the onset of cigarette smoking, that is, preventing the transition from nonsmoking to smoking. Eventually, the onset of alcohol and illicit drug use was targeted as well. Most studies have targeted junior high school students, generally beginning with seventh graders. Fewer studies include elementary school students, partly because substance use rates are very low, and it is difficult to demonstrate behavioral effects in this age group. Social resistance skills programs generally teach students how to recognize situations in which they will have a high likelihood of experiencing peer pressure to smoke, drink, or use drugs so that these high-risk situations can be avoided. In addition, students are taught how to handle situations in which they might experience peer pressure to engage in substance use. Typically, this includes teaching students not only what to say (i.e., the specific content of a refusal message), but also how to deliver it in the most effective way possible. Material has also generally been included in these programs to combat the perception that substance use is widespread because adolescents typically overestimate the prevalence of smoking, drinking, and using certain drugs. These beliefs can be challenged by simply providing students with the prevalence rates of substance use among their age mates in terms of national survey data or conducting classroom or schoolwide surveys, which can be organized and directed by students participating in the program. Resistance skills training programs also typically include a component designed to increase students' awareness of the techniques used by advertisers to promote the sale of tobacco products or alcoholic beverages and to teach techniques for formulating counterarguments to the messages used by advertisers.

Perhaps the best known application of the social resistance skills training model is Project DARE (Drug Abuse Resistance Education), which is being used in approximately 60% of the classrooms in America. A unique aspect of DARE, and one that undoubtedly has contributed to its adoption by many schools, is that it is conducted by police officers. Although DARE has been remarkably successful with respect to being adopted by a large number of schools and in promoting an awareness of drug abuse, the results of DARE are disappointing. Although DARE has been repeatedly evaluated, many outcome studies have been of limited scientific value because of weak research designs (e.g., posttest only), poor sampling and data collection procedures, inadequate measurement strategies, and problems in data analysis approaches (31). Several evaluation studies of DARE using more scientifically rigorous designs (i.e., large samples, random assignment, and longitudinal follow-up) show that DARE has little or no impact on drug use behaviors, particularly beyond the initial posttest assessment (32–34).

While DARE is not effective in changing behavior, several studies have documented that well-designed and rigorously implemented social resistance skills programs can prevent substance use in adolescence. In a comprehensive meta-analysis of school-based smoking prevention programs, 23 randomized controlled trials (RCTs) were identified that met rigorous inclusion criteria for research design and execution quality, and 13 of these were categorized as social resistance programs (24). The main outcome variable was prevalence of nonsmoking at follow-up among those students not smoking at the baseline assessment. Of 13 RCTs of social resistance programs rated as most valid in terms of research design, 9 were found to produce positive intervention effects on smoking prevalence; four RCTs showed no effects on smoking behavior. In general, the positive behavioral effects of social resistance smoking prevention programs were relatively short term. A separate review of the smoking prevention literature compared studies comparing social influence programs to no intervention control group conditions. Findings indicated that mean differences in smoking across conditions ranged from 5% to 60% with durations of 1 to 4 years (35). The authors concluded that the most effective school-based smoking prevention programs are those with sustained application, booster sessions over several years, and reinforcement in the community including the involvement of parents and/or the mass media, and those that are part of a comprehensive school health promotion program.

In general, results from long-term follow-up studies of school-based social influence approaches indicate that these prevention effects are typically not maintained. While this has led some to conclude that school-based prevention approaches may not be powerful enough to produce lasting prevention effects, others have argued that the apparent failure of studies testing resistance skills training approaches to produce long-term prevention effects may have to do with factors related to either the type of intervention tested in these studies or the way these interventions were implemented. Resnicow and Botvin (36) argue that the absence of long-term prevention effects in these studies should not be taken as an indictment of school-based prevention; instead, the lack of effects in several long-term follow-up studies may have occurred because (a) the length of the intervention may have been too short (i.e., the prevention approach was effective, but the initial prevention "dosage" was too low to produce a long-term effect), (b) booster sessions were either inadequate or not included (i.e., the prevention approach was effective, but it eroded over time because of the absence or inadequacy of ongoing intervention), (c) the intervention was not implemented with enough fidelity to the intervention model (i.e., the correct prevention approach was used, but it was implemented incompletely, improperly, or both), and/or (d) the intervention was based on faulty assumptions, was incomplete, or was otherwise deficient (i.e., the prevention approach was ineffective). Indeed, it now appears that these factors played a role in the negative findings of long-term follow-up studies with prevention approaches based on the resistance skills training model. School-based prevention programs that are powerful enough to have a durable impact on adolescent substance use need to focus on a broad and comprehensive set of skills-building activities, have a strong initial dosage and include at least two additional years of (booster) intervention, and be implemented in a manner that is faithful to the underlying intervention model.

Competence Enhancement

Since the end of the 1970s and up to the present, considerable research has also been conducted with a prevention approach that teaches general personal and social skills either alone (37) or in combination with components of the social resistance skills model (38). These competence enhancement approaches are more comprehensive than either traditional cognitive–affective approaches or the more recent resistance skills model. In addition to recognizing the importance of social learning processes such as modeling, imitation, and reinforcement, competence-enhancement approaches posit that youth with poor personal and social skills are not only more susceptible to influences that promote drug use, but also motivated to use drugs as an alternative to more adaptive coping strategies (38). They are based on social learning theory (30) and problem behavior theory (17). Substance abuse is conceptualized as a socially learned and functional behavior, resulting from the interplay of social and personal factors. Substance use behavior is learned through modeling and reinforcement and is influenced by cognition, attitudes, and beliefs.

Personal and social skills training prevention approaches typically teach two or more of the following:

- General problem-solving and decision-making skills
- General cognitive skills for resisting interpersonal or media influences
- Skills for increasing self-control and self-esteem
- Adaptive coping strategies for relieving stress and anxiety through the use of cognitive coping skills or behavioral relaxation techniques
- General social skills
- General assertive skills

These skills are taught using a combination of instruction, demonstration, feedback, reinforcement, behavioral rehearsal (practice during class), and extended practice through behavioral homework assignments. The intent of these programs is to teach the kind of generic skills for coping with life that will have a relatively broad application. This is in contrast to the resistance skills training approaches, which are designed to teach skills with a problem-specific focus. Personal and social skills training programs emphasize the application of general skills to situations directly related to substance use and abuse (e.g., the application of general assertive skills to situations involving peer pressure to smoke, drink, or use drugs). These same skills can be used for dealing with many of the challenges confronting adolescents in their everyday lives, including, but not limited to, smoking, drinking, and drug abuse.

Although prevention approaches that emphasize the development of general personal and social skills have a broader focus compared to approaches designed to teach skills for resisting social influences to use drugs, the most effective prevention approaches appear to combine the features of both. Indeed, evidence suggests that broad-based competence enhancement approaches may not be effective unless they also contain some resistance skills training material. A prevention approach with both components will help teach students to apply generic personal and social skills to situations related specifically to preventing substance abuse and may also serve to increase antidrug norms.

Evaluation studies testing a combined social influence and competence enhancement skills training approach have demonstrated significant behavioral effects on alcohol, tobacco, and other drug use. A series of evaluation studies has been conducted over the past 30 years examining the effectiveness of the Life Skills Training (LST) program, a universal school-based prevention approach that teaches general personal and social skills training combined with drug-refusal skills and normative education. Studies range from small-scale efficacy studies to large-scale randomized trials. These studies consistently show that the LST approach produces positive behavioral effects on alcohol, tobacco, and other drug use.

The focus of the initial evaluation research of the LST program was on cigarette smoking and involved predominantly white middle-class populations. Several early small-scale efficacy studies demonstrated that this prevention approach effectively reduces cigarette smoking among youth receiving the program, as compared to a control group that does not. Additional studies examined its effectiveness with different delivery formats, different program providers, and different substances; these studies found that the prevention approach was made more effective by the inclusion of booster sessions after the initial year of intervention; that it is equally effective when taught by teachers, peer leaders, and health educators; and that it produced behavioral effects on alcohol and marijuana. These initial studies were among the first school-based prevention studies to show consistent behavioral effects on adolescent substance use (see Ref. (39) for a review).

More recent evaluation research on the LST approach has focused on the intervention's long-term effects on drug use, effects on more serious levels of drug involvement including illicit drug use, and its impact on hypothesized mediating variables, and has increasingly focused on effects when used with inner-city minority populations. The evaluation designs have become increasingly sophisticated with time, including two large-scale multisite randomized prevention trials with long-term follow-up. The first of these randomized controlled prevention trials focused on a predominantly white, suburban sample of youth. Beginning in 1985, this prevention trial examined the short- and long-term effects of the LST approach among close to 6000 students from 56 junior high schools in New York State. Students in the prevention condition received the intervention in the seventh grade and booster sessions during the eighth and ninth grades. Significant prevention effects were found among intervention participants at the end of the ninth grade in terms of cigarette smoking, marijuana use, and immoderate alcohol use (40), as well as at the end of the 12th grade (41). In the latter follow-up study, there were significantly fewer smokers, heavy drinkers, marijuana users, and polydrug users among students who received the prevention program relative to controls. The strongest prevention effects were produced for the students who received the most complete implementation of the prevention program. A related study using data from a confidential and random subsample of these students ($N = 447$) found that there were lower levels of overall illicit drug use and lower levels of use for hallucinogens, heroin, and other narcotics in the intervention group relative to controls (42).

A large-scale prevention trial tested the LST approach among inner-city minority youth in New York City. The sample was predominantly African American (61%) and Hispanic (22%) and consisted of students ($N = 3621$) in 29 urban middle schools. Results at the posttest and 1-year follow-up indicated that those who received the prevention program reported less smoking, drinking, drunkenness, inhalant use, and polydrug use relative to those in the control group who did not receive the intervention (43). Additional studies using data from this large-scale trial focused on prevention effects of the intervention program in terms of cigarette smoking onset and binge drinking. The first of these studies examined the effectiveness of the prevention program in reducing the initiation and escalation of smoking in a subsample of girls from the larger study (44). One-year follow-up data indicated that girls who participated in the intervention condition were significantly less likely to initiate smoking relative to controls, and 30% fewer participants escalated to monthly smoking relative to students in the control group. A second study showed that this intervention approach had protective effects in terms of binge drinking (five or more drinks per drinking occasion) among inner-city, middle school boys and girls (45). In this study, the proportion of binge drinkers was more than 50% lower in those who received the prevention program relative to the control group at both 1- and 2-year follow-up assessments. Finally, a study of a subset of students from the larger sample examined the effectiveness of the prevention program among youth at high risk for substance use initiation and found that those students who had poor grades in school and friends that engaged in substance use were less likely to engage in smoking, drinking, inhalant use, or polydrug use than were similarly matched controls that did not receive the intervention (46). Taken together, the results from several large-scale randomized prevention trials provide strong evidence of the effectiveness of the competence enhancement plus resistance skills prevention approach, with both suburban white youth and inner-city minority youth. A major strength of the evaluation studies conducted with the broader personal and social skills training approaches such as LST is that they also have a demonstrated impact on variables hypothesized to mediate the effect of the prevention programs in a direction consistent with nonsubstance use. These include significant changes in knowledge and attitudes, assertiveness, locus of control, social anxiety, self-satisfaction, decision making, and problem solving.

Together, the results of these studies provide compelling evidence supporting the efficacy of broad-spectrum prevention strategies focusing on general personal and social skills development combined with drug-specific social resistance skills. Thus, this prevention approach has been demonstrated to produce reductions in substance use (relative to controls), as well as changes in several hypothesized mediating variables in a direction consistent with reduced substance abuse risk.

SUMMARY AND CONCLUSION

A number of substance abuse prevention approaches have been developed and tested over the years. The most common approaches to tobacco, alcohol, and drug abuse prevention are those that focus on providing factual information about the adverse consequences of using these substances, with some approaches including a mix of scare tactics and moral messages. Other commonly used approaches to substance abuse prevention have used affective education and alternatives approaches. The existing evaluation literature shows rather conclusively that these are not effective prevention strategies when the standard of effectiveness concerns the ability to influence substance use behavior. On the other hand, research shows that the most effective prevention approaches are based on an understanding of the etiology of substance abuse supported by a sound theoretical model. Contemporary school-based substance abuse prevention programs that focus on social resistance and competence enhancement skills are effective in large part because their assumptions about the causes of substance use are consistent with more recently conducted etiologic research.

The large body of research on school-based prevention contains a number of findings regarding the key components and characteristics of effective substance use prevention programs (47,48). Programs should be based on a comprehensive theoretical framework that addresses multiple risk and protective factors. Program content should be developmentally appropriate and include information relevant to the target age group and the important life transitions they face. The material should include skills training exercises to help young people recognize and resist pressures to use drugs, as well as comprehensive skills training to enhance personal and social competence skills, and other skills to build resilience and help participants navigate developmental tasks. Programs should provide accurate information regarding rates of drug use to reduce the perception that it is common and normative. They should be delivered using interactive methods—including facilitated discussion, structured small group activities, and role-playing scenarios—to stimulate participation and promote the acquisition of skills. Interventions must be culturally sensitive and incorporate relevant language and audiovisual content familiar to the target audience. They should include adequate dosage to introduce and reinforce the material, including booster sessions in subsequent years. Program providers should participate in comprehensive interactive training sessions to generate enthusiasm, increase implementation fidelity, and give providers a chance to learn and practice new instructional techniques. Published meta-analytic studies indicate that competence enhancement and social influence approaches are more effective than traditional didactic approaches and that attitude and behavior change is most substantial in high intensity, multicomponent programs implemented with booster sessions after the initial intervention. To be effective, school-based interventions need to be more comprehensive, have a stronger initial dosage, include at least two additional years of (booster) intervention, and be implemented in a manner that is faithful to the underlying intervention model. Generally social resistance prevention programs are effective with a broad range of adolescents including high- and low-risk individuals and urban, suburban, and rural students. These studies indicate that the inclusion of additional intervention components produces stronger prevention effects than the school-based intervention alone. Peer-led programs have been found to frequently be more effective than adult-led programs (25), particularly when peer leaders assist adult program providers and have specific and well-defined roles.

Over the past two to three decades, there have been a number of significant developments in the field of substance abuse prevention. Yet despite the promise offered by these approaches, future research is needed to further refine current prevention models and to develop new ones. Given the urgency and importance of dealing with the problem of substance abuse, it seems prudent to proceed on two simultaneous tracks: one involving further prevention research and the other involving the dissemination of the most promising existing prevention approaches. This is particularly important in view of the fact that the most widely utilized prevention approaches continue to be those that have already been found either to be ineffective or to lack any scientifically defensible evidence of their efficacy.

The problem of substance abuse is still very prevalent. However, for the first time in the history of its prevention, evidence now exists from a number of rigorously designed evaluation studies that specific school-based and community-based prevention models are effective. It is now incumbent upon health care professionals, educators, community leaders, and policy makers to move expeditiously toward wide dissemination and use of these approaches. It is equally important for private and governmental agencies to provide adequate funding for the important research necessary to further refine existing prevention models and to increase our understanding of the causes of substance abuse.

REFERENCES

1. Newcomb MD, Locke T. Health, social, and psychological consequences of drug use and abuse. In: Sloboda, Z, ed. *Epidemiology of Drug Abuse*. New York: Springer; 2005:45–59.
2. Paglia A, Room R. Preventing substance use problems among youth: a literature review and recommendations. *J Prim Prev.* 1999;20:3–50.
3. Petraitis J, Flay BR, Miller TQ. Reviewing theories of adolescent substance use: organizing pieces in the puzzle. *Psychol Bull.* 1995;117:67–86.
4. Hawkins JD, Catalano RF, Miller JY. Risk and protective factors for alcohol and other drug problems in adolescence and early adulthood: implications for substance abuse prevention. *Psychol Bull.* 1992;112:64–105.
5. Johnston LD, O'Malley PM, Bachman JG, et al. *Monitoring the Future National Survey Results on Drug Use, 1975–2008. Volume I: Secondary School Students* (NIH Publication No. 09-7402). Bethesda, MD: National Institute on Drug Abuse; 2009.
6. Substance Abuse and Mental Health Services Administration. *The NSDUH Report: Misuse of Over-the-Counter Cough and Cold Medications among Persons Aged 12 to 25*. Rockville, MD: Office of Applied Studies; 2008.
7. Wang LW, Crossett LS, Lowry R, et al. Cost-effectiveness of a school-based tobacco-use prevention program. *Arch Pediatr Adolesc Med.* 2001;155:1043–1050.
8. Swadi H. Individual risk factors for adolescent substance use. *Drug Alcohol Depend.* 1999;55:209–224.
9. Hartel CR, Glantz MD. *Drug Abuse: Origins and Interventions*. Washington, DC: American Psychological Association; 1997.
10. Andrews J, Hops H. The role of peers and family as predictors of drug etiology. In: Scheier LM, ed. *Handbook of Drug Use Etiology*. Washington, DC: American Psychological Association; 2010.
11. McCool JP, Cameron LD, Petrie KJ. Adolescent perceptions of smoking imagery in film. *Soc Sci Med.* 2001;52:1577–1587.
12. Snyder LB. Substance use and the media. In: Scheier LM, ed. *Handbook of Drug Use Etiology*. Washington, DC: American Psychological Association; 2010.
13. Piko B. Smoking in adolescence: do attitudes matter? *Addict Behav.* 2001;26:201–217.
14. Simons-Morton B, Haynie DL, Crump AD, et al. Expectancies and other psychosocial factors associated with alcohol use among early adolescent boys and girls. *Addict Behav.* 1999;24:229–238.
15. Khantzian EJ. The self-medication hypothesis of substance use disorders: a reconsideration and recent applications. *Harv Rev Psychiatry.* 1997;4:231–244.
16. Saal D, Dong Y, Bonci A, et al. Drugs of abuse and stress trigger a common synaptic adaptation in dopamine neurons. *Neuron.* 2003;37:577–582.
17. Jessor R, Jessor SL. *Problem Behavior and Psychosocial Development: A Longitudinal Study of Youth*. New York: Academic Press; 1977.

18. Donovan JE, Jessor R. Structure of problem behavior in adolescence and young adulthood. *J Consult Clin Psychol.* 1985;53:890–904.
19. Resnicow K, Ross-Gaddy D, Vaughan RD. Structure of problem and positive behaviors in African-American youth. *J Consult Clin Psychol.* 1995;63:594–603.
20. Kandel D. *Stages and Pathways of Drug Involvement: Examining the Gateway Hypothesis.* New York: Cambridge University Press; 2002.
21. Steinberg L, Morris AS. Adolescent development. *Ann Rev Psychol.* 2001;52:83–110.
22. Piaget J. *The Moral Judgment of the Child.* New York: Collier; 1962.
23. Institute of Medicine. *Reducing Risks for Mental Disorders: Frontiers for Preventive Intervention Research.* Washington, DC: National Academy Press; 1994.
24. Thomas R, Perera R. School-based programmes for preventing smoking. *Cochrane Database Syst Rev.* 2006;(3). Art. No.: CD001293. DOI: 10.1002/14651858.CD001293.pub2.
25. Faggiano F, Vigna-Taglianti FD, Versino E, et al. School-based prevention for illicit drugs use: a systematic review. *Prev Med.* 2008;46:385–396.
26. Collingwood TR, Sunderlin J, Reynolds R, et al. Physical training as a substance abuse prevention intervention for youth. *J Drug Educ.* 2000;30(4):435–451.
27. Evans RI. Smoking in children: developing a social psychological strategy of deterrence. *Prev Med.* 1976;5:122–127.
28. McGuire WJ. The nature of attitudes and attitude change. In: Lindzey G, Aronson E, eds. *Handbook of Social Psychology.* Reading, MA: Addison-Wesley; 1968:136–314.
29. Evans RI, Rozelle RM, Mittlemark MB, et al. Deterring the onset of smoking in children: knowledge of immediate physiological effects and coping with peer pressure, media pressure, and parent modeling. *J Appl Soc Psychol.* 1978;8:126–135.
30. Bandura A. *Social Learning Theory.* Englewood Cliffs, NJ: Prentice-Hall; 1977.
31. Rosenbaum DP, Hanson GS. Assessing the effects of school-based drug education: a six-year multilevel analysis of Project D.A.R.E. *J Res Crime Delinquency.* 1998;35:381–412.
32. Lynam DR, Milich R, Zimmerman R, et al. Project DARE: no effects at 10-year follow-up. *J Consult Clin Psychol.* 1999;67(4):590–593.
33. Ennett ST, Tobler NS, Ringwalt CL, et al. How effective is drug abuse resistance education? A meta-analysis of project DARE outcome evaluations. *Am J Public Health.* 1994;84:1394–1401.
34. Clayton RR, Cattarello AM, Johnstone BM. The effectiveness of Drug Abuse Resistance Education (Project D.A.R.E.): five-year follow-up results. *Prev Med.* 1996;25:307–318.
35. La Torre G, Chiaradia G, Ricciardi G. School-based smoking prevention in children and adolescents: review of the scientific literature. *J Public Health.* 2005;13:285–290.
36. Resnicow K, Botvin GJ. School-based substance use prevention programs: why do effects decay? *Prev Med.* 1993;22:484–490.
37. Caplan M, Weissberg RP, Grober JS, et al. Social competence promotion with inner-city and suburban young adolescents: effects on social adjustment and alcohol use. *J Consult Clin Psychol.* 1992;60:56–63.
38. Botvin GJ. Preventing drug abuse in schools: social and competence enhancement approaches targeting individual-level etiological factors. *Addict Behav.* 2000;25:887–897.
39. Botvin GJ, Griffin KW. Life Skills Training: empirical findings and future directions. *J Prim Prev.* 2004;25:211–232.
40. Botvin GJ, Baker E, Dusenbury L, et al. Preventing adolescent drug abuse through a multimodal cognitive-behavioral approach: results of a three-year study. *J Consult Clin Psychol.* 1990;58:437–446.
41. Botvin GJ, Baker E, Dusenbury L, et al. Long-term follow-up results of a randomized drug abuse prevention trial in a white middle-class population. *JAMA.* 1995;273:1106–1112.
42. Botvin GJ, Griffin KW, Diaz T, et al. Preventing illicit drug use in adolescents: long-term follow-up data from a randomized control trial of a school population. *Addict Behav.* 2000;5:769–774.
43. Botvin GJ, Griffin KW, Diaz T, et al. Drug abuse prevention among minority adolescents: one-year follow-up of a school-based preventive intervention. *Prev Sci.* 2001;2:1–13.
44. Botvin GJ, Griffin KW, Diaz T, et al. Smoking initiation and escalation in early adolescent girls: one-year follow-up of a school-based prevention intervention for minority youth. *J Am Med Wom Assoc.* 1999;54:139–143.
45. Botvin GJ, Griffin KW, Diaz T, et al. Preventing binge drinking during early adolescence: one- and two-year follow-up of a school-based preventive intervention. *Psychol Addict Behav.* 2001;15:360–365.
46. Griffin KW, Botvin GJ, Nichols TR, et al. Effectiveness of a universal drug abuse prevention approach for youth at high risk for substance use initiation. *Prev Med.* 2003;36:1–7.
47. Cuijpers P. Peer-led and adult-led school drug prevention: a meta-analytic comparison. *J Drug Educ.* 2002;32(2):107–119.
48. Tobler NS, Stratton HH. Effectiveness of school-based drug prevention programs: a meta-analysis of the research. *J Prim Prev.* 1997;18:71–128.

CHAPTER 55
Harm Reduction: New Drug Policies and Practices

Ernest Drucker ■ Robert G. Newman ■ Ethan Nadelmann ■ Dr. Alex Wodak ■ Daniel Wolfe ■ David C. Marsh ■ Eugene Oscapella ■ Jennifer Mcneely ■ Yujiang Jia ■ Kasia Malinowska-Sempruch

OVERVIEW

In this chapter, we review the conceptual basis and scientific evidence for harm reduction (HR) drug policies and document their applications in practice worldwide. We begin with the public health model for many HR methods that are some of its signature applications (i.e., syringe exchange, safe injecting sites, overdose [OD] prevention). We then discuss HR approaches to drug treatment (especially opioid substitution methods) and introduce some of the more innovative HR drug policies (such as heroin maintenance and medical marijuana). A section on China is included as a current case study in the development of a national HR program. We conclude by examining how these prevention and intervention strategies affect individual and public health outcomes, such as the HIV epidemic, and the more general HR goals of human rights, improvements in global security, and the protection of public health and safety in civil societies.

THE PROBLEM

The production, distribution, and sale of illicit drugs are among the world's leading industries. Approximately 200 million people (4.8% of the world's population) use illicit drugs each year (75% of that cannabis)—an economy estimated at $400 to $500 billion annually by the World Bank, U.S. Drug Enforcement Agency (DEA), United Nations International Drug Control Program (UNDCP), and Interpol (1) (Table 55.1). This unprecedented scale and worldwide nature of today's international drug markets has profound social, public health, and political implications, confronting us with a potent new version of a very old problem—the globalization of drugs.

Our apparent inability to contain illicit drugs and their harms challenges old ways of thinking about drugs and forces us to reconsider the fundamental ideas and policies we employ for their control. Additionally, with its many links to the HIV/AIDS pandemic, drug use is now one of the most urgent public health problems facing the world (1). The HR model is an outgrowth of these contemporary realities (2). Well before AIDS, the Dutch undertook HR as "normalization" of drug policies to increase users' contact with social, treatment, health, and other community services. The realization that people shared needles, spreading the human immunodeficiency virus (HIV) and other infectious diseases (e.g., hepatitis C), created powerful new reasons for establishing new public health goals for drug policy. In the 1980s, public health officials in the United Kingdom declared: "HIV is a greater threat to public and individual health than drug misuse" (3) (a sentiment echoed in Australia, Canada, Switzerland, and many other countries) (4). By 2009, some 74 countries explicitly supported HR as a basis of their national drug policies.

REFRAMING THE ISSUE

HR concepts and measures share two underlying assumptions:

1. It is better (for both society and the individual) to reduce the risks and harms of drug use, rather than to focus solely on the utopian goal of making people (or the world) "drug free."
2. Drug control policies based primarily on the criminalization of drug use and drug users should be replaced with policies that produce demonstrable reductions in the adverse consequences of continued drug use worldwide.

HR concepts and policies address the harms of drug policies as well as those of drugs themselves, offering pragmatic public health-oriented alternatives to the unachievable goals of drug prohibition—"a drug-free society" (5)—through a new model and set of pragmatic approaches intended to address the following significant challenges:

How can we reduce the likelihood of people who use drugs contracting and spreading blood-borne infections (HIV, hepatitis), and other infectious diseases (e.g. tuberculosis), suffering fatal overdoses, and developing other drug use–related medical problems?

How can we reduce the likelihood that people who use drugs will engage in criminal and other undesirable behaviors?

How can we increase the likelihood that people who use drugs will be good citizens, act responsibly toward others in their communities, take care of their families, complete their education or training, and become legally employed?

How can we develop drug policies that are both effective (at reducing adverse outcomes) and humane, while improving quality and access to effective prevention, treatment, and rehabilitation services? and

TABLE 55.1	Extent of drug use (annual prevalence[a]) estimates 2005/2006 (or latest year available)					
	Cannabis	Amphetamine-type stimulants		Cocaine	Opiates	Heroin
		Amphetamines	Ecstasy			
(Million people)	158.8	24.9	8.6	14.3	15.6	11.1
In % of global population aged 15–64	3.8	0.6	0.2	0.3	0.4	0.3

[a]Annual prevalence is a measure of the number/percentage of people who consumed an illicit drug at least once in the 12-month period preceding the assessment.

Data from the United Nations Office on Drugs and Crime. The World Drug Report 2007. Available at: http://www.unodc.org/unodc/en/data-and-analysis/WDR-2007.html.

How can we minimize the harms associated with prohibition drug policies and the criminalization of drug users?

DRUG USE, PUBLIC HEALTH, AND HUMAN RIGHTS

The HR model grows from the clinical and preventive medicine framework of public health (6), whose goals include reducing morbidity and mortality in populations by using the tools of primary, secondary, and tertiary prevention. In HR, rather than focusing on the reduction of drug use per se, primary prevention seeks to reduce the harms of drugs and drug control policies (i.e., rates of addiction and other hazards of drug use, including infectious diseases, and OD deaths) and the risks of illicit drug markets (with their violence and corruption). Secondary prevention aims to limit the prevalence and severity of these individual psychologic harms and medical disorders associated with continued drug use and addiction (i.e., effective treatment and rehabilitation, HIV programs). Tertiary prevention involves limiting collateral medical and social consequences of drug use, drug markets, and addiction for individuals, families, and communities—once drug use has become a prevalent and chronic condition.

This is a shift of viewpoint: one where drug use and drug problems are not seen as based on a model of individual psychologic, moral, or legal deficiencies. Rather, HR recognizes that many of the most destructive consequences and refractory problems of illicit drug use are not only attributable to the ingestion of drugs but are the result of the methods of use (e.g., injection leading to HIV, HCV) or uncontrolled dependence on drugs of unknown purity and potency (OD and poisoning). Others are linked to the failure of the drug policies employed to control them—especially harsh enforcement of their prohibition and criminalization of drug users. Combined with the irrepressible global demand for mood-altering drugs, this must inevitably increase their value, foster aggressive trafficking, and spread drug use. Criminalization also undermines drug users' ability to protect themselves, their families and communities, setting the stage for collateral public health and social damages (e.g., epidemics of blood-borne diseases, violent drug wars in communities, and mass incarceration (7).

Drug use and drug policies are also a matter of human rights: abuses committed in the name of drug policy violate international conventions ratified by the member states of the United Nations. Human rights considerations focus on protecting people who use drugs from discrimination, individuals rights violations, and disproportionate punishment—including arrest and incarceration for positive urine tests or possession of drugs for personal use, deprivation of due process (e.g., internment in forced labor camps with no right of appeal), and police abuses such as extortion of monies from drug users threatened with arrest, the use of withdrawal symptoms to coerce confessions, or use of medical records to subject patients to repeated stop-and-frisk procedures. Additionally, human rights advocates support "positive obligations" to promote the health of people who use drugs, arguing against bans on methadone treatment, needle exchange, or provision of medical care. Jurisprudence, rather than peer-reviewed scientific studies, is often cited in support of these positions. Regional human rights courts and leading human rights officials have affirmed with increasing force that drug users do not forfeit their human rights just because they use illicit drugs and questioned the legality of punitive drug control practices (8).

THREE CAVEATS

Analysis of HR efforts and their outcomes must be qualified by three important caveats:

1. Drug prohibition policies remain the context for all HR efforts: In most countries HR programs and policies must coexist in tension with (and are usually dominated by) the "War on Drugs" and the international drug prohibition regime. The rise of HIV infection rates has created competing discourses based on international public health and human rights, but these do not have the force of law. HR programs therefore continue to struggle with largely hostile mechanisms of drug law enforcement and criminalization.

2. The limits of research and science: Illicit drug use and behavior are shaped by so many societal influences that it is extremely difficult and sometimes impossible to isolate and determine the precise impact of specific measures on drug-related behavior. Data collection and analysis regarding generally hidden and highly stigmatized illicit behavior are inherently difficult (making the subject very difficult to study), and governments vary in how they collect and categorize data on illicit drug use and related public health and criminal justice information—making cross-national comparisons problematic.

3. The importance of different cultural contexts: Most societies in which HR policies (e.g., syringe availability or substitution treatment) were first implemented are advanced industrialized social democracies. Some HR programs now exist in most countries of the former Soviet Union and multiple countries in East and Southeast Asia; for example, methadone treatment is currently operative in more than 65 countries but not in Russia or India. Naturally these programs vary sharply in their scale, quality, and auspice (private, church, government). Even in countries of the developing world, HR models and practices may also be quite different—for example, do they support community outreach or prefer stationary, clinic-based approaches; do they acknowledge or reject a role for people who use drugs in the formation and operation of programs and policies?

HARM REDUCTION IN THE UNITED STATES

While there are exceptions, most American politicians and public officials have publicly rejected many HR premises and ignored the evidence supporting HR, even as drug policy in the United States remains officially blind to abundant evidence of its own failures. While Europeans and Australians established and expanded such programs in the 1980s (often in response to the all-too-apparent American catastrophe of HIV among injection drug users [IDUs]), the United States resisted needle syringe programmes (NSPs) arguing that syringe distribution encourages illicit drug use and "sends the wrong message." Bitter confrontations blocked public and governmental action during the crucial early phase of the U.S. HIV/AIDS epidemic. It is now estimated that more than 4300 HIV infections (and perhaps as many as 9000 to 10,000 infections, depending on estimates of NSPs effectiveness) could have been prevented between 1987 and 1995, had an effective program of needle exchange been implemented and approximately 20,000 IDUs are still being infected with HIV in the United States each year (9).

In 1988, Congressional amendments first banned the use of federal funds for needle and syringe programs (because they could "promote drug use"). Until 2008, the very term "harm reduction" was banned from government vocabulary and from federal grant applications. HR policies (e.g., medical marijuana) have been attacked by U.S. government officials as "surrender in the War on Drugs" and stepping-stones to "drug legalization" (10). President Barack Obama's campaign pledged support for needle exchange, and in 2009, officials agreed to rein in federal officers threatening California's medical marijuana program (with over 250,000 registrants). As of this writing (2010), the federal ban on funding of needle exchange has been lifted, but federal health officials remain unwilling to endorse HR more broadly.

HARM REDUCTION AS PREVENTION: NEW MODELS AND SERVICES FOR ACTIVE DRUG USERS

Syringe Exchange Programs

Early in the HIV/AIDS epidemic, the sharing of syringes was clearly linked to HIV transmission. By 1995, about half of the new HIV infections in the United States (now estimated by the CDC as 55,000 per year (9,10)) were attributed directly or indirectly to drug use. The institution of NSPs was the first well-organized and explicit HR program in the United States (11) and in many European and Asian countries and had a marked impact—by 2007, less than one third of newly reported AIDS cases in the United States and Western Europe were among IDUs or their sexual partners. However, in many countries NSPs still meet with strong opposition and are not implemented at levels adequate to affect the spread of blood-borne pathogens.

The positive effects of NSPs on syringe sharing and a wide range of other behaviors linked to HIV/AIDS risk were well documented in the United States, Great Britain, the Netherlands, and Australia by the early 1990s. Both previous and more recent reviews NSPs (12) found more than half of the programs were associated with reductions in syringe sharing. In Connecticut, the sharing of needles among IDUs dropped by 40% after that state changed its paraphernalia laws in 1992 to allow for purchase, possession, and sale of up to 10 syringes without a prescription. The results of this change were a decrease in IDUs marginalization (11,13), better access to social and legal services and drug treatment, as well as increased referrals to medical care (e.g., for tuberculosis [TB] and HIV). A few showed an increase in HIV (e.g., in Montreal and Vancouver among populations involved in very high-risk cocaine injecting), but study designs precluded adequate comparisons to non-NSP users (13,14).

Referral to drug treatment is a major accomplishment of SEPs in practice. Since 1991, a Tacoma, Washington NSP has been the largest single source of recruitment to methadone-maintenance programs in the region. Of the first 569 clients in New Haven, Connecticut's NSP, 188 (33%) requested drug treatment, and 107 (57%) of those clients were placed in treatment programs. In the United Kingdom, where almost 60% of new NSP clients have no contact with other treatment or HIV prevention services, many clients are subsequently referred to such services. NSPs are well suited for disseminating information on HIV/AIDS risks and users take such information seriously; the claim that drug injectors will not alter their behavior to reduce the risks of contracting HIV and other infections has consistently been refuted. In cities that implemented SEPs in the mid-1980s, there is evidence of lower HIV prevalence among IDUs than in cities that did not offer SEPs until later in the HIV/AIDS epidemic. In Australia and the United Kingdom, where NSPs were instituted in the mid-1980s, HIV seroprevalence in drug injectors has remained lower than in most other countries (15).

Needle and Syringe Programs in the United States

Despite very favorable early reports on the public health impact of NSPs worldwide and endorsements by national commissions (i.e., *the National Commission on Acquired Immune Deficiency Syndrome, the Centers for Disease Control and Prevention, the General Accounting Office, the National Academy of Sciences' Institute of Medicine, and the Office of Technology Assessment*) (13–15), implementation of NSPs faced daunting challenges throughout their American history: funding shortages, continued police harassment, and, in some cities, criminal prosecution for activists caught distributing syringes. Many American NSPs operate without the legal sanction of local authorities, and all sanctioned SEPs operate under strict rules—which may include limits on the number of syringes that can be dispensed to individual clients, restrictions on where NSPs can be located and what hours they are open—requirements hindering their ability to achieve maximum effectiveness (16). U.S. federal support for even the evaluation of NSPs did not occur until 1992, the 11th year of the AIDS epidemic. And (until 2009) the United States prohibited the use of federal funds to pay for NSPs either in America or overseas. It is the private sector, charitable foundations, and community volunteers and activists, along with state and local officials, which provide the funds and personnel for many NSPs in the United States. Today only 10% to 15% of U.S. drug injectors have access to NSPs, of which there were 101 (including Puerto Rico). Some local laws prohibit the sale or possession of syringes without a prescription, and all but five states have drug paraphernalia laws that criminalize the possession or distribution of syringes except for "legitimate medical purposes" (16).

In 2000, New York State began a pilot program under which 2500 community pharmacists could sell syringes under a waiver of paraphernalia laws (15); this program has been evaluated and found to produce positive outcomes. Circulation time of used syringes is minimized by encouraging or requiring drug injectors to return used syringes for clean ones and by providing multiple disposal sites for used syringes. But even where over-the-counter sale is permitted, pharmacists may be prohibited or discouraged from selling syringes to anyone they suspect of illicit drug use. Paraphernalia laws also dissuade users from returning syringes to the exchanges, because they could be arrested if police find them in possession of syringes (16).

Needle and Syringe Programs Outside the United States

Unlike the United States, most countries in Western Europe, and many elsewhere, never enacted prescription or paraphernalia laws, and two that did—France (17) and Austria—revoked

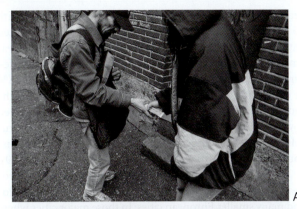

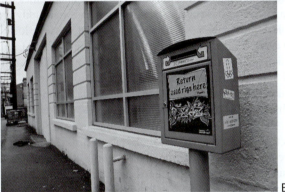

Figure 55.1. A: Sterile needle distribution, Vancouver, BC. **B:** Safe needle disposal. (Photo courtesy of Urban Health Research Initiative, BC Centre for Excellence in HIV/AIDS, St. Paul's Hospital, Vancouver, BC, Canada.)

them during the mid-1980s when HIV/AIDS came on the scene. By the late 1980s, virtually all developed countries allowed legal access to sterile injection equipment through syringe exchanges, over-the-counter sales, or both (Fig. 55.1). Most NSPs abroad are strongly supported by government officials at the national and local levels, most law enforcement officials, and a substantial majority of public opinion. Most public health authorities agree on the importance of reaching as many drug injectors as possible and minimizing the circulation of used syringes through aggressive syringe exchange and distribution efforts. Syringes are available around the clock, from pharmacies (18), vending machines, and even police stations. NSPs are now commonplace throughout the world: they are found in the Netherlands, Britain, Switzerland, and Australia and are present in dozens of cities in Europe.

The first exchanges were established in 1981 in the Netherlands and rapidly expanded in response to the threat of HIV later in the decade. In the United Kingdom, political support for syringe exchange arose in 1986 in response to evidence from Scotland that a shortage of syringes in Edinburgh had facilitated the spread of HIV. More than 200 NSPs now operate in England and two thirds of all drug agencies maintain some syringe distribution or exchange scheme. In Australia, NSPs began in 1986, initially with a pilot program that was illegal. Since 1996, all eight Australian states provide NSPs—distributing 30 million sterile needles and syringes yearly—about the same number as the United States with 15 times the number of injectors. A British study analyzed data from 103 cities worldwide and found that HIV prevalence increased an average of 8% in cities without needle–syringe exchange programs and declined an average of 18% in cities with NSPs. Applying these results to Australia, the independent evaluators estimated that NSPs have saved (by 2000) 25,000 HIV infections, 21,000 hepatitis C virus (HCV) infections, at least a $1.6 billion (at 5% annual discount), and (by 2010) 4500 AIDS and 90 HCV deaths (13,19).

NSPs are now commonplace in most large cities in European countries (e.g., Vienna, Madrid, Bologna, Dublin, Oslo) and many smaller European cities. In those major cities where no exchanges have been established, syringes are readily available in pharmacies. NSPs now operate in at least one location in every country of Central and Eastern Europe and Central Asia (except Turkmenistan) as well as in multiple countries of South, Southeast, and East Asia, including Nepal, India, Pakistan, Cambodia, Vietnam, Malaysia, Indonesia, and China (20).

Services at NSPs extend far beyond the distribution of injecting equipment (e.g., alcohol swabs, sharps containers, medicinal ointments, bleach, cookers, cotton, sterile water, and usually condoms) and collection and safe disposal of used paraphernalia. Clients may be shown how to inject less hazardously so as to avoid complications (such as abscesses, septicemia, and endocarditis), and programs often provide access to primary health services and more generic advice on maintaining good health. The ethos is sympathetic to users, and drug injectors are not harassed about their drug use, although they are informed of, and on request referred to, drug-treatment programs and other alternatives (20).

Peer Outreach and Education

Most needle and syringe exchange programs rely on active drug users such as outreach workers and volunteers. Their HIV prevention efforts engage the highest risk groups for OD and new-onset HIV infection—active drug users not in treatment—through street outreach in local drug scenes, drop-in centers, and social service settings. Rather than aiming solely to direct people who use drugs into treatment, they focus most of their energies on minimizing drug-related harms outside formal treatment settings. Some use vans or buses, while others have drop-in centers with support services, but importantly for the most marginal users, they have amenities such as laundries, showers, and food. These organizations typically offer information about safer drug use and safer sex, provide a link between people who use drugs and social and/or medical services, distribute needles and condoms, and prove indispensable in collecting information about recent developments in the drug scene. A growing number of programs are initiated and promoted by current and former drug users and employ users as street outreach workers, program staff, leaders of peer counseling groups, and the like (18,20,21).

NSPs also provide outreach services with mobile vans and pedestrian distributors to homes or street corners. In Zurich and Vienna, sterile syringes can be obtained around the clock via a network of distribution points, a "syringe van," mobile medical teams, pharmacies, and vending machines (20). In Amsterdam, police stations will provide clean syringes in return for dirty ones. In Liverpool, all pharmacies can sell injecting equipment and, of these, 20 operate free syringe exchanges. In New Zealand, by 1990, 16% of all retail pharmacies were involved in syringe distribution and exchange (19); today that figure is 60%. Automated syringe exchange machines, which deliver a clean syringe when a used one is deposited, can now be found in more than a dozen European and Australian cities (19). These machines are inexpensive and available 24 hours a day. The synergy of NSPs and expanded access to methadone appears to be especially effective in controlling HIV (20), and many countries that averted or controlled epidemics of HIV among IDUs explicitly accepted HR strategies and vigorously implemented both needle–syringe exchange programs and methadone.

OTHER PUBLIC HEALTH STRATEGIES FOR ACTIVE USERS

Overdose Prevention

In many areas of the world, where HIV has been controlled by HR programs, drug OD is the leading cause of death among IDUs. Since the 1990s, a series of OD prevention programs have evolved (21): educational programs using both popular media and underground publications; better emergency medical services and police response systems; and new models for the distribution of injectable narcotic antagonists that reverse OD symptoms (naloxone [Narcan]) as well as cardiopulmonary resuscitation (CPR) training for users' networks; and formation of groups of victims' families who work with local authorities to improve response to OD emergencies. These programs are now being piloted and studied in the United Kingdom, Australia, and parts of Europe as well as in U.S. cities including Chicago, Boston, San Francisco, and New York. Naloxone distribution has also been initiated, although on a limited basis, in countries including Tajikistan, China, Kyrgyzstan, Kazakhstan, and Russia. Such programs and many others described below are facilitated by the development of drug user eductational organizations and the community involvement of drug users and their advocacy organizations in OD prevention (19–21).

Other Initiatives Supporting Safer Drug Use

HR efforts also seek to reduce the damage resulting from drugs of unknown purity or potency, which is especially important as new drugs (e.g., ecstasy and other club drugs) arrive in a country that has little history of experience with their effects. Some syringe exchanges have taken the initiative and distributed information gained from users about which street drugs are particularly potent or have dangerous adulterants.

This information, however, tends to be erratic, comes only after a hazardous batch of drugs hits the street, and reaches only a small fraction of users. Recognizing this need (and opportunity), Dutch public health authorities identified that one of the greatest dangers associated with the sudden expansion of the "rave scene" (gatherings, often at dance clubs, where young people consume methylenedioxymethamphetamine [MDMA] and other stimulants and hallucinogens while dancing to high-energy music) was the sale of adulterated and unexpectedly high-potency drugs. Private organizations, which later gained government support, responded by employing drug analysis units at raves where illicit drugs could be tested prior to consumption. Some cities in Germany (e.g., Berlin and Hanover) maintain silent or unspoken agreements between HR groups and officials, allowing for inconspicuous drug analysis of MDMA and methylenedioxyethylamphetamine (MDE) as well as heroin in the context of "fixer rooms" (see below). Such initiatives resemble the earliest HR attempts in the United States—the Analysis Anonymous drug-testing service in the United States, created by PharmChem Laboratories, Inc. in 1972 to provide a similar service to people who mailed in samples of illicit drugs.

Drug Consumer Groups

Organized and subsidized self-help groups of people who use drugs have played a modest but important role in the formulation and implementation of drug control policies in the Netherlands, Germany, and Australia and have begun to exercise some influence in Switzerland and the United States (22). The Rotterdam "junkie union" began the first Dutch syringe exchange in response to the hepatitis B epidemic. Amsterdam's junkie union was decisive in initiating free SEPs in 1983 to 1984, after a major pharmacist in the central inner city "copping" area refused to sell needles to people who use drugs. Similar groups in Canberra, Rotterdam, Groningen, Basel, Bern, and Bremen have worked with local public health officials on SEPs and other HR initiatives. Although these groups tend to be short-lived and dependent on one or two highly motivated individuals, they play an important role in articulating the sentiments and perceptions of precisely those citizens who are most affected by local policies. They also offer valuable conduits between local policy makers and underground populations. Most of these groups also produce publications (often comic books or "zines") targeted at people who use illicit drugs with information on reducing drug-related harms, kicking the habit, and identifying treatment alternatives. Drug user groups also operate throughout Asia and the former Soviet Union, with activities including public protests against limited drug treatment and criminal penalties, information exchanges, and internet posting on daily realities.

Municipal Zoning Policies and Open Drug Scenes (23)

In large part, public opposition to certain forms of drug use relates to their visible presence in the community, that is, to public appearance of intoxicated individuals and to open drug dealing scenes with their associated loitering, violence, and disorderly conduct. Such open drug scenes are deeply embarrassing to city officials, especially in cities that pride themselves on maintenance of public order, underscoring the need to work collaboratively with local police. Like prostitution, homelessness, and public consumption of alcohol, they challenge community morals, appear disorderly or threatening, and effectively resist all attempts to be suppressed. This is in contrast to alcohol use, which is generally accepted in private spaces (i.e., bars, restaurants, and homes), and public intoxication, which is tolerated under a broad (though declining) range of circumstances, from the office party to public sporting events.

The use of illicit drugs is viewed quite differently when it occurs in public. Although public cannabis use is viewed benignly in many cities, the use and sale of hard drugs is often seen as a sharp challenge to authority. Open drug dealing broadcasts to community residents that law enforcement has been displaced from power. Public consumption—particularly injection—of illicit drugs communicates a clear breakdown of public order and social control. Both attract political attention and create pressure for change that frequently—in the context of prohibition and its enforcement—takes the form of short-term solutions that do little more than conceal drug scenes or shift them to a different locale. In the United States, this spawned the "shooting gallery," a place where people who use drugs could buy drugs and rent injecting equipment in a locale somewhat insulated from the view of the law, and which played a key role in the explosive growth of HIV in many U.S. cities in the 1980s. European and Australian police and public health officials, aware of this relationship early in the HIV/AIDS epidemic, officially tolerated certain spaces where drug use could be contained and health risk reduced while meeting the social requirements of drug law enforcement.

Under this concept, "open drug scenes" were allowed to develop in a few restricted areas. Early experiences with open scenes were sometimes adverse, as in Zurich's Platzspitz of the late 1980s and early 1990s, which became notorious as "Needle Park," but was instructive for later attempts at steering the use of drugs to less publicly offensive locations and for the need to establish many small scenes rather than one central "supermarket." In Rotterdam, police briefly allowed and supervised an open drug scene next to the central railway station, known as "Platform Zero," with syringe exchange services and a mobile methadone unit readily available. In Frankfurt, open heroin scenes emerged during the 1970s and 1980s in two adjacent parks, the Gallusanlage and the Taunusanlage, when top police officials decided that their decade-long efforts to suppress the local drug scenes had failed to halt their growth and merely shifted them from one neighborhood to another. Local authorities in Frankfurt established three crisis centers in the vicinity of the drug scenes, stationed a mobile ambulance to provide syringe exchange services and emergency medical assistance, offered first aid courses, and established a separate bus to provide services for drug users in commercial sex work. These initiatives were combined with efforts to lure users away from the exclusive involvement in the drug scene by providing night lodgings, daytime residences, and methadone treatment centers in neighborhoods removed from the city center. In conjunction with these measures, the open drug scene in the park was shut down in late 1992, and the new policies that grew from that experience are believed to be responsible for significantly reducing the number of homeless people who use drugs, drug-related robberies, and drug-related deaths in the city (23).

"Safe Spaces" for People Who Use Drugs (24)

Low-threshold facilities known as "contact centers," "street rooms," "health rooms," "harm reduction centers," "supervised consumption facilities," and "safe injecting rooms," where active users congregate, are now officially tolerated (and sometimes even government sponsored) in many European cities. Another innovation worth noting is the "apartment dealer" arrangement, adopted informally in Rotterdam, whereby police and prosecutors refrain from arresting and prosecuting apartment dealers—including sellers of heroin and cocaine—as long as they do not cause problems for their neighbors. This arrangement is viewed as part and parcel of broader "safe neighborhood" plans in which police and residents collaborate to keep neighborhoods safe, clean, and free of nuisances. Both toleration and regulation of open drug scenes and safe spaces for people who use drugs represent forms of informal zoning controls similar to those long employed in Europe and Asia to regulate commercial sex work.

Safe injecting facilities challenge norms but are regarded as preferable to the two most likely alternatives: open injection of illicit drugs in public places, which is widely regarded as distasteful and unsettling to most urban residents, or consumption of drugs in unsanctioned "shooting galleries," which are often dirty, sometimes violent, frequently controlled by drug dealers, and where needle sharing is often the norm. A few "fixing rooms" were quietly tolerated within some drug agencies in England during the 1960s, and during the late 1970s a number of "drug cafes" for heroin users were established in Amsterdam, but they were later shut down when drug dealers effectively displaced social workers from control of the daily course of events. In Switzerland, the first Gassenzimmer ("fixer rooms") were established by private organizations in Bern and Basel during the late 1980s. By late 1993, eight were in operation, with most under the direct supervision of city officials: two in Bern, two in Basel, one in Lucerne (in City Hall), and three in Zurich. An evaluation of the three Gassenzimmers in Zurich after their first year of operation concluded that they were effective in reducing the transmission of HIV and the risk of OD. Three "injection rooms" have been in place in Frankfurt since 1995. By 2003, over 60 supervised consumption facilities were operating in Europe, and the number of sites and countries involved has continued to expand.

Building on the European experiences, medically supervised safer injection facilities (SIFs) have opened as scientific research pilots in Sydney, Australia (25), and Vancouver, Canada (26). In 2001, local health authorities in Sydney, Australia, opened a "medically supervised injecting centre" (MISC), after a long debate successfully gained community support (25). The MISC is linked to a well-established full service Harm Reduction (HR) program (the Kirketon Road Centre) located in the Kings Cross area of the city—well known for its open drug and sex scene—the site now sees about 200 drug injectors per day i.e. > 70,000/year and "aims to reduce harm associated with illicit drug use by supervising injecting episodes that might otherwise occur in less safe circumstances such as public places or alone and has documented its capacity to "reduce the risk of morbidity and mortality associated with drug ODs and transmission of blood-borne infections" and getting active users more "engaged with the health and social welfare system." The trial of the Sydney MISC has now been successfully concluded and the program is set to become a regular part of the states public health service apparatus.

In Canada, a supervised injection facility known as "InSite" was opened in Vancouver in 2003 (Fig. 55.2), although its continued operation is under threat from Canada's current federal government. The federal government has (so far) unsuccessfully appealed a 2008 constitutional decision (25) that confirmed the facility's right to operate. These are places where drug users can meet, pick up injection equipment and condoms, and obtain simple medical care, advice, help with domestic problems, access a public washroom or laundry, and sometimes a place to sleep. Most facilities allow users to remain anonymous, many have qualified medical staff present, and some provide a "fixer room" where drug injectors can consume illicit drugs in a relatively hygienic environment.

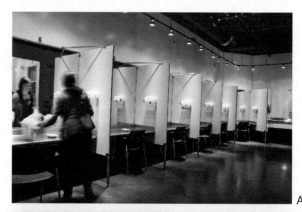

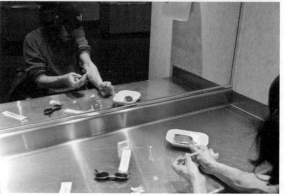

Figure 55.2. A: InSite—safe injecting site, Vancouver, BC. **B:** InSite client. (Photo courtesy of Urban Health Research Initiative, BC Centre for Excellence in HIV/AIDS, St. Paul's Hospital, Vancouver, BC, Canada.)

Both of these programs have been subjected to very close oversight and rigorous evaluations. The results published in leading peer-reviewed medical and public health journals (25,26) have demonstrated a range of positive impacts—including reduction in HIV risk behavior, successful intervention in the event of OD, and improved public order around the site. Drug users attending a supervised site have the opportunity for regular contact with health care professionals and addiction counselors that leads to increased admissions to addiction treatment. Drug-related crime did not increase around the SIF. Of note, following the opening of the Vancouver site, no detrimental impact was found on IDUs enrolled in a preexisting cohort study in terms of prolonging their use of drugs or increasing relapse for those who had stopped. Modeling the impact of the Vancouver site based on published studies suggests that 2 to 12 OD deaths and over 100 HIV infections are prevented annually through the operation of the supervised injecting site, leading to health care savings of $2 million per year (25).

ADDICTION TREATMENT AS HARM REDUCTION

HR views problematic drug use (including self destructive chronic use and valid diagnoses of addiction) as only one possible outcome of even significant levels of drug use. Vaillant and Zinberg (26) have noted that the majority of drug users (of tobacco, opiates, and alcohol) do not develop serious problems from that use—modulating its level and generally reducing and terminating use over time. They argue further that most who do develop problems manage to resolve them without formal treatment, especially many cigarette smokers and heavy alcohol drinkers—although this appears to be less so of heavy stimulant use. However, many illicit drug users living under punitive prohibition regimes also face serious psychologic, social, and medical problems (as well as serious legal difficulties) that are attributable to the criminalization of their addictions, for example, the destabilizing effects of recurrent criminal justice involvement (especially multiple arrests and prison recidivism) on their ability to reestablish stable homes and family ties. Accordingly, much treatment of addiction often represents "tertiary prevention," occurring many years after initiation of use, and compounded by its neglect and mistreatment, as well as the adverse effects of criminalization of users, their families, and their communities. In many countries, long involuntary internment for drug dependence is a common practice (1–8).

In the HR model, the pathologies of addiction and challenges of drug treatment are seen as inseparable from prohibitionist drug policies, and these policies' collateral damages must be addressed in all treatment and HR programs (27). The recent advent of HR-oriented drug treatment (28) also acknowledges a different set of goals than those of conventional treatment (i.e., total abstinence) and may even include the wishes of the clients to continue some forms of safer drug use at lower levels (i.e., "controlled drug use") and certainly not to make continued drug use a basis of termination of treatment. "Low-threshold" treatment models may also address users other real and perceived needs (e.g., for health care, housing, and legal assistance) as pathways to engaging clients, placing only minimal demands regarding cessation of all drugs. A pillar of HR approaches to drug treatment for many years has been for the medical prescriptions of "substitution" medications, especially of opiates, on a long-term basis as "maintenance treatment," which has now become an integral part of HR policy and practice worldwide.

Drug Substitution and Maintenance Treatment

Drug substitution, drug replacement therapies, and maintenance treatment are an essential part of HR strategies in many countries (see also Chapters 28 and 29 on methadone and buprenorphine treatment). But substitution treatments have a long and complex history (28,29). Despite strong medical and public health evidence for their effectiveness, these approaches still encounter opposition in many societies that consider them to violate the goal of a "drug-free society." A crucial factor is the right of physicians to prescribe maintenance drugs for their addicted patients. Drug maintenance was first pioneered in Great Britain (where doctors have long had the authority to gradually detoxify or maintain addicts by prescribing their drugs of choice). When AIDS struck in the mid-1980s, Britain was able to rapidly increase prescription of maintenance medications—mostly oral methadone (which was increased 10-fold) accompanied by other HR efforts, including opening over 100 needle and syringe exchanges within medical and public health services. This and similar HR approaches have effectively contained the HIV epidemic in the United Kingdom, Australia, and New Zealand—where HIV rates among drug injectors have remained at low levels for 20 years or more.

But in the United States, where morphine was prescribed to more than 10,000 chronic dependent users from 1900 to 1925, the drug maintenance approach was soon overwhelmed by the militant temperance movement and by federal and state drug enforcement agents hostile to opiate maintenance. By 1925, organized medicine and the U.S. courts had rejected drug maintenance, largely silenced its proponents, and led American medicine to all but abandon not only the maintenance treatment but also the entire field of addiction medicine—conceding the problem to law enforcement (28,29). It was not until the early 1960s, with the pioneering work of Drs. Vincent Dole and Marie Nyswander (see chapter 28) that the concept of addiction treatment using the prescription of maintenance drugs was reintroduced in the United States (30,31).

Methadone

There are hundreds of studies of the effects and outcomes of methadone maintenance treatment (MMT) (see Chapter 28). Positive outcomes include the complete elimination of or large reductions in daily heroin use and injecting, reductions in criminal behavior and arrests, reductions in death rates, and increased employment (32–34). The public health significance of MMT soon became apparent as the rate of HIV infection among those in MMT was found to be inversely proportional to the time in treatment. Thus, although 20% to 30% of New York City's injectors were HIV positive by 1995, those in MMT since 1978 were virtually free of the virus.

Despite this result and the overwhelmingly positive findings for MMT (most of them initially from American studies), the United States has fallen far behind other Western nations when it comes to its effective utilization. For three decades methadone was the most tightly regulated drug in the U.S. pharmacopoeia (35) and could only be dispensed in licensed "programs," subject to strict federal and state regulations governing matters typically left to the discretion of physicians. This has had a chilling effect on the normalization and accessibility of MMT programs (MMTPS) in America.

Although it is acknowledged that many patients do not totally cease drug use while receiving MMT, most programs have not integrated HR interventions that recognize that reality, for example, are providing access to sterile syringes, OD prevention, or education on safer drug use. Recently some US MMT programs do provide access to sterile syringes via needle and syringe programs and pharmacies, and provide safe syringe disposal on-site. But in the United States, many more remain "patient unfriendly," expelling clients who use drugs illegally or who otherwise violate program requirements (e.g., failure to attend "counseling sessions"). In addition, the large public MMTPs with hundreds of patients (a scale dictated by regulatory and cost considerations) are no one's favorite neighbor, and the NIMBY (Not In My Back Yard) phenomenon serves to further constrict access to care. Accordingly, the United States has failed to expand MMT to the scale required to effectively respond to the needs of the estimated 1 million heroin-dependent individuals, plus 2 to 3 million additional opioid-dependent Americans who have received prescribed opiate analgesics, which they may, in some cases, misuse or sell (30,34).

Furthermore, the therapeutic efficacy of many MMTPs in the United States has eroded as standards of clinical practice have deteriorated (31). There is widespread ignorance of the proper use of this treatment and often hostility toward methadone among many of those working in MMTPs. Problems include administration of inadequate doses and a misguided orientation toward abstinence, not just from illegal drugs but also from methadone itself, as a universal treatment goal. The failure to relax counterproductive regulatory constraints and the continued punitive posture of some local drug enforcement authorities regarding MMT have taken a once successful modality of addiction treatment and driven it to the margins of American medical and public health practice (30–34).

Despite methadone's proven clinical effectiveness over millions of patient-years of positive experience using this treatment, punitive prohibitionist attitudes and policies have had a huge adverse impact on public health by restricting access to this treatment, in the United States and elsewhere (30). One striking example of this failure is AIDS, where the epidemic continues to infect over 20,000 injecting drug users and their sex partners each year in the United States (34). Only 20% of the 1 million heroin-dependent individuals, and an even smaller portion of the growing prescription opioid–dependent population, receive maintenance treatment. In many American states, methadone regulations conflict with sound medical and public health practices regarding dosage ceilings (often self-imposed by the programs), prohibition of take-home medication, and arbitrary restrictions on the number of methadone clinics allowed within a certain area (e.g., Tennessee allows no more than one clinic within a 100-mile radius). As of 2009, five states—Idaho, Mississippi, Montana, North Dakota, and South Dakota—still had no methadone-maintenance programs. In California and elsewhere, privatization and limitations on the duration of publicly funded treatment have raised barriers to MMT.

There have been many efforts to correct these problems in the United States, but they continue largely unabated today (35). In 1996, the Institute of Medicine issued a series of studies and a report calling for the expansion and modification of methadone treatment, and in 1997, a National Institutes of Health (NIH) Consensus Conference reasserted the conceptualization of opiate addiction as a medical disorder. It called for "effective medical treatment of opiate addiction" through the reduction of "misperceptions and stigma," improved medical training, assurance of greater access to methadone, and the reduction of "unnecessary regulations" that restrict the availability and quality of methadone treatment. In 2000, the Drug Abuse Treatment Act (DATA) was passed by Congress, expanding the possibilities of employing new models of opioid-maintenance treatment with buprenorphine—an alternative to methadone. Buprenorphine and a buprenorphine–naloxone combination via community-based physicians became available in the United States in 2003.

Buprenorphine's safety and efficacy are well established (38), but it remains underutilized due to slow uptake of prescribing among office-based physicians. While current buprenorphine treatment guidelines advance a treatment model substantially less intense than that of conventional methadone maintenance, they still go far beyond the level of care and monitoring standard in treating other chronic conditions such as diabetes, depression, or HIV/AIDS. As of 2008, 13,000 physicians had been certified (following completion of the federally required training) to prescribe buprenorphine, yet only an estimated 67% were actually treating patients. Even among addiction treatment specialists, just over half (58%) of those with waivers to prescribe it had done so in the first year after its approval. Important barriers identified by practitioners include the guidelines' recommendations regarding three components of treatment "intensity": in-clinic (observed) induction, frequent visits, and the ability to provide ancillary behavioral health services. Though covered by many insurance providers, buprenorphine itself is priced at several times the (very low) price of methadone and results in outpatient buprenorphine costs (in private practice) now comparable to "full service" methadone clinic treatment ($3000 to $5000 per year).

International Developments in Maintenance Treatment

Despite the lags in treatment availability in the United States (where many drug-free treatment advocates remain hostile to medication-assisted treatment), public health and medical authorities in a number of other countries have greatly expanding access to substitution treatment. They have also altered their intervention strategies to accommodate a greater number and wider spectrum of patients. Much of this expansion has been achieved through the use of primary care practitioners to prescribe opioid-agonist medication within office-based practices. Today in Europe, Canada, and the Asian-Pacific Region, more than 250,000 patients are prescribed opioids by a general practitioner in health clinic settings (38,39), and this model of addiction medicine is gaining popularity and application worldwide. But despite the adoption of buprenorphine for patients in the United States, except for some "medical maintenance" experiments, American pharmacists and doctors in general medical practice still are barred by federal regulations from playing any role in methadone maintenance.

With the growing international awareness of AIDS risks and the potential role of maintenance treatment in limiting its spread, most countries in the developed world initiated or have greatly expanded maintenance treatment. Australia increased its MMT capacity 10-fold between 1985 and 1994. In Germany, methadone was outlawed as late as 1987, but today more than 70,000 patients receive it (the great majority from generalist, community-based practitioners) without other comorbidities being a requirement. In France, in 1995, there were only 52 patients who were maintained on methadone in the entire country; a decade later, approximately 10,000 patients were being treated with methadone, and an additional 80,000 were prescribed buprenorphine through general practitioners (36,38).

In combination with NSPs, opiate substitution treatments have contained and reduced new HIV infections among injecting drug users in many countries. While availability remains minimal in Eastern Europe and Central Asia, several Asian countries—including Iran, China, and Malaysia—have moved beyond pilots and are scaling up services. Outside the United States, some of methadone's expansion has been achieved within "mainstream" medical practice (39). Thousands of general practitioners in community-based practices throughout Europe, Australia, New Zealand, and Canada are involved in methadone maintenance. In Belgium, Germany, France, Australia, Canada, Ireland, Scotland, and Croatia, this is the principal means of methadone distribution. In the Netherlands and, to a lesser extent, Switzerland, methadone is available in public and private health clinics and other government facilities. In Copenhagen, Amsterdam, and Rome, methadone is available at police stations for drug users who have been arrested.

Low-Threshold Maintenance

Low-threshold maintenance treatment does not "require" ancillary services (such as counseling) nor does it make retention in treatment contingent upon total abstinence from eroin and/or other drugs. Accordingly, it can accommodate a far broader segment of addicts in the community for a longer period of time. These programs frequently provide fewer ancillary services, although referrals are usually offered to relevant sources available to the general population. Many do not demand regular attendance, urine tests, or regular counseling contacts, all of which are standard requirements in U.S. methadone clinics. Support for low-threshold programs is based on their relatively low cost; the relative ease of establishment on a large scale; their proven success in establishing contact with people who use illicit drugs but are put off by programs with more rigorous requirements; and the fact that, as expected, their patients have been shown to fare better than drug users not enrolled in any programs (39). The Dutch were pioneers in deploying low-threshold "methadone buses"—mobile facilities that carry previously prescribed doses, free of charge, for a list of 100 or more patients who may meet the bus at any one of several predesignated locations daily, an innovation that has been adopted in Barcelona and, in the United States, in Baltimore and Boston. Low-threshold programs also now operate in several cities in Europe and Australia, and in Hong Kong.

Methadone in Correctional Settings (see also Chapter 65)

The injection of heroin within correctional facilities has been documented in many countries and continues to exist, notwithstanding vigorous attempts to deter and detect the importation of drugs and injecting equipment into these facilities. Although episodes of drug injecting inside these facilities generally are far less frequent than in the community, adverse consequences (including HIV infection) are well documented. The use of methadone in jails and prisons—in the United States—has generally been restricted to brief detoxification programs, although there are exceptions. For over 25 years, New York City's Rikers Island jail has operated a methadone-maintenance program with 3000 annual admissions, and there are now small pilot prison and jail programs in Puerto Rico and New Mexico. However, elsewhere in the United States, there is still no methadone maintenance for the 2 million longer-term state and federal inmates. By contrast, as of January 2008, methadone maintenance has been implemented in prisons in at least 29 countries or territories, with the proportion of all prisoners in care ranging from less than 1% to over 14% (39). In Canada, any methadone maintenance patient who is incarcerated is maintained on methadone throughout their time in custody and many heroin users are started on methadone during a period of federal incarceration. In Eastern Europe and Central Asia, Moldova and Kyrgyzstan now offer methadone maintenance in prison, and the Republic of Georgia has initiated a short course of methadone-to-detoxification program in a pretrial detention facility.

Other Drug Substitution Initiatives

Despite its unparalleled effectiveness, some who receive oral methadone-maintenance treatment either drop out or continue to use illicit drugs in addition to the prescribed medication. Stimulated by the need to control the spread of HIV/AIDS, maintenance treatment is entering a new phase of clinical experimentation. Accordingly, several countries have expanded drug-maintenance programs and practices beyond oral methadone and sublingual buprenorphine to include prescribed injectable methadone and, most recently, injectable heroin, which many considered revolutionary. But, in fact, this approach has a long history (40,41).

In the United States from 1919 to 1923, several morphine- and heroin-assisted therapy clinics were in operation until their termination by the government (29). British physicians prescribed injectable opiates early in the 20th century and in a controlled trial in the 1970s; a small morphine-maintenance program was initiated in 1983 in the Netherlands and was deemed modestly successful in improving the health and functioning of most of the addicts and in reducing their involvement in criminal activities. Another program, operated by the Municipal Health Department in Amsterdam, prescribed injectable methadone and dextromoramide tartrate (Palfium)—an opioid that can be taken orally—to a group of long-term heavy opioid users, the latter medication did not gain user acceptance and was difficult to administer. In Italy during the late 1970s, a number of physicians dissatisfied with the quality of care for heroin addicts began providing addicts with injectable morphine on an outpatient basis. The Italian government legalized this prescribing experiment in 1980, but approval was abruptly withdrawn a few years later. No comprehensive evaluation of the program was ever conducted, although it is estimated that as many as 4000 patients were participating in 1982. Years earlier, in Canada, in 1972, the LeDain Commission recommended the implementation of a heroin prescription trial for addicts who could not be attracted into conventional forms of opioid addiction treatment.

In Austria, physicians have always been free to prescribe any legally available drug to addicts. In 1993, in addition to widespread availability of oral methadone, approximately a dozen addicts were receiving prescriptions for injectable morphine or methadone, and many others had prescriptions for codeine and other synthetic opioids. One study substituted oral morphine sulfate for methadone and found the morphine preferable for some patients who experienced negative methadone side effects. In Australia, until the mid-1950s, physicians could prescribe maintenance doses of opioids, principally morphine, and did so for a small numbers of white, middle-class patients and to aging Chinese opium smokers. In Queensland, a small injectable methadone program has operated for decades.

More flexible prescribing practices also emerged in Edinburgh in 1988, a few years after authorities realized that the prevalence of HIV infection (more than 50%) among local heroin users was the highest in the United Kingdom. Community-based physicians responded with more liberal prescription of methadone, as well as oral versions of other drugs in common use (e.g., dihydrocodeine, diazepam). This policy, combined with the rapid expansion of needle distribution and exchange, is believed to have played an important role in reducing needle use and sharing, the rate of new HIV infections, and drug-related criminality. Experimentation with oral opioids other than methadone includes the use of long-acting codeine (dihydrocodeine) in Germany (1), and ethylmorphine in the Czech Republic. Even where there is ready access to methadone, however, it is clearly desirable that medical practitioners have the freedom to prescribe different opioids for different patients, depending on circumstances, and that researchers be able to responsibly try to identify more effective treatments without excessive constraints from policy makers.

During the 1970s, numerous proposals to prescribe heroin for addiction treatment were advanced in the United States: as a lure and stepping-stone to oral methadone maintenance; as a supplement to oral methadone; and as a distinct program to attract heroin addicts unwilling to enter methadone or drug-free treatment programs. Each of these proposals was rejected, mostly on political rather than scientific grounds, and to date, none has been implemented in the United States.

Recent Studies of Heroin-Assisted Treatment (41)

In the 1990s, Switzerland and the Netherlands both initiated major studies examining the effectiveness of heroin prescription in the treatment of opioid addiction. The 3-year multisite Swiss study (1994 to 1997) provided injectable opioids to more than 1000 opioid-dependent individuals who had a history of long-term heroin injection and multiple unsuccessful treatment attempts. This naturalistic cohort study produced important feasibility results for prescribed injection opioid maintenance, with on-site nursing supervision of every dose and a rich package of primary care, mental health treatment, and social services. Benefits demonstrated included retention of 69% of the original sample of chronic, previously treatment-resistant patients in treatment throughout the 18-month study period; more than half of the dropouts switched to other treatments or went drug free, and no deaths occurred as a direct consequence of the opioid drugs prescribed. Analysis of 12-month retention rates showed that among the heroin-assisted treatment group, the retention rate was twice that of either methadone maintenance or residential drug-free treatment samples from other studies in Switzerland. The majority of those leaving heroin-assisted treatment switched to abstinence-based therapy (22%) or methadone maintenance (37%). Importantly, self-reported drug use decreased dramatically during the first 18 months of treatment. The proportion of patients reporting no illicit heroin use increased from 18% at entry to 91% at 6 months and 94% at 18 months.

Participants experienced marked improvements in physical and social health (e.g., social functioning, employment, decrease in illegal activities, housing). The overall death rate was 3%; a rate comparable to other reported death rates in cohorts of regular injection heroin users. The proportion of participants with unstable housing fell from 43% on admission to 21% at 18 months. The rate of unemployment fell from 73% to 45%. Arrests and illegal income generation decreased substantially from 69% to 11%, and there was a greater than 50% reduction in criminal offenses registered by the police over the time of the study. A subsequent cost:benefit analysis of the study suggested that, despite the considerable research and treatment costs of the trial, the outcomes were cost-effective at a ratio of almost 2:1. Furthermore, the study demonstrated the feasibility of implementing and operating a heroin-assisted treatment program without disorder, misconduct, and/or diversion of heroin supply. In 1997 in two referenda, 71% of the Swiss voted in favor of continuing the trial as an ongoing program for more than 1000 patients. In addition, a World Health Organization (WHO) evaluation of the Swiss study issued a call for continued investigation of the effectiveness of heroin-assisted therapy.

Although evaluated favorably by the WHO commission, there were several methodological limitations identified in the Swiss study, whose observational design and lack of a randomized control group may have allowed uncontrolled biases into the study. However, the Geneva arm of the study used a randomized controlled design and had similar findings to the rest of the national study. In addition, the Swiss program provided extensive psychiatric and social services making it less clear to what degree the heroin-assisted therapy versus the psychosocial interventions caused the positive changes in the program participants. Subsequent studies include a more rigorous selection methodology and controlled design with randomization and are finding similar results.

In response to these limitations, the Dutch government commissioned a multisite randomized control trial of heroin-assisted treatment that began in July 1998. In contrast to the Swiss design, the Dutch conducted two randomized clinical trials, one examining injectable heroin and the other heroin smoked off foil, the most common mode of use in the Netherlands. Both trials had similar designs, consistent outcome measures based on well-validated instruments, and a single a priori definition of both response and effect. Because of the wide availability of maintenance treatment in the Netherlands, the Dutch trials were targeted at patients in methadone-maintenance treatment who continued to use illicit drugs. In both the injection and inhalation trial, the Dutch found significantly greater improvements in drug use, physical and mental health, and social function in those receiving heroin prescription in combination with methadone, than in those randomized to continue on oral methadone alone, with 56% of the heroin-assisted group compared with 31% of the control group meeting response criteria. Despite the higher costs of heroin-assisted treatment, the additional benefits produced savings of €12,793 per patient per year when compared with methadone maintenance. The Dutch results persuasively demonstrate the effectiveness of heroin-assisted treatment for those whose response to methadone maintenance was deemed poor. However, because of their focus on patients currently on methadone and the very different treatment system in place in the Netherlands, there are limitations on the generalizability of their findings to other localities.

The large German clinical trial of heroin-assisted treatment extended the Dutch results through randomly assigning 1015 patients to heroin-assisted treatment or methadone maintenance and to one of two manualized psychosocial treatments. Participants had long-term heroin injection but were not required to currently be in methadone treatment at study enrollment. Treatment retention was greater in heroin-assisted treatment (67.2%) than methadone maintenance (40%). Heroin-assisted treatment patients were more likely to meet criteria for improved physical and/or mental health (OR = 1.41; CI = 1.05 to 1.89; $p = 0.023$) and reduced illicit drug use (OR = 1.85; CI = 1.43 to 2.40; $p < 0.001$). Heroin has subsequently been approved as a medication for the treatment of addiction in Switzerland, Germany, and the Netherlands and forms an increasingly integrated component of the comprehensive treatment system. Heroin-assisted treatment studies have also been conducted in Spain and the United Kingdom with efforts ongoing to expand access to this treatment option to other countries in Europe.

Therefore, to investigate heroin-assisted therapy suited to their own settings, Germany and Spain have started heroin trials. In 2008 Canada completed a 3-year randomized controlled clinical trial, the North American Opiate Medication Initiative (NAOMI), and is scheduled to begin another, the Study to Assess Longer-term Opioid Medication Effectiveness (SALOME) in 2011 to test the efficacy of hydromorphone as a treatment option.

Recently, the NAOMI trial of heroin-assisted treatment has been completed in Canada (41). The NAOMI study demonstrated the effectiveness of heroin-assisted treatment in a setting with less comprehensive social services than Western Europe, high rates of unstable housing, and pervasive dependence on cocaine. Heroin-assisted treatment patients were more likely to meet predefined criteria for treatment retention (88.7% vs. 54.1%) and treatment response (67% vs. 47.7%) than those on methadone maintenance. In addition, the inclusion of a small group of participants treated with injection hydromorphone on a double-blind basis suggested that this widely available pain medication might be a viable alternative for countries where prescription of injection heroin as addiction treatment may not be politically feasible.

Prescription of Nonopioid Drugs (42)

Methadone is not a treatment for primary addiction to cocaine, amphetamine, alcohol, and other nonopioid drugs, although use of these drugs by heroin addicts in MMT will often decline over time. But opioid-maintenance programs do not directly address the consumption of nonopioid drugs such as amphetamines and cocaine. This is an increasingly important limitation, given the dramatic growth since the late 1970s in cocaine and multidrug consumption, notably the use of "crack" cocaine and "cocktail" combinations of cocaine and heroin known as "speedballs," and the recent rise in use of amphetamine-type substances worldwide.

In the United Kingdom, where some physicians reason that legal maintenance with prescribed stimulants is preferable to illegal "maintenance" with illicit drugs, the practice of prescribing stimulants, typically in combination with heroin and/or methadone, has persisted for decades (43). An initiative in Britain to prescribe injectable amphetamine during the amphetamine epidemic of 1968 was deemed a failure, but recent attempts to prescribe oral amphetamine appear more successful. A 3-year study of a small oral amphetamine-prescribing program in Portsmouth found that more than half of the 26 study participants (all daily amphetamine injectors on entry) stopped injecting and that all decreased their sharing of injecting equipment and used less illicit amphetamine. The program was popular among users: it retained 67% of those who entered for at least 15 months, and of those who dropped out, two had stopped amphetamine use. The program also precipitated an increase in the number of primary amphetamine users presenting to treatment services in the area. Treatment services in Exeter, and a larger program in Cornwall, also achieved substantial drops in illicit amphetamine use and injecting with similar programs of oral amphetamine prescription. Using oral and injectable methadone, oral amphetamine, codeine, and benzodiazepine prescription, and a drug team that integrates needle exchange, prenatal and primary care health services, and mental health care, the Cornwall service exemplifies the flexible HR-oriented approach that is the legacy of the British system. In Australia, researchers demonstrated the feasibility of establishing a clinical trial model for amphetamine maintenance for both cocaine and amphetamine users, and are now planning full trials (42).

DRUG POLICY REFORM AS HARM REDUCTION

Although addiction treatment innovations and expanded access, preventive interventions such as SEPs, environmental changes to make drug use safer, and OD prevention programs play a crucial role in reducing the harms associated with drug use under prohibition, it is changes in drug control policy that offer the best chance for minimizing drug-related harm. By reducing the association of drug use with criminal prosecution, a system that drives drug use and people who use drugs to the most dangerous margins of society, the reform of punitive legal policies can produce clear benefits in the realm of public health and social order. Marijuana, the most widely used illicit drug, has been a special target for such law reform.

Marijuana Policies

In the United States in the 1970s, the movement to decriminalize marijuana was driven by the realization that criminal sanctions created greater harm than marijuana use itself. During the 1970s, 11 states decriminalized marijuana, effectively reducing the punishment for possession of small amounts to sanctions other than imprisonment (43). The impact on marijuana consumption and related problems was negligible, but decriminalization did reduce the number of marijuana arrests and prosecutions. California saved an estimated $1 billion in the decade following the 1976 Moscone Act decriminalizing marijuana. While total drug arrests increased almost every year throughout the 1980s, arrests for marijuana consistently declined, leading many to suggest the drug had been effectively decriminalized. However, in response to harsher drug policies, marijuana arrests have risen in recent years in the United States (more than 800,000 in 2001). In contrast, significant drug law reform has been undertaken in several European countries and Australia in direct response to perceived public health needs and humanitarian concerns, starting with de facto decriminalization of marijuana. The case of Dutch regulation of cannabis is the most impressive example of this approach, both for its longevity (more than 35 years) and its apparent success.

Dutch Cannabis Policy and the Separation of Markets (44)

The Netherlands decriminalized cannabis at the national level in 1976, when The Baan Commission, a national drug policy working group, said that drug laws should not be more damaging to an individual than the use of the drug itself and argued that the tendency of some cannabis users to move on to illicit opiate use could be reduced by separating the "soft-drug" and "hard-drug" markets. The national Opium Law was revised to increase penalties for heroin and cocaine trafficking and to cut penalties for the sale and consumption of small amounts of cannabis to misdemeanor offenses. Prosecutorial and police guidelines were also revised to de-emphasize enforcement of cannabis laws. The result was the creation of a relatively normalized, essentially non-criminal, and easily accessible cannabis distribution system in most Dutch cities. A clear-cut distinction was made between people who use drugs and traffickers, and between "hard" illegal drugs, with so-called "unacceptable health risks" (e.g., heroin, cocaine), and cannabis products (44).

The Netherlands permits the retail trade of cannabis products in hundreds of local "coffee shops" under very specific conditions, that is, no advertising, no hard drugs, no disturbance of public order, no sale to minors (under 18 years of age), and strict limits on the amount that can be sold to each customer. Enforcement of these guidelines falls to local "Triangle Committees" composed of the mayor, chief of police, and district attorney of each city. Today, the domestic Dutch market is a well-established commercial structure operating in a "gray economy" with legal tolerance and even some taxation. An estimated half-million regular customers are supplied by many small to midsize local producers plus a number of larger importers. So far there has been little evidence of organized crime in the coffee shop operations, and virtually no violence associated with the domestic trade of cannabis in the Netherlands.

This tolerant policy toward the retail trade and use of cannabis for recreational purposes has had a positive effect in the Netherlands. Cannabis consumption among Dutch teenagers has increased somewhat over the decades (as it has in most other countries), but the rate of regular cannabis users in the Netherlands has remained significantly below U.S. levels. Rates of cocaine and heroin consumption among Dutch citizens are similarly modest, although the relatively high quality and low price of the drugs have attracted "drug tourists" from elsewhere in Europe. Dutch authorities express some concern about organized criminal involvement in wholesale production and sale of cannabis, and they contend with complaints from authorities in neighboring Germany, Belgium, and, lately, France, but by and large, the policy is supported by most of the public, politicians, and law enforcement officials. Cases of problematic cannabis use are rare, but cannabis users (like all Dutch citizens) who do develop problems have ready access to diverse and comprehensive treatment facilities based in the public health sector. Because of international pressures and some local discontent with the rapid growth in coffee shops, the Dutch government has cut back the number of coffee shops (in some cities by as much as 50%) and reduced the amount of cannabis allowed to be purchased at any given time by each customer from 30 to 5 g.

Other governments have also moved toward decriminalization of cannabis. During the 1970s, national drug commissions in many countries recommended cannabis decriminalization. In Australia in 1987 (46), the South Australian government introduced a Cannabis Expiation Notice system that allows individuals apprehended with small quantities of cannabis (up to 100 g) to have their offense discharged, with no record of a criminal conviction, upon payment of a fine. A similar scheme was introduced in the Australian Capital Territory in 1992, and later in two other jurisdictions. Although there has been a small consistent increase in cannabis use since 1985 (prior to the expiation system), an analysis of the first 2 years of the expiation system by the South Australian Office of Crime Statistics found little evidence of any impact on the number or type of people detected using cannabis. Its principal recommendation was that steps be taken to ensure that notice recipients pay their fines promptly to avoid court appearances.

In Switzerland, the Federal High Court decided in 1991 that penalties for dealing cannabis were unduly harsh and needed to be revised, given increasing evidence that the health hazards of cannabis consumption were relatively modest. A number of lower courts in Germany have ruled similarly, finding cannabis prohibition laws in conflict with the German constitution. A German Supreme Court decision in May 1994 removed criminal penalties for possession of small amounts of cannabis, furthering an earlier decision that had given states the option not to prosecute for possession of small amounts of any drug. Although some states (e.g., Bavaria) responded by decreasing the amount necessary to trigger a "large amount" charge, many other state officials announced that they would no longer arrest people for possessing small amounts of any drug. The state of Hessen initiated federal legislation in the Second Chamber (equivalent to the German senate), requesting the legalization of cannabis and its regulation by way of state monopoly. The state of Schleswig-Holstein received consent from the majority of state health ministers to dispense marijuana in pharmacies but withdrew in the face of opposition from the Federal Agency in Berlin. Spain decriminalized private use of cannabis in 1983 but has since tightened its laws. Italy decriminalized possession of "moderate amounts for personal use" of any drug in 1975, toughened penalties in 1990, and then abolished criminal sanctions for illicit drug use altogether in April 1993. Although no government has advocated outright repeal of cannabis prohibition, an increasing number now favors decriminalization.

Most recently, Canada, Australia , and the United Kingdom have taken significant steps toward the decriminalization of cannabis (46). Although Canada's federal Liberal government introduced successive bills between 2003 and 2005 to remove the possibility of incarceration for possession or production of small quantities of cannabis, it backed away from calling the measure "decriminalization," and none of the bills became law. The Conservative Party that won the 2006 Canadian federal election, and that has governed since, remains strongly opposed to decriminalizing cannabis. In 2007, it introduced a bill to increase penalties for some cannabis offenses, including provisions for mandatory minimum prison terms in some situations. That bill died when an election was called, but the re-elected government introduced a nearly identical bill in 2009. At the time of this writing, the bill had been passed by Canada's House of Commons but not by the Senate, which was undertaking a thorough, and often critical, review of the bill.

Medical Marijuana—A Special Case (47)

Many patients have found marijuana to be a relatively safe, well-tolerated, and rapidly effective way to deal with some medical conditions: reducing nausea in chemotherapy; intraocular pressure in glaucoma; muscle spasms and chronic pain; stimulating appetite; relieving the symptoms of HIV/AIDS; cancer and chemotherapy; multiple sclerosis; and epilepsy. The hostility to this use of marijuana (especially by federal officials in the United States, where the campaign for medical marijuana has been most vigorous) has made it almost impossible to gain support for rigorous research to confirm (or disprove) these widespread beliefs. Polls indicate that a majority of Americans believe marijuana should be medically available, and numerous organizations, including the American Public Health Association and the American Federation of Scientists, have issued resolutions in support of medical marijuana. In 1988, a Drug Enforcement Administration administrative law judge ruled that marijuana should be moved to Schedule II, making it available for medical purposes, but the agency refused to comply. Thus, marijuana remains a Schedule I drug, meaning that in the eyes of the U.S. government, it has no legitimate medical use, and further research on its medical properties has been stifled. Hundreds of individuals received marijuana for medical purposes in the 1980s, but this federal program was discontinued, and all but eight of the original recipients have either died or been cut from the program.

In the meantime, there have been moves to provide marijuana to medical patients through "cannabis buyers' clubs," which are illegal but often tolerated by local police. Buyers' clubs, which supply marijuana to patients who have a doctor's prescription for marijuana, have sprung up across the country in recent years. Many of the clubs are private, underground operations, but others have achieved national attention. Many of those who grow marijuana for such clubs have been arrested and prosecuted. Additionally, antiparaphernalia laws ban the use, possession, and sale of items used to consume illegal substances. Included in those laws are vaporizers, heating devices that deliver the medically useful components of marijuana without burning the plant material. Because the smoking of any organic substance can deposit tars and other harmful substances in the lungs, vaporizers are extremely useful tools for medical patients.

Nonetheless, an increasing number of doctors and patients view marijuana as a legitimate medicine that can be effective in reducing the nausea associated with cancer chemotherapy, stimulating appetite for AIDS patients suffering from wasting syndrome, and reducing the intraocular pressure of glaucoma. It is also commonly used as an anticonvulsant, muscle relaxant, and mild pain reliever for menstrual cramps and certain types of chronic pain. In May 2001, the U.S. Supreme Court ruled that so-called medical marijuana "buyers' clubs," which operate legally under California state law, cannot use a "medical necessity" defense to federal marijuana charges. Such clubs, which offer varying potencies and varieties of marijuana to patients certified to use it under California law, have experienced continual harassment from federal authorities since that ruling, and others have shut down preemptively, effectively depriving thousands of patients of their medicine. But the issue remains open in the United States: in an important ruling in 2003, the U.S. Supreme Court upheld a lower court's opinion that the federal Drug Enforcement Agency could not continue to threaten doctors who advised their patients that marijuana might be beneficial with loss of licensure.

Despite decades of prosecution of marijuana users in the United States (e.g., 300,000 in prison; 800,000 arrests in 2000), no state ballot initiative dealing only with medical marijuana has ever failed, and an October 2002 *Time* magazine poll showed that 80% of the American public supports legal access to medical marijuana. Since 1996, a majority of voters in Alaska, Arizona, California, Colorado, the District of Columbia, Maine, Nevada, Oregon, and Washington have voted in favor of ballot initiatives to remove criminal penalties for seriously ill people who grow or possess medical marijuana. Hawaii has passed a medical marijuana bill through its state legislature. Nonetheless, the federal government continues to fight against state laws that accept the medical value of marijuana.

Medical Marijuana in Canada (45)

Although Canada's Controlled Drugs and Substances Act (CDSA), the central law on illegal drugs, prohibits possession, cultivation, trafficking, and importing and exporting of marijuana, the Minister of Health is authorized to grant exemptions from the Act for a medical or scientific purpose, or if it would be otherwise in the public interest. In 1997, a small

---

Box 55.1   Harm Reduction in China—A National Case Study

China faces the dual challenge of drug use and HIV/AIDS. Proximity to the Golden Triangle and the Golden Crescent contributes to trafficking and ready availability of heroin to residents along drug trafficking routes. Heroin is the main illicit drug used in China, with amphetamine and polydrug use on the rise. Needle sharing has been the major transmission route of HIV in China, since the first indigenous outbreak was identified in 1989 among IDUs in Yunnan Province in southwestern China (48). China reported in 2008 that HIV/AIDS was the nation's leading infectious disease killer, continuing its spread among IDUs. Nearly half of the new HIV cases in 2007 were transmitted through IDU (49). This recent history serves as the baseline of a case study of China that will teach us much about the outcome of HR efforts in such a large and important society. Recognizing the efficacy of HR strategies, the Chinese government has committed significant resources and energy to addressing these epidemics (50). As a result, they have built HR services at an unprecented rate, with over 600 methadone programs and 900 needle syringe programs (NSPs).

In 2004, the first eight MMT clinics opened in five provinces (Guangxi, Guizhou, Sichuan, Yunnan, and Zhejian) (51). By the end of 2006, there were 320 MMT clinics operating in 22 provinces. By the end of 2008, over 600 MMT clinics were operating in China; 178,684 heroin users had cumulatively been served, and 93,773 clients were being served (52). An expansion of NSPs is underway despite their common perception as "condoning and encouraging" drug use. Nonetheless, government officials have agreed that NSPs should be the work of health professionals and non-government organizations (NGOs), not that of law enforcement agencies. In 2004, China had 93 needle-exchange service points. By 2006, this number had increased to 790, of which 392 were supported by the government. By the end of 2008, there are 897 NSPs operating monthly and serving 360,000 IDUs, on average, each month (52).

The government has also scaled up HIV testing throughout the country; there were 6077 free HIV testing sites in operation by the end of 2008 (52). Expansion of these services has been concentrated in venues with a high prevalence of HIV and thus has become increasingly available to drug users. However, uptake of these services has been disappointingly low. Nearly 70% of HIV-infected adults in China are unaware of their infection status, despite outreach efforts. Barriers, for example, stigma and discrimination, contribute to both low testing rates and low utilization of HIV services, especially among IDUs.

China is a country with such a vast population and highly autonomous provincial governments, a large population of drug users confined in geographically disparate rural areas, and only a recent recognition of the efficacy of HR. Thus, the implementation of HR programs, while massive in quantity, needs to mature in quality. Programs are still unevenly and inconsistently conducted nationwide. Mere access to HR services is insufficient to ensure adequate uptake, adherence, and impact. So scaling up the response to drug use and HIV remains an enormous challenge, if HR services are to be effective and reach a majority of drug users such that their public health impact is assured.

group of Ottawa lawyers and physicians applied unsuccessfully on behalf of an AIDS patient for medical access to cannabis, However, the minister introduced a narrow exemption from the Act for medical cannabis in 1999, and by May 2002, 658 exemptions had been granted under this program. Access to medical marijuana was initially permitted to a small number of applicants in the late 1990s through such a ministerial exemption, and formal regulations followed in 2001, driven by a successful constitutional challenge to the marijuana laws. As of June 2009, 4029 individuals were authorized to possess marijuana under the regulations (45). The Canadian government is now exploring ways to permit both the cultivation and possession of cannabis for therapeutic reasons.

CONCLUSIONS

The HR paradigm has made great progress during the last decade. A public health conception of drug use, the foundation of HR, is now generally far better understood than previously, although often still willfully misinterpreted by its opponents. Nonetheless, in an increasing number of countries and regions of the world, HR is now regarded as mainstream drug policy (e.g., virtually throughout all countries of Western Europe), while zero tolerance supporters are growing ever more isolated and marginalized as their failure and its high cost become evident. This sea change is driven by genuine national concerns, including a new interest in the implications of drug addiction, AIDS, and the huge illicit drug markets for human rights and the potent effects of HIV epidemics on regional and global security (54), fueled by high levels of opium production in Afghanistan (destined for European markets), a growing drug trade in China, and a vicious power struggle over the U.S. drug markets now occurring in Mexico (53).

Several countries have now also explicitly endorsed HR as national drug policy, including the United Kingdom, the Netherlands, Australia, Canada (until a recent change in the federal government), France, Switzerland, Spain, Germany, New Zealand, many countries in Central and Eastern Europe, Iran, and several countries in Asia (Nepal, Vietnam, Indonesia, and China) and South America (Brazil and Argentina). HR has also been endorsed in recent years by an increasing number of United Nations agencies (including WHO and UNAIDS) and by organizations such as the International Red Cross.

Although HR programs continue to spread, their availability and scale are still well below levels required to achieve the public health goals that we should be setting in the drugs area. Thus, zero tolerance and the basic premises of the "War on Drugs" remains the stated drug policy in the United States. And while the US is the most important and most influential opponent to HR, it is not the only country to bitterly oppose these policies. Other countries that oppose HR policies are Russia, Japan, and Sweden, which play vocal roles in setting UN drug policies—with a Russian chosen in 2010 to head the powerful UNODC. In Canada, the federal government had a national drug strategy since the late 1980s that—at least on paper—identified drug use as primarily a health rather than an enforcement issue. But now, it has moved away from this philosophy with the election of a new government that promises more punitive drug legislation, has aborted the NAOMI heroin trial and tried to reverse Vancouver's successful supervised injection facility INSITE, although (as of this writing) this has been held off by court rulings.

But the surge in interest in HR around the world in the last two decades has been most powerfully stimulated by the urgent need, first recognized in the early 1980s, to control HIV among people who use drugs. With 25 million deaths to date, 42 million people currently living with HIV infection, and HIV estimated to infect additional millions each year, HIV/AIDS is now the most serious threat to global public health since the Black Death and is widely seen as a threat to national security. In most regions of the world, drug injecting has played a central role in the ignition of HIV outbreaks that rapidly made the transition from small, localized epidemics to extensive, generalized regional ones, buttressed by sexual transmission and amplified by widespread unsterile medical injections and unsafe blood transfusions throughout the developing world (53). Violent drug markets and drug injection are now emerging in sub-Saharan Africa (54) and undoubtedly will open a new chapter in the monstrous epidemic that now grips that region, challenging both the theory and practice of HR in unprecedented ways.

Thus, although the growth in support for new drug policies and programs is gratifying, HIV continues to spread faster than HR programs are being established or expanded to meet the need. The struggles to spread HR in the developing world (with its majority of the world's population) are especially important, and acceptance of HR in principle is insufficient to avert disaster. For example, although HR programs were introduced early enough in Nepal, they failed to avert an HIV epidemic there because they were not expanded rapidly enough. And the growing popular and professional commitment to HR in many countries is often thwarted by a strong national commitment to traditional control methods and a culture of corruption that surrounds all illicit drug markets: the more intense the repressive drug policies, the more they undermine effective HR.

Nonetheless, there continues to be strong growth in HR institutions worldwide. By 2010, there had been 21 annual meetings of the International Conference on the Reduction of Drug-Related Harm, the leading international meeting on drug policies and innovations in the field. These conferences, attracting a growing body of delegates from an increasing number of countries, have now been held in developing and transitional countries several times. The International Harm Reduction Association (IHRA) was established in 1996 and has grown rapidly. It now has a constitution, elects new members to its Executive Council, has a vigorous publication division (producing a hard copy journal, electronic newsletter, and Web site), and held its 21st annual meeting in Liverpool, where it first met in 1990. Increasingly, the IHRA plays an active advocacy role for HR with other organizations and within the UN system and is expanding its scope beyond illicit drugs to alcohol and tobaccos. The International Harm Reduction Development Program was established in 1995 as part of the Open Society Institute (OSI) and Soros Foundation. It operates in Eastern Europe and Asia to protect the health and human rights of drug users and has supported the promotion of HR policies and programs in more than 26 countries. The Centre for Harm Reduction (CHR) in Australia was established in 2001 to conduct research and disseminate research findings, provide training, and advocate for HR. Six regional HR networks (including Eurasia, Asia, Latin America, North America, the Caribbean, and Africa) have been established with significant international support. There is even an online peer review academic journal dedicated to the subject (www.HarmReductionJournal.com) devoted to HR studies. These developments represent a growing trend toward the building of HR institutions throughout the world and the normalization of HR practices. Although HR continues to face formidable opposition, it is now clear that this new approach to policy and practice, based on public health and human rights, is becoming the mainstream approach for dealing with the global nature and broad implications of illicit drugs and their many consequences.

REFERENCES

1. United Nations Office on Drugs and Crime (UNODC). 2007 World Drug Report. Available at: https://www.unodc.org/pdf/research/wdr07/WDR_2007.pdf; Mann J, Tarantola D. *AIDS in the World-2*. Harvard: Oxford University Press, 1998; Turner CF, Miller HG, Moses LE. *AIDS, Sexual Behavior, and Intravenous Drug Use*. Washington, DC: National Academy Press, 1989; Stimson GV. The global diffusion of injecting drug use: implications for HIV infection. *Bull Narc*. 1993;45:3–17; National Commission on Acquired Immune Deficiency Syndrome. *The Twin Epidemics of Substance Use and HIV*. Washington, DC: National Commission on Acquired Immune Deficiency Syndrome, 1991; UNAIDS. *2008 Report on the Global AIDS Epidemic*. Geneva: UNAIDS.
2. O'Hare P, Newcombe R, Matthews A, et al. *The Reduction of Drug Related Harm*. New York, NY: Routledge, 1992; Heather N, Wodak A, Nadelmann EA, et al., eds. *Psychoactive Drugs and Harm Reduction: From Faith to Science*. London: Whurr Publishers, 1993:49–54; Drucker E. Harm Reduction: A Public Health Strategy. *Curr Issues Public Health*. 1995;1:64–70; Hunt N, Ashton M, Lenton S, et al. *Forward Thinking on Drugs: A Review of the Evidence Base for Harm Reduction Approaches to Drug Use*. London: International Harm Reduction Association, 2003.
3. Advisory Council on the Misuse of Drugs. *AIDS and Drug Misuse, Part I: Report of the Advisory Council on the Misuse of Drugs*. London: Her Majesty's Stationery Office, 1988; Grund JP, Stern LS, Kaplan EH, et al. Drug use contexts and HIV consequences: the effect of drug policy on patterns of everyday drug use in Rotterdam. *Br J Addict*. 1992;87:381–392.
4. Wodak A. HIV infection and injecting drug use in Australia: responding to a crisis. *J Drug Issues*. 1992;22(3):549–562; Netherlands Ministry of Health Welfare and Sports, Netherlands Ministry of Justice. *Drug Policy in the Netherlands: Continuity and Change*. The Hague, the Netherlands: Ministry of Health, Welfare and Sports, 1995; Erickson P, Drucker E. Harm reduction: a public health strategy. *Curr Issues Public Health*. 1995;1:64–70; Advisory Council on the Misuse of Drugs. *AIDS and Drug Misuse, Part I: Report of the Advisory Council on the Misuse of Drugs*. London: Her Majesty's Stationery Office, 1988; Interdepartmental Stuurgroep Alcohol en Drugbeleid. *Drugbeleid in beweging: naar een normalisering van de drugproblematiek*. The Hague: Ministerie van Welzijn, Volksgezondheid en Culture, 1985; Staples P. Reduction of alcohol- and drug-related harm in Australia: a government minister's perspective. In: Heather N, Wodak A, Nadelmann EA, et al., eds. *Psychoactive Drugs and Harm Reduction: From Faith to Science*. London: Whurr Publishers, 1993:49–54; van de Wijngaart GF. The Dutch approach: normalization of drug problems. *J Drug Issues*. 1990;20(4):667–678.
5. U.S. Office of National Drug Control Policy. Washington, DC, 2003; UN Drug and Crime Control Program, Vienna, 2000.
6. Last JM, Wallace RB. *Maxcy-Rosenau-Last Public Health and Preventive Medicine*. 13th ed. Norwalk, CT: Appleton & Lange, 1992; Drucker E. Harm reduction: a public health strategy. *Curr Issues Public Health*. 1995;1:64–70. Mann J, Tarantola D. 1998. op cit.
7. Drucker E. Drug prohibition and public health: 25 years of evidence. *Public Health Rep*. 1999;114:14–29; Drucker E. *A Plague of Prisons: The Epidemiology of Mass Incarceration in America*. New York, NY: The New Press, 2010.
8. Bewley-Taylor DR. *The United States and International Drug Control, 1909–1997*. London/New York: Continuum, 2001; Bewley-Taylor DR. Challenging the UN drug control conventions: problems and possibilities. *Int J Drug Policy*. 2003;14:171–179 (ref, e.g., within the UN system such as the High Commissioner on Human Rights, the Special Rapporteur on the Right to the Highest Attainable Standard of Mental and Physical Health, and the Special Rapporteur on Torture and Cruel, Inhumane and Degrading treatment).

    International prohibition policies are founded on United Nations (UN) treaties and conventions: the Single Convention on Narcotic Drugs (1961), the Convention on Psychotropic Substances (1971), and the 1988 United Nations Convention Against Illicit Traffic in Narcotic Drugs and Psychoactive Substances, which have been ratified by more than 95 percent of United Nations member states. The Single Convention on Narcotic Drugs (1961). U.S. Department of State Office of the Legal Adviser Treaty Affairs Staff. *Treaties in Force: A List of Treaties and Other International Agreements of the United States in Force as of January 1, 1995*. Washington, DC: U.S. Department of State, 1995; Nadelmann EA. Global prohibition regimes: the evolution of norms in international society. *Int Organ*. 1990;44(4):479–526; Stares PB. *Global Habit: The Drug Problem in a Borderless World*. Washington, DC: Brookings Institution, 1996; Nadelmann EA. *Cops Across Borders: The Internationalization of U.S. Criminal Law Enforcement*. University Park, PA: Pennsylvania State University College Press, 1993; Drucker E. Drug prohibition in America: a human rights perspective. In: Minot A, Francois J, eds. *Drogues et les Droits de L'Homme* (Drugs and Human Rights). Geneva: Swiss League of Human Rights, 1992.
9. Lurie P, Drucker E. An opportunity lost: HIV infections associated with lack of a national needle-exchange programme in the USA (commentary). *Lancet*. 1997;349:604–608; Stancliff S. Syringe access and HIV incidence in the United States. *JAMA*. 2008;300(20):2370; Des Jarlais D. The first and second decades of AIDS among injecting drugs users. *Br J Addict*. 2006;87(3): 347–353; Hall H, Song R, Rhodes P, et al. Estimation of HIV incidence in the United States. *JAMA*. 2008;300(5):520–529.
10. Bayer R, Oppenheimer GM. *Confronting Drug Policy*. New York, NY: Cambridge University Press, 1993; Drucker E. Harm reduction: a public health strategy. *Curr Issues Public Health*. 1995;1: 64–70; Nadelmann EA. Thinking seriously about alternatives to drug prohibition. *Daedalus*. 1992;121(3):85–132; MacCoun RJ,

Saiger AJ, Kahan JP, et al. Drug policies and problems: the promise and pitfalls of cross-national comparison. In: Heather N, Wodak A, Nadelmann EA, et al., eds. *Psychoactive Drugs and Harm Reduction: From Faith to Science*. London: Whurr Publishers, 1993:103–117.

11. Kaplan EH. Probability models of needle exchange. *Oper Res*. 1995;43:558–569.

12. Stimson GV. Syringe exchange programs for injecting drug users. *AIDS*. 1989;3:253.

13. Lurie P, Reingold AL. *The Public Health Impact of Needle Exchange Programs in the United States and Abroad*. Berkeley, CA: University of California, Institute for Health Policy Studies, 1993; Drucker E, Lurie P, Alcabes P, et al. Measuring harm reduction: the effects of needle and syringe exchange programs and methadone maintenance on the ecology of HIV. *AIDS*. 1998; 12(suppl A):S217–S230.

14. Drucker E. Drug prohibition and public health: 25 years of evidence. *Public Health Rep*. 1999;114:4–29; National Commission on Acquired Immune Deficiency Syndrome. *The twin epidemics of substance use and HIV*. Washington, DC: National Commission on Acquired Immune Deficiency Syndrome, 1991; Lurie P, Reingold AL. *The public health impact of needle exchange programs in the United States and abroad*. Berkeley, CA: University of California, Institute for Health Policy Studies, 1993; Needle Exchange Programs: Research Suggests Promise as an AIDS Prevention Strategy HRD-93-60 March 23, 1993; Lurie P. Policy experts unanimous: needle-exchange programs effective [letter]. *AIDS Wkly*. 1996:29; O'Hare P, Newcombe R, Matthews A, et al. *The Reduction of Drug Related Harm*. New York, NY: Routledge, 1992; Case P, Meehan T, Jones ST. Arrests and incarceration of injection drug users for syringe possession in Massachusetts: implications for HIV prevention. *J Acquir Immune Defic Syndr Hum Retrovirol*. 1998;18(suppl 1):S71–S75; Arrest of needle-exchange workers draws national attention: New Brunswick, New Jersey Chai project. *Alcohol Drug Abuse Wkly*. 1996;8(19):3; New Jersey panel's support of needle exchange stirs debate. *Alcohol Drug Abuse Wkly*. 1996;8(14):1; Arnao G. Italian referendum deletes criminal sanctions for drug users. *J Drug Issues*. 1994;24(3):483–487; Australian Government. *Inter-governmental Report on AIDS: A Report on HIV/AIDS Activities in Australia, 1990–1991*. Canberra: Australian Government Publishing, 1992; Barreras R. *Social Policy, Science and Activism in the History of Needle Exchange in NYC*. Unpublished PhD Thesis, City University of NY, March 2004.

15. Drug Policy Alliance: Fourteen Article Abstracts on Needle and Syringe Exchange, 2004. Available at: http://www.drugpolicy.org/library/lipp14.cf.; Moss AR. Epidemiology and the politics of needle exchange [comment]. *Am J Public Health*. 2000;90: 1395–1396; NY State Department of Health, Report on Syringe Exchange Programs. Available at: http://www.health.state.ny.us/diseases/aids/workgroups/aac/docs/syringeaccess.pdf. Accessed 2005.

16. Gostin LO. The legal environment impeding access to sterile syringes and needles: the conflict between law enforcement and public health. *J Acquir Immune Defic Syndr Hum Retrovirol*. 1998;18(suppl 1):S60–S70; Burris S. Needle exchange knowledge asset. Web site created by the Robert Wood Johnson Foundation's Substance Abuse Policy Research Program; January 2009. Available at: http://saprp.org/knowledgeassets/knowledge_detail.cfm.

17. Serfaty A. HIV infection drug use in France: trends of the epidemic and governmental responses. In: Reisinger M, ed. *AIDS and Drug Addiction in the European Community*. Brussels: Commission of the European Communities, European Monitoring Centre on Drugs and Drug Addiction, 1993:61–70.

18. Van Santen GW. Exchange of expertise in Europe: the Frankfurt experience. In: Reisinger M, ed. *AIDS and Drug Addiction in the European Community*. Brussels: Commission of the European Communities, European Monitoring Centre on Drugs.

19. Lungley S, Baker M. *The Needle and Syringe Exchange Scheme in Operation*. Wellington: New Zealand Department of Health, 1990; Steketee H. *Needle-Exchange Programs Have Curbed HIV, Hepatitis C Among IDUs In Australia, Should Be Expanded*. The Australian, February 23, 2006.

20. International Harm Reduction association (IHRA). *Global State of Harm Reduction*. Liverpool: International Harm Reduction Association, 2009.

21. Overdose prevention: Curtis M, Guterman L. International Harm Reduction Development Program of the OSI. Overdose Prevention and Response: A Guide for People Who Use Drugs and Harm Reduction Staff in Eastern Europe and Central Asia, June 2009. Harm Reduction Coalition, 2009. Available at: http://www.harmreduction.org/index.php; Drucker E, ed. Drug overdose. *Special Issue of Addiction Research and Theory*. 2001; 9(5); Bigg D, Maxwell S, Stanczykiewicz K. Use of Narcan to prevent overdose. Paper presented at: APHA Annual Conference, Chicago Recovery Alliance, October 2003; Deitze P, Fry C, Rumbold G, et al. Context management and prevention of heroin overdose in Victoria, Australia. *Addict Res Theory*. 2001;9(60): 437; Ali R. Australia OD campaign. *Drug Alcohol Rev*. 2001. See also http://www.anypositivechange.org/res.html.

22. Grund JP, Blanken P, Adriaans FP, et al. Reaching the unreached: targeting hidden IDU populations with clean needles via known user groups. *J Psychoactive Drugs*. 1992;24(1):41–47; Friedman SR, De Jong W, Wodak A. Community development as a response to HIV among drug injectors. *AIDS*. 1993;7(suppl 1): S263–S269; Crofts N. A history of peer-based drug-user groups in Australia. *J Drug Issues*. 1993;25:599–616; Jürgens R. "Nothing About Us Without Us": Greater, Meaningful Involvement of People Who Use Illegal Drugs: A Public Health, Ethical, and Human Rights Imperative. International edition. Toronto: Canadian HIV/AIDS Legal Network, International HIV/AIDS Alliance, Open Society Institute, 2008; Broadhead RS, Heckathorn DD, Altice FL, et al. Increasing drug users' adherence to HIV treatment: results of a peer-driven intervention feasibility study. *Soc Sci Med*. 2002;55(2):235–246.

23. Fromberg E, Jansen F. Rave drug monitoring system. *Verslag*. 1993;1(7). Netherlands Institute on Alcohol and Drugs (NIAD) Utrecht. Drug Consumer Groups: Grund JP. *Drug Use as a Social Ritual: Functionality, Symbolism and Determinants of Self regulation*. IVO series 4. Rotterdam: IVO, 1996. Municipal Zoning Policies and Open Drug Scenes: See Nadelmann E, McNeely J, Drucker E. International perspectives. In: Lowinson J, Ruiz P, Millman, RB, et al., eds. *Comprehensive Textbook of Substance Abuse*. 4th ed. Willliams & Wilkins, 1995.

24. Dolan K, Kimber J, Fry C, et al. Drug consumption facilities in Europe and the establishment of supervised injecting centres in Australia. *Drug Alcohol Rev*. 2000;19:337–346; Christie T, Wood E, Schechter M, et al. Regulating supervised Injection site in Canada. *Int J Drug Policy*. 2004;15(1):66–73; Wright NMJ, Tompkins CNE. Supervised injecting centres. *BMJ*. 2004;328:100–102. Available at: http://bmj.bmjjournals.com/cgi/content/full/328/7431/100; Strang J, Fortson R. Supervised fixing rooms, supervised injectable maintenance clinics-understanding the difference.

BMJ. 2004;328: 102–103. Available at: http://bmj.bmjjournals.com/cgi/content/ full/328/7431/102; Burton, B. Supervised drug injecting room trial considered a success. *BMJ.* 2003;327:122. Available at: http:// bmj.com/cgi/content/full/327/7407/122-a (Dance Safe: http:// www.dancesafe.org/); also see Holland J, ed. *Ecstacy: The Complete Guide. A Comprehensive Look at the Risks and Benefits of MDMA.* Rochester, NY: Inner Traditions, 2003; EMCDDA. EMCDDA Annual Report, 2004. Luxembourg: Office for Official Publications of the European Communities.

25. Safe Injecting Sites: Australia: Van Beek I. *The Eye of the Needle.* Allen & Unwin, 2004; NDARC, Final Report of MISC Evaluation, 2003. Available at: http://www.druginfo.nsw.gov.au/_data/page/1229/NDARC_final_evaluation_report; Wood E, Tyndall MW, Montaner JS, et al. Summary of findings from the evaluation of a pilot medically supervised safer injecting facility. *Can Med Assoc J.* 2006;175(11):1399–1404. Findings from the Evaluation of Vancouver's Pilot Medically Supervised Safer Injection Facility—Insite. Report prepared by the Urban Health Research Initiative of the British Columbia Centre for Excellence in HIV/AIDS. Available at: http://uhri.cfenet.ubc.ca/images/Documents/insite_report-eng.pdf; Wood E, Kerr T, Tyndall MW, et al. The Canadian government's treatment of scientific process and evidence: inside the evaluation of North America's first supervised injecting facility. *Int J Drug Policy.* 2008;19(3):220–225.

26. Zinberg NE. *Drug, Set, and Setting: The Basis for Controlled Intoxicant Use.* New Haven, CT: Yale University Press, 1984; Zinberg NE, Harding WM. Control and intoxicant use: a theoretical and practical overview. *J Drug Issues.* 1979;9:121–143. Vallaint GE. *The Natural History of Alcoholism.* Cambridge, MA: Harvard University Press, 1983; Vallaint GE, Hiller-Sturmhöfel S. The natural history of alcoholism. *Alcohol Health Res World.* 1996; 20(3):152–161.

27. Tatarsky A. *Harm Reduction Psychotherapy: A New Treatment for Drug and Alcohol Problems.* Northvale, NJ: Jason Aronson, 2002; Denning P. *Practicing Harm Reduction Psychotherapy: An Alternative Approach to Addictions.* New York, NY: Guilford Press, 2002; Marlatt AG, ed. *Harm Reduction: Pragmatic Strategies for Managing High-Risk Behaviors.* London: Guilford Press, 2002; Ruefli T, Rogers S. How do drug users define their progress in harm reduction programs? Qualitative research to develop user-generated outcomes. *Harm Reduct J.* 2004;1:8. Available at: http://www.harmreductionjournal.com/content/1/1/8; Rosenberg H, Phillips KT. Acceptability and availability of harm reduction interventions for drug abuse in American substance abuse treatment agencies. *Psychol Addict Behav.* 2003;17(3): 203–210; McNeely J, Arnsten JH, Langrod JG, et al. Response to a program to improve access to sterile syringes and safe syringe disposal for injection drug users in a methadone maintenance treatment program. Presented at the American Public Health Association Conference; November 2003; San Francisco, CA.

28. Musto DF. *The American Disease: Origins of Narcotic Control.* New York, NY: Oxford University Press, 1987; Stimson GV, Oppenheimer E. *Heroin Addiction: Treatment and Control in Britain.* London: Tavistock, 1982; Chapter by Musto in Lowinson; American Public Health Association. *Resolution for Access to Therapeutic Marijuana/Cannabis.* Washington, DC: American Public Health Association, 1995; Mino A. *Analyse scientifique de la literature pour la remise controlee d'heroine ou de morphine.* Geneva: Office Federal de la Sante Publique, 1990; Drucker E. From morphine to methadone. In: Inciardi J, Harrison L, eds. *Harm Reduction: A Textbook.* Thousand Oaks, CA: Sage, 2000; Picard E. Legal action against the Belgian Medical Association's restrictions of methadone treatment. In: Reisinger M, ed. *AIDS and Drug Addiction in the European Community.* Brussels: Commission of the European Communities, European Monitoring Centre on Drugs and Drug Addiction, 1993:41–49; and Drug Addiction, 1993:169–173; Fleming PM. Prescribing policy in the UK: a swing away from harm reduction? *Int J Drug Policy.* 1995;6:173–177; Recent Scotch and UK problems.

29. Drucker E, Wodak A, eds. Re-inventing methadone: critical studies. Special Issue of *Addict Res.* 1996;3(4).; Drucker E. From morphine to methadone. In: Inciardi J, Harrison L, eds. *Harm Reduction: A Textbook.* Thousand Oaks, CA: Sage, 2000; Newman RG. *Methadone Treatment in Narcotic Addiction.* New York, NY: Academic Press, 1977; MMTP positive outcomes include decreases in heroin use; Ball JC, Ross A. *The Effectiveness of Methadone Maintenance Treatment.* New York, NY: Springer-Verlag, 1991; Hubbard RL. *Drug Abuse Treatment: A National Study of Effectiveness.* Chapel Hill, NC: University of North Carolina Press, 1989; Nadelmann E, McNeely J. Doing methadone right. *Public Interest.* 1996;123:83–93; U.S. Office of Technology Assessment. *The Effectiveness of AIDS Prevention Efforts.* Washington, DC: U.S. Government Printing Office, 1995; Caplehorn JRM, Bell J. Methadone dosage and retention of patients in maintenance treatment. *Med J Aust.* 1991;154:195–199; Cooper JR. Ineffective use of psychoactive drugs: methadone treatment is no exception. *JAMA.* 1992;267(2):281–282; D'Aunno T, Vaughn T. Variations in methadone treatment practices: results from a national study. *JAMA.* 1992;267(2):253–258; Hargreaves WA. Methadone dose and duration for maintenance treatment. In: Cooper JR, ed. *Research on the Treatment of Narcotic Addiction: State of the Art.* Rockville, MD: National Institute on Drug Abuse, 1983; Caplehorn JRM. A comparison of abstinence-oriented and indefinite methadone maintenance treatment. *Int J Addict.* 1994;19:1361–1375; U.S. Department of Health and Human Services Center for Substance Abuse Treatment. *State Methadone Treatment Guidelines.* Rockville, MD: U.S. Department of Health and Human Services, Center for Substance Abuse Treatment, 1993; D'Aunno T, Pollack HA. Changes in methadone treatment practices: results from a national panel study, 1988–2000. *JAMA.* 2002;288(7):850–856; Cunningham C, Drucker E, Meissner P, et al. The perceived need for buprenorphine treatment at a primary care clinic in the South Bronx: a market survey. *Addict Disord Their Treat.* 2005;4(4):125–126.

30. Institute of Medicine. *Federal Regulation of Methadone Treatment.* Washington, DC: National Academy Press, 1995.

31. Australian Government. *Inter-Governmental Report on AIDS: A Report on HIV/AIDS Activities in Australia, 1990–1991.* Canberra: Australian Government Publishing, 1992; Bammer G. *Report and Recommendations of Stage 2 Feasibility Research into the Controlled Availability of Opioids.* Canberra: Australian Institute of Criminology, National Centre for Epidemiology and Population Health, 1995; World Health Organization Programme on Substance Abuse Drug Substitution Project. *Report of WHO Consultation, Geneva, 15–19 May 1995.* Geneva: World Health Organization, 1996. Australian Government. *Inter-Governmental Report on AIDS: A Report on HIV/AIDS Activities in Australia, 1990–1991.* Canberra: Australian Government Publishing, 1992; Ball JC, Ross A. *The Effectiveness of Methadone Maintenance Treatment.* New York, NY: Springer-Verlag, 1991; Bammer G. *Report and Recommendations of Stage 2 Feasibility Research Into the Controlled Availability of Opioids.* Canberra: Australian Institute of Criminology, National Centre for Epidemiology and Population Health, 1995; Bammer G, Dance P, Stevens A, et al.

Attitudes to a proposal for controlled availability of heroin in Australia: is it time for a trial? *Addict Res.* 1996;4(1):45–55; Darke S, Hall W, Heather N, et al. The reliability and validity of a scale to measure HIV risk taking behavior among intravenous drug users. *AIDS.* 1991;5(2):181–185; Selwyn PA, Feiner C, Cox CP, et al. Knowledge about AIDS and high risk behavior among intravenous drug users in New York City. *AIDS.* 1987;1(4):247–254.

32. Joseph H. The criminal justice system and opiate addiction: an historical perspective. In: Leukefeld CG, Tims FM, eds. *Compulsory Treatment of Drug Abuse: Research and Clinical Practice.* Rockville, MD: National Institute on Drug Abuse, 1988:106–125; Newman RG, Peyser NP. Methadone treatment: experiment and experience. *J Psychoactive Drugs.* 1991;23:115–121.

33. PH gains of MMTP HIV: Gibson DR, Flynn NM, McCarthy JJ. Effectiveness of methadone treatment in reducing HIV risk behavior and HIV seroconversion among injecting drug users [editorial]. *AIDS.* 1999;13:14, 1807–1818.

34. Institute of Medicine. *Federal Regulation of Methadone Treatment.* Washington, DC: National Academy Press, 1995; Dole VP. Hazards of process regulations: the example of methadone maintenance. *JAMA.* 1992;267(16):2234–2235; Dole VP, Nyswander ME. Methadone maintenance treatment: a ten year perspective. *JAMA.* 1976;235(19):2117–2119; Ball JC, Ross A. *The Effectiveness of Methadone Maintenance Treatment.* New York, NY: Springer-Verlag, 1991.

35. Webster LR. Methadone related deaths. *J Opioid Manag.* 2005;1:(4):211–217; Joseph H, Springer E. Methadone maintenance treatment and the AIDS epidemic. Chap 23. In: Platt, JJ. editor. The effectiveness of drug abuse treatment: Dutch and American perspectives. Malabar (FL): Robert E. Krieger; 1990. pp. 261–274. Center for Substance Abuse Treatment. Clinical Guidelines for the Use of Buprenorphine in the Treatment of Opioid Addiction. Treatment Improvement Protocol (TIP) Series 40. Rockville, MD: Substance Abuse and Mental Health Services Administration; 2004. (DHHS Publication No. (SMA)04-3939.): Substance Abuse and Mental Health Services Administration. The Determinations Report: A Report on the Physician Waiver Program Established by the Drug Addiction Treatment Act of 2000 ("DATA"). Rockville, MD; 2006. Available from: http://buprenorphine.samhsa.gov/SAMHSA_Determinations_Report.pdf (Accessed Jan. 24, 2009).; Kissin W, Mcleod C, Sonnefeld J, Stanton A. Experiences of a National Sample of Qualified Addiction Specialists Who Have and Have Not Prescribed Buprenorphine for Opioid Dependence. Journal of Addictive Diseases 2006;25(4):91–103; Joseph H, Springer E. Methadone maintenance treatment and the AIDS epidemic. Chap 23. In: Platt, JJ. editor. The effectiveness of drug abuse treatment: Dutch and American perspec-tives. Malabar (FL): Robert E. Krieger; 1990. pp. 261–274.

36. Buprenorphine Substance Abuse and Mental Health Services Administration. The Determinations Report: A Report on the Physician Waiver Program Established by the Drug Addiction Treatment Act of 2000 ("DATA"). Rockville, MD, 2006. Available at: http://buprenorphine.samhsa.gov/SAMHSA_Determinations_Report.pdf. Accessed January 24, 2009; Kissin W, Mcleod C, Sonnefeld J, et al. Experiences of a national sample of qualified addiction specialists who have and have not prescribed buprenorphine for opioid dependence. *J Addict Dis.* 2006;25(4):91–103; Auriacombe M. Buprenorphine use in France background and current use. In: Ritter A, Kutin J, Lintzeris N, et al., eds. *Expanding Treatment Options for Heroin Dependence in Victoria Buprenorphine, LAAM, Naltrexone and Slow-Release Oral Morphine. New Pharmacotherapies Project—Feasibility Phase.* Fitzroy: Victoria Turning Point Alcohol and Drug Center Inc., 1997:73–80; Auriacombe M, Franques P, Bertorelle V, et al. Use of buprenorphine for substitution treatment a French experience in Bordeaux and Bayonne. *Res Clin Forum.* 1997;19:47–50; Auriacombe M, Franques P, Martin C, et al. Economic impact of methadone and buprenorphine treatments. A tentative approach. In: 59th *Annual Scientific Meeting of the College on Problems of Drug Dependence, Nashville, TN, 1997;* Auriacombe M, Tignol J. Buprenorphine use in France quality of life and conditions for treatment success. *Res Clin Forum.* 1997;19:25–32; Fhima A, Henrion R, Lowenstein W, et al. Two-year follow-up of an opioid-user cohort treated with high-dose buprenorphine (Subutex). *Ann Med Interne (Paris).* 2001;152:26–36; Lepĉre B., Gourarier L., Sanchez M, et al. Reduction in the number of lethal heroin overdoses in France since 1994. *Annal de Med Interne (Paris).* 2001;152:5–12.

37. Roberts K, Hunter C. A comprehensive system of pharmaceutical care for drug misusers. *Harm Reduct J.* 2004;1(1):6; Tommasello AC. Substance abuse and pharmacy practice: what does the community pharmacist need to know about drug abuse and dependence? *Harm Reduct J.* 2004;1(1):3; The American Society of Health-System Pharmacists (ASHP). ASHP Statement on the Pharmacist's Role in Substance Abuse Prevention, Education, and Assistance. *Am J Health Syst Pharm.* 2003;60(19):1995–1998; Sheridan J, Strang J, eds. *Drug Misuse and Community Pharmacy.* London: Taylor & Francis, 2002; Tuchman E, Gregory C, Simson MJ, et al. Office-based opioid treatment (OBOT)—practitioner's knowledge, attitudes and expectations in New Mexico. *Addict Disord Their Treat.* 2005;4(1):11–19; Drucker E, Rice S, Ganse G, et al. The Lancaster office based opiate treatment program: a case study and prototype for community physicians and pharmacists providing methadone maintenance treatment in the US. *Addict Disord Their Treat.* 2007;6(3):121–135.

38. Picard E. Legal action against the Belgian Medical Association's restrictions of methadone treatment. In: Reisinger M, ed. *AIDS and Drug Addiction in the European Community.* Brussels: Commission of the European Communities, European Monitoring Centre on Drugs and Drug Addiction, 1993:41–49; and Drug Addiction, 1993:169–173; Fleming PM. Prescribing policy in the UK: a swing away from harm reduction? *Int J Drug Policy.* 1995;6:173–117; Farrell M. *Methadone Treatment in the European Union.* London: Oxford University Press, 1999; Verster A, Buning E. *Key Aspects of Substitution Treatment for Opiate Dependence.* Amsterdam: Euro Methwork, 2003; Amsterdam Advisory Council on the Misuse of Drugs. *AIDS and Drug Misuse, Part I: Report of the Advisory Council on the Misuse of Drugs.* London: Her Majesty's Stationery Office, 1988; Bell J. Alternatives to nonclinical regulation: training doctors to deliver methadone maintenance treatment. *Addict Res.* 1986;3:297–315; Buning EC. Involving G.P.'s in Paris. *Euro-methwork.* 1996;8:3–4; Byrne A, Wodak A. Census of patients receiving methadone in a general practice. *Addict Res.* 1986;3:323–341; Greenwood J. Creating a new drug service in Edinburgh. *Br Med J.* 1990;300:587–589; Pearson G. Drug-control policies in Britain. *Crime Justice Rev Res.* 1991;14:167; Picard E. Legal action against the Belgian Medical Association's restrictions of methadone treatment. In: Reisinger M, ed. *AIDS and Drugs Addiction in the European Community.* Brussels: Commission of the European Communities, European Monitoring Centre on Drugs and Drug Addiction, 1993:41–49; Reisinger M. *AIDS and Drug Addiction in the European Community.* Brussels: Commission of the European Communities, European Monitoring Centre on Drugs and Drug Addiction,

1993; Stimson GV. AIDS and injecting drug use in the United Kingdom, 1988–1993: the policy response and the prevention of the epidemic. Unpublished manuscript, 1994; Van Brussel GHA. Methadone treatment in Amsterdam: the critical role of the general practitioners. *Addict Res.* 1986;3:363–369; Buning EC, Van Brussel GHA, Van Santen GW. The "Methadone by Bus" project in Amsterdam. *Br J Addict.* 1990;85(10):1247–1250; Gossop M, Grant M. *The Content and Structure of Methadone Treatment Programs: A Study in Six Countries.* Geneva: WHO, Programme on Substance Abuse, 1990; Klingemann HKH. Drug treatment in Switzerland: harm reduction, decentralization and community response. *Addiction.* 1996; 91:723–736; Plomp HN, van der Hek H, Ader HJ. The Amsterdam dispensing circuit: genesis and effectiveness of a public health model for local drug policy. *Addiction.* 1996;91(5):711–721; Pompidou Group Co-operation Group to Combat Drug Abuse and Illicit Trafficking in Drugs. *Multi-City Study: Drug Misuse Trends in Thirteen European Cities.* Strasbourg: Council of Europe Press, 1994; Ward J, Mattick RP, Hall W. *Key Issues in Methadone Maintenance Treatment.* Kensington, Australia: New South Wales University Press, 1992; Newman RG. Narcotic addiction and methadone treatment in Hong Kong. *J Public Health Policy* (South Asian edition) 1985;6:526–538; Pompidou Group Co-operation Group to Combat Drug Abuse and Illicit Trafficking in Drugs. *Multi-City Study: Drug Misuse Trends in Thirteen European Cities.* Strasbourg: Council of Europe Press, 1994.

39. Dole VP, Robinson JW, Orraca J, et al. Methadone treatment of randomly selected criminal addicts. *N Engl J Med.* 1969;280:1372–1375; Dolan KA, Wodak A. An international review of methadone provision in prisons. *Addict Res.* 1996;4(1):85; CDC. *Prevention and Control of Infections with Hepatitis Viruses in Correctional Settings.* Atlanta: Centers for Disease Control and Prevention, 2003. Morbidity and Mortality Weekly Report 24:19; Crofts N, Stewart T, Hearne P, et al. Spread of blood borne viruses among Australian prison entrants. *Br Med J.* 1995;310:285–288; Magura S, Rosenblum A, Lewis C, et al. The effectiveness of in-jail methadone maintenance. *J Drug Issues.* 1993;23(1):75–99; Dolan KA, Shearer JD, MacDonald M, et al. A randomised controlled trial of methadone maintenance treatment versus wait list control in an Australian prison. *Drug Alcohol Depend.* 2003;72:59–65; Levasseur L, Marzo J-N, Ross N, et al. Frequency of re-incarcerations in the same detention centre: role of substitution therapy. A preliminary retrospective analysis. *Ann Med Interne.* 2002;153(3):1S14–1S19; Kinlock TW, Battjes RJ, Schwartz RP, et al. TMP. A novel opioid maintenance program for prisoners: preliminary findings. *J Subst Abuse Treat.* 2002;22:141–147; Bellin E, Wesson J, Tomasino V, et al. High dose methadone reduces criminal recidivism in opiate addicts. *Addict Res.* 1999;7(1):19–29; McKay D, Jail Site of Health Service. *Albuquerque Journal.* 2004:1.

40. Hartnoll RL, Mitcheson MC, Battersby A, et al. Evaluation of heroin maintenance in controlled trial. *Arch Gen Psychiatry.* 1980;37:877–884; Battersby M, Farrell M, Gossop M, et al. "Horse trading": prescribing injectable opiates to opiate addicts. A descriptive study. *Drug Alcohol Rev.* 1992;11:35–42.

41. Swiss Drugs Policy, September 2000, Bern; Swiss Federal Office of Public Health Heroin Assisted Treatment, 2002, Bern; Drucker E, Vlahov D. Controlled clinical evaluation of diacetyl morphine for treatment of intractable opiate dependence (commentary). *Lancet.* 1999;353:1543–1544; Rehm J, Gschwend P, Steffen T, et al. Feasibility, safety and efficacy of injectable heroin prescription for refractory opiate addicts: a follow-up study. *Lancet.* 2001;358:1417–1420; Drucker E. Injectable heroin substitution treatment for opiate dependency (commentary). *Lancet.* 2001;358:1385; Central Committee on the Treatment of Heroin Addicts (CCBH). *Investigating the Medical Prescription of Heroin.* Utrecht, Netherlands: Central Committee on the Treatment of Heroin Addicts, 1997; van den Brink W, Hendriks VM, Blanken P, et al. Results of the Dutch Heroin Trial. Addictions (www.ccbh.nl). *BMJ.* 2003; Uchtenhagen A, Gutzwiller F, Dobler-Mikola A. eds. *Medical Prescription of Narcotics Research Programme: Final Report of the Principal Investigators.* Zurich: Institute for Social and Preventive Medicine at the University of Zurich: Zurich, 1998; Bammer G, Dobler-Mikola A, Fleming PM, et al. The heroin prescribing debate: integrating science and politics. *Science.* 1999;284(5418):1277–1278; Report of the WHO External Panel on the Evaluation of the Swiss Scientific Studies of Medically Prescribed Narcotics to Drug Addicts. WHO Report, April 1999; Frei A, Greiner R, Mehner A, et al. *Socioeconomic Evaluation of the Trials for the Medical Prescription of Opiates, Final Report.* HealthEcon: Basel, 1997 (translated June 1998); Drucker E, Vlahov D. Controlled clinical evaluation of diacetyl morphine for treatment of intractable opiate dependence. *Lancet.* 1999;353(9164):1543–1544; Farrell M, Hall W. The Swiss heroin trials: testing alternative approaches: prescribed heroin is 1ikely to have a limited role. *BMJ.* 1998;316(7132):639; Fischer B, Rehm J. The case for a heroin substitution treatment trial in Canada. *Can J Public Health.* 1997;88(6):367–370; Cooper-Mahkorn D. German doctors vote to prescribe heroin to misusers. *BMJ.* 1998;316:1037; North American Opiate Medication Initiative (NAOMI). *Status Report*, October 2008. Available at: http://www.naomistudy.ca/pdfs/NAOMI; Oviedo-Joekes E, Brissette S, Marsh DC, et al. Diacetylmorphine versus methadone for the treatment of opioid addiction. *N Engl J Med.* 2009;361:777–786; Lintzeris N. Prescription of heroin for the management of heroin dependence. *CNS Drugs.* 2009;23(6):463–476.

42. Prescription of Non Opiates: Bradbeer TM, Fleming PM, Charlton P, et al. Survey of amphetamine prescribing in England and Wales. *Drug Alcohol Rev.* 1998;17(3):299–304; Fleming PM, Roberts D. Is the prescription of amphetamine justified as a harm reduction measure? *J R Soc Health.* 1994;114(3):127–131; Fleming PM. Prescribing amphetamine to amphetamine users as a harm reduction measure. *Int J Drug Policy.* 1998; 9(5):339–344; Mattick RP, Darke S. Drug replacement treatments: is amphetamine substitution a horse of a different colour? *Drug Alcohol Rev.* 1995;14:389–394; Merrill J. Evaluation of prescribing dexamphetamine in the treatment of amphetamine dependence. Unpublished document, 1998; Myles J. Treatment for amphetamine misuse in the United Kingdom. In: Klee H, ed. *Amphetamine Misuse: International Perspectives on Current Trends.* Amsterdam, Netherlands: Harwood Academic, 1997:69–79; Sherman JP. Dexamphetamine for "speed" addiction. *Med J Aust.* 1990;153(5):306; Strang J, Sheridan J. Prescribing amphetamines to drug misusers: data from the 1995 National Survey of Community Pharmacies in England and Wales. *Addiction.* 1997;92(7):833–838; Kingston S, Conrad M. Harm reduction for methamphetamine users. 2004 Focus: UCSF AIDS Health Project. 19, 1; Shearer J, Wodak A, van Beek I, et al. Related Article Links: Pilot randomized double blind placebo-controlled study of dexamphetamine for cocaine dependence. *Addiction.* 2003;98(8):1137–1141.

43. Marijuana Policies: Kaplan S. *Marijuana: The New Prohibition.* New York, NY: Pocket Books, 1970; Anderson P. *High in America: The True Story Behind NORML and the Politics of Marijuana.*

New York, NY: Viking Press, 1981; see also Nadelmann, Ethan, et al. Marijuana Regulation Bibliography. Drug Policy Alliance website, January 2010. Available at: http://www.drugpolicy.org/marijuana/medical/.

44. International Cannabis Policies: Cohen P. Building upon the successes of Dutch drug policy. *Int J Drug Policy.* 1988;2(2):22–24; Cohen P. The case of the two Dutch drug policy commissions. An exercise in harm reduction 1968–1972. In: Erickson P, Riley DM, Cheung YW, et al., eds. *New Public Health Policies and Programs for the Reduction of Drug Related Harm.* Toronto: University of Toronto Press, 1997; Cohen P, Arjan S. Cannabis use, a stepping stone to other drug use? The case of Amsterdam. In: Böllinger L, ed. *Cannabis Science/Cannabis Wissenschaft.* Frankfurt Am Main: Peter Lang Publishing, 1997:49–82; de Kort M. The Dutch cannabis debate 1968–1976. *J Drug Issues.* 1994; 24(3):417–427; Engelsman EL. Dutch policy of the management of drug-related problems. *Br J Addict.* 1989;84:211–218; Grapendaal M, Leuw E, Nelen H. Legalization, decriminalization and the reduction of crime. In: Leuw E, Haen Marshall I, eds. *Between Prohibition and Legalization: The Dutch Experiment in Drug Policy.* New York, NY: Kugler Publications, 1996:233–253; Jansen ACM. The development of a "legal" consumers' market for cannabis: the "coffee shop" phenomenon. In: Leuw E, Haen Marshall I, eds. *Between Prohibition and Legalization: The Dutch Experiment in Drug Policy.* New York, NY: Kugler Publications, 1996:169–181; Korf DJ. Cannabis retail markets in Amsterdam. *Int J Drug Policy.* 1990;2(1):23–27; Korf DJ. Twenty years of soft drug use in Holland: a retrospective view based on twenty years of prevalence studies. *Dutch J Alcohol Drugs Other Psychotropic Subst.* 1988;14(3):81–89; Lap M, Drucker E. Recent changes in the Dutch cannabis trade: the case for regulated domestic production. *Int J Drug Policy.* 1994;5(4): 249–252; Leuw E, Haen Marshall I, eds. *Between Prohibition and Legalization: The Dutch Experiment in Drug Policy.* Amsterdam, New York: Kugler Publications, 1994; Leuw E. Drugs and drug policy in the Netherlands. In: Tonry M, ed. *Crime and Justice: A Review of Research.* Chicago, IL: University of Chicago Press, 1991; Leuw E. Recent reconsiderations in Dutch drug policy. In: Böllinger L, ed. *Cannabis Science: From Prohibition to Human Right [Cannabis Wissenschaft: Von der Prohibition zum Recht auf Genuβ].* Frankfurt, Germany: Peter Lang, 1997:153–168; Netherlands Ministry of Health, Welfare and Sports; Netherlands Ministry of Justice. *Drug policy in the Netherlands: Continuity and Change.* The Hague, Netherlands: Ministry of Health, Welfare and Sports, 1995; Ossebaard HC. Netherlands cannabis policy [letter]. *Lancet.* 1996;347(9003):767–768; Scheerer S. The new Dutch and German drug laws: social and political conditions for criminalization and decriminalization. *Law Soc Rev.* 1978;12(4): 585–606; Silvis J. Enforcing drug laws in the Netherlands. In: Leuw E, Haen Marshall I, eds. *Between Prohibition and Legalization: the Dutch Experiment in Drug Policy.* New York, NY: Kugler Publications, 1996:41–58.

45. Addiction Research Foundation. *Cannabis, Health and Public Policy.* Toronto, Canada: Addiction Research Foundation, 1997; Canada: Commission of Inquiry into the Non-medical Use of Drugs. *Cannabis: a report of the Commission of Inquiry into the non-medical use of drugs [also known as the LeDain report].* Ottawa, Canada: Information Canada, 1972. *Note:* especially chapter 5, "The law" (pp. 209–261) and chapter 6, "Conclusions and recommendations of Gerald LeDain, Heinz Lehmann, J. Peter Stein" (pp. 265–316); Canadian Centre on Substance Abuse (CCSA), National Working Group on Addictions Policy. *Cannabis control in Canada: Options Regarding Possession.* Ottawa, Canada: Canadian Centre on Substance Abuse (CCSA), 1998; Dupuis T, MacKay R. Bill C-15: An Act to amend the Controlled Drugs and Substances Act and to make related and consequential amendments to other Acts, Second Session, Fortieth Parliament, 57–58 Elizabeth II, 2009.

46. Australia: Atkinson L, McDonald D. Cannabis, the law and social impacts in Australia. Trends and Issues in Crime and Criminal Justice. 1995, no. 48; Christie P. *The Effects of Cannabis Legislation in South Australia on Levels of Cannabis Use.* Parkside, Australia: Drug and Alcohol Services Council, 1991; Christie P, Ali R. The operation and effects of the cannabis laws in South Australia. In: McDonald D, Atkinson L, eds. *Social Impacts of the Legislative Options for Cannabis in Australia (phase 1 research): A Report to the National Drug Strategy Committee.* Canberra, Australia: Australian Institute of Criminology, 1995; Criminal Justice Commission. *Report on Cannabis and the Law in Queensland.* Brisbane, Australia: Criminal Justice Commission, 1994.

47. Medical Marijuana: Grinspoon L, Bakalar J. *Marijuana: Forbidden Medicine.* Yale: Yale U press New Haven, 1997; Zimmer L, Morgan J. *Marijuana Myths, Marijuana Facts.* New York, NY: The Lindesmith Center, 1997; Joy JE, Watson SJ, Benson JA, eds. *Marijuana and Medicine: Assessing the Science Base.* Washington, DC: Division of Neuroscience and Behavioral Health, Institute of Medicine, National Academy Press, 1999; Earleywine M. *Understanding Marijuana: A New Look at the Scientific Evidence.* New York: Oxford University Press, 2002. Current Sites: http://www.marijuanainfo.org/ popup .php?Source_ID=138&Source_Tbl=Info OR http://www .mpp.org/USA/news_1919.html OR http://www.mpp.org/ 10statepoll/index.html; Medical Marijuana in Canada: S.C. 1996, c. 19. R. v. Parker (2000), 49 O.R. (3d) 481. S.O.R./2001 227. Hitzig v. Canada [2003] O.J. No. 12 (Ontario Superior Court, Lederman J.) January 9, 2003.

48. Jia Y, Sun J, Fan L, et al. Estimates of HIV prevalence in a highly endemic area of China: Dehong Prefecture, Yunnan Province. *Int J Epidemiol.* 2008;37:1287–1296; Jia Y, Lu F, Sun X, et al. Sources of data for improved surveillance of HIV/AIDS in China. *Southeast Asian J Trop Med Public Health.* 2007;38:1041–1052.

49. China Ministry of Health and UN theme Group on HIV/AIDS in China. A Joint Assessment of HIV/AIDS Prevention, Treatment and Care in China (2007). Beijing, 2008. Available at: http://www.chinaids.org.cn/n443289/n443292/6438.html. Accessed on October 31, 2009.

50. Mesquita F, Jacka D, Ricard D, et al. Accelerating harm reduction interventions to confront the HIV epidemic in the Western Pacific and Asia: the role of WHO (WPRO). *Harm Reduct J.* 2008;5:26.

51. Sullivan SG, Wu Z. Rapid scale up of harm reduction in China. *Int J Drug Policy.* 2007;18:118–128.

52. China CDC. AIDS prevention and treatment work progress report. The National Conference on HIV/STD Treatment and Prevention in 2009. Beijing, 2009.

53. Lyman A. Council on Foreign Relations (US) Addressing the HIV/AIDS Pandemic: A U.S. Global AIDS Strategy for the Long Term 2006; AIDS Epidemic Update for the former soviet union: December 2002. The report notes, "In recent years, the Russian Federation has experienced an exceptionally steep rise in reported HIV infections. In less than eight years, HIV/AIDS epidemics have been discovered in more than 30 cities and 86 of the country's 89 regions." in Torrey Clark, "Counting the Cost of AIDS on GDP." *Moscow Times,* May 16, 2002, A1. The estimate of the number of Ukrainians living with HIV is from Oleksander Yaramenko, the director of the Ukrainian Institute for

Social Research, who quoted this figure in November 2002 in a speech at a conference in Crimea. The estimate is based on research his organization carried out for the British Council. Also quoted in "Every 10th Ukrainian Lives with HIV," November 11, 2002: NEWSru.com, online in Russian.UNAIDS, AIDS Epidemic Update, December 2002. See also Rhodes T, Sarang A, Bobrik A, et al. HIV transmission and prevention associated with IDU in the Russian Federation. *Int J Drug Policy*. 2004;15(1):1–16; Human Rights: Csete J. Rights and lessons scorned: human rights and HIV/AIDS in Russia and Eurasia. In: Twigg JL, ed. *HIV/AIDS in Russia and Eurasia*. Vol 1. New York, NY: Palgrave Macmillan, 2006:165–180; Csete J. Rhetoric and reality: HIV/AIDS as a human rights issue. In: Harris, PG, Siplon P, eds. *Global Politics of AIDS*. Boulder, CO: Lynne Rienner, 2007:247–262;2007; Mathers BM, Degenhardt L, Phillips B, et al. Global epidemiology of injecting drug use and HIV among people who inject drugs: a systematic review. *Lancet*. 2008; 372(9651):1733–1745.

54. Sub-Saharan Africa: Becker JU, Drucker E. A paradoxical peace: HIV in post-conflict states. *Med Confl Surviv*. 2008;24(2):101–106; Csete J, Gathumbi J, Wolfe D, et al. Lives to save: PEPFAR, HIV, and injecting drug use in Africa. *Lancet*. 2009;373 (9680):2006–2007; Drucker E, Alcabes PG, Marx PA. The injection century: massive unsterile injecting and the emergence of human pathogens. *Lancet*. 2001;358:1989–1992; Madhava V, Burgess C, Drucker E. The epidemiology of chronic of Hepatits C infection in sub Saharan Africa. *Lancet Infect Dis*. 2002; 2(5):293–302; Schneider W, Drucker E. The role of blood transfusions in the early decades of AIDS in Sub-Saharan Africa. Paper Presented at the American Association of the History of Medicine, May 2004; Beckerleg S. How "cool" is heroin injecting at the Kenya Coast. *Drug Educ Prev Policy*. 2004;11:67–77; Beckerleg S, Telfer M, Hundt GL. The rise of injecting drug use in east Africa: a case study from Kenya. *Harm Reduct J*. 2005;2:12. Available at: http://www.harmreductionjournal.com/content/2/1/12; Reid SR. Injection drug use, unsafe medical injections, and HIV in Africa: a systematic review. *Harm Reduct J*. 2009;6:24. Available at: http://www.harmreductionjournal.com/content/6/1/24.

CHAPTER 56 Work Setting

Paul F. Engelhart ■ Cindy Taormina

THE VALUE OF WORK IN THE RECOVERY PROCESS

Some of us may be uncomfortable with Thomas Carlyle's poetic assertion that "the whole soul of man is composed into a kind of harmony the instant he sets himself to work" (1). Still, we cannot deny the significant role that work can play, both in the disease progression of alcohol and drug addiction and in the recovery process. Clients in substance abuse treatment programs realize the contribution that employment makes to their recovery. Research indicates that many recovering substance abusers express a need for greater vocational services than they are presently receiving (2).

Personality theorists from the early psychoanalysts to the more recent existential analysts have identified love and work, Freud's *liebe und arbeit*, as two of the most basic principles of human existence. Their absence can destroy a person's life and, just as powerfully, their presence can save it. Involvement in meaningful relationships and contribution to the tasks of society are crucial to the development of a healthy sense of self (3).

While not denying the equally important role that love plays, this chapter focuses on the role that work plays in the recovery process. Though the entry or return to employment can have many benefits, recovering substance abusers may face many problems when returning to the workplace, and therefore there is a need for a coordinated range of services for facilitating their success.

Work may be defined as purposeful effort expended to positively alter one's environment. Traditionally, work has been seen as a central component of one's identity. Standard adult social introductions usually begin with responses to two coupled questions: "What's your name?" and "What do you do for a living?" Young children are repeatedly asked about their future worker identity: "What do you want to be when you grow up?" Older adults can find adjustment to retirement difficult not only because of a reduction in established activities, but also because of a loss of their specific occupational identity.

American culture extols the virtues of work and assigns a stigma to the unemployed. In our society, employment is a sign of maturity and considered necessary for the independence associated with adulthood. Moreover, our society assigns degrees of respect to people based on the type of work they do.

Although there are different theories on how an individual determines a specific worker identity for himself or herself, most occupational psychologists agree that vocational identity is attained through a developmental process. If we agree with this perspective, then it is easy to see how a disability like substance abuse could deprive an individual of the experiences necessary for a transformation from a nonworking child into a working adult. Substance abuse is a disability that begins before or during early adulthood or that removes a worker from employment for a significant period during later adulthood.

There are two basic groups of recovering substance abusers in the treatment setting: those who, as a consequence of their abuse or other environmental or family factors, have never worked and those who have worked and been suspended from their jobs or fired as a consequence of substance abuse. The first group is looking to enter the workforce for the first time and the second group is looking to return. Although there are similarities between the two, care must be taken to fully understand the unique dynamics influencing each group's movement toward work.

Recovering substance abusers entering the labor force for the first time may be confronted with poor, inadequate, or unrealistic concepts of what work is and who they are and can be as workers. Individuals who grew up in disadvantaged or unstable homes because of poverty, generational substance abuse, or family conflict may never have worked formally or been raised with close "worker" role models. Employment may be seen by recovering substance abusers as foreign and unknown, creating feelings of inadequacy and fear. Many of their lifestyle patterns and habits are maladaptive and not conducive to work. Adolescents and young adults whose lives have focused on drug or alcohol addiction have not experienced many of the stresses and fears that most people gradually confront in high school educational programs or their first part-time or summer jobs.

In addition to not experiencing these feelings early on, substance abusers may have missed the opportunities to develop effective coping skills and strengths, to make mistakes in less-significant vocational responsibilities, and to learn from these mistakes, integrating healthy social and personal management skills into their sense of self (4,5). They lack concrete experiences in exploring specific occupational fields, as well as the general expectations and unwritten rules associated with employment. As a result, many have false and immature expectations of what to expect from a job or of the necessary elements to build a career. They may also lack awareness of their own values, interests, and abilities.

These individuals arrive at the job market overwhelmed by the enormity of the task of entering the "straight" world and meeting employers' expectations that they have already completed the more basic vocational development tasks. Still, a position in the labor force is attractive, because it offers to place them into a recognized position in society for the first time in their lives.

Other individuals coming from the mainstream with an intact background may have come to accept their chemical addiction only when their substance abuse destroyed their ability to work. They were removed from the labor market for one or more periods of employment. Paradoxically, they may now question their ability to handle work demands sober and drug free. They face discrimination because of employment gaps and poor previous work references. They may lack a career plan because of the unstable and interrupted patterns of their prior employment. Employment for these people is a sign of their restored health and a return to their place in society.

As a result of the current economic downturn, the current job market is characterized by keen competition and advanced skills requirements for even entry-level jobs. Regretfully, both of these groups of recovering abusers are often further handicapped by a lack of marketable educational and occupational skills. Either they never developed these skills, or they have been absent from the workforce for so long that their developed skills are obsolete. Many of these individuals may also suffer additional discrimination because of a history of legal convictions.

Obviously, recovering men and women have many needs as they seek to enter or return to work and re-establish themselves in the community. Comprehensive, specialized services are needed to help them make this transition.

VOCATIONAL REHABILITATION

Rehabilitation can be simply defined as the series of steps taken by a disabled person to achieve fulfillment in life. The process that specifically addresses an individual's work fulfillment and remuneration is referred to as vocational rehabilitation. A further distinction in terms is important because of the specific needs of recovering substance abusers. The process for many who are characterized by a late onset of substance abuse, or who have worked before and are returning to competitive employment, may appropriately be termed vocational "rehabilitation." These individuals are being restored to a former level of functioning. However, for those recovering people who have lived on the fringe of society, never having worked before, vocational "habilitation" provides a more accurate understanding of their need to learn what work is about and to establish for the first time effective work behaviors. Having made this distinction, the term *rehabilitation* is used in this chapter to refer to both concepts.

There are three basic vocational rehabilitation strategies (6). The first and most desirable strategy is to remedy the cause of the person's disability by restoring or developing functional ability. For example, a recovering person who is impaired by the lack of current marketable job skills may "cure" this handicap by completing an appropriate occupational skills training program. The second strategy is to enhance the individual's other vocational/educational attributes so that the person can compensate for the disability. For example, a recovering substance abuser may need to outweigh a lack of past employment by obtaining significant positive references from volunteer positions the individual has held. The third strategy is to adapt the work environment so that the person's disability is not a functional impairment. This tactic is least feasible because the provision of specialized tools or techniques or making physical changes in a workstation usually does not effectively rectify the consequences of a recovering substance abuser's disability. However, an example of this strategy might be the alteration of a regular work schedule to allow a recovering person to keep ongoing counseling support appointments.

The ultimate guideline for all rehabilitation and vocational rehabilitation is to provide help so that the recovering individual becomes less dependent on external resources and more independent by making changes in himself or herself. With this as one of our guiding principles, we can now examine the components of an effective vocational rehabilitation program for recovering substance abusers: assessment, counseling and referral, and placement and follow-up.

Assessment

The first and most crucial component of vocational rehabilitation for any disabled group is assessment. The fourth step of the Alcoholics Anonymous recovery program is a "searching and fearless moral inventory" (7). A similar vocational inventory needs to be undertaken by recovering individuals to develop their vocational plans. They must be evaluated in four key areas: Is the recovering substance abuser ready to enter or return to work? If so, for which specific employment position is the individual best suited? If not, what is the client lacking to effectively obtain and maintain a job? And, finally, where and how can these needs be addressed?

The question of readiness for work is multifaceted. As a result, the assessment must be ongoing in terms of evaluating the client initially in relation to work in general and then later in the process in relation to a specific job's demands. Obviously, a person's understanding of and attitude toward work must be evaluated. Often, as a consequence of their lack of exposure to healthy worker models and their own absence from the labor force, many substance abusers develop an inaccurate concept of what a job will require or provide. Frequently, recovering substance abusers see employment as a panacea. Obtaining a job, they believe, will solve all their problems, help them stay "straight," and move them into the mainstream. Their concept of employment is a fantasy: wearing a suit, having a secretary, going to lunch, and getting a paycheck.

Motivation is a crucial ingredient and, unless properly assessed and addressed, will lead to resistance from the client and frustration for the counselor later in the process. If the client is not able to progress to a point where the client is keeping appointments on time and demonstrating initiative and choice in selecting from available vocational options, then the client's motivation is questionable. Certainly, a criterion for evaluating motivation, as well as overall work readiness, is the client's chemical abuse status. If the individual is neither drug and alcohol free nor stabilized on a prescribed medication like methadone, then the client is unable to be endorsed for employment. Moreover, a vocational/educational assessment battery would have little value if the client was abusing drugs or alcohol when involved in the testing.

If the recovering substance abuser has an accurate understanding of what employment involves, is expressing a desire to work, and showing some evidence of this motivation, the next issue is evaluating the client's ability to work. Specifically is the client physically, psychologically, occupationally, socially, and placement ready (8)?

First, is the client physically ready? Are there any medical problems that would either rule out employment or restrict job options? For example, a client affected by acquired immunodeficiency syndrome (AIDS) may be able to work full-time, part-time, or only on a temporary basis depending on the status and progression of the disease. In some cases, health problems can be remedied. Still, care must be taken to allow adequate time and logical service provision so that the client is not expected to engage in vocational pursuits before stable health has been established. Further physical considerations include issues such as the possession of a stable residence, the availability of childcare if necessary, and realistic travel time to and from a job.

Second, is the client emotionally and psychologically ready? Has the client developed adequate coping skills to handle the frustration, rejection, and criticism associated with looking for, obtaining, and keeping a job? If clinical issues such as denial, transference, or projection are present, have they been adequately addressed? Is the client mature enough to appreciate the short-term benefits of a realistic vocational step as opposed to focusing on the long-term "ideal" job, which may be serving as a fantasized panacea? If further psychological support is necessary, does it preclude further vocational steps or can it be offered in conjunction with the progressive steps toward employment?

Third, is the client occupationally ready? Does the client have a job goal? Appropriate vocational interest assessment can be accomplished through a combination of psychometric testing and individual research. The combination of the two provides an opportunity for a client to be actively involved in the process with greater responsibility for the outcome. Based on John Holland's trait–factor theory of occupational choice, the Career Assessment Inventory, Strong Vocational Interest Inventory, and Self-Directed Search are some of the available standardized interest-testing measures. Other tests such as the Career Occupational Preference System (COPS), the Career Orientation Placement and Evaluation Survey (COPES), and the Barriers to Employment Success Inventory are available to help clients clarify their values and preferences and understand obstacles to their job attainment. Computerized programs such as the System of Interactive Guidance and Information Plus (SIGI^3) and CareerZone help clients obtain an integrated occupational profile of their interests and values. SIGI^3 integrates self-assessment with in-depth and current career information and provides users with a realistic view of the best educational and career options. CareerZone provides information on more than 800 occupations from the National Occupational Information Network (O'Net). Up-to-date job postings provide data on the labor market, and the resume builder helps users prepare the tools needed for a successful job search. Many of these tests are available in Spanish and have forms for clients with lower reading levels.

Individualized research can be done in the *Occupational Outlook Handbook* (OOH) and the *Dictionary of Occupational Titles* (DOT), published by the United States Department of Labor. The OOH is a reference work that describes the nature, qualifications, employment outlook, and promotional opportunities for general job groupings. The DOT is a specific classification system for the breakdown of general job groupings with descriptions of the exact efforts, techniques, and tools needed to accomplish the typical work tasks. Both the OOH and the DOT can be accessed online. O'Net is a full-access online version of the occupational network database and can be linked to Career One Stops. It is designed to assist individuals in planning and preparing for the transition to work.

In addition to an interest focus, an occupationally ready client should possess the specific aptitudes, general intelligence, and appropriate math, reading, and writing skills to adequately meet the job demands. General and specific assessment tools are available to help clients with limited awareness of their abilities to determine their strengths as well as to verify perceived abilities. The Differential Aptitude test, the Career Ability Placement Survey (CAPS), the Bennett Mechanical Comprehension Test, and SIGI^3 are examples of assessment tools. Work Keys, the assessment system component of KeyTrain, assists users in measuring and improving the common skills required for success in the workplace. An important component of this program is job profiling, the process of determining the basic skills that a person needs to do a specific job successfully.

A client's level of educational skills, particularly in the areas of reading and math, should also be assessed using measures such as the Adult Basic Learning Examination, the Test of Adult Basic Education, and the Wide Range Achievement Test 4. As with the interest tests, versions in Spanish and those for different ages or skill levels are available to obtain a more accurate picture of an individual's functioning. Undiagnosed learning disabilities may be at the root of some clients' development of a substance abuse problem, and therefore, screening should be incorporated into all educational evaluations. Educational remediation services are available through the ProLiteracy, the Learning Disabilities Association of America, local school districts, and specialized diagnostic and tutorial agencies.

If the client possesses the basic aptitudes for an occupation, does the client also possess sufficient relevant experience, academic degrees, training certificates, or licenses to meet hiring standards and compete in the job market? Does the client have any legal convictions that would be a bar to the desired employment goal? If the client has impairments in any of these areas, referrals for educational remediation, vocational, or legal assistance should be made. A way of responding to the complex needs of a client is the provision of wraparound services. Recent studies have indicated a positive association between wraparound services and treatment outcomes (9). Assistance with childcare, housing, transportation, and medical issues is provided directly or by referral as part of the client's total treatment plan.

A fourth area to evaluate is the client's social readiness. Remembering that a significant percentage of recovering substance abusers have been living in a "subculture" with little or no exposure to a work environment underscores the importance of this assessment. Can the client communicate effectively, speaking as well as listening? Does the client know how to dress appropriately for a specific job environment, neither underdressing nor overdressing, and dressing neither to attract attention nor to make a statement? Has the client evidenced the ability to interact appropriately with coworkers, supervisors, and employment authority figures? Observations of a client's interaction with his or her peers and treatment staff may provide excellent insight into this ability. Does the client possess sufficient self-management and planning skills to ask questions when unclear about instructions and to notify an employer when unable to meet a commitment? A supportive family and involvement in a 12-step program are important factors in determining social readiness.

Finally, the client needs to be evaluated in terms of the ability to job-hunt effectively. Can the client complete a job application or resume? Is the client capable of presenting marketable job qualities and a positive work attitude in an employment interview? Is the client able to address an employer's possible questions about work gaps and conviction history, or possibly past substance abuse, in a way that will relieve the employer's fears about hiring someone with negative elements in his or her background? Special attention must be paid to the level of work readiness skills in the counseling process.

It should be clear that comprehensive vocational assessment of the recovering substance abuser may require a significant commitment of time and resources. It is essential that adequate time be allowed lest undiagnosed deficiencies surface later in the vocational rehabilitation process. Not only could this significantly delay or disrupt the progress that the client is making, but it could also cause the client to become discouraged and lose confidence in his or her abilities, thereby diminishing motivation. Proper assessment should determine the scope, timing, and logical sequence of the client's rehabilitation steps and services delivery.

Counseling and Referral

The basic goal of counseling is accelerated learning. As a result of a proper assessment, a counselor should be able to depict what a client needs to know and clues for helping the client learn what he or she needs to know. A basic epistemological principle applies, helping a client understand the unknown by examining what the client already knows.

Vocational counseling has four classic elements: developing a positive self-concept, obtaining occupational information, expressing the self in occupational terms, and learning job-seeking skills (10).

The starting point for all counseling is the client, and more specifically, the perception that the client has of himself or herself. A fundamental task for rehabilitation counselors is to help clients remove the stigma of disability that many have internalized. Vocational rehabilitation with recovering substance abusers must address this issue. Many of these clients believe the label that society has assigned them, more convinced of what they cannot do than confident of what they can do. Their histories of failures become a projection for the future, a self-fulfilling prophecy rooted in a negative self-concept or, at best, low self-esteem.

With histories of missed opportunities and nonsuccess, recovering substance abusers need to be reminded by their counselors of the obstacles that they overcame and the progress made in treatment. Vocational rehabilitation counselors can further boost their clients' self-concepts by extracting from their "past" experiences transferable job skills. For example, experience caring for an elderly relative could transfer to nursing aide skills in health facilities.

Recovering substance abusers in vocational counseling will generally present one of four major needs. The first group of clients possess no occupational goals and will therefore need assistance in establishing goals. The second group has inappropriate or unrealistic goals and will need help in developing more achievable goals. The third group has appropriate goals but needs support in planning the steps and obtaining the resources needed to achieve the goals. The fourth group sees no value in working. Values clarification activities must be the foundation of this group's vocational counseling (10).

Counselors need to help clients integrate their self-concepts, interest assessments, values clarifications, aptitude evaluations, and the realities of the job market into a concrete employment goal. Additional assistance may be required by clients to locate the necessary resources and to plan the specific achievable steps to the desired goal. Empowering the client to choose is a central theme in the vocational counseling relationship. Clients will invest energy only in goals that they have had responsibility for selecting. Among the materials available to help clients achieve this integration and empowerment is the *Adkins Life Skills Program: Career Development Series* created at Columbia University's Institute for Life Coping Skills in New York. The institute is currently located in Stamford, Connecticut.

Referrals to resource agencies for aptitude assessment, educational remediation, or occupational skills training may augment a client's strengths and may serve as gradual steps in the transition to employment. However, initially such referrals may also threaten a weakened self-concept. Returning to the classroom can rekindle the feelings of insecurity and self-doubt that a client experienced in school. Apprehensions about testing, competition, and acknowledgment of mistakes will need to be addressed by the counselor prior to and during a client's attendance at such programs. In light of these considerations it is important that a counselor develop a client's ability to evaluate not only the general efficacy of such a program but also the appropriateness of the program to the client's individual needs. Is a large or small program better for the client? Is a teaching approach with more hands-on lab experience more appropriate to the client's needs or is one with more classroom lecture?

Obtaining employment is a major challenge for even the most mentally, physically, and emotionally capable person. The basic skills necessary to look for and secure a job must be either learned or relearned by the recovering substance abuser. Moreover, because of their disability, specialized techniques and strategies must be used for the job-hunting process to be successful. The importance of counseling support at this juncture cannot be overemphasized.

The seemingly simple task of completing a job application or resume can be overwhelming for clients. If they have never worked before, they may feel intimidated by the extensive questions about past employment and education. Even if they have worked before, many clients have poor memory and limited records of the training and job experiences during their periods of substance abuse. Moreover, some clients report that during the compilation of necessary work data, they become overwhelmed by negative feelings associated with the failures and incomplete undertakings that were consequences of their abuse.

In general, job hunting for clients with employment gaps and other stigmatized background elements is a very frustrating process. Equipping clients to handle the rejections and disappointments of a job search, offering them healthy outlets to vent their feelings, and providing them with coping strategies are necessary components of placement preparation.

Placement and Follow-up

The National Association on Drug Abuse Problems (NADAP) is a private nonprofit organization based in New York City that provides placement assistance to recovering substance abusers. NADAP has found that for many recovering persons it is necessary to augment the individual vocational rehabilitation counseling with specialized group workshops. These workshops have been designed as "groups" because work is public and requires socialization. As members of these groups, clients can be further assessed in terms of their ability to interact appropriately. The workshops also provide clients with opportunities to learn and practice job-related social skills.

The presence of other clients who are also searching job helps each client realize that they are not alone in their rejections and frustrations. Also, they realize that they are not alone in their ignorance of aspects of the work world and job-hunting skills. They learn from others' mistakes and are encouraged by others' successes. The shared disability of the members allows for more direct peer critique of individual obstacles and assistance in breaking their goals into short-term concrete steps. The group often, very practically, serves as a networking resource for employment leads.

The skills-building exercises in the NADAP workshops incorporate role playing, videotaping, and the involvement of employer representatives. Through role playing and videotaping, a client is able to see very clearly the strengths and weaknesses of his or her interviewing behaviors. The corporate personnel recruiters who participate in the role-plays provide an excellent "dress rehearsal" for the client's real interview, directly represent employers' expectations of job applicants, and offer clients suggestions on how they can better present their marketable traits and such negative elements in their background as legal convictions, job dismissals, and periods of unemployment.

Appropriately addressing these elements of the application and in an interview is a major task for recovering substance abusers. Guidelines for the presentation of confidential information are also addressed in the workshops. Clients learn through group exercises that the way information is presented is as important as what the information is. First, clients are encouraged not to volunteer negative data unless it is specifically requested (11). Second, they are trained to couple their admittance of past negative experiences with at least one positive step or change that has occurred as a result of their substance abuse treatment.

Depending on the client's individual background and chosen employment direction, the client may require consultations with agencies such as the Legal Action Center and the state Human Rights Office. Through such resources, recovering substance abusers learn their employment rights; eliminate unrealistic employment options; access bonding, licensure, or certification alternatives; and challenge employment discrimination.

Participation in such workshops helps a client develop not only specific skills but also a self-evaluation ability that will help to improve presentations on successive interviews and enhance their job performance. Research has demonstrated that recovering substance abusers who participate in job-hunting groups are more likely to secure and retain employment (12). Faced with discrimination and impairments, clients looking for work have to try different strategies and use as many employment resources as possible: community, city, county, state, and federal agencies, as well as specialized placement services such as NADAP.

NADAP advocates with large and small employers for competitive job opportunities for recovering substance abusers. In 2008, NADAP placed more than 50% of the clients who entered the program who were job-ready (13).

To enhance a client's success in employment, NADAP provides retention and career advancement services. A NADAP staff member is available to clients and their employers to resolve problems that might arise during the initial adjustment to a job. Follow-up, aftercare, and ongoing support issues are important from a vocational rehabilitation, as well as a clinical, perspective.

Support services in the form of group or individual counseling should be available to employed clients. Issues of anxiety, self-confidence, socialization, communication, basic attendance, and punctuality are usually greater determinants of job terminations for recovering substance abusers than lack of adequate skills or inability to learn quickly enough. Clients may need continued opportunities to role-play problem situations on the job and concrete exercises addressing assertive as opposed to aggressive behaviors.

Being a "worker" puts a client in a new role with family and friends. These significant others may be threatened by the client's progress and attempt to sabotage job retention. Coupled with a new job, budgeting money, scheduling leisure pursuits, and attending to daily living needs may also create new stresses for a client who previously had never worked or had been unemployed for a long time. After securing an entry-level position, clients will need career-planning assistance so that they can develop appropriate long-term goals, strategies, and timetables.

Given adequate rehabilitation time, comprehensive assessment, and appropriate services, recovering substance abusers can succeed in securing employment. The New York State Office of Vocational and Educational Services for Individuals with Disabilities (VESID) provides this proper climate and has established a history of helping disabled individuals achieve employment. Historically, the VESID office rehabilitated consumers with histories of substance abuse at a higher rate than consumers with other disabilities. VESID spent only slightly more money to help a recovering substance abuser secure employment than to rehabilitate most of the other disability groups it serves (14).

A final consideration in analyzing the placement of recovering substance abusers is how these individuals compare with other employees on the job. Two research studies indicate that there are no significant differences between recovering substance abusers and their peers on the job in terms of job retention, absenteeism, punctuality, performance, promotions, dismissals, and resignations (15,16).

Illustrative Cases

Jane

Jane was a 34-year-old woman who had been raised in an alcoholic home and had a history of 11 years of heroin addiction. She had been stabilized on methadone for 18 months after four unsuccessful detoxification attempts. Recently divorced from her husband, she was responsible for supporting herself and her 7-year-old son.

Jane was a high school graduate who had managed a retail business with her husband for 6 years. She had been unemployed for the past 2 years. Motivated by her desire to provide for her son, she entered into vocational rehabilitation counseling at her outpatient clinic. Her counselor referred her to an employment exploration and skills development group and helped her complete some occupational research. As a result of these undertakings, Jane decided that she was interested in pursuing a career in computer programming. However, she lacked confidence in her academic skills and knew that her goal would require college-level training. She feared that with her existing childcare responsibilities, therapy appointments, and necessary dental treatments, she would not have sufficient time to devote to school. She was concerned that employment would reduce her welfare benefits for herself and her son. She also felt isolated from others because of her "addict" stigma and was afraid of entering into new social situations.

An initial educational assessment revealed basically strong reading and math skills, although weak algebraic ability. As such ability would be needed for computer training, Jane was referred to a part-time evening tutoring program. She also decided to participate in a half-day vocational aptitude assessment program to address some of her other fears.

Jane made progress in her math tutoring and demonstrated the necessary aptitudes and work behaviors to consider a referral to the state office of vocational rehabilitation. This agency agreed to fund Jane for a 1-year computer certificate program at the local community college. This was in keeping with welfare reform regulations and was approved by her local Department of Social Services. Because of her age and childcare responsibilities the college granted her special student status. This gave her priority in registering for courses and allowed her to design a class schedule that ensured that even though she was taking a full course load, she could be home for most of the times when her son was not in school. Daycare for her son was provided at a licensed center through social services.

Initially after starting college, Jane maintained contact with her tutor for assistance with her first math classes. She also continued in primary therapy for support with her single-parenting issues and socialization needs. Jane graduated from college and was able to secure a job with a company that provided her with additional in-house programming training.

John

John was a 24-year-old polydrug abuser. He had dropped out of high school and was living at home, supporting himself on his earnings as a semiprofessional athlete. The death of his girlfriend because of cancer was the catalyst for his involvement in counseling. His bereavement counselor noted John's need for substance abuse treatment. While attending outpatient treatment, John realized the need for vocational rehabilitation services.

Because John had no consistent work record, specific occupational interest, or sense of his abilities, his vocational counselor referred him to an aptitude assessment and work adjustment program. While there, John received occupational interest testing. The testing revealed John's preferences for health and computer activities. Additional occupational exploration helped John focus on a position in medical billing. The assessment indicated that he possessed the necessary aptitudes for such work, but his math skills were not sufficient to pass the entrance exam for the appropriate training schools. Moreover, a high school diploma was required to meet the hiring standards of most of the employers in the medical billing field.

John investigated the three local trade schools offering medical billing training. He decided to attend the longest and most advanced course because of the increased career opportunities it would afford him. John's counselor helped him see that this choice meant more homework than the other programs required and additional efforts on his part because of his math deficiencies. John rose to the challenge and enrolled in a part-time educational program offering preparation for the high school, General Equivalency Diploma (GED), and math tutoring.

As a result, he was able to raise his math skills sufficiently to pass the training program's entrance exam. He applied for and received government-sponsored financial aid to cover most of the tuition costs. Once in training, he transferred the discipline he had developed as an athlete into his new endeavor. John established a specific study schedule and took advantage of every "extra help" session his training instructors offered him. He secured a part-time, evening maintenance job to meet his general expenses and the tuition costs not covered by his financial aid. He continued his outpatient counseling to help him resolve his grief and relationship issues.

On his first attempt prior to the end of his medical billing training, John passed the GED exam. He graduated from training and secured a position as a medical biller for a small group practice. After 2 years he left his first job for a more advanced position at a health clinic. At the new firm he received specialized training on a unique piece of technology and became a troubleshooter and trainer of new staff.

IMPEDIMENTS TO VOCATIONAL REHABILITATION SERVICE DELIVERY

The federal government has joined with state and local governments in endorsing the connection between work and recovery. This is evident in their policy developments and antidiscrimination legislation. This extends to funding provisions for training and job opportunities for recovering substance abusers (17). Certainly the Rehabilitation Act of 1973 serves as a cornerstone for the legal rights and public opportunities available to individuals with disabilities (18).

However, it is naive to believe that this support alone guarantees vocational rehabilitation services to those who need and desire it. There are three major categories of hindrances to effective provision and use of these services by recovering substance abusers: the clients themselves, the programs that treat them, and the society to which they return (19).

Clients who have been addicted to drugs and/or alcohol typically suffer with multiple impairments: poor health, HIV/AIDS or AIDS-related complex (ARC), psychological limitations, educational deficits, vocational development deficiencies, conviction records, family problems, daycare needs, and/or public assistance dependency. These factors affect the nature, pace, scope, and objectives of a client's vocational rehabilitation. As has already been outlined, careful, comprehensive assessment and appropriate remediation, compensation, or adaptation require significant commitments of time and energy to overcome these various problems. Some clients are too discouraged and alienated to persist in the process.

Treatment program obstacles can be examined in terms of the themes of philosophy and staffing. Historically, vocational rehabilitation, if considered at all by substance abuse treatment programs, has been seen as an adjunct, ancillary part of the recovery process. This is indicative of the low priority and concern that treatment professionals in general have for this component of treatment (20).

Many believe that the basic premise of most treatment programs is that if a client stops abusing drugs and alcohol, everything will fall into place and all things are possible. This principle is much too simplistic. Regretfully, clients accept this false expectation and find themselves returning to their communities without the knowledge and skills needed to function independently and achieve stability. Vocational rehabilitation is the treatment that helps these individuals develop much of this knowledge and many of these skills.

Unfortunately, a philosophic orientation toward vocational rehabilitation that downplays its contribution to the treatment process has translated into reduced staff resources available for such services. The drug and alcohol treatment field in general suffers from staff shortages and high turnover. The low-pay, insufficient advancement opportunities and the frustrations and burnout associated with serving multidisabled clients have reduced the appeal of positions in substance abuse treatment (21). Faced with this reality, treatment program administrators knowingly or unknowingly diminish the status of vocational rehabilitation services. If they can afford the time, effort, and funds to hire a vocational rehabilitation counselor, it is usually a last priority in their hiring hierarchy, offering lower salaries than most clinical positions, unrealistic caseloads, less than full-time opportunities, or combined responsibilities, for example, general program intake and vocational counseling.

As a consequence of these factors, personnel with limited vocational rehabilitation skills may be hired. Research shows that less trained rehabilitation counselors provide less efficient, less cost-effective, and less successful delivery of vocational rehabilitation services (22). Certainly the multiple disabilities with which many recovering substance abusers suffer require highly trained counseling staff. Without such staff the integrity of the rehabilitation services provided to recovering substance abusers is compromised.

Societal obstacles are probably the most difficult to overcome because of the prevalent ignorance and fear that are at their roots. Recovering substance abusers suffer from the same degrees of employment discrimination as many other disabled individuals and ex-offenders.

The discrimination that recovering substance abusers confront in the employment market is discouraging enough. Regretfully, they are also frequently faced with discrimination and misunderstanding by agencies in the social services system that supposedly exist to help them. This includes the disincentives to competitive employment imposed by public assistance guidelines as well as insensitive, illogical, and often contradictory eligibility criteria for counseling, educational remediation, training, and job placement assistance.

Is formal entry-level employment with limited or no fringe benefits attractive to a recovering substance abuser if it means surrendering the Medicaid, which covers the cost of his or her treatment as well as the health insurance costs of his or her family? Substance abusers with psychiatric histories are often refused entry into substance abuse treatment programs because these programs do not provide psychiatric counseling and supervision. These same clients are refused entry into psychiatric facilities because of their substance abuse.

A similar, if not more extreme, situation exists for physically disabled substance abusers who are often rejected by substance abuse treatment programs that cannot accommodate some of their special needs and are uneasy about how to treat these clients. Rehabilitation treatment programs for the physically disabled are just beginning to acknowledge that they may have clients with substance abuse problems and often cannot provide adequate substance abuse treatment for them.

Pregnant abusers are also ineligible for many programs because they are not designed to handle the needs of expectant mothers. There are limited treatment programs for women with children. This can force mothers with a substance abuse problem to have to choose between treatment and placing their children in foster care. Even clients who are functioning appropriately on monitored methadone dosages find it difficult to access many of the support services available to other substance abusers because they are not considered "drug free."

Against such obstacles, even the most motivated client may lose hope that he or she can succeed in his or her employment recovery.

IMPROVING VOCATIONAL REHABILITATION SERVICES

The past four decades of providing vocational rehabilitation services to men and women recovering from drug and alcohol abuse point to three guidelines for improving these services: understanding, expansion, and coordination.

Regretfully, there will probably always be new drugs surfacing that carry with them certain unique vocational impairments. These impairments will need to be examined as they become evident and new rehabilitation strategies and resources will need to be developed to address them. However, we now have an understanding of the depth and scope of the effect that substance abuse has on an individual's vocational development and of the basic rehabilitation principles to apply. Most recovering substance abusers can make progress if they are allowed to do so in a slow, gradual manner with a full complement of support services. Although it may be too strong to say that relapse is frequently part of the recovery process, we know that it is a reality for many clients. This is true in terms of a client's vocational development as well. It is not necessarily a neat progression but one that may be characterized by false starts and occasional steps backward. For some, because of the chronic nature of their substance abuse histories and the multiple handicaps they have, competitive or full-time employment may not be a realistic goal. For others, it will be appropriate only as a very long term goal.

In keeping with these characteristics we must adopt more of a mental health model of rehabilitation as opposed to a medical one. We must acknowledge this understanding in the design of vocational programs and in the expectations about working that we communicate to clients.

The second theme for future vocational rehabilitation is expansion. This means adding new services, but it also means expanding existing roles to involve more segments of society in the delivery of vocational rehabilitation services. If we acknowledge the need of recovering substance abusers for gradual movement from not working to working, then we must provide more work adjustment and transitional employment opportunities. These may include noncompetitive sheltered or semisheltered workshops that are available to other disability groups. Supported work programs for recovering substance abusers increase levels of employment and income and reduce arrests and jail time (23,24). New programs alone, however, are insufficient to meet the vocational rehabilitation needs of recovering substance abusers.

Employers in the United States are confronting a shrinking labor force of educated, skilled workers. Certainly the drug crisis is contributing to this deficit. Employers must respond with programs that offer alternatives to substance abuse and nourish the vocational development of recovering individuals who are looking for new positions or for a healthy return to their former jobs. Included must be nondiscriminatory hiring practices, business-sponsored training, transitional and noncompetitive work opportunities, and job maintenance and support services. At the very least, employers must be willing to abide by the current legislation addressing these issues. The Americans with Disabilities Act (ADA) specifically extends antidiscrimination treatment and employment policies to individuals with drug and alcohol problems and to those affected by the AIDS virus. While not protecting current users of illegal drugs, the ADA generally safeguards individuals with a history of substance abuse who have completed or are enrolled in treatment. For example, the ADA dictates that accommodations be made in the work schedule of a recovering individual to allow that person to attend a treatment program, unless such an accommodation would create undue hardship for the employer (25).

Researchers, as well, must become more involved in examining the vocational rehabilitation of recovering substance abusers. They can help to better delineate specific needs of these individuals and enhance the design of effective interventions and strategies.

Finally, for there to be effective vocational rehabilitation of recovering substance abusers, there needs to be increased coordination of relevant services. Drug and alcohol prevention programs need to include career exploration, educational remediation, occupational skills training, and work adjustment experiences into their services. Treatment programs must integrate comprehensive educational/vocational services into the early, middle, and late stages of their clinical treatment. Staff of these programs should familiarize themselves with existing vocational rehabilitation resources and adapt their program procedures to allow clients to avail themselves of these services. Just as a placement specialist working with a recovering person must be aware of the client's clinical needs and progress, so must a treatment counselor be aware of the client's vocational impairments and efforts at remedying or compensating for them. Treatment staff must be trained in the basic principles of vocational assessment so that while clients are in their care they can at least refer them to appropriate agencies that can prepare them for employment and independent living outside treatment.

In addition to the expected increases in employment, it appears from recent research that vocational rehabilitation programs are one of the psychosocial support services that can be effective in reducing drug use (26). Moreover, employment, specifically, can be an effective reinforcement for abstinence (27,28). Clearly such an outcome justifies the costs associated with integrating these components into substance abuse treatment programs. Both because of what it demands from an individual in recovery and because what it provides for that individual, sustained employment is a significant component of successful treatment (29).

Work dignifies us as human beings. Unless we provide men and women recovering from substance abuse with support and opportunities to achieve this dignity, to earn a place in society, we should not fault them for taxing our welfare system, straining our criminal justice system, and perpetuating a destructive subculture.

REFERENCES

1. Carlyle T. *Past and Present*. London: JM Dent & Sons; 1960:189.
2. Brewington V, Deren S, Arella L, et al. Obstacles to vocational rehabilitation: the client's perspective. *J Appl Rehabil Counsel*. 1990;21(2):27.
3. Stump W. Love, work and recovery. *NADAP News Rep*. 1973;14(4):3.
4. Neff WS. *Work and Human Behavior*. 2nd ed. Chicago: Aldine; 1977:264.
5. Adkins WR. Life skills education: a video-based counseling/learning delivery system. In: Larson D, ed. *Teaching Psychological Skills: Models for Giving Psychology Away*. Monterey, CA: Brooks/Cole; 1984:57.
6. Wright GN. *Total Rehabilitation*. Boston: Little, Brown; 1980:5.
7. Alcoholics Anonymous. *Twelve Steps and Twelve Traditions*. New York: Author; 1979.
8. Robinson H, Texeira M. *Vocational Rehabilitation*. 2nd ed. New York: Narcotic & Drug Research; 1990:154–156.
9. Pringle JL, Edmondston LA, Holland CL, et al. The role of wrap around services in retention and outcome in substance abuse treatment: findings from wrap around services impact study. *Addict Disord Their Treat*. 2002;1(4):109–118.
10. Reichman W, Levy M, Herrington S. Vocational counseling in early sobriety. *Labor Manage Alcohol J*. 1979;8:193.
11. Beale AV. A replicable program for teaching job interview skills to recovering substance abusers. *J Appl Rehabil Counsel*. 1988;19(1):5.
12. Hall S, Loeb P, Coyne K, et al. Increasing employment in ex-heroin addicts II: methadone maintenance sample. *Behav Ther*. 1981;12:443–460.
13. National Association on Drug Abuse Problems. *2008 NADAP Placement Statistics*. New York; 2009.
14. New York State Education Department. The vocational and educational services for individuals with disabilities. *Case Service Dollar Report*. 4/1/1994–3/31/1995.
15. Graham R, Gottcent R. Restoration of drug abusers to useful employment. In: Smith D, Anderson S, Buton M, et al., eds. *A Multicultural View of Drug Abuse*. Cambridge, UK: G.K. Hall/Schenkman; 1978:463.
16. Wijting JP. Employing the recovered drug abuser-viable? Personnel. 1979;56(3):56-63.
17. Strategy Council on Drug Abuse. *Federal Strategy for Drug Abuse and Drug Traffic Prevention*. Washington, DC: U.S. Government Printing Office; 1979:24.
18. The Rehabilitation Act of 1973, Public Law 93–112, sections 503 and 504.
19. Deren S, Randell J. The vocational rehabilitation of substance abusers. *J Appl Rehabil Counsel*. 1990;21(2):5.
20. Rudner S. *The Role of Vocational Rehabilitation in the Treatment of Substance Abusers*. Nassau County, NY: Department of Drug and Alcohol Addiction; 1982:5–6.
21. Simeone RS, Kott A, Torrington W. *Summary Report on the DSAS Personal Services Survey*. Albany, NY: New York State Division of Substance Abuse Services; 1989:3–10.
22. Szymanski EM, Parker RM. Relationship of rehabilitation client outcome to the level of rehabilitation counselor education. *J Rehabil*. 1989;10:35.
23. Friedman L. *The Wildcat Experiment: An Early Test of Supported Work*. New York: Vera Institute of Justice; 1978.
24. Hollister RG Jr, Kemper P, Maynard RA, eds. *The National Supported Work Demonstration*. Madison: University of Wisconsin Press; 1984.
25. Legal Action Center. The Americans with Disabilities Act: a summary of alcohol and drug and AIDS provisions. *Action Watch*. 1990;10:2.
26. Kleinman P, Millman R, Lesser M, et al. The comprehensive vocational enhancement program: results of a five year research/demonstration project. In: Tims F, Inciardi J, Fletcher B, et al., eds. *The Effectiveness of Innovative Approaches in the Treatment of Drug Abuse*. Westport: Greenwood Press; 1997:219–232.
27. Silverman K, Wong CJ, Needham M, et al. A randomized trial of employment-based reinforcement of cocaine abstinence in injection drug users. *J Appl Behav Anal*. 2007;40(3):387–410.
28. Magura S, Staines GL, Blankertz L, et al. The effectiveness of vocational services for substance abusers in treatment. *Subst Use Misuse*. 2004;39(13–14):2165–2213.
29. Tsui E, Rukow L. An integrated approach to recovery from drug addiction: creating linkages between drug treatment and employment services in Baltimore. First Place, Abell Award in Urban Policy Competition; 2007.

SECTION 9 ■ LIFE CYCLE

CHAPTER 57 Adolescent Substance Abuse

Robert Milin ■ Selena Walker

INTRODUCTION

This chapter focuses on enhancing knowledge and comprehension of adolescent substance abuse by addressing the following areas: epidemiology, vulnerability and developmental course, comorbidity, assessment, and treatment/outcome. The areas of prevention and early intervention are addressed more thoroughly in the section on Models of Prevention. The goal of the chapter is not a critical analysis of the literature, but rather a discussion of the preponderance or balance of the evidence. Over the last two decades there has been significant growth in number of studies and an advance in the knowledge related to adolescent substance abuse, yet much remains to be learned. In this manner, only original and review articles that specifically relate to this topic and population will be included here, distinguishing itself from the adult literature.

The focus of this chapter is on adolescents, as preadolescent substance abuse is uncommon and there are few studies and/or comprehensive reports on such use. Substance abuse in adolescence continues to present as a major challenge. It is a serious mental health and social problem with its significant association with morbidity and mortality. Substance abuse has progressed from the more antisocial, risk-taking, and marginal groups of the population to the mainstream of society and dramatically to younger populations, reinforcing and expanding the boundaries of at-risk populations for substance abuse. The transitional period of adolescence presents itself as an especially critical and vulnerable time for the onset of substance use disorders (SUDs) (1–4).

EPIDEMIOLOGY

The Monitoring the Future survey has been annually measuring the prevalence rates of substance use in adolescents attending school across the United States in a nationally representative sample for more than three decades. Substance use (alcohol and illicit drugs) in general, across all grade levels 8, 10, and 12, has shown a steady and considerable decline over a decade or more, though with some exceptions. Rates appear to have stabilized in recent years. Marijuana, in contrast, has shown an increased trend in use over the last 2 to 3 years affecting the rate of illicit drug use, whereas illicit drug use other than marijuana has more or less held steady or declined. This recent rise in marijuana use has been associated with an even longer decline in adolescents' perceived risk of regular marijuana use. Annual prevalence rates for 2009 of any illicit drug use in grades 8, 10, and 12 stand at 15%, 30%, and 37%, respectively, which remain relatively high. It is almost without exception that substance use increases with the next higher grade level or age in adolescents. Inhalant use, on the other hand, shows the reverse prevalence, being most common in 8th graders and heroin use being equally distributed across the grades, though annual prevalence rates remain nominal at less than 1% in any of the three grades. However, narcotic use other than heroin has remained elevated at 9% in grade 12 students for many years. By far, the two most common substances used by adolescents are alcohol and marijuana, with annual rates for senior high school (grade 12) students of 66% and 33% in 2009. However, marijuana has been the most common substance of daily use among adolescents for more than a decade, with rates over 50% higher than for alcohol. The prevalence of daily marijuana use for the past 5 years in senior high school students has ranged from 5.0% to 5.4% as compared to alcohol at 2.5% to 3.1%. Binge drinking has hovered at 25% for the past several years in grade 12 students. Prescription drug misuse among high school seniors remains a concern at approximately 15% per annum. Included in this group are narcotic analgesics (vicodin and oxycontin), stimulants used for treatment of attention-deficit hyperactivity disorder (ADHD) (Adderall and Ritalin), and sedatives/tranquilizers.

Prevalence rates of substance use do not provide one with comparable rates of SUDs in general and especially in adolescents, barring the controversy with respect to the applicability of DSM-IV-TR SUD criteria, developed for adults, to adolescents (5). Substance experimentation among adolescents is highly prevalent, though the vast majority of these adolescents do not develop an SUD, even with some of these adolescents engaging in more regular use for a period of time, though the latter does increase the likelihood of developing an SUD (1,2,5). These patterns of substance use, as it would relate to alcohol and marijuana use seen in adolescents, appear for some to be within normative behavior and part of the maturation process of adolescence, but for others may lead to significant substance abuse (1,6).

Community samples of adolescents have found lifetime rates of SUD to range from approximately 10% to 30% with rates of alcohol use disorders (AUD) and drug use disorders (predominantly cannabis) similar, apart from one study. This wide range in SUD rates may be attributed to differences in methodology and categorization of SUD. Several common themes are identified in these studies in that SUD rates increase with age, appear to be greater in males, and are quite infrequent for ages 13 and younger (7–10).

Prevalence rates have also been examined for higher risk groups of adolescents, specifically those receiving services in the public sectors of alcohol and drug, juvenile justice, school-based services for severely emotionally disturbed youth, child welfare, and mental health. An overall prevalence rate of 24% was found for SUD in the past year (11).

Community studies have also shown that lifetime SUD rates are notably greater than current rates for adolescents, indicating some movement in and out of SUD through adolescence. The U.S. National Survey on Drug Use and Health (12) provides estimates of SUD for youth 12 to 17 years of age as well as for young adults 18 to 25 years of age. The most recent report on the 2008 findings showed an SUD rate of 7.6% that was significantly less from findings in 2004 (8.8%). The highest rate of SUD was found in the young adult group at 20.8%, whereas the greatest proportion with illicit drug use disorders was in the adolescent group at 60.6%, in comparison to 37.4% for young adults. An interesting finding that may be reflective of the survey was that females were somewhat more common than males in the youth group with SUD. This is in contrast to community samples of adolescents and adult findings. However, it would suffice to say that females are definitely in greater proportion in adolescents with SUD than in adults.

In summary, despite the overall decline in substance use and SUD in adolescents, the prevalence remains high and is the greatest with older adolescents. As well, it is important to recognize the historical cyclic pattern of substance use and abuse rates. One can also surmise that cannabis would appear to be the most significant and the most common substance of dependence in adolescents with alcohol being the predominant substance of abuse (13).

DEVELOPMENT AND COURSE OF DISORDER

Adolescence is a time of major risk for the onset of substance abuse. The peak age of onset for both alcohol and drug use disorders is in late adolescence/early adulthood, between the ages of 18 to 20 (1,14). Adolescence, as seen from a developmental perspective, represents a time of convergence of significant neurobiologic, cognitive, behavioral, emotional and social changes with continuity of risk from earlier developmental stages, providing a unique period of heightened vulnerability and susceptibility for SUD (1,3). Brown and colleagues (1) reflect on these interrelated developmental factors, the changes that occur during adolescence, and its influence on individual alcohol use trajectories and risk for problem drinking. Their narrative highlights the increasing evidence that adolescents are particularly vulnerable to the adverse effects of heavy alcohol use both in the biological and social domains and that the consequences of drinking appear to differ between adolescents and adults. They also identify that problem drinking has the potential to redirect the normative course of adolescent development in a manner that not only increases the risk of alcohol use disorders but also of mental health and social problems.

Schepis and coauthors (3) in their review of the neurobiological processes involved in the etiology of adolescent SUD emphasize the significance of maturational changes of the central nervous system that occur in adolescence; the foremost of these being synaptic pruning, myelination, and neurotransmitter system modification. Adolescents overall appear to have greater neurological bases for risk-taking behavior with attenuated suppressive and regulatory controls on behavior. The authors surmise that the abnormal neurological markers of those at risk for the development of SUD may best correspond to disinhibition and/or negative affect. Adolescents appear more vulnerable to the effects of many substances that are most likely mediated by increased neuroplasticity and the effects of stress. It is likely that substance-induced neurobiological changes enhance drug use behaviors. These attributes reinforce the progression to SUD in adolescents.

An abundance of risk factors have been, and continue to be, identified in the prediction of substance abuse in adolescence/young adulthood. These various risk factors may be conceptualized into four domains: (a) culture and society (e.g., laws and availability of substances); (b) interpersonal (e.g., peers and family including attitudes); (c) psychobehavioral (e.g., early/persistent behavioral problems, poor school performance, rebelliousness, early onset of substance use, personality characteristics such as temperament and affect); and (d) biogenetic (e.g., inherited susceptibility and psychophysiologic vulnerability to the effects of substances) (2,14,15).

It appears that social factors, particularly peer influence, are the strongest determinants of initiation of substance use, whereas psychological factors and self-reinforcing effects of the substance are more closely associated with substance abuse (16).

There is little evidence on distinguishing the relative importance of risk factors and their specificity in the development of adolescent substance abuse. It is the cumulation of risk factors, rather than any one factor, that is predictive of substance abuse. Many of these risk factors overlap with those related to the onset of other adolescent psychiatric disorders (2,16).

Protective factors are those that reduce the likelihood and level of substance use. Multiple protective factors have been identified which include a positive temperament (absence of depression)/self-acceptance, intellectual ability/academic performance, supportive family/home environment, caring relationship with at least one adult, external support system (e.g., religion/church) that encourages prosocial values, and law abidance/avoidance of delinquent peer friendships

(2,16,17). Newcomb and Felix-Ortiz (18) in the analysis of their longitudinal prospective study of drug use in early adolescence found several important relationships for multiple protective and risk factors. Again, it is not one particular protective factor but, rather, the number of protective factors that have the most influence on reducing the likelihood of adolescence substance abuse. For example, those adolescents with five or more protective factors were over 20 times less likely to develop cannabis abuse than the general sample. They also found a moderating effect of protective factors on risk for involvement and most notably that high protective indices had their greatest impact on those at high risk for greater drug involvement. One variable that has been identified above others as protective of substance use, and not per se SUD, is having early academic success (19). The strongest predictor of current substance use in late adolescence and young adulthood is past use (20,21). The early onset of substance (alcohol and marijuana/illicit drugs) use in adolescence predicts a considerably greater likelihood of developing later SUD and a more rapid progression to substance dependence, at least for cannabis. These findings are most robust for initiation of substance use by age 15 or younger, thereafter other variables may come into play (12,22–25). Adolescent SUD has been found to be a strong homotypic (refers to a disorder predicting itself over time) predictor of young adult SUD (25). The regular weekly use of cannabis by adolescents appears to be a threshold marker for the risk of cannabis dependence in young adulthood (26).

A widely held concept contends that there are developmental stages in the progression of substance use through adolescence into young adulthood; this concept has been derived, in part, from epidemiologic studies (27). The sequence of stages defines a temporal relationship progressing from legal to illegal and softer to harder drug use, with each stage acting as a potential "gateway" to the initiation of the next stage (27,28). The use of one substance increases the likelihood of initiation of the second substance. For example, very few individuals who have tried cocaine and heroin have not already tried marijuana, the majority having previously used alcohol or cigarettes. However, the use of one substance does not invariably lead to the use of other substances. Many youth will stop at a certain stage and do not progress further or may return to an earlier stage of substance use (27). It is typical to carry over substance use from one stage to the next versus substitution. This carryover effect has clinical relevance in the application of the polysubstance dependence diagnosis for adolescents. The causal effect of the gateway hypothesis is more open to debate and specifically as it relates to cannabis use and other drugs. However, a clear association has been well established for cannabis use and the use of other illicit drugs (29). Further to this, regular or heavy cannabis use has been significantly associated with other illicit drug use and abuse/dependence. The relationship is especially strong during adolescence and declines with age. These findings add support to the potential causal role of cannabis use on the development of other illicit drug use disorders, though the actual causal mechanisms, whether direct or indirect, remain unclear (30,31). Adolescents have shown a greater likelihood of developing drug dependence (cannabis) than adults across levels of use (32).

Substance abuse in adolescence is clearly associated with significant negative consequences in the developmental tasks' multiple life areas including behavioral, emotional, social, and academic/vocational problems (1,33,34).

In summary, the onset of substance abuse in adolescence with its biopsychosocial determinants is a serious problem, with a direct impact on development and a strong link to future SUD.

COMORBIDITY OF SUD

The association of SUD and mental health disorders is well established. In clinical and treatment studies of adolescent SUD, elevated rates of comorbid mental health disorders have been found across settings from hospitalized/residential to outpatient status with prevalence rates ranging from 55% to 80% (35–38). Prevalence rates of comorbid disorders are significantly greater than community control samples of non-SUD adolescents. Adolescent SUD patients often present with more than one comorbid disorder. Clinical studies, however, may typically suffer from Berkson's bias where it is probable that an adolescent with a particular disorder such as SUD seeking treatment will have a higher likelihood of a second disorder, thus confounding the ability to generalize results. Only a handful of studies have examined the psychiatric comorbidity of adolescent SUD in general community samples. Two such studies have found similar results of elevated rates of comorbidity as seen in clinical studies. Comorbidity rates were two to three times greater in adolescents with SUD than those without SUD for any anxiety, mood, or disruptive behavior disorders (DBD). In comparison to adult studies, comorbidity rates of psychiatric disorders are similar for lifetime SUD and may be higher for current SUD in adolescents (7,39). These reported higher rates of psychiatric comorbidity in adolescents with SUD are most likely reflective of the greater number of DBD (Axis I) diagnoses available for adolescents that are either not applicable or not routinely assessed in adult SUD populations. There is some evidence to support the idea that comorbidity of mental health disorders increases with progression of substance use diagnosis and is associated with more severe substance use (40,41). In terms of gender relationship to comorbidity, males and females share far greater similarities than any meaningful differences, especially when gender differences seen in the general population of such disorders as conduct disorder (CD) and major depressive disorder (MDD) are considered (35,42).

Prospective studies suggest that early and more frequent substance use through adolescence is associated with, and may predict, later psychiatric disorders in particular depressive disorders in young adulthood (43–45). Analysis of retrospective data for the National Comorbidity Survey Replication found the age of onset of DBD and anxiety disorders to preceed the onset of substance dependence (46).

The most common comorbid psychiatric disorder seen in community studies of adolescent SUD are the DBD, in particular CD, with these disorders showing a prevalence range of 25% to 50% and a median of four times greater likelihood of co-occurrence with SUD than without. This is followed by depression with a prevalence range of 20% to 30% and a median of over twice the likelihood of co-occurrence (42). These findings are relatively consistent with clinical studies, though there is a fair degree of variability in prevalence rates between studies, depending on the clinical population sample. SUD, on the other hand, is a common comorbid disorder in clinical studies of youth that present with serious emotional disturbances or mental health disorders (47–50).

In this section of comorbidity, we will take a closer look at selected aspects of the relationship of the more prominent comorbid psychiatric disorders and SUD.

Conduct Disorder

CD and SUD are strongly associated, with CD typically preceding the onset of SUD (51–53). This relationship, however, appears to be reciprocal with each condition heightening the expression of the other. In such a manner, CD may influence the early adolescent development of SUD and the severity of CD has been found to predict the severity of SUD. Early-onset substance use has been associated with later criminality. Furthermore, if substance use or drug dealing is reduced, there is a subsequent decrease in criminality (54). Reebye and colleagues (55) in their clinical study of CD and SUD found the rapid development of substance abuse and substance dependence in adolescents with CD, on average taking about 9 and 18 months, respectively, after initiation of drug use. Gender differences have been found such that adolescent girls with CD progress more rapidly to SUD following first use than boys (56).

Juvenile offenders with comorbid SUD have shown greater additional psychopathology than juvenile offenders without SUD. It is also important to recognize that no relationship with early conduct problems has been found for the onset of SUD in adulthood (57).

Attention-Deficit Hyperactivity Disorder

ADHD has been found to be a common comorbid disorder in clinical studies of adolescents with SUD, with large outpatient clinical studies reporting a range of 17% to 38%; however, similar findings have not been found in community samples (36,37,42,58).

The significance of comorbid ADHD appears to lie with its association with CD in adolescents. The clustering of ADHD, CD, and SUD has been found in several studies of adolescents (58–60). Together, longitudinal prospective studies of ADHD into adolescence, in comparison to normal controls, and a large population-based study examining the relationship of ADHD, CD, and SUD in adolescents provide consensus that ADHD as a risk factor for SUD is strongly mediated by its association with CD and/or externalizing disorders of oppositional defiant disorder (ODD)/CD. In essence, ADHD when not associated with another DBD is not generally seen as a significant independent risk factor for the development of SUD in adolescence (58–61). The severity of ADHD may have an impact on the risk for development of SUD in adolescence (62,63).

Adolescents with ADHD have shown an earlier age of onset of SUD and a more rapid progression of SUD from abuse to dependence than normal controls; as well, adolescents with SUD and comorbid ADHD have exhibited more severe substance abuse than those without ADHD (59,61). No significant gender differences have been found in the effects of ADHD on SUD in adolescents (58,59). The persistence of ADHD into young adulthood has been shown to be an independent risk factor for the development of SUD (64).

It is important to recognize that both well-designed prospective longitudinal studies and a meta-analysis provide sound evidence that stimulant treatment of children and adolescents with ADHD does not increase the risk of developing an SUD in either adolescence or young adulthood (65–68). There is also some evidence to suggest that stimulant treatment of children with ADHD actually significantly reduces the risk of developing SUD in adolescence by several fold (67,69). However, these protective findings of stimulant treatment of children and adolescents with ADHD appear to wane and become nonsignificant as they continue on into young adulthood (66).

The relationship between ADHD, CD, and SUD remains complex in adolescence and may represent a worse prognosis for the persistence of antisocial behaviors and substance abuse.

Depressive Disorders

Depressive disorders frequently co-occur with adolescent SUD and are the second most common comorbid disorder. The association of depressive and substance use disorders in adolescents is more frequent than one would expect and has been more widely studied than other comorbidities. It is also noteworthy that adolescents with a history of MDD show an elevated rate of SUD than those without a history of depression (12,70). Rao and Chen (71) in a comprehensive review of this topic proposed that common genetic, environmental, and neurobiologic factors may possibly mediate the relationship between depressive and substance use disorders in adolescents, constituting a basis for their linkage. The authors recognized the limitations of the neurobiologic findings and by design, the selectivity of various risk mechanisms examined.

In adolescents with SUD, the onset of MDD most often follows the onset of SUD (secondary MDD). Secondary MDD is considerably more common than MDD preceding the onset of SUD (primary MDD) (72,73). In the majority of cases, irrespective of whether it is primary or secondary, comorbid MDD has not been found to spontaneously remit with abstinence and/or early treatment (excluding pharmacotherapy) by the third week in adolescents. This finding appears to differentiate adolescent SUD from that found in adults with elevated rates of acute remission (72). As would be expected, comorbid MDD has been found to be more prevalent in girls with adolescent SUD than in boys, with the girls showing an earlier age of onset of depression (73). Adolescents with depressive symptoms and SUD on admission in residential treatment have shown poor substance use outcome (74).

In adolescents with depression, comorbid SUDs are associated with earlier onset of and more severe substance abuse. Comorbid SUD in adolescents with depression appears to have a negative impact on the phenomenology and course of illness with greater behavioral and CD problems, longer duration of depressive episodes, and increased psychosocial (school, family, and legal) impairment (70,71,74–76). Recently, it has also been shown that simply a greater severity of substance use in adolescents with treatment-resistant MDD and without comorbid SUD is associated with increased severity of depression and comorbid ODD and CD. Adolescents with low substance-related impairment at the end of treatment for depression demonstrated the best response (77).

SUD in adolescents has been linked to an increase in suicidal behaviors including ideation, attempts (frequency, recurrence, and seriousness), and completed suicide. However, the risk for suicide is most significant when comorbid with MDD (78–80). A history of recent interpersonal separations and family dysfunction has been found to be more common in adolescents who attempt suicide with depression and comorbid SUD than without. Alcohol abuse has been most often associated with increased risk, though the number of substances used may be a more important predictive factor (81).

The comorbidity of substance use and depressive disorders appears to be interactive and has at least an additive, if not a synergistic effect on the burden of illness of these disorders, carrying a significant morbidity and mortality.

Psychotic and Bipolar Disorders

There is a paucity of studies that report the incidence of comorbid primary psychotic disorders (PPD)/schizophrenia related disorders and bipolar disorders (BD) in the adolescent SUD population. This absence of reporting may be a reflection of the severity of the illnesses, with those adolescents who experience the onset of these disorders being more likely to present to psychiatric services for assessment irrespective of whether they have an SUD or not. In that comorbid PPD and BD are not commonly or reliably reported in the adolescent SUD population, a detailed discussion of their association is beyond the scope of this chapter. Apart from a few general comments, the interested reader is referred to a comprehensive review on the topic of comorbid SUD with PPD and BD in adolescents/young adulthood by Milin and colleagues (82).

A strong association has been found for comorbid SUD with both PPD and BD in clinical studies involving adolescents/young adults as well as first-episode psychosis (FEP) or mania. The presence of comorbid SUD has been associated with a more debilitating course of illness, poorer clinical and treatment outcomes, as well as greater functional impairment in patients with FEP and BD (including preliminary evidence in first episode mania and adolescents) than without comorbid SUD. Comorbid SUD has been linked to an earlier age at onset of schizophrenia and BD with its clinical implication on prognosis. In the majority of cases, SUD typically precedes the onset of psychosis/schizophrenia, whereas the onset of BD often precedes that of SUD. The most common SUD is that of cannabis in FEP and first-episode/ early-onset BD.

Cannabis use has been found to be an independent risk factor for the development of psychosis/schizophrenia in young adulthood. The risk for this outcome increases in a dose-dependent manner and is greater with the onset of use in adolescence and especially in vulnerable individuals. Cannabis-induced psychotic disorder has been found to be a cogent marker in the vulnerability for developing PPD. In essence, adolescents and young adults should be counseled that cannabis use may increase their likelihood of developing a PPD (82).

Other Comorbid Disorders

There is considerably less extant literature on the relationship of other comorbid disorders in adolescents with SUD. Elevated rates of anxiety disorders, including social and generalized anxiety disorders and posttraumatic stress disorder (PTSD), have been noted in clinical studies (37,83–86). From these studies, social anxiety disorders (SAD) and PTSD have been identified as the most clinically significant of the anxiety disorders. SAD precedes the onset of SUD and inherently may have an impact in SUD treatment that is oriented toward group therapy. Those with SAD may best be served initially through individual cognitive behavior–oriented SUD treatment.

The importance of PTSD in this population has significant relevance, given the high rate of physical and sexual abuse (57% of girls and 31% of boys) identified in a clinical sample across treatment settings (residential, inpatient, and out/day patient programs) (87). In a cross-sectional community sample of adolescents, a strong association was found for the comorbidity of SUD and PTSD with a significant impact on psychosocial impairment. The findings suggested multiple pathways leading to comorbid SUD and PTSD (86).

No consistent association has been found in adolescents for comorbid SUD and eating disorders (ED). There is some clinical evidence to suggest a possible relationship of SUD with bulimia (88).

ASSESSMENT OF ADOLESCENT SUBSTANCE USE DISORDERS

The importance of screening and assessing SUDs in adolescents is underscored by the recommendation of the inclusion of such screening as a part of mental health assessments of older children and adolescents (5). Despite the importance of screening adolescents for substance use, most physicians/pediatricians feel uncomfortable screening for drug and alcohol use and even fewer feel comfortable completing a comprehensive assessment or referring adolescents for drug and alcohol treatment (89). Reasons for failure to screen adolescents for substance use and abuse include lack of training and familiarity with screening tools, lack of time to complete the assessment, need to triage competing medical problems, unfamiliarity with treatment options and resources, and issues with confidentiality and disclosure due to parents who will not leave the room (89).

Screening tools are brief self-reports or interviews often used as the initial step in assessing for adolescent substance use and related problems. The outcome of screening may determine the need for further evaluation and a more comprehensive assessment. The next step would entail a comprehensive assessment that examines the nature and severity of substance use and related problems (frequency, quantity, duration, number of substances used and circumstances, etc., problem-related consequences of substance use and treatment needs in multiple life domains (90)). The appropriateness of the instrument is dependent upon the setting for the assessment and the purpose of the assessment (91). Winters and Kaminer (90) identified and reviewed several preferred measures for screening and assessing adolescent SUD in clinical populations. Their selection of instruments was comprised of two screening tools, the CRAFFT and the Personal Experience Screening Questionnaire, and three comprehensive assessment instruments, the Global Appraisal of Individual Needs (GAIN), the Teen Severity Addiction Index, and the Personal Experience Inventory. These instruments were guided by a combination of robust psychometrics and user-friendliness. The features they examined included the strength of psychometric properties, simplicity of scoring, efficient length of administrations, and the degree of user training required. The measures were also found suitable for periodic use in re-evaluation of treatment outcome. The authors recommend that clinicians working with youth should receive training in at least one screening and one comprehensive assessment instrument, ideally during their formal years of education. For a more comprehensive review of available assessment instruments for adolescent substance use disorders, the reader is referred to a recent review of the topic by Winters and colleagues (92).

Urine drug testing is an objective measure to screen for recent drug use in a time-limited manner. However, a positive urine screen is not diagnostic of an SUD and does not provide information on substance-related problems. Echoing the findings from studies investigating the concordance between objective, self-, and collateral reports of substance use in adolescents (93,94), Winters and Kaminer (90) advocate that the use of self-report and collateral information may be the most reliable measure in many instances of assessing adolescent substance use and disorders. Nevertheless, urine drug analysis may be beneficial when screening those who fear the consequences of reported substance use and abuse or those who are concerned about confidentiality and therefore may not respond validly. As well, it may be helpful in promoting clinical feedback to the adolescent in treatment.

Further to the instruments identified, we would like to provide additional information on three tools that may be clinically useful in screening for adolescent SUD in different settings.

The CRAFFT (95) is a six-item questionnaire designed to be given orally by the clinician during a routine interview of the adolescent patient. Responding yes to two or more of the questions indicates further assessment is required. It has been found to be predictive of SUDs (96). The CRAFFT is suitable for use in primary care settings.

The Adolescent Alcohol and Drug Involvement Scale (AADIS) (97) is a 14-item self-report instrument designed to screen for alcohol and drug abuse in adolescents, and to assess the extent to which substance use is interfering with the adolescent's psychological, social, and family functioning. A significant total score suggests alcohol and/or drug use which may reach DSM-IV criteria for an SUD, thus indicating the need for comprehensive assessment. The AADIS has reasonable psychometric properties, including moderate to good internal consistency (Cronbach's alpha from 0.42 to 0.94) and test–retest reliability ($r = 0.91$) (97). The AADIS is a suitable screening tool for clinical mental health programs and may be used as a repeated measure.

The Global Appraisal of Individual Needs-Short Screener (GAIN-SS) (98) was adapted from the GAIN. It is a brief interview questionnaire that can be self-administered and is designed to identify youth with internalizing, externalizing, substance use, and criminality problems and to triage them to the appropriate level of services and comprehensive assessment in a timely manner. Dennis and fellow researchers (98) report that the GAIN-SS is highly correlated with the GAIN, has high internal consistency, and is able to discriminate between those with and without psychiatric disorders with excellent sensitivity and specificity. The GAIN-SS is highly suitable for screening by clinicians in addiction centers or in the community to help identify comorbid mental health issues in those who present with substance use problems.

The significance of screening and assessing for SUD in adolescents using multiple sources is brought to bear by findings from a study of adolescents seeking mental health treatment (50). The study found an SUD prevalence of approximately 17% on a self-report structured measure, whereas clinicians identified less than half (45%) of these adolescents with SUD. The researchers suggested that the gap between the need and access to SUD treatment services may have contributed to poorer outcomes for youth with comorbid SUD. They also realized the important clinical consideration that clinicians should continue to screen/assess for SUD throughout treatment in that confidence to disclose this behavior may be enhanced with the establishment of a therapeutic relationship with the adolescent patient and family.

In summary, there is convincing evidence that all adolescents presenting for treatment of either substance-use or mental health problems should, at minimum and in an ongoing manner, receive screening and as warranted more comprehensive assessment for comorbidity of substance use and mental health disorders. Assessment should include diverse sources where possible and cover multiple life domains leading to identifying the appropriate treatment sources to meet the needs of the adolescent.

TREATMENT

Treatment of adolescent SUD starts for all intents and purposes with the process of a biopsychosocial/multidimensional assessment. The American Society of Addiction Medicine Patient Placement Criteria (ASAM-PPC) for the Treatment of Substance-Related Disorders (99) sets forth consensus criteria and guidelines for adolescents with many distinguishing features from that of adults. The six dimensions identified for assessment include (a) intoxication and withdrawal potential, (b) medical conditions and complications, (c) emotional, behavioral, and cognitive condition (includes stages of development) and complications, (d) readiness for change, (e) relapse, continued use, or problem potential, and (f) recovery environment. The third dimension is further expanded into subdomains to underscore the significance of broad functional impairments that are associated with both SUD and mental health problems/psychiatric comorbidity. These subdomains are composed of dangerous/lethality, interference with addiction recovery efforts, social functioning (including educational or vocational responsibilities), ability for self-care, and course of illness. The evaluation of these key clinical domains is intended to help guide the clinician with treatment planning and toward matching the adolescent patients to the appropriate level of care. ASAM-PPC has become a standard in the addiction field in the United States. Unfortunately, only preliminary work has been done in the study and operationalization of the adolescent PPC. The reader can consult Fishman (100) for a further discussion of this topic specific to adolescents.

An area often previously overlooked in adolescents is the presence of substance withdrawal and its impact. Two recent studies support that cannabis withdrawal is common and of clinical significance in adolescents with cannabis dependence (101,102).

The treatment of adolescent SUD may occur at one of several levels of care, across a range of settings reflecting the intensity of treatment and level of supervision/restriction of environment (5). These treatment settings mainly encompass outpatient, partial hospitalization/day treatment, and inpatient or residential care. There continues to be a significant gap between adolescents who need treatment for SUD and those who receive treatment in a specialty facility. It is likely that two major factors play a role in this marked deficit of treatment: they did not seek treatment or they were unable to access treatment for various reasons (12).

As of date, there has been a proposed shift away from large-scale outcomes–based performance measurements as they may be impractical where outcomes may be reflective of case-mix, and between program differences may be small, for identifying quality of care indicators for adolescent SUD treatment programs (103). In this vein, Brannigan and colleagues (104) identified several key elements of effective adolescent drug treatment through literature review and expert panel consensus. The key elements identified were (a) assessment and treatment matching, (b) comprehensive integrated treatment approach, (c) family involvement, (d) developmentally appropriate program in treatment, (e) engaging and retaining teens in treatment, (f) qualified staff, (g) gender and cultural competence, (h) continuing care, and (i) treatment outcomes. However, no weighting was assigned to these key elements. In a subsequent survey of highly regarded adolescent SUD treatment programs across a range of settings in the United States, most were found to be insufficiently undertaking the key elements of effective adolescent SUD treatment in their programs. The elements with the poorest quality performance were assessment and treatment matching, engaging and retaining teens in treatment, gender and cultural competence, and treatment outcomes. The authors concluded that there is a considerable need to expand the awareness of effective elements in treating adolescent SUD, and that this will heighten program improvement and also serve as a measurement of progress in the field.

In reviews of the literature on adolescent SUD treatment outcomes, it has been deduced that treatment is better than no treatment (5). The largest follow-up study to date of over 1000 adolescent patients, SUD treatment outcomes across different treatment modalities, [outpatient, short-term inpatient, and residential care] showed significant improvements in the domains of substance use, psychological adjustment, school performance, and criminal behavior at one year post treatment than in the year prior to treatment. Also, a longer duration of treatment was associated with reduced rates of substance use and arrested following treatment. This finding is similar to that in adult SUD evaluation research as well as the finding that different treatment modalities appeared to reflect different levels of problem severity (105).

Psychosocial Treatments

Waldron and Turner (106) undertook a comprehensive review and meta-analysis of specific psychosocial outpatient treatment modalities for adolescent SUD with the purpose of establishing evidence-based practice guidelines. They identified three approaches to be considered as well-established interventions: the first two being family-based approaches, Multidimensional Family Therapy (MDFT) and Functional Family Therapy, and the third being group Cognitive Behavioral Therapy (CBT). The authors also found other family models, including Multisystemic Therapy, Brief Strategic Family Therapy, and Behavioral Family Therapy, as most likely efficacious pending further exploration by independent researchers. Both Adolescent Community Reinforcement Approach (ACRA) and other individual CBT models appear promising but require further research. They also concluded that none of the treatment approaches emerged as being superior over another. Waldron and Turner also identified Winters and colleagues' (107) evaluative study of the Minnesota Model 12-step approach for treatment of adolescent SUD as promising, with favorable substance use outcomes and worthy of further research to establish the effectiveness of this treatment approach. The Minnesota Model has been reported to be the most widely used approach in the United States for the treatment of severe SUD/substance dependence in adolescents which is typically taken within a short-term (28 days/admission to a specialized) inpatient hospital or residential care setting (107). Although, an intensive outpatient program employing the Minnesota model was included as part of Winters and colleagues' (107) study which showed similar treatment outcome findings to short-term residential care.

To date, the largest randomized adolescent SUD treatment comparison study has been the Cannabis Youth Treatment (CYT) Study (36). This multisite study ($N = 600$) was comprised of two interrelated randomized trials of five short-term psychosocial treatment interventions for outpatient adolescents with cannabis use disorders (46% met criteria for a substance dependence diagnosis). All interventions were designed to be developmentally appropriate. The study included an extended period of naturalistic follow-up of more than 8 months posttreatment, with study completion at 12 months postrandomization to treatment. All five CYT interventions, including brief psychotherapy of five sessions in total, were found to be effective, demonstrated by significant improvements in the days of abstinence by an average of 24% and the percent of adolescents in recovery (no substance use or abuse/dependence problems) averaging 24% across the 12-month duration of the study. Clinical outcomes were similar across treatment sites and interventions, with no significant differences between conditions on these outcome measures. Despite the findings of clinical improvements, more than 50% of adolescents went in and out of recovery or relapse one or more times posttreatment. The majority were still reporting substance use or related problems at 12 months. These results lead the authors to suggest a need to consider the potential role of continuing care for a significant segment of adolescents entering outpatient treatment for SUD.

Treatment Outcome Parameters

A substantive concern has been the high rates of attrition reported in adolescent SUD treatment that ranges from 20% to greater than 50% across program types (108,109). This high rate of treatment dropout is greater than that seen in adults and is likely related to the adolescents' typically low motivation for treatment and the absence of perceiving their substance use as a problem. The CYT study (41) reported that only 20% of adolescents who entered treatment viewed their substance use as a problem. There has been no thorough examination of motivation as a moderator of treatment outcome in adolescents. However, along this line of thinking, several psychosocial interventions for adolescent SUD have specifically incorporated individual motivational enhancement therapy (MET) as part of treatment (106). Recent studies have demonstrated in several modes of treatment that formation of early therapeutic alliance predicts the likelihood that adolescents will stay in treatment and that they will have better clinical outcomes on measures of drug use as well as internalizing and externalizing behaviors (106,110).

Most adolescent SUD treatment programs advocate a primary goal of achieving and maintaining substance abstinence. The maintenance of abstinence has been linked to positive long-term psychosocial functioning in treated youth (111). Reviews of adolescent treatment outcome studies identify relatively low rates of continuous abstinence following treatment with over 50% of adolescents showing relapse of substance use by 3 months posttreatment (108,112). In comparison to adults, the rates and timing of relapse to any substance use posttreatment appear to be similar. However, the most common context for initial relapse differs between adolescents and adults. Adolescents most commonly report a social situation or peer influence such as socializing with pretreatment friends as context for initial relapse, whereas adults most commonly report negative intra- or interpersonal states (108).

Follow-up treatment studies that examine the patterns of substance use suggest fluctuations in use and problems with an overall reduction of clinical symptoms in youth who have received treatment (108). The reduction in substance use and improvement in related problems are appropriate measures of treatment outcome. Predictors of adolescent SUD treatment outcome have been historically categorized into pretreatment, in-treatment, and posttreatment determinants.

Pretreatment factors, in general, represent background and personal characteristics that, upon entering treatment, may be associated with outcome. Multiple pretreatment characteristics have been identified as potential variables that may have an impact on outcome, but study findings and the manner of reporting factors associated with treatment outcomes are inconsistent. However, a few pretreatment determinants are worth consideration, these being severity of substance use, school functioning, and social supports. Demographic characteristics of gender and ethnicity, overall, have not been found to predict outcome.

The in-treatment factors most consistently associated with favorable treatment outcomes are treatment completion, with its correlation to programs that provide comprehensive services and longer time in treatment. Posttreatment factors include a wide range of psychosocial and environmental variables that occur following treatment that may influence outcomes. Posttreatment factors most consistently related to positive outcome include, but are not limited to, participation in aftercare treatment, peer/parental social support, and prosocial activities. Posttreatment factors, as one may have expected, have been found to be the most important determinant of clinical outcomes (5,108,112,113). More recently, the literature on adolescent SUD treatment has emphasized the need for evaluation of both moderators and mediators of specific treatment interventions that may affect outcome. Moderators are pretreatment characteristics that influence the association between treatment intervention or other independent variables and treatment outcome. Mediators are intervening determinants that may account for the association between a treatment intervention and outcome (106).

A better understanding of the impact of risk and protective factors on substance-related outcomes improves the ability to enhance treatment and relapse prevention programs (113). For example, in an adolescent treatment outcome study, persistent cigarette smokers and smoking initiators during the follow-up period of 1 year were found to be significantly at greater risk for relapse of any substance than those who quit smoking or were nonsmokers. The implications of this study would be to incorporate smoking cessation treatment in the context of adolescent SUD treatment and relapse prevention programs (114).

Several adolescent SUD studies have identified the deleterious impact of psychiatric comorbidity on treatment outcomes across treatment modalities (residential, short-term inpatient/residential care, and outpatient programs). In general, those adolescents with mixed comorbidity of both internalizing and externalizing disorders or with a greater number of comorbid psychiatric disorders showed an increased rate/level of substance relapse/use. Findings from certain studies have supported a more rapid time to relapse of substance use than those adolescents without comorbidity at treatment follow-up of 6 or 12 months (40,115–117). The majority of adolescents with comorbidity in these treatment studies presented with both comorbid internalizing and externalizing disorders. In an adolescent SUD treatment study that investigated the impact of internalizing and externalizing behaviors on clinical outcomes over both short-term (1 year) and long-term (4 and 5.5 years) follow-up, it was found that adolescents with externalizing behaviors had significantly more rapid and higher rates of substance relapse as well as lower treatment retention than those with internalizing behaviors. The authors concluded that these results suggest poorer prognostic treatment outcomes for youth who show core features of delinquency or deviant behavior (92).

Comorbid CD has been implicated in poorer SUD treatment outcomes. Kamon and colleagues (118), in an open study involving a family-based contingency management model including individual CBT provided support for the feasibility and potential for improved retention, substance use outcomes, and reduction of conduct problems in adolescents with SUD (all met criteria for cannabis use disorder), who received this intervention.

Aftercare Treatment

There is a paucity of studies examining the effectiveness of continuing care (CC) in adolescents who have received SUD treatment. Godley and colleagues (119) provided preliminary evidence in their randomized study to support the role of assertive continuing care (ACC) involving case management and ACRA over referral to CC as usual for adolescents discharged from residential SUD treatment. Adolescents who received ACC were more likely to show greater initiation and retention in CC and improved short-term substance use outcomes in comparison to those referred for CC as usual. Adolescents who receive residential SUD treatment often have the most serious SUD and are at high risk for relapse.

Kaminer and colleagues (120) conducted the first and what would appear to be the *only* published prospective randomized controlled trial (RCT) of active aftercare intervention (five in-person or brief telephone sessions) in outpatient adolescents with AUD. The adolescents were identified for the study as having alcohol use disorders (AUD) and completed outpatient group CBT treatment for SUD with aftercare intervention being delivered in the first 3 months posttreatment. Adolescents who received aftercare were significantly less likely to experience relapse to alcohol use versus those who did not receive aftercare, despite the overall significant increase in relapse occurrence at the end of aftercare compared to the end of treatment. The authors concluded that active aftercare posttreatment was relatively efficacious but that the dose of aftercare may not have been sufficient to maintain treatment gains.

Pharmacotherapy

The role of psychopharmacology in the treatment of adolescent substance abuse has not been adequately investigated. Barriers include the lack of safety and efficacy information for the use of psychotropic medications in younger populations and a general reluctance in the consideration of psychopharmacology to treat adolescent SUD. A review of the literature investigating psychopharmacologic treatment of adolescent SUD, with or without comorbid psychiatric disorders, revealed a paucity of studies (121). However, clinical studies have reported high rates of medication use by adolescents receiving SUD treatment, though on the other hand many treatment studies will omit altogether the reporting of medication use in this population. When pharmacotherapy is used in the treatment of adolescent SUD, it is typically for comorbid psychiatric symptoms or disorders and not directly for the SUD.

Pharmacotherapy for SUD

Open-label studies of buprenorphine treatment for adolescents with opioid addiction (122), naltrexone treatment for adolescents with alcohol dependence (123), and ondansetron treatment for youth with alcohol dependence (124) have shown a reduced frequency of substance use.

Randomized clinical trials of 28 days of buprenorphine treatment (125) and 12 weeks of buprenorphine–naloxone treatment (126) in youth with opioid dependence reported significantly greater treatment retention and greater abstinence than comparison treatments of clonidine for detoxification and short-term detoxification with buprenorphine–naloxone, respectively.

An RCT ($N = 26$) of acamprosate treatment for 90 days in adolescents with alcohol dependence reported the number of youth continuously abstinent and the number of continuous days abstinent was greater in the acamprosate group than those in the placebo group (127).

All of these studies reported pharmacotherapy in the context of concurrent psychosocial or behavioral therapies for SUD. The exact role of each therapy cannot be determined definitively. Furthermore, due to methodologic differences in research studies, results may not be replicable and are not directly comparable, rendering it difficult to assess the preference of one pharmacotherapy over another. Nevertheless, the research suggests an advantage for those using pharmacotherapy in the treatment of adolescent substance dependence, in conjunction with either psychosocial or behavioral therapy.

In a case series study by Duffy and Milin (101) of withdrawal syndrome in adolescents with cannabis dependence, the authors commented on the clinical utility of using trazodone 50 to 100 mg at bedtime to assist with withdrawal insomnia. Since then, our center has also found quetiapine 50 to 100 mg at bedtime to be helpful for cannabis withdrawal insomnia in outpatients. Research studies are required to investigate whether selective pharmacotherapy may be beneficial in the management of cannabis withdrawal symptoms and enhance rates of discontinuation of cannabis dependence in adolescents.

Pharmacotherapy for Comorbid Disorders

A randomized, controlled pilot study of sertraline in a small number of outpatient adolescents with alcohol dependence and comorbid clinical depression showed that both groups (sertraline and placebo) experienced a reduction in number of drinking days, a reduction in depression scores, and no significance between group differences. These results may have been due, at least in part, to the requirement that all subjects received CBT regardless of group membership, suggesting the potential effectiveness of CBT in treating MDD and alcohol dependence (128).

In a small open trial of fluoxetine in adolescents with comorbid MDD, SUD, and CD who were in residential treatment for SUD, found promising results. Subjects were included in the study if their depression persisted after at least 1 month of residential care and they were abstinent from substance use (129). The findings showed an improvement of depressive symptoms and functioning. Cornelius and colleagues (130) examined the effectiveness of fluoxetine, in an acute open-label trial and 5-year naturalistic follow-up study of a small group of adolescents with comorbid AUD and MDD who also received treatment as usual, individual psychotherapy, over the acute phase of the study. The acute-phase study results showed a significant reduction (improvement) in depression symptoms and alcohol use. In the 5-year follow-up phase of the study, the subjects (who were now young adults) continued to maintain improvements in depressive symptoms although recurrent episodes were common, and comorbid AUD continued to improve over the course of follow-up.

To date, the largest published RCT of pharmacotherapy in adolescents with comorbidity ($N = 126$) evaluated the efficacy of fluoxetine and individual CBT for SUD in adolescents with MDD, SUD, and CD (131). Riggs and coauthors reported that fluoxetine combined with CBT had demonstrated greater efficacy on one of two depression response measures with a significantly greater reduction in depressive symptoms than placebo and CBT. Both treatment groups demonstrated a higher-than-expected rate of treatment response, which suggested to the researchers that CBT may have contributed to this occurrence with mixed efficacy results. There was an overall decrease in substance use and CD symptoms in both conditions but no between group differences were found. It was also reported that those adolescents who experienced remission of MDD had a greater proportion of negative results on weekly urine drug screens and self-reported days of drug use in the past month, compared to those without remission, irrespective of treatment group assignment. In terms of clinical implications, the authors proposed that the study findings showed that in the context of CBT for SUD, comorbid depression may improve or remit without antidepressant pharmacotherapy. However, if depression does not appear to be improving early in the course of SUD treatment with CBT, then fluoxetine treatment should be considered even if the adolescent is not abstinent, with careful follow-up monitoring of adherence and progress in treatment.

A subsequent RCT in adolescents ($N = 50$) with comorbid MDD and AUD also investigated the efficacy of fluoxetine treatment with all subjects receiving individual manualized CBT for the treatment of MDD and AUD, and manualized MET for SUD. Cornelius and colleagues (132) found no significant treatment outcome differences between the fluoxetine and placebo treatment groups. Both treatment groups showed significant improvements in alcohol use and depressive symptoms over the duration of the study, with having received a course of CBT/MET therapy. The number of heavy drinking days was significantly associated with the lack of remission of self-reported depressive symptoms. The study results lead the researchers to consider various reasons for their findings including limited medication efficacy, small sample size, the efficacy of CBT/MET psychotherapy and to some extent, depressive symptoms may have been alcohol/substance induced. They suggested that psychological intervention should be the first line of treatment in this adolescent comorbid MDD/AUD population with pharmacotherapy afforded to those adolescents who do not respond to psychosocial intervention alone (132). In commentary, the findings of these two RCTs of fluoxetine/placebo and CBT add to the evidence of the effectiveness of individual CBT as a treatment intervention for adolescents with SUD and especially for those adolescents with comorbid MDD.

Only one RCT study of adolescents with BD and comorbid SUD has been conducted. Geller and colleagues (133) in a small RCT ($N = 25$) examined the efficacy of acute lithium treatment in outpatients presenting with bipolar spectrum disorders and comorbid substance dependence with all subjects receiving interpersonal therapy. The lithium treatment group demonstrated a reduced number of positive drug urine screens and an improvement of general psychopathology on a measure of global assessment in comparison to those receiving placebo. However, no between group differences were found on measures of mood or substance dependence symptoms. Nevertheless, the authors concluded that lithium was an effective treatment for both disorders. Though often reported in the literature, this study has numerous limitations and there have been no further published trials to replicate or build on the findings.

In an open-label study, Riggs and colleagues investigated the effectiveness buproprion (134) in a small group of adolescent males with comorbid ADHD, SUD and CD, who were attending a residential SUD treatment program. They reported an improvement in ADHD symptoms and in overall functioning for those adolescents receiving buproprion treatment. However, the effectiveness of buproprion treatment on SUD or CD symptoms could not be evaluated as these variables were well controlled within the residential setting (134). Solhkhah and colleagues (135) also reported positive findings in a retrospective chart review of outpatient adolescents who had presented with comorbid ADHD, mood disorders and SUD and received naturalistic treatment with buproprion sustained release (SR). The adolescents showed improvement of substance use, ADHD symptoms, depressive symptoms and the severity of these disorders at 6 months of treatment. Buproprion SR was well tolerated.

In a community study, adolescents with ADHD and comorbid SUD and CD participated in an RCT ($N = 69$) to evaluate the effectiveness of pemoline treatment (136). The study results demonstrated a significant improvement in the severity of ADHD symptoms for the pemoline group as compared to the placebo group. No significant differences were found between the two groups on measures of substance use or conduct symptoms that did not differ from baseline scores. This study was unique as no concurrent psychosocial SUD treatment was provided. The authors concluded that pemoline was efficacious for ADHD but lacked effect on symptoms of CD and SUD in the absence of specific treatments for SUD supporting the clinical importance of treating comorbid ADHD in the context of concurrent SUD treatment.

A small 6-week crossover ($N = 16$) in adolescents with ADHD and SUD who received treatment with methylphenidate-SODAS, a long-acting formulation, demonstrated a significant reduction in ADHD symptoms and improvement of clinical global functioning versus placebo. There was no significant treatment effect on substance use including no increase in substance use with this long-acting treatment (137).

In a larger RCT ($N = 70$) of atomoxetine for ADHD in adolescents with SUD where all subjects received MET/CBT for SUD, no between group differences were found for ADHD or substance use. However, both groups, atomoxetine plus MET/CBT and placebo plus MET/CBT, showed a significant reduction in ADHD symptoms. The authors concluded that MET/CBT and/or a placebo response contributed to a high treatment response in the placebo group for ADHD, although substance use findings were more equivocal (138).

Riggs and colleagues have recently completed a multisite community-based RCT of OROS methylphenidate an extended release formulation, in adolescents with SUD and comorbid ADHD and the results await publication (139). An important clinical consideration in the selection of these medications for the treatment of comorbid ADHD in adolescents with SUD has been the understanding that they carry low abuse lability.

In summary, over the last decade there have been significant advances in the development of evidence-based psychosocial treatments for adolescent SUD in outpatient settings. These fall within the broad categories of family-based interventions and developmentally appropriate CBT as well as the assimilation of MET as part of these interventions. There is accumulating evidence that supports the benefit of adolescent SUD treatment programs across different settings, including residential, short-term residential/inpatient, partial hospitalization/day treatment and outpatients, as well as some promising findings with respect to aftercare.

It is well defined that treatment of comorbid psychiatric disorders in adolescent SUD remains a priority and a necessity to enhance treatment effectiveness. Pharmacotherapy for the treatment of adolescent SUD remains a work in progress, especially with respect to the direct treatment of substance dependence. At this point, the effectiveness of pharmacotherapy for such common comorbid disorders as MDD and ADHD has not been established in the context of adolescents with active substance dependence. There are mixed findings whether concurrent pharmacotherapy of these comorbid disorders may be beneficial from the onset of treatment in the framework of evidence based psychosocial therapy for adolescents presenting with SUD.

The current clinical implication being that concurrent pharmacotherapy for comorbid disorders may be best served for those adolescents engaged in SUD treatment who show persisting symptoms of MDD or ADHD with significant reduction in substance use/abstinence. Apart from the need for larger treatment studies, there is also the need for extended or maintenance pharmacotherapy trials in adolescents with SUD and comorbid disorders.

CONCLUSION

SUD is a complex and serious problem in the adolescent population with a significant impact on normal development, future SUD and thereby for society in general. Adolescent SUD must be viewed through a developmental lens with adolescence being a period of major risk for the development of SUD. It is closely interrelated with other mental health disorders and social problems requiring comprehensive assessment and an integrated developmentally appropriate treatment approach in working with the adolescent and their family. Significant advances have occurred in determining evidence based treatments for adolescent SUD. There is a strong case that can be made for the need to provide psychiatric care for adolescents in SUD treatment with psychiatric comorbidity being more the rule rather the exception (37). The intervention needs of comorbid youth may best be served by an integrated treatment approach focusing both on SUD and comorbid psychiatric disorders in order to enhance treatment for these conditions. The implementation of treatment specific for adolescent SUD is paramount to an integrated approach. One must consider both the chronicity of SUD in some adolescent populations and the self-limited nature of substance use and related problems in others (5). Defining the adolescent SUD population better such as in terms of substance dependence and substance abuse versus the general category of SUD or employing a standard measure of substance use severity may assist in the development of more specific evidence-based treatment approaches.

ACKNOWLEDGMENT

The authors would like to gratefully acknowledge the assistance of Natasha Ferrill, BA, for all her hard work in the completion of this book chapter.

REFERENCES

1. Brown SA, McGue M, Maggs J, et al. A developmental perspective on alcohol and youths 16 to 20 years of age. *Pediatrics.* 2008;21(4):S290–S310.
2. Gilvarry E. Substance abuse in young people. *J Child Psychol Psyc.* 2000;41(1):55–80.
3. Schepis TS, Adinoff B, Rao U. Neurobiological processes in adolescent addictive disorders. *Am J Addict.* 2008;7:6–23.
4. Johnston LD, O'Malley PM, Bachman JG, et al. Teen marijuana use tilts up, while some drugs decline in use. University of *Michigan News Service.* Ann Arbor, MI: 2009.
5. American Academy of Child and Adolescent Psychiatry (AACAP). Practice parameter for the assessment and treatment of children and adolescents with substance use disorders. *J Am Acad Child Adolesc Psychiatry.* 2005;44:609–621.
6. Shedler J, Block J. Adolescent drug use and psychological health: a longitudinal inquiry. *Am Psychol.* 1990;45(5):612–630.
7. Kandel DB, Johnson JG, Bird HR, et al. Psychiatric comorbidity among adolescents with substance use disorders: findings from the MECA study. *J Am Acad Child Adolesc Psychiatry.* 1999;38(6):693–699.
8. Reinherz HZ, Giaconia RM, Lefkowitz ES, et al. Prevalence of psychiatric disorders in a community population of older adolescents. *J Am Acad Child Adolesc Psychiatry.* 1993;32(2): 369–377.
9. Lewinsohn PM, Hops H, Roberts RE, et al. Adolescent psychopathology: I. Prevalence and incidence of depression and other DSM-III-R disorders in high school students. *J Abnorm Psychol.* 1993;102(1):133–144.
10. Young SE, Corley RP, Stallings MC, et al. Substance use, abuse and dependence in adolescence: prevalence, symptom profiles and correlates. *Drug Alcohol Depen.* 2002;68:309–322.
11. Aarons GA, Brown SA, Hough RL, et al. Prevalence of adolescent substance use disorders across five sectors of care. *J Am Acad Child Adolesc Psychiatry.* 2001;40(4):419–426.
12. Substance Abuse and Mental Health Services Administration. *Results from the 2008 National Survey on Drug Use and Health: National Findings (Office of Applied Studies, NSDUH Series H-36, HHS Publication No. SMA 09-4434).* Rockville, MD: Office of Applied Studies, Substance Abuse and Mental Health Services Administration, U.S. Department of Health and Human Services 2009.
13. Dennis M, Babor TF, Roebuck C, et al. Changing the focus: the case for recognizing and treating cannabis use disorders. *Addiction.* 2002;97(1):4–15.
14. Compton WM, Thomas YF, Stinson FS, et al. Prevalence, correlates, disability, and comorbidity of DSM-IV drug abuse and dependence in the United States. *Arch Gen Psychiat.* 2007; 64:566–576.
15. Hawkins JD, Catalano RF, Miller JY. Risk and protective factors for alcohol and other drug problems in adolescence and early adulthood: implications for substance abuse prevention. *Psychol Bull.* 1992;112(1):64–105.
16. Newcomb MD. Identifying high-risk youth: prevalence and patterns of adolescent drug abuse. In: Rahdert E, Czechowicz D, eds. *Adolescent Drug Abuse: Clinical Assessment and Therapeutic Interventions.* Rockville, MD: National Institute on Drug Abuse; 1995:7–37.
17. Fergusson DM, Lynskey MT. Adolescent resiliency to family adversity. *J Child Psychol Psyc.* 1996;37(3):281–292.
18. Newcomb MD, Felix-Ortiz M. Multiple protective risk factors for drug use and abuse: cross-sectional and prospective findings. *J Pers Soc Psychol.* 1992;63(2):280–296.
19. Upadhyaya HP. Routinely assess substance use disorders (SUDs). *J Am Acad Child Adolesc Psychiatry.* 2008;47(6):610.
20. Boyle MH, Offord DR, Racine YA, et al. Predicting substance use in late adolescence: results from the Ontario Child Health Study follow-up. *Am J Psychiat.* 1992;149(6):761–767.
21. Kandel DB, Davies M, Karus D, et al. The consequences in young adulthood of adolescent drug involvement. *Arch Gen Psychiat.* 1986;43:746–754.
22. Anthony JC, Petronis KR. Early-onset drug use and risk of later drug problems. *Drug Alcohol Depen.* 1995;40:9–15.
23. Chen CY, O'Brien MS, Anthony JC. Who becomes cannabis dependent soon after onset of use? Epidemiological evidence from the United States: 2000–2001. *Drug Alcohol Depen.* 2005; 79:11–22.
24. DeWit DJ, Adlaf EM, Offord DR, et al. Age at first alcohol use: a risk factor for the development of alcohol disorders. *Am J Psychiatry.* 2000;157:745–750.
25. Copeland WE, Shanahan L, Costello EJ, et al. Childhood and adolescent psychiatric disorders as predictors of young adult disorders. *Arch Gen Psychiatry.* 2009;66(7):764–772.
26. Coffey C, Carlin JB, Lynskey M, et al. Adolescent precursors of cannabis dependence: Findings from the Victorian Adolescent Health Cohort Study. *Br J Psychiatry.* 2003;182:330–336.
27. Kandel DB. Stages in adolescent involvement in drug use. *Science.* 1975;190:912–914.
28. Kandel DB, Yamaguchi K, Chen K. Stages of progression in drug involvement from adolescence to adulthood: further evidence for the gateway theory. *J Stud Alcohol.* 1992;53:447–457.

29. Kandel DB. Does marijuana use cause the use of other drugs? *J Amer Med Assoc.* 2003;289(4):482–483.
30. Fergusson DM, Boden JM, Horwood LJ. Cannabis use and other illicit drug use: testing the cannabis gateway hypothesis. *Addiction.* 2006;101:556–569.
31. Fergusson DM, Boden JM, Horwood LJ. Testing the cannabis gateway hypothesis: replies to Hall, Kandel et al. and Maccoun (2006). *Addiction.* 2006;101:474–476.
32. Chen K, Kandel DB, Davies M. Relationships between frequency and quantity of marijuana use and last year proxy dependence among adolescents and adults in the United States. *Drug Alcohol Depen.* 1997;46:53–67.
33. Macleod J, Oaskes R, Copello A, et al. Psychological and social sequelae of cannabis and other illicit drug use by young people: a systematic review of longitudinal, general population studies. *Lancet.* 2004;363:1579–1588.
34. Newcomb MD. Psychosocial predictors and consequences of drug use: a developmental perspective within a prospective study. *J Addict Dis.* 1997;16(1):51–88.
35. Clark DB, Pollock N, Bukstein O, et al. Gender and comorbid psychopathology in adolescents with alcohol dependence. *J Am Acad Child Adolesc Psychiatry.* 1997;36(9):1195–1203.
36. Dennis M, Godley SH, Diamond G, et al. The Cannabis Youth Treatment (CYT) study: main findings from two randomized trials. *J Subst Abuse Treat.* 2004;27:197–213.
37. Sterling S, Weisner C. Chemical dependency and psychiatric services for adolescents in private managed care: implications for outcomes. *Alcohol Clin Exp Res.* 2005;29(5):801–809.
38. Stowell RJ, Estroff TW. Psychiatric disorders in substance-abusing adolescent inpatients: a pilot study. *J Am Acad Child Adolesc Psychiatry.* 1992;31(6):1036–1040.
39. Rohde P, Lewinshohn PM, Seeley JR. Psychiatric comorbidity with problematic alcohol use in high school students. *J Am Acad Child Adolesc Psychiatry.* 1996;35(1):101–109.
40. Grella CE, Hser YI, Joshi V, et al. Drug treatment outcomes for adolescents with comorbid mental and substance use disorders. *J Nerv Ment Dis.* 2001;189(6):384–392.
41. Tims FM, Dennis ML, Hamilton N, et al. Characteristics and problems of 600 adolescent cannabis abusers in outpatient treatment. *Addiction.* 2002;97(1):46–57.
42. Armstrong TD, Costello EJ. Community studies on adolescent substance use, abuse, or dependence and psychiatric comorbidity. *J Consult Clin Psych.* 2002;70(6):1224–1239.
43. Brook DW, Brook JS, Zhang C, et al. Drug use and the risk of major depressive disorder, alcohol dependence, and substance use disorders. *Arch Gen Psychiat.* 2002;59:1039–1044.
44. Brook JS, Cohen P, Brook DW. Longitudinal study of co-occurring psychiatric disorders and substance use. *J Am Acad Child Adolesc Psychiatry.* 1998;37(3):322–330.
45. Hayatbakhsh MR, Najman JM, Jamrozik K, et al. Cannabis and anxiety and depression in young adults: a large prospective study. *J Am Acad Child Adolesc Psychiatry.* 2007;46(3):408–417.
46. Glantz MD, Anthony JC, Berglund PA, et al. Mental disorders as risk factors for later substance dependence: estimates of optimal prevention and treatment benefits. *Psychol Med.* 2009;39:1365–1377.
47. Deas D. Adolescent substance abuse and psychiatric comorbidities. *J Clin Psychiat.* 2006;67(7):18–23.
48. Greenbaum PE, Prange ME, Friedman RM, et al. Substance abuse prevalence and comorbidity with other psychiatric disorders among adolescents with severe emotional disturbances. *J Am Acad Child Adolesc Psychiatry.* 1991;30(4):575–583.
49. Grilo CM, Becker DF, Walker ML, et al. Psychiatric comorbidity in adolescent inpatients with substance use disorders. *J Am Acad Child Adolesc Psychiatry.* 1995;34(8):1085–1091.
50. Kramer TL, Robbins JM, Phillips SD, et al. Detection and outcomes of substance use disorders in adolescents seeking mental health treatment. *J Am Acad Child Adolesc Psychiatry.* 2003;42(11):1318–1326.
51. Costello EJ, Mustillo S, Erkanli A, et al. Prevalence and development of psychiatric disorders in childhood and adolescence. *Arch Gen Psychiaty.* 2003;60:837–844.
52. Grilo CM, Becker DF, Fehon DC, et al. Conduct disorder, substance use disorders, and coexisting and substance use disorders in adolescent inpatients. *Am J Psychiatry.* 1996;153(3):914–920.
53. Sung M, Erkanli A, Angold A, et al. Effects of age at first substance use and psychiatric comorbidity on the development of substance use disorders. *Drug Alcohol Depen.* 2004;75:287–299.
54. Stein LA, Hesselbrock V, Bukstein OG. Conduct disorder and oppositional defiant disorder and adolescent substance use disorders. In: Kaminer Y, Bukstein OG, eds. *Adolescent Substance Abuse Psychiatric Comorbidity and High-Risk Behaviors.* New York, NY: Routledge Taylor & Francis Group; 2008:163–194.
55. Reebye P, Moretti MM, Lessard JC. Conduct disorder and substance use disorder: comorbidity in a clinical sample of preadolescents and adolescents. *Can J Psychiat.* 1995;40:313–319.
56. Mezzich AC, Moss H, Tarter RE, et al. Gender differences in the pattern and progression of substance use in conduct-disordered adolescents. *Am J Addict.* 1994;3:289–295.
57. Milin R, Halikas JA, Meller JE, et al. Psychopathology among substance abusing juvenile offenders. *J Am Acad Child Adolesc Psychiatry.* 1991;30(4):569–574.
58. Disney ER, Elkins IJ, McGue M, et al. Effects of ADHD, conduct disorder, and gender on substance use and abuse in adolescence. *Am J Psychiat.* 1999;156(10):1515–1521.
59. Horner BR, Scheibe KE. Prevalence and implications of attention-deficit hyperactivity disorder among adolescents in treatment for substance abuse. *J Am Acad Child Adolesc Psychiatry.* 1997;36(1):30–36.
60. August GJ, Winters KC, Realmuto GM, et al. Prospective study of adolescent drug use among community samples of ADHD and non-ADHD participants. *J Am Acad Child Adolesc Psychiatry.* 2006;45(7):824–832.
61. Biederman J, Wilens T, Mick E, et al. Is ADHD a risk factor for psychoactive substance use disorders? Findings from a four-year prospective follow-up study. *J Am Acad Child Adolesc Psychiatry.* 1997;36(1):21–29.
62. Molina BS, Pelham WE Jr. Childhood predictors of adolescent substance use in a longitudinal study of children with ADHD. *J Abnorm Psychol.* 2003;112(3):497–507.
63. Barkley RA, Fischer M, Smallish L, et al. Young adult follow-up of hyperactive children: antisocial activities and drug use. *J Child Psychol Psyc.* 2004;45(2):195–211.
64. Biederman J, Wilens T, Mick E, et al. Psychoactive substance use disorders in adults with attention deficit hyperactivity disorder (ADHD): effects of ADHD and psychiatric comorbidity. *Am J Psychiat.* 1995;152(11):1652–1658.
65. Mannuzza S, Klein RG, Truong NL, et al. Age of methylphenidate treatment initiation in children with ADHD and later substance abuse: prospective follow-up into adulthood. *Am J Psychiat.* 2008;165(5):604–609.

66. Biederman J, Monuteaux MC, Spencer T, et al. Stimulant therapy and risk for subsequent substance use disorders in male adults with ADHD: a naturalistic controlled 10-year follow-up study. Am J Psychiat. 2008;165(5):597–603.
67. Wilens TE, Faraone SV, Biederman J, et al. Does stimulant therapy of attention-deficit/hyperactivity disorder beget later substance abuse? A meta-analytic review of the literature. Pediatrics. 2003;111(1):179–185.
68. Barkley RA, Fischer M, Smallish L, et al. Does the treatment of attention-deficit/hyperactivity disorder with stimulants contribute to drug use/abuse? A 13-year prospective study. Pediatrics. 2003;111(1):97–109.
69. Katusic SK, Barbaresi WJ, Colligan RC, et al. Psychostimulant treatment and risk for substance abuse among young adults with a history of attention-deficit/hyperactivity disorder: a population-based, birth cohort study. J Child Adol Psychop. 2005;15(5):764–776.
70. Rao U, Ryan ND, Dahl RE, et al. Factors associated with the development of substance use disorder in depressed adolescents. J Am Acad Child Adolesc Psychiatry. 1999;38(9):1109–1117.
71. Rao U, Chen LA. Neurobiological and psychosocial processes associated with depressive and substance-related disorders in adolescents. Curr Drug Abuse Rev. 2008;1:68–80.
72. Bukstein OG, Glancy LJ, Kaminer Y. Patterns of affective comorbidity in a clinical population of dually diagnosed adolescent substance abusers. J Am Acad Child Adolesc Psychiatry. 1992;31(6):1041–1045.
73. Deykin EY, Buka SL, Zeena TH. Depressive illness among chemically dependent adolescents. Am J Psychiat. 1992;149(10):1341–1347.
74. Subramaniam GA, Stitzer MA, Clemmey P, et al. Baseline depressive symptoms predict poor substance use outcome following adolescent residential treatment. J Am Acad Child Adolesc Psychiatry. 2007;46(8):1062–1069.
75. King CA, Ghaziuddin N, McGovern L, et al. Predictors of comorbid alcohol and substance abuse in depressed adolescents. J Am Acad Child Adolesc Psychiatry. 1996;35(6):743–751.
76. King CA, Naylor MW, Hill EM, et al. Dysthymia characteristic of heavy alcohol use in depressed adolescents. Biol Psychiatry. 1993;33:210–212.
77. Goldstein BI, Shamseddeen W, Spirito A, et al. Substance use and the treatment of resistant depression in adolescents. J Am Acad Child Adolesc Psychiatry. 2009;48(12):1182–1192.
78. Crumley FE. Substance abuse and adolescent suicidal behavior. J Amer Med Assoc. 1990;263(22):3051–3056.
79. Brent DA, Perper JA, Moritz G, et al. Psychiatric risk factors for adolescent suicide: a case-control study. J Am Acad Child Adolesc Psychiatry. 1993;32(3):521–529.
80. Esposito-Smythers C, Spirito A. Adolescent substance use and suicidal behavior: a review with implications for treatment research. Alcohol Clin Exp Res. 2004;28(5):77s–88s.
81. Borges G, Walters EE, Kessler RC. Associations of substance use, abuse, and dependence with subsequent suicidal behavior. Am J Epidemiol. 2000;151(8):781–789.
82. Milin R, Walker S, Duffy A. Assessment and treatment of comorbid psychotic disorders and bipolar disorder. In: Kaminer Y, Winters K, eds. Clinical Manual of Adolescent Substance Abuse Treatment. Arlington, VA: APPI. 2010.
83. Clark DB, Bukstein OG, Smith MG, et al. Identifying anxiety disorders in adolescents hospitalized for alcohol abuse or dependence. Psychiatr Serv. 1995;46(6):618–620.
84. Hovens JG, Cantwell DP, Kiriakos R. Psychiatric comorbidity in hospitalized adolescent substance abusers. J Am Acad Child Adolesc Psychiatry. 1994;33(4):476–483.
85. Abrantes AM, Brown SA, Tomlinson KL. Psychiatric comorbidity among inpatient substance abusing adolescents. J Child Adoles Subst. 2003;13(2):83–101.
86. Giaconia RM, Reinherz HZ, Carmola Hauf A. Comorbidity of substance use and post-traumatic stress disorders in a community sample of adolescents. Am J Orthopsychiat. 2000;70(2):253–262.
87. Rounds-Bryant JL, Kristiansen PL, Fairbank JA, et al. Substance use, mental disorders, abuse, and crime: gender comparisons among a national sample of adolescent drug treatment clients. J Child Adolesc Subst Abuse. 1998;7(4):19–20.
88. Von Ranson KM, Iacono WG, McGue M. Disordered eating and substance use in an epidemiological sample: I. Associations within individuals. Int J Eat Disord. 2002;31:389–403.
89. Van Hook S, Harris SK, Brooks T, et al. The "Six T's": barriers to screening teens for substance abuse in primary care. J Adolesc Health. 2007;40:456–461.
90. Winters KC, Kaminer Y. Screening and assessing adolescent substance use disorders in clinical populations. J Am Acad Child Adolesc Psychiatry. 2008;47(7):740–744.
91. Samet S, Waxman R, Hatzenbuehler M, et al. Assessing addiction: concepts and instruments. Addict Sci Clin Pract. 2007;40:19–31.
92. Winters KC, Stinchfield RD, Latimer WW et al. Internalizing and externalizing behaviors and their association with the treatment of adolescents with substance use disorder. J Subst Abuse Treat. 2008;35:269–278.
93. Burleson JA, Kaminer Y. Adolescent alcohol and marijuana use: concordance among objective-, self-, and collateral-reports. J Child Adoles Subst. 2006;16(1):53–68.
94. Gignac M, Wilens TE, Biederman J, et al. Assessing cannabis use in adolescents and young adults: what do urine screen and parental report tell you? J Child Adolesc Psychopharmacol. 2005;15:742–750.
95. Knight JR, Shrier LA, Braveder TD, et al. A new brief screen for adolescent substance abuse. Arch Pediatr Adolesc Med. 1999;153:591–596.
96. Knight JR, Sherritt L, Shrier LA, et al. Validity of the CRAFFT substance abuse screening test among adolescent clinic patients. Arch Pediatr Adolesc Med. 2002;156:607–614.
97. Moberg DP. Screening for Alcohol and Other Drug Problems Using the Adolescent Alcohol and Drug Involvement Scale (AADIS). Madison, WI: University of Wisconsin, Center for Health Policy and Program Evaluation; 2003.
98. Dennis ML, Chan Y-F, Funk R. Development and validation of the GAIN Short Screener (GSS) for internalizing, externalizing and substance use disorders and crime/violence problems among adolescents and adults. Am J Addict. 2006;15:80–91.
99. American Society of Addiction Medicine (ASAM). ASAM PPC-2R: ASAM Patient Placement Criteria for the Treatment of Substance-Related Disorders. 2nd ed. revised. Chevy Chase, MD: American Society of Addiction Medicine, Inc. 2001.
100. Fishman M. Treatment planning, matching, and placement for adolescents with substance use disorders. In: Kaminer Y, Bukstein OG, eds. Adolescent Substance Abuse, Psychiatric Comorbidity and High-Risk Behaviors. New York, NY: Taylor & Francis; 2008:87–110.

101. Duffy A, Milin R. Case study: Withdrawal syndrome in adolescent chronic cannabis users. *J Am Acad Child Adolesc Psychiatry.* 1996;35(12):1618–1621.
102. Cornelius JR, Chung T, Martin D, et al. Cannabis withdrawal is common among treatment-seeking adolescents with cannabis dependence and major depression, and is associated with rapid relapse to dependence. *Addict Behav.* 2008;33:1500–1505.
103. Morral AR, McCaffrey DF, Ridgeay G, et al. The relative effectiveness of 10 adolescent substance abuse treatment programs in the United States. Santa Monica, CA: RAND Drug Policy Research Center; 2006.
104. Brannigan R, Schackman BR, Falco M, et al. The quality of highly regarded adolescent substance abuse treatment programs. Results of an in-depth survey. *Arch Pediatr Adolesc Med.* 2004; 158:904–909.
105. Hser Y, Grella CE, Hubbard RL, et al. An evaluation of drug treatments for adolescents in 4 US cities. *Arch Gen Psychiatry.* 2001;58:689–695.
106. Waldron HB, Turner CW. Evidence-based psychosocial treatments for adolescent substance abuse. *J Clin Child Adolesc Psychol.* 2008;37(1):238–261.
107. Winters KC, Stinchfield RD, Opland E, et al. The effectiveness of the Minnesota Model approach in the treatment of adolescent drug abusers. *Addict.* 2000;95(4):601–612.
108. Chung T, Maisto SA. Relapse to alcohol and other drug use in treated adolescents: review and reconsideration of relapse as a change point in clinical course. *Clin Psychol Rev.* 2006;26: 149–161.
109. Monti PM, Barnett NP, O'Leary TA, et al. Motivational enhancement for alcohol-involved adolescents. In: Monti P, Colby SM, O'Leary TA, eds. *Adolescents, Alcohol, and Substance Abuse.* New York, NY: Guilford Press; 2001:145–182.
110. Diamond GS, Liddle HA, Wintersteen MB, et al. Early therapeutic alliance as a predictor of treatment outcome for adolescent cannabis users in outpatient treatment. *Am J Addict.* 2006;15:26–33.
111. Brown SA, D'Amico EJ, McCarthy DM, et al. Four-year outcomes from adolescent alcohol and drug treatment. *J Stud Alcohol.* 2001;62:381–388.
112. Williams RJ, Chang SY. A comprehensive and comparative review of adolescent substance abuse treatment outcome. *Clin Psychol-Sci Pr.* 2000;7:138–166.
113. Anderson KG, Ramo DE, Schulte MT, et al. Substance use treatment outcomes for youth: integrating personal and environmental predictors. *Drug Alcohol Depen.* 2007;88:42–48.
114. de Dios MA, Vaughan EL, Stanton CA, et al. Adolescent tobacco use and substance abuse treatment outcomes. *J Subst Abuse Treat.* 2009;37:17–24.
115. Rowe CL, Liddle HA, Greenbaum PE, et al. Impact of psychiatric comorbidity on treatment of adolescent drug abusers. *J Subst Abuse Treat.* 2004;26:129–140.
116. Tomlinson KL, Brown SA, Abrantes A. Psychiatric comorbidity and substance use treatment outcomes of adolescents. *Psychol Addict Behav.* 2004;18(2):160–169.
117. Shane PA, Jasiukaitis P, Green RS. Treatment outcomes among adolescents with substance abuse problems: the relationship between comorbidities and post-treatment substance involvement. *Eval Program Plann.* 2003;26:393–402.
118. Kamon J, Budney A, Stanger C. A contingency management intervention for adolescent marijuana abuse and conduct problems. *J Am Acad Child Adolesc Psychiatry.* 2005;44(6):513–521.
119. Godley MD, Godley SH, Dennis ML, et al. Preliminary outcomes from the assertive continuing care experiment for adolescents discharged from residential treatment. *J Subst Abuse Treat.* 2002;23:21–32.
120. Kaminer Y, Burleson JA, Burke RH. Efficacy of outpatient aftercare for adolescents with alcohol use disorders: a randomized controlled study. *J Am Acad Child Adolesc Psychiatry.* 2008; 47(12):1405–1412.
121. Waxmonsky JG, Wilens TE. Pharmacotherapy of adolescent substance use disorders: a review of the literature. *J Child Adolesc Psychopharmacol.* 2005;15(5):810–825.
122. Gandhi DH, Jaffe JH, McNary S, et al. Short-term outcomes after brief ambulatory opioid detoxification with buprenorphine in young heroin users. *Addiction.* 2003;98:453–462.
123. Deas D, May K, Randall C, et al. Naltrexone treatment of adolescent alcoholics: an open-label pilot study. *J Child Adolesc Psychopharmacol.* 2005;15(5):723–728.
124. Dawes MA, Johnson BA, Ait-Daoud N, et al. A prospective, open-label trial of ondansetron in adolescents with alcohol dependence. *Addictive Behav.* 2005;30:1077–1085.
125. Marsch LA, Bickel WK, Badger GJ, et al. Comparison of pharmacological treatments for opioid-dependent adolescents: a randomized controlled trial. *Arch Gen Psychiatry.* 2005;62: 1157–1164.
126. Woody GE, Poole SA, Subramaniam G, et al. Extended vs short-term buprenorphine-naloxone for treatment of opioid-addicted youth: a randomized trial. *JAMA.* 2008;300(17): 2003–2011.
127. Neiderhofer H, Staffen W. Acamprosate and its efficacy in treating alcohol dependent adolescents. *Eur Child Adolesc Psychiatry.* 2003;12:144–148.
128. Deas D, Randall CL, Roberts JS, et al. A double-blind, placebo-controlled trial of sertraline in depressed adolescent alcoholics: a pilot study. *Hum Psychopharmacol Clin Exp.* 2000;15: 461–469.
129. Riggs PD, Mikulich SK, Coffman LM, et al. Fluoxetine in drug-dependent delinquents with major depression: an open trial. *J Child Adolesc Psychopharmacol.* 1997;7(2):87–95.
130. Cornelius JR, Clark DB, Bukstein OG, et al. Acute phase and five-year follow-up study of fluoxetine in adolescents with major depression and a comorbid substance use disorder: a review. *Addict Behav.* 2005;30:1824–1833.
131. Riggs PD, Mikulich-Gilbertson SK, Davies RD, et al. A randomized controlled trial of fluoxetine and cognitive behavioural therapy in adolescents with major depression, behavior problems, and substance use disorders. *Arch Pediatr Adoelsc Med.* 2007;161(11):1026–1034.
132. Cornelius JR, Bukstein OG, Wood S, et al. Double-blind placebo-controlled trial of fluoxetine in adolescents with comorbid major depression and an alcohol use disorder. *Addict Behav.* 2009;34:905–909.
133. Geller B, Cooper TB, Sun K, et al. Double-blind and placebo-controlled study of lithium for adolescent bipolar disorder with secondary substance dependency. *J Am Acad Child Adolesc Psychiatry.* 1998;37(2):171–178.
134. Riggs PD, Leon SL, Mikulich SK, et al. An open trial of bupropion for ADHD in adolescents with substance use disorders and conduct disorder. *J Am Acad Child Adoesc Psychiatry.* 1998;37(12):1271–1278.
135. Solhkhah R, Wilens T, Daly J, et al. Bupropion SR for the treatment of substance abusing outpatient adolescents with

attention-deficit/hyperactivity disorder and mood disorders. *J Child Adol Psychop.* 2005;15(5):777–786.
136. Riggs PD, Hall SK, Mikulich-Gilbertson SK, et al. A randomized controlled trial of pemoline for attention-deficit/hyperactivity disorder in substance-abusing adolescents. *J Am Acad Child Adolesc Psychiatry.* 2004;43(4):420–429.
137. Szobot CM, Rohde LA, Katz B, et al. A randomized crossover clinical study showing that methylphenidate-SODAS improves attention-deficit/hyperactivity disorder symptoms in adolescents with substance use disorder. *Braz J Med Biol Res.* 2008; 41(3):250–257.
138. Thurstone C, Riggs PD, Salomonsen-Sautel S, et al. Randomized, controlled trial of atomoxetine for attention-deficit/hyperactivity disorder in adolescents with substance use disorder. *J Am Acad Child Adolesc Psychiatry.* 2010;49(6): 573–582.
139. Yan, Y. Stimulant abuse doesn't aggravate substance abuse. *Psychiatric News.* 2010;45(3):3.

CHAPTER 58: The Older Drug Abuser

Bennett W. Fletcher ■ Wilson M. Compton

Older adults in the United States have experienced a period of rapid cultural change unlike any other in history. This period saw the United States become embroiled in a long and bloody war in Southeast Asia that fueled the rise of a youth culture of acceptance and widespread use of illicit drugs, especially marijuana. Other illicit drugs, notably heroin, also saw epidemic use in the 1960s, but that period and the decades following were characterized by the misuse of many types of illicit drug use, including use of hallucinogens and prescription medications (stimulants, depressants, and synthetic opiates), as well as cocaine and heroin. Many older adults in the United States have had personal experience with use of illicit drugs at some point in their lives. The 2008 National Survey on Drug Use and Health (NSDUH) estimated that 40% to 60% of those between the ages of 45 and 64 had used illicit drugs at some point in their lives (1). Throughout their youth and adult lives, all older adults have lived with an awareness that illicit drug use is a significant societal problem.

Some older adults who began drug use in their earlier years became addicted and continued use over time. Drug abuse in early years affects health and well-being later in life. The chronic misuse of certain drugs, particularly stimulants, is associated with neurodevelopmental abnormalities that can impair cognitive function during early to middle age (2), and that may interact with aging to speed the onset and progression of degenerative brain processes such as dementia and Alzheimer disease (3).

Other older adults who used illicit drugs may have discontinued use for long periods for the sake of family or employment. There is a concern that as their situation changes—with retirement, from social isolation following the departure of children or friends, or with the onset of a chronic illness—some older individuals may return to drug use. Chronic illness has a higher prevalence rate in older populations. Many of these illnesses are treatable, but patients with histories of illicit drug use may be susceptible to relapse, medication misuse, or harmful drug interactions if misuse is ongoing. Individuals who initiated heroin, cocaine, or hallucinogen use before the age of 30 were estimated to be three times more likely to use drugs when 50 or older (4). Projections of drug abuse in 2020 estimate a doubling of the number of adults age 50 or higher who report misuse or abuse of illicit drugs compared to 1999 to 2001 (from 1.6 million to 3.5 million), as a result of both increasing size of the older population and the higher rates of illicit drug use in this segment of the population.

The United States experienced a large increase in the number of babies born between 1946 and 1964. This "Baby Boom" cohort will begin to turn 65 in 2011. In addition, populations in the United States and many industrialized countries are becoming older as a result of increased life expectancies coupled with declining fertility rates (5). The U.S. Census Bureau estimates that in 2010 about 32% of the U.S. population, or 98.6 million residents, will be 50 years of age or older. The proportion will grow to nearly 37%, or about 161.1 million, by 2050.

The misuse and abuse of psychotropic drugs by older adults is a matter of great concern, both for the health of the individual patient and for public health. The prevalence of illicit drug abuse by those 50 and older is projected to increase in the coming years, and this will create problems for those individuals, for their families, and for a health care system that is not presently oriented toward screening, assessing, or providing care for the older drug abuser.

The purpose of this chapter is to provide an overview of the research and clinical implications for drug abuse in the older adult population, defined as adults who are age 50 or above. The topics that we review include the epidemiology of drug abuse and addiction in older adults; the implications of living in a time of widespread illicit drug use for the "baby boomer" generation; the emerging neurobiology research in two areas, aging and addiction, and how these may intersect; the impact of comorbid and chronic illnesses on drug use in the older adult population; and research on the treatment of drug abuse and addiction in the older adult.

EPIDEMIOLOGY OF DRUG ABUSE AND ADDICTION IN OLDER ADULTS

Increasing Prevalence of Illicit Drug Use

Rates of illicit drug use peak in the general population around ages 18 to 25 and decline with increasing age. Rates of illicit drug use among adults aged 65 or older have historically been quite low. However, as the baby boom generation has aged, the prevalence of illicit drug use among older adults has increased. In the 2008 NSDUH, a national household survey conducted annually by the U.S. Substance Abuse and Mental Health Services Administration (SAMHSA), 40% to 60% of those between the ages of 45 and 64 had used illicit drugs at some point in their lives (1).

Some individuals simply continue to use illicit drugs as they grow older. Han, Gfroerer, and Colliver (6) analyzed the NSDUH to explore whether the increase in use of illicit drugs by older adults was from new users (those who initiated drug use after age 50) or from resumption of illicit use after a period of abstinence, or whether use was continued over time. Continuing use was defined as past-year use (use in the 12 months prior to the survey) coupled with use in the 13 to 24 months prior to the survey. For marijuana use, the researchers found that continuing use described about 82% of current marijuana users over 50, and about 17% represented a resumption in prior use following abstinence. Only about 1% were new initiates to marijuana use; about nine tenths of those reporting lifetime illicit drug use initiated use before the age of 30. Together with the growing size of the baby boomer population, it is not surprising that the prevalence of current drug use (use of drugs in the past month) by adults aged 50 to 59 has increased in recent years, to 5% in the 2007 NSDUH, compared with 2.7% in 2002 and about 1% in 2000 (when the survey was called the National Household Survey on Drug Abuse).

Marijuana and nonmedical use of prescription drugs comprise the majority of illicit drug use by older adults, but the average age of injection drug use has also increased over time (7). Based on NSDUH surveys, the mean age of participants who had injected drugs in the past year increased from 21 years in 1979 to 36 years in 2002. From 1979 to 2002, the average age of respondents who had ever used injection drugs increased from 26 to 42 years. Injection drug use by younger adults has trended downward over the same time period. As the baby boom cohort ages, older adults will be more likely to have a lifetime history of injection drug use than younger adults. It is recommended that clinicians should routinely ask patients about present and past drug use in order to prevent public health consequences of blood-borne viruses (7).

The National Comorbidity Survey Replication (NCS-R) is a nationally representative, multistage weighted household survey of English-speaking household respondents interviewed in 2001 to 2003. The NCS-R has been used to examine the cumulative incidence of alcohol and illicit drug use in four age groups—those aged 18 to 29, 30 to 44, 45 to 59, and 60 to 98 years (8). The incidence of illicit drug use in the 45 to 59 year baby boomer cohort, those born during 1943 to 1957, was much more like that of the younger cohorts than of the oldest cohort, those born between 1904 and 1942. Another study of a general household sample of adults, the National Epidemiologic Survey on Alcohol and Related Conditions (NESARC), found similar results. Nonmedical lifetime use of prescription drugs by those aged 45 to 64 was significantly higher than by those 65 or older, but did not differ significantly from prevalence rates in younger ages (9). Depending on the drug category (sedatives, tranquilizers, opioids, or amphetamines), lifetime nonmedical use of prescription drugs in the 45 to 64 age cohort ranged from 3.3% to 4.9% in the general population.

Projected Need for Drug Abuse Treatment by Older Adults

Admissions to substance abuse treatment are counted in the United States by SAMHSA through their Drug and Alcohol Services Information System and reported in the Treatment Episode Data Set (TEDS). TEDS is an annual census of admissions to specialty treatment providers receiving public funding. While it does not include private practice providers or treatment provided by federal agencies such as the Bureau of Prisons or Veterans Administration, it provides useful trend information. The data show an upward trend in admissions to substance abuse treatment for older adults.

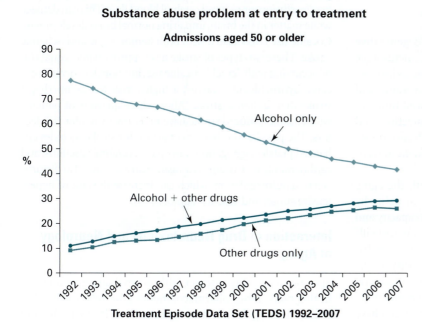

Figure 58.1. Changes over time in the percentage of admissions (age 50 years and old) reporting alcohol-only problem, alcohol problem with another drug problem, or drug problem without an alcohol problem. (Data from US Dept Health & Human Services, Substance Abuse and Mental Health Services Administration, Office of Applied Studies. *Treatment Episode Data Set (TEDS) Highlights–2007 National Admissions to Substance Abuse Treatment Services*. OAS Series #S-45, HHS Publication No. (SMA) 09-4360, Rockville, MD; 2009.)

Across all ages, substance abuse treatment admissions have increased over time. Total admissions to treatment reported to TEDS for a drug problem or a combined drug and alcohol problem (excluding admissions for alcohol alone) increased from 932,300 in 1992 to 1,356,802 in 2007 (10). Individuals aged 50 or older have grown from 20,383 (2.2%) admissions in 1992 to 114,561 (8.4%) in 2007 (10). There has also been a shift away from admissions for alcohol alone toward illicit drugs alone or in combination with alcohol (Fig. 58.1). In 1992, admissions for problems with alcohol made up only about 77% of all admissions for people aged 50 and higher. By 2007, over half (55%) of all older admissions were for drugs alone or in combination with alcohol, reflecting the increasing upward trend in older admissions for problems with multiple substances (11).

Estimates of future numbers of older adults using illicit drugs take account of the increasing population and the increased illicit drug use by this aging cohort. Projections suggest that the number of individuals 50 year or older who use illicit drugs will more than double in the 20 years between 2000 and 2020, from an estimated 1.6 million with past-year illicit drug use in the interval 1999 to 2001 to about 3.5 million in 2020 (4). (Note that this does not include the number who might need treatment for alcohol problems.) The number of past-year marijuana users aged 50 or higher is projected to increase by about 355% (from 719,000 to 3.3 million) in this period, and the increase projected for the nonmedical use of prescription psychotherapeutics is about 190%, from 911,000 in 1999 to 2001 to about 2.7 million in 2020.

Some of these aging individuals will develop a substance use disorder, resulting in a projected increase in demand by older adults for substance abuse treatment. Han et al. estimate that there may be 5.7 million older adults who would need treatment for alcohol or illicit drug use in 2020 (12).

EFFECTS OF DRUG USE ON HEALTH

Increased Risk of Physical Problems

Aging can be considered a set of progressive degenerative changes that cumulatively affect an individual's neurologic and physiologic capacities. The normal aging process involves a loss of brain cells, reductions in muscular volume and strength, reduced cardiovascular function, reduced function in body organs, increased vulnerability to infection and chronic illnesses, and increased risk of mental health disorders. How a given individual ages depends on genetic and environmental factors.

Drug abuse and addiction can interact with the aging brain and body to increase the apparent rate of aging by speeding the decline in cognitive and functional capacity and by increasing the vulnerability to both chronic and acute illnesses. Individuals in their 50s who have a substance use disorder may be more similar in their medical morbidity profile to non-drug-using individuals in their 60s in terms of general health, physical and social functioning, bodily pain, and mortality risk (11). Chronic misuse of addictive drugs can have serious clinical effects. Cocaine, for example, may result in clinical problems in the following areas: cardiac, pulmonary, psychiatric, neurologic, gastrointestinal, and endocrinologic function; other physical problems (head and neck problems, optic neuropathy, thrombosis); as well as infections from intravenous use (13).

Neurotoxicity, Neuroprotective Effects

Normal aging processes interact with the neurobiologic systems implicated in drug abuse. Drugs of abuse act on the dopaminergic, serotonergic, and glutamatergic systems of the brain. It has been demonstrated, for example, that both heroin and cocaine reduce the number of dopaminergic receptors in the brain and that these changes persist for significant periods of time after cessation of drug use (14,15). The dopaminergic, serotonergic, and glutamatergic systems also change as part of normal brain aging (16). Changes associated with aging include decreases in dopamine receptor binding in the striatum and in extrastriatal regions (including the frontal cortex, anterior cingulate gyrus, temporal insula, and thalamus) that can affect motor and cognitive functions. The nature of the interactions between aging and drug misuse is an important area for further research.

Aging increases susceptibility to the neurotoxic effects of some illicit drugs, particularly methamphetamine. Aging may compound the effects of methamphetamine-induced neurotoxicity, which is associated with reductions in dopaminergic function. Chronic cocaine use at younger ages can impair the maturation of white matter—myelinated nerve axons—in the brain's temporal and frontal lobes (2). Neural transmission is related to axon diameter and thickness of the myelin sheath, and white matter is thus implicated in higher neurocognitive processing functions. Although more research is needed, cocaine use may exacerbate the loss of white matter volume, which begins to decline around age 50 as part of the natural aging process. Chronic cocaine use results in frequent and persistent hypoperfusion, or reduced cerebral blood flow. This can damage white matter in the brain, impairing normal brain development. Cocaine use is associated with both hemorrhagic and ischemic stroke. These two types of stroke have approximately equal risk of occurring with "crack" cocaine use, but powder cocaine (cocaine hydrochloride) carries a higher risk for hemorrhagic stroke than ischemic stroke. About three quarters of patients with cocaine-induced stroke have no known vascular risk factors. The possible mechanism of action for stroke includes enhanced platelet aggregation, vasospasm, cerebral vasculitis, and cardioembolism. Cocaine is a vasoconstrictor and also disturbs cerebral autoregulation, which can increase the risk of hypertensive surges and vascular rupture (13).

Interaction of Drug Neurotoxicity and Neurology of Aging

Specific drugs may interact with normal aging to increase health risks. Drug pharmacokinetics (the relationship between the drug dose and its concentration in the body) and pharmacodynamics (the relationship between the concentration of a drug in the body and the pharmacologic response to it) change as the body ages (17). Individuals older than 65 react differently to a number of drugs (and to alcohol); of particular note are drugs affecting the central nervous system (CNS), particularly benzodiazepines and opioids. Although the mechanisms for these functional changes are not well understood, it is known that some CNS drugs may penetrate the blood–brain barrier more readily with advancing age, neurotransmitters and receptors change with age, glucose metabolism slows as cerebrovascular function declines, and hormone levels change with age.

Increased Risk of Mortality

Illicit drug use increases several premature death risk factors, and these risk factors tend to increase as an individual ages. Direct risks include the immediate consequences of drug use, including poisoning (overdose) and increased risk of an accident while intoxicated, such as falling or having a traffic accident. Indirect risks include those associated with the illicit nature of drug abuse, including criminal activity, physical trauma, arrest, and incarceration. Indirect risks also include contracting substance abuse–related illnesses, including chronic infectious diseases such as the human immunodeficiency virus (HIV) and hepatitis C, through sharing of unsanitary injection equipment. Smoking is prevalent among those who use illicit drugs and is associated with higher rates of many chronic illnesses (such as cardiovascular disease) as well as cancer.

A 14-year follow-up of a household survey of mental health in Baltimore found that those with a drug dependence diagnosis had nearly a threefold increased risk of death compared with nonusers. Using illicit drugs only a few times (that is, less than five times over a lifetime) was not associated with increased mortality, but exceeding this threshold resulted in a twofold increase in mortality risk (18). The authors estimated that individuals with a drug use disorder died on average 22.5 years earlier than those without such a diagnosis. This is comparable to findings on premature death (defined as death before age 65) in a cohort of 581 heroin addicts followed over a 33-year timespan from 1962 to 1964 to 1996 to 1997. The authors estimated that on average, Whites and Hispanics lost about 19 years, and African Americans about 9 years, to premature death (19). At the end of the 33-year follow-up, 282 subjects (48.5%) had died. The mean age at death was 46.9 years. Overdose deaths, liver disease, and fatal accidents or injuries were the three most frequent causes of premature death.

A longitudinal prospective study of a community sample of adolescents and their fathers found that fathers with a substance use disorder (about 44% of the 769 fathers) had a mortality rate about 2.5 times higher than in fathers with no substance use disorder (20). At death, the mean age of the fathers with substance use disorders was 50.7; most deaths were caused by medical problems rather than drug-related causes.

CHRONIC ILLNESSES AND USE OF MEDICATIONS: IATROGENIC ADDICTION OR ABUSIVE MISUSE

Use of Psychotropic Medications by Older Population

Psychotropic medications are commonly prescribed for older adults. It has been estimated that one third of all such psychotropic medications are prescribed for those aged 65 or older (21). Epidemiologic surveys show that increased age is associated with a higher likelihood of prescriptions for antipsychotics, antidepressants, and/or hypnotics. Women are more likely to be prescribed medications than men. These prescriptions are often for multiple indications and for long periods of time. Older adults are at risk for unintentional or "inadvertent" nonmedical use, which can result in adverse health consequences, toxicity, cognitive impairment, falls, and motor vehicle accidents. Prescription medications may also be misused. The inappropriate use of prescription drugs includes sharing medications, using higher doses for longer durations than prescribed, recreational use, and of course, persistent abuse and dependence (22).

Many psychotropic medications prescribed for older adults, including tricyclic antidepressants and benzodiazepine sedatives, can lead to a variety of cognitive impairments, including effects on attention, executive function, language, memory, and perception (23). Cognitive impairment may be reversible once the drug is discontinued (21). Benzodiazepines, either used by prescription or misused without a prescription, may cause drowsiness or cognitive impairment, increasing the possibility of falling (causing hip and thigh fractures) and of vehicle accidents.

Use of Pain Medications

Opioid analgesics are increasingly prescribed for chronic pain, and there is ongoing concern that opioids prescribed for pain management may evolve into misuse or addiction (24). Persistent pain is common among older patients, including among patients who are dependent on opioids (25). Even patients with a history of substance use disorders are more likely to be prescribed opioid medications for pain than in past years (26).

Patients prescribed opioid medications are at higher risk for opioid misuse problems, especially patients with co-occurring depressive and anxiety disorders (27). Pain can be treated successfully using opioid medications, but physicians must balance the risks and benefits of pain medication (28,29).

Pain medicine physicians would benefit from better screening methods, better ways to recognize and intervene if opioid treatment for pain shifts from benefit to harm, and better ways to screen for co-occurring mental disorders such as depression. Passik, Kirsh, and Casper provide a review of instruments that might be useful for screening pain patients (30).

A number of tools have been developed to evaluate the risk of opioid misuse with chronic pain patients. Examples include the DIRE (Diagnosis, Intractability, Risk, and Efficacy) Score for rating patient suitability for long-term opioid analgesic treatment (31), the Screener and Opioid Assessment of Pain Patients-Revised (SOAPP-R) (32), and the STOPP (Screening Tool of Older Person's Prescriptions) (33). Of these, only the STOPP was developed specifically for older patients. The STOPP is comprehensive and covers potentially inappropriate prescribing for several of the body's systems, including the cardiovascular, central nervous, gastrointestinal, respiratory, musculoskeletal, urogenital, and endocrine systems. Sections that may be of particular interest with regard to potential drug problems include use of analgesic medications, drugs that adversely affect those at risk of falling, and identification of duplicate drug classes.

Medications and Interactions with Illicit Substances

Aging results in a progressive decline in the functional reserve of body organs and physiologic systems. Drug effects, both medical and nonmedical, can be altered by the effects of aging, including delayed renal excretion, delayed gastrointestinal absorption, increased body fat and decreased proportion of body water, and reduced basal metabolic rate (34,35). There is a decline in the functionality of the circulatory, gastrointestinal, and hepatic systems. Older adults are also much more likely to suffer from chronic illnesses such as diabetes, cardiovascular diseases, and hypertension. These diseases may have a greater impact than age per se on the level of impairment in body system functionality.

Physiologic changes associated with aging can alter drug metabolism and drug pharmacokinetics. With aging, the metabolism of many drugs is slowed, increasing their bioavailability compared to physiologically younger individuals (36). This reduced drug tolerance can contribute to accidental drug overdose or adverse drug interactions in older adults. Older adults may also reduce their level of use since the effects of illicit drug and alcohol use persist for longer periods.

Older adults are more likely to suffer from a variety of chronic physical and mental disorders than younger adults, and this likelihood increases with age. A study of a national random sample of 1.2 million Medicare beneficiaries found that 65% had multiple chronic conditions. It is estimated that prescription medications are used by 60% to 78% of older adults. Individuals 65 and older consume about 30% of all prescription medications (37). Although it has been suggested that the most common type of drug misuse is underuse, polypharmacy—prescribing multiple medications—is also common for older patients. Since the likelihood of adverse drug interactions increases with the number of medications prescribed, older adults are more susceptible to adverse drug effects simply because they are prescribed more medications than younger adults. In a sample of 626 Iowa Medicare beneficiaries, over half had received at least one potentially inappropriate medication, including drugs contraindicated for older patients, drug–drug interactions, drug–disease interactions, and therapeutic duplications (38). Those with inappropriate medication use were twice as likely to report having experienced an adverse drug effect in the past year compared with patients who had no inappropriate use. However, determining the optimal prescription of medications for older adults is complex, and the various approaches that have been tested to improve prescribing practices have met with mixed success (39).

The number of prescribed psychotropic medications (antidepressants, antipsychotics, mood stabilizers, and sedative-hypnotics) has trended upward over time. Data from the National Ambulatory Medical Care Surveys show an increase in visits with two or more psychotropic medications from 42.6% in 1996 to 1997 to 59.8% in 2005 to 2006 (40). Individuals aged 45 to 64 were more likely to be prescribed two or more of these types of medications than either younger or older patients, and were also more likely to be prescribed combinations of antidepressants + antipsychotics and antidepressants + sedative-hypnotics. Multiple drug prescriptions over long periods of time and from multiple providers increase the chance of adverse drug interactions. Adverse drug interactions are more likely for older adults because of a higher level of prescribed drugs, more psychotropic drugs prescribed (especially for women), and changing pharmacokinetics, physiology, and neurophysiology in older adults (41). Drug misuse—using medications in ways other than prescribed, sharing medications, using higher doses or using for longer durations than prescribed, and of course, recreational use or abuse—can result in harmful interactions between illicit drugs and prescribed drugs. Drug or alcohol misuse may also impair the patient's ability to adhere to prescribed medications.

Many older adults drink, some in excess of recommended limits. While not a focus of this chapter, it must be noted that alcohol interacts adversely with many prescribed medications. Acute alcohol use can inhibit hepatic enzyme production, prolonging drug bioavailability and increasing potentially adverse side effects. Conversely, the efficacy of many oral medications is reduced when they are consumed with substances (including chronic alcohol use, tobacco, and barbiturates) that induce the production of liver and lower intestine enzymes, which speed medication metabolism (36,42). Alcohol use is contraindicated for a large number of prescribed and over-the-counter medications, including antihistamines; anti-infectives; antineoplastics; autonomic drugs; many cardiovascular drugs; many CNS drugs; electrolytic agents; antitussives; eye, ear, nose, and throat drugs; gastrointestinal drugs; hormones; antidiabetic drugs; and smooth muscle relaxants (43). In addition to altered efficacy, bioavailability, and drug or alcohol metabolism, adverse outcomes can include liver toxicity, gastrointestinal inflammation or bleeding, sedation and delirium, and disulfiram-like reactions (44).

Symptoms of substance abuse in the older patient may include confusion, fatigue, irritability, insomnia, forgetfulness, or emotional instability. These symptoms may be mistaken for conditions common in old age, presenting the potential

TABLE 58.1 Warning signs for prescription drug abuse

Patient behavior	Comment/example
Overreporting symptoms	Drug-seeking behavior to obtain prescriptions for controlled medications[a]
Multiple or vague somatic complaints	Pain of unclear origin, anxiety, insomnia
Insistence on specific medications	More concerned about the drug than the complaint
Refusal of generic equivalents	Trade-name prescription drugs more valuable than generics when diverted
Arguments about pharmacology	Display of sophisticated knowledge of particular drugs
Insistence on controlled prescriptions on first visit	Visit to emergency department rather than primary physician
Flattery or veiled threats followed by prescription request	"You are the only one who can help me"
Symptom complexes that seem to indicate need for multiple controlled drugs	Diagnostic/symptomatic criteria for two or more controlled drug prescriptions are rare
Self-asserted multiple medication sensitivities or high tolerance	"It is the only thing that works …"
Scams to obtain prescriptions or refills, more potent or higher formulations, or controlled drug alternatives	"Lost" prescriptions or medications; "the dog ate it"; "but you filled it before …"; prescription alterations or forgeries
Obtaining prescriptions for controlled drugs from two or more physicians	"Doctor shopping" to obtain prescription drugs; calling clinic after hours or when primary physician is unavailable

[a]Controlled drugs most often implicated in prescription abuse include opioid analgesics, benzodiazepines, stimulants, barbiturates, and sedative-hypnotics.
Data from Ref. (45) and Isaacson et al. (46).

for misdiagnosis and inappropriate prescribing. Patients may play an active role in medication misuse. The prescription medications that are most likely to be intentionally misused or abused by older adults include sedative-hypnotics (benzodiazepines and barbiturates), anxiolytics, and opioid analgesics. These medications are often prescribed for insomnia, anxiety, and chronic pain, which are conditions common in older patients (42). In turn, older patients may seek to take these because of their psychoactive effects (that is, reinforcement and reward). Prescribing clinicians should closely monitor the patient for adverse side effects, inappropriate use, or use of medications for longer periods or in higher dosages than planned. Parran (45) cautions that clinicians should be alert to strategies that drug-dependent patients may use to obtain prescribed medications (Table 58.1). He catalogs a variety of these drug-seeking behaviors; examples include insistence on specific medications (particularly on the first visit); reporting vague symptom complexes involving pain, anxiety, and insomnia; and overreporting of multiple somatic symptoms. Parran also provides guidance for physicians who encounter a patient engaging in drug-seeking behavior. Clinicians should not underestimate the importance of family members; particularly if they are in caregiver roles, they may be able to provide information about their elders' history and status with regard to substance abuse, addiction, and drug-seeking behavior.

HIV, Aging, and Drug Abuse

HIV, the virus that causes AIDS, is most commonly contracted through sexual contact with an infected individual or through sharing contaminated syringes or other injection drug use components. Until about 1995, adults over the age of 50 comprised about 10% of the cumulative number of AIDS cases, but the number of newly diagnosed HIV infections among older adults has increased in recent years (47).

In 2005, about 19% of newly diagnosed AIDS cases were 50 or older. Given the relatively long latency period of AIDS, it is likely that many individuals live with undetected HIV infection for a number of years, and HIV infection is diagnosed only when symptoms begin to appear in later years. It is also likely that some of the increase in new cases results from higher HIV testing rates, following the revised recommendations of the U.S. Centers for Disease Control and Prevention (CDC) (48). The CDC estimated that in 2006, about 10% individuals with HIV were age 50 or older when they were infected (49).

It is estimated that by 2015 about half of all HIV-seropositive individuals will be 50 or older (50). The HIV exposure category of injection drug use has declined from its peak in the mid-1990s. In the nationally representative HIV Cost and Service Utilization Study (HCSUS), 23% of HIV cases in those over 50 were attributed to injection drug use (51). As the baby boom cohort ages, the number of adults over 50 with an injection drug use history can also be expected to increase (52). Older adults who use illicit drugs appear to be less likely to engage in risky injection drug use behavior than those under age 50, but they appear to be as likely as their younger counterparts to engage in risky sexual behavior (53). However, because of medical advances in the prevention and treatment of HIV infection, older adults who began heroin use in their later years appear to be at lower risk for HIV and other health disorders than those who began using heroin before age 30.

Although individuals with treated HIV are living longer as a result of advances in antiretroviral treatment, the time from HIV infection to the development of AIDS decreases with age, and HIV can accelerate the development of many age-related chronic illnesses. Older patients with HIV are more likely to report symptoms such as weight or hair loss and peripheral neuropathy, but may underreport other symptoms, including headaches, depression, white oral patches, and diarrhea (54). Compared with whites, older nonwhites may underreport HIV symptoms (54). Older patients tend to have better adherence to antiretroviral treatment, but CD4+ T cell restoration and immune recovery are poorer in older patients. Among those with HIV diagnoses, age and injection drug use appear to contribute independently to increased mortality measured as average years of life lost compared to life expectancies among similar individuals in the general population (55).

For a number of reasons, HIV-infected injection drug users are less likely to be prescribed antiretroviral therapy than nondrug users. Some research suggests that while older patients have better adherence to HIV medications than younger patients, ongoing illicit drug use has been associated with lower rates of antiretroviral adherence. Hinkin et al. (56) found that about half of the patients older than 50 achieved 95% adherence to highly active antiretroviral therapy (HAART), compared with only about a quarter of the younger patients. Neurocognitive impairment, which may be related both to aging and to AIDS, reduces the likelihood of good adherence and may be a more important determinant of adherence than ongoing drug use (57). Many older drug users also have hepatitis C, acquired through injection drug use or other risky behavior in prior years (58). Antiretroviral therapy can interact with methadone medication, and while more study is needed, there is some indication that HAART may increase the risk of hepatic failure and cirrhosis in those coinfected with HIV and hepatitis (59). Despite concerns about treating HIV-infected drug users, mortality rates in patients on HAART do not appear to be associated with a history of injection drug use (60).

TREATING SUBSTANCE ABUSE IN OLDER ADULTS

The number of individuals 50 and older admitted to drug abuse treatment in 2007 (208,910, or 11.5%) was more than double the number admitted in 1992 (102,705, or 6.6%). Alcohol, long the primary problem at treatment admission among older adults, has been supplanted as the primary problem by drugs alone and by combined drugs and alcohol for those aged 50 and older (Fig. 58.1) (11). Based on a household survey of drug use in the general (noninstitutionalized) population, it was estimated that about 4.4 million individuals 50 years or older would need treatment for drug or alcohol abuse in 2020 (61). A national survey of drug abuse treatment services for older adults found that about 18% of the 13,749 responding facilities were designed for older adults (those aged 65 or more). These tended to be associated with hospitals, especially those with psychiatric inpatient units. The number of these facilities in the states was lower than the need based on the size of the state's older population (62).

Screening and Assessment

Screening for substance use disorders is an important first step in identifying the need for preventive interventions or drug treatment in older adults. Many symptoms of substance abuse and withdrawal (such as mild cognitive impairment, irregular heartbeat, and tremor) are seen in many aging individuals. It is important for medical providers to have a high "index of suspicion" and to understand the symptoms of substance abuse and dependence in order to be able to properly diagnose, treat, and refer the older patient.

There are a number of instruments to screen and assess alcohol and drug use disorders in the general population, but many of these have shortcomings that limit their utility for clinical applications, and few have been validated for use with older adults. The Michigan Alcohol Screening Test—Geriatric Version (MAST-G) (63) and the CAGE (64) are two screening tools that have been tested with older populations. The MAST-G is a 24-item screener for alcohol problems that has good psychometric properties. A shorter, 10-item version (the SMAST-G) is also available (65). Although there is a parallel drug abuse version of the MAST, no version of the Drug Abuse Screening Test (DAST) (66) has been developed for the older individual.

The CAGE is a four-item screener that has been tested in clinical substance abuse treatment patients aged 50 and older (67). The CAGE-AID version (CAGE-Adapted to Include Drugs) (68) has four items: (a) Have you felt you should Cut down on your drinking or drug use? (b) Have people Annoyed you by criticizing your drinking or drug use? (c) Have you ever felt bad or Guilty about your drinking or drug use? and (d) Have you ever had a drink or used drugs first thing in the morning (Eye-opener) to steady your nerves or to get rid of a hangover? Its reviewers suggest that the specificity of the instrument may be improved for the older patient by omitting the first, "cut down," item (67).

The Alcohol, Smoking and Substance Involvement Screening Test (ASSIST) was developed by the World Health Organization to identify substance use problems in primary care settings. The ASSIST compares favorably with a number of drug abuse screening tools in samples from several countries (69), but it has not been validated on adults older than 45 years.

Current standardized criteria for diagnosing substance use disorders were developed and validated using young and middle-aged populations. They may not be appropriate for older or elderly populations because the diagnostic criteria are oriented toward adverse consequences in a younger population (70). Diagnostic criteria based on failure to meet role obligations or adverse social, legal, or interpersonal consequences may miss older adults with substance use disorders. Older and elderly adults are more likely to be socially isolated and are less likely to be employed, married, have minor children, or have legal involvement. The criteria for increased tolerance leading to increased levels of consumption do not consider the pharmacodynamic changes that lower drug tolerance in the elderly (71). Tolerance or withdrawal symptoms may not create problems for individuals who do not have major role obligations and whose performance is therefore not closely observed. Drug and alcohol abuse and dependence rates are often very low in the older population. In the National Comorbidity Survey-Revision (NCS-R), a nationally representative sample of community-dwelling adults, only 1.5% of those aged 45 to 64 had a substance abuse disorder in the year preceding the NCS-R interview, and virtually no one aged 65 and older in this survey met criteria for past-year drug abuse (72). Rates for lifetime drug abuse were 6.0% in the 45 to 64 year age group and near zero for those 65 or older. (Dependence rates were not reported in this study because of a controversial decision to skip collection of dependence criteria unless at least one abuse criterion was reported.) Medical and psychiatric problems are more common consequences of drug misuse in the older adult (73). Thus, for the older patient, clinicians may be advised to pay more attention to quantity and frequency of use than to diagnostic cutoff scores for abuse or dependence (74).

Prevention of Illness

Drug abuse treatment can be considered primary prevention because it reduces the incidence of chronic illnesses associated with misuse of drugs. For example, for those 50 years and above, smoking cessation interventions are primary prevention: they can increase longevity and, by avoiding the cost of treating chronic illness associated with smoking, can also reduce health care costs over the life of the individual. Models of smoking cessation suggest that it could add over 3 years to life depending on the effectiveness of the smoking cessation intervention (75).

Access to Medical Care

Because of illnesses associated with aging, the older drug abuser often has a connection with a primary care provider. This medical provider can play an important role in screening, diagnosing, and assessing substance use disorders, and in recommending and referring the patient to appropriate treatment. It is also important for physicians to recognize the risk of prescription drug abuse in their elderly patients (76).

Older Offenders

Criminal justice involvement is common among users of illicit drugs, including older adults. About a quarter of older adults admitted to treatment are referred by the criminal justice system (77). Approximately half of the individuals incarcerated in jails, state prisons, or federal correctional institutions meet criteria for drug abuse or dependence (78). In the 2008 National Survey of Drug Use and Health, a survey of the civilian noninstitutionalized population, it was estimated that over 18% of adults on parole/supervised release and about 24% of those on probation were current illicit drug users (1). These rates compare with about 7.5% of the adult population not under criminal justice supervision who were current illicit drug users.

Like the general population, the offender population is aging. From 1992 to 2001, the number of state and federal inmates aged 50 or older increased by over 170%, from 41,586 to 113,358. At least one state (Florida) has established a prison for geriatric inmates. Apart from demographic trends, this increase in the number of older offenders stems from stricter laws mandating long-term determinate sentencing for certain felonies and offender classes such as substance abusers, and the elimination of parole at the federal level and in many states.

It has been estimated that about 70% of older offenders—those aged 50 or older—have a substance use disorder. Alcohol-only disorders are more common among older inmates. Relatively few older inmates have received drug abuse treatment (79). Although some correctional administrators suggest that incarceration speeds the aging process and the general deterioration of health, others suggest that the prevalence of health problems among older inmates is similar to or only somewhat higher than those of the aging adult in the general population. These problems include dementia, cancer, stroke, incontinence, arthritis, ulcers, hypertension, chronic respiratory ailments, chronic gastrointestinal problems, prostate problems, heart disease, and deteriorating kidney functions (80). Higher rates of offender health problems may, in part, be attributed to the long-term consequences of smoking, drug and alcohol use, and other risky and unhealthy behaviors (81).

Treatment Outcomes

Despite earlier concerns that elderly substance abuse patients might not fare well in treatment (70), many recent studies have found that older patients in treatment for substance use disorders have outcomes that are similar to or better than those of younger patients (82,83). Patients aged 55 or older do have more medical problems than younger patients, but they may have better substance abuse outcomes and comparable or better levels of functioning in mental health, family, and legal domains.

Older adults treated in the private health care system may have more favorable treatment outcomes than younger adults (84). At 5 years posttreatment, 52% of adults over 55 years of age (older adults) in a private managed care program reported total abstinence in the month prior to the interview, compared to 40% of younger adults (those aged 18 to 39). Older adults also had significantly longer periods of total abstinence, averaging nearly 2 years, compared with 1.33 years for younger adults. Older adults tended to stay in treatment longer and to have a social support network that discouraged substance abuse. Older women had somewhat more favorable outcomes than older men (or younger women), but this was explained in part by their better retention in treatment.

The service needs of methadone patients change with age. A clinical sample of methadone maintenance patients over the age of 50 ($N = 140$) was studied to determine their physical and mental health status (85). Over half the sample indicated having a mental health problem in the past year, with the most common being major depressive episode, generalized anxiety disorder, and posttraumatic stress disorder. Physical health problems were found as well; over half the sample indicated their health was fair or poor. Common complaints included arthritis and hypertension. Drug treatment may reduce medical and lifestyle risk factors associated with illicit drug use in the older patient, but older drug treatment patients may still have a higher incidence of chronic illness and other lifestyle risk factors compared to the general population (86).

SUMMARY

An increasing overall population of older Americans combined with an increasing prevalence of drug abuse and addiction in this population suggests the need for greater clinical attention to the drug abuse–related problems of aging. Specific concerns are especially rooted in the interaction of drugs of abuse with an aging body. The normal complexities and consequences of aging are accentuated in the face of drug abuse and addiction. Clinicians will need to increase their vigilance about drug abuse and addiction in their older patients.

REFERENCES

1. Substance Abuse and Mental Health Services Administration. Office of Applied Studies. *Results from the 2008 National Survey on Drug Use and Health: National Findings.* Rockville, MD: US Department of Health and Human Services; 2009. Available at: www.samhsa.gov. Accessed June 2010.
2. Bartzokis G, Beckson M, Lu PH, et al. Brain maturation may be arrested in chronic cocaine addicts. *Biol Psychiatry.* 2002;51(8):605–611.
3. Fein G, Di Sclafani V. Cerebral reserve capacity: implications for alcohol and drug abuse. *Alcohol.* 2004;32(1):63–67.
4. Colliver JD, Compton WC, Gfroerer JC, et al. Projecting drug use among aging baby boomers in 2020. *Ann Epidemiol.* 2006;16:257–265.
5. Christensen K, Doblhammer G, Rau R, et al. Ageing populations: the challenges ahead. *Lancet.* 2009;374(9696):1196–1208.
6. Han B, Gfroerer JC, Colliver JD. *OAS Data Review: An Examination of Trends in Illicit Drug Use among Adults Aged 50 to 59 in the United States.* Rockville, MD: US Department of Health and Human Services; 2009. Available at: www.samhsa.gov. Accessed June 2010.
7. Armstrong GL. Injection drug users in the United States 1979–2002–an aging population. *Arch Intern Med.* 2007;167(2):166–173.
8. Degenhardt L, Chiu WT, Sampson N, et al. Epidemiological patterns of extra-medical drug use in the United States: evidence from the national Comorbidity Survey Replication, 2001–2003. *Drug Alcohol Depend.* 2007;90(2–3):210–223.
9. Huang BJ, Dawson DA, Stinson FS, et al. Prevalence, correlates, and comorbidity of nonmedical prescription drug use and drug use disorders in the United States: results of the National Epidemiologic Survey on Alcohol and Related Conditions. *J Clin Psychiatry.* 2006;67(7):1062–1073.
10. United States Department of Health and Human Services. Substance Abuse and Mental Health Services Administration, Office of Applied Studies. *Treatment Episode Data Set–Admissions (TEDS-A), 2007* [Computer file]. ICPSR24280-v3. Ann Arbor, MI: Inter-university Consortium for Political and Social Research; 2009. Available at: www.icpsr.umich.edu/SAMHDA. Accessed June 2010.
11. Lofwall MR, Schuster A, Strain EC. Changing profile of abused substance by older persons entering treatment. *J Nerv Ment Dis.* 2008;196:898–905.
12. Han B, Gfroerer JC, Colliver JD, et al. Substance use disorder among older adults in the United States in 2020. *Addiction.* 2009;104(1):88–96.
13. Treadwell SD, Robinson TG. Cocaine use and stroke. *Postgrad Med J.* 2007;83(980):389–394.
14. Koob GF, Volkow ND. Neurocircuitry of addiction. *Neuropsychopharmacology.* 2010;35(1):217–238.
15. Volkow ND, Hitzemann R, Wang GJ, et al. Long-term frontal brain metabolic changes in cocaine abusers. *Synapse.* 1992;11(3):184–190.
16. Dowling GJ, Weiss SRB, Condon TP. Drugs of abuse and the aging brain. *Neuropsychopharmacology.* 2008;33(2):209–218.
17. Bowie MW, Slattum PW. Pharmacodynamics in older adults: a review. *Am J Geriatr Pharmacother.* 2007;5(3):263–303.
18. Neumark YD, Van Etten ML, Anthony JC. "Drug dependence" and death: survival analysis of the Baltimore ECA sample from 1981 to 1995. *Subst Use Misuse.* 2000;35(3):313–327.
19. Smyth B, Hoffman V, Fan J, et al. Years of potential life lost among heroin addicts 33 years after treatment. *Prev Med.* 2007;44(4):369–374.

20. Cornelius JR, Reynolds M, Martz BM, et al. Premature mortality among males with substance use disorders. *Addict Behav*. 2008; 33(1):156–160.
21. National Institute on Drug Abuse. *Prescription Drugs–Abuse and Addiction. Research Report Series*. Rockville, MD: U.S. Department of Health and Human Services; 2005. Available at: www.drugabuse.gov. Accessed June 2010.
22. Simoni-Wastila L, Yang HK. Psychoactive drug abuse in older adults. *Am J Geriatr Pharmacother*. 2006;4(4):380–394.
23. Brooks JO, Hoblyn JC. Neurocognitive costs and benefits of psychotropic medications in older adults. *J Geriatr Psychiatry Neurol*. 2007;20(4):199–214.
24. Denisco RA, Chandler RK, Compton WM. Addressing the intersecting problems of opioid misuse and chronic pain treatment. *Exp Clin Psychopharmacol*. 2008;16(5):417–428.
25. Rosenblum A, Joseph H, Fong C, et al. Prevalence and characteristics of chronic pain among chemically dependent patients in methadone maintenance and residential treatment facilities. *JAMA*. 2003;289(18):2370–2378.
26. Weisner CM, Campbell CI, Ray GT, et al. Trends in prescribed opioid therapy for non-cancer pain for individuals with prior substance use disorders. *Pain*. 2009;145(3):287–293.
27. Edlund MJ, Sullivan M, Steffick D, et al. Do users of regularly prescribed opioids have higher rates of substance use problems than nonusers? *Pain Med*. 2007;8(8):647–656.
28. Ballantyne JC, LaForge KS. Opioid dependence and addiction during opioid treatment of chronic pain. *Pain*. 2007;129(3): 235–255.
29. Gallagher RM, Rosenthal LJ. Chronic pain and opiates: balancing pain control and risks in long-term opioid treatment. *Arch Phys Med Rehabil*. 2008;89(suppl 1):S77–S82.
30. Passik SD, Kirsh KL, Casper D. Addiction-related assessment tools and pain management: instruments for screening treatment planning and monitoring compliance. *Pain Med*. 2008; 9(suppl 2):S145–S166.
31. Belgrade MJ, Schamber CD, Lindgren BR. The DIRE Score: predicting outcomes of opioid prescribing for chronic pain. *J Pain*. 2006;7(9):671–681.
32. Butler SF, Budman SH, Fernandez KC, et al. Cross-validation of a screener to predict opioid misuse in chronic pain patients (SOAPP-R). *J Addict Med*. 2009;3(2):66–73.
33. Gallagher P, O'Mahony D. STOPP (Screening Tool of Older Persons' potentially inappropriate Prescriptions): application to acutely ill elderly patients and comparison with Beers' criteria. *Age Ageing*. 2008;37(6):673–679.
34. Raffoul PR, Cooper JK, Love DW. Drug misuse in older-people. *Gerontologist*. 1981;21(2):146–150.
35. Klotz U. Pharmacokinetics and drug metabolism in the elderly. *Drug Metab Rev*. 2009;41(2):67–76.
36. Herrlinger C, Klotz U. Drug metabolism and drug interactions in the elderly. *Best Pract Res Clin Gastroenterol*. 2001;15(6):897–918.
37. Williams CM. Using medications appropriately in older adults. *Am Fam Physician*. 2002;66(10):1917–1924.
38. Chrischilles EA, VanGilder R, Wright K, et al. Inappropriate medication use as a risk factor for self-reported adverse drug effects in older adults. *J Am Geriatr Soc*. 2009;57(6):1000–1006.
39. Spinewine A, Schmader KE, Barber N, et al. Appropriate prescribing in elderly people: how well can it be measured and optimised? *Lancet*. 2007;370(9582):173–184.
40. Mojtabai R, Olfson M. National trends in psychotropic medication polypharmacy in office-based psychiatry. *Arch Gen Psychiatry*. 2010;67(1):26–36.
41. Mallet L, Spinewine A, Huang A. The challenge of managing drug interactions in elderly people. *Lancet*. 2007;370(9582): 185–191.
42. Reid MC, Anderson PA. Geriatric substance use disorders. *Med Clin N Am*. 1997;81(4):999–1016.
43. Pringle KE, Ahern FM, Heller DA, et al. Potential for alcohol and prescription drug interactions in older people. *J Am Geriatr Soc*. 2005;53(11):1930–1936.
44. Adams WL. Interactions between alcohol and other drugs. *Int J Addict*. 1995;30(13–14):1903–1923.
45. Parran T. Prescription drug abuse–a question of balance. *Med Clin N Am*. 1997;81(4):967–978.
46. Isaacson JH, Hopper JA, Alford DP, et al. Prescription drug use and abuse: Risk factors, red flags, and prevention strategies. *Postgrad Med*. 2005;118(1):19–26.
47. Mack KA, Ory MG. AIDS and older Americans at the end of the twentieth century. *J Acquir Immune Defic Syndr*. 2003;33(suppl 2): S68–S75.
48. Centers for Disease Control and Prevention. Revised recommendations for HIV testing of adults, adolescents, and pregnant women in health-care settings. *MMWR*. 2006;55(RR-14):1–17.
49. Centers for Disease Control and Prevention. *HIV/AIDS Surveillance Report, 2007*. Vol 19. Atlanta, GA: U.S. Department of Health and Human Services, Centers for Disease Control and Prevention; 2009. Available at: www.cdc.gov/hiv/topics/surveillance/resources/reports/. Accessed June 2010.
50. Effros RB, Fletcher CV, Gebo K, et al. Workshop on HIV infection and aging: what is known and future research directions. *Clin Infect Dis*. 2008;47(4):542–553.
51. Zingmond DS, Wenger NS, Crystal S, et al. Circumstances at HIV diagnosis and progression of disease in older HIV-infected Americans. *Am J Public Health*. 2001;91(7):1117–1120.
52. Lieb S, Rosenberg R, Arons P, et al. Age shift in patterns of injection drug use among the HIV/AIDS population in Miami-Dade County, Florida. *Subst Use Misuse*. 2006;41(10–12):1623–1635.
53. Kwiatkowski CF, Booth RE. HIV risk behaviors among older American drug users. *J Acquir Immune Defic Syndr*. 2003; 33(suppl 2):S131–S137.
54. Zingmond DS, Kilbourne AM, Justice AC, et al. Differences in symptom expression in older HIV-positive patients: the veterans aging cohort 3 site study and HIV cost and service utilization study experience. *J Acquir Immune Defic Syndr*. 2003;33 (suppl 2):S84–S92.
55. Harrison KM, Song R, Zhang X. Life expectancy after HIV diagnosis based on national HIV surveillance data from 25 states, United States. *J Acquir Immune Defic Syndr*. 2010;53: 124–130.
56. Hinkin CH, Hardy DJ, Mason KI, et al. Medication adherence in HIV-infected adults: effect of patient age, cognitive status, and substance abuse. *AIDS*. 2004;18(suppl 1):S19–S25.
57. Ettenhofer ML, Hinkin CH, Castellon SA, et al. Aging, neurocognition, and medication adherence in HIV infection. *Am J Geriat Psychiatry*. 2009;17(4):281–290.
58. Dienstag JL. Hepatitis C: a bitter harvest. *Ann Intern Med*. 2006; 144:770–771.
59. Neuman MG, Monteiro M, Rehm J. Drug interactions between psychoactive substances and antiretroviral therapy in individuals infected with human immunodeficiency and hepatitis viruses. *Subst Use Misuse*. 2006;41(10–12):1395–1463.
60. Wood E, Hogg RS, Lima VD, et al. Highly active antiretroviral therapy and survival in HIV-infected injection drug users. *JAMA*. 2008;300(5):550–554.

61. Gfroerer J, Penne M, Pemberton M, et al. Substance abuse treatment need among older adults in 2020: the impact of the aging baby-boom cohort. *Drug Alcohol Depend.* 2003;69(2):127–135.
62. Schultz SK, Arndt S, Liesveld J. Locations of facilities with special programs for older substance abuse clients in the US. *Int J Geriatr Psychiatry.* 2003;18(9):839–843.
63. Blow FC, Brower KJ, Schulenberg JE, et al. The Michigan Alcohol Screening Test–Geriatric Version (MAST-G): a new elderly specific screening instrument. *Alcohol Clin Exp Res.* 1992;16(2):372.
64. Ewing JA. Detecting alcoholism: the CAGE questionnaire. *JAMA.* 1984;252(14):1905–1907.
65. Johnson-Greene D, McCaul ME, Roger P. Screening for hazardous drinking using the Michigan Alcohol Screening Test–Geriatric Version (MAST-G) in elderly persons with acute cerebrovascular accidents. *Alcohol Clin Exp Res.* 2009;33(9):1555–1561.
66. Skinner HA. The drug abuse screening test. *Addict Behav.* 1982;7(4):363–371.
67. Hinkin CH, Castellon SA, Dickson-Fuhrman E, et al. Screening for drug and alcohol abuse among older adults using a modified version of the CAGE. *Am J Addict.* 2001;10(4):319–326.
68. Brown RL, Rounds LA. Conjoint screening questionnaires for alcohol and other drug abuse: criterion validity in a primary care practice. *Wisc Med J.* 1995;94(3):135–140.
69. Humeniuk R, Ali R, Babor TF, et al. Validation of the alcohol, smoking and substance involvement screening test (ASSIST). *Addiction.* 2008;103(6):1039–1047.
70. Patterson TL, Jeste DV. The potential impact of the baby-boom generation on substance abuse among elderly persons. *Psychiatry Serv.* 1999;50(9):1184–1188.
71. Jeste DV, Blazer DG, First M. Aging-related diagnostic variations: need for diagnostic criteria appropriate for elderly psychiatric patients. *Biol Psychiatry.* 2005;58(4):265–271.
72. Gum AM, King-Kallimanis B, Kohn R. Prevalence of mood, anxiety, and substance-abuse disorders for older Americans in the National Comorbidity Survey Replication. *Am J Geriatr Psychiatry.* 2009;17(9):769–781.
73. Miller NS, Belkin BM, Gold MS. Alcohol and drug-dependence among the elderly–epidemiology diagnosis and treatment. *Compr Psychiatry.* 1991;32(2):153–165.
74. King CJ, Van Hasselt VB, Segal DL, et al. Diagnosis and assessment of substance-abuse in older adults: current strategies and issues. *Addict Behav.* 1994;19(1):41–55.
75. Goldman DP, Zheng Y, Girosi F, et al. The benefits of risk factor prevention in Americans aged 51 years and older. *Am J Public Health.* 2009;99(11):2096–2101.
76. Morgan M, Brosi WA. Prescription drug abuse among older adults: a family ecological case study. *J Appl Gerontol.* 2007;26(5):419–432.
77. Substance Abuse and Mental Health Services Administration. Office of Applied Studies. *The DASIS Report: Adults Aged 65 or Older in Substance Abuse Treatment: 2005.* Rockville, MD: U.S. Department of Health and Human Services, 2007. Available at: www.samhsa.gov. Accessed June 2010.
78. Chandler RK, Fletcher BW, Volkow ND. Treating drug abuse and addiction in the criminal justice system: improving public health and safety. *JAMA.* 2009;301(2):183–190.
79. Arndt S, Turvey CL, Flaum M. Older offenders, substance abuse, and treatment. *Am J Geriatr Psychiatry.* 2002;10(6):733–739.
80. Reimer G. The graying of the U.S. prisoner population. *J Correct Health Care.* 2008;14(3):202–208.
81. Kuhlmann R, Ruddell R. Elderly jail inmates: problems, prevalence and public health. *Californian J Health Promot.* 2005;3(2): 49–60.
82. Brennan PL, Nichol AC, Moos RH. Older and younger patients with substance use disorders: outpatient mental health service use and functioning over a 12-month interval. *Psychol Addict Behav.* 2003;17(1):42–48.
83. Firoz S, Carlson G. Characteristics and treatment outcome of older methadone-maintenance patients. *Am J Geriatr Psychiatry.* 2004;12(5):539–541.
84. Satre DD, Mertens JR, Arean PA, et al. Five-year alcohol and drug treatment outcomes of older adults versus middle-aged and younger adults in a managed care program. *Addiction.* 2004;99(10):1286–1297.
85. Rosen D, Smith ML, Reynolds CF. The prevalence of mental and physical health disorders among older methadone patients. *Am J Geriatr Psychiatry.* 2008;16(6):488–497.
86. Fareed A, Casarella J, Amar R, et al. Benefits of retention in methadone maintenance and chronic medical conditions as risk factors for premature death among older heroin addicts. *J Psychiatr Pract.* 2009;15(3):227–234.

SECTION 10 ■ SPECIAL POPULATIONS

CHAPTER 59 — African Americans: Alcohol and Substance Abuse

William B. Lawson ■ Jessica Herrera ■ Robert G. Lawson

INTRODUCTION

Alcohol and drugs of abuse are popular and their related disorders are common, as noted in other chapters in this volume. They are a source of substantial health care costs, morbidity, and mortality (1). The neurobiologic factors, psychological factors, and socioeconomic conditions that contribute to their widespread use and destructive capacity are well documented. These issues are true for the African American community, but there are unique factors that exacerbate both their use and outcomes. The problem of health disparities for African Americans is well documented. The Surgeon General's Report noted that African Americans had significantly greater morbidity and mortality for general medical conditions and added mental and substance abuse disorders to that list (1,2). The disparity in the prevalence of substance abuse disorders appeared to be a consequence of socioeconomic factors, lifestyle, and the disparities in care from limited access to information and services (1). In a supplement, *Mental Health: Culture, Race, and Ethnicity,* they reaffirmed these findings for mental and substance abuse disorders for racial and ethnic minorities. These and subsequent reports showed that African Americans often always were more likely to have these disorders, but not consistently so. However, they reliably carried a greater disease burden that was often a consequence of limited access to services (2,3). We will show that the life experiences and culture of the African American community both protect against and exacerbate the risk of substance abuse. However, cultural factors, limited access to services, and a focus on a correctional approach have led to a greater individual and community burden. This burden extends beyond the substance abusers and impacts others through family disintegration, loss of employment, failure in school, domestic violence, child abuse, and other crimes (3). Moreover, mental disorders are often undertreated and unrecognized in the African American community (4). The combination of mental disorders and substance abuse reinforces the consequences and risk of both conditions and worsens the outcome. Substance abuse is known to contribute to general medical disorders (1). Many of the disparities in health in general are to a large part due to substance abuse. Finally, some individuals face a triple whammy: mental disorders, substance abuse, and chronic disease burden with such disorders as AIDS. These individuals are all too common and greatly strain the service delivery system and community burden.

We will discuss the pervasive impact of substance abuse and show its effect on social forces and health issues that extend beyond the individual and often the African American community. We will also discuss the development of new prevention and treatment approaches that when available show great promise in addressing substance abuse. The result may be a reduction in the health disparities seen in African Americans, and moreover, these treatments not only impact substance abuse, but also provide hope for many of the disorders that disproportionately kill African Americans.

Sociocultural Factors

Clearly, socioeconomic factors are important. Substance abuse costs the country over half a trillion dollars per year in direct costs, including $181 billion for illicit drugs, $168 billion for tobacco, and $185 billion for alcohol (5). African American families are more likely to have incomes below the poverty level, and they are more likely to be uninsured (2). Moreover, they are often the first or second generation able to accumulate wealth. As a result, family wealth is only a fraction of that of their white counterparts (6). Consequently, there is simply not enough resources within the family to address the need for treatment services. Moreover, the stigma attached to treatment, the barriers related to racism, and the tendency to criminalize substance abuse greatly limit the willingness of the public sector to provide treatment resources (3). As a consequence, economic factors alone could contribute to the disparities seen in substance abuse consequences and lack of access to treatment. However, the Surgeon General's Reports showed that disparities in outcome persisted even when income or insurance status was controlled (1,2). Subsequent studies have shown that poverty is important, but the consequences of substance abuse extend beyond what socioeconomic factors would predict (3). Clearly, socioeconomic factors interact with sociocultural and political issues to greatly increase the burden of substance abuse on communities that often have to struggle with the effects of poverty and limited resources.

Epidemiology

African Americans are often stigmatized as being at greater risk of becoming substance abusers (2). The evidence, however, paints a more complex picture. Prevalence of overall substance abuse disorders is indeed greater (7). However, these global statistics often hide findings that show the opposite, depending on age of use, gender, residence, and type of drug. The household survey of youth consistently shows that African American youth are less likely to abuse many types of drugs and alcohol (2). Among teenagers, Caucasians are more likely to drink or use some drugs than African American youth (8). African Americans tended to begin drinking and to use marijuana at an older age than other ethnic groups and are less likely to smoke. As a consequence, African Americans are less likely to suffer from alcohol-related problems. Designer drugs are rare among African American youth (3). The peak age for injected heroin use is higher for African Americans than for Caucasians (9).

Some drugs are used heavily by African American youth. Crack cocaine is used at the same rate as or greater than in other ethnic groups (3). Most importantly, as we will show, the consequences of drug abuse are more devastating. Nevertheless, the later age of onset is worth investigating and suggests preventive factors in the lifestyle of African Americans. Overall these findings show the importance of examining the patterns of usage rather than the volume or quantity of use to better understand ethnic differences.

Preventive and Risk Factors

Multiple factors contribute to the ethnic differences in use patterns. As noted above, socioeconomic factors are important. They are important not only because the cost of a drug may determine its use, but also because income can determine where one resides. Drugs of abuse may be more easily accessible in inner city and marginalized areas. Moreover, residents in many of these areas see themselves as trapped and unable to move due to poverty and other social factors such as redlining (3).

Place of residence also adds to economic and cultural determinants. African Americans who live in the same locations as Caucasians consequently have the same use pattern. Regardless of race, the same access to drugs tend to show the same abuse pattern both in the type of drug used and in the prevalence of abuse.

The type of neighborhood also can determine the risk of exposure to trauma. Traumatic experiences are a risk factor for substance abuse even when they do not lead to post traumatic stress disorder. It is well documented that individuals in inner city neighborhood are more likely to be exposed to traumatic events (10). African Americans are especially at risk, given their residence pattern, which is often not because of choice (3).

Education and positive role models are associated with drug use. Academic achievement and peer drug use have been consistently shown to have protective effects. In a recent study, they were shown to be significant predictors of alcohol and marijuana use among high-risk African American youth (11). Religiosity and spirituality have been proposed as protective factors (12). One way in which these factors may work in inner city youth may be through preventing posttraumatic stress disease or other complications of trauma exposure (10). Understanding the mechanisms by which religion might influence substance use and the reasons why these mechanisms may vary by race and ethnicity may provide clues to implementing effective prevention programs.

Social Consequences

Drug abuse is known to be associated with family and personal violence. Adults who were abused were often done so by an intoxicated parent leading to increased risk of drug abuse and abusive behavior. The increased risk of child abuse in African American communities can be attributed to the interaction of drug abuse with other risk factors in inner city settings. Drug abuse contributes to behaviors such as personal conflicts, poverty, poor maternal care, and other factors that increase the risk of abusive behavior (2,3).

Dealing drugs of abuse is potentially lucrative. For a low-income individual, the benefits may outweigh the risks and have the added value of giving the dealer status. Such individuals may appear altruistic to the community—as one who has the power and income to distribute resources to improve the life of everyone. However, any wealth accumulated by dealers does not offset the tremendous costs to the community of drugs of abuse. Also the dealer runs the very high risk of being incarcerated or a homicide victim as a result of turf wars (13).

The problem of gang violence is well known as a risk factor for the high rate of adolescent assaults and the extremely high homicide rate in African Americans. Unsafe communities and worsening poverty make such areas unattractive to businesses. Drug abuse is clearly a factor (3). Drug use can lead to violent turf wars, and serve as a justification for violent crimes. Even illicit but less lucrative drugs such as marijuana can contribute to gang formation and criminal activity in African American youth. In fact, alcohol and marijuana are often the most commonly used drugs (14).

One of the other consequences of drug abuse is involvement with the criminal justice system. African American substance abusers are far more likely to be referred to the correctional system than for treatment. Moreover, African Americans arrested for possession are more likely to be incarcerated than their white counterparts. These observations are significant because 40% of those in the correctional system have alcohol use and 20% have substance abuse at the time of offense, with two third actively involved in drugs prior to admission to jail (13). Incarceration means that as many as 14% of African American males can no longer vote as a result of criminal conviction. Those who have served time can be excluded from public assistance, subsidized housing programs, and college financial aid. Many are also barred from employment in certain professions, including education, childcare, and nursing home service provision.

In an effort to remedy the negative consequences of drug abuse, legislatures across the country de-emphasized treatment and addressed drug abuse exclusively as a correctional problem with stringent penalties including mandatory minimum sentences. Crack cocaine users received especially harsh sentences, while distributors of the parent drug, cocaine, were able to escape with less punishment. This legislation had the consequence of further exacerbating the disparity in incarceration seen for African Americans since they and others in poverty settings were far more likely to use crack cocaine (3).

Thus, while African Americans do not reliably use drugs more often than other ethnic groups, drug use itself interacts with other risk factors that contribute to violence and other risky behaviors. African Americans may be in fact at lower risk of drug abuse if all other factors were kept equal (15). A legacy of discrimination, poverty, and social adversity contributes to a drug abuse problem that in turn worsens the impact of drug use on both the individual and the larger society.

Medical Comorbidity

Alcohol- or substance-abusing African Americans compared to other ethnic groups have worse outcomes in mental health, physical health, and social outcomes when socioeconomic factors are controlled (1,2). These agents adversely affect health outcome irrespective of race. African Americans, however, seem to have a worse morbidity and mortality.

African American alcohol-, heroin-, or cocaine-dependent persons are less likely to have primary medical care, but more likely to have a chronic illness, prior medical hospitalizations, and more emergency room visits (15). Moreover, such findings indicate the problem of lack of access to services, since emergency room visits can be considered a proxy for limited access to treatment programs. The result is that medical comorbidities are worsened due to inadequate preventive and follow-up care.

Substance abuse also contributes to mortality. The Surgeon General's Report and other previous reports have noted the consistently lower life expectancy in African Americans in comparison to other racial and ethnic groups (1,2).

One of the most important comorbid conditions is AIDS. African Americans experience striking disparities in HIV infection rates compared with other populations, and they are at particularly high risk for developing AIDS (16). African Americans make up just 13% of the U.S. population, but more than half of the total AIDS cases diagnosed in 2004. Moreover, African American females accounted for 68% of the female HIV/AIDS diagnoses from 2001 through 2004, while white females accounted for 16% and Hispanic females 15%. Although African Americans in the 13 to 19 age group represent only 15% of U.S. teenagers, they account for 66% of new AIDS cases reported among teens. HIV infection has become the leading cause of death for African American women aged 25 to 34. Nora Volkow, director of the National Institute on Drug Abuse (NIDA), has concluded that HIV/AIDS is now a pandemic that has literally put the world at risk. NIDA has established that drug abuse treatment *is* one of the most effective means of HIV prevention (17).

While intravenous drugs are well known as agents for the spread of AIDS, less recognized is the role that drug abuse plays more generally in the spread of HIV by increasing the likelihood of high-risk sex with infected partners. As a consequence, while the use of illicit substances by injection has featured prominently in the epidemic, the recent tendency to use agents intranasally such as opiates has not diminished the risk. Noninjecting drugs such as cocaine, marijuana, methamphetamine, and even alcohol are also significant cofactors that affect HIV transmission as well as the course and outcome of the disease.

Mental Illness Comorbidity

Substance abuse is often comorbid with mental disorders as well. Persons diagnosed with mood or anxiety disorders were about twice as likely to suffer also from a drug use disorder (abuse or dependence) as respondents in general. Similarly, persons diagnosed with drug disorders were roughly twice as likely to suffer also from mood and anxiety disorders (18). This observation has important implications for African Americans.

First, comorbidity may contribute to the misdiagnosis of mental disorders. It has been established in multiple studies that African Americans with mental disorders are often misdiagnosed or never diagnosed (4). As a consequence, they are often never treated or overmedicated, or not offered treatment by mental health professionals. Because drugs of abuse affect similar brain circuits or receptor mechanisms proposed for mental disorders, they can cause abusers to experience one or more symptoms of mental illness. The result is misdiagnosis and inappropriate treatment of those without a mental disorder. Second, mental illnesses can lead to drug abuse (18). In addition, individuals with overt, mild, or even subclinical mental disorders may abuse drugs as a form of self-medication. As a result, the mental disorder is ignored or considered yet another symptom of substance abuse. Treatment for mental disorder is delayed or never provided. This treatment deferral or delay is often seen in African Americans with mental disorders (2). Because drug use disorders and other mental illnesses are caused by overlapping factors such as underlying brain deficits, genetic vulnerabilities, and/or early exposure to stress or trauma, the very factors that we described earlier as risk factors for substance abuse also increase the risk of mental disorders. Finally, the combination of substance abuse and mental disorders adds greatly to the burden of illness (2). Treatment is more difficult. Services are less available, and the burden on the individual, family, and community is far greater.

Often African Americans face a triple burden as both disorders are important risk factors for general medical conditions such as HIV. In a recent study, individuals were assessed for psychiatric diagnoses, substance abuse, and HIV risk behavior using structured clinical interviews and self-report questionnaires. The majority (75%) were sexually active in the past 6 months and reported high rates of sexual risk behaviors, including unprotected intercourse (69%), multiple partners (39%), sex with prostitutes (24%, men only), and sex trading (10%). Recent manic episode and greater drug severity were independent predictors of total HIV risk. Cocaine dependence was associated with increased risk of sex trading (19). Mental disorders and substance abuse, therefore, can interact to increase the risk for HIV.

Prevention

The paradigms of primary and secondary prevention are applicable, but they must be tailored to specific minority groups. Further exploration in this area is critical. The problem of awaiting the availability of treatment programs continues the devastating rates of HIV, violence, and incarceration for the African American population. However, a focus on a correctional approach, paucity of culturally competent providers, as well as an assumption of homogeneity in this population are barriers to the development of prevention programs.

As noted above, protective and risk factors can be identified that may impact on drug use. Such a strategy can be used to develop prevention interventions for high-risk youth. Prevention strategies indeed work. These can include parental monitoring and supervision. They may also include drug education and information for parents or caregivers. In addition, brief, family-focused interventions for the general population can positively change specific parenting behavior that can reduce later risks of drug abuse. These programs are particularly effective when culture is taken into account (19). In fact, studies have found that African American adolescents who endorse positive attitudes about being African American report more antidrug attitudes and less substance abuse (20). Therefore, enhancing racial identity may be one area that may prove beneficial for those at risk.

As noted previously, spirituality can have a protective effect (12). Spirituality has been found to be especially influential in substance abuse prevention and treatment for African Americans. Spirituality is often found to be incorporated into activities with the African American community, and most of these events are centered around the Black Church. In fact, spirituality and perceived social support were found to serve as protective factors for smoking and alcohol use among African American college students (21). Given these findings, involvement in the church may be especially salient for African Americans at risk for abuse.

Treatment

There is now little doubt that treatment can work, and it works for a variety of substances, across ethnicity, and in a variety of settings (5). Treatment programs, especially if they address cultural needs, are effective and have strong participation by ethnic minorities. Moreover, effective treatment also can mean reductions in behaviors that increase the risk of HIV (22).

Racial disparities in treatment participation and access are well documented. African Americans have more unmet needs than other ethnic groups (23). They have less access to specialty substance abuse treatment services (24). Income and poverty are certainly important factors. As a result, African Americans have to depend on the availability of public facilities, which are sensitive to the political climate, and willingness to provide funding for treatment versus the correctional system. Also there is a perception among many African Americans that treatment programs are not culturally congruent or insensitive. However, differences persist even when income is controlled and culture is taken into account (24). Part of the disparity may be related to the unwillingness of African Americans to accept treatment. In fact, African Americans may discontinue treatment sooner, leading to a poorer outcome (25). Family privacy, lack of knowledge regarding treatment, and concerns about stigma and about medication have been reported as substantial barriers to accessing treatment. This finding is complicated by the fact that African Americans are less likely to receive outpatient care. When access to outpatient care was controlled for statistically, racial differences in residential care and overall treatment retention disappeared (26). Americans tend to have less access to professional services and more likely to include 12-step meetings, rehabilitation programs, and church-related support in their treatment (27). As a consequence, African Americans may have less access to newer treatment approaches.

The problem of access to service is further complicated by the type of services available in a given locale. In one study a city's racial composition is found to influence treatment center characteristics and services available, but the pattern is complex in that there are inequalities in treatment for certain types of services but not in others. For instance, cities with high percentages of Latinos and African Americans provide more treatment options, such as employment and domestic violence counseling or programs for gay/lesbian clients. However, minority cities have fewer integrated treatment centers that provide comprehensive assessment for substance abuse and mental health problems (28). Thus, the problem is not simply the quantity of services but the quality of services, which may greatly impact the poor and the underserved.

African Americans with substance abuse problems are more likely to be incarcerated. However, correctional settings for African Americans are more likely to be punitive rather than rehabilitative. Moreover, the limitations in personal freedom after incarceration further limit access to treatment (3,29).

African Americans have been found to have less access to newer, more effective treatment approaches in mental health services (4). The same appears to be true for substance abuse (27). For example, buprenorphine is a long-acting partial agonist that acts on the same receptors as heroin and morphine, relieving drug cravings without producing the same intense "high" or dangerous side effects. The Congress passed the Drug Addiction Treatment Act (permitting qualified physicians to prescribe narcotic medications [Schedules III to V]) for the treatment of opioid addiction. This legislation created a major paradigm shift by allowing access to opiate treatment in a medical setting or private office rather than limiting it to federally approved Opioid Treatment Programs. Buprenorphine was found to be effective in reducing opiate abuse and is an effective tool in AIDS prevention (30). African Americans were as accepting of this treatment as other ethnic groups, yet the vast majority of those who have access to buprenorphine are white males (31).

Clearly, barriers exist that limit access to treatment. However, recent approaches to treatment have greatly improved access to care for African Americans. Untreated substance-abusing offenders are more likely to relapse to drug abuse and return to criminal behavior. This can bring about rearrest and reincarceration, jeopardizing public health and public safety and taxing the criminal justice system resources. Successful drug abuse treatment in the criminal justice system can help reduce crime as well as the spread of HIV/AIDS, hepatitis, and other infectious diseases. Introducing treatment to the correctional system improves treatment availability for African Americans because they are substantially overrepresented in this setting. Drug treatment is extremely effective in this setting in the correctional system (32). Treatment cuts drug abuse rates by half and reduces criminal activity and arrests. African Americans previously without access to treatment can have more treatment availability and avoid reincarceration. Moreover, such treatment also reduces the spread of HIV, which has been related to individuals in corrections returning to the community. Additional efforts such as drug courts to avoid incarceration and legislative changes that would make it easier for inmates to expunge a criminal record if substance use or possession is the only crime would go a long way to reduce the factors that contribute to involvement in the correctional system (3).

The notion of culturally relevant and culturally competent prevention and treatment programs has been supported by several studies. In an analysis of African American Youth in the National Cross-Site Evaluation, it was found that higher levels of satisfaction and improved outcomes were seen with culturally specific versus nonculturally specific programs (26). These studies underscore the importance of cultural aspects in the treatment of African Americans because they show a greater willingness to accept treatment and to be retained in the treatment program. There is widespread agreement that implementing an Afrocentric approach in prevention and treatment programs could prove beneficial for some communities (32).

CONCLUSION

Alcohol and substance abuse disorders greatly impact the African American community. While the prevalence of substance use is not substantially different from other ethnic groups, the burden to individuals and the community is greater. Drug abuse is clearly a problem that exacerbates the consequences of discrimination and poverty. Most importantly, substance abuse contributes to the disparities in morbidity and mortality seen in the general health in African Americans and accounts for some of the excessive disease burden seen with mental disorders. On the other hand, there are clearly protective factors in African American culture. Moreover, advances have been made in understanding the behavior and neurobiology of addiction that has led to effective ways of detection, prevention, and treatment. These interventions work for African Americans when they have access to them and when they are culturally appropriate. The challenge is to create the public and political will to shift the addiction focus to prevention and treatment, to reduce disparities, and to improve treatment accessibility in African American communities.

REFERENCES

1. U.S. Department of Health and Human Services. *Mental Health: A Report of the Surgeon General.* Rockville, MD: U.S. Department of Health and Human Services, Substance Abuse and Mental Health Services Administration; 1999.
2. U.S. Department of Health and Human Services. *Mental health: Culture, Race, and Ethnicity—A Supplement to Mental Health: A Report of the Surgeon General.* Rockville, MD: U.S. Department of Health and Human Services, Substance Abuse and Mental Health Services Administration; 2001.
3. Primm BJ, Hewitt WW, Primm AB, et al. Addicted populations. In: Ruiz P, Primm A., eds. *Disparities in Psychiatric Care.* Baltimore, MD: Lippincott Williams & Wilkins; 2010.
4. Lawson, WB. Mental health issues for African Americans. In: Guillermo B, Trimble JE, Burlow AK, et al., eds. *Handbook of Racial and Ethnic Minority Psychology.* Thousand Oaks, CA: Sage Publications Inc.; 2002.
5. National Institute of Drug Abuse. *InfoFacts.* Available at: http/www.drugabuse.gov. Accessed June 2010.
6. Lawson WB, Kennedy C. Role of the severely mentally ill in the family. In: Lewis-Hall F, Williams TS, Panetta JA, et al., eds. *Psychiatric Illness in Women: Emerging Treatments and Research.* Washington, DC: American Psychiatric Association Press; 2002.
7. Keyes KM, Hatzenbuehler ML, Alberti P, et al. Service utilization differences for Axis I psychiatric and substance use disorders between white and black adults. *Psychiatr Serv.* 2008;59:893–901.
8. Horton EG. Racial differences in the effects of age of onset on alcohol consumption and development of alcohol-related problems among males from mid-adolescence to young adulthood. *J Ethn Subst Abuse.* 2007;6:1–13.
9. Broz D, Ouellet LJ. Racial and ethnic changes in heroin injection in the United States: implications for the HIV/AIDS epidemic. *Drug Alcohol Depend.* 2008;94:221–233.
10. Alim TN, Feder A, Graves RE, et al. Trauma, resilience, and recovery in a high-risk African-American population. *Am J Psychiatry.* 2008;165:1566–1575.
11. Clark TT, Belgrave FZ, Nasim AJ. Risk and protective factors for substance use among urban African American adolescents considered high-risk. *Ethn Subst Abuse.* 2008;7:292–303.
12. Wallace JM Jr, Delva J, O'Malley PM. Race/ethnicity, religiosity and adolescent alcohol, cigarette and marijuana use. *Soc Work Public Health.* 2007;23:193–213.
13. Department of Justice. *Prison and Jail Inmates at Midyear 2001.* Washington, DC: Bureau of Justice Statistics; 2001.
14. Gil AG, Vega WA, Turner RJ. Early and mid-adolescence risk factors for later substance abuse by African Americans and European Americans. *Public Health Rep.* 2002;117(suppl 1):S15–S29.

15. De Alba I, Samet JH, Saitz R. Burden of medical illness in drug and alcohol dependent persons without primary care. *Am J Addiction*. 2004;13:33–45.
16. Kang SY, Goldstein MF, Deren S. Health care utilization and risk behaviors among HIV positive minority drug users. *J Health Care Poor Underserved*. 2006;17:265–275. DOI: 10.1353/hpu.2006.0063.
17. National Institute of Drug Abuse. *Research Report Series*. Available at: http://www.drugabuse.gov/ResearchReports/HIV/hiv.html. Accessed June 2010.
18. Conway KP, Compton W, Stinson FS, et al. Lifetime comorbidity of DSM-IV mood and anxiety disorders and specific drug use disorders: results from the National Epidemiologic Survey on Alcohol and Related Conditions. *J Clin Psychiatry*. 2006;67:247–257.
19. Meade CS, Graff FS, Griffin ML, et al. HIV risk behavior among patients with co-occurring bipolar and substance use disorders: associations with mania and drug abuse. *Drug Alcohol Depend*. 2008;92:296–300.
20. Szapocznik J, Prado G, Burlew AK, et al. Drug abuse in African American and Hispanic adolescents: culture, development, and behavior. *Annu Rev Clin Psychol*. 2007;3:77–105.
21. Turner-Musa J, Libscomb L. Spirituality and social support on health behaviors of African American undergraduates. *Am J Health Behav*. 2007;31(5):495–501.
22. Sterk CE, Theall KP, Elifson KW. Effectiveness of a risk reduction intervention among African American women who use crack cocaine. *AIDS Educ Prev*. 2003;15:15–32.
23. Wells K, Klap R, Koike A, et al. Ethnic disparities in unmet need for alcoholism, drug abuse, and mental health care. *Am J Psychiatry*. 2001;158:2027–2032.
24. Alegria M, Canino G, Rios R, et al. Inequalities in use of specialty mental health services among Latinos, African Americans, and non-Latino whites. *Psychiatr Serv*. 2002;53:1547–1555. DOI: 10.1176/appi.ps.53.12.1547.
25. Jacobson JO, Robinson PL, Bluthenthal RN. Racial disparities in completion rates from publicly funded alcohol treatment: economic resources explain more than demographics and addiction severity. *Health Serv Res*. 2007;42:773–794.
26. Bluthenthal RN, Jacobson JO, Robinson PL. Are racial disparities in alcohol treatment completion associated with racial differences in treatment modality entry? Comparison of outpatient treatment and residential treatment in Los Angeles County, 1998 to 2000. *Alcohol Clin Exp Res*. 2007;31:1920–1926.
27. Perron BE, Mowbray OP, Glass JE, et al. Differences in service utilization and barriers among blacks, Hispanics, and whites with drug use disorders. *Subst Abuse Treat Prev Policy*. 2009;4:3. DOI: 10.1186/1747-597X-4-3.
28. Vélez MB, Campos-Holland AL, Arndt S. City's racial composition shapes treatment center characteristics and services. *J Ethn Subst Abuse*. 2008;7:188–199.
29. Chaddock GR. U.S. notches world's highest incarceration rate. *Chris Sci Monitor*. 2003;(August 18):2.
30. Sullivan LE, Barry D, Moore BA, et al. A trial of integrated buprenorphine/naloxone and HIV clinical care. *Clin Infect Dis*. 2006;43(suppl 4):S184–S190.
31. Cicero T, Inciardi J. Potential for abuse of buprenorphine in office-based treatment of opioid dependence. *N Engl J Med*. 2005;353:1863–1865.
32. Wechsberg WM, Zule WA, Riehman KS, et al. African-American crack abusers and drug treatment initiation: barriers and effects of a pretreatment intervention. *Subst Abuse Treat Prev Policy*. 2007;2:10.

CHAPTER 60 Hispanic Americans

Pedro Ruiz

INTRODUCTION

Despite the recent advances in the biopsychosocial treatment of addictive disorders, addiction to drugs and alcohol continues to be a major challenge among the different Hispanic American groups who reside in the United States. Additionally, disparities within the field of addiction are a major factor insofar as the lack of substantial progress among Hispanic American addicts who reside in this country is concerned. Racial and ethnic discrimination, excessive poverty, lack of parity between medical and addiction care, excessive emphasis on criminalization-oriented policies, lack of universal access to health care, insufficient preventive efforts, and the like all contribute to the current crisis faced in the United States insofar as access to care, full rehabilitation, and the biopsychosocial aspects of prevention of the Hispanic American addicts is concerned. As a result of this failure within the addiction system of care that currently prevails in the United States, a very large number of Hispanic American addicts do not receive appropriate treatment, and a very large number of Hispanic American addicts drop out from treatment prematurely (1). Among these previously eluded barriers to appropriate care for the Hispanic American addicts, the lack of medical insurance stands as a formidable one. Recent data originated from the National Household Survey on Drug Abuse depicts that 38% of Americans lack behavioral health coverage or do not know about their coverage (2). Among them, Hispanics, Asians, young adults between 18 and 25 years of age, adults in the lowest income levels, and less educated adults were the most likely groups to be uninsured. Obviously, untreated addictive disorders and conditions, as well as psychiatric disorders, are a major challenge to society in the United States in the 21st century. Policy makers across this country, whether it is at the local, state, or federal government, must reverse the current negative trend vis-à-vis mental health services that have prevailed in this country for several decades if not centuries. Our socially disadvantaged subgroups, especially the ethnic and minority populations, deserve to be given parity and much more attention from every sector of society (3).

Lack of culturally oriented manpower, insufficient cross-cultural expertise, lack of sensitivity toward ethnic, racial, and other minority groups, lack of appropriate educational levels, and excessive poverty levels are all contributing to the lack of preventive programs, quality of care, lack of access, insufficient psychosocial treatments, and inadequate research efforts vis-à-vis the Hispanic American addicts who reside in this country, and we can also add to all ethnic, racial, and minority groups who reside in this country (4–6).

It is within this biopsychosocial context that in this chapter we plan to address all relevant factors pertaining to the Hispanic American substance abuser. In this respect, we plan to (a) define the population; (b) describe the relevant epidemiologic trends of the Hispanic American substance abuse groups; (c) focus on the role of migration and acculturative stress and sociocultural factors vis-à-vis substance abuse trends and rates; (d) discuss the most salient characteristics of the different Hispanic American groups who reside in this country within the realm of addictive behaviors; (e) depict the most relevant factors with respect to the minority connotations of the Hispanic American addicts; and finally (f) advance appropriate recommendations directed to effectively solve the most challenging issues within the Hispanic American addiction dilemma.

DEFINITION OF THE POPULATION

The number of Hispanics continues to grow in the United States, whether it is internal growth within the U.S. territory or via migration from Central America and the Caribbean, South America, or the Iberian Peninsula (7–9). As depicted in Table 60.1, the Hispanic population in the United States grew from 29.3 million (9%) in 1990 to 35.3 million (12.5%) in year 2000. This number does not include the Hispanic illegal aliens who are currently estimated to be about 11 million (7–9).

As seen in Table 60.2, the growth of the Hispanic population during the decade of 1990 to 2000 surpassed any other ethnic group living in the United States. Hispanics grew during this decade at a rate of 58%. In contrast, Asians grew 50%, Native Americans grew 17%, Blacks grew 16%, and the Whites grew only 3% (7,8).

The U.S. Census Bureau report, 2000 showed some very relevant data pertaining to the status of the structure of the families in the United States (8). As described in Table 60.3, 24.4% of the Hispanic families and 46.7% of the Black families living in the United States in the year 1997 were headed by women. Moreover, 39.4% of the Puerto Rican families were headed by women.

Another factor that needs to be taken into consideration with respect to the multiple ethnic and minority groups that reside in the United States is the U.S. median family income levels.

TABLE 60.1 U.S. population

	2000	1990
	N (% of total)	N (% of total)
Total	281.4 (100)	248.8 (100)
Whites	194.6 (69.2)	188.3 (75.7)
Hispanics	35.3 (12.5)	22.4 (9.0)
Blacks	33.9 (12.1)	29.3 (11.8)
Asians	10.5 (3.7)	7.0 (2.8)
Native Americans	2.1 (0.7)	1.8 (0.7)
Other	0.5 (0.2)	N/A (N/A)
Two or more races	4.6 (1.6)	N/A (N/A)

Data from Refs. 7 to 9.

TABLE 60.2 Population growth from 1900 to 2000

Ethnic group	Population growth (%)
Hispanics	58
Asians	50
Native Americans	17
Blacks	16
Whites	3

Data from Refs. 7 to 8.

TABLE 60.3 U.S. household status in 1997

Women	Married (%)	Headed (%)
Whites	80.9	14.2
Asians	78.5	13.2
Blacks	45.5	46.7
Hispanics	68.2	24.4
Mexican Americans	72.2	20.2
Puerto Ricans	54.3	39.4
Cuban Americans	76.9	16.9
Central and South Americans	65.2	26.8

Data from the 2000 U.S. Census (www.census.gov/main/www/cen2000.html.).

As noted in Table 60.4, the median family income level for Hispanics who reside in the United States, in accordance with the U.S. Census Bureau report, 2000, was $30,735, in comparison to $51,205 for Asian families, $44,366 for White families, $30,784 for Native American families, and $27,910 for Black families.

Given this level of median family income in accordance with the U.S. Census Bureau report, 2000, the percentage of the U.S. population below the poverty level as delineated in Table 60.5 was 10.2% for the total U.S. population, 22.7% for the Black population, 21.7% for the Hispanic population, 9.6% for the Asian population, and 5.7% for the Native American population (8).

From a different although important perspective, when defining the Hispanic population who reside in the United States, we should also address the uninsured population. In accordance with the U.S. Census Bureau report, 2000, as underlined in Table 60.6, 43.6% of illegal aliens in the United States were uninsured from a medical point of view; also, 34.2% of the foreign-born aliens were also medically uninsured; additionally, 18.2% of the naturalized U.S. population was medically uninsured, and, finally, 14.2% of the U.S. native-born population was medically uninsured (8).

TABLE 60.4 U.S. median family income in 1999

Ethnic group	Income (US$)
Asians	51,205
Whites	44,366
Native Americans	30,784
Hispanics	30,735
Blacks	27,910

Data from the 2000 U.S. Census (www.census.gov/main/www/cen2000.html).

TABLE 60.5 U.S. population below poverty level ($17,029 for a family of four) in 1999

	Population (%)
Total population[a]	10.2
Blacks	22.7
Hispanics	21.7
Asians	9.6
Whites	5.7
Native Americans	N/A

[a]32.3 million of 273.5 million.

Data from the 2000 U.S. Census (www.census.gov/main/www/cen2000.html).

TABLE 60.6 U.S. uninsured population in 1997

Origin	Population (%)
Native born	14.2
Naturalized	18.2
Foreign-born alien	34.2
Illegal alien	43.6

Data from the 2000 U.S. Census (www.census.gov/main/www/cen2000.html).

TABLE 60.7 U.S. uninsured population in 1997

Working full time	16.8%
Working part time	24.1%
Unemployed	26.2%

Data from Refs. 8 and 9.

TABLE 60.8 U.S. uninsured population in 1999

Ethnic group	Population (%)
Hispanics	33.4
Blacks	21.2
Asians	20.8
Whites	11.0
Others	13.6

Data from Refs. 8 and 9.

Likewise, as portrayed in Table 60.7, 26.2% of the unemployed population in the United States is medically uninsured, as against 24.1% of the part-time U.S. working population and 16.8% of the full-time U.S. working population (8,9).

According to the U.S. Census Bureau report, 2000, deeper analysis of the U.S. medically uninsured population, as depicted in Table 60.8, demonstrates that 33.4% of the total U.S. Hispanic population is medically uninsured, as against 21.2% of the U.S. Black population, 20.8% of the Asian population, and 11% of the White population (9).

Finally, Table 60.9 describes, in accordance with the U.S. Census Bureau report, 2000, the level of the medically uninsured among the poor population of the United States (8). In this context, 43.7% of the poor Hispanics, 41.7% of the poor Asians, 28.1% of the poor Blacks, and 28% of the poor Whites who resided in the United States were medically uninsured.

TABLE 60.9 U.S. health uninsured population in 1999[a]

Population	Million	%
Total uninsured population	42.6	15.5
Total uninsured poor population	10.4	32.2
Ethnicity	%	% Poor
Whites	11.0	28.0
Blacks	21.2	28.1
Asians	20.8	41.7
Hispanics	33.4	43.7
Origin	%	% Poor
Native born	13.5	28.4
Foreign born	33.4	56.1

[a] Total population: 274.1 million; total poor population: 32.3 million.
Data from the 2000 U.S. Census (www.census.gov/main/www/cen2000.html).

CURRENT SUBSTANCE ABUSE TRENDS AMONG HISPANICS

Hispanics are currently the highest growing segment of the U.S. population. Similarly, 13% of the admissions in the Treatment Episode Data Set (TEDS) in 1999 were Hispanics (9). Likewise, in 1999, among Hispanic admissions to TEDS, 42% were Mexicans, 35% Puerto Ricans, 2% Cubans, and 21% other Hispanics (10). TEDS in this context represents those admitted for substance abuse treatment. TEDS also represents admissions for substance abuse treatment in facilities that receive some public funding. In 1999, in accordance with TEDS, the Hispanic gender distribution of substance abuse admissions was 69.6% Hispanic men and 31% Hispanic women. Also in 1999, the most common substances of abuse among Hispanics were alcohol (36%), opiates (32%), and marijuana (14%); other substances used by Hispanics were cocaine (11%) and stimulants (4%). The states with the largest percentages of substance abuse admission among Hispanics in 1999 according to TEDS are outlined in Table 60.10 (10).

By 2003, the gender difference with respect to Hispanic admissions for substance abuse treatment was 78% for men and 22% for women (11). Also in 2003, the Hispanic admission levels for substance abuse treatment in accordance with TEDS was 36% for alcohol, 28% for opiates, 15% for marijuana, 10% for cocaine, 9% for stimulants, and 2% for other substances. In 2003, the percentage of substance abuse treatment admissions among Hispanics between the ages of 25 and 34 was 27% for Mexicans, 31% for Cubans, and 35% for Puerto Ricans.

From a worldwide perspective, it is important to note that globally 4.4% of the burden of diseases is attributable to alcohol consumption; likewise, neuropsychiatric disorders due to alcohol use and abuse, including alcohol dependence, account for 34% of the burden of disease and disability that is attributable to alcohol (12). Additionally, in some countries of the Americas and Eastern Europe, the estimated prevalence of disorders due to alcohol use is around 10% (12). Alcohol consumption is causally related to more than 60 international classifications of disease codes; among them liver damage, pancreatic damage, suicides, unintentional injuries, and hormonal disturbances are the prominent ones (12). In addition, disorders due to the use and abuse of alcohol also affect social services, fiscal sector, services related to law enforcement and criminal justice, fire services, transport, traffic regulations, the alcohol industry, the agricultural sector, tourism, hospitality, and the entertainment industry (12). Despite that the worldwide use of alcohol predominates among men, women are seriously affected by "alcohol use" and "alcoholism," for instance, as a causative factor in domestic violence (12).

Within the same context, 200 million people worldwide were estimated to have used illicit drugs in the period 2005 to 2006. Among developed countries, the economic cost of illicit drug use has been estimated to be 0.2% to 2% of the gross domestic product (12). Illicit use of opioids was estimated to account for 0.7% of global DALYs in 2000 (12). The estimated number of injecting drug users worldwide is about 13 million. Cannabis is the most widely used illicit drug; that is, it is being used by 3.8% of the global population older than 15 years. Cannabis use accounts for about 80% of the illicit drug used worldwide (12). Along these lines, dependent heroin users have an increased risk of premature death from drug overdoses, violence, suicide, and causes related to alcohol. Additionally, 5% to 10% of new HIV infections worldwide are attributable to use of drugs intravenously or as a result of sharing contaminated equipment. Moreover, disorders due to use of illicit drugs are associated with an increased risk of other infectious diseases such as hepatitis B and C (12).

TABLE 60.10	States with the largest percentages of substance abuse admission among Hispanics in 1999
Ethnicity/States	**Substance abuse (%)**
Mexican	
California	49
Colorado	14
Texas	12
All other states	25
Total	100
Puerto Rican	
New York	44
Connecticut	14
Massachusetts	13
All other states	29
Total	100
Cuban	
Florida	48
New York	13
California	11
All other states	28
Total	100
Other Hispanics	
New York	22
California	22
Florida	9
All other states	47
Total	100

Data from Ruiz P. Psychopathology and migration. In: "Psiquiatria 2006": III Symposium Admirall; "Libro de Resumenes", Vol 1. Barcelona, Spain; 2004:47–60.

Finally, disorders due to the use of illicit drugs affect social services, the criminal justice system, educational sectors, and road traffic safety (12).

Undoubtedly, these worldwide examples and implications related to alcohol use and abuse, as well as substance use and abuse, have major negative impacts in a large number of Hispanics, not only in those Hispanics who live in the United States, but worldwide as well. Therefore, it is important that they are noted here and addressed fully in this chapter.

SOCIOCULTURAL CONSIDERATIONS

In recent years, a major emphasis and priority have been accorded to investigational and clinical efforts focusing on the basic social and cultural structures and processes that influence directly or indirectly health in general, and mental health in particular, including addictive behavior. In general, social and cultural factors influence health and mental health outcomes, affecting exposure and vulnerability to illnesses, risk-taking behaviors, the efficacy of health promotion efforts, as well as access to, and availability of, health and mental health care, including addiction services, and the quality of such services. The factors that link the sociocultural environment to health or mental health outcomes is of utmost importance. In this context, socioeconomic status, social class, gender-related issues, and ethnic and racial factors all relate to potential disparities in the health and mental health care systems. Undoubtedly, social policies and cultural norms have unique linkages to human behavior and personal health.

The influence of social and cultural factors with respect to coping strategies are intrinsically related to illness and disability, as well as the well-being of individuals, families, and community at large. Improving sociocultural conditions also have a direct impact on prevention and health promotion. In this context, many community-based practices might produce protective mechanisms against substance abuse in some populations via its influence on the structure and process of people's interpersonal relationships, as well as its impact on individuals' psychology and behavior (13). Likewise, it has been emphasized that stressors associated to cultural transmutation may exert particular pressures on Latino men, in particular to third-generation Latinos vis-à-vis substance use and abuse (14). In this study, lifetime psychiatric disorder prevalence estimates were 28.1% for men and 30.2% for women. Puerto Ricans, however, had the highest overall prevalence rate among the Latino ethnic groups assessed. Increased rates of psychiatric disorders were observed among U.S.-born, English language-proficient, and third-generation Latinos (14). This type of studies and their outcomes can certainly have an impact on clinical practice and also appropriately guide the program development.

In a recent survey conducted by the U.S. National Alcohol Survey in 2005, an attempt was made to assess the adverse impact of social disadvantages on the health status of minority populations and also, along these lines, on the relationship of social disadvantages and alcohol problems (15). The outcome of this very important survey demonstrated that Hispanic Americans and Blacks reported greater exposure to social disadvantage than Whites. Greater disadvantage in this context meant greater poverty, unfair treatment, racial/ethnic stigma, and cumulative degree of disadvantage. Additionally, the survey also showed that in all the racial and ethnic groups (Hispanic Americans, Blacks, and Whites) exposure to social disadvantage was fully correlated to problem drinking; moreover, frequent unfair treatment, high levels of racial stigma vis-à-vis Hispanic Americans and Blacks, and multiple sources of extreme social disadvantage were directly related to an increased, in the range of twofold to sixfold greater, risk of alcohol problems. This seriously detrimental outcome could be partially explained by psychological distress.

This finding is of great importance with respect to the role of sociocultural factors vis-à-vis substance use and/or abuse. Obviously, the result of this relevant survey strongly suggests that future research efforts should be dedicated to better assess causal directions in the relationships among social and economic hardships, level of stress, and alcohol problems.

On a different study, an attempt was made to assess whether ethnic and racial disparities in public-funded alcohol treatment completion are due to racial differences in attending outpatient or residential treatment (16). The outcome of this study showed that Hispanic patients were significantly less likely to complete treatment as compared with White patients. It is, therefore, expected that a reduction in racial disparities will certainly lead to an increase in enrollment of Hispanic patients who suffer from alcoholism into a residential alcohol treatment programs. A similar expectation will also hold true for Black patients. Obviously, more research is warranted insofar as the impact of disparities in alcohol treatment among ethnic and racial minorities.

From a similar viewpoint, another study focusing on Hispanic and African American adolescents who suffered from alcoholism problems demonstrated that culturally sensitive substance abuse intervention could have a positive impact in this patient population, particularly with those who demonstrate a tendency to delinquent behavior (17). In this context, cultural factors, such as ethnic orientation and ethnic mistrust, constitute influential factors among U.S.-born Hispanic youth with lower level of acculturation. This type of youth respond better to culturally sensitive methods of intervention to treat juvenile delinquency from multiethnic populations who suffer from alcoholism.

In another interesting study, it was depicted that outcome expectancy is associated with more alcohol problems based on the particular meaning of the outcome; this meaning, in turn, depends upon an individual's particular sociocultural perspective (18). These perspectives are, indeed, associated with gender and ethnicity; for instance, anticipated loss of control due to drinking excessively was more negatively related to Puerto Ricans and female alcohol problems than it was to Irish and male alcohol problems.

Ethnic identity and spirituality have both been evaluated with respect to their potential influences vis-à-vis treatment outcomes among Hispanic American addicts in treatment with methadone (19). This study showed that while spirituality has no influence vis-à-vis the increase of drug use and abuse at follow-up with methadone maintenance, ethnic identity definitely demonstrated to be related to a greater number of drugs used at follow-up with methadone maintenance treatment programs. No significant effects were found for spirituality.

In a statewide household survey of substance abuse conducted in New York State by the Division of Substance Abuse Services, Alcoholism, and Alcohol Abuse, it was demonstrated that certain correlates between culture and illicit substance use among Hispanics existed (20). For example, findings for Hispanics show that the stronger the ties to the Hispanic culture, the less likely the use of drugs is to occur; conversely, the stronger the ties to the American culture, the more likely is the drug use. Fifty-three percent of Hispanics born in the United States reported using more illicit drugs during their lifetime, as compared to only 25% of those born in Puerto Rico and 11% of Hispanics born in other Hispanic countries. Along the same lines, 45% of Hispanics who spoke only English or mostly English had used some illicit drugs during their lifetime, whereas only 8% of those Hispanics who spoke Spanish or mostly Spanish did so. Puerto Ricans, as well as Mexican Americans, Cuban Americans, and other Hispanics who recently migrated to the United States, also must confront the additional disadvantage of a language barrier. This language barrier further complicates the acculturation process, thus increasing vulnerability to substance abuse.

To counteract these negative influences, Puerto Rican migrants who are older or have better economic resources frequently visit Puerto Rico and, thus, attempt to maintain their traditional values and customs. In contrast, younger Puerto Ricans identify more often with the "Anglo" mainland society and therefore are under greater pressure to reject their Hispanic cultures in favor of the "Anglo" majority culture. Many of them are caught between cultures, having given up or forgotten most of the cultural traditions of Puerto Rico, while not yet having developed a strong identification with the American way of life. This group is certainly very vulnerable to drug abuse. Indeed, the incidence of substance abuse among Hispanics, particularly Puerto Ricans, is higher among the youth.

In the case of Cuban Americans, there have been, so far, very limited opportunities to visit Cuba, a situation that has contributed to a stronger sense of survival within the United States. Fortunately for Cuban Americans, however, the process of acculturation has resulted in integration rather than assimilation, separation, or marginalization. The integration process has had a very positive impact insofar as substance abuse is concerned. Cuban Americans have fostered strong relations with the members of the majority "Anglo" culture, while preserving their Cuban cultural traditions and heritage. This has resulted in much less alienation and identity confusion among Cuban Americans than among other Hispanic subgroups that have migrated to the United States. Furthermore, it has assisted Cuban Americans to achieve economic success and independence in the United States.

The previously discussed sociocultural issues lead to a series of key questions concerning substance abuse among Hispanic populations. For instance, how do specific sociocultural factors common to all Hispanics affect types of drug use, patterns of abuse, and treatment needs? Despite all Hispanic subgroups having some common characteristics, such as the Spanish language, a Catholic background, Indian and/or African traits, or an Iberian heritage, they differ in the incidence and type of substance abuse. How can we account for the differences? Do Hispanics born and raised in the United States have different treatment outcomes than Hispanics born and raised outside of the United States and who later migrate to this country? If so, why? For instance, it has already been reported in the medical literature that different ethnic groups, including Hispanics, vary in terms of response to drug dosages, side effects, and metabolism of certain psychotherapeutic medications (21). To what extent could this be physiologically caused and to what extent could this be culturally determined? These types of questions need to be investigated further so that the answers can be incorporated into the health care and substance abuse treatment armamentarium.

Also of great importance, particularly from a prevention point of view, are gender differences in current substance abuse trends. For instance, substance abuse among young Hispanic women in Puerto Rico and in the United States is on the rise, particularly for certain substances. The fact of female emancipation must be considered in the analysis of these trends, as well as the unnecessary prejudice and discrimination this emancipating process creates. Culturally determined family dynamics could also play a major role in the increased incidence of substance abuse among Hispanic women (22). Furthermore, a large number of Hispanic women in the United States are head of households and therefore are forced to function in a variety of different social roles. Undoubtedly, these situations lead to additional stress and thus to increased vulnerability to substance abuse.

Along these same lines, we must also address the special treatment needs of Hispanic female addicts. First of all, they must be treated with equality and respect. Personal and sexual issues must be addressed sensitively and with understanding, particularly when the counselors and therapists are men. The employment of Hispanic female staff is certainly indicated in programs with a large Hispanic female clientele.

In addition, the involvement of the family in the treatment process is critically important. Hispanic families have excellent networking systems, and these systems can play a positive role in both the treatment process and primary prevention. For instance, Hispanic families with no father figure are said to be more vulnerable to addiction. In these cases, the individual roles of all family members must be understood, respected, and utilized appropriately in treatment setting (1). Each member of the family plays a unique role in the dynamics of the family. For example, grandparents are respected for their wisdom, fathers for their authority, mothers for their devotion, children for their future role, and godparents ("padrinos") for their potential available support in times of need.

At times, however, cultural values and norms may impact adversely upon the fight against substance abuse. For instance, it is well known that fatalism is an important trait among Hispanics. "Que sea lo que Dios quiera" (God willing) is an attitude frequently expressed by Hispanics (4). This posture can play a negative influence by leading an individual to avoid seeking assistance or drop out of a treatment program. We must combat, educate, persuade, and break those negative attitudes that are caused by poverty, feelings of hopelessness, and powerlessness. Conversely, key Hispanic cultural values such as dignity, respect, and love (dignidad, respeto, y cariño), which represent the core triangle of the Hispanic culture, can all be positively used in both treatment and prevention (1). At times, migration can play a negative role in the fight against substance abuse because it could lead to a breakdown of the family network system, thus making the members who migrate, as well as those who remain behind, very vulnerable to sociocultural stressors and therefore to addiction (20). Frequent visits to the native country, telephone calls, and correspondence between family members can all minimize these negative influences. In this regard, reinforcement of new networking systems, which could include treatment staff, should be maximized. This should be accomplished without fears of transferential and other related psychodynamic issues.

These problems can also be addressed through the use of group therapy approaches. Group discussions with a focus on historical and/or patriotic themes, when skillfully used, could lead to improvement of individual self-esteem. In this regard, the role of church affiliation, such as Catholic, Pentecostal, and Jehovah's Witness, or other nonorthodox religious beliefs, such as Spiritism, Santeria, Brujeria, and Curanderismo, could play a major positive role in the development of networking systems, treatment compliance, and primary prevention (16). On certain occasions, it is quite appropriate to develop linkage and liaisons between substance abuse treatment programs and religious institutions for the specific purpose of implementing preventive strategies, whether primary, secondary, or tertiary (1). These approaches have proved to be beneficial in other areas of health care, as well as in mental health, and thus could also be applied to the field of substance abuse treatment and prevention (1). Along these lines, it is important to recognize that Mexican Americans have a strong Indian heritage derived from the Aztec and Mayan cultures; thus, they share a widespread belief in Curanderismo. Similarly, Cuban Americans and Puerto Ricans have been highly influenced by the European Spiritist philosophy of Alan Kardec. Similarly, Cuban Americans, in common with many other Hispanic Caribbean populations, also believe in Santeria and Brujeria. Santeria and Brujeria are syncretistic religious beliefs that were brought to the Caribbean from Africa during the period of slavery (1).

As previously discussed and documented, sociocultural factors could play a major role in the prevention and treatment of substance abuse among Hispanics and are critically important to the development of comprehensive programs for the treatment of the substance abusers in the United States.

ETHNIC AND RACIAL CONSIDERATIONS

The term "Hispanic" describes a population that includes several ethnic subgroups representing different countries of origin. In accordance with the Drug and Alcohol Services Information System, in 2003 about 238,000 TEDS admissions were Hispanics; of this number, 41% were Mexican, 34% Puerto Rican, 3% Cuban, and 22% other Hispanic subgroups (11). It has also been advanced that Hispanics have similarities and also differences with respect to biologic factors related to drug abuse and addiction (23). Women from Hispanic origin also need to be taken into consideration with respect to addictive behavior; an estimated 1% of Hispanic women aged 12 years and older have injected drugs for addictive purposes on at least one occasion; additionally, intravenous drug use is 4.6 to 6.5 times more often among 18- to 44-year-old Hispanic women in comparison to 12- to 17-year-old Hispanic women (24). With respect to drinking patterns among men, Mexicans report the most frequent and also the most heavy drinking, as well as the greatest prevalence of drunkenness and alcohol-related problems. Cubans report the lowest and Puerto Ricans and other Hispanic subgroups are in between Mexicans and Cubans (25).

Mexicans who migrate to the United States are considered to have a better mental health profile than do U.S.-born Mexican Americans; perhaps, this difference is due to a protective effect of traditional family networks and a lower level of expectations about what really constitutes "success" in Americans among Mexicans who migrate to the United States; however, the high rates of psychopathology among U.S.-born Mexican Americans may also be related to their easier access to abused substances and their elevated frequency of substance abuse (26,27).

In another study, it was demonstrated that smoking interventions for people of Mexican descent should be tailored in accordance with gender, nativity, and level of acculturation, as well as targeted to all ages, not just persons (28). In this study, smoking rates among Mexican-born women were lower than reported rates for Hispanics, non-Hispanic Whites, and African Americans. Among U.S.-born people, older age, male gender, a higher level acculturation, more than a high school education, and residing in a census tract with a higher median age predicted a history of smoking.

In a similar study focusing on Mexicans and Mexican Americans, men had higher rates of drug use than women for every drug; urban rates were higher than rural rates for both men and women; however, the combined effect of U.S. nativity and acculturation vis-à-vis drug use was greater among women than among men. Obviously, in this study, acculturation and U.S. nativity were risk factors for illicit drug use among Mexican origin men and women; however, women had increased vulnerability compared with men (29–31).

With respect to Puerto Ricans, a recent study has shown that Hispanic drug-using women in Puerto Rico and in New York City are exposed to severe drug treatment disparities (6). Additionally, in terms of HIV risk behavior among Puerto Rican injection drug users (IDUs), despite the decrease in the AIDS incidence in Puerto Rico, the prevalence of HIV risk behaviors in Puerto Ricans is very high (32). Another interesting study focusing on Puerto Rican addicts demonstrated that similar patterns of substance use were found for Hispanic youth living in Puerto Rico in comparison with Hispanic youth residing in the United States (33). Similarly, another study examined whether the place of residency is a factor associated with the reporting of positive HIV/AIDS, Hepatitis C (HCV), or sexually transmitted disease (STD) status in a sample of 400 IDUs residing in Puerto Rico and in the United States (Western Massachusetts). Additionally, this study showed that the Capacity Enhancement Model was successful in reducing drug use, HIV/AIDS, HCV, and STDs among Puerto Ricans living in both Puerto Rico and Western Massachusetts (34). Along these lines, another study focusing on the role of acculturation vis-à-vis needle-sharing behavior among Puerto Rican IDUs demonstrated that incarceration could be a significant risk factor in the spread of HIV among intravenous drug users; for instance, Puerto Rican IDUs born in the mainland United States are 2.1 times more likely to share needles than their counterparts born in Puerto Rico, after controlling for gender, age, education, drug overdose, incarceration history, and psychiatric status (35–37).

PUBLIC POLICY CONSIDERATIONS

In discussing the subject of substance abuse among the different Hispanic populations residing in the United States, one must also address issues related to public policy development and implementation. To begin with, we recommend and expect that Hispanics be directly involved and fully participate in the design and implementation of such policies. This type of involvement will ensure identification with these policies and, more importantly, compliance with them. Hispanic consumers must also be involved at all levels of this process because they will be the recipients of the impact of these policies. Hispanics based on their clinical skills and cultural knowledge can better plan and design culturally sensitive program models geared to the treatment of Hispanic patients. In doing so, they can also serve as ideal role models for future generations of Hispanic mental health professionals.

An important public policy issue has to do with the development of an appropriate national database for Hispanics. So far, efforts in this regard have been limited. The collection of reliable data at a national level will be a positive step toward its application to public policy development. It was only recently that Hispanics began to be classified according to their country of origin, and that attention was given to this very important issue. Reliable national data is very powerful in calling attention to public health problems and thus leading to their solution.

Another issue that requires attention is the development of preventive and educational programs. While patient care is important, efforts directed at prevention are also essential. The spiraling costs of health care in this nation have negatively affected prevention efforts. However, the most effective method of reducing health care cost is to prevent illnesses.

We should also focus on the legal system in relation to public policy formulations. In this regard, drug legalization and decriminalization deserve consideration and attention. In analyzing legalization of drugs, we must focus on the pros and cons of drug prohibition policies. The total U.S. antidrug expenditure in 1990 was $9.5 billion (38). Because legalization or decriminalization could lead to a reduction in the cost of the government's antidrug expenditures, it could also lead to a redistribution of expenditures in the direction of treatment and prevention. Additionally, because legalization or decriminalization would result in lowering the cost of illicit drugs, it would also result in a decrease in drug-related criminal activities. This reduction in drug-related criminal activities would also further reduce the cost of the criminal justice system. In this regard, methadone maintenance programs represent a limited form of drug legalization and decriminalization. While the connection between drugs and crime could be seen as coincidental, it is nevertheless important. For instance, a survey conducted in 1986 among inmates of state prisons revealed that 43% were using illegal drugs on a daily basis (39). Furthermore, it is a well-accepted fact that some illicit drugs influence people to commit crimes by reducing inhibitions and increasing aggressiveness. Cocaine, for instance, is a drug that has gained this reputation in recent years. However, opponents of legalization or decriminalization claim that such measures would certainly increase drug availability, decrease their price, and remove the deterrent power of the criminal sanctions, thus leading to an increase in drug use and abuse. However, the use of tobacco has decreased in recent years as a result of educational and prevention efforts.

Undoubtedly, legalization or decriminalization of illicit drugs contains some risks. However, our current laws and policies have not yet yielded much permanent benefit. We must objectively evaluate all of our options, including legalization or decriminalization alternatives. Not doing so will help maintain the status quo and will further contribute to the deterioration on the living conditions of our ethnic minority ghetto populations, particularly Hispanics.

CONCLUSION

For decades, the substance abuse problem has been devastating for the Hispanic population residing in the United States. However, not enough attention has been given to this problem, particularly with respect to preventive approaches, epidemiologic research, culturally sensitive clinical interventions, treatment outcome studies, and public policy formulations. Additionally, program development and fiscal allocations have not been commensurate with the size of these problems. Recently, however, the substance abuse and HIV epidemics have extended into the White population of this country. As a result of this shift, the government, particularly at the federal level, has been forced to pay more attention to the substance abuse problem. Generally, traditional agencies and government bureaucracy have overlooked the need for basic awareness of the characteristics, conditions, and circumstances surrounding the Hispanic substance abuser.

Unfortunately, most of the non-Hispanic staff currently employed in substance abuse treatment programs servicing Hispanics are unprepared in terms of (a) Spanish language ability, (b) an understanding of the Hispanic substance abusers' socioeconomic background, and (c) awareness of the Hispanic culture and heritage. Undoubtedly, these critical gaps have had a negative impact on service effectiveness, positive treatment outcomes, and, even more importantly, prevention strategies. If Hispanic substance abusers are to be rehabilitated effectively, program designers and treatment staff must understand not only the values and norms inherent in the Hispanic cultures, but also those circumstances which threaten that culture.

This chapter is aimed to shed light upon these problems and to present data to support our observations. Hopefully, through increased research efforts and appropriate financial support, we will eventually conquer this major tragedy that is currently faced by the Hispanic families.

REFERENCES

1. Ruiz P, Langrod JG. Hispanic Americans. In: Lowinson JH, Ruiz P, Millman RB, et al., eds. *Substance Abuse: A Comprehensive Textbook*, 4th ed. Philadelphia, PA: Lippincott Williams & Wilkins; 2005:1103–1112.
2. Wu L, Schlenger WE. Private health insurance coverage for substance abuse and mental health services, 1995 to 1998. *Psychiatr Serv*. 2004;55(2):180–182.
3. Ruiz P. Presidential address: addressing patient needs: access, parity and humane care. *Am J Psychiatry*. 2007;164(10): 1507–1509.
4. Alvarez LR, Ruiz P. Substance abuse in the Mexican American population. In: Straussner SLA, ed. *Ethnocultural Factors in Substance Abuse Treatment*. New York, NY: Guilford Press; 2001:111–136.
5. Rothe EM, Ruiz P. Substance abuse among Cuban Americans. In: Straussner SLA, ed. *Ethnocultural Factors in Substance Abuse Treatment*. New York, NY: Guilford Press; 2001:97–110.
6. Robless RR, Matos TD, Deren S, et al. Drug treatment disparities among Hispanic drug-using women in Puerto Rico and New York City. *Health Policy*. 2006;75(2):159–169.
7. U.S. Census Bureau, 1990 Census. Available at: http://www.census.gov/main/www/cen1990.html. Accessed June 1, 2010.
8. U.S. Census Bureau, 2000 Census. Available at: http://www.census.gov/main/www/cen2000.html. Accessed June 1, 2010.
9. Ruiz P. Psychopathology and migration. In: "Psiquiatria 2006": III Symposium Admirall; "Libro de Resumenes", Vol 1. Barcelona, Spain; 2004:47–60.
10. Substance Abuse and Mental health Services Administration (SAMHSA): The DASIS Report, September 20, 2002.
11. Office of Applied Studies, Substance Abuse and Mental Health Services Administration (SAMHSA): The DASIS Report, August 19, 2005.
12. World Health Organization (WHO). Mental Health Gap Action Programme: Scaling up care for mental, neurological, and substance use disorders. World Health Organization, 2008.
13. Wallace JM Jr. The social ecology of addiction: race, risk, and resilience. *Pediatrics*. 1999;103(5):1122–1127.
14. Alegria M, Mulvaney-Day N, Torres M, et al. Prevalence of psychiatric disorders across Latino subgroups in the United States. *Am J Public Health*. 2007;97(1):68–75.
15. Mulia N, Ye Y, Zemore SE, et al. Social disadvantage, stress, and alcohol use among Black, Hispanic, and White Americans: findings from the 2005 U.S. National Alcohol Survey. *J Stud Alcohol Drugs*. 2008;69:824–833.
16. Bluthental RN, Jacobson JO, Robinson PL. Are racial disparities in alcohol treatment completion associated with racial differences in treatment modality entry? Comparison of outpatient treatment and residential treatment in Los Angeles, County, 1998 to 2000. *Alcohol Clin Exp Res*. 2007;31(11):1920–1926.
17. Gil AG, Wagner EF, Tubman JG. Culturally sensitive substance abuse intervention for Hispanics and African American adolescents: empirical examples from the Alcohol Treatment Targeting

Adolescents in Need (ATTAIN) project. *Addiction*. 2004;99(suppl 2):140–150.
18. Johnson PB, Glassman M. The moderating effects of gender and ethnicity on the relationship between effect expectancies and alcohol problems. *J Stud Alcohol*. 1999;60(1):64–69.
19. Wong EC. Ethnic identity, spirituality, and self-efficacy influences on treatment outcome among Hispanic American methadone maintenance clients. *J Ethn Subst Abuse*. 2008;7(3):328–340.
20. State Division of Substance Abuse Services. Statewide Household Survey of Substance Abuse, 1986: Illicit Substance Use among Hispanic Adults in New York State. State Division of Substance Abuse Services; 1988.
21. Ruiz P, Varner RV, Small DR, et al. Ethnic difference in the neuroleptic treatment of schizophrenia. *Psychiatr Q*. 1999;70(2):163–172.
22. Gfroerer J, De La Rosa M. Protective and risk factors associated with drug use among Hispanic youth. *J Addict Dis*. 1993;12(2):87–107.
23. Trujillo KA, Castañeda E, Martinez D, et al. Biological research on drug abuse and addiction in Hispanics: current status and future directions. *Drug Alcohol Depend*. 2006;84(suppl 1):S17–S18.
24. Delva J, Furr CF, Anthony JC. Personal characteristics associated with injecting drug use among Latinas in the United States of America. *Rev Panam Salud Publica*. 1998;4(5):341–345.
25. Nielsen AL. Examining drinking patterns and problems among Hispanic groups: results from a national survey. *J Stud Alcohol*. 2000;61(2):301–310.
26. Escobar JI, Nervi CH, Gara MA. Immigration and mental health: Mexican Americans in the United States. *Harv Rev Psychiatry*. 2000;8:64–72.
27. Farley T, Galves A, Dickinson LM, et al. Stress, coping and health: a comparison of Mexican immigrants, Mexican-Americans, and non-Hispanic whites. *J Immigr Health*. 2005;7(3):213–220.
28. Wilkinson AV, Spitz MR, Strom SS, et al. Effects of nativity, age at migration, and acculturation on smoking among adult Houston residents of Mexican descent. *Am J Public Health*. 2005;95:1043–1049.
29. Vega WA, Alderete E, Kolody B, et al. Illicit drug use among Mexicans and Mexican Americans in California: the effects of gender and acculturation. *Addiction*. 1998;93(12):1839–1850.
30. Ruiz P, Matorin AA. Factores determinantes de la adiccion en la comunidad hispana de los estados unidos. *Psychline*. 2002;4(2):21–28.
31. Ruiz P. Spanish, English, and mental health services. *Am J Psychiatry*. 2007;164(8):1133–1135.
32. Reyes JC, Robles RR, Colon HM, et al. Severe anxiety symptomatology and HIV risk behavior among Hispanic injection drug users in Puerto Rico. *AIDS Behav*. 2007;11(1):145–150.
33. Maldonado-Molina MM, Collins LM, Lanza ST, et al. Patterns of substance use onset among Hispanics in Puerto Rico and the United States. *Addict Behav*. 2007;32(10):2432–2437.
34. Lopez LM, Zerden LS, Fitzgerald TC, et al. Puerto Rican injection drug users: prevention implications in Massachusetts and Puerto Rico. *Eval Program Plann*. 2008;31(1):64–73.
35. Cuadrado M, Lieberman L. Traditionalism in the prevention of substance misuse among Puerto Ricans. *Subst Use Misuse*. 1998;33(14):2737–2755.
36. Epstein JA, Botvin GJ, Diaz T. Linguistic acculturation associated with higher marijuana and polydrug use among Hispanic adolescents. *Subst Use Misuse*. 2001;36(4):477–499.
37. Estrada AL. Drug use and HIV risks among African Americans, Mexican-Americans, and Puerto Rican Drug injectors. *J Psychoactive Drugs*. 1998;30(3):247–253.
38. U.S. News & World Report; December 24, 1990, p. 12.
39. Nadelmann EA. Drug prohibition in the United States: cost, consequences, and alternatives. *Science*. 1989;245:939–946.

CHAPTER 61

Asian Americans and Pacific Islanders

John W. Tsuang ■ Edmond H. Pi

INTRODUCTION

Recent research findings have shown that biologic, psychological, and social/cultural factors affect the onset and course of substance abuse. Coinciding with the increasing numbers of Asian Americans and Pacific Islanders (AA/PIs) in the United States, there are increasing efforts to evaluate substance use issues among them. However, factors that influence substance abuse among AA/PIs remain multifaceted. This chapter reviews the available data related to the use of substances among AA/PIs, focusing on demographics, epidemiology, biopsychosocial factors, treatment, and prevention.

EPIDEMIOLOGY

AA/PIs are diverse in ethnicity, as well as their historical experiences in the United States. They represent heterogeneous groups differing in language, religion, culture, immigration pattern, generation, socioeconomic status, and the degree of acculturation into the mainstream American culture. However, despite all these differences, most epidemiologic studies have clustered all Asians and PIs into one grouping. Recent studies have shown a tremendous growth in the number of AA/PIs, with data suggesting that the percentage growth of the Asian population within a certain period was the highest in any ethnic group (1). This rapid growth has made existing data extremely complex, while also confusing. Thus, to simplify the issue, for the epidemiologic portion, we will summarize results for Asians and PIs as a group first and then discuss the subgroups subsequently.

The estimated number of U.S. residents in July 2007 who said they were Asian alone or Asian in combination with one or more other ethnic group was 15.2 million (1). This group comprised about 5% of the total U.S. population. Between 2006 and 2007, the percentage growth of the Asian population was 2.9%, the highest of any ethnic group during that time period (1). The increase in the Asian population during the period totaled 434,000. In 2007, there were 5 million self-identified Asians in California, the state with the largest Asian population. California also had the largest numerical increase from 2006 to 2007 at 106,000 (1). New York (1.4 million) and Texas (915,000) followed in population. Texas (44,000) and New York (33,000) followed in numerical increase. In Hawaii, Asians made up the highest proportion of the total population (55%), with California (14%) and New Jersey and Washington (8% each) next. Asians were the largest minority group in Hawaii and Vermont. The estimated number of U.S. residents in July 2007 who said they were Native Hawaiian and Other Pacific Islander, either alone or in combination with one or more other ethnic groups, was 1 million (1). This group comprised 0.3% of the total population. In 2007, Hawaii had the largest population (269,000) of Native Hawaiians and Other Pacific Islanders (either alone or in combination with one or more other races), followed by California (262,000) and Washington (50,000). California had the largest numerical increase (2900) of people of this group, with Texas (2500) and Florida (1100) next (1). In Hawaii, Native Hawaiians and Other Pacific Islanders comprised the largest proportion (21%) of the total population, followed by Utah (1%) and Alaska (0.9%). Between 2006 and 2007, the percentage growth of the Native Hawaiian and Other Pacific Islander population was 1.6%. The increase in the Native Hawaiian and Other Pacific Islander population during the period totaled 16,000 (1).

In 2007, the major Asian groups in the United States were Chinese (3.54 million), followed by Filipinos (3.05 million), Asian Indians (2.77 million), Vietnamese (1.64 million), Koreans (1.56 million), and Japanese (1.22 million). Other Asian groups (13%) include Burmese, Cambodian, Hmong, Laotian, Thai, and Tongan. These estimates represented the number of people who were either of a particular Asian group only or of that group in combination with one or more other Asian groups or races. The major PI groups were Native Hawaiian—the largest Asian group—followed by Samoan, Guamanian or Chamorro, and other Pacific Island groups (1).

During the 1990s, the Substance Abuse and Mental Health Services Administration (SAMHSA) sponsored a series of national household surveys to measure the prevalence of illicit drug and alcohol use among Americans. AA/PIs were classified in the "other" category until 1999, when Asian and Native Hawaiian or Other Pacific Islander was separated (2). In the 2000 SAMHSA survey, 2654 AA/PIs were interviewed. It was estimated that 0.4 million (5.2%) of AA/PIs "used illicit drugs in the past year" and 0.2 million (2.7%) "used an illicit drug in the past month" (3). AA/PIs had the lowest rate of illicit drug use in comparison to the general population and to other ethnic subgroups (3). However, contrary to the popular myth of being the "model minority," data showed that AA/PIs do use illicit drugs.

The SAMHSA survey showed that AA/PIs are more likely to drink alcohol and smoke cigarettes than to use illicit drugs (3). It was estimated that 2.3 million AA/PIs (28%) had "used alcohol in their lifetime," and in the 18- to 25-year-old age group, 3.2 million (39.4%) had consumed alcohol. Three million AA/PIs (38.8%) had "used cigarettes in their lifetime," and 3.4 million (41.9%) in the 18- to 25-year-old age group had smoked in their lifetime (3). AA/PIs ranked the lowest among all racial subgroups in terms of proportions that drank alcohol or smoked cigarettes. However, the gap between AA/PIs and the next racial group (African Americans), in terms of smoking (41.9% vs. 50.2%) or drinking (39.4% vs. 43.9%), was much smaller than the differences in illicit drug use (3).

The survey showed a drop in illicit drug and alcohol use by AA/PIs when comparing data from 1999 to 2000. "Illicit drug use in the last year" went from 20.2% to 18.8%, and "any alcohol use" went from 30.7% to 28% (3). However, there were some disturbing trends in this study, as well as in others. The rates of heavy alcohol use by Asian youth (five binges in the last month) doubled from 1999 to 2000 (0.5% to 0.9%). Others researchers found that AA/PI high school students who met criteria for heavy drinking consumed more alcohol per day when they did drink (1.46 ounces/day) than did whites (0.86 ounces/day) (4). The SAMHSA survey showed that in the age group 26 years and older, Vietnamese Americans had the highest percentage of current marijuana use (2.8%). The "past-month hallucinogen use" for Asian youth was 1.4%, which is equal to the highest rates of hallucinogen use. Finally, AA/PI youths' abuse of prescription drugs had more than tripled from 1999 to 2000 (5). One particularly concerning trend, though, is the evidence showing elevated rates of methamphetamine abuse and dependence among AA/PIs. These rates have been shown to be as high as 9% in some studies (6).

National treatment surveys showed that AA/PIs represent 4% of population, but less than 1% of them were admitted to Treatment Episode Data Set (TEDS, which is a compilation of data on those admitted to substance abuse treatment [DASIS]) (7). But the trend is changing; between 1994 and 1999, the number of AA/PI admissions increased by 37% (9800 to 13,400), while total admissions decreased by 3%. For AA/PIs, alcohol abuse counted for 34% of all admissions followed by marijuana (19%), stimulants (19%), opiates (15%), and cocaine (11%). At the time of admission, Asians were younger (average age 30 years) than the general population (average age 33 years), and a greater proportion of them were in treatment for the first time (51% vs. 36%, respectively). This increase in the number entering into substance abuse treatment might reflect more substance abuse by AA/PIs or the greater acceptance of need for treatment among Asians (7,8).

Critics have argued about the inaccuracy of national survey studies. In the SAMHSA study, results from the Native Hawaiian or Other Pacific Islanders were not reported because only 545 people were surveyed. This was unfortunate as PIs have high rates of substance abuse and alcohol use (9). By excluding them, the numbers of substance abusers among AA/PIs were artificially lowered. In addition, underreporting of substance abuse problems is prominent among AA/PIs (8).

Some Asian cultures incorporate substances use into their religious practices or daily accepted activities; thus, their uses are often not mentioned. Other issues, such as types of people surveyed, cultural and language barriers, and culturally insensitive questions, all can contribute to the lower rates of substance abuse (10). In summary, AA/PIs do have the lowest rates of illicit drug, alcohol, and cigarette use among all different ethnic subgroups. However, there is concern about increasing substance abuse among AA/PI adolescents and other high-risk groups. More current nationwide survey studies on substance abuse by different ethnic minorities need to be done.

Another behavioral addiction gaining more attention among AA/PIs is pathologic gambling. Recent community surveys have shown that approximately 30% of the AA/PI casino patrons surveyed met criteria for pathologic gambling that is strikingly high (11). Gambling problem is a century-old issue among certain Asian subgroups. However, little is known about the etiology and treatment of gambling addiction among AA/PIs. There are investigators attempting to study this area, but more attention is required.

PREVENTION

Various people have written about prevention strategies against substance abuse for AA/PIs, but the effectiveness of these measures has not been studied. Most authors agree with the thought that culturally responsive prevention strategies should be linked into the natural support systems of that particular Asian Pacific community, for example, in the Filipino community, using the church as a forum for prevention work. Prevention should provide Asian parents with the skills they need to help their children assimilate into American culture, such as helping them with their roles in the educational and recreational processes. Programs should develop strategies to minimize shame and loss of face in AA/PIs. One example of how this can be done is by using a community intermediary to manage interpersonal conflicts between parents and youth. Finally, community education programs might use more personalized contacts for prevention, such as a door-to-door education campaign in the high-risk community (8).

A family-oriented approach in which an extended family is included in issues of prevention, intervention, and treatment will have the best chance of success in the Asian community. One needs to address issues of denial, underreporting, and the need for getting outside help. It is very important to preserve the family unit as a hedge against substance use (12). Other strategies can include the use of media campaigns in their native languages and the use of high-profile community role models to advertise against substance abuse. One should also promote self-esteem and culturally appropriate life-skills building for Asian youth, and engage culturally specific human service networks for prevention process. It is imperative to understand that inclusion of family members in prevention of addiction among AA/PIs is extremely important. However, one needs to not forget the issues of acculturation among the younger generation of the population, where society and peer values may triumph over family values. In such case, not only will the family need to be involved, but peer education in school as well as in the community will also be necessary. Needless to say, all of these recommendations on prevention approaches should be studied for their effectiveness (10).

TREATMENT

Despite the growing body of evidence that shows that addictive disorders in AA/PIs are significant, there remain many barriers to treatment. These barriers include cultural, individual, and practical issues (13). Studies have shown that AA/PIs have poor access to medical and psychiatric health care as well as to addiction treatment (14,15). This occurs despite the fact that AA/PI and non-AA/PI substance abusers do not differ in terms of treatment retention and outcome once they have received treatment (16). As seen from the TEDS data, an increasing number of AA/PIs are entering substance abuse treatment; however, they are still greatly underrepresented in various addiction treatment settings (7,17). This underrepresentation of AA/PIs in treatment may result from many factors (13,18). As for the cultural factors, the traditional way to "handle" an Asian addict is to either deny the problem or attempt to handle the issue within the family structure. Family members often rescue and enable the patient and try to solve the problem internally to maintain the appearance of normality. The strategy is to "save face," which often causes the family to delay confrontation of the patient. By the time the addiction process becomes unmanageable, both a strong sense of failure and family shame have occurred. Thus, when an AA/PI patient is referred to a drug/alcohol treatment program, typically all other alternatives have been exhausted and they are further along in their addiction process. The family wants a "quick fix" from the treatment program, but the client is still reluctant to receive treatment. Often, abandonment of the patient can occur at this time when family support is most essential. Consequently, AA/PIs see entrance into drug and alcohol treatment programs as the last resort, while the addicts are often angry and feel abandoned, which makes their treatment even more difficult (19,20).

There are other cultural barriers facing AA/PIs for entering into a substance abuse treatment program. They include the stigma of suffering from addiction to drugs and/or alcohol, the lack of recognition of addiction as a medical disorder, the language and cultural barriers, and a sense of mistrust for the U.S. health care system. AA/PI clients also face the problem of openly acknowledging personal problems, the double standard for women, and the religious belief of fate and need for suffering. AA/PIs are also racially and culturally heterogeneous; they don't all fit well in just one type of treatment program. They probably will benefit much more from culturally sensitive and specific programs (8,19).

There are practical barriers to the delivery of care to the AA/PI population. Issues such as cost, lack of awareness that such treatment exists, or lack of addiction treatment services are all potential limiting factors. Those who do not have access to care include those who do not speak English, recent immigrants, and the uninsured (14). Also, a critical system issue is the lack of culturally competent services tailored to specific AA/PI language, cultural beliefs, and values. Finally, the lack of evidence-based treatment program and the misinterpretation of "a cure" in substance abuse treatment, all make these important contributing factors deterring AA/PIs from entering into treatment.

Many authors have recommended strategies to overcome barriers, and understanding the cultural and practical barriers that exist is the first step to reducing them. Some have suggested that treatment programs for AA/PIs should be multicultural and multilingual (8,10,19). These services should be delivered from community-based sites with community inputs. The inpatient treatment should include a therapeutic community in residential treatment and the use of cognitive–behavioral treatment. The program should follow the traditional Alcoholics Anonymous (AA)/Narcotics Anonymous (NA) treatment strategies of combining 12-step approaches with meeting locations that are close to the local community. However, there should be some alterations to the "one-treatment-fits-all" approach. These modifications, specifically for AA/PIs, should include the strategy of reducing confrontation initially, so individuals can decrease the embarrassment, shame, and loss of face upon entering a treatment program. Additionally, having a trusted member of the Asian community present at these support groups might be helpful. Counseling approaches and peer groups should be supportive and educational, less confrontational. Family engagement, counseling, and support from the community will be crucial to the individual's recovery (8). Working with family members, even before the clients enter into treatment, might be beneficial in reducing enabling behaviors and negative emotions. Having bilingual meetings, help of local community cultural expert, and use of a medical approach that simultaneously treats medical and addiction issues might also improve acceptability of the treatment. Finally, any outside factors to increase motivation, such as court involvement (i.e., drug court), or to get the encouragement of the patriarchal member of the family will be helpful (19). Future tools to reduce barriers should be studied, and this should include collaborative efforts between the local Asian communities with the federal, state, and county agencies.

In addition to reducing barriers to substance abuse treatment for AA/PIs, one also needs to be aware of the high prevalence of mental illness among those suffering from addictive disorders. The presence of mental disorders can be a major obstacle to obtaining appropriate treatment. Studies have shown that more than half of people who meet a lifetime history of a *Diagnostic and Statistical Manual of Mental Disorders, Third Edition, Revised (DSM–III–R)* mental disorder diagnosis also have a concurrent substance abuse diagnosis, so-called co-occurring disorder patients (21,22). Given the growing evidence that mental disorders and substance abuse problems frequently co-occur, mental health assessment among AA/PIs seeking substance abuse treatment should be conducted. Though there are no studies addressing the specific issues of treating AA/PIs with co-occurring disorders, most patients suffering from dual-diagnosis issues should be treated in an integrated treatment program for maximum benefit (23,24).

The state-of-the-art treatment for addictive disorders should include using psychosocial treatment combined with psychopharmacology. Several new pharmacotherapy agents have been developed to provide relief from acute withdrawal symptoms as well as relapse prevention and maintenance treatments. Agents for treatment of acute withdrawal are most relevant to dependence on alcohol and opioids. These include benzodiazepines, beta-blockers, barbiturates, valproate/carbamazepine for alcohol withdrawal, and buprenorphine, clonidine, and methadone for opiates (25,26). Prevention and maintenance treatments can be either blocking agents or substitution agents. In the United States, the Federal Drug Agency (FDA) has approved four agents for the treatment of alcoholism—disulfiram, naltrexone, acamprosate, and vivitrol (IM naltrexone) (25). As for opiates, FDA has approved methadone and buprenorphine for maintenance treatment (26). Unfortunately, no studies have been done for using these agents in the AA/PI populations. Thus, despite the approval of these addictive medications for treatment in the general population, their effectiveness in the ethnic Asian minority groups has not been established. One interesting side note is the fact that using pharmacotherapy for treatment of addictive disorders is not well accepted in the general substance abuse treatment community because of the belief of the need to be totally abstinent, the fear of medications, and the general distrust for the medical community. For AA/PIs, the use of medications might actually be more likely to be accepted by them, as some of the AA/PIs are more likely to associate the use of medication with treatment of medical disorders. Often they may look down upon psychosocial treatment only, and if it can combine with a legitimate medication, it might make the treatment more palatable. Thus, an unintended effect could be the better acceptance of medications and improved compliance of using them for treatment of addictive disorders.

FACTORS INFLUENCING SUBSTANCE USE IN THIS POPULATION

Genetic/Biologic Factors

Although multiple factors, including genetics, have been proposed to affect the addiction process, there is a striking lack of information between genetics and drugs of abuse in the AA/PI population. Yet the best genetic data came from the twin studies of alcohol abuse, so we use this as a model for much of the discussion that follows. Most recently, new findings have come out of China linking genetics to opioid addiction among Han Chinese. This exciting new discovery will be discussed at the end of this section.

The best-studied area is still the genetic contribution to the development of alcoholism. Family and adoption studies have found a significant hereditary contribution in alcoholism, although these data were not derived from the AA/PI population (27,28). For Asians, the transmission of alcohol genes and the mechanism for impaired alcohol metabolism are areas of special interests.

Approximately 50% of northeast Asians (Chinese, Japanese, and Koreans) have a genetically defined deficiency in the liver enzyme, aldehyde dehydrogenase (ALDH2) (29,30). This deficiency is inherited through one mutant ALDH2*2 allele, a dominant mutation that disrupts the function of the subunit polypeptide and reduces enzyme activity (31). The ALDH2*2 allele is prevalent among northeast Asians but is rare in non-Asians (32). Asians with ALDH2*2 alleles have slower oxidation of acetaldehyde during alcohol metabolism, resulting in the accumulation of acetaldehyde, and subsequently the exhibition of a "flushing reaction" after ingestion of alcohol (33,34). This response is accompanied by increased heart rate, visible redness, and feelings of warmth (35) that are presumably mediated through histamines and other vasoactive compounds (36). This genetically determined flushing reaction is thought to be one factor related to the reduction in alcohol consumption among Asians (37,38). Individuals with ALDH2*2 alleles (ALDH2*1/2*2 heterozygotes or ALDH2*2/2*2 homozygotes) drink less alcohol (37,39,40) and have lower rates of alcohol dependence (41,42) when compared with those with the ALDH2*1/2*1 homozygous genotype. Conversely, most patients with alcoholic liver diseases have the ALDH2*1/2*1 homozygous genotype (40,42).

Also 85% to 90% of northeast Asians possess an "atypical" alcohol dehydrogenase enzyme (ADH2) that can increase the capacity to convert alcohol into acetaldehyde, further contributing to the flushing reaction after alcohol ingestion (43). The ADH2 is a functional polymorphism of the alcohol dehydrogenase gene that protects against heavy drinking and alcoholism (36). To date, ALDH2 is the enzyme that is most likely to influence drinking behaviors, and it might be a protective factor for AA/PIs from alcohol dependence (30,36,40–42).

Illicit drug use and its genetic transmission is not well understood. Some researchers suggest that AA/PIs with certain genetic variations and metabolic differences might be at decreased risk for illicit drug use. For example, a recent study found that ALDH2 might be associated with the reduction in substance abuse behavior among Asians (30). Other factors such as the cytochrome P450 (CYP) system is involved in the metabolism of commonly used substances (36,44,45). Nicotine is metabolized to cotinine principally by the CYP2A6 enzyme. Individuals carrying the null (inactive) CYP2A6*2 or CYP2A6*3 alleles have impaired nicotine metabolism compared to the active CYP2A6*1 and show reduced smoking and nicotine dependence (46). Genetic deficiency in CYP2D6 metabolism, which converts codeine to morphine derivatives, provides protection against oral opiate dependence (47). AA/PIs may show some polymorphisms in the cytochrome enzymes that are responsible for this conversion. Thus, among AA/PIs, there are people who are extensive metabolizers (EMs) and others who are poor metabolizers (PMs) or slow metabolizers (SM), which can account for the fact that substances can be broken down in different rates. The relationship between genetic variations and the different rates of breaking down substances may all contribute to the lower rates of substance abuse by AA/PIs, and one needs to study this interaction further.

Other researchers have found evidence to suggest that genetic influences contribute to a common vulnerability for abusing marijuana, sedatives, stimulants, heroin or opiates, and psychedelics (48). In addition to this shared vulnerability, each drug has its own genetic vulnerability. For some abused drugs, there might be a stronger genetic impact on vulnerability than for other drugs (48). Results from the Wave Two study of genome-wide linkage of heroin-dependent Han Chinese found evidence for linkage at marker D17S1880, which maps to 53.4cM on chromosome 17q11.2. This has become the most strongly implicated locus for opiate addiction in this population (49). Other loci on chromosomes 1, 2, 4, 12, 16, and X also displayed significant evidence for linkage. As opioid dependence is considered a complex disorder, it is possible that other genes will make contributions to the overall risk for the development of opioid dependence. This is the strongest data thus far in the Han Chinese population that implicates a strong genetic contribution to the development of an addictive disorder. Other linkage studies are needed to find other loci as risk factors for the development of opioid and other substance abuse disorders not only in the general population but particularly among the AA/PIs.

Nonbiologic Factors

The genetic studies have made a major impact on our understanding of the inheritance of alcoholism. Even with this biologic predisposition, however, the expression of alcoholism can be affected by environmental, social, and psychological factors (40). It is difficult to disentangle the specific environmental factors that affect drinking, but for the purpose of discussion, we separate them into family/cultural, acculturation, and psychological factors.

Family/Cultural Factors

Family unity and other cultural factors play a significant role in the development of substance abuse issues. It was suggested that the relatively late age of onset of alcohol use for Asian American youth than for non-Asian American youth might be a result of parental modeling or cultural influences (30). Asian American students, who had a more abstinence-promoting environment than their European–American counterparts, were less likely to drink alcohol. Asian students were less likely to have "adult and peer influences to use alcohol or cigarettes," "less offers of alcohol," and "increased likelihood of having an intact family." It was concluded that a strong family connection and the lower prevalence of parents and peer use might reduce Asian's alcohol use (35).

The importance of norms and values in Asian cultures may moderate drinking by AA/PIs. One study proposed that attitudes about drinking, such as lack of negative feelings about alcohol by Chinese and Jewish communities, might be related to reduced alcohol consumption (50,51). Other cultural factors, such as responsibility to others, prescribed behaviors, interdependence, restraint, and group achievement, all may reduce drinking (52). Additional factors such as cultural traditions; Asian religions; respect for authority; Asians' belief in order, propriety, and harmony; as well as concerns with shame and losing face can affect alcohol consumption (53). Some Asian cultural beliefs validate habitual alcohol and substance use. Many traditional medicines are alcohol based and are taken for energy boost (gelatin from tiger bones dissolved in alcohol) or for pain relief (opium in alcohol). Others, such as chewing of the betel quid or stimulant leaf, are done to produce euphoria (20,12,54). Use of sleeping pills to alleviate stress is also considered a culturally acceptable practice among some AA/PIs as a means of re-establishing equilibrium (12,54).

Other researchers have shown that peer pressure, acculturation, and family discord are the major factors associated with marijuana and cocaine use among AA/PIs (55). Factors related to a higher lifetime use of cigarettes, alcohol, and marijuana by high school students of Vietnamese and Chinese descent included poor school performance, low subjective well-being, lack of parents' or peers' disapproval of substance use, perceived tensions at school, and being male (55). At this time, although significant, not much is known about the environmental influences on illicit drug use by AA/PIs.

Acculturation Factors

The degree of acculturation into mainstream America has correlated significantly with the development of addictive disorders. This is the case not only for AA/PIs but also for Hispanics and some African Americans. The definition of the acculturation process varies, but some have based it on a number of generations residing in the United States and the ability to speak English and/or their ethnic languages. One study found that Asians who did not speak English well reported drinking less than those who did speak it well (56). It was also reported that alcohol consumption was related to generation status and birthplace. Third- and fourth-generation Asians in the United States reported more drinking than did first- and second-generation Asians. There appeared to be significant group differences in alcohol consumption between foreign-born Asians and Asians born in America (56). This was the case for Hawaiian residents of Chinese and Japanese ancestry who had lower mean levels of alcohol use if they were born in Asia than if they were born in Hawaii (57). Hawaiian residents of white ancestry had lower mean levels of alcohol use if they were born in Hawaii than if they were born on the mainland. For Hawaiians, whom many considered to be more acculturated than other AA/PI groups, alcohol use is intermediate between the lower levels found in Asia and the higher levels found in the United States. Some studies found that assimilation of recently arrived immigrant groups is associated with increases in alcohol use. These results were found in Hispanic Americans (58), Mexican Americans (59), as well as in AAs (56,60). However, not all studies concurred with the idea that increased acculturation into Western culture will increase the amount of alcohol consumed (61,62). Nevertheless, it does appear that the acculturation process plays a role in the consumption of alcohol by AA/PIs. Some studies were done in the past to address the relationship between acculturation and addictive process, but more studies are required to better define acculturation and systematically determine the relationship between the degree of acculturation and alcohol and illicit substance use.

Psychological Factors

Psychological factors tend to be ignored by AA/PIs in the past, especially relating to addiction. Stress has been imputed to be a precursor to alcohol abuse in non-Asians as well as in Asians now (52,61,63). In general, psychological factors such as self-esteem, self-confidence, and assertiveness are related to alcohol use among adolescents (64). Psychological maladjustment was a significant factor associated with alcohol use among a sample of Chinese and Filipino youth (65). Other factors associated with risk for alcohol use among AA/PIs included pressure to succeed and a feeling of shame (10). For some Asians, the impact of immigration and accompanied psychological symptoms increased the risk for alcohol abuse (19). These immigrants suffered from feelings of personal failure and loss of control, which can lead to alcohol abuse (66). For example, Vietnamese and Highland Laotian (Hmong) immigrants reported using more alcohol as a means of coping with pain, insomnia, and alleviation of distress (20,63,67). The impact of stress and other psychological factors among people in general is obvious, and its effect on addictive process is particularly pertinent. For AA/PIs, many psychological reasons have been linked to increased alcohol abuse. However, this area continues to be poorly studied, and the degree of psychological impact on the precipitation and maintenance of alcoholism and illicit drug use among AA/PIs needs to be more intensely examined.

In summary, among AA/PIs, family and peer attitude, degree of assimilation, and psychological stresses, as well as cultural factors, appear to play a significant role in alcohol consumption. Although biologic/genetic factors are important, one must not forget the contributions of nonbiologic factors to explain racial/ethnic differences in alcohol consumption. Unfortunately, some of these studies had methodologic weaknesses, making it difficult to determine the extent of psychological/social/cultural influences on the onset and course of alcohol consumption; consequently, more studies are needed. In addition, more studies focusing on the relationships between environmental factors and illicit drug uses are needed.

CONCLUSIONS

With the rapid growth of the AA/PI populations in the United States, there is an increased need to address substance abuse issues among these populations. The limited epidemiologic data suggests that, in general, AA/PIs are at a relatively lower risk for substance use than other ethnic groups. However, it also suggests that rates of alcohol use, smoking, and use of some illicit drugs may not be as low as generally assumed. Recent finding of a strong genetic contribution to the development of opioid addiction among Han Chinese supports the biologically mediated process in addiction but also the severity of the problem in China. We also know that environmental influences can also play a role in contributing to substance use patterns. Past findings of AA/PIs infrequently use substance treatment services, which have led to a misperception as a lack of need for services by them. In fact, AA/PIs who entered treatment are younger and appeared in treatment for the first time, suggesting an increased need and acceptance for treatment. At present, there is a paucity of empirical information on the effectiveness of treatment and prevention programs targeting AA/PIs. Professionals who treat ethnically and culturally diverse AA/PI populations with substance abuse should be aware of the issues described in this chapter, so that they can tailor therapeutic regimens to be "culturally responsive," to assure high quality of care, and to meet the needs of population served. Because biologic, environmental, and cultural differences exist among different Asian ethnic groups, understanding similarities and differences between them can play an important role in ensuring that AA/PIs receive optimum substance abuse treatment.

REFERENCES

1. AsianWeek Newspaper (2008). Available at: Http://www.asianweek.com/2008/05/01/asian-american-population-surpasses-15-million/
2. U.S. Department of Health and Human Services, SAMHSA (1999). *National Household Survey on Drug Abuse Series: H-12. Summary of Findings from the 1999 National Household Survey on Drug Abuse*. NHSDA Series H-12, DDHS Publication No. (SMA) 01-3549. Rockville, MD: Office of Applied Studies.
3. U.S. Department of Health and Human Services, SAMHSA (2000). Summary of Findings from the 2000 Household Survey on Drug Abuse. NHSDA Series: H-13, DHHS Publication No. (SMA) 01-3549. Rockville, MD: Office of Applied Studies.
4. Welte J, Barnes GM. Alcohol use among adolescent minority groups. *J Stud Alcohol*. 1987;48:329–336.
5. U.S. Department of Health and Human Services, NCADI, SAMHSA. Asian/Pacific Islander Americans and substance abuse. *Prev Alert*. 2002;5:7.
6. Nemoto T, Operario D, Soma T. Risk behaviors of Filipino methamphetamine users in San Francisco: implications for prevention and treatment of drug use and HIV. *Public Health Report*. 2002;117:S30–S80.
7. Office of Applied Studies, Substance Abuse and Mental Health Services Administration. *The DASIS Report. Asians and Pacific Islanders in Substance Abuse Treatment: 1999*; 2002.
8. Zane N, Kim JH. Substance use and abuse. In: Zane N, Takeuchi D, Young K, eds. *Confronting Critical Health Issues of Asian and Pacific Islander Americans*. Thousand Oaks, CA: Sage Publications; 1994:316–343.
9. McLaughlin PG, Raymond JS, Murakami SR, et al. Drug use among Asian Americans in Hawaii. *J Psychoactive Drugs*. 1987;19:85–94.

10. Kuramoto F, Nakashima J. Developing an ATOD prevention campaign for Asian and Pacific Islanders: some considerations. *J Public Health Manage Pract.* 2000;6:57–64.
11. Fong TW, Campos MJ, DeCastro V, et al. Prevalence of problem and pathological gambling in a sample of casino patrons. *J Gambl Stud.* DOI 10.1007/s10899-010-9200-6. (Published online 12 June 2010).
12. D'Avanzo CE. Southeast Asians: Asian Pacific Americans at risk for substance misuse. *Subst Use Misuse.* 1997;32:829–848.
13. Fong TW, Tsuang JW. Asian-Americans, addictions, and barriers to treatment. *Psychiatry.* 2007;4(11):51–59.
14. Ta VM, Juon HS, Gielen AC, et al. Disparities in use of mental health and substance abuse services by Asian and native Hawaiian/other Pacific Islander women. *J Behav Health Serv Res.* 2008; 35(1):20–36. (Epub 2007 Jul 24).
15. Agency for Healthcare Research and Quality. *National Healthcare Disparities Report, 2004.* Available at: www.ahrq.gov/qual/nhdr04/nhdr04.htm. Accessed June 2010.
16. Niv N, Wong EC, Hser YI. Asian Americans in community-based substance abuse treatment: service needs, utilization, and outcomes. *J Subst Abuse Treat.* 2007;33(3):313–319. [Epub 2007 Mar 21].
17. James WH, Kim GK, Armijo E. The influence of ethnic identity on drug use among ethnic minority adolescents. *J Drug Educ.* 2000;30(3):265–280.
18. Sakai JT, Ho PM, Shore JH, et al. Asians in the United States: substance dependence and use of substance-dependence treatment. *J Subst Abuse Treat.* 2005;29(2):75–84.
19. Ja D, Aoki B. Substance abuse treatment: cultural barriers in the Asian-American community. *J Psychoactive Drugs.* 1993;25: 61–71.
20. Westermeyer JC. Native Americans, Asians, and new immigrants. In: Lowinson JH, Ruiz P, Millman RB, eds. *Substance Abuse: A Comprehensive Textbook.* 3rd ed. Baltimore: Williams & Wilkins; 1997:712–715.
21. Regier DA, Farmer ME, Rae DS, et al. Comorbidity of mental disorders with alcohol and other drug abuse: results from the epidemiologic catchment area (ECA) study. *JAMA.* 1990;264: 2511–2518.
22. Kessler RC, McGonagle KA, Zhao S, et al. Lifetime and 12-month prevalence of *DSM–III–R* psychiatric disorders in the United States: results from the National Comorbidity Survey. *Arch Gen Psychiatry.* 1994;51:8–19.
23. Tsuang J, Ho A, Eckman T, et al. Dual diagnosis treatment for patients with schizophrenia who abuse psychostimulants: rehab rounds [Invited article]. *J Psychiatric Serv.* 1997;48(7): 887–889.
24. Ho A, Tsuang J, Liberman R, et al. Achieving effective treatment of patients with chronic psychotic illness and comorbid substance dependence. *Am J Psychiatry.* 1999;156:1765–1770.
25. Leikin, J. Substance-related disorders in adults. *Dis Mon.* 2007; 53(6):315–335.
26. Vocci FJ, Acri J, Elkashef A. Medication development for addictive disorders: the state of the science. *Am J Psychiatry.* 2005;162(8):1432–1440.
27. Goodwin DW, Schulsinger F, Hermansen L, et al. Alcohol problems in adoptees raised apart from alcoholic biological parents. *Arch Gen Psychiatry.* 1973;28:238–243.
28. Schuckit MA, Goodwin DW, Winokur G. A study of alcoholism in half-siblings. *Am J Psychiatry.* 1972;128:1132–1136.
29. Wolff PH, Shea SH, Cha KK, et al. Vasomotor sensitivity to alcohol in diverse Mongoloid populations. *Am J Hum Genet.* 1973;25:193–199.
30. Wall TL, Shea SH, Chan KK, et al. A genetic association with the development of alcohol and other substance use behavior in Asian Americans. *J Abnorm Psychol.* 2001;110:173–178.
31. Crabb DW, Edenberg HJ, Bosron WF, et al. Genotypes for aldehyde dehydrogenase deficiency and alcohol sensitivity: the inactive ALDH2(2) allele is dominant. *J Clin Invest.* 1989; 83:314–316.
32. Goedde HW, Agarwal DP, Fritze G, et al. Distribution of ADH2 and ALDH2 genotypes in different populations. *Hum Genet.* 1992;88:344–346.
33. Shibuya A, Yasunami M, Yoshida A. Genotypes of alcohol dehydrogenase and aldehyde dehydrogenase loci in Japanese alcohol flushers and nonflushers. *Hum Genet.* 1989;82:14–16.
34. Wall TL, Thomasson HR, Ehlers CL. Investigator-observed alcohol-induced flushing but not self-report of flushing is a valid predictor of ALDH2 genotype. *J Stud Alcohol.* 1996;57: 267–272.
35. Au JG, Donaldson SI. Social influences as explanations for substance use differences among Asian American and European American adolescents. *J Psychoactive Drugs.* 2000;32:15–23.
36. Li TK. Pharmacogenetics of responses to alcohol and genes that influence alcohol drinking. *J Stud Alcohol.* 2000;61:5–12.
37. Tu GC, Israel Y. Alcohol consumption by Orientals in North America is predicted largely by a single gene. *Behav Genet.* 1995;25:59–65.
38. Wall TL, Thomasson HR, Schuckit MA, et al. Subjective feelings of alcohol intoxication in Asians with genetic variations of ALDH2 alleles. *Alcohol Clin Exp Res.* 1992;16:991–995.
39. Takeshita T, Morimoto K. Self-reported alcohol-associated symptoms and drinking behavior in three ALDH2 genotypes among Japanese university students. *Alcohol Clin Exp Res.* 1999; 23:1065–1069.
40. Yoshida A. Genetic polymorphisms of alcohol-metabolizing enzymes related to alcohol sensitivity and alcoholic diseases. In: Lin KM, Poland RE, Nakasaki G, eds. *Psychopharmacology and Psychobiology of Ethnicity.* Washington, DC: American Psychiatric Press; 1993:169–183.
41. Chen CC, Lu RB, Wang MF, et al. Interaction between the functional polymorphisms of the alcohol-metabolism genes in protection against alcoholism. *Am J Hum Genet.* 1999;65: 795–807.
42. Thomasson HR, Edenberg HJ, Crabb DW, et al. Alcohol and aldehyde dehydrogenase genotypes and alcoholism in Chinese men. *Am J Hum Genet.* 1991;48:667–681.
43. Agarwal DP, Goedde HW. *Alcohol Metabolism, Alcohol Intolerance and Alcoholism: Biochemical and Pharmacogenetic Approaches.* Berlin: Springer-Verlag; 1990.
44. Karlow W. Pharmacogenetics: past and future. *Life Sci.* 1990;47: 1385–1397.
45. Pi EH, Gray GE. A cross-cultural perspective on psychopharmacology. *Essential Pharmacol.* 1998;2:233–260.
46. Pianezza LM, Sellers EM, Tyndale RF. Nicotine metabolism defect reduces smoking. *Nature.* 1998;393:750.
47. Tyndale RF, Droll KP, Sellers EM. Genetically deficient CYP2D6 metabolism provides protection against oral opiate dependence. *Pharmacogenetics.* 1997;7:375–379.
48. Tsuang M, Lyons MJ, Meyer JM, et al. Co-occurrence of abuse of different drugs in men. *Arch Gen Psychiatry.* 1998;55:967–972.
49. Glatt SJ, Lasky-Su JA, Zhu SC, et al. Genome-wide linkage analysis of heroin dependence in Han Chinese: results from Wave Two of a multi-stage study. *Drug Alcohol Depend.* 2008;98: 30–34.

50. Peele S. A moral vision of addiction: how people's values determine whether they become and remain addicts. *J Drug Issues*. 1987;17:187–215.
51. Peele S. The limitations of control-of-supply models for explaining and preventing alcoholism and drug addiction. *J Stud Alcohol*. 1987;48:61–77.
52. Sue D. Use and abuse of alcohol by Asian Americans. *J Psychoactive Drugs*. 1987;19:57–66.
53. Johnson RC, Nagoshi CT. Asians, Asian Americans and alcohol. *J Psychoactive Drugs*. 1990;22:45–52.
54. Flaskerud JH, Kim S. Health problems of Asian and Latino immigrants. *Nurs Clin North Am*. 1999;34:359–380.
55. Sasao T. Identifying at-risk Asian American adolescents in multiethnic schools: implications for substance abuse prevention interventions and program evaluation. In: *Identifying At-Risk Asian American Adolescents in Multiethnic Schools: Implications for Substance Abuse Prevention Interventions and Program Evaluation*, DHHS Publication No. (SMA) 98-3193. Rockville, MD: U.S. Department of Health and Human Services; 1999:143–167.
56. Sue S, Zane N, Ito J. Alcohol drinking patterns among Asian and Caucasian Americans. *J Cross-Cult Psychol*. 1979;10:41–56.
57. Johnson RC, Nagoshi CT, Ahern FM, et al. Cultural factors as explanations for ethnic group differences in alcoholism in Hawaii. *J Psychoactive Drugs*. 1987;19:67–75.
58. Caetano R. Acculturation and attitudes toward appropriate drinking among U.S. Hispanics. *Alcohol Alcohol*. 1987;22:427–433.
59. Caetano R, Medina Mora ME. Acculturation and drinking among people of Mexican descent in Mexico and the United States. *J Stud Alcohol*. 1988;49:462–471.
60. Kitano HH, Hatanake H, Yeing WT, et al. Japanese-American drinking patterns. In: Bennett LA, Ames GM, eds. *The American Experience with Alcohol: Contrasting Cultural Perspectives*. New York: Plenum Press; 1985:335–357.
61. Sue S, Kitano H, Hatanaka H, et al. Alcohol consumption among Chinese in the United States. In: Bennett L, Ames G, eds. *The American Experience with Alcohol: Contrasting Cultural Perspectives*. New York: Plenum Press; 1985:359–371.
62. Klatsky AL, Siegelaub AB, Landy C, et al. Racial patterns of alcoholic beverage use. *Alcohol Clin Exp Res*. 1983;7:372–377.
63. Yee BWK, Thu ND. Correlates of drug use and abuse among Indochinese refugees: mental health implications. *J Psychoactive Drugs*. 1987;19:77–83.
64. Bhattacharya G. Drug use among Asian Indian adolescents: identifying protective/risk factors. *Adolescence*. 1998;33:169–184.
65. Zane N, Park S, Aoki B. The development of culturally valid measures for assessing prevention impact in Asian American communities. In: *The Development of Culturally Valid Measures for Assessing Prevention Impact in Asian American Communities*, DHHS Publication No. (SMA) 98-3193. Rockville, MD: U.S. Department of Health and Human Services; 1999:61–89.
66. Kim S, McLeod JH, Shantzis C. Cultural competence for evaluators working with Asian American communities: some practical considerations. In: Orlandi MA, ed. *Cultural Competence for Evaluators: A Guide for Alcohol and Other Drug Abuse Prevention Practitioners Working with Ethnic/Racial Communities*. Rockville, MD: U.S. Department of Health and Human Services; 1992:203–260.
67. D'Avanzo CE. The Southeast Asian client and alcohol and other drug abuse: implications for health care providers. *Subst Abuse*. 1994;15:109–113.

CHAPTER 62

American Indians and Alaska Natives

Daniel Dickerson, D.O., M.P.H.

INTRODUCTION

Living in balance and harmony has been highly valued traditional belief constructs among American Indians/Alaska Natives (AI/ANs) for many centuries. However, the introduction of the recreational use of alcohol to American Indians by English colonists hallmarked a deleterious change in the harmony and overall well-being of Indigenous groups residing in North America. Although some AI tribes fermented berries and grains to create alcohol prior to European contact, alcohol was used mostly for ceremonial activities. The first reports of overuse of alcohol among American Indians were associated with fur trading between American Indians and English colonists. The use of alcohol as a bargaining tool in fur trading by English colonists was substantial. For example, Charles Stewart, an agent to a tribe located within the colonies, believed that alcohol consisted of approximately 80% of the trade goods purchased by this tribe in 1770 (1). Consequently, many AI/ANs overindulged in drinking, which resulted in an immediate effect on tribal communities including widespread reports of violent behavior, fighting, and homicides (2). Furthermore, the effects of alcoholism in Indian communities were reported to endanger "the general Peace and Tranquility" of southern Indians (3). As a result, various ordinances and limits to alcohol trading were enacted in attempts to decrease drinking among American Indians. For example, in 1633, provincial officials in the Massachusetts Bay ordered that "noe man shall sell or give any stronge water to any Indean. [sic]" Although attempts were made to decrease drinking among American Indians during the U.S. colonial period, many have suggested that the introduction of alcohol and dysregulation of excessive trading of alcohol to American Indians for furs may have hallmarked the initial degradation and exploitation of North America's Indigenous population and subsequent injustices experienced by this population.

Alaska Natives were introduced to alcohol in 1741 by Russian fur traders (4), in a similar fashion to American Indians. Fur traders relied upon rum and whiskey in their negotiations with Alaska Natives. Insofar as that, even the shrewdest traders or those who sought maximum profit refused to trade with a sober native (4). The demand for alcohol by Alaska Natives became significant and most likely contributed to the development of a concoction called *hoochinoo*, a fermented alcoholic beverage made from dried fruit, berries, flour, and yeast (4). This drink was made by Alaska Natives when alcohol usually supplied by Russians was not available. Alcohol use during the 1700s and 1800s throughout AN villages was significant, resulting in the prohibition of alcohol in the Territory of Alaska, which was under the jurisdiction of the U.S. War Department during this period.

The majority of AI/ANs do not experience significant substance abuse problems. However, continuing challenges exist today with regard to substance abuse in AI/AN communities. For example, compared to other racial/ethnic groups in the United States, the Indigenous populations have the highest rates of all drugs of abuse (5,6). Various reasons for significant substance abuse problems among AI/ANs include low socioeconomic status, traumatic exposure, family history of substance abuse, urbanicity, and co-occurring mental health problems (7). In addition, historical factors affecting AI/AN communities including forced relocations from native homelands and issues associated with loss of cultural identity have had profound effects among AI/ANs and may contribute to higher levels of stress and substance abuse.

Although AI/ANs have experienced significant substance abuse problems throughout the U.S. history, promising strategies for addressing the substance abuse prevention, treatment, and research needs of this population are evident and may assist in providing a comprehensive approach toward addressing this challenging public health issue. A resurgence of cultural pride and tribal recognition may also assist in addressing the many challenges associated with substance abuse in the AI/AN population.

EPIDEMIOLOGY

The study of epidemiology among AI/ANs with substance abuse is inherently challenging. Since the AI/AN population comprises 562 federally recognized tribes, characterizing substance abuse in this population as one distinct category is not possible because each tribe has its own unique history, culture, language, and traditions. In addition, there may be differences biologically as different tribal groups may have historical origins from various regions of the continent. In fact, from an anthropologic sense, AI/ANs are a part of a worldwide population of *Indigenous peoples*.

Limited information exists with regard to the epidemiology of substance abuse in AI/AN communities. The majority of studies and surveys performed have been conducted among specific tribal groups and specific regions in the United States. However, studies have demonstrated that AI/ANs have the highest rates of marijuana, cocaine, and hallucinogen use disorders (5) and the second highest rates of methamphetamine rates, only behind another Indigenous group, Native Hawaiians (6). According to a Substance Abuse and Mental Health Services Administration (SAMHSA) survey, from 2002 to 2005, with regard to alcohol use and alcohol use disorders, a lower likelihood of using alcohol at least once in the past year was observed among AI/ANs aged 12 or older than among members of other racial groups (60.8% vs. 65.8%), but a higher likelihood of having a past-year alcohol use disorder was observed (10.7% vs. 7.6%) (5). Also according to this SAMHSA survey, from 2002 to 2005, a higher likelihood of having used an illicit drug at least once in the past year (18.4% vs. 14.6%) and having a past-year illicit drug use disorder (5.0% vs. 2.9%) was observed among AI/ANs aged 12 or older than among members of other racial groups. Also, according to the SAMHSA report, with regard to specific illicit drug use, past-year heroin use and nonmedical use of sedatives, pain relievers, and tranquilizers were similar between AI/ANs aged 12 or older and other racial groups. However, AI/ANs had a higher likelihood of using all other drugs analyzed. With regard to illicit drug use disorders, rates of past-year tranquilizer, stimulant, inhalant, pain reliever, and sedative use disorders were similar between AI/ANs and members of other racial groups, but rates were higher among AI/ANs for cocaine, hallucinogen, and marijuana use disorders. Past-year heroin use disorders were less common among AI/ANs than among members of other racial groups. Of note, anecdotal evidence suggests a rise in prescription pain medication and over-the-counter (OTC) medication abuse among AI/ANs. To date, studies analyzing prescription pain medication and OTC medication abuse among AI/ANs are very limited.

Death rates attributable to alcoholism are significant. For example, deaths attributable to alcoholism among individuals aged 15 to 24 are more than 15 times higher compared to a combined all-races group of the same age group in the United States (8). Also, death certificate data retrieved from 2001 to 2005 found that 11.7% of all AI/AN deaths were accounted for by alcohol-attributable deaths (AADs) (9). Motor vehicle accidents were identified as the leading acute cause of AADs (9). The largest number of AADs occurred in the Northern Plains (494), followed by the South West region (315), Pacific Coast region (23), and Alaska (86). Data from this analysis also found that alcoholic liver disease was the leading chronic cause of alcohol-related deaths (21.2%).

Psychiatric disorders may be significant factors among some AI/ANs with substance abuse problems. For example, high rates of comorbid psychiatric and substance use problems have been reported among American Indians (10). In a study conducted by Walker et al., among AI women with a history of alcohol dependence, higher rates of depression, anxiety, hostility, phobic anxiety, paranoid ideations, psychoses, and obsessive-copulative behaviors have been found than among AI women without a history of alcohol dependence (10,11). Also, in a study conducted by Novins et al., among AI/AN adolescents in residential treatment, psychiatric comorbidities were reported including depression, antisocial behavior, previous suicide attempts, and number of psychiatric symptoms (12). In addition, in a study conducted by Dickerson et al., significant psychiatric and substance use disorder comorbidites were found among a sample of AI veterans with nicotine dependence (13).

Various reports of traumatic exposure have been documented among AI/ANs with substance abuse problems. For example, American Indians with a history of childhood trauma have been shown to be more likely to use alcohol and drugs as adults. Also, an increased risk of alcohol and other drug dependence has been demonstrated among a sample of Northern Plains Indians with a history of childhood physical abuse (14). Also, among a sample of AI adolescents and young adults living on or near two closely related AI reservations, severe traumatic exposure was associated with increased odds of having an alcohol use disorder (15).

SAMHSA utilized data combined from 2002 and 2003 in its SAMHSA's National Survey on Drug Use and Health to evaluate risk factors for substance use among three categories (individual/peers, family, and school) (16). Risk factors were compared between AI/AN youth and other racial/ethnic groups among 46,310 individuals between 12 and 17 years of age. Findings revealed that AI/ANs were more likely than youths from other racial/ethnic groups to perceive moderate to no risk associated with substance use, to believe that all or most of the students in their school get drunk at least once a week, and to perceive their parents as not strongly disapproving of their substance use. In addition, AI/AN youths were less likely than youths from other racial/ethnic groups to participate in youth activities and to attend religious services regularly. However, parents of AI/AN youth were as likely to discuss with their children about the dangers associated with substance use, to praise the youth when they had done a good job and to let them know that they were proud of something they had done, to set limits with regard to the amount of watching TV, and to expect their youth to do chores around the house.

Studies analyzing predictors of relapse for AI/ANs have been limited. However, one study conducted among AI women enrolled in residential substance abuse treatment found that intrapersonal factors were the strongest predictors of relapse, followed by proximal and distal factors (17). Proximal factors are defined as factors that occur close in time to the relapse event and precipitate substance use. Distal factors are factors that occur farther back in the patient's history. Significant factors associated with alcohol relapse in the short term (6 months following entry into residential treatment) included being around individuals who use alcohol and drugs (proximal factors) and craving alcohol or drugs (intrapersonal factors). Significant factors associated with drug use relapse in the short term included having conflicts with other people at intake and within the proximal timeframe, the number of years that the client had used more than one drug regularly (not including alcohol), and being around others using alcohol or drugs. Significant factors associated with alcohol use relapse in the long term (12 months following entry into residential treatment) included reported family conflicts at intake (distal), being around individuals who use alcohol or drugs (proximal), and craving alcohol (interpersonal). Predictors of drug use in the long term included having conflicts with family at intake, using polydrugs, being around others who use alcohol or drugs, and craving drugs. In addition, these authors found various factors associated with a reduced probability of alcohol use at 6 months, including having drug treatment experience, using drugs with family members, having a father who had warned about alcohol and drugs, having a positive rating in perceived physical health, and having a high self-efficacy score.

SOCIOCULTURAL CONSIDERATIONS

Studies analyzing how childhood characteristics are associated with the stage of substance use in adulthood have also been limited. However, in a study conducted by O'Connell et al. in 2007, utilizing data obtained from the American Indian Service Utilization, Psychiatric Epidemiology, Risk and Protective Factors Project (AI-SUPERPFP), investigators sought to analyze childhood characteristics associated with adulthood stage of substance use (18). In a sample consisting of two closely related Northern Plains tribes (NP) and a Southwestern tribe (SW), four correlates of substance abuse based on hierarchical stages were used including lifetime abstinence (Stage 0), use of alcohol only (Stage 1A), use of marijuana/inhalants with or without alcohol (stage 1B), and use of other illicit drugs with or without the previously listed substances (Stage 2). Findings revealed that SW females were more likely to report Stage 1 rather than Stage 0 substance use than SW males. Also, in this study, a history of sexual abuse significantly increased the odds of Stage 1B versus Stage 1A substance use. Witnessing family violence increased the odds of Stage 1A versus Stage 0 use among NP individuals, and significantly increased the odds of Stage 1B versus Stage 1A substance use in both tribes combined. Also, adolescent conduct problems resulted in a significant increase in the likelihood of higher stage substance use.

A study conducted by Stiffman et al. in 2007 sought to analyze the trajectory or path of substance use among AI/AN adolescents (7). In this study among 401 urban and reservation youth, data was analyzed from 2001 to 2004 to model behavior change trajectories, with psychological and environmental variables. Five trajectory groups were identified: (a) very high chronic, (b) high chronic, (c) high improving trajectory, (d) low stable, and (e) low improving. High improving group had sixfold higher proportion of reservation youths, less school problems, only about one-tenth depression symptoms, much less thoughts about attempting suicide, only half as many parents with mental health problems, and lower family conflict compared to the very high chronic group. Various reasons for improved treatment outcomes were considered. First, many changes to the reservation including a new casino, more community programs, and more jobs were observed. The community also added more service providers in schools, courts, and jails; more family-oriented social treatment and prevention programs; as well as family programs for youths in treatment. In addition, the community also focused on programs for youth including recreational, physical, social, and employment programs. Urban areas did not have any service changes or new interventions between 2001 and 2004 in this study. Results from this study may suggest a need for a greater role of community/environment in AI/AN substance abuse treatment.

Findings in Stiffman's study mirror trends observed in other studies where lower substance use rates have been observed among SW tribes in comparison to NP tribal groups (18,19). For example, in the previously described study by O'Connell, the identified SW tribe was postulated to have larger and stronger social networks and low cultural stress due to fewer changes in culture, economy, and diet over the past 200 years (18). In addition, the SW tribal group was identified as a matrilineal society, with females having an expectation to conform to cultural norms more, thus possibly attributing to lower substance abuse among SW women. Thus, some cultural characteristics reported in these studies may have contributed to lower alcohol/drug problems among SW tribal groups.

Participation in cultural and traditional activities and traditional ceremonies has been an important area of research as it relates to AI/ANs with substance abuse problems. Culturally based treatments are utilized in numerous substance abuse programs serving AI/ANs. However, formalized studies analyzing the potential effects of traditional activity participations on substance abuse behavior are relatively limited. To date, studies conducted have found both positive and negative associations with cultural identity and traditional activity participation among AI/ANs with substance abuse problems. With regard to benefits, one study analyzing inhalant abuse among AI/ANs found a significant positive effect with participation in tribal activities among nonusers compared to users (20). Also, another study found that American Indians with a low orientation toward traditional culture were more than 4.4 times as likely to be heavy drinkers as more culturally oriented adults (21). Also, in a study among a sample of four AI reservations in the upper Midwest and five Canadian First Nation reserves, participation in traditional activities and traditional spirituality were positively associated with alcohol cessation, while cultural identity was not significantly associated with alcohol cessation in a multivariate analysis (22). However, the authors in this study caution that the data is cross-sectional and does not indicate directions of effects, warranting further longitudinal studies.

Cultural indicators have also been reported to be negatively associated with substance abuse treatment outcomes. For example, in a study analyzing tobacco use among AI adolescents, being more connected to AI culture increased the odds of cigarette use (23). Also, in a study conducted among AI/AN adolescents in Wisconsin and Minnesota, attendance at cultural events was positively correlated with marijuana and cigarette use. Participation in tribal ceremonies was weakly correlated with cigarette use and more strongly correlated with marijuana use among males. Another study analyzing data among AI/AN youth participating in a substance abuse prevention program found males who rated the importance of Indian identity highly were more likely to use marijuana, and females who rated the importance of Indian identity highly were less likely to use alcohol (24).

PREVENTION

Preventing the initiation of alcohol, drugs, and tobacco has been known to assist in decreasing overall substance abuse rates in various populations. Implementing effective prevention protocols for AI/ANs is critical since AI/ANs are known to have earlier onset of illicit drug and alcohol use and more negative consequences compared to other racial/ethnic groups.

Identification of potential protective factors is important in implementing effective prevention programs. For example, potential protective factors that may be associated with tobacco nonuse may be related to family structure. In a study conducted by Beebe et al., higher rates of tobacco nonuse were found among AI/AN youth who lived in a two-parent households compared to AI/AN youth from one-parent households (25). Also in this study, having a nonparental adult role model was associated with not using alcohol. In addition, AI/AN youth with a family communication asset was associated with not using drugs. Families that demonstrated effective communication may suggest more family cohesiveness and family bonding. Bebe and colleagues emphasized the potential value of extended families and sense of collectivism that exists in many AI communities. Also, religion asset was found to be associated with drug nonuse and was observed to be potentially valuable in building traditional resilience.

A theme commonly observed among drug and alcohol prevention programs for AI/ANs throughout the United States is the integration of cultural strengths identified in the culture. For example, enhancing cultural identity through integration of various cultural activities and events in AI/ANs has been implicated as a vital approach toward decreasing the likelihood of alcohol and drug use. Adequate teaching and mentoring programs providing lessons in traditionally held beliefs and principles may provide foundations that may be conclusive to drug and alcohol abstinence.

Since approximately two thirds of AI/ANs reside in urban areas, creating and analyzing substance abuse prevention programs in the urban setting is important. The *Seventh Generation Program* is an urban after-school alcohol prevention program designed for youth in Colorado. The program blends general prevention approaches with culturally appropriate interventions including an emphasis on core AI/AN values and concepts associated with the *Medicine Wheel* of the Northern Plains (26). In a study conducted by Moran and Bussey in 2007, this approach was compared between a group of AI/ANs receiving this intervention and a no-intervention comparison group (26). Results revealed significant effects in areas of alcohol beliefs, social support, locus of control, and depression, and demonstrated increased benefits over time among participants enrolled in the *Seventh Generation Program* in comparison to the nonintervention condition. An additional finding in this study demonstrated the benefits of booster sessions. Six booster sessions reviewed the basic content of this 13-week afterschool-hour program.

A focus on bicultural competence among AI adolescents has been another substance abuse prevention strategy developed. Schinke and colleagues utilized concepts related to a bicultural approach, indicating that AI youth need to acquire skills to be able to function in both AI/AN and non-AI/AN settings (27). This application involves 10 group intervention sessions to learn bicultural competence skills and social learning principles. Communication skills; coping skills; discriminations skills; and school, family, and reservation resources are utilized. In a study conducted by Schinke et al. in 1988, AI youth who received the bicultural competence skills approach improved more than an AI adolescent no-intervention control sample (27).

Public health strategies and legislations have also played a role in addressing substance abuse in AI/AN communities. In addition, utilization of these strategies appears to be increasing. For example, tribes with statutes that permit alcohol increased from 29.2% to 63.5% from 1975 to 2006 (28). Some potentially useful alcohol control polices include changes in liquor sales regulations, a local alcohol excise tax, and alcohol server training (28). Tobacco public health policies also have significant potential to decrease smoking rates in AI/AN communities. Strict clean air laws, cigarette taxes, and community-tailored prevention programs may assist in decreasing smoking rates among AI/ANs. However, further knowledge about community support with regard to these tobacco control policies is needed.

Another proposed substance abuse prevention strategy is utilizing effective treatment strategies currently used in the general U.S. population with appropriate cultural modifications (29). This suggestion was proposed due to similar drug, alcohol, and tobacco use trends observed between AI/ANs and the general population. It is postulated that utilizing current proven effective substance abuse prevention strategies that have been shown to work in the general U.S. population may also be effective among AI/ANs with appropriate cultural modifications capitalizing on the inherent strengths of the culture in addition to increasing the acceptability of the approaches in the community.

TREATMENT

Need for Culturally Relevant Treatment Approaches for American Indians/Alaska Natives

Incorporating traditional aspects of healing has been recognized as being important in the development of effective treatment strategies for AI/ANs. For example, the Tribal Participatory Research (TPR) model, created by Philip Fisher and Thomas Ball, highlights the need for culturally specific interventions that allow for the incorporation of traditional practices and concepts and create the potential for testing indigenous models of health and well-being (30). Furthermore, identifying substance abuse treatments that will be both beneficial and acceptable among AI/ANs may assist in higher treatment retention and completions rates and ultimately decrease substance abuse rates.

Developing culturally relevant substance abuse treatment approaches for AI/ANs has the potential to enhance treatment protocols in addition to a renewed sense of personal and cultural identity. For example, previous studies have observed themes of feeling renewed pride in their cultural heritage, feeling motivated to learn more about it, and coming to feel "worthy" of participating in it (31). It also appears to be true that many American Indians strongly believe that their problems with alcohol stem from their sudden disconnection with traditional AI culture (32). Furthermore, various researchers have reported that denying American Indians the opportunity to rely on those mechanisms may have increased the likelihood that American Indians would rely on less adaptive coping mechanisms such as excessive alcohol consumption (32).

Although the incorporation of cultural elements into substance abuse treatment and prevention is recognized as being particularly important among AI/ANs, some studies have found that currently provided substance abuse treatments without cultural adaptations may be effective. For example, results of a study conducted by Evans et al. in 2005 comparing alcohol and drug treatment outcomes between a sample of California American Indians and a non-AI comparison group utilizing the California Treatment Outcome Project (CalTOP) revealed that American Indians and non-American Indians demonstrated a similar level of severity before treatment in all seven domains measured by the Addiction Severity Index (ASI)—alcohol, drug, medical, psychiatric, family, legal, and employment—and demonstrated similar levels of improvement in all seven ASI domains (33). Also, another study observed no treatment outcomes differences between a sample of 279 AI/ANs and a non-AI/AN comparison group at 12 months posttreatment based on legal, employment, medical, and psychiatric measures (34). Results of these studies highlight the need for improving access to community-based AI/ANs since currently available substance abuse treatment may be beneficial for AI/ANs with substance abuse problems. However, various barriers exist with regard to AI/ANs receiving substance abuse treatment, which may limit their likelihood of receiving treatment, including low socioeconomic status, transportation barriers, a shortage of integrated substance abuse treatment models, and stigma associated with substance abuse in AI/AN communities. Thus, further attention is needed to ensure that AI/ANs with substance abuse problems have adequate access to substance abuse services since they may benefit from currently provided substance abuse treatment services.

Numerous studies have suggested a comprehensive treatment approach for AI/ANs. For example, in a study analyzing treatment outcomes among AI/ANs and a matched comparison group conducted by Evans et al. (2006), a more intense level of services addressing various problems among American Indians receiving substance abuse services in addition to American Indians receiving more group sessions addressing psychiatric problems was identified (33). In this study, additional family-related and abuse-related services were received by AI/ANs compared to a matched comparison group, and may have assisted in addressing specific treatment needs of AI/ANs with substance abuse resulting in similar improvements when compared to non-AI/ANs. These results mirror many other reports of a significant association between substance abuse and traumatic experiences, abuse, and psychiatric comorbidities among AI/ANs with substance abuse problems (11–14). Thus, individual and group trauma-related treatments and community-based healing may especially be needed among AI/AN individuals in substance abuse treatment.

Cultural Considerations in Evidence-Based Substance Abuse Treatments for AI/ANs

Currently available psychotherapeutic interventions include motivational interviewing, cognitive–behavioral therapy, 12-step facilitation, psychodynamics, contingency management, network therapy, group therapy, and family therapy, which have been shown to be effective in various studies. However, their effectiveness and cultural relevancy among AI/ANs are relatively unknown. Currently available evidence-based treatments have not been thoroughly tested among various ethnic/minority groups; thus the assumption that these substance abuse treatments are effective among all patients is not valid. Although consisting of various distinct tribes, AI/ANs share many cultural characteristics including similarities in behavior patterns, lifestyle, values, beliefs, views, and attitudes. Thus, adequate attention to these factors is critical when providing evidence-based treatments to AI/ANs.

Motivational Interviewing for Native Americans

In 2006, Venner, Feldstein, and Tafoya developed a motivational interviewing (MI) manual culturally tailored for Native Americans—*Native American Motivational Interviewing: Weaving Native American and Western Practices* (35). This manual provides counselors a thorough overview of MI with particular attention toward relevant Native American cultural ideals and traditions including spirituality, community, and cultural identity. In addition to providing a fundamental overview of the MI treatment approach, relevant considerations with regard to how to incorporate these cultural elements into the delivery of this treatment strategy to AI/ANs are provided. Information utilized in this culturally tailored treatment approach was retrieved from focus groups among community members possessing knowledge regarding Native American communication styles and behavior health providers, which are meant to guide the practice of MI in Native American communities.

Another treatment approach that has been culturally adapted for AI/ANs with substance abuse problems is the Matrix Model. It is a multielement package of evidence-based practices delivered in a 16-week intensive outpatient program (36). The Native American adapted version was created by UCLA Integrated Substance Abuse Programs (ISAP) in collaboration with Friendship House, a residential treatment facility for AI/ANs in San Francisco through feedback obtained from elders and

Native American cultural experts to provide a treatment approach utilizing relevant cultural elements and culturally designed worksheets and diagrams and culturally appropriate quotes and references to AI/AN culture (37). Currently, this treatment approach has been widely accepted and utilized in many tribal communities across the United States.

Knowledge with regard to the utilization and acceptance of evidenced-based substance abuse treatments for AI/AN is limited. However, studies are being performed analyzing the use, acceptance, and implementation of evidence-based treatment strategies in AI/AN communities. For example, Douglas Novins, MD, University of Colorado at Denver and Health Sciences Center, is currently analyzing the use of specific evidence-based treatments in substance abuse programs serving AI/AN communities and is seeking to understand the factors associated with the implementation of evidence-based treatments in these programs and to identify methods for more effective dissemination of Evidence Based Practices (EBPs) to substance abuse programs serving AI/AN communities. In addition, Traci Rieckmann, PhD, Oregon Health Sciences University, is seeking to increase our understanding with regard to the use of evidence-based treatments in clinics providing substance abuse services to AI/ANs through an analysis of the utilization and adoption of EBPs in community-based treatment programs across the United States.

Medicine Wheel and 12 Steps

One of the most widely revered and utilized substance abuse treatment strategies utilized in many AI/AN substance abuse treatment programs is the *Medicine Wheel and 12 Steps*, by Don Coyhis of White Bison, Inc. (38). This program utilizes the fundamental philosophies and practices of Alcoholics and Narcotics Anonymous with a particular focus on the fundamental concepts of the Native American Medicine Wheel. The Medicine Wheel is a representation of Native American philosophy originated among the Northern Plains Indians. Particular attention is directed toward a focus on the culture as being an integral part of overcoming addictions among AI/ANs with substance abuse problems. The *Medicine Wheel and 12 Steps* approach states that the principles of Alcoholics Anonymous parallels many Native American cultural beliefs. The 12 steps are recognized as being interconnected and a process of natural order that assists AI/ANs with substance abuse problems and a process to establish or re-establish order within their own lives. This approach also teaches that "injured seeds" need a "Healing Forest," illustrating that sobriety and the healing of an individual are not separate from the healing of the family and the tribal community.

Utilization of Traditional Healing Methods for AI/ANs with Substance Abuse Disorders

Traditional healing continues to be a highly valued form of treatment for urban and reservation-based AI/ANs with a variety of health problems, including addiction. Although a variety of definitions and opinions exist with regard to what constitutes Native American traditional healing, traditional healing can be thought of as a spectrum of activities from participation in traditional activities including drumming, bead making, and attendance of powwows to participation in specific traditional ceremonies. Commonly used traditional treatments used in substance abuse facilities servicing AI/ANs include smudging ceremonies, sweat lodge participation, and talking circles, a traditionally founded form of group therapy. Participation in these ceremonies may contribute to a renewed elevated sense of self- and cultural pride, thus serving as a potential protective factor for substance abuse problems.

Providing traditional healing services necessitates that providers, community members, and cultural elders assist in ensuring that they are delivered in an appropriate culturally relevant manner. Exploitation of various forms of Native American traditional healing services may be considered offensive and disrespectful since these activities are considered sacred and private by tribal communities. Although traditional healing services may be especially useful for AI/ANs with substance abuse problems, particular attention must be paid toward protecting and respecting the use of traditional forms in order to protect the history and dignity of native cultures.

The integration of traditional healing with Westernized care as it relates to substance abuse treatment among AI/ANs has gained further recognition among treatment service delivery programs across the United States. Although traditional healing continues to be utilized among many AI/AN tribes within the clinical setting, established systems of an integrated system have been less common. Nonetheless, there are specific health care systems in AI/AN communities providing an integrated treatment model. For example, the Navajo Nation has developed an integrated model whereby AI/ANs have access to traditional healing and traditional healers. In addition, an integrated model has been recognized at the Southcentral Foundation in Anchorage, Alaska. Momentum for an integrated treatment approach for both substance abuse and mental health problems among AI/ANs in Los Angeles County through a project coordinated with the Los Angeles County Department of Mental Health has also been recognized. Some of the challenges with regard to successful implementation of an integrated treatment model may include reimbursement issues, "evidence" of effectiveness, and a process to validate the legitimacy of traditional healers within a community.

Medications to Treat Addiction for AI/ANs

Advancements with regard to the utilization of evidence-based pharmacologic treatments for addiction also hold tremendous promise toward addressing the treatment needs of AI/ANs with addictive diseases (i.e., naltrexone for alcohol dependence, buprenorphine for opioid dependence, and nicotine replacement therapy). However, information with regard to the utilization and effectiveness of these medications among AI/ANs is significantly limited. However, one study conducted by O'Malley et al. in 2008 analyzed the effectiveness of naloxone, a Federal Drug Administration (FDA)–approved medication for alcoholism, among a sample of Alaska Natives ($n = 68$) (39). This study found naloxone to be effective in this population in addition to demonstrating its potential usefulness in Alaska Natives residing in both rural and urban areas. This trial also highlighted the potential benefits of pharmacologic treatment for AI/ANs with alcoholism. Further attention addressing significant logistical and financial barriers to receiving pharmacologic treatments for substance use disorders for AI/ANs is needed.

FACTORS INFLUENCING SUBSTANCE USE AMONG AI/ANs

Historical Trauma

Various historical and cultural factors may explain why substance abuse rates are high among AI/ANs. A growing body of literature, however, has cited various perpetuating psychosocial stressors experienced by AI/ANs as being ongoing risk factors. Specifically, the theory of "historical trauma," developed by Maria Yellowhorse Brave Heart, postulates that various injustices impounded on AI/ANs have had a perpetuating, intergeneral traumatic effect throughout the U.S. history and have been responsible for setting the foundation for community stress, impoverishment, loss of cultural identity, and a sense of traumatic loss in the AI/AN population (40,41). Some traumatic events include the forced removal of AI/ANs from homelands, removal of religious freedom, and forced placement of children into boarding schools away from original homelands, in addition to numerous broken treaties between the U.S. government and tribal groups. These events have "laid the groundwork" for a host of potential risk factors for substance abuse problems and consequences associated with substance use. Furthermore, these effects associated with historically based trauma have been implicated as a causative factor for substance abuse among AI/ANs (42). The results of these traumatic events may be contributing to high rates of poverty, unemployment, high school dropout rates, and very limited access to comprehensive culturally appropriate substance abuse treatment services in both rural and urban settings. Thus, a significant risk for significant substance abuse problems among AI/ANs may be due to these intergenerational effects resulting in ongoing substance abuse problems among AI/ANs.

Genetics

It has been a widely held popular belief that "the reason" for high rates of alcoholism and substance abuse among AI/ANs is a genetic predisposition. However, to date, limited data exists that posits that genetic characteristics are significant risk factors for a wide variety of substance use disorders among AI/ANs. For example, in a study conducted among Southwest California Indians, results revealed that heritability of the initiation of substance use may be similar to other population samples (43). Furthermore, another study analyzing genetic variations among Finns and American Indians concluded that there are likely to be independent, complex contributions among chromosomal regions (44). Nonetheless, studies analyzing the role of genes and gene–environment interactions may assist in furthering our understanding of substance abuse problems among AI/ANs.

SPECIAL CONSIDERATIONS

Human Immunodeficiency Virus/Acquired Immunodeficiency Syndrome (HIV/AIDS)

HIV/AIDS has become an emergent health problem among AI/ANs. Native Americans have the third highest rates compared to other racial/ethnic groups in the United States, behind African Americans and Hispanics (45). Furthermore, urban American Indians may be at greater risk for HIV infection than American Indians residing on reservations due to significant risk factors known to exist in urban areas. These risk factors include the tendency to trade sex for money or drugs, and unsafe sexual practices (46). In addition, various health-related disparities known to exist among AI/ANs may contribute to an increased risk of HIV/AIDS including limited access to culturally appropriate HIV/AIDS prevention and treatment programs, limited access to adequate health care, and decreased access to proper medical management.

An additional challenge with regard to providing effective HIV/AIDS prevention and treatment programs in AI/AN populations is the stigma associated with HIV/AIDS and homosexuality in many native communities. HIV/AIDS is often not seen as an "Indian problem" in many urban and rural AI/AN communities. Thus, further attention to the HIV/AIDS prevention and treatments needs of the AI/AN lesbian, gay, bisexual, and transgender (LGBT) community is needed. One innovative prevention approach is the *Red Circle Project*, developed by Elton Naswood, to target Native American Two Spirit/Gay Men in the Los Angeles area. The project provides resources, referrals, and information about HIV to the urban Native American community. In addition, this strategy provides a support group curriculum comprised of six workshops to address issues such as decision making, skills building, healthy image/body fitness, HIV/AIDS and STD information, risk reduction information, and storytelling.

Intravenous drug abuse (IVDA) is a significant risk factor for HIV/AIDS. Although studies with regard to IVDA among AI/ANs have been limited, recent reports have demonstrated noticeable trends of IVDA among some AI/AN groups. For example, AI/ANs aged 12 or older had the higher rates of injection drug use (0.24%) compared to any other single racial/ethnic group in the United States, with the highest rates being among "two or more races" (0.35%) (47). This is especially noteworthy due to the known significant rise in methamphetamine drug abuse among AI/ANs over the last decade. Thus, further HIV/AIDS prevention efforts targeting at-risk groups inclding AI/AN who abuse intravenous drugs may assist in decreasing this trend.

Methamphetamine

The effects associated with methamphetamine abuse have exacerbated many significant psychosocial problems known to exist among AI/ANs. For example, methamphetamine has been associated with increased domestic violence crimes, burglary, assault and battery, and child neglect/abuse among AI/ANs. In a 2006 Bureau of Indian Affairs survey of 96 tribal law enforcement agencies, 74% ranked methamphetamine as the drug that poses the greatest threat to their community, 64% indicated increases in domestic violence and assault/battery, and 48% reported an increase in child neglect/abuse cases due to recent increases in methamphetamine use (48). Methamphetamine abuse has also been reported as a significant substance abuse problem among AI/AN groups residing in urban areas. For example, in a study conducted by Spear et al., in Los Angeles County, methamphetamine was shown to be the drug most abused by AI women and the second most abused drug among AI men (49).

Due to the significant effects of methamphetamine in tribal communities, the National Congress of American Indians (NCAI), in a coordinated effort with SAMHSA, and the leadership provided by Dale Walker, MD and the Association of American Indian Physicians (AAIP), a set of comprehensive strategies to combat methamphetamine abuse in tribal communities was created. Assembled in a creatively decorated box, the toolkit includes a variety of materials and educational information for tribal providers and health care leaders to use in their communities. The contents include an educational overview of methamphetamine basics in Indian country, tribal code-policy examples, public service announcements, preventative posters and flyers tailored to specific audiences, educational presentations, and "fun youth items" created to provide youth with an antimethamphetamine message.

Nicotine

While alcohol was introduced to AI/ANs by Europeans, tobacco was introduced to colonists by American Indians. Tobacco has been used by AI and other Indigenous groups throughout North and South America for religious and ceremonial purposes for at least 2000 years and possibly up to 7000 years. However, AI/ANs have the highest smoking rates compared to any other racial or ethnic group in the United States (50) and are at higher risk for many tobacco-related health problems. Various risk factors for smoking among AI/ANs include lower socioeconomic status and high rates of unemployment and poverty. These factors may also influence access to smoking cessation prevention interventions and prevention programs. Finally, high levels of stress exist in many AI/AN communities as evidenced by high rates of suicide, homicide, violence, accidents, and unresolved historically based traumas that may impede smoking cessation.

Urban AI/ANs

A significant number of AI/ANs currently reside in urban areas (two thirds). However, unique challenges exist with regard to providing the much needed culturally relevant treatment services. A significant shortage of comprehensive substance abuse services exists in the urban setting. In addition, many individuals who reside in urban areas may be unaware that clinics providing substance abuse services specifically for AI/ANs exist. In addition, challenging dilemmas exist with regard to understanding the "community of urban AI/ANs." More aggressive outreach efforts are needed in order to increase AI/ANs who may require substance abuse treatments. Coordinating comprehensive substance abuse treatment and prevention programs for AI/ANs may be especially challenging since the most promising treatment and prevention strategies entail that a coordinated effort among various entities including mental health professionals, medical facilities, recreation and social networks, education systems, and the legal system is implemented. Within large metropolitan areas, such as Los Angeles and New York City, where the largest populations of AI/ANs reside, this effort may be especially challenging.

CONCLUSION

Substance abuse has significantly impacted the AI/AN population. Due to a variety of complicating factors including historically based traumas and various health-related disparities, a comprehensive approach to prevention and treatment programs should be considered. In addition, recognizing the need for blending currently available evidence-based treatment approaches with the incorporation of culturally relevant approaches is essential for optimizing potentially useful prevention and treatment programs. Also, due to the growing population of AI/ANs residing in urban areas, further understanding is needed with regard to providing effective prevention and treatment programs to this population. Furthermore, recognition of comorbid psychiatric issues may assist in optimizing treatment outcomes among AI/ANs with substance use disorders.

REFERENCES

1. Mancall PC. "The bewitching tyranny of custom": the social costs of Indian drinking in colonial America. *Am Indian Cult Res J.* 1993;17:15–42.
2. Mail PD, Heurtin-Roberts S, Martin SE, et al., eds. *Alcohol Use among American Indians and Alaska Natives.* Bethesda: U.S. Department of Health and Human Services; 2002.
3. Thomas Bosworth to Mr. Elsinor, 23 December 1752, and Lachland McGillivray to Glen, 14 April 1754. In: *Colonial Records of South Carolina: Documents Relating to Indian Affairs, May 21, 1750–August 7, 1754* [hereafter CRSC: *Indian Affairs, 1750–1754*], William L. McDowell, Jr., ed. Columbia, SC: South Carolina Archives Department; 1958:325, 502.
4. Anderson TI, Alaska State Office of Alcoholism and Drug Abuse, eds. *Alaska Hooch: The History of Alcohol in Early Alaska.* Fairbanks: Hoo-Che-Noo; 1988.

5. USDHHS, SAMHSA, Office of Applied Statistics. *The NSDUH Report: Substance Use and Substance Use Disorders among American Indians and Alaska Natives.* Rockville, MD: U.S. Department of Health and Human Services; 2007.
6. USDHHS, SAMHSA, Office of Applied Statistics. *The NSDUH Report: Substance Use and Substance Use Disorders among American Indians and Alaska Natives.* Rockville, MD: U.S. Department of Health and Human Services; 2005.
7. Stiffman AR, Alexander-Eitzman B, Silmere H, et al. From early to late adolescence: American Indian youth's behavior trajectories and their major influences. *J Am Acad Child Adolesc Psychiatry.* 2007;46:849–858.
8. Mitchell CM, Beals J, Whitesell NR, et al. Alcohol use among American Indian high school youths from adolescence and young adulthood: a latent Markov model. *J Stud Alcohol Drugs.* 2008;69:666–675.
9. Centers for Disease Control and Prevention (CDC). Alcohol-attributable deaths and years of potential life lost among American Indians and Alaska Natives-United States, 2001–2005. *MMWR Morb Mortal Wkly Rep.* 2008;57(34):938–941.
10. Walters KL, Simoni JM, Evans-Campbell T. Substance use among American Indians and Alaska Natives: incorporating culture in an "Indigenist" stress-coping paradigm. *Public Health Rep.* 2002;117(suppl 1):S104–S117.
11. Walker RD, Lambert MD, Walker PS, et al. Alcohol abuse in urban Indian adolescents and women: a longitudinal study for assessment and risk evaluation. *Am Indian Alsk Native Ment Health Res.* 1996;7:1–47.
12. Novins DK, Beals J, Shore JH, et al. Substance abuse treatment of American Indian adolescents: comorbid symptomatology, gender differences, and treatment patterns. *J Am Acad Child Adolesc Psychiatry.* 1996;35:1593–1601.
13. Dickerson DL, O'Malley SS, Canive J, et al. Nicotine dependence and psychiatric and substance use comorbidities in a sample of American Indian male veterans. *Drug Alcohol Depend.* 2009; 99:169–175.
14. Libby AM, Orton HD, Novins DK, et al. Childhood physical and sexual abuse and subsequent depressive and anxiety disorders for two American Indian tribes. *Psychol Med.* 2005;35:329–340.
15. Boyd-Ball AJ, Manson SM, Noonan C, et al. Traumatic events and alcohol use disorder among American Indian adolescents and young adults. *J Trauma Stress.* 2006;19:937–947.
16. USDHHS, SAMHSA, Office of Applied Statistics. *The NSDUH Report: Risk and Protective Factors for Substance Use among American Indian or Alaska Native Youths.* Rockville, MD: U.S. Department of Health and Human Services; 2004.
17. Chong J, Lopez D. Predictors of relapse for American Indian women after substance abuse treatment. *Am Indian Alsk Native Ment Health Res.* 2008;14:24–48.
18. O'Connell JM, Novins DK, Beals J, et al. Childhood characteristics associated with stage of substance use of American Indians: family background, traumatic experiences, and childhood behaviors. *Addict Behav.* 2007;32:3142–3152.
19. Nez Henderson PH, Jacobsen C, Beals J. Correlates of cigarette smoking among selected southwest and northern plains tribal groups: the AL-SUPERPFP study. *Am J Public Health.* 2005; 95:867–872.
20. Thurman PJ, Green VA. American Indian adolescent inhalant use. *Am Indian Alsk Native Ment Health Res.* 1997;8:24–40.
21. Herman-Stahl M, Spencer DL, Duncan JE. The implications of cultural orientation for substance use among American Indians. *Am Indian Alsk Native Ment Health Res.* 2003;11:46–66.
22. Stone RA, Whitbeck LB, Chen X, et al. Traditional practices, traditional spirituality, and alcohol cessation among American Indians. *J Stud Alcohol.* 2006;67:236–244.
23. LeMaster PL, Connell CM, Mitchell CM, et al. Tobacco use among American Indian adolescents: protective and risk factors. *J Adolesc Health.* 2002;30:426–432.
24. Petoskey EL, Van Stelle KR, De Jong JA. Prevention through empowerment in a Native American community. *Drugs Soc.* 1998;12:147–162.
25. Beebe LA, Vesely SK, Oman RF, et al. Protective assets for non-use of alcohol, tobacco and other drugs among urban American Indian youth in Oklahoma. *Matern Child Health J.* 2008; 12(suppl 1):S82–S90.
26. Moran JR, Bussey M. Results of an alcohol prevention program with urban American Indian youth. *Child Adolesc Social Work J.* 2007;24:1–21.
27. Schinke SP, Orlandi MA, Botvin GJ, et al. Preventing substance abuse among American-Indian adolescents: a bicultural competence skills approach. *J Couns Psychol.* 1988;35:87–90.
28. Kovas AE, McFarland BH, Landen MG, et al. Survey of American Indian alcohol statutes, 1975–2006: evolving needs and future opportunities for tribal health. *J Stud Alcohol Drugs.* 2008;69: 183–191.
29. Beauvais F, Jumper-Thurman P, Burnside M. The changing patterns of drug use among American Indian students over the past thirty years. *Am Indian Alsk Native Ment Health Res.* 2008;15: 15–24.
30. Fisher PA, Ball TJ. Tribal participatory research: mechanisms of a collaborative model. *Am J Community Psychol.* 2003;32:207–216.
31. Prussing E. Reconfiguring the empty center: drinking, sobriety, and identity in Native American women's narratives. *Cult Med Psychiatry.* 2007;31:499–526.
32. Spillane NS, Smith GT. A theory of reservation-dwelling American Indian alcohol use risk. *Psychol Bull.* 2007;133:395–418.
33. Evans E, Spear SE, Huang Y-C, et al. Outcomes of drug and alcohol treatment programs among American Indians in California. *Am J Public Health.* 2006;96:889–896.
34. Dickerson D, Spear S, Marinelli-Casey P, et al. American Indians/Alaska Natives and substance abuse treatment outcomes: positive signs and continuing challenges. Submitted for publication.
35. Venner K, Feldstein S, Tafoya N. *Native American Motivational Interviewing: Weaving Native American and Western Practices. A Manual for Counselors in Native American Communities.* 2006. Retrieved September 23, 2010, from http://quantumunitsed.com/ceus/ceu31/index/.htm.
36. Rawson RA, Obert JL, McCann MJ. *The Matrix Model for the Treatment of Opiate Addiction with Naltrexone.* Beverly Hills, CA: Matrix Institute; 1992.
37. Matrix Institute. *Matrix Model; Culturally Designed Client Handouts for American Indians/Alaskan Natives.* Los Angeles: Matrix Institute; 2006.
38. White Bison, Inc. Colorado Springs, CO: Welcome to White Bison. Retrieved July 20, 2010, from: http://www.test.whitebison.org/
39. O'Malley SS, Robin RW, Levenson AL, et al. Naltrexone alone and with sertraline for the treatment of alcohol dependence in Alaska natives and non-natives residing in rural settings: a randomized controlled trial. *Alcohol Clin Exp Res.* 2008;32:1271–1283.
40. Weaver H, Brave Heart MYH. Examining two facets of American Indian identity: exposure to other cultures and the influence of historical trauma. *J Hum Behav Soc Environ.* 1999;2(1/2):19–33.
41. Johnson CL. An innovative healing model: empowering urban native Americans. In: Witko T, ed. *Mental Health Care for Urban*

Indians: Clinical Insights from Native Practitioners. Washington, DC: American Psychological Association; 2006:189–204.

42. Nebelkopf E, Phillips M. Morning star rising: healing in Native American communities. *J Psychoactive Drugs.* 2003;35:1–5.
43. Ehlers CL, Wall TL, Corey L, et al. Heritability of illicit drug use and transition to dependence in Southwest California Indians. *Psychiatr Genet.* 2007;17:171–176.
44. Enoch MA, Hodgkinson CA, Yuan Q, et al. GABRG1 and GABRA2 as independent predictors for alcoholism in two populations. *Neuropsychopharmacology.* 2009;34:1245–1254.
45. Centers for Disease Control and Prevention. *HIV/AIDS among American Indians and Alaska Natives*; 2008. Available at: http://www.cdc.gov/hiv/resources/factsheets/PDF/aian.pdf. Accessed June 2010.
46. Stevens SJ, Estrada AL, Estrada BD. HIV drug and sex risk behaviors among American Indian and Alaska Native drug users: gender and site differences. *Am Indian Alsk Native Ment Health Res.* 2000;9:33–46.
47. Substance Abuse and Mental Health Services Administration, Office of Applied Studies. *The NSDUH Report: Injection Drug Use and Related Risk Behaviors.* Rockville, MD: SAMHSA; 2009.
48. National Congress of American Indians. *Methamphetamine in Indian Country: An American Problem Uniquely Affecting Indian Country*; 2006. Available at: http://methpedia.org/pdf/Meth%20in%20Indian%20Country%20Fact%20Sheet.pdf
49. Spear S, Crevecoeur DA, Rawson RA, et al. The rise in methamphetamine use among American Indians in Los Angeles county. *Am Indian Alsk Native Ment Health Res.* 2007;14: 1–15.
50. American Lung Association. *Smoking and American Indians/Alaska Natives Fact Sheet*; 2007. Retrieved October 10, 2007, from http://www.lungusa.org/site/pp.asp?c=dvLUK9O0E&b=35999.

CHAPTER 63 Women and Addiction

Shelly F. Greenfield ■ Sudie E. Back ■ Katie Lawson ■ Kathleen T. Brady

EPIDEMIOLOGY

Substance use disorders are highly prevalent in our society. Data from the National Epidemiologic Survey on Alcohol and Related (NESARC; $N = 43,093$), the largest and most recent study of substance use and other psychiatric disorders, estimates the 12-month prevalence rate of alcohol use disorders to be 8.5% and drug use disorders to be 2.0% (1,2). Similarly, data from the 2006 National Survey on Drug Use Disorders (NSDUH) found that approximately 22.6 million people (9.2% of the population aged 12 and older) met criteria for past year substance abuse or dependence (3).

Significant gender differences in rates of substance use disorders have been consistently observed in both the general population and treatment-seeking samples. In comparison to women, men have been shown to demonstrate significantly higher rates of substance use, abuse and dependence (2,4–6). However, recent epidemiologic surveys demonstrate that the gender difference in prevalence of alcohol use disorders has narrowed in recent decades. Surveys in the early 1980s estimated a male-to-female ratio of alcohol use disorders as five-to-one (7), whereas recent NESARC data found that men were 3.1 times more likely than women to meet criteria for an alcohol use disorder (2.3 times more likely to have alcohol abuse and 2.6 times more likely to have alcohol dependence) (8). Findings from two cross-sectional analyses of drinking across birth cohorts demonstrated little variation in lifetime drinking histories among men from different birth cohorts compared at similar ages. By contrast, women born between 1954 and 1963 had significantly more lifetime drinking than those born in the previous cohort of women between 1944 and 1953 (9). Increases were particularly significant among white and Hispanic women—beginning with those born in the United States after World War II (9).

Compared with alcohol use disorders, the gender difference in drug use disorders is somewhat less pronounced. NESARC data showed that men were 2.3 times more likely than women to meet criteria for a drug use disorder, 2.2 times more likely to have drug abuse and 1.9 times more likely to have drug dependence (4). Data regarding the use of prescription drugs is less consistent. Some data suggest that rates of nonmedical prescription drug use are higher among women than men, particularly for narcotic analgesics and tranquilizers (10). Other, more recent studies of nonmedical prescription opioid use report gender equivalent rates (3,11–13) or higher rates among men as compared to women (14–17). Gender differences in nicotine use and dependence are also substantially less than for other substances of abuse (18).

TELESCOPING

The phenomenon of "telescoping" has been consistently observed in investigations of gender and substance use disorders. Telescoping is a term used to describe an accelerated progression found in women from the initiation of substance use to the onset of dependence and first admission to treatment (19,20). In particular, women are more likely than men to show an accelerated progression between regular use and treatment seeking for opioids, cannabis and alcohol (19). Thus, when women enter treatment for substance use disorders, they typically present with more severe clinical profiles (e.g., more medical, behavioral, psychological, and social problems characteristic of substance use disorders), despite having used the substance for a shorter period of time.

BIOLOGICAL ISSUES

Sex differences in the neurobiological correlates of substance use disorders have been elucidated in a growing number of studies over the past decade. In particular, sex differences related to responsivity to drugs of abuse and to relapse have been demonstrated in animal models and human studies in three areas: (a) neuroactive gonadal steroid hormones, as well as fluctuations of these hormone levels across the menstrual cycle; (b) sex differences in stress reactivity and relapse to substance abuse; and (c) sex differences in neurobiologic correlates evident from neuroimaging studies.

Neuroactive Gonadal Steroid Hormones

Animal models have demonstrated that neuroactive gonadal steroid (e.g., estradiol, testosterone, and progesterone) affect the reinforcing properties of drugs under numerous conditions (21). Neuroactive steroid hormones can have excitatory and inhibitory effects on the brain (22) and may influence the saliency of drug effects. These gonadal steroid hormones are linked in mediating neurobehavioral processes related to the reward system (21) and can mediate reinforcing effects of abused drugs. Ovarian steroid hormones (e.g., estrogen and progesterone), metabolites of progesterone, and negative allosteric modulators of the GABA-A receptor such as dehydroepiandrosterone (DHEA) are neuroactive and can influence the behavioral effects of drugs (21). In animal models, for example, DHEA reduces self-administration and cocaine seeking in rats (23). Changes are also evident in brain function and neurochemistry across the phases of the menstrual cycle that are likely correlated with fluctuating levels of estrogen and progesterone (21), and these fluctuations have been correlated with the reinforcing properties of drugs of abuse in women.

In human studies, the follicular phase of the menstrual cycle is associated with greatest responsivity to stimulants such as cocaine (24,25). A number of studies indicate that during the follicular phase, when estradiol levels are high and progesterone low, the effects of stimulants are increased compared to the luteal phase when both estradiol and progesterone levels are elevated (24,26,27). It is unclear whether these effects are attributable to estradiol or progesterone (28). For example, in one study investigating response to cocaine administration, sex and menstrual cycle effects, women in the luteal phase reported lower ratings of feeling "high" than did women in the follicular phase of their cycle or men (24). It is not clear whether sex differences in response to stimulants is accounted for by enhancing effects of estradiol or attenuating effects of progesterone. However, a study of oral progesterone administration to males as well as to females in both phases of the menstrual cycle indicated that progesterone attenuates the subjective response to smoked cocaine in women but not men (28). Heart rate and subjective effects in response to smoked cocaine were greater in the follicular than luteal phase among female cocaine smokers (27).

In addition to menstrual phase cycle differences and the effects of gonadal hormones on response to cocaine administration, studies of alcohol and nicotine also demonstrate potential greater saliency for these substances in the luteal phase of the cycle (21,29–31). An early study of smoking cessation demonstrated that women in the luteal phase reported more fatigue, irritability, anxiety and depression symptoms in response to nicotine withdrawal than did women in the follicular phase (30). Other studies have replicated the finding that women have greater nicotine withdrawal symptoms and craving if they quit smoking in the luteal versus follicular phase (21,29).

The effect of gonadal steroids on behavioral and subjective responses to alcohol is less clear than for other substances of abuse. Animal studies have found no difference in the effect of alcohol across menstrual phases (32). One study examined the subjective and behavioral effects of alcohol in healthy women across the early follicular, late follicular, midluteal, and late-luteal phases of the menstrual cycle and found that the effects of alcohol did not vary across the cycle (33). Other research in women with and without premenstrual syndrome showed that alcohol infusion suppressed allopregnanolone serum concentrations in the late-luteal phase but had no effect during the follicular phase (34).

While opioids directly affect the hypothalamic–pituitary–gonadal system by inhibiting the release of luteinizing hormone releasing hormone, few human studies have examined the role of gonadal steroid hormones in sex differences in response to opioids. Human studies have examined sex differences in response to pain, including pain thresholds across the menstrual cycle (35) and found that pain thresholds are the highest during the follicular phase and lower during luteal and premenstrual phases. Animal studies have yielded inconsistent results examining the effects of opioids on behavioral outcomes (21).

Overall, accumulating evidence from animal and human studies demonstrate sex differences in the role of neuroactive steroid hormones on drug abuse, but the findings vary depending on the drug studied, the species, and the specific outcome measured.

Sex Differences in Stress Reactivity and Relapse to Substance Abuse

In a related area of investigation regarding sex differences in the neurobiologic correlates of substance use disorders, the hypothalamic–pituitary–adrenal (HPA) axis controls gonadotropin and gonadal steroid hormone release through a complex feedback mechanism. The HPA axis is also the neuroendocrine pathway for the stress response. Sex differences in neuroendocrine adaptations to stress and reward systems can function as a mediator for susceptibility to drug abuse and relapse in women (36). Stressors and drug-related cues are important in facilitating drug seeking and drug reinforcement behaviors in humans and animals (36). Sex differences in neuroendocrine adaptations to stress and reward have been elucidated, including sex differences in stress-symptom neuroadaptations in substance-dependent men and women (36), the impact of sex hormones on stress response (27), attenuating effects of progesterone on stress response and drug craving (37,38) among other studies (39).

Human laboratory studies have examined sex differences in stress response and relapse to substance abuse (40–42), including sex differences in emotional and autonomic differences in response to stress and cues (36). Human studies, among cocaine-dependent subjects demonstrate greater stress response in men than women, with higher ACTH and cortisol levels following exposure to stress and drug cues (43). This HPA dysregulation in women may be associated with greater emotional intensity at lower levels of HPA arousal than men (38) and may be one key to enhanced vulnerability to use substances in response to negative affect among women. Similar results have been found in alcohol (44,45) and nicotine dependence (46).

Neuroimaging and Neurobiologic Correlates

Neurobiological correlates of substance use disorders can be assessed with neuroimaging techniques, such as functional magnetic resonance imaging (fMRI), which can measure information processing in discrete brain circuits that may not be behaviorally observed but may be connected with manifestations of alcohol or drug use disorders (47). Sex differences in neural activity have been demonstrated using fMRI techniques including the response of medial prefrontal cortex for drug reward anticipation and receipt, and stress- and cue-induced craving (48,49). Another line of work indicates the possibility of neural correlates of sex differences in treatment outcome. For example, sex hormones may regulate the ventromedial prefrontal cortex, which is involved in extinction memory (50). In one study, men had greater recall of extinction memory than women in the late, but not early, follicular phase of the menstrual cycle (51). While observed correlations between BOLD fMRI findings in limbic areas and gene–gene interactions suggest endophenotypes that may be useful in exploring disease processes (47), the degree to which such processes may be associated with prognosis or treatment outcomes remains unclear (47). Translational research in this area might be targeted at understanding the way in which sex differences in the neurobiological correlates of substance use disorders are associated with prognosis and substance abuse treatment outcomes.

ROLE OF CO-OCCURRING DISORDERS

Mood and Anxiety Disorders

Mood and anxiety disorders are some of the most common co-occurring psychiatric conditions among women with substance use disorders (52). Epidemiologic studies utilizing the NCS and the NESARC data (53,54) show that lifetime rates of mood and anxiety disorders among individuals with substance use disorders are significantly higher among women than men. For example, among individuals with substance use disorders, rates of major depression range from 30.1% to 48.5% among women versus 9.0% to 30.1% among men. Rates of simple or specific phobia range from 28.2% to 30.7% among women versus 5.9% to 13.9% among men. Similar gender differences have been observed in the general population, as well (1).

A recent study by Goldstein (55) investigated 12-month prevalence, comorbidity, and treatment utilization rates for substance use, mood, and anxiety disorders among women in the Wave 1 NESARC ($n = 24,575$) (1,56), which was conducted in 2001 to 2002 by the National Institute on Alcohol Abuse and Alcoholism (NIAAA). Goldstein found that the 12-month prevalence rates of mood and anxiety disorders among women with substance use disorders were 29.7% and 26.2%, respectively. The most common mood disorder among women with alcohol or drug use disorders was major depressive disorder (15.4%) and the most common anxiety disorder was specific phobia (15.6%).

The order in which co-occurring psychiatric conditions develop may help elucidate the etiology as well as help determine the best treatment approach. Some individuals manifest depression prior to the development of a substance use disorder (i.e., primary depression), while others manifest depression following the development of a substance use disorder (i.e., secondary depression). A third group of individuals develop depression and the substance use disorder simultaneously. Of these three potential orders of onset pathways, the most common is secondary depression (57). Furthermore, women are more likely than men to present with secondary depression, and therefore may be more likely to respond to depressive symptoms by "self-medicating" with alcohol and drugs (58,59). In fact, one study found that the risk of developing heavy drinking was 2.6 times greater for women with, as compared to without, a history of depression (60).

Given the high prevalence of co-occurring mood and anxiety disorders among women with substance use disorders, a comprehensive psychiatric assessment at treatment entry is critical. Because substances of abuse have profound effects on neurotransmitter systems involved in the pathophysiology of mood and anxiety disorders, chronic alcohol or drug use may unmask a vulnerability or lead to organic changes that manifest as a mood or anxiety disorder. One of the best ways to differentiate substance-induced, transient symptoms from a disorder that warrants treatment is through observation of symptoms during a period of abstinence from alcohol or drugs. Transient substance-induced symptoms will improve with time. The duration of abstinence necessary for accurate diagnosis should be based on the diagnosis being assessed and the substance used. For example, drugs with a longer half-life (e.g., some benzodiazepines, methadone) may require several weeks of abstinence for withdrawal symptoms to subside, but drugs with a shorter half-life (e.g., alcohol, cocaine, short half-life benzodiazepines) require less abstinence to make a valid diagnosis. A family history of mood or anxiety disorders, the onset of symptoms before the development of the substance use disorder, and sustained symptoms during lengthy periods of abstinence all suggest an independent mood or anxiety disorder (61).

Following a comprehensive assessment, women should receive or be referred to evidence-based treatments that will adequately address both conditions, especially given the fact that many women use substances in response to co-occurring psychiatric symptoms. Unfortunately, the large majority (91%) of women with substance use disorders and a co-occurring mood or anxiety disorder do not seek treatment (55). In particular, women with alcohol use, as compared to drug use, disorders demonstrate very low rates of treatment seeking. The highest treatment-seeking rates are seen among women with substance use disorders and co-occurring major depression, dysthymia, or panic disorder (55).

To date, few investigations have examined gender differences in response to psychotherapeutic or pharmacotherapeutic treatments for mood and anxiety disorders among individuals with co-occurring substance use disorders. The use of agents targeting substance use, such as naltrexone or disulfiram, as add-on treatment for individuals with co-occurring mood or anxiety disorders is under-explored. In one study of 254 alcohol-dependent outpatients with a variety of co-occurring psychiatric disorders, Petrakis and colleagues (62) investigated the efficacy of disulfiram and naltrexone, or their combination and found that active treatment with either medication was associated with improved frequency and severity of alcohol consumption. Among 100 (52 men, 48 women) alcohol-dependent outpatients, Pettinati and colleagues (63) examined gender differences in the effectiveness of sertraline among Type A and B alcoholics, many of whom had current (up to 57.9%) or lifetime (up to 78.9%) major depression. Findings showed that Type A alcoholic men, but not women, responded more favorably to sertraline than placebo (i.e., longer time to relapse, fewer days drinking, fewer drinks per drinking day). No differences were seen with Type B alcoholics. More recently, Pettinati et al. (64) examined gender differences in response to a higher-than-typical dose of naltrexone (150 mg/day) among 164 individuals (116 and 48 women) with dependence on cocaine and alcohol. This dose was found to be effective in men, but not in women. In fact, among women the higher dose was associated with increased cocaine use. In this study, psychosis and mania were the only Axis I conditions excluded. None of the above studies, however, examined the effects of specific co-occurring psychiatric disorders.

Eating Disorders

Eating disorders (EDs) occur more frequently among women than men (65) with a lifetime prevalence in women estimated to be 2 to 3 times higher than in men (66). The large majority (90%) of the cases of Anorexia Nervosa (AN) and Bulimia Nervosa (BN) are found in women (67). In contemporary Western cultures, thinness in women has come to signify attractiveness, competence, success, and self-control and may negatively affect the development and perception of women's body image (65).

The *DSM-IV* (67) classifies EDs into three main categories: (a) AN, (b) BN, and (c) EDs not otherwise specified (ED NOS). A new ED subtype, Binge Eating Disorder (BED), is also included in the *DSM-IV* as a research category and is classified under the ED NOS category. Of the three categories, AN is the least common and BED is the most common (68). Lifetime prevalence rates of AN and BN are estimated to be 0.5% and 2%, respectively (67).

Women with substance use disorders demonstrate higher rates of EDs, in particular the purging subtypes of bulimia, than women in the general population (69–71). In their review, Holderness and colleagues (70) found that lifetime ED behaviors co-occurred with substance use disorders in up to 40% of women in clinical populations. More recently, the NCS-R estimated that rates of lifetime alcohol use disorders occurred in up to 34% of individuals with EDs, which is significantly higher than rates of alcohol use disorders in the general population. Rates of co-occurring lifetime drug use disorders up to 26% among individuals with EDs have been reported (66). Among women with BN, in particular, and co-occurring substance use disorders, there is also a high reported rate of severe childhood sexual abuse (72). Similarly, among women with BN or BED, rates of substance abuse are greater among those with, compared to those without, a history of sexual or physical abuse (73).

Evidence-based behavioral treatments for EDs include cognitive–behavioral therapy and interpersonal therapy. Psychopharmacotherapy for EDs has focused on antidepressant medications. Given the biological, psychological, and social factors involved in the development of EDs, treatment is complex and requires a multidisciplinary approach. For example, in addition to behavioral and pharmacological treatment, nutritional counseling and medical supervision are indicated (74). Individual, group, and family modalities of treatments are also often utilized to treat EDs, with or without co-occurring substance use disorders. Even though research suggests that treatment for EDs is most effective when addressed in the context of programs specializing in the treatment of EDs (75), most ED patients tend to receive treatment in a general medical setting (66). At present, no integrated, evidence-based treatments for EDs and substance use disorders are available and few treatment programs provide integrated treatment for co-occurring eating and substance use disorders (69). Like many co-occurring psychiatric conditions, individuals with substance use disorders and EDs are usually treated in programs specializing in either substance use disorders or EDs, but do not receive services for both disorders. A recent review of screening and treatment practices at 351 addiction treatment programs revealed that only half (51%) screen for EDs at intake or assessment (69). Furthermore, only 29% of addiction programs admit patients who screen positive for EDs. Overall, fewer than 1 in 6 addiction programs (17%) attempt to treat co-occurring EDs and only 3% have a formal referral arrangement for patient to receive ED-focused treatment.

Posttraumatic Stress Disorder

Posttraumatic stress disorder (PTSD) is a syndrome marked by symptoms of intense horror, helplessness, or fear following exposure to a distressing event that involves real or perceived threat to physical integrity (67). PTSD typically results from an extreme, catastrophic, or overwhelming experience (e.g., sexual assault, natural disaster, combat exposure) and is characterized by the following three symptom clusters: (a) re-experiencing the event through flashbacks, nightmares, and intrusive memories, (b) avoidance of stimuli (e.g., people, places, thoughts, feelings) associated with the event, and (c) increased arousal, such as, hypervigilance, trouble sleeping and concentrating, and increased irritability (67). Among victims of sexual assault, prevalence estimates of PTSD range from 14% to 80% and, among victims of physical assault, from 13% to 23% (76–78). Notably, interpersonal victimization is more likely than noninterpersonal traumas, such as serious accidents and natural disasters, to lead to the development of PTSD (79,80).

Among individuals with substance use disorders, the prevalence of PTSD is 1.4 to 5 times higher compared to those without substance use disorders (81). Rates of physical or sexual abuse among treatment-seeking women as high as 99% have been reported (82–84). Repeated forms of trauma, such as, domestic violence and revictimization are also common (85). Among men with substance use disorders and PTSD, exposures to crime victimization (e.g., being physically assaulted or mugged) or combat-related traumas are common.

Consensus is lacking regarding the best approach to treat co-occurring PTSD and substance use disorders; however, an emerging body of clinical treatment research demonstrates the efficacy of integrated interventions (83,85,86). This is in contrast to earlier concerns that PTSD treatment may be too stressful for substance use disordered patients and may induce relapse (87,88). The studies that have been conducted to date on integrated treatments for co-occurring PTSD and substance use disorders show good tolerability and efficacy, including significant reductions in both PTSD symptoms and alcohol and drug use severity (83,89–91). Unfortunately, most individuals with PTSD and substance use disorders receive addiction treatment only (92). For those patients who do receive treatment for both the PTSD and substance use disorders, most receive a sequential form of therapy. That is, they first receive addiction treatment, while the trauma/PTSD related issues are deferred. It is unclear how many patients who are later referred for PTSD treatment actually seek and obtain it following the completion of addiction treatment. Insofar as abuse of alcohol and drugs occurs in response to PTSD symptoms, addressing trauma-related symptoms first, or early in treatment, may provide opportunity for improved likelihood of recovery from substance use disorders (86,89,93).

Although selective serotonin reuptake inhibitors (SSRI's) are the pharmacological treatments of choice for PTSD, only three published studies have examined their use among patients with co-occurring alcohol or drug use disorders, and all of those studies tested sertraline (94–96). There was a trend for the sertraline group to show less severe PTSD symptoms, particularly in intrusion and hyperarousal symptoms. Follow-up cluster analyses identified that the medication-responsive group tended to have earlier PTSD (i.e., primary PTSD). A secondary analysis of the Brady et al. (95) data found that the presence of a second anxiety disorder or depression did not detract from treatment response to sertraline (96).

Personality Disorders

Personality disorders (PDs) are serious mental disorders characterized by inflexible patterns of thoughts and actions that are pervasive across situations and that begin during adolescence or early adulthood (67). Individuals with PDs demonstrate impaired functioning in at least two major areas, such as interpersonal functioning and affectivity. Prevalence rate across genders for any PD is approximately 14.8% (1). According to the *DSM-IV* (67), there are 10 categories of PDs, divided into three clusters:

Cluster A (odd or eccentric): paranoid personality disorder, schizoid personality disorder, schizotypal personality disorder

Cluster B (dramatic, erratic, emotional): borderline personality disorder, antisocial personality disorder, narcissistic personality disorder, histrionic personality disorder

Cluster C (anxious and fearful): avoidant personality disorder, obsessive compulsive personality disorder, dependent personality disorder

Some studies have found that among individuals with substance use disorders, especially drug use disorders, the prevalence of co-occurring Axis II disorders is higher than that of Axis I disorders (97–100). For example, among individuals with an alcohol use disorder, one study in the general population found that 28.6% had at least one PD, and among those with a drug use disorder, 47.7% had at least one PD (1). Clinical samples reveal an even stronger association between PDs and substance use disorders (99,101).

Among both men and women, Cluster B and C PDs are the most prevalent co-occurring PDs among individuals with substance use disorders (100,102). The co-occurrence of specific PDs, however, differs by gender. For example, women with substance use disorders demonstrate a greater prevalence of co-occurring borderline personality disorder (BPD) than men (99,103), while the prevalence of antisocial personality disorder (ASPD) is greater among men than women with substance use disorders (99,104).

Individuals with co-occurring personality and substance use disorders are more likely to have greater severity and, earlier age of onset of their substance use disorders, as well as higher rates of polydrug use, and more use of illicit drugs (105–107). High rates of self-harm and suicidal behaviors are common in women with co-occurring personality and alcohol and drug use disorders, requiring careful assessment and close monitoring (105,108). Finally, women with co-occurring personality and substance use disorders present with many complex problems and urgent needs. A specialized cognitive–behavioral therapy intervention, Dialectical Behavior Therapy (DBT) created by Dr. Marsha Linehan, includes a variety of treatment modalities (e.g., individual therapy, skills group, telephone coaching, therapist consultation team) and was originally designed for suicidal patients with BPD. Over the past decade, DBT has been adapted to address problems associated with co-occurring substance use and BPD (109). The four core DBT skills include: (a) mindfulness, (b) distress tolerance, (c) emotion regulation, and (d) interpersonal effectiveness. These core skills are relevant to both substance abuse and other problem behaviors. Several randomized controlled trials indicate that DBT is associated with superior substance use outcomes, maintenance of treatment gains, and good retention among women with BPD and substance use disorders (110,111).

Another treatment for co-occurring personality and substance use disorders is Dual Focused Schema Therapy (DFST) developed by Samuel Ball (112). It represents an adaptation of Young's Schema Focused Therapy (113). In addition to targeting the maladaptive schemas related to self, others, and events that are assumed to be learned in childhood and that organize a person's beliefs and behaviors, DFST includes specific interventions to target maladaptive schemas and specific relapse prevention techniques to address substance abuse (e.g., coping with cravings and urges to use). A recent, 24-week randomized controlled trial compared DFST to standard 12-Step

Drug Counseling in a sample of 52 opioid-dependent, homeless individuals with co-occurring PDs and substance use disorders (114). Individuals in the DFST group attended more individual sessions, but low retention rates across both groups (40%) limited the researcher's ability to compare other treatment outcomes by group.

SPECIFIC SUBSTANCES

Alcohol

Gender and Epidemiology

In general, men consume and misuse alcohol at significantly higher rates than women (115). However, this gender gap has decreased over time due to women's increased use of alcohol (116). This phenomenon, known as the "convergence hypothesis," is well documented in several large epidemiological studies. For example, data collected from over 42,000 participants in the 2001 to 2002 National Epidemiological Survey on Alcohol and Related Conditions (NESARC) indicated that sex differences in rates of alcohol use and abuse or dependence were smallest for younger cohorts (with cohorts ranging from 1913 to 1932 to 1968 to 1984) (117). Similarly, examination of changes in the age of initiation of alcohol use over the past 50 years shows significant narrowing of the gender gap (9). Whereas the male to female ratio of initiation in the 10 to 14 year old age group was 4:1 in the 1950s, it was one-to-one by the early 1990s. Finally, epidemiologic data show that while males aged 12 and older demonstrate significantly higher rates of alcohol dependence, examination of 12- to 17-year-olds show no significant difference. Some researchers propose that women's increase in alcohol consumption can be explained by sociocultural factors, such as society's increased acceptance of women's use of alcohol (9).

Telescoping Effect

Compared to men, women experience shorter time intervals between the initiation of alcohol use and the onset of significant alcohol-related problems (e.g., medical, social) and entrance into addiction treatment (19,118,119). This accelerated course of alcohol dependence, or "telescoping" may be attributed to a variety of biological, socioeconomic, psychologic, and cultural factors. Women may be more adversely affected than men by alcohol due to the lower percentage of total body water, decreased first pass metabolism because of lower levels of alcohol dehydrogenase in the gastric mucosa, and slower rates of alcohol metabolism (20). Sociocultural factors, such as the negative stigma associated with women and heavy drinking, economic barriers such as lack of insurance and lack of childcare, may cause women to wait until symptoms are more severe before entering treatment (120).

Triggers for Alcohol Use

Gender differences in triggers for alcohol use have been observed. In general, women are more likely than men to consume alcohol in response to stress and negative emotions, whereas men are more likely than women to consume alcohol to enhance positive emotions or to conform to a group (121,122). These differences in drinking motives should be considered when designing prevention and treatment plans for men and women with alcohol use disorders (123). As compared to men, women with alcohol use disorders are significantly more likely to have co-occurring psychiatric disorders, including EDs (specifically BN) (124,125) BPD (103), depression (1), and anxiety disorders, such as, PTSD (54). It is important to address co-occurring psychiatric conditions among women with alcohol use disorders, as these conditions may serve to impede substance use treatment efforts.

Treatment

Women are less likely than men to seek treatment, and some data indicate that once in treatment women are more likely to drop out or attend fewer sessions (126,127). These differences may be affected by gender differences in factors such as childcare responsibilities, transportation, financial status, and social stigma. Offering childcare, prenatal care, women-only admission, and services specific for women's issues may be particularly effective in getting women to initiate and continue treatment (128). To enhance women's treatment retention rates, researchers have developed and implemented interventions specifically designed for women-only groups. Early results are promising, indicating that women not only experience fewer relapses in women-only treatment groups, but also gave higher satisfaction ratings for the treatment (129,130).

Stimulants

Gender and Epidemiology

In contrast to alcohol, rates of stimulant use are similar among men and women (131). However, both preclinical (132–135) and clinical studies (136,137) suggest that women may be particularly vulnerable to the reinforcing effects of stimulant drugs. In the past, women may have evidenced lower prevalence rates of stimulant drug use (138), however, societal changes are altering the "protective factors" (e.g., social stigma) that once lowered the rates of drug use. Because women may be more susceptible to the reinforcing effects of stimulants and "protective factors" are diminishing, women may be particularly at risk for using stimulants (139).

More recently, public health monitoring has indicated that methamphetamine use in the United States and worldwide has been on the rise with an estimated 5.8% of individuals age 12 and older in the United States having endorsed use at least once in their lifetime (3). The Treatment Episode Data Set (TEDS) documents that treatment admissions for methamphetamine as the primary substance use problem have more than doubled from 3.7% to 9.2% between 1995 and 2005 (140). A recent population-based study of noninstitutionalized adults ($N = 4297$) aged 18 to 49 in the United States in 2005 found that the overall prevalence of current nonmedical methamphetamine use was estimated to be 0.27% with lifetime use estimated to be 8.6% (141). There were no significant gender differences in current use rates (0.32% for men and 0.23% for women) although the 3-year prevalence rate for men (3.1%) was higher than in women (1.1%). In 1994, among pregnant women admitted to federally funded substance abuse treatment centers, 8% were admitted for treatment of methamphetamine dependence, whereas in 2006, that proportion had risen to 24% leading the study's authors to conclude that methamphetamine is the primary substance of abuse for which women seek care during pregnancy (142). A 2005 study conducted in four states in the western United States, found that 5.2% of pregnant women living in these areas were affected by methamphetamine use (140). Other research has indicated that the relative rise of women in the criminal justice system is in part accounted for by the rise of methamphetamine use (143).

Hormones

Hormones may play an important role in the reinforcing effects of stimulant drugs for women. Both basic and clinical studies indicate that estrogen increases the reinforcing effects of stimulants for women (26,132–135), whereas progesterone decreases the reinforcing effects (144,145). In response to cocaine administration, women have been found to report increased subjecting feelings of "high" and increased heart rate during the follicular phase, when levels of estrogen are elevated and progesterone levels are low, as compared to the luteal phase, when levels of progesterone and estrogen are low (24,28). Furthermore, exogenous administration of progesterone has also been shown to result in attenuated subjective responses to cocaine administration among women (28).

Treatment

Preclinical studies suggest that women may have a harder time quitting stimulants than men (146,147). Elman, Karlsgodt, and Gastfriend (148) hypothesize that gender differences in response to drug cues may help explain this difference. Research suggests that cognitive–behavioral therapy is as effective in treating stimulant use disorders among women as men (149,150). One study focusing on 359 women methamphetamine-using offenders who were treated in a modified therapeutic community program ($n = 234$) or standard outpatient treatment ($n = 125$) found that both treatment groups improved on psychosocial measures with a greater effect size seen in the modified therapeutic community (143).

Currently, there are no approved pharmacotherapy treatments for cocaine dependence. However, preclinical studies suggest that baclofen, a GABA-ergic drug, may be more effective in reducing cocaine use for women than men. In one study, female rats injected with baclofen self-administered cocaine significantly fewer times than male rats injected with baclofen (151). Clinical studies using naltrexone to reduce cocaine use (64) and bupropion to decrease methamphetamine use (152) indicate that these pharmacotherapies may be more effective in treating men than women.

OPIOIDS

Prescription Opioids

Gender and Epidemiology

In 2006, 5.2 million Americans reported using prescription opioids for nonmedical purposes (3). A 141% increase in prescription opioid abuse was reported from 1992 to 2003 (153). There are a number of potential explanations for this increase: prescription opioids are relatively easy to obtain from a variety of sources (e.g., primary care physicians, the Internet), less social stigma is attached to prescription drug use as opposed to the use of "harder" drugs like cocaine or heroin, and prescription opioids are less closely monitored by law enforcement than other illicit drugs (153,154).

Research on gender differences in rates of nonmedical prescription opioid use is inconclusive. Although two large epidemiological surveys found that women use prescription opioids nonmedically more often than men (10), other studies suggest that rates of use are similar between men and women (3,12), or that men use prescription opioids nonmedically more than women (17). Furthermore, some studies indicate that gender differences in prescription opioid use may occur within specific age groups. For example, data from the 2002 to 2004 National Surveys on Drug Use and Health (NSDUH) show that compared to men women aged 12 to 17 report higher rates of prescription opioid abuse and dependence, whereas women aged 18 to 25 report lower rates of abuse and dependence (155).

Triggers for Nonmedical Prescription Opioid Use

Carise and colleagues (14) found that 86% of individuals in treatment programs used prescription opiates to "get high" or "get a buzz." Among college students, McCabe et al. (13) found that women were significantly less likely than men to report using prescription opioids for "experimentation" (18.4% vs. 35.3%) or to "get high" (24.4% vs. 39.4%). Among chronic pain patients, women have also been found to be more likely to engage in particular "aberrant" drug taking behaviors, such as, hoarding unused medications, and using additional drugs (e.g., sedatives) to enhance the effectiveness of prescription opioids (156).

Comorbidity

Compared to nonopioid users, individuals who have used prescription opioids nonmedically and/or are dependent on opioids are more likely to suffer from anxiety disorders, affective disorders, or other substance use disorders (157,158). Men are more likely to be diagnosed with co-occurring substance use disorders (157) and ASPD (158), whereas women are more likely to be diagnosed with an affective disorder (e.g., major depressive disorder) (158,159) and suffer from more severe occupational, economic, or medical problems (19,157,158).

Heroin and Intravenous Drug Abuse (IVDA)

Gender and Epidemiology

Data from the 2008 NSDUH indicates that 0.2% of the U.S. population aged 12 and older has used heroin (131). Using data collected from a community sample, one study ($N = 408$) found that in comparison to men, women use smaller amounts of the heroin, use heroin for a shorter period of time, and are less likely to inject heroin (59% of women heroin users endorsed a history of injecting vs. 76% of the men) (160). Among injection drug users only, no sex differences in the duration or amount of use were revealed. In general, IV users report more instability in employment, more problematic use, and more health problems (e.g., hepatitis C, HIV, cirrhosis) than non-IV users (161). A recent analysis of NESARC data explored gender differences among 578 individuals with opioid disorders (159) and found that women were twice as likely to have a mood or anxiety disorder. Women were also more likely to have a paranoid personality disorder and men were more likely to have ASPD. Women had a significantly higher risk of having several co-occurring psychiatric disorders compared with men who had greater odds of having other substance use disorders.

Triggers for Heroin and IVDA

As compared to men, women's injection of drugs may be more influenced by their sexual partner's injection risk behavior (162). For example, Powis and colleagues (160) found that women who injected heroin were significantly more likely than men to have a sexual partner who also injected heroin (96% vs. 82%). Female users are also more likely than male users to be introduced to injection by their sexual partners (160,163). For example, in Powis and colleagues' (160) research, 51% of the female heroin users were first injected by their male sexual partner, whereas 90% of men were injected the first time by a friend. Compared to men who inject, women who inject also report being more influenced by social pressure and by sexual partner encouragement (163). In another study of older individuals with heroin dependence, women were more likely to describe the adverse consequences of their addiction on their families but both men and women expressed concerns about hepatitis C and mental health issues (164).

Adverse Consequences of Needle Sharing

Individuals with IVDA who share needles or preparation equipment are at increased risk for numerous physical diseases, including hepatitis B and C (HBV, HCV), as well as HIV (163). Research to date is inconsistent as to whether sex differences in injection risk behaviors occur. Frajzyngier and colleagues (163) found no sex differences in sharing needles during the first injection, but women were significantly more likely to share preparation equipment than men. Other results suggest that although women are more likely to share needles (165–167), they are also more likely to engage in protective behaviors such as carrying clean syringes (166).

Treatment

Less than one fourth of individuals with opioid use disorders receive treatment (56). Potential reasons for low rates of treatment include the belief that using opioids is not as serious as using other illicit drugs since they are prescribed by physicians (11). For individuals with co-occurring chronic pain, they may fear that the pain will return or be exacerbated if opioid use ceases. To date, little research has investigated gender differences in the treatment of opioid use disorders. Preliminary findings for a manual-based, 12-session group treatment specifically designed for women using methadone suggests this may be an effective way to treat opioid dependence in women (168).

With regard to opioid agonist therapies, methadone maintenance therapy has been associated with reduced heroin use and improvements in psychiatric, medical, and legal problems (169–171). Jones, Fitzgerald, and Johnson (172) found that both men and women remained in treatment for a significantly longer period of time when given methadone as opposed to LAAM and that women given methadone remained in treatment longer than women given buprenorphine (115 vs. 105 days), although this finding did not reach statistical significance. Although buprenorphine, LAAM, and methadone reduced drug use for all participants, results suggest that sex differences may occur in the effectiveness of these pharmacologic agents. For women, buprenorphine was associated with significantly fewer positive urine samples and less self-reported opioid use than methadone. For men, LAAM was associated with less drug use than burprenorphine.

Cannabis

Gender and Epidemiology

According to the 2004 National Survey on Drug Use and Health (NSDUH), approximately 96.6 million Americans (40.2%) have tried marijuana, with 25.4 million (10.6%) having used within the last year, making it the most commonly used illegal drug in the United States (173). Among individuals who used marijuana within the past year, approximately 35.6% abused or were dependent on marijuana (174).

In comparison to women, men are more likely to use marijuana daily (2.0% vs. 0.7%) (175), have more initial opportunities to use marijuana (176), and initiate marijuana use at a younger age (16.4 years vs. 17.6 years) (177). Men and women may also differ in their risk of becoming dependent on marijuana (174). For women, there is approximately a 1% chance of becoming dependent during the first 5 years after initial use. For men, during the first year there is a 1% chance of becoming dependent, but for the following 2 years, there is a 4% chance per year that men will become dependent on marijuana (6). Research suggests that women enter treatment for marijuana use disorder after significantly fewer years of use than men do (i.e., telescoping effects) (19).

Hormones

Unlike other substances (e.g., stimulants), no relationship between the menstrual phase and women's use of (178), or response to, marijuana (e.g., mood and pulse rate) (179) has been observed. However, marijuana use may be related to the menstrual cycle for women who have severe premenstrual syndrome (PMS) or premenstrual dysphoric disorder (PMDD) (179).

Negative Effects of Marijuana Use

Marijuana use may affect attention processes and memory up to 7 days after use (180) and the effects of marijuana use on neuropsychological processes may differ for men and women. When comparing heavy marijuana users to light users, Pope and colleagues (181) found that visual–spatial memory was impaired for women who smoked heavily as compared to women who were light smokers. For men, however, no such difference was observed.

Comorbidity

When compared to individuals without marijuana dependence, those with dependence are significantly more likely to have co-occurring psychiatric disorders (90% vs. 55%) (182). In particular, marijuana dependence has been found to be associated with conduct disorder, ASPD, alcohol dependence (183), mood disorders, anxiety disorders (182), depression (184,185), posttraumatic stress disorder (186), and social phobia (182,53). Although gender differences in rates of comorbidity have not been thoroughly explored, there is some evidence that differences may exist. For example, one study found that social anxiety disorder was correlated with marijuana use for women but not men (187).

Treatment

Due to low numbers of women in treatment, no studies have been published regarding gender differences in the effectiveness of treatment for marijuana use disorders. However, research (with predominately male participants) suggests that cognitive–behavioral therapy, contingency management treatments, motivational enhancement therapies, and administering oral THC and nefazodone are effective treatments for marijuana dependence (188–191).

Nicotine

Gender and Epidemiology

In 2008, approximately 70.9 million Americans (28.4%) reported currently using nicotine. This includes people who smoke cigarettes and cigars, use smokeless tobacco, and use pipes to smoke tobacco. Males use nicotine at higher rates than females (34.5% vs. 22.5%) (131).

While most people understand the serious consequences of nicotine use, few are aware that women may be at an increased risk for health problems caused by smoking. Compared to men, women who smoke are twice as likely to have a heart attack (192), experience faster lung deterioration, and are at increased risk for chronic obstructive pulmonary disease (193) and lung cancer (194). Furthermore, smoking may cause women to commence menopause earlier, experience increased menstrual bleeding, have difficulty becoming pregnant, or experience spontaneous abortion (195). The children born to women who smoke while pregnant are at increased risk for sudden infant death syndrome (SIDs), death or severe complications caused by lung impairment, or low birth weight (196).

Triggers for Nicotine Use

Both pharmacological and nonpharmacological factors influence nicotine use and dependence. Nicotine is the main pharmacological factor in tobacco that plays a key role in the acquisition and maintenance of use. Nonpharmacological factors are stimuli that are often paired with nicotine, which can be both proximal (e.g., the smell of a cigarette) and distal (e.g., people associated with smoking) (197). Compared to men, women may be influenced less by nicotine factors (198,199) and more influenced by proximal cues (200). These gender differences in underlying motivations or triggers for use may help inform gender-sensitive treatment approaches.

Treatment

Women may have more difficulty quitting smoking than do men. Data from the Centers for Disease Control and Prevention (2006), which surveys over one hundred thousand U.S. citizens, indicates that over a million fewer women than men over the age of 35 are able to quit smoking (201). Menstrual cycle phase may be associated with women's success at smoking cessation (21,30). Women who attempt to quit during the first 14 days of their menstrual cycle (e.g., the follicular phase) may be more likely to be successful in their attempt than women who attempt to quit in the second half of the cycle (e.g., the luteal phase) and that women have greater nicotine withdrawal symptoms and craving if they quit smoking in the luteal versus follicular phase (21).

Nicotine Replacement and Nonnicotine Medication Research is inconclusive as to whether there are sex differences in the efficacy of nicotine replacement therapy (NRT). In 2004, a meta-analysis of 11 placebo-controlled NRT patch trials indicated that NRT is equally effective for men and women (202). More recently, however, Perkins and Scott (203) added three additional placebo-controlled trials to this meta-analysis and the results indicated that NRT is significantly more effective for men than women. Nonnicotine medication (bupropion and varenicline) are equally effective in men and women up to 12 weeks after treatment (204,205). However, no research has examined the abstinence rates following longer periods of time after treatment (206).

Behavioral Treatments Although medications are the standard approach to help individuals quit smoking, therapy and counseling generally enhance the efficacy of medication treatment and appear to be more effective in women than men (206). There are a number of approaches to counseling that may specifically help women address obstacles to quitting. For example, interventions that teach women how to cope with cues (e.g., distracting oneself from cues), since research suggests women respond more to nonnicotine factors (200) may be particularly helpful. In addition, interventions that address co-occurring mood and anxiety disorders may help decrease women's susceptibility to smoking cigarettes in order to cope with negative affect. Bupropion, which has been found to be equally effective for both men and women, may be a particularly effective method for women because it has been found to also help relieve depression (205).

Another obstacle to cessation is women's concern about weight gain. Women worry twice as much about weight gain caused by smoking cessation than men (207), and relapse three times more often than men because of weight gain (208). Cognitive–behavioral therapy designed to address women's concern about weight gain has been found to be more effective than standard cessation counseling alone (200).

Smoking during pregnancy is another issue of concern for women. This is a complicated issue because of the social stigma attached to smoking during pregnancy. Often women report abstinence when they are still smoking (209). Behavioral treatment approaches are particularly important for smoking cessation during pregnancy, because many medications are contraindicated in pregnancy. Therapy should be modified specifically for pregnant women (e.g., incentives for cessation, such as vouchers that can be exchanged for baby supplies) both while women are pregnant and after delivery, since approximately 65% of women who quit while pregnant relapse within 6 months of delivery (210).

Treatment Outcome for Women with Substance Use Disorders

Treatment Seeking and Utilization

The Treatment Episodes Data System (TEDS) captures data on national treatment admission rates and provides information on the extent to which women participate in substance abuse treatment. Based on the TEDS data, the overall proportion of men to women within the treatment system has remained fairly constant (e.g., from 1995 to 2005) at 2:1 (211).

A recent review of the literature between 1975 and 2005 examining characteristics associated with treatment outcome in women with substance use disorders concluded that over their lifetime, women are less likely to enter treatment compared with men (212). However, once women enter treatment, gender itself is not a predictor of treatment retention, completion, or outcome (212). While gender itself does not necessarily predict outcome, there are a number of gender-specific predictors of outcome and patient characteristics and treatment approaches can affect outcomes differentially by gender (212).

A number of barriers to treatment entry affect women more significantly than men. The role of children in women's lives can be central to seeking treatment as well as recovery. The majority of women who enter substance abuse treatment are mothers, and at least half have had contact with child welfare (213). Thus, the relationship with and responsibility for their children is likely a central influence on women's decision whether or not to enter treatment. One study of women entering methadone maintenance treatment found that women who were residing with their children were significantly more likely than women not residing with their children to enter treatment (214). For some women, however, residing with their children may serve as an impediment to entering treatment if they fear it may lead to the loss of custody of their children (215). Studies show that, once in treatment, women who were able to keep their children with them while in residential drug treatment or who retain custody of their infants while in intensive day treatment are more likely to stay in treatment (216).

Gender differences in sources of referral to treatment have been shown, highlighting the varying pathways by which women and men enter substance abuse treatment facilities. Overall, more men than women are referred to treatment through the criminal justice system (40% men vs. 28% women), whereas about twice as many women as men (15% women vs. 6% men) are referred from other community agencies, such as, welfare, mental health and other health care providers (209,217). One potential site for screening and referral of women is reproductive health services, such as obstetrics and gynecology (218). A study of eight obstetrics clinics demonstrated the feasibility of screening for alcohol use problems by using a brief screener in waiting rooms (219). The study found that 13% of pregnant women scored above the cutoff, indicating at-risk alcohol use, defined as binge drinking or more than one standard drink per week. At-risk use was predicted by earlier stage of pregnancy, indicating the feasibility of intervening early in pregnancies to reduce subsequent harm to the developing fetus. The criminal justice system is increasingly becoming more relevant to the lives of women with substance use disorders as the number of female prisoners in the United States is growing substantially (e.g., 53% since 1995), due largely to changes in sentencing for drug-related charges which have disproportionately affected women, particularly women of color (220).

Finally, differences in the sources of payment for substance abuse treatment have also been found, with a significantly greater proportion of men reporting self-pay (26% men vs. 18% women) and more women than men being dependent upon public insurance (26% women vs. 12% men) (211). This finding highlights how gender differences in economic and employment status are associated with gender differences in pathways to treatment, and suggest that women may be more vulnerable to changes in insurance-related benefits and coverage because of their greater reliance upon public insurance to pay for treatment.

In addition to financial and childcare issues, other factors may present as impediments to treatment seeking and utilization for women. For example, social stigma and labeling, lack of awareness of the range of treatment options, concerns about confrontational approaches that were pervasive in traditional substance abuse treatment, co-occurring mental disorders and/or a history of trauma and victimization, as well as homelessness all present possible barriers for women (221).

Once in treatment, some studies indicate that women may be more vulnerable than men to drop out of substance abuse treatment (222–224). However, other studies suggest that men are more likely to drop out of treatment (225) or that rates of treatment completion are equivalent among men and women (226,227). Finally, larger, population-based investigations provide a convergence of results showing few or no gender differences in treatment retention (130,228,229). Even though no consistent gender differences in treatment retention has been observed, some characteristics have been shown to be associated with more favorable outcomes for both men and women, such as greater financial resources, fewer mental health problems, and less severe drug problems (212,226,227). Studies in women-only samples have found associations between certain characteristics and retention, including better psychological functioning, higher levels of personal stability and social support, lower levels of anger, treatment beliefs, and referral source (230–234).

Gender-Specific Treatment for Women with Substance Use Disorders

Historically, the majority of substance abuse treatment models have been designed for men and based predominantly on male norms (116,130,235,236). More recently, however, gender-specific interventions are beginning to emerge. Gender-specific interventions and services for women are designed specifically to provide information and services that are tailored for women. Gender-specific and gender-sensitive treatments have emerged in response to mixed-gender programs, which often fail to address women's specific needs, such as childcare assistance, pregnancy, parenting, domestic violence, sexual trauma and victimization, housing, income support, and social services (227–242). Furthermore, only a minority of women (7%) believe there is no difference between mixed-gender and women-only programs (241). Despite this, data from the most recent National Survey of Substance Abuse Treatment Services (N-SSATS), which collects data on both public and private treatment centers, indicates that only a third (33%) of treatment facilities offer special programs for women and only 14% offer programs for pregnant or postpartum women (173).

Arguments in support of gender-specific treatment include differences in interaction styles and men's traditional societal dominance, which might negatively affect women in mixed-gender programs (136,243–246). In addition, women may not respond well to confrontational therapy styles (247), but rather they may benefit more from less structured and rigid styles (236). Moreover, women and men with substance use disorders differ significantly in terms of risk factors, co-occurring psychiatric conditions, motivations for treatment, and risks for relapse (236,248). Gender-sensitive treatments can address these issues directly for women in treatment for substance use disorders and may help to improve treatment-seeking and retention rates, as well as treatment satisfaction.

With regard to outcome of gender-specific treatments, the findings remain unclear (128,243,244,249,250). However, only a few randomized clinical trials have examined the relative effectiveness of comparable women-only versus mixed-gender interventions (130,212). In a meta-analysis examining single-gender substance abuse treatment for women, Orwin et al. (239) concluded that single-gender treatment was effective, however its strongest impact was on pregnancy outcomes, psychological well-being, attitudes/beliefs, and HIV risk reduction. Only modest improvements in alcohol and drug use, or criminal activity were revealed (239). It is important to note that only a few of the studies compared gender-sensitive or gender-specific treatment to mixed-gender programs, which limits the interpretation of the findings (239).

Mixed results have been reported among studies comparing women-only versus mixed-gender programs. One study that randomized women ($N = 1573$) to women-only versus mixed-gender treatment failed to show treatment group differences in attrition (251). In contrast, another study that randomized crack cocaine-dependent women with infants to either a specialized women-only day treatment program or a traditional mixed-gender outpatient program found that participants in the women-only program had significantly higher retention rates at 4 months (60.2% vs. 46.1%) (252). In a more recent study, treatment outcomes and costs of women-only and mixed-gender day treatment programs were compared among 122 women randomized to a women-only program with gender-specific programming, or one of three standard mixed-gender programs (253). Participants in the women-only program demonstrated significantly lower total abstinence during the follow-up period as compared to the hospital-based program (OR = 0.17), but the hospital-based program cost twice as much. Limitations included a small sample size and the focus on only day treatment programs (253).

In a recent Stage I Behavioral Development Trial, Greenfield et al. (130) developed a manual-based, 12-session Women's Recovery Group (WRG) and compared WRG to mixed-gender Group Drug Counseling (GDC), an effective manual-based treatment for Substance use disorders. Women were randomized to WRG ($n = 16$) or GDC ($n = 7$). The WRG was equally effective as the mixed-gender GDC in reducing substance use during the 12-week in-treatment phase, but demonstrated significantly greater improvement in reductions in drug and alcohol use over the 6-month posttreatment follow-up phase. In addition, while satisfaction with both groups was high, women were significantly more satisfied with WRG than GDC (130). Secondary analyses of these data found a significant three-way interaction effect of treatment condition, time and baseline Brief Symptom Inventory scores, and found that women with greater baseline psychiatric severity made greater reductions in substance use during 12 weeks of group therapy and in the 6-month follow-up if they were assigned to the WRG rather than the mixed-gender GDC condition (254). Furthermore, women with low self-efficacy were more likely to have better treatment outcomes if assigned to WRG than mixed-gender group treatment (255).

Results from nonrandomized studies have shown mixed results (256–258). Comparisons of data from publicly funded residential women-only and mixed-gender drug treatment programs show that women-only programs have significantly longer lengths of stay (87.4 vs. 74.0 days) and higher rates of completion (16.9% vs. 7.6%) than women in mixed-gender programs.

A number of studies have shown greater success with treatments addressing problems more common to women with substance use disorders. Those include, for example, services for pregnant women leading to reduction of alcohol use (259), contingency management to increase abstinence from cocaine in pregnant women (260), a comprehensive services model for pregnant women (261), parenting skills for methadone-maintained mothers (262), relapse prevention for women with co-occurring PTSD (263,264), relapse prevention for women with marital distress and alcohol dependence (265), DBT for women with co-occurring BPD and drug dependence (266), and prison-based single-gender drug treatment for women offenders (248). Even though more data, in particular from randomized controlled trials, are needed, the results indicate that gender-specific interventions may lead to improved outcomes for specific subgroups of women.

Behavioral Couples Treatment

Dyadic conflict and relationship stress appears to affect the substance use of men and women differently. For example, studies show that women are more vulnerable than men to consuming alcohol subsequent to marital discord, divorce, negative emotional states, and interpersonal conflict (267,268). Furthermore, having a partner that abuses alcohol or drugs is more strongly related to relapse for women than for men (213).

Because relationships and family discord play a critical role in women's substance use problems, treatment interventions designed specifically to address these issues may be particularly beneficial. One such treatment approach is Behavioral Couples Therapy (BCT), which has been shown in numerous studies to lead to reduced drinking and positive dyadic adjustment among men with substance abuse problems, decreased IPV (269). BCT is founded upon two fundamental assumptions: (1) family members, specifically spouses or other intimate partners, can reward abstinence and (2) a reduction of relationship distress and conflict leads to improved substance use outcomes by reducing possible antecedents to relapse and heavy use. Compared to traditional individual-based treatments (IBTs), participation in BCT results in significantly less partner violence, lower substance use severity, higher rates of marital satisfaction, greater improvements in psychosocial functioning of children living with parents, and better cost-benefit and cost-effectiveness (269,270). In one trial (271), participants ($N = 138$) who were married or cohabiting women were randomly assigned to one of three interventions: (a) BCT, (b) IBT, or (c) a psychoeducational attention control treatment (PACT) condition. In comparison to women who received IBT or PACT, women who received BCT reported significantly fewer days drinking and higher levels of dyadic adjustment during a 12-month posttreatment follow-up period.

ADDITIONAL ISSUES

Pregnancy and Substance Abuse

Alcohol Use in Pregnancy

Data from the 2008 National Survey on Drug Use and Health indicates that approximately 10.6% of pregnant women use alcohol, while 4.5% report binge drinking (131). Alcohol use during pregnancy may cause pregnancy-related complications (e.g., preterm labor, spontaneous abortions) and negatively affect the fetus. Approximately 1 in 300 to 1 in 1000 children born per year in the United States are diagnosed with a fetal alcohol spectrum disorder (FASD) (272). Children with FASD experience physical abnormalities (e.g., malformed ears, flattened midface) (273), cognitive and behavioral changes (e.g., impulse control problems, ADHD) (274), and psychiatric disorders (e.g., mood disorders, conduct and behavior disorders) (275).

Four main treatment interventions are used to treat/prevent alcohol use in pregnant women: (a) primary care treatment of women of childbearing age who meet criteria for alcohol use disorders, (b) detoxification, (c) follow-up programs for women who used alcohol while pregnant, and (d) brief interventions. Research suggests that brief motivational interventions may be particularly effective in reducing the use of alcohol during pregnancy (276). A recently conducted randomized trial of a single session brief intervention for 304 pregnant women and their partners demonstrated that drinking reductions were greatest among pregnant women with the highest levels of alcohol use (277). Research studies conclude that there should be consistent screening for prenatal alcohol use, followed by diagnostic assessment when screening results are positive, and if diagnosis of alcohol use is confirmed, interventions such as a patient–partner brief intervention for the heaviest drinkers is indicated (277).

Nicotine Use in Pregnancy

Past month prevalence rates indicate that 16.4% of pregnant women report using nicotine (131). Research indicates that using nicotine during pregnancy may cause maternal complications (e.g., vitamin and mineral deficiencies, pregnancy-induced hypertension) (278,279), neonatal complications (e.g., low birth weight, congenital malformations, and intrauterine growth restriction) (280,281), and long-term consequences for the children (e.g., cognitive deficits) (282). Although research suggests that bupropion (283) and behavioral interventions (284) are effective treatments for smoking cessation in women, nicotine replacement therapy (NRT) may increase negative birth outcomes (285) but studies indicate that it is unclear whether associated low birth weight is a direct effect of the NRT or rather the associated heavy smoking among women referred for NRT (286). More research in this area is strongly needed to help enhance effective behavioral treatments for smoking cessation during pregnancy as well as to advance safe pharmacotherapy options for pregnant women wanting to quit smoking during pregnancy.

Marijuana Use in Pregnancy

Data from the 2001 Maternal Lifestyle Study indicates that 11.1% of pregnant women use marijuana (3,287). The use of marijuana during pregnancy can lead to maternal complications (e.g., negative effects on duration of pregnancy, implantation) (288), complications for the neonate (e.g., intrauterine growth retardation, acute myeloblastic leukemia) (289), and long-term effects on the children (e.g., slower motor development, increased depressive symptoms) (290,291). To date, no research has investigated specific treatment interventions for pregnant women using marijuana.

Opioid Use in Pregnancy

Approximately 7000 children born each year in the United States are exposed to opioids prenatally (292). Both the mother and fetus are at risk for overdosing, which can lead to complications such as, coma, hypothermia, and circulatory collapse (293). The use of opioids during pregnancy can also cause the fetus to develop neonatal abstinence syndrome, which includes symptoms such as irritability, temperature disregulation, and seizures (294). Treatment options for pregnant women using opioids include methadone maintenance and detoxification (292,295). Studies suggest that treatment of pregnant opioid-dependent women and their children in specialized treatment programs can help enhance maternal and child outcomes (239).

Cocaine Use in Pregnancy

A multisite study of university hospitals found a 10% rate of cocaine use among pregnant women using illicit drugs (296). Cocaine use during pregnancy can cause significant maternal complications (e.g., pneumonitis and placental abruption) (297,298) and put the fetus at risk for adverse outcomes (e.g., HIV and harm fetal–placental circulation) (299). Since withdrawal is not life threatening for the mother or fetus, treatment to support cessation of use and ongoing relapse prevention and abstinence are indicated for cocaine use in pregnant women (300). Anticraving medications, for which effectiveness studies are inconclusive, are typically avoided, since the FDA has not approved the medications for pregnant women (301).

Cultural Issues

Epidemiology

Approximately 98 million minorities live in the United States (33% of the U.S. population) (302). Rates of illicit drug use vary by race/ethnicity, with rates being estimated as follows (from smallest to largest): Asian Americans (3.6%), Hispanics (6.2%), Native Hawaiians or other Pacific Islanders (7.3%), European Americans (8.2%), Native Americans or Alaska Natives (9.5%), African Americans (10.1%), and individuals reporting more than one race (14.7%). Rates of substance abuse or dependence also vary by race/ethnicity, with rates being estimated as follows (from smallest to largest): Asian Americans (4.2%), African Americans (8.8%), European Americans (9.0%), Hispanics (9.5%), individuals reporting more than one race (9.8%), and Native Americans or Alaska Natives (11.1%) (122).

Risk Factors for Diverse Women

In order to effectively counsel diverse women with substance use disorders, it is imperative that clinicians are knowledgeable about cultural histories, norms, practices, and environments. Common correlates of substance use disorders are found among women from diverse ethnic/racial groups. Many women with substance use disorders may also experience other at-risk behaviors and conditions such as high-risk sexual behaviors (303), co-occurring psychiatric disorders (304), physical and medical problems (e.g., HIV/AIDS) (303), traumatic histories and victimization (e.g., rape, loss of children) (303,305), functional problems (e.g., unemployment) (306), incarceration histories (307), and experiences of racism (308).

Treatment

There is limited research available that addresses the treatment of substance use disorders among specific ethnic groups, due mainly in part to the strict criteria and guidelines in clinical research (309). Therefore, it is best practice at this time to use evidence-based treatment modalities and programs (e.g., cognitive–behavioral therapy) (303) modified to address common correlates found among diverse women with substance use disorders. For example, treatment programs should address co-occurring disorders (e.g., PTSD caused by trauma histories) or other functional problems in diverse women's lives.

Sexual-Minority Issues

Epidemiology

Limited research has been conducted to date on sexual-minority women and substance use disorders. Within these studies, definitions of sexual-minority women have varied, making the interpretation and generalizability of the results difficult. For example, while some studies define women as either "heterosexual" or "homosexual," other studies develop additional categories to adequately assess sexual behaviors and identity (e.g., "women who reported having sex with other women" (WSW) (310). Research suggests that using only two categories may cause researchers to overlook differences within the sexual-minority female population (311).

Compared to heterosexual women who report only having sex with men, sexual-minority women (including lesbians, bisexual women, and WSW) use alcohol at higher rates and have more alcohol-related problems (310,312,313). Lesbians and bisexual women were also found to be more likely to meet criteria for alcohol dependence and/or participate in treatment than heterosexual women (311). Sexual-minority women are also more likely than heterosexual women who reported having sex only with men to use marijuana, analgesics, nicotine, and to meet criteria for substance dependence (314–318).

Risk Factors

Compared to heterosexual women, sexual-minority women report significantly higher rates of traumatic events, such as, discrimination, and verbal and physical attacks from peers, parents, and partners (319–321). Sexual-minority women also report higher rates of mood and anxiety disorders (322,323), suicidality (310,322,324), and psychological distress (325). Discrimination, traumatic events, and psychological problems may put sexual-minority women at increased risk for substance use disorders. Furthermore, social structures within the United States may also place sexual-minority women at risk for developing substance use disorders. Bars are one of the few social outlets that exist in the United States where sexual minorities feel free from ostracism or scrutiny, which may lead to higher rates of alcohol use among lesbian and bisexual women (326).

Treatment

Although homosexuality has not been considered a clinical disorder in the *Diagnostic and Statistical Manual of Mental Disorders* (327) for more than 25 years, some clinicians still support conversion therapy, designed to convert homosexuals to heterosexuals (328). Early research on substance use disorder treatment of sexual-minorities indicates that many programs either refused treatment to sexual-minorities, focused on "converting" the patients to heterosexuals, or had limited experience and training in treating substance use disorders among sexual minorities (329,330). A more current study conducted by Eliason (331) also found that many counselors are not trained to work with sexual minorities and are unaware of legal and family issues for sexual minorities.

Although little research has investigated the effectiveness of addiction programs for sexual minorities, treatment recommendations have been proposed. For example, it may be beneficial for clinicians to be trained and supervised in "culturally sensitive treatment for LGBT clients and patients" (p. 484), nondiscrimination literature should be placed in waiting rooms, and group therapies should be supervised in a way to create a supportive environment for everyone (332).

Legal Issues

Drug Use and Civil Law

Over the last 20 years, states have criminally prosecuted pregnant women using illicit drugs in an attempt to protect fetuses (333), which has led to women's incarceration and the loss of custody of children (334). Limitations to the punitive approach include the fact that it may cause pregnant women using illicit drugs to choose an abortion or avoid medical care altogether (335).

Research shows that mothers who abuse substances are more likely to have their children placed in out-of-home care (336). Mothers using substances who lost the custody of their children experienced more psychological and functional impairments, homelessness, victimization experiences, higher frequencies of drug use, and engaged in more risky sex practices, as compared to mothers using substances who did not lose custody of their children (337,338). However, custodial mothers are less likely to start treatment for substance use disorders (337), and if started they are more likely to drop out of treatment, possibly due to childcare responsibilities (339). One line of research offering promise for effective treatment for pregnant and parenting women with substance use disorders reported that 61% percent of women who attended a residential substance abuse program for pregnant and parenting women were completely drug- and alcohol-free throughout the 6-month follow-up period (340).

Drug Use and the Criminal Justice System

Nearly 1.9 million individuals are arrested each year for drug abuse violations (341,342). Approximately 17% of crimes are committed for drug money and between 25% and 33% of crimes are committed under the influence of drugs (343). Within state prison facilities, 60% of the women (vs. 40% of men) were committed for property or drug crimes (344). It is estimated that 80% of incarcerated women used substances in the past and that approximately 60% of women met criteria for drug dependence (345).

Research indicates that correctional facilities are not adequately treating women and men with substance use disorders (346). Approximately 18% of local jail inmates with substance use disorders receive treatment while incarcerated (343). Research also indicates that addiction treatment programs within correctional facilities do not adequately address the histories of women in correctional facilities, including high rates of trauma, abuse, and co-occurring psychiatric disorders (343,347), which may help explain why treatment within correctional facilities may be effective only for men (347). Future research examining the effectiveness of gender-specific treatment programs within correctional facilities is needed (248).

CONCLUSIONS AND FUTURE DIRECTIONS

Over the last decade there has been an increasing number of studies focusing on gender differences in substance use disorders, as well as gender-specific treatments and outcomes for women with substance use disorders. Current research supports that there are important gender differences in biologic, psychological, cultural, and socioeconomic factors that affect the initiation, use patterns, disease acceleration, and help-seeking patterns in women, as well as gender-specific predictors of substance abuse treatment entry, retention, and outcomes for women. Further research will enhance our understanding of basic biological mechanisms that underlie these gender differences in substance use vulnerability, responsiveness, and neurobiologic correlates of addiction. There is also a concomitant need to understand gender differences in response to standard behavioral and pharmacologic treatments, to identify characteristics of women who can benefit from single-gender versus mixed-gender treatments, and to develop and test effective treatments for specific subgroups of women with substance use disorders. Further research will also improve our understanding effectiveness and cost-effectiveness of gender-specific versus standard treatments.

ACKNOWLEDGMENTS

The authors acknowledge support from Grant K24DA019855 (to Shelly F. Greenfield), K23DA021228 (Sudie E. Back) and K24 DA00435 from the NIH/NIDA (Kathleen T. Brady), and P50 DA016511 (Kathleen T. Brady) from NIAMS/ORWH.

REFERENCES

1. Grant BF, Stinson F, Dawson D, et al. Co-occurrence of 12-month alcohol and drug use disorders and personality disorders in the United States. *Arch Gen Psychiatry.* 2004;61: 361–368.
2. Stinson FS, Grant BF, Dawson DA, et al. Comorbidity between DSM-IV alcohol and specific drug use disorders in the United States: results from the National Epidemiologic Survey on Alcohol and Related Conditions. *Drug Alcohol Depend.* 2005; 80(1):105–116.
3. Substance Abuse and Mental Health Services Administration. *Methamphetamine Use.* In the NSDUH report. Rockville, MD: Office of Applied Studies, 2007.
4. Compton WM, Thomas YF, Stinson FS, et al. Prevalence, correlates, disability, and comorbidity of DSM-IV drug abuse and dependence in the United States: results from the National Epidemiologic Survey on Alcohol and Related Conditions. *Arch Gen Psychiatry.* 2007;64:566–576.
5. Kessler RC, Chiu WT, Demler O, et al. Prevalence, severity, and comorbidity of 12-month DSM-IV disorders in the National Comorbidity Survey Replication. *Arch Gen Psychiatry.* 2005; 62(6):617–627.
6. Wagner FA, Anthony JC. Male-female differences in the risk of progression from first use to dependence upon cannabis, cocaine, and alcohol. *Drug Alcohol Depend.* 2007;86:191–198.
7. Helzer JE, Burnam A, McEvoy LT. Alcohol abuse and dependence. In: Robins LN, Regier DA, eds. *Psychiatric Disorders in America: The Epidemiological Catchment Area Study.* New York City: The Free Press; 1992:81–115.
8. Hasin DS, Stinson FS, Ogburn E, et al. Prevalence, correlates, disability, and comorbidity of DSM-IV alcohol abuse and dependence in the United States: results from the National Epidemiologic Survey on Alcohol and Related Conditions. *Arch Gen Psychiatry.* 2007;64(7):830–842.
9. Grucza RA, Norberg K, Bucholz KK, et al. Correspondence between secular changes in alcohol dependence and age of drinking onset among women in the United States. *Alcohol Clin Exp Res.* 2008;32(8):1493–1501.
10. Simoni-Wastila L. The use of abusable prescription drugs: the role of gender. *J Women's Health Gend Based Med.* 2000;9(3):289–297.
11. Blanco C, Alderson D, Ogburn E, et al. Changes in the prevalence of non-medical prescription drug use and drug use disorders in the United States: 1991-1992 and 2001-2002. *Drug Alcohol Depend.* 2007;90(2-3):252–260.
12. Zacny J, Bigelow G, Compton P, et al. College on problems of drug dependence taskforce on prescription opioid non-medical use and abuse: position statement. *Drug Alcohol Depend.* 2003; 69(3):215–232.
13. McCabe SE, Cranford JA, Boyd CJ, et al. Motives, diversion and routes of administration associated with nonmedical use of prescription opioids. *Addict Behav.* 2007;32(3):562–575.
14. Carise D, Dugosh KL, McLellan AT, et al. Prescription Oxycontin abuse among patients entering addiction treatment. *Am J Psychiatry.* 2007;164(11):1750–1756.
15. Cicero TJ, Inciardi JA, Munoz A. Trends in abuse of Oxycontin and other opioid analgesics in the United States: 2002-2004. *J Pain.* 2005;6(10):662–672.
16. Huang B, Dawson DA, Stinson FS, et al. Prevalence, correlates, and comorbidity of nonmedical prescription drug use disorders in the United States: results of the National Epidemiologic Survey on Alcohol and Related Conditions. *J Clin Psychiatry.* 2006;67(7):1062–1073.
17. Tetrault JM, Desai RA, Becker WC, et al. Gender and non-medical use of prescription opioids: results from a National US survey. *Addiction.* 2008;103:258–268.
18. Grant BF, Hasin DS, Chou SP, et al. Nicotine dependence and psychiatric disorders in the United States. *Arch Gen Psychiatry.* 2004;61(11):1107–1115.
19. Hernandez-Avila CA, Rounsaville BJ, Kranzler HR. Opioid-, cannabis-, and alcohol-dependent women show more rapid progression to substance abuse treatment. *Drug Alcohol Depend.* 2004;74(3):265–272.
20. Brady KT, Randall CL. Gender differences in substance use disorders. *Psychiatr Clin North Am.* 1999;22:241–252.
21. Newman JL, Mello NK. Neuroactive gonadal steroid hormones and drug addiction in women. In: Brady KT, Back SE, Greenfield SF, eds. *Women and Addiction: A Comprehensive Handbook.* New York City: Guildford Press; 2009:35–64.
22. Rupprecht R. Neuroactive steroids: Mechanisms of action and nueropsychopharmacological properties. *Psychoneuroendocrinology.* 2003;28:139–168.
23. Doron R, Fridman L, Gispan-Herman I, et al. DHEA, a neurosteroid, decreases cocaine self-administration and reinstatement of cocaine-seeking behavior in rats. *Neuropsychopharmacology.* 2006;31(10):2231–2236.
24. Sofuoglu M, Dudish-Poulsen S, Nelson D, et al. Sex and menstrual cycle differences in the subjective effects from smoked cocaine in humans. *Exp Clin Psychopharmacol.* 1999; 7(3):274–283.
25. Evans SM. The role of estradiol and progesterone in modulating the subjective effects of stimulants in humans. *Exp Clin Psychopharmacol.* 2007;15:418–426.
26. Justice AJ, de Wit H. Acute effects of estradiol pretreatment on the response to *d*-amphetamine in women. *Neuroendocrinology.* 2000;71(1):51–59.
27. Evans SM, Haney M, Foltin RW. The effects of smoked cocaine during the follicular and luteal phases of the menstrual cycle in women. *Psychopharmacology.* 2002;159(4):397–406.
28. Evans SM, Foltin RW. Exogenous progesterone attenuates the subjective effects of smoked cocaine in women, but not in men. *Neuropsychopharmacology.* 2006;31(3):659–674.
29. Perkins KA, Levine M, Marcus M. Tobacco withdrawal in women and menstrual cycle phase. *J Consult Clin Psychol.* 2000;68(1): 176–180.
30. Craig D, Parrott A, Coomber JA. Smoking cessation in women: effects of the menstrual cycle. *Int J Addict.* 1992;27:697–706.

31. Mello NK, Mendelson JH, Lex BW. Alcohol use and premenstrual symptoms in social drinkers. *Psychopharmacology.* 1990;101(4):448–455.
32. Green KL, Azarov AV, Szeliga KT, et al. The influence of menstrual cycle phase on sensitivity to ethanol-like discriminative stimulus effects of GABA(A)-positive modulators. *Pharmacol Biochem Behav.* 1999;64(2):379–383.
33. Holdstock L, de Wit H. Effects of ethanol at four phases of the menstrual cycle. *Psychopharmacology.* 2000;150:374–382.
34. Nyberg S, Andersson A, Zingmark E, et al. The effect of a low dose of alcohol on allopregnanolone serum concentrations across the menstrual cycle in women with severe premenstrual syndrome and controls. *Psychoneuroendocrinology.* 2005;30: 892–901.
35. Riley JL, Robinson ME, Wise EA, et al. A meta-analytic review of pain perception across the menstrual cycle. *Pain.* 1999;81(3): 225–235.
36. Sinha R. How does stress increase risk of drug abuse and relapse? *Psychopharmacology.* 2001;142:343–351.
37. Sinha R, Fox H, Hong KI, et al. Sex steroid hormones, stress response, and drug craving in cocaine-dependent women: implications for relapse susceptibility. *Exp Clin Psychopharmacol.* 2007;15(5):445–52.
38. Fox HC, Hong KA, Paliwal P, et al. Altered levels of sex and stress steroid hormones assessed daily over a 28-day cycle in early abstinent cocaine-dependent females. *Psychopharmacology.* 2008; 195(4):527–536.
39. Fox H, Sinha R. Stress, neuro-endocrine response and addiction in women. In: Brady KT, Back SE, Greenfield S, eds. *Women and Addiction: A Comprehensive Handbook.* New York City: Guildford Press; 2009:65–83.
40. Sinha R, Lacadie C, Skudlarski P, et al. Neural activity associated with stress-induced cocaine craving: a functional magnetic resonance imaging study. *Psychopharmacology.* 2005;183(2): 171–180.
41. Back SE, Brady KT, Jackson JL, et al. Gender differences in stress reactivity among cocaine-dependent individuals. *Psychopharmacology.* 2005;180(1):169–176.
42. Kelly MM, Tyrka AR, Anderson GM, et al. Sex differences in emotional and physiological responses to the Trier Social Stress Test. *J Behav Ther Exp Psychiatry.* 2008;39(1):87–98.
43. Fox H, Garcia M, Kemp K, et al. Gender differences in cardiovascular and corticoadrenal response to stress and drug cues in cocaine dependent individuals. *Psychopharmacology.* 2006;185: 348–357.
44. O'Malley S, Krishnan-Sarin S, Farren C, et al. Naltrexone decreases craving and alcohol self-administration in alcohol-dependent subjects and activates the hypothalamo-pituitary-adrenocortical axis. *Psychopharmacology.* 2002;160: 19–29.
45. Adinoff B, Junghanns K, Kiefer F, et al. Suppression of the HPA axis stress-response: implications for relapse. *Alcohol Clin Exp Res.* 2005;29(7):1351–1355.
46. Back SE, Waldrop AE, Saladin ME, et al. Effects of gender and cigarette smoking on reactivity to psychological and pharmacological stress provocation. *Psychoneuroendocrinology.* 2008;33(5): 560–568.
47. Schumann G. Okey Lecture 2006: identifying the neurobiological mechanisms of addictive behavior. *Addiction.* 2007;102(11): 1689–1695.
48. Potenza, M.N., et al. (2009). Neural correlates of stress-induced and cue-induced craving: influences of sex and cocaine dependence. *Am J Psychiatry* (under revision).
49. Kilts CD, Gross RE, Ely TD, et al. The neural correlates of cue-induced craving in cocaine-dependent women. *Am J Psychiatry.* 2004;161(2):233–241.
50. Quirk GJ, Mueller D. Neural mechanisms of extinction learning and retrieval. *Neuropsychopharmacology.* 2008;33(1):56–72.
51. Milad MR, Goldstein JM, Orr SP, et al. Fear conditioning and extinction: influence of sex and menstrual cycle in healthy humans. *Behav Neurosci.* 2006;120:1196–1203.
52. Brady KT, Back SE, Greenfield S, eds. *Women and Addiction: A Comprehensive Handbook.* New York City: Guilford Press; 2009.
53. Conway KP, Compton W, Stinson FS, et al. Lifetime comorbidity of DSM-IV mood and anxiety disorders and specific drug use disorders: results from the National Epidemiologic Survey on Alcohol and Related Conditions. *J Clin Psychiatry.* 2006;67:247–257.
54. Kessler RC, Crum RM, Warner LA, et al. Lifetime co-occurrence of DSM-III-R alcohol abuse and dependence with other psychiatric disorders in the National Comorbidity Survey. *Arch Gen Psychiatry.* 1997;54:313–321.
55. Goldstein RB. Comorbidity of substance use with independent mood and anxiety disorders in women: results from the National Epidemiologic Survey on Alcohol and Related Conditions. In: Brady KT, Back SE, Greenfield SF, eds. *Women and Addiction: A Comprehensive Handbook.* New York City: Guilford Press; 2009:173–192.
56. Grant BF, Moore TC, Shepard J, et al. *Source and accuracy statement for Wave 1 of the 2001-2002 National Epidemiologic Survey on Alcohol and Related Conditions.* Bethesda, MD: National Institute on Alcohol abuse and Alcoholism; 2003.
57. Schuckit MA, Tipp JE, Bergman M, et al. Comparison of induced and independent major depressive disorders in 2,945 alcoholics. *Am J Psychiatry.* 1997;154(7):948–957.
58. Moscato BS, Russell M, Zielezny M, et al. Gender differences in the relation between depressive symptoms and alcohol problems: a longitudinal perspective. *Am J Epidemiol.* 1997;146(11): 966–974.
59. Wilsnack RW, Klassen AD, Wilsnack SC. Retrospective analysis of lifetime changes in women's drinking behavior. *Adv Alcohol Subst Abuse.* 1986;5(3):9–28.
60. Dixit AR, Crum RM. Prospective study of depression and the risk of heavy alcohol use in women. *Am J Psychiatry.* 2000; 157(5):751–758.
61. Greenfield SF. Assessment of mood and substance use disorders. In: Westermeyer J, Weiss RD, Ziedonis D, eds. *Integrated Treatment for Mood and Substance Use Disorders.* Baltimore: Johns Hopkins University Press; 2003;432–467.
62. Petrakis IL, Poling J, Levinson C, et al. Naltrexone and disulfram in patients with alcohol dependence and comorbid post-traumatic stress disorder. *Biol Psychiatry.* 2005;60:777–783.
63. Pettinati HM, Dundon W, Lipkin C. Gender differences in response to sertraline pharmacotherapy in Type A alcohol dependence. *Am J Addict.* 2004;13(3):236–247.
64. Pettinati HM, Kampman KM, Lynch KG, et al. Gender differences with high-dose naltrexone in patients with co-occurring cocaine and alcohol dependence. *J Subst Abuse Treat.* 2008;34(4): 378–390.
65. Cohen LR, Gordon SM. Co-occurring eating and substance use disorders. In Brady KT, Back SE, Greenfield SF, eds. *Women and Addiction: A Comprehensive Handbook.* New York, NY: Guilford Press; 2009:225–241.
66. Hudson JI, Hiripi E, Pope HG, et al. The prevalence and correlated of eating disorders in the National Comorbidity Survey Replication Study. *Biol Psychiatry.* 2007;61:348–358.

67. American Psychiatric Association. *Diagnostic and Statistical Manual of Mental Disorders DSM-IV-TR*. Washington, DC: American Psychiatric Association; 2000.
68. Nielsen S. Epidemiology and mortality of eating disorders. *Psychiatr Clin N Am*. 2001;24:201–214.
69. Gordon SM, Johnson JA, Greenfield SF, et al. Assessment and treatment of co-occurring eating disorders in publicly funded addiction treatment programs. *Psychiatr Serv*. 2008;59:1056–1059.
70. Holderness CC, Brooks-Gunn J, Warren MP. Co-morbidity of eating disorders and substance abuse: review of the literature. *Int J Eat Disord*. 1994;16:1–34.
71. Schuckit MA, Tipp JE, Anthenelli RM, et al. Anorexia nervosa and bulimia nervosa in alcohol-dependent men and women and their relatives. *Am J Psychiatry*. 1996;153:74–82.
72. Deep AL, Lilenfeld LR, Plotnicov KH, et al. Sexual abuse in eating disorder subtypes and control women: the role of comorbid substance dependence in bulimia nervosa. *Int J Eat Disord*. 1999;25:1–10.
73. Dohm FA, Striegal-Moore R, Wilfley DE, et al. Self harm and substance use in a community sample of black and white women with binge eating disorders or bulimia nervosa. *Int J Eat Disord*. 2002;32:389–400.
74. Bowers WA, Andersen AE, Evans K. Management of eating disorders: inpatient and partial hospital programs. In: Brewerton TD, ed. *Clinical Handbook of Eating Disorders: An Integrated Approach*. New York City: Marcel Dekker, Inc; 2004:349–376.
75. Wonderlich SA, Connolly KM, Stice E. Impulsivity as a risk factor for eating disorder behavior: assessment implications with adolescents. *Int J Eat Disord*. 2004;36(2):172–182.
76. Breslau N, Davis G, Andreski P, et al. Traumatic events and posttraumatic stress disorder in an urban population of young adults. *Arch Gen Psychiatry*. 1991;48:216–222.
77. Kilpatrick DG, Saunders BE, Veronen LJ, et al. Criminal victimization: lifetime prevalence, reporting to police, and psychological impact. *Crime Delinq*. 1987;33:479–489.
78. Norris FH. Epidemiology of trauma: frequency and impact of different potentially traumatic events on different demographic groups. *J Consult Clin Psychol*. 1992;60:409–418.
79. Freedy JR, Kilpatrick DG, Resnick HS. Natural disasters and mental health: theory, assessment, and intervention. *J Soc Behav Pers*. 1993;8:49–103.
80. Resnick HS, Kilpatrick DG, Dansky BS, et al. Prevalence of civilian trauma and posttraumatic stress disorder in a representative national sample of women. *J Consult Clin Psychol*. 1993;61(6):984–991.
81. Cottler LB, Compton WM, Mager D, et al. Post-traumatic stress disorder among substance users from the general population. *Am J Psychiatry*. 1992;149:664–670.
82. Back SE, Dansky BS, Coffee SF, et al. Cocaine dependence with and without Post-traumatic Stress Disorder: a comparison of substance use, trauma history, and psychiatric comorbidity. *Am J Addict*. 2000;9(1):51–62.
83. Brady KT, Dansky BS, Back SE, et al. Exposure therapy in the treatment of PSTD among cocaine-dependent individuals: preliminary findings. *J Subst Abuse Treat*. 2001;21:47–54.
84. Fullilove MT, Fullilove RE, Smith M, et al. Violence, trauma and post-traumatic stress disorder among women drug users. *J Trauma Stress*. 1993;6(4):533–543.
85. Back SE, Dansky BS, Carroll KM, et al. Exposure therapy in the treatment of PTSD among cocaine-dependent individuals: description of procedures. *J Subst Abuse Treat*. 2001;21(1):35–45.
86. Hien DA. Trauma, posttraumatic stress disorder and addiction among women. In: Brady KT, Back SE, Greenfield SF, eds. *Women and Addiction: A Comprehensive Handbook*. New York City: Guilford Press; 2009;242–256.
87. Nace EP. Posttraumatic stress disorder and substance abuse. Clinical issues. *Recent Dev Alcohol*. 1988;6:9–26.
88. Pitman RK, Altman B, Greenwald E, et al. Psychiatric complications during flooding therapy for posttraumatic stress disorder. *J Clin Psychiatry*. 1991;52(1):17–20.
89. Back SE, Brady KT, Sonne SC, et al. Symptom improvement in co-occurring PTSD and alcohol dependence. *J Nerv Ment Dis*. 2006;194(9):690–696.
90. Hien DA, Litt L, Cohen LC, et al. *Reclaiming Pandora: Integrating Trauma Services for Women in Addictions Treatment*. New York: American Psychological Association Press; (in press).
91. Najavits LM. *Seeking safety: a treatment manual for PTSD and substance abuse*. New York City: Guilford Press; 2002.
92. Najavits LM, Sullivan TP, Schmitz M, et al. Treatment utilization by women with PTSD and substance dependence. *Am J Addict*. 2004;13(3):215–224.
93. Ouimette PC, Ahrens C, Moss RH, et al. Posttraumatic stress disorder in substance abuse patients: relationship to one-year posttreatment outcomes. *Psychol Addict Behav*. 1997;11:34–47.
94. Brady KT, Sonne SC, Roberts JM. Sertraline treatment of co-morbid posttraumatic stress disorder and alcohol dependence. *J Clin Psychiatry*. 1995;56:502–505.
95. Brady KT, Sonne S, Anton RF, et al. Sertraline in the treatment of co-occurring alcohol dependence and posttraumatic stress disorder. *Alcohol Clin Exp Res*. 2005;29(3):395–401.
96. Labbate LA, Sonne SC, Randal CL, et al. Does comorbid anxiety or depression affect clinical outcomes in patients with posttraumatic stress disorder and alcohol use disorders? *Compr Psychiatry*. 2004;45(4):304–310.
97. Koenigsberg H, Kaplan R, Gilmore M, et al. The relationship between syndrome and personality disorder in DSM-III: experience with 2,462 patients. *Am J Psychiatry*. 1985;14:207–212.
98. Seivewright N, Daly C. Personality disorder and drug use: a review. *Drug Alcohol Rev*. 1997;16:235–250.
99. Verheul R, van den Brink W, Hartgers C. Prevalence of personality disorders among alcoholics and drug addicts: an overview. *Eur J Addict Res*. 1995;1:166–177.
100. Warshaw MG, Dolan RT, Keller MB. Suicidal behavior in patients with current or past panic disorder: five years of prospective data from the Harvard/Brown Anxiety Research Program. *Am J Psychiatry*. 2000;157:1876–1878.
101. Sher KJ, Trull TJ. Substance use disorder and personality disorder. *Curr Psychiatry Rep*. 2002;4:25–29.
102. Rounsaville BJ, Kranzler HR, Ball S, et al. Personality disorders in substance abusers: relation to substance use. *J Nerv Ment Dis*. 1998;186:87–95.
103. Trull TJ, Sher KJ, Minks-Brown C, et al. Borderline personality disorder and substance use disorders: a review and integration. *Clin Psychol Rev*. 2000;20:235–253.
104. Chapman AL, Cellucci T. The role of antisocial and borderline personality features in substance dependence among incarcerated females. *Addict Behav*. 2007;32:1131–1145.
105. Darke S, Williamson A, Ross J, et al. Borderline personality disorder, antisocial personality disorder and risk-taking among heroin users: fundings from the Australian Treatment Outcome Study (ATOS). *Drug Alcoh Depend*. 2003;74:77–83.

106. Kosten TA, Kosten TR, Rounsaville BJ. Personality disorders in opiate addicts show prognostic specificity. *J Subst Abuse Treat.* 1989;6:163–168.
107. Skodol AE, Oldham JM, Gallaher PE. Axis II Comorbidity of substance use disorders among patients referred for treatment of personality disorders. *Am J Psychiatry.* 1999;156:733–738.
108. Nace EP, Saxon JJ, Shore N. A comparison of borderline and nonborderline alcoholic patients. *Arch Gen Psychiatry.* 1983;40: 54–56.
109. Linehan MM, Dimeff LA. *Dialectical Behavior Therapy Manual of Treatment Interventions for Drug Abusers with Borderline Personality Disorder*. Seattle, WA: University of Washington; 1997.
110. Linehan MM, Dimeff LA, Reynolds SK, et al. Dialectical behavior therapy versus comprehensive validation therapy plus 12-step for the treatment of opioid dependent women meeting the criteria for borderline personality disorder. *Drug Alcoh Depend.* 2002;67:13–26.
111. Verheul R, van den Bosch LMC, Koeter M, et al. Dialectical behaviour therapy for women with borderline personality disorder: 12-month randomised clinical trial in The Netherlands. *Br J Psychiatry.* 2003;182:135–140.
112. Ball SA. Manualized treatment for substance abusers with personality disorders: dual focus schema therapy. *Addict Behav.* 1998;23:83–891.
113. Young J. *Cognitive Therapy for Personality Disorders: A Schema-Focused Approach*. Sarasota, FL: Professional Resource Exchange; 1990.
114. Ball SA, Cobb-Richardson P, Connolly A, et al. Substance abuse and personality disorders in homeless drop-in center clients: symptom severity and psychotherapy retention in a randomized clinical trial. *Compr Psychiatry.* 2005;46:371–379.
115. Wilsnack RW, Volgetanz ND, Wilsnack SC, et al. Gender differences in alcohol consumption and adverse drinking consequences: cross-cultural patterns. *Addiction.* 2000;95:251–265.
116. Greenfield S. Women and alcohol use disorders. In: Pearson KH, Rosenbaum JF, eds. *Women's Health and Psychiatry*. Philadelphia: Lippincott Williams & Wilkins; 2002;67–75.
117. Keyes KM, Grant BF, Hasin DS. Evidence for a closing gender gap in alcohol use, abuse, and dependence in the United States population. *Drug Alcohol Depend.* 2008;93:21–29.
118. Johnson PB, Richter L, Kleber HD, et al. Telescoping of drinking-related behaviors: Gender, racial/ethnic, and age comparisons. *Subst Use Misuse.* 2005;40:1139–1151.
119. Piazza NJ, Vrbka JL, Yeager RD. Telescoping of alcoholism in women alcoholics. *Int J Addict.* 1989;24:19–28.
120. Blankfield A. Female alcoholics: the expression of alcoholism in relation to gender and age. *Acta Psychiatr Scand.* 1990;81:448–452.
121. Annis HM, Graham JM. Profile types on the inventory of drinking situations: implications for relapse prevention counseling. *Psychol Addict Behav.* 1995;9:176–182.
122. Schall M, Weede T, Maltzman I. Predictors of alcohol consumption by university students. *J Alcoh Drug Educ.* 1991;37:72–80.
123. Stewart SH, Gavric D, Collins P. Women, girls, and alcohol. In: Brady KT, Back SE, Greenfield SF, eds. *Women & Addiction*. New York City: Guilford Press; 2009;341–359.
124. Dunn EC, Larimer MA, Neighbors C. Alcohol and drug-related negative consequences in college students with bulimia nervosa and binge eating disorder. *Int J Eat Disord.* 2002;32:171–178.
125. Stewart SH, Brown CG, Devoulyte K, et al. Why do women with alcohol problems binge eat? Exploring the connections between binge eating and heavy drinking in women receiving treatment for alcohol problems. *J Health Psychol.* 2006;11:409–425.
126. Brennan PL, Moos RH, Kim JY. Gender differences in the individual characteristics and life contexts of late-middle-aged and older problem drinkers. *Addiction.* 1993;88:781–790.
127. Mammo A, Weinbaum DF. Some factors that influence dropping out from outpatient alcoholism treatment facilities. *J Stud Alcohol.* 1993;54:92–101.
128. Ashley OS, Marsden ME, Brady TM. Effectiveness of substance abuse treatment programming for women: a review. *Am J Drug Alcohol Abuse.* 2003;29:19–53.
129. Dahlgren L, Willander A. Are special treatment facilities for female alcoholics needed? A controlled 2-year follow-up study from a specialized female unit (EWA) versus a mixed male/female treatment facility. *Alcohol Clin Exp Res.* 1989;13:499–504.
130. Greenfield SF, Trucco EM, McHugh RK, et al. The Women's Recovery Group Study: a Stage I trial of women-focused group therapy for substance use disorders versus mixed-gender group drug counseling. *Drug Alcohol Depend.* 2007;90:39–47.
131. Substance Abuse and Mental Health Services Administration (SAMHSA). *Results from the 2008 National Survey on Drug Use and Health: National Findings* (Office of Applied Studies, NSDUH Series H-36, HHS Publication No. SMA 09-4434). Rockville, MD: US Department of Health and Human Services; 2009.
132. Becker JB, Hu M. Sex differences in drug abuse. *Front Neuroendocrinol.* 2008;29:36–47.
133. Carroll ME, Lynch WJ, Roth ME, et al. Sex and estrogen influence drug abuse. *Trends Pharmacol Sci.* 2004;25(5): 273–279.
134. Lynch WJ. Sex differences in vulnerability to drug self-administration. *Exp Clin Psychopharmacol.* 2006;14(1):34–41.
135. Lynch WJ, Roth ME, Carroll ME. Biological basis of sex differences in drug abuse: preclinical and clinical studies. *Psychopharmacology.* 2002;164:121–137.
136. Griffin ML, Weiss RD, Mirin SM, et al. A comparison of male and female cocaine abusers. *Arch Gen Psychiatry.* 1989;46(2): 122–126.
137. Westermeyer J, Boedicker AE. Course, severity, and treatment of substance abuse among women versus men. *Am J Drug Alcohol Abuse.* 2000;26(4):523–535.
138. Copeland J. A qualitative study of barriers to formal treatment among women who self-managed change in addictive behaviours. *J Subst Abuse Treat.* 1997;14(2):183–190.
139. Lynch WJ, Potenza MN, Cosgrove KP, et al. Sex differences in vulnerability to stimulant abuse: A translational perspective. In: Brady KT, Back SE, Greenfield SF, eds. *Women & Addiction*. New York City: Guilford Press; 2009;407–418.
140. Della Grotta S, LaGasse LL, Arria AM, et al. Patterns of methamphetamine use during pregnancy: results from the infant development, environment, and lifestyle (IDEAL) Study. *Matern Child Health J.* 2009.
141. Durell TM, Kroutil LA, Crits-Christoph P, et al. Prevalence of nonmedical methamphetamine use in the United States. *Subst Abuse Treat Prev Policy.* 2008;3:19.
142. Terplan M, Smith EJ, Kozoloski MJ, et al. Methamphetamine use among pregnant women. *Obstet Gynecol.* 2009;113:1285–1291.
143. Rowan-Szal GA, Joe GW, Simpson DD, et al. During treatment outcomes among female methamphetamine using offenders in prison-based treatments. *J Offender Rehabil.* 2009;8: 388–401.
144. Jackson LR, Robinson TE, Becker JB. Sex differences and hormonal influences on acquisition of cocaine self-administration in rats. *Neuropsychopharmacology.* 2006;31(1):129–138.

145. Sofuoglu M, Mitchell E, Kosten TR. Effects of progesterone treatment on cocaine responses in male and female cocaine users. *Pharmacol Biochem Behav.* 2004;78(4):699–705.
146. Fuchs RA, Evans KA, Mehta RH, et al. Influence of sex and estrous cyclicity on conditioned cue-induced reinstatement of cocaine-seeking behavior in rats. *Psychopharmacology.* 2005;179(3):662–672.
147. Kerstetter KA, Aguilar VR, Parrish AB, et al. Protracted time-dependent increases in cocaine-seeking behavior during cocaine withdrawal in female relative to male rats. *Psychopharmacology.* 2008;198(1):63–75.
148. Elman I, Karlsgodt KH, Gastfriend DR. Gender differences in cocaine craving among non-treatment-seeking individuals with cocaine dependence. *Am J Drug Alcohol Abuse.* 2001;27(2):193–202.
149. Hser YI, Evans E, Huang YC. Treatment outcomes among women and men methamphetamine abusers in California. *J Subst Abuse Treat.* 2005;28(1):77–85.
150. Westhuis DJ, Gwaltney L, Hayashi R. Outpatient cocaine abuse treatment: predictors of success. *J Drug Educ.* 2001;31(2):171–183.
151. Campbell UC, Morgan AD, Carroll ME. Sex differences in the effects of baclofen on the acquisition of intravenous cocaine self-administration in rats. *Drug Alcohol Depend.* 2002;66(1):61–69.
152. Elkashef AM, Rawson RA, Anderson AL, et al. Bupropion for the treatment of methamphetamine dependence. *Neuropsychopharmacology.* 2008;33(5):1162–1170.
153. Center on Addiction and Substance Abuse at Columbia Univeristy (2005, July). Under the counter: the diversion and abuse of controlled prescription drugs in the U.S. Retrieved September 15, 2008, from http://www.casacolumbia.org/absolutenm/articlefiles/380-Under%20the%20Counter%20-%20Diversion.pdf.
154. Compton WM, Volkow ND. Major increases in opioid analgesic abuse in the United States: concerns and strategies. *Drug Alcohol Depend.* 2006;81(2):103–107.
155. Colliver JD, Kroutil LA, Dai L, et al. *Misuse of prescription drugs: data from the 2002, 2003, and 2004 National Surveys on Drug Use and Health* (DHHS Publication No. SMA 06-4192, Analytic Series A-28). Rockville, MD: Substance Abuse and Mental Health Services Administration, Office of Applied Studies; 2006.
156. Back SE, Payne R, Waldrop AE, et al. Prescription opioid aberrant behaviors: a pilot study of gender differences. *Clin J Pain.* 2009;25:477–484.
157. Fach M, Bischof G, Schmidt C, et al. Prevalence of dependence on prescription drugs and associated mental disorders in a representative sample of general hospital patients. *Gen Hosp Psychiatry.* 2007;29(3):257–263.
158. Jones HE, Johnson RE, Bigelow G, et al. Differences at treatment entry between opioid-dependent and cocaine-dependent males and females. *Addict Disord Their Treat.* 2004;3(3):110–121.
159. Grella CE, Mitchell PK, Wardna US, et al. Gender and comorbidity among individuals with opioid use disorders in the NESARC study. *Addict Behav.* 2009;34:498–504.
160. Powis B, Griffiths P, Gossop M, et al. The differences between male and female drug users: community samples of heroin and cocaine users compared. *Subst Use Misuse.* 1996;31(5):529–543.
161. Callaghan RC, Cunningham JA. Intravenous and non-intravenous cocaine abusers admitted to inpatient detoxification treatment: a 3-year medical-chart review of patient characteristics and predictors of treatment re-admission. *Drug Alcohol Depend.* 2002;68:323–328.
162. Bryant J, Treloar C. The gendered context of initiation to injecting drug use: evidence for women as active initiates. *Drug Alcohol Rev.* 2007;26:297–293.
163. Frajzyngier V, Neaigus A, Gyarmathy VA, et al. Gender differences in injection risk behaviors at the first injection episode. *Drug Alcohol Depend.* 2007;89:145–152.
164. Hamilton AB, Grella CE. Gender differences among older heroin users. *J Women Aging.* 2009;21:111–214.
165. Breen C, Roxburgh A, Degenhardt L. Gender differences among regular injecting drug users in Sydney, Australia, 1996-2003. *Drug Alcohol Rev.* 2005;24:353–358.
166. Montgomery SB, Hyde J, De Rosa CJ, et al. Gender differences in HIV risk behaviors among young injectors and their social network members. *Am J Drug Alcohol Abuse.* 2002;28(3):453–475.
167. Sherman SG, Latkin CA, Gielen AC. Social factors related to syringe sharing among injecting partners: A focus on gender. *Subst Use Misuse.* 2001;36(14):2113–2136.
168. Najavits LM, Rosier M, Nolan AL, et al. A new gender-based model for women's recovery from substance abuse: results of a pilot outcome study. *Am J Drug Alcohol Abuse.* 2007;33(1):5–11.
169. Fareed A, Casarella J, Amar R, et al. Benefits of retention in methadone maintenance and chronic medical conditions as risk factors for premature death among older heroin addicts. *J Psychiatr Pract.* 2009;15(3):227–234.
170. Kinlock TW, Gordon MS, Schwartz RP, et al. A randomized clinical trial of methadone maintenance for prisoners: results at 12 months postrelease. *J Subst Abuse Treat.* 2009;37(3):277–285.
171. White J, Bell J, Saunders JB, et al. Open-label dose-finding trial of buprenorphine implants (Probuphine0 for treatment of heroin dependence. *Drug Alcohol Depend.* 2009;103(1-2):37–43.
172. Jones HE, Fitzgerald H, Johnson RE. Males and females differ in response to opioid agonist medications. *Am J Addict.* 2005;14:223–233.
173. Substance Abuse and Mental Health Services Administration (SAMHSA). *National Survey of Substance Abuse Treatment Services (N-SSATS).* Rockville, MD: Department of Health and Human Services; 2005.
174. Compton WM, Grant BF, Colliver JD, et al. Prevalence of marijuana use disorders in the United States, 1991-1992 and 2001-2002. *J Am Med Assoc.* 2004;291:2114–2121.
175. Substance Abuse and Mental Health Services Administration. *The NSDUH Report: Daily Marijuana Users* (Based on the 2003 *National Survey on Drug Use and Health: National Findings* (Office of Applied Studies, NSDUH Series H-25, DHHS Publication No. SMA 04-3964). Rockville, MD: U.S. Department of Health and Human Services; 2004.
176. Van Etten ML, Anthony JC. Comparative epidemiology of initial drug opportunities and transitions to first use: marijuana, cocaine, hallucinogens, and heroin. *Drug Alcohol Depend.* 1999;54:117–125.
177. Gfroerer JC, Wu LT, Penne MA. *Initiation of Marijuana use: trends, Patterns, and Implications* (Analytic Series: A-17, DHHS Publication No. SMA 02-3711). Rockville, MD: Substance Abuse and Mental Health Administration, Office of Applied Studies; 2002.
178. Griffin ML, Mendelson JH, Mello NK, et al. Marijuana use across the menstrual cycle. *Drug Alcohol Depend.* 1986;18:213–224.

179. Terner JM, de Wit H. Menstrual cycle phase and responses to drugs of abuse in humans. *Drug Alcohol Depend.* 2006;84:1–13.
180. Pope HG, Gruber AJ, Hudson JI, et al. Neuropsychological performance in long-term cannabis users. *Arch Gen Psychiatry.* 2001;58:909–915.
181. Pope HG, Jacobs A, Mialet JP, et al. Evidence for a sex-specific residual effect of cannabis on visuospatial memory. *Psychother Psychosom.* 1997;66:179–184.
182. Agosti V, Nunes E, Levin F. Rates of psychiatric comorbidity among U.S. residents with lifetime cannabis dependence. *Am J Drug Alcohol Abuse.* 2002;28:643–652.
183. Pederson W, Mastekaasa A, Wichstrom L. Conduct problems and early cannabis initiation: a longitudinal study of gender differences. *Addiction.* 2001;96:415–431.
184. Bovasso GB. Cannabis abuse as a risk factor for depression. *Am J Psychiatry.* 2001;158:2033–2037.
185. Troisi A, Pasani A, Saracco M, et al. Psychiatric symptoms in male cannabis users not using other illicit drugs. *Addiction.* 1998;4:487–492.
186. Vlahov D, Galea S, Resnick H, et al. Increased use of cigarettes, alcohol, marijuana among Manhattan, New York, residents after the September 11th terrorist attacks. *Am J Epidemiol.* 2002;155:988–996.
187. Buckner JD, Mallott MA, Schmidt NB, et al. Peer influence and gender differences in problematic cannabis use among individuals with social anxiety. *Anxiety Disord.* 2006;20:1087–1102.
188. Budney AJ, Higgins ST, Radonovich PL, et al. Adding voucher-based incentives to coping skills and motivational enhancement improves outcomes during treatment for marijuana dependence. *J Consult Clin Psychol.* 2000;68:1051–1061.
189. Budney AJ, Vandery RG, Hughes JR, et al. Oral delta-9-tetrahydrocannabinnol suppresses cannabis withdrawal symptoms. *Drug Alcohol Depend.* 2007;86:22–29.
190. Copeland J, Swift W, Roffman R, et al. A randomized controlled trial of brief cognitive-behavioral interventions for cannabis use disorder. *J Subst Abuse Treat.* 2001;21:55–64.
191. Marijuana Treatment Project Research Group. Brief treatments for cannabis dependence: findings from a randomized multisite trial. *J Consult Clin Psychol.* 2004;72:455–466.
192. Prescott E, Hippe M, Schnohr P, et al. Smoking and risk of myocardial infarction in women and men: longitudinal population study. *Br Med J.* 1998;316:1043–1047.
193. Dransfield MT, Davis JJ, Gerald LB, et al. Racial and gender differences in susceptibility to tobacco smoke among patients with chronic obstructive pulmonary disease. *Respir Med.* 2006;100:1110–1116.
194. International Early Lung Cancer Action Program Investigators. Women's susceptibility to tobacco carcinogens and survival after diagnosis of lung cancer. *J Am Med Assoc.* 2006;296:180–184.
195. Hornsby PP, Wilcox AJ, Weinberg CR. Cigarette smoking and disturbance of menstrual function. *Epidemiology.* 1998;9:193–198.
196. DiFranza JR, Aligne CA, Weitzman M. Prenatal and postnatal environmental tobacco smoke exposure and children's health. *Pediatrics.* 2004;113(suppl.):1007–1015.
197. Conklin CA. Environments as cues to smoke: Implication for human extinction-based research and treatment. *Exp Clin Psychopharmacol.* 2006;14:12–19.
198. Perkins KA, Jacobs L, Sanders M, et al. Sex differences in the subjective and reinforcing effects of cigarette nicotine dose. *Psychopharmacology.* 2002;163:194–201.
199. Perkins KA, Doyle T, Ciccocioppo M, et al. Sex differences in the influence of nicotine and dose instructions on subjective and reinforcing effects of smoking. *Psychopharmacology.* 2006;184:600–607.
200. Perkins KA, Gerlach D, Vender J, et al. Sex differences in the subjective and reinforcing effects of visual and olfactory cigarette smoke stimuli. *Nicotine Tob Res.* 2001;3:141–150.
201. Rodu B, Cole P. Declining mortality from smoking in the United States. *Nicotine Tob Res.* 2007;9:781–784.
202. Munafo M, Bradburn M, Bowes L, et al. Are there sex differences in transdermal nicotine replacement therapy patch efficacy? A meta-analysis. *Nicotine Tob Res.* 2004;6:769–776.
203. Perkins KA, Scott J. Sex differences in long-term smoking cessation rates due to nicotine patch. *Nicotine Tob Res.* 2008;10:1245–1251.
204. Gonzales D, Rennard SI, Nides M, et al. Varenicline, an a4b2 nicotinic acetylcholine receptor partial agonist, vs. sustained-release bupropion and placebo for smoking cessation. *J Am Med Assoc.* 2006;296:47–55.
205. Scharf D, Shiffman S. Are there gender differences in smoking cessation, with and without bupropion? Pooled and meta-analyses of clinical trials of bupropion SR. *Addiction.* 2004;99:1462–1469.
206. Cepeda-Benito A, Reynoso JT, Erath S. Meta-analysis of the efficacy of nicotine replacement therapy for smoking cessation: differences between men and women. *J Consult Clin Psychol.* 2004;72:712–712.
207. Pirie PL, Murray DM, Luepker RV. Gender differences in cigarette smoking and quitting in a cohort of young adults. *Am J Public Health.* 1991;81:324–327.
208. Swan GE, Ward MM, Carmelli D, et al. Differential rates of relapse in subgroups of male and female smokers. *J Clin Epidemiol.* 1993;46:1041–1053.
209. England LJ, Grauman A, Qian C, et al. Misclassification of maternal smoking status and effects on an epidemiologic study of pregnancy outcomes. *Nicotine Tob Res.* 2007;9:1005–1013.
210. Parker DR, Windsor RA, Roberts MB, et al. Feasibility, cost, and cost-effectiveness of a telephone-based motivational intervention for underserved pregnant smokers. *Nicotine Tob Res.* 2007;9:1043–1051.
211. Office of Applied Studies, Substance Abuse and Mental Health Services Administration. *Treatment Episode Data Set (TEDS) highlights—2005 national admissions to substance abuse treatment services: 1995-2005.* Rockville, MD, 2006. Retrieved November 8, 2007 from http://oas.samhsa.gov/teds2k5/TEDSHi2k5.htm
212. Greenfield SF, Brooks AJ, Gordon SM, et al. Substance abuse treatment entry, retention, and outcome in women: a review of the literature. *Drug Alcohol Depend.* 2007;86:1–21.
213. Grella CE, Scott CK, Foss MA, et al. Gender differences in drug treatment outcomes among participants in the Chicago Target Cities Study. *Eval Program Plan.* 2003;26:297–310.
214. Lundgren LM, Schilling RF, Fitzgerald T, et al. Parental status of women injection drug users and entry to methadone maintenance. *Subst Use Misuse.* 2003;38(8):1109–1131.
215. Haller DL, Miles DR, Dawson KS. Factors influencing treatment enrollment by pregnant substance abusers. *Am J Drug Alcohol Abuse.* 2003;29(1):117–131.
216. Chen X, Burgdorf K, Dowell K, et al. Factors associated with retention of drug abusing women in long-term residential treatment. *Eval Program Plan.* 2004;27:205–212.

217. Schmidt L, Weisner C. The emergence of problem-drinking women as a special population in need of treatment. In: Galanter M, ed. *Recent Developments in Alcoholism: Alcoholism and Women.* New York: Plenum Press; 1995:309–334.
218. Morse B, Gehshan S, Hutchins E. *Screening for Substance Abuse During Pregnancy: Improving Care, Improving Health.* Arlington, VA: National Center for Education in Maternal and Child Health; 1997.
219. Flynn HA, Marcus SM, Barry KL, et al. Rates and correlates of alcohol use among pregnant women in obstetrics clinics. *Alcohol Clin Exp Res.* 2003;27(1):81–87.
220. Harrison PM, Beck AJ. *Prisoners in 2004* (BJS Bulletin, NCJ 210677). Washington, DC: Bureau of Justice Statistics, U.S. Department of Justice; 2005. Retrieved October 10, 2006, from http://www.ojp.usdoj.gov/bjs/abstract/p04.htm.
221. Padgett DK, Hawkins RL, Abrams C, et al. In their own words: trauma and substance abuse in the lives of formerly homeless women with serious mental illness. *Am J Orthopsychiatry.* 2006;76(4):461–467.
222. Arfken CL, Klein C, di Menza S, et al. Gender differences in problem severity at assessment and treatment retention. *J Subst Abuse Treat.* 2001;20:53–57.
223. King AC, Canada SA. Client related predictors of early treatment drop out in a substance abuse clinic exclusively employing individual therapy. *J Subst Abuse Treat.* 2004;26:189–195.
224. Sayre SL, Schmitz JM, Stotts AL, et al. Determining predictors of attrition in an outpatient substance abuse program. *Am J Drug Alcohol Abuse.* 2002;28:55–72.
225. Hser YI, Huang D, Teruya CM, et al. Gender differences in treatment outcomes over a three-year period: a PATH model analysis. *J Drug Issues.* 2004;34:419–439.
226. Green CA, Polen MR, Dickinson DM, et al. Gender differences in predictors of initiation, retention, and completion in an HMO-based substance abuse treatment program. *J Subst Abuse Treat.* 2002;23:285–295.
227. Mertens JR, Weisner CM. Predictors of substance abuse treatment retention among women and men in an HMO. *Alcohol Clin Exp Res.* 2000;24:1525–1533.
228. Hser Y, Grella C, Hubbard R, et al. An evaluation of drug treatments for adolescents in 4 US cities. *Arch Gen Psychiatry.* 2001;58:689–695.
229. Joe GW, Simpson DD, Broome KM. Retention and patient engagement models for different treatment modalities in DATOS. *Drug Alcohol Depend.* 1999;57:113–125.
230. Davis S. Drug treatment decisions of chemically dependent women. *Int J Addict.* 1994;29:1287–1304.
231. Huselid RF, Self EA, Gutierres SE. Predictors of successful completion of a halfway-house program for chemically-dependent women. *Am J Drug Alcohol Abuse.* 1991;17:89–101.
232. Kelly PJ, Blacksin B, Mason E. Factors affecting substance abuse treatment completion for women. *Issues Ment Health Nurs.* 2001;22:287–304.
233. Knight DK, Hood PE, Logan SM, et al. Residential treatment for women with dependent children: one agency's approach. *J Psychoactive Drugs.* 1999;31:339–351.
234. Loneck B, Garrett J, Banks SM. Engaging and retaining women in outpatient alcohol and other drug treatment: The effect of referral intensity. *Health Soc Work.* 1997;22:38–46.
235. Greenfield SF, Grella CE. Alcohol & drug abuse: what is "women-focused" treatment for substance use disorders? *Psychiatr Serv.* 2009;60:880–882.
236. Hodgins DC, el-Guebaly N, Addington J. Treatment of substance abusers: single or mixed gender programs? *Addiction.* 1997;92:805–812.
237. Comfort M, Kaltenbach KA. Predictors of treatment outcomes for substance-abusing women: a Retrospective Study. *J Subst Abuse.* 2000;21:33–45.
238. Greenfield SF, Pirard S. Gender-specific treatment for women with substance use disorders. In: Brady KT, Back SE, Greenfield SF, eds. *Women and Addiction: A Comprehensive Handbook.* New York City: Guildford Press; 2009:289–306.
239. Orwin RG, Francisco L, Bernichon T. *Effectiveness of women's substance abuse treatment programs: a meta-analysis.* Arlington, Virginia: Center for Substance Abuse Treatment, SAMHSA; 2001.
240. Nelson-Zlupko L, Dore M, Kauffman E, et al. Women in recovery: their perceptions of treatment effectiveness. *J Subst Abuse Treat.* 1996;13:51–59.
241. Swift W, Copeland J. Treatment needs and experiences of Australian women with alcohol and other drug problems. *Drug Alcohol Depend.* 1996;40:211–219.
242. Volpicelli J, Markman I, Monterosso J, et al. Psychosocially enhanced treatment for cocaine-dependent mothers: evidence of efficacy. *J Subst Abuse Treat.* 2000;18:41–49.
243. LaFave LM, Echols LD. An argument for choice. An alternative women's treatment program. *J Subst Abuse Treat.* 1999;16:345–352.
244. Schliebner CT. Gender-sensitive therapy. An alternative for women in substance abuse treatment. *J Subst Abuse Treat.* 1994;11:511–515.
245. Welle D, Falkin GP, Jainchill N. Current approaches to drug treatment for women offenders. Project WORTH. Women's Options for Recovery, Treatment, and Health. *J Subst Abuse Treat.* 1998;15:151–163.
246. Wilke D. Women and alcoholism: how a male as norm bias affects research, assessment, and treatment. *Health Soc Work.* 1994;19:29–35.
247. Kauffman E, Dore MM, Nelson-Zlupko L. The role of women's therapy groups in the treatment of chemical dependence. *Am J Orthopsychiatry.* 1995;65:355–363.
248. Pelissier BMM, Camp SD, Gaes GG, et al. Gender differences in outcomes from prison-based residential treatment. *J Subst Abuse Treat.* 2003;24(2):149–160.
249. Nelson-Zlupko L, Kauffman E, Dore MM. Gender differences in drug addiction and treatment: implications for social work intervention with substance-abusing women. *J Soc Work.* 1995;40:45–54.
250. Smith WB, Weisner C. Women and alcohol problems: a critical analysis of the literature and unanswered questions. *Alcohol Clin Exp Res.* 2000;24:1320–1321.
251. Condelli WS, Koch MA, Fletcher B. Treatment refusal/attrition among adults randomly assigned to programs at a drug treatment campus. The New Jersey Substance Abuse Treatment Campus, Seacaucus, NJ. *J Subst Abuse Treat.* 2000;18:395–407.
252. Strantz IH, Welch SP. Postpartum women in outpatient drug abuse treatment: correlates of retention/completion. *J Psychoactive Drugs.* 1995;27:357–373.
253. Kaskutas LA, Zhang L, French MT, et al. Women's programs versus mixed-gender day treatment: results from a randomized study. *Addiction.* 2005;100:60–69.
254. Greenfield SF, Potter JS, Lincoln MF, et al. High psychiatric severity is a moderator of substance abuse treatment outcomes among women in single vs. mixed gender group treatment. *Am J Drug Alcohol Abuse.* 2008;34:594–602.

255. Cummings A, Kuper L, Gallop R, et al. Self-efficacy and substance use outcomes for women in single gender versus mixed-gender group treatment. *J Groups Addict Recover.* (in press).
256. Bride BE. Single-gender treatment of substance abuse: effect on treatment retention and completion. *Soc Work Res.* 2001;25:223–232.
257. Copeland J, Wayne H, Didcott P, et al. A comparison of a specialist women's alcohol and other drug treatment service with two traditional mixed-sex services: client characteristics and treatment outcome. *Drug Alcohol Depend.* 1993;32:81–92.
258. Claus RE, Orwin RG, Kissin W, et al. Does gender-specific substance abuse treatment for women promote continuity of care? *J Subst Abuse Treat.* 2007;32:27–39.
259. Reynolds KD, Coombs DW, Lowe JB, et al. Evaluation of a self-help program to reduce alcohol consumption among pregnant women. *Int J Addict.* 1995;30:427–443.
260. Elk R, Schmitz J, Spiga R, et al. Behavioral treatment of cocaine-dependent pregnant women and TB-exposed patients. *Addict Behav.* 1995;20:533–542.
261. Jansson LM, Svikis D, Lee J, et al. Pregnancy and addiction. A comprehensive care model. *J Subst Abuse Treat.* 1996;13:321–329.
262. Luthar SS, Suchman NE. Relational Psychotherapy Mothers' Group: a developmentally informed intervention for at-risk mothers. *Dev Psychopathol.* 2000;12:235–253.
263. Hien DA, Cohen LR, Miele GM, et al. Promising treatments for women with comorbid PTSD and substance use disorders. *Am J Psychiatry.* 2004;161:1426–1432.
264. Najavits LM, Weiss RD, Shaw SR, et al. "Seeking safety": outcome of a new cognitive-behavioral psychotherapy for women with posttraumatic stress disorder and substance dependence. *J Trauma Stress.* 1998;11:437–456.
265. Kelly AB, Halford WK, Young RM. Maritally distressed women with alcohol problems: the impact of a short-term alcohol-focused intervention on drinking behaviour and marital satisfaction. *Addiction.* 2000;95:1537–1549.
266. Linehan MM, Schmidt H, Dimeff LA, et al. Dialectical behavior therapy for patients with borderline personality disorder and drug-dependence. *Am J Addict.* 1999;8:279–292.
267. Lemke S, Brennan PL, Schutte KK. Upward pressures on drinking: exposure and reactivity in adulthood. *J Stud Alcohol Drugs.* 2007;68:437–445.
268. Connors GJ, Maisto SA, Zywiak WH. Male and female alcoholics' attributions regarding the onset and termination of relapses and the maintenance of abstinence. *J Subst Abuse.* 1998;10:27–42.
269. Fals-Stewart W, O'Farrell TJ, Birchler GR, et al. Behavioral couples therapy for alcoholism and drug abuse: Where we've been, where we are, and where we're going. *J Cogn Psychother.* 2005;30:1479–1495.
270. Winters J, Fals-Stewart W, O'Farrell TJ, et al. Behavioral couples therapy for female substance-abusing patients: effects on substance use and relationship adjustment. *J Consult Clin Psychol.* 2002;70:344–355.
271. Fals-Stewart W, Birchler GR, Kelley ML. Learning sobriety together: a randomized clinical trial examining behavioral couples therapy with alcoholic female patients. *J Consult Clin Psychol.* 2006;74:579–591.
272. Calhoun F, Attilia ML, Spagnolo PA, et al. National Institute on alcohol abuse and alcoholism and the study of fetal alcohol spectrum disorders. The International Consortium. *Ann Ist Super Sanita.* 2006;42(1):4–7.
273. Chudley AE, Kilgour AR, Cranston M, et al. Challenges of diagnosis in fetal alcohol syndrome and fetal alcohol spectrum disorder in the adult. *Am J Med Genet.* 2007;145(3):261–272.
274. Manning MA, Hoyme HE. Fetal alcohol spectrum disorders: a practical clinical approach to diagnosis. *Neurosci Biobehav Rev.* 2007;31(2):230–238.
275. Langbehn DR, Cadoret RJ. The adult antisocial syndrome with and without antecedent conduct disorder: comparisons from an adoption study. *Compr Psychiatry.* 2001;42(4):272–282.
276. Floyd RL, Sobell M, Velasquez MM, et al. Project CHOICES Efficacy Study Group. *Am J Prev Med.* 2007;32(1):1–10.
277. Chang G, McNamara TK, Orav EJ, et al. Brief intervention for prenatal alcohol use: a randomized trial. *Obstet Gynecol.* 2005;105:991–998.
278. Bolisetty S, Naidoo D, Lui K. Postnatal changes in maternal and neonatal plasma antioxidant vitamins and the influence of smoking. *Arch Dis Child Fetal Neonatal Ed.* 2002;86(1):F36–F40.
279. Yang Q, Wen SW, Smith GN, et al. Maternal cigarette smoking and the risk of pregnancy-induced hypertension and eclampsia. *Int J Epidemiol.* 2006;35(2):288–293.
280. Andres RL, Day MC. Perinatal complications associated with maternal tobacco use. *Semin Neonatol.* 2000;5(3):231–241.
281. Meyer KA, Williams P, Hernandez-Diaz S, et al. Smoking and the risk of oral clefts: exploring the impact of study designs. *Epidemiology.* 2004;15(6):671–678.
282. Mortensen EL, Michaelsen KF, Sanders SA, et al. A dose-response relationship between maternal smoking during late pregnancy and adult intelligence in male offspring. *Paediatr Perinat Epidemiol.* 2005;19(1):4–11.
283. Chan B, Einarson A, Koren G. Effectiveness of bupropion for smoking cessation during pregnancy. *J Addict Dis.* 2005;24(2):19–23.
284. Kilby JW. A smoking cessation plan for pregnant women. *J Obstet Gynecol Neonatal Nurs.* 1997;26(4):397–402.
285. Pollak K, Oncken C, Lipkus P, et al. Nicotine replacement and behavioral therapy for smoking cessation in pregnancy. *Am J Prev Med.* 2007;33(4):297–305.
286. Gaither K, Brunner Huber LR, Thompson ME, et al. Does the use of nicotine replacement therapy during pregnancy affect pregnancy outcomes? *Matern Child Health J.* 2009;13:497–504.
287. Lester BM, ElSohly M, Wright LL, et al. The Maternal Lifestyle Study: drug use by meconium toxicology and maternal self-report. *Pediatrics.* 2001;107(2):309–317.
288. Taylor AH, Ang C, Bell SC. The role of the endocannabinoid system in gametogenesis, implantation and early pregnancy. *Hum Reprod Update.* 2007;13(5):501–513.
289. Wilson PD, Loffredo CA, Correa-Villasenor A, et al. Attributable fraction for cardiac malformations. *Am J Epidemiol.* 1998;148(5):414–423.
290. Astley SJ, Little RE. Maternal marijuana use during lactation and infant development at one year. *Neurotoxicol Teratol.* 1990;12(2):161–168.
291. Grey KA, Day NL, Leech S. Prenatal marijuana exposure: effect on child depressive symptoms at ten years of age. *Neurotoxicol Teratol.* 2005;27(3):439–448.
292. Luty J, Nikolau V, Beam J. Is opiate detoxification unsafe in pregnancy? *J Subst Abuse Treat.* 2003;24(4):363–367.
293. LoVecchio F, Pizon A, Riley B, et al. Onset of symptoms after methadone overdose. *Am J Emerg Med.* 2007;25(1):57–59.
294. Kuschel C. Managing drug withdrawal in the newborn infant. *Semin Fetal Neonatal Med.* 2007;12(2):127–133.

295. Wang EC. Methadone treatment during pregnancy. *J Obstet Gynecol Neonatal Nurs*. 1999;28(6):615–622.
296. Bauer CR, Shankaran S, Bada HS, et al. The maternal lifestyle study: drug exposure during pregnancy and short term maternal outcomes. *Am J Obstet Gynecol*. 2002;186(3):487–495.
297. Little BB, Gilstrap LC, Cunningham FG. Social and illicit substance use during pregnancy. In: Cunningham G, McDonald PC, Gant NF, eds. *Williams Obstetrics*. 18th ed. Norwalk, CT: Appleton and Lange; 1990.
298. O'Donnell AE, Mappin FG, Sebo TJ, et al. Interstitial pneumonitis associated with "crack" cocaine abuse. *Am Coll Chest Physicians*. 1991;100(4):1155–1157.
299. Storen EC, Wijdicks EF, Crum BA, et al. Moyamoya-like vasculopathy from cocaine dependency. *Am J Neuroradiol*. 2000;21(6):1008–1010.
300. Gardner TJ, Kosten TR. Therapeutic options and challenges for substances of abuse. *Dialogues Clin Neurosci*. 2007;9(4):431–445.
301. Kampman KM. Medications for cocaine abuse. *Psychiatr Times*. 2005;22(2):38–46.
302. United States Census Bureau News. (2007). *Minority population tops 100 million*. Retrieved from http://www.census.gov/PressRelease/www/releases/archives/population/010048.html
303. Wallace BC. *Making Mandated Treatment Work*. New York: Jason Aronson Publishers; 2005.
304. Handmaker N, Packard M, Conforti K. Motivational interviewing in the treatment of dual disorders. In: Miller WR, Rollnick S. eds. *Motivational interviewing: Preparing People for Change*. 2nd ed. New York City: The Guilford Press; 2002:362–376.
305. Ouimette P, Brown PJ, eds. *Trauma and Substance Abuse: Causes, Consequences, and Treatment of Comorbid Disorders*. Washington, DC: American Psychological Association; 2003.
306. Riggs DS, Rukstalis M, Volpicelli JR, et al. Demographic and social adjustment characteristics of patients with comorbid posttraumatic stress disorder and alcohol dependence: potential pitfalls to PTSD treatment. *Addict Behav*. 2003;28(9):1717–1730.
307. Drucker EM. Incarcerated people. In: Levy BS, Sidel VW, eds. *Social Injustice and Public Health*. Oxford: Oxford University Press; 2006.
308. Sue DW, Capodilupo CM, Torino GC, et al. Racial microaggressions in everyday life: implications for clinical practice. *Am Psychol*. 2007;62(4):271–286.
309. Marlatt G. From hindsight to foresight: a commentary on Project MATCH. (1999). *Changing Addictive Behavior: Bridging Clinical and Public Health Strategies*. New York City: The Guilford Press; 1999:45–66.
310. Cochran SD, Mays VM. Relation between psychiatric syndromes and behaviorally defined sexual orientation in a sample of the U.S. population. *Am J Epidemiol*. 2000;151:516–523.
311. Drabble L, Trocki K. Alcohol consumption, alcohol-related problems, and other substance use among lesbian and bisexual women. *J Lesbian Stud*. 2005;9(3):19–30.
312. Diamant AL, Wold C, Spritzer K, et al. Health behaviors, health status, and access to and use of health care: a population-based study of lesbian, bisexual, and heterosexual women. *Arch Fam Med*. 2000;9(10):1043–1051.
313. Valanis BG, Bowen DJ, Bassford T, et al. Sexual orientation and health: comparisons in the women's health initiative sample. *Arch Fam Med*. 2000;9(9):843–853.
314. Aaron DJ, Markovic N, Danielson ME, et al. Behavioral risk factors for disease and preventive health practices among lesbians. *Am J Public Health*. 2001;91(6):972–975.
315. Cochran SD, Ackerman D, Mays VM, et al. Prevalence of nonmedical drug use and dependence among homosexually active men and women in the US population. *Addiction*. 2004;99:989–998.
316. Diamant AL, Wold C. Sexual orientation and variation in physical and mental health status among women. *J Women's Health*. 2003;12(1):41–49.
317. Gruskin EP, Hart S, Gordon N, et al. Patterns of cigarette smoking and alcohol use among lesbians and bisexual women enrolled in a large health maintenance organization. *Am J Public Health*. 2001;91(6):976–979.
318. Mays VM, Yancey AK, Cochran SD, et al. Heterogeneity of health disparities among African American, Hispanic, and Asian American women: unrecognized influences of sexual orientation. *Am J Public Health*. 2002;92(4):632–639.
319. Balsam KF, Beauchaine TP, Mickey RM. Mental health of lesbian, gay, bisexual, and heterosexual siblings: Effects of gender, sexual orientation, and family. *J Abnormal Psychol*. 2005;114(3):471–476.
320. Rivers I, D'Augelli AR. The victimization of lesbian, gay, and bisexual youths. In: D'Augelli AR, Patterson CJ, eds. *Lesbian, Gay, and Bisexual Identities, and Youth: Psychological Perspectives*. New York City: Oxford University Press; 2001:199–223.
321. Mays VM, Cochran SD. Mental health correlates of perceived discrimination among lesbian, gay, and bisexual adults in the United States. *Am J Public Health*. 2001;91(11):1869–1876.
322. Gilman SE, Cochran SD, Mays VM, et al. Risk of psychiatric disorders among individuals reporting same-sex sexual partners in the National Comorbidity Survey. *Am J Public Health*. 2001;91(6):933–939.
323. Sandfort TG, de Graaf R, Bijl RV, et al. Same-sex sexual behavior and psychiatric disorders: findings from the Netherlands Mental Health Survey and Incidence Study (NEMESIS). *Arch Gen Psychiatry*. 2001;58(1):85–91.
324. Paul JP, Catania J, Pollack L, et al. Suicide attempts among gay and bisexual men: Lifetime prevalence and antecedents. *Am J Public Health*. 2002;92(8):1338–1345.
325. Warner J, McKeown E, Griffin M, et al. Rates and predictors of mental illness in gay men, lesbians and bisexual men and women: results from a survey based in England and Wales. *Br J Psychiatry*. 2004;185:479–485.
326. Heffernan K. The nature and predictors of substance use among lesbians, *Addict Behav*. 1998;23:517–528.
327. Spitzer RL. The diagnostic status of homosexuality in DSM-III: a reformulation of the issues. *Am J Psychiatry*. 1981;138:210–215.
328. Nicolosi J. Objections to AAP Statement on Homosexuality and Adolescence. *Pediatrics*. 1994;93(4):696.
329. Hellman RE, Stanton M, Lee J. Treatment of homosexual alcoholics in government-funded agencies: provider training and attitudes. *Hosp Community Psychiatry*. 1989;40:1163–1168.
330. Weathers B. Alcoholism and the lesbian community. In: Eddy MC, Ford J, eds. *Alcoholism and Women*. Dubunque, IA: Kendall/Hunt; 1980.
331. Eliason MJ. Substance abuse counselors' attitudes regarding lesbian, gay, bisexual, and transgender clients. *J Subst Abuse*. 2000;12(3):311–328.
332. Irwin TW. Substance use disorders among sexual-minority women. In: Brady KT, Back SE, Greenfield SF, eds. *Women & Addiction*. New York City: Guilford Press; 2009:475–489.
333. Minkoff H, Paltrow LM. Melissa Rowland and the rights of pregnant women. *Obstet Gynecol*. 2004;104(6):1234–1236.

334. Paltrow LM. Perspective of a reproductive rights attorney. *Future Child.* 1991;1(1):85–92.
335. Linder EN. Punishing prenatal alcohol abuse: the problems inherent in utilizing civil commitment to address addiction. *Univ Ill Law Rev.* 2005;3:873–902.
336. Sarkola T, Kahila H, Gissler M, et al. Risk factors for out-of-home custody child care among families with alcohol and substance abuse problems. *Acta Paediatr.* 2007;96(11): 1571–1576.
337. Lam WKK, Wechsberg W, Zule W. African-American women who use crack cocaine: a comparison of mothers who live with and have been separated from their children. *Child Abuse Negl.* 2004;28 (11):1229–1247.
338. Minnes S, Singer LT, Humphrey-Wall R, et al. Psychosocial and behavioral factors related to the post-partum placements of infants born to cocaine-using women. *Child Abuse Negl.* 2008; 32(3):353–366.
339. Scott-Lennox J, Rose R, Bohlig A, et al. The impact of women's family status on completion of substance abuse treatment. *J Behav Health Serv Res.* 2000;27(4):366–379.
340. Porowski AW, Burgdorf K, Herrell JM. Effectivenss and sustainability of residential substance abuse treatment programs for pregnant and parenting women. *Eval Program Plan.* 2004;27: 191–198.
341. Federal Bureau of Investigation. Uniform Crime Report: crime in the United States 2004, Appendix II: Offenses in Uniform Crime Reporting. Washington, DC: United States Department of Justice, 2005. Retrieved on May 30, 2008, from www.fbi.gov/ucr/cius_04/appendices/appendix_02.html.
342. Federal Bureau of Investigation. Uniform Crime Report: crime in the United States 2006. Washington, DC: United States Department of Justice, 2007. Retrieved on May 30, 2008, from ww.fbi.gov/ucr/cius2006/arrests/index.html.
343. United States Department of Justice Bureau of Justice Statistics (USDOJ). Drugs and Crime Facts, Report NCJ 165148, United States Department of Justice, 2007. Retrieved May 21, 2008, from http://www.ojp.usdoj.gov/bjs/dcf/contents.htm.
344. The Sentencing Project. *Women in the Criminal Justice System* (Briefing Sheets). Washington, DC: The Sentencing Project; 2007.
345. Center for Disease Control (CDC). *Women, Injection Drug Use, and the Criminal Justice System* 2001. Retrieved on May 21, 2008, from www.cdc.gov/idu/facts/cj-women.pdf
346. Gendel MH. Substance misuse and substance-related disorders in forensic psychiatry. *Psychiatr Clin N Am.* 2006;29:649–673.
347. Messina N, Burdon W, Prendergast M. Prison-based treatment for drug-dependent women offenders: treatment versus no treatment. *J Psychoact Drugs.* 2006;(SARC Suppl. 3):333–343.

CHAPTER 64 Gays, Lesbians, and Bisexuals

Robert Paul Cabaj

Gay men, lesbians, and bisexual men and women are a special population with specific needs and concerns—a population defined not by traditionally understood cultural and ethnic minority criteria, but, rather, by having a sexual orientation that is different from the majority. A culturally competent approach is essential for working with gay, lesbian, and bisexuals (GLB) who have substance use or abuse concerns. Such competencies come from knowledge about and experience in working with GLB persons. To help with the knowledge component, this chapter discusses the nature of homosexuality and bisexuality; gay men, lesbians, and bisexuals themselves; the substance use and abuse concerns in this population; and the specific treatment\issues that need to be addressed when working with people who are gay, lesbian, or bisexual. (Transgender people require a special focus on their behavioral health concerns and will not be featured in this chapter.)

Nearly all studies and reviews (1–3), and the experiences of most clinicians working frequently and extensively with GLB persons (3), estimate an incidence of substance abuse of all types at approximately 30%—with ranges of 28% to 35%, in contrast to an incidence of 10% to 12% for the general population. One study noted bisexuals might have even higher rates than gay men and lesbians (4).

The GLB population is benefiting from newer studies and research, often with a focus on a subpopulation. For example, recent reviews of GLB youth indicate the same higher rates, noted above, that persist into adulthood (5,6). Studies that focus on minority GLB persons also indicate higher rates of alcohol and drug use and abuse (7,8).

Rather than just report on the higher incidence, studies now try to address the reasons behind the higher rates and look into the risk factors. Some risk factors have been noted that differ between non- or light users from frequent or binge drinker. These factors include: race/ethnicity; gay bar attendance; depression; sensation seeking; peer risk behaviors; and age of alcohol initiation (9). Co-occurring problems are also being studied, one of the most important being the combination of substance use/abuse and suicide attempts, mirroring the very high rates of suicidal thinking and behaviors among GLB youth (1,4,8,9).

Some studies have focused exclusively on lesbian substance abuse noting both higher rates of use overall as well as higher abuse patterns as compared to the general population (10,11). A commonly noted risk factor is early exposure to alcohol in school and persistence into adulthood, as also noted above for minorities (9,12).

Currently, no study specifically focuses exclusively on the drug or alcohol use of bisexual men or women, although many such people are included in some of the studies already described. Most of the concepts in this chapter can apply to bisexuals, however, because the key roles of external and internalized homophobia, as will be described below, apply to this population as well.

Alcohol abuse has been the primary focus of most studies. No specific studies of injecting drug use (IDU) and the gay population are currently available. The annual Centers for Disease Control and Prevention (CDC) report on acquired immunodeficiency syndrome (AIDS) and human immunodeficiency virus (HIV) infections clearly indicate a subgroup of IDU gay and bisexual men, and one of the routes of HIV infection for lesbians is via IDU (12). One survey (13) did review the use of all types of abusable substances among gay men and lesbians, noting a greater use of cigarettes, marihuana, and alcohol than in the general population.

In the last decade or more, the use and abuse of methamphetamine (also known as "speed," "crystal," "tina," "crank," and other names) has emerged as a particular problem for gay men especially in urban areas on the West Coast, the South, and the Northeast Coast. Though use is not exclusive to gay men (adolescents across the country and urban younger Asian and Latina women are also noted to be high users), the problem has multiple psychological and medical concerns for gay men in particular. The frequent route of use is intravenous (i.v.), but it can also be inhaled/snorted or swallowed. Combined with its disinhibiting effect and sexual stimulating effect, the i.v. gay male users of methamphetamine are at extremely high risk for HIV infection via sharing needles and engaging in sexual activity that may last for hours and may not always follow safer sex guidelines. The use of the drug is highly associated with sexual activity and is popular at "circuit parties" where large numbers of gay men gather for partying, dancing, and sexual activity (often accompanied by drugs use) and with men seeking sexual partners over the internet ("party and play") (14,15). Additional focus of crystal meth will be in the treatment section of this chapter.

SEXUAL ORIENTATION IN GENERAL

Homosexuality, as a term, is subject to some controversy. It was first used when homosexuality was considered a clinical, pathologic condition. Because the term "gay" is less prejudicial and has a long accepted history, this chapter refers to gay men, lesbians, and bisexuals as people, and homosexuality and bisexuality in reference only to certain types of behavioral activities or orientations.

The understanding of certain terms is crucial to understanding homosexuality; failure to have clear definitions and understanding has led to much of the confusion in the literature about homosexuality and sexuality in general, and certainly has contributed to some of the prejudicial feeling about homosexuality. It is important to recognize the difference between sexual orientation and sexual behavior, as well as the differences between sexual orientation, gender identity, and gender role. Sexual orientation refers to the desire for sex, love, and affection, and/or sexual fantasies from or with another person, whereas sexual behavior is strictly sexual activities and may not coincide with primary sexual orientation. Gender identity is the sense of self as male or female, with no reference to sexual orientation or gender role. Gender role refers to behaviors and desires to behave that are viewed as masculine or feminine by a particular culture. Behavior that a particular culture may label as masculine or feminine is not necessarily a reflection of gender identity, but it is common to call behavior, styles, or interests shown by a male that are associated with women as "effeminate" (boys are often labeled "sissies") and the equivalent by a woman as "being like a man" or "butch" (girls are often labeled "tomboys").

Using both the pioneering scientific and psychological evidence collected by Dr. Evelyn Hooker that gay men were as psychologically healthy as matched heterosexuals (16) and subsequent research, the American Psychiatric Association (APA), in 1973, removed homosexuality per se as a mental illness from its list of disorders. Some psychiatrists who mistakenly thought the removal was a response to political pressure challenged this decision, but the APA supported its scientifically based decision via a vote by the membership and support by APA leadership. There was, however, a "political" compromise, with the creation of a nonscientific diagnosis called "ego-dystonic homosexuality." In 1987, the APA recognized this error and removed that label from the *Diagnostic and Statistical Manual of Mental Disorders*, 3rd ed., revised (*DSM–III–R*) (17). The current *Diagnostic and Statistical Manual of Mental Disorders*, 4th ed., text revision (2000) (*DSM–IV–TR*) followed the same revisions.

This nonjudgmental, nonprejudicial framework on homosexuality has led to new thinking and revisions on homosexual behavior and on gay men, lesbians, and bisexuals, as well as an awareness of the heterosexist bias in earlier research (18,19). New literature founded on work with gays in psychotherapy and substance-abuse counseling continues to be generated (3,20–22). American psychoanalytic thinking has been extremely persistent in trying to view homosexuality as pathologic even at one point trying to assert "repressed" homosexuality was a cause of alcoholism, but most current psychoanalytical literature has been able to review and revise some traditional, conservative views on homosexuality (23).

HOMOSEXUAL BEHAVIOR AND BISEXUALITY

Homosexual Behavior

Besides the work of Dr. Hooker noted above, the famous Kinsey report helped put homosexual behavior *itself* in perspective (24). Although somewhat dated and challenged over representativeness, the extensive survey reported that 67% of American men have had at least one homosexual experience to orgasm after adolescence; 30% have had more than one experience; 5% to 7% have bisexual experiences but prefer homosexual ones; and 4% to 5% have homosexual experiences exclusively as adults. The often used estimate that 10% of the male population is primarily or exclusively homosexual in terms of sexual behavior is based on this data from 1948. These data point out the widespread occurrence of male homosexual behavior, not necessarily the numbers of self-identified gay men. People may engage in same-sex sexual behavior but not self-identify as gay or lesbian respectively. Many people who do self-identify as gay, lesbian, or bisexual may not be open to all about their orientation—especially in a medical or research setting—thus making the true measure of the numbers of GLB persons difficult.

Gay and bisexual people and homosexual and bisexual behavior are found in almost all societies and cultures around the world and throughout history (25). Tolerance and acceptance has varied throughout history, and varies from country to country, culture to culture, and community to community. Anyone may be gay, lesbian, or bisexual. Gay and bisexual men and women do not have uniform ways of behaving nor do they live uniform lifestyles.

Gay people are found in all segments of society and in all minority and ethnic groups, may be of any age, and may have any occupation or career. Most gay people are not readily identifiable, in spite of persistent stereotypes. Sexual behavior and sexual orientation itself are not necessarily fixed in an individual and may change over time. Intense homosexual longings in young adulthood or adolescence may change as one grows older, and, conversely, some heterosexuals may discover gay feelings later in life.

Bisexuality

Many people are clearly bisexual in behavior—being able to sexually function with either sex—but often prefer one sex to the other. The above noted Kinsey report (24) devised the Kinsey scale to describe this range of behavior: from 0 for exclusive heterosexual behavior to 6 for exclusive homosexual behavior. This classification puts the majority of men in a bisexual range, based on sexual experiences. As will be discussed, bisexuality and bisexual behavior are especially important in HIV infection prevention work, because many men have gay sexual experiences, without informing their spouses or other female partners. Many lesbians have had, and do have, sex with men. For many minority populations, bisexuality, but not homosexuality per se, is acceptable (or at least admitted to) in surveys and interviews. A recent survey in New York City noted nearly 10% of men who reported sex exclusively with other men did not identify as gay—usually describing themselves as heterosexual or bisexual (26).

There are no specific studies of bisexuals and substance abuse, although with the focus on men who have sex with men as a risk factor for HIV infections, more information will no doubt be forthcoming. The issues that face men and women who are bisexual, especially if relating more strongly to the homosexual longings, will be the same issues that men who identify as gay and women who identify as lesbian will face.

GAY SEXUAL ORIENTATION

Gay men and lesbians are remarkably like everyone else. There are three major differences, however, which may be of help in understanding the high incidence of substance abuse: (a) having a sexual orientation expressed by the desire to have affectional, sexual, sexual fantasy, and/or social needs met mostly by a same-sex partner rather than an opposite-sex partner; (b) negotiating a process of self-identity and self-recognition as a gay person, different from the majority, known as "coming out"; and (c) confronting a widespread and insidious dislike, hatred, and/or fear of gay and lesbian people, homosexual activity, and homosexual feelings, known as "homophobia" or "anti-gat bias." This last factor forms the largest barrier to gays and lesbians obtaining quality health care and substance-abuse treatment, and may be the primary factor in explaining the widespread incidence of substance abuse in gay populations. Homophobia is a result of societal heterosexism, that is, the perspective that the majority situation—heterosexuality—is the "norm" or superior in some way. Homophobia is parallel to such societal forces as racism and sexism (27).

In trying to understand the nature of homosexuality, there have been new insights into sexuality in general and in the nature of gender identity. In looking at the etiology of homosexuality, most new research indicates that a homosexual orientation is not learned and not a result of any family or social patterns. The "classic" psychoanalytical description of a close, seductive mother and absent, distant father does not occur more frequently in the backgrounds of gay men; in fact, it may occur more often in heterosexuals (28). New research continues to point out familial patterns that may indicate a genetic component (29) and/or biologic and biochemical factors (30). Such knowledge and awareness about the origins of sexual orientation may help to relieve both the patients who are having difficulty accepting their homosexuality and the families of patients who are gay or lesbian who may feel guilty, as if they had done something "wrong" to "cause" the sexual orientation.

Coming Out

Coming out is a complex process that may occur throughout the entire life cycle (31). The best way to conceptualize coming out is to view it as a series of steps that an individual negotiates at his or her own time and pace, with periodic steps forward and backward. The individual must first become aware of his or her own sexual orientation as "different" from that of the majority. The next step is to accept the awareness and begin to integrate it into a self-concept and grapple with the negative feelings associated with homosexuality. Next, the individual may choose to act on the feelings (although some gay people with strong gay feelings do not engage in sex with others of the same sex, such as celibate priests or others). Finally, the person makes a series of lifelong decisions about whether to let others know and whom to let know, such as friends, family, work colleagues, peers, teachers, and medical providers. Some gay people only come out to selected people and not to everyone at once; some may come out, then deny it later or not continue to let new friends or people at new workplaces know. The bias and prejudice against people with AIDS and the often automatic, but mistaken, association of AIDS and gay men, rather than the association of HIV infection and behaviors that may lead to infection, may lead some men to "return to the closet" or hesitate in continuing the coming out process.

Homophobia and Heterosexism

Homophobia, both internalized and externalized, combined with heterosexism are the major forces that gays and bisexuals must deal with in our society (32). Almost all gay people develop some degree of internalized homophobia, having been brought up in a homophobic society that tends to promote prejudicial myths about gay people or, from the heterosexist concentric point of view, to just ignore gay and bisexual people in general. The coming out process may be delayed or undergo great difficulties depending on the intensity of internalized homophobia (if the person believes homosexuality is a sin, an illness, unnatural, evil, or will only lead to sadness, loneliness, and isolation) and may well require the help of psychotherapy.

Externalized homophobia is found at every level in our society: legal, medical, scientific, religious, political, social, educational, and judicial. Violent attacks on gay people, ranging from verbal threats to outright physical attacks and murder, are usually fueled by homophobia. Heterosexist thinking and homophobia and the fear of what others will do if they know an individual is gay or even think an individual is gay, are major factors in the difficulty of getting accurate data about gays and lesbians for scientific investigations (19). It follows that in undertaking research surveys, gay and bisexual people hesitate to disclose sexual orientation, even with great assurances of confidentiality. Gathering information on gay and bisexual people, therefore, is extremely difficult and contributes to the skewed samples, as already noted in the studies on substance abuse and the gay community.

Gay people also face many additional challenges that majority populations escape. There are many issues generated by two people of the same gender forming a relationship such as: finding comfortable and safe living quarters; financial concerns; legal battles over insurance and wills; acknowledgment of benefits; and, ability to marry which varies from state to state.

Because there is such a high incidence of substance abuse, there are many codependent relationships or relationships between two active substance abusers.

Gay and lesbian adolescents are a population of serious concern. Many studies indicate a much higher suicide attempt rate in these youth—30% versus 10% to 12% in the general population; a more volatile type of substance abuse than is seen in other adolescents, especially combinations of drugs and alcohol; and hesitancy to follow HIV infection risk-reduction guidelines (1,4,5,33). Older gays and lesbians face the same problems as other older adults, with added isolation, loneliness, and possible senses of hopelessness and resignation about substance abuse (34).

Lesbian Issues

Lesbians have some specific issues that need to be highlighted. As described previously, the incidence of substance abuse is equally high among gay men and lesbians. In general, lesbians may have additional social struggles and concerns. Compared to gay men, they are more likely to have lower incomes (as do women in general, when compared with men); lesbians are more likely to be parents (about one-third of lesbians are biologic parents); lesbians face the prejudices aimed at women, as well as those for being gay, including the stronger reaction against (and willingness to ignore) female substance abusers; lesbians are more likely to come out later in life (about 28 years of age vs. 18 years of age in men); and lesbians are more likely to have bisexual feelings or experiences, so that they are still at risk for HIV infection via a sexual route as well as possible i.v. drug use (11,13,28,35).

According to surveys noted above, lesbians are somewhat more likely to be in a long-term relationship than are the comparable gay men, so there needs to be a clear focus on relationships, parenting, and family concerns in working with lesbian substance abusers. Lesbians are also subject to the increase in violence, both verbal and physical, against gays; and, as is true with anyone, including gay men, they are subject to domestic violence. This latter fact is often ignored. Because there are correlations with domestic violence and substance abuse, clinicians need to be aware of this possibility in working with lesbians.

SUBSTANCE ABUSE AND GAY IDENTITY FORMATION

Many factors contribute to the prominent role of substance use and abuse in gay men, lesbians, and bisexuals. The two most important factors are genetic or biologic contributions, as well as the psychological effects of heterosexism and homophobia.

New research continues to support, in great part, genetic, biologic, and biochemical origins for the diseases of alcoholism and substance abuse. As already noted, there is continuing and growing evidence that homosexual orientation may have—at least in part—genetic, biologic, and biochemical components. Such parallel contributions to both sexual orientation and substance abuse has led to some speculation of a possible chromosomal link between the genetic contributions to substance abuse and sexual orientation. Such a direct genetic link between sexual orientation and the propensity to substance abuse, however, is unlikely. The studies cited indicate that male homosexuality and female homosexuality may be different phenomena, with differing familial patterns. Substance abuse appears to have equal incidence among gay men and women.

Societal, cultural, and environmental factors, however, may lead to a greater expression of any genetic predisposition. By analogy, there has been an increase in the incidence of alcoholism in women since the beginning of the twentieth century. Although partially explained by better data collection, and awareness of the hidden homebound female alcoholic, the increase can also be explained by social factors. In the early 1900s, women were prohibited from drinking in public by societal pressures. As the social acceptability of drinking increased, more women drank, thus increasing the likelihood of exposure to alcohol, which, in turn, could trigger the genetic predisposition to alcoholism.

Gay men, lesbians, and bisexuals have faced great societal prohibitions, not only on the expression of their sexual feelings and behavior, but also around their very existence. Societal homophobia or heterosexism could well create enough stress that gay men, lesbians, and bisexual persons turn to alcohol and other substances for "relief." This increased exposure could, in turn, lead to the higher degree of expressivity of the genetic potentials for substance abuse in gay men, lesbians, and bisexuals.

In addition, it is well known that societies or cultures in turmoil or undergoing social change have higher rates of alcoholism. Gay people can be seen as experiencing almost continuous stress and social change for most of the twentieth century. Societal pressures forced most gay people to remain "in the closet," hiding their sexual orientation or not acting on their feelings. Responding to societal expectations rather than personal desire, some gay, lesbian, and bisexual people may marry someone of the opposite sex and raise a family, creating a potentially stressful situation. Legal prohibitions on homosexual behavior, overt discrimination, and the failure of society to accept or even acknowledge gay people have limited the types of social outlets available to gay men and lesbians to bars, private homes, or clubs where alcohol and other drugs often played a prominent role. The role models for many young gay men and lesbians just coming out may be gay people using alcohol and other drugs, who are met at bars or parties. Continuing societal homophobia, as well as the impact of HIV on gay men, lesbians, and bisexuals, further adds to the stress (36).

Some gay and bisexual men and women cannot imagine socializing without alcohol or other mood-altering substances. Gay men, lesbians, and bisexuals are brought up in a society that says they should not exist and certainly should not act on their feelings. Such homophobia is internalized. Many men and women have had their first homosexual sexual experiences while drinking or being drunk to overcome their internal fear, denial, anxiety, or even revulsion about gay sex. For many men and women, this linking of substance use and sexual expression persists and may become part of coming out and the development of a personal and social identity. Many gay people continue to feel self-hatred. The use of mood-altering substances temporarily relieves, but then reinforces, this self-loathing in the drug-withdrawal period. Alcohol and many other drugs can cause depression, leading to a worsening of self-esteem and the "erosion of spirit" so well described by many of the 12-step recovery programs.

Given the state of acceptance of homosexuality and bisexuality in our society at this time, the stages of developing a gay, lesbian, or bisexual identity, influenced by such societal reactions, may be intimately involved with substance use. Although some substance abusers appear to have a genetic predisposition to substance abuse—supporting an illness model with psychosocial manifestations—not all people with such a genetic predisposition develop alcoholism or substance abuse in their lifetimes. Intrapsychic, psychological, and psychodynamic factors, influenced by psychosocial and parental upbringing, may lead certain people to turn to substance use and, therefore, potentiate a genetic predisposition for substance abuse.

The link between the psychodynamic forces in developing a gay, lesbian, or bisexual identity and the use or abuse of substances becomes clear in examining the early development and the progression through the life cycle for a gay person. Parents reward what is familiar and acceptable to them and discourage or de-emphasize behavior or needs they do not value or understand. Harm, of course, occurs when a parent is too depressed, preoccupied, or narcissistic to respond to the actual child and the actual needs and wants of the child. Children eventually learn to behave the way parents expect to get rewards, and to hide or deny the longings or needs that are not rewarded.

Many gay and bisexual men and women are aware of being different early in life—being aware, however subtly, of affectional and sexual needs and longings that are different from the majority of people around them. Some male children who will grow up to be gay may desire a closer, more intimate relationship with their father; this desire is not encouraged or even understood in our society. The prehomosexual child learns to hide such needs and longings, creating a false self. Real needs are often suppressed, or repressed, and rejected as wrong, bad, or sinful. Dissociation and denial, therefore, become major defenses to cope with internal feelings.

Some studies of familial patterns (29) point out that gay men have a greater-than-normal chance of having an alcoholic father and a greater chance of having a mother with a major affective disorder—either or both situations likely leading to growing up with emotionally unavailable parents. Therefore, the psychological, as well as genetic and emotional, backgrounds in the families of many gays and lesbians already predispose them to substance abuse.

The psychology of being different and learning to live in a society that does not accept difference readily shapes the sexual identity development as the child emerges from childhood and the latency period. With the rewards for the "false self," the child suppresses their more natural feelings. The child has no clear role models about how to be gay or lesbian; teachers usually cannot reveal their sexual orientation and there is still limited positive media attention for gays and lesbians. In latency, children who will become gay or bisexual—especially boys who may be effeminate—may fear other children, feel even more different, and become more isolated.

In adolescence, the gay sexual feelings emerge with great urgency, but with little or no context or permission. Conformity is certainly encouraged, further supporting denial and suppression of gay feelings. Adolescents often reject and isolate those who are "different." The gay adolescent further develops dissociation and splitting off of affect and behavior. These various factors may help to explain the many problems facing gay youth (33). For example, gay youth may be subject to sexual abuse and violence, and sometimes are introduced to sex via hustling or prostitution, or get "used" sexually by others. The extreme difficulty many gay men and women have in coming out and integrating sexuality and personal identity makes sense from this perspective.

Substance use serves as an easy relief, can provide acceptance, and, more importantly, mirrors the comforting dissociation developed in childhood. Alcohol and other drugs cause a dissociation of feelings, anxiety, and behavior, and may mimic the emotional state many gay people had to develop in childhood to survive. The "symptom-relieving" aspects help fight the effects of homophobia; it can allow "forbidden" behavior, allow for social comfort in bars or other unfamiliar social settings, and, again, provide comfort through the familiar experiences of dissociation and isolation.

The easy availability of alcohol and drugs at gay bars or parties and the limited social options other than those bars and parties certainly encourages the use of substances early in the coming out and gay or lesbian socialization process. For gay men especially, sex and intimacy are often split off—dissociated. Again, substance use allows for acting on feelings long suppressed or denied, but also mirrors the dissociative experience and makes it harder to integrate intimacy and love. There is an easy relief of longings and needs, with sex and/or substance use, and the more challenging needs for love and intimacy may be ignored. Substances help many gay people brace themselves for rejection by others—either as a gay person coming out to friends or family, or from potential dates and sexual partners.

Substance use enhances denial and can even cause "blackouts" around sexual behavior. It can certainly make "living in the closet" with its built-in need for denial and dissociation easier or even possible (the "I-was-so-drunk-I-didn't-know-what-I-did-last-night" scenario often used in high school and college). Because so many gay people are adult children of alcoholics, they are even more skilled at denying their own self and their own needs.

Finally, the internal state that accompanies internalized homophobia and that occurs with substance abuse are very similar—the "dual oppression" of homophobia and abuse (3).

The following traits are seen in both: denial; fear, anxiety, and paranoia; anger and rage; guilt; self-pity; depression, with helplessness, hopelessness, and powerlessness; self-deception and development of a false self; passivity and the feeling of being a victim; inferiority and low self-esteem; self-loathing; isolation, alienation, and feeling alone, misunderstood, or unique; and fragmentation and confusion. These close similarities make it very difficult for gay men or lesbians who cannot accept their sexual orientation to recognize or successfully treat their substance abuse. Self-acceptance of one's sexual orientation thus appears to be crucial to recovery from substance abuse.

The pervasive internal and social pressures to use mood-altering substances and the difficulty in creating or finding currently existing non–substance-using social situations certainly contributes to the greater expression of the alcohol and other drug-dependence potentials in gay men and women. One wonders if the rate of substance abuse in the general population would not be much greater if everyone in the United States was subject to such pressures. Possibly, there is no greater genetic predisposition to substance abuse in gays, but an increased potentiation of expression due to greater use and presence of such substances in gay society.

HOMOSEXUAL BEHAVIOR, SUBSTANCE ABUSE, HIV INFECTIONS, AND AIDS

Men-who-have-sex-with-men continues to be the largest "at-risk" group for current and new HIV-related infections and cases of AIDS in the United States. Although most clinicians and researchers attribute the spread of HIV in this population to certain highly risky unsafe sexual practices, the role of i.v. drug use is significant. The same CDC report noted that a good percentage of all adult cases were men who both had sex with men *and* i.v. drug users. Many men in the CDC statistics "i.v.-drug-users-only" category are also gay or bisexual, but fail to report this additional risk category for the reasons already discussed.

Besides the obvious potential spread of HIV through the i.v. drug-using segments of the gay population via needle sharing, substance abuse plays a not-so-obvious role in spreading the virus through sexual practices. In most reviews of gay men and safer sex practices, men who were knowledgeable about safer sex but failed to practice it uniformly report being under the influence of some substance, such as alcohol or other drugs, at the times they failed to follow the guidelines. In addition, some gay men seek to enhance and prolong sexual activity through the use of drugs such as amyl nitrite (known as "poppers"), alcohol, marihuana, ecstasy, and especially methamphetamines, or a combination of these substances (14,15,37–39).

The phenomena of "circuit parties" (this is a highly organized series of parties across the world that emphasize sex and drugs) and the club scene at local bars and dance clubs are not exclusive to gay men and lesbians, but both have taken hold of a significant number of gay people. Drugs are extremely frequently used in those settings—especially the so-called club drugs such as ecstasy, special K, and methamphetamines (38). The drugs are used to enhance the dancing and party experience but are also frequently used to enhance sexual activity, with the same consequences as noted above.

Judgment is clearly suspended or altered during even the moderate, let alone heavy, use of alcohol and other substances. There is definitely a higher risk for exposure to HIV with larger numbers of sexual partners, but the risk is also higher in any one particular encounter when safer sex guidelines are not followed—whether because of suspended judgment with substance use, pressure by the partner to not bother, or having highly charged sexual feelings. Furthermore, there is clear evidence that many abused substances alter the immune system, which may well compromise the immune system's initial reaction to exposure to HIV in men engaged in risky sexual practices under the influence of substances. With the widespread use of such agents and such conditions in the gay community, it appears that substance use and abuse, especially of methamphetamines, is a definite cofactor in the spread of HIV through sexual practices.

ADDED FOCUS ON METHAMPHETAMINE USE AND ABUSE

Why gay men in particular are more likely to use and abuse methamphetamine may be tied to the sexual enhancement aspect of the drug in and of itself, but there appear several additional reasons, including the impact of internalized homophobia, for example, and lower self-esteem and social awkwardness many gay men experience. The situations described such as sex clubs and circuit parties for many gay men are tied to expectations of peak sexual performance, certainly enhanced by use of methamphetamines. Gay men of color are also at risk for use of methamphetamines, including a population that usually is not associated with great substance use—Asian and Pacific Islanders (40,41).

There are many routes of administration, including oral inhalation, nasal insufflation, absorption through the rectal mucosa, and i.v. use. Methamphetamine is experienced as heightening sexual feelings and duration of sexual activity—as well as sexual disinhibition, allowing some men to have sex for 12 hours or more. There are risks for increased exposure to HIV with multiple sexual partners and unprotected anal intercourse (sex without condoms) and IDU—all of which are associated with methamphetamine use (42,43). Some men who specifically wish to become infected with HIV (for a variety of psychological reasons) find using methamphetamine and unprotected sex a particularly successful route to accomplish their goal (44). Those gay men who prefer to have unprotected anal sex with all of its risks (known as "barebacking") are also more likely to use methamphetamines (45).

The use of methamphetamines has clearly been linked to a higher risk for HIV infection due to the many factors already discussed. One study focused on gay male HIV-positive methamphetamine users who are sexually compulsive and the high rates of unsafe sexual activity that puts so many others at risk (46). Other studies look at the use of sildenafil (Viagra®) and methamphetamine as contributing to the higher HIV-risk (since many users of methamphetamines have transient erectile dysfunction so use sildenafil in addition)(47).

Many urban areas have started to address the concerns specific to gay men and some treatment programs are emerging for gay methamphetamine abusers. Who is likely to seek treatment is not clear since many of the gay men who use use with others and there are often social pressures to stay using even when problems develop. Many men enter treatment only after suffering great financial consequences or major health problems (48).

Several types of treatments have been studies, and more studies are looking specifically at gay men. Contingency-management types of behavioral modifications are showing promise as successful interventions (49). In San Francisco, a program called PROP (Positive Reinforcement Opportunity Project), a variation of contingency management with rewards for staying clean, is meeting the specific needs for some gay men and may well be used successfully elsewhere (50). The role of outpatient treatment alone or in combination with other interventions also needs additional study. Traditional 12-step programs are increasing with a focus specific to methamphetamine in many urban areas and Methamphetamine Anonymous (or Crystal Anonymous) groups are forming.

SPECIAL TREATMENT CONCERNS FOR GAY PEOPLE

Evaluation and Treatment Issues

Treatment must focus on both recovery from substance abuse and from the consequences of homophobia. To reverse and treat the denial and dissociation, the patient will need to address his or her own acceptance of self as a gay or bisexual person. Although no one should be forced to come out to any one, self-acceptance appears to be crucial to recovery. Treatment needs to be at least gay-sensitive if not gay-affirmative, as will be discussed. Many gay people, once in solid recovery, will need to deal with the grief and rage associated with mourning the loss of the "false self" and must learn how to get his or her own real needs met.

In the assessment of a gay man, lesbian, or bisexual person presenting for mental health services, clinicians need to be aware of the higher incidence of substance abuse in this population and, accordingly, routinely screen for symptoms of alcoholism or other substance abuse. In formulating a treatment plan for gay men, lesbians, or bisexuals determined to have a substance-abuse problem, the personalized treatment plan needs to include the influences and effects of the following for each individual: the stage in the life cycle; the degree and impact of internalized homophobia; the stage in the coming-out process and the experience of coming out; the support and social network available; current relationship, if any, including married spouses and the history of past relationships; the relationship with the family of origin; comfort with sexuality and expression of sexual feelings; career and economic status; and health factors, including HIV status.

Homophobia is the major consideration in meeting the treatment needs of gay men and lesbians with substance-abuse problems, as well as the proper care and prevention of HIV-related infections. Few inpatient or outpatient detoxification and rehabilitation programs have knowledge about homosexuality and are often unaware that they have gay and lesbian patients, who may be too frightened to "come out" to the staff. Attitudes of the staff and treating clinicians about homosexuality are crucial in the success of treatment for gays and lesbians (51). Many gay and lesbian staff are afraid to come out because of administrative reaction and are not able to either serve as role models or to provide a more open and relaxed treatment.

Gay-sensitive programs—programs that are aware of, knowledgeable about, and accepting of gay people in a nonprejudicial fashion—are opening up around the country. Most current and well-established programs are training staff about gay concerns, although many centers still fail to even ask about sexual orientation or address it as a specific topic. The Center for Substance Abuse Treatment has put out a guideline on working with gay, lesbian, bisexual, and transgender substance abusers, an extremely helpful and resourcefull guide.

Programs are also available across the country that are gay-affirmative, that is, actively promoting self-acceptance of a gay identity as a key part of recovery. Discussed above, substance abuse and sexual identity formation are often tightly woven together, and it is difficult to imagine much success in treating the gay or lesbian substance abuser without addressing sexual orientation and homophobia.

Aftercare may be a major problem. Twelve-step recovery programs and philosophies are the mainstays, of course, in recovery and in staying clean and sober. There may be no gay-sensitive therapists or counselors in the patients' communities. AA, although open to all, is still a group of people at any individual meeting that may reflect the perceptions and prejudices of the local community and not be open to or accepting of openly gay members. Most communities now have gay and lesbian AA, Narcotic Anonymous (NA), and Al-Anon meetings, and AA as an organization clearly embraces gays and lesbians, as it embraces anyone concerned about a substance-abuse problem.

Some gay people in recovery, however, may not have come out or may not feel comfortable in such meetings, especially if a discussion of sexual orientation was not part of the early recovery. Some groups parallel and similar to AA have formed to meet the needs of these gays and lesbians, such as Alcoholics Together, and many large cities sponsor "roundups," large 3-day-weekend gatherings focused on AA, NA, lectures, workshops, and drug- and alcohol-free socializing.

Although 12-step programs such as AA and NA recommend avoiding emotional stress and conflicts in the first 6 months of recovery, for the gay man, lesbian, or bisexual in such programs, relapse is almost certain if the gay or bisexual person cannot acknowledge and accept his or her sexual orientation. Discussion about the conflicts around acknowledging sexual orientation and ways to learn to live comfortably as a gay or bisexual person are essential for recovery, even if these topics are emotionally laden and stressful.

Many localities now have gay, lesbian, and bisexual health or mental health centers, almost all with a focus on recovery and substance-abuse treatment. National organizations, such as the National Association of Lesbian and Gay Addictions Professionals, the Association of Gay and Lesbian Psychiatrists, the Gay and Lesbian Medical Association, the Association of Lesbian and Gay Psychologists, and the National Gay Social Workers, can help with appropriate referrals.

Some of the suggestions and guidelines of AA and NA and most treatment programs may be difficult for some gay men, lesbians, and bisexuals to follow. For example, giving up or avoiding old friends, especially fellow substance users, may be difficult when the gay or bisexual person has limited contacts that relate to him as a gay person. Staying away from bars or parties may be difficult if they are the only social outlets; special help on how to not drink or use drugs in such settings may be necessary. Many gay people mistakenly link AA and religion; because many religious institutions denounce or condemn homosexuality, gay men, lesbians, and bisexuals may be resistant to trying AA or NA. Harm reduction models and relapse prevention techniques are especially useful approaches.

Specific Additional Factors to Consider

Gay men, lesbians, and bisexually identified minorities who abuse substances must also deal with homophobia—often from within the same self-identified ethnic or cultural groups—in addition to possible racism and other prejudices in seeking recovery (6,8). Culturally competent services must address not just race, culture, and ethnicity, but also gender, gender identity, and sexual orientation.

HIV infections and AIDS are much better understood, especially routes of transmission and therapeutic interventions, and can be treated as chronic conditions without the old fear of imminent death at diagnosis. Substance-abuse treatment centers and programs, though, may still be frightened to work with HIV-positive individuals, despite the clear CDC guidelines, or may resist talking about safer sex because it is uncomfortable to talk about such matters or it is viewed as detracting from recovery issues. All one needs to do is remember that AIDS prevention education is just as lifesaving an intervention for a substance abuser.

There are many additional difficult clinical issues facing a substance-abusing gay man who is HIV-positive or who has AIDS, whether actively using substances or in recovery, such as suicidality, dementia, negotiating safer sex, and legal issues concerning wills and powers-of-attorney. Some communities now have AA groups with a special focus on HIV-positive individuals or people with AIDS, such as the Positively Sober groups.

Other factors affect the treatment of lesbians, gay men, and bisexuals. As noted above, many gay men, lesbians, and bisexuals are in long-term relationships, and treatment for these individuals must clearly focus on relationships, parenting, and family concerns. Again, gay men, lesbians, and bisexuals are also subject to an increase in violent attacks because of their sexual orientation, both verbal and physical. Reaction to such an attack may include a relapse to drug or alcohol use in a person in recovery or an increase in use by someone currently using or abusing substances. In addition, many gay men, lesbians, and bisexuals are victims of domestic violence. Because there are correlations with domestic violence and substance abuse, clinicians need to be aware of this possible combination.

Additional treatment issues facing all people in recovery, which have special impact on gays and lesbians and are beyond the scope of this brief review chapter, include learning how to have safer sex while clean and sober; learning how to adjust to clean and sober socializing without the use of alcohol or drugs to hide social anxiety; dealing with employment problems and adjusting to the impact of being out as a gay person at work; working with the family of origin regarding their acceptance of the sexual orientation of their gay, lesbian, or bisexual child; helping couples adjust to the damaging effects substance use may have had over the years and embrace a recovery that will avoid the negative impact of codependent relationships; maintaining confidentiality in record keeping, especially around discussion in the medical record of sexual orientation or HIV status; dealing with child custody issues when necessary; diagnosing and treating additional medical problems; and coping with the effects of legal problems.

Clinicians and counselors must be aware of their own personal attitudes regarding homosexuality. If a health care provider is homophobic and cannot get help in working out these attitudes with a supportive colleague or supervisor, the patient would be better off if he or she was referred to another staff member for help (5). Gay men and women facing recovery from substance abuse should not have to fight homophobia in a health care system to get quality care.

CONCLUSION

Taking a culturally competent approach to working with GLB persons provides the best way to help those dealing with issues of substance use or abuse. The knowledge that substances and alcohol can play a significant role in the lives of many GLB people and that there is indeed a higher incidence of use and abuse can alert the provider to add a more intensive review of substance use history and the possible consequences of such use on a person's life when starting to work with a new client. Knowing that some drugs are more likely to be used in some populations—such as methamphetamines with urban gay men—will also help the provider gather information needed to determine the most helpful interventions and treatment planning.

Understanding the unique social issues many GLB people face can also help shape a treatment plan tailored to the client and improve outcomes. Recognizing the profound impact of homophobia and the developmental issues unique to most GLB people will also improve care and outcomes. The various types of treatments and interventions are not unique—12-step, motivational interviews, contingency management, pharmacology where appropriate, and so on—but the context in which such care is offered can be unique and very helpful. The gay-sensitive and gay-affirmative approaches are the most helpful and usually create a welcoming environment that helps the client address issues and work towards recovery. Openness and acceptance by the provider to all the issues facing GLB persons sets the frame for improved care.

Extended recovery is more likely to happen—indeed, may only be possible—if a gay man, lesbian, or bisexual person is able to accept his or her sexual orientation, address internalized homophobia, and discover how to live clean and sober without fearing or hating his or her real self. Providers less familiar with issues around differing sexual orientations will benefit from consultation with knowledgeable sources but may also wish to refer GLB clients to gay-specific service if available.

REFERENCES

1. King M, Semlyem J, Tai SS, et al. A systematic review of mental disorder, suicide, and deliberate self harm in lesbian, gay and bisexual people. *BMC Psychiatry.* 2008;8(Aug 18):70.
2. McCabe SE, Hughes TL, Bostwick WB, et al. Sexual orientation, substance use behaviors and substance dependence in the United States. *Addiction.* 2009;104(8):1333–1345.
3. Finnegan DG, McNally EB. *Dual Identities: Counseling Chemically Dependent Gay Men and Lesbians.* Center City, MN: Hazelden; 1987.
4. Meyer IH, Dietrich J, Schwartz S. Lifetime prevalence of mental disorders and suicide attempts in diverse lesbian, gay and bisexual populations. *Am J Public Health.* 2008;98(6):1004–1006.
5. Marshal MP, Friedman MS, Stall R, et al. Sexual orientation and adolescent substance use: a meta-analysis and methodological review. *Addition.* 2008;103(4):546–556.
6. Hatzenbuehler ML, Corbin WR, Fromme K. Trajectories and determinants of alcohol use among LGB young adults and their heterosexual peers: results from a prospective study. *Dev Psychol.* 2008;44(1):81–90.
7. Harawa NT, Williams JK, Ramamurthi HC, et al. Sexual behavior, sexual identity, and substance abuse among low-income bisexual and non-gay-identifying African American men who have sex with men. *Arch Sex Behav.* 2008;37(5):748–762.
8. Cochran SD, Mays VM, Alegria M, et al. Mental health and substance use disorders among Latino and Asian American lesbian, gay, and bisexual adults. *L Consult Clin Psychol.* 2007;75(5):785–794.
9. Wong CF, Kipke MD, Weiss G. Risk factors for alcohol use, frequent use, and binge drinking among young men who have sex with men. *Addict Behav.* 2008;33(8):1012–1020.
10. Bloomfield K. A comparison of alcohol consumption between lesbians and heterosexual women in an urban population. *Drug Alcohol Depend.* 1993;33(3):257–269.
11. Parks CA, Hughes TL, Kinnison KE. The relationship between early drinking contexts of women "coming out" as lesbian and current alcohol use. *J LGBT Health Res.* 2007;3(3):73–90.
12. Centers for Disease Control and Prevention. *HIV/AIDS Surveillance Report* 2007;19:1–61.
13. Skinner WF. The prevalence and demographic predictors of illicit and licit drug use among lesbians and gay men. *Am J Public Health.* 1994;84:1307–1310.
14. Halkitis PN, Solomon TM, Moeller RW, et al. Methamphetamine use among gay, bisexual and non-identified men-who-have-sex-with-men: an analysis of daily patterns. *J Health Psychol.* 2009;14(2):222–231.
15. Reback CJ, Shoptaw S, Grella CE. Methamphetamine use trends among street-recruited gay and bisexual males, from 1999 to 2007. *J Urban Health.* 2008;85(6):874–879.
16. Hooker E. The adjustment of the male overt homosexual. *J Proj Tech.* 1957;21(1):18–31.
17. Cabaj RP. Strike while the iron is hot: science, social forces, and ego-dystonic homosexuality. *J Gay Lesbian Mental Health.* 2009;13(2):87–93.
18. Marmor J, ed. *Homosexual Behavior: A Modern Reappraisal.* New York: Basic Books; 1980.
19. Morin SF. Heterosexual bias in psychological research on lesbianism and male homosexuality. *Am Psychol.* 1977;32:629–36.
20. Cabaj RP. Substance abuse in gay men, lesbians, and bisexual individuals. In: Cabaj RP, Stein TS, eds. *Homosexuality and Mental Health: A Comprehensive Review.* Washington, DC: American Psychiatric Press; 1996:783–799.
21. Guss JR, Drescher J, eds. *Addictions in the Gay and Lesbian Community.* New York: Huntington Medical Press; 2000.
22. Division 44/Committee on Lesbian, Gay, and Bisexual concerns joint task force on guidelines for psychotherapy with lesbian, gay and bisexual clients. *Am Psychol.* 2000;55(12):1440–1451.
23. Drescher J. A history of homosexuality and organized psychoanalysis. *J Am Acad Psychoanal Dyn Psychiatry.* 2008;36(3):443–460.
24. Kinsey AC, Pomeroy WB, Martin CE. *Sexual Behavior in the Human Male.* Philadelphia: WB Saunders; 1948.
25. Herdt G. Issues in the cross-cultural study of homosexuality. In: Cabaj RP, Stein TS, eds. *Homosexuality and Mental Health: A Comprehensive Review.* Washington, DC: American Psychiatric Press; 1996:65–82.
26. Pathela P, Hajat A, Schillinger J, et al. Discordance between sexual behavior and self-reported sexual identity: a population-based survey of New York City men. *An Int Med.* 2006;145:416–425.
27. Herek GM. Heterosexism and homophobia. In: Cabaj RP, Stein TS, eds. *Homosexuality and Mental Health: A Comprehensive Review.* Washington, DC: American Psychiatric Press; 1996:101–113.
28. Bell AP, Weinberg MS, Hammersmith SK. *Sexual Preference: Its Development in Men and Women.* Bloomington, IN: Indiana University Press; 1981.
29. Pillard RC. Homosexuality from a familial and genetic perspective. In: Cabaj RP, Stein TS, eds. *Homosexuality and Mental Health: A Comprehensive Review.* Washington, DC: American Psychiatric Press; 1996:115–128.
30. Byne W. Biology and homosexuality: implications of neuroendocrinological and neuroanatomical studies. In: Cabaj RP, Stein TS, eds. *Homosexuality and Mental Health: A Comprehensive Review.* Washington, DC: American Psychiatric Press; 1996:129–146.
31. Cass V. Sexual orientation identity formation: a Western phenomenon. In: Cabaj RP, Stein TS, eds. *Homosexuality and Mental Health: A Comprehensive Review.* Washington, DC: American Psychiatric Press; 1996:227–251.

32. Amadio DM. Internalized heterosexism, alcohol use, and alcohol-related problems among lesbians and gay men. *Addict Behav.* 2006;31:1153–1162.
33. Rotheram-Borus MJ, Rosario M, Reid H, et al. Predicting patterns of sexual acts among homosexual and bisexual youth. *Am J Psychiatry.* 1995;152(4):588–595.
34. Addis S, Davies M, Greene G, et al. The health, social care and housing needs of lesbian, gay, bisexual and transgender older people: a review of the literature. *Health Soc Care Community.* 2009;17(6):647–658.
35. Corliss HL, Grella CE, Mays VM, et al. Drug use, drug severity and help-seeking behaviors of lesbian and bisexual women. *J Womens Health.* 2006;15:555–568.
36. McKirman D, Peterson PL. Psychological and cultural factors in alcohol and drug abuse: an analysis of a homosexual community. *Addict Behav.* 1989;14:555–563.
37. Jerome RC, Halkitis PN, Siconolfi DE. Club drug use, sexual behavior, and HIV seroconversion: a qualitative study of motivations. *Subst Use Misuse.* 2009;44(3):431–447.
38. Halkitis PN, Jerome RC. A comparative analysis of methamphetamine use: black gay and bisexual men in relation to men of other races. *Addict Behav.* 2008;33(1):83–93.
39. Halkitis PN, Parsons JT, Stirratt MJ. A double epidemic: crystal methamphetamine drug use in relation to HIV transmission among gay men. *J Homosex.* 2001;41(2):17–35.
40. Choi KH, Operario D, Gregorich SE, et al. Substance use, substance choice, and unprotected anal intercourse among young Asian American and Pacific Islander men who have sex with men. *AIDS Educ Prev.* 2005;17:418–429.
41. Nemoto T, Operario D, Soma T. Risk behaviors of Filipino methamphetamine users in San Francisco: implications for prevention and treatment of drug use and HIV. *Public Health Rep.* 2002;117(suppl 1):S30–S38.
42. Mansergh G, Colfax GN, Marks G, et al. The Circuit Party Men's Health Survey: findings and implications for gay and bisexual men. *Am J Public Health.* 2001;91:953–958.
43. Mansergh G, Purcell DW, Stall R, et al. CDC consultation on methamphetamine use and sexual risk behavior for HIV/STD infection: summary and suggestions. *Public Health Rep.* 2006; 121:127–132.
44. Halkitis PN, Wilton L, Drescher J, eds. *Barebacking: Psychosocial and Public Health Approaches.* Binghamton, NY: Haworth Medical Press; 2006.
45. Mansergh G, Marks G, Colfax GN, et al. "Barebacking" in a diverse sample of men who have sex with men. *AIDS.* 2002;16:653–659.
46. Semple SJ, Zians J, Grant I, et al. Sexual compulsivity in a sample of HIV-positive methamphetamine-using gay and bisexual men. *AIDS Behav.* 2006;10:587–598.
47. Fisher DG, Malow R, Rosenberg R, et al. Recreational viagra use and sexual risk among drug abusing men. *Am J Infect Dis.* 2006; 2:107–114.
48. Cochran BN, Cauce AM. Characteristics of lesbian, gay, bisexual, and transgender individuals entering substance abuse treatment. *J Subst Abuse Treat.* 2006;30:135–146.
49. Shoptaw S, Reback CJ, Peck JA et al. Behavioral treatment approaches for methamphetamine dependence and HIV-related sexual risk behaviors among urban gay and bisexual men. *Drug Alcohol Depend.* 205;78:125–134.
50. Strona FV, McCright J, Hjord H, et al. The acceptability and feasibility of the Positive Reinforcement Opportunity Project, a community-based contingency management methamphetamine treatment program for gay and bisexual men in San Francisco. *J Psychoactive Drugs.* 2006;Suppl 3:377–383.
51. Cochran BN, Peavy KM, Cauce AM. Substance abuse treatment providers' explicit and implicit attitudes regarding sexual minorities. *J Homosex.* 2007;53(3):181–207.

CHAPTER 65 Incarcerated Populations

Timothy W. Kinlock ■ Michael S. Gordon ■ Robert P. Schwartz

INTRODUCTION

Substance abuse is a significant problem among individuals incarcerated in jails and prisons throughout the world. Substantial research evidence from many countries has indicated that jail and prison inmates have a higher prevalence of preincarceration substance abuse compared to the general population. This is particularly evident with regard to illicit opioids (primarily heroin), cocaine, and the abuse of multiple substances—patterns of substance abuse that are most closely associated with adverse health and criminogenic consequences. Some inmates continue to use substances during incarceration, and most such individuals do not receive substance abuse treatment while incarcerated or upon release. As a consequence, substance abuse either continues or resumes quickly after release to the community, placing such individuals at increased risk for death from drug overdose, human immunodeficiency virus (HIV), and hepatitis B and C infections, increased criminal activity, and reincarceration. Correctional health officials, treatment providers, and policy makers need innovative, effective, and cost-beneficial approaches to help inmates with substance abuse histories successfully transition to the community following release from incarceration.

The impact of substance abuse among inmates, both during incarceration and upon release to the community, is exacerbated by the large numbers of individuals imprisoned throughout the world. According to the latest available estimate of the number of persons incarcerated and the rate of incarceration in 218 countries (1), there were 9.8 million individuals incarcerated in prisons throughout the world, with the United States having the highest number of prisoners and the highest rate of incarceration. Furthermore, in 71% of these countries, prison populations have been increasing (1), and this trend is expected to continue (2). Because of these circumstances, it is crucial that effective interventions designed to address substance abuse be developed, implemented, and evaluated.

To understand the context in which the above topics are discussed, it is important to understand the distinction between jails and prisons, which is most pronounced in the United States. Jails typically hold individuals who are awaiting trial or sentencing or are serving shorter sentences for less serious offenses (typically less than 1 year). Prisons typically confine individuals who have been convicted of more serious crimes and thus are serving longer sentences.

This chapter begins with a discussion of the epidemiology of substance abuse among incarcerated populations. Next, prevention strategies are examined. This is followed by a discussion of the availability and effectiveness of various substance abuse treatment interventions for incarcerated individuals. Afterward, the focus of the chapter turns to sociocultural considerations and factors influencing substance use in this population. A discussion of special considerations for jail and prison inmates and overall conclusions, respectively, comprise the final sections of this chapter.

EPIDEMIOLOGY

Epidemiologic studies have consistently found a higher prevalence of substance use, abuse and/or dependence among jail and prison inmates than the general population (2–5). This has been the case independent of nationality, gender, the measure(s) used to assess an individual's consumption of substances (e.g., use, abuse, and/or dependence), and the criteria used to assess substance abuse and/or dependence. A recent nationwide study in the United States (5) reported that only 2% of the general U.S. population met standardized diagnostic criteria (DSM-IV) of drug abuse or dependence in the last 12 months compared with 52% of state inmates and 44% of federal prisoners in the year prior to incarceration.

One of the most comprehensive reports of the prevalence of substance abuse and dependence among incarcerated individuals, a review of 13 epidemiologic studies (4), involved 7563 prisoners (4293 men and 3270 women). Nine of the studies were conducted in the United States; two took place in Ireland, and one each in England and New Zealand. Each of these studies, published between 1988 and 2001, used standardized diagnostic criteria (four studies used DSM-III criteria, four other studies used DSM-IIIR criteria, and five others employed DSM-IV) and assessed substance abuse and dependence with regard to the year prior to incarceration. Results indicated that the prevalence of substance abuse and dependence varied considerably across the studies. The prevalence of alcohol abuse and dependence at prison entry ranged from 18% to 30% in men and from 10% to 24% in women. The corresponding findings for drug abuse and dependence ranged from 10% to 48% for men and from 30% to 60% in women. The authors noted that while both male and female prisoners displayed estimated prevalence rates of substance abuse and dependence that were higher than their counterparts in the general population, the discrepancy was even greater among women.

Furthermore, incarcerated individuals are also substantially more likely than the general population to have patterns of substance abuse that are most closely associated with adverse health and crime-related consequences, such as heroin and/or cocaine addiction and abuse of multiple substances (2,3). Long-term abuse of heroin, particularly by injection, along with abuse of multiple substances, strongly contributes to disproportionately high rates of HIV and hepatitis infection (2,3) as well as higher risk of death from overdose among newly released prisoners (3). Regarding the regular use of heroin, in the United States, recent studies have reported inmates' lifetime prevalences ranging from 12% to 15% (5,6). In each of these studies, regular use of heroin was defined as having used heroin once a week or more frequently for at least a month (5,6). An epidemiologic study of prisoners in England and Wales (7) found that 23% reported being dependent on heroin during the 4 weeks prior to prison entry. A similar study of new entrants to prisons in Italy (8) reported that 28% of prisoners indicated that they had used heroin on a daily basis at any time in their lives before the index incarceration. The comparable figure for use of heroin at least weekly was 33%.

Moreover, most epidemiologic studies of substance abuse among jail and prison inmates report on preincarceration behavior, either lifetime or the year prior to incarceration. Relatively few studies examine the prevalence of substance abuse during incarceration. A survey of male prisoners in England and Wales (9) found that 6% of these inmates reported acutely problematic use (defined as using cannabis more than once a day and/or any other drug four times per week or more) during incarceration compared with 65% in the year prior to prison entry. A review of studies of heroin-dependent prisoners in various European nations (10) reported that the percentage of such individuals who continue to inject during incarceration ranges from 16% to 60%, although a more recent report from Germany (11) indicated that 75% of injectors continued this behavior during incarceration. Estimates of the prevalence of in-prison drug use in the United States as detected by urine testing and hair testing were typically less than 10%, although one estimate reported 27% (12).

Finally, as emphasized below, most jail and prison inmates do not receive treatment for substance abuse, and without such treatment, jail and prison inmates are likely to return to drug abuse and crime shortly after return to the community (13,14), and rates of postrelease criminal activity among such individuals are very high (13). Among incarcerated individuals, those with preincarceration heroin addiction typically become re-addicted within a month of release from incarceration (14). Because of these circumstances, as well as the increased threat of HIV and hepatitis infection and overdose death, treatment interventions that begin during incarceration and continue in the community are urgently needed for such individuals (3,14,15).

PREVENTION

Prevention strategies can be classified in three different ways. Primary prevention involves prevention of new onset drug use, secondary prevention intends to prevent the progression from drug use to symptomatic drug abuse or dependence, and tertiary prevention is concerned with reducing the adverse consequences for those with drug abuse or dependence (16). Ideally, given that substance abuse is a major contributor to suicide, criminal behavior, injuries, overdose death, and many types of infectious disease, perhaps the most promising approach would involve preventing the onset of use in childhood or early adolescence through a combination of interventions including those that enhance protective factors and reduce risk factors, as well as regulatory approaches (16). Examples of the former type of intervention would involve collaboration among parents, educators, physicians, and community leaders, whereas the latter strategy would include laws, policies, and enforcement to reduce supply and demand. These interventions have also been shown to prevent or at least delay the onset of delinquent and criminal activity as well, thus substantially reducing the risk for incarceration (16). However, many such interventions involving enhancement of protective factors and reduction of risk factors have not been evaluated in real-world settings (16). Moreover, a recent nationwide survey conducted in the United States indicated that teachers often do not have adequate time to provide such interventions, and parents' priorities have focused on economic concerns and survival, limiting their ability to devote sufficient time and energy to substance abuse prevention initiatives (17). Furthermore, given that over 80% of incarcerated individuals in both Great Britain (18) and the United States (5) and well over half of such individuals overall in the European Union (19) have been estimated to have a history of illicit drug *use*, in addition to the high prevalence of substance *abuse* reported above, perhaps the most feasible prevention strategy would involve harm reduction—decreasing the risk for life-threatening consequences (3)—more in line with tertiary prevention approaches defined above (16).

Among the most frequent and severe consequences resulting from drug abuse, specifically drug injection, in prison, are HIV and viral hepatitis infections (2,3). Increased risk of these diseases among prisoners has been documented in 16 countries, with injecting drugs and sharing injection equipment being major contributors to such circumstances (3). Unfortunately, most nations do not have adequate prevention services for incarcerated persons despite the fact that the Council of Europe and the World Health Organization have developed guidelines emphasizing that inmates have the right to the same prevention and treatment services to those available in the community (3). Furthermore, corrections officials at times have denied that substance use and drug injection occur in their facilities, and this circumstance, together with budgetary constraints and overcrowding, can contribute to the lack of services for infection prevention (3).

Harm reduction services include the provision of information and education with regard to drug-related disease, voluntary testing and counseling concerning HIV and hepatitis, and interventions designed to reduce risky sexual and injection-related behaviors (20). Such procedures have been implemented in several European nations, Canada, and

Australia (20). A major harm reduction intervention targeted toward reducing HIV and hepatitis infections in prison are needle exchange programs. Only a small number of countries have implemented these programs, starting with Switzerland in 1992 (3). A review of the literature on the effectiveness of prison-based needle exchange programs reported that they have substantially reduced the sharing of injection equipment, with no increases in injecting or drug use (21).

TREATMENT

Challenges to Implementation and Evaluation

Prisons and jails provide a significant opportunity to enlist individuals with histories of substance dependence into treatment (3,4,15). The provision of effective treatment in correctional settings has the opportunity to not only reduce the health- and crime-related impact of substance abuse postrelease, but also has the potential of decreasing the frequency and severity of facility management problems as more inmates become enrolled in treatment (3). However, in many countries, scarce resources are devoted to substance abuse treatment in correctional facilities, where security is the primary concern (3). Security concerns are increased when inmates need to be moved to different areas of the facility for treatment, and some corrections personnel may be opposed to certain types of treatment, particularly opioid agonist therapy, particularly in the United States (3,14,15). As a consequence, many incarcerated individuals with histories of substance abuse do not receive treatment, and the range of modalities offered is often quite limited. For example, in the United States, less than 20% of inmates with substance abuse histories receive treatment during incarceration (5,6), with drug education being the most common service provided (15). Furthermore, while the results of a recent survey of correctional programs and organizations in the United States indicated that most correctional agencies provide some type of substance abuse treatment, the median proportion of offenders with access to such treatment at any given time is under 10% (22).

Another challenge to the development, implementation, and evaluation of new correctional substance abuse treatment programs involves the different priorities, agendas, and beliefs about inmates on the part of treatment personnel and correctional employees (14,15). Treatment staff tend to view inmates with substance abuse histories as persons with some type of illness who are in need of help. In contrast, correctional personnel may view such inmates as individuals in need of punishment and control. Thus, establishing and maintaining new programs resulting from recent justice system/treatment collaborations has been challenging. Progress in this regard has been slow and gradual over the past several decades in creating novel initiatives that combine criminal sanctions with rehabilitation, such as residential drug-abuse treatment programs for incarcerated individuals and corrections-based therapy, including opioid agonist therapy, for inmates with opioid addiction histories (14). Ongoing cooperation among diverse correctional, treatment, and research organizations is crucial for such new programs to operate continuously. Sufficient jurisdictional and/or correctional funding is also needed for the continuous operation of new substance abuse treatment programs (3).

It also needs to be emphasized that, given the diversity among incarcerated individuals with substance abuse histories with regard to severity of addiction, criminality, psychological functioning, and other relevant dimensions, a single approach is not likely to be effective for all individuals. Therefore, a persistent challenge to treatment providers, corrections officials, and researchers, has been to determine what types of treatment work best for what types of individuals. While this question has dominated the substance abuse treatment field for many years, achieving progress has been slow (4,14).

Furthermore, many correctional substance abuse treatment programs have never been rigorously evaluated, and most published reports on the effectiveness of substance abuse treatment for incarcerated populations are anecdotal and descriptive (14). Meta-analyses of correctional substance abuse treatment have consistently reported that most studies have major methodologic problems (23–25). Caution is advised in interpreting the results of a number of evaluations of substance abuse interventions because of limitations such as short postrelease follow-up periods, low postrelease assessment rates, infrequent use of comparison groups, multivariate methods, standardized assessment instruments, and appropriate control variables (14,26). Nevertheless, there have been some well-controlled studies of corrections-based substance abuse treatment which are discussed below.

Modalities

Therapeutic Community (TC)

The therapeutic community (TC) modality in a correctional setting operates on the premise that inmates with long histories of severe substance abuse must change their attitudes and thinking patterns to reduce the influences of lifestyles condoning violence, manipulation, and irresponsibility found in the prison environment (26). Because of these circumstances, inmates in TC treatment reside apart from other inmates in order to minimize such negative influences and to develop a sense of community in which the community members themselves serve as therapeutic agents. Inmates residing in the TC rely on their group leader, typically a recovering person, and peers to provide rewards and sanctions. TC members support and reward abstinence from substance abuse and crime and the adoption and maintenance of prosocial attitudes and values. Confrontation and sanctions are employed as a response to negative behaviors and positive feedback is employed as a response to positive behaviors.

There are challenges to the implementation and operation of TCs in the correctional setting (3,14). Similar to other substance abuse treatment programs conducted within prisons and jails, TCs require strong, consistent commitment to the program on the part of correctional administrators and staff. Furthermore, a considerable amount of space within the facility needs to be devoted to provide TC members with housing, food service, and rooms to conduct group treatment sessions. As a result, TCs can be expensive to operate.

In their 1999 meta-analysis, Pearson and Lipton (23) concluded that there was evidence of effectiveness of in-prison treatment in terms of reducing readdiction and/or crime only for a TC approach, while rigorous research regarding other approaches was either insufficient and/or of poor methodologic quality to allow for firm conclusions regarding their effectiveness. More recently, Mitchell, Wilson, and MacKenzie (25), in a 2007 meta-analysis of 66 evaluations of incarceration-based treatment, 58 of which were conducted in the United States, found that the most consistent evidence with regard to reducing both postrelease criminal recidivism and relapse to drug use came from evaluations of TC programs, and that this result was robust to variations in method, sample, and program features. However, the positive effects of correctional TC treatment may be much smaller without the provision of postrelease aftercare (3,23,27).

There is evidence that offenders who receive a three-stage TC approach administered in a U.S. prison, in work release during the transition from the institution to the community, and in combination with aftercare involving outpatient individual counseling, group therapy, and reinforcement sessions had lower rates of postrelease relapse to drug use and criminal recidivism at 5 years postrelease than offenders who receive little or no treatment (26). Other long-term, methodologically rigorous follow-up studies conducted in the United States using comparison or control groups have reported similar results for incarceration-based TC treatment followed by community-based aftercare (27,28).

Among the most comprehensive evaluations of TC results was the one conducted by Inciardi and colleagues (26). In this study, 60-month postrelease outcomes were examined. Consistent with previous research involving 18- and 42-month postrelease follow-up periods, this long-term evaluation employed multivariate methods and multiple outcome measures. In addition, the two main outcome variables, drug-free and arrest-free status, were conservatively defined. In order to be determined drug-free, the respondent must have reported no drug use and have tested negative for drug use according to urine screening at each follow-up point. Similarly, the criteria for arrest-free status involved no self-report of arrest along with no official arrest records for new offenses since release from incarceration. Findings showed that treatment participation was a major predictor of both drug-free and arrest-free status. More specifically, examination of four comparison groups of research participants indicated that individuals who had completed prison treatment and had received aftercare were most likely to be both drug-free and arrest-free. Individuals who had completed prison treatment without aftercare had the second best outcomes, followed by those who were TC treatment dropouts. Individuals with no treatment were least likely to be both drug-free and arrest-free. While the authors noted that their results were somewhat limited in that major control and confounding variables were not modeled and differences between voluntary versus mandatory supervision were not addressed, they concluded that the findings provide evidence for the value of providing a continuum of care from incarceration to aftercare in the community. Specifically, the transitional programming provided in this intervention served as a critical bridge spanning the prison and re-entry into society by offering assistance for reducing the many psychological, social, and legal barriers that lead to greater vulnerability for relapse to substance dependence and criminal recidivism among newly released inmates.

Similarly, another of the most rigorously conducted evaluations of TC treatment involved a 5-year postrelease follow-up of 715 male prison inmates who were randomly assigned to either TC treatment or a control (no treatment) condition (27). Results of this study, conducted by Prendergast and colleagues in the United States (27), found that while over 75% of the sample had been reincarcerated, inmates assigned to the TC group had significantly lower reincarceration rates than controls, with no group differences reported for relapse to heavy drug use. Prendergast et al. also found that completion of prison treatment followed by aftercare was significantly associated with reduced rates of reincarceration, but was not related to reductions in relapse to heavy drug use.

Cognitive–Behavioral Interventions

Because of the influence of substance-abusing peers and the multiple demands of housing, legitimate employment, and family are significantly diminished during incarceration, greater opportunity exists for focused, comprehensive treatment that intends to change patterns of behavior, thinking, and feeling that contribute to substance abuse and criminality. Some clinicians and researchers have contended that cognitive–behavioral treatment programs are among the most promising for reducing relapse to substance abuse and criminal recidivism because they focus on internal client factors and predispositions contributing to deviant behavior. Furthermore, cognitive–behavioral interventions are less expensive than therapeutic communities to operate as they place fewer demands on correctional staff and require less space.

Although cognitive–behavioral programs have been widely used throughout the world for over two decades, they have been subject to relatively few controlled evaluations (23–25).

Pearson and Lipton (23), in their 1999 meta-analysis of correctional substance abuse treatment, mentioned above, noted that although cognitive–behavioral approaches showed some favorable results with both offenders and substance abusers in general, very few rigorous evaluations had been conducted with incarcerated substance abusers. Subsequently, in a meta-analysis of 69 evaluations of corrections-based cognitive–behavioral treatment, Pearson et al. (24) reported that such treatment was generally superior to standard correctional programming in reducing re-arrest. However, these authors rated the methodologic rigor of 45 (65%) of these studies as either "poor" or "fair," pointing out the lack of specific details regarding the training and supervision of treatment staff, frequency of sessions, and treatment program duration. Furthermore, there were far more evaluations of the impact of corrections-based cognitive–behavioral treatment on postrelease arrest and reincarceration than on postrelease substance abuse (24,29).

Among the few more methodologically rigorous evaluations of prison-based cognitive–behavioral treatment was a multisite evaluation involving over 2000 inmates (30). Three-year postrelease outcomes, analyzed separately for men and women, indicated that while both male and female program participants had lower rates of re-arrest and drug use than their counterparts in the comparison group, the findings were only significant for males. Subsequently, a 1-year postrelease analysis of a cognitive–behavioral treatment program for women prisoners found that treated women had significantly less drug use and arrests than a comparison group (31).

Boot Camps

Boot camp programs, which primarily operate in the United States, are highly structured and are patterned after military basic training. They involve vigorous exercise (including obstacle courses), military drill, ceremony, and discipline. Inmates are required to wear uniforms and are subject to confrontation and sanctions on the part of drill instructors for rule violations. Proponents of boot camps claim that such interventions instill self-discipline needed to avoid relapse to substance abuse and criminal recidivism. Pearson and Lipton (23) and Mitchell et al. (25), in meta-analyses of correctional substance abuse treatment programs mentioned above, found no evidence for the effectiveness of boot camp programs with regard to reducing substance use and criminal recidivism.

Opioid Agonist Maintenance

The use of opioid agonists such as methadone and buprenorphine for the treatment of opioid dependence in the community is among the most rigorously and frequently studied of all the drug-abuse treatment modalities (32). These medications have been found effective in numerous randomized controlled trials (32) and are on the World Health Organization's list of essential medications because of their extensively documented ability to reduce heroin use and HIV-risk behaviors (33). These medications act by occupying the opioid receptor and blocking the euphoric effects of self-administered heroin or other opioids (32). Forty years of research evidence in community-based settings throughout the world has found that opioid agonist therapy, primarily involving the provision of methadone maintenance, is highly effective in reducing heroin addiction, criminal activity, and HIV-related risk behavior (3,14,32,34). In addition, methadone maintenance treatment has been found superior to other types of substance abuse treatment in retaining patients in treatment (14,32). Treatment retention is crucial to successful treatment outcome; research results have consistently reported that regardless of modality, greater treatment duration is related to reduced substance abuse and crime (14).

However, despite its effectiveness, opioid agonist maintenance treatment is underutilized in jail and prison settings, particularly in the United States (14,15). In contrast to the United States, a number of other countries have routinely offered it to incarcerated populations, including nearly all nations in the European Union, Canada, and Australia (34). In jails, opioid agonists can be used to detoxify newly incarcerated inmates from dependence on heroin or prescription opioids, to maintain methadone or buprenorphine patients whose treatment is interrupted by incarceration, or can be started and maintained for individuals in opioid withdrawal in order to link them to community-based treatment upon release. In prisons, it can be used to treat ongoing drug dependence (as it would be used in the community) or as a re-entry strategy. These aspects of corrections-based opioid agonist treatment are described below in more detail.

Jail-Based Agonist Treatment

a. *Detoxification*: Jails bear the brunt of dealing with opioid withdrawal of newly incarcerated individuals. While there are many methods of providing opioid detoxification, methadone is a low-cost medication that is highly effective in resolving withdrawal symptoms. Detoxification with methadone while medically appropriate, humane, and preferred by some inmates (as compared to maintenance) is not highly effective in keeping individuals from relapsing upon release and does expose re-entering prisoners to the heightened risk of overdose death upon resumption of heroin use postrelease (34).

b. *Initiating maintenance therapy upon incarceration*: An alternative to detoxification for newly incarcerated inmates who are opioid dependent is to initiate and continue maintenance therapy and then connect patients to community-based treatment upon release. This has been the practice at few facilities in the United States. The Rikers Island jail program in New York City has been in continuous operation since 1987, and treatment in this program has been found to facilitate community-based treatment entry as well as to reduce reincarceration (35,36). It has been estimated that the Rikers Island facility provides methadone maintenance and/or detoxification to over 4000 inmates annually (37). The rate of continuation in the community with this approach has been reported to be 75% (37). It is important to have arrangements with community-based providers to accept released individuals seamlessly (3). For those individuals who receive prison sentences and must be transferred to a facility which does not have the capability of providing opioid agonist therapy, a gradual dose taper is appropriate.

With the availability of buprenorphine, there is now a choice between methadone and buprenorphine for this purpose. There has been one study comparing the two medications initiated in a jail recently conducted by Magura and colleagues in the Rikers Island jail in New York City (38). Results showed that patients started on buprenorphine as compared to methadone while in opioid withdrawal at the start of their incarceration were more likely to enter and remain in community-based treatment at 3 months postrelease although the rates of self-reported measures of relapse to drug use, re-arrest, reincarceration, and severity of crime committed did not differ between the two groups.

c. *Maintaining existing patients*: It is crucial that jail inmates who were on methadone or buprenorphine treatment just prior to incarceration in the community be maintained on their medication, as they would be if they were on any other medication. Should they be released from jail, arrangements need to be made to return them to their treating clinician or clinic. Should they receive a long incarceration sentence and need to be transferred to a prison without opioid agonist treatment capability, they should be gradually tapered off medication over the course of a few weeks (depending on their dosage). This is the standard practice at Rikers Island.

d. *Initiating maintenance therapy postdetoxification*: Some individuals who are detoxified at the start of their incarceration may wish to resume methadone or buprenorphine treatment prior to release to permit re-entry to community-based treatment and to prevent relapse to heroin use and overdose death. Dole et al. (39) studied just such an approach in New York City in a randomized trial in which 12 inmates were started on methadone approximately 10 days before release. At 7 to 10 months postrelease, these 12 inmates had lower rates of readdiction and reincarceration than 16 untreated controls. Because the patients had previously undergone detoxification while incarcerated and had lost tolerance to opioids, Dole started patients at a low dose (10 mg) and gradually increased the dose to a target of 35 mg over the course of 10 days. Patients who are initiated in this manner need to be carefully monitored by medical and nursing staff for oversedation and constipation and the dosage reduced and/or the dose increase schedule slowed as necessary. There have been no published studies to date of such an approach with buprenorphine, although the present authors are conducting a randomized clinical trial study in a prerelease prison with buprenorphine.

Prison-Based Agonist Treatment

In prisons in which there is a relatively high rate of illicit opioid use, prison-based agonist treatment can be used in a manner similar to opioid agonist treatment in the community. For example, in Puerto Rico, in a study using buprenorphine–naloxone, such an intervention was found to be feasible and facilitated community-based postrelease treatment entry (40). Similarly in France, there have been reports of prison-based buprenorphine maintenance treatment, found to be effective in reducing heroin use and reincarceration (41). Perhaps the most rigorously evaluated of these programs has been the one that began in a prerelease prison in Australia in 1986 by the New South Wales Department of Correction for inmates with heroin dependence. Over 80% of participants either reported using heroin in prison a month before study entry and/or had morphine-positive hair test results upon admission to the study. Methadone maintenance began at 30 mg with 5 mg increases every five days until 60 mg was achieved. A randomized controlled trial of this methadone program compared to the wait-list for the prison program indicated that heroin use was lower among treated inmates during a 4-month, in-prison follow-up (42). At 4-year follow-up, greater treatment duration was associated with decreased mortality, reincarceration, and hepatitis C infection (43). Regarding mortality, no participants died while actively enrolled in methadone maintenance treatment, while 17 died while out of treatment. The risk of reincarceration was lowest during periods of methadone treatment lasting 8 months or longer, although methadone maintenance treatment of 2 months or less was associated with the highest risk of reincarceration (43).

However, there are circumstances in which inmates would have met the criteria of opioid agonist treatment prior to their index incarceration but who have been completely or largely abstinent from heroin use while in a controlled environment. These individuals may be at high risk of relapse upon release to the community and may wish to be on agonist treatment prior to re-entry. They may have had the experience of relapsing to heroin use every time they were released from prison or jail and not wish to repeat the same outcome. Since they are no longer tolerant to opioids, it is essential that such individuals be started at low doses of opioids (e.g., 5 mg of methadone or 1 mg of buprenorphine). Dose induction should proceed more slowly (especially at the lower doses) than for tolerant patients, in our experience at 5 mg of methadone or 1 mg of buprenorphine per week.

To our knowledge, there has been only one randomized controlled trial of this type of prerelease methadone treatment fashioned on the study by Dole et al. (39) in the prerelease jail.

The present authors conducted the first randomized clinical trial in the United States to examine the effectiveness of prison- (as opposed to jail-) initiated methadone treatment.

It was undertaken to examine the extent to which beginning methadone maintenance in prison prior to release with continued treatment in the community would be more effective than initiating methadone maintenance in the community or providing counseling only in prison with passive referral to community treatment upon release. Participants met criteria for methadone maintenance in the community for the year prior to their incarceration. They were started at 5 mg methadone daily for the first week and doses were increased in 5 mg increments weekly until a target of 60 mg was achieved.

Short-term results at 1 and 3 months postrelease (44,45) and longer-term findings at 6 months postrelease (46) found that prison-initiated and community-initiated methadone treatment were more effective than counseling only regarding heroin use and treatment entry. Subsequent results at 12 months postrelease (47) found that prison-initiated

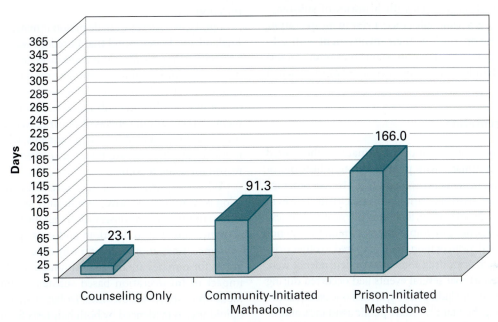

Figure 65.1. Mean days in community-based substance abuse treatment, 12 months postrelease. (Data from Kinlock TW, Gordon MS, Schwartz RP, et al. A randomized clinical trial of methadone maintenance for prisoners: results at 12-months postrelease. *J Subst Abuse Treat.* 2009;37:277–285.)

methadone had superior outcomes to the other two treatment conditions with regard to community-based treatment duration (see Fig. 65.1) and heroin use. Regarding self-reported crime and any reincarcerations, outcomes favored prison-initiated methadone compared to counseling only at 3 months postrelease. Results at 6 months postrelease regarding the number of days of self-reported crime also favored prison-initiated methadone over counseling only, although there were no group differences concerning the number of days reincarcerated. However, no differences among treatment conditions were found at 12 months postrelease on either the number of days of self-reported crime or the percentage of participants arrested.

SOCIOCULTURAL CONSIDERATIONS

It is strongly recommended that interventions for incarcerated individuals be tailored to the inmates' specific sociocultural needs. Individual characteristics of inmates may influence drug-use behavior and therefore the types of interventions that may be most promising for reducing drug use and its disastrous public health and public safety consequences (2–4,14). Ideally, all services to be provided to incarcerated populations need to be based on an assessment of individual inmate needs (3,4,15). The greater prevalence of substance abuse among women than men, both overall and compared to their counterparts in the general population, suggests that the gender of the inmate be one dimension that needs to be strongly considered in the development of appropriate interventions for inmates with histories of drug abuse (4). In addition to gender, nationality, ethnicity, and rural/urban status are likely to be factors that have a bearing on one's pattern of drug use and thus the type(s) of treatment that may be most appropriate (2).

In addition, many individuals enter jails and prisons with poor health in addition to drug abuse, often brought on by socioeconomic conditions such as unsanitary living conditions and lack of access to affordable health care (20). These circumstances are typically exacerbated by the prison environment, where overcrowding, poor nutrition, and poor ventilation are commonplace along with violence, unprotected sex, and drug use and injection (2,20). These circumstances, in turn, can lead to the development of many infectious diseases, including HIV and hepatitis (20).

Furthermore, individual inmate differences in response to various types of drug-abuse treatment interventions have not been frequently reported (14). Because there are considerable individual differences among inmates with histories of drug abuse with respect to criminality, psychological functioning, and motivation for treatment (14), as well as types of drugs abused and route of injection (9), among other factors, a single treatment modality is not likely to be effective for all inmates with drug-abuse histories. Moreover, research on the processes of matching inmate needs with treatments needs to be significantly improved, and all too often funds are not available for services to be delivered (14). Because the failure to adequately match inmates to interventions could result in increased substance abuse and its attendant health- and crime-related consequences, funding appropriate services and assessment needs to be emphasized (14).

FACTORS INFLUENCING SUBSTANCE ABUSE

Since incarcerated individuals with histories of substance abuse typically begin using substances prior to incarceration, and many relapse or continue their involvement with substances following release, it is important to examine factors influencing such individuals' substance abuse during each of these periods.

Prior to Incarceration

A recent nationwide survey of prison inmates in the United States found that inmates with preincarceration histories of drug abuse and/or dependence were more likely than other inmates to report experiencing various adverse circumstances in their lives prior to incarceration, including physical and/or sexual abuse, homelessness, unemployment, parental substance abuse, and parental incarceration (5). Compared to other prisoners, inmates with prior drug abuse and/or dependence were more likely to report that several events had occurred during their formative years, including having at least one parent abuse substances, having their family receive public assistance, and/or having lived in a single-parent household. While the inmates were not asked whether any or all of the adverse circumstances they experienced prior to incarceration had caused the onset or continuation of substance abuse, previous research has established that these factors are among the antecedents of substance abuse and dependence (16).

Furthermore, Borrill et al. (48), in a survey of female prisoners in England and Wales, compared the backgrounds of inmates who had been drug dependent prior to incarceration with that of other inmates. Prisoners who had been drug dependent were significantly more likely than other prisoners to report dropping out of school during their formative years as well as being unemployed in the year prior to incarceration. Prisoners with drug-dependence histories were also significantly more likely than other prisoners to report experiencing or witnessing a physical assault at some point in their lives prior to incarceration. Similarly, inmates with prior drug dependence were significantly more likely than other prisoners to have experienced unwanted sexual contact, including sexual assault. While prisoners were not asked directly if these events had led to their substance abuse, such factors have been frequently identified by previous research as antecedents of substance abuse (16).

During Incarceration

Relatively few studies have examined the factors contributing to the use of substances during incarceration. A review of the literature by Dolan et al. (3) reported that the prison environment has a significant impact on inmate substance use and abuse in that corrections officials continually attempt to stop drugs from entering the prison, which often leads to inmates stopping or reducing use. However, these authors also reported that placing so many offenders with preincarceration substance abuse histories in close proximity with one another with little constructive activity often leads to boredom, which, in turn, increases the likelihood of substance use, including injection (3).

Similarly, a survey of male prison inmates incarcerated in England and Wales found that boredom was a major reason why the inmates used various substances, including cannabis, heroin, and/or tranquilizers (9). The need for relaxation was another frequently cited reason as to why the inmates used one or more of the three substances mentioned above. Enjoyment and the calming effects of the drug were additional reasons inmates provided for using cannabis, whereas the need to block out their situation was also given as an important reason for using heroin.

While the prevalence of substance abuse during incarceration is, as indicated above, significantly less than that found in the community, the observation that the lack of productive activities can lead to boredom and subsequently to inmate substance use is another reason why effective treatment programs for inmates are needed. Although most studies of the impact of incarceration-based substance abuse treatment focus on postrelease outcomes, Dolan et al. found that illicit opioid use, as evidenced by both hair tests for morphine and self-reported heroin use, was lower at 4-month during-prison follow-up among methadone maintenance patients than untreated controls (42). Furthermore, treated participants reported significantly lower rates of drug injection and syringe sharing at follow-up. However, no group differences with regard to incidence of HIV or hepatitis C infections were found.

Following Release to the Community

It has been well documented that upon release from incarceration, individuals with histories of substance abuse typically experience multiple stressors that substantially increase their risk of relapse (14,15,26,28). Prominent among these factors are the need for stable housing and legitimate employment (14,15,26), the stigma of being labeled an ex-offender (15), poor or conflictual relationships with family members (14,26), and meeting multiple requirements regarding criminal justice supervision (14,15). In the United States, the escalation of parole and probation caseloads has made it increasingly difficult for parole and probation agents to effectively monitor and supervise their clients' behavior (14). Finally, as indicated previously, most newly released inmates do not receive drug-abuse treatment upon re-entry to the community.

Furthermore, many newly released inmates return to neighborhoods where drug abuse is rampant (15). Such individuals frequently encounter friends, neighbors, former drug business associates, and/or family members who are drug dependent and often pressure or otherwise encourage the former inmate to relapse (49). Such areas generally lack opportunities for legitimate employment as well (49).

In addition, there are neurobiologic factors associated with such environments that strongly influence the likelihood of relapse (15). Considerable research evidence indicates that addiction is a chronic brain disease greatly influenced by both genetic and environmental factors (15). Repeated exposure to drugs in persons who are vulnerable as a result of genetic and/or individual factors leads to neuroadaptations in the brain that, in turn, lead to compulsive drug use and loss of control over behaviors related to drugs (15). Because environments in which many newly released prisoners with prior substance abuse return typically serve as triggers or cues for the individual to use drugs, the individual's reward/motivational processes are activated, leading to intense desires or cravings for drug use (15).

SPECIAL CONSIDERATIONS

Given the multiple stressors facing newly released inmates with substance abuse histories upon return to the community, as well as the high rates of relapse involved, it is crucial that jail- and prison-based treatment programs provide a continuum of care in the community (3,14,15,26,27,45,46). As emphasized above, the benefits of incarceration-based treatment are greatly enhanced by the provision of community-based aftercare. Perhaps the most promising programs for reducing relapse and recidivism may be corrections-treatment partnerships in which a single treatment team or primary counselor takes primary responsibility for provision of services, both during incarceration and in the community (26).

However, successfully developing and implementing such programs, independent of the modality involved, is a very challenging task because it involves frequent collaboration between various agencies (corrections and substance abuse treatment) with different, and often conflicting, priorities and agenda (3,14,15). It is helpful in this regard to first conduct a pilot, or exploratory study to alleviate interagency tensions and develop feasible procedures (14). It is strongly recommended that both treatment and corrections staff be equally involved in planning the intervention, with responsibilities of various agency personnel specified in advance. In addition, differences with respect to logistics and space need to be reconciled so that treatment procedures do not interfere with routine security and other procedures in the jail or prison.

CONCLUSIONS

From the above, there is considerable research evidence to indicate that jail and prison inmates have substantially higher rates of substance abuse than the general population. This is particularly evident with regard to patterns of use found to be most closely associated with adverse health- and crime-related consequences, such as addiction to opioids (primarily heroin), cocaine, and/or multiple substances, as well as drug injection. While substance abuse tends to be more frequent prior to incarceration than during incarceration, substance use, including injection, is not uncommon in jails and prisons. Unfortunately, most inmates with substance abuse histories do not receive treatment while incarcerated, and either relapse or continue substance abuse upon release, greatly increasing the likelihood of HIV and hepatitis infections, overdose death, criminal activity, and reincarceration.

As documented previously, there are a number of treatment interventions that can be effective in reducing substance use and its attendant health and criminogenic effects for incarcerated individuals. However, it is important to recognize that the benefits of incarceration-based substance abuse treatment may diminish following release to the community. Therefore, it is advised that a continuum of treatment spanning incarceration and the community be implemented to further help interrupt the pernicious cycle of relapse, recidivism, and reincarceration.

Furthermore, one of the effective treatment interventions reviewed herein, opioid agonist maintenance, is underutilized in jail and prison settings. Consistent with the recommendations of others (3,15,34,37), expanding the availability of such treatment in prisons and jails has several potential benefits, including reduction of heroin use and injection in facilities where such behaviors are common, alleviating withdrawal symptoms among newly arrived, opioid-dependent inmates, and reducing readdiction, transmission of blood-borne viruses, and overdose death following release. Therefore, in keeping with the longstanding positions of the World Health Organization (3) and the National Institutes of Health (37), we recommend that opioid agonist treatment be expanded in correctional settings.

It also needs to be emphasized that achieving long-term recovery from substance abuse for incarcerated persons is an exceptionally challenging endeavor. As Latessa (50) noted, "for those who have tried to lose weight, quit smoking, eat fewer sweets, or exercise more, it is not easy" (p. 548). Latessa went on to say that researchers often like to present their findings as logical reasons for behavioral change. However, he remarked that when one observes that 80% is the median rate for noncompliance with recommended health care practices by health care professionals, researchers' expectations that their results alone can convince inmates to change and correctional agencies to support their research agendas is too simplistic. Therefore, researchers need to make their findings understandable in a manner that assists potential clients and practitioners understand the value of the results and their potential benefits (50). Similarly, it is well documented that even in interventions where there is considerable research evidence for effectiveness in reducing relapse and recidivism, many clients continue to experience periods of relapse and recovery following the end of a treatment episode (14). The presence of such circumstances provides additional support for Latessa's contention that positive behavioral changes result from hard work and occur in small increments.

Another challenge to the successful development and implementation of effective and innovative incarceration-based substance abuse treatment programs is that agencies with different and sometimes conflicting priorities and agenda need to be in constant collaboration (14,15). It is crucial that both treatment and corrections staff establish and maintain an equal partnership with regard to planning the intervention, with responsibilities of various agency staff defined in advance. Furthermore, potential conflicts concerning logistics and the allocation of space for treatment-related activities need to be reconciled so that intervention procedures do not interfere with routine security and other procedures in the jail or prison.

Moreover, both correctional and treatment personnel need to recognize individual diversity among jail and prison inmates with histories of substance abuse (3,14,15). It needs to be emphasized to practitioners, administrators, and policy makers, that no single intervention is effective for all clients. In view of the observation that failure to adequately match inmates to interventions may lead to increased substance abuse and its attendant health- and crime-related consequences, funding appropriate services and assessment needs to be emphasized (3,4,14,15).

Finally, the urgency of the need to provide effective substance abuse treatment to jail and prison inmates with histories of substance abuse needs to be emphasized. As documented earlier, without such treatment, the lives of not only the newly released inmates themselves, but also those of others are threatened given the increased likelihood of relapse, primarily to heroin and/or cocaine addition and drug injection, patterns of use associated with overdose death and exposure to HIV and hepatitis infections. In addition to adverse health consequences, there are also public safety consequences in that relapse to the above-mentioned substance abuse patterns are related to an increase in the frequency of criminal behavior. These circumstances are exacerbated by the observation that increases in the worldwide prison population are expected to continue (1,2).

REFERENCES

1. Walmsley R. *World Prison Population List.* 8th ed. King's College, London: International Centre for Prison Studies; 2009.
2. Kanato M. Drug use and health among prison inmates. *Curr Opin Psychiatry.* 2008;21:252–254.
3. Dolan K, Khoei EM, Brentari C, et al. *Prisons and Drugs: A Global Review of Incarceration, Drug Use and Drug Services.* Report 12. Oxford: Beckley Foundation; 2007.
4. Fazel S, Bains P, Doll H. Substance abuse and dependence in prisoners: a systematic review. *Addiction.* 2008;101:181–191.
5. Mumola CJ, Karberg JC. *Drug Use and Dependence, State and Federal Prisoners, 2004.* (NCJ 213530). Washington: U.S. Department of Justice, Bureau of Justice Statistics; 2006.
6. Karberg JC, James J. *Substance Dependence, Abuse, and Treatment of Jail Inmates, 2002.* (NCJ 209588). Washington: U.S. Department of Justice, Bureau of Justice Statistics; 2005.
7. Stewart D. Drug use and perceived treatment need among newly sentenced prisoners in England and Wales. *Addiction.* 2008;104:243–247.
8. Rezza G, Scalia Tomba G, Martucci P, et al. Prevalence of the use of old and new drugs among entrants in Italian prisons. *Ann 1st Super Sanita.* 2005;41:239–245.
9. Bullock T. Changing levels of drug use before, during, and after imprisonment. In: Ramsay M, ed. *Prisoners' Drug Use and Treatment: Seven Research Studies.* London: Home Office Research, Development, and Statistics Directorate; 2003:71–95.
10. Stover H. *An Overview Study: Assistance to Drug Users in European Union prisons.* Lisbon: European Monitoring Centre for Drugs and Drug Addiction (EMCDDA); 2001.
11. Stark K, Herrmann U, Ehrhardt S, et al. A syringe exchange programme in prison as prevention strategy against HIV infection and hepatitis B and C in Berlin, Germany. *Epidemiol Infect.* 2006;134:814–819.
12. Prendergast M, Campos M, Farabee D, et al. Reducing substance use in prison: the California Department of Corrections drug reduction strategy project. *Prison J.* 2004;84:265–280.
13. Hough M. Drug user treatment within a criminal justice context. *Subst Use Misuse.* 2002;37:985–996.
14. Kinlock TW, Gordon MS. Substance abuse treatment: new research. In: Bennett LA, ed. *New Topics in Substance Abuse Treatment.* New York: Nova Science Publishers; 2006:73–111.
15. Chandler RK, Fletcher BW, Volkow N. Treating drug abuse and addiction in the criminal justice system: improving public health and safety. *J Am Med Assoc.* 2009;301:183–190.
16. Toumborou JW, Stockwell T, Neighbors C, et al. Interventions to reduce harm associated with adolescent substance use. *Lancet.* 2007;369:1391–1401.
17. Anderson P, Aromaa S, Rosenbloom D. *Prevention Education in America's Schools: Findings and Recommendations From a Survey of Educators.* Boston: National Center on Addiction and Substance Abuse at Columbia University; 2007.
18. Boys A, Farrell M, Bebbington P, et al. Drug use and initiation in prison: results from a national prison survey in England and Wales. *Addiction.* 2002;97:1551–1560.
19. Zurhold H, Stover H, Haasen C. *Female Drug Users in European Prisons—Best Practice for Relapse Prevention and Reintegration.* Hamburg: Centre for Interdisciplinary Addiction Research, University of Hamburg UNODC Annual Report; 2005.
20. Mair JS. Reducing harm in prisons: lessons from the United States and worldwide. In: Beyrer C, Pizer HF, eds. *Public Health and Human Rights: Evidence-Based Approaches.* Baltimore: Johns Hopkins University Press; 2007:103–124.
21. Stover H, Nelles J. Ten years of experience with needle and syringe exchange programmes in European prisons. *Int J Drug Pol.* 2003;14:437–444.
22. Taxman FS, Perdoni ML, Harrison LD. Drug treatment services for adult offenders: the state of the state. *J Subst Abuse Treat.* 2007;32:239–254.
23. Pearson FS, Lipton DS. A meta-analytic review of the effectiveness of corrections-based treatments for drug abuse. *Prison J.* 1999;79:384–410.
24. Pearson FS, Lipton DS, Cleland CM, et al. The effects of behavioral/cognitive-behavioral programs on recidivism. *Crime Delinq.* 2002;48:476–496.
25. Mitchell O, Wilson DB, MacKenzie DL. Does incarceration-based drug treatment reduce recidivism? A meta-analytic synthesis of the research. *J Exp Criminol.* 2007;3:353–375.
26. Inciardi JA, Martin SS, Butzin CA. Five-year outcomes of therapeutic community treatment of drug-involved offenders after release from prison. *Crime Delinq.* 2004;50:88–107.
27. Prendergast M, Hall E, Wexler H, et al. Amity prison-based therapeutic community: five-year outcomes. *Prison J.* 2004;84: 36–60.
28. Knight K, Simpson DD, Hiller ML. Three-year reincarceration outcomes for in-prison therapeutic community treatment in Texas. *Prison J.* 1999;79:337–351.
29. Landenberger N, Lipsey MW. The positive effects of cognitive-behavioral programs for offenders: a meta-analysis of factors associated with effective treatment. *J Exp Criminol.* 2005;1:451–476.
30. Pelissier B, Camp SD, Gaes GG, et al. Gender differences in outcomes from prison-based residential treatment. *J Subst Abuse Treat.* 2003;24:149–160.

31. Hall EA, Prendergast ML, Wellisch J, et al. Treating drug-abusing women prisoners: an outcomes evaluation of the forever free program. *Prison J.* 2004;84:81–105.
32. Kleber HD. Methadone maintenance 4 decades later: thousands of lives saved but still controversial. *J Am Med Assoc.* 2008;300: 2303–2305.
33. Herget G. Methadone and buprenorphine added to the WHO list of essential medicines. *HIV AIDS Policy Law Rev.* 2005;10: 23–24.
34. Stallwitz A, Stover H. The impact of substitution treatment in prisons—a literature review. *Int J Drug Pol.* 2007;18:464–474.
35. Magura S, Rosenblum A, Lewis C, et al. The effectiveness of in-jail methadone maintenance. *J Drug Issues.* 1993;23:75–99.
36. Tomasino V, Swanson AJ, Nolan J, et al. The key extended entry program (KEEP): a methadone treatment program for opiate-dependent inmates. *Mt Sinai J Med.* 2001;68:14–20.
37. Parrino MW. Providing access to treatment for opioid addiction in jails and prisons in the United States. In: Henningfield JE, Santora PB, Bickel WK, eds. *Addiction Treatment: Science and Policy for the Twenty-First Century.* Baltimore: Johns Hopkins University Press; 2007:120–125.
38. Magura S, Lee JD, Hershberger J, et al. Buprenorphine and methadone maintenance in jail and post-release: a randomized clinical trial. *Drug Alc Depend.* 2009;99:222–230.
39. Dole VP, Robinson JW, Orraga J, et al. Methadone treatment of randomly selected criminal addicts. *N Engl J Med.* 1969; 280:1472–1475.
40. Garcia CA, Caraballo Correa C, Hernandez Viver A, et al. Buprenorphine-naloxone treatment for pre-release opioid-dependent inmates in Puerto Rico. *J Addict Med.* 2007;1: 126–132.
41. Levasseur L, Marzo JN, Ross N, et al. Frequence des reincarcerations dans une meme maison d'arret: role des traitements de substitution. *Ann Med Interne.* 2002;153:S14–S19.
42. Dolan KA, Shearer J, McDonald M, et al. A randomized controlled trial of methadone maintenance treatment versus wait list control in an Australian prison system. *Drug Alc Depend.* 2003;72:59–75.
43. Dolan KA, Shearer J, White B, et al. Four-year follow-up of imprisoned male heroin users and methadone treatment: mortality, re-incarceration, and hepatitis C infection. *Addiction.* 2005;100:820–828.
44. Kinlock TW, Gordon MS, Schwartz RP, et al. A randomized clinical trial of methadone maintenance for prisoners: results at 1-month post-release. *Drug Alc Depend.* 2007;91:220–227.
45. Kinlock TW, Gordon MS, Schwartz RP, et al. A study of methadone maintenance for male prisoners: 3-month post-release outcomes. *Crim Justice Behav.* 2008;35:34–47.
46. Gordon MS, Kinlock TW, Schwartz RP, et al. A randomized clinical trial of methadone maintenance for prisoners: findings at 6-months post-release. *Addiction.* 2008;103:1333–1342.
47. Kinlock TW, Gordon MS, Schwartz RP, et al. A randomized clinical trial of methadone maintenance for prisoners: results at 12-months post-release. *J Subst Abuse Treat.* 2009;37:277–285.
48. Borrill J, Maden A, Martin A, et al. Substance abuse among white and black/mixed race prisoners. In: Ramsay M, ed. *Prisoners' Drug Use and Treatment: Seven Research Studies.* London: Home Office Research, Development, and Statistics Directorate; 2003:49–70.
49. Petersilia J. *When Prisoners Come Home: Parole and Prisoner Re-Entry.* New York: Oxford University Press; 2003.
50. Latessa EJ. The challenge of change: correctional programs and evidence-based practices. *Criminol Publ Pol.* 2004;3:547–560.

CHAPTER 66

Substance Use Disorders among Health Care Professionals*

J. Wesley Boyd ■ John R. Knight

INTRODUCTION

The Greek philosopher Plato believed that if we had knowledge about any matter, then proper action would follow. If Plato were correct, then given their knowledge of medications and addiction, health care professionals would never abuse psychoactive substances. When it comes to this problem, Plato was wrong. Health care professionals know better than the general population just how dangerous psychoactive substances can be, but their overall rates of substance abuse are roughly equivalent to the general population (1). However, health care professionals' patterns of use differ from the general population.

Physicians who abuse substances often self-prescribe them and choose different substances than the general population. Nurses, who are often on the front lines of health care delivery, can easily divert medications from patients for their own use. Pharmacists, having perhaps the greatest direct access to psychoactive drugs of all health care professionals, are also prone to self-medication (2). Finally, dentists who are prone to addiction often turn to nitrous oxide, given its easy access for them (3,4).

EPIDEMIOLOGY

Lifetime rates of substance use disorders among health care providers are in the 11% to 14% range (5–9). The 1992 Physician Substance Use Survey (PSUS), which polled 9600 physicians about their own use of alcohol and other drugs, is the most extensive survey of physician substance use performed in the United States to date (1). The PSUS reported a lower rate of substance use disorders than other surveys: 8% lifetime rate for physicians. However, it relied on physician self-report and may have underestimated actual prevalence. Like physicians, the prevalence of substance abuse among nurses is comparable to that in the general public (10,11).

Health care professionals are more likely to abuse benzodiazepines and opiates other than heroin, more likely to abuse alcohol, and less likely to abuse recreational street drugs such as marijuana and cocaine than the general public (1,12). One older study found that pharmacy students were abusing drugs at alarmingly high rates: up to 62% abused drugs at some point in the past and 19% were using a substance regularly (13). As recently as 2006, the American Nurses Association estimated that 6% to 8% of nurses practiced while impaired by alcohol or other drugs (14).

Among physicians, psychiatrists, emergency physicians, and anesthesiologists are at the highest risk of abusing substances (1,15,16). Conversely, pediatricians, pathologists, radiologists, and obstetrician-gynecologists have the lowest reported rates of substance abuse (16,17). Among physicians who misuse drugs, emergency medicine physicians tend to use more illicit drugs, anesthesiologists tend to misuse narcotic analgesics, and psychiatrists are more likely to misuse benzodiazepines. It is likely that availability and familiarity are contributing risk factors for medical specialists.

RISK FACTORS

A substantial number of health care professionals with substance use disorders report a family history of substance abuse, significant stress at both work and home, emotional problems, and sensation-seeking behaviors (12). When health care professionals do misuse substances—whether alcohol, tranquilizers, or other substances of abuse—they often do so for reasons of "self-treatment." Physicians often work long hours, beyond any standard job description, and may find self-treatment an expedient alternative to taking the time to make and keep appointments with physician colleagues.

Being a female health care professional may also increase risk. Compared to their male counterparts, female physicians who have an identified substance abuse disorder are younger, more likely to have coexisting psychiatric or medical illness, and more likely to have suicidal ideation and/or to have attempted suicide while intoxicated (12,18). Furthermore, compared to men, once they had achieved initial sobriety, women physicians had significantly shorter time to first relapse (16,19).

Younger age may also increase risk. One study (20) found that older health care professionals are significantly less likely to suffer from a substance use disorder than their younger colleagues.

---

*We dedicate this chapter to the memory of Dr. Michael B., who shared his experience, strength, and hope with many physicians until his sudden, untimely death from a dissecting aneurysm. He died clean and sober, before the miracle of his recovery could be even half-completed. We will always miss him.

PREVENTION

Education on physician health and the risks of self-treatment should be a standard component of physician education at all levels, from medical school, to residency and fellowship, and throughout continuing medical education. Similar educational interventions are appropriate for nurses, pharmacists, dentists, and veterinarians. Every state in the United States except one has a physician health program, which may be an ideal agency to provide continuing education through presentations at hospital grand rounds.

Hospital chiefs, practice managers, administrators, and other health care leaders should consider substance abuse, among other health problems, when staff exhibit performance problems. Also, since health care workers may begin misusing substances in an attempt to treat their own physical or emotional discomfort, we recommend that all medical professionals have a primary care physician, resist the temptation to self-diagnose, and never self-prescribe. Seeking medications from colleagues—even a few painkillers here or there—is a bad practice that jeopardizes the career of the prescriber and the well-being of the person obtaining such medications. Physicians prescribing medications for another health care professional should do so only in the course of their usual medical practice, and always generate a note into an appropriate medical record indicating the reason for the medication and the dosing details.

With the possible exception of true emergencies, we recommend that health care professionals not prescribe for family or friends or bring drugs home from office supplies or samples. Many states limit or prohibit prescribing for self and family.

Health care professionals should attend to their own health and wellness. Studies have shown that physicians who exercise, do not smoke, eat well, drink in moderation, and are otherwise attuned to their own health are better caregivers across all measures (21,22). This may also be true for other health care professionals.

SIGNS AND SYMPTOMS

Initial signs of substance misuse among health care professionals almost always appear outside of the workplace. By the time problems arise at work, the substance use disorder may be quite advanced. One study concluded that physicians received treatment for substance abuse an average of 6 to 7 years after problem onset (23).

Initial warning signs of substance use disorders include difficulties at home, loss of interest in activities previously enjoyed, disrupted family relationships, vehicle crashes, accidents, and injuries. Behavioral symptoms are nonspecific, but include apathy, anxiety, lack of self-discipline, strained communications with others, personality changes, and abrupt mood swings (12).

Physical signs include change in eating habits and weight, poor self-care, a generalized deterioration in appearance, dilated pupils, watery eyes, smelling of alcohol, slurred speech, conjunctival injection, dilated or constricted pupils, falling asleep at odd times, and, rarely, needle marks, bruises, or bandages. Health care providers who abuse IV drugs often inject themselves in areas of their body that are not exposed to view, such as lower extremity veins or those in the genital area.

Sometimes, health care professionals with substance use disorders will make direct statements of distress. These may include expressing constant sadness or tearfulness, excessive anxiety or irritability, unprovoked anger or hostility, expressions of hopelessness or worthlessness, and feeling or acting isolated.

When signs of substance misuse become manifest in the workplace, symptoms may include deterioration in the quality of work, repeatedly showing up late for meetings and appointments, recurring absences, continually seeking special accommodations, repeatedly having trouble in getting along with staff and patients, or not responding to pages when on call. While none of these warning signs alone confirm a diagnosis, taken together with other symptoms they may indicate the need for an evaluation.

The level of impairment by health care professionals varies according to pattern of use (e.g., morning vs. evening, weekday vs. weekend), onset and duration of action of the specific substance, the amount consumed, and the degree of tolerance. Some individuals with tolerance will tend to show symptoms when they are in withdrawal, whereas others will show more prominent signs when intoxicated (24).

INTERVENTION

The first step in helping a colleague who may have a problem is having him evaluated. One approach to a directive intervention is summarized by the acronym "FRAMER" (Fig. 66.1). The first step is to gather the **facts**. These facts should include written documentation of any oral complaints about the colleague. For example, if another staff member tells you he has seen signs and symptoms suggesting substance use, record them in a confidential e-mail or as private notes kept locked in your desk. These should state the facts and observations, and avoid drawing any conclusions.

The second step is ascertaining one's own **responsibility** for reporting a colleague who is suspected of having a problem. Are there mandatory reporting requirements by the state licensing board? Health care providers in Massachusetts are required to report any physician to the licensing agency if they have a reasonable basis to believe that the individual may be impaired by alcohol or other substances. Massachusetts also allows for a waiver of the report if the physician has not broken any laws, placed any patients at risk of harm, and enters a treatment program within 30 days of the problem being discovered. Hospital rules and regulations, medical staff bylaws, and other regulations might also mandate a certain course of action. Regardless of law, health care providers may also have an ethical obligation

PRINCIPLES OF DIRECTIVE INTERVENTIONS

F	Gather all of the **FACTS**.
R	Determine your **RESPONSIBILITY** for reporting; consult confidentially with medical and legal experts.
A	Bring in **ANOTHER PERSON**.
M	Begin the meeting with a **MONOLOGUE**, in which you present the facts and summarize your responsibility.
E	Insist on a comprehensive **EVALUATION**. Refrain from giving a diagnosis.
R	Insist on a **REPORT BACK**, and signed releases allowing all parties to freely communicate.

Figure 66.1. Principles of directive interventions. (Reprinted with permission from Knight JR. A 35-year-old physician with opioid dependence. *J Am Med Assoc.* 2004;292:1351–1357.)

to intervene with a colleague before he or she can harm patients, a family member, or self.

The third principle is to have **another person** present at the initial meeting with the colleague. This person can serve as a witness to what you discuss and also might act as a buffer if things begin to heat up. Ideally, this other person should be a member of the hospital's wellness program, the department chief, or an addiction specialist. If you do not have administrative authority over the target physician, bring someone else who does.

The meeting should begin with a **monologue**, during which you list the observations that have led to your concern. The purpose of this monologue is to state facts, which are not open to debate. Avoid drawing conclusions, which may lead to arguing about details or having the individual spend all his time refuting each and every point of concern.

If the individual admits to having a substance abuse problem, then the colleague should be thanked for his or her honesty and referred to treatment immediately. If the individual denies any problems, insist on an independent **evaluation**. If the evaluation concludes that a substance use disorder is present, then the evaluation should be followed by appropriate treatment. The individual should be placed on immediate leave from all professional responsibilities and not allowed to return until the evaluation and any needed treatments are completed.

Finally, tell the individual that you will expect a **report** back from the evaluating or treating entity. This report should specify requirements for aftercare, a plan for re-integration into practice, any workplace restrictions, and any recommendations for continuous monitoring.

EVALUATION

The initial evaluation of any health care worker with a possible substance use disorder should begin with a discussion about any limits of confidentiality. In certain situations, licensing boards of other authorities may require evaluation records or treatment discharge summaries as a condition of return to practice. Ideally, a full history and physical examination should occur. When assessing the health care professional's substance use, evaluators should gather as much detail as possible about what drugs were abused and how the drugs were procured (were they self-prescribed, diverted from patients, samples stolen from an office), whether tolerance and withdrawal symptoms are present, whether they were used during working hours or in other dangerous situations (i.e., before driving, while tending to children, etc.), when use began, and what the peak amount ever used was. Evaluators must, however, exercise discretion in how much of this information to include in reports that may ultimately go to others.

Collateral history from family members can be helpful. However, family members may downplay problems in an effort to protect the professional. Also, asking family members for collateral information can potentially strain family relationships. It should be done only when essential and then as delicately as possible. Information should also be obtained from a small number of professional colleagues. Care should be taken to protect the health care professional's confidentiality to the greatest extent possible. An inadvertent misstep by the evaluator might result in significant harm to the individual once she or he is ready to return to work.

When the individual denies using substances, we recommend obtaining laboratory testing immediately. Some substances of abuse (e.g., cannabis) may be detectable for weeks after cessation of chronic use. However, alcohol and many pharmaceuticals have a fairly narrow detection window in a blood or urine sample (12 to 72 hours). Hair samples can provide detection windows of up to 3 months and may be useful in certain circumstances. However, they are controversial for detecting smoked drugs, because passive exposure can contaminate the hair and cause a false positive result (25).

We recommend consultation with a toxicologist before collecting the specimen for testing. Every specimen should be collected under the federally mandated protocol (26). Given the significant legal and professional sanctions that health care professionals face, specimens must be handled properly and laboratories should use chain-of-custody procedures.

TREATMENT

If the evaluation of the health care professional confirms a substance use disorder, we recommend entry into a structured treatment program. This may be inpatient or outpatient; typical programs last between 2 weeks and 4 months. The American Society on Addiction Medicine has treatment placement guidelines, which may be helpful. Individuals who remain in treatment do better than those who drop out, but we could find no studies supporting a specific length of treatment for health care professionals. Residential facilities often provide medical stabilization of drug-dependent individuals, followed by an intensive psychosocial treatment program that includes group therapy, individual therapy, family meetings, psychopharmacologic evaluation, psychological evaluation, and 12-step fellowship meetings. Some programs offer aftercare plans which can include reunion gatherings for successful graduates.

Residential treatment can be quite costly ($8000 to over $50,000 per month) and insurance usually covers only a fraction, if any, of this cost. This expense may be prohibitive for younger professionals, especially those in training. Outpatient programs, or partial hospitalization, may be available closer to home, allow for greater family participation, may accept insurance benefits, and can be much more affordable.

MONITORING

Every hospital is mandated by the Joint Commission (formerly the Joint Commission on Accreditation of Health Care Organizations, or JCAHCO) to have a process apart from discipline by which physicians and other professionals can seek confidential help for health-related matters. However, not every hospital has such a committee, and those that exist have varying degrees of experience and expertise. Some situations regarding health care professional substance use may warrant immediate attention from a state's physician health program, nursing wellness committee, or some other nondisciplinary agency. The goals of these entities are to identify, assess, refer for treatment, and monitor health care providers with substance use disorders (and other impairing conditions). They can also provide guidance to individual health care professionals, hospital administrators, and department chiefs, about treatment resources and licensing regulations. Given that these entities also monitor health care professionals, they can also provide advocacy for health care practitioners with documented recovery to licensing boards, insurance companies, and hospitals (27).

Comparing efficacy of various monitoring entities is often difficult because of differences in the criteria they assess and monitor. Variables include length of follow-up, total abstinence versus relative abstinence, ability to resume work, and others. Despite their differences, most professional monitoring programs report success rates in the 75% to 85% range, far better than those reported for the general population (16,28–30) (Table 66.1).

One large study of U.S. physicians who were monitored by 16 different state physician health programs found that 80.7% of physicians being monitored for alcohol and drug use successfully completed their respective state physician health programs (39). Of this group, 78.7% were working as physicians 5 years after successfully completing monitoring; 10.4% had either died, retired, or were lost to follow-up; and 10.8% had had their licenses revoked. These high success rates are likely related to the highly structured nature of the treatment and monitoring programs, along with accountability: the rewards of maintaining sobriety are great and the costs of relapse are quite high.

SOCIOCULTURAL CONSIDERATIONS

Because health care professionals are often among the socioeconomic elite, those outside of the profession may see them as immune from problems—including substance abuse. Within the professions, a culture of denial has sometimes turned a blind eye to substance use disorders. This blindness might stem from the fact that many health care providers do not see addiction as a treatable brain disease (41–43). Fortunately, this seems to be changing.

Some who fail to intervene with professional colleagues might do so for fear of triggering a disciplinary action, thereby preventing their colleague from being able to practice again. A few have advocated that, because patients' lives are at stake and the risk of relapse is too great, any health care professional who has had a substance abuse disorder should never be allowed to return to practice (44). However, the actual risk to patients by impaired physicians is quite low (45), and the likelihood of recovery is very high (16). We therefore recommend that health care professionals who are recovering from substance abuse disorders continue to practice, provided they accept close supervision, random drug screens, and are fully compliant with monitoring by the appropriate professional entity.

LEGAL CONSIDERATIONS

Many states mandate health care professionals to report professional colleagues who they suspect of being impaired because of substance abuse. (Some states, such as Massachusetts,

TABLE 66.1 Outcome of physician treatment and monitoring programs

Author	Intervention	Sample size	Outcome measure (definition of success)	Method	Follow-up interval (months)	Success rate
Gualtieri, 1983 (31)	Individualized treatment program and multiple-level monitoring system	117 participants in California diversion program	Able to continue practice	Not specified	Not specified	93%
Morse, 1984 (32)	3–6 weeks inpatient hospital program	53 physicians who completed treatment	Abstinence or 1 brief relapse	Self-report	1–5 years	83%
Crowley, 1986 (33)	Individualized treatment and laboratory testing	15	No drug use	Self-report, collateral report, laboratory testing	5–41 months	47%
Shore, 1987 (34)	Comprehensive initial evaluation and required adherence with individualized treatment plan	63 physicians on probation with Oregon Board	Engaged in medical practice, stable professional, and interpersonal relationships	Systematic record review	0–96 months	75%
Geyser, 1988 (35)	At least 4 weeks inpatient treatment followed by individual therapy, attendance at AA/NA meetings, and random testing	49 participants in Arizona state program	"Successfully rehabilitated"	Not specified	2–3 years	88%
Smith, 1991 (36)	Inpatient treatment for 2–3 months Inpatient treatment for 4–6 weeks Other	I. 47 II. 65 III. 21	Abstinence from alcohol/drug use	Record review	Not specified	I. 83% II. 31% III. 19%
Gallegos, 1992 (37)	Completion of initial treatment followed by individualized treatment plan, attendance at AA/NA meetings, and random testing	100 participants with Georgia Impaired Physicians Program	Complete abstinence from alcohol/drug use	"Reports from many sources," random laboratory testing	20 months	77%

Study	Intervention	N	Outcome	Method	Follow-up	Result
Reading, 1992 (38)	Individualized treatment plan	80	No use of alcohol/drugs by self-report, collateral report, laboratory testing	Survey	24 months	84%
Knight, 2007	Comprehensive initial evaluation and required adherence with individualized treatment plan including individual psychotherapy, attendance at AA/NA meetings, and random testing	120	No use of alcohol/drugs by self-report, collateral report, laboratory testing	Electronic database extracted	9 years 36–60 months	74% 75%
McLellan, 2008 (39)	Monitoring of substance use by 16 different state programs	904	Licensed and working	Systematic review	5 years	78.7%
DuPont, 2009 (40)	Monitoring of substance use by 42 different state programs	All physicians in the state programs	Negative tests while being monitored; successful completion of monitoring program, as well as licensed and employed	Survey of individual state programs	5 years	78% with all negative tests while being monitored; 71% licensed and employed at 5 years

Adapted from Knight JR. A 35-year-old physician with opioid dependence. *J Am Med Assoc.* 2004;292:1351–1357.

also mandate reporting colleagues suspected of impairment due to physical or mental instability as well.) Given the extensive professional scrutiny that can result, such a report should only occur after careful consideration of the facts, discussion with colleagues, and consultation with an attorney familiar with state licensing regulations. Individuals and health care entities that fail to report a colleague in these circumstances risk disciplinary action themselves.

These reporting regulations may include a waiver of the reporting requirement when referral is made to a professional health program for treatment and monitoring, provided the health care professional complies with all treatment and monitoring recommendations. This avenue is commonly referred to as a "diversion program," because the report is diverted away from the licensing agency and made instead to a professional health program. Our experience is that physicians almost never refuse a referral to the state physician health program when they understand the alternative is a board report.

To support their addiction, some health care professionals may engage in illegal acts, such as self-prescribing, diverting medications, stealing medications, or prescribing for family members or fictional patients. These individuals should obtain legal counsel from an attorney who is experienced in dealing with health care professionals, hospitals, and licensing entities.

A final legal consideration is whether to self-report information to the licensing board about a possible infraction of their rules and, if so, how much information to disclose. Health care providers must honestly answer all questions on license renewal and other credentialing forms. Failure to answer questions honestly can result in sanctions that are more severe than those that might have occurred if the health care professional had disclosed the information initially. However, health care professionals should be cautious about providing unnecessary detail, which could lead to unwelcome scrutiny or disciplinary procedures. We recommend consultation with an attorney prior to disclosing any information about substance use treatment or monitoring.

ETHICAL CONSIDERATIONS

Ethical dilemmas arise when basic principles are in conflict with one another, which may occur when dealing with a colleague who has a substance use disorder. For example, we have a basic duty to respect the *autonomy* of others. However, when a health care professional is actively misusing psychoactive substances, this duty often directly competes with other guiding principles such as *justice*, *beneficence* (defined as "doing good"), and *nonmaleficence* (alternately defined as "preventing harm" and/or "not inflicting harm on others").

These conflicts and tensions may be most pronounced when we are not certain about the cause of a colleague's unusual behavior, when we might have suspicions about substance use but little confirmatory evidence. The peril here is failure to act, which may result in harm to the health care professional or others, versus false accusations that could result in the health care professional being forced out of work and numerous patients being left without their physician.

Ethical issues also arise because state physician health programs by their very structure are often coercive. Physicians are not free to refuse evaluation, treatment, or monitoring when the alternative is a report to the state licensing agency. Coerced treatment is effective, but should be applied cautiously and with ethical oversight (46–48). For example, physician health programs commonly require independent evaluations as a condition of initial evaluation, or when the meaning of a positive laboratory is in dispute. These evaluations can cost thousands of dollars. Programs have an ethical obligation to ensure that the physician they are referring for such an evaluation has the financial means to obtain it.

Furthermore, many centers that specialize in evaluating health care professionals also provide treatment at the same site. If a health care professional is sent to one of these sites for a 1- to 5-day evaluation and the recommendation is made for a 4- to 12-week stay (at even greater expense), can we be sure that financial incentives did not play a role in the recommendation? Once such a recommendation is made, it is often hard if not impossible for the state program to overrule it.

Further ethical questions arise because our testing for substances of abuse has become exceedingly sensitive, but serious questions remain regarding specificity of those same laboratory tests and the positive predictive value of their results. For example, many monitoring programs are now checking urine specimens not only for ethanol itself (which has a window of detection up to about 12 hours) but also for ethyl glucuronide (EtG), a metabolite of ethanol with a detection window of approximately 3 days, which can be positive at very low levels. We have seen low-level positive EtG results in individuals who have used alcohol hand wash or asthma inhalers (some of which contain alcohol as a propellant) but who have not purposely ingested alcohol or otherwise relapsed. The Substance Abuse and Mental Health Services Administration has issued an advisory cautioning that EtG testing be used for clinical purposes only, and not used solely as the basis of reports in forensic programs (49).

Given that reporting a positive EtG result can have significant deleterious ramifications for the health care provider, it may be that monitoring agencies should not use this test at all or, if ordered for clinical purposes, not report all positive results to licensing agencies and employers. Reporting all positive EtG results to the licensing board is ethically indefensible. Even if the board does not impose a sanction, the process of investigation has substantial economic and emotional costs for the monitored physician.

SPECIAL CONSIDERATIONS

How should a health care professional inform a potential employer about a history of substance use treatment? We generally counsel professionals to wait to make a disclosure until they know that they are interested in the position, and to make the disclosure in a face-to-face interview. We also advise them to have a short, factual statement prepared and practice it several times before friends or a sponsor. The statement should briefly state that they had a problem with a substance, that they completed a treatment program and entered a continuing care program that includes laboratory monitoring, what they have learned from this experience, and how it has changed them for the better.

How should professional health programs respond when professionals who are being monitored suffer from conditions such as attention-deficit/hyperactivity disorder (ADHD), anxiety, or chronic pain that warrant treatment with psychostimulants, benzodiazepines, or narcotic analgesics? Most monitoring programs insist on abstinence from all intoxicating substances, including alcohol, illicit drugs, and psychoactive prescription drugs. However, many will allow health care professionals to receive appropriate treatment as long as it is provided by a usual treatment provider who is knowledgeable about the history of substance abuse. This course of action is appropriate. Those with co-occurring substance use disorders and ADHD can be treated safely with stimulant medications (50–53), and that those with co-occurring substance use disorders and chronic pain can safely be treated with narcotic analgesics (54–57).

And finally, medications such as naltrexone, methadone, and buprenorphine may have an important role in managing addictions in health care professionals. Some health care professionals who have had histories of opioid use have been allowed back to practice contingent upon taking daily naltrexone. We are also aware of health care professionals who lost their licenses because of opiate abuse and were eventually allowed to return to practice on buprenorphine maintenance therapy, with the full knowledge of the licensing board. In addition, we are aware of a small number of opioid-dependent physicians who are on methadone maintenance therapy, but as of this writing we are not aware of any who have returned to practice on this medication. We believe that there is merit in allowing health care professionals to return to work either while taking or contingent upon taking medications such as these. In some cases, including those in which healthcare professionasl are taking methadone or buprenorphine, a careful neuropsychological assessment and addiction treatment consultation should guide any decisions about return to practice. Just as in general addiction practice, it is unclear when, if ever, these individuals should be weaned off maintenance therapy.

CONCLUSION

Health care professionals are neither immune from substance use disorders nor at higher risk for them. However, professionals' patterns of use often reflect both the availability and knowledge of psychoactive prescription medications. Everyone in the healing profession can facilitate early detection and treatment by helping to educate staff members about these matters, knowing how to refer a colleague for assistance without fear of hurting his or her career, and by ensuring that the colleague receives appropriate workplace support and accommodation.

Health care professionals whose lives have been affected by substance use can and do recover, and they usually can return to work safely and effectively. Early intervention is best, but intervention needs to occur whenever possible. Most states offer treatment and monitoring programs for physicians, nurses, and other health care professionals. Health care professionals in recovery from substance abuse have high success rates. Great care must be taken to ensure that these professional health programs operate under the highest ethical standards.

REFERENCES

1. Hughes PH, Brandenburg N, Baldwin DC Jr, et al. Prevalence of substance use among US physicians [erratum in: *JAMA*. 1992;268(18):2518] [see comments]. *J Am Med Assoc*. 1992; 267(17):2333–2339.
2. Dabney DA. Onset of illegal use of mind-altering or potentially addictive prescription drugs among pharmacists. *J Am Pharm Assoc (Wash)*. 2001;41(3):392–400.
3. Cedarholm B. Nitrous oxide becomes the vice of dentists. *Dentistry*. 1990;10(3):13–22.
4. Blanton A. Nitrous oxide abuse: dentistry's unique addiction. *J Tenn Dent Assoc*. 2006;86(4):30–31.
5. McAuliffe WE, Rohman M, Wechsler H. Alcohol, substance use, and other risk-factors of impairment in a sample of physicians-in-training. *Adv Alcohol Subst Abuse*. 1984;4(2):67–87.
6. Brewster J. Prevalence of alcohol and other drug problems among physicians [Review]. *J Am Med Assoc*. 1986;255(14): 1913–1920.
7. Clare AW. The alcohol problem in universities and the professions. *Alcohol Alcohol*. 1990;25(2–3):277–285.
8. Blondell RD. Impaired physicians. *Prim Care*. 1493;20(1): 209–219.
9. Skipper GE. Treating the chemically dependent health professional. *J Addict Dis*. 1997;16(3):67–73.
10. Trinkoff AM, Eaton WW, Anthony JC. The prevalence of substance abuse among registered nurses. *Nurs Res*. 1991;40(3): 172–175.
11. Dunn D. Substance abuse among nurses—defining the issue. *AORN J*. 2005;82(4):573–582, 585–588, 592–596; quiz 599–602.
12. Baldisseri MR. Impaired healthcare professional. *Crit Care Med*. 2007;35(2 suppl):S106–S116.
13. McAuliffe WE, Santangelo SL, Gingras J, et al. Use and abuse of controlled substances by pharmacists and pharmacy students. *Am J Hosp Pharm*. 1987;44(2):311–317.
14. Pavlovich-Danis SJ. The impaired nurse, 2000. Available at: Retrieved Oct 6, 2010, from http://ce.nurse.com/CE153-60/The-Impaired-Nurse/
15. Mansky PA. Physician health programs and the potentially impaired physician with a substance use disorder. *Psychiatr Serv*. 1996;47(5):465–467.
16. Knight JR, Sanchez LT, Sherritt L, et al. Outcomes of a monitoring program for physicians with mental and behavioral health problems. *J Psychiatr Pract*. 2007;13(1):25–32.
17. Hughes PH, Storr CL, et al. Physician substance use by medical specialty. *J Addict Dis*. 1999;18(2):23–37.
18. Wunsch MJ, Knisely JS, Cropsey KL, et al. Women physicians and addiction. *J Addict Dis*. 2007;26(2):35–43.
19. Schernhammer E. Taking their own lives—the high rate of physician suicide. *N Engl J Med*. 2005;352(24):2473–2476.
20. Kenna GA, Lewis DC. Risk factors for alcohol and other drug use by healthcare professionals. *Subst Abuse Treat Prev Policy*. 2008;3:3.
21. Abramson S, Stein J, Schaufele M, et al. Personal exercise habits and counseling practices of primary care physicians: a national survey. *Clin J Sport Med*. 2000;10(1):40–48.

22. Frank E, Bhat Schelbert K, Elon L. Exercise counseling and personal exercise habits of US women physicians. *J Am Med Womens Assoc.* 2003;58(3):178–184.
23. Brooke D, Edwards G, Taylor C. Addiction as an occupational hazard: 144 doctors with drug and alcohol problems. *Br J Addict.* 1991;86(8):1011–1016.
24. American Psychiatric Association. *Diagnostic and Statistical Manual of Mental Disorders.* 4th ed. Washington DC: American Psychiatric Association; 1994.
25. DuPont R, Griffin D, Siskin BR, et al. Random drug tests at work: the probability of identifying frequent and infrequent users of illicit drugs. *J Addict Dis.* 1995;14(3):1–17.
26. Vogl W, ed. *Urine Specimen Collection Handbook for Federal Workplace Drug Testing Programs.* DHHS Publication No. (SMA) 96-3114. Rockville, MD: Center for Substance Abuse Prevention, Substance Abuse and Mental Health Services Administration, U.S. Department of Health and Human Services; 1996.
27. Knight JR. A 35-year-old physician with opioid dependence. *JAMA.* 2004;292:1351–1357.
28. Baggaley MR, Morgan-Jones D. Long-term follow up study of military alcohol treatment programme using post-treatment career as an outcome measure. *J R Army Med Corps.* 1993; 139(2):46–48.
29. Eklund C, Melin L, Hiltunen A, et al. Detoxification from methadone maintenance treatment in Sweden: long-term outcome and effects on quality of life and life situation. *Int J Addict.* 1994;29(5):627–645.
30. Noda T, Imamichi H, Kawata A, et al. Long-term outcome in 306 males with alcoholism. *Psychiatry Clin Neurosci.* 2001;55(6): 579–586.
31. Gualtieri AC, Consentino JP, Becker JS. The California experience with a diversion program for impaired physicians. *J Am Med Assoc.* 1983;249(2):226–229.
32. Morse RM, Martin MA, Swenson WM, et al. Prognosis of physicians treated for alcoholism and drug dependence. *J Am Med Assoc.* 1984;251(6):743–746.
33. Crowley TJ. Doctors' drug abuse reduced during contingency-contracting treatment. *Alcohol Drug Res.* 1986;6:299–307.
34. Shore JH. The Oregon experience with impaired physicians on probation. *J Am Med Assoc.* 1987;257(21):2931–2934.
35. Geyser MR. The impaired physician: the Arizona experience. *Federation Bull.* 1988;75(3):77–80.
36. Smith PC, Smith JD. Treatment outcomes of impaired physicians in Oklahoma. *J Oklahoma State Med Assoc.* 1991;84(12):599–603.
37. Gallegos KV, Lubin BH, Bowers C, et al. Relapse and recovery: five to ten year follow-up study of chemically dependent physicians—the Georgia experience. *Md Med J.* 1992;41(4):315–319.
38. Reading EG. Nine years experience with chemically dependent physicians: the New Jersey experience. *Md Med J.* 1992;41(4): 325–329.
39. McLellan AT, Skipper GS, Campbell M, et al. Five year outcomes in a cohort study of physicians treated for substance use disorders in the United States. *Br Med J.* 2008;337:a2038.
40. DuPont RL, McLellan AT, Carr G, et al. How are addicted physicians treated? A national survey of Physician Health Programs. *J Subst Abuse Treat.* 2009;37(1):1–7.
41. Leshner AI. Addiction is a brain disease, and it matters [see comments]. *Science.* 1997;278(5335):45–47.
42. Comerci GD, Schwebel R. Substance abuse: an overview. *Adolesc Med.* 2000;11(1):79–101.
43. Wise RA. Addiction becomes a brain disease. *Neuron.* 2000; 26(1):27–33.
44. Berge KH, Seppala MD, Lanier WL. The anesthesiology community's approach to opioid- and anesthetic-abusing personnel: time to change course. *Anesthesiology.* 2008;109(5):762–764.
45. Skipper GE, DuPont RL. Anesthesiologists returning to work after substance abuse treatment. *Anesthesiology.* 2009;110(6): 1422–1423; author reply 1426–1428.
46. Lawental E, McLellan AT, Grissom GR, et al. Coerced treatment for substance abuse problems detected through workplace urine surveillance: is it effective? *J Subst Abuse.* 1996;8(1): 115–128.
47. Miller NS, Flaherty JA. Effectiveness of coerced addiction treatment (alternative consequences): a review of the clinical research. *J Subst Abuse Treat.* 2000;18(1):9–16.
48. Caplan AL. Ethical issues surrounding forced, mandated, or coerced treatment. *J Subst Abuse Treat.* 2006;31(2):117–120.
49. Center for Substance Abuse Treatment. The role of biomarkers in the treatment of alcohol use disorders. *Subst Abuse Treat Adv.* 2006;5(4):1–7. Available at: http://www.kap.samhsa.gov/products/manuals/advisory/pdfs/0609_biomarkers.pdf. Accessed December 21, 2009.
50. Schubiner H, Saules K, Arfken CL, et al. Double-blind placebo controlled trial of methylphenidate in the treatment of adults ADHD Patients with comorbid cocaine dependence. *Exper Clin Psychopharmacol.* 2002;10:286–294.
51. Riggs PD, Hall SK, Mikulich-Gilbertson SK, et al. A randomized controlled trial of pemoline for attention-deficit/hyperactivity disorder in substance-abusing adolescents. *J Am Acad Child Adolesc Psychiatry.* 2004;43(4):420–429.
52. Levin FR, Evans SM, Brooks DJ, et al. Treatment of methadone-maintained patients with adult ADHD: double-blind comparison of methylphenidate, bupropion and placebo. *Drug Alcohol Depend.* 2006;81(2):137–148.
53. Levin FR, Evans SM, Brooks DJ, et al. Treatment of cocaine dependent treatment seekers with adult ADHD: double-blind comparison of methylphenidate and placebo. *Drug Alcohol Depend.* 2007;87(1):20–29.
54. Kennedy JA, Crowley. TJ. Chronic pain and substance abuse: a pilot study of opioid maintenance. *J Subst Abuse Treat.* 1990;7(4):233–238.
55. Dunbar SA, Katz NP. Chronic opioid therapy for nonmalignant pain in patients with a history of substance abuse: report of 20 cases. *J Pain Symptom Manage.* 1996;11(3):163–171.
56. Jamison RN, Raymond SA, Slawsby EA, et al. Opioid therapy for chronic noncancer back pain. A randomized prospective study. *Spine.* 1998;23(23):2591–600.
57. Jovey RD, Ennis J, et al. Use of opioid analgesics for the treatment of chronic noncancer pain—a consensus statement and guidelines from the Canadian Pain Society 2002. *Pain Res Manage.* 2003;8(A):3A–14A.

CHAPTER 67 The Homeless

Jacqueline Maus Feldman

INTRODUCTION

To understand the interaction between homelessness and substance abuse requires unraveling multiple strands of a very tangled condition. Statistically defining homelessness can offer some insight into the risk factors for problems with alcohol and drugs, but further elaboration of the myriad stressors of being homeless begin to shed light on the condition, on treatment, and barriers to abstinence. There is agreement that people who are homeless are at an increased risk for substance abuse and dependence. One condition does not automatically cause the other, but each can complicate problems associated with the other. Those who use or abuse substances are more likely to become chronically homeless, have difficulty accessing and receiving treatment for their multitude of problems, including addiction, and difficulty establishing and sustaining sobriety. Ethnicity, gender, and age influence drug of choice and treatment acceptance and success. Interestingly, homeless women substance abusers seem to respond in a more positive fashion to treatment; homeless youth are particularly difficult to treat. Philosophy regarding treatment has evolved from putting supports in place to minimizing the impact of a system that contributes to homelessness, to a focus on and assumption of individual pathology. The literature is replete with multiple treatment modalities that have been developed, although research reflects a gap between research and practice, and their limited success on the homeless substance-abusing population. Recognition and amelioration of the life-challenges, as well as collaboration among community providers to provide support, are imperative to prevent and minimize the disruption and devastation wrought by substance abuse and dependence in this vulnerable population. Ultimately the approach to successful treatment means embracing a more broad world view: Dr Larry Meredith, originator of Treatment on Demand in San Francisco, observed, "If we are going to make a difference with the substance abuse problem, then we have to realize that drug abuse is related to housing is related to health care is related to joblessness is related to poverty. You can't deal with any one of those without dealing with all of them." (1).

EPIDEMIOLOGY

Homelessness and substance abuse problems can be intertwined. Defining and discussing the prevalence of both situations will allow a better understanding of the interaction between the two. There are approximately 2.5 to 3.5 million homeless people in the United States. Of these, 23% were reported to be chronically homeless. Temporary homelessness caused by disasters or evictions is different from episodic homelessness, and it is thought that *chronic* homelessness poses the most significant burden on those who experience it (2). Fifteen percent to 57% of those homeless in urban areas are considered chronically homeless. In a 2006 U.S. Conference of Major 23 City survey on hunger and homelessness, the population demographics of homeless were reported: Whites (39%); Hispanics (13%), Asians (2%); African Americans (42%); Native Americans (4%). Twenty-six percent of them were reported to have substance abuse problems, 16% mental health problems. Thirty percent were family with children, 51% single men, and 17% single women. Causes of homelessness reported from this survey included poverty, unemployment, lack of affordable housing, lack of needed services for substance abuse and mental illness, job loss, domestic violence, and prisoner re-entry (3).

Prevalence of substance abuse problems in those who are homeless has been notoriously difficult to establish because of different definitions, methodologies, and tools for assessment. However, it is generally agreed that about 20% to 35% of those who are chronically homeless have alcohol or drug problems (although some claim it is as high as 50%, with 23% reporting problems with alcohol and 27% with drugs). An additional 10% to –20% have dual-diagnoses (mental illness and substance use disorders) which may exacerbate their life difficulties. In a survey of adult homeless shelter users, Culhane et al. found that *two-thirds of those queried* admitted to mental health or substance abuse problems some time in their life (4). Problems with alcohol use are three times more common in homeless men than homeless women; crack-cocaine dependence is reportedly more common in urban homeless African American men and women. The prevalence of seeking and/or receiving treatment by those who are homeless with substance abuse problems has been poorly studied, although it is suggested they have significantly limited success in accessing services (5). Intriguingly one article reports that in their study 30% of their homeless population reported using more substances when homeless, 71% reported using less, with 50% of those using less because they were in recovery, while 22% reported using less because they simply could not afford the drugs (6).

Men are two times more likely than women to receive treatment. Those aged 18 to 25 are thought to have the highest rate of treatment need, *but* the lowest rate of treatment receipt. About 18% of those homeless who have substance abuse problems receive substance abuse treatment from a specialty facility. Of those who are admitted for inpatient substance abuse treatment, those there for first admission report marijuana as their drug of choice; those with greater than four admissions report their drug of choice is opioids, and are more likely (24% vs. 8%) to be homeless (7). Thirteen percent of those in substance abuse treatment were homeless at the time of admission (this translates into >120,000 admissions for substance abuse treatment by persons who were homeless) (8). It is reported that one-fourth of the homeless admitted for substance abuse treatment had co-occurring disorders (mental health and substance abuse), and that one-third to one-half of homeless vets have co-occurring disorders. Among jail detainees with mental illness, 72% had co-occurring disorders (3). Homeless addicts also impact on other systems of care. A recent study reviewed over 5000 acute hospitalizations of those who were admitted because of suicide and substance abuse (substance-induced suicide syndrome). These folks were more likely to be homeless, unemployed, uncooperative, have shorter lengths of stay, and have more rapid improvement in their symptoms. This study concluded there is a need for intensive addition component to outpatient care and additional outpatient services to care for suicidal substance-abusing patients (9).

Those who are homeless are at risk for being substance abusers. Risk for substance abuse as predicted by gender, length of time afflicted with substance dependence, and ethnicity can be powerful reflections of the need for services. Co-occurring disorders are common (and discussed in another chapter). It is readily apparent from the extant literature that these people are living disrupted lives and are in desperate need of support and treatment.

SOCIOCULTURAL CONSIDERATIONS

There are numerous sociocultural risk factors to consider in understanding the development of substance use/abuse in the homeless population. Osher and Dixon (10) declared there were three factors contributing to the link between substance abuse and housing problems:

1. *Systems issues* (like the restricted eligibility for housing for those who used substances and the exclusion of those with dual diagnosis to access to public housing)
2. *Legal issues* (limitations of providing SSI for those with substance abuse, those with criminal records not eligible for public housing)
3. *Clinical factors*. For example, people with substance abuse often have histories of social awkwardness, psychotic behavior, poor hygiene, daytime sleep (with nighttime wandering), smoking in undesignated areas (or leaving doors unlocked for easy outside access to smoke), or violence. Landlords view these behaviors as unacceptable and are considerably less likely to rent to people with these kinds of behaviors.

Other comorbid conditions predict homelessness as well: poor treatment compliance, medical problems, poor money management skills, and greater use of crisis services (11).

SAMHSA (Substance Abuse Mental Health Service Administration, a federal oversight organization that coordinates setting of federal standards, monitoring, and research funding) notes other challenges for those with substance abuse and homelessness that can complicate their lives:

1. *Inadequate access* to appropriate screening
2. *Fragmented services*
3. *Lack of appropriate discharge planning*
4. *Poor integration of care*
5. *Insurance coverage limitations*
6. *Stigma and discrimination* (6)

Individual characteristics can also interfere in treatment considerations and delay engagement by the consumer into treatment: these include disaffiliation/social isolation, distrust of caregivers and authority, mobility, and multiplicity of needs (6). Although society and governmental and funding agencies may be distressed by homeless people with substance abuse problems, some of these homeless people do *not* view substance abuse treatment as a high priority, or even important. A recent survey asked homeless persons what they needed urgently. They responded: finding a job (42%), help finding permanent housing (30%), and assistance paying expenses. The *13th* most frequent response was treatment for use of alcohol or drugs; only 5% mentioned detoxification (12).

Other social/cultural considerations are extant as well. Men are more likely to report alcohol- and drug-related problems, while homeless women are more likely to report higher rates of mental illness. Koegel and Sullivan found substance abuse service use was predicted not by need but by other factors (race/ethnicity, location, perceived social support, health insurance). Women need child care; once offered, this enhances positive outcomes for women in treatment. Research reflects that there are more positive results in treatment of homeless women with substance abuse, perhaps because programs take into account physical and sexual abuse and motherhood (13). In a group of adolescents studied for several years, it was noted that ultimately about 5% become homeless. Risk factors associated with this included poor family functioning, few financial supports, and separation from parents or caregiver. These observations might have an impact on decisions for early intervention (14).

And finally, conceptualization of substance use and abuse as in issue of individual responsibility has influenced the development of treatment protocols. In lieu of addressing individual needs for housing, stable funding, work, social skills development, substance abuse often is considered, by policy makers and funders, to be a disease of choice, and treatment philosophy embraces addressing individual pathology instead. System level features (how and which services are provided, how access to services is structured) affect how homeless people with substance abuse problems access the care they need.

FACTORS INFLUENCING SUBSTANCE USE IN PEOPLE WHO ARE HOMELESS

Numerous factors contribute to the development and maintenance of substance abuse in the homeless population. *Access to care* remains a huge obstacle for those who are homeless and have substance abuse. But access must be more broadly drawn; a wide variety of services are necessary to keep people supported once they are housed, and access to these services is critical: "health care, mental health care, money management, benefits assistance, job training, transportation, parenting skills" (15).

Funding of mental health and substance abuse services is often along separate funding streams, with discrete lines for monitoring, reporting, standards, and accountability. As such, patients needing access to both kinds of treatment may find themselves treated by two sets of clinicians who often have opposed therapeutic skills sets and different established goals and expectations of outcomes.

Funding for housing must always be a salient consideration. While Section 8 housing is often refused for consumers with a known history of substance abuse, other federal resources have been made available: Community Development Block Grants (CDBG) and the McKinney-Vento Act in 2000 have authorized federal homeless assistance programs to provide transitional and permanent house to the homeless; access to stable housing is paramount in the battle for sobriety (15).

The concept of *treatment matching* (matching patient needs and characteristics) with specific treatments has been studied, but not supported by research. Exploration of what types of clinician "treater styles" work most effectively with what kind of patients is an intriguing research paradigm, but one that is as yet unexplored.

TREATMENT

Before turning to an explicit discussion of models of care, it is important to consider defining successful outcomes: these can include complete sobriety, graduation from treatment programs, attainment of life skills objectives (employment, school, money management, housing), change in psychological realms, improvement in interpersonal relationships, ability to cope with problems and stress, and a global improvement in one's life. Which goals are pursued and achieved will depend on a variety of factors, including the system of care and personal attributes of the individual. For now, present research seems to focus mainly on treatment program completion.

Different models of care have been proffered for the treatment of homeless persons with substance abuse problems. A survey has reported that the *most frequent* inpatient treatment for homeless persons with substance abuse is hospital detoxification, and the most likely outpatient treatment is a 12-step recovery program. Interestingly, however, most research has been done on day treatment and therapeutic communities.

Models of care include the medical model, the social model, 12-step recovery, harm reduction, intensive outpatient, day treatment, case management, and contingency management interventions.

The *medical model* (particularly medical detoxification) was an early focus in the treatment of addiction; however, only about 5% of people with alcohol dependence need acute medical intervention. A consistent finding in research effectiveness treatment is the connection between length of time spent in treatment and positive treatment outcomes; unfortunately dropout rates can be as high as two-thirds. Brief interventions have not been found to be useful in the homeless substance abuse population (5). As such, an acute care model like the medical model is typically insufficient for someone with chronic homelessness.

The rise of the *social model* reflected the different needs of a chronically ill population; its key characteristics include

1. *Use of nonprofessional staff* often in the midst of their own recovery, who do not make diagnoses, but instead act as role models;
2. *Open admissions* with less record keeping and no standardized assessment;
3. A *reliance on natural recovery* (vs. therapeutic treatment)
4. A *focus on experiential knowledge* and spiritual understanding (compared to formal diagnoses and professionally driven treatment plans) (16).

While both models are typically noninstitutional, and view alcoholism as a treatable disease that requires personal responsibility for recovery, the social model is considered more cost-effective, and as such, primarily serves indigent populations. Unfortunately, there are no reports of randomized clinical trials for efficacy of social model patients followed longitudinally.

12-step recovery programs, which include self-help and peer support, are the dominant approach to treatment of alcoholism in the United States. There is some support for the effectiveness of this treatment (17), but little research on the efficacy of this approach with homeless substance abusers per se, although there is speculation that it might be helpful in addressing the need to connect with a supportive community (5). The focus on sobriety may not meet the total needs of the homeless individual (which include affordable housing and stable employment), which would leave them at risk for relapse.

Another model of substance abuse treatment is known as *harm reduction*, which is designed to provide a variety of services to meet the individual needs of *each* drug abuser; instead of demanding users conform to rigid program requirements, treatment is designed to meet the individualized needs of persons with substance abuse problems (5).

Results of treatment may differ depending on client makeup (solely substance abuse vs. dual diagnoses), model of delivery, and availability to and intensity of additional services (5). Treatment for this challenging population must include addressing *both* the homelessness *and* the substance abuse. As noted above, multiple programs exist to address housing. Once established in housing, many individuals, with supports, are able to remain housed, are less likely to use crisis services or hospitals, or end up detained by law enforcement (15). *Housing First models* (see discussion below) seem to enhance users' acceptance of treatment, as well as retention, particularly if wrap-around high-intensity services are proffered.

Given the statistics above, it is apparent that those who are homeless have an increased need for treatment but will probably face more difficulty in accessing it. Multiple models of care have been developed and efficacy research performed. Unfortunately, considerable flaws in design and execution, as well as small sample size and ethical concerns, have conspired to limit interpretation of results as well as replicability. Issues regarding dropout rates must be addressed; dropout rates as high as two-third are common, so the occurrence of relapse (and the offer of relapse prevention) must be expected, and hopefully used as opportunities for growth and change via *nonjudgmental* intervention (6). Predictors of poor housing stability include assaultiveness, self-destructiveness, and medication noncompliance.

A variety of housing modalities have been offered and studied (6):

1. *Supportive housing* (either scattered site or congregate)
2. *Housing ready* (compliant contingency, stay if sober, ready to occupy housing, psychiatric stability, sobriety, willingness to comply)
3. *Housing First* (placement in housing regardless of clinical status or receipt of mental health or substance abuse services). As per Dr Tsemberis, "Once housed, individuals' priorities shift from ensuring their survival to improving the quality of their lives, and that's when they become interested in other services." Studies show that those enrolled in Housing First had 80% housing retention compared to 23% in usual care group; a significant reduction in hospitalization was also reported (18).
4. *Wet housing*: where substance use is discouraged but allowed without consequence on site; abstinence may be an unrealistic standard for most dually diagnosed residents during the engagement and pretreatment stages.
5. *Damp housing*: where substance use is discouraged, not allowed on site, but tolerated off-site.
6. *Dry housing*: where substance abuse is not allowed; any use results in dismissal from the program.
7. *Transitional housing*: location in housing that is stable, but temporary; occupancy changes as one advances through program.
8. *Permanent housing*: stable housing considered an end point (no further moves necessary); typically associated with wrap-around services (learning social skills, activities of daily living, help with transportation to appointments, accessing medication) that help the patient remain in independent living. Of note, the strongest predictor of program completion is the existence of social supports.
9. *Therapeutic communities*: where substance abuse is conceptualized as a disorder of the whole person, with problems not just with drugs or alcohol but also in conduct, attitudes, moods, emotional management, and values. Therapeutic communities promote sobriety, and set goals of eliminating antisocial behavior and facilitate a change in lifestyle, including attitudes and values (19).

Stabilization of housing should always be part of the consideration in the overall treatment plan. As noted above, numerous housing models have been attempted with mixed results. A recent meta-analysis of 30 studies on housing models for persons with mental illness examined 44 different housing situations; the results reflect that more stable housing results if the patient participates in a program that assumes a model of care (vs. nonmodel housing). Permanent supported housing (where a consumer is established permanently and offered considerable support to remain in independent living) has the largest effect on stabilizing housing, but there was no statistical difference between the housing models (permanent supported housing, residential) (20).

Linkage to services necessary to survive being homeless also plays a huge role in the recovery of homeless people with substance abuse problems. The need for an integrated, comprehensive, community-based system of care has been shown numerous times. These services can lead to employment, permanent housing, decrease in legal problems, decreases in substance abuse, and improved mental health (6). To meet the challenges for this population, multiple supports should be offered: aggressive outreach, permanent housing, treatment environment, strategies to increase motivation, family-based therapy, and peer leadership.

This *Linkage Model* is somewhat diffuse and less demanding, and may be the only form tolerated by those who are actively using (5).

Others have come forward noting that linkage to services, while important, misses a major consideration: the individual. Mueser et al. have written extensively on the use of the *Integrated Model* to approach housing instability in those with dual diagnoses. The basic guidelines of treatment approach by Mueser et al. include (21):

1. *No wrong door* (the patient can enter services via housing, substance abuse, or mental health treatment door)
2. *Shared decision making*
3. *Treatment that is comprehensive and assertive*
4. *Less focus on negative consequences*
5. *Time unlimited*
6. *Multiple therapies offered*
7. *Culturally sensitive*

Mueser et al. encourage clinicians to remain "invested and optimistic" (p. 309), avoiding, if they can, blaming clients for their addiction.

In Mueser's paradigm of Integrated Treatment, it is understood that individuals possess variable levels of motivation to begin treatment and become sober. As such, a process of assessing, inviting, and strengthening motivation is key and includes multiple steps.

Engagement

This is the first step in treatment. A working relationship is established, typically via outreach to the patient in his or her own environment, or in a safe, nonthreatening environment. Practical assistance is offered, including crisis intervention, support, stabilizing medical and mental health problems, reducing legal issues, and encouraging family involvement. A study of homeless dually diagnosed men and women reflected that men say themselves as forced into treatment; as such, it has been suggested that motivational interviewing might enhance the men's need for control and as such might be particularly effective for this subset of the population (22).

Persuasion

The patient slowly becomes aware that substance abuse is creating problems in his life. The individual and family begin to meet, and group meetings discuss the pros and cons of substance abuse. Nonsubstance abuse social skills are encouraged (how to get together in nonsubstance abuse venues). Structured activities are offered, including social and recreational outlets. Damp housing is considered, and a focus on psychiatric stabilization ensues. The patient is approaching a time when they understand the consequences of their substance use, and are sufficiently engaged and supported to move into active treatment.

Active Treatment

Active treatment is comprehensive. It includes outreach and case management. It is interesting that Mueser et al. caution against reliance on self-report, because even at this stage, consumers notoriously underreport or do not report substance use. Hopefully, substance use begins to abate, and the consumer is offered strategies to reduce substance abuse, like social skills to resist peer pressure. Self-help groups like AA (Alcoholics Anonymous), NA (Narcotics Anonymous), and Recovery Anonymous are encouraged. Individual therapy is offered and patients learn to substitute healthy activities for substance using activities. Medications (disulfuram [an alcohol antagonist], naltrexone [an opioid antagonist]) are considered to help maintain sobriety. Dry housing can be offered, as well as techniques for coping with stress.

Maintenance/Relapse Prevention

Maintenance and extended recovery are the focus. Interpersonal social skills are honed, as are problem-solving skills. Lifestyle improvement can be tackled (smoking cessation, improved diet, and exercise). Independent housing can be attempted and the consumer can offer himself or herself as a role model for those in earlier stages of recovery.

Efficacy of Integrated Treatment has been a focus of research. The following results have been reported (integrated treatment vs. usual care): increased retention (55%), decreased substance use (40%), employment (40%), stable housing (60% vs. 50%), money for basic needs (70% vs. 45%), $6000 per individual in criminal justice savings from fewer arrests, and fewer hospitalizations.

Beyond Integrated Treatment, other forms of treatment reported in the literature include

1. *Intensive outpatient treatment* to homeless people (23) should include linkages to shelter and/or public housing; provision of food, medical care and social services, case management, long-term rehab, and strategies to engage chronically homeless.
2. *Day treatment* found to be useful in homeless cocaine abusers (17). This includes active programming each day (6 to 8 hours), including community meetings, psycho education (relapse prevention, assertiveness, medical awareness, relaxation, 12 steps, and job training), and individual and group counseling, with eventual transition to aftercare programs for relapse prevention (24).
3. *Assertive outreach*: case managers diligently and robustly reach out to potential consumers with the hope of engaging them in treatment.
4. *Modified therapeutic communities* seek to incorporate additional services to address the needs of those who are homeless (education, jobs, legal, housing); they are somewhat more flexible than traditional therapeutic communities and often last 18 to 24 months. Research reflects they are a viable treatment option for homeless mentally ill consumers.
5. *Contingency management interventions* where housing/work placement are contingent on provable sobriety. There is little research to support the concept's usefulness.
6. *Intensive case management*: includes "outreach, assessment, treatment planning, linkages, monitoring and evaluation, client advocacy, crisis advocacy, system advocacy, supporting counseling, practical support, and program linkage." (5) This form of support seems particularly challenging with a homeless population who suffers with issues of control and trust (as they may have a fear of being watched or monitored and dislike intrusiveness and drug testing). While its general efficacy has not been established by research, it definitely decreases hospitalization and emergency department visits.
7. *Residential programming* where the intent is to stabilize housing so that access is gained to the patient to begin engagement in treatment.
8. *Lottery*: for allotted time periods of sobriety or completing therapeutic tasks, patients earn "lottery" tickets that offer them a chance to win prizes.
9. *Payeeships* where a person besides the recipient of a disability check is named to supervise the use of the check. Research shows those involved have fewer days of homelessness, but there were no positive substance abuse outcomes.

A wide variety of treatment models have been tried, proved effective with some individuals, but overall, no statistical significance between treatment modalities has been reported in the literature. One key issue does resonate: treatment must be long-term. Brief interventions have been reliably demonstrated to have no long-lasting effects when utilized with those who are homeless and have substance abuse problems.

Experience has demonstrated that interagency collaboration is imperative. People who are homeless and have substance abuse problems have complex multiple needs that require responses from a wide variety of agencies. Linkage to said agencies is imperative. Unfortunately, there are funding limits, limits in information technology, lack of available services, lack of political will, and legislative/political opposition (6).

Unfortunately, there have been sustained limits and/or decreases in funding. For example, CSAT funding dropped 10 million over 3 years (2005 to 2008) to 91 million. This occurred even in the face of positive results from CSAT treatment for homeless program that showed an increase from 50% to 72% of participants in terms of sobriety from drugs and alcohol. In addition, homeless families have benefited from CSAT treatment (1600 families studied and placed in treatment, illegal drug use dropped from 25% to 14% over 14 months of treatment). Regardless, funding has been capped for many substance abuse treatment programs.

In spite of gloomy economic times and possible further cutbacks, efficacy research still occurs and is being published. Use of case management has been researched with some positive effects (25) reflecting statistically significant decreases in psychosocial problems, homelessness, health insurance, and SSI, emergency room use and cost. Okin et al. (26) also reported efficacy in the use of case managers. Fifty three high-service utilizers were studied (pre and post case management). With intensive case management, median emergency room visits dropped from 15 to 9, and costs were significantly reduced because of fewer admission. Homelessness dropped by 257%. Alcohol use dropped by 22%, and drug use by 26%. Every dollar invested yielded $1.44 reduction in hospital costs.

Retaining patients in treatment is a core issue (recall the correlation between the length of stay in treatment program and successful outcomes). Retention is more difficult in the homeless population than those in stable housing. Provision of housing increases retention but as research reports these gains are negated when housing is bundled with *high*-intensity services. People do leave programs for a variety of reasons; perhaps if programs discern the patient's concerns the program might be able to do a mid-process correction that will entice the consumer to stay. People quit because of "A lack of motivation, a desire to return to outside world, a delay in starting treatment, dissatisfaction with degree of program structure, dissatisfaction with program environment, difficulty with transportation, and failure to see value." (27).

In one study it was demonstrated that homelessness dropped 43% over 3 years; the most consistent predictor of failure (more risk of homelessness) was crack as drug of choice. Less risk (or more likely success of sustaining housing) was associated with others depending for food/shelter on the identified homeless person with substance abuse problems. Unfortunately, specific treatment factors did *not* predict outcomes (28). It has been demonstrated that crack-abusing homeless persons who were enrolled in an abstinent-contingency work/therapy/housing program could successfully complete the program. Certainly postdetox stabilization is associated with improved outcomes for homeless addicted person, demonstrating the treatment modality might slow the "revolving door phenomenon of relapse" after detoxification among homeless people (29).

Limits of research into treatment efficacy include concerns about the validity of patient self-report and ethical constraints of placing homeless people in randomized experiments.

In spite of these barriers, ultimately it would appear that programs that are the most effective are ones that address homeless client's tangible needs (housing, employment) as well as their addiction, are initially flexible and nondemanding, are targeted to specific needs of sub-populations (gender, age, diagnoses), and provide long-term continuous interventions (5).

Meyer and Schwartz note (30): "In practice, despite the conceptual understanding of the role of structural causes of homelessness, homelessness has been studied as if it were a disease, an outcome defined as residing in the individual." As such, the federal response has been to support programs to halt alcohol and drug abuse rather than address issues regarding housing markets and urban economies. Studies and services focused on individual pathology models might have minimal impact on the structural issues that "exacerbate or even cause these individual pathologies; substance abuse problems among homeless individuals and their treatment needs should be viewed from a structural perspective as one piece of a much bigger societal problems." (5). A focus on tangible needs of the homeless (housing, money, employment) is certainly necessary, but to date, in the research literature specific *treatment* modality does not appear to differentially affect outcomes. Certainly, "global" treatment has positive effects, but even these diminish over time if treatment is not sustained.

REFERENCES

1. Shavelson L. *Hooked: Five Addicts Challenge our Misguided Drug Rehab System*. New York, NY: The New Press; 2001.
2. National Alliance to End Homelessness. Homelessness counts report 2007. Available at: http://www.naeh.org. Accessed June 4, 2010.
3. The U.S. Conference of Mayors. Hunger and Homelessness Survey: a status report on hunger and homelessness in America's cities. U.S. Conference of Mayors; 2006. Available at: www.usmayors.org/uscm/hungersurvey/2006/report06.pdf. Accessed June 4, 2010.
4. Culhane DP, Avery JM, Hadley TR. Prevalence of treated behavioral disorders among adult shelter users: a longitudinal study. *Am J Orthopsychiatry*. 1998;68:63–72.

5. Zerger S. Substance abuse treatment: What works for homeless people. A review of the literature. Report for translating research into practice Subcommittee. National Health Care for the Homeless Council; 2002.
6. SAMHSA Office of Applied Studies. Results of 2008 National Survey on drug use and health: national findings (Office of Applied Studies NSDUH Series H-3, HHS Publication No. SMA 09-4434). Rockville, MD: SAMHSA Office of Applied Studies; 2008.
7. O'Toole T, Gibbon JL, Hanusa BH, et al. Self-report changes in drug and alcohol use after being homeless. *Am J Public Health.* 2004;94:830–835.
8. The DASIS Report: Characteristics of Homeless Admissions to Substance Abuse Treatment. Drug and Alcohol Services Information System (DASIS). Rockville, MD: SAMHSA, OAS; 2002.
9. Ries RK, Yuodelis-Flores C, Comtois KA, et al. Substance-induced suicidal admissions to acute psychiatric services: characteristics and outcomes. *J Subst Abuse Treat.* 2008;34:72–79.
10. Osher FC, Dixon LB. Housing for persons with co-occurring mental and addictive disorders. In: Drake RE, Mueser KT, eds. *Dual Diagnosis of Major Mental Illness and Substance Abuse. Vol 2: New Directions for Mental Health Services.* San Francisco, CA: Jossey-Bass; 1996.
11. Dixon L. Dual diagnosis of substance abuse in schizophrenia; prevalence and impact on outcomes. *Schizophr Res.* 1999;35:93–100.
12. Acosta O, Toro P. Let's ask the homeless people themselves: a needs assessment based on a probability sample of adults. *Am J Community Psychol.* 2000;28:343–366.
13. Koegel P, Sullivan G. Utilization of mental health and substance abuse services among homeless adults in Los Angeles. *Med Care.* 1999;33:306–317.
14. Shelton KH, Taylor PH, Bonner A, et al. Risk factors for homelessness—evidence from a population based study. *Psychiatr Serv.* 2009:465–472.
15. SAMHSA. Blueprint for exchange: ending chronic homelessness for persons with serious mental illnesses and/or co-occurring disorders, DHHS Pub No. SMA-04-3870. Rockville, MD: SAMHSA; 2003.
16. Borkman TJ, Kaskutas LE, Barrows D. *The Social Model: A Literature Review and History.* Rockville, MD: Center for Substance Abuse Treatment; 1999.
17. National Institute on Alcohol Abuse and Alcoholism (NIAAA). 10th Special Report to the US Congress on Alcohol and Health: Highlights from Current Research. Washington, DC: U.S. Department of Health and Human Services; June 2000:444–453.
18. Stefancic A, Tsemberis S. Housing First for long-term shelter dwellers with psychiatric disabilities in a suburban county. *J Prim Prev.* 2007;28:265–279.
19. Rawlings B, Yates R, eds. *Therapeutic Communities for the Treatment of Drug Abusers.* London: Jessica Kingsley Publishers; 2001.
20. Leff HS, Chow CM, Pepin R, et al. Does one size fit all? What we can and can't learn from a meta-analysis of housing models for persons with mental illness. *Psychiatr Serv.* 2009;60: 478–482.
21. Mueser KT, Noordsy DL, Drake RE. *Integrated Treatment for Dual Diagnosis: A Guide to Effective Treatment.* New York, NY: Guilford Press; 2003.
22. Watkins KE, Shaner A, Sullivan G. The role of gender in engaging the dually diagnoses in treatment. *Community Ment Health J.* 1999;35:115–126.
23. NIH. 2001. *Intensive outpatient treatment for alcohol and other drug abuse.* Treatment Improvement Protocol Series 8. Rockville, MD: National Institute of Health; 2001.
24. Schumacher JE, Milby JE, Dunning J, et al. Linking practice and science in the substance abuse treatment of homeless persons. *J Appl Behav Sci.* 2000;36:297–313.
25. Shumway M, Boccellari A, O'Brien K, et al. Cost effectiveness of clinical case management for emergency department frequent users: results of a randomized trial. *Am J Emerg Med.* 2008; 26:155–164.
26. Okin RL, Boccellari A, Azocar F, et al. Efficacy of clinical case management on hospital service use among ED frequent users. *Am J Emerg Med.* 2000;18:603–608.
27. Orwin RG, Garrison-Mogen R, Jacobs ML. Retention of homeless clients in substance abuse treatment: findings from the National Institute of Alcohol Abuse and Alcohol Cooperative Agreement Program. *J Subst Abuse Treat.* 1999;17: 45–66.
28. Orwin RG, Scott CK, Arieira C. Transitions through homelessness and factors that predict risk: three year treatment outcomes. *J Subst Abuse Treat.* 2005;28:523–539.
29. Kertesz SG, Horton NJ, Friedmann PD, et al. Slowing the revolving door: stabilization programs reduce homeless persons' substance abuse after detoxification. *J Subst Abuse Treat.* 2003; 24:197–207.
30. Meyer IH, Schwartz S. Social issues as public health: promise and peril. *Am J Public Health.* 2000;90:1189–1191.

CHAPTER 68

Disability, Impairment, and Addiction

Stuart Gitlow

INTRODUCTION

The status of disability, a legal finding, is based upon an individual's level of impairment as determined through medical examination. Clarity in the field of impairment and disability can be difficult to achieve. A patient with 20/20 vision is less able to see distant items than an individual with 20/10 vision, but is the patient impaired? Would the answer differ if the patient himself had previously enjoyed 20/10 vision? What if the patient's occupation is "sharpshooter," a position dependent upon his having 20/10 vision? Impairment and disability may be assessed in comparison to the average abilities inherent in the general population, the average abilities of a population of individuals of similar age and heritage, or to a baseline level of ability for a given individual. In another example, an individual has occasional but rare seizures; how common must the seizures be for this person to be impaired through a restriction from driving? And would the person be permanently restricted from driving, or would the restriction be time-limited based upon the date of the most recent seizure? Would we change our assessment if the vehicle being driven were a school bus or ambulance rather than a personal car? Would the restriction be determined based upon population epidemiologic studies, or would it be based instead on an educated opinion from the treating physician? How do we weigh risk to the individual and to society as a whole versus the potential individual productivity and societal benefit? Whole textbooks exist to focus upon these issues, yet such texts have given minimal attention to the topic of addiction.

Under the 1990 American Disabilities Act (ADA), drug addiction is included among the list of physical and mental impairments. An individual with addictive disease is noted to be disabled if the addiction "substantially limits one or more major life activities," if the past addiction was limiting, or if the individual is "regarded" as having addictive illness. The law then makes an exception, excluding those engaged in illegal use of drugs, such as underage use of alcohol, use of controlled substances without prescription, or use of illicit substances. This exception underscores the role of the legal system in the determination of disability: two individuals with equivalent addictive disease, where one uses alcohol and the other marijuana, may have equivalent medical findings and impairments but one is found disabled and the other not.

In 2001, the World Health Organization (WHO) endorsed the International Classification of Functioning, Disability, and Health (ICF) (1). The ICF recognizes that disability is a universal experience in which every individual will at some point likely have a decline in health and thereby experience some degree of disability. Disability is therefore no longer perceived only as a medical or biologic dysfunction. That said, there are multiple working definitions of impairment and disability applied throughout industry for purposes of Social Security, worker's compensation, and insurance coverage. The earlier 1980 WHO construct is an approach still sometimes applied in industry:

"A disease, disorder, or injury produces an impairment causing a change to ordinary functioning. Impairment refers to … loss or abnormality of psychological, physiological or anatomical structure or function. A disability refers to the resulting reduction or loss of ability to perform an activity in the manner considered normal for a human being…." (2)

More recent WHO statements indicate impairments as "problems in body function or structure such as a significant deviation or loss" (3). Other models include the United Kingdom's Disability Discrimination Act of 1995, which indicates that individuals are disabled if they have "a physical or mental impairment which has a substantial and long-term adverse effect on her or his ability to carry out normal day to day activities" (4). The Act contains guidance as to how to interpret terms such as "normal" contained within the text.

In essence then, impairment is often defined as an alteration in function from the population normal, not from the individual's premorbid state. However, there are times when impairment would be present without departure from the population normal. Imagine that dementia has caused degradation of IQ in a specific individual from 140 to 100. The individual now has normal IQ but can no longer perform the same tasks as he could formerly perform, at the same pace, or with the same degree of accuracy. This might result in decline in his ability to litigate as a lawyer, to play on stage in an improvisation, or to win at gambling. While this individual is not impaired when compared to the population norm, his own inherent abilities to do what he once did have deteriorated. Rather than looking at impairment as being the abnormality of structure or function, it could be defined as the deterioration of structure or function, with disability as one potential consequence of such impairment.

Just as an individual can be suffering from severe illness without resulting impairment, an individual can be impaired without being disabled. An example of impairment could be a decline in IQ from 140 to 125 after a head injury. But perhaps this same individual shows that he can still interact socially, play guitar, and carry out the usual activities of his daily life and work as he did in the past. Impairment is present—a measurable and objective decline in function as a result of a medical event—but there is no resulting adverse effect of the impairment, and therefore no disability.

Returning to the 2001 ICF brings up two additional terms of interest: limitations and restrictions. Disability is referred to as limitations of activity, those actions that an individual is *unable* to carry out. Handicap now is covered as restrictions in participation, those actions an individual *should not* carry out. Differentiating limitations from restrictions is a frequently encountered section within disability forms filled out by clinicians. A mildly intoxicated person may be able to drive, but should not drive due to the loss of coordination and potential risk to self and others; that person would therefore be *restricted* from driving. At higher blood levels of substance, the level of intoxication would be so high that the person would be unable to walk to the car, open the door, get in, or start the car. At this point, the person would be *limited* with respect to ability to drive. Occupational limitations are often tied directly to the type of limitations that are present. It is therefore inappropriate for the clinician to indicate simply that a patient is unable to work unless the clinician is aware of the diagnosis, impairments secondary to that diagnosis, the resulting limitations, and the degree to which those limitations would directly impact the patient's ability to carry out the activities inherent in his or her occupation.

It is evident by now that determination of disability secondary to an impairment is more than a question of science. Moral and policy issues have therefore been explored in the literature in depth (5).

PRIMARY INFORMATION SOURCES

Several sources of disability information are available; each has a somewhat different perspective and different purpose but can be used together to gather information related to disability secondary to most given illnesses or conditions.

- Guides to the Evaluation of Permanent Impairment (6)
- Occupational Medicine Practice Guidelines (7)
- Official Disability Guidelines (8)

The current edition of the *Guides to the Evaluation of Permanent Impairment* has a chapter dedicated to mental and behavioral disorders, but no separate section related to addictive diseases. The mental disorders chapter provides a method of evaluating psychiatric impairment, perhaps the closest the text comes to evaluating addiction-related impairment. There is broad recognition within the text that the presence of a psychiatric illness does not necessarily reflect the presence of impairment or related limitations. For example, an individual might be so depressed as to commit suicide, yet a retrospective analysis of that individual's life might reveal him to have been carrying out all of his usual activities without any apparent difficulties. That individual would have potentially had severe psychiatric illness, yet no impairment. Conversely, a tractor-trailer driver following an accident might have only mild anxiety when seen in the physician's office upon examination, yet could be markedly limited with respect to his ability to function occupationally due to findings which would only arise while at work.

The *Guides* indicates four domains within which psychiatric function can be assessed:

- Activities of Daily Living
- Social Functioning
- Concentration, Persistence, and Pace
- Deterioration or Decompensation in Complex or Worklike Settings

Depending upon findings within these areas, a degree of severity may then be applied to impairment within each domain, chosen from these categories: none, mild, moderate, marked, and extreme. Finally, dependent upon the number of domains in which one has significant severity, an assessment may be made regarding the degree of overall impairment and resulting limitation.

The *Official Disability Guidelines*, unlike the *Guides*, specifically addresses issues of addictive disease. This text focuses on the duration for which an individual with a given illness is likely to remain limited in terms of his ability to carry out his occupational function. For addiction, whether to alcohol or other drugs, these guidelines indicate that patients are no longer impaired after approximately 1 month—at worst. Patients who do not require inpatient care or rehabilitation are presumed to be unimpaired after only several days. Since addictive disease is a chronic lifelong illness, it seems reasonable that these guidelines are focused upon an individual who is actively using substances, then stops, with the number of days starting at the time of abstinence. This, however, is an assumption on our part and is not specifically stated within the guidelines.

The *Occupational Medicine Practice Guidelines*, while it currently has reference to stress-related disability, does not contain addiction-related information specifically.

DISABILITY AND ADDICTION

Within the *Diagnostic and Statistical Manual of Mental Disorders* (DSM-IV), the diagnosis of substance dependence may include the criterion, "important social, occupational, or recreational activities are given up or reduced because of substance use" (9), suggesting impairment. But the diagnosis can be met without that specific criterion being met. This is not the case in some primary psychiatric diagnoses such as major depression, which require that "…symptoms cause clinically significant distress or impairment in social, occupational, or other important areas of functioning." As a result, the simple presence of a diagnosis of substance dependence differs from some psychiatric diagnoses in that it does not, by itself, indicate the presence of impairment. Axis V of the multiaxial diagnostic system refers to the Global Assessment of Functioning scale. The title of this scale implies that the score for any given individual is a direct reference to that individual's level of function, thereby suggesting that any provided score can be interpreted as the clinician's assessment regarding impairment. *DSM-IV-TR*, however, is quite specific that the scale be used to indicate "symptom severity OR level of functioning." As a result, individuals can be accurately given a score of 41 if they have serious symptoms of substance dependence, even if they have no significant impairment in any domain. The GAF therefore cannot be used alone as an indication of impairment level when substance use disorders are present.

For the purposes of disability, one can look at addictive disease as having several phases (Figure 68.1). In phase I, an individual has a sense of discomfort and lack of coping skills necessary to address the discomfort. We can ascribe the discomfort to the genetic aspect of addiction while the lack of coping skills results from the environmental underpinnings of the disease. In phase II, the individual has discovered that use of psychoactive substances leads to acute but impermanent relief of discomfort. The psychoactive substance use therefore represents a coping mechanism, albeit an imperfect one, with which the patient deals with the existing discomfort. In phase III, the individual is using the psychoactive substances to his or her own detriment. In phase IV, the individual has stopped using psychoactive substances and is essentially back at phase I but for the knowledge that discomfort can be relieved temporarily by psychoactive substances. A relapse would lead back to phase III or recovery leads to phase V, in which an individual leaves the circular cycle by discovering new coping strategies (perhaps as addressed within 12-step programs) or by relieving the original sense of discomfort, potentially with pharmacologic or other therapeutic input. Each phase carries with it the potential for differing restrictions and/or limitations with potentially resulting disability.

Phase I

Traditional diagnostic approaches unfortunately do not yet allow for the diagnosis of addiction prior to the onset of substance use itself. Given that addictive disease is not caused by the psychoactive substance involved, it is reasonable to suspect that it exists prior to the initiation of substance use. What is likely to be observed during this time are difficulties with respect to anxiety, or mood variation beyond normal parameters. Since the psychiatric diagnostic approach is largely based upon observed characteristics and subjective reports rather than upon neurochemical studies, patients in phase I of addictive disease, if diagnosed with any disease, are likely to be diagnosed with a primary psychiatric illness. It is unknown whether treatment of the psychiatric symptoms at this stage results in a reduced likelihood of eventual substance use or dependence or whether treatment in these cases has the same degree of efficacy as it does in actual primary psychiatric disease cases. Ultimately, some of these patients may have two disease states, but Occam's razor would suggest that what we are observing is a single disease state not yet fully expressed, comparable to prediabetes or prehypertension. This issue is important as patients will often state that their substance use represents "self-medication" of underlying distress. Their perspective may therefore be that they are treating a primary non-substance-related disease, but objectively this is what addictive disease represents. An individual without addiction, when experiencing a primary psychiatric illness, would not self-medicate with psychoactive substances over an extended period of time. Since, during this phase, addiction is not yet diagnosed, any measurable dysfunction and related disability would be caused by what is diagnosed as a primary psychiatric illness.

Phase II

Here, our theoretical patient has discovered psychoactive substances. Typically, this is a youthful individual who is using alcohol or marijuana, but a middle-aged individual prescribed opioids for the first time is another common scenario. Other substances are frequently involved, often depending upon the geographic region in which the patient resides. Some areas have a high incidence of heroin use, while in others methamphetamine is widespread. LSD and psychedelics are commonly used in some parts of the world as well. During this phase, substance dependence might not be diagnosed. Rather, the user might be placed in a category of substance "misuse" or "heavy use." If patients are first encountered when in this phase, psychiatric symptoms might be ascribed to the substance use itself, as in an alcohol-induced mood disorder.

VIGNETTE 1

Melissa is a 20-year-old college student. She began drinking with her friends on weekends while in high school, never with any resulting difficulties. She graduated in the top quarter of her class and went on to college. Melissa has never experienced any psychiatric issues though she was briefly in therapy after her parents divorced. She now presents to the psychiatric emergency room with a distant gaze and apparent responsiveness to internal stimuli. She is accompanied by a friend who refuses to give his name but who states, "Two days ago, on Saturday, Melissa took a hit of LSD. She said she hadn't tried it before. It looked

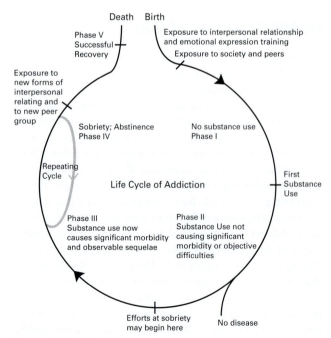

Figure 68.1. Life Cycle of Addiction.

like she was feeling good when we all went to sleep early Sunday morning. No one saw her on Sunday, but on Monday when she didn't show up for any of her classes, we had the dorm manager open her room. We found her there—like this." The patient is admitted to the hospital. Three weeks later, after treatment with antipsychotics, Melissa has shown some improvement but is still delusional, slow to respond to questioning, and showing significant signs of an ongoing thought disorder.

Vignette 1 is a slightly altered actual case from the late 1980s. In disability cases, there are two initial questions—is there impairment, and if there is impairment, is it the result of a medical process? In some legal contexts, those questions may be reversed: Is there a medical process, and if so, is it causing impairment? As we will see later, a third question is often posed: is the medical process involved an addictive illness? In Vignette 1, there is clearly impairment with resulting adverse effects: our patient is unable to think clearly, respond normally within social situations, focus or attend to conversation, or carry out simple instructions. The cause, however, is not clear. Prior to the single use of LSD, Melissa had no history of a substance use disorder or of psychiatric illness. Following one use of LSD, Melissa now has a psychotic disorder. Perhaps Melissa was predisposed to the development of psychotic illness, and in this case the illness was triggered by the effects of LSD. Or perhaps the LSD was contaminated by a substance that led to organic brain damage. In the first few days after LSD use, we might most appropriately determine that impairment is secondary to the acute effects of LSD. Now that several weeks have passed, we might instead find that impairment is due to a primary psychotic disorder. In both cases, LSD represents the likely cause, but the disability determination is different, and can therefore lead to a different final decision in related legal cases.

Another example for clarification would be that of a heavy smoker who develops chronic obstructive pulmonary disease with related impairments. Barring other causes of COPD, the smoking in such a case is a likely cause of the pulmonary disease. In such a case, the pulmonary disease would now be the proximate cause of impairment despite its having arisen as a result of an underlying addiction. Tobacco use or nicotine dependence, taken alone, is not described in any resource as a source of impairment or disability. So looking again at Melissa, the cause of her psychotic disorder is not germane to a finding of impairment as the impairment would be a direct result of the psychosis independent of the etiology of the psychotic state.

Use of substances that is independent of addictive disease may be confusing as such use can lead to impairment. For example, a patient might have three glasses of wine over the course of each evening for many years, then present with insomnia, anxiety in the morning, and low mood. The insomnia may cause difficulties with attention and focus to such an extent that impairment is present. Advising the patient to discontinue alcohol use, if it leads to successful cessation, is an indicator that alcohol dependence was not present; if symptoms remit, that would suggest that alcohol-induced impairment had been present. So one can have substance-induced difficulties without having a substance use disorder. Further, substance use alone, where such use is independent from addictive illness, can lead to brief periods of impairment secondary to acute intoxication or to the acute withdrawal effects that follow. Acute impairment is not generally a consideration in disability determination. Longer periods of withdrawal with related impairment would generally be found only after extended periods of substance use, more likely found in phase III.

Phase III

Within this phase, individuals are actively using substances despite their best interest. Note that frequency and quantity of use are not related to whether a person falls into this category. Individuals might therefore vary widely from one another: the 75-year-old who has fallen while intoxicated twice, breaking a rib and hip as a result, yet still drinks from time to time; the 25-year-old drinking a pint a day despite losing several jobs as a result; the 18-year-old who does not go to class without first smoking marijuana, despite failing two classes the previous semester; the 30-year-old snorting cocaine on weekends, despite having used up her savings as a result. It is this phase of addictive disease to which the *Official Disability Guidelines* appears to refer.

VIGNETTE 2

Rebecca is a 30-year-old who has been using cocaine for about 5 years. At age 27, she sought medical care for worsening mood variability, with the presence of periods of irritability, depression, and anxiety. She was diagnosed with bipolar disorder and started on a mood stabilizer. A retrospective review of the early medical record reveals that Rebecca had failed to be forthcoming about her cocaine use. Her physician had not done a complete workup for nonpsychiatric causes of mood variability and no drug screen was ever performed. The mood stabilizer failed to have any efficacy and Rebecca's medications have been changed several times in the years since. She now presents to a new physician on an atypical antipsychotic, still having mood variability, but now also having increased weight and worsening results of fasting blood sugar tests. She claims that she cannot work as a result of her symptoms of bipolar disorder and wants disability paperwork filled out. A complete history, obtained from the patient and family members, suggests significant difficulties with social functioning. Further, family members indicate that Rebecca has become unreliable due to her disorganization and lack of focus. She sometimes stays in bed for days and fails to participate in many of her activities of daily living without assistance or encouragement. The new physician performs a urine drug screen and finds a positive cocaine result. Rebecca initially denies any use of cocaine but over the course of early treatment, and following another positive urine screen, acknowledges that she has been spending hundreds of dollars per week for cocaine for years.

In this case, Rebecca most likely was suffering from cocaine dependence and a cocaine-induced mood disorder. The mood variability was due to both the acute effects of cocaine and to its withdrawal effects. Unlike the case of Melissa in

Vignette 1, where the psychiatric symptoms persisted long after a single use of LSD, in this case the psychiatric symptoms have been present only during the ongoing use of cocaine. The proximate cause of any resulting impairment is therefore the cocaine dependence. Naturally, arguments can be made to the contrary. One could speculate that Rebecca has a pre-existing bipolar disorder being self-medicated with cocaine, although even so, there would be no evidence that the pre-existing bipolar disorder was impairing absent the addition of cocaine use. One might also argue that Rebecca was predisposed to development of bipolar disorder, which then arose coincidentally during the time in which Rebecca was using cocaine actively. Again, though, it would not be clear that the bipolar disorder is impairing in the absence of cocaine use, since no such time period has yet taken place.

If we view impairment as a medical question, and disability as a legal one, it is clear in this case that Rebecca is impaired, but the cause of disability must be demonstrated to a legal rather than a medical standard. Two potential sources of information would be necessary to demonstrate that the impairment in this case is not secondary to cocaine use. The first source would be the existence of a medical record prior to the initial substance use while the second would be an evaluation performed after the direct and withdrawal effects of cocaine have passed. Difficulties are present in both situations. Few patients with addictive disease are forthcoming about their substance use, especially during the early phases of their illness. It can be difficult, if not impossible, to accurately determine the initial date of substance use or to determine if early medical records reflect substance-induced disease rather than a primary psychiatric illness. Difficulties with the second possibility, the evaluation after cocaine use has been terminated, arise due to the long period of time that passes before brain function returns to its original or new baseline. It is also critical from both legal and medical perspectives that ongoing urine drug screens be regularly collected. These, if negative, will serve the legal requirement of representing an objective measure of the absence of cocaine-induced disorders, as well as the medical requirement of ensuring that the proper disease is receiving ongoing treatment. Long-term withdrawal effects are possible not only with cocaine but with other drugs such as alcohol, where sleep, for example, takes many months to return to baseline, potentially resulting in impairment for an extended duration.

Phase IV

Impairment resulting from the acute effects of substance use is no longer present by this phase, and patients here are abstinent from substance use. They are not participating in an active recovery program, but psychiatric symptoms are minimal and mental status exams will often reveal no significant findings. Treatment for the substance use disorder is often terminated after the completion of rehabilitation despite the lifelong nature of addiction. The patient in this phase is therefore still suffering from an ongoing illness, but denies any symptoms on history and indeed has no significant objective findings on exam.

VIGNETTE 3

Don is a 48-year-old bartender who was diagnosed 10 years ago with alcoholism. He went through rehabilitation at the time of diagnosis, then returned to his family and his occupation. Three years later, he relapsed, drinking steadily for 12 months though continuing in his position as bartender. He went through rehabilitation a second time, was discharged, and returned to his prior life. Again, he remained abstinent for several years. Finally, however, he relapsed again last year. He presented for treatment, this time with hepatic abnormalities on lab studies, went through medical and addiction treatment, and now presents for follow-up. His liver enzymes are back to baseline, within the normal range. There are no abnormalities on mental status examination. Don has remained sober for 2 months and feels ready to return to work. He is active at home, carrying out all his regular activities without difficulty. He is able to drive and often spends part of his day caring for his young children, again without difficulty. There are no signs of impairment present.

Don is not impaired and therefore is not limited. There remains a significant question as to whether Don should be restricted. That is, is it in Don's best interest to return to his job as bartender? Or should Don be restricted from working in occupations where there is frequent exposure to alcoholic beverages? There is no scientific literature upon which to draw a conclusion. The literature contains references to relationships between work-related stress in general and alcohol use behavior, but does not contain specific studies dedicated to determining the ability of alcoholics to return to a workplace where alcohol is used. One could make the argument that this would be akin to having the fox guarding the henhouse, that the exposure to alcohol on a daily basis would eventually lead to a lack of willpower on the part of the patient who would therefore inevitably succumb. However, one could also posit that alcohol is omnipresent in society, available in every corner liquor store, advertised and promoted in billboards and on television, and that the slight added convenience imposed through work in a bar would not necessarily prove devastating.

A middle ground could be developed that would look at available information:

- Number of years in which the patient was actively using the drug
- Number of years in which the patient has been sober
- Family history (degree of genetic loading)
- Recovery participation and ongoing treatment
- Medical and psychiatric comorbidities
- Number of prior relapses following treatment

This information could then be used to essentially calculate the odds ratio of relapse comparing a return to bartending versus an entrance into another occupation. If indeed it is found that the odds are against the patient should he return to bartending, that alone would not be sufficient for a restriction to be in place. Indeed one might find that the odds of having alcohol-related disease are higher for anyone bartending versus not bartending. For a restriction to be imposed, the odds ratio would have to be significantly worse for the addictive disease population than it would be for the control population. Otherwise, the entire population would be restricted from this type of work. And again, there are no data available to demonstrate such a comparative odds ratio finding.

Phase V

In this phase, the patient's addictive illness is still present, but the patient no longer has evident symptoms of the disease. The patient is actively participating in a recovery program, regularly sees his physician, and has his health monitored with respect to his substance use disorder. Urine drug screens, liver function tests, and other quantitative studies are performed in addition to collection of subjective reports in order to ensure or support those reports. Direct effects of former drug use are now minimal, though there may be some continued nonimpairing difficulty with sleep, motivation, and mood stability depending on the original drug of choice and assuming no comorbidities.

VIGNETTE 4

Mary is a 41-year-old anesthesiologist who was caught using Fentanyl while in the OR. She was turned in to the state's physician health board and her license to practice medicine was suspended. Three years have passed. Her license to practice has been returned. She has been abstinent from all addictive substances for 3 years. She has been attending 12-step programming regularly. She currently has no psychiatric or medical symptoms. History reveals that Mary had been using Fentanyl on an intermittent basis while in the hospital for 2 years. Her use began after she had been prescribed opioid pain relievers for lower back pain. Prior to that time, there was no relevant addiction history. There have been no relapses of opioid use and Mary indicates that her back pain is now well controlled with OTC pain relievers.

VIGNETTE 5

Robert is a 37-year-old anesthesiologist who had been using opioids since high school. His use was minimal at first as his drug of choice was marijuana. However, after becoming an anesthesiologist, the ready access to narcotics led to increased use of those substances preferentially. Robert went into treatment at the encouragement of his family, returned to the OR where he relapsed. This cycle occurred twice. Robert was then referred to the State Board of Professional Medical Conduct and was placed into an Impaired Physician program. Five years have now passed. Robert works at home as a medical reviewer. He is considering a return to the practice of medicine, but in another specialty. He has anxiety and fears that if he returns to anesthesiology, he would relapse. Robert participates actively in a 12-step program, sees his addiction specialist physician every 2 weeks, and shows no evidence of ongoing impairment in any domain.

Both Mary and Robert are socially active, can carry out their daily activities without deficit, and are able to focus and concentrate on any reasonable task. They therefore have no limitation. Are they restricted, however, from returning to their original occupation, as a result of their addiction? These two cases have similarities, but they differ significantly in terms of the severity of the addiction itself. One may speculate, using some of the specifiers described in the phase IV discussion, that Robert would be more likely than Mary to relapse upon returning to work as an anesthesiologist. A paucity of literature addressing this topic led me to bring this question to several experts in fields of pain medicine and addiction medicine. Some said that neither of these individuals should return to anesthesiology. Their relapse risk would be higher than it would be should they engage in some other occupation, they said. Other experts disagreed, pointing out that re-engagement in work when accompanied by active and ongoing treatment has not been demonstrated as having higher risk, though studies did not focus precisely upon anesthesiologists with a history of opioid use. One study that did focus on this group was Domino's 2005 work in which 11 years of outcome data from the Washington Physicians Health Program was reviewed; this study noted that anesthesiologists have a higher rate of abuse of opioids than do other physicians (10).

Domino indeed noted that the risk of relapse of substance use was increased in health care professionals if they had used a major opioid, if they had a coexisting psychiatric illness, or if there was a family history of substance use disorder. Research has demonstrated a high mortality rate among anesthesia residents relapsing upon opioid use (11). Berge, Seppala, and Lanier indicate in their 2008 discussion of the topic that there appears "to have been a national consensus that narcotic-dependent anesthesia personnel in recovery should be allowed to return to the practice" of anesthesiology "in a closely monitored setting" once they are in recovery (12). The authors of that essay suggest that such individuals be directed to lower risk occupations, either within medicine or outside the field, though they agree that data to support the potential of lower risk through such a maneuver do not exist. They conclude that "sometimes we do not need time-consuming prospective studies to do the right thing…." But what is right may be dependent upon one's perspective, one's desires, one's history, and a restriction may be the correct answer in general, but might stop an individual who possibly has a low risk, such as Mary, from returning to her desired profession. Indeed, it might be that there is such a high risk of opioid dependence among anesthesiologists that the risk is actually lower in the population of closely monitored recovered physicians than it would be among the general group. In that case, which group should be restricted?

IMPAIRMENT SECONDARY TO ADDICTIVE SUBSTANCES

In phase II, above, we specifically noted the potential for impairment secondary to substance use that falls short of addictive illness. An individual can suddenly die in response to a single use of cocaine. If the use of cocaine was not part of a distinctive pattern of substance use, then the death would not be the result of addiction but rather of a single event in which the individual was, perhaps, irresponsible. Thus far, there have been only the two potential origins of the substance use and resulting impairment: addiction and social use. The social use may be licit or illicit, but there are no significant medical differences between an individual using alcohol at age 20 and another individual using alcohol at age 21, or between a marijuana user in Pittsburgh and a marijuana user in Amsterdam. The question of legality is therefore eliminated from issues of medical impairment. But there is indeed a third potential origin of substance use and impairment, that of prescribed substances.

Opioid prescribing patterns have changed markedly over the past two decades (13). From 1993 to 2003, there has been a 32% increase in the visit rate for opioid prescriptions in medical offices. The American Medical Association's Council on Science and Public health noted in a recent report that hydrocodone-combination products are the most commonly prescribed medication in the United States with more than 110 million prescriptions issued in 2007 alone (14). At the same time as this increased demand for opioids has arisen, physicians have been encouraged to adequately relieve pain. There have been many guidelines recommending use of opioids in appropriate patients who have chronic noncancer pain (15,16). The AMA report concurs that the current practice environment is "...more conducive to managing acute nociceptive pain in patients suffering from cancer, terminal illness, and [HIV]." Opioids are also recognized within these same guidelines and consensus statements as being related to potentially serious adverse effects including addiction.

The APS-AAPM Clinical Guidelines for the Use of Chronic Opioid Therapy in Chronic Noncancer Pain specifically note that there are short-term adverse events secondary to opioid prescription, but none fall within the mental health rubric except sedation and somnolence. There are no significant data to indicate the presence of any long-term mental health harm secondary to ongoing prescription of opioids. There are also no randomized or controlled trials that look directly at the use of prescribed long-term opioids in patients who have an addiction history.

As a result, an individual may have opioid addiction and related impairment as described earlier, but when excluding patients with addictive illness, there is little if any evidence to indicate that mental impairment arises from long-term opioid prescribing. This conclusion is markedly dissimilar from the situation with long-term use of sedative-hypnotics.

Benzodiazepines and nonbenzodiazepine sedative agents are also widely prescribed agents, generally used for brief, intermittent, relief of anxiety. Therapeutic doses lead to physiologic dependence, as with the opioids, but with the sedative class of medication, symptoms are often present between doses as a result of rebound effects. Cognitive impairment, psychomotor retardation, and impairment of memory have also been noted in patients taking sedative-hypnotics for an extended period of time (17,18). The American Psychiatric Association Task Force report noted that such risks are greater in patients receiving sedatives for longer than 4 months, in those of advanced age, and in those receiving higher potency and shorter half-life substances.

Ashton, in 1987, reported a case study of 50 consecutive patients who presented for discontinuation of prescribed benzodiazepines (19). On presentation, all the patients had symptoms that included incapacitating agoraphobia, irritable bowel syndrome, poor memory and concentration, and panic attacks. Many of the symptoms were such that clinicians might be tempted to increase the sedative dose in an effort to obtain what might be seen as an efficacious dose. Long-term benzodiazepine use was found to be associated with considerable morbidity. Ashton demonstrated that, apparently paradoxically, the majority of the patients had a positive response to sedative discontinuation.

The paradox is solved by recognizing that all sedatives, including alcohol, have two pharmacologic effects:

- Effect 1 is a brief period of sedation, the amplitude of which is controlled by the dose and the duration of which is controlled by the half-life of the drug.
- Effect 2 is a longer period of agitation, the amplitude of which is less than that of the amplitude of the previous sedation, but the duration of which is almost four times longer than the duration of the first effect.

The effects add upon one another with the ultimate result being that if sedatives are taken over a long enough period of time, the symptoms being treated are primarily those arising from Effect 2 rather than from the original morbidity. The patient is now not only uncomfortable from the original illness but from side effects of medication.

As a result, the potential for impairment from sedatives, including the benzodiazepines, the barbiturates, the so-called "Z-Drugs," meprobamate, and the prototypic sedative, alcohol, is always present even when no addictive disease is present.

VIGNETTE 6

Mark is seen regularly at the community mental health center. He acknowledges drinking a pint each day and receives ongoing treatment for depression. He occasionally is admitted for detoxification but relapses almost immediately after discharge. He lives with friends, who let him sleep in the basement, but is more often homeless and staying in shelters. He has tried to work on several occasions in the last 2 years, but inevitably is let go as he fails to show up to work in a timely manner. He reports that he lacks the energy and motivation to go to work. He tends instead to spend the day in bed. His physician opines that he suffers from major depression and prescribes an antidepressant in addition to recommending that he stop his alcohol intake. One of Mark's friends offers him a diazepam tablet, indicating that it will help him stop drinking. Within a short period of time, Mark indeed stops drinking alcohol but is now using a variety of solid sedative agents which he obtains on the street. His difficulties with depression persist and he applies for Social Security Disability Insurance (SSDI).

John has a nearly identical history to Mark's. John, however, is prescribed a combination of diazepam and zolpidem. John also stops drinking alcohol. His difficulties with depression persist and the dosages of sedatives are gradually being increased by his physician. John therefore applies for SSDI.

Both John and Mark have a sedative-induced mood disorder. Mark has alcoholism as well. Mark's sedative-induced mood disorder is the result of illicit substance use, while John's is the result of poor medical care. The legal disability determination may be significantly different for these two individuals despite the similarities from a medical perspective. One could make the argument that Mark's illness is the result of his addictive disease while John's is the result of side effects of prescribed medical care, and it is not the disability determination system's role to play arbiter with respect to whether the provided medical care represents the standard of care or follows currently acceptable guidelines. Since John is not actively using psychoactive drugs as part of his addictive illness—and recognizing that this is arguable as well—it is possible that he will be found eligible for SSDI while Mark will not.

SOCIAL SECURITY DISABILITY INSURANCE

In 1996, over 200,000 individuals were receiving SSDI or Supplemental Security Income (SSI) benefits secondary to addictive illness (20). Such recipients were required to be in treatment with monitored compliance. They were also required to have a representative payee. Benefits were available under such a program for up to 3 years as a result of 1994 legislation limiting the duration of benefits for addictive disease. In 1996, Congress terminated the provision of SSDI to claimants disabled by drug addiction, including alcoholism, through Public Law 104-121, effective the following January. Prior to January 1, 1997, beneficiaries disabled by addiction were granted benefits under both SSDI and SSI programs. Claimants who had received such benefits were allowed to apply for recertification, but only two thirds of those eligible did so, and only half of those cases were resolved in favor of the claimant (21). One study revealed that "many of those who lost benefits had significant self-reported psychiatric problems in the absence of active substance abuse" (22). In 2004, Hanrahan reported that the 1996 law change had adverse effects on other vulnerable populations, notably those with psychiatric disorders (23). Staff interviews in that study suggested that those needing the benefits most were the ones least able to follow through with the reapplication process. In 2005, the Centre for Addiction and Mental Health in Canada explored the sensibility of a new policy in Ontario in which those with substance dependence would no longer be eligible for welfare (24). The review led to the conclusion that this was an "ill-advised policy for Ontario" and that its continuation was not recommended. This was based upon the scientific view of addiction as a chronic illness, the fostering of stigma by exclusionary social policies, and negative impact upon mental health and homeless status. A 2006 study at Yale explored whether receipt of SSI or SSDI was associated with increased drug and alcohol use (25). Although such use was measured by self-report and clinician ratings rather than by more reliable objective measures, the hypothesis that disability benefits facilitate drug use was not supported by longitudinal data.

Under Social Security law, evaluation of disability on the basis of mental disorders, including addiction, requires (26):

1. Documentation of a medically determinable impairment. This documentation must be from an accepted medical source. The documentation must include more than subjective description of symptoms. Rather, objective findings are necessary, whether resulting from psychological testing, urine drug test results, or mental status exams, again as conducted by an accepted medical source. Acceptable medical sources are licensed physicians and psychologists. Therapists and other allied medical professionals *may* be referenced, but only to demonstrate severity of impairment and impact upon work (27).
2. Consideration of the degree of limitation such impairment may impose on the individual's ability to work.
   a. Activities of Daily Living—marked impairment is defined by the nature and overall degree of interference with function and indicates that the individual has serious difficulty performing ADLs without supervision, in a suitable manner, or on a consistent, useful, and routine basis without undue interruptions or distractions.
   b. Social Functioning—marked impairment is defined by the nature and overall degree of interference with function.
   c. Concentration, Persistence, or Pace—marked impairment is noted to some extent by clinical findings, but these data must wherever possible be supplemented by other available evidence. An emphasis is given upon how independently, appropriately, and effectively a claimant is able to complete tasks on a sustained basis. Deficiencies apparent only in performance of complex procedures or tasks do not fall into the marked impairment category.
   d. Episodes of Decompensation—three episodes within 1 year, each lasting for at least 2 weeks, represents the equivalent of a marked level of severity for this category.
3. Consideration of whether these limitations have lasted or are expected to last for a continuous period of at least 12 months.

Disability is then defined as the inability to "engage in any substantial gainful activity by reason of any medically determinable physical or mental impairment which can be expected to result in death or which has lasted or can be expected to last for a continuous period of not less than 12 months" (28).

Substance addiction disorders are defined within Social Security as behavioral or physical changes associated with regular use of substances that affect the central nervous system. If the changes are primarily behavioral, they are then evaluated under listings for organic mental disorders, depressive syndrome, anxiety disorders, or personality disorders.

VIGNETTE 7

Lisa is seen for treatment of depression and anxiety by a therapist. She receives medication from a nurse clinician with whom the therapist regularly works. Lisa is noted on the initial history to use marijuana on a daily basis. The diagnoses written in the record by the treating therapist are major depression and generalized anxiety. No further reference is made to the marijuana use. No toxicology report is present in the record. Two years later, Lisa applies for SSDI due to ongoing depressive and anxiety-related symptoms. The state Disability Determination Service (DDS) sends Lisa to a psychiatric consultant for an examination. Lisa tells the consultant that she uses marijuana on a daily basis and has done so for many years. She is noted by the consultant to have marked impairment in multiple areas of function. The consultant reflects upon the ongoing use of marijuana and diagnoses the claimant with marijuana dependence and marijuana-induced mood and anxiety disorders. He reflects that the claimant might have primary mood and anxiety disorders but that these have not been demonstrated due to the ongoing substance use. Lisa fails to qualify for SSDI.

This case highlights two features of Social Security related disability. The first is that the therapist and nurse clinician do not meet the criteria for being a medically acceptable source of diagnostic information. The second is that the burden of proof of disability is, as a matter of law, upon the claimant. The claimant's records must therefore substantiate the presence of not only impairment, but of the impairment being related to a mental disorder *other than* addiction. Once the chart indicated that there was use of a psychoactive substance, the potential that addiction was the cause of impairment had to be ruled out. From a medical perspective, we are uncertain; from a legal perspective, this uncertainty may amount to the claimant's not meeting her burden of proof.

SSDI DISCUSSION

The Social Security Administration has several potential sources of clinical information for each disability applicant:

- Clinical records are gathered and submitted for review.
- A treating physician report can be requested by the state DDS. Within these reports, the clinician is asked to opine specifically about impairment resulting from diagnosed illness.
- A consultative exam (CE) can be requested by the state DDS or by the administrative law judge (ALJ) reviewing a case for the Office of Disability Adjudication and Review.
- A medical expert (ME) can be requested by the ALJ. The ME reviews the entire file, including treating physician reports and CE's, if any, and presents the case either in live testimony, through written interrogatory, or through telephonic review.

Treating physicians and ME's composing reports should be aware of these issues:

- Initial diagnostic formulation should be the result of an evaluation by a physician or a psychologist. Although in many states, other clinicians are eligible to make diagnoses or to compose treatment plans, these sources remain outside the boundaries of "acceptable" under Social Security law. Of note, the American Medical Association maintains policy stating that diagnosis of disease constitutes the practice of medicine (Resolution 904, I-06).
- Medical records thereafter should include ongoing evaluations by a physician. These evaluations must include documentation of objective measures demonstrating functional capacity or lack thereof.
- A patient statement in the initial evaluation that no drug- or alcohol-related difficulties are present does not represent an objective finding. Given the high percentage of psychiatric symptoms caused by addictive substances and the high prevalence of addictive substance use in the population overall, a urine drug screen is an appropriate part of a full psychiatric workup. Such a screen also prevents the entire diagnostic formulation from being disregarded from a legal standpoint should other records in the case demonstrate the presence of substance use.
- If the patient applying for disability is abstinent from substance use, document that abstinence through objective measures. Regular urine drug screens represent the best such measure for drugs other than alcohol. Documentation that the applicant has been attending AA/NA regularly, that he has a sponsor, that he is a sponsor, or that he is otherwise participating actively in recovery programming are helpful in demonstrating that addictive disease is no longer the impairing factor. Note, however, that such documentation also suggests that there is no or minimal impairment in social function.
- If the patient is not abstinent from substance use, document how the diagnosis of a primary psychiatric disorder was determined, perhaps during a period of extended and objectively demonstrated abstinence, and describe the impairments that were present during that specific period.
- A treating physician report stating simply that substance use is not material to either the diagnosis or the impairments, when the overall record indicates otherwise, is not likely to lead to a favorable outcome for the disability applicant (29).
- Ensure that the applicant is not being prescribed addictive substances. Besides simply being a wise approach to the treatment of addictive illness, an ongoing prescription of addictive substances blurs the picture as to whether the patient is able to prove impairment secondary to a psychiatric disorder rather than to a substance-induced disorder. If opioid prescriptions are medically necessary for treatment of pain, this should be well documented in the record.
- Be particularly savvy about use of an electronic medical record. Many such records carry over information from one entry to the next. If the majority of such entries are identical with unchanging treatment, the record will reflect overall stability and a low level of overall severity. Higher levels of severity usually result in treatment intensity increases, changes of medication, or other modality of treatments being initiated.
- Do not exaggerate the degree of impairment present. Indicating that the patient has marked impairment of

concentration, persistence, and pace is illogic if that patient is also described elsewhere in the record as driving long distances to visit family members. Note that driving is a complex task that requires sustained attention, something that would not be possible in an individual with marked impairment in this domain. Exaggeration of impairment levels can lead to an entire conclusion being disregarded. Ensure that the degree of impairment which you are indicating is supported by objective findings in your serial mental status examinations.

A final point must be considered not only for Social Security cases but for all cases:

- The role of treating physicians is not to obtain disability benefits for their patients, but to honestly and appropriately document the presence of a specific disease state first, and second, any restrictions or limitations arising as a direct result of that disease state. It is then the role of the insurance carrier, or state or federal agency to determine whether disability benefits are warranted.

REFERENCES

1. World Health Organization. *International Classification of Functioning, Disability, and Health*. Geneva: World Health Organization; 2001.
2. World Health Organization. *International Classification of Impairments, Disabilities, and Handicaps (ICIDH)*. Geneva: World Health Organization; 1980.
3. World Health Organization. *Towards a Common Language for Functioning, Disability, and Health*. Geneva: World Health Organization; 2002.
4. United Kingdom Disability Discrimination Act 1995 Chapter 50.
5. Wasserman D. Addiction and disability: moral and policy issues. *Subst Use Misuse*. 2004;39(3):461–488.
6. American Medical Association. *Guides to the Evaluation of Permanent Impairment*. 6th ed. Chicago, IL: American Medical Association; 2008.
7. *Occupational Medicine Practice Guidelines: Evaluation and Management of Common Health Problems and Functional Recovery in Workers*. 2nd ed. Elk Grove Village, IL: American College of Occupational and Environmental Medicine; 2008.
8. *Official Disability Guidelines*. Encinitas, CA: Work Loss Data Institute; 2009.
9. *Diagnostic and Statistical Manual of Mental Disorders*, Fourth Edition, Text Revision (DSM-IV-TR). Washington DC: American Psychiatric Association; 2000.
10. Domino KB, Hornbein TF, Polissar NL, et al. Risk factors for relapse in health care professionals with substance use disorders. *J Am Med Assoc*. 2005;293:1453–1460.
11. Fry RA. Chemical dependency treatment outcomes of residents. *Anesth Analg*. 2006;103:1588.
12. Berge KH, Seppala MD, Lanier WL. The anesthesiology community's approach to opioid- and anesthetic-abusing personnel: time to change course. *Anesthesiology*. 2008;109(5): 762–764.
13. Mendelson J, Flower K, Pletcher MJ, et al. Addiction to prescription opioids: characteristics of the emerging epidemic and treatment with buprenorphine. *Exp Clin Psychopharmacol*. 2008; 16(5):435–441.
14. American Medical Association Council on Science & Public Health. Improving Medical Practice and Patient/Family Education to Reverse the Epidemic of Nonmedical Prescription Drug Use and Addiction. November 2008 Report. Chicago, IL: American Medical Association.
15. Trescot AM, Boswell MV, Altiuri SL, et al. Recommendations for using opioids in chronic non-cancer pain. *Eur J Pain*. 2003;7(5):381–386.
16. Guideline for the Use of Chronic Opioid Therapy in Chronic Noncancer Pain. The American Pain Society, The American Academy of Pain Medicine. *J Pain*. 2009;10(2):113–130.e22.
17. American Psychiatric Association Task Force. *Benzodiazepine Dependence, Toxicity, and Abuse*. Washington, DC: American Psychiatric Association Task Force; 1990.
18. Uhlenhuth EH, Balter MB, Ban TA, et al. International study of expert judgment on therapeutic use of benzodiazepines and other psychotherapeutic medications: IV. Therapeutic dose dependence and abuse liability of benzodiazepines in the long-term treatment of anxiety disorders. *J Clin Psychopharmacol*. 1999; 19(suppl 2):23S–29S.
19. Ashton CH. Benzodiazepine withdrawal: outcome in 50 Patients. *Br J Addict*. 1987;82:655–671.
20. Gresenz CR, Watkins K, Podus D. SSI, DI, and substance abusers. *Community MHJ*. 1998;34(4):337–350.
21. Social Security Administration. *Highlights of Summary Report of Drug Addiction and Alcoholism Implementation*. Washington, DC: Social Security Administration; 1997.
22. Watkins KE, Wells KB, McLellan AT. Termination of social security benefits among Los Angeles recipients disabled by substance abuse. *Psychiatr Serv*. 1999;50:914–918.
23. Hanrahan P, Luchins DJ, Cloninger L, et al. Medicaid eligibility of former SSI recipients with drug abuse or alcoholism disability. *Am J Pub Health*. 2004;94(11):46–47.
24. Erickson PG, Callaghan RC. The probable impacts of the removal of the addiction disability benefit in Ontario. *Can J Commun Ment Health*. 2005;24(2):99–108.
25. Rosen MI, McMahon TJ, Lin H, et al. Effect of Social Security payments on substance abuse in a homeless mentally ill cohort. *Health Serv Res*. 2006;41(1):173–191.
26. Disability Evaluation Under Social Security, September 2008. SSA Office of Disability Programs. Washington DC: Social Security Administration Office of Disability Programs.
27. US Code of Federal Regulations. 20 CFR 404.1513(d).
28. US Code of Federal Regulations. 42 USC 423(d)(1)(A). 2006.
29. Carol L. Blais, Plaintiff v. Michael J. Astrue, Commissioner, Social Security Administration, Defendant. CA 08-119 ML; 2009 US Dist LEXIS 64919.

CHAPTER 69: New Immigrants and Refugees

Joseph Westermeyer

HISTORICAL AND CULTURAL BACKGROUND

Immigrants

Since its inception as a nation more than 200 years ago, the U.S. population has often consisted of 10% to 20% foreign-born people. In the 2000 census, 31,107,889 people were foreign born, and an additional 3,527,551 people were born outside of the United States in various territories (e.g., Puerto Rico, Virgin Islands). Together these two groups comprise 12.3% of the total 281,421,906 people counted in the census. A conservative estimate of 3 million illegal residents in the United States (1) brings the total to around 38 million, or approximately 13.5% of the total population. In addition, the United States has several million visitors per year, including foreign students, visitors, temporary workers, tourists, entertainers, and representatives of foreign governments (military, embassy staff). Immigrants, refugees, and these special categories of visitors all include individuals who seek services for substance abuse in the United States.

From 1980 to 2000, the number of counted foreign-born people in the United States rose by 224%. Although Canada and Australia also have man foreign-born residents, the number of immigrants to the United States has exceeded the number of immigrants entering all other countries of the world in recent years (2). In sum, clinicians in the United States must be prepared to address substance abuse problems within immigrant and refugee groups.

In the 2000 census, the continent-wide origins of foreign-born people in the United States were as follows: the Americas, 16,916,416; Asia, 8,226,254; Europe, 4,915,557; Africa, 881,300; and Oceania, 168,046. National origins of the most numerous immigrants included the following: Mexico, 9,177,487; China, 1,518,652; Philippines, 1,369,070; India, 1,022,552; Korea, 864,125; Canada, 820,771; El Salvador, 817,336; and United Kingdom, 677,751. Immigrants bring new types of substance use and abuse to the United States, including opium smoking, betel nut chewing, and qat chewing. These traditional substances may involve drugs or modes of administration unfamiliar to American clinicians.

Refugees

Unlike other immigrants, most refugees would have preferred to remain in their country of origin. Refugees have fled their homeland to avoid prejudice, incarceration, or even death for their political or religious beliefs, or their ethnic affiliation. Although people have fled war and social tumult throughout human history, the number of people involved in such flight has dramatically increased. A United Nations report estimated that 45 million people had left their homelands between 1945 and 1967 (3)—a trend that continues annually (4). This recent trend has greatly increased the number of people coming from underdeveloped countries, from which many arrive poorly prepared for life in the United States.

There are several definitions of refugees, ranging from strict United Nations definitions to lay terms such as "economic refugees." For immigration and legal purposes in the United States, a refugee is defined as such by the federal government. The status extends special privileges to anyone so labeled. As clinicians, we may identify someone as seeking refuge, but the person may not have federal status as a refugee in the United States. Likewise, some legal refugees may resemble immigrants in that they have experienced no trauma and have left the home country willingly to come to the United States for personal reasons.

From a health perspective, refugees can pose a special challenge in view of their exposure to war or other trauma. This group is at special risk to numerous health problems. Drug trafficking and substance abuse sometimes accompany war and civil unrest—factors that can haunt a resettlement country (5).

CLINICAL ASSESSMENT

Working with Translators

In the 2000 census, 9.5 million inhabitants of the United States reported that they spoke English either "not well" (6.3 million) or "not at all" (3.2 million). The greatest proportion was Spanish speaking, accounting for 4.1 million. The second largest group was Asian–Pacific Islanders, with 1.6 million. Indo-Europeans comprised 1.3 million, with the remainder coming largely from Africa. Patients with inadequate skills in English will need a translator for an adequate assessment, unless the clinician speaks the patient's language.

Prior to working with a translator, the clinician should have a model for understanding the process of interpreting the clinician's queries and the patient's and family's responses. Three models common to the clinical context are as follows (6):

- The "black box" model. The clinician views the translator as a magical "black box" in which all queries and responses are accurately and completely translated. This model does not function well with psychiatric or substance use interviews.
- The "junior clinician" model. The clinician views the translator as a junior assistant clinician, whose task is to obtain the relevant clinical data being sought by the clinician. This model may work well if the translator is also a trained clinician whose work is being supervised by an experienced clinician-educator.
- The "three partners" model. The clinician, translator, and patient share the difficult task of informing one another regarding various queries and responses. This task is rendered complex through the absence of shared language and shared culture between clinician and patient. Typically, the translator has extensive experience in both languages and cultures but not in clinical assessment and care. The task is further complicated by a three-sided series of transference and counter-transference relationships. Despite its challenges for the clinician, this model lends itself best to psychiatric and substance use interviews.

Training the translator to this task requires more than a brief orientation. The translator's own views and attitudes toward substance use disorder can obstruct the clinician–patient relationship in a myriad of ways. The translator's own lay attitudes, use of substances, and choice of words can either enhance communication or seriously undermine it.

Case Example
An Asian foreign student, trained as a translator in a nonclinical setting, developed a personal relationship with a patient outside of the clinical setting. She did not initially reveal this to the clinic staff. As this friendship developed, the patient became less open and at ease in clinical setting. When asked about this change, the patient revealed his hesitance to express himself openly without first considering the effect it would have on his deepening friendship with the translator. Following this explanation, another translator was assigned to the case. The original translator received additional training regarding the special ethical, legal, and professional boundaries needed when working in a clinical setting.

Obtaining a Substance Use History

Substance use and abuse manifest many similarities across cultures. Through a supportive, informed, and empathetic approach, the clinician can usually obtain a complete picture of the patient's substance-related problem. At times, the clinician may have to seek help from the literature if the substance, route of administration, or pattern of use is unfamiliar. PubMed and other Internet-based sources can assist in bringing a broad published literature to the service of the patient abusing unfamiliar drugs, and consuming them in an unfamiliar way.

The chronologic sequence of substance use vis-a-vis migration should be established. Did the patient begin use in the country of origin? Or in the United States? Or in another country? How was the patient introduced to the experience? What were the patient's circumstances at the time? Was the initial use of the substance a culturally deviant or syntonic activity?

Case Example
A veteran-immigrant born and raised in Latin America returned from a combat rotation with the American Army in Iraq, where he served with a combat unit. His combat experienced included killing the enemy (although distinguishing bystanders with combatants was at times unclear), injury and death of members of his combat unit, and an open arm wound with a brief period of unconsciousness from an explosion. While he was overseas, his mother died of a drug overdose, and his father died of AIDS. A member of his unit, who had been threatening suicide, shot himself in the head in the patient's presence. Although he had not abused drugs previously, upon discharge from the military he began to abuse opioid and sedative medications prescribed for his arm injury. When Veterans Administratio (VA) physicians would no longer prescribe opioids for him, he began to purchase opiates on the street. He entered treatment when he developed an abscess in his forearm from injecting drugs. With abstinence from opioids, posttraumatic stress disorder (PTSD) symptoms emerged.

Establishing the family or community attitude toward drug use is health care generally. For example, in this case most of the patient's family members abused opioid drugs. Moreover, obtaining illicit opioids for one's personal use was commonplace in his community of origin. Had his VA physicians been aware of these early experiences, they might have monitored his opioid treatment more judiciously.

Culturally Competent Evaluation

In most respects, the evaluation continues largely as it would for other patients from indigenous ethnic groups. Review of systems should emphasize specific queries regarding psychological symptoms (e.g., anorexia, weight or sleep changes, fatigue, crying spells, fears, chronic pain, headache, bowel changes, anhedonia, hearing or seeing things not perceived by others), since foreign-born patients might not spontaneously report such symptoms to a nonkin person. While taking a family history, the clinician should be alert to patriarchal or matriarchal kin systems, because patients may not consider nonkin to be relatives in the biogenetic sense. A social history should reflect the patient's former life in the country of origin, as well as the past and present life in the country of immigration.

Mental status should be culturally informed because orientation in time and space can be affected by culture (e.g., Buddhist and Islamic calendars, differences in counting floors of a building). Education can affect the ability to do arithmetic or replicate figures with paper and pencil. English fluency and literacy can affect naming, reading, writing, and enunciating. To interpret proverbs, the patient needs to consider a proverb familiar to the patient's culture. Ability to discern similarities in unlike objects depends upon education and familiarity with the objects.

The final step consists of putting the entire story together into a coherent, integrated whole. This process should provide information regarding the patient's cultural identity, his or her explanation or understanding of the disorder, and sociocultural factors that favor recovery or chronicity. The clinician should consider the cultural aspects of the doctor–patient relationship. Finally, cultural factors that might support or impede the diagnosis and care plan should be considered.

Acquiring the Migration History

Immigrants and refugees come from every corner of the world, from the largest and most sophisticated cities to the most remote and undeveloped of rural villages. Inquiry into this premigration phase of the patient's life can enhance the clinician's understanding of the patient and the presenting clinical problem. This dialogue also enables the patient to inform the clinician regarding that unknown portions of the patient's past life.

During this exercise, the clinician can inquire into the patient's early exposure to substance use and abuse in the country of origin. In turn, this can lead to a family history of substance use and other psychiatric disorders. Models of treatment or recovery from substance abuse in the former country can lead to recommendations familiar to the patient and family.

Many immigrants and refugees do not come directly to the United States. The patient may not report these peregrinations if not asked about them. Inquiry may elicit important circumstances regarding the genesis of substance use.

A premigration history informs the clinician regarding the patient's competence, accomplishments, losses, and stressors before reaching the United States. This history provides a history of the individual within the culture of origin, or in countries of first refuge for refugees. Typically, early successes forecast subsequent successes. This is not always the case, however. An occasional person who did well in the homeland does miserably in the United States, and vice versa.

Special Comorbidity Risks

Refugees are at special risk to diverse posttraumatic psychiatric disorders, which can accompany substance use disorder (SUD). The latter include PTSD, major depressive disorder, phobic disorder, generalized anxiety disorder, and panic disorder (7). Somatization and somatic presentations are also highly prevalent among migrants (8). These disorders may predate SUD, occur around the same time, or appear after SUD has been successfully treated.

PTSD may affect not only refugees, but also some immigrant groups (9). Ruling PTSD out may not be easily accomplished, as the migrant may be alexithymic vis-a-vis perceived emotional distress, denying or suppressing past traumatic events, somatizing the emotional distress, or embarrassed or ashamed to reveal the trauma and its consequences (10). Rapport sets the groundwork for gentle probing of traumatic experiences. Inquiry regarding nightmares, intrusive thoughts, or hypervigilance can also suggest past trauma. Pansystem somatic symptoms (e.g., frequent headache, dizziness or faintness, appetite change, sleeping problems) can reflect past trauma (11). Missed grieving or delayed grieving may also co-occur in situations where traumatic experiences involved the deaths of friends or family members (12). Addictive disorders can contribute to delayed or missing grieving.

Other externalizing disorders besides SUD may also accompany SUD. Externalizing disorders in adulthood include pathologic gambling, eating disorders, tobacco dependence, antisocial personality disorder, compulsive shopping, and kleptomania (13). Prolonged insecurity (14) or numerous negative life events (15) during childhood or adolescence may contribute to these disorders in refugees and some immigrants coming from insecure areas. Mechanisms include possible prolonged cortisol elevation due to stress (16) and/or prolonged nicotine exposure (17)—both common in certain premigration circumstances. Loss of traditional values can also favor externalizing disorders (18). International adoptees have shown an increased risk to the externalizing disorders (19).

Physical problems can serve as a clue to comorbid problems that may not improve with sobriety alone. For example, chronic pain may be a clue to PTSD (20). Mild to moderate brain damage is prevalent in some refugee groups (21).

INTERPRETATION OF FINDINGS

Acculturation

The "melting pot" in the United States has introduced new models and methods of substance use. European Americans not schooled in the ceremonial use of tobacco, developed tobacco dependence along with its myriad biomedical disorders. Some young Somali refugees, with no exposure to alcohol use in their Islamic families, have chosen weekend drunkenness as an "American" recreational form.

Cultural changes can include changes in traditional substance use. For example, the Hmong, a refugee group from Southeast Asia, formerly had a rigid protocol for alcohol drinking, with few problems (22). However, in the United States, many of the animistic Hmong converted to abstinence-oriented Christianity. This social change undermined the former stability in drinking practices, resulting in diversity from those who drank nothing to those who drank in a secular and sometimes dissocial fashion, that is, at times and in amounts that they choose (23). Another example is the traditional use of qat in Somalia, Ethiopia, and nearby countries (24), where groups largely used it under socially controlled circumstances. However, some refugees from these groups have become addicted to qat when using it to relieve physical or emotional symptoms following migration. In contexts of rapid sociocultural change, old traditions of use can give way to new patterns of use adopted.

Other changes also modify the drinking or drug use context following relocation to a new society. For example, the nature of work, transportation, and other technology can increase the risk associated with even mild intoxication or morning-after hangovers. Increased access to high-speed vehicles, complex machinery, and the smooth interaction and coordination of many workers can render intoxication newly risky for the immigrant. In addition to the individual, society at large bears the cost of vehicular and industrial accidents (25).

As a consequence of these changes, alcohol and/or other drugs can become a virtual scourge for certain subgroups in the United States. For them, substance abuse is a major cause of child neglect, family disruption, divorce, vehicular accidents, injury, and death.

Case Example

A 36-year-old Asian refugee had fled his country of origin a decade earlier with his military unit, leaving family behind. In the United States, he drank heavily and episodically with ethnic peers, much as he had done as a young soldier in Asia. During one of these episodes, he was involved in a serious accident in which a friend was killed and he sustained a traumatic brain injury. Treatment was not provided for either the alcohol abuse or the brain injury. Subsequently, he married an American woman and had three children. His episodic heavy drinking persisted, primarily on weekends and holidays, but at times after work. Following a long weekend holiday of drinking with American friends, he killed his wife, three children, and mother-in-law while they were asleep. In the morning, discovering with horror the massacre, he called the police, who established beyond doubt that he had murdered his family, apparently during one of many alcoholic "black outs" that he had been having.

Cultural Diversity within Groups

Groups of immigrants to the United States differ greatly. The same is true of individuals within these groups, for whom the new country presents many choices and alternatives. Some immigrants remain staunchly traditional to their country of origin. Others assimilate to a considerable extent with the "mainstream" American culture. Years following relocation, immigrant groups often manifest greater differences among themselves than were previously manifest in the country of origin.

Failure to acculturate successfully to the new country can increase the risk of substance abuse. Successful acculturation can be identified by the immigrant's ability to speak English, hold a job, use the social institutions of the receiving society (e.g., banks, libraries, health care), access the mass media, and establish relationships outside of the immigrant's own group. Acculturation failure is manifest by dependence on others, declining mental health, social isolation, ignorance of social forces at play in the community, confusion regarding how to plan one's future life, and increasing lack of control over one's life.

Substance abuse may provide an alternative to young immigrants caught between the "old country" culture and the new culture. Some of the superficial accouterments of American culture, for example, fast cars and drug or alcohol use, may substitute for a more fundamental acculturation. Petty crime or drug trafficking may be pursued as a means of paying for this apparent "American" lifestyle (26).

Migratory History and Onset of Substance Abuse

Some cases of substance abuse begin after migration. However, most cases among adult migrants involve continuation of premigration substance abuse or dependence, rather than new cases. The following case exemplifies this pattern.

Case Example

A 26-year-old Palestinian graduate student had become a heroin addict in his native Palestine. Formerly a good student, he was unable to obtain a job consistent with his education. Berated by his father for his inability to support the extended family despite his education, he found solace in spending his time with a group of unemployed college graduates. Exposed to heroin in this group, he was soon addicted. His father arranged for him to attend graduate school in the United States, following detoxification in Israel. For 6 months he did well academically and socially. Exposed to the opportunity to use heroin, however, he soon became readdicted. Failing academically, he sought treatment for his addiction (as he had done previously in Israel). However, he was unable to maintain his grades at that point, was dropped from school, and returned to Palestine.

Krupinski studied the appearance of new cases of substance abuse among post–World War II immigrants from East Europe to Australia (27). Most immigrants abused alcohol. Typically, these immigrants were in Australia for several years before heavy drinking began, and then several years more before seeking treatment for alcoholism. This chronologic pattern was unlike postmigration mood, anxiety, or psychotic disorders, which tended to appear within months to several years following relocation. Factors that may delay onset of substance disorder following migration include the following:

- Immigration officials screen out obvious cases of alcoholism or addiction.
- Purchasing alcohol or drugs requires disposable income, so years may pass before the immigrant has sufficient funds to purchase alcohol or drugs.
- On average it requires about 3 years of heavy cocaine or heroin abuse before initial treatment seeking, and about a decade of alcohol or opium abuse before initial treatment seeking (25).

Analysis of an opium smoking epidemic among refugees in the United States revealed two groups of addicts, that is: (1) those who became readdicted in the United States and (2) those who became addicted for the first time in the United States (28). Of relevance to Krupinski's observations, the first use of opium in the United States did not appear in this refugee group until they had been in the United States for several years. At that time a large-scale smuggling operation developed to bring opium from Mexico and Asia to the United States, along with some local poppy production.

These studies from Australia and the United States indicate that older immigrants are most likely to abuse substances traditional in the country of origin. Young immigrants may also abuse the traditional substance if they remain ensconced within the immigrant community, as occurred among the young Hmong opium addicts. However, young immigrants may abuse substances that are not traditional within the immigrant community, but are substances abused within American society, in an abortive attempt to join, or at least emulate the majority society.

High-Risk Immigrant Groups

As a nation composed largely of immigrants and refugees, we tend to idealize these groups as harking back to our own origins. However, idealization should not render us blind to subgroups at high risk to substance abuse. The propensity of foreign countries to "dump" their problematic citizens in the United States (and other immigrant countries) was first recognized more than 150 years ago, when several European countries sent prisoners and debtors to the United States at public expense as a means of being rid of them (29).

Immigration laws have removed this historical trend to a considerable extent, because foreign countries are liable for the return of their mentally disabled citizens at their own expense. Nonetheless, refugee groups can include individuals at high risk to substance disorders. Perhaps the most flagrant modern example was President Carter's acceptance of thousands of criminals in the "Mariel" flight from Cuba (Mariel referred to the prison from which the refugees originated). Although many of the 120,000 participants in this flight were not addicted or criminal, thousands of "Mariel refugees" appeared in jails and treatment facilities across the United States soon after their arrival.

Case Example

A 36-year-old Mariel refugee had been a petty criminal and alcohol abuser in Cuba. Upon arrival in the United States, he discovered that his contacts in the Hispanic community gave him access to cocaine trafficking. He became a street trader, buying from smugglers and selling on the streets. He soon became addicted to cocaine himself, resulting in his "cutting" his product with inert substances. This practice led to a conflict with a client, as a result of which he shot the client. He is now serving a sentence in the United States for murder.

Another general category at risk consists of young, single men who were members of defeated armies allied with the United States. Often illiterate or poorly educated, they may not have sufficient skills to sustain them in the United States. Unfortunately, the United States has not provided veterans' benefits nor acculturation training and education for these high-risk young men.

Case Example

A refugee had been a soldier from the age of 17 years in his homeland, coming to the United States at age 26 years when his national army was defeated. He fled without his wife and daughter, whom he has never been able to locate. Although he was literate in his own language and had risen to the rank of noncommissioned officer, his former achievements did not predict success in the United States. A shrapnel wound to his forehead followed by several hours of unconsciousness suggested a possible head injury. Unable to learn English, he worked principally as a dishwasher and unskilled laborer. His recreational activities consisted entirely of gambling and drinking in the company of men similar to himself. At the age of 44 years he was incarcerated for killing an ethnic peer in a fight that occurred in a context of drinking and cannabis use.

TREATMENT AND RECOVERY

"Mainstream" Treatment Modalities

Addicted persons of virtually any ethnic background accept care in detoxification centers, emergency rooms, and inpatient hospital units. The challenge to continued treatment begins beyond this acute phase. Once beyond the pain of withdrawal or other health emergency, the addicted person may become more selective about continued care.

The "three A's" integral to successful rehabilitation following early acute care are as follows:

- Availability: The treatment must be reasonably close at hand, so that the person can participate in the recovery-centered endeavors. Telemedicine services can greatly facilitate services to rural areas or ethnic neighborhoods.
- Access: The patient must have access to the program; lack of insurance or language barriers can prevent entry.
- Acceptance: The patient and the program must accept each other.

An analysis of barriers in one health care system revealed four categorical sources of cultural barriers to mental health care (30). Two of these general barriers lay on the health care side, that is, the clinicians and the health care system. The other two categories consisted of the patient barriers (e.g., antitherapeutic attitudes, ignorance, lack of resources) and the patient's family and community (e.g., not supportive, do not understand).

Self-Help in Recovery

Some self-help activities can occur regardless of ethnic affiliation, such as avoiding people and places associated with use (31). However, other forms of self-help may differ across cultures. These differences can be due to cultural values, customs, or institutions.

Alcoholics Anonymous can change form and content considerably when translated across culture and language (32). Entire communities can engage in self-help, through eliminating substance abuse and associated problems (33).

For example, in cultures that view self-disclosure as self-centered, "confession" of addiction-related "sins" may prove unacceptable.

Religious Conversion and Recovery

Conversion to abstinence-oriented religion has alleviated addictive disorders for many around the world. For example, Hispanics throughout the Americas have joined abstinence-oriented fundamentalist Christian religions as a means of achieving sobriety and resisting invitations to drink (34). Buddhist monasteries have served as places of recovery, especially when a charismatic abbot leads the way (35). Galanter described the "large-group psychotherapy" that may attend membership in an abstinence-oriented or recovery-oriented religious group (36). Some programs, such as involvement in the Native American Church, may be restricted to members of the ethnic groups sponsoring them (37). Even without conversion efforts, spirituality and religiosity tend to increase during the early months of sobriety (38), providing a rationale for the efficacy of religious conversation in fostering recovery.

Previous Exposure to Treatment

We sometimes assume that treatment for addiction is available only in a few industrialized societies. However, treatment exists virtually wherever addiction occurs (39). Inquiry into previous treatments in the country of origin can provide important information.

Treatment can include community sings, herbal medications, and sweat lodges. Often these modalities possess a ritual or ceremonial dimension (39). Ceremonies can be useful in engendering social support for the recovering person, establishing a new social persona, and fostering new attitudes toward a sober lifestyle (40). Inquiry about traditional modalities can aid in appreciating the patient's understanding of addiction treatment.

Psychotherapies

English literacy or advanced education is not necessary for successful psychotherapy. Supportive counseling can be applied in any setting; it can be especially efficacious if the immigrant patient is seeking an advisor for successful adjustment to the new society. Cognitive-behavioral therapy (CBT) and behavioral modification can apply to members of any group. Examples include desensitization for phobic disorder or PTSD.

Family therapy may involve special considerations, depending on the family structure and traditions in the patient's culture and family. In family therapy, the explicit family hierarchy will often hold sway, so that family members do not typically confront a matriarch or patriarch in front a therapist. This special challenge is not a rationale for circumventing the family, however. Whenever possible, the family should be involved in the patient's assessment and care (41), as well as other members of the patient's social network who are committed to the patient's recovery (42). Elements of interpersonal psychotherapy and psychodynamically oriented psychotherapy can also have their place in cross-cultural care.

As indicated above, delayed or missed grieving may appear once the addicted person becomes sober. Bereavement may involve the deaths of friends and family members. Especially in the case of refugees, bereavement may involve other losses (9), such as:

- Separation from family and friends, still alive in the home country
- Loss of home, community, work, familiar recreation, and nation
- Rejection by the country of origin
- Failure of the family, religion, or homeland to provide safety and security
- Shame at behaviors needed to survive (e.g., theft, lying, duplicity, prostitution, abandoning relatives or friends, killing)
- Inability to discharge one's responsibilities to family, friends, or society.

Pharmacotherapy and Culture

Medications are often thought of as mechanistic modalities that affect neurotransmitter systems, but have no cultural relevance. To some extent, this may be true. For example, one does not have to understand the pharmacotherapy of diazepam (Valium) to obtain relief in the midst of alcohol withdrawal.

Medications can also play important social and cultural roles. For example, disulfiram (Antabuse) and naltrexone (ReVia) have provided an excuse for recovering alcoholics to refuse friendly invitations by peers to go out drinking or drug using (43). The following case of a refugee demonstrates the principle.

Case Example

A 42-year-old immigrant from Puerto Rico had difficulty refusing his peers' invitations to drink on weekends, despite his strong intent to remain sober. His relatives and neighbors accused him of trying to act better than them, or of abandoning their long relationship. A recovered neighbor told him to ask his doctor for disulfiram (Antabuse), as this could provide an acceptable excuse for not drinking. The patient did request and received disulfiram from his physician. As the neighbor indicated, his weekend drinking buddies took this as an acceptable excuse. They knew that the man could not drink on Antabuse, and they accepted the doctor's authority and knowledge providing an acceptable rationale.

Acculturation Therapy

By the time an immigrant has been failing in acculturation and has become an SUD patient, it is unlikely that simple referral to job training, education, or other local forms of rehabilitation will succeed. Special programs for those failing in the acculturation task are required.

An "acculturation failure" group should include individuals from a variety of cultures and languages. Combining a culturally diverse clientele into a single large group offers certain economies of scale. Because all clients are unlikely to require all elements of such a program, a "smorgasbord" approach should permit each client to engage in those aspects of the program that the client needs. Elements of such a program may include

- Taking English-as-a-second language (ESL) instruction
- Training in elemental aspects of community life (e.g., shopping, taking public transportation, food preparation, accessing health services, obtaining police protection, using financial services)
- Knowing the history, government, laws, and cultural values and norms of the United States
- Child raising and family laws in the United States
- Acquiring job skills and learning how to acquire job
- Learning how to keep a job and progress in employment
- Participating in recreational activities that do not require substance use
- Coping with bias, prejudice, and racism.

Return to the Culture of Origin

Forcible removal to the culture of origin, while not a therapy per se, sometimes becomes an undesired but inevitable disposition. Those working with immigrants must accept this as potential outcome in some cases. Clinical considerations rarely dissuade immigration officials from a deportation decision.

Return to the culture of origin may produce clinical improvement in the substance abuse. The largest naturalistic study involved American military in Vietnam. Among those who abused opiates in Vietnam, few ever returned to opiate abuse in the United States (44). Many expatriate opiate addicts in Laos did well upon return to their respective countries of origin in Europe, North America, and elsewhere (45).

PREVENTION

Religious affiliation with groups that forbid any use of alcohol or other recreational drugs has been effective as prevention, as well as a treatment. Abstinence-oriented religion also provides easier access to leadership as compared to religions that require clergy to study for many years before becoming leaders; immigrants themselves have become the leaders and clergy in fundamentalist sects. Community consensus against alcohol abuse or use of illicit drugs may evolve from these church enclaves. A danger is that the abstinence-oriented sect may ultimately turn against addicted people, lumping the persona with the drug.

Prevention among refugees and immigrants can be fostered by making culturally sensitive medical and psychiatric care available to immigrants and refugees as a means of preventing self-treatment with alcohol and dependence-producing drugs. Immigrating individuals and families can be educated to the early signs and symptoms of substance abuse in family members, and to methods of supportive confrontation of drug and alcohol abuse. Awareness of enabling and rescuing behaviors by family members, and their detrimental effects on the course of substance abuse, should be promulgated.

To reduce the availability of illicit drugs in immigrant communities, expatriate police officers must be represented on the local police force. As with health care, the civil security network must be available to expatriate social networks.

Immigrant groups bring their unique histories and traditions to the societal mainstream in the United States. In addition to their rich customs, they also bring their vulnerabilities to psychoactive substances, whether traditional substances from the past or new substances. In a few instances, they bring new substances to the United States. American society and its institutions should recognize its contributions to immigrant use and abuse of substances, and its responsibility in supporting prevention. Likewise, immigrant groups should realize their role in contributing to the well being of the society at large. Prevention requires the efforts of both the mainstream society and the immigrant groups.

For immigrants themselves, brief-but-repeated introspection can prove valuable in maintaining function, helping planning, and avoiding malfunction such as alcohol and drug abuse. One method fostered by Australian aborigines struggling to adapt to the surrounding Australian society has been to consider and discuss with others the following three questions:

Who am I?
Where do I come from?
How is my life meaningful?

Part of the task lies in figuring out the questions. Queries that are so broad and open-ended do not make for obvious answers. Discussing the query with others helps to clarify the nature of the question for one's self. Each question can be freestanding, but they also have underlying unities. Thus, responding in considerable detail to the earlier query facilitates addressing the subsequent query. And finally, the responses are dynamic and changing for the immigrant, who is changing over time. Since recovery from SUD also entails numerous changes, these three queries contribute to the recovery process.

REFERENCES

1. Crockcroft JD. *Outlaws in the Promised Land*. New York: Grove Press; 1986.
2. Bacon KH. Population and power: preparing for change. *Wall St J*. January 7, 1988.
3. United Nations High Commissioner for Refugees. *United Nations: Refugee Report*. Geneva: United Nations High Commissioner for Refugees; 1969.

4. United Nations High Commissioner for Refugees. *United Nations: Refugee Report*. Geneva: United Nations High Commissioner for Refugees; 2009.
5. Westermeyer J, Lyfoung T, Westermeyer M, et al. Opium addiction among Indochinese refugees in the U.S.: characteristics of addicts and their opium use. *Am J Drug Alcohol Abuse*. 1991;17:267–277.
6. Westermeyer J. Working with an interpreter in psychiatric assessment and treatment. *J Nerv Ment Dis*. 1990;178:745–749.
7. Fazel M, Wheeler J, Danesh J. Prevalence of serious mental disorder in 7000 refugees resettled in Western countries: a systematic review. *Lancet*. 2005;365:1309–1314.
8. Hinton DE, Hinton SD, Loeum RJR, et al. The 'multiplex model' of somatic symptoms: application to tinnitus among traumatized Cambodian refugees. *Transcult Psychiatry*. 2008;45:287–317.
9. Cervantes R, Salgado-de-Snyder VN, Pakilla AM. Posttraumatic Stress in immigrants from Central America and Mexico. *Hosp Community Psychiatry*. 1989;40:615–619.
10. Westermeyer J, Wahmenholm K. Assessing the victimized psychiatric patient. *Hosp Community Psychiatry*. 1989;40:245–249.
11. Westermeyer J, Bouafuely M, Neider J. Somatization among refugees: an epidemiological study. *Psychosomatics*. 1989;30:34–43.
12. Munoz L. Exile as bereavement: socio-psychological manifestations of Chilean exiles in Great Britain. *Br J Med Psychol*. 1980;53:227–232.
13. Chan YF, Dennis ML, Funk RR. Prevalence and comorbidity of major internalizing and externalizing problems among adolescents and adults presenting to substance abuse treatment. *J Subst Abuse Treat*. 2008;34:14–24.
14. Allen JP, Porter M, McFarland C, et al. The relation of attachment security to adolescents' paternal and peer relationships, depression, and externalizing behavior. *Child Dev*. 2007;78:1222–1239.
15. Button TM, Lau JY, Maughan B, et al. Parental punitive discipline, negative life events and gene-environment interplay in the development of externalizing behavior. *Psychol Med*. 2008;38:29–39.
16. Alink LR, van Ijzendoorn MH, Bakermans-Kranenburg MJ, et al. Cortisol and externalizing behavior in children and adolescents: mixed meta-analytic evidence for the inverse relation of basal cortisol and cortisol reactivity with externalizing behavior. *Dev Psychobiol*. 2008;50:427–450.
17. Gatzke-Koop LM, Beauchaine TP. Direct and passive nicotine exposure and the development of externalizing psychopathology. *Child Psychiatry Hum Dev*. 2007;38:255–269.
18. Gonzales NA, German M, Kim SY, et al. Mexican American adolescents' cultural orientation, externalizing behavior and academic engagement: the role of traditional cultural values. *Am J Community Psychol*. 2008;41:151–164.
19. Harf A, Taieb O, Moro MR. Externalizing behaviour problems of internationally adopted adolescents: a review. *Encephale*. 2007;33:270–276.
20. Buchwald D, Goldberg J, Noonan C, et al. Posttraumatic stress disorder and pain in American Indians. *Pain Med*. 2005;8:72–79.
21. Ta K, Westermeyer J, Neider J. Physical disorders among Southeast Asian refugee outpatients with psychiatric disorders. *Psychiatr Serv*. 1996;47:975–979.
22. Westermeyer J. *Poppies, Pipes and People: Opium and Its Use in Laos*. Berkeley, CA: University of California Press; 1982.
23. Westermeyer J. Hmong drinking practices in the United States: the influence of migration. In: Bennett L, Ames G, eds. *The American Experience with Alcohol*. New York: Plenum Press; 1985:373–391.
24. Griffiths P, Gossop M, Wickenden S. A transcultural pattern of drug use: Qat (khat) in the U.K. *Br J Psychiatry*. 1997;170:281–248.
25. Arif A, Westermeyer J, eds. *A Manual for Drug and Alcohol Abuse: Guidelines for Teaching*. New York: Plenum Press; 1988.
26. Westermeyer J. Substance use disorders among young minority refugees: common themes in a clinical sample. *NIDA Res Monogr*. 1993;130:308–320.
27. Krupinski J, Stoller A, Wallace L. Psychiatric disorders in Eastern European refugees now in Australia. *Soc Sci Med*. 1973;7:31–45.
28. Westermeyer J, Lyfoung T, Neider J. An epidemic of opium dependence among Asian refugees in Minnesota: characteristics and causes. *Br J Addict*. 1989;84:785–789.
29. May JV. Immigration as a problem in the state care of the insane. *Am J Insanity*. 1912;69:313–322.
30. Westermeyer J, Canive J, Garrard J, et al. Perceived barriers to mental health care for American Indian and Hispanic veterans: reports by 100 VA staff. *Transcult Psychiatry*. 2002;39:516–530.
31. Westermeyer J, Myott S, Aarts R, et al. Self-help strategies among substance abusers. *Am J Addict*. 2001;10:249–257.
32. Jilek-Aal L. Alcohol and the Indian-White relationship: a study of the function of Alcoholics Anonymous among coast Salish Indians. *Confin Psychiatr*. 1978;21:195–233.
33. Taylor V. The triumph of the Alkali Lake Indian band. *Alcohol Health Res World*. 1987;11:57.
34. Kearny M. Drunkenness and religious conversion in a Mexican village. *Q J Stud Alcohol*. 1970;31:248–249.
35. Westermeyer J. Two neo-Buddhist cults in Asia: the influence of the founder and the social context on religious movements. *J Psychological Anthro*. 1980;3:143–152.
36. Galanter M, Westermeyer J. Charismatic religious experience and large-group psychology. *Am J Psychiatry*. 1980;137:1550–1552.
37. Albaugh B, Anderson P. Peyote in the treatment of alcoholism among American Indians. *Am J Psychiatry*. 1974;131:1247–1256.
38. Robinson EAR, Cranford JA, Webb JR, et al. Six-month change in spirituality, religiousness, and heavy drinking in a treatment-seeking sample. *J Stud Alcohol Drugs*. 2007;68:282–290.
39. Jilek WG. Indian healing power: indigenous therapeutic practices in the Pacific Northwest. *Psychiatr Ann*. 1974;4:13–21.
40. Jilek WG. *Indian Healing: Shamanistic Ceremonialism in the Pacific Northwest Today*. Surrey, Canada: Hancock House; 1982.
41. Catalano RF, Morrison DM, Wells EA, et al. Ethnic differences in family factors related to early drug initiation. *J Studies Alcohol*. 1992;53:208–217.
42. Galanter M. *Network Therapy for Alcohol and Drug Abuse*. New York: Basic Books; 1993.
43. Savard RJ. Effects of disulfiram therapy in relationships within the Navaho drinking group. *Q J Stud Alcohol*. 1968;29:909–916.
44. Robins LN, Davis DH, Goodwin GW. Drug use by U.S. Army enlisted men in Vietnam: a follow-up on their return home. *Am J Epidemiol*. 1974;99:235–249.
45. Berger LJ, Westermeyer J. "World Traveler" addicts in Asia: II. Comparison with "Stay at Home" addicts. *Am J Drug Alcohol Abuse*. 1977;4:495–503.

CHAPTER 70: Substance Use in the Armed Forces

Robert M. Bray ■ Michael R. Pemberton

INTRODUCTION

Substance use and abuse, including heavy alcohol use, illicit drug use, and tobacco use, have long been associated with military life. The armed services have experienced problems with alcohol abuse from the earliest days of military service, in part because heavy drinking has been an accepted custom and tradition that continues today (1–4). In the past, alcohol was thought to be necessary for subsistence and morale and as such was provided as a daily ration to sailors and soldiers. There are numerous early documented accounts of alcohol abuse among military personnel, for example, in the British army in the 18th century (5) and during the U.S. Civil War in the 1860s (6). Within the predominantly male U.S. military population, heavy drinking and being able to "hold one's liquor" have served as tests "of suitability for the demanding masculine military role" (7). A common stereotype has been to characterize hard-fighting soldiers as hard-drinking soldiers. Alcoholic beverages have been available to military personnel at reduced prices at military outlets and, until recently, during "happy hours" on base (7,8). In addition, alcohol has become part of the military work culture and has been used to reward hard work, to ease interpersonal tensions, and to promote unit cohesion and camaraderie (4,9).

Similar to alcohol, illicit drugs (including illegal drugs as well as prescription drugs used nonmedically) have been used by soldiers since they discovered that certain herbs reduced pain, lessened fatigue or increased alertness, or helped them cope with times of boredom or panic that accompany battle. During the U.S. Civil War, medical use of opium resulted in addiction among some soldiers. In the modern U.S. military, drug use was not a notable problem until the Vietnam War in the late 1960s and early 1970s. Heroin and opium were widely used among U.S. military personnel in Vietnam, in part as a way to tolerate the difficulties of war and cope with a threatening environment. Approximately 20% of Vietnam War veterans reported having used narcotics on a weekly basis, and 20% also were considered to be addicted based on reported symptoms of dependence (10). Although few personnel continued using heroin when they returned home, there were concerns about addiction. This finding, along with the subsequent discovery in the 1980s that drug use was more widespread among military personnel (11,12), led the Department of Defense (DoD) to develop policies and approaches to reduce it (13).

Tobacco use has also been common among military personnel and its use was sanctioned in the U.S. military beginning in the early years of the 20th century. Although there was initial debate in the armed forces about whether cigarettes were in keeping with proper military discipline, the onset of World War I gave rise to widespread encouragement of tobacco use in the military (14). A turning point for easy access and encouragement of tobacco use came in response to the famous plea by General Pershing: "You ask me what we need to win this war. I answer tobacco as much as bullets" (15). The response was organized efforts by volunteer groups such as the YMCA and the Salvation Army to raise funds to buy and distribute cigarettes to the troops. Despite these well-meaning efforts, supporters found it difficult to ensure delivery to all servicemen. Amidst complaints of uneven distribution of tobacco by volunteers, in 1918 the War Department assumed responsibility for equitable distribution and did so by issuing tobacco rations. This action made tobacco readily accessible and implied strong organizational support for its use. Indeed, the sharing of a cigarette symbolized the camaraderie of war. This sentiment continued during World War II with widespread radio and print cigarette advertisements praising service members (16). Cigarettes continued to be included as part of the K-rations and C-rations and sometimes became more valuable for trading or selling than the food items in the rations (16).

Currently, alcohol abuse (i.e., binge or heavy drinking), illicit drug use, and tobacco use are strongly discouraged within U.S. armed forces because of their negative effects on the health and well-being of military personnel and because of their detrimental effects on military readiness and the maintenance of high standards of performance and military discipline (17). In the U.S. military, alcohol abuse is defined as alcohol use that has adverse effects on the user's health or behavior, family, community, or the DoD, or that leads to unacceptable behavior. Drug abuse is defined as the wrongful use, possession, distribution, or introduction onto a military installation of a controlled substance (e.g., marijuana, heroin, cocaine), prescription medication, over-the-counter medication, or intoxicating substance (other than alcohol). Tobacco use is defined as use of cigarettes, cigars, pipes, snuff, or chewing tobacco and is discouraged because of its negative effects on performance and association with disease.

DEVELOPMENT OF MILITARY SUBSTANCE USE POLICY

The Vietnam War and the resulting reports of substance abuse from returning servicemen led to the development of DoD policy on substance use and abuse. In 1967, DoD convened a task force to investigate drug and alcohol abuse in the military and in 1970 formulated a drug and alcohol abuse policy based on task force recommendations. The policy emphasized the prevention of drug and alcohol abuse through education and law enforcement procedures focusing on detection and early intervention (18,19). However, treatment was provided for problem users with an emphasis on returning them to service.

In response to continuing public concern about reports of serious drug addiction among U.S. forces in Southeast Asia, President Nixon in 1971 directed DoD to take additional measures to address the drug problem. The result was the establishment of a urinalysis testing program that initially consisted of mandatory testing for service members leaving Southeast Asia and grew to include mandatory, random urinalysis for all U.S. forces worldwide. The program experienced problems in the mid-1970s due to a legal challenge that the Fifth Amendment protection against self-incrimination was being violated (20). Subsequently, Congress discouraged use of wide-scale drug testing as not cost-effective, which resulted in the program becoming dormant from 1976 to 1981. During this period, there were reports of increased drug use among U.S. military personnel, especially those stationed in the Federal Republic of Germany, which kept attention focused on the problem.

In 1981, the crash of a jet on the aircraft carrier *Nimitz* riveted public attention on the military's drug abuse problem, particularly marijuana use. Autopsies of the 14 Navy personnel killed in the crash showed evidence of marijuana use among 6 of the 13 sailors and nonprescription antihistamine use by the pilot. As a result of this incident and other concerns about drug use in the active-duty services, the military reinstituted urine testing for drugs, and the Navy launched its War on Drugs in 1981. New breakthroughs in drug-testing confirmation procedures and more rigorous chain-of-custody procedures for tracking urine samples were adequate to overcome earlier legal objections. Urine tests, which are conducted either randomly or when an individual is suspected of using drugs, have become a major tool for the detection and deterrence of illicit drug use in the military (17).

Beginning in 1986 and continuing into the 1990s, policies on drug and alcohol abuse were placed in the broader perspective of a coordinated, comprehensive policy on health promotion that recognizes the value of good health and healthy lifestyles for military performance and readiness. A 1986 directive defined health promotion as those activities designed to support and influence individuals in managing their health through lifestyle decisions and self-care (21). Smoking prevention and cessation, as well as alcohol and drug abuse prevention, physical fitness, nutrition, stress management, and prevention of hypertension, were included in the directive. Smoking prevention and cessation programs were to include information on the health consequences of smoking provided at initial entry and permanent change of station. The health promotion strategy was developed to encourage changes in lifestyle to make healthy behaviors the norm and thereby foster the belief that unhealthy behaviors, such as smoking and drug and alcohol abuse, were incompatible with military service.

During this period, DoD also examined the impacts of the sale of tobacco in the military, including the impact of increasing prices of tobacco products. The resulting report clearly recognized the negative health impacts of smoking and the importance of individual choice (22). In 1986, the Secretary of Defense issued a memorandum calling for an intensive antismoking campaign with an emphasis on the negative health impacts of smoking. Smoking rates and effects on health continued to be monitored, and positive steps were taken to reduce the impact of "passive smoking," including restrictions on smoking in certain common areas and prohibition of smoking by medical personnel in the presence of patients (23,24). All of the services now prohibit smoking on base except in designated smoking areas and offer smoking cessation programs to encourage smokers to quit (25,26).

U.S. military substance use policy continues to be updated periodically and has focused mainly on illicit drug use and alcohol abuse (13,27). Current DoD policy requires the following with regard to drug and alcohol abuse programs and resources:

- Education and training on DoD policies for drug and alcohol abuse and/or dependency, and on effective measures to alleviate problems associated with drug and alcohol abuse and/or dependency
- Prevention programs designed to deter substance abuse to include Drug Demand Reduction (DDR), a urinalysis testing program, mandated across the services supported by a program manager at the installation level to oversee urinalysis testing and outreach programs
- Treatment and/or rehabilitation for military personnel who abuse alcohol
- Periodic assessment of the nature and extent of drug and alcohol abuse in DoD

EPIDEMIOLOGY

Health Behavior Surveys

To help monitor the extent of substance use, DoD initiated a series of comprehensive health behavior surveys among active duty military personnel in the Army, Navy, Marine Corps, and Air Force. The first survey was conducted in 1980 (28) with subsequent surveys conducted in 1982, 1985, 1988, 1992, 1995, 1998, 2002, 2005, and 2008; the Coast Guard was added in 2008 (12,29). The goal of the surveys has been to provide data to help assess the prevalence, correlates, and consequences of substance abuse and other health behaviors in the military.

The surveys have all been conducted using similar methods. Civilian researchers first randomly selected a sample of approximately 60 military installations to represent the armed forces throughout the world. At these designated installations, the civilian researchers randomly selected men and women of all ranks to represent all active duty personnel. Personnel were omitted from consideration if they were recruits, academy students, undergoing a permanent transfer to a new location, or absent without leave. Civilian research teams administered printed questionnaires anonymously to selected personnel in classroom settings on military bases or aboard ships. Personnel who were unable to attend the group sessions (e.g., those who were on leave, sick, or temporarily away from the base) were mailed questionnaires and asked to complete and return them. Participants answered questions about their use of alcohol, tobacco, illegal drugs (e.g., marijuana, cocaine, tranquilizers, heroin), their misuse of prescription drugs (e.g., stimulants, tranquilizers), and problems resulting from their drug or alcohol use. These data collection procedures yielded from 12,000 to 28,000 completed questionnaires for the various surveys. From 59% to 84% of those eligible to take part actually did so. After participants completed the surveys, the data were weighted to represent the eligible population of the active duty force.

Substance Use Definitions

Heavy alcohol use was defined as five or more drinks per typical drinking occasion at least once per week. Any illicit drug use was defined as the use of marijuana/hashish, cocaine, inhalants, hallucinogens, or heroin, or nonmedical use of prescription-type drugs, including stimulants, sedatives, tranquilizers, or analgesics one or more times during the past 30 days. Any cigarette use was defined as having smoked one or more cigarettes in the past 30 days and having smoked at least 100 cigarettes in the lifetime.

Sociodemographic Characteristics of Active Duty Personnel

Table 70.1 presents estimates of the distribution of sociodemographic characteristics among military personnel in selected survey years—1980, 1988, 1998, 2002, 2005, and 2008. Because of the omission of some personnel from the surveys (i.e., recruits, service academy students, people absent without official leave, and people who had been transferred to a new base at the time of data collection), these estimates may differ slightly from the characteristics of the total active force but are still very close approximations. As shown, the military population in all survey years was predominantly male, white, and concentrated in pay grades E4–E6. When looking at the profile pattern across the 28-year period, the proportion of women, Hispanic and other racial/ethnic groups, college-educated personnel, and personnel aged 35 years or older increased significantly between 1980 and 2008, and for some characteristics nearly doubled. The demographic profile for 2008 is quite similar to the profile for 2005.

Trends in Substance Use

Figure 70.1 presents the trends from 1980 to 2008 of the percentage of active duty military personnel who engaged in heavy alcohol use, illicit drug use, and cigarette use during the 30 days prior to the survey. Coast Guard data were omitted from analyses of the 2008 survey estimates to provide comparable data across survey years. As shown, heavy alcohol use decreased between 1980 and 1988, showed some fluctuations between 1988 and 1998, increased significantly from 1998 to 2002, and remained at about that same level in 2005 (19%) and 2008 (20%). The heavy drinking rate for 2008 (20%) was not significantly different from when the survey series began in 1980 (21%), although use increased during the past decade (from 15% to 20%).

The prevalence of any reported illicit drug use (including prescription drug misuse) during the past 30 days declined sharply from 28% in 1980 to 3% in 2002. In 2005, the prevalence of illicit drug use for the past 30 days was 5% and in 2008 it was 12%. Improved question wording in 2005 and 2008 may partially account for the higher observed rates, which are largely attributable to reported increases in misuse of prescription pain medications. Because of wording changes, data from 2005 and 2008 are not comparable to data from prior surveys and are not included as part of the trend line. An additional line from 2002 to 2008 shows estimates of illicit drug use excluding prescription drug misuse. As shown, those rates were very low (2% in 2008) and did not change across these three iterations of the survey.

The percentage of military personnel who smoked cigarettes in the past 30 days decreased significantly from 51% in 1980 to 30% in 1998. It increased significantly from 1998 (30%) to 2002 (34%), and has been slowly trending downward since then, such that the rate in 2008 (30.5%) was similar to the rate in 1998.

Despite the significant downward trends in illicit drug use, cigarette use, and heavy drinking (in the earlier years), the question arises as to whether these changes are due to military programs and policies or to other factors. One possible explanation for the changes could be shifts in the demographic composition of the armed forces noted in Table 70.1. From 1980 to 1998, demographic changes were favorable to lower levels of use in that military members were more likely to be older, to be officers, to be married, and to have more education (all groups with lower rates of use). In contrast, the increases in cigarette use and heavy drinking between 1998 and 2002 could be associated with a shift toward younger personnel joining the military in response to the events of September 11, 2001. Bray and Hourani (11) examined this issue and found that the differences across the years were still evident even after adjusting for the demographic differences. This suggests that the sociode-

TABLE 70.1 Estimated sociodemographic characteristics of active duty military personnel in selected survey years

Sociodemographic characteristic	Survey year					
	1980 (N = 15,268)	1988 (N = 18,673)	1998 (N = 17,264)	2002 (N = 12,756)	2005 (N = 16,146)	2008[a] (N = 24,690)
Gender						
Male	91.2 (0.7)	88.8 (1.0)	86.3 (0.7)	83.1 (0.8)	85.2 (0.7)	85.7 (0.8)
Female	8.8 (0.7)	11.2 (1.0)	13.7 (0.7)	16.9 (0.8)	14.8 (0.7)	14.3 (0.8)
Race/ethnicity						
White, non-Hispanic	70.7 (1.4)	69.4 (0.9)	64.5 (0.9)	67.3 (1.3)	64.4 (1.2)	64.0 (1.0)
African American, non-Hispanic	18.8 (1.3)	18.5 (0.8)	17.6 (0.8)	20.7 (1.4)	17.6 (1.0)	16.7 (0.8)
Hispanic	4.6 (0.4)	8.0 (0.6)	10.8 (0.5)	7.1 (0.4)	8.8 (0.5)	10.4 (0.4)
Other	5.8 (0.4)	4.1 (0.3)	7.1 (0.4)	5.0 (0.5)	9.2 (0.6)	8.9 (0.5)
Education						
High school diploma or less	53.9 (1.6)	42.9 (1.5)	31.3 (1.2)	36.0 (1.6)	33.9 (1.5)	32.8 (1.4)
Some college	30.4 (1.2)	34.7 (0.9)	46.3 (1.0)	44.3 (1.2)	44.1 (1.3)	45.0 (0.8)
College degree or more	15.7 (1.2)	19.4 (1.4)	22.4 (1.4)	19.7 (1.6)	22.0 (1.7)	22.3 (1.6)
Age						
20 or younger	21.3 (1.4)	13.8 (1.1)	10.2 (0.6)	13.8 (1.0)	14.1 (1.1)	14.7 (1.0)
21–25	35.2 (1.1)	30.4 (1.2)	28.4 (0.9)	32.9 (1.2)	32.6 (1.2)	32.2 (1.4)
26–34	27.8 (1.1)	34.4 (1.0)	34.4 (0.7)	28.8 (0.7)	30.3 (1.0)	29.3 (0.7)
35 or older	15.6 (1.1)	21.4 (1.4)	27.0 (1.0)	24.5 (1.7)	23.1 (1.4)	23.8 (1.4)
Family status						
Not married	47.1 (1.4)	39.3 (1.9)	39.9 (0.7)	44.3 (1.2)	45.8 (1.4)	45.7 (1.1)
Married	52.9 (1.4)	60.7 (1.9)	60.1 (0.7)	55.7 (1.2)	54.2 (1.4)	54.3 (1.1)
Rank						
E1–E3	27.2 (1.5)	21.0 (1.4)	18.9 (0.9)	22.0 (1.6)	24.0 (1.7)	21.0 (1.3)
E4–E6	50.2 (1.0)	51.9 (1.0)	52.5 (1.2)	51.9 (1.0)	49.6 (1.8)	51.7 (2.4)
E7–E9	8.2 (0.6)	10.4 (0.6)	10.8 (0.4)	10.8 (0.8)	9.7 (0.8)	10.2 (0.5)
W1–W5	1.1 (0.2)	1.0 (0.1)	1.2 (0.1)	1.2 (0.2)	1.0 (0.1)	1.4 (0.7)
O1–O3	8.3 (0.6)	9.6 (0.7)	9.5 (0.8)	8.3 (0.5)	9.4 (1.0)	9.3 (0.7)
O4–O10	5.0 (0.7)	6.1 (0.7)	7.2 (0.7)	5.8 (1.1)	6.3 (0.8)	6.4 (0.8)

Note: Table entries are column percentages (with standard errors in parentheses).
[a]2008 sociodemographic characteristics omit the Coast Guard.
Source: DoD Surveys of Health Related Behaviors Among Active Duty Military Personnel, 1980 to 2008. Table reprinted with permission from Military Medicine: International Journal of AMSUS. Vol 175 (8), 2010.

mographic changes in the makeup of the military were not sufficient to explain the trends in Figure 70.1. Other factors such as changes in military culture, norms, and attitudes resulting from military programs and policies as well as possible differences in smoking patterns of civilians selecting to join the military were more likely to account for these changes.

Characteristics of Substance Users

Table 70.2 allows us to gain a better understanding of the sociodemographic characteristics of the heavy alcohol, illicit drug, and cigarette users from the 2008 survey. It presents the prevalence and the odds ratios (i.e., the odds that persons are

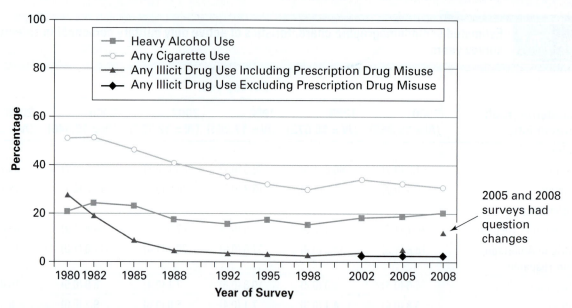

Figure 70.1. Trends in past 30-day substance use, total DoD, 1980–2008. Heavy alcohol use is defined as five or more drinks on the same occasion at least once a week in the past 30 days. Any illicit drug use including prescription drug misuse is defined as the use of marijuana, cocaine (including crack), hallucinogens (PCP/LSD/MDMA), heroin, methamphetamine, inhalants, GHB/GBL, or nonmedical use of prescription-type amphetamines/stimulants, tranquilizers/muscle relaxers, barbiturates/sedatives, or pain relievers. Any illicit drug use excluding prescription drug misuse is defined as the use of marijuana, cocaine (including crack), hallucinogens (PCP/LSD/MDMA), heroin, methamphetamine, inhalants, or GHB/GBL.

Source: DoD Surveys of Health Related Behaviors Among Active Duty Military Personnel, 1980 to 2008. Figure reprinted with permission from Military Medicine: International Journal of AMSUS. Vol 175 (6), 2010.

users compared with a reference group) adjusted for all of the other characteristics in the table. As shown, the overall adjusted prevalence of heavy drinkers was 20%. Although a number of subgroups were significantly higher than the specific reference group, the higher rates of heavy alcohol users occurred among persons who were serving in the Marine Corps or Army, were men, were white or Hispanic, had less than a college degree, were single or married but unaccompanied by their spouse, and were of any rank (pay grade) except senior officers (O4–O10). The overall prevalence of illicit drug use (excluding prescription drug misuse) was very low at 2.2%. Drug users were more likely to be serving in the Army, Navy, or Marine Corps relative to the Air Force, and were more likely to be men and to be single or married but unaccompanied by their spouse. Cigarette use prevalence was 30.7%. Smokers were more likely to be serving in the Army, Navy, or Marine Corps, and were more likely to be men, to be white non-Hispanic, to have less than a college degree, to be single, to be enlisted (especially pay grades E1–E6), and to be stationed outside the continental United States (OCONUS). The findings for demographic characteristics are highly similar for heavy alcohol users and cigarette users.

Military and Civilian Comparisons

To help gauge the progress of substance use policies and programs, military leaders often use the civilian population as a comparison benchmark. To make this comparison, military data were drawn from the 2008 health behavior survey and civilian data from the 2007 National Survey on Drug Use and Health (NSDUH), a nationwide survey of substance use. Military and civilian data sets were equated for age and geographic location of respondents, and civilian substance use rates were standardized (adjusted) to resemble the demographic distribution of the military. Comparisons were made for four age groups: those aged 18 to 25, 26 to 35, 36 to 45, and 46 to 64.

Results shown in Figures 70.2 and 70.3 indicate that the patterns varied by substance and by age groups. As shown in Figure 70.2, military personnel aged 18 to 25 or aged 26 to 34 were significantly more likely than civilians in those age groups to have engaged in heavy drinking, whereas this pattern was reversed for those aged 46 to 64. Rates of past month cigarette use were lower for military personnel aged 36 to 45 or aged 46 to 64 than for civilians in those age groups, whereas there was no significant difference between military personnel and civilians in younger age groups. As shown in Figure 70.3, service members aged 18 to 25 were less likely than civilians in that age group to engage in illicit drug use, whereas this pattern was reversed for service members aged 36 to 45 or aged 46 to 64. Note that this higher prevalence of illicit drug use among these older age groups is due to the misuse of prescription drugs; when looking just at illicit drug use excluding prescription drugs, the rates were lower for service members than for civilians in each age group.

The findings indicate that substance use patterns in the military do not simply mirror similar use among civilians. The lower rates of drug use (excluding prescription misuse)

TABLE 70.2 Sociodemographic correlates of substance use, past 30 days, 2008

Sociodemographic characteristics	Heavy alcohol use		Any illicit drug use excluding prescription drug misuse		Any cigarette use	
	Adjusted prevalence	Adjusted odds ratio[a,b]	Adjusted prevalence	Adjusted odds ratio[a,b]	Adjusted prevalence	Adjusted odds ratio[a,b]
Service						
Army	21.6	1.49*	3.1	3.85*	33.5	1.62*
Navy	17.9	1.16	1.8	2.20*	31.2	1.44*
Marine Corps	25.2	1.84*	2.3	2.85*	32.3	1.53*
Air Force	15.9	1.00	0.8	1.00	24.5	1.00
Gender						
Male	21.8	2.97*	2.4	1.71*	31.9	1.61*
Female	8.9	1.00	1.4	1.00	23.3	1.00
Race/ethnicity						
White, non-Hispanic	21.6	1.00	2.2	1.00	35.3	1.00
African American, non-Hispanic	14.3	0.59*	2.3	1.06	19.6	0.42*
Hispanic	20.7	0.94	2.5	1.16	23.4	0.53*
Other	17.4	0.75*	2.4	1.10	29.4	0.74*
Education						
High school or less	23.4	1.98*	2.7	1.60	36.5	2.60*
Some college	19.6	1.56*	1.9	1.10	29.9	1.89*
College graduate or higher	13.8	1.00	1.7	1.00	19.0	1.00
Family status						
Not married	24.3	1.83*	2.7	1.99*	31.7	1.14*
Married, spouse not present	20.9	1.50*	2.8	2.11*	32.2	1.16
Married, spouse present	15.3	1.00	1.4	1.00	29.3	1.00
Pay grade						
E1–E3	18.8	2.27*	3.3	3.74	33.6	5.02*
E4–E6	22.6	2.92*	2.3	2.51	34.7	5.28*
E7–E9	16.2	1.88*	0.4	0.45	23.6	2.97*
W1–W5	17.3	2.05*	1.3	1.43	14.5	1.59
O1–O3	16.7	1.95*	0.2	0.20	16.5	1.86*
O4–O10	9.5	1.00	+	1.00	9.8	1.00
Region						
CONUS[c]	19.4	0.89	2.3	1.07	29.6	0.85*
OCONUS[d]	21.2	1.00	2.1	1.00	32.8	1.00
Total	20.0		2.2		30.7	

Note: Prevalence estimates are percentages among military personnel in each sociodemographic group that reported heavy alcohol use, any illicit drug use excluding prescription drug misuse, and any cigarette use in the past 30 days. Adjusted prevalence is a model-based, standardized estimate. The main effects of service, gender, race/ethnicity, education, family status, pay grade, and region were included in the standardization model. Heavy alcohol use is defined as consumption of five or more drinks on the same occasion at least once a week in the past 30 days. Any illicit drug use excluding prescription drug misuse is defined as the use of marijuana, cocaine (including crack), hallucinogens (phencyclidine [PCP], lysergic acid diethylamide [LSD], methylenedioxymethamphetamine (this is ecstacy)[MDMA], and other hallucinogens), heroin, inhalants, or gamma hydroxybutyrate /gamma butyrolactone [GHB/GBL]. Any cigarette use is defined as any use of cigarettes in the past 30 days.

[a] Odds ratios were adjusted for service, gender, race/ethnicity, education, family status, pay grade, and region.

[b] An asterisk "*" beside an estimate indicates that the estimate is significantly different from the reference group.

[c] Refers to personnel who were stationed within the 48 contiguous states in the continental United States.

[d] Refers to personnel who were stationed outside the continental United States or aboard afloat ships.

Source: DoD Surveys of Health Related Behaviors Among Active Duty Military Personnel, 1980 to 2008. Table reprinted with permission from Military Medicine: International Journal of AMSUS. Vol 175 (8), 2010.

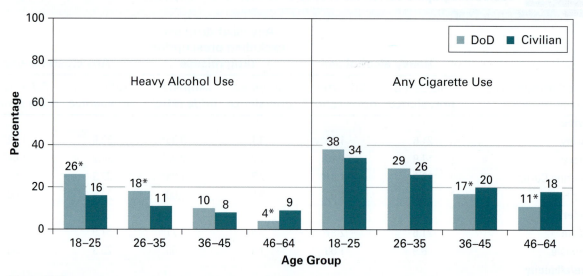

Figure 70.2. Standardized comparisons of DoD and civilians, heavy alcohol use and past 30-day smoking, by age group, 2008. *Statistically significant from civilian at 0.05 level. Military data source: DoD Survey of Health Related Behaviors Among Active Duty Military Personnel, 2008. Civilian data source: National Survey on Drug Use and Health, 2007. Civilian data were standardized to the U.S.-based 2008 military data by gender, age, education, race/ethnicity, and marital status.

among military personnel compared with civilians suggest either that military policies and practices deter drug use in the military or that military personnel hold attitudes and values that discourage substance use. Because of the military's stringent policy prohibiting drug use and the urinalysis testing program to enforce it, it seems likely that the difference in drug use prevalence between military personnel and civilians results from military policies and practices. In contrast, the higher rates of heavy drinking among younger military personnel suggest that certain aspects of military life may foster heavy drinking or that those military policies and programs directed toward reducing these substances have not been as effective as similar efforts among civilians. The comparable or lower smoking rates in the military relative to civilians suggests that military and societal factors both are likely playing a role in smoking behavior. Unfortunately, nearly a third of these populations still smoke cigarettes at least monthly.

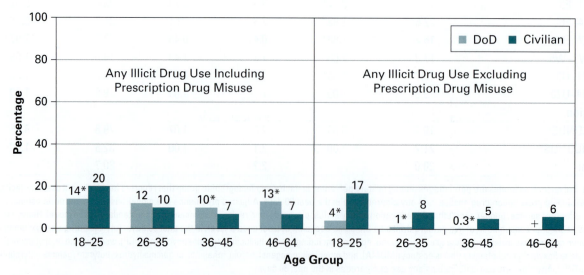

Figure 70.3. Standardized comparisons of DoD and civilians, past 30-day illicit drug use, by age group, 2008. *Statistically significant from civilian at 0.05 level. +Data not reported. Low precision. Military data source: DoD Survey of Health Related Behaviors Among Active Duty Military Personnel, 2008. Civilian data source: National Survey on Drug Use and Health, 2007. Civilian data were standardized to the U.S.-based 2008 military data by gender, age, education, race/ethnicity, and marital status.

PREVENTION, INTERVENTION, AND TREATMENT

To help address the challenges of military life, especially during periods of conflict, the military has implemented prevention, intervention, and treatment programs that address substance use issues. These programs have changed over time to adapt to the changing social and military environment and vary by service, but they typically share common models and elements. Substance abuse programs take a community approach that encourages responsible choices based on leadership involvement, individual responsibility, base installation community participation, and local community partnerships. Other programs are tailored to fit the severity of the problem.

Prevention

All services include drug abuse prevention information as part of general military training, ranging from the earliest days of recruit training to other times during their career. Education includes information on the hazards of drug use, administrative and punitive consequences, responsible decision making, and healthy alternatives to drug use. Many commands use drug detection dogs to periodically search barracks and vehicles at installation gates. Selected high-risk target groups, such as units preparing to deploy to areas where drug use is prevalent, often receive tailored drug abuse prevention information and education.

The military also has a drug-testing program, commonly referred to as urinalysis, that plays a key role in drug use prevention. The purpose of drug testing is to deter service members from using drugs and to permit commanders to detect drug abuse and assess the security, readiness, and discipline of their commands. Drug testing is conducted under a number of different situations, including random testing at least once per year, probable cause searches, during inspections, and during any valid medical examination, including emergency room treatment.

Prevention of alcohol abuse has also been a key component of military substance abuse programs. Each service stresses the importance of alcohol abuse prevention through various training and education classes. These include providing members with basic information on alcohol and alcohol abuse, and emphasizing early detection and early intervention as critical in the prevention of alcohol abuse. A member's on-base driving privileges are revoked if the member is convicted of driving while intoxicated (DWI). Many commands offer safety stand-downs and red ribbon campaigns prior to holidays and the vacation season, reminding members of the dangers of drinking and driving. National Drunk and Drugged Driving Awareness week is another opportunity that commands use to make members aware that "drinking and driving don't mix." Commands encourage their personnel to use designated drivers for situations where alcohol will be available, and most bases provide server training for employees of on-base clubs and restaurants that serve alcohol. It is common for bases to set up driving mazes at gates and other checkpoints to detect intoxicated drivers, especially on weekends. Alcohol deglamorization campaigns stress the importance of food and nonalcoholic beverages at command-sponsored social events. In addition, the armed forces emphasize personal responsibility and caring for your "buddy." Designated drivers often receive free nonalcoholic beverages from various clubs and restaurants. Supervisory personnel are expected to lead by example and be role models for junior personnel, both on and off duty.

A comprehensive effort to address tobacco prevention in the armed forces was launched in 1999 by DoD's Alcohol and Tobacco Advisory Committee (ATAC), which developed a tobacco use prevention strategic plan that is still in effect. The plan set forth a series of goals and tasks, metrics and objectives, requirements for policy, programs, practices, and resources, along with a timeline for achieving the goals. The goals of the plan were and are to (a) reduce the smoking rate and smokeless tobacco rates, (b) promote a tobacco-free lifestyle and culture through education and leadership, (c) educate commanders on how to promote healthy lifestyles, (d) promote the benefits of not smoking and provide tobacco counter-advertising, (e) decrease accessibility, (f) identify users and provide targeted interventions, (g) provide effective cessation programs, and (h) continue to assess best practices in tobacco use prevention.

Intervention and Treatment

Through the years, DoD and the services have developed and implemented intervention and treatment programs that address alcohol, tobacco, and illicit drug abuse issues. These programs have changed over time to adapt to the changing social and military environment. Early intervention services are provided for personnel at risk of developing substance-related problems; outpatient services treat service members' level of clinical severity to help achieve permanent changes; intensive outpatient treatment/partial hospitalization includes education and treatment while allowing patients to apply newly acquired skills; and inpatient services provide a planned regimen of care in a 24-hour live-in setting.

The following are examples of efforts that DoD has implemented. The Air Force Alcohol Drug Abuse Prevention and Treatment (ADAPT) program and DDR program provide services that support the wellness of airmen and their families. A key component is the Culture of Responsible Choices initiative that involves a community-based working group to provide leadership, encourage individual responsibility, and involve the base and local communities. The Air Force also utilizes additional prevention programs, such as the "That Guy" media campaign and the Enforcement of Underage Drinking Laws (EUDL) to combat underage drinking.

Navy programs address varying levels of substance abuse. The Level 0.5 is an early intervention service for specific individuals who, for a known reason, are at risk of developing substance-related problems or for those for whom there is not yet sufficient information to document a substance use disorder. Level I programs provide outpatient services to treat an individual's level of clinical severity and to help the individual achieve permanent changes in his or her alcohol-using behavior and mental functioning. These services address major lifestyle, attitudinal, and behavioral issues that have the potential to undermine the goals of treatment. Level II programs provide intensive outpatient treatment/partial hospitalization. The program provides essential education and treatment components while allowing patients to apply their newly acquired skills within "real-world" environments. The program provides comprehensive biopsychosocial assessments and individualized treatment plans. Level III programs encompass organized services staffed by designated addiction treatment and mental health personnel who provide a planned regiment of care in a 24-hour live-in setting. This level of treatment provides for individuals who need safe and stable living environments in order to develop their recovery skills. Level IV provides medically managed intensive inpatient detoxification at a major medical treatment facility.

DoD requests that all commands provide their personnel with effective tobacco cessation programs. Lectures, films, pamphlets, and other forms of health promotion incorporate the latest available medical research information on tobacco, smoking, health, and treatment. Tobacco cessation programs take many different forms, and local installation commanders are authorized to implement activities that are appropriate to their sites and populations. Most bases offer some form of tobacco cessation classes, generally presented by personnel from the installation hospital or clinic, substance abuse counseling facility, health promotion office, or family service center. Physicians and other health care providers are expected to evaluate all their patients for use of tobacco products and, where indicated, to recommend appropriate cessation activities. When clinically determined as safe and appropriate, nicotine replacement therapy (NRT) is prescribed. This includes the use of nicotine gum or a nicotine patch. NRT is most effective when used in combination with other cessation activities, including counseling/social support and skills training that enable one to achieve and maintain abstinence.

Despite the regulations, directives, and programs the military has put into place, DoD and the military branches have provided only limited assessment and evaluation of the effectiveness of these prevention, intervention, and treatment programs (30). Some of the programs, such as urinalysis testing, are likely having their desired effect of reducing illicit drug use. Others, however, may not, and although they may appear to have face validity, they need to be evaluated to determine if they demonstrate evidence-based best practices for confronting and dealing with substance use issues.

FACTORS INFLUENCING SUBSTANCE USE IN THE MILITARY

There are a number of complex factors that contribute to substance use and misuse in the armed forces, including individual, social, cultural, and environmental influences. Individual factors include demographic, genetic, and psychological components. Individual factors such as age and genetic makeup are also possible risk factors for substance use. For example, as shown in Table 70.2, young adults and males are more likely to engage in substance use than their older or female counterparts. Genetic makeup also plays a role in addiction. Drugs such as heroin and nicotine are well known for their addictive properties. Psychological components include individuals' beliefs, attitudes, intentions, and values, some of which lead to higher risk for substance use and some persons with substance use problems self-selecting into the military. Bray et al. (31) found evidence of selection as a partial explanation for heavy alcohol use in the military.

Social factors include family, friends, and norms or shared expectations about desired behavior. Peer pressure to fit in with friends (an example of normative influence) may lead service members to engage in the heavy drinking, drug use, or smoking habits of their buddies. Haddock et al. (32) found that social factors are strong predictors of tobacco use and that service members are at increased risk of becoming smokers if they have friends who smoke and view smoking positively. Social factors identified with initiation of smoking soon after joining the Navy were curiosity, friends smoking, and wanting to be "cool" (33). Similarly, Bray et al. (31) found that socialization about the regulations and normative expectations regarding substance use helped explain lower rates of heavy drinking among military personnel in regular units compared with rates of heavy drinking by recruits prior to joining the military.

Cultural factors include perceptions about traditions and acceptable practices, and acceptance, support, and tolerance for use. As suggested in the introduction to this chapter, over the years a culture and resulting stereotype has developed of the military being composed of heavy-smoking, hard-drinking, adventuresome service members (16). Indeed, there is evidence suggesting that military culture could be encouraging tobacco use (34). Clearly, many positive steps have been taken since then to modify this stereotype (e.g., the ban on tobacco use during basic training, smoke-free federal buildings, the introduction of alcohol treatment programs), but some of this perception remains. Incidents such as the Tailhook scandal in 1991, in which excessive drinking resulted in rapes and misconduct by many Navy and Marine officers, serve as a reminder of the magnitude of the negative impacts of alcohol abuse. The findings that heavy alcohol use and tobacco use rates are higher than those in the civilian population (at least among young adults—see Figure 70.2) indicate some level of acceptance, tolerance, and/or lack of enforcement of policies among some services, installations, or commanders.

Environmental factors include such things as high availability and easy access to substances, advertising that encourages use, and lack of enforcement of policies to control use. With the exception of basic training, where substance use is banned, alcohol and tobacco are readily available to service members and priced favorably (at least tobacco), and use is encouraged via advertising (e.g., tobacco and alcohol advertisements in military news publications such as *Army and Navy Times*) (35). Illicit drugs may be less available generally, but pockets of use suggest that users have internal networks that allow them to gain access. These factors may contradict and interfere with some policies and programmatic efforts to reduce substance use in the military. However, drug use policy appears as a positive example of what can be achieved with a rigorous and clear protocol that is strongly encouraged and closely monitored at all DoD levels.

CONCLUSIONS

Heavy alcohol use, illicit drug use, and cigarette smoking constitute significant detriments to the health, productivity, and welfare of military personnel. Substance abuse is a major contributor to mortality and morbidity and also adversely affects work performance. To address these issues, DoD has set forth a series of policies designed to decrease the impact of substance abuse on military personnel. Alcohol abuse, drug abuse, and smoking policies are now included in a broader health promotion framework that encourages healthy lifestyles to promote high-level military performance and readiness. Current policies include prevention, intervention, and treatment components and have been the genesis for a wide range of programs to address substance abuse issues. Although the programs appear to have face validity, more research is needed to demonstrate their efficacy and effectiveness.

Assessment of substance use patterns indicates that the military has made steady and notable progress in combating illicit drug use and cigarette use, particularly during the 1980s and 1990s. Illicit drug use has shown dramatic declines since 1980, and in 2008, rates of use among military personnel (omitting prescription misuse) were lower than those among civilians. Although cigarette use has shown declines over the last 25 years, over 30% of military personnel are current smokers. In contrast, the military has made less progress in reducing heavy drinking. In 2008, heavy drinking affected one in five active duty personnel and was significantly higher than among civilians.

Despite impressive progress, more remains to be done. A variety of individual, social, cultural, and environmental factors within the armed services contribute to continued substance use and need to be addressed to further reduce substance use, especially heavy drinking and tobacco use.

ACKNOWLEDGMENTS

The 2008 DoD health behavior survey was supported by Contract No. GS-10F-0097L, Task Order No. W81XWH-07-F-0538 for the Assistant Secretary of Defense (Health Affairs) and Task Order No. HSCG23-07-F-PMD047 for the U.S. Coast Guard. This chapter was prepared by internal funds from RTI International. The views, opinions, and findings contained in this chapter are those of the authors and should not be construed as an official Department of Defense position, policy, or decision, unless so designated by other official documentation. The authors acknowledge the editorial assistance of Justin Faerber and the assistance of Michael Witt with statistical analysis of these data.

REFERENCES

1. Bryant CD. *Khaki-Collar Crime*. New York, NY: Free Press; 1979.
2. Schuckit MA. Alcohol problems in the United States armed forces. *Military Chaplain's Review: Alcohol Abuse*. 1977;(winter): 9–19.
3. Ames GM, Baraban EA, Cunradi CB, et al. *A Longitudinal Study of Drinking Behavior Among Young Adults in the Military*. Paper presented at: Research Society on Alcoholism Annual Scientific Meeting; June 2004; Vancouver, BC.
4. Ames GM, Cunradi CB. Alcohol use and preventing alcohol related problems among young adults in the military. *Alcohol Res Health*. 2004/2005;28(4):252–257.
5. Kopperman PE. The "cheapest pay": alcohol abuse in the eighteenth-century British army. *J Mil Hist*. 1996;60(3): 445–470.
6. Selcer R. Fighting under the influence. *America's Civil War*. 1998;10(6):38–43.
7. Bryant CD. Olive-drab drunks and GI junkies: alcohol and narcotic addiction in the U.S. Military. In: Bryant CD, ed. *Deviant Behavior*. Chicago, IL: Rand McNally; 1974:129–145.
8. Wertsch ME. *Military Brats: Legacies of Childhood Inside the Fortress*. New York, NY: Harmony Books; 1991.
9. Ingraham LH. *The Boys in the Barracks*. Philadelphia, PA: Institute for the Study of Human Issues; 1984.
10. Robins LN, Helzer JE, Davis DH. Narcotic use in Southeast Asia and afterward: an interview study of 898 Vietnam Returnees. *Arch Gen Psychiatry*. 1975;32:955–961.
11. Bray RM, Hourani LL. Substance use trends among active duty military personnel: findings from the United States Department of Defense health related behavior surveys, 1980–2005. *Addiction*. 2007;102(7):1092–1101.
12. Bray RM, Pemberton M, Hourani LL, et al. *2008 Department of Defense Survey of Health Related Behaviors Among Military Personnel*. Final Report [prepared under Contract No. GS-10F-0097L, Task Order No. W81XWH-07-F-0538 for the Assistant Secretary of Defense (Health Affairs) and Task Order No. HSCG23-07-F-PMD047 for the U.S. Coast Guard]. Research Triangle Park, NC: Research Triangle Institute; 2009.
13. Bray RM, Marsden ME, Mazzuchi JF, et al. Prevention in the military. In: Ammerman RT, Ott PJ, Tarter RE, eds. *Prevention and Societal Impact of Drug and Alcohol Abuse*. Mahwah, NJ: Lawrence Erlbaum Associates; 1999.
14. Brandt AM. *The Cigarette Century*. New York, NY: Basic Books; 2007.
15. Sobel R. *They Satisfy: The Cigarette in American Life*. Garden City, NY: Anchor Books; 1978.
16. Conway, TL. Tobacco use and the United States military: a longstanding problem. *Tob Control*. 1998;7:219–221.
17. Department of Defense. *Directive No. 1010.4: Alcohol and Drug Abuse by DoD Personnel*. 1010.4 supersedes and cancels August 25, 1980, version of Directive No. 1010.4 and September 23, 1985, version of Directive No. 1010.3. Washington, DC: Department of Defense; September 3, 1997.
18. Department of Defense. *Directive No. 1300.11: Illegal or Improper Use of Drugs by Members of the Department of Defense*. Washington, DC: Department of Defense; October 23, 1970.
19. Department of Defense. *Directive No. 1010.2: Alcohol Abuse by Personnel of the Department of Defense*. Washington, DC: Department of Defense; March 1972.
20. U.S. v. Ruiz. 23 U.S. Court of Military Appeals 181. *Court Martial Reports*. 1974;48:797.

21. Department of Defense. *Directive No. 1010.10: Health Promotion*. Washington, DC: Department of Defense; March 1986.
22. Department of Defense. *Smoking and Health in the Military*. Washington, DC: Department of Defense; 1986.
23. Ballweg JA, Bray RM. Smoking and tobacco use by U.S. military personnel. *Mil Med.* 1989;154:165–168.
24. Department of Defense. *1987 Department of Defense Updated Report on Smoking and Health in the Military*. Prepared by the Office of the Assistant Secretary of Defense (Health Affairs). Washington, DC: Department of Defense; 1987.
25. Department of Defense. 1994, March 7. *Instruction No. 1010.15: Smoke-Free Workplace*. Washington, DC: Department of Defense; March 7, 1994.
26. Kroutil LA, Bray RM, Marsden ME. Cigarette smoking in the U.S. military: findings from the 1992 Worldwide Survey. *Prev Med.* 1994;23:521–528.
27. Bray RM, Marsden ME, Herbold JR, et al. Progress toward eliminating drug and alcohol abuse among U.S. military personnel. In: Stanley J, Blair JD, eds. *Challenges in Military Health Care: Perspectives on Health Status and the Provision of Care*. New Brunswick, NJ: Transaction Publishers; 1993:33–53.
28. Burt MR, Biegel MM, Carnes Y, et al. *Worldwide Survey of Nonmedical Drug Use and Alcohol Use Among Military Personnel: 1980*. Bethesda, MD: Burt Associates, Inc.; 1980.
29. Bray RM, Hourani LL, Rae Olmstead KL, et al. *2005 Department of Defense Survey of Health Related Behaviors Among Military Personnel*. Final Report [prepared for the Assistant Secretary of Defense (Health Affairs), US Department of Defense, Cooperative Agreement no. DAMD17-00-2-0057, RTI/7841/106-FR]. Research Triangle Park, NC: Research Triangle Institute; 2006.
30. Institute of Medicine (IOM). *Combating Tobacco Use in Military and Veteran Populations*. Washington, DC: The National Academies Press; 2009.
31. Bray RM, Brown JM, Pemberton MR, et al. Alcohol use after forced abstinence in basic training among United States navy and air force trainees. *J Stud Alcohol Drugs.* 2010;71:15–22.
32. Haddock CK, Klesges RC, Talcott GW, et al. Smoking prevalence and risk factors for smoking in a population of United States Air Force basic trainees. *Tob Control.* 1998;7(3):232–235.
33. Cronan TA, Conway TL, Kaszas SL. Starting to smoke in the Navy: when, where and why. *Soc Sci Med.* 1991;33:1349–1353.
34. Cronan TA, Conway, TL. Is the military attracting or creating smokers. *Mil Med.* 1998;153:175–178.
35. Haddock CK, Parker LC, Taylor JE, et al. An analysis of messages about tobacco in military installation newspapers. *Am J Public Health.* 2005;95:1458–1463.

SECTION 11 ■ TRAINING AND EDUCATION

CHAPTER 71

Medical Education on Addiction

Karen Drexler

BACKGROUND

Although Benjamin Rush, MD, America's first Surgeon General, referred to drunkenness as a disease (1), alcoholism and other addictions have not been widely recognized as warranting medical attention. The American Medical Association (AMA) first formally recognized alcoholism in 1956 (2). That declaration heralded a movement to improve medical education in the treatment of alcoholism and other addictions that continues to the present time.

The need for physicians and other health professionals to have competence in detecting and treating alcohol dependence and other addictions is clear from the magnitude of their negative impact on human health and well-being. In the United States, tobacco, alcohol, and illicit drug use represent 3 of the top 10 actual causes of death, accounting for 537,000 deaths in 2000 (22.3% of all deaths) (3). In 1995, the total cost of alcohol and drug abuse to society in the United States was estimated to be $276.4 billion (or 3.7% of total gross domestic product) (4).

Screening and brief intervention in health care settings reduce smoking, hazardous drinking, and medical consequences of alcohol and tobacco use (5). Reduction in drinking is associated with improved health and quality of life (6). Behavioral interventions and medications are effective for treating substance use disorders (7).

Despite the significant effect of alcohol and drug use on public health and the availability of effective prevention and treatment strategies for health care professionals, physicians have been slow in implementing evidence-based screening, brief intervention, and treatment. Numerous surveys of physicians and other health care professionals across the globe and across several decades indicate these professionals' lack of confidence in the ability to deal with patients with addiction (8–11). Physicians and other health professionals fail to detect alcohol use disorders in routine patient encounters (11). When intoxication or problems with alcohol use are detected, few physicians follow up with appropriate intervention and referral (12). House staff in internal medicine and family medicine score significantly better on management of hypertension than of alcoholism (13). Approximately one third of medical students endorse personally consuming more alcohol than guidelines recommend for safe alcohol consumption, exceeding rates for employed individuals (14).

Physician ownership of prevention and treatment has been slowly improving in the area of smoking cessation where the number of patients receiving advice to stop smoking has doubled since the mid-1990s. Consequently, success in quitting has improved such that the number of former smokers has surpassed the number of current smokers (15). Physicians' rates of smoking are far less than that of the general population in the United States, Japan, and the United Kingdom (16). There is recent evidence that physicians' skills in screening and brief intervention for at-risk alcohol use are also improving, but treatment of alcohol use disorders and detection and management of other substance use disorders still lag (17).

This chapter will review the history, current state of the art, and evidence-based best practices in medical education on alcohol and other drug (AOD) use and addiction.

HISTORY

Recognition of drunkenness as a disease by Dr. Rush (1) was not widely accepted by American physicians in the 18th century. Physicians had noted for centuries the utility of opium and alcohol for pain relief. Some noted the risk of repeated use leading to addiction, but the greater concern was that using opium to relieve pain would mask an underlying serious illness (18). In the early- to mid-19th century, prominent physicians extolled the benefits of opium, morphine, and cocaine for treating a variety of diseases, and their use became widespread (18). In the late 19th century, some prominent physicians began publishing papers on the devastating effects of addiction to these substances, but there was a widespread belief that the risk of addiction was limited to lower socioeconomic classes, those of weak moral fiber, and psychopaths (18). With increasing availability, Civil War veterans and upper class citizens increasingly became addicted and medical attention increased. The concept of a vice disease (i.e., one that was easily acquired, progressively damaging, and difficult to cure) became widely accepted for opium addiction, alcoholism, and syphilis. Some physicians practiced maintenance treatment for narcotic addiction, but many regarded this as immorally keeping patients addicted for the physician's monetary gain (18). In the late 1800s and early 20th century, governments began to restrict the availability of narcotics and alcohol in hopes to reduce the costs of addiction to society. Overly optimistic claims of cure by nonphysicians together with significant legal penalties for physicians prescribing narcotics to patients for maintenance treatment essentially eliminated maintenance treatment by physicians. In 1929, the U.S. Congress established two "narcotic farms" or prison hospitals for the treatment of narcotic addiction (19). Disappointment in the high relapse rates after detoxification (reported to be about 75%) led physicians to ignore addiction treatment (18).

In the mid-20th century, increasing optimism in the effectiveness of Alcoholics Anonymous, of in-patient rehabilitation, and of medically managed alcohol withdrawal led to increasing interest by some physicians in medical treatment for alcoholism. In 1954, the New York City Medical Society on Alcoholism (NYCMSA) held its first scientific meeting with one of its goals to improve medical education on alcoholism (20). In 1956, the AMA recognized alcoholism as an illness warranting treatment and advocated that hospitals not deny admission to patients with alcoholism (2). By 1966, the AMA had established a Committee on Alcoholism (21), which drafted a report on alcoholism as a disease. In 1967, the NYCMSA became the American Medical Society on Alcoholism (AMSA), with one of its goals to improve physician education on alcoholism (20). In that same year, the Cooperative Commission on the Study of Alcoholism published *Alcohol Problems: A Report to the Nation* (22), which noted that

> There has been a virtual disregard of problem drinking in the curricula of professional institutions. Medical schools along with schools of nursing and social work have virtually ignored it.

The 1970s witnessed a historic growth in physician education and interest in addiction treatment. In 1972, the AMA Council on Mental Health and the Committee on Alcoholism and Drug Dependence issued a position statement (23), stating that it was "not appropriate at this time to suggest a specific plan or a model for a program on psychoactive drug dependence," but emphasizing a biopsychosocial concept of addiction, pharmacology of psychoactive drugs, iatrogenic drug abuse, and special risk of physicians to development of addiction.

Recognizing alcoholism as "the Number One Public Health Problem of the United States," the National Council on Alcoholism (NCA) sponsored a conference in 1970 on "Professional Training on Alcoholism," which brought together experts in the field to share "experience, strength, and hope" in improving education on the treatment of alcoholism. Surveys of health care personnel identified negative attitudes toward alcoholic patients as a major barrier to providing appropriate treatment. Many conference speakers noted that negative attitudes of role models presented a major barrier to effective education. In his opening remarks, Dr. Seixas noted,

> … We not only have neglected alcoholism, but, by precept and example, by gesture and joke, have given the medical student an antieducation in the subject.

There was lively debate over the best strategy to improve physician attitudes—whether improved diagnostic and treatment techniques would lead to improvement in attitudes or whether current treatments were sufficient and efforts should focus primarily on changing attitudes (24). The conferees recommended specific strategies to improve professionals' education on alcoholism:

1. Increased grant support and change in research to focus more on pathophysiology and treatment of the primary disorder (25)
2. Clinical resources and treatment facilities affiliated with medical schools so that trainees could participate in clinical rotations and observe positive responses to treatment
3. Coordination of the curriculum to develop a cohesive plan (25)
4. Research into effective teaching strategies for the addictions

In 1971, the National Institutes of Health (NIH) launched the Career Teacher Program in the Addictions, providing faculty development grants to 63 of the 124 medical schools (26). This program provided salary support for a career teacher at 59 medical schools (27), conferences where career teachers were able to collaborate and share best practices, and significant advances in the quantity and quality of medical education (20). Career teachers faced significant barriers in changing the traditional allocation of training hours, but succeeded in increasing academic attention to addiction education over the 10-year program. Among the career teachers' accomplishments were

1. Quantitative surveys of medical education on the addictions (28).
2. Increases in the number of required hours in medical school curricula. Schools with career teachers realized larger gains, but the total number of required hours devoted to addiction remained less than 1% of the total curriculum time (28,29).
3. Founding of the Association for Medical Education and Research in Substance Abuse (AMERSA) in 1976 to expand and improve medical education on the addictions (20).
4. The NIDA task force working with the National Board of Medical Examiners (NBME) developed an examination on drug and alcohol use disorders for medical students. Six hundred twenty-nine medical students scored more poorly on this exam than on traditional content of the NBME exam. They scored better in areas of pharmacology, Alcoholics Anonymous, and treatment of delirium tremens (30).
5. Results of this examination informed development of curriculum guides for medical schools on addiction.

Private foundations and the NIH also supported development of model curricula as a means of enhancing medical education on addiction. In 1977, Dartmouth Medical School received a large grant from the Kroc Foundation (Project Cork) to develop a model medical school curriculum on alcohol and alcoholism. Its primary emphasis was to increase attention on alcohol throughout the curriculum. For example, cardiology expanded from one mention of alcoholism in a lecture on cardiomyopathy to include alcohol's effects on hypertension and hyperlipidemia and appropriate use of alcohol by heart patients. Similarly, the psychiatry course expanded from a brief mention of alcohol's effects on psychotropic medications to include diagnosis and treatment of alcohol use disorders. Clerkships included medical management of alcoholism (8). In 1984, Johns Hopkins launched a comprehensive training program on alcoholism detection, management, and referral for all levels of practitioners—medical students, house staff, and attending physicians (31). Georgetown University School of Medicine introduced exposure of medical students to panels of recovering physicians (8).

Also starting in the early 1970s, several independent initiatives began to improve physician competency in addiction treatment through postgraduate certification. In 1972, in response to a new California law, the California Society for the Treatment of Alcoholism and Other Drug Dependencies (CSTAODD) was incorporated to focus on medical education and to certify physician competency in the addictions (20). In 1975, G. Douglas Talbott organized the American Academy of Addictionology in Atlanta, Georgia, to certify physicians in the practice of addiction medicine. In the 1970s, the first postgraduate fellowships in addiction medicine were established (27). In 1983, the Kroc Foundation sponsored a meeting to encourage collaboration between the various organizations devoted to improving physician education in addiction treatment. The American Medical Society on Alcoholism and Other Drug Dependencies (AMSAODD) became the umbrella organization and accepted the task of developing continuing medical education (CME) courses and administering a national examination for competency in addiction medicine (32). Conferees debated the merits of pursuing specialty or subspecialty recognition for addiction medicine, but decided that the addiction medicine certification should be separate and distinct from the American Board of Medical Specialties (ABMS) certification process.

The 1980s and 1990s witnessed unprecedented growth and maturity of specialist training in addiction treatment. In 1985, the American Academy of Psychiatrists in Alcoholism and Addiction (AAPAA) was formed with one of its missions to improve competency of psychiatrists and allied health care professionals in treating addictions and to pursue this in part through subspecialty ABMS board certification (33). In 1996, the organization renamed itself the American Academy of Addiction Psychiatry (AAAP). Also in 1985, the Accreditation Council on Graduate Medical Education (ACGME) added a requirement for training in addictions to the general psychiatry residency training requirements (34). In 1986, AMSAODD accepted its first applications for the addiction medicine certificate. Family practice (32%) and psychiatry (28%) constituted the two largest areas of specialty among the applicants and were overrepresented compared to the distribution of these specialties among practising physicians. Internal medicine constituted the third largest group at 24%, similar to their proportion among practicing physicians. The majority of the applicants were board certified in their primary specialty (26). AMSAODD renamed itself the American Society of Addiction Medicine (ASAM), and from 1986 until 2008, the organization certified over 4200 physicians in addiction medicine.

In 1989, the New York University Center for Medical Fellowships in Alcoholism and Drug Abuse was established with the support from AMERSA and AAPAA. Its goal was to promote postgraduate training in the addictions by developing standards for medical training in the addictions, disseminating information on existing fellowships, and facilitating establishment of new programs (35,36). By 1989, there were 27 addiction fellowships training 44 fellows each year, with two thirds of fellowships accepting physicians from all disciplines (34). In 1991, the American Board of Psychiatry and Neurology (ABPN) received ABMS approval to offer certification in addiction psychiatry. In 1993, ABPN offered the first certification examination (37). In 1997, the ACGME accredited the first addiction psychiatry residency training programs (38). These 12-month, fifth postgraduate year (PGY-5) clinical training programs were designed to prepare board-eligible psychiatrists for ABMS subspecialty certification in addiction psychiatry. By 2000, there were 38 ACGME-accredited addiction psychiatry residency training programs offering 83 positions. In addition, there were four non-ACGME addiction fellowships. However, 23 positions were unfilled in 1999, prompting calls to expand postgraduate training in addiction to include other medical specialties (27).

Beginning in the 1980s and continuing through the 1990s, there was continued steady progress in formalizing addiction treatment training for all health care professionals. Noting that physicians' negative attitudes toward alcoholics represented a major barrier to effective assessment and treatment and the limited time in the medical school curriculum, Nocks recommended a 6-hour course aimed at changing medical students' negative attitudes toward patients with substance use disorders (39). In 1984, the Society of Teachers of Family Medicine published a residency training curriculum guide on addiction treatment, and in 1985, the American College of Physicians published a position paper on the subject (20). Also in 1985, AMERSA, NIAAA, NIDA, the Betty Ford Center, and the Annenberg Center cosponsored a consensus conference on the knowledge, skills, and abilities that physicians needed to diagnose and care for patients with substance use disorders (20). Out of this conference grew specialty societies in internal medicine, family practice, pediatrics, and psychiatry as well as NIAAA and NIDA contracts to develop and implement model curricula. One of these, Project ADEPT (Alcohol and Drug Education for Physician Training in primary care), began at Brown University to develop routine integration of drug and alcohol training throughout the primary care curriculum through trained faculty in six departments—internal medicine, family medicine, pediatrics, psychiatry, community health, and obstetrics and gynecology (20). NIAAA and the Center for Addiction Research and

Education (CARE) at the University of Wisconsin developed a model curriculum for training primary care providers in screening and brief intervention (40). Another model curriculum was developed at the University of Toronto, which included both didactic and clinical curriculum throughout the second and third years of medical school. Goals of the curriculum were that students would have the knowledge, skills, and abilities to identify and address alcoholism in patients treated in their chosen fields and that they would avoid personal difficulties with substances (41).

In 1990, the Institute of Medicine (IOM) issued a report, "Broadening the base of treatment for alcohol problems," that called for increasing the types and availability of alcohol treatment and for research to determine appropriate treatment matching (42). In 1996, the College of Family Physicians of Canada Alcohol Risk Assessment and Intervention (ARAI) project began providing national and regional trainings and a resource material packet for CME (43). In 1997, the Residency Review Committee on Internal Medicine instituted a requirement for "instruction in the diagnosis and treatment of alcoholism and other substance abuse" (27).

In the early 21st century, previous trends continued. Further maturation of specialty practice in addiction treatment progressed at a rapid pace. Under the leadership of Elizabeth Howell, the ASAM formed the Medical Specialty Action Group (MSAG) in 2006 to investigate ABMS recognition for addiction medicine. The MSAG recommended formation of an independent American Board of Addiction Medicine (ABAM) separate from ASAM, and in 2007, ABAM was formed with the goal to pursue ABMS recognition for addiction medicine (44). More information is available through the ABAM website http://www.abam.net/about/default.aspx or the ASAM website http://www.asam.org/abam.html.

Gains in general medical education on addiction continued at a slower pace than that of specialty training due to a variety of factors. In the late 1990s, experts continued to note that practising physicians' skills in detecting and managing substance use disorders lagged behind their skills in managing other chronic diseases (45) and that the historical gap in addiction education resulted in a lack of skills in medical school faculty that was likely to persist for some time (46). In 2000, a survey of select residency training directors in multiple specialties including internal medicine, pediatrics, family medicine, obstetrics and gynecology, psychiatry, and emergency medicine found that 56% of programs had required training on substance use disorders (ranging from 38.1% in pediatrics to 95% in psychiatry). The median number of curricula hours ranged from 3 (emergency medicine and pediatrics) to 12 (family medicine). Overall, 47% of the graduate medical education programs surveyed reported a required rotation in addiction treatment, ranging from 12% of programs in obstetrics and gynecology to 74% in psychiatry. The authors concluded that primary care medical training in the diagnosis and management of substance use disorders remained inadequate (47). McAvoy noted that there were multiple guidelines for evidence-based management of alcohol problems in primary care, but few evidence-based best practices for teaching these skills and no systematic plan for implementation (48). Other factors contributing to a lack of enthusiasm for physician management of substance use problems included lack of reimbursement for these activities by third-party payers and a denial of coverage for another illness if it was deemed to be substance related.

Evidence demonstrating that screening and brief intervention in primary care is a cost-effective means of reducing high-risk substance use began mounting in the early 2000s (49). Recognizing the importance of the physician's role in demand reduction for drugs, the Office of National Drug Control Policy (ONDCP) took a leadership role in bringing together federal stakeholders and medical educators through a series of National Leadership Conferences on Medical Education in Substance Abuse. The first of these conferences convened in 2004, the second in 2006, and the third in 2008. Among the recommendations were calls for champions in each medical school and a list-serve to improve communication and sharing of best practices; for the ACGME and ABMS to add requirements and exam questions regarding screening, assessment, and brief intervention to all graduate medical education programs and specialty exams; and for continuing education for all medical specialties to increase competency in these areas perhaps through Web-based trainings (50). Through the dialogue at these conferences, ONDCP recognized financial disincentives for physicians to embrace "screening, brief intervention, and referral to treatment" (SBIRT) and began advocating for Medicare procedure codes for screening and brief intervention for hazardous substance use. The National Institute on Alcohol Abuse and Alcoholism published a Web-based training on screening, brief intervention, referral, and treatment of at-risk alcohol use and alcohol use disorders—the *Clinician's Guide for Helping Patients Who Drink Too Much* (51)—available at http://www.niaaa.nih.gov/Publications/EducationTrainingMaterials/VideoCases.htm.

With the passage of the Drug Addiction Treatment Act of 2000, the Substance Abuse and Mental Health Services Administration (SAMHSA) initiated training for physicians in the office-based practice of buprenorphine maintenance through its Center for Substance Abuse Treatment (CSAT). SAMHSA/CSAT (along with the manufacturer of buprenorphine) supported CME buprenorphine training courses through the American Psychiatric Association (APA), ASAM, the American Osteopathic Association (AOA), and the AAAP. CSAT also supported an innovative program called the Physician Clinical Support System (PCSS), which provided ongoing mentoring of new practitioners in addiction treatment (52). Although many physicians completed the training and obtained a waiver, significant barriers prevented more widespread availability of treatment including lack of institutional support, lack of reimbursement by third-party payers, and lack of demand among current caseloads of patients (53).

The IOM published two reports, which highlighted attention to alcohol and other substance use and addiction. The IOM report on improving neuroscience and behavioral health education in medical schools noted that using tobacco, being overweight, and having excessive alcohol use together

TABLE 71.1 AMERSA Project Mainstream: critical core competencies in substance abuse education for physicians

Level I: All physicians with clinical contact should:
1) Be able to perform age, gender, and culturally appropriate substance abuse screening.
2) Be able to provide brief interventions to patients with substance use disorder (SUD).
3) Be able to use effective methods of counseling patients to help prevent SUD.
4) Be able to refer patients with SUD to treatment settings that provide pharmacotherapy for relapse prevention.
5) Recognize and treat or refer comorbid medical and psychiatric conditions in patients with SUD.
6) Be able to refer patients with SUD to appropriate treatment and supportive services.
7) Be aware of the ethical and legal issues around physician impairment from SUD and of resources for referring potential impaired colleagues, including employee assistance programs, hospital-based committees, state physician health programs, and licensure boards.
8) Identify the legal and ethical issues involved in the care of patients with SUD.

Level II: All physicians co-ordinating care for patients with SUD in addition should:
1) Use effective methods to assess patients with SUD.
2) Provide pharmacologic withdrawal to patients with SUD.

Level III: All physicians providing specialty services to patients with SUD in addition should:
1) Provide pharmacotherapy for relapse prevention in patients with SUD.
2) Provide, or refer for, psychosocial counseling for relapse prevention in patients with SUD.

accounted for half of the deaths each year in the United States and recommended greater attention in medical school to "patient behaviors" leading to morbidity and mortality (54). In 2006, *Improving the Quality of Health Care for Mental and Substance-Use Conditions* recommended that

> The health care workforce has the education, training, and capacity to deliver high-quality care for mental and substance-use conditions (55).

Meanwhile, AMERSA broadened its focus to include multidisciplinary health care professional education with the initiation of Project Mainstream and the publication of its *Strategic Plan* (56). The knowledge and skills recommended for all health care professionals mirrored those of other guidelines and included the following:

1. All health professionals should receive in their basic core curricula knowledge that substance use disorders are disorders for which appropriate treatment can lead to improved health and well-being.
2. All health professionals should have a basic understanding of substance use disorders and their effects on the patient, family, and community. Each professional should have an understanding of the evidence-based principles of universal, selected, and indicated prevention strategies as outlined by the IOM.
3. All health care professionals should be aware of the benefits of screening for potential and existing substance-related problems and of the benefits of intervention.
4. All health care professionals should possess basic knowledge of treatment and be able to initiate treatment or refer for appropriate assessment and treatment. At a minimum, all heath professionals should be able to communicate an appropriate level of concern and the requisite skills to be able to offer information, support, follow-up, or referral to an appropriate level of services (57).

Core competencies for physicians were included in the strategic plan and are outlined in Table 71.1.

CURRENT MEDICAL EDUCATION REQUIREMENTS

There currently are requirements for education regarding substance use and addiction at each level of medical education in the United States. The Liaison Committee on Medical Education (LCME), a collaboration between the Association of American Medical Colleges (AAMC) and the AMA, accredits U.S. medical schools. The LCME refrains from proscribing a specific curriculum or minimum time spent on any given topic; however, its accreditation standards include requirements for training in six clinical disciplines including psychiatry and in "behavioral and socioeconomic subjects, in addition to basic science and clinical disciplines." "Substance abuse" is included as one of 33 "behavioral and socioeconomic subjects" (58). In 2005, the AAMC reported that of the 131 accredited MD-granting U.S. medical schools, 122 included

TABLE 71.2	ACGME-required addiction psychiatry curriculum content

Residents must acquire knowledge and skills in the following areas:

1) Knowledge of the signs and symptoms of the use and abuse of all of the major categories of substances enumerated in V.B.3.b (i.e., alcohol; opioids; cocaine and other stimulants; cannabis and hallucinogens; benzodiazepines; other substances of abuse, including sedatives, hypnotics, or anxiolytics; and miscellaneous/unusual drugs, e.g., nutmeg, designer drugs, and organic solvents/inhalants) as well as knowledge of the types of treatment required for each.

2) Knowledge of the signs of withdrawal from these major categories of substances, knowledge and experience with a range of options for treatment of the withdrawal syndromes, and the complications commonly associated with such withdrawal.

3) Knowledge of the signs and symptoms of overdose, the medical and psychiatric sequelae of overdose, and experience in providing proper treatment of overdose.

4) Management of detoxification: in-patient management of substance-related disorders; experience in working collaboratively with specialists in the emergency department and intensive care units in the diagnosis and management of acute overdose symptoms.

5) Knowledge of the signs and symptoms of the social and psychological problems as well as the medical and psychiatric disorders that often accompany the chronic use and abuse of the major categories of substances.

6) Experience in the use of psychoactive medications in the treatment of psychiatric disorders often accompanying the major categories of substance-related disorders.

7) Experience in the use of techniques required for confrontation of and intervention with a chronic substance abuser, and in dealing with the defense mechanisms that cause the patient to resist entry into treatment.

8) Experience in the use of the various psychotherapeutic modalities involved in the ongoing management of the chronic substance abusing patient, including individual psychotherapies (e.g., cognitive–behavioral therapy), couples therapy, family therapy, group therapy, motivational enhancement therapy, and relapse prevention therapy.

9) Experience in working collaboratively with other mental health providers and allied health professionals, including nurses, social workers, psychologists, nurse practitioners, counselors, pharmacists, and others who participate in the care of patients with substance-related disorders.

10) Knowledge and understanding of the special problems of the pregnant woman with substance-related disorders and of the babies born to these women.

11) Knowledge of family systems and dynamics relevant to the etiology, diagnosis, and treatment of substance-related disorders.

12) Knowledge of the genetic vulnerabilities, risk and protective factors, epidemiology, and prevention of substance-related disorders.

13) Familiarity with the major medical journals and professional-scientific organizations dealing with research on the understanding and treatment of substance-related disorders.

14) Critical analysis of research reports, as resented in journal clubs and seminars.

15) Experience in teaching and supervising clinical trainees in the care of patients with substance-related disorders.

16) Understanding of the current economic aspects of providing psychiatric and other health care services to the addicted patient.

17) Knowledge of quality assurance measures and cost-effectiveness of various treatment modalities for substance-related disorders.

"substance abuse" in a required course and 62 offered elective training in this area (59).

In order to practice medicine in any U.S. state or territory, physicians must pass the United States Medical Licensing Examination (USMLE). This examination consists of three parts: Step 1 assesses knowledge of sciences basic to the practice of medicine, Step 2 assesses clinical knowledge essential to the supervised practice of medicine, and Step 3, taken after 1 year of postgraduate training, assesses clinical skills necessary for the independent practice of medicine. All three steps include content related to substance use and addiction including content on prevention, detection, and diagnosis (60). However, specific requirements regarding treatment including screening and brief intervention or medications (e.g., naltrexone, bupropion, nicotine, varenicline, buprenorphine) for treatment of substance use disorders are not mentioned.

The ACGME is responsible for accrediting postmedical school medical training programs in the United States (38). Residency training program requirements are developed by Residency Review Committees (RRC) for each medical specialty. Requirements for postgraduate training in emergency medicine, family medicine, pediatrics, psychiatry, and obstetrics and gynecology specifically include recognition of substance abuse or addiction. Requirements for anesthesiology, internal medicine, neurology, and pain medicine refer to recognition of co-occurring psychiatric conditions or behavioral aspects of care, but not specifically substance abuse or addiction. Preventive medicine, physical medicine, and rehabilitation and surgery have no references to required knowledge of substance use disorder detection, prevention, or treatment. Psychiatry is the only medical specialty with a minimum length of time devoted to a clinical rotation in addictions treatment—1 month (or 2% of clinical rotation time).

The ACGME RRC requirements for addiction psychiatry are specific. The RRC defines addiction psychiatry as

> ... the psychiatry subspecialty that focuses on the prevention, evaluation, and treatment of Substance-related Disorders as well as related education and research. In addition, the addiction psychiatrist will be fully trained in techniques required in the treatment of the larger group of patients with dual diagnoses of addictive disorders and other psychiatric disorders.

In order to be eligible for the program, candidates must have "satisfactorily completed an ACGME accredited general psychiatry residency prior to entering the program" (38). The duration of clinical addiction psychiatry training must be 12 months. The curriculum must contain 17 specific aspects of addiction psychiatry (see Table 71.2). Clinical experiences must include evaluation, consultation, and management of patients with substance-related disorders related to the following substances: alcohol; opioids; cocaine and other stimulants; cannabis and hallucinogens; benzodiazepines; other substances of abuse, including sedatives, hypnotics, or anxiolytics; and miscellaneous/unusual drugs (e.g., nutmeg, designer drugs, and organic solvents/inhalants). Specific program requirements can be found at the ACGME website www.acgme.org.

The ABPN is an ABMS member whose mission is "to serve the public interest and the professions of psychiatry and neurology by promoting excellence in practice through certification and maintenance of certification processes" (37). The ABPN provides certification and maintenance of certification examinations in addiction psychiatry. It publishes its exam content outlines on its website http://www.abpn.com/content_outlines.htm.

The Accreditation Council on Continuing Medical Education (ACCME) accredits CME for activities by U.S. physicians in independent practice. All states require continuing education for renewal of licensure to practice medicine. The ACCME does not prescribe specific content for CME; rather it emphasizes that CME content address important "practice gaps"—differences between current medical practice and evidence-based best practices particularly those that have a major impact on public health. In 2008, the ONDCP partnered with ACCME to address important practice gaps in physician management of patients with high-risk substance use and addiction as a prototype for bridging gaps in health care quality that would apply to physicians in all medical specialties. A video primer on addressing a practice gap on screening and brief intervention is available online at http://education.accme.org/video/accme-interviews/addressing-substance-abuse-cme-part-1-2. More detailed information on the specifics of screening and brief intervention is available at http://sbirt.samhsa.gov/about.htm.

EVIDENCE-BASED BEST PRACTICES IN MEDICAL EDUCATION ON SUBSTANCE USE AND ADDICTION

The evidence base for medical education in substance use and addiction has been growing in volume and sophistication since the career teachers began the first quantitative analyses of medical education in the 1970s. Studies range from surveys of educational offerings and physician opinion and self-reported practices to knowledge tests before and after an intervention to randomized controlled trials of different educational interventions with and without cost–benefit analyses.

CAREER TEACHER OR CHAMPION MODEL

In 1978, Pokorny and colleagues published the results of a survey on the state of U.S. medical education on drug abuse 5 years after implementation of the Career Teacher Program (61). The survey was sent to all 117 medicine schools, and 90% of schools responded. Twelve of these received a site visit to verify their responses (10 of 12 site visits agreed with survey: 83% accuracy). Required hours devoted to addiction teaching ranged from 0 (9 schools) to 126 hours (mean = 25.7 hours). Most of the basic science hours (mean = 7.6 hours) were spent in teaching pharmacology (mean = 4.7 hours). Most of the clinical science hours (mean = 17.7 hours) were spent in teaching psychiatry (mean = 12.0 hours). The percentage of required hours devoted to addictions ranged from 0% to 3.1% (mean = 0.6%). Schools with career teacher had significantly more hours of instruction on addictions (mean = 36.3 hours) than those without a career teacher (mean = 19.8 hours). Eighty percent of schools had one or more addiction treatment programs in their affiliated hospitals. Forty-nine percent of the schools indicated that there was no instruction in addiction treatment in their residency programs; 31% indicated it was taught in one program; 19% reported 2 to 6 programs included addiction treatment teaching. Seventeen percent indicated that they offered CME related to addictions. The authors concluded that compared to previous reports, teaching on addictions was improving. The richness of experience could be gauged by three factors—the number of required hours, the number of elective courses, and the presence of an affiliated treatment program.

Compared to the prevalence of the disorder, teaching on the subject was far too little, leaving graduating physicians feeling unprepared to deal with their patients' substance use disorders. In 1983, the authors published results of a follow-up survey to measure the impact of the Career Teacher Program (28). The follow-up survey was abbreviated to include only the questions that gave the most useful data in the first survey, and the sample was also limited. Schools were divided into four groups—"rich" (those reporting the most hours of addiction instruction) and "limited" programs (those falling in the lowest third in addition instruction on the first survey), with and without a career teacher. On average, the number of hours in required addictions teaching increased by 5.8 hours with poor schools experiencing the greatest increase and rich schools remaining unchanged whether or not a career teacher was present. The largest increases in didactic and clinical rotation hours were in psychiatry and family practice departments. The presence of a career teacher had a significant positive impact on the number of elective opportunities. In 1992, Australian medical schools implemented a faculty-training program based on the career teacher model from the United States. Nine of ten schools implemented a drug and alcohol co-ordinator, and those schools realized a 158% increase in required teaching hours related to addictions and a 383% increase in electives opportunities (62).

UNDERGRADUATE MEDICAL EDUCATION

Some of the early quantitative research on medical school education in addiction involved examining participants' responses to novel educational activities. In 1983, Siegal and Rudisill reported on medical student reactions to their participation in educating DUI (driving under the influence) arrestees in a weekend intervention program, which provided "an intense exposure to alcohol and drug dependent individuals' intervention and treatment." Students rated the experience as "highly enjoyable and effective" (63). Viewing of a video montage of commercially available films and training videos on the signs and symptoms of substance intoxication and withdrawal was rated as helpful by over 90% of students (64). Teaching of specific interviewing skills and use of role-plays were rated as "highly acceptable" by both students and teachers (65) and were better predictors of clinical performance than attitudes toward alcoholic patients (66). Medical students assigned by convenience to complete a Web-based training module ($N = 82$) or a lecture ($n = 81$) on alcohol use disorders then evaluated a standard patient with an alcohol use disorder. Students completing the Web-based module scored significantly higher on specific elements of screening and brief intervention (67).

Randomized trials of teaching interventions have shown significant improvement in skills using standardized patients from before to after the intervention. In one study, 76 medical students were randomized to receive a 3-hour workshop on problem drinking (intervention) or depression (control). All students then participated in eight simulated office visits (Objective Structured Clinical Examination [OSCE] stations). Those who had the training scored significantly higher on checklist scores for assessment and management of high-risk alcohol use than those in the control condition (68). In a second study, 55 medical student volunteers were randomized into one of two teaching conditions. Both participated in standardized patient interviews before and after training. Both received a detailed 35-page reading on the subject, a traditional lecture, and videotape demonstration interview. The experimental group also recorded a 20-minute simulated patient interview and received feedback on their performance in a small group setting. Both groups demonstrated significant improvement in their interview skills from before to after training with no significant difference between groups (69). Finally, in a third study, replacing 1 week of a 6-week psychiatry clerkship with an experience on an addiction treatment unit resulted in increased tolerance and positive regard for patients with alcoholism. Knowledge of psychiatry based on end-of-course exams was not changed from before to after the intervention (70).

GRADUATE MEDICAL EDUCATION

Educational interventions on the diagnosis and treatment of substance use disorders are associated with increased knowledge and skills among house staff and more positive attitudes toward patients with substance use disorders. Family medicine residents indicated a high level of satisfaction with a new 20-hour course on alcoholism that included didactics, supervised intake assessments, and participation in group sessions (71). Implementation of a longitudinal didactic series over a 3-year internal medicine residency mitigated the usual negative effect of graduate medical education on attitudes toward patients with high-risk alcohol use and alcoholism (72). Pediatric residents receiving an AOD curriculum that included interactive didactics, participation in a community-based adolescent AOD program, role-playing practice, and interview skill sessions performed significantly better than untrained controls on tests of knowledge, skills, and abilities in assessing and managing AOD disorders (73). Participants in a Chief Resident Immersion Training Program demonstrated significantly improved knowledge, skills, and confidence related to addiction treatment than nonparticipating peers at 6- and 11-month follow-up (74).

Measurement of physician behaviors from before to after a clinically supervised addiction education activity resulted in improved performance by resident physicians. Introduction of an in-patient rotation on an addiction treatment unit corresponded to a significant increase in the diagnosis of substance use disorders by family medicine residents as indicated by chart reviews (75). Education on alcohol use disorders increased the diagnosis of alcohol dependence from 2.5% to 4.1% by internal medicine residents and nurse practitioners in a primary care clinic (76). Increased clinical supervision training on the use of the CAGE questionnaire (have you felt you should *Cut* down on your drinking, *Annoyed* by people criticizing your drinking, felt bad or *Guilty* about your drinking, used an *Eye*-opener in the morning?) to screen for alcoholism and incorporation of the CAGE questions into clinic forms increased screening with the CAGE from 5.9% to 76.7%, and asking about the quantity/frequency of alcohol use increased from 26.5% to 93% (77). Introduction of a drug and alcohol treatment unit rotation was associated with a 10-fold increase in the number of interns' emergency department notes that addressed alcohol use and a significant increase in appropriate prescribing of benzodiazepines (78).

Education on SBIRT (screening, brief intervention, and referral to treatment) results in improved skills from before to after the intervention. A 4-hour didactic, video-based, and skills-based training program significantly increased emergency medicine residents' knowledge scores and practice in screening and intervention for alcohol from 17% before to 58% after the intervention and compared to a control group (79). Internal medicine residents who received clinical supervision on NIAAA recommended guidelines for screening and brief intervention increased the frequency of asking about alcohol use twofold and of counseling threefold (80). Implementation of a staged screening and brief intervention protocol in a family medicine residency clinic using the AUDIT-C was associated with increased screening rates. Nurses followed up a positive AUDIT-C with a full AUDIT, and residents provided counseling and referral if needed. Screening rates increased significantly from before to after the intervention (81). Primary care residents randomized to receive an 8-hour interactive training on a brief alcohol intervention (BAI) were significantly more likely to explain safe drinking limits and to elicit the patients' opinions about their drinking than controls who received training on lipid management; however, BAI-trained residents implemented an average of only 2.4 of the 15 elements of BAI (82). Adherence to national guidelines on quantifying alcohol intake and screening for drug use increased modestly from a high baseline after a 2.5 day SBIRT training (83). Surgical interns demonstrated significant improvement from baseline and compared to a control group in SBIRT skills using standardized patients 5 weeks after an 8-hour interactive training course on SBIRT. Trained surgical interns showed significant improvement in asking permission to discuss drinking, informing the patient of blood alcohol level and recommended limits, using less closed-answer questions, offering hope, encouragement and a menu of options. They also were less likely to engage in arguments over referral to treatment (84).

CONTINUING MEDICAL EDUCATION

CME interventions for addictions have been associated with mixed results.

Brief experiential training aimed at improving optimism and attitudes toward patients with addiction has had mixed results. Brief training on alcoholism and the implementation of a brief questionnaire to assess drinking resulted in modest improvement in alcohol histories and no change in smoking histories based on in-patient chart review (85). A learner-centered, experiential training program increased the confidence of faculty (80% internal medicine) in diagnosing and managing patients with substance use disorders and increased their optimism about patient outcome (86). Primary care multidisciplinary teams demonstrated a significant change in attitude after a 2-day experiential training on alcohol use disorders, whereas trained emergency medicine teams and control teams demonstrated no change in attitudes (87). General practitioners and nurses in a primary care clinic received training and supervision for a 3-month period in alcohol screening (CAGE and MAST) and referral. Both reported increased optimism about alcoholism treatment and improvement in the frequency of asking about alcohol problems (88). Interactive training sessions teaching general practitioners to use the drink-less brief intervention package significantly increased practitioners' confidence in implementing the elements of screening (49% to 90%) and brief intervention (40% to 92%) for high-risk alcohol use (89).

Brief training aimed at teaching new clinical skills is associated with improved implementation of these skills. Patients of general practitioners who volunteered for university-based training with ongoing supervision to implement a protocol for primary care–based management of patients with alcohol use disorders were more likely to attempt abstinence, to repeat attempts at abstinence, and to have more days of abstinence than patients of physicians who did not volunteer for the training (90). A 2-hour skills-based training on a brief negotiation interview (BNI) was effective in teaching emergency physicians. Ninety-one percent passed the proficiency examination and performed the BNI in an average of 7.75 minutes (91).

Web-based training programs on Alcoholics Anonymous (92) and on Network Therapy and naltrexone (46) have demonstrated feasibility with access by both specialists and generalists. The majority of website visitors who completed a questionnaire reported that the training was useful (70%) and that it would improve their management of patients on naltrexone (67%) (46,93).

Brief training and office support is associated with improved implementation of evidence-based SBIRT. Primary care providers with enhanced training in SBIRT and office support were significantly more likely to talk with their patients about alcohol use and were more likely to provide evidence-based counseling. This difference persisted throughout the 32-month follow-up phase (94). Physicians and mid-level practitioners were randomized to receive training in the management of a maintenance phase of care for alcohol dependence. Trained providers received an initial 2.25-hour training, a booster session, study materials, and chart-based prompts. Of 164 patients, 67% saw intervention providers. Intervention patients were significantly more likely than controls to report that their provider asked about alcohol use (95).

Studies that have examined comparative cost-effectiveness of training have found mixed results. Three different methods for disseminating training in screening and brief intervention for family practitioners were compared for effectiveness and cost-effectiveness. Telemarketing was significantly more effective than mailing print media and more cost-effective than academic detailing (96). Relative cost-effectiveness of four forms of training (academic detailing, interactive continuing education, computerized reminders, and targeted payments) was compared for their efficacy in decreasing risky drinking in the patients of Australian general practitioners. Academic detailing and computerized reminders were the most effective. Targeted payments were least cost-effective, whereas cost-effectiveness of the other three was comparable (97).

In their review of teaching methods for SBIRT, Polydorou and colleagues concluded that interactive teaching methods that enable skill demonstration, practice, and assessment have been shown to be most effective (98).

CONCLUSION

Tobacco, alcohol, and other substance use continue to take a tremendous toll on health. Physicians have the potential for significant positive impact in preventing and treating high-risk substance use and substance use disorders. Medical education has not kept pace with advances in prevention and treatment of substance use disorders such that many physicians are unprepared to effectively manage patients with high-risk substance use and addiction. Ongoing efforts to address this significant practice gap include training of addiction specialist champions for medical school faculty, development of model curricula, and updating requirements at every stage of medical training to include appropriate training for physicians in every patient care specialty. Empirical data support novel educational approaches to improve physician competency in screening, brief intervention, and treatment of at-risk substance use and substance use disorders. Continued efforts to refine educational approaches and reduce institutional barriers such as lack of reimbursement or other institutional support are needed to further improve medical education in addiction prevention and treatment.

REFERENCES

1. Rush B. *An Inquiry into the Effects of Ardent Spirits upon the Human Body and Mind*. 8th ed. Boston, MA: James Loring; 1823:36.
2. AMA. Reports of officers: hospitalization of patients with alcoholism. *JAMA*. 1956;162(8):750.
3. Mokdad AH, Marks JS, Stroup DF, et al. Actual causes of death in the United States, 2000. *JAMA*. 2004;291(10):1238–1245.
4. NIDA and NIAAA. In: N.I.o.H. Department of Health and Human Services, ed. *The Economic Costs of Alcohol and Drug Abuse in the United States*. Bethesda, MD: DHHS, NIH; 1998.
5. Babor TF, Kadden RM. Screening and interventions for alcohol and drug problems in medical settings: what works? *J Trauma*. 2005;59(3 suppl):S80–S87. [discussion S94–S100]
6. LoCastro JS, Youngblood M, Cisler RA, et al. Alcohol treatment effects on secondary nondrinking outcomes and quality of life: the COMBINE study. *J Stud Alcohol Drugs*. 2009;70(2):186–196.
7. Room R, Babor T, Rehm J. Alcohol and public health. *Lancet*. 2005;365(9458):519–530.
8. Holden C. The neglected disease in medical education. *Science*. 1985;229(4715):741–742.
9. Roche AM, Parle MD, Campbell J, et al. Substance abuse disorders: psychiatric trainees' knowledge, diagnostic skills and attitudes. *Aust N Z J Psychiatry*. 1995;29(4):645–652.
10. Koopman FA, Parry CD, Myers B, et al. Addressing alcohol problems in primary care settings: a study of general medical practitioners in Cape Town, South Africa. *Scand J Public Health*. 2008;36(3):298–302.
11. Johansson K, Bendtsen P, Akerlind I. Early intervention for problem drinkers: readiness to participate among general practitioners and nurses in Swedish primary health care. *Alcohol Alcohol*. 2002;37(1):38–42.
12. Terrell F, Zatzick DF, Jurkovich GJ, et al. Nationwide survey of alcohol screening and brief intervention practices at US level I trauma centers. *J Am Coll Surg*. 2008;207(5):630–638.
13. Lasswell AB, Liepman MR, McQuade WH, et al. Comparison of primary care residents' confidence and clinical behavior in treating hypertension versus treating alcoholism. *Acad Med*. 1993;68(7):580–582.
14. Varga M, Buris L. Drinking habits of medical students call for better integration of teaching about alcohol into the medical curriculum. *Alcohol Alcohol*. 1994;29(5):591–596.
15. Fiore MC, Jaén CR, Baker TB, et al. *Treating Tobacco Use and Dependence: 2008 Update*; 2008. Available at: http://www.ncbi.nlm.nih.gov/bookshelf/br.fcgi?book=hsahcpr&part=A28163.
16. Ohida T, Sakurai H, Mochizuki Y, et al. Smoking prevalence and attitudes toward smoking among Japanese physicians. *JAMA*. 2001;285(20):2643–2648.
17. Fucito L, Gomes B, Murnion B, et al. General practitioners' diagnostic skills and referral practices in managing patients with drug and alcohol-related health problems: implications for medical training and education programmes. *Drug Alcohol Rev*. 2003;22(4):417–424.
18. Musto DF. *The American Disease: Origins of Narcotic Control*. 3rd ed. Oxford, England: Oxford University Press; 1999.
19. Lewis DC, Niven RG, Czechowicz D, et al. A review of medical education in alcohol and other drug abuse. *JAMA*. 1987;257(21):2945–2948.
20. Lewis DC. Medical education for alcohol and other drug abuse in the United States. *CMAJ*. 1990;143(10):1091–1096.
21. Annual reports: Committee on Alcoholism and Addiction. *JAMA*. 1966;198(4):177.
22. Plaut T, ed. *Alcohol Problems: A Report to the Nation*. New York: Oxford University Press; 1967.
23. Medical school education on abuse of alcohol and other psychoactive drugs. *JAMA*. 1972;219(13):1746–1749.
24. Ewing J. Professional training on alcoholism. Workshop 4: changing student and faculty attitudes toward alcoholic patients. *Ann NY Acad Sci*. 1971;178:87–91.
25. Hughes HE. Professional training an alcoholism. Annual dinner address. *Ann NY Acad Sci*. 1971;178:13–16.
26. Galanter M, Bean-Bayog M. A study of physicians certified in alcohol and drug dependence. *Alcohol Clin Exp Res*. 1989;13(1):1–2.
27. Galanter M, Dermatis H, Calabrese D. Residencies in addiction psychiatry: 1990 to 2000, a decade of progress. *Am J Addict*. 2002;11(3):192–199.
28. Pokorny AD, Solomon J. A follow-up survey of drug abuse and alcoholism teaching in medical schools. *J Med Educ*. 1983;58(4):316–321.
29. Galanter M. Postgraduate certification in alcohol and drug dependence. *Alcohol Clin Exp Res*. 1985;9(5):387–389.
30. Griffin JB Jr, Hill IK, Jones JJ, et al. Evaluating alcoholism and drug abuse knowledge in medical education: a collaborative project. *J Med Educ*. 1983;58(11):859–863.
31. Hanlon MJ. A review of the recent literature relating to the training of medical students in alcoholism. *J Med Educ*. 1985;60(8):618–626.

32. Bean-Bayog M, Galanter M, Halikas J, et al. Special report: AMSAODD: plan for certification of members, 1985–1986. *Alcohol Clin Exp Res*. 1985;9(5):390–392.
33. American Academy of Addiction Psychiatry. 2009. Available at: http://www2.aaap.org/.
34. Galanter M, et al. The current status of psychiatric education in alcoholism and drug abuse. *Am J Psychiatry*. 1989;146(1):35–39.
35. Galanter M. Subspecialty training in alcoholism and drug abuse. *Am J Psychiatry*. 1989;146(1):8–9.
36. Division of Alcoholism and Drug Abuse, Center for Medical Fellowships. 2008. Available at: http://www.med.nyu.edu/substanceabuse/cendes.html.
37. ABPN (American Board of Psychiatry and Neurology). 2009. Available at: http://www.abpn.com/home.htm.
38. ACGME (Accreditation Council on Graduate Medical Education). 2009. Available at: http://www.acgme.org/acWebsite/home/home.asp.
39. Nocks JJ. Instructing medical students on alcoholism: what to teach with limited time. *J Med Educ*. 1980;55(10):858–864.
40. Murray M, Fleming M. Prevention and treatment of alcohol-related problems: an international medical education model. *Acad Med*. 1996;71(11):1204–1210.
41. Rankin JG. The development of medical education on alcohol- and drug-related problems at the University of Toronto. *CMAJ*. 1990;143(10):1083–1091.
42. Broadening the base of treatment for alcohol problems. Institute of Medicine, 1990.
43. Peters C, Wilson D, Bruneau A, et al. Alcohol risk assessment and intervention for family physicians. Project of the College of Family Physicians of Canada. *Can Fam Physician*. 1996;42:681–689.
44. American Board of Addiction Medicine. 2009. Available at: http://www.abam.net/.
45. Klamen DL. Education and training in addictive diseases. *Psychiatr Clin North Am*. 1999;22(2):471–480, xi.
46. Galanter M, Keller DS, Dermatis H. Using the internet for clinical training: a course on network therapy for substance abuse. *Psychiatr Serv*. 1997;48(8):999–1000, 1008.
47. Isaacson JH, Fleming M, Kraus M, et al. A national survey of training in substance use disorders in residency programs. *J Stud Alcohol*. 2000;61(6):912–915.
48. McAvoy BR. Alcohol education for general practitioners in the United Kingdom—a window of opportunity? *Alcohol Alcohol*. 2000;35(3):225–229.
49. Solberg LI, Maciosek MV, Edwards NM. Primary care intervention to reduce alcohol misuse ranking its health impact and cost effectiveness. *Am J Prev Med*. 2008;34(2):143–152.
50. ONDCP. *Third National Leadership Conference on Medical Education in Substance Abuse*. Washington, DC: George Washington University School of Medicine; 2008.
51. NIAAA. *Clinician's Guide for Helping Patients Who Drink Too Much*. 2006. Available at: http://www.niaaa.nih.gov/Publications/EducationTrainingMaterials/VideoCases.htm.
52. SAMHSA. *Buprenorphine*. 2002. Available at: http://buprenorphine.samhsa.gov/.
53. Barry DT, Irwin KS, Jones ES, et al. Integrating buprenorphine treatment into office-based practice: a qualitative study. *J Gen Intern Med*. 2009;24(2):218–225.
54. Cuff PA, Vanselow NA, B.o.N.a.B.H.o.t. IOM, eds. *Improving Medical Education: Enhancing the Behavioral and Social Science Content of Medical School Curricula*. Washington, DC: The National Academies Press; 2004:148.
55. IOM, B.o.H.S.o.t., ed. *Improving the Quality of Health Care for Mental and Substance-Use Conditions*. Quality Chasm Series, ed. C.o.C.t.Q.C.A.t.M.H.a.A.D. BHCS. Washington, DC: The National Academies Press; 2006.
56. Haack M, Adger H. Strategic plan and recommendations for HRSA, AMERSA, SAMHSA/CSAT interdisciplinary faculty development. *Subst Abus*. 2002;23(2):123.
57. AMERSA. Strategic plan for interdisciplinary faculty development: arming the nation's health professional workforce for a new approach to substance use disorders. In: Haack MR, Adger H, eds. Providence, RI: Association for Medical Education and Research in Substance Abuse (AMERSA); 2002.
58. Liaison Committee on Medical Education. 2009. Available at: http://www.lcme.org/.
59. AAMC. *Number of US Medical School Teaching Selected Topics*. Washington, DC. 2005:2.
60. USMLE (United States Medical Licensing Examination). 2009. Available at: http://www.usmle.org/.
61. Pokorny A, Putnam P, Fryer J. Drug abuse and alcoholism teaching in U.S. medical and osteopathic schools. *J Med Educ*. 1978;53(10):816–824.
62. Roche AM. Drug and alcohol medical education: evaluation of a national programme. *Br J Addict*. 1992;87(7):1041–1048.
63. Siegal H, Rudisill JR. Teaching medical students about substance abuse in a weekend intervention program. *J Med Educ*. 1983;58(4):322–327.
64. Welsh CJ. OD's and DT's: using movies to teach intoxication and withdrawal syndromes to medical students. *Acad Psychiatry*. 2003;27(3):182–186.
65. Frith J. The use of role plays in teaching drug and alcohol management. *Aust Fam Physician*. 1996;25(4):532–533.
66. Saunders JB, Roche AM. Medical education in substance use disorders. *Drug Alcohol Rev*. 1991;10(3):263–275.
67. Lee JD, Triola M, Gillespie C, et al. Working with patients with alcohol problems: a controlled trial of the impact of a rich media web module on medical student performance. *J Gen Intern Med*. 2008;23(7):1006–1009.
68. Kahan M, Wilson L, Midmer D, et al. Randomized controlled trial on the effects of a skills-based workshop on medical students' management of problem drinking and alcohol dependence. *Subst Abus*. 2003;24(1):5–16.
69. Walsh RA, Sanson-Fisher RW, Low A, et al. Teaching medical students alcohol intervention skills: results of a controlled trial. *Med Educ*. 1999;33(8):559–565.
70. Christison GW, Haviland MG. Requiring a one-week addiction treatment experience in a six-week psychiatry clerkship: effects on attitudes toward substance-abusing patients. *Teach Learn Med*. 2003;15(2):93–97.
71. Confusione M, Leonard K, Jaffe A. Alcoholism training in a family medicine residency. *J Subst Abuse Treat*. 1988;5(1):19–22.
72. Heiligman RM, Nagoshi CT. A longitudinal study of family practice residents' attitudes toward alcoholism. *Fam Med*. 1994;26(7):447–451.
73. Kokotailo PK, Fleming MF, Koscik RL. A model alcohol and other drug use curriculum for pediatric residents. *Acad Med*. 1995;70(6):495–498.
74. Alford DP, Bridden C, Jackson AH, et al. Promoting substance use education among generalist physicians: an evaluation of the Chief Resident Immersion Training (CRIT) program. *J Gen Intern Med*. 2009;24(1):40–47.

75. Mulry JT, Brewer ML, Spencer DL. The effect of an inpatient chemical dependency rotation on residents' clinical behavior. *Fam Med*. 1987;19(4):276–280.
76. Cowan PF. An intervention to improve the assessment of alcoholism by practicing physicians. *Fam Pract Res J*. 1994;14(1):41–49.
77. Lawner K, Doot M, Gausas J, et al. Implementation of CAGE alcohol screening in a primary care practice. *Fam Med*. 1997;29(5):332–335.
78. Gaughwin M, Dodding J, White JM, et al. Changes in alcohol history taking and management of alcohol dependence by interns at the Royal Adelaide Hospital. *Med Educ*. 2000;34(3):170–174.
79. D'Onofrio G, Nadel ES, Degutis LC, et al. Improving emergency medicine residents' approach to patients with alcohol problems: a controlled educational trial. *Ann Emerg Med*. 2002;40(1):50–62.
80. Wilk AI, Jensen NM. Investigation of a brief teaching encounter using standardized patients: teaching residents alcohol screening and intervention. *J Gen Intern Med*. 2002;17(5):356–360.
81. Seale JP, Shellenberger S, Tillery WK, et al. Implementing alcohol screening and intervention in a family medicine residency clinic. *Subst Abus*. 2005;26(1):23–31.
82. Chossis I, Lane C, Gache P, et al. Effect of training on primary care residents' performance in brief alcohol intervention: a randomized controlled trial. *J Gen Intern Med*. 2007;22(8):1144–1149.
83. Gunderson EW, Levin FR, Owen P. Impact of a brief training on medical resident screening for alcohol misuse and illicit drug use. *Am J Addict*. 2008;17(2):149–154.
84. MacLeod JB, Hungerford DW, Dunn C, et al. Evaluation of training of surgery interns to perform brief alcohol interventions for trauma patients. *J Am Coll Surg*. 2008;207(5):639–645.
85. Rowland N, Maynard AK, Kennedy PF, et al. Teaching doctors to take alcohol histories: a limited success story. *Med Educ*. 1988;22(6):539–542.
86. Bigby J, Barnes HN. Evaluation of a faculty development program in substance abuse education. *J Gen Intern Med*. 1993;8(6):301–305.
87. Gorman DM, Werner JM, Jacobs LM, et al. Evaluation of an alcohol education package for non-specialist health care and social workers. *Br J Addict*. 1990;85(2):223–233.
88. Bendtsen P, Akerlind I. Changes in attitudes and practices in primary health care with regard to early intervention for problem drinkers. *Alcohol Alcohol*. 1999;34(5):795–800.
89. Proude EM, Conigrave KM, Haber PS. Effectiveness of skills-based training using the drink-less package to increase family practitioner confidence in intervening for alcohol use disorders. *BMC Med Educ*. 2006;6:8.
90. Malet L, Reynaud M, Llorca PM, et al. Impact of practitioner's training in the management of alcohol dependence: a quasi-experimental 18-month follow-up study. *Subst Abuse Treat Prev Policy*. 2006;1:18.
91. D'Onofrio G, Pantalon MV, Degutis LC, et al. Development and implementation of an emergency practitioner-performed brief intervention for hazardous and harmful drinkers in the emergency department. *Acad Emerg Med*. 2005;12(3):249–256.
92. Sellers B, Galanter M, Dermatis H, et al. Enhancing physicians' use of Alcoholics Anonymous: internet-based training. *J Addict Dis*. 2005;24(3):77–86.
93. Galanter M, Keller DS, Dermatis H, et al. Use of the internet for addiction education. Combining network therapy with pharmacotherapy. *Am J Addict*. 1998;7(1):7–13.
94. Adams A, Ockene JK, Wheller EV, et al. Alcohol counseling: physicians will do it. *J Gen Intern Med*. 1998;13(10):692–698.
95. Friedmann PD, Rose J, Hayaki J, et al. Training primary care clinicians in maintenance care for moderated alcohol use. *J Gen Intern Med*. 2006;21(12):1269–1275.
96. Gomel MK, Wutzke SE, Hardcastle DM, et al. Cost-effectiveness of strategies to market and train primary health care physicians in brief intervention techniques for hazardous alcohol use. *Soc Sci Med*. 1998;47(2):203–211.
97. Shanahan M, Shakeshaft A, Mattick RP. Modelling the costs and outcomes of changing rates of screening for alcohol misuse by GPs in the Australian context. *Appl Health Econ Health Policy*. 2006;5(3):155–166.
98. Polydorou S, Gunderson EW, Levin FR. Training physicians to treat substance use disorders. *Curr Psychiatry Rep*. 2008;10(5):399–404.

RESOURCES

Model Curricula

Association for Medical Education and Research in Substance Abuse (AMERSA): http://www.amersa.org/

Project Mainstream: http://www.projectmainstream.net/project-mainstream.asp?cid=21

Lecture Handouts, Slide Sets, and Other Resources

Research Society on Alcoholism Lecture Series: http://www.rsoa.org/lectures/

Alcohol Medical Scholars Program: http://www.alcoholmedicalscholars.org/

National Institute on Alcohol Abuse and Alcoholism publications for clinicians: http://www.niaaa.nih.gov/Publications/EducationTrainingMaterials/

Clinician's Guide for Helping Patients Who Drink Too Much: http://www.niaaa.nih.gov/Publications/EducationTrainingMaterials/guide.htm

National Institute on Drug Abuse: Principles of Drug Addiction Treatment—A Research-Based Guide: http://www.drugabuse.gov/PDF/PODAT/PODAT.pdf

Center of Excellence for Physician Education: http://www.drugabuse.gov/coe/topic.htm

American Academy of Addiction Psychiatry: http://www2.aaap.org

American Society of Addiction Medicine: http://www.asam.org

College on Problems of Drug Dependence: http://www.cpdd.vcu.edu/index.html

American Psychiatric Association: http://www.psych.org

CHAPTER 72 Psychologists: Training and Education

D. Baron ■ C.J. Combs ■ A.P. Wells

Psychologists are uniquely trained to assess and treat disorders that frequently co-occur with substance abuse and substance dependence, and the treatment of the co-occurring disorders enhances an individual's chances of recovery. Despite these unique skills, few psychologists themselves are adequately trained in the assessment and treatment of substance use disorders (SUDs), thus limiting their effectiveness within this population. Research conducted by Alcoholics Anonymous (AA) reveals that 60% of AA membership sought some form of psychological counseling prior to their joining a 12-step program and treatment was discontinued due to dissatisfaction with the care provided by the psychologist (1).

In the general U.S. population, approximately 1 in 10 individuals has an SUD (2). In psychiatric in-patient facilities, the prevalence rate climbs as high as 1 in 2 (3), and 90% of offenders entering prison meet diagnostic criteria for an SUD (4). With prevalence rates this high, adequate training and education of psychologists in the assessment and treatment of SUDs can no longer be elective or absent entirely from training curricula.

Each year, drug and alcohol abuse contributes to the deaths of more than 120,000 Americans. SUDs cost taxpayers in excess of $360 billion annually in preventable health care costs, extra law enforcement, auto accidents, crime, and lost productivity (5). A sizable portion of the general population uses psychoactive substances in response to anxiety or depressive disorders (6), both areas in which evidence-based practices have excelled. Adding a core SUD education and training component to skills already inherent in quality psychology programs would place psychologists in a uniquely qualified position to effectively treat SUDs.

The President's New Freedom Commission on Mental Health (2003) highlighted the importance in cross-training practitioners in the treatment of psychiatric and SUDs. The expert panel noted, "A key challenge to developing integrated treatment programs is overcoming the traditional separation between mental health and substance abuse treatment . . . much remains to be accomplished" (p. 65). They went on to advocate that both mental health and SUDs should be considered primary disorders, and endorsed the 5-year blueprint for action contained with the Substance Abuse and Mental Health Services Administration's (2002) *Report to Congress on the Prevention and Treatment of Co-occurring Substance Abuse Disorders and Mental Disorders*, which recommended the co-ordinated treatment of mental and substance abuse disorders in a manner "seamless to the client" (p. 113). While the latter report suggested that such co-ordinated treatment could be conducted among different collaborating providers, it would clearly be advantageous to have clinicians available who are trained in both disorders to minimize the possibility of patient attrition when treatment is received from two (or more) providers when each disorder is addressed separately.

The existing literature that examines the training in substance abuse for doctoral-level psychologists is scarce. A survey of rehabilitation psychologists (7) found that while most treated patients with alcohol and drug abuse issues, few felt adequately trained to intervene with such patients, with a majority rating their training as poor. Twenty percent reported receiving no formal training in substance abuse. Of those having received some training in this area, most had either completed a graduate course where substance abuse was discussed (42%) or participated in a continuing education or postgraduate workshop on substance abuse (40%). Only one in five reported having completed a graduate course fully devoted to substance abuse.

In another survey (8), this one of doctorate psychology programs accredited by the American Psychological Association (APA), only 38% of programs offered at least one course in alcohol or substance abuse, and 95% of these were elective, not required, courses. On the other hand, 62% of schools indicated that substance abuse was part of some course in their curriculum, with 78% of these courses being required ones. It was estimated that about 10% of the time in these latter courses was devoted to alcohol or drug abuse, suggesting that substance abuse was typically incorporated into a broad course on psychopathology. To our knowledge, there has not been a more recent survey of doctoral psychology programs than this one, which was conducted in 1991 to 1992.

Harwood and colleagues (2004) surveyed a large sample of behavioral health practitioners, including psychologists, about their education and training in substance abuse. Not surprisingly, substance abuse counselors reported receiving the most formal coursework in substance abuse, although even here, the 69% of substance abuse counselors endorsing such coursework seems low, given the concentrated focus of their role. About half of other practitioners, such as marital and family therapists and professional counselors, reported formal coursework in the addictions, while only 30% of psychologists reported such coursework. Thus, it was more common for practitioners at the predoctoral (i.e., master's) level to have taken coursework in substance abuse than psychologists, most of whom are required to obtain a doctoral degree. The authors concluded, "Continuing education, including seminars and workshops, is the primary mechanism through which these behavioral health practitioners received training in substance abuse treatment" (p. 200). With respect to psychologists, however, it would be difficult to argue that their training in substance abuse treatment, mainly through continuing education, is truly "continuing," given their lack of initial training in this area during graduate school and internship.

To get a sense of the current state of training in the addictions, we examined the online curricula and course offerings of 33 doctoral psychology programs sampled from the APA's list of accredited programs with functioning websites in the summer of 2009. These programs included both Ph.D. and Psy.D. programs and schools from different regions across the United States and Canada. Of our sample, only three programs required a course in substance abuse or chemical dependency, while seven programs offered elective coursework in substance abuse. One university-based program offered a practicum in motivational interviewing for advanced students. Thus, fewer than half of the programs examined had coursework in the addictions available to their students. Of the three schools mandating a course in substance abuse, all were professional schools offering the Psy.D. degree.

What can account for this dearth of training in the addictions? As Harwood and colleagues (2004) noted, "The low rate of formal training in substance abuse among professionals such as psychologists is due, at least in part, to the curriculum design of graduate education programs" (p. 193). Indeed, the available survey and anecdotal evidence suggests that any substance abuse education at the graduate school level is likely to occur in the context of a broader survey course in psychopathology or the biologic underpinning of behavior. Students with an interest in the addictions, or the foresight to realize that they will likely encounter many such patients, are left to seek out an elective course, if one is available. It is quite plausible that many, if not most, students graduate from doctoral-level psychology programs with one or two lectures comprising their entire education on SUDs.

Historically, training in the treatment of mental (nonaddictive) disorders has focused on lectures and formal, structured clinical experiences that are found in university-based programs, which are often bastions for scientific research in the diagnosis and treatment of these disorders. In this sense, graduate student training is similar to that received by their counterparts in medicine and allied health. In contrast, training in the treatment of addictive disorders has been traditionally more concentrated on the apprentice model, where practitioners learn by observing model teachers (9,10). This may be, in part, based on the widespread notion within the field of addictions that only former addicts can truly understand and, thus, assist the substance-abusing patient, and this may explain the popularity and endorsement of 12-step programs over other treatments with a stronger base of empirical support.

Although there is no empirical evidence to bear on this question, it also appears to be the case that graduate students have limited exposure to patients with co-occurring substance abuse disorders during the supervised training in their program's affiliated training clinic. Such clinics often screen out for referral such patients with co-occurring disorders, as they are deemed too difficult or complex for student therapists just beginning to train in psychotherapy. It may also be the case that a lack of supervisors with proper training, experience, or interest in the addictions would prevent training clinics from accepting such patients for their students, as these patients would then fall outside the professional competence of the responsible supervisor.

As a result, many students reach the internship phase of their training with little, if no, experience with substance-abusing patients, despite the prevalence of such patients in general clinical practice. One suspects that students gain greater exposure to these patients at the internship level, as the internship is considered the capstone clinical experience before the conferral of the doctoral degree with a corresponding emphasis on direct clinical work. The directory of internship programs of the Association of Psychology Postdoctoral and Internship Centers (APPIC) listed 257 predoctoral internship programs offering substance abuse disorders as a "major rotation," or a primary focus, of training. However, it is unclear whether the nature of these major rotations involves simply the exposure to patients with co-occurring addictive disorders or actual coursework and specific training in empirically based treatment approaches for such patients. The same can be said for postdoctoral placements, which are fewer in number than internships, as they are not a requirement to complete the doctoral degree. It is hard to envision strong, evidence-based training in treating the addictions for students at the internship and postdoctoral levels, except for placements at Veterans Administration Centers and the few specialized substance treatment sites. The limiting factor in providing this training is almost certainly the lack of supervisors at all levels of the graduate school–internship–postdoctoral chain who are properly trained themselves. This dearth of qualified supervisors in the area of addictions not only prevents patients with co-occurring disorders from receiving integrated treatment, but also curtails the training of students who can go on to train others in a "train the trainer" model (11), which will be critical in exponentially increasing the number of competent practitioners needed to meet this clinical demand.

Given this data and the high prevalence of SUDs across patient populations, it is imperative that psychologists be proficient in the assessment and appropriate referral of individuals with SUDs through knowledge obtained about the disease of addiction, the use and interpretation of assessment materials, and clinical training as a requirement to graduate from any institution conferring a degree of doctorate of philosophy or psychology preparing students to practice in the field of psychology.

Box 72.1 is a syllabus outlining an example of the education and training that should be received by psychology students enrolled in any doctoral-level program. This course could be placed in the school curriculum subsequent to or in

> **Box 72.1** **Substance Use Disorders: Education and Training—Sample Syllabus**

Course Description

This course introduces and examines basic concepts in the neurobiology, assessment, treatment, and appropriate referral of patients with substance use disorders (SUDs). Lectures, small group discussions, demonstrations, and videos will be incorporated in the presentation of topics. Opportunities for experiential learning—e.g., attendance at an open AA meeting—will be expected. Students will have an opportunity to research a specific topic in the addiction literature and complete a term paper outlining their findings, and explore personal views and biases via electronic submission of weekly one- to two-page essays.

Course Objectives and Philosophy

This course is designed to provide doctoral-level psychology students with a working knowledge of research trends and findings in the treatment of SUDs. Students will be challenged to explore the difference between traditional treatment approaches and current research findings. Emphasis is placed on empirically based or empirically supported treatments.

This course will provide:

1. Cogent and comprehensive coverage of what is now known to be crucial in understanding and treating SUDs
2. Understanding of the trends in pharmacotherapy
3. Assessment of the biologic, psychological, and sociocultural contributors to the addictive process
4. Understanding and evaluation of the complexities of the addictive processes, including co-occurring disorders and relapse prevention
5. Development of an understanding of commonly used assessment tools in the addiction field and hands-on practice with these instruments
6. Understanding of the key techniques for integrating therapy with 12-step programs and their relevance in addiction counseling today
7. Development of an understanding of the key concepts of Motivational Interviewing and Harm Reduction Therapy models
8. Demonstration of familiarity with appropriate referral sources and the process of effective referral of patients for specialized treatment

Course Requirements

Required texts

Miller WR, Carroll KM. *Rethinking Substance Abuse: What the Science Shows, and What We Should Do About It*. New York: Guilford Press; 2006.

Daley DC, Marlatt GA. *Overcoming Your Alcohol or Drug Problem: Effective Recovery Strategies (Treatments That Work)*. 2nd ed. New York: Oxford University Press; 2006.

Alcoholic Anonymous. *Twelve Steps and Twelve Traditions*. New York: AA World Services, Inc; 2002.

Methods of Evaluation

Weekly essays: The student will submit a one- to two-page essay each week. The essays are to include thoughts regarding class discussions, reading assignments, and personal opinions. The essays will be used as a basis for class discussion and will be submitted via e-mail 2 hours in advance of class time.

Exams: There will be two exams. Each in-class exam will cover the preceding section of the course, including the content of the lectures, discussions, and reading assignments. The format of the exam will include 40 multiple-choice questions and two essay questions.

Term paper: A formal paper is due at the end of the term. The purpose of this assignment is to give the student an opportunity to explore a specific issue/area within the addictions. Suggested paper topics include

- Why do 12-step programs work for some people and not for others?
- What resources are available for young people with an SUD?
- How do we manage countertransference in the assessment of individuals with SUDs?

Term papers will be a minimum of 10 pages to a maximum of 15 pages in length. Topic must be selected by the student and approved by the professor prior to the 11th week of the course.

Alcoholics Anonymous meeting attendance: The student will be provided a list of suggested Big Book and/or Step meetings to attend. The student must be transparent, asking the leaders consent for their presence at the time of the meeting. Students will use the weekly essay to discuss their experience.

Grade Computation:

- Essays and participation = 15%
- Exam I = 35%
- Exam II = 35%
- Term paper = 15%

Course Outline

Week 1: Introduction to SUDs; need for training and education

- Handouts
- Harwood HJ, Kowalski J, Ameen A. The need for substance abuse training among mental health professionals. *Adm Policy Ment Health*. 2004;32:189–205.

(Continued)

Box 72.1 Continue

- Commonly abused drugs: http://www.drugabuse.gov/PDF/CADChart.pdf
- Selected prescription drugs with potential for abuse: http://www.drugabuse.gov/PDF/PrescriptionDrugs.pdf
- Gifford E, Humphreys K. The psychological science of addiction. *Addiction*. 2006;102:352–361.

Week 2: Neurobiological factors

- Readings:
- Miller WR, Carroll KM. *Rethinking Substance Abuse: What the Science Shows, and What We Should Do About It*. New York: Guilford Press; 2006:1–77.
- Gilpin NW, Koob GF. Neuroscience: pathways to alcohol dependence. Part 1: overview of the neurobiology of dependence. *Alcohol Res Health*. 2008;31(3). Available at: http://pubs.niaaa.nih.gov/publications/arh313/toc31-3.htm.

Week 3: Psychological factors

- Readings:
- Miller WR, Carroll KM. *Rethinking Substance Abuse: What the Science Shows, and What We Should Do About It*. New York: Guilford Press; 2006:81–150.
- Bierut LJ, Dinwiddie SH, Begleiter H, et al. Familial transmission of substance dependence: alcohol, marijuana, cocaine, and habitual smoking. *Arch Gen Psychiatry*. 1998;55:982–988. Available at: http://archpsyc.ama-assn.org/cgi/reprint/55/11/982.
- Vaillant GE. A 60-year follow-up of alcoholic men. *Addiction*. 2003;98:1043–1051. Available at: http://www.ncbi.nlm.nih.gov/pubmed/12873238.

Week 4: Social factors

- Readings:
- Miller WR, Carroll KM. *Rethinking Substance Abuse: What the Science Shows, and What We Should Do About It*. New York: Guilford Press; 2006:153–219.
- Galvan FH, Caetano R. *Alcohol Use and Related Problems among Ethnic Minorities in the United States*; 2003. Available at: http://pubs.niaaa.nih.gov/publications/arh27-1/87-94.htm.
- Tonigan JS. Project Match treatment participation and outcomes by self reported ethnicity. *Alcohol Clin Exp Res*. 2003;27:1340–1344. Available at: http://www.ncbi.nlm.nih.gov/pubmed/12966335.

Week 5: Assessment; Part I: The face of abuse and withdrawal

- Readings:
- Lesher AI. *The Essence of Drug Addiction*. National Institute of Drug Abuse; 2001. Available at: http://www.nida.nih.gov/Published_Articles/Essence.html.
- TIP 45—Detoxification and Substance Abuse Treatment Executive Summary. Available at: http://www.ncbi.nlm.nih.gov/books/bv.fcgi?rid=hstat5.section.85311

Week 6: Assessment; Part II: Application of common assessment measures

- Readings:
- *Substance Abuse Services for Primary Care Clinicians: A Concise Desk Reference Guide*—TIP 24, pp. 1–16. Available at: http://www.ncbi.nlm.nih.gov/books/bv.fcgi?rid=hstat5.chapter.45293.
- *Addiction Severity Index (ASI)*. 5th ed. Available at: http://pubs.niaaa.nih.gov/publications/Assesing%20Alcohol/InstrumentPDFs/04_ASI.pdf.
- CRAFT. Available at: http://www.hpssat.org/pdfs_of_cards/CAGE_CRAFFT.pdf.
- NET. Available at: http://www.niaaa.nih.gov/publications/net.htm.
- Structured Clinical Interview for DSM Disorders-Axis I. Available at: http://www.scid4.org/revisions/download_pdf.html.

Week 7: Pharmacotherapy of SUD

- Readings:
- Miller WR, Carroll KM. *Rethinking Substance Abuse: What the Science Shows, and What We Should Do About It*. New York: Guilford Press; 2006:240–256.
- Sammons MT, Schmidt NB. *Combined Treatments for Mental Disorders: Pharmacological and Psychotherapeutic Strategies for Intervention*. Washington, DC: American Psychological Association Press; 2001.
- Kosten TR, O'Connor PG. Management of drug and alcohol withdrawal. *N Engl J Med*. 2003;348(18):1786–1795.

Week 8: Exam I

Week 9: Behavior therapies

- Readings:
- Miller WR, Carroll KM. *Rethinking Substance Abuse: What the Science Shows, and What We Should Do About It*. New York: Guilford Press; 2006:223–239.
- Carroll KM, Onken LS. Behavioral therapies for drug abuse. *Am J Psychiatry*. 2005;162:1452–1460.
- Griffith JD, Rowan-Szal GA, Roark RR, et al. Contingency management in outpatient methadone treatment: a meta-analysis. *Drug Alcohol Depend*. 2000;58:55–66.

Week 10: Twelve-step programs

- Joan Ellen Zweben demonstrates integrating therapy with 12-step programs. Available at: http://psychotherapy.net/video/Zweben_Addictions (to be viewed in class).
- AA meeting attendance deadline
- Readings:
- Miller WR, Carroll KM. *Rethinking Substance Abuse: What the Science Shows, and What We Should Do About It*. New York: Guilford Press; 2006:257–274.

- Alcoholic Anonymous. *Twelve Steps and Twelve Traditions.* New York: AA World Services, Inc; 2002.
- *What Is a Twelve Step Program?* Available at: http://www.12step.org.

Week 11: Motivational interviewing

- William R. Miller demonstrating motivational interviewing techniques. Available at: http://psychotherapy.net/video/miller_motivational_interviewing?gclid=CPqk56aRwJwCFdND5godBi_0mw (to be viewed in class).
- Term paper topic approval due
- Readings:
- NIDA. *A Cognitive-Behavioral Approach: Treating Cocaine Addiction. Manual 2.* Available at: http://www.nida.nih.gov/TXManuals/CBT/CBT9.html.
- NIDA. *A Brief Encounter with Peer Educator Can Motivate Abstinence.* Available at: http://www.drugabuse.gov/NIDA_notes/NNvol20N3/Brief.html.
- *What Is Motivational Interviewing?* Available at: http://www.motivationalinterview.org/clinical/whatismi.html.
- Miller WR, Rose GS. Toward a theory of motivational interviewing. *Am Psychol.* 2009;64:527–537.

Week 12: Treatment of co-occurring depression

- Readings:
- *Managing Depressive Symptoms in Substance Abuse Clients During Early Recovery (TIP 48).* Available at: http://www.ncbi.nlm.nih.gov/books/bv.fcgi?rid=hstat5.chapter.91408.

Week 13: Relapse prevention

- G. Alan Marlatt demonstrating harm reduction techniques. Available at: http://psychotherapy.net/video/marlatt_harm_reduction (to be viewed in class).
- Readings:
- Daley DC, Marlatt GA. *Overcoming Your Alcohol or Drug Problem: Effective Recovery Strategies (Treatments That Work).* 2nd ed. New York: Oxford University Press; 2006.
- Havassy BE, Hall SM, Wasserman DA. Social support and relapse: commonalities among alcoholics, opiate users and cigarette smokers. *Addict Behav.* 1991;16:235–246. Available at: http://www.ncbi.nlm.nih.gov/pubmed/1663695.

Week 14: Referrals: What's out there; what's needed?

- Readings:
- Miller WR, Carroll KM. *Rethinking Substance Abuse: What the Science Shows, and What We Should Do About It.* New York: Guilford Press; 2006:275–292.
- *Substance Abuse Services for Primary Care Clinicians: A Concise Desk Reference Guide*—TIP 24, pp. 17–22. Available at: http://www.ncbi.nlm.nih.gov/books/bv.fcgi?rid=hstat5.chapter.45293.
- http://www.drug-rehabs.org/withdrawal-symptoms.htm.

Week 15: The challenge to psychologists

- Term paper due
- Readings:
- Miller WR, Carroll KM. *Rethinking Substance Abuse: What the Science Shows, and What We Should Do About It.* New York: Guilford Press; 2006:293–311.
- Carroll KM, Rounsaville BJ. A vision of the next generation of behavioral therapies research in the addictions. *Addictions.* 2007;102:850–862.
- SAMHSA: *Implementing Change in Substance Abuse Treatment*—TAP 31. Available at: http://download.ncadi.samhsa.gov/prevline/pdfs/SMA09-4377.pdf.

Week 16: Exam II

Resources for practicing professionals:

- American Psychological Association, College of Professional Psychology—www.apa.org/college
- American Psychological Association, Division on Addictions—http://www.apa.org/divisions/div50/
- Consumer Organization and Networking Technical Assistance Center (CONTAC)—www.contac.org.
- National Empowerment Center—www.power2u.org
- National Institute on Alcohol Abuse and Alcoholism—www.niaaa.nih.gov
- National Institute on Drug Abuse (NIDA)—www.nida.nih.gov
- National Mental Health Association—www.nmha.org
- Substance Abuse and Mental Health Services Administration (SAMHSA), Co-occurring Center for Excellence (COCE)—www.coce.samhsa.gov
- Substance Abuse and Mental Health Services Administration (SAMHSA), Center for Substance Abuse Treatment (CSAT)—http://csat.samhsa.gov

conjunction with psychopathology, psychopharmacology, and/or the biologic bases of behavior. This information is best presented as a stand-alone course, consisting of two-and-one-half hour, weekly classes, with assigned readings, examinations, and experiential learning opportunities.

Within psychology there is a well-kept secret: post-licensure, the APA's College of Professional Psychology offers a Certificate of Proficiency in the Treatment of Alcohol and Other Psychoactive Substance Use Disorders. The College of Professional Psychology is a professional certification entity of the APA Practice Organization; it is not involved with graduate or undergraduate education in psychology. They offer a 3-hour exam that consists of 150 multiple-choice questions that can be taken by computer at more than 200 locations. The exam gauges a practitioner's knowledge in such areas as clinical pharmacology and epidemiology of psychoactive substances, causes of substance use disorders, prevention, screening, diagnosis, treatment, ethical concerns, and issues specific to certain populations. Postcertification, practitioners are required to maintain 18 hours of continuing-education credits every 3 years in order to maintain certification. This certification has been in existence since 1996, and offers the national credentialing necessary for psychologists to practice independently within the field of addiction. Information on this APA certification can be found online at www.apapractice.org/apo/insider/professional/college.html.

The reality of SUD treatment today is that few licensed psychologists qualify to sit for this certification exam due to the lack of education and clinical experience. Implementing the suggested SUD Education and Training course would begin the education process, but clearly, clinical training opportunities need to be made available in order for psychologists to effectively practice in this area. Addiction subspecialties, internships, and postdoctoral positions in the assessment and treatment of SUDs need to be created. Clinical training should be an integral part of the subspecialties, internship, and postdoctoral opportunities in the addictions and could be created via collaborative relationships between psychology programs and local substance abuse treatment centers.

CONCLUSION

The overarching goal of every graduate training program is to provide students with the requisite knowledge, attitudes, and skills to be successful in their professional careers. For the behavioral sciences, as in many other fields of study, this task is complicated by the ever-growing body of knowledge in the discipline. Advances in neuroscience, particularly neuroimaging and neurogenetics, have created new challenges for educators responsible for keeping an up-to-date, relevant curriculum. Given the finite period of time available to train students, difficult decisions must be made on what to teach and what to leave out of the didactic and clinical course of study.

What factors should determine the content of the curriculum covered? It would seem logical that highly prevalent conditions and those with the greatest potential impact on the patient and society should be at the top of the list. Unfortunately, this does not appear to be the case when it comes to addictive disorders. SUDs—including alcohol, tobacco, and other drugs of abuse—are arguably near the top of any list of behavioral problems that create a significant negative impact on a person's life, his or her family, and society. Yet formal training in the etiology, diagnosis, and treatment of these disorders is marginal to virtually nonexistent in most graduate training programs in psychology. The dearth of well-trained addiction mental health professionals worldwide underscores the need to have this be an integral component of all graduate psychology training programs.

The reason for its exclusion may be related to an ongoing prejudice toward patients with SUDs, or merely a lack of trained faculty in the field available to teach this subject. Likely, it is a combination of both. Despite available federal grants for training in the field of addictions, few programs offer comprehensive training. The availability of funds has not translated into better training. As noted above, it's been our experience that graduate training clinics routinely screen out for referral patients with co-occurring SUDs, deeming these clients too technically complex for beginning psychotherapists. The consequence of this practice is that it virtually eliminates any opportunity for a meaningful clinical exposure to these patients. The federal government, especially NIDA, is keenly aware of this problem and has recommended that SUDs be considered as important as mood and anxiety disorders in terms of public mental health importance.

In this chapter we have reviewed the current state of affairs regarding training of psychology students in SUDs. We have attempted to highlight the critical need for additional well-trained mental health professionals to care for patients and their families with addictive disorders. Finally, we have developed a model curriculum for consideration by training directors at the graduate, internship, or postdoctoral level. We hope that providing the structure of a course on SUDs targeted directly at psychology students will make the provision of such training less daunting.

Given the current available training grants, the problem does not appear to be strictly financial. Whatever the underlying cause, the need to incorporate didactic and clinical training in addictions into all graduate psychology training programs cannot be overstated. In no small way, the future of public mental health demands it.

REFERENCES

1. Flores PJ. *Group Psychotherapy with Addicted Populations: An Integration of Twelve Step and Psychodynamic Theory*. New York: Haworth Medical Press; 1997.
2. Grant BF, Stinson FS, Dawson DA, et al. Prevalence and co-occurrence of substance use disorders and independent mood and anxiety disorders: results from the National Epidemiologic Survey on alcohol and related disorders. *Arch Gen Psychiatry*. 2004;61:807–816.
3. Alexander MJ, Craig TJ, MacDonald J, et al. Dual diagnosis in a state psychiatric facility. *Am J Addict*. 1994;3:314–324.
4. Easton CJ, Devine S, Scott M, et al. Commentary: implications for assessment and treatment of addictive and mentally disordered offenders entering prisons. *J Am Acad Psychiatry Law*. 2008;36:35–37.
5. Levit KR, Kassed CA, Coffey RM, et al. *Projections of National Expenditures for Mental Health Services and Substance Abuse Treatment, 2004–2014*. SAMHSA Publication No. SMA 08-4-326. Rockville, MD: Substance Abuse and Mental Health Services Administration; 2008.
6. American Psychological Association (APA) [press release]. *Mental Illness and Drug Addiction May Co-occur Due to Disturbance in the Brain's Seat of Anxiety and Fear*; December 2, 2007.
7. da Silva Cardoso E, Pruett SR, Chan F, et al. Substance abuse assessment and treatment: the current training and practice of APA division 22 members. *Rehabil Psychol*. 2006;51:175–178.
8. Chiert T, Gold S, Taylor J. Substance abuse training in APA-accredited doctoral programs in clinical psychology: a survey. *Prof Psychol Res Pr*. 1994;25:80–84.
9. Kerwin ME, Walker-Smith K, Kirby KC. Comparative analysis of state requirements for the training of substance abuse and mental health counselors. *J Subst Abuse Treat*. 2006;30:173–181.

10. Miller WR, Carroll KM. *Rethinking Substance Abuse: What the Science Shows, and What We Should Do About It.* New York: Guilford Press; 2006.
11. Carroll KM, Rounsaville BJ. A vision of the next generation of behavioral therapies research in the addictions. *Addictions.* 2007;102:850–862.

SUGGESTED READINGS

Bierut LJ, Dinwiddie SH, Begleiter H, et al. Familial transmission of substance dependence: alcohol, marijuana, cocaine, and habitual smoking. *Arch Gen Psychiatry.* 1998;55:982–988.

Brown S. *Treating the Alcoholic: A Developmental Model of Recovery.* Hoboken, NJ: Wiley; 1996.

Carroll KM, Onken LS. Behavioral therapies for drug abuse. *Am J Psychiatry.* 2005;162:1452–1460.

Center for Substance Abuse Treatment. *Substance Abuse: Clinical Issues in Intensive Outpatient Treatment.* Treatment Improvement Protocol (TIP) Series 47. DHHS Publication No. (SMA) 06-4182. Rockville, MD: Substance Abuse and Mental Health Services Administration; 2006.

Center for Substance Abuse Treatment. *Substance Abuse: Administrative Issues in Outpatient Treatment.* Treatment Improvement Protocol (TIP) Series 46. DHHS Publication No. (SMA) 06-4151. Rockville, MD: Substance Abuse and Mental Health Services Administration; 2006.

Combs RH, ed. *Addiction Recovery Tools: A Practical Handbook.* Thousand Oaks, CA: Sage; 2001.

Compton WM, Volkow ND. Abuse of prescription drugs and the risk of addiction. *Drug Alcohol Depend.* 2006;83S:S4–S7.

Daley DC, Marlatt GA. *Overcoming Your Alcohol or Drug Problem: Effective Recovery Strategies.* New York: Oxford University Press; 2006.

Edmundson E, McCarty D, eds. *Implementing Evidence-Based Practices for Treatment of Alcohol and Drug Disorders.* Binghamton, NY: Haworth Medical Press; 2005.

Emmelkamp PMG, Vedel E. *Evidence-Based Treatment for Alcohol and Drug Abuse: A Practitioner's Guide to Theory, Methods, and Practice.* New York: Taylor & Francis Group; 2006.

Encrenaz G, Kovess-Masféty V, Jutand MA, et al. Use of psychoactive substances and health care in response to anxiety and depressive disorders. *Psychiatr Serv.* 2009;60:351–357.

Erickson CK. *The Science of Addiction: From Neurobiology to Treatment.* New York: W.W. Norton and Company, Inc; 2007.

Finley JR, Lenz BS. *The Addiction Counselor's Documentation Sourcebook.* 2nd ed. Hoboken, NJ: Wiley; 2005.

Finley JR. *Integrating the 12 Steps into Addiction Therapy. A Resource Collection and Guide for Promoting Recovery.* Hoboken, NJ: Wiley; 2004.

Finley JR, Lenz BS. *Addiction Treatment Homework Planner.* Hoboken, NJ: Wiley; 2006.

Galvan FH, Caetano R. Alcohol use and related problems among ethnic minorities in the United States. Retrieved September 26, 2009, from http://pubs.niaaa.nih.gov/publications/arh27-1/87-94.htm; 2003.

Gibson M, Freeman A. *Overcoming Depression: A Cognitive Therapy Approach for Taming the Depression BEAST.* New York: Oxford University Press; 1999.

Gifford E, Humphreys K. The psychological science of addiction. *Addiction.* 2006;102:352–361.

Gilpin NW, Koob GF. Neuroscience: pathways to alcohol dependence. Part 1—overview of the neurobiology of dependence. *Alcohol Res Health.* 2008;31:(3).

Gordon T, Edwards WS. *Making the Patient Your Partner: Communication Skills for Doctors and Other Caregivers.* Westport, CT: Auburn House; 1995.

Gorski TT, Trundy AB. *Relapse Prevention Counseling Workbook: Practical Exercises for Managing High-Risk Situations.* Independence, MO: Herald House/Independence Press; 2006.

Griffith JD, Rowan-Szal GA, Roark RR, et al. Contingency management in outpatient methadone treatment: a meta-analysis. *Drug Alcohol Depend.* 2000;58:55–66.

Harwood HJ, Kowalski J, Ameen A. The need for substance abuse training among mental health professionals. *Adm Policy Ment Health.* 2004;32:189–205.

Havassy BE, Hall SM, Wasserman DA. Social support and relapse: commonalities among alcoholics, opiate users and cigarette smokers. *Addict Behav.* 1991;16:235–246.

Hofmann SG, Tompson MC, eds. *Treating Chronic and Severe Mental Disorder: A Handbook of Empirically Supported Interventions.* New York: Guilford Press; 2002.

Imhof JE. Overcoming countertransference and other attitudinal barriers in the treatment of substance abuse. In: Washton AM, ed. *Psychotherapy and Substance Abuse: A Practitioner's Handbook.* New York: Guilford Press; 1995.

Kosten TR, O'Connor PG. Management of drug and alcohol withdrawal. *N Engl J Med.* 2003;348:1786–1795.

Lesher AI. *The Essence of Drug Addiction. National Institute of Drug Abuse.* Retrieved September 26, 2009, from http://www.nida.nih.gov/Published_Articles/Essence.html.

Margolis RD, Zweben JE. *Treating Patients with Alcohol and Other Drug Problems: An Integrated Approach.* Washington, DC: American Psychological Association; 1998.

Marlatt GA, Gordon JR. *Relapse Prevention.* New York: Guilford Press; 1985.

McKay M, Wood JC, Brantley J. *The Dialectical Behavior Therapy Skills Workbook: Practical DBT Exercised for Learning Mindfulness, Interpersonal Effectiveness, Emotion Regulation and Distress Tolerance.* Oakland, CA: New Harbinger Publications, Inc; 2007.

Miller WR, Rollnick S. *Motivational Interviewing: Preparing People for Change.* 2nd ed. New York: Guilford Press; 2002.

Miller WR, Zweben A, DiClemente CC, et al. *Motivational Enhancement Therapy Manual: A Clinical Research Guide for Therapists Treating Individuals with Alcohol Abuse and Dependence.* DHHS Pub. No. ADM 94-573. Washington, DC: U.S. Department of Health and Human Services; 1996.

Miller WR, Rollnick S. *Motivational Interviewing: Preparing People to Change Addictive Behavior.* New York: Guilford Press; 1991.

Miller WR, Brown SA. Why psychologists should treat alcohol and drug problems. *Am Psychol.* 1997;52:1267–1279.

Miller WR, Rose GS. Toward a theory of motivational interviewing. *Am Psychol.* 2009;64:527–537.

Miller WR, Benefield RG, Tonigan JS. Enhancing motivation for change in problem drinking: a controlled comparison of two therapist styles. *J Consult Clin Psychol.* 1993;61:455–461.

Miller WR, Sorenson JL, Selzer JA, et al. Disseminating evidence-based practice in substance abuse treatment: a review with suggestions. *J Subst Abuse Treat.* 2006;31:25–39.

Mueser KT. *Integrated Treatment for Dual Disorders: A Guide to Effective Practice.* New York: Guilford Press; 2003.

Najavits LM. *Seeking Safety: A Treatment Manual for PTSD and Substance Abuse.* New York: Guilford Press; 2002.

National Institute on Alcohol Abuse and Alcoholism. *Motivational Enhancement Therapy Manual.* Vol. 2. Project Match. NIH

Publication No. 94-3723. Washington, DC: U.S. Department of Health and Human Services; 1994.

National Institute on Drug Abuse. *Beyond the Therapeutic Alliance: Keeping the Drug-Dependent Individual in Treatment.* Washington, DC: U.S. Department of Health and Human Services; 1997.

Parrott A, Morinan A, Moss M, et al. *Understanding Drugs and Behavior.* Hoboken, NJ: Wiley; 2004.

Pourmand D, Kavanagh DJ, Vaughan K. Expressed emotion as predictor of relapse in participants with co-morbid psychoses and substance use disorder. *Aust N Z J Psychiatry.* 2005;39:473–478.

Quello SB, Brady KT, Sonne SC. Mood disorders and substance use disorder: a complex co-morbidity. *Sci Pract Perspect.* 2005;3(1):22–24.

Reiger DA, Farmer ME, Rae DS, et al. Co-morbidity of mental disorders with alcohol and other drug abuse. *JAMA.* 1990;264:2511–2518.

Robinson TE, Berridge KC. The psychology and neurobiology of addiction: an incentive–sensitization view. *Addiction.* 2002;95:91–117.

Rollnick S, Miller WR. What is motivational interviewing? *Behav Cogn Psychother.* 1995;23:325–334.

Rotgers F, Morgenstern J, Walter ST, eds. *Treating Substance Abuse: Theory and Technique.* 2nd ed. New York: Guilford Press; 2003.

Sammons MT, Schmidt NB. *Combined Treatments for Mental Disorders: Pharmacological and Psychotherapeutic Strategies for Intervention.* Washington, DC: American Psychological Association Press; 2001.

Spiga R, Wells A. Functional analytic structured systemic treatment: treatment manual. In: Smith DS, ed. Philadelphia, PA: P.M. Gordon Associates, Inc; 2007.

Spiga R, Wells A. Functional analytic structured systemic treatment: participant workbook. In: Smith DS, ed. Philadelphia, PA: P.M. Gordon Associates, Inc; 2007.

Spiga R, Wells A. Functional analytic structured systemic treatment: Spanish version of participant workbook. In: Alvarez I, Romero MH, eds. & trans. Philadelphia, PA: P.M. Gordon Associates, Inc; 2007.

Substance Abuse and Mental Health Services Administration. *Report to the Congress on the Prevention and Treatment of Co-occurring Substance Abuse and Mental Disorders.* Rockville, MD: U.S. Department of Health and Human Services; 2002.

Tonigan JS. Project Match treatment participation and outcomes by self reported ethnicity. *Alcohol Clin Exp Res.* 2003;27:1340–1344.

Vailiant GE. A 60-year follow-up of alcoholic men. *Addiction.* 2003;98:1043–1051.

Van Humbeeck G, Van Audenhove Ch, Storms G, et al. Expressed emotion in the patient-professional dyad: a comparison of three expressed emotion instruments. *Eur J Psychol Assess.* 2004;4:237–246.

Washton AM. *Why Psychologists Should Know How to Treat Substance Use Disorders.* Washington, DC: American Psychological Association Press; 2001.

Washton AM, ed. *Psychotherapy and Substance Abuse: A Practitioner's Handbook.* New York: Guilford Press; 1995.

Witkiewitz K, Marlatt GA. *Therapist's Guide to Evidence-Based Relapse Prevention.* Burlington, MA: Academic Press; 2007.

CHAPTER 73
Nursing Education in Addictions and Substance Abuse

Betty D. Morgan ■ Donna M. White ■ Colleen T. LaBelle

Nursing as a profession is focused on understanding the patient/person on individual, family, and community levels. The nursing paradigm concerns itself with four constructs: person, environment, health, and nursing. A variety of nursing theories have demonstrated how these concepts interact in health and illness and the role of nursing in caring for persons with potential and actual health problems.

Nursing practice exists on a continuum from preventive care to provision of care in the treatment of specific illnesses. "The essence of nursing practice is the nurse-patient relationship that embodies beliefs about the nature of the person and the nature of nursing" (1). Nursing uses knowledge, theory, and evidence-based practice to guide the delivery of care and to promote change in patients, families, systems, the environment, and the policy arenas, to care for individuals and the health of society (1).

Nurses are educated in a variety of programs in the United States. Registered nurses may complete their initial nursing education in a 2-year community college for an associate degree in nursing, or a 4-year university program for a Bachelor of Science degree in nursing. Three-year hospital-based nursing diploma programs have become rare in the United States. Advanced practice nurses (APNs) are educated in university settings at the graduate level and receive either a Master of Science degree or a Master of Science in Nursing degree. Typically these programs are 2 years in length and prepare nurses to be nurse practitioners, nurse midwives, clinical nurse specialists, or nurse anesthetists. APNs have advanced education in pharmacology, pathophysiology, and physical assessment, as well as courses that are related to their specialty area. Many APNs also have prescriptive authority; requirements for collaboration with medical physicians for prescriptive authority vary from state to state; however, some APNs are able to practice independently. Additionally, many schools have recently begun to educate people with a college degree in another field, allowing them to become nurse practitioners after completing a 3-year intensive program.

In each of these programs, students study the care of adults, children, pregnant women, medical and surgical illnesses, and psychiatric/mental health. Addictions issues are often addressed as part of the mental health course; many schools have integrated mental health concepts throughout the nursing curriculum instead of having a separate course dealing with mental health concepts. Addiction issues may be encountered in any health care setting, and therefore, this approach may make sense; however, the danger is that the topic may not be discussed in full detail and therefore may not be given the importance needed to prepare nurses to deal with this complicated disease. All nurses use a problem-solving approach to assess patients and identify problems, and plan, implement, and evaluate interventions. Knowledge of generalized nursing care as well as specialized knowledge of addictions is essential to provide effective care for people with addictive disorders.

"Addictions nursing is a distinct specialty practice that integrates the biological, behavioral, environmental, psychological, social, and spiritual aspects of human responses to the illness of addiction into the nursing care provided to those affected by this disorder/disease, regardless of the clinical setting" (2). Addictions nurses provide direct care, consult with other health care providers, shape policy, and advocate for patients. Nurses provide care to individuals, families, communities, or special populations and use evidence-based, holistic strategies to formulate this care. With a point of care that may exist anywhere in the wellness–illness continuum, addictions nurses focus care on specific phenomena of concern as identified in the *Scope and Standards of Addictions Nursing Practice* (2004):

- Conditions that increase vulnerability to or risk for addiction
- Consequences and impairment that occur when people use those substances or behaviors
- Responses of people to dependence on addictive substances or behaviors
- Conditions that affect recovery and rehabilitation (2, p. 16)

Within these concerns the following issues are considered:

- Physiologic effects
- Psychological effects
- Spiritual effects
- Cognitive effects
- Impact on families and community
- Workplace effects
- Legal consequences

This chapter will provide information on the history of addictions nursing and the development of training and education programs in addictions nursing. Nursing licensure and certification will be described in terms of both general and specialty nursing as it relates to addictions treatment. The role of the specialty addictions nurse in a variety of settings will be presented.

Additional topics such as stigma and nursing attitudes toward those with addictive disorders will be included.

HISTORY OF ADDICTIONS NURSING

Although nurses have cared for people with addictions from the early years of nursing, there has been little description of this care in the literature. The first article related to addiction in the *American Journal of Nursing* was published in 1931, and concerned a patient with delirium tremens. Other early articles focused on case reports and discussion of the role of the nurse in caring for people with both alcohol and drug addiction (3). The first example of use of research findings in relation to the nursing care of alcoholic patients occurred in 1956, and this same author was the first in nursing to identify alcoholism as a disease (4).

"Educational preparation for addictions nursing practice has lagged behind education for other nursing specialties" (2, p. 26). Several groups have supported models of curricula for both undergraduate and graduate nursing education, including the National Institute on Alcohol Abuse and Alcoholism (NIAAA), the National Institute on Drug Abuse (NIDA), and the Office for Substance Abuse Prevention (now the Center for Substance Abuse Prevention) (2).

The lack of evidence-based content about addictions in nursing curricula has contributed to the stigma and negative attitudes that have been demonstrated among nursing personnel. Howard and Chung (5) reviewed the literature of the past three decades on nurses' attitudes toward those with a chemical dependency. They found that there have been some improvements in attitudes in that time period; however, compared to the attitudes of other professional groups (physicians, psychologists, social workers, and addiction providers), nurses were more negative and punitive and had more authoritarian orientations toward those with a problem with addictive disorders. Hutton and Treisman (6) contrasted the personality characteristics of persons with an addictive disorder problem and HIV disease, and the characteristics of health care providers. Persons with an addictive disorder problem were described as being oriented, present focused, impulsive, and engaging in risky behaviors. In contrast, health care professionals were described as having opposite characteristics such as a future orientation, low risk taking, and the ability to make long-range plans rather than act impulsively. These differing ways of operating in the world may heighten the professionals' negative attitudes toward, and communication with, those with addictive disorders.

Stigma is associated with substance abuse (7–9). Corley and Goren (10) discussed the "dark side of nursing" and examined the effects of stigmatizing, labeling, and stereotyping of patients by nurses, on the quality of patient care and on the nurses, themselves. Nurses have reported psychological stress and feelings of guilt, shame, and grief over their irrational responses and unprofessional judgmental behaviors (10,11). Johnson and Webb (12) found that nurses spent less time with patients that they viewed negatively, providing only physical care and not talking much with the patients.

Nursing Education

Prior to World War II there were no advanced programs in addictions nursing in the United States. The first university-based program was located at Yale University at the Yale Center of Alcohol Studies Summer School. This program was later relocated to Rutgers University. In 1971 the NIAAA provided funding for nursing educational programs on alcoholism, and in 1974 the University of Washington established the first graduate nursing program focused on alcoholism. In 1983 the American Nurses Association Council on Psychiatric and Mental Health Nursing Practice recommended that addictions nursing be recognized as a specialty area of nursing (3). A recent review of existing schools of nursing in the United States that provide a specific curriculum addressing behavioral, genetic, and biopsychosocial components of the disease of addiction revealed a paucity of programs.

Addiction nursing education is currently focused on patients with addiction and their treatment; it is important that all undergraduates have some clinical experiences in caring for patients who have problems related to their addictive disorder. Model curricula have been developed and include content related to neuroanatomy and neurochemistry as it relates to addiction, assessment for early signs of risk behaviors, brief intervention skills, assessment and treatment of withdrawal symptoms, harm reduction, and trauma informed care. All of these topic areas should be included in nursing education about addictive disorders. Pharmacology of addictive substances, etiology of abuse and dependence on substances, care of affected family, and mobilization of community resources should also be included in educational programs. Nursing education should also include information about the risk for addiction among nursing and other health care professionals (3). Ideally, addictions content should be included throughout the nursing curricula since addictions issues occur in all stages of health and disease and throughout all of the different specialties in nursing.

Graduate education for practice in the specialty of addictions nursing needs to include theory and research, evidence-based content on addictions, as well as development of clinical skills such as assessment, differential diagnosis, and interventions or treatment of individuals and families dealing with addictive disorders (3). All APNs need basic skills in assessment of addictive disorders and the need for referral for specialty care.

Addictions Nursing Specialty Organizations

The first U.S. specialty gathering in addictions nursing took place at the 1975 National Council on Alcoholism (NCA). This group was initially known as the National Nurses Society on Alcoholism (NNSA). In 1978 the Drug and Alcohol Nursing Association (DANA) was formed by a group of nurses who objected to the NNSA's sole focus on alcohol. The NNSA separated from the NCA in 1981 and became the National Nurses Society on Addictions (NNSA) to reflect the broader scope of the practice of its members (3). In 1985 this group expanded to become the International Nurses Society on Addictions (IntNSA). IntNSA sponsors an annual conference and has published an addiction nursing journal since 1989 and other publications on addictions nursing. It has published a core curriculum on addiction nursing, and has worked with the American Nurses Association (ANA) to develop Scope and Standards for Addictions Nursing Practice. Impaired nursing practice and approaches to caring for the impaired nurse have been a major focus of this organization. Development of certification exams on a generalist and specialist level has been undertaken with other nursing organizations (13).

THE ROLE OF THE CERTIFIED PROFESSIONAL ADDICTIONS NURSE

In 1989, the NNSA sought to create a separate specialty of nursing that reflected a specific body of knowledge and related skill sets and competencies (14). In addition, another organization, the National Consortium of Chemical Dependency Nurses (NCCDN), also was developing a similar goal. These organizations shared a common goal recognizing the need to develop a theoretical body of knowledge and promote research in the work of addictions nursing.

Currently, the organizations that have the ability to credential a nurse in the field of addictions nursing are the IntNSA and the Consortium of Behavioral Health Nurses and Associates (CBHNA). IntNSA offers the Certified Addictions Registered Nurse (CARN) at the generalist level and the CARN-AP for the APN. The Consortium of Behavioral Health Nurses Association offers the chemical dependency (CD) credential. Both certifications assure that the nurse is certified as knowledgeable in the field of addictions nursing, and this credential serves as a benchmark of expertise.

The role of the professional nurse providing treatment to individuals who suffer from addictive disorders requires a specialized knowledge base, skill set, and core competencies. Completion of the certification process validates that a nurse has expertise in specific domains of practice and provides a standard that the nurse adheres to as a part of his/her professional ethical mandates in health care (15).

Various agencies emerged to address the interest of nurses who were employed in or interested in this area of clinical practice. Although the ANA recommended that addictions nursing be considered a clinical specialty, several other organizations developed certification processes. The DANA, the NNSA, and the NCCDN were organizations that, by their evolutionary processes, all had similar goals and objectives toward this area. As drug addiction became more problematic as a societal issue in the United States, the role of the nurse addressing critical issues related to care of the person with addiction became increasingly important (16). However, emergence as a specialty evolved through changes in various organizations, and eventually led to a single organization, the IntNSA, that offers certification at the basic and advanced levels of preparation.

In the late 1980s the NCCDN offered an exam to both registered nurses and licensed practical nurses that provided certification as a certified chemical dependency nurse, designated as a CD credential by this organization. NCCDN evolved into the CBHNA and now only recertifies nurses who currently have the credential. Thus, the IntNSA has emerged as the leading professional organization that credentials nurses in the clinical specialty of addictions nursing. In 1989, the IntNSA first offered a certification exam that specifically addressed core areas of chemical addictions and behavioral compulsions leading to the Certified Addictions Registered Nurse (CARN) credential (17). Since that time, the certification process has evolved into a basic generalist and advanced practitioner level. This generalist level credential was the initial comprehensive certification offered in the clinical specialty of addictions nursing practice. The exam is framed in the nursing process format and comprises 200 multiple-choice questions. IntNSA defines two objectives in the CARN examination:

1. "… to determine the nurse's ability to apply knowledge from nursing and related disciplines in the care of persons with problems resulting from patterns of abuse, dependence and addiction, and to determine the nurse's knowledge of principles of prevention of addiction."
2. "… to determine the nurse's ability to synthesize the nursing process in the care of persons with potential or actual problems resulting from patterns of abuse, dependence, and addiction." (18)

Issues addressed in the exam to meet the established objectives are included in Table 73.1. A score of 95 is required to pass the CARN examination (19). One unique advantage to this credential is that in some states, the CARN is recognized as an addiction treatment provider (19).

In 1985, The NNSA changed its name to IntNSA to reflect the broader picture of addictions. This change reflected the broadening awareness of the national and global problem of drug use, abuse, dependence, and related health issues and sequelae. Thus, nurses who were members of this organization viewed the diseases of all drug-related disorders and behavioral compulsions and viewed the problem from an international perspective. These changes reflect the evolution of science-based research that study the neurobiologic etiology of the disease and related terminology used in clinical work. Subsequent to these changes, IntNSA is now considered the leading organization that defines the clinical specialty of addictions nursing (20,21).

Consistent with the organization's commitment to further the role of addictions nursing as a recognized and valued specialty, IntNSA developed the credential for APNs (22). This level of certification is offered to nurses who are prepared at the graduate level. It may encompass the role of a nurse practitioner or a clinical nurse specialist. The advanced level credential offered is a Certified Addictions Registered Nurse—Advanced Practice (CARN-AP). Eligibility to apply and sit for the advanced practice level of certification is built on the completion of the generalist CARN certification process with preparation at the master's level of education in addition to supervised direct patient care contact. The CARN-AP credential certifies

TABLE 73.1	Areas of knowledge included in the CARN certification examination
Diagnostic and Statistical Manual criteria for substance dependence disorders
Definition and characteristics of addictive disorders
Assessment and treatment of physiologic, social, and psychological problems
Application of the nursing process and standards of care
Use of appropriate screening tools
Assessment techniques
Neurobiology of addiction
Acute abstinence syndromes (withdrawal states)
Pharmacologic effects of drugs of abuse
Nursing interventions to ameliorate painful withdrawal states and symptoms associated with addictions
Treatment modalities—pharmacologic and nonpharmacologic
Prevention strategies
Relapse prevention
Outcome evaluation

that the nurse is a recognized professional with a level of expertise that is broadened to consultation, counseling, teaching, and research. The core areas of testing at this level encompasses "biological, psychosocial, cognitive and spiritual problems resulting from concurrent diagnoses: depressant, stimulant and hallucinogenic substances: and process addictions" (20).

Certification in the field of addictions nursing provides the professional credential as a recognized expert in the area of addictions nursing clinical practice. It offers an assurance that states the nurse adheres to parameters of competence and retains a specific knowledge base rooted by a commitment to ethical mandates. Various studies that examine the usefulness as well as the role of certification in health care support the premise that the certified practitioner provides increased accountability with expertise in a specific area of clinical practice (23,24). "The ANA posits that professional self-regulation through certification is important to ensure safe, high-quality services" (3,25). In a White Paper published by IntNSA as part of the *CARN Examination Manual* (19), the association states "Specialty certification also provides advantages to nurses, including self-verification of specialty knowledge, increased self-esteem, and increased pay and job security." As the profession continues to create uniformity of standards in the clinical practice of addictions nursing, certification ensures the value and worth of the specialty itself and the professional recognition due to those who achieve the credential.

THE ROLE OF THE NURSE IN ADDICTION TREATMENT

Nurses have an important role in providing addiction treatment to patients in both acute care setting and outpatient setting. Patients present in all treatment settings with diagnosed and undiagnosed disease and fear of disclosure due to concerns of being "labeled," undertreated, or poorly treated. Nurses have a critical role in engaging the patient in treatment and acknowledging their disease with compassion and empathy. The nurse can obtain a good substance abuse history both with thorough physical exam and with nonjudgmental, thoughtful interviewing. Often the diagnosis of addiction is missed because no one asks the questions, the questions are asked in a judgmental manner, or toxicology testing does not occur. Toxicology testing should be utilized as a tool to assist the nurse and the patient in identifying and addressing substance use. Toxicology screening allows for a dialogue if it is presented in a nonthreatening, nonaccusatory manner.

Professionals often forget to ask the important questions regarding substance use. When seeing a provider, a person may be asked whether they wear a seat belt and whether they smoke cigarettes, but how often are they asked about alcohol or illicit drug use? Medical providers need to begin the dialogue to provide a safe place for patients to discuss these issues and to provide an opportunity for the health care provider to intervene at a place where the patient is willing to begin. Research has shown that screening and brief intervention (SBI) in primary care is effective in reducing hazardous alcohol use, tobacco use, and illicit drug use (26,27). The health care provider can raise awareness about risks of substance use and enhance the patient's motivation to change unhealthy drinking and/or drug use patterns.

ADDICTION TREATMENT SETTINGS

Addiction treatment has taken place in traditional inpatient detoxification units, self-help meetings such as AA and NA, emergency settings, and inpatient units, but has not typically been a part of primary care. Methadone maintenance has been in existence since the 1960s. However, it has been and continues to be a separate system from mainstream medical care, other than when a patient is admitted to the hospital and medication and dosage need to be confirmed by the inpatient medical staff and maintained until discharge. In the inpatient setting the nurse is involved in many components of addiction treatment including medical management of withdrawal, detoxification, and maintenance therapy with prescribed medication-assisted treatment, pain management, and patient advocacy for appropriate management of addiction and pain. In the outpatient setting the nurse again may find herself/himself addressing detoxification issues, assisting with placement or referral, and medication-assisted treatment.

NURSING AND METHADONE TREATMENT

Medication-assisted treatment (MAT) is any treatment for opioid dependence that includes a medication (e.g., methadone, buprenorphine, and naltrexone) approved by the U.S. Food and Drug Administration (FDA) for opioid addiction detoxification or maintenance treatment. Methadone is dispensed for opioid dependence under the federal regulations for an outpatient treatment program (OTP) (28).

> OTPs must ensure that opioid agonist treatment medications are administered or dispensed only by a practitioner licensed under the appropriate State law and registered under the appropriate State and Federal laws to administer or dispense opioid drugs, or by an agent of such a practitioner, supervised by and under the order of the licensed practitioner. This agent is required to be a pharmacist, registered nurse, or licensed practical nurse, or any other health professional authorized by Federal and State law to administer or dispense opioid drugs. (28)

Since 1971, when this practice was implemented, nurses have been able to dispense methadone, if their state allows them to do so, to patients treated at an OTP (27). Most patients are dosed daily, and others may earn take home doses for between 1 and 28 days of methadone. Nurses play a central role in methadone administration in an OTP: for daily assessments, triage, dosing, dose evaluation, and education, and often as a patient's social support.

NURSING AND BUPRENORPHINE TREATMENT

Major advances in the science of addiction treatment have brought more options to patients and practitioners in caring for patients with addiction. The NIDA and NIAAA have been at the forefront of advances that have brought medication treatment options for tobacco, alcohol, and opioid dependence. All of these medications can be prescribed by physicians, as well as nurse practitioners and physician assistants with prescribing privileges, with the exception of those that fall under the Drug Addiction Treatment Act (DATA, 2000) (29). DATA 2000 allows physicians to prescribe and dispense scheduled III, IV, and V medications approved by the FDA specifically for the purpose of opioid addiction. At this time this can only be done by an MD or a DO who meets certain requirements and obtains a special DEA number. Nurse practitioners and physician assistants are not allowed to prescribe under DATA 2000 at this time. This regulation has allowed patients to now seek treatment for opioid dependence in traditional medical settings such as a primary care practitioner office, further removing the stigma of addictions treatment and allowing patients to concurrently engage in other medical care. MAT with a scheduled III, IV, or V opioid in an office-based program or an OTP has dramatically changed the management of patients and their addictions by moving treatment into the primary care setting and allowing physicians to manage patients' opioid dependence. Thus far the only licensed medication for this purpose is buprenorphine, which is a partial opioid agonist that treats withdrawal and cravings. Buprenorphine has a ceiling effect, which makes it safer and less likely to be diverted.

MAT has evolved from methadone maintenance in OTPs to office-based treatment for opioid dependence with DATA 2000. Even though nurse practitioners cannot prescribe under DATA 2000, registered nurses and APNs play a critical role in the integration and management of MAT in primary medical care settings. The APNs are often the initial point of contact for many patients seen in a primary care office, and therefore have the unique opportunity to address drug and alcohol use and to educate patients about treatment options, including medications that can be prescribed under DATA 2000. The APN can serve as an educator, an advocate, and a support in engaging someone into treatment. Although the APN cannot prescribe, he/she is often critical in performing the physical exam and lab work and providing referrals and follow-up care.

Having the support of an educated nurse to assist the physician in this process is likely to allow for the seamless integration of MAT in outpatient settings. Models of care utilizing nurses are proving to be an effective strategy in integrating addiction treatment, improving access for patients, and encouraging more physicians to take this on. The Baltimore Buprenorphine Initiative expanded access to treatment by engaging treatment settings, substance abuse agencies, and social service supports. This initiative then built treatment capacity by training physicians to become wavered buprenorphine prescribers (30). The Bureau of Substance Abuse Services in Massachusetts, in conjunction with the Boston Medical Center, piloted a nurse care manager model of care to expand buprenorphine treatment access and then further expanded this with grant-funded models across Massachusetts, utilizing a nurse care manager model of care. This allowed for the expansion of buprenorphine treatment by having nurses working with waivered physicians and taking a primary role in the education, screening, assessment, induction, stabilization, and maintenance of patients requiring MAT. In the first 2 years after the development of this model, over 2000 patients received treatment in community settings awarded grant funding (31).

In the Boston Medical Center treatment model, nurses serve as the initial point of contact for patients seeking treatment, performing a screening assessment, evaluating appropriateness, and then arranging for the patient to come in for a more detailed assessment, education, and plan. Screening and assessment of patients assist in identifying drug, alcohol, mental health, and social issues. On intake the nurse obtains a medical history, assessment, and standard laboratory tests, and provides education on MAT for opioid dependence. A treatment plan is formulated, program expectations are reviewed, and a treatment agreement and consents are signed. Admission lab work includes a CBC; hepatitis A, B, and C serologies; RPR; LFTs; a pregnancy test for women; and a urine toxicology test to include at a minimum opiates, cocaine, benzodiazepines, methadone, buprenorphine, and oxycodone. Additional tests may be added depending on the drug use of the specific region. It is often beneficial to patient's treatment if they wait to start buprenorphine until they screen negative for all substances other than opioids and/or buprenorphine. Some patients may benefit from an inpatient detoxification to assist them in this process. Treatment consents and treatment agreements should be reviewed with the patient so the expectations for treatment are clear, in order to avoid initiating treatment when a patient is not able or willing to adhere to the program requirements.

All patients prescribed buprenorphine must meet *DSM-IV* criteria for opioid dependence prior to initiation of therapy; this must be documented in the patient's chart (32). This information should all be collected and passed along to the approved physician to then further assess and clear for treatment. This treatment model allows physicians to easily integrate complicated patients into their already busy medical practices with the support of a nurse with advanced-level skills. Once the physician sees the patient, agrees with the treatment plan, and confirms the diagnosis of opioid dependence, he/she would communicate with the nurse and generate the prescription, which serves as the induction for the patient about to begin buprenorphine treatment. The patient is then scheduled to follow up with the nurse for induction onto buprenorphine. It is important that the nurse and the patient have established a relationship of trust. Together they schedule a date and time to start the early phase of withdrawal, and dispose of all opioids, paraphernalia, and contacts with active users. This requires a great deal of trust by the patient; however, it is important in helping the patient move forward by eliminating the social components and environmental triggers of his/her addiction.

The induction process has caused many providers to shy away from this treatment because the patient should be in the early stages of withdrawal prior to induction with buprenorphine. Buprenorphine is a partial agonist and therefore will cause a precipitated withdrawal if taken too early after the administration of a short- or long-acting opioid. To avoid this, the patient should come in to see the provider in the early stages of withdrawal. For short-acting opioids, this means 8–12 hours since last use; for long-acting opioids, it is 48–72 hours and sometimes longer. In the Boston Medical Center model, the nurse does a clinical assessment using the Clinical Opioid Withdrawal Scale (COWS) (32) to ensure the patient is in mild-to-moderate withdrawal and therefore safe for administration of buprenorphine. If the patient meets criteria for withdrawal, they begin with a small dose of buprenorphine with the support of the nurse, who ensures that it is taken sublingually and tolerated without side effects or interactions. Patients usually wait in the waiting room or go outside and return 30–60 minutes later or sooner if in need of further assessment. On return after receiving their first dose, patients often feel much better as withdrawal symptoms begin to resolve. A follow-up plan is arranged, and patients are then monitored with frequent phone contacts until stable, followed by weekly nursing and counseling visits under the direction of the licensed physician. Ongoing visits focus on MAT education, administration techniques, and management of side effects, which might include insomnia, taste perversion, constipation, and headaches.

Follow-up appointments either remain weekly or are adjusted depending on the patient's stability and adherence. This is determined at nursing follow-up, and by negative urine screens, engagement in counseling and psychiatric treatment if warranted, and social stability. Patients need to be scheduled to see the buprenorphine-prescribing physician at a minimum of every 3–6 months for evaluation of their opioid dependence and sooner if needed. In some treatment settings the physician sees the patient more frequently; in other settings the nurse is the point of frequent contact, with the physician involved in treatment planning through verbal and written communication. As patients progress in their treatment to maintenance, it is important to continue to assist them in moving forward in their recovery. Patients should be encouraged to maintain social and psychiatric supports, attend self-help meetings and identify sponsors, and engage in weekly counseling in either a group or an individual setting.

Counseling is an integral component in treating the disease of addiction; the federal guidelines state that "in order to qualify to prescribe Suboxone, physicians must have the capacity to provide or to refer patients for necessary ancillary services such as psychosocial therapy" (28). Many different forms of counseling are available and may be selected or combined based on the patient's needs, including individual counseling, group counseling, self-help, cognitive–behavioral therapy (CBT), and buprenorphine/naloxone (Suboxone) specific groups. Close assessment of the patient's mental health is critical, both at the start of treatment and as the patient reaches a state of abstinence. Often when patients stop using drugs, psychiatric diseases that had been self-medicated may present themselves. Therefore, engagement into services for full evaluation and treatment is essential to the recovery process.

SPECIAL POPULATIONS AND MEDICATION-ASSISTED TREATMENT

Special consideration may be needed in caring for HIV-positive patients, homeless patients, and pregnant women seeking addiction treatment. HIV-positive patients are frequently treated with antivirals that, like buprenorphine and methadone, are metabolized by the cytochrome P450 inhibitor; fewer drug interactions have been seen with buprenorphine than with methadone (33,34). There have been reports of liver toxicity issues as buprenorphine is metabolized by the liver, so patients with abnormal transaminases or liver complications should be monitored closely (33,34). Pregnancy is a critical time to engage women into care as data have shown that outcomes are greatly improved when pregnant women are managed on medication-MAT. Limited data have shown that treatment with buprenorphine during pregnancy may be safe and efficacious; however, methadone remains the standard of care in pregnancy (35). Use of buprenorphine in pregnancy is off-label and requires careful review, education, and a detailed consent and release of liabilities (35). Methadone should be considered as the first option and has the advantage of daily, observed dosing and assessment, which may be a safer option for some women who may be entering care only due to pregnancy and may benefit from this level of monitoring. Homelessness is another issue that may require special considerations. Treatment utilizing buprenorphine in the homeless population had not been reported until recently. When implemented with additional supports, including more frequent nursing follow-up visits and weekly prescriptions, buprenorphine treatment for this population was as successful as it was for housed, socially stable patients. Methadone is a very effective treatment option for the homeless as there are no concerns regarding storage, administration, or assessment of the medication. A homeless patient would likely benefit from the daily observed dosing offered in an OTP setting by licensed personnel.

Office-based opioid treatment with buprenorphine has opened many doors for patients, allowing them the ability to treat their addiction in a safe, confidential setting with the support of a medical team of providers. Some patients may never have sought out care if it was not for the ability to receive this treatment outside of traditional detoxification settings. Engaging the nurse in this process to further support, educate, treat, and assist patients will allow for further integration, and expansion of treatment to patients who may never have sought the care they needed or had the option to do so.

NURSING AND NICOTINE ADDICTION TREATMENT

Nurses can also play a critical role in treating nicotine dependence. When a patient comes to the hospital and is screened for tobacco dependence, the nurse can educate the patient and offer supportive therapies such as: nicotine replacement therapies, counseling, groups, and CBT. These treatments can begin inpatient and continue on discharge with a follow-up plan. In the outpatient setting when the nurse engages with the patient, he/she can intervene and offer the patient treatment options such as support groups, harm reduction, and nicotine replacement therapy, which comes in patch, gum, tablet, and lozenges.

CONCLUSION

Nurses can play an important role in treatment for addiction to cocaine, alcohol, nicotine, opioids, and other drugs. Screening is a natural fit as nurses are often the providers who spend the most direct, hands-on time with the patient—triaging, screening, assessing, educating, supporting, and assisting with specific service needs. Caring for patients with opioid dependence involves a great deal of hands-on care by the nurse, and treating patients with opioid dependence can have good outcomes with the support of an educated nurse. The nurse can assist the patient in looking at his/her disease, agreeing to an intervention and assisting in this process. Interventions could range from brief motivational interviews to assistance with detoxification, aftercare, or medication-assisted options.

Currently there is no other disease for which less than 2% of patients get treatment (36). Nurses need to address this disparity by educating themselves, talking with patients, and engaging all members of the medical team. In this way nurses can help eliminate the stigma of addiction and its devastating consequences. All nurses should treat with dignity persons with addictions!

REFERENCES

1. *Consensus Statement on Emerging Nursing Knowledge: A Value-Based Position Paper Linking Nursing Knowledge and Practice Outcomes*. USA Nursing Knowledge Conference, 1998, Boston, MA. http://www.bc.edu/bc_org/avp/son/theorist/roy.pdf. Accessed June 2010.
2. *Scope and Standards of Addictions Nursing Practice*. Washington, DC: American Nurses Association; 2004:16, 26.
3. *The Core Curriculum of Addictions Nursing*. 2nd ed. Text Revision. Columbus, OH: International Nurses Society on Addictions; 2006.
4. Golder GM. The nurse and the alcoholic patient. *Am J Nurs*. 1956;56:436–438.
5. Howard MO, Chung SS. Nurses' attitudes toward substance misusers. I. Surveys. *Subst Use Misuse*. 2000;35(3):347–365.
6. Hutton H, Treisman GJ. Personality characteristics and their relationship to HIV-risk behavior, compliance and treatment. *Prim Psychiatry*. 1999;6(5):65–68.
7. Morris DB. Sociocultural and religious meanings of pain. In: Gatchel RJ, Turk DC, eds. *Psychosocial Factors in Pain: Critical Perspectives*. New York: The Guilford Press; 1999.
8. Walters GD. *The Addiction Concept: Working Hypothesis or Self-Fulfilling Prophecy?* Boston: Allyn and Bacon; 1999.
9. Younger JB. The alienation of the sufferer. *Adv Nurs Sci*. 1995;17(4):53–72.
10. Corley MC, Goren S. The dark side of nursing: impact of stigmatizing responses on patients. *Sch Inq Nurs Pract*. 1998;12(2):99–122.
11. Fisher A. The ethical problems encountered in psychiatric nursing practice with dangerous mentally ill persons. *Sch Inq Nurs Pract*. 1995;9:193–208.
12. Johnson M, Webb C. Rediscovering unpopular patients: the concept of social judgment. *J Adv Nurs*. 1995;21:466–475.
13. Cary AH. Certified registered nurses: results of the study of the certified work force. *Am J Nurs*. 2001;101(1):44–52.

14. American Nurses Association, National Nurses Society on Addictions, and Drug and Alcohol Nurses Association. *Care of Clients with Addictions: Dimensions of Nursing Practice.* Kansas City, MO: American Nurses Association; 1987.
15. Miller P, Boyle D. Nursing specialty certification: a measure of expertise. *Nurs Manag.* 2008;October, 10–16.
16. National Institute on Drug Abuse (NIDA). *Principles of Drug Addiction Treatment: A Research-Based Guide.* Bethesda, MD: National Institutes of Health; 1999.
17. Baird, C. Addictions nursing certification: twenty years strong. *IntNSA Today.* 2008–2009;13(2):3.
18. *American Nurses Association (ANA) Response to PEW Commission Report 1997.* Available at: http://nursingworld.org/readroom/pew.htm#recommendations. Accessed April 27, 2002.
19. *Preparation Manual for the CARN Examination.* Columbus, OH: International Nurses Society on Addictions; 2002.
20. *Preparation Manual for the CARN Examination.* Columbus, OH: International Nurses Society on Addictions; 2007.
21. Handley SM *Addictions Nursing. Frontline*; 2009. Available at: http://addictionrecov.org/paradigm/P_PR_F98/FrontLine.html.
22. Baird C. Specialty certification: is it for you? *J Addict Nurs.* 2007; 18(4):217–218.
23. Finnell D, Garbin M, Scarborough J. Advanced practice nursing specialty certification. *J Addict Nurs.* 2004;15:37–40.
24. Shirey MR. Celebrating certification in nursing: forces of magnetism in action. *Nurs Adm Q.* 2005;29(3):245–253.
25. Stromberg MF, Niebuhr B, Prevost S, et al. Specialty certification. *Nurs Manag.* 2005;36(5):36–46.
26. Madras BK, Compton WM, Avula D, et al. Screening, brief interventions, referral to treatment (SBIRT) for illicit drug and alcohol use at multiple healthcare sites: comparison at intake and 6 months later. *Drug Alcohol Depend.* 2009;99(1–3):280–295.
27. Babor TF, McRee BG, Kassebaum PA, et al. Screening, brief intervention, and referral to treatment (SBIRT): toward a public health approach to the management of substance abuse. *Subst Abuse.* 2007; 28(3):7–30.
28. TIP 43. *Medication-Assisted Treatment for Opioid Addiction in Opioid Treatment Programs: U.S. Department of Health and Human Services.* Rockville, MD: Substance Abuse and Mental Health Services Administration Center for Substance Abuse Treatment; 2005.
29. Drug Addiction Treatment Act of 2000. Public Law No. 106–310, Title XXXV. http://www.buprenorphine.samhsa.gov/fulllaw.htm. www.buprenorphine.samhsa.gov/fulllaw.html.
30. *Baltimore Buprenorphine Initiative Newsletter 2008*, volume IV. Baltimore, MD: Baltimore Health Care Access.
31. LaBelle CT. Dissemination of buprenorphine treatment for opioid dependence into community settings utliization of a state funded nurse care manager model (abstract). In Association of medical education and research in substance abuse. Annual Conference, Washington DC, 2008.
32. American Psychiatric Association. *Diagnostic and Statistical Manual of Mental Health Disorders, Fourth Edition, Text Revision.* Washington, DC; American Psychiatric Association; 2000.
33. Bruce RD, Altice FL, Gourevich MH, et al. Pharmacokinetic drug interactions between opioid agonist therapy and antiretroviral medications: implications and management for clinical practice. *J Acquir Immune Defic Syndr.* 2006;41:563–572.
34. Chang Y, Mooody DE, McCance-Katz EF. Novel metabolites of buprenorphine detected in human liver microsomes and human urine. *Drug Metab Dispos.* 2006;34:440–448.
35. Jones HE, Johnson RE, Jasinki DR, et al. Buprenorphine versus methadone? In the treatment of pregnant opioid-dependent patients: effects on the neonatal abstinence syndrome. *Drug Alcohol Depend.* 2005;79:1–10.
36. U.S. Department of Health and Human Services, Substance Abuse and Mental Health Services Administration, Office of Applied Studies. Rockville, MD: *National Survey for Drug Use and Health*; 2008. [Figure 7.10]

CHAPTER 74

Social Worker Education and Training in the Care of Persons with Substance Use Disorders

Michelle Tuten

BACKGROUND

Substance misuse is a common occurrence in the United States and throughout much of the rest of the world. According to the 2008 National Survey on Drug Use and Health, an estimated 20.8% of U.S. residents aged 18 and above met criteria for substance abuse or dependence (1). Competent assessment and treatment of substance use disorders is paramount in the helping professions. Social workers provide services across a range of agencies, populations, and geographic locales; as such, they routinely assess, treat, and refer patients affected by substance use disorders. According to the Bureau of Labor Statistics, 21% of social workers were employed in mental health and substance abuse positions in 2006 (2). The prevalence and wide-reaching effects of substance misuse underscore the importance of specialized education and ongoing training among social workers in the treatment of this vulnerable population.

The historical role in the treatment of substance use disorders by social workers has been described as "reluctant" (3); social workers—along with other helping professionals—have experienced difficulty shedding negativistic and moralistic attitudes about individuals with substance use disorders (4). However, there are notable, important exceptions. This chapter provides a brief history of the treatment of substance use disorders in the field of social work, describes the education and training needs of social workers in addiction treatment, and summarizes recommendations for social work's role in the treatment of addictions, including the important step of embracing the evidence-based practice movement. Lastly, a summary of some of the available resources on evidence-based practices and interventions is provided.

U.S. HISTORY OF ALCOHOL AND DRUG USE TREATMENT BY SOCIAL WORKERS

Social workers have played a role in the treatment of substance use disorders since the days of Charity Organization Societies (COS) and the settlement house movement of the late 1800s (5). At the time, the prevailing attitude toward addictions was that such disorders represented a moral deficit in the individual. A notable social work figure and prominent COS leader, Mary Richmond, however, rejected the moral model, and promoted the notion that "inebriety" was a disease in need of early identification and treatment. In her seminal work, *Social Diagnosis*, Ms. Richmond describes the "inebriate" as a patient and not a "culprit" (6), emphasizing the importance of treating rather than blaming patients with substance use disorders. In the early days of the social work profession, assistance was generally offered through educational activities associated with the growing temperance movement; however, few direct services were offered to individuals with substance use disorders. In fact, many individuals with substance use disorders were confined to institutions or incarcerated because of the prevailing moral model and the lack of knowledge regarding substance use disorders on the part of helping professionals, including social workers (7).

Social workers also contributed to the treatment of alcohol use disorders—and to a lesser extent, substance use disorders—following the repeal of prohibition in 1933 and during the Second World War. In the 1940s, Gladys Price, a social worker at the Washingtonian Center for Addictions in Boston, developed the first alcoholism-focused field placement for social work students. Social workers also were represented on the interdisciplinary team of providers at the Yale Plan Clinics founded in 1944. The Yale Clinics included inpatient treatment for alcoholism and served as precursors to modern-day inpatient treatment (6). In 1955, the Yale Summer School of Alcohol Studies organized the first training seminar for social workers focused on alcoholism. In the 1960s, Margaret Bailey, a social worker and author of *Alcoholism and Family Casework*, headed an alcoholism training project that included three family casework agencies. In 1969 she also established the Alcoholism Committee under the New York City Chapter of the National Association of Social Workers (NASW). The committee, now entitled the Addictions Committee, remains in existence and has expanded its scope to include drug use disorders (6).

In the 1970s several factors led to the expansion of the role of social workers in the treatment of substance use disorders. The Hughes Act of 1970 led to the founding of the National Institute on Alcohol Abuse and Alcoholism (NIAAA) and the National Institute on Drug Abuse (NIDA). These agencies provided legitimacy and financial assistance to students pursuing careers focused on substance use disorders (5). During the 1970s, the NIAAA funded several demonstration projects to train students across the helping professions to work in the area of alcohol use disorders. An important focus of these demonstration projects was to improve practitioners' perceptions of individuals with alcohol use disorders (8). The Hughes Act also provided funding for treatment programs, primarily for alcoholism treatment.

The role of social work in the treatment of drug use has been more limited than the focus on alcoholism (6). From 1935 to 1971 the U.S. government operated large treatment programs, commonly referred to as "federal farms," which were actually federal prisons focused on the treatment of drug use disorders, including detoxification services (6,9). In the late 1950s and 1960s, the therapeutic community (TC) movement grew. TCs espoused a grassroots approach to the treatment of drug addiction, and are very much alive today. It is unclear to what extent social workers were involved in the grassroots movement of the TCs (6). It was not until the 1980s—when media and public attention focused on the crack cocaine "epidemic"—that social workers began to take on more prominent roles in the treatment of substance use disorders as well as roles in program management and administration. The growing attention and awareness of HIV and AIDS also has led social workers to take on more prominent roles in harm reduction strategies and prevention programs, many of which focus on substance use disorders (6). The founding of the Substance Abuse and Mental Health Services Administration (SAMHSA) in 1994 also has increased the pool of federal funds—along with funding provided by NIAAA and NIDA—to prepare students, including social workers, for work in the substance abuse field. See Figure 74.1 for a timeline of factors affecting social work involvement in the treatment of substance use disorders.

LICENSURE AND CERTIFICATION OF SOCIAL WORKERS

All states have licensing, certification, or registration requirements for the practice of social work. Typically, there are four categories of practice that jurisdictions may legally regulate: (a) *bachelor's*: the baccalaureate social work degree, which is granted upon completion of a 4-year degree, (b) *master's*: the MSW degree in social work without post-MSW experience, (c) *advanced generalist*: the MSW degree with 2 years of supervised post-master's work experience, and (d) *clinical*: MSW with 2 years of post-master's clinical social work practice. State Boards of Social Work require that social work degrees are granted by programs accredited by the Council on Social Work Education (CSWE) (from the Association of Social Work Boards [ASWB] website: http://www.aswb.org/SWL/licensingbasics.asp).

GENERAL EDUCATION AND TRAINING

A bachelor's degree in social work (BSW) is typically the minimum requirement for entry-level social work positions; however, the MSW degree has become the standard for many positions and is required for independent clinical practice. As of 2006, the CSWE accredited 458 bachelor's programs and 181 master's programs (2). Doctoral education in the United States has grown considerably in recent years (10). In 1957 there were only 10 social work doctoral programs, in 1990 there were 47, and in 2003 there were 72. The growth in doctoral programs is largely the result of a growing emphasis on research, publication, and grant funding (11).

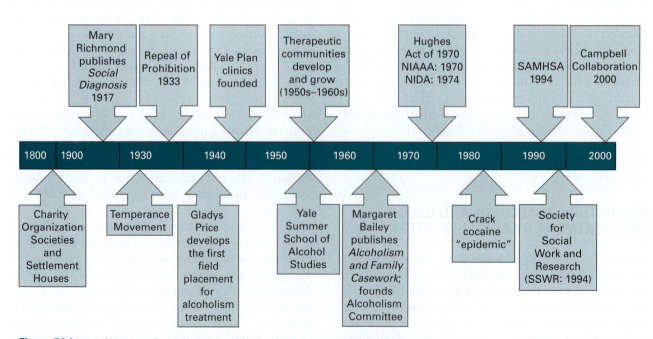

Figure 74.1. Brief history of social work in addictions treatment. (Adapted, in part, from Straussner S. The role of social workers in the treatment of addictions: a brief history. *J Soc Work Pract Addict*. 2001;1:3–9.)

SUBSTANCE ABUSE TREATMENT SERVICES PROVIDED BY SOCIAL WORKERS

According to a 2000 survey of NASW members, 71% of respondents reported activities related to the diagnosis or treatment of patients with substance use disorders in the past 12 months; however, only 2% of the sample identified substance abuse as their primary area of practice (12). The sample reported a mean of 35.4 hours spent in professional development training during the past year; however, the number of hours spent in substance abuse–related training was only 4.4 hours for the same 12-month period. Although the majority of the respondents (81%) reported lifetime training in substance abuse (primarily through continuing education courses), only 1% of the sample had completed a substance abuse certification program (12). The findings from the NASW survey seem to suggest that although social workers routinely assess and treat substance use disorders, only a few treatment agencies and/or practitioners have embraced substance use disorders as a specialty area of primary practice. There also appears to be disproportionate availability and/or interest in training related to substance abuse disorders. Given the high prevalence of substance use disorders among patients treated by social workers, the survey highlights the need for increased coursework focused on substance abuse in social work programs, as well as increased continuing education opportunities related to substance abuse (12).

EDUCATION AND TRAINING IN SUBSTANCE USE DISORDERS

It has been long agreed that social work programs are primarily responsible for training social workers to effectively treat substance use disorders (3). However, there is a large gap between science and practice in the addiction field. This gap may be the result of values and models gained through professional training (13). However, despite the prevalence of substance use disorders among patients being treated by social workers, substance abuse specialties and coursework is limited in schools of social work. Consequently, social workers enter the field with little or no training in the area of substance use and related issues. Bina et al. (14) conducted a survey of a random sample of social work programs (30% of the 187 accredited programs in 2007 to 2008) and found that none of the programs surveyed offered a substance abuse specialization. Furthermore, 52% did not offer a single substance abuse–specific course. Not surprisingly, the majority of social workers (54%) report the need for more training in the area of substance abuse assessment and treatment (15). The paucity of training provided to social workers is associated with a lack of practitioner knowledge of substance use disorders, more negative attitudes toward patients with substance use problems, and decreased effectiveness and quality of treatment provided (16).

Substance abuse training and education, on the other hand, has been shown to have a positive impact on social work practice. Lemieux and Schroeder (3), in a sample of foundation and advanced year MSW students, showed that training curricula in substance abuse resulted in greater knowledge of substance use disorders, fewer negative experiences in substance abuse–related internships, and more proactive assessment of patients for substance use disorders. Amodeo, Fassler, and Griffin (4) compared the behavioral outcomes of MSW-level practitioners who completed postgraduate substance abuse training to a comparison group of MSW practitioners without postgraduate substance abuse training. They found that social workers with specialized training were more likely to provide substance abuse training in their own agencies, to receive training and supervision in substance abuse outside of their agency settings, to engage in substance abuse community service, to present at conferences on substance abuse topics, and to treat significant others with substance use disorders.

EVIDENCE-BASED PRACTICE (EBP) IN ADDICTIONS

There is growing emphasis on the use of EBP in the field of social work (10), as researchers and practitioners alike advocate for the highest quality care for patients. This increased momentum is underscored by the growing number of publications on EBP across social work disciplines, including mental health services, health, and social welfare. There also has been an increase in the number of social work textbooks dedicated to the topic of EBP, as well as meta-analyses and systematic reviews of EBPs—all of which make EBPs more accessible to academicians and practitioners (17). Although EBPs are becoming more widely advertised and disseminated, practitioners remain ambivalent about embracing EBPs. There remains a large gap between processes that are supported by science and the processes used by social work practitioners. The translation time from the scientific world to the "real world" of practice, in fact, is estimated at between 15 and 20 years, and some empirically supported practices never translate into community practice (Balas and Boren, as cited in Ref. (18)). Given the large body of literature in substance abuse treatment, including the growth of several evidence-based interventions, social workers need to remain abreast of the current treatments to ethically and most effectively treat their patients.

Social work is in a good position to embrace the EBP movement, rather than continue to lag behind scientific advances, and to increase the profession's credibility in the process (10). For this reason, academicians have suggested a new pedagogy for social work education that focuses on a framework of EBP (19). Howard et al. (19) suggest social work education curricula for MSW students that focus on seven key objectives. According to these curricula, graduates should be able to

a. Understand and value the evidence-based perspective;
b. Select empirically tested interventions or practice methods supported by the best available scientific evidence;

c. Appreciate the degree to which leading social work theories and polices are research based;
d. Effectively deliver micro-, mezzo-, and macropractice interventions with the strongest empirical support in their fields of practice;
e. Adapt the recommendations of practice guidelines, treatment manuals, and systematic reviews for use with specific client populations and in diverse agency settings;
f. Evaluate the effectiveness of their own practice efforts; and
g. Identify their information needs as they arise in varied practice settings, define searchable questions with which to query relevant scientific databases, and locate, critically appraise, and apply interventions based on the evidence they judge valid and pertinent (19, p. 242).

Woody, D'Souza, and Dartman (20), in a survey of deans and directors of 66 MSW programs, found that informal faculty commitment to the teaching of evidence-supported interventions (ESIs), a term often used interchangeably with evidence-based practices, was significantly greater than that of program commitment. Only 31 of the programs surveyed endorsed teaching specific ESIs, and only 26 had designated courses to teach ESI content. Further research is needed to evaluate the manner in which social work programs are responding to the growing emphasis on science as a guide for practice decisions in social work.

Although EBP has received increased attention in the helping professions, there remain considerable barriers to defining these practices and encouraging practitioners and programs to adopt them. There are many, often divergent, definitions of EBP, making consensus regarding what constitutes EBP elusive. Some researchers define EBP as a set of processes that the practitioner uses when providing clinical care. Sackett et al. (21) define EBP as "the conscientious, explicit, and judicious use of current evidence in making decisions about the care of individual patients" (21, p. 71). The EBP process is further described by a set of activities, including posing relevant searchable questions, accessing and critically analyzing evidence, evaluating the applicability of the evidence to the client, and evaluating outcomes (22,23).

In other research, EBP is defined as the use of specific empirically validated *interventions* (e.g., use of cognitive–behavioral treatment) rather than the use of processes. The implementation of these interventions is more accurately described as *evidence-based interventions*. However, the terms *evidence-based practice*, *evidence-based treatment*, and *evidence-based interventions* are often used interchangeably, a methodological flaw in the literature that makes comparisons across the studies using process activities versus specific interventions difficult. Research is needed to evaluate to what extent process activities, such as posing questions and searching the literature, actually lead to the implementation of specific recommended interventions. In other words, it is unclear whether engaging in the process of looking up information, for example, actually leads to the implementation of the empirically validated interventions suggested in the literature. It is also unclear what factors may impede the use of EBP when process-oriented activities are utilized by practitioners. For example, the practitioner may have difficulty accessing information on EBPs, either because information is not readily available for a particular population/problem area or because the practitioner does not have the knowledge about how best to access them. It may also be that the practitioner is able to access the information but does not implement the intervention because he/she does not agree with the interventions suggested. In fact, personal attitudes about EBI—including perceived flexibility and the perceived requirements of the practice—may have greater influence on practitioner behavior than the weight of scientific evidence (18).

RESOURCES AVAILABLE ON EBPs AND EBIs

Fortunately, there are a growing number of resources available to aid practitioners in identifying EBPs and interventions for mental health and substance abuse prevention and treatment. The SAMHSA maintains the National Registry of Evidence-Based Programs and Practices (NREPP, http://www.nrepp.samhsa.gov). Practitioners can enter search terms to determine which programs and/or practices are effective for particular populations (e.g., gender, age, and problem area). Another SAMHSA resource is the Addiction Technology Transfer Centers (ATTCs), which provide valuable information on EBPs as well as videos, pamphlets, and other instructional tools on how to implement these practices (see http://www.attcnetwork.org/aboutus/index.asp).

The NIDA is another useful resource for accessing information on EBPs. NIDA published a guide to effective treatment entitled "Principles of Drug Addiction Treatment: A Research Based Guide" to disseminate information on basic principles of the treatment of substance use disorders and to identify research-based treatments (NIH Publication No. 09-4180, 2009; see http://www.nida.nih.gov/podat/ Evidence.html). The interventions identified by NIDA include two main categories: (a) pharmacologic treatments for opiate, nicotine, and alcohol abuse and (b) behavioral treatments for a range of substance use disorders. A number of comprehensive treatment manuals specific to cocaine addiction also are available online.

The Campbell Collaboration, a sibling organization to the Cochrane Collaboration, was founded in 2000 to promote access to systematic reviews in the areas of education, crime and justice, and social welfare. The Campbell Collaboration website provides a keyword search for systematic reviews at http://www.campbellcollaboration.org/.

RESOURCES ON SUBSTANCE USE DISORDERS

Journals

The first social work journal dedicated to the topic of alcohol and drug abuse, *Social Work Practice in the Addictions*, was published in 2001 (5). Today, there are a growing number of journals in social work and related disciplines devoted to the topic of substance use disorders, including *Addiction, Addictive Behaviors, Addictive Disorders and Their Treatment, Alcohol and Alcoholism, The American Journal on Addictions, The American Journal of Drug and Alcohol Abuse, Drug and Alcohol Dependence, Journal of Child and Adolescent Substance Abuse, Journal of Groups in Addiction and Recovery,* and *Journal of Substance Abuse Treatment.*

Websites

Online resources also are available to educate and assist practitioners working in the field of addictions. SAMHSA's *The National Clearinghouse for Alcohol and Drug Information* is a repository of information on a wide range of topics related to substance use disorders. Information on drug classes and other addiction-related educational materials, including fact sheets, posters, statistics, and videos/DVDs is available to practitioners and their patients. The ATTCs, NIAAA, NIDA, and the Center for Substance Abuse Treatment (CSAT; http://csat.samhsa.gov/) websites (see also the section "Resources Available on EBPs and EBIs") also serve as repositories of information and educational materials for patients and practitioners alike.

The NASW is the largest organization for social workers, with a current membership of approximately 150,000 (from http://www.socialworkers.org/nasw/default.asp). The NASW website provides information on NASW-approved continuing education courses, including those related to substance use disorders. For NASW members at the MSW level specializing in alcohol, tobacco, and other drug use disorders, the NASW offers a specialty credential, the Certified Clinical Alcohol, Tobacco, and Other Drugs Social Worker (C-CATODSW).

SUMMARY

Historically, social workers have played key roles in the assessment, treatment, and understanding of substance use disorders. Given the large numbers of individuals impacted by substance use disorders, and the growth of programs to treat them, social workers will continue to be among frontline staff in addictions treatment. As such, social workers have considerable influence on the prevailing attitudes toward individuals with substance use disorders and the type and quality of treatments available to them. There is promising momentum for an increased emphasis in the field of social work on the use of evidence-based and best practices to more effectively treat patients. To the extent that social workers embrace this movement, the field as a whole serves to gain tremendous credibility as an equal partner in the helping professions. Social work programs can facilitate the adoption of an EBP framework by teaching future practitioners, academicians, and administrators about how to critically analyze research literature, how to implement evidence-based practices, and how to disseminate practices in community agencies.

REFERENCES

1. Substance Abuse and Mental Health Services Administration. *Results from the 2008 National Survey on Drug Use and Health: National Findings.* NSDUH Series H-36, HHS Publication No. SMA 09-4434. Rockville, MD: Office of Applied Studies; 2009.
2. United States Bureau of Labor Statistics. United States Department of Labor. *Occupational Outlook Handbook: An Up-To-Date Guide To Today's Job Market.* New York, NY: Skyhorse Publishing. 2009.
3. Lemieux CM, Schroeder J. Seminar of addictive disorders: an exploration of students' knowledge, attitudes, and behavior. *J Soc Work Pract Addict.* 2004;4:3–21.
4. Amodeo M, Fassler I, Griffin M. MSWs with and without substance abuse training: agency, community, and personal outcomes. *Subst Abus.* 2002;23:3–16.
5. DiNitto DM. The future of social work practice in addictions. *Adv Soc Work.* 2005;1:202–209.
6. Straussner S. The role of social workers in the treatment of addictions: a brief history. *J Soc Work Pract Addict.* 2001;1:3–9.
7. DiNitto, DM and McNeese, CA. Addictions and social work practice. In: DiNitto, DM and McNeese, CA, eds. *Social Work Issues and Opportunities in a Challenging Profession.* Chicago, IL: Lyceum Books, Inc. 2008:171–192.
8. Kilty KM, Feld A. Professional education in understanding and treating alcoholism. A demonstration project. *J Stud Alcohol.* 1979;11:929–942.
9. Rowe T. *Federal Narcotics Law and the War on Drugs: Money down a Rat Hole.* Binghamton, NY: The Hawthorn Press, Inc.; 2006.
10. Thyer BA. The quest for evidence-based practice? We are all positivists! *Res Soc Work Pract.* 2008;18:339–345.
11. Harold R. Tradition, continuity, legacy: the role of doctoral programs in social work education and the profession. *Keynote Address, Fifteenth National Symposium on Doctoral Research in Social Work;* Ohio State University School of Social Work, Columbus, OH. 2003.
12. Smith M, Whitaker T, Weismiller T. Social workers in the substance abuse treatment field: a snapshot of service activities. *Health Soc Work.* 2006;31:109–115.
13. Miller WR, Sorensen JL, Selzer JA, et al. Disseminating evidence-based practices in substance abuse treatment: a review with suggestions. *J Subst Abuse Treat.* 2006;31:25–29.
14. Bina R, Harnek Hall DM, Mollette A, et al. Substance abuse training and perceived knowledge: predictors of perceived preparedness to work in substance abuse. *J Soc Work Edu.* 2008;44:7–20.
15. Weismiller T, Whitaker T, Smith M. Practice research network III: final report; 2005. Retrieved November 2, 2009, from www.socialworkers.org/naswprn/surveyThree/report0205.pdf.
16. Amodeo M. The therapeutic attitudes and behavior of social MSW clinicians with and without substance abuse training. *Subst Use Misuse.* 2000;35:1319–1348.
17. Rubin A, Parrish D. Views of evidence-based practice among faculty in master of social work programs: a national survey. *Res Soc Work Pract.* 2007;17:110–122.
18. Nelson TD, Steele RG, Mize JA. Practitioner attitudes toward evidence-based practice: themes and challenges. *Adm Policy Ment Health.* 2006;33:398–409.
19. Howard MO, McMillen CJ, Pollio DE. Teaching evidence-based practice: toward a new paradigm for social work education. *Res Soc Work Pract.* 2003;13:234–259.

20. Woody JD, D'Souza HJ, Dartman R. Do master's in social work programs teach empirically supported interventions? A survey of deans and directors. *Res Soc Work Pract.* 2006;16:469–479.
21. Sackett DL, Richardson WS, Rosenberg W, et al. *Evidence-Based Medicine: How to Practice and Teach EBM.* New York: Churchill Livingstone; 1997.
22. Gibbs L. *Evidence-Based Practice for the Helping Professions: A Practical Guide with Integrated Multimedia.* Pacific Grove, CA: Brooks/Cole; 2003.
23. Sackett, Straus, Richardson, Rosengerg, & Haynes, *Evidence-Based Medicine: How to Practice and Teach EBM,* 2nd ed. London, UK: Churchill Livingstone, 2000.

CHAPTER 75: Counselor Training and Education

Gregory S. Brigham ■ Natasha Slesnick ■ Grant Schroeder

INTRODUCTION

The majority of substance abuse treatment in the United States is provided in addiction specialty care centers. Counselors comprise the greater part of the work force in these centers and they provide most of the behavioral treatments (1). In the broader context of behavioral health care, counselors are a distinct professional group with a defined academic and training curriculum, competency, and licensure standards. In the addiction treatment field, the term counselor is used as a job title for individuals with a wide range of backgrounds who provide counseling services. These counseling positions are occupied by individuals with a variety of backgrounds including professional counselors, social workers, or individuals who enter the addiction workforce due to life experiences rather than academic and professional training. Historically, many of the counselors working in addictions are themselves recovering from alcohol and/or drug dependence. Proponents of a recovering addiction treatment workforce suggest that recovering persons may possess a special empathy for drug-dependent patients that makes them particularly effective in working with this population. Critics of this view claim that many of these "recovering" professionals may hold strong bias as a result of their own experience, insisting that their approach is the only or the best, which may limit their effectiveness. Just as the patients presenting for addiction treatment are a diverse population so are the environments in which treatment is provided and so also is the counseling workforce that provides a great deal of that treatment.

Training and development of addiction counselors has traditionally favored an apprentice model over the more common academic model for professional counselors. The "on-the-job training" approach presents some unique challenges for the dissemination of new information to the workforce. The science of addiction treatment has made numerous advances in the development of both behavioral therapies and medications for the treatment of addiction. While these advances have made some impact in the treatment delivery system, there remains a gap between the state of addiction science and the treatment services that patients are likely to receive (2). In addition to the gap in knowledge between scientists and practitioners, due in part to the prevalence of the on-the-job training model, the addiction treatment system itself has been chronically underfunded and suffers from numerous barriers to its advancement including the vulnerability of treatment facilities to closure due to fiscal problems and the large staff turnover in centers that remain open (3). The prevalence of the apprentice training model for addiction counselors, the gap between addiction treatment science and practice, and the unreliable resources supporting addiction treatment all have significant implications for the training of the addictions counseling workforce.

HISTORY

The addiction counselor workforce has long been thought of as a dichotomy consisting of recovering counselors on the one hand and counselors who have come into the field of addictions through academic training on the other. In his 1996 review of the addiction treatment workforce, Barry Brown (4) noted that while the educational qualifications of drug abuse counselors were increasing, the majority were paraprofessionals who relied heavily on their personal experiences. While this dichotomous view is somewhat outdated, it represents an important historical trend in addictions counseling. We say this view is outdated because the trend toward increasing educational qualifications noted by Brown has continued and, recovering individuals themselves often possess graduate level training in counseling and both state and national certifications, as well as licensing efforts, have progressively professionalized the counseling workforce. In a 2003 report, Mulvey et al. (5) described the addiction treatment workforce based on surveys and interviews of 3267 respondents, of whom 37% were counselors, 31% were program directors, and 30% were clinical supervisors. They found that counselors in the sample were well educated: 74% held at least a bachelor's degree, 42% held graduate degrees, and 72% were certified or licensed as substance abuse/mental health professionals.

The development of substance abuse counselor certification and licensure is closely linked to the history of the substance abuse treatment system. Federal funds for community-based alcoholism treatment were first authorized in 1967. In the following year, the Alcoholic Rehabilitation Act of 1968 described alcoholism as a major community health problem, encouraged community-based treatment and prevention, and authorized federal funds for construction and staffing of services in community mental health centers. With the availability of federal funding and state legislative action pressuring many insurance companies to offer substance abuse treatment in their policies, states began to license both the facilities and the individuals that could provide care for persons with substance use disorders (6).

In the late 1970s and early 1980s, three states in the Midwest of the United States established a small consortium to develop some common standards for certification of alcoholism or addiction counselors. Using the Birch and Davis Report (7), based on a survey of critical job functions and skills of active alcoholism counselors, the first national competencies for alcoholism and drug abuse counselors were developed. The *twelve core functions of the addiction counselor* were defined as consisting of screening, intake, orientation, assessment, treatment planning, counseling, case management, crisis intervention, client education, referral, report and record keeping, and consultation with other professionals. Many certification and licensure boards now require that applicants seeking substance abuse counseling credentials document that they have at least the minimum number of hours of experience required in each of the core functions. Boards requiring oral examination, in addition to written examination, may use the core functions in a Case Presentation Method (CPM) in which the candidates must present a case that demonstrates their competence in each of these core functions. Competence in each of these areas is evaluated using a set of criteria referred to as the "Global Criteria." John Herdman (8) provides a detailed history of the development of substance abuse certification and the CPM. Table 75.1 provides definitions of the Twelve Core Functions and the respective Global Criteria used to evaluate a certification or licensure candidate's competence in them.

In 1993, the Addiction Technology Transfer Center (ATTC) Network created by the Center for Substance Abuse Treatment (CSAT) of the Substance Abuse and Mental Health Services Administration (SAMHSA) set out to improve the preparation of addiction counselors. The ATTC established the National Curriculum Committee to evaluate criteria and establish priorities for curriculum development. From these efforts, the Addiction Counseling Competencies

TABLE 75.1 The 12 core functions and global criteria

Core function	Definition	Global criteria
Screening	The process by which the client is determined appropriate and eligible for admission to a particular program	1) Evaluate psychological, social, and physiological signs and symptoms of alcohol and other drug use and abuse 2) Determine the client's appropriateness for admission or referral 3) Determine the client's eligibility for admission or referral 4) Identify any coexisting conditions (medical, psychiatric, physical, etc.) that indicate need for additional professional assessment and/or services 5) Adhere to applicable laws, regulations, and agency policies governing alcohol and other drug abuse services
Intake	The administrative and initial assessment procedures for admission to a program	6) Complete required documents for admission to the program 7) Complete required documents for program eligibility and appropriateness 8) Obtain appropriately signed consents when soliciting from or providing information to outside sources to protect client confidentiality and rights
Orientation	Describing to the client the general nature and goals of the program; rules governing client conduct and infractions that can lead to disciplinary action or discharge from the program; the hours during which services are available; costs to be borne by the client, and client rights	9) Provide an overview to the client by describing program goals and objectives for client care 10) Provide an overview to the client by describing program rules, and client obligations and rights 11) Provide an overview to the client of program operations

Core function	Definition	Global criteria
Assessment	The procedures by which a counselor/program identifies and evaluates an individual's strengths, weaknesses, problems, and needs for the development of a treatment plan	12) Gather relevant history from client including, but not limited to, alcohol and other drug abuse using appropriate interview techniques 13) Identify methods and procedures for obtaining corroborative information from significant secondary sources regarding clients' alcohol and other drug abuse and psychosocial history 14) Identify appropriate assessment tools 15) Explain to the client the rationale for the use of assessment techniques in order to facilitate understanding 16) Develop a diagnostic evaluation of the client's substance abuse and any coexisting conditions based on the results of all assessments in order to provide an integrated approach to treatment planning based on the client's strengths, weaknesses, and identified problems and needs
Treatment planning	Process by which the counselor and the client identify and rank problems needing resolution; establish agreed upon immediate and long-term goals; and decide upon a treatment process and the resources to be utilized	17) Explain assessment results to the client in an understandable manner 18) Identify and rank problems based on individual client needs in the written treatment plan 19) Formulate agreed upon immediate and long-term goals using behavioral terms in the written treatment plan 20) Identify the treatment methods and resources to be utilized as appropriate for the individual client
Counseling	(Individual, group, and significant others): The utilization of special skills to assist individuals, families, or groups in achieving objectives through exploration of a problem and its ramifications; examination of attitudes and feelings; consideration of alternative solutions; and decision making	21) Select the counseling theory(ies) that apply(ies) 22) Apply technique(s) to assist the client, group, and/or family in exploring problems and ramifications 23) Apply technique(s) to assist the client, group, and/or family in examining the client's behavior, attitudes, and/or feelings if appropriate in the treatment setting 24) Individualize counseling in accordance with cultural, gender, and lifestyle differences 25) Interact with the client in an appropriate therapeutic manner 26) Elicit solutions and decisions from the client 27) Implement the treatment plan
Case management	Activities that bring services, agencies, resource, or people together within a planned framework of action toward the achievement of established goals	28) Coordinate services for client care 29) Explain the rationale of case management activities to the client
Crisis intervention	Those services that respond to an alcohol and/or other drug abuser's needs during acute emotional and/or physical distress	30) Recognize the elements of the client crisis 31) Implement an immediate course of action appropriate to the crisis 32) Enhance overall treatment by utilizing crisis events

Continued

TABLE 75.1	The 12 core functions and global criteria (*Continued*)	
Core function	**Definition**	**Global criteria**
Client education	Provision of information to individuals and groups concerning alcohol and other drug abuse and the available services and resources	33) Present relevant alcohol and other drug use/abuse information to the client through formal and/or informal processes 34) Present information about available alcohol and other drug services and resources
Referral	Identifying the needs of a client that cannot be met by the counselor or agency and assisting the client to utilize the support systems and community resources available	35) Identify need(s) and/or problem(s) that the agency and/or counselor cannot meet 36) Explain the rationale for the referral to the client 37) Match client needs and/or problems to appropriate resources 38) Adhere to applicable laws, regulations, and agency policies governing procedures related to the protection of the client's confidentiality 39) Assist the client in utilizing the support systems and community resources available
Reports and recordkeeping	Charting the results of the assessment and treatment plan, writing reports, progress notes, discharge summaries, and other client-related data	40) Prepare reports and relevant records integrating available information to facilitate the continuum of care 41) Chart pertinent ongoing information pertaining to the client 42) Utilize relevant information from written documents for client care
Consultation with other professionals in regard to client treatment/services	Relating with in-house staff or outside professionals to assure comprehensive, quality care for the client	43) Recognize issues that are beyond the counselor's base of knowledge and/or skill 44) Consult with appropriate resources to ensure the provision of effective treatment services 45) Adhere to applicable laws, regulations, and agency policies governing the disclosure of client-identifying data 46) Explain the rationale for the consultation to the client, if appropriate

Adapted from *Twelve Core Functions of the Alcohol and Other Drug Abuse Counselor* provided to member boards by the IC&RC. Available at: http://www.ocdp.ohio.gov/forms/Twelve%20Core%20Functions.pdf (30).

(ACC), covering 121 specific areas of competency, were established. In 1998, SAMHSA published the ACC as Technical Assistance Publication 21 (TAP 21), which was reviewed and updated in 2005 (9). The ACC is divided into two sections. The first contains Transdisciplinary Foundations organized into four dimensions covering the *basic knowledge and attitudes* necessary for caregivers in the addiction field. These include understanding addictions, treatment knowledge, application to practice, and professional readiness. The eight dimensions of the second section focus on the *practice* of addiction counseling and include clinical evaluation; treatment planning; referral; counseling; client, family, and community education; documentation; and professional and ethical responsibilities.

LICENSURE AND CERTIFICATION ISSUES

While legal requirements and standards for credentialing of substance abuse and mental health counselors in the United States are established at the individual state government level, there are national and international efforts to support the adoption of ACC and to standardize certification testing for substance abuse counselors. The International Certification and Reciprocity Consortium (IC&RC) was formed in 1981, with a mission to advance reciprocal competency standards for substance abuse professionals and to support the member certification/licensure boards. The IC&RC currently reports that over 37,000 alcohol and drug abuse counselors are certified by over 73 member certification boards (10). In 2007, the

IC&RC board voted to stop using the oral Case Presentation Method and instead revised the written examination to cover questions of competency in the core functions, which were previously addressed in the CPM.

The National Association for Addiction Professionals was founded in 1972, as the National Association of Alcoholism Counselors and Trainers (NAACT), and later became the National Association for Alcoholism and Drug Abuse Counselors (NAADAC) in 1982. The primary objective of NAADAC is to develop a field of counselors with professional qualifications and backgrounds. In 1990, concerned with the lack of national standards and the confusion caused by numerous acronyms used by state certification boards, NAADAC developed a national certification that required applicants to be certified at the state level, pass a national examination, and have an academic degree. This was the first time in the addiction counselor credentialing process that academic degrees were paired with competencies as a basis for certification. They now offer three levels of national certification for addiction counselors, which are commensurate with education, hours of work experience, contact hours, and length of supervised experience. They also offer a Tobacco Addiction Specialist (TAS) certification (11).

While the efforts to define core functions, describe competencies, and develop common minimum certification/licensure requirements have served to advance the professionalism of substance abuse counselors, there remains a lower academic standard for substance abuse counselors when compared with counselors working in other areas of behavioral health. For example, there are notable differences in the requirements for credentialing of substance abuse treatment counselors versus those for mental health professionals. These differences reflect a continuation of the historical trend of a reliance on personal experience and an apprentice model of professional development for addiction counselors. According to a 2006 report by Kerwin et al. (12), only 67% of state governments either offered or required certification or licensure for substance abuse counselors, while 96% offered or required the same for mental health counselors. Of the 48 states with a minimum degree requirement for mental health counselors, 98% required a graduate degree. Of the 31 states with a minimum degree requirement, only 10% require graduate degrees for substance abuse counselors. While these states have lower degree requirements for substance abuse counselors compared with mental health counselors, they tend to require more hours of supervised work experience for substance abuse counselors. For substance abuse counselors, the mean minimum required supervised work experience was 3819 hours, whereas that for mental health counselors was 2801 hours.

The primary function of certification and licensing boards is to protect the public by ensuring providers of substance abuse counseling services meet at least a minimum standard of training and competence. Most states license behavioral health-related professionals such as psychologists, counselors, and social workers, and in many states, these professionals may provide substance abuse treatment services within the scope of those licenses. Specialized addiction certifications or licensure provide an avenue for addiction counselors, who do not have a general license, to practice in a restricted fashion with substance abuse related patients only. Addiction certifications or licenses may also be held by professionals with other behavioral health licenses in order to demonstrate addiction-specific expertise or to privilege themselves to perform functions that have been restricted to those who hold addiction-specific certification or licensure. For instance, in some states, only individuals with an addiction-specific licensure or certification can supervise addiction counselors.

APPROACHES TO TRAINING AND EDUCATION

Given the widely acknowledged gap between empirically supported substance abuse treatment interventions and community-based practice, research efforts are beginning to focus on identifying successful methods of dissemination (2,13,14). In the field of behavioral substance abuse treatment, this is a relatively nascent area of study. Compared to Oxman et al.'s (15) review conducted 15 years ago, which identified 102 randomized clinical trials focused on improving aspects of professional medical practice, Walters et al. (16) identified only 17 studies focused on evaluating behavioral treatment training methods for community-based practitioners. The pharmaceutical industry employs several strategies to disseminate information about new pharmacologic treatments including training sessions, promotional materials, and incentives offered to health care providers (17). Effective mechanisms for disseminating behavioral treatments, which often require more complex skill acquisition, are not yet identified. However, studies offer preliminary information to guide future efforts in this area.

Currently, Motivational Interviewing (MI) is the most frequently taught method, followed by Cognitive–Behavioral Treatment (CBT), network therapy, and other brief interventions (16). While these manualized treatments are evidence based, a small cadre of literature also indicates that subsequent patient outcomes for treatment as usual, as provided by community substance abuse treatment programs, can perform similarly to the intervention approaches developed in randomized controlled trials (18,19). As the primary goal of training clinicians in empirically supported interventions is to improve patient outcomes above that of treatment as usual, it is important to ensure that the intervention has not only proven efficacious in a controlled environment but that it has also proven to be more powerful than interventions currently used by the community agencies (i.e., proven effective). Otherwise, training efforts are premature. Even so, Miller and Wilbourne (20) identified several treatment approaches utilized by many community-based substance abuse treatment programs, which lack evidence for their effectiveness. These approaches include educational lectures and films, general counseling, confrontational approaches, and milieu therapy.

Some have suggested that community-based substance abuse counselors prefer 12-step interventions over other empirically based interventions such as CBT, since most community treatment programs are based upon a 12-step approach (18). Also, manualized-based treatments might be less acceptable to community providers, given the perceived inflexibility of manualized intervention components. These assumptions have not been supported by research. In particular, Morgenstern et al. (18) concluded the opposite, that many counselors actively seek new skills to improve patient outcomes and that counselors appreciate the structure and specificity of manuals. However, unmotivated clinicians, or those mandated to trainings (vs. actively seeking training), might benefit from a focus on increasing their motivation to learn and apply new clinical skills (13).

Training procedures used in clinical trials differ from those used to train frontline clinicians. Among trials, therapist training often involves (a) selecting experienced therapists committed to the treatment approach, (b) a 2- to 3-day didactic seminar with role play and practice, and (c) ongoing supervision (usually audio- or videotape) of cases until the clinician shows adequate skill and fidelity with the intervention (17). In contrast to the rigorous therapist training procedures used in controlled trials, the most frequently used methods for dissemination of treatments to community-based clinicians, who have a range of education and practice experience, include distribution of treatment manuals and/or a brief didactic training without ongoing supervision (16,17). As noted below, the most commonly used strategy to train clinicians has shown limited success in translating to changes in patient behavior.

Although the extant training studies report changes in therapist behavior, attitude, and/or skills associated with many training procedures, concomitant change in patient outcomes is less studied. The exception has been the work conducted by Miller and colleagues. Miller and Mount (21) found that clinicians' practice behaviors significantly changed subsequent to a 2-day training workshop (without ongoing supervision), but in-session patient behavior did not change. Miller et al. (13) suggested that more intensive, ongoing training that includes empirically grounded learning aids—systematic feedback and reinforced practice—was needed in order to impact complex clinician behaviors, and that this would positively impact patient behavior. As such, a follow-up study (13) evaluated MI training in five formats with clinicians randomly assigned to (a) workshop alone, (b) workshop plus telephone coaching, (c) workshop plus feedback on audio-recorded sessions, (d) workshop plus individual feedback and coaching, or (e) a waitlist control. The findings support a "more is better" hypothesis. Those receiving feedback and/or coaching more fully retained their clinical proficiency in MI than those who received the workshop alone. However, only patients whose clinicians received the workshop, feedback, and coaching sessions showed in-session changes in behavior.

Clinicians in the workshop-only condition showed initial gains in skill but these degraded over time, which is consistent with other research findings (17,22). That is, a discrete training workshop is associated with a short-term increase in knowledge and skills, but these gains do not lead to long-term changes in clinician skills (16). Similarly, self-guided training using the MI book and training videotapes produced no increase in clinician skill. Self-study and one-time workshops are common methods that clinicians seek to acquire new skills (13). Although adding additional contact to workshop training appears to improve clinician skill, the length and amount of training needed to sustain clinician improvement, as well as concomitant patient improvement, is not known.

To date, training methods target the clinician alone without consideration of institutional barriers, which could impact the clinician's utilization of new found skills. Incompatibility of the new treatment approach with the underlying philosophy of the program is a potential barrier to the widespread adoption of empirically supported treatments. For example, Miller et al. (13) reported that several newly trained clinicians in their research study left their positions of employment because the collaborative, autonomy-respecting style of MI was incompatible with their practice setting. These clinicians sought practice settings more compatible with their new found skills and therapeutic approach. Possibly, clinicians unable to secure alternative employment may not be supported to implement new found techniques if those techniques are incompatible with the agency's overall philosophy.

Another institutional barrier is that the intensive clinician training, which has a mounting evidence suggesting its superiority over less intensive methods, requires expert trainers' time, clinician time, and concomitant expense. The financial burden can be a significant barrier for many agencies that struggle to maintain their programs and staff in an economy of dwindling resources. Overall, institutional factors that affect the successful adoption of new intervention practices require more attention (13,16). An important consideration is that the clinician is not an isolated organism within a systemic vacuum but instead is powerful in his/her ability to influence and be influenced by his/her social ecology.

Innovative and practical solutions to high training costs are under investigation. For example, computer and web-based training can be a less expensive method for training large numbers of clinicians and might be more feasible than face-to-face training (17). In fact, preliminary support for teleconferencing supervision (23) and web-based training methods (17,24) has begun to appear in the literature. The use of technology in new and creative ways has the potential to overcome logistical barriers such as physical distance between expert trainers and clinicians, as well as reduce the costs associated with trainer time.

Overall, the necessary components of clinician training, which translate into improved patient outcomes, have not been identified. Research has not deciphered whether training methods need to focus on diminishing old habits rather than simply teaching new behaviors as suggested by Miller et al. (13), and which principles of learning are most salient for different therapeutic techniques. Some of the more complicated techniques such as complex reflections used in MI or family-systems-based techniques might require a range of strategies to ensure clinician skill including systematic shaping of behaviors, role play practice, modeling, immediacy of feedback, and even cognitive shifts among clinicians themselves. Alternatively, clinical techniques such as contingency management might only require an initial workshop with follow-up phone consultation. However, some tentative conclusions are possible based upon the small number of studies conducted to date. It appears that a workshop training alone can improve clinician skill, but without continued supervision or support, skills degrade with time. Studies suggest that a core training workshop, manuals, and ongoing video or audiotaped supervision appear to be the current "gold standard" of training methods. However, the context of training (face-to-face vs. technology-based, tape review vs. live supervision), its intensity and duration, and how to engage institutional supports to maintain change are among the areas requiring more research. This information will certainly be integral for narrowing the research–practice gap.

ROLE OF THE SPECIALTY IN ADDICTION TREATMENT AND TRAINING WITHIN AND ACROSS SPECIALTIES

As the addiction treatment delivery system changes, the roles, skills, and knowledge required by counselors will also change. There are current efforts focused on broadening the availability of addiction treatment services beyond the specialty care settings. Primary care physicians have a unique opportunity to identify substance abuse in individuals who are seeking care for other medical problems. Traditionally, physicians have been reluctant to address these issues due in part to the lack of resources to treat substance abuse problems once they are identified. Increasingly substance abuse services such as identification, referral, and monitoring are being addressed in primary care settings by having counselors available in the primary care setting or by developing close collaborative relationships to provide linkage to those services off-site. These settings require new knowledge and skills to address early detection and motivating nontreatment-seeking individuals. These practices are significant because they show considerable promise for extending the benefits of substance abuse treatment to populations that currently do not access treatment (25).

SPECIAL CONSIDERATIONS

There are numerous subpopulations of individuals with substance dependence problems for which counselors may require specialized training to achieve competence. The subpopulations may be based on demographic characteristics such as gender, cultural background, or developmental stages as in adolescents, or they may be based on clinical characteristics such as criminal justice populations or co-occurring substance abuse with other psychiatric disorders.

Women generally have more barriers to seeking treatment and are more likely to seek treatment in gender-specific settings or primary care medical settings. In general, although women face more difficulties accessing treatment and have more complications to cope with in comparison with men, they tend to have better treatment outcomes than men. Even though women are more likely to seek treatment in gender-specific programs, there is no clear evidence that gender-specific programs are more effective than mixed-gender treatment. Although there are no specific training curriculums for counselors to specialize in the treatment of women, the interventions that are considered useful would suggest that additional competencies in assessment of victims of sexual and violent trauma, and arranging comprehensive services such as housing, transportation, education, and income support (26) are desirable.

Individuals presenting for the treatment of substance use disorders are culturally diverse and this diversity has implications for treatment. Cultural competence is increasingly viewed as an important aspect of substance abuse counselor competence. While no single approach to developing cultural competence has emerged as superior, it is generally accepted that cultural competence should be addressed as an important component in any addiction professional training curriculum.

Treating adolescents with substance abuse problems requires knowledge and skills unique to the treatment of this population. Adolescents who present for treatment are often involved in multiple medical and social systems reflecting their diverse health, legal, and social problems. In addition, the reasons adolescents use substances may differ from adults and require unique counselor competencies to address them (27). The most effective treatments for this population often involve systems approaches that require specialized training and supervision.

The incidence of other mental disorders co-occurring with substance use disorders is high in both adult and adolescent populations. There is general consensus that the best practice is to provide concurrent treatment for both the mental health diagnosis and the substance use disorder. This type of treatment requires specialized training for the recognition, diagnosis, and treatment of mental disorders. Numerous counselor-training curriculums have been developed to provide this specialized training. CSAT develops treatment improvement protocols (TIPs), which are best-practice guidelines for the treatment of substance use disorders. CSAT's TIP 42 focuses on substance abuse treatment for persons with co-occurring disorders, and an in-service training protocol has been developed to accompany the TIP (28).

CONCLUSIONS

Counselors play a critical role in the delivery of addiction care. The distinction *counselor* has developed more as a job than as a profession within the substance abuse field and the training and certification standards reflect this vocational emphasis. Much of the required training for substance abuse counselors is based on a job analysis of the functions performed by individuals in these positions and historically less emphasis has been placed on specialized knowledge. While the SAMHSA TIP 21 provides a comprehensive guide to the development of training for addiction counselors, it also documents the substantial gap between these standards and the actual and needed competences of addictions professionals in the field. State, national, and international efforts to develop and evaluate uniform minimum competency standards have helped the addiction counselor job progress into a profession. However, the gap between science and practice in addiction care highlights a critical challenge presented by the lingering apprentice model of addiction counselor development. Academic preparation and professional training activities for addiction counselors will need to become more comprehensive and provide greater continuity to develop the capacity to integrate science-based improvements into the treatment of addiction (29).

REFERENCES

1. Substance Abuse and Mental Health Services Administration. *National Drug and Alcoholism Treatment Unit Survey (NDATUS): 1991 Main Findings Report*. Rockville, MD: U.S. Department of Health and Human Services, Substance Abuse and Mental Health Services Administration; 1993.
2. Institute of Medicine. *Bridging the Gap Between Practice and Research: Forging Partnerships with Community-Based Drug and Alcohol Treatment*. Washington, DC: National Academy of Sciences Press; 1998.
3. McLellan TA, Carise D, Kleber HD. Can the national addiction treatment infrastructure support the public's demand for quality care? *J Subst Abuse Treat*. 2003;25:117–121.
4. Brown BS. Staffing patterns and services for the war on drugs. In: Egerston JA, Fos DM, Leshner AI, eds. *Treating Drug Abusers Effectively*. Malden, MA: Blackwell Publishers; 1996.
5. Mulvey KP, Hubbard S, Hayashi S. A national study of the substance abuse treatment workforce. *J Subst Abuse Treat*. 2003;24: 51–57.
6. McCarty D, Argeriou M, Mulligan D. *State and Federal Policy Influences on Alcohol Treatment Services*. Available at: http://addictionmanagement.org/mccarty_et_al_on_policy%20062204%20(2).doc. Accessed November 1, 2009.
7. Birch & Davis, Inc. *Development of Model Professional Standards for Counselor Credentialing*. Rockville, MD: National Institute on Alcohol Abuse and Alcoholism; 1984.
8. Herdman, J. *Global Criteria: The 12 Core Functions of the Substance Abuse Counselor*. 3rd ed. Holmes Beach, FL: Learning Publications, Inc.; 2001.
9. Center for Substance Abuse Treatment. *Addiction Counseling Competencies: The Knowledge, Skills, and Attitudes of Professional Practice*. Technical Assistance Publication (TAP) Series 21. DHHS Publication No. (SMA) 08-4171. Rockville, MD: Substance Abuse and Mental Health Services Administration, 2006, reprinted 2007 and 2008.
10. International Certification & Reciprocity Consortium. *Candidate Guide: International Certification Examination for Alcohol and Other Drug Abuse Counselors, 2008*. Available at: http://www.icrcaoda.org/PDFs/2008%20AODA%20Candidate%20Guide.pdf. Accessed November 1, 2009.
11. National Association for Alcoholism and Drug Abuse Counselors. Available at: http://www.naadac.org/index.php?option=com_content&view=article&id=396&Itemid=61. Accessed November 1, 2009.
12. Kerwin ME, Walker-Smith K, Kirby KC. Comparative, analysis of state requirements for the training of substance abuse and mental health counselors. *J Subst Abuse Treat*. 2006;30:173–181.
13. Miller WR, Yahne CE, Moyers TB, et al. A randomized trial of methods to help clinicians learn motivational interviewing. *J Consult Clin Psychol*. 2004;72:1050–1062.
14. Miller RW, Sorensen JL, Selzer JA, et al. Disseminating evidenced-based practices in substance abuse treatment: a review with suggestions. *J Subs Abuse Treat*. 2006;31:25–39.
15. Oxman AD, Thompson MA, Davis DA, et al. No magic bullets: a systematic review of 102 trials of interventions to help health care professionals deliver services more effectively and efficiently. *Can Med Assoc J*. 1995;153:1423–1431.
16. Walters ST, Matson SA, Baer JS, et al. Effectiveness of workshop training for psychosocial addiction treatments: a systematic review. *J Subst Abuse Treat*. 2005;29:283–293.
17. Scholomskas DE, Syracuse-Siewert G, Rounsaville BJ, et al. We don't train in vain: a dissemination trial of three strategies of training clinicians in cognitive–behavioral therapy. *J Consult Clin Psychol*. 2005;73:106–115.
18. Morgenstern J, Morgan TJ, McCrady BS, et al. Manual guided cognitive–behavioral therapy training: a promising method for disseminating empirically supported substance abuse treatments to the practice community. *Psychol Addict Behav*. 2001; 15:83–88.
19. Najavits LM, Harned MS, Gallop RJ, et al. Six-month treatment outcomes of cocaine-dependent patients with and without PTSD in a multisite national trial. *J Stud Alcohol Drugs*. 2007; 68: 353–361.
20. Miller WR, Wilbourne PL. Mesa Grande: a methodological analysis of clinical trials of treatments for alcohol use disorders. *Addiction*. 2002;97:267–277.
21. Miller WR, Mount KA. A small study of training in motivational interviewing: does one workshop change clinician and client behavior? *Behav Cogn Psychother*. 2001;29:457–471.
22. Baer JS, Rosengren DB, Dunn CW, et al. An evaluation of workshop training in motivational interviewing for addiction and mental health clinicians. *Drug Alcohol Depend*. 2004;73: 99–106.
23. Smith JL, Amrhein PC, Brooks AC, et al. Providing live supervision via teleconferencing improves acquisition of motivational interviewing skills after workshop attendance. *Am J Drug Alcohol Abuse*. 2007;33:163–168.
24. McPherson TL, Cook RF, Back AS, et al. A field test of a web-based substance abuse prevention training program for health promotion professionals. *Am J Health Promot*. 2006;20: 396–400.
25. Madras BK, Compton WM, Avula D, et al. Screening, brief interventions, referral to treatment (SBIRT) for illicit drug and alcohol use at multiple healthcare sites: comparison at intake and 6 months later. *Drug Alcohol Depend*. 2009;99:280–295. doi: 10.1016/j.drugalcdep.2008.08.003.
26. Green CA. Gender and use of substance abuse treatment services. *Alcohol Res Health*. 2006;29:55–62.
27. Schubert K, Pond A, Kraft M, et al. The adolescent addiction treatment workforce: status, challenges, and strategies to address their particular needs. *J Psychoactive Drugs*. 2004;36(4):483–488.
28. Center for Substance Abuse Treatment. *Substance Abuse Treatment for Persons with Co-Occurring Disorders Inservice Training*. DHHS Publication No. (SMA) 07-4262. Rockville, MD: Substance Abuse and Mental Health Services Administration; 2007.
29. Knudsen HK, Roman PM. Modeling the use of innovations in private treatment organizations: the role of absorptive capacity. *J Subst Abuse Treat*. 2004;26:51–59. doi: 10.1016/S0740-5472 (03)00158-2.
30. International National Certification Reciprocity Consortium. *Twelve Core Functions of the Alcohol and Other Drug Abuse Counselor*, 1995. Available at: http://www.ocdp.ohio.gov/forms/Twelve%20Core%20Functions.pdf. Accessed December 2, 2009.

CHAPTER 76 Other Mental Health Professionals

E. Akerele ■ N. Nahar ■ J. Cerimele

INTRODUCTION

In general when we think of treatment of individuals with substance use disorders (SUDs), the primary focus is on the role of physicians. However, the treatment of individuals with SUDs requires a complex coordinated team, a multidisciplinary group. This team includes a significant number of nonphysicians. Psychologists, counselors, social workers, nurses, and other allied health care providers play essential roles in promoting the biopsychosocial well-being of individuals with SUDs. In order to maximize the professional team's efficiency and efficacy, it is vital that the role of each member of the group is structured and understood.

There is minimal research literature on the role of nonphysician professionals in the substance abuse treatment team. Addressing their role requires an in-depth understanding of the type of standardized training that exists for these professionals. Only then is it possible to suggest modalities for improving the contribution of individual professional groups and that of the overall team. The range of settings in which treatment is provided further complicates the professional roles. These range from the emergency room, acute inpatient detoxification, to 2-year treatment facilities in therapeutic communities. Furthermore, the role of these nonphysician health professionals may vary with setting. They probably play a major role in community settings. This is likely due to the difficulty of recruiting physicians in community clinics (1). It is important that all members of these professional groups are provided with the right balance of mental health and substance abuse training for their level and range of practice. Therefore, the field must provide high-quality appropriate training within each profession. The role of these professionals is not limited to treatment and a number of them, especially psychologists, contribute to the development of biological and behavioral interventions for SUDs. For example, psychologists play a major role in medication development from basic science to clinical trials. However, it is beyond the scope of this chapter to address the research role of other professionals.

There is no standard homogeneous education/training available to educate and train other addiction health professionals. However, there are limited fellowship, workshops, and training available for the other professionals in the field of addiction. Some of this training or certification are recommended or approved by specific state or professional organizations. Some institutes offer fellowship or other training for all other professionals—psychologists, social workers, occupational therapists, nurses, and chaplains. For example, the Veterans Affairs Medical Center at Seattle developed an interdisciplinary program (2), which trains professionals in details of substance abuse treatment using biopsychosocial model. Other institutions offer 1-year advanced fellowship training in substance abuse treatment for psychologists, social workers, occupational therapists, nurses, and chaplains.

In this chapter, we attempt to review the existing data on nonphysician providers' roles in substance abuse treatment. We will present each professional group, define each scope of practice, and examine the current roles in treatment. Lastly, we will address future directions within each professional group.

PSYCHOLOGISTS

Definitions

The American Psychological Association (APA) policy on the use of the title "psychologist" is contained in the General Guidelines for Providers of Psychological Services, which define the term "Professional Psychologist" as "Psychologists have a doctoral degree in psychology from an organized, sequential program in a regionally accredited university or professional school." There are many different types of psychologists, as reflected by the 56 different divisions of the APA. Psychologists are generally described as being either "applied" or "research" oriented. This major division is also described as the difference between scientists and practitioners or scholars and professionals. The training models endorsed by the APA require that practitioners be trained as both scholars and professionals and to possess advanced degrees.

A *clinical psychologist* has a Ph.D. or a Psy.D., and has successfully completed an internship in clinical psychology. Clinical psychologists are qualified to diagnose and treat psychological disorders and perform psychological testing. In some cases, after additional training, they may prescribe medication in some medical settings.

A *counseling psychologist* has either a Ph.D. or an Ed.D., and has completed an internship in counseling psychology. Like a clinical psychologist, a counseling psychologist can perform psychological testing. In addition, he or she may assess and provide therapy for routine problems of life.

A *school psychologist* may have a Ph.D., an Ed.D., or a master's degree, in addition to an internship in school psychology.

Along with psychological testing, a school psychologist can assess and treat school (and other related) problems in children and adolescents.

Education and Training

The APA has certification program in addiction proficiency (3). The *Certificate of Proficiency* (Certification for Licensed Psychologists in Substance Abuse Treatment) is a uniform national credential offered exclusively to licensed psychologists who meet the following criteria:

Possess a current state or provincial license in good standing to engage in the independent practice of psychology.
Have treated alcohol and other psychoactive SUDs as a licensed psychologist for at least 1 year during the last 3 years.
Have provided health services in psychology.
Have successfully completed the *College of Professional Psychology* examination in the treatment of alcohol and other psychoactive SUDs.
Have provided alcohol- or substance abuse treatment for at least 5 of the last 8 years.
Following the above criteria, a psychologist must take a 3-hour computerized examination of 150 multiple-choice questions. This exam measures the psychologist's knowledge in several areas including epidemiology of psychoactive substances, etiologies of SUDs, prevention, screening, diagnosis, treatment, ethical concerns, and matters specific to certain populations

The APA Practice Organization, College of Professional Psychology's Certificate of Proficiency provides certification for 3 years. To maintain certification, recipients must then take 18 hours of continuing education during each 3-year period of Certification and to submit verification that his/her state or provincial license continues in good standing (4).

The *Certificate of Proficiency* assists the public in identifying licensed psychologists whose scope of practice includes the treatment of patients with alcohol and SUDs. A growing number of state agencies (Georgia, Hawai, Indiana, New Hampshire, North Carolina, Vermont, Wisconsin) have encouraged addiction psychologists to obtain the *Certificate of Proficiency.*

Other psychology program like internships and fellowships (clinical and research) make psychologist work with credential in the field of addiction offered by many institutions and Universities (5,6). Many graduate and postdoctoral programs have concentration on addiction. There are also graduate and postdoctoral fellowships available for the psychologist in different institutes (7). However, there are no mandatory requirements for a psychologist to fulfill to work in the field of addiction.

Role and Scope of Practice

Scope of Practice is a terminology used by state licensing boards for various professions that define the procedures, actions, and processes that are permitted for the licensed individual. The scope of practice is limited to that which the law allows for specific education and experience, and specific demonstrated competency. Each state has laws, licensing bodies, and regulations that describe requirements for education and training, and define scope of practice.

Psychologists work in teaching, research, social service in schools, clinics, government agencies, and private industry. About 34% of psychologists were self-employed in 2006 among 166,000 psychologist jobs (8). Educational institutions employed about 29% of psychologists in positions other than teaching, such as counseling, testing, research, and administration. About 21% were employed in health care, primarily in offices of mental health practitioners, hospitals, physicians' offices, and outpatient mental health and substance abuse centers. Advancement depends on many factors, including education, experience, and other personal qualities. Psychologists can expand their private practices or move into high-level jobs in research, teaching, counseling, or administration. Some psychologists advance by serving as consultants to government or industry or by writing about their special fields.

There is increasing emphasis by psychologist educators and advocates to involve psychologists in the treatment of addiction-related disorder (9) over the past decade. According to advocates, psychologists should treat SUDs by recognizing that these disorders are fundamentally behavioral and psychological in nature (10). They argue that SUDs respond to many of the same psychotherapeutic principles and interventions that apply to other mental health problems. The efficacy of addiction treatment approaches based on behavioral and other psychotherapeutic techniques is well documented. Included among these are motivation-enhancement strategies based on Rogerian principles of client-centered therapy (11); relapse prevention strategies based on principles of cognitive-behavioral therapy (12); solution-oriented and other brief therapy techniques (13); and harm reduction approaches (14). Miller and Brown et al. (10) assert that practicing psychologists are particularly well qualified by their training and expertise to treat SUDs.

NURSES/NURSE PRACTITIONERS

Definition

Registered nurses provide care in hospitals, private clinics, long-term health care centers and other medical facilities. A registered nurse is qualified to administer medication, provide therapies and treatments to patients, and consult with practicing physicians on patient care. Registered nurses also provide patients with explanations of test results and treatment options.

Nursing practice involves autonomous and collaborative care of individuals of all ages, families, groups, and communities, in many settings. Nurses also promote health and disease screening, prevention of illness. Furthermore, some nurses have roles in patient advocacy, promotion of a safe environment, research, health policy, health systems management, and education. Addiction nurses need an understanding of both general nursing along with a specialized knowledge of addictions in order to provide effective care.

Education and Training

Subsequent to high school graduation, an individual may apply to nursing programs at accredited colleges and universities. Some individuals first earn an associate's degree in nursing (an AND). Bachelor's degree programs in nursing (BSN) are granted only from accredited 4-year universities. These programs often combine nursing course work with several hours of clinical experience. BSN students have 2 years of general college courses before entering the nursing major, including behavioral and physical science courses. In each program, nursing students study the care of adults, children, pregnant women, mental health nursing and community health nursing. Although addiction issues are addressed in all nursing specialty areas, basic knowledge in addiction nursing is often taught as part of the mental health course. Addiction nurses can gain advanced education through workshops, specialty journals, and graduate programs.

There is little data about nursing education and training in the field of addiction. Pillon et al. (15) conducted a study on nurses in Brazil and demonstrated that 70% of the participants had received little or no information on physical, family, and social problems related to alcohol use. Furthermore, 87% of participants had received little or no information on high-risk behaviors in specific populations and 95% of participants had received little or no information on nursing procedures for alcohol-abuse patients.

The National Nurses Society on Addictions (NNSA) sponsors an annual conference on addiction nursing, an addiction nursing journal, and other publications on addiction nursing. NNSA is currently the largest professional nursing organization representing addiction nursing. It has published a core curriculum on addiction nursing, and has worked with the American Nurses Association to define the dimensions of addiction nursing and develop standards. Advance Practice Nurses (APNs) are prepared at the graduate level and receive a Master of Science Degree in Nursing (MS or MSN) as either nurse practitioners or clinical nurse specialists. APNs have advanced education in pharmacology, pathophysiology, and courses related to their area of specialization. In many states, APNs also have prescriptive privileges. There are several graduate nursing programs with a specialty in addictions nursing; other programs include addiction nursing as a subspecialty of mental health nursing.

Over the last decade there have been some initiatives (government and nongovernment) and advocacy for training and education of nurses in the field of addiction that emphasizes the skills that the nurse must possess to intervene effectively with the substance abuser (16–22). The International Nurses Society on Addictions (IntNSA) publishes *Journal of Addictions Nursing*: this journal offers continuing education credits for nursing addiction professionals.

Certification as an Addiction Nurse

In 1989, the *Addictions Nursing Certification Board* (ANCB) offered the first certification for addictions Registered Nurses (CARNs). A similar certification became available for advanced practice nurses in the year 2000 (the CARN-NP) (23). These certifications ensure consistent basic training in addiction nursing among certified nurses. The applicant for the CARN-AP must be an RN holding a master's degree or higher degree with documented clinical practice hours at the advanced practice level. The American Nurses Association describes that professional certification helps ensure delivery of safe, high-quality services (24). Nurses generally must complete the following requirements to become an addiction nurse (CARN or CARN-NP):

State's guidelines for becoming an addictions nurse.
Mental health nursing curriculum
Attending conferences for addiction rehabilitation and counseling
Postgraduate nursing programs. Many certifications require a minimum of a bachelor's degree and some require up to a doctorate.
Volunteer in rehabilitation centers or clinics.
Familiarize with the current trends in substance abuse by visiting sites such as the one ran by the National Association for Addiction Professionals.
At least 3 years of work as an RN, and a minimum of 4000 hours (2 years) of nursing related to addictions (for instance on a dual diagnosis unit).

Specialty certification in addiction nursing provides several advantages to nurses including self-verification of specialty knowledge, increased self-esteem, increased pay and job security, and increased confidence (25). Furthermore, certification may help reduce health care errors, demonstrate nurses' commitment to state-of the-art care, and improve retention of nurses in the workforce.

Some nursing programs offer nurses roles in addiction research. The University of Washington School of Nursing has been awarded funding by the National Institute on Drug Abuse (NIDA) for nursing research training in substance abuse (26).

Role and Scope of Practice

Nurses with advanced training in addiction have several skill sets including knowledge of general nursing and details of common addiction behaviors. Because behavioral health units in hospital settings often combine addiction and mental health programs, many addiction nurses routinely use both skill sets. Specific nursing activities include counseling patients, educating patients and their families, facilitating group therapy sessions, and working closely with other staff members.

Nurses may choose to work in hospitals, outpatient facilities, and community care centers. Some nurses pursue managing interests and may develop skills to serve as a nurse case manager (27). The addiction nurse's role depends on the setting as well as the expertise and interests of the nurse. On an inpatient unit, addiction nurses are involved in the full range of patient care. They are involved in the detoxification phase of treatment and maintain ongoing monitoring of the patient's health status using protocols such as the Clinical Institute Withdrawal Assessment (CIWA) scale. Some outpatient settings are experimenting with outpatient detoxification based on nursing assessment and monitoring via intermittent contact and a paging system.

Addiction nurses provide a variety of therapeutic modalities. Nurses often develop and maintain a therapeutic environment to promote recovery and both personal and interpersonal growth. Nurses also facilitate group activities, talk with patients' family members, and contribute observations to the interdisciplinary treatment team. Furthermore, nurses directly observe patients around the clock and may gather an in-depth view of the patient's behavior and relationships.

The addiction nurse's role in outpatient settings also includes telephone consultations with patients. Nurses may also be involved in intake evaluations of new patients. Some participate in administrative activities in the role of nurse supervisor or manager within the nursing department or within an organizational environment. Nursing roles also exist outside of traditional treatment settings. Occupational health nursing, school nursing, and community and home health nursing are all areas in which a substantial amount of addiction nursing is practiced. Some general hospitals employ nurses to assist in substance use screening for all hospitalized patients. These nurses help determine which patient would benefit from further evaluation of substance use.

Addiction nurses, particularly those with advanced degrees, are often involved in addiction research. This may occur through individual or group research projects. Several university schools of nursing currently receive grants to fund postdoctoral study in addiction research.

Nursing emphasizes disease prevention and health promotion through education and other appropriate means, and also recognizes the importance of the patient's family as part of recovery. Individualized care plans are developed collaboratively between the patient and the nurse.

PHYSICIAN ASSISTANTS

Definition

A physician assistant (PA) is a midlevel medical practitioner who works under the supervision of a licensed physician. The PA came about in the 1960s as a response to the need for more clinicians (there was a shortage of family physicians) and to improve access to care. The first PA program was developed by Dr. Eugene Stead, chairman of the Department of Medicine at Duke University, to train PAs for rural areas with dwindling numbers of physicians and nurses. Although there is not yet a requirement to hold a degree beyond the bachelor's level, most PAs have a master's degree.

Education and Training

The National Commission on Certification of Physician Assistants accredits PA training programs. Each state in the United States has its own specific licensing and practicing restrictions for PAs. Most states require PAs to pass the certification examination of the National Commission on Certification of Physician Assistants.

To practice as a PA, most states require a master's degree and a degree from an accredited PA program. Candidates must meet state requirements pertaining to a PA.

Most PA programs have little training in the area of addiction. During their clinical rotation series, students usually train for 6 to 10 weeks in the area of behavioral science, which may or may not include addiction medicine. PA students must often use elective time during school to obtain training in addiction principles. PAs interested in addiction medicine may require extra training in addiction prior to encountering patients. Few PA programs offer specific postgraduate training in addiction medicine, complicating a PA's path to becoming involved in addiction treatment. Some national courses exist to train PAs in addiction principles (28). A national society for PAs involved in addiction medicine offers opportunities for continuing education and networking (29).

Role and Scope

PAs evaluate patients under the supervision of a licensed physician. Although the physician need not be present during the time the PA performs his or her duties, there must be a method of contact between the supervising physician and the PA at all times. The PA must be competent in the duties he or she is performing and the physician for whom the PA is working must also be licensed and trained to perform the relevant duties. Examples of the duties of a general PA include:

Medical histories and physical examinations: a PA can usually perform histories and physical examinations that do not go beyond a particular level.
Laboratory tests: a PA can order any test which he or she is competent to interpret and provide the appropriate treatment.
Follow-up: PAs follow patients through their hospital course, their course of treatment in a clinic setting, and so on.

Many private insurers and health plans sometimes require advanced degrees and/or certifications for PA specifically in behavioral health as a prerequisite for payment. Some companies do not pay for services delegated to PAs, even if the delegated service is within the PA's legal scope of practice (30).

SOCIAL WORKERS

Definition

The International Federation of Social Workers states, "social work bases its methodology on a systematic body of evidence-based knowledge derived from research and practice evaluation, including local and indigenous knowledge specific to its context. It recognizes the complexity of interactions between human beings and their environment, and the capacity of people both to be affected by and to alter the multiple influences upon them including biopsychosocial factors. The social work profession draws upon theories of human development and behavior and social systems to analyze complex situations and to facilitate individual, organizational, social and cultural changes."

Training in psychotherapy and techniques of managing various mental health and daily living problems to improve overall functioning are necessary to qualify as a licensed clinical social worker. Furthermore, social workers hold a masters degree in social work and have studied sociology, growth and development, mental health theory and practice, human behavior/social environment, psychology, and research methods. In addition to a minimum of a master's degree in social work (M.S.W), additional course work and training to pass accreditation tests as a licensed clinical social worker (L.C.S.W.) is necessary. Social workers may diagnose and treat psychological disorders. They often assist with the identification of supportive community services frequently working in conjunction with institutions such as hospitals.

A licensed professional counselor (L.P.C.) also has a master's degree, as does a marriage and family therapist. They focus primarily on private practice and may specialize in relationships, day-to-day life problems, and/or psychological disorders.

Generally, those who hold a professional degree in social work are considered professional workers. They usually have a license or some other professional registration.

Education and Training

Social work education programs usually award a bachelor of social work (BA, BSc, or BSW) degree. However, some also offer postgraduate degrees such as masters (MA, MSc, or MSW) or doctorates (PhD or DSW).

Despite the long history and importance of social service in the field of addiction, there is no uniform standard curriculum in addiction social worker education. Some states make recommendations and regulations regarding the training of social workers in the addiction field; however, no nationwide standards exist.

SUDs may be overlooked in many social worker training programs. In 1989, all Certificate of Qualification in Social Work (CQSW) courses in the British Isles were included in a survey of the training offered to social work students on responding to psychoactive substance misuse (31). There was a 74% response rate. Eleven percent of the courses that responded provided no formal substance misuse training. Those that offered training provided a median of 8 hours, with over 70% of students receiving less than 11 hours, indicating that many students were being given the briefest of overviews. Outside of four or five centers of excellence, social workers received less than the recommended amount of preparation to work with people with alcohol- and drug-related problems, despite evidence that these patients account for a large and growing proportion of their caseloads.

Social workers may receive little training in addiction in the United States as well. In 2000, the results by Hall et al. (32) of an assessment of the substance abuse treatment training needs of social workers working in randomly selected substance abuse treatment facilities in New England revealed that clinical supervision related to substance abuse treatment had not been available to a significant percentage of the respondents throughout their careers. Despite limited previous training experience and considerable barriers to current training, social workers surveyed in this study reported considerable interest in additional substance abuse treatment training.

In 2006, Smith et al. (33) studied the results of the first Practice Research Network (PRN) survey conducted by the National Association of Social Workers, a collaborative project funded by the Center for Substance Abuse Treatment. The objectives of the PRN survey were to develop broad knowledge about social work practices and more specific knowledge about social workers' involvement with substance abuse services. Although 71% of the employed social workers reported taking some action related to substance abuse diagnosis and treatment in the preceding 12 months, 53% reported receiving no training in substance abuse during the same period. More than 25% of the clients seen by the sample were reported to have either a primary or a secondary SUD, yet only 2% of the respondents reported addictions as their primary practice area. The results of the survey indicate a need to further assess social workers' role in substance abuse services and to identify training opportunities for the profession.

Recent initiatives aim to increase interest in the field of addiction (34–37). Various organizations provide different programs available in several states. Interested social workers may take courses in addiction and substance use to obtain advances certification. These programs generally require graduate level education prior to enrollment.

The Department of Social Work at the University of North Dakota provides an Addiction Counselor Training Program sponsored by the North Dakota Board of Addiction Counseling Examiners. Students successfully completing the course of study, the clinical training requirements, and the licensure examination are eligible for licensing as addiction counselors in the State of North Dakota. Students are admitted to this training on two levels. The first level includes social work majors who also complete the minor in Chemical Use/Abuse Awareness (required courses for licensing in addiction counseling, or their equivalent) and the 9-month practicum in a certified addiction facility. Students must meet all requirements for a social work major in addition to the minor requirements and the addiction practicum requirement. This generally involves a 5-year program of study. The second level relates to graduate students in counseling who must meet the required graduate program of study, the required addiction courses, and the 9-month practicum (38).

The National Institute on Alcohol Abuse and Alcoholism (NIAAA) has developed a social worker training program for those seeking a career in the service of patients with alcohol and other SUDs. The program's main goals are to teach motivational interviewing skills in managing coordinated care systems and the techniques for assisting special populations.

Role and Scope of Practice

Social workers play a significant role in serving individuals with SUDs (39). The data suggest that adding social services to public sector programs significantly improves the treatment outcomes in addiction (40).

Professional social workers provide a variety of services that include case management (linking clients with agencies and programs that will meet their psychological needs), counseling, medical social work, human services management, social welfare policy analysis, policy and practice development, community organizing, advocacy, teaching (in schools of social work), and social science research. Other settings in which professional social workers are active include advocacy organizations, hospices, community health agencies, schools, international organizations, employee assistance, philanthropy, and the military. Social workers also assist in a number of therapeutic groups, playing a key role in the interdisciplinary management of individuals with SUDs.

COUNSELORS

Definition

A *licensed chemical dependency counselor* (L.C.D.C.) provides counseling and education for substance abuse problems, but may not diagnose or provide official treatment.

Education and Training Requirements

A high school diploma is usually required to work in this field. Counselors generally are trained on the job. Training programs vary in length from 6 weeks to 2 years. Some colleges also offer training programs for counselors. These programs usually last 2 years and include courses on the effects of alcohol and other drugs. Students may also learn crisis intervention—a way of handling emergency situations. Graduates are usually awarded an associate's degree. Students may also obtain certification from the National Board for Certified Counselors. For some positions, a bachelor's degree or higher in sociology, psychology, or a related field may be required. An increasing number of substance abuse counselors are obtaining master's degrees in mental health counseling.

OASAS-CASAC Credentialing

The New York State Office of Alcoholism and Substance Abuse (OASAS) offers CASAC (Credentialed Alcoholism and Substance Abuse Counselor certification), which is intended for individuals who provide alcoholism and substance abuse COUNSELING services in approved work settings.

In order to become certified as a CASAC, the individual must have specific ethical and competency, work experience, education, and training and pass the International Certification and Reciprocity Consortium/Alcohol Drug Abuse (ICRC/AODA) written examination. Furthermore, the individual must be at least 18 years old, have earned either a high school diploma or a General Equivalency Diploma (GED), have lived or worked in New York at least 51% of the time.

Evaluation of Competency and Ethical Conduct

The individual signs an affidavit to abide by the Canon of Ethical Principles and arranges to have three individuals complete an Evaluation of Competency and Ethical Conduct on his/her behalf. All evaluators must have direct knowledge of his/her work experience observed for a minimum of 6 months. One evaluator must be the individual's current clinical supervisor, one must be a CASAC or hold reciprocal-level credential issued by another member of the ICRC/AODA. The third evaluator must be a Qualified Health Professional with at least 1 year of experience in substance abuse treatment.

Work Experience

The individual must document a minimum of 6000 hours (approximately 3 years) of supervised, full-time equivalent experience in an approved work setting as a provider or supervisor of direct patient services. A minimum of 2000 hours must be paid. The work experience must have been obtained within 10 years prior to submission of application and include 18 consecutive months during the 5 years leading up to the application. The individual must have performed professional tasks including but not limited to, diagnostic assessment, evaluation, intervention, referral, substance abuse counseling in both individual and group setting. Furthermore, there is a need for a minimum weekly, on-site, and documented clinical supervision by a Qualified Health Professional; must include a minimum of 300 hours of supervised practical training in 12 core functions performed for a minimum of 10 hours, under the supervision of a Qualified Health Professional. OASAS strongly recommends the majority of your work experience be devoted to the practice of substance abuse counseling.

In addition, the following academic degree substitutions may be claimed toward satisfying the 6000 hour work experience requirement:

- A master's (or higher) degree in an approved Human Services field from an accredited college or institution may be substituted for the remaining 4000 hours of work experience, provided that the 2000 hours of paid work experience occurred within 5 years prior to submission of the application.
- A Bachelor's Degree in an approved Human Services field from an accredited college or institution may be substituted for 2000 hours of work experience. A maximum of 2000 hours of full-time equivalent voluntary or other

nonpaid work experience (including a formal internship or formal field placement) that occurred within 5 years prior to submission of the application may also be claimed, providing it involved appropriately supervised direct patient services in an approved work setting.

If an academic degree substitution is not being claimed toward satisfying the 6000 hour work experience requirement, a maximum of 2000 hours of full-time equivalent voluntary or other nonpaid work experience (including a formal internship or formal field placement) that occurred within 5 years prior to submission of the application may be claimed, providing it involved appropriately supervised direct patient services in an approved work setting. A formal internship or formal field placement may be claimed as work experience OR education and training, but not both. You should calculate the need to claim a formal internship or formal field placement as either work experience or education and training. Work experience claimed may not include any experience gained as part of, or required under, participation as a patient in a formal alcoholism and/or substance abuse treatment/aftercare program and/or plan.

Education and Training

The individual must document education and a total of 350 hours of training. The minimum requirements include hours ranging from 45 to 150 in Knowledge of Alcoholism and Substance Abuse; training with focus on Alcoholism and Substance Abuse Counseling, Assessment; Clinical Evaluation; Treatment Planning; Case Management; and Patient, Family and Community Education; and Professional and Ethical Responsibilities. All these must have occurred within 10 years prior to date of submission of the application. Long-distance learning is acceptable as long as the institution is OASAS approved. However, no more than 30 hours of training through participation in conferences by professional organizations is acceptable. A formal internship or formal field placement may be claimed as work experience or education and training based on the academic credit associated with completion, but not both. One should calculate the need to claim a formal internship or formal field placement as either work experience or education and training.

Addiction counselor students may obtain training and certification from the National Association of Addiction Counselor (NAADAC). NAADAC certifications vary by amount and type of clinical experience and are graded as follows: National Certified Addiction Counselor (NCAC) Level 1, NCAC Level 2, and Master Addiction Counselor (MAC). Other training exists in age-group specific areas (such as the Adolescent Specialist Endorsement) and spiritual-belief areas (Certificate in Spiritual Caregiving to Help Addicted Persons and Families).

The NCAC I certificate requires 6000 hours of supervised experience in counseling, current licensure as a counselor, and 270 hours of education in SUD counseling subjects. The NCAC II certificate requires a bachelor's degree in a subject emphasizing counseling, 10,000 hours of supervised experience, and 450 hours of education in SUD counseling. The MAC certificate requires a master's degree in an area emphasizing counseling, current state licensure, 6000 hours of supervised experience, and 500 hours of education in substance use topics.

California also provides a Training Institute for Addiction Counselors (TIAC). This provides training in addiction counseling to meet state requirements for certification in drug and alcohol counseling. Students completing the TIAC program will be prepared to apply for the Certified Alcohol and Drug Abuse Counselor (CADC) certification and others. This is a CAADAC and a CAADE Continued Education Unit (CEU) Provider (41).

Role and Scope of Practice

Substance abuse counselors help people who have problems related to alcohol and other drugs. They counsel patients with SUDs. Counselors also help the families, friends, and loved ones of patients.

Addiction counselors usually help with practical problems. For example, a counselor might help a former addicted person find a job. Counselors do not prescribe medicine or provide medical or psychological therapy. Doctors, psychologists, or social workers often supervise substance abuse counselors.

Some counselors work in halfway houses. Counselors may also work in outpatient clinics where people come in on a regular basis for treatment. Other counselors work in hospitals, treatment centers, or human service agencies. Sometimes counselors have personal histories of substance misuse and use their experiences to help others. Many counselors host group meetings to discuss the common complications involved in managing SUDs.

CONCLUSION AND FUTURE DIRECTION

Many disciplines serve within the substance use field; however, no standard/uniform curriculum, policies, or strategies exist to train professionals in the field of addiction. Fellowships and certification trainings are available; however, these programs do not necessarily follow any standard. These uncertain credentialing practices may contribute to the variable practice standards in addiction.

The APA has developed a nationwide certification program. This program assists clinical and research psychologists in pursuing advanced training in SUDs and research methods. Social workers commonly assist in the management of patients with SUDs. Not all social workers working in the addiction field have specialized training in addiction. Perhaps a standardized training program can be developed to provide more structured and nationally standardized addiction training for social workers during their undergraduate years. PA training in addiction is limited, although the potential for PA service in the field is large. As is common among physician-extenders, PAs usually gain experience in this field through their regular encounter with addiction population. The in-school training in addiction for PAs and the opportunities for postgraduate training could be expanded and standardized to prepare PAs to work in the addiction field. Some addiction counselors receive education and training; however, standards vary from state to state in credentialing. Some standardized certificates exist, but most counselors remain uncertified. Statewide or nationwide certification practices could ensure that addiction counselors receive adequate basic training in counseling before encountering individuals with SUDs.

The primary concern across all fields is that there is no requirement for addiction education prior to entering the field. There is a dearth of outcome data on the services these professionals provide, further complicating picture. Inefficient or potentially dangerous practices may continue within if most professionals remain without adequate training and education, and the field requires regulation and quality control measures. Considering the staggering social and economic costs of addiction and the great concern to society, increasing and developing other professionals' involvement could improve the effectiveness and decrease the cost of addiction treatment. Furthermore, ongoing patient supervision during acute and maintenance phases of treatment could be provided by well-trained nonphysician professionals. Developing standardized policies and training curriculum could improve the quality and contribution of these professionals to the field of addiction treatment.

REFERENCES

1. Rosenblatt RA, Andrilla CH, Curtin T, et al. Shortages of medical personnel at community health centers: implications for planned expansion. *JAMA*. 2006;295:1042–1049.
2. Addictions Treatment Center at the Seattle VAMC. U.S. Veteran Affairs Administration. Addictions Psychiatry Fellowship: Positions are available for Psychologists, Social Workers, Chaplains, and Nurses. Available at: http://www.uwpsychiatry.org/education/addiction_psychiatry.html and http://depts.washington.edu/adai/training/uwgrad.htm. Accessed on June 30, 2010.
3. The College of Professional Psychology. Certification for Licensed Psychologists in Substance Abuse Treatment. Available at: http://www.apapracticecentral.org/ce/courses/certificate-proficiency-guide.pdf. Accessed on June 30, 2010.
4. The College of Professional Psychology. APA Online. APA Practice Organization. Available at: http://www.apapracticecentral.org/ce/courses/certificate-proficiency-guide.pdf. Accessed on June 30, 2010.
5. Centre for Addiction and Mental Health (CAMH), University of Toronto. Fellowships, Internships & Post-Graduate Studies. Available at: http://www.camh.net/education/Fellowships_internships_postgraduate/index.html. Accessed on June 30, 2010.
6. Alcohol and Drug Addiction Treatment Center, Hazelden Foundation. Postdoctoral Psychology Fellowship. Available at: http://www.hazelden.org/web/public/postdoctoral.page. Accessed June 30, 2010.
7. Department of Psychology, Psychiatry and Behavioral Science Department of Medicine and Pharmacology. University of Washington School of Medicine. Psychology Training in Alcohol Research (PTAR) Fellowship; Postdoctoral Training in Molecular Pharmacology of Abused Drugs. Available at: http://www.uwpsychiatry.org/education/ptar.html and http://faculty.washington.edu/cchavkin/training.html. Accessed June 30, 2010.
8. United States Department of Labor. Bureau of Labor Statistics. *Occupational Outlook Handbook, 2008–09 Edition: Psychologist*. Available at: http://www.bls.gov/oco/ocos056.htm#training. Accessed June 30, 2010.
9. Washton AM. Why psychologist should know how to treat substance use disorder. *New Jersey Psychologist*, Spring, 2001. Washton, AM. *NYS Psychologist* (Jan. 2002); Vol. 14(1);9–13.
10. Miller WR, Brown SA. Why psychologists should treat alcohol and drug problems. *Am Psychol*. 1997;52:1269–1279.
11. Miller WR, Rollnick S. *Motivational Interviewing: Preparing People to Change Addictive Behavior*. New York, NY: Guilford Press; 1991.
12. Marlatt GA, Gordon JR. *Relapse Prevention*. New York, NY: Guilford Press; 1985.
13. Hester RK, Bien TH. Brief treatment. In Washton AM, ed. *Psychotherapy and Substance Abuse: A Practitioner's Handbook*. New York, NY: Guilford Press; 1995.
14. Denning P. *Practicing Harm Reduction Psychotherapy: An Alternative Approach to Addictions*. New York, NY: Guilford Press; 2000.
15. Pillon SC, Laranjeira RR. Formal education and nurses' attitudes towards alcohol and alcoholism in a Brazilian sample. *Sao Paulo Med J*. 2005;123:175–180.
16. McRee B, Babor TF, Church OM. *Instructor's Manual for Identifying Drug Abusers*. Project NEADA. Rockville, MD: US Department of Health and Human Services/NIDA/SAMHSA's National Clearinghouse for Alcohol and Drug Information; 2002.
17. Neagle MA, ed. *Substance Abuse Education in Nursing. Project SAEN*. vol. 1–3. New York, NY: National League for Nursing; 1993.
18. Jack L, ed. *Nursing Care Planning with the Addicted Client, Volumes I and 11*. Skokie, IL: National Nurses Society on Addictions; 1989–1990. Vol. I, 155pp.; Vol. II, 215pp.
19. Burns E, Thompson A, Ciccone J, eds. *An Addictions Curriculum for Nurses and Other Helping Professionals*. Columbus, OH: Ohio State University Press; 1991. Distributed by Springer Publishing Company.
20. Lock CA, Kaner E, Lamont S, et al. A qualitative study of nurses' attitudes and practices regarding brief alcohol intervention in primary health care. *J Adv Nurs*. 2002;39:333–342.
21. Mistral W, Velleman R. Are practice nurses an underused resource for managing patients having problems with illicit drugs? A survey of one health authority area in England. *J Subst Use*. 1999;4:82–87.
22. Happell B, Taylor C. In-service drug and alcohol education for generalist nurses: are they interested? *J Subst Use*. 2000;4(4):164–169.
23. Finnell DS. Certification in Addictions Nursing Promoting and Protecting the Health of the Public. April 27, 2002. Available at: http://www.intnsa.org/pdfs/intnsa-VHYjpC.pdf. Accessed June 30, 2010.
24. Cary AH. Certified Registered Nurses: results of the study of the certified workforce. *Am J Nurs*. 2001;101(1):44–52.
25. Brady C, Becker K, Brigham LE, et al. The case for mandatory certification. *J Nurs Adm*. 2001;31(10):466–467.
26. University of Washington School of Nursing. Graduate Training in Substance Abuse & Addiction Research. Nursing Research Training in Substance Abuse. Available at: http://www.son.washington.edu/departments/pch/training.asp. Accessed June 30, 2010.
27. Roose RJ, Kunins HV, Sohler NL, et al. Nurse practitioner and physician assistant interest in prescribing buprenorphine. *J Subst Abuse Treat*. 2008;34:456–459.

28. American Academy of Physician Assistants. Education and Certification. Available at: http://www.aapa.org/. Accessed June 30, 2010.
29. Society of Physician Assistants in Addiction Medicine. Retrieved 6/16/09, 2009, from http://www.spaam.net/. Accessed June 30, 2010.
30. American Academy of Physician Assistants. Available at: http://www.psychpa.com/. Accessed June 30, 2010.
31. Harrison L. Substance misuse and social work qualifying training in the British Isles: a survey of CQSW courses. *Addiction*. 2006;87:635–642.
32. Hall MN, Amodeo M, Shaffer HJ, et al. Social workers employed in substance abuse treatment agencies: a training needs assessment. *Soc Work*. 2000;45:141–155.
33. Smith MJ, Whitaker T, Weismiller T. Social workers in the substance abuse treatment field: a snapshot of service activities. *Health Soc Work*. 2006;31:109–115.
34. Stein JB. Attitudes of social work students about substance abuse: can a brief educational program make a difference? *J Soc Work Pract Addict*. 2003;3:77–90.
35. Kranz KM. Development of the alcohol and other drug self-efficacy scale. *Res Soc Work Pract*. 2003;13:724–741.
36. Mullen EJ, Bledsoe SE, Bellamy JL. Implementing evidence-based social work practice. *Res Soc Work Pract*. 2008;18(4):325–338.
37. Amodeo M, Litchfield L. Integrating substance abuse content into social work courses: effects of intensive faculty training. *Subst Abuse*. 1999;20:5–16.
38. University of North Dakota. Addiction Counselor Training Program. Available at: http://www.und.edu/dept/socialwo/html/bssw.html#addictioncounselor. Accessed June 30, 2010.
39. Straussner, SLA. The role of social workers in the treatment of addictions. *J Soc Work Pract Addict*. 2001;1(1):3–9.
40. Mclellan AT, Hagan TA, Levine M, et al. Supplemental social services improve outcomes in public addiction treatment. *Addiction*. 2002;93:1489–1499.
41. Training Institute for Addiction Counselors (TIAC). Family Intervention Center & Services. Available at: http://www.addictioncounselors.org/. Accessed June 30, 2010.

SECTION 12 — POLICY ISSUES

CHAPTER 77: Drug Policy: A Biological Science Perspective

Robert L. DuPont ■ Bertha K. Madras ■ Per Johansson

INTRODUCTION

Drug policy is often politicized, sometimes passionately. This reflects the fact that drug use can be interpreted as derivative of other contentious issues, from poverty and racism to mental illness and crime. Moreover, the phrase *the war on drugs* can be seen as a dehumanizing assault on drug users. The reality is simpler. The root of the drug problem is found in the human brain, specifically the brain's reward centers that control behavior. Humans, in a relentless exploration of our environments, have discovered—and more recently invented—a variety of chemicals that hijack the brain's reward system, thus *rewarding* drug-taking behavior. The negative behavioral consequences of drug use—including intoxication and addiction—are collateral damage from the powerful brain reward that results from the use of these chemicals.

The goal of drug policy is to limit drug use and the damage to individuals and society from the negative effects of drug use by taking actions that recognize the serious consequences of drug use while remaining consistent with the society's values and laws. The drug policy debate is how best to achieve this goal. Although drug addiction is rooted in biology, the drug problem reflects a wide range of issues from economic to cultural, all of which determine the level of exposure of people to drugs and the environments in which they make decisions to use or not to use them. There are few issues more complex and fascinating than drug policy, and not many that are more important to human health and welfare.

A *policy* is a course of action selected from among alternatives to guide present and future decisions regarding goals and procedures. Public policy usually refers to government actions, and in particular plans at the highest level of government. Policy is closely related to politics which also focuses on the actions of governments but often on issues of broader impact than specific policies. Most drug policy issues are not captured by partisan politics but a few are, if only briefly. For example, it is not easy to define a Democratic or a Republican drug abuse policy, nor is it possible to identify methadone maintenance or Alcoholics Anonymous as liberal or conservative. Nevertheless when drug issues come up in legislatures, partisan conflicts are often evident. Rather than seeing drug policies as consistently partisan it is more accurate to note that parties in a democracy often disagree. The positions of the two parties in the United States on drug policies are often more easily distinguished by which party is in power than by which one is conservative or liberal.

When considering drug policies the question is not only, what is a policy, but also, what is a *drug*? In this chapter, we define a drug as a dependence-producing illegal drug of abuse, or the nonmedical sale or use of a legal dependence-producing drug, such as oxycodone. The focus on brain reward which is at the heart of the modern science of drug abuse has identified a wide range of behaviors and substances that produce brain reward. This perspective leads to a wider definition of a drug including not only alcohol and tobacco but also addicting behaviors such as gambling, playing video games, and unhealthy eating (1). In this chapter, we stick to the most restrictive definition of a drug, namely dependence-producing drugs—which mostly means *controlled substances* listed in the Controlled Substances Act as administered by the Food and Drug Administration (FDA) and the Drug Enforcement Administration (DEA). In short, this definition means illegal drugs used nonmedically, such as smoking marijuana, snorting cocaine, shooting heroin, or illegally using a prescribed controlled substance such as an opiate, stimulant, or sedative-hypnotic.

In response to the dramatic increase in heroin addiction, the drug policy response resulted in the approval of methadone as a treatment for heroin addiction in December 1972 (37 FR 26790) by the FDA and the DEA. This approval became effective in March 1973 (2). In 1987, another policy decision created more severe criminal penalties for crack cocaine compared to powdered cocaine in response to the emergent crack epidemic. An even larger drug policy decision came in 1971 when for the first time the federal government made massive investments in treatment, prevention, and research on a level similar to the investments in law enforcement that had characterized the federal government's approach to drug policy for the previous half century (3).

Drug policy is sometimes debated in the mass media and may engage the political processes, as did these three policies. Many drug policies can be considered as either relatively permissive of drug use or relatively restrictive (4).

Drug abuse is the only health issue, and one of few problems of any kind, to which a White House Office is devoted. The United States federal government has had a White House *drug czar* since June 17, 1971 when President Richard M. Nixon appointed research psychiatrist, Jerome H. Jaffe as the nation's first drug czar and declared drug abuse to be the nation's *public enemy number one*. Each year since 1973 this office has published a National Strategy detailing the government's drug policies. Since 1988 the White House drug office has been called the Office of National Drug Control Policy (ONDCP) making clear in its name that this agency leads the federal government's drug policy. Year-in and year-out Congress has supported retaining the White House drug policy office with its director held responsible for the Executive Branch's multifaceted drug control efforts (5).

Over the past four decades, 12 separate drug czars have served 8 presidents. These drug czars all have testified at hearings held by the United States House of Representatives and the United States Senate. Both of these houses of Congress have changed hands between political parties many times over these decades. While there have been a few truly partisan disputes, the drug policies of the federal government have evolved with striking stability and bipartisanship over this prolonged period of time. In this chapter, we explore why drug abuse policy has occupied this uniquely prominent position in the federal government and what the major evolving drug policies have been. To better inform drug policy decisions, the federal government's investment in research has created the explosive increase in understanding of the biology of brain reward, the biology that creates the public health and public safety consequences of drug use.

Sometimes, both in the United States and around the world, the high priority given over the last four decades to policies dealing with illegal drugs is criticized as misguided. To understand why drug abuse has sustained a unique position of prominence in the public policy debate of recent decades, it is helpful to understand why the modern drug abuse epidemic is different from the ancient use of these same substances. It has been argued that drug use is both old, and relatively trivial, and that the intense focus on drug policy in recent decades is *A Signal of Misunderstanding*, the title of the 1972 initial report of the National Commission on Marijuana. The Commission's second, and final, report in 1973 was titled *Drug Use in America: Problem in Perspective* to show that the Commission thought the politicians, and the voting public, did not have the drug problem "in perspective" (6,7).

Both within the domestic policy debate in the United States and in the world there are abundant and enduring policy conflicts. Many commentaries on drug policy have failed to recognize that the modern drug abuse epidemic is profoundly different from earlier skirmishes. Four characteristics distinguish the modern drug abuse epidemic even though many of the drugs themselves are truly ancient (8–10).

First, the modern drug abuse epidemic is not limited to the oral route of administration. For example, smoked cocaine is not to be confused with chewing coca leaves. Smoked marijuana is not similar to the earlier cannabis remedies that were low dose oral preparations. Even smoking opium, a terrible health problem which first emerged in the 16th century when smoking was introduced as a route of drug administration with the introduction of tobacco outside the Western hemisphere, is not comparable to intravenous heroin use. To make this same point with another old drug, it was the invention of the cigarette at the end of the 19th century that created a health crisis as a result of tobacco use. Changing the route of administration and the dose profoundly changed the health consequences of nicotine, just as shifting from snorting to smoking changed the health consequences of cocaine use in the late 1980s. The preferred routes of administration of modern drug users are smoking, snorting, and intravenous injection, all of which produce dramatically enhanced brain reward. It is no accident that once adopted, these new routes of administration become the preferred methods of illegal drug use. New brain science has shown that these routes of administration produce far more intense brain reward than do the old methods that fail to deliver rapidly rising high levels of drugs to the brain.

Secondly, the modern drug epidemic involves multiple, often simultaneous drug use often at far higher doses than did the earlier, single use of some of these same drugs. Third, for the most part in earlier exposures to drugs, the drug-using populations were relatively small segments of total populations. Today drug use involves large populations exposed to a wide range of potent drugs by intensely rewarding routes of administration. Fourth, the modern drug epidemic is characterized by initiation to drug use at very young ages when the human brain is especially vulnerable to addiction.

Not only are these four characteristics of drug use new in the world, but also there is a compounding factor in the growth of new sophisticated, globalized drug distribution networks. Moreover, the use of drugs of abuse, for example marijuana and heroin, has been justified by significant political and cultural movements as consciousness expansion, self-medication, and as a legitimate legally protected expression of individual choice. The modern drug epidemic, as new as the computer, is continuing to evolve. This evolution, facilitated by the Internet and increasingly sophisticated and globalized drug trafficking, is moving toward higher doses and wider access to drugs.

This new epidemic began in the United States and quickly became worldwide. Previously isolated cultures and peoples saw a dramatic shift in values with a decline in traditional controls over behavior and a correspondingly sharp increase in the perceived value of personal control over behavior and the importance of immediate pleasure. Delayed gratification, restraint, and traditional controls over behavior, whether from religion or law, became passé, especially for the young. The modern drug abuse epidemic first took hold in youth because young people are disproportionately affected by these changed values and because the adolescent brain is uniquely vulnerable to brain reward. While there remains much debate about the reasons for and the meaning of the cultural change that ushered in the world's modern drug abuse epidemic, one fact is clear: it occurred when the baby boom generation entered adolescence. Suddenly with this demographic shift, a heretofore stable cultural balance shifted as well (11). The baby boom was a global phenomenon, resulting from delayed fertility in the developed world due to first the great depression then to World War II, and in the developing world to the dramatic fall in infant mortality.

To understand the potential health impact of this epidemic of illegal drug use it is important to recognize the unprecedented investments that have been made over the past four decades in the United States and abroad to curtail illegal drug traffic and limit illegal drug use. In addition, powerful cultural forces have been marshaled to curb illegal drug use. As a result of these twin efforts, the current levels of illegal drug use have been kept relatively low. In contrast, alcohol and tobacco are relatively unrestricted legally and culturally, with resulting relatively high levels of use compared to the illegal drugs. In 2007, the most recent year for which data is available, there were 126.8 million Americans who drank alcohol in the prior 30 days (defined by epidemiologists as "current use"), 60.1 million who smoked cigarettes, and only 19.9 million who used any illegal drug (12). The social costs of either alcohol use ($166.5 billion) (13) or tobacco use ($193 billion) (14) alone exceed the social costs of all of the illegal drugs combined ($109.8 billion) (13). Another useful comparison is that in 2006, the number of illegal drug-induced deaths totaled 38,396 in the United States, while alcohol-induced deaths totaled 22,073 and tobacco-related deaths topped 400,000. The proportion of health-related costs is far greater for legal drugs and the criminal justice costs are far greater for illegal drugs. These data lead to an important policy conclusion: while making drugs illegal reduces the levels of use of those drugs and reduces resulting health costs, it increases criminal justice costs. However, making drugs illegal leads to smaller combined social costs. Regardless, the currently illegal drugs are today a major cause of preventable illness and death. The impact of the currently illegal drugs on the developing world is profound, and rapidly growing.

There are few public policy issues on which almost everyone has an opinion. Drug policy is one of those issues. In discussions about drug policy, sometimes heated and politically cast, the contrasting positions are often reduced to the simplest terms as either being pro- or antidrug. According to David Musto, an eminent historian of drug abuse, national and even global drug policy has swung between periods of permissiveness and restriction over the past century (4). Such simplification of often complex and finely nuanced policy conflicts is common in political discourse because complex issues need to be reduced to simple terms to be transmitted in the modern media and to find resonance in partisan politics. The same simplification—and regrettable but inevitable distortion—takes place in other significant public policy disputes for the same reasons.

The two poles of contemporary drug policy can be variously described. For example, the current United States *balanced policy* is made up of supply reduction (or law enforcement) and demand reduction (either prevention, treatment, or a combination of the two). This balanced policy can be described as a *restrictive drug policy*. The objective of a balanced and restrictive policy is the reduction of illegal drug use. When it is demeaned, it is usually called *prohibition* to conjure up the image of alcohol prohibition which is widely seen to have failed. In contrast to the balanced and restrictive policy, the other pole of drug policy can be called *harm reduction or a permissive* policy. A policy of harm reduction accepts illegal drug use as inevitable and seeks to reduce the "harms" caused both by drug use and by the policies designed to reduce drug use (especially those involving the criminal justice system). In reality most drug policies have features of both approaches and many serious issues (such as setting the legal drinking age for alcohol at 18 or 21, or establishing parity for substance abuse treatment) are not easily characterized in this politicized and caricatured drug policy dichotomy (15).

Influencing drug policy, which many people want to do, is a bit like trying to change the direction of a slow-moving aircraft carrier by nudging it with a rowboat. While no single rowboat can have any measurable effect there is no doubt that millions of rowboats can nudge the biggest aircraft carriers. From time to time the change of course of major national drug abuse policy is dramatic and sudden. As an example, the course of American drug policy took a dramatic new turn in the early 1970s when the national drug policy which had been focused almost exclusively on law enforcement for half a century was suddenly balanced by a huge new investment in treatment, research, prevention, and training (3). This policy change balanced traditional supply reduction by a similar-sized investment in demand reduction.

To have an impact on national or even local drug policies, first it is necessary to team up with lots of other rowboats to do the nudging. Second, it is easier to slightly change the direction of the moving aircraft carrier than it is to start it moving in an entirely new direction. So, as practical steps, drug policy advocates need to find individuals and organizations that share their views. They are most likely to have success when they are able to catch a strong policy momentum that is either growing or already established on specific drug policies.

A good place to start learning about drug policy is the annual report of the ONDCP which can be found on its web site http://www.whitehousedrugpolicy.gov. Good resources also can be found on the web sites of nongovernmental organizations (NGOs) dealing with substance abuse problems. An example of an NGO is the American Society of Addiction Medicine (http://www.asam.org) with 165 published policy positions on its web site ranging from statements on underage drinking to drugged driving and from parity to buprenorphine. Most other organizations in the substance abuse field take active positions to influence drug policy that often focus on areas of their own self-interest, for example supporting greater funding for their activities. But all organizations also focus on less obviously self-interested aspects of drug policy. (For a recent scholarly review of drug policy see *An Analytic Assessment of US Drug Policy* by David Boyum and Peter Reuter.) (16).

With this overview in mind, we turn to a review of the history of drug policy initially in the context of an earlier drug epidemic in the United States at the end of the 19th century and the response to it both in the United States and around the world. We then look at the modern epidemic and the major drug policies of the past four decades.

Following that discussion, the chapter next explores the science of drug abuse and the central place of brain reward in this story, looking closely at lessons that can be taken from rapidly evolving and very promising research to inform drug policy.

Following after the information about brain science and policy, the chapter describes the public health and safety dimensions of drug policy from an international perspective.

The chapter concludes with a description of the major drug policy issues facing the United States and other countries today, and speculates about issues likely to be confronted in the decades ahead.

THE CONTEXT OF DRUG POLICY

While drug policy, like drug use, can be traced back to the beginning of history when alcohol use already was widespread, the modern era of drug policy started in the 19th century when the chemicals responsible for drug effects were first identified and when injection became an available route of administration. Although global distribution of drugs was a factor for centuries, in the 19th century the global supply of all commodities, including the drugs that are now illegal, become far more common. By the end of the 19th century there was a significant drug epidemic in the United States and in some other areas of the world, especially in Asia where opium consumption had created havoc ever since the Opium War in 1842. As a result of losing that war China was forced, along with other Asian countries, to open their markets to opium brought mostly from India by the British. Compounding world drug problems, in 1898 the Bayer Company introduced a semisynthetic opiate, heroin, to the global market as a cough medicine. It was especially popular in that era because of the high prevalence of tuberculosis. This was the era in which patent medicines in the United States often contained alcohol, morphine, and cocaine and when a popular soft drink introduced in a pharmacy in Atlanta adopted the trade name "Coke" to make unmistakable the origin of its stimulating effects.

Most of these preparations, including Coca-Cola, were sold with medicinal claims. In reaction to this open market in what now are known to be addicting drugs, there was a powerful grassroots progressive backlash that urged new legislation to restrict access to these substances. The first of several laws passed during this infant era of modern drug policy, the Food and Drug Act of 1906, did not prohibit the sale of these drugs but required them to be clearly labeled. The next legislation was the Harrison Narcotics Act of 1914 which restricted the use of opiates through the federal government's power of taxation. In 1919, using a similar mechanism to restrict the sale of alcohol, the Volstead Act, also known as the *18th amendment*, became law. These laws were not only bipartisan but they were central parts of the agenda of the then triumphant progressive era. From a drug policy perspective, it is important to recognize that these were all restrictive laws.

They all were passed in response to the rapidly escalating and serious problems created by the open market in addicting drugs.

This progressive movement's focus on addicting drugs was not limited to domestic policy within the United States. In 1909, the Shanghai Conference targeted the global opium trade by invoking international cooperation. The United States played a key role at this international meeting. It brought to the table experience with its polyglot population made up of immigrants with drug-using habits from every part of the globe, its distinctive culture and laws that promoted individual freedom and limited government interventions on behavior, and its recent legislative measures restricting the availability of abused substances.

These events, in this first drug abuse epidemic, are well described in many fascinating histories of drug abuse and drug policy (4,8–10,17,18). Even in this short review it is important to notice the origins and characteristics of the responses to this epidemic. While there was little government investment in treatment during that time, William White has shown that in the early years of the 20th century there were significant nongovernmental developments in substance abuse treatment even though they were small by comparison with what was to follow half a century later (19).

The initial law enforcement effort to restrict access to drugs of abuse was backed by the strong support of large majorities in the United States. At the time there were few voices from any part of the political spectrum raised to support drug use or individual rights to use drugs, including privacy rights. These early efforts to contain drug abuse with near exclusive reliance on law enforcement were remarkably effective, but not without problems. They did not end drug or alcohol use although from today's perspective it is remarkable how successful they were in reducing drug use and reducing the negative consequences of that use—despite their modest size.

Following these events, there was a flurry of interest in what happened to the drug addicts themselves, leading in 1925 to Congressional hearings and ultimately in 1935 to the first investment of the federal government in what would today be called *demand reduction*—the science of addiction and treatment of addicted individuals. The Narcotics Farm and later the Addiction Research Center (ARC) in Lexington Kentucky were born, the organizations that would later spawn both the National Institute for Mental Health (NIMH) in 1946 and the National Institute on Drug Abuse (NIDA) in 1973.

In the first half of the 20th century, some voices were raised against the government's balanced and restrictive drug policy. Some concerns were heard from the medical community, but the medical establishment, led by the American Medical Association, was strongly supportive of this approach. The results spoke for themselves as these decades were remarkable for a generally low level of drug and alcohol use (20). In contrast to the continuing support for restrictive drug laws, the 18th amendment to the Constitution was repealed in the 21st amendment as one of the first acts of economic stimulation by Franklin Roosevelt in 1933. Prohibition of alcohol sale was the only Constitutional amendment to be repealed. President Roosevelt explained his dramatic action mainly as an effort to promote jobs in the alcohol industry but also as a way of helping working people cope with the suffering of the depression. The rationale of curbing organized crime was later offered as a significant factor, but in 1933 this was far down the list of reasons for repeal. While repeal did deprive organized crime of one source of revenue, few claimed in the 1930s that the repeal of alcohol prohibition reduced the serious threats posed by organized crime.

Prohibition dramatically reduced drinking and many of the most serious effects of excessive drinking (21). Nevertheless as the years went by the support for alcohol prohibition waned until the Depression shifted the political balance in favor of repeal. After the end of alcohol prohibition, the *per capita* consumption of alcohol in the United States rose steadily from the lowest levels in the nation's history during prohibition until the mid-1980s. Since that time it has declined modestly. The highest level of *per capita* consumption of alcohol occurred in the early years of the 19th century, creating the push for prohibition which by the later half of the 19th century had become one of the three major popular movements in the country. (The others were the abolition of slavery and women's suffrage.) Today few people know that in the 19th century, the *temperance movement* attracted more support than either of the other two big policy ideas or that Maine in 1851 was the first state to prohibit alcohol. By the time the 18th Amendment became federal law, most states were already *dry*. When alcohol prohibition in the United States ended in 1933, there was no interest in removing the restrictive laws on illegal drugs.

The second drug epidemic in the United States, the modern drug abuse epidemic, began with an increase in illegal drug use that had incubated in the late 1940s and throughout the 1950s only to spring to life as a major national threat to public health and public safety in the late 1960s.

In 1962, only 4% of Americans 18 to 25 years old had ever used an illegal drug. That number rose to a peak of 68% in 1979. That is evidence of the massive impact of the modern drug abuse epidemic. Since that time the levels of illegal drug use have changed profoundly over relatively short periods of time. This is in contrast to the smoother, more consistent trend lines showing the use of alcohol and tobacco, both of which have declined from recent peaks and show signs of continuing to do so, with drops in alcohol use being much more modest than those of tobacco in recent decades.

Figure 77.1 shows the national rates of use of marijuana over the past three decades for students in the 8th, 10th, and 12th grades. While data on individual drugs show some variability, over this long period of time marijuana has remained the most commonly used illegal drug. Most other illegal drugs have shown trends similar to those shown here for marijuana. The dramatic escalation of illegal drug use that started in the mid-1960s peaked in 1978 when the highest levels of illegal drug use in the United States were recorded. Between 1973 and 1978, ten states signaled a change in drug policy when they *decriminalized* marijuana. This drug policy activity was associated with the more permissive side of the drug policy debate. The long decline in illegal drug use between 1978 and 1991 was widely attributed to the impact of the *Parents Movement* and other efforts to restrict drug use, all of which were clearly reactions to the dramatic increase in drug use in the prior decade. After 1978 no state decriminalized marijuana and two states rescinded their earlier decriminalization efforts.

Both the rise in drug use from the 1960s to 1978 and the subsequent drop from that high point to the low in 1991 cannot be explained by changes in brain biology or any change in the drugs that generally were in use during those years. Instead these changes are most plausibly explained by shifts in the environment in which drugs and human brains come in contact. The upsurge in illegal drug use was the result of an

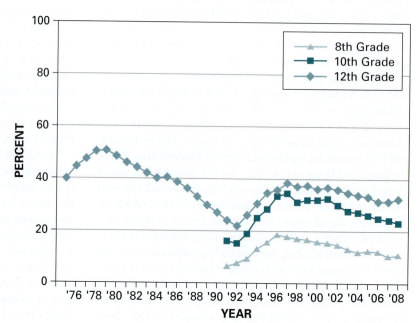

Figure 77.1. Marijuana: trends in annual use, grades 8, 10, and 12. Percentage who used in the last 12 months. (Data from Johnston LD, O'Malley PM, Bachman JG, et al. *Teen Marijuana Use Tilts Up, While Some Drugs Decline in Use*. Ann Arbor, MI: University of Michigan News Service; 2009. Retrieved 04/27/2010 from http://www.monitoringthefuture.org.)

attitude of permissiveness and even a widespread appreciation for the positive effects of illegal drugs, especially marijuana and the hallucinogens. The subsequent fall in national levels of illegal drug use is explained by the widespread counterreaction to this sharp rise. In both cases marijuana use and perceptions regarding that use were at the center of the trends. This is clearly seen in the data from Monitoring the Future (22) which has shown the inverse relationship between perceived risk and drug use: The more the perceived risk the less the use, the less the perceived risk the more the use. On the other hand perceived availability showed a less dramatic correlation with levels of marijuana use over time.

Since 1991 the battles over drug policy have intensified. The critics of the balanced and restrictive strategy of national drug policy received an infusion of new funding in the early 1990s, fueling a resurgence of the debate. This debate over drug policy had been largely muted if not absent from 1978 to 1991, the era of declining drug use. The renewed battlegrounds include medical marijuana, needle exchange programs, and the cultivation of hemp on the one hand and random student drug testing and tough enforcement of drugged driving laws on the other. Central to this drug policy debate have been issues such as the health risks versus the safety of marijuana use and the role of the criminal justice system. This critique of the restrictive drug policy has been widely labeled *reform*, a word that has become a code word for the more permissive drug policies of harm reduction.

While Figure 77.1 shows the trends in marijuana use over recent decades, with the current level far below the peak level in 1979, note in Figure 77.2 that the drug overdose deaths have shown no decline over that time. Instead the drug-related deaths indicate a dramatic and continuing escalation. How can those two trends be rationalized? Why does drug use show powerful changes over relatively short periods of time while deaths show a steady escalation? This is one of the many mysteries of current drug epidemiology, mysteries that are important for the development of better drug policies (23).

Figure 77.1 suggests that the balanced drug policies have contained the use of illegal drugs and that the level of use of illegal drugs in the United States has declined since the peak in 1978. In contrast, Figure 77.2 implies that the illegal drug problem is continuing to escalate.

One of the foci of political discussions of drug policy is the role of the criminal justice system. Critics of the current balanced and restrictive strategy of drug abuse prevention contend that law enforcement is abusive, counterproductive, and not *evidence based*. Supporters of the current balanced policies are more likely to defend the role of the criminal justice system. Similarly, critics of current balanced drug policies point to evidence that *the war on drugs* has failed, while defenders of this policy see progress in drug prevention. In sorting out these conflicting views it is helpful to ask, "compared to what?" As stated earlier in this chapter, the criminal justice costs of illegal drugs exceed the criminal justice costs of alcohol and tobacco, for example but the health costs of alcohol and tobacco (and their rates of use) are far larger than the costs of all the illegal drugs combined. What would be the potential rate of use of the currently illegal drugs if they were legalized? Opponents of current policies generally perceive the United States to be saturated already with drug availability and doubt there would be an increase in use if the drugs were legalized. Supporters of the current policies expect increases in use of the currently illegal drugs to levels now seen for alcohol and tobacco were these drugs to be legalized. Many critics of current policies focus only on the criminal justice costs of the currently illegal drugs ignoring the health and other social costs related to their use, while supporters of current policies are more apt to emphasize these costs. As an example, they point to the vastly larger health costs from the currently legal drugs, alcohol, and tobacco.

An ominous new trend in drug use confounds many of these formerly common policy conflicts. The rise in the abuse of prescription drugs such as oxycodone (OxyContin), alprazolam (Xanax), and dextroamphetamine (Adderall) has

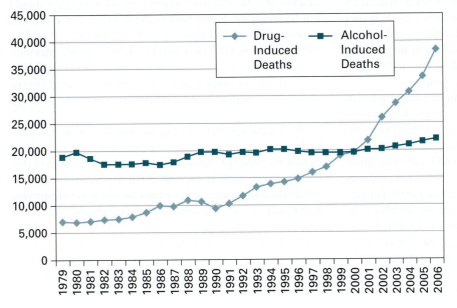

Figure 77.2. Drug- and alcohol-induced deaths, 1979–2006. (Data from CDC National Vital Statistics Report, Vol. 58, No. 14.)

provided useful evidence about the fundamental nature of the public health problems of drug abuse and addiction. Since 2005 more Americans have first used a prescription opiate nonmedically each year than have first used marijuana, the most popular of the illegal drugs. There now is more death in the United States from the nonmedical use of prescribed opiates than from heroin and cocaine combined. These tough facts impact the drug policy debate. In prescription drug abuse, there is no Mafia and no actively enforced prohibition. Instead the vast majority of the prescription drug supply flows directly from physician prescriptions to medical patients at which point they are diverted and/or used in a nonmedical pattern of abuse. The old-fashioned debates on drug policy are moot when it comes to this growing problem, a problem that leads back to the brain and the uniquely powerful reinforcing effect of these drugs, whatever their source. The recent dramatic rise in prescription drug abuse not only reflects the huge increase in the use of controlled substances in medical treatments over the past decade (and thus the increasing availability of these drugs), but it also shifts the policy picture from a focus on global drug traffic as the force driving drug use to a focus on the role of a unique group of chemicals in brain reward. Prescription drug abuse is pushing the perspective back to brain biology as the fundamental problem to be addressed by future drug policies.

A valuable, and often overlooked, source of evidence that can inform drug policy is found in the common experiences of families confronting drug problems. Just as whole societies are often taken aback by drug problems and come to recognize them long after they are firmly entrenched, so it is with most families. Drug addiction has two salient features. The first is dishonesty. Most drug users hide their use from those who care about them, and they lie about it if confronted. Moreover, the drug user does not want to stop using. The second characteristic feature of drug use is its continuation despite the serious and even devastating problems flowing from it. Such paradoxical behavior can be compared to that of an abusive love affair. In this case, the lover is the drug in the user's brain. Those associated with the addicted individual try to discourage return to the chemical lover but the drug user repeatedly believes the next time will be different and will not lead to painful consequences. The distortion in the thinking of the drug-dependent person is striking. This individual's brain has been hijacked by the chemical lover.

Many families reluctantly emerge from a long period of not knowing about the drug use to face the problem initially with compassion and love, expressed by tolerant behaviors that are widely seen in the drug treatment community to be *enabling*. Only when this initial approach fails do most families turn to *tough love*. Tough love is characterized by determined efforts to make continued participation in the benefits of the family conditional on stopping drug use, sometimes by getting into and sticking with substance abuse treatment. The seductive pull of the chemical lover is intense. The challenge of recovery is great. But with help, and often that includes the 12-step programs of Alcoholics Anonymous and Narcotics Anonymous, it can be achieved and maintained. This is a joyous outcome for all involved. Addiction is modern, chemical slavery. Recovery is emancipation (24).

Analogous to this common experience, communities and entire nations confront the problems flowing from nonmedical drug use first with denial, then with enabling, and typically only belatedly with tough love. It is vital to maintain compassion and respect in the context of such a struggle.

THE SCIENCE OF DRUG USE AND ADDICTION

The Magnitude of the Public Health Problem

The brain science of addiction is rooted in public health. Individuals, families, societies, and nations bear a heavy burden from the use of drugs for nonmedical purposes. Potentially life-changing consequences range from accidents, trauma, compromised health, cognition and education, unplanned pregnancies, failure to meet commitments, high job turnover, psychotic reactions, and drug-induced violence. The devastating end point of nonmedical drug use—addiction—has the dubious distinction of being among the leading causes of preventable deaths and chronic illness during the prime of life, and among the most prevalent, most costly, and deadliest of neuropsychiatric disorders (23,25). In the United States, over 22 million people (8.9% of the population over 12 years) are estimated to harbor a medical diagnosis of alcohol or illicit drug abuse/addiction (26). More than double this number (estimated at 46 million) are engaged in risky, problematic alcohol, and other drug use and are at risk for addiction with medical, psychiatric, social, and emotional consequences of substance abuse (27). An emerging concern is the blurred boundaries between illicit and prescription drug abuse. Prescription drug abuse now ranks second, after marijuana in number of users, first among new initiates of drug use (numerically, but not statistically), second among those dependent on illicit drugs, and first among causes of drug-related deaths (26).

Advocates for decriminalization or legalization of drugs frequently argue that as a victimless activity, drug use should not be regulated. Numerous medical, social, and economic reasons argue against this stance. Consider that 8.3 million children (11.9% of all children) live in the United States with at least one parent who is dependent on, or abuses alcohol or an illicit drug during the past year, with an estimated 70% of child abuse/neglect cases involving parental use of drugs (28,29).

Biological research of drug use and addiction has clarified specific events that can compromise the function of our brains, the repository of our humanity. We have learned that certain drugs, such as cocaine, methamphetamine, ecstasy, inhalants, and alcohol, can be toxic to the brain, destroying nerve cells or nerve endings and interrupting normal blood supply (30,31). Even without inducing frank toxicity, drugs can promulgate adaptive changes in cell structure, metabolism, brain signals, and circuitry, leading to behavior consistent with addiction (31–33). As addiction sets in, survival behaviors (waking up, washing, eating, dressing, attending work or school, and focusing on personal and work commitments and goals) become secondary, as the brain increasingly focuses on a narrow set of compulsive, uncontrollable goals—to seek and consume drugs despite adverse consequences. The addicted brain converts normal behavior into a drug-centered existence. Those motivated to become and sustain abstinence can endure drug cravings months or years after withdrawal symptoms have ceased, cravings that can trigger relapse at vulnerable periods. A number of treatment approaches (cognitive–behavioral therapy, medication-assisted therapy) effectively assist people in overriding these biological changes (34).

The biological science of drug use and addiction provides an essential framework for shaping clinical, social policies and programs for prevention, intervention, and treatment. Yet, biological understanding is a daunting quest: how can a simple ingested chemical imprint itself on the brain, create sensations that surpass, suppress, or supplant natural rewards, transform personality, and usurp the pursuit of fundamental human priorities: survival, food, safety, shelter, family, and health? What brain systems does it invade? What brain systems does it change? How does this chemical enable the addicted brain to tolerate doses that, in a drug-naive person, would be lethal? How can a simple molecule leave such a strong imprint on the brain and body that when it clears the system dysphoria or severe withdrawal symptoms surface? How can drug craving reoccur years after the last dose of the drug? These questions drive neuroscientists to create a biological roadmap, the starting point a simple chemical, the end points being hedonistic sensations, powerful memories, behavioral and personality changes, addiction, craving, and relapse. Within the triad of risk factors—the environment, the individual, and the drug—most environmental and individual factors cannot be faithfully replicated in preclinical laboratory settings as models and for further scrutiny at a molecular level. By and large, our knowledge relies on incomplete human studies using a paucity of noninvasive techniques, or imperfect animal research. Despite these limitations, evidence-based risk factors and the underlying biology that influence the behavioral trajectories of new drug initiates and susceptibility to addiction are increasingly understood.

Risk Factors: The Environment

Chaotic homes with ineffective parents, inadequate bonding with parents, parent or sibling drug use or acceptance of drug use as a rite of passage, stress, sexual and physical abuse, posttraumatic stress disorder, the need for social acceptability, peer pressure, initiation of alcohol and smoking, and the media are all recognized as risk factors for initiation and sustaining drug use. Public misinformation or no information on the physical and mental health risks of specific drugs (e.g., prescription drugs are harmless or safer than street drugs) is another risk factor, highlighting the need to survey the knowledge base of the public and address these voids. Countering these influences are unequivocal negative attitudes and stances on drugs conveyed by parents and communities. Other factors countering the pressure to use drugs are views of friends, schools, religious authorities, the media, affiliations and participation in social and religious organizations, and laws enforced by the criminal justice system. Evidence-based risk factors need adequate representation in prevention programs.

Risk Factors: The Individual, Genetics

As with other neuropsychiatric disorders, certain individuals are more vulnerable to addiction, with genetic influences penetrating every dimension of human drug response. Strong evidence from family, twin, and adoption studies indicate that genetic and environmental factors play equally important roles in the development of addiction. For example, siblings of abusers are more likely to use drugs. Likewise, adopted children with histories of substance abuse in their biological families are more likely to become abusers themselves, even if the current environment is devoid of drugs. Identical twins have a higher propensity to share drug histories than fraternal twins, with a genetic component greater for drugs with higher addictive potential (e.g., heroin). It is now feasible to scan multiple genes at the same time—500,000 gene snippets (SNPs or single nucleotide polymorphisms) simultaneously—to seek genetic differences between nonaddicted and addicted populations. More than 100 candidate genes for addiction susceptibility have emerged from this approach, indicating that genetic influences are complex and arise, not as a result of a single anomaly, but of convergence of multiple genes. Genome-wide association studies reveal a complex polygenic (multiple genes) influence on addiction vulnerability, which distinguish addicts of different ethnicities from matched controls. Intriguingly, susceptibility genes overlap for different drugs (36). Scientists can infer from these findings that addictive processes are likely to converge on common molecular events and neural networks in the brain, even though the starting point of addiction, activation of diverse brain receptors is unique to each drug class. Molecular, anatomical, and brain imaging research lends credence to this model of "biological convergence of addictive processes" (see below). Prominent among susceptibility genes are those encoding cell adhesion molecules and other genes involved in learning, memory, and cognition, implying that memory/salience play a critical role in compulsive drug seeking and drug craving (35). Also, inherited traits for vulnerability to addiction are shared with other common heritable neuropsychiatric disorders (e.g., bipolar disorder, cognitive ability, Alzheimer disease). Accordingly, prevention, diagnosis, and treatment of addictions should be viewed in the context of the neuropsychiatric profile of people at risk for addiction. The promising genetic approach portends a future of genetically based personalized prevention and treatment approaches (35).

Other individual factors with high predictive value for drug abuse are psychiatric comorbidity, personality disorders, poor school performance, inappropriate school behavior, or early drug use. For those enduring posttraumatic stress disorder, anxiety and depression, drug use has been interpreted as a form of maladaptive chemical coping. Severe emotional shocks, such as child abuse, the death of a parent, or alcoholic or drug-addicted parents, can increase drug use. Age of onset of first drug use is the most significant risk factor for progressing to addiction, another important rationale for promoting prevention in youthful populations. All of these risk factors have one thing in common, they make individuals more willing to try drugs and they make individuals more willing to ignore the risks, and the warning of risks, from escalating drug use. In other words, these risk factors generally make individuals more vulnerable to the biology of brain reward which itself is ubiquitous in the human brain.

Risk Factors: The Developing Brain in the Adolescent

Adolescent drug use is a unique public health challenge, warranting aggressive prevention and intervention policies in this population: (a) age of onset of drug use is declining; (b) during adolescence, initiation of one drug accelerates the use of other drugs; (c) the younger the drug initiation, the higher the probability of progressing to addiction; (d) psychiatric symptoms are higher in adolescent users; (e) drug use is associated with risk-seeking behavior, delinquency, and criminal behavior; (f) adolescent drug use is associated with a higher likelihood of injury or death; (g) adolescent use is associated with lowered academic performance, absenteeism, higher school drop-out rates, gang membership, and later involvement in criminal behaviors.

Initiation of drug use is largely an adolescent phenomenon, with at least 60% of new initiates falling below the age of 18, and even a higher percentage for tobacco and alcohol use (26). Onset of prescription drug abuse is later and more likely to emerge in the third decade of life often in association with earlier use of alcohol and other drugs. Drug initiation during the early phase of adolescence, in contrast with adult onset of use, confers a much higher risk for developing addiction during adolescence or later in adulthood. Risk analyses demonstrate considerably higher rates of addiction with early onset of use of marijuana, cocaine, other psychostimulants (e.g., amphetamines), hallucinogens, opioids, inhalants, alcohol use, smoking, prescription drugs (stimulants, opioid analgesics, sedatives, tranquilizers, anxiolytics) (36–41). Progression to addiction is higher, if involvement with drugs occurs prior to 18 years of age (36,42,43). With each year of delay of onset of use, the likelihood of lifetime drug abuse and dependence is reduced significantly (36), and the odds of developing prescription drug abuse decreases 5% with each year of delay of nonmedical use (44).

The alarmingly high risk of the adolescent becoming addicted can be attributed to the underdeveloped adolescent brain which is uniquely vulnerable to addiction. The adolescent brain undergoes extensive linear (age-dependent) neurodevelopment, primarily in regions associated with motivation, impulsivity, and addiction (45). Brain regions that serve attention, reward evaluation, emotional responses, and goal-directed behaviors undergo structural and functional reorganization throughout late childhood and early adulthood (46–48). Magnetic resonance imaging of living brain reveals critical anatomical and functional changes in brain development, beginning in utero and *ending at age 24* (47,48). The most robust changes are a linear increase in white matter volume as a function of age, and peak increases in grey matter volume during late childhood or early adolescence. The back of the brain, evolutionarily the oldest part of brain, matures more quickly than the frontal cortex, the most recent addition to mammalian brain. The higher-order cortices, involved in decision-making, inhibiting impulses are developmentally immature in the adolescent compared with adult brains and reach adult form only after brain regions involved in interpreting sensory and visual stimuli are formed. This may account for the activities favored by adolescents, the sensory, physical, impulsive, risk-seeking over cognitive, impulse control, and executive functions of the adult brain. The later maturation of the prefrontal cortex is paralleled by increased abilities in abstract reasoning, attentional shifting, response inhibition, and processing speed (46).

At the cellular and molecular level, brain development is an exquisitely regulated progression of formation of circuits and connections. Consider that the brain contains over 100 billion nerve cells and each cell may have a few or more of 10,000 connections with other cells. With meticulous precision, a family of proteins designated axonal guidance molecules, steers the complex formation of neural circuits, some by lengthening, others by stopping or directing the wires (axons) that connect nerve cells. In the adult brain, these proteins also regulate neuroadaptive changes, by shaping the morphology of nerve cells (dendrites), modulating the strength of memory processing, and regulating the genesis of nerve cells. Drugs can modulate the expression of neurodevelopmental proteins in brain and in cell cultures, resulting in altered levels or ratios of expression (49,50). Conceivably, the introduction of drugs during adolescence, a period of rapid neurodevelopment, may change the concentrations of axon guidance molecules, modifying neural circuitry, signaling, and neurogenesis. These processes may alter the normal trajectory of adolescent brain development, leading to a much higher vulnerability to addiction.

Risk Factors: The Drug

Addictive drugs can elicit powerful, subjective responses, embedded in their unique chemistry and chemical formulation (e.g., salt, free base). The impact of the drug is partly engineered by the dose, dosing regimen, route of administration (intravenous, inhalation–smoking, insufflation, subcutaneous, oral), how fast it combines with its brain targets, and user response. Self-reports of "high" are greater when heroin or cocaine is administered intravenously compared with insufflation, potentially increasing the desire for more drug and heightening addictive potential (51).

Are some drugs more addictive than others? Overall, drugs directly targeting brain dopamine or opioid systems (e.g., cocaine, heroin) have higher addictive potential, progress from initial use to addiction. The prevalence of addiction among users of cocaine, heroin, amphetamines, or marijuana is higher than for 3,4-methylenedioxy-methamphetanine (MDMA), or inhalants (52). Higher still is the percent of smokers who manifest addictive symptoms, but this is a questionable comparison, as nicotine delivery systems are legal, inexpensive, socially acceptable in certain domains, and widely available. Predicting the relative addiction potential of drugs on an individual basis is even more daunting, considering the unique individual experiences of environment, genetics, and psychiatric comorbidity.

These variables are of minimal significance in a homogeneous population of laboratory animals matched for genetic backgrounds, environment, and stress levels. Animals self-administer all the same drugs that humans compulsively seek, including marijuana, cocaine, heroin, ecstasy (MDMA), amphetamine, methamphetamine, phencyclidine (PCP), nicotine, and alcohol. These findings reflect a fundamental property of the mammalian, and even the bird brain. (Pigeons will consistently poke at a lever to receive cocaine.) Drugs elicit hedonic, rewarding responses in mammalian brain; the responses are not unique to a few susceptible individuals or to humans. This fundamental observation implicates drugs and associated drug addiction as a universal risk and support the limitations on drug availability as a sound public health response.

Mammalian species, from mice to monkeys, rapidly learn to self-administer cocaine and opioids, with cocaine reportedly causing inevitable death in primates that are given free, uncontrolled access to it. The relative addiction potential of the majority of drugs can be measured by various tests; the rate at which they acquire self-administration, whether the drug requires coupling with another re-enforcer or a priming agent to initiate drug-taking behavior (e.g., adding sugar to alcohol), the amount of effort expended to acquire a single dose, and how much effort is exerted before subjects give up, whether self-administration persists despite an adverse consequence, and how quickly a single dose, stress, or environmental cue reinstates drug administration during abstinence. These procedures have not been systematically applied in uniform experiments to assess the relative addictive potential of a wide range of drugs.

Brain Biology

Addiction biology refers to complex biological adaptations in the brain that reflect a sequence of progressive behaviors manifest as addiction: initial use, escalation of dose and frequency, transition to loss of control and compulsive use, withdrawal, craving, and relapse (31). Current models, although rudimentary, provide important insights that are crucial for infusing prevention programs with sound scientific discoveries and for providing biochemical leads to develop effective medications and other treatment strategies.

The Immediate Targets of Drugs in the Brain: Receptors

In complex organisms, communication within the brain is the key to survival. It is intriguing to consider the value of communication to human survival, as at least 15% of the human genome encodes proteins involved in communication. All addictive drugs target proteins that are critical for the complex communication system of the brain. From the instant a drug encounters its protein target, it inserts itself into the communication system of the brain, triggering a prodigious array of molecular and cellular changes to affect brain function and behavior. At the core of this communication system are an estimated 100 billion nerve cells (neurons) and even higher numbers of infrastructural cells, glia, which are also implicated in facilitating communication. Neurons accumulate information from sensory systems in the body, from other brain regions and from the environment, attribute a priority and salience (value) to this information, develop a response, communicate the response, and memorize the sequence of events for future use. Reduced to the molecular level, when a sensation originates, for example, from visual, auditory, tactile, pain, temperature sensors, or drugs, it is propagated through the axons (wires) of nerve cells to target cells that receive and interpret the signal, to generate a response. Neurons communicate this signal with their neighboring cells by releasing quantal amounts of chemical messengers, *neurotransmitters* (over 100 different types), into a gap. The transmitter diffuses across the space to adjacent neurons to convey the message. On these adjacent neurons, transmitters bind to interpreters (receptors) which not only decipher the chemical signal but propagate it, by an elegantly regulated sequence of events. This reflects the critical role of communication in maintaining homeostasis and the viability of an organism.

Transmitters and their receptors are made by specific neurons in specific brain regions. The transmitter/receptor signaling partners can initiate movement (dopamine), suppress pain (opioids), engender tranquility or fear (serotonin), imprint or erase memories (dopamine, glutamate, acetylcholine, anandamide), produce arousal, pleasurable or unpleasant sensations (dopamine, endorphins, norepinephrine, serotonin, dynorphin), induce paranoia, regulate heart rate (catecholamines), respiration (opioids), and a myriad of other functions. Of core relevance to addiction, specific signaling systems and circuits alert the brain to natural rewards that are necessary for human survival, for example, food, water, safety, relationships, and sex. Drug structures resemble, but are not identical to the structures of endogenous transmitters produced by the brain. The "imposters" (cocaine, amphetamine, and ecstasy) have structural similarities to dopamine, serotonin, and norepinephrine; Δ9-tetrahydrocannabinol (THC) the major psychoactive constituent of the marijuana plant resembles the brain's cannabinoids (anandamide, 2-arachidonylglycerol); heroin shares structural overlap with the brain's opioids (endorphins, enkephalins); lysergic acid diethylamide (LSD) resembles the neurotransmitter serotonin. As structural analogs of neurotransmitters, the drugs become embedded in the communication system and they trigger signals. But the similarities end here: drugs do not replicate, with fidelity, communication by brain neurons. Communication is an exquisitely regulated series of events, designed for chemicals produced by the brain and not for drugs. Normal brain transmitters are produced in highly circumscribed brain regions by specialized nerve cells, and released in carefully controlled amounts. In contrast, drugs access all brain regions at concentrations the brain cannot regulate. Drugs may activate multiple receptor targets simultaneously, with receptor activation differing from natural transmitters. Drugs may generate signals of unusually long duration, that are irregular, and that change the rhythm of normal tonic or phasic signals which maintain homeostasis or alert the brain to a natural reward. Termination of signals, an essential step in normal communication and to maintain homeostasis, is also affected by drugs. A critical step in terminating communication and resetting the system is removal of the transmitter by rapid transport and storage in storage vessels (vesicles). Most transporters cannot accommodate the unusual structures (shapes and charges) of psychoactive drugs (e.g., LSD, morphine, cocaine, marijuana), again enabling drugs to trigger persistent signals, at abnormally high strength for abnormally prolonged periods of time, and in inappropriate brain regions.

Researchers have identified the immediate target proteins of most drugs of abuse in the brain (31), isolated and expressed (cloning) the genes that encode these proteins, and documented a prodigious array of molecular and cellular adaptive events triggered from the moment the drug and its receptor target in the brain meet and bond.

The effects of all drugs are unique, with each binding to a unique spectrum of receptors, which under normal conditions, are activated by the transmitters that drugs resemble. LSD produces hallucinations via serotonin receptors; marijuana magnifies sensory perception, distorts time, reduces coordination, and interferes with working memory through cannabinoid receptors. Cocaine indirectly activates dopamine receptors to produce powerful stimulant and euphoriant sensations. Heroin induces a measure of tranquility combined with euphoria by activating opioid receptors. All drugs have highly distinctive sensory effects on the body that contribute to their emotional value. With repeated use, the brain and body adapt, which is manifested dramatically during withdrawal. Yet as complex, unique, and diverse as these acute and adaptive responses may be, addictive drugs also activate convergent neuronal circuits, circuits that signal changes in homeostasis.

The Brain Reward System

Although drugs elicit a wide spectrum of sensations, through multiple circuits in the brain, they all propagate one common biological response: the release of dopamine in the nucleus accumbens. Dopamine is not a hedonic signal, but a signal for learning and motivated behavior. Dopamine is also released in anticipation of, or during, natural rewards (e.g., food) and even in response to aversive stimuli, serving as the brain's "adrenaline," to alert the body of novel, meaningful rewarding or aversive stimuli and of pending appearances of a stimulus associated with a hedonic reward. Signals that alert the brain of natural rewards differ from drug-induced rewards. Drugs release dopamine at concentrations and for periods of time grossly exceeding dopamine release and clearance times triggered by natural rewards. This focal, unregulated dopamine signal fans out to brain circuits, alerting other regions of a novel, motivating, positive experience, recruiting other transmitter systems, primarily glutamate, along the way. Glutamate, one of the transmitters implicated in mediating short- and long-term memory, most likely encodes the specific details of the drug experience and stores these details (53). These complex signals carry the message to specialized circuits and brain regions (54) that interpret and consolidate memories of the liking and cued associations of the experience (hippocampus, amygdala), that learn to repeat the behaviors involved in acquiring these rewards (dorsal striatum, nucleus accumbens), that assign a priority or relative value for response to these awards (orbital prefrontal cortex), and that imprint cognitive control over rewarding behaviors (prefrontal cortex, striatum, thalamus). Although natural rewards and drugs share some common alerting circuits and memory processes, the natural rewards benefit the individual by rousing conscious and unconscious behaviors for survival and reproduction. In contrast, the extraordinary hedonic signals propagated by drugs overpower signals of natural rewards, suppress the salience (value) of essential rewards, and eventually supplant the drive for essential, natural, rewarding behavior, and draws the person into a deleterious state. Drug craving and drug seeking evolves into a compulsion that can persist for months or years after the last dose of a drug (55).

With repeated abnormal signaling, other transmitters are recruited. Adaptive processes at the molecular level trigger biological sequences to change the structure of nerve cells and reconfigure neural circuitry. This may result in a biochemical and functional disease of the brain. Understanding these processes is of fundamental relevance for identifying objective biological criteria for the disease of addiction and the state of recovery, for defining reversibility or irreversibility of adaptive states, for identifying genetic susceptibility, and developing leads for psychological or pharmacological treatment of addiction. Equally fascinating and ultimately practical is the development of a comprehensive view of how the brain assigns value for competing rewards and rewarding behaviors, how it learns and stores reward-related experiences to motivate behavior, how environmental stressors and the developing brain heighten susceptibility for addiction, and whether the transition or "switch" to addictive behavior is discernable at a biological level. We remain at a rudimentary stage in resolving these questions.

Transition to the Disease of Addiction

DSM-IV criteria separate abuse (adverse consequences) from addiction (adverse consequences coupled with loss of control, compulsive use, neuroadaptation), but objective data increasingly do not sustain a clear division between abuse and addiction. On a population basis, the transition from use to addiction is time, age of onset, and drug specific. Approximately 23% of heroin users meet the criteria for lifetime dependence. Corresponding values for cocaine (16.7%), other stimulants (11%), marijuana (9%), hallucinogens (4.9%), and inhalants (3.7%) are lower, with alcohol and tobacco dependence (15% and 32%) possibly reflecting their legal, acceptable social status, and availability (38). A subpopulation progresses rapidly to addiction; 4% to 6% of recent onset users of cocaine or other stimulants (methamphetamine, amphetamines, methylphenidate) become addicted within 24 months, a lower level with marijuana. In general, marijuana and alcohol display a slower, more insidious onset of addiction (38,52,56–58). Is there biological evidence of a brain switch, one that propels a user from controllable use to compulsive, involuntary drug-seeking and -using behavior? (59).

With repeated and frequent use, the brain adapts to and compensates for abnormal reward signals by altering production of gene copies and proteins, leading to profound changes in every dimension of brain biology and function. Some adaptive changes, of unpredictable reversibility, can be visualized in human brain, and are manifest as suppressed glucose metabolism, dopamine release, and altered blood supply. Activation or suppression of unique brain regions, particularly those involved in judgment and impulse control, follow exposure to drugs or drug cues and during abstinence. The insula, a brain region ignored for years, has recently been designated the "hidden island of addiction," as it may play a crucial role in the conscious urge to take drugs (60). Uniquely, this brain region alone is activated in human subjects during urges to use a large array of drugs (cocaine, heroin, alcohol, and cigarettes). Intriguingly, addicted smokers with lesioned or destroyed insula (but not populations with other damaged brain regions) readily quit smoking without relapse, and lose the urge to smoke (61). This brain region is viewed as a key location for integrating stimuli arising from the body, arousing conscious awareness of these feelings, attributing a value to them, and integrating a response to them. Accordingly, signals from the insula may override the prefrontal cortex, subverting its function as a reasoning center for impulse control. Conversely, the impaired insula may permit the prefrontal cortex to reassume impulse control, executive function, and judgment. Conceivably, medications that interrupt insula function may dampen the conscious urge to seek and consume drugs during the abstinence phase.

In experimental animals, repeated administration of a drug leads to an excess of, and diminished expression of many genes in various brain regions, in conjunction with abnormal production of proteins. The findings provide powerful clues for clarifying how the brain adapts to drug-induced activity and sensations, as well as leads for designing drug therapies to treat addiction. In brains of animals exposed to repeated cocaine, a restructuring of neural circuitry is visible, and correlates with altered behavior and motor function (33). Brain signaling systems, gene function and expression (62), protein production (49), cell structure (32) change. But do these changes constitute a molecular switch, a biochemical process that switches behavior from controllable to uncontrollable use? (63) Theoretically, this switch would have to persist for months or years after the drug is withdrawn, to sustain and reinstate drug-seeking behavior on a whim, a cue, stress, or re-exposure to the drug. The transcription factor deltaFosB is one candidate for this molecular switch. Transcription factors turn on or off genes that encode proteins, the critical drivers of brain function. Intriguingly, deltaFosB accumulates within the nucleus accumbens and dorsal striatum (brain regions highlighted above as relevant to addiction), not immediately, but after repeated administration of many kinds of drugs of abuse. Once induced, it is stable and remains in these brain regions for long periods of time, possibly triggering the expression of a panoply of genes/proteins implicated in addiction, long after the drug has cleared the body. Accordingly, Nestler et al. (59) have designated deltaFosB as a sustained "molecular switch" that functions as a transducer to convert sustained drug exposure into complex adaptive responses. It is premature to conclude that deltaFosB is the critical or only molecular switch responsible for changes in brain and behavior that characterize addiction.

The Toxic Effects of Specific Drugs

Certain drugs are frankly toxic to the brain and cause cell damage or death, either directly or by interrupting blood supply. Cocaine promotes vasospasm and loss of normal blood flow in human brain (30). Frequent exposure to amphetamine, methamphetamine, and ecstasy produce cell-specific toxicity and damage. Heavy alcohol or inhalant use (e.g., toluene) can produce profound irreversible toxic effects that are manifest as shrinkage of brain grey matter and enlargement of the fluid-filled spaces of the brain's drainage system.

Withdrawal

Upon withdrawal from the drug, the adapted brain is no longer at the original set point as in the predrug state, requiring the drug for "normal function." During drug withdrawal, anxiety, irritability, dysphoria, stress, and other psychological or physical (tremors, flu-like symptoms) discomforts emerge. Abrupt withdrawal from drugs such as alcohol and heroin unmask the adapted brain and produce wrenching physical symptoms. Withdrawal from marijuana, nicotine, cocaine, amphetamine generate a spectrum of symptoms, including anxiety, irritability, dysphoria, insomnia or hypersomnia, aches, craving, and other drug-specific effects.

Craving and Relapse

With prolonged abstinence, the addicted brain can generate intense craving and suppress efforts to control compulsive drug seeking. Craving leads to relapse, and the addict can rotate through compulsive use, withdrawal, and relapse several times, unless the cycle is finally broken. Yet craving can persist for months or decades, causing vulnerable people to relapse and revert to addictive behavior, especially if they encounter stress, drug cues, or are primed by a single dose of the addicting drug or another drug.

Policy Lessons from Modern Brain Biology

The science of drug use and addiction can inform and shape drug policies, in the realm of demand reduction and supply reduction. Without agreed upon biological markers for addiction in humans, the science remains at a rudimentary state. Nevertheless, research has yielded a number of fundamental principles with core relevance to drug policy. (a) The rewarding effects of drugs of abuse are universally sensed by mammalian brain (even the fruit fly!) and not only by small subpopulations of humans. Control of drugs is a necessary public health measure, to prevent an array of adverse consequences with the potential to derail individual lives, from in utero to old age. (b) Drugs produce a cluster of biochemical, cellular, physiological, behavioral, and psychological effects that can propel individuals into the detrimental state of addiction. A disease model of the brain is justified, on the basis of these findings and so is the shift to a public health domain. A disease model should also motivate medical professionals to contribute to diagnosis and treatment of substance use disorders. (c) Adolescents and persons with psychiatric disorders are at high risk for use and addiction, and warrant specific prevention and intervention policies and programs. (d) All drugs of abuse produce psychological or physiological withdrawal signs, indicative of altered, adapted brain and body biochemistry. The availability of medications to provide assistance to suppress or reverse adaptive responses that trigger drug craving should be an integral component of research and treatment.

Prevention

Federal funding for national drug control policies expended on prevention in the United States falls into several categories. State Prevention block grants provide states with discretionary funds for prevention, while other grant programs are designed to create community coalitions to formulate local solutions to local drug problems. The Department of Education issues grants for safe and drug-free schools, and the national Media Anti-drug Campaign is targeted primarily to youth. Adolescence is a critical risk factor for progression to addiction to all drugs and prevention in this population is of paramount importance. Evidence-based prevention programs targeted to parents, a critical factor in youth drug use, and to youth are likely to be among the most effective and cost-effective use of public funds. As indicated above, each year delay in onset of drug use can reduce addiction potential by a significant percent, notwithstanding a host of other adverse consequences that can accumulate in the drug-using adolescent population. This is not to suggest that 18 to 25 year olds, the highest consumers of all drugs, are immune to the adverse consequences of drug use or to addiction. On the contrary, it is necessary to address this population of users within their unique environments, including colleges, workplace and specific jobs at higher risk for use, as well as the unemployed and the homeless.

Intervention

The goals of prevention are to stop the initiation to drug use, while the goals of intervention are to prevent progression to addiction or to reverse the behavioral patterns associated with risky, problematic use. Interventions to prevent progression to addiction, improve health and parenting, reduce medical costs, reduce transmission of infectious diseases such as AIDS, and to reduce crime, will benefit the health and welfare of individuals (27). It is estimated that over 46 million people engage in risky, problematic drug use. Paradoxically, the health care system does not address this issue aggressively, which leads to burgeoning health problems (e.g., trauma, injuries, infections, depression) and escalating health care costs.

Substantial evidence indicates that brief behavioral interventions are effective when used by clinicians who are not specialists in substance abuse treatment, especially when enhancing entry to more intensive substance abuse treatment. Equally relevant, a significant proportion of drug users (as many as 50%) have underlying psychiatric problems that should be diagnosed and treated concurrently with drug treatment. For adolescents, brief interventions that include feedback on risks, an emphasis on personal responsibility, and alternatives for change have proven effectiveness. Calls for universal screening (verbal, written, electronic) for a full spectrum of drug use and providing brief interventions or referrals to specialty treatment constitutes an exquisite convergence of prevention, intervention, and treatment policies (27).

Why screen universally for risky use in health care settings? (a) Early detection among youth is crucial, especially as early onset of use is among the highest risk factors for progression to addiction. (b) Screening of pregnant women can identify at-risk fetuses: exposure to heavy alcohol, drugs in utero can cause harmful developmental, behavioral, and physical effects. (c) It is routine for physicians to inquire about all patients' medications (drugs), to prevent drug interactions and compromised effectiveness of prescribed medications, yet physicians do not routinely inquire about all nonmedical substance use. (d) Prescription drug misuse and abuse is a growing problem. (e) Prescription drug abuse is considerably more common in alcohol and illicit drug abusers, justifying universal screening for all drugs. (f) Overdose deaths due to prescription drug misuse are higher than at any time period in recent history, and far exceed deaths due to heroin or cocaine. (g) Drug intoxication is associated with higher Emergency Room and Trauma Center use. (h) Injuries are more common and clinical outcomes are worse in the alcohol and drug-abusing population. (i) Substance use disorders increase health care costs (e.g., HIV-AIDS, injuries, and trauma).

Treatment

A fundamental premise of neuroscience is the view of addiction as a brain disease (64). The biological evidence that drugs forge a diseased state of the brain is based primarily on drug-induced brain remodeling, visualized in living human brain by imaging, and in preclinical research by a variety of techniques. Dictionaries define disease as: "an alteration in the state of the body or of some of its organs, interrupting or disturbing the performance of the vital functions, and causing or threatening pain and weakness and characterized by an identifiable group of signs or symptoms"; "a pathological condition of a part, organ, or system of an organism resulting from various causes, such as infection, genetic defect, or environmental stress." Drug addiction can be viewed as a chronic, relapsing disease, characterized by compulsive, uncontrollable use despite adverse consequences. The neurobiology, however, should not supplant the role of personal responsibility in propagating this behavior. Within the construct of a disease model, patients are urged to assume responsibility for compliance with treatment, comparable to patients with asthma, hypertension, and diabetes.

Notwithstanding the progress in the biology of addiction, the DSM-IV criteria for addiction—compulsive, uncontrollable use despite adverse consequences—appear retrogressive, based as they are on loss of voluntary control (65). The medical diagnostic criteria not only eschew the mountain of biological evidence but minimize older definitions that highlight symptoms of biological adaptation, namely drug tolerance and withdrawal. Based primarily on alcohol and heroin, early biological hallmarks of addiction were thought to be reflected by diminished pharmacological effects of a fixed drug dose (tolerance) and frank physical signs of withdrawal during initial abstinence. In DSM-IV, these traditional criteria were retained but diluted by the preponderance of other criteria emphasizing loss of behavioral control and adverse consequences. The diminishing value of these specific physical signs is justified, as they are not uniformly relevant to all addictive drugs. For example, withdrawal from cocaine and nicotine is not manifest by physical signs (e.g., vomiting, pain, diarrhea, tremors, piloerection, hand tremor, fever, or convulsions). Patients treated with high doses of opioids for acute pain, can, upon drug cessation, display profuse sweating, nausea and vomiting, similar to moderate withdrawal from heroin without manifesting the signs of the disease of addiction. Prescription drugs with low abuse potential also can engender tolerance and withdrawal symptoms. Taken together, neuroadaptation that is manifest as withdrawal or tolerance is not a hallmark of addiction but one of many components that drive behavioral change for addictive drugs. Unfortunately, as there is no consensus on valid biological markers for the disease of addiction, behavioral terminology prevails. Nevertheless, positioning addiction in the category of a biological disease offers a framework to accelerate treatment research, reduce stigmatization by professionals, focus on problem solving, increase treatment availability for the populations in general and those involved in the criminal justice system, and medicalize this public health challenge. According to the latest National Survey on Drug Use and Health, over 20 million people in the United States harbor a medical diagnosis of abuse/addiction yet do not seek treatment and remain unidentified (28).

Treatment effectiveness can be measured by a range of outcome measures including reduced drug use, improved physical and mental health, employment, family relationships, reduced mortality, crime, and diminished medical, legal, social services, employment, and educational costs to society. By all these measures, numerous studies have demonstrated positive outcomes of treatment (34,66). A variety of treatment approaches is necessary to accommodate the needs of substance abusers, who present with varying social skills, economic status, underlying psychiatric disorders, criminal activity, age, and family support systems. The majority of residents of the United States who had an alcohol or illicit drug problem in 2002 did not receive treatment. Nearly all who needed treatment (dependent on or abuse of drugs or alcohol) but did not receive it, reported they did not feel a need for treatment. This may partially reflect a conscious or biologically based loss of judgment that gradually prevents drug users from understanding their predicament and supports the need for external intervention. Outpatient drug-free, outpatient methadone, long-term residential, and short-term inpatient programs reduce drug use. The cost-effectiveness for treating compared with the cost of not treating is variable. Some reports indicate a cost savings equivalent to a 1:3 ratio, whereas others report much higher ratios. Medications development offers a powerful rationale for clarifying the mechanisms underlying drug rewards and the progression to addiction.

Yet there is a dearth of effective medications to reduce drug cravings, prevent relapse, and facilitate recovery, one of several reasons why health care professionals do not universally screen for addiction. Although not universally effective or enduring, over 25 different medication formulations are available for smoking cessation and more than 3 for alcoholism. In contrast, approved medications to treat addictions to illicit drugs are available to less than 30% of the estimated 6.8 million people addicted to any illicit drug. Only those addicted to heroin or prescription opioids can avail themselves of approved medications (methadone, buprenorphine, naltrexone, and naloxone) to assist in recovery. Treatment of prescription opioid abuse/addiction (25% of total) with medications traditionally used for heroin addiction, is still in the experimental phase. Yet the heroin-addicted population is but a fraction, 3%, of the population estimated to harbor DSM-IV signs of abuse/addiction to illicit drugs. The remaining populations (marijuana: 57%; cocaine: 24%; other stimulants: 6%) do not have the benefit of medications-assisted recovery (28). The dearth of medications alone justifies the quest to understand the underlying biological processes of addiction and relapse and identify novel leads for medications development.

INTERNATIONAL PERSPECTIVE

On June 24, 2009 in Washington DC the Executive Director of drug abuse prevention efforts for the United Nations, Antonio Maria Costa, released The World Drug Report in collaboration with R. Gil Kerlikowske, the newly appointed Director of the White House ONDCP (67). The report concluded that global markets for cocaine, opiates, and cannabis were in "steady decline, while production and use of synthetic drugs is feared to be increasing in the developing world." Further, the report "offers several recommendations on how to improve drug control. These include universal access to drug treatment, international agreements against organized crime and greater efficacy in law enforcement."

A decade earlier, the United National General Assembly Special Session (UNGASS) had called on governments to reduce drug production and consumption greatly within 10 years. The World Drug Report, representing an independent and scholarly study of that decade-long effort concluded that "the demand for drugs in the world has stabilized mainly as a result of the interaction of epidemic forces, culture and economic development." This study found that the supply of drugs "has become more concentrated and the menu of drugs has changed surprisingly slowly." Further, the study reported that "The most prominent innovations under discussion have limited potential effects (heroin maintenance), have been unproductive policy interventions ("addition is a brain disease") or have no political appeal (legalization)." On a more optimistic note this report concluded that "The option with the most scope is increased effort at diverting arrested drug users out of the criminal justice systems."

In commenting on the report, ONDCP Director Kerlikowske summarized his approach to the drug problem. He stated, "In the United States, we are moving away from divisive drug war rhetoric and focusing on employing all the tools at our disposal to get help to those who need it. We recognize that addiction is a disease and are seeking public health solutions. My top priority is to intensify efforts to reduce the demand for drugs which fuels crime and violence around the world."

While there are widely varied rates of drug use in the world, there are no populations without drug problems. Most, if not all, countries have seen significant increases in drug use in recent decades, despite the most recent stabilization of drug use rates in some countries. Those populations most exposed to modern values which emphasize individual freedom and pursuit of pleasure and which have correspondingly lower levels of traditional or religious control over behavior have higher rates of drug use. Since these values are characteristic of much of the modern world, it is easy to see why the vulnerability to drug abuse has increased worldwide since the 1960s.

The drug problem was recognized as global in the early years of the 20th century when the first international efforts were made to curtail drug supply. The modern drug epidemic beginning in the 1960s has become truly global and is a major threat not only in developed nations but also in developing nations.

The United States was early in experiencing a serious drug problem for many reasons including the fact that the country is made up of people from all parts of the globe who brought with them to their new homes their drug-using behaviors related to religion and ritual, but not their cultural intolerance of these behaviors for pleasure and in excess. The United States has been characterized by diversity of values and behaviors and by a tolerance for this diversity that has been unique in the world. This vulnerability led to serious alcohol abuse problems that peaked in the first two decades of the 19th century. There was a strong grassroots reaction in the United States to this problem, made more cohesive and effective by newly emerging indigenous religious movements that were strongly opposed to alcohol use. The temperance movement was a powerful influence against alcohol as well. By the close of the 19th century other drugs of abuse emerged in the United States, including cocaine and heroin, resulting in a correspondingly strong antidrug movement focused on law enforcement, and new legislation passed by the United States Congress, as described in the first section of this chapter. In both the 19th and 20th centuries the American drug experience led to significant worldwide efforts to reduce alcohol and drug problems.

These efforts culminated in a series of international treaties that codified the commitment to curbing illegal drug use worldwide. Through leadership by the United Nations, the Single Convention on Narcotic Drugs in 1961 focused on the agriculturally produced drugs specifically cocaine and opiates (especially the semisynthetic heroin). In 1971, the Convention on Psychotropic Drugs focused on the completely synthetic newer drugs of abuse including the synthetic opiates, the stimulants, the depressants, and others. These meetings resulted in treaties that were widely ratified and managed effectively by the United Nations. The United Nations system of drug control includes the Office of Drugs and Crime (UNODC) established in 1997, the International Narcotics Control Board (INCB) established in 1968, and the Commission on Narcotic Drugs (CND) established in 1946. In the United States, the drug laws were updated in the Controlled Substance Act of the 1970s as amended over time (68).

Among the dramatic differences in drug use rates globally, those in Europe are noteworthy because of the wide differences between similar countries and the generally high quality of data available about drug use in these countries. Some countries can be characterized as having low drug use while others have higher drug use. The former countries generally have more restrictive drug policies (see the first part of this chapter) and the latter more tolerant, permissive drug policies. According to a recent UN report, for example, the percentage of students in the low use European countries that reported use of marijuana or hashish in the prior 30 days was: Sweden 1%, Turkey 2%, Greece 2%, and Iceland 4%, while the percentage of students reporting prior 30-day use in the more tolerant countries was: Spain 23%, France 22%, United Kingdom 20%, and the Netherlands 13% (69). More striking still is the contrast in student drug use in Malmo, Sweden, and Copenhagen, Denmark, twin cities across a bridge in the Baltic Sea. The rates of ever use in Copenhagen are three times higher than those in Malmo, and the rates of use in the last 30 days are five times higher in Copenhagen than in Malmo.

While the future of drug policy is increasingly being debated in Europe and elsewhere in the world, the experience in Sweden offers an especially instructive lesson.

THE SWEDISH DRUG POLICY EXPERIENCE

In the early 1960s, Sweden was among the first countries in Western Europe to experience a large-scale drug problem among young people. The origins of the Swedish drug epidemic date back to the late 1940s when abuse was limited to tiny bohemian circles in Stockholm and only later spread to individuals with criminal lifestyles. Gradually, a wider segment of young people was introduced to nonmedical drug use at which time the media began reporting the Swedish drug epidemic.

Central nervous system stimulants of the amphetamine-type then dominated the illegal drug market in Sweden. Because these drugs were seen as nonaddicting and had widespread clinical use at the time, it is not hard to understand why many Swedish physicians were attracted to the idea of prescribing drugs in order to keep individuals from obtaining them through illegal sources. This idea was quickly adopted by some health and law enforcement authorities. Between 1965 and 1967 nonmedical drug users in Stockholm could obtain their favorite drugs including not only stimulants, but also opiates, with a prescription from a handful of doctors who took part in a special program sanctioned by the National Board of Health. Initially, around 110 drug-addicted patients were enrolled in the program for whom more than 4 million doses were prescribed. Out of those, about 3.4 million doses were stimulants; most of the rest were opiates. Unsurprisingly, a large percentage of these legally prescribed drugs were resold or given away, flooding the city with drugs and spreading the drug epidemic in Sweden rather than limiting it as the program's sponsors naively expected. This legal prescription experiment came to an abrupt end in June of 1967 2 years after it started, following the tragic and widely publicized death of a 17-year-old girl who had been offered drugs by one of the patients in the prescription program.

As a psychiatrist working with the Stockholm police, Nils Bejerot was one of the few physicians in Sweden at this time with firsthand experience of drug addiction. Bejerot's work with criminals since the 1950s in Stockholm gave him a unique perspective with regard to the National Board of Health's drug policy experiment. He tried in vain to stop this legal prescription experiment by offering his expertise and experience to the authorities. Out of frustration and in the hope that this initial experiment would never be restarted, in 1965 he initiated a study of drug injection marks among arrestees at the Remand Prison in Stockholm. He later linked the changes in the frequency of injection marks to the changes in the Swedish drug policy (70). In 1969 he founded the National Association for a Drug-free Society (abbreviated RNS in Swedish) in order to promote the idea of restrictive drug policy by educating both the public and his medical colleagues.

In 1968 Bejerot published his first book—later to become a series of books—about the drug problem under the title, *The Drug Issue and Society* (71). He presented his analysis of the drug problem as a response to the diametrically opposed, and widely influential, analysis of drug policy that had been presented a few years earlier by the American sociologist Alfred Lindesmith in his book, *The Addict and The Law* (72).

One of Bejerot's major contributions to the understanding of the drug problem was his classification of different types of drug abuse, presented in his 1968 book. At that time most classifications were focused on the various drugs or types of drugs that people used nonmedically. Bejerot took a different approach to classification in which he categorized the various patterns of abuse based on how the drug was introduced to individual drug users. In his early models he described six different patterns of drug abuse. Over the next two decades he refined his model, settling on three main types: therapeutic, cultural or endemic, and epidemic types.

The therapeutic type of illicit drug use occurs when a patient in medical care becomes addicted to drugs, knowingly or unknowingly, when using the drugs prescribed by a physician. Medical staff who become addicted because drugs are available to them at work are also included in this group. Addicts of this type differ from other types because women dominate the group. They are relatively old when first introduced to drugs and use them initially for medical purposes. Bejerot found that these addicts tended to be secretive about their addiction and very seldom introduced others to drug abuse.

The cultural type of drug use occurs when the drug use/abuse is culturally accepted in society, for example, alcohol use/alcoholism in the Western world. This pattern of drug use is more or less part of becoming an adult in most parts of the world. It can even be considered antisocial behavior not to use alcohol in certain settings. Cigarette smoking is similar in that it is culturally and legally accepted in many societies not only to use but even to be addicted to nicotine. Other endemic drugs are the chewing of coca leaves among native Bolivians and khat leaves in Somalia and Yemen.

The epidemic type of drug addict was described by Bejerot as a type of substance use which is not socially accepted generally in the society at large and is often illegal. Novices are introduced through intimate contact with someone, usually a close friend, who recently has been introduced to nonmedical, prohibited drug use. These relatively new drug users have enough experience to pass on to initiate other new drug users, while they do not yet exhibit the negative consequences of the drug use that might protect a nonuser from trying the drug. Bejerot had observed that early in the epidemic, especially vulnerable individuals were overrepresented among drug users of this type. However, as the drug epidemic grew in Sweden, people with little or no social or psychological problems became active drug abusers.

Based on his analysis Bejerot wrote many articles and books (71,73–76) and acted through RNS to promote a drug policy that focused for two reasons on small-scale drug crimes and early intervention to reduce the epidemic type of drug use:

1. The spread of drug abuse from person to person usually occurs early after onset of the illicit drug use. Bejerot described this period as the honeymoon of drug abuse, when almost everything is positive about the drug use, encouraging the

newcomer to introduce his friends as a generous gesture of friendship. Bejerot concluded that if society wants to stop drug abuse from spreading it must intervene early to interrupt this malignant and rapid spread of nonmedical drug use.

2. Once addiction is established the prognosis for the individual to become drug free is substantially worsened. Drug addiction, once entrenched in an individual and in society, is difficult to stop. The willingness of drug addicts to go into treatment usually occurs only after many years of abuse and after an accumulation of many painful experiences and losses. For this reason, for a policy to be effective in reducing the prevalence levels of drug use in a society, Bejerot concluded that the society must prevent young people from starting to use drugs altogether.

While evidence-based and persistently expressed, Professor Bejerot's views on drug policy initially were not universally accepted in Sweden. There was a strong counter argument based on the belief that medicalizing nonmedical drug use would reduce not only drug use but also the many serious and even fatal problems that drug use created. This view was attractive to many Swedish health officials because it appeared to be more compassionate and humane. During the 1970s the debate about drug policy in Sweden picked up momentum gradually. Official drug prevention policy at that time directed the police to concentrate on trafficking and smuggling and not arrest the drug users for drug possession and street peddling on the presumption that this would make it more attractive for them to voluntarily seek treatment and other help from social services providers or hospitals. During those years in Sweden it was legally safe for drug users to possess up to 20 g of hashish for personal use. Naturally the street pushers never had more than this legal limit. This legal practice was criticized by Bejerot and RNS for several years. Public debates, demonstrations, and media debates were organized and finally achieved results. The Swedish Prosecutor General issued a directive to all prosecutors in January 1980 that waivers of prosecution for small amounts of narcotic drugs would not be allowed any longer. Overnight, this announcement changed Swedish drug policy as a practical matter. It was the tipping point, when Swedish drug policy swung from being a permissive to a restrictive drug policy. The restrictive policy has continued to the present time.

Based on this newly articulated drug policy, the Swedish police changed its priorities to focus on small crimes of possession, making small-scale trafficking of drugs a much riskier business. Unsurprisingly, the number of drug crimes rose initially while at the same time drug use surveys showed a consistent decline all through the 1980s. In those years, the economy in Sweden was good. The city councils were generally willing to fund drug treatment and antidrug prevention activities in schools. The general debate in society about drug policy receded as all parties adopted the restrictive policy, which was an important inspiration to everyone working professionally with the drug problem.

In 1983, the Supreme Court of Sweden ruled that the Narcotic Drugs Act did not cover the act of consuming illegal drugs. Simply speaking, it was forbidden to have any drug of abuse in your pocket or in your possession in any other way, but to smoke, eat, inhale, or inject drugs was not illegal. The following year RNS began campaigning to make the consumption of illegal drugs itself a crime. An opinion poll in 1984 showed that 95% of the public were in favor of this change in the law. The debate went on for several years, engaging all of Sweden's political parties in the Parliament. In 1988, the Swedish law was changed so that consumption of narcotic drugs was made illegal. Initially the law did not allow the police to take a urine or blood test as evidence of use. The law was rewritten in 1993 so that the police could use drug tests for evidence of drug consumption.

During 2008 approximately 35,000 drug tests were taken by Swedish police based on suspicion of illegal consumption. Over 10,000 tests were taken on suspicion of drugged driving. The punishment for illegal consumption is a monetary fine related to the offender's income. Drugged driving can lead to imprisonment, depending on the circumstances.

If the 1980s were the Golden Age of drug prevention in Sweden, then the 1990s were the Dark Age. Sweden was hit by a severe economic crisis in the early part of the decade, a crisis that took the rest of the decade to sort out. Virtually all segments of Swedish society experienced an economic decline, or ground to a halt. Since the drug problem, especially among the young, was at such a low level at the beginning of the 1990s, drug policy did not receive much attention from those with political power. As a consequence, antidrug efforts declined in the 1990s, and drug treatment became much harder to obtain. For these same economic reasons, schools did not focus on the drug problem in the 1990s. It is not surprising that drug abuse levels in Sweden went up during this decade, although they never again reached the levels seen in the late 1960s and early 1970s. However by the end of the 1990s, drug abuse was again serious enough for the government to take action to rectify this trend.

In 1998, the Government appointed a Narcotics Commission which put forth many suggestions for action and change. With the general debate about the drug problem heating up, funding for various types of projects was made available by the government. During the first years of the new century the rise in illegal drug use rates among the young flattened out and gradually declined (Figure 77.3).

There are many in Sweden who believe there are further challenges in the nation's efforts to curtail illegal drug use. However, with unusually low rates of drug use, Sweden compares very favorably to other developed nations. Since 1971 the Swedish Council for Information in Alcohol and other Drugs (CAN) has administered drug use surveys among teenagers during the year they have their 16th birthday. The model used in these surveys was adopted from a European survey conducted in 1995 in 26 countries, the European School Survey Project on Alcohol and other Drugs (ESPAD). The latest ESPAD survey was presented in February 2009 and shows data from 2007.

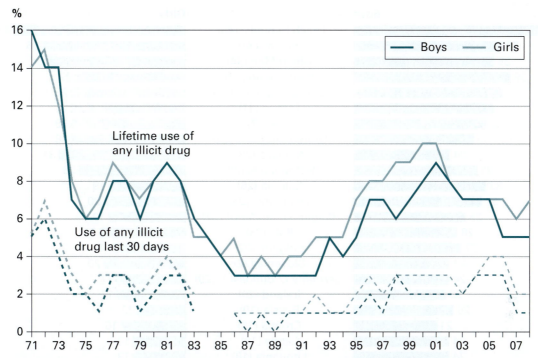

Figure 77.3. Lifetime use of any illicit drug and use of any illicit drug during last 30 days (data not availabe, 1983–1985), by gender, 1971–2008. (Data from Hvitfeldt T, Nystrom S. *Skolelevers Drogvanor 2008*. Stockholm, Sweden: Swedish Council for Information on Alcohol and other Drugs; 2009.)

Figure 77.4 shows a comparison among self-reported lifetime marijuana and hashish use by 16-year-olds from 35 European countries. The reported drug use of boys can be found in the left-side graphs, while the reported drug use of girls appears in graphs on the right. The average of the reported use of the boys and girls combined can be found as a number to the right of the country name. The differences in self-reported use of cannabis are very large between the European countries with the lowest and the highest prevalence levels. Several comparisons of other countries with Sweden are of interest. There is a striking difference between Sweden and the United Kingdom even though the modern drug epidemic started at about the same time in both countries and even though both are liberal welfare states with high levels of economic development. In another comparison, it is interesting to note the reported drug use between teenagers in Sweden and in the Netherlands. During the 1970s Sweden, after a heated internal debate, began enforcing stricter drug laws. The Netherlands in 1976 decided to go the opposite way by passing the Opium Act, making a distinction between the permissive enforcement of *soft* drug use and a more restrictive enforcement of *hard* drugs. It is helpful to consider the impact of significant change in a country's political structure and the resulting impact on drug policy when viewing these data. For example, a number of these countries endured harsh and repressive experiences of dictatorship. It can be inferred that some of these countries, such as the Czech Republic, Slovak Republic, Spain, and Estonia, having became democratic, include the freedom to use illegal drugs in their concept of freedom. However, this is not a uniform experience, as other countries, such as Greece, have had a similar historical experience yet the country maintains a restrictive drug policy and experiences low levels of drug use among its teenagers. Portugal, which became a democracy in 1974, has adopted a less stringent policy, with resulting reported teenage use approximately midway between the data reported by teens in Spain and Greece. From this ESPAD scale, it is possible to infer the presence of quite permissive drug policy associated with the increased prevalence levels of illegal drugs.

The authors of the ESPAD survey concluded in their summary that in the 2007 data there are apparent associations between the aggregate use of different substances at the country level. In countries where teenagers drink more, they also tend to use illegal drugs more. A nation's drug policy reflects a cultural set of values, beliefs, and behaviors, and its associated laws result in normative actions on the part of its citizens. People, especially young people, adapt quickly to laws that impact on behavior related to the use of illegal drugs.

One of the common stereotypes in global drug policy debates is that successful welfare states adopt permissive drug policies as part of their commitment to compassion and tolerance of diversity. Sweden, a country noted for its liberal views, stands out as an exception to this stereotype and offers a model for a more restrictive drug policy, not because it is repressive politically but because it promotes the public health and lowers both drug use and the harms caused by drug use (77,78).

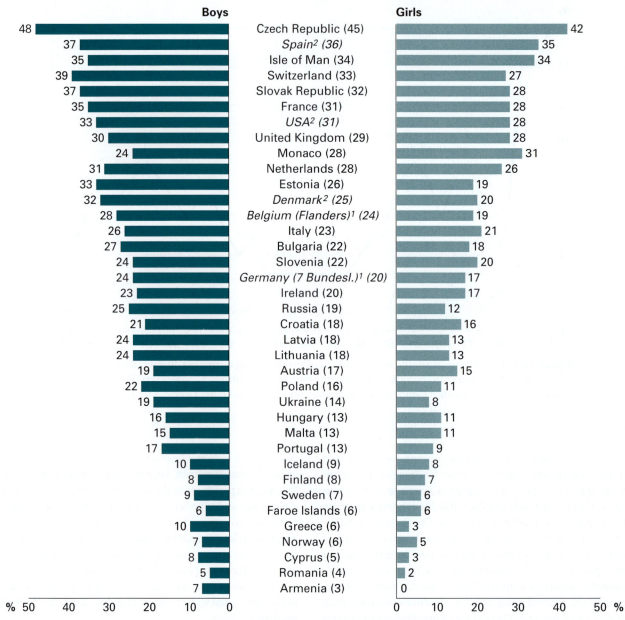

Figure 77.4. Lifetime use of marijuana or hashish by gender, 2007. (1) Belgium and Germany: Limited geographical coverage. (2) Denmark, Spain, and the United States: Limited comparability. (Data from Hibell B, Guttormsson U, Ahlstrom A, et al. *The 2007 ESPAD Report: Substance Abuse Among Students in 35 European Countries*. Stockholm, Sweden: Swedish Council for Information on Alcohol and other Drugs; 2009.)

THE CENTRAL DRUG POLICY ISSUES TODAY

During recent years, a short, and still evolving list of highly charged drug policy issues has been prominent in the mass media. One group of these issues has included medical marijuana, needle exchange programs, injection rooms (where addicts can inject government-provided heroin, cocaine, and other drugs), and hemp cultivation. Another group springing from a different view of drug policy has included random student drug testing and more vigorous drugged driving enforcement. Until the past few years the media chatter pitted arguments about the merits of harm reduction versus abstinence. More recently new support has emerged for the legalization of marijuana or even of all currently illegal drugs—a proposal rarely articulated in public debate even a few years ago. The argument for legalization rests on the belief that most of the costs of illegal drug use are not from the drug use itself but from the efforts to prohibit illegal drug use such as arrests and imprisonment for both the use and sale of illegal drugs. The supporters of legalization advocate making these currently illegal substances available just as tobacco and alcohol are available, regulated, and taxed in a similar manner. Considerations of the health cost of such a measure is absent from this proposal.

Entirely separate from these often heated media debates are a wide range of practical drug policy questions ranging from the coverage of substance use disorders by private and public health insurance—focused on efforts to achieve *parity* for substance abuse with other disorders—to issues of the proper goals of drug testament programs (pharmacotherapy maintenance vs. abstinence, for example).

Separate from both the sensationalized media and practical policy discussions are innovations that quietly contribute to the solution of important problems. One example can be found in the terrible epidemic of escalating use of prescribed controlled substances especially the opiates, but also the benzodiazepines and the stimulants. There are important, ongoing discussion regarding the policies needed to curb this massive problem and how those proposed efforts impact on the legitimate medical treatment of serious medical disorders including pain, anxiety, and attention deficit-hyperactivity disorder (ADHD)? This is a policy issue that has no political traction and rarely engages the traditional drug policy debate. One of the most promising strategies to reduce prescription drug abuse without inhibiting legitimate medical treatment of diseases is widespread use of abuse-resistant formulations, an innovation of biomanufacturing (78). Another example is a socio-legal innovation that links the criminal justice system to treatment in creative ways that reduce incarceration and improve treatment outcomes (80). These are examples of out-of-the-box innovations that can impact upon the future of drug policy. They are utterly absent from the static, politicized debates about drug policy that preoccupy the media and party politics.

Resuming the consideration of hot topics in today's drug policy debates, what are appropriate goals for drug abuse prevention efforts? By one side the primary goal is seen as reducing the use of the currently illegal drugs in the society. On the other side, this use is regarded as protected by privacy rights and the appropriate goal is reducing the harm produced by drug use, especially heavy use. Prevention efforts advocated by proponents of harm reduction include teaching young people how to use drugs more safely, clean needle giveaway programs for intravenous drug users to limit the spread of HIV-AIDS, with optional treatment opportunities offered as well, and the distribution of Narcan-containing syringes to intravenous opiate users for treatment for themselves and their friends for opiate overdose.

As stated earlier in this chapter, the complex issues of drug policy provoke strong opinions. Almost everyone is an expert on drug policy. Readers no doubt recognize these intense reactions and opinions in themselves and in others of their acquaintance. This all but universal response reflects the importance of the illegal drug problem in the modern world and in particular, the unsettled nature of the response to the problems associated since the dramatic rise in illegal drug use since the 1960s. If the solution were entirely clear there would be no debate. The drug policy will endure for some time to come. However, the questions over time will be shaped and reshaped by changes in values, experience, and lessons learned as policies evolve. The fact that the illegal drug epidemic has become global insures that there will be a variety of responses from countries all over the world and that diverse experiences will provide useful data to inform and enrich drug policy considerations. This is a subject that invites active engagement with these highly visible policy disputes but at the same time requires respect for the adversarial process. While there are life-and-death issues at stake it is not reasonable to deny the legitimacy of the other side of these issues. Civility can result in greater productivity, understanding, and the possibility of resolution and even agreement on many drug policies.

Perhaps more important in the long run than the settling of these fundamental drug policy disputes is the fact that most drug policy issues never get to the mass media and are not captured by partisan politics. Instead they are worked out by individuals, by programs, and by communities. Here are a few examples of the drug policy issues that are flying below the media radar: What should a substance abuse treatment program do about continuing nonmedical drug use by patients? How often should patients be drug tested and what drugs should they be tested for? What should drug treatment programs do—if anything—about patients continuing to use alcohol and tobacco? With regard to *evidence-based* policies, what is the evidence showing the most effective and humane goals of substance abuse treatment? Even well-conducted studies (and most of the most important policy disputes produce little controlled research), are fraught with caveats and limitations. They are never definitive. The most common outcome of research is the need for more research. Experience and research is likely to be the foundation of future drug policies.

THE FUTURE OF UNITED STATES AND INTERNATIONAL DRUG POLICY

The future will rise from current drug policies. One of the principal goals of future drug policy is for the criminal justice system to work better with the treatment system so that together they can achieve results that neither alone can achieve. While the common way of expressing the fundamental drug policy debate is to ask whether one supports the criminal justice system (and prison) *or* drug treatment, the reality is that nearly half of those people in drug treatment today are there *because* of the criminal justice system. That fact alone leads to the conclusion that one of the challenges to drug policy lies in finding better, more cost-effective ways to link the criminal justice system and treatment.

With respect to the debate about pharmacotherapy versus abstinence-based treatment, it seems clear that most drug abusers, however ambivalently and inconstantly, seek to be drug free. The future rests with long-term outcome studies that show how various approaches to substance abuse and dependence contribute to long-term favorable outcomes which, for most patients, means abstinence from the use of abused drugs. To date most treatment evaluations are short term. The most common findings of treatment research are first, that a large percentage of substance abuse patients prematurely terminate treatment and second, after-treatment relapses to drug use are common—often quickly after leaving treatment. Of course these findings on outcome studies are far from unique to substance abuse treatment. Noncompliance with treatment, especially behaviorally oriented treatment, is common across the spectrum of medical care. The use of coerced abstinence linked to prolonged treatment for substance abuse is a possible model for other behavior-related health problems (81–86).

Drug abuse prevention will also be a major area of development as new approaches to education and intervention, including random student drug testing and efforts to curb drugged driving, become more prominent. The future will almost certainly explore more actively the environment in which the choice to use or not to use drugs takes place including the role of coercive actions like random student drug testing and active and prolonged monitoring for alcohol and drug use after treatment (81–86).

Most striking will be the worldwide response to the problems of both drug supply and drug use. The drug problem is a human problem that knows no political, economic, demographic, or geographic boundaries. Because the drug problem is global, the solutions to the drug problem must also be global. Any country that fails to contain drug users and drug sellers is a threat to every other nation. No country is or will be without both drug users and drug sellers. Surely in the enduring words of Walt Kelly's beloved cartoon character, Pogo, when it comes to drug problems "We have met the enemy and they are us."

CONCLUSIONS

The experience of health care professionals with individual drug abusers will continue to be the foundation for the evolution of new drug policies. Across the political spectrum there is a rapidly growing conviction that the future of drug policy lies in linking the supply side activities with those on the demand side. Increasingly the global drug prevention policy focus has shifted toward greater emphasis on demand reduction. This shift reflects the knowledge coming from the experience of those who have worked with addicts over long periods of time, new information from brain science, and a growing body of public health research.

In their recent review of United States drug policy, Boyum and Reuter conclude by summarizing their recommendations, "We have offered a series of suggestions for reducing the damage that drug use and drug control inflict upon American society: fewer incarcerations, better and more treatment, elimination of criminal penalties for marijuana possession, and implementation of coerced abstinence for drug-involved offenders are the most prominent. For none of them can we offer strong empirical evidence of substantial effectiveness" (16). This summary strikes a fine balance in drug policy and links it to a thoroughly appropriate humility about the state of the research evidence about what works and what does not when it comes to drug policy in the United States and throughout the world.

Drug problems and the risk for their significant escalation are ubiquitous in the modern world. Drug policies are needed to mitigate that risk to the extent that they are compatible with modern values, and are affordable and effective. There is no silver bullet, no simple correct answer. No policy will end drug problems, although some policies clearly make them worse while others make them better. Rather than being a signal for resignation, this complexity and this ubiquity of risk are challenges to scientists, policy-makers, and those most dedicated to the public interest. There are few human problems more fascinating, complex, rewarding, and challenging than these.

REFERENCES

1. Gold MS, Graham NA, Cocores JA, et al. Food addiction? *J Addict Med*. 2009;3(1):42–45.
2. Institute of Medicine. *Federal Regulation of Methadone Treatment*. Washington, DC: The National Academies Press; 1995.
3. Massing M. *The Fix*. Berkeley, CA: University of California Press; 2000.
4. Musto DF. *The American Disease*. New York, NY: Oxford University Press; 1999.
5. Office of National Drug Control Policy. National drug control strategy, 2009. Washington, DC: Author; 2009.
6. National Commission on Marihuana and Drug Abuse. Marihuana: A signal of misunderstanding. Washington, DC: U.S. Government Printing Office; 1972.
7. National Commission on Marihuana and Drug Abuse. Drug abuse in America: Problem in perspective. Washington. DC: U.S. Government Printing Office; 1973.
8. Courtwright D. *Forces of Habit: Drugs and the Making of the Modern World*. Cambridge, MA: Harvard University Press; 2001.
9. Courtwright DT. *Dark Paradise: A History of Opiate Addiction in America*. Cambridge, MA: Harvard University Press; 2001.
10. Jonnes J. *Hepcats, Narcs and Pipe Dreams*. Baltimore, MD: JHU Press; 1999.
11. Wilson JQ, DuPont RL. The sick sixties. *Atlantic Monthly*. 1973(Oct):91–98.
12. Substance Abuse and Mental Health Services Administration. *Results from the 2007 National Survey on Drug Use and Health: National Findings*. (NSDUH Series H-34, DHHS Publication No. SMA 08-4343). Rockville, MD: Office of Applied Studies; 2008.
13. National Institute on Drug Abuse, National Institute on Alcohol Abuse and Alcoholism. *The Economic Costs of Alcohol and Drug Abuse in the United States*. Rockville, MD: U.S. Department of Health and Human Services; 1998. Available at: http://www.nida.nih.gov/EconomicCosts/Chapter1.html#1.10. Accessed July 2, 2010.
14. Targeting Tobacco Use: The Nation's Leading Cause of Death: At a Glance; 2008. Available at: http://www.cdc.gov/nccdphp/publications/aag/osh.htm. Accessed July 2, 2010.
15. Babor TF, Caulkins JP, Edwards G, et al. Drug Policy and the Public Good. Oxford University Press: Oxford; 2010.
16. Boyum D, Reuter P. *An Analytic Assessment of U.S. Drug Policy*. Washington, DC: American Enterprise Institute for Public Policy Research; 2005.
17. Musto DF, Korsmeyer P, Maulucci TW. *One Hundred Years of Heroin*. Santa Barbara, CA: Greenwood Publishing Group, Incorporated; 2002.

18. Musto DF. *Drugs in America*. New York, NY: New York University Press; 2002.
19. White WL. *Slaying the Dragon: The History of Addiction Treatment and Recovery in America*. Bloomington, IL: Chestnut Health Systems/Lighthouse Institute; 1998.
20. Lindesmith AR. *Addiction and Opiates*. Piscataway, NJ: Aldine Transaction; 1968.
21. Moore M. Actually, prohibition was a success. *The New York Times*. October 16, 1989.
22. Johnston LD, O'Malley PM, Bachman JG, et al. *Monitoring the Future National Results on Adolescent Drug Use: Overview of Key Findings, 2008 (NIH Publication No. 09-7401)*. Bethesda, MD: National Institute on Drug Abuse; 2009.
23. Leonard J. Paulozzi. *Trends in Unintentional Drug Overdose Deaths*. Quote from U.S. Congress. Senate Subcommittee on Crime & Drugs Committee on the Judiciary and the Caucus on International Narcotics Control. March 12, 2008.
24. DuPont RL. *The Selfish Brain: Learning from Addiction (Revised and updated)*. Center City, MN: Hazelden; 2000.
25. Uhl GR, Grow RW. The burden of complex genetics in brain disorders. *Arch Gen Psychiatry*. 2004;61(3):223–229.
26. National Survey on Drug Use and Health, 2009. Results from 2008. Available at: http://oas.samhsa.gov/nsduh/2k8nsduh/2k8Results.pdf. Accessed July 2, 2010.
27. Madras BK, Compton WM, Avula D, et al. Screening, brief interventions, referral to treatment (SBIRT) for illicit drug and alcohol use at multiple healthcare sites: comparison at intake and 6 months later. *Drug Alcohol Depend*. 2009;99(1–3):280–295.
28. The NSDUH Report Children Living with Substance-Dependent or Substance-abusing Parents: 2002–2007. Available at: http://www.oas.samhsa.gov/2k9/SAparents/SAparents.htm. Accessed July 2, 2010.
29. National Center on Addiction and Substance Abuse. No safe haven: Children of substance-abusing parents. New York, NY: Author; 1999.
30. Kaufman MJ, Levin JM, Ross MH, et al. Cocaine-induced cerebral vasoconstriction detected in humans with magnetic resonance angiography. *JAMA*. 1998;279(5):376–380.
31. Madras BK. Introduction; Cocaine. In: Madras BK, Colvis CM, Pollack JD, et al., eds. *Cell Biology of Addiction*. Cold Spring Harbor, NY: Cold Spring Harbor Laboratory Press; 2006:1–12.
32. Robinson TE, Kolb B. Structural plasticity associated with exposure to drugs of abuse. *Neuropharmacology*. 2004;47(suppl 1):33–46.
33. Saka E, Goodrich C, Harlan P, et al. Repetitive behaviors in monkeys are linked to specific striatal activation patterns. *J Neurosci*. 2004;24(34):7557–7565.
34. Treatment approaches for drug addiction. National Institute on Drug Abuse. Available at: http://www.nida.nih.gov/PDF/InfoFacts/Treatment08.pdf. Accessed July 2, 2010.
35. Uhl GR, Drgon T, Johnson C, et al. Molecular genetics of addiction and related heritable phenotypes: genome-wide association approaches identify "connectivity constellation" and drug target genes with pleiotropic effects. *Ann NY Acad Sci*. 2008;1141:318–381.
36. Grant BF, Dawson DA. Age of onset of drug use and its association with DSM-IV drug abuse and dependence: results from the National Longitudinal Alcohol Epidemiologic Survey. *J Subst Abuse*. 1998;10(2):163–173.
37. Anthony JC, Petronis KR. Early-onset drug use and risk of later drug problems. *Drug Alcohol Depend*. 1995;40(1):9–15.
38. Wagner FA, Anthony JC. From first drug use to drug dependence; developmental periods of risk for dependence upon marijuana, cocaine, and alcohol. *Neuropsychopharmacology*. 2002;26(4):479–488.
39. Storr CL, Westergaard R, Anthony JC. Early onset inhalant use and risk for opiate initiation by young adulthood. *Drug Alcohol Depend*. 2005;78(3):253–261.
40. McCabe SE, West BT, Morales M, et al. Does early onset of non-medical use of prescription drugs predict subsequent prescription drug abuse and dependence? Results from a national study. *Addiction*. 2007;102(12):1920–1930.
41. Chen CY, Storr CL, Anthony JC. Early-onset drug use and risk for drug dependence problems. *Addict Behav*. 2009;34(3):319–322.
42. Stone AL, Storr CL, Anthony JC. Evidence for a hallucinogen dependence syndrome developing soon after onset of hallucinogen use during adolescence. *Int J Methods Psychiatr Res*. 2006;15(3):116–130.
43. Palmer RH, Young SE, Hopfer CJ, et al. Developmental epidemiology of drug use and abuse in adolescence and young adulthood: Evidence of generalized risk. *Drug Alcohol Depend*. 2009;102(1–3):78–87.
44. McCabe SE, Knight JR, Teter CJ, et al. Non-medical use of prescription stimulants among US college students: prevalence and correlates from a national survey. *Addiction*. 2005;100(1):96–106.
45. Chambers RA, Taylor JR, Potenza MN. Developmental neurocircuitry of motivation in adolescence: a critical period of addiction vulnerability. *Am J Psychiatry*. 2003;160(6):1041–1052.
46. Yurgelun-Todd D. Emotional and cognitive changes during adolescence. *Curr Opin Neurobiol*. 2007;17(2):251–257.
47. Giedd JN, Lalonde FM, Celano MJ, et al. Anatomical brain magnetic resonance imaging of typically developing children and adolescents. *J Am Acad Child Adolesc Psychiatry*. 2009;48(5):465–470.
48. Gogtay N, Giedd JN, Lusk L, et al. Dynamic mapping of human cortical development during childhood through early adulthood. *Proc Natl Acad Sci USA*. 2004;101(21):8174–8179.
49. Bahi A, Dreyer JL. Cocaine-induced expression changes of axon guidance molecules in the adult rat brain. *Mol Cell Neurosci*. 2005;28(2):275–291.
50. Jassen AK, Yang H, Miller GM, et al. Receptor regulation of gene expression of axon guidance molecules: implications for adaptation. *Mol Pharmacol*. 2006;70(1):71–77.
51. Samaha AN, Robinson TE. Why does the rapid delivery of drugs to the brain promote addiction? *Trends Pharmacol Sci*. 2005;26(2):82–87.
52. Anthony JC, Warner LA, Kessler RC. Comparative epidemiology of dependence on tobacco, alcohol, controlled substances and Inhalants: basic findings from the national comorbidity Survey. *Exp Clin Psychopharm*. 1994;2:244–268.
53. Kalivas PW. The glutamate homeostasis hypothesis of addiction. *Nat Rev Neurosci*. 2009;10(8):561–572.
54. Koob GF, Volkow ND. Neurocircuitry of addiction. *Neuropsychopharmacology*. 2009; Aug 26 [Epub ahead of print].
55. Koob GF. Neurobiological substrates for the dark side of compulsivity in addiction. *Neuropharmacology*. 2009;56(suppl 1):18–31.
56. Chen CY, O'Brien MS, Anthony JC. Who becomes cannabis dependent soon after onset of use? Epidemiological evidence from the United States: 2000–2001. *Drug Alcohol Depend*. 2005;79(1):11–22.
57. O'Brien MS, Anthony JC. Risk of becoming cocaine dependent: epidemiological estimates for the United States, 2000–2001. *Neuropsychopharmacology*. 2005;30(5):1006–1018.

58. Reboussin BA, Anthony JC. Is there epidemiological evidence to support the idea that a cocaine dependence syndrome emerges soon after onset of cocaine use? *Neuropsychopharmacology*. 2006;31(9):2055–2064.
59. Nestler EJ, Barrot M, Self DW. DeltaFosB: a sustained molecular switch for addiction. *Proc Natl Acad Sci USA*. 2001;98(20):11042–11046.
60. Naqvi NH, Bechara A. The hidden island of addiction: the insula. *Trends Neurosci*. 2009;32(1):56–67.
61. Naqvi NH, Rudrauf D, Damasio H, et al. Damage to the insula disrupts addiction to cigarette smoking. *Science*. 2007;315(5811):531–534.
62. Nestler EJ. Review. Transcriptional mechanisms of addiction: role of DeltaFosB. *Philos Trans R Soc Lond B Biol Sci*. 2008;363(1507):3245–3255.
63. Nestler EJ. Molecular mechanisms of drug addiction. *Neuropharmacology*. 2004;47(suppl 1):24–32.
64. Leshner AI. Addiction is a brain disease, and it matters. *Science*. 1997;278(5335):45–47.
65. Hyman SE. The neurobiology of addiction: implications for voluntary control of behavior. *Am J Bioeth*. 2007;7(1):8–11.
66. McLellan AT, Kemp J, Brooks A, et al. Improving public addiction treatment through performance contracting: the Delaware experiment. *Health Policy*. 2008;87(3):296–308.
67. United Nations Office on Drugs and Crime. World Drug Report 2009. Vienna, Austria: Author; 2009.
68. 21 U.S.C. 812(c), Schedule I(c)(10).
69. The Swedish Council for Information on Alcohol and Other Drugs. The 2007 ESPAD report: Substance use among students in 35 European countries. Stockholm, Sweden: Modintryckoffset AB; 2009.
70. Bejerot N. Drug abuse and drug policy: an epidemiological and methodological study of drug abuse of intravenous type in the Stockholm police arrest population 1965–1970 in relation to changes in drug policy. *Acta Psychiatrica Scandinavica Supplementum*. 1975;256:3–277.
71. Bejerot N. *Addiction and Society*. Springfield, IL: Ch. Thomas; 1970.
72. Lindesmith AR. *The Addict and the Law*. Bloomington, IN: Indiana University Press; 1965.
73. Bejerot N. A theory of addiction as an artificially induced drive. *Am J Psychiatry*. 1972;128(7):842–846.
74. Bejerot N. The six day war in Stockholm. *New Scientist*. 1974;61(886):486–487.
75. Bejerot N. Addiction: Its nature, spread and treatment. *Isr Ann Psychiatr Relat Discip*. 1971;9(2):155–169.
76. Bejerot N. Premises for the treatment of addiction. *Br J Addict Alcohol Other Drugs*. 1969;64(1):87–93.
77. United Nations Office on Drugs and Crime. Sweden's successful drug policy: A review of the evidence. Vienna, Austria: Author; 2007.
78. Hartelius J. *Narcotic Drug Control Policy in Sweden: The Post-War Experience*. Stockholm: Fri Förlag; 2008.
79. Coleman JJ, Bensinger PB, Gold MS, et al. Can drug design inhibit abuse? *J Psychoactive Drugs*. 2005;37(4):343–362.
80. Caulkins JP, DuPont RL. Is 24/7 Sobriety a good goal for repeat driving under the influence (DUI) offenders? [Editorial]. *Addiction*. 2010;105:575–577.
81. DuPont RL, McLellan AT, Carr G, et al. How are addicted physicians treated? A national survey of physician health programs. *J Subst Abuse Treat*. 2009;37:1–7.
82. DuPont RL, McLellan AT, White WL, et al. Setting the standard for recovery: Physicians Health Programs evaluation review. *J Subst Abuse Treat*. 2009;36(2):159–171.
83. McLellan AT, Skipper GE, Campbell MG. et al. Five year outcomes in a cohort study of physicians treated for substance use disorders in the United States. *Br Med J*. 2008;337:a2038.
84. DuPont RL. Addiction in medicine. *Trans Am Clin Climatol Assoc*. 2008;119:227–241.
85. Skipper GE, DuPont RL. Substance abuse among physicians and other health professionals. In: Korsmeyer P, Kranzler HR, eds. *Encyclopedia of Drugs, Alcohol and Addictive Behaviors*. 3rd ed. 2008:242–251.
86. White WL, DuPont RL, Skipper GE. Physician health programs: what counselors can learn from these remarkable programs. *Counselor*. 2007;8(2):42–47.

CHAPTER 78: Substance Abuse Policy and Payment

Anita Everett

Throughout US history, there has been significant public policy debate on substance use and abuse. Policies on alcohol and other substances of abuse have included a wide variety of federal, state, and local government agencies. This has included taxation, law enforcement, armed services, highway transportation, prisons, courts, parks and recreation, social services, education, labor safety, health care delivery, disease surveillance, and more recently behavioral health care. Initially public policies related to substance abuse were more centered on containment of supply and appropriate taxation. Priority in policy development has gradually shifted toward limiting the untoward impact of alcohol and other substance abuse on others including family members and coworkers. More recent policy debate has centered on access to treatment and rehabilitation. The growing literature in support of prevention as viable and effective has had recent increasing prominence in public policy. Funding for substance abuse services and drug control programs has come from a variety of sources including private health insurance, as well as federal, state and local government sources. By far, the single biggest payer for treatment and drug control is the US Federal Government.

This chapter is written in two major parts. The first section provides a basic familiarity with public policy development. The second section outlines several federal government entities, particularly the federal entities that have had and continue to have a role in policy development and implementation. The first section will incorporate an example of an actual event and will explore several potential outcomes in policy development and implementation of strategies in response to a substance abuse–related event. Core knowledge regarding a basic definition, formation, and implementation of public policy on substance abuse will also be provided. This section is intended to demonstrate the complex interplay between various groups that influence and develop public substance abuse policy.

The goal of the second section is to highlight the history and role of several prominent government entities that are involved in developing and implementing substance abuse policy. The section includes entities that are responsible for drug control as well as treatment and prevention. This section will emphasize the sometimes competing interests of drug control with prevention and treatment. Throughout both sections, information on relative budgets and changes in budget over time will be included. This is intended to provide a broad perspective as to the relative investment US citizens have in substance abuse policy development and implementation.

POLICY DEVELOPMENT

Policy and policy development often moves in a nonlinear and in what may appear to be an illogical, reactionary, and disorderly fashion. This is a fundamental reality that it is critical for students of American Substance Abuse Policy to understand. Rational and science-based individuals who are more comfortable in a world where rational solutions are provided to solve problems of the greatest impact, are often frustrated by the process of the politics that invariably become involved with developing and implementing policy in a mature democracy such as the US government. A goal of this chapter is to provide an orientation to public policy development so that students and practitioners in the field of substance abuse are better equipped to work to influence good public policy development. Often in policy development, relative priorities have to be considered and appropriate resources are not applied to the most important problems. Understanding enough about how a process works is necessary in order to be able to effectively impact the process.

In this chapter, we will consider policy to be a collection of principles and ideas that are organized for the purpose of addressing a problem and with the intent that action will be taken to resolve the problem that is consistent with the policy. Steps in a public policy development process generally include a *problem definition,* consideration of *alternative solutions, policy development,* and *policy implementation.* In an ideal situation, the problem is a high-impact problem, all alternative solutions are considered and deliberated by experts, the best rational and most just or fair policy is developed and articulated, and logical steps are implemented that will resolve the problem. Problem-resolving steps can include a wide array of activities which often include new laws, financial resources, new staff, shifting of priorities in enforcement, treatment or prevention, new procedures, public awareness campaigns, etc. This four-element process is a foundation of policy development. The following event will serve as an example for discussion of policy development.

On Thursday March 20, 2008, the Modesto Bea ran a story entitled: *Huge amount of alcohol killed teen, coroner says.* In this article, writer Michael Shea reported that the body of 16-year-old Julia Gonzalez was found in a local park. On autopsy she had a blood alcohol level of 0.52 which is 6.5 times the legal limit in California. Shea reported that at 100 lbs and only 5 feet 2 in. tall, this would likely mean that she had consumed the equivalent of about one pint of 86 proof alcohol in an hour. Julia was reported to have lived with her grandmother and to have run away on two prior occasions. She left her home at 7 PM with friends and her body was found at 5 AM the following morning. At the time of the article, the exact circumstances of her death were unclear and friends who may have been with her were not providing further information regarding where and with whom she had been drinking. Police Detective Brandon Bertram stated that there could have been a crime associated with her death and that "manslaughter in cases like this is difficult to establish because of the difficulty in proving that the victim was forced to drink alcohol." Chief Deputy District Attorney Dave Harris related that the prosecution of adults who provide alcohol to minors is difficult and is a "nuanced area of the law." This article was accessed at the Modesto Bea site, at the following link on 1-8-2010 (http://alcoholism.about.com/gi/o.htm?zi=1/XJ&zTi=1&sdn=alcoholism&cdn=health&tm=181&gps=252_1564_990_535&f=10&su=p284.9.336.ip_p736.8.336.ip_&tt=2&bt=0&bts=0&zu=http%3A//www.modbee.com/local/story/244848.html). This incident will be used to illustrate the various potential entities and issues involved with substance abuse policy on treatment, prevention, and enforcement. The four-element process as described above (problem, solutions, policy, and implementation) will be used to explore a variety of potential outcomes from this incident.

Problem Definition

There are numerous ways a single incident like this can be used as a basis for problem formation. On one level this incident could be seen as the isolated and accidental death of one person, that is, a small and isolated incident that is not representative of a social problem or failure of existing policy and practice. On another level this incident could be framed as representing a serious problem of high risk with high consequences in the US teen population that was not able to be brought to justice due to inadequate underage drinking laws, inadequate law enforcement, inadequate park security or police patrolling, and inadequate alcohol and drug prevention and treatment programs in the community and schools, that is, a single incident that represents a problem of tremendous magnitude and social significance.

In addition to the facts, the context and attention an incident or problem receives can shape the relevant priority a problem is given. Contemporary media often serves to highlight or raise the profile of a problem. If this story became the subject of a Cable News Network (CNN) expose on a media outlet such as the Nancy Grace Show, it might draw a great deal of attention and raise public awareness regarding teen death by alcohol intoxication as a broad public problem effecting many communities that requires immediate remedy. Similarly the association with a high-profile individual can serve to expedite public concern about an incident. If Julie Gonzales were a family member of a Modesto area celebrity resident such as Star Wars producer George Lucas, the incident might become a prominent problem in terms of public interest.

Advocacy groups can be very influential in raising public awareness and opinion as to the severity of a problem. Several different advocacy groups might be interested in this event as an example of a problem that their group works to address. Examples of primary advocacy groups would include: *Students Against Drugs and Alcohol* (SADA, http:// www.sada.org) and *Students Against Destructive Decisions* (SADD) which was founded as *Students Against Driving Drunk* in 1981. Currently SADD includes over 10,000 chapters throughout the United States (information from website retrieved 1-10-2010, http://www.sad.org).

Mothers Against Drunk Driving (MADD, http://www.madd.org) is another advocacy organization with a primary interest in underage drinking. MADD has been described by author Malcolm Gladwell (1) in his bestseller, *Tipping Point*, as one of our nation's most successful advocacy organizations. Gladwell describes MADD as having catalyzed a national tipping point in American society such that it is no longer socially acceptable to drive under the influence of alcohol. This group has been extremely successful since its origin in 1980 in influencing public policy centered on the core problem of driving while under the influence of alcohol. MADD focuses advocacy on three priority areas, drunk driving, support for the victims of drunk driving, and underage drinking. This organization has strongly supported the creation and enforcement of strict penalties for Driving Under the Influence charges. Thus MADD might be instrumental in highlighting this tragic alcohol intoxication death as a representative example of the consequences of underage drinking. Other types of groups that might play a role in publicizing the significance of the problem of underage drinking on a local or national scale might include professional organizations such as the American Academy of Pediatrics (AAP), the California Chapter of the AAP (in their role as advocates for the health and safety of children and adolescents), the National Association of Medical Examiners (advocacy for reduction in preventable deaths), law-enforcement organizations such as the Fraternal Order of Police (FOP), the Parent Teacher Associations (PTA), or other local civic groups.

Solution Deliberation

Once the problem is identified and takes form, a general next step in policy process is the consideration of various solutions that would remedy the problem. Proposed solutions can come from a wide variety of sources and often include scientific expertise as well as consultation with individuals who have had direct experience with the problem. This might include input from a senior level of advisors or cabinet members, community members, opinion editorials, individual experts, or special advisors. A common approach to the generation of a solution in a political arena is to convene a "blue ribbon" panel of experts that deliberate aspects of a problem and create a report that includes recommendation for resolution of the problem.

Generally a blue ribbon panel has some degree of independence from government and is set up to impartially deliberate the problem and make recommendations for policy. In this case, a possible scenario might have been the mayor, county board of commissioners, county school board, a California state legislator, a governor or other elected official convening such a panel or commission. Blue ribbon panels are comprised of experts as well as stakeholders with vested interest in the problem. Membership of a blue ribbon panel in the situation of underage drinking might include local elected officials, representatives of the PTA, student body, local city council or school board, parents or other prominent community members. Generally a series of presentations and testimony is organized to inform the panel regarding the current status of the problem as well as to provide expert opinion regarding potential solutions to the problem. Thus there might be presentations from the county school system drug and alcohol prevention coordinator so that the current content and status of prevention curriculum could be considered. Existing state laws and local ordinances regarding the provision of alcohol to underage individuals might be reviewed for the panel and the level of evidence required for prosecuting manslaughter or other potential crimes under current laws might be reviewed. Individuals from other states with more aggressive laws or school prevention programs might be consulted to provide their data and experience with similar problems. Researchers might be invited to provide testimony that summarizes current literature regarding effective prevention and law-enforcement programs.

The work of a panel often culminates in a report that includes at a minimum, a listing of recommendations or potential solutions to the problem. Advocacy groups themselves are very often involved with advocating for panels to be set up to focus attention to a specific problem. Advocacy groups often provide testimony and resources to panel members on their particular aspect of the problem. Blue ribbon panels can be a very effective mechanism for assembling a set of possible recommendations or solutions to a problem in the political policy formation process. Panels have the advantage of being independent from an elected government official and thereby have independence in the types of policy and recommendations they make.

Policy Development

The policy itself may be a clearly written document that articulates the problem and solutions that are to be taken to remedy the problem, or it may be much less formal. In this particular case, there may be recommendations that are oriented around drug and alcohol control and there may be recommendations oriented around increased access to treatment and preventive services. An elected official, with a candidacy based on a platform of being tough on crime, might be more likely to support policy that prioritizes law enforcement and includes tightening of any gaps in the laws so that law enforcement is more able to make arrests and so that prosecutors are more likely to successfully prosecute. In our example situation, a resultant policy might be to assure that youth who appear intoxicated in public can be detained; to create laws so that it becomes a criminal act to facilitate the provision of alcohol or other illicit substance of abuse to minors even if they did not force the minor to use the substance; or to strengthen the enforcement of laws regarding the illegal retail sale of alcohol to underage individuals. On the other hand, an individual or party elected on a broad policy in support of harm reduction and treatment of individuals with substance abuse problems might be much more oriented toward strengthening prevention curriculum in schools, increasing access to adolescent treatment centers, providing hot lines and community escort services for inebriated youth and individuals, and community education of involved adults such as teachers and peers so that excessive and risky drinking and substance abuse behaviors can be identified and addressed early.

Implementation

Implementation and execution are an important component of the policy development process. How a policy is executed, that is how it is codified and enforced is critical to success. Codification is the clear articulation and/or passage of a written procedure, law, act, ordinance, or regulation itself. Enforcement is the actual plan for assurance that the policy is followed as intended. Codification for prevention could include school board policy that mandates prevention classes for all high school freshmen, budget revisions that provide a prevention staff for every high school, etc. Enforcement of mandated prevention could include no passing to 10th grade without prevention classes or budget and staffing audits to assure that schools have complied. Codification of actual laws could come from a review of existing laws and passage of amendments and new laws that make any act that enables an underage person to have access to alcohol or illicit drugs to be able to be arrested and convicted. Enforcement could come from priorities established with local law enforcement to make arrests of adults that are involved with enabling underage access to alcohol or other drugs.

In this section, four steps in the process of the development and implementation of policy have been presented and discussed. These steps are not always linear and orderly, however, these four steps are generally seen with public policy development. Factors that are commonly involved with problem definition, alternative consideration, policy development, and pursuant implementation were presented. The goal of this section is to provide a basic foundation as to how policy is developed and implemented.

FEDERAL POLICY AGENCIES

The historical and policy context of several entities that are involved with substance abuse policy and funding will be presented in this section. One cannot understand contemporary substance abuse policy without a basic understanding as to the rich historical context of alcohol and substances of abuse in American history. A thorough review of substance abuse history is beyond the scope of this chapter, however, a few prominent highlights of early American history as well as a basic summary of the historical political origin of several substance abuse–related government and advocacy agencies will provide readers with a basic foundation as to the importance of substance abuse policy in American history.

Alcohol has been integrally involved with American history since before government was created. In *The Spirits of America: A Social History of Alcohol*, Eric Burns, writes that General George Washington was a strong believer in the necessity of spirits for his troops. Burns recounts General Washington's distress when shipments of alcohol for his troops were disrupted. In a letter to the president of the Continental Congress, Washington wrote: "The benefits arising from the moderate use of strong liquor have been experienced in all armies and are not to be disrupted" (2). Thus at the very outset of American history, a founding father asserted a policy that alcohol was essential for his soldiers and must be included as a component of the proper provisioning for his troops. The requested alcohol provision was 4 ounces per man per day.

Following the Revolutionary War, many US colonial farms and plantations, including George Washington's Mount Vernon, operated highly profitable distilleries. Alcohol was also included as an essential component of provisions for the Discovery Corps for the Lewis and Clark Expedition. Throughout early American history, distilled spirits in the form of rum have been an important part of the economy as a product for trade with Caribbean farmers for sugar cane and slaves from Africa.

As the young federal government developed, one of the first challenges in sustaining credibility as a viable government was to repay revolutionary war debt. Initially, the federal government had no authority to levy taxes, even to pay for federal government functions such as maintaining an army. A policy for funding federal government functions was developed and one of the first taxes was a tax on imported spirits. A special office was created to collect these taxes and today this office is known as the Bureau of Alcohol, Tobacco, Firearms, and Explosives (ATF).

Many federal agencies that are involved with substance abuse were formed as a part of the implementation step in response to public pressure that resulted in policy development. In the following section, several of these agencies will be reviewed in terms of the historical problem they were designed to solve as well as the current role in substance abuse policy. The Office of National Drug Control Policy (ONDCP) as well as several agencies that have been designed to control the supply of drugs and alcohol and several agencies that have been designed to control the use or demand for drugs and alcohol.

The ONDCP is the national coordinating entity for all federal drug policy. The ONDCP was formed as a component of the Anti-Drug Abuse Act in November of 1988 during the Reagan administration. The Anti-Drug Abuse Act also created the Drug Free Workplace rules that require workplaces to maintain a drug-free workplace as a condition of receiving federal funding for contracts and/or grants. The phrase "just say no" was coined by first lady, Nancy Reagan, as a component of President Regan's crusade against drug use in America. The ONDCP was formed to solve the problem of rising drug and cocaine abuse in the early 1980s as well as to align widespread variability in the approach to substance abuse policy within the executive branch of the federal government. With central coordination and alignment of all the federal entities and agencies that are involved with substance abuse there is a much greater likelihood of success in addressing the adverse impact that licit and illicit substance use has on society.

The ONDCP is within the Executive Office of the president and a chief function is to produce the National Drug Control Strategy, which is the chief policy document that is designed to align all federal activities that are related to substance abuse policy, enforcement, research, prevention, and treatment. This strategy outlines a budget as well as guidelines for coordination and cooperation among federal state and local entities. The ONDCP also evaluates and advises the president on international anti-drug policy. The ONDCP tracks and coordinates all federal spending on substance abuse. A detailed review of the functions of the ONDCP can be found on the website: http://www.whitehousedrugpolicy.gov/about/index.html.

The two broad policy priority areas that ONDCP considers include drug control and drug demand. Drug demand, that is, demand for drugs by drug abusers, includes policy and activities that address treatment and prevention. Treatment and prevention reduce demand. Policies that relate to the control of drug availability include domestic law enforcement and international counter drug enforcement.

Table 1 from the 2010 ONDCP budget (http://www.ondcp.gov/publications/policy/10budget/index.html) represents the administrative budget requests for the federal 2010 budget. This provides aggregated information from across cabinets and agencies that enable a broad comparison of the relative federal expenditures on drug demand versus drug control expenditures. This table demonstrates that over the last several years, approximately twice as many federal dollars have been allocated for drug control and law enforcement as opposed to funding for treatment and preventionservices.

The federal entities that are included within the substance abuse demand realm include the Departments of Health and Human Services, Interior, Veterans Affairs, Education, and the Small Business Administration. The federal entities that are counted as being within the drug supply control realm include the Departments of Defense, Homeland Security, Justice, State, Transportation, and Treasury. Each of these federal demand and control entities was created to address an aspect of public substance abuse policy. In the following section, several important federal entities will be discussed. Sections will include a discussion of the historical policy problem that the agency was formed to address as well as provide information about the current budget and active programs.

DRUG CONTROL AGENCIES

The ATF was created as an agency of the Department of Justice in January 2003 under the Homeland Security Act. This agency had previously been within the Treasury Department and was known as the Bureau of Alcohol, Tobacco and Firearms, which was also designated by the same three-letter acronym, ATF. The ATF is the oldest of the federal agencies related to drug control and has origins in federal policy on tax collection. In 1789, congress imposed a national tax on imported spirits in order to help repay debt associated with the Revolutionary War. Accountants were trained to be investigators to function within the Department of Treasury to enforce the collection of taxes on alcohol. Similar federal taxes were enacted on tobacco products and the task of enforcing these taxes was given to a group of special agents within the office of Internal Revenue.

In response to growing public concern that alcohol consumption had grave impact on American families, prohibition was passed as the 18th amendment to the Constitution in 1919 and it resulted in laws that made it illegal to manufacture, sell, or transport alcohol. The Office of Internal Revenue was a major force of the federal attempt to enforce these laws. The term "revenuers" was coined from this era and describes internal revenue agents from the Treasury Department who were responsible for the investigation of illegal production of alcohol (moonshine) thus resulting in tax evasion. A special unit called the Prohibition Unit was formed from the expertise of the revenuers which today is part of the historic legacy of the ATF. Prohibition lasted for 14 years until it was repealed in 1933 with the ratification of the 21st amendment. In response to public concern regarding firearms exposure that was present throughout prohibition, the national firearms act was passed in 1934 which added firearms regulatory responsibilities to the ATF precursor. Duties regarding explosives were added to the ATF in the 1970s and the most recent reorganization of ATF moved it from treasury and into the Department of Homeland Security in 1998 (http://www.atf.gov/about/history/atf-from-1789-1998.html).

Today the ATF employs about 5000 people and in 2009 had a budget of just over 1 billion dollars. In the Fiscal year 2010 Congressional Budget Submission, the ATF lists its mission as "the U.S. law enforcement agency dedicated to protecting our Nation from the illicit use of firearms and explosives in violent crime and acts of terrorism. ATF protects our communities from violent criminals and criminal organizations by investigating and preventing the illegal use and trafficking of firearms, the illegal use and improper storage of explosives, acts of arson and bombings, and the illegal diversion of alcohol and tobacco products" (ATF congressional Budget Report, accessed on January 20, 2010 at http://www.justice.gov/jmd/2010justification/pdf/fy10-atf.pdf). Whereas this agency has its origins in alcohol and tobacco control, it now currently focuses predominantly on violent crime and gun and explosives control.

The Drug Enforcement Administration or DEA was established by congress in 1973 during the Nixon Administration and was started in response to growing concern about illicit drug use in the United States in the 1960s to 1970s. In a speech in 1971, President Nixon declared drug abuse as "public enemy number one." Of particular concern at that time was the importation of Mexican cannabis as well as heroin. President Nixon coined the term "War on Drugs," and strengthened the role of the federal government considerably in the coordination of the control of illicit drugs.

A brief description of the historic lineage of the DEA helps to demonstrate the complexity and far reaching involvement of the federal government in substance abuse policy. In 1968, President Johnson formed the US Bureau of Narcotics and Dangerous Drugs (BNDD) from two agencies: the Bureau of Narcotics in the Treasury Department which was responsible for the control of marijuana and heroin (illicit drugs), with the Bureau of Drug Abuse Control, in the Department of Health, Education, and Welfare, which was responsible for the control of dangerous drugs. The BNDD was then placed under the Department of Justice which is primarily concerned with law enforcement. Five years later in 1973 and during the Nixon Administration, the DEA was developed in order to create a stronger federal agency that could better enforce domestic federal drug laws as well as address the growing sophistication of international drug traffickers primarily from Europe and South America. The DEA was formed from the BNDD, the US Customs Department, the Office of National Narcotics Intelligence, and the Office of Drug Abuse Law Enforcement. At the outset, the DEA had 1470 Special Agents with a budget of 74.9 million dollars. Currently there are over 5000 DEA agents and the annual budget is just over 2 billion dollars. The DEA operates as an agency within the US Department of Justice (http://www.justice.gov/dea/pubs/history/1970-1975.pdf).

Today an important function of the DEA is the enforcement of the legal prescribing of narcotics. This function has its origins in the Harrison Narcotic Act. The Harrison Narcotic Act was passed in 1914 and required prescriptions for narcotics and mandated record keeping for physicians and pharmacists who dispense narcotics. The Harrison Narcotic Act was passed to solve the problem of uncontrolled growth in the use of narcotics as well as the use of heroin and cocaine. This act followed US participation in the Shanghai Opium Commission of 1909 which was the first international conference convened to address worldwide the problem of drug abuse, most particularly heroin. With growing concern regarding the abuse and nonmedical use of prescription drugs as reported in the National Survey on Drug Use and Health in 2009, DEA has worked with state government drug control agencies to develop more coordinated policy that enhances the capacity to identify and control prescription drug abuse (3).

The Federal Bureau of Investigation (FBI) has its origins in 1908 during the presidency of Theodore Roosevelt. This agency was created to provide investigative ability to the US Attorney General in the Department of Justice. The FBI does not have a primary mission in the investigation of drug-related crime; however, much of the crime that the FBI investigates involves or is funded by drug-related criminal activity such as terrorism, organized crime, money laundering, and gangs. The FBI works with other local, federal, and international law enforcement to investigate drug crimes. The FBI started 100 years ago with 34 investigators and a budget of several million dollars. Currently there are nearly 30,000 employees and the budget is over 7 billion dollars (http://www.fbi.gov/homepage.htm).

The Food and Drug Administration (FDA) is currently within the federal Health and Human Services agencies and is considered to have been founded on June 30, 1906 when the Pure Food and Drugs Act was signed into law by President Theodore Roosevelt. This act restricted interstate commerce in misbranded and adulterated foods, drinks, and drugs. The original bureau responsible for this act was in the Department of Agriculture (http://www.fda.gov/AboutFDA/WhatWeDo/History/Milestones/ucm128305.htm). The FDA has a role in regulating the safety of the production of prescription narcotics but does not directly regulate the legal use of addicting medications.

FEDERAL DEMAND DEPARTMENTS AND AGENCIES

The federal departments that operate programs designed to limit the demand for substances of abuse include the Department of Health and Human Services (DHHS), Interior, Veterans Affairs, Education, and the Small Business Administration. In general, programs that are designed to provide treatment are more recent than programs that control supply. The DHHS receives the single largest amount of federal funding for substance abuse of any of the other federal cabinet-level departments. This funding includes funding for treatment that is administered by the Center for Medicare and Medicaid (CMS), funding for treatment and prevention programs that are operated by the Substance Abuse and Mental Health Services Administration (SAMHSA) and the Indian Health Service. The National Institutes of Health (NIH) includes two institutes that address problems related to drugs and alcohol as a primary mission. These are the National Institute on Drug Abuse (NIDA) and the National Institute on Alcohol Abuse and Alcoholism (NIAAA). The Federal Drug Administration (FDA) which is also within DHHS, regulates the safety of licit domestic drugs but does not have a direct role in addressing supply or abuse of addicting medications.

In 1992, the Alcohol and Drug Abuse, Mental Health Administration (ADAMHA) was divided into several research agencies including NIDA, NIAAA, and NIMH. At this time the SAMHSA was created to operate and administer federal substance abuse and mental health programs and services grants. This role is conceptually distinct from research entities that have some degree of intellectual independence from treatment program administration. SAMHSA is divided into three principal offices: the Center for Mental Health Services (CMHS), the Center for Substance Abuse Treatment (CSAT), and the Center for Substance Abuse Prevention (CSAP).

NIDA and NIAAA are the two primary substance abuse research entities in NIH. These institutes have distinct histories and have been maintained as two entities on the conceptual grounds that alcohol is a legal substance of potential abuse which can be used safely, and other drugs of abuse are illegal. It is likely that this separation has a historical association with prohibition and the subsequent repeal of prohibition in 1933 with the passage of the 21st amendment. Clearly there are inconsistencies in policy that separates alcohol on the grounds that it is a legal substance from other legal and addictive substances such as prescription pain medications and in some states, medical cannabis.

The NIDA budget has more than doubled since it origin in 1992 and in 2008 was just over a billion dollars. The NIAAA budget as well has more than doubled in this period with a budget in 2008 of just under 500 million dollars. This represents tremendous federal investment in research on the underlying causes and treatment of drug use and alcohol abuse. At its core, research is the unbiased discovery of new facts. While research produces new knowledge and information that influences policy and public policy, the scientific knowledge that is produced should be free from bias. In our four-step paradigm of public policy development (problem, identification of potential solutions, policy formation, implementation) NIDA and NIAAA would not be involved in advocacy for a problem rather they would be involved with the provision of scientific information that would help to delineate the problem as well as potential best solutions. Additionally, increased funding for research on a particular problem is often done as an implementation step in response to public policy that is created to solve a societal problem.

A recent example of this would be the problem of rural use of methamphetamine, "crystal meth" in the United States. Methamphetamine has been used in the United States for over a century, however, in the early 1980s methods for easy home manufacturing from common inexpensive household products became widely known. The use of crystal meth has spread primarily from the west to the east coast and may have origins in Japan. The manufacture of crystal meth has increasingly become identified as a significant problem in rural areas. Rural areas are attractive for crystal meth because manufacturing results in large quantities of waste that must be hidden or dispersed and also because the ingredients are inexpensive and readily available. Although there are regional differences in the penetration of the problem, crystal meth use has progressively become defined as a nationally significant problem. As is common in substance abuse policy, the range of potential solutions generally includes both control measures through tighter laws and law enforcement and reducing the demand for the substance through treatment and prevention.

Because crystal meth is a relatively new problem, and not much is known about the relative efficacy of potential treatments, prevention techniques and/or long-term impact of abuse and/or addiction, NIDA has been involved as a component of a national policy action to reduce the adverse impact of crystal meth on our nation. In this case NIDA was funded by the president and congress to create a series of projects that are designed to provide information on the epidemiology of the problem, best treatment methods, medications and immunizations that may reduce or eliminate craving and abuse as well as to study the impact of high exposure to crystal meth on human bodies and particularly the central nervous system. This research is designed to increase knowledge about the problem so that iterative policy can be developed and implemented that is more able to accurately eliminate the problems associated with crystal meth use. Thus, the federal research institutes are involved with generating science that informs public policy and the budgets of these institutions is impacted by what problems policymakers decide to solve. Research institutes are not generally directly involved in advocacy or in making public policy.

Other entities within the federal government that provide health and substance use information that informs policy development are the US HHS Center for Disease Control (CDC) and the National Highway Traffic Safety Administration (NHTSA). The CDC conducts numerous nationally based disease and health-related surveys that include substance abuse. Two examples of this within the CDC are the Behavioral Risk Factor Surveillance Survey (BRFSS, http://www.cdc.gov/brfss/about.htm) which monitors general health behaviors that includes substance abuse, and the National HIV Behavioral Surveillance System (NHBS, http://www.cdc.gov/hiv/topics/surveillance/index.htm) which includes statistical information on IV drug abuse and its relationship to trends in HIV/AIDS.

The NHTSA maintains national statistics on highway safety and on motor vehicle accidents and has been a significant source of information for advocacy groups such as the aforementioned MADD which apply pressure to prioritize the problem of driving while under the influence.

The federal government has a large investment in the provision of substance abuse treatment to Americans. The primary agencies that are involved with treatment funding include Medicaid and Medicare. Both of these programs are administered by the Center for Medicare and Medicaid Services (CMS). An additional federal entity that provides funding for treatment includes the federal substance abuse block grant which is administered by CSAT within SAMHSA. Other entities such as the Veterans Administration and the Department of Defense also provide substance abuse treatment for armed services soldiers and employees.

Medicare was formally created in the Johnson administration in 1965. Medicare was enacted after 20 years of pressure in congress and various incremental programs that were designed to solve the problem of health care access for elderly and retired individuals. Elderly individuals were no longer employed and did not have access to employee-based health insurance. They were often living on meager pensions and in poverty. In 1972 Medicare was expanded to include individuals with long-term disability. In 2003, according to the SAMHSA Behavioral Health Care Expenditures Report, Medicare comprised 5% of total national expenditures on substance abuse treatment (4). The majority of substance abuse–related Medicare expenditures were for inpatient hospital-based detoxification. The benefits that are covered under Medicare are determined by CMS payment policy as well as regulations that are created in response to congressional legislation. A Medicare Evidence Development and Coverage Advisory Committee exists to provide recommendations from experts regarding changes in coverage to include new developments in treatment and to eliminate payment for ineffective treatments.

Medicaid is the second major federal health insurance program that is administered by CMS. Medicaid was enacted just after Medicare and is a significant funder of substance abuse treatment services. Medicaid is a state and federal partnership wherein states provide just under half of the funds. Each state makes determinations regarding the type of substance abuse benefit that its Medicaid program will cover and state programs vary widely regarding coverage of treatment of substance abuse treatment. Medicaid is principally designed to provide health insurance for children and adults in poverty. According to the SAMHSA health care expenditure report, in 2003 Medicaid paid for 18% of all expenditure on substance abuse treatment (4).

Although this chapter focuses primarily on the role of federal government entities that are involved in developing substance abuse policy and in funding control and treatment, state and local government have significant roles in the development of parallel local and regional state policy on substance abuse control and demand. In considering overall sources of funding for substance abuse treatment nationally, state and local government provides 40% of the total US substance abuse treatment expense. In comparison, the national figures for the amount that private insurance pays are only about 10% of all expenditures on substance abuse treatment. This has reduced considerably since 1993, when private insurance paid for 14% of the total substance abuse treatment expenditures (4).

The CSAT within SAMSHA administers the Substance Abuse Block Grant which as of 2003 provides 8% of all monies that are spent on substance abuse treatment (3). This grant is distributed to substance abuse treatment providers through state government recipients.

CONCLUSION

This chapter was written to provide a foundation for understanding the elements in policy development in the area of substance abuse. It is not possible within the confines of a chapter to review the entire history of US substance abuse policy development. Numerous examples were woven into the chapter to demonstrate the basic policy process: problem identification, alternatives consideration, policy development, and implementation. Substance abuse problems are of great social concern and have tremendous capacity to adversely impact individuals, families, communities, and our entire nation. Policies on substances of abuse have been embedded in US government function throughout the entire history of our nation. A wide variety of government and federal agencies are involved in the provision of drug control enforcement and drug abuse treatment and prevention. In general, the US federal government allocates twice as much funding for drug control activity as it does for activity that would reduce drug demand. The mission of the ONDCP is to coordinate all federal agencies and activities that are related to substance abuse policy. Many other entities are involved with policy implementation. It is essential for stakeholders involved with advocating for substance abuse treatment and prevention to understand the foundations of policy development so that effective solutions can be implemented to reduce the adverse impact of substance abuse on our families and society.

REFERENCES

1. Gladwell M. *The Tipping Point: How Little Things Can Make a Big Difference.* New York: Little, Brown and Company; 2000.
2. Burns E. *The Spirits of America: A Social History of Alcohol.* Philadelphia, PA: Temple University Press; 2004.
3. Substance Abuse and Mental Health Services Administration, Office of Applied Studies (February 5, 2009). *The NSDUH Report: Trends in Nonmedical Use of Prescription Pain Relievers: 2002 to 2007.* Rockville, MD (http://www.oas.samhsa.gov/2k9/painRelievers/nonmedicalTrends.cfm).
4. Mark TL, Levit KR. *National Expenditures for Mental Health Services and Substance Abuse Treatment 1993–2003.* Substance Abuse and Mental Health Administration Publication No. SMA 07-4227. Rockville, MD: Substance Abuse and Mental Health Services Administration; 2007.

CHAPTER 79 Forensics

Ihsan M. Salloum

The interface between forensic and addiction psychiatry is rich and spans both clinical and legal arenas within the civil and criminal areas. This chapter is a synoptic overview and is intended to serve as a practical guide to *criminal* forensic practice for the addiction specialist. In this chapter, we will highlight conceptual questions arising from the interaction between the law and addiction medicine and we will provide references to primary legal sources, textbooks, reviews, and commentaries for the interested reader. We will also discuss issues related to the applicability of *DSM-IV-TR* (*Diagnostic and Statistical Manual of Mental Disorders*. 4th ed., text revision) criteria in the courtroom, the relevance of intoxication to intent, and residual effects of substance use following discontinuation of such use.

This chapter is divided into six main sections. In the first section, we summarize the fundamental legal principles and procedures governing expert testimony about the "mental" elements in the criminal law. In the second section, we examine the potential roles for the addiction expert in criminal proceedings. In the third section, we discuss the relevance of the effects of intoxicant substance use on criminal responsibility, considering defenses as well as mitigation based on intoxication, dependence, and withdrawal. (For heuristic purposes, unless otherwise qualified, the term *intoxicant* refers to *substances*, i.e., *drugs*.)

In the remaining sections, we will discuss issues raised by the "addictive processes," with primary focus on pathologic gambling (fourth section), and we will consider the vexing problem of the credibility of the testimony of intoxicant-involved witnesses (fifth section). In the sixth and final section of this chapter, we will address regulatory and administrative matters related intoxicant substances, with particular emphasis on the implications of the concept of "impairment" and the regulatory problems of long-term opioid therapy in private practice.

THE ADDICTION MEDICINE SPECIALIST AS A FORENSIC EXPERT

Clinical Experts in the Criminal Law

The addiction specialist's role as expert in forensic matters has grown significantly over the past decades reflecting the growth of the accredited specialty of addiction psychiatry and addiction medicine and of the maturation of this subspecialty in general. Addiction specialists are being preferentially sought after by attorneys for consultation and expert testimony about the effects of intoxicant use instead of continuing to resort to general psychiatrists, psychologists, or other mental health professionals. The emergence of a body of "facts" in the specialty of addiction medicine, about which there is little or no difference of opinion in the field, as analyzed by Burglass and Shaffer (1–3), has contributed significantly to this shift. Burglass and Shaffer critically review the state of knowledge in the addictions field, including theory, research, and practice (1–3).

Being Qualified as an Expert

Although there are federal and state standards that govern expert testimony, there is little consistency between and within jurisdictions about the qualifications of expert witnesses. Determining who should be an expert witness for "psychologic" matters has been a difficult task for the courts. Often, decisions regarding who qualifies as an "expert" are made on pragmatic rather than jurisprudential grounds. Some courts have permitted (or precluded) a wide range of individuals, including case workers (4,5), police officers (6–8), and even lay witnesses (9,10), to testify about a variety of psychologic issues (including the question of sanity). Other courts have been unwilling to recognize the expertise of psychiatrists, physicians, psychologists, and others, and have refused to admit their testimony in selected matters. Examples include compulsive gambling (11,12), the effects of drugs on witness credibility (13,14), and satanic ritual murder (15).

With rare exceptions, psychiatrists, physicians who specialize in mental (neurologic and psychologic) disorders, and doctoral-level clinical psychologists are qualified as experts. Although professional associations in psychiatry (16) and psychology (17) have developed guidelines for determining forensic expertise and practice, these criteria have not been adopted as authoritative by the courts. For the most part, courts have been reluctant to admit psychologic evidence tending to favor an accused (18). For a comprehensive review of the determination and utilization of expertise in mental matters in the federal and state jurisdictions, see Ref. 19 (§2:2–11).

Rationale for the Admission of Expert Testimony

The Federal Rule of Evidence 702 provides that "if scientific, technical, or other specialized knowledge will assist the trier of fact [judge or jury] to understand the evidence or to determine a fact in issue, a witness qualified as an expert by knowledge, skill, experience, training, or education, may testify thereto in the form of an opinion or otherwise" (20). Most states have a rule of evidence that parallels the Federal Rule of Evidence 702, although a few states have adopted different and confusing rules on this point. The states also have tended to follow Federal Rule of Evidence 704, which limits expert testimony to an explanation of the defendant's diagnosis and the characteristics of the disease or defect. This rule specifically precludes expert opinion on "whether the defendant did or did not have the mental state or condition constituting an element of the crime charged or of a defense thereto" (20). This question (referred to in the law as the "ultimate issue") is for the jury to decide. The trial judge makes the final decision regarding expertise and the admissibility of expert testimony, despite the prevailing rules of evidence (11,12,21–24).

In practice, if satisfactory evidence of knowledge, skill, experience, or training in the diagnosis and/or active treatment (but not mere research) of intoxicant-involved patients is provided, it is likely that expert qualification in the areas of addiction and the effects of intoxicants will be recognized by the court. Although qualified as an expert by the court, the admissibility of expert testimony into evidence is a separate question to be argued by counsel. Ultimately, all decisions regarding the qualification of experts and the admissibility of their testimony are made at the discretion of the trial judge (25–29).

How the Law Views Expert Testimony

Under prevailing rules of evidence, the testimony of expert witnesses is presented to the court in the form of expert opinion. As such it does not enjoy the same privileged status as "fact" testimony. It is up to the judge or the jury (the trier of fact) to evaluate the credibility, reliability, relevance, and applicability of any expert testimony introduced. Thus, even what is considered accepted medical "fact" is considered only "opinion" when expressed in expert testimony and as such it may be accepted, discounted, or rejected in whole or in part. When testifying, any lapse of awareness of this crucial distinction may result in the expert being perceived as argumentative, defensive, sanctimonious, condescending, or hostile. This always compromises the expert's credibility and undermines the power of the testimony as evidence, which may prove fatal to the client's case.

THE ROLE OF THE EXPERT IN ADDICTION MEDICINE

The professional mandate as an expert witness is to assist the court. It is important to remember that the role of the expert witness is not that of an advocate. The expert testimony responsibility is to provide the judge and jury with information that is truthful, intelligible, and clear and to offer the opinions that are unbiased, carefully reasoned, and based on the expert's understanding of the facts in evidence. The expert witness is more likely to be engaged by the defense than the by persecution, as it rarely serves the interest of the prosecution's case to introduce expert testimony in support of exculpating or mitigating mental defenses. Thus, the following discussion may seem to express a defense bias. The prosecution, on the other hand, may call experts to rebut testimony introduced by defense experts and the expert should be willing to appear for either side.

The Pretrial Phase

The addiction specialist activities in the pretrial phase involve several areas. The addiction specialist can assist the attorney by reviewing the initial discovery materials (e.g., police reports, arrest forms, affidavits of investigating agencies, waivers of rights, medical examiner reports, toxicology screens, statements of witnesses and/or the accused, confessions, the formal complaint, information, or indictment) to identify any immediate or potential issues related to intoxicants. Furthermore, attorneys may seek assistance in managing a difficult, compromised, or dangerous client. It may be necessary to immediately evaluate and refer the client for primary treatment or stabilization so that the client can adequately assist counsel in the preparation of the case. Determination of competency to stand trial is a separate matter, both clinically and legally.

The addiction specialist should make a preliminary assessment of all available background materials of prospective witnesses to identify any possible clinical (i.e., medical, neuropsychiatric, or addiction) issues that require investigation. The addiction specialist can also help the attorney to prepare for depositions by (a) drafting specific questions to be posed, (b) doing content and psycholinguistic analyses of taped or written evidence (e.g., statements or depositions made by the defendant or witnesses), and (c) suggesting strategies and tactics for conducting interviews or depositions. It is often important to interview family members, friends, former teachers, or others who may have particular knowledge or a different perspective of the defendant or witness (30).

The cornerstone of the addiction specialist's evaluation of the defendant is a comprehensive addiction history. The addiction specialist must aggressively inquire about every aspect of use and experience with intoxicants of all classes and all of the addictive processes. The addiction specialist must take a lifetime neuropsychiatric history, exploring every sign or symptom reported, suggested, implied, or suspected. Also, complete medical (including all responses to prescription and over-the-counter medications), psychosocial, developmental, educational, relational, and vocational histories must be taken. History or indicia of psychologic, sexual, or physical abuse must also be aggressively sought and explored.

The addiction specialist and the attorney work closely together during the pretrial phase with reciprocal responsibilities. The addiction specialist's responsibility to the attorney is to identify, analyze, develop, and explain facts or issues relating to the use or effects of intoxicants. The attorney's responsibility to the addiction specialist is to analyze and explain the laws of the jurisdiction that (a) govern the nature and scope of admissible expert testimony, (b) define the required mental "elements of the offense" for the crime charged, and (c) determine the availability of defenses or mitigation based upon the use and/or effects of intoxicants. This interaction between the disciplines of law and medicine, unfettered by the legal rules of the courtroom, is invariably a stimulating and instructive experience for both the attorney and the addiction specialist. This collaboration will result in the formulation of potential clinical approaches to the defense of the case, and in time, they will develop agreement upon a strategy for the clinical component of the defense and set the general contour of the addiction specialist testimony.

Once the clinical and legal issues are clarified and resolved, the addiction specialist should draft the actual questions that the attorney should ask the addiction specialist on direct examination. At the very least, the addiction specialist must frame the questions that establish his or her expertise and any questions required to elicit the predicate facts and issues to be introduced into evidence as the basis for the addiction specialist testimony and opinions. This is a tedious and time-consuming task; however, it cannot be done by the attorney. Only the expert in addiction medicine can fully appreciate the relevance and implications of the clinical subtleties and distinctions and can identify and illuminate the clinical concepts likely to confuse the judge or jury. And only the addiction specialist can anticipate the pitfalls that loom on the narrow plateau of accommodation between the restrictive rules of legal discourse and the broad latitude required in complex clinical explanations. There is no more frustrating or unsettling experience for an expert than being put or left in a compromised position on the witness stand as a result of having been asked ill-framed questions by an inadequately prepared attorney.

The addiction specialist also can assist the attorney if the other side will be calling an addiction expert by (a) evaluating that expert's credentials, (b) anticipating the nature of the testimony, (c) analyzing the strengths and weaknesses of both expert positions, and (d) drafting appropriate questions for the attorney to ask in cross-examination.

The Trial Phase

The two most common types of cases in which an addiction specialist will be engaged in are those in which a person either is accused of having committed a crime while drug involved (i.e., while experiencing the acute, subacute, chronic, or residual effects of previous intoxicant use, dependence, or withdrawal), or is on trial as the result of statements made to law enforcement officers or testimony given by witnesses who themselves are or have been drug involved. Typically, the first type of case requires testimony about the nature and effects of intoxicant use on the defendant. Common issues include the impact of specific intoxicants on (a) the physical and mental ability to have committed the crime, (b) the state of mind required for the offense charged, or (c) the formation of the requisite intent. Other questions may involve the special issues of diminished capacity or insanity. The second type of case usually involves testimony about the effects of acute and/or chronic intoxicant use on cognition and memory, and how such use might affect the credibility of witnesses.

In some jurisdictions, the fact pattern of a specific case and/or the local rules may preclude an expert witness from commenting or offering an opinion on any aspect of the mental state of the defendant. An addiction expert, even in such circumstances, will usually be permitted to "assist the trier of fact" by giving the jury a basic education about the intoxicants involved in the case. Such basic education on intoxicants might include (a) general pharmacology; (b) modes, methods, patterns, and demographics of use; (c) interaction with antecedent or concurrent neuropsychiatric or medical conditions; and (d) specific effects on cognition, emotion, and behavior.

The Postconviction Phase

Usually defenses involving intoxicants do not prevail which may be difficult to accept, even in cases where colleagues in the field would find the clinical evidence supportive of the defense position. Long-standing biases in the criminal law, public opinion, and political factors often have greater influence on the outcome of a case than does the clinical evidence. Although most of the expert clients will be convicted, the expert testimony may result in conviction for a lesser offense, which carries a lesser penalty. It is important to remember that the addiction expert testimony in every case can make a meaningful difference to what eventually happens to the defendant.

The postconviction phase, at sentencing, often offers the opportunity for the addiction expert's most valuable contribution to a case. During the sentencing phase, the rules governing the nature, content, form, and scope of expert testimony are far more liberal at this phase than at trial and most jurisdictions permit the defense to present evidence (including expert testimony) in support of mitigation during the sentencing process. At sentencing, an expert may be permitted to (a) discuss the defendant's entire intoxicant history, (b) comment on the influence of intoxicant use on the acts constituting the crime charged, (c) make prescriptive treatment recommendations, or (d) propose an alternative sentencing plan, such as providing for dispositions, for example, supervised release probation, community control (home confinement), or community service. In offering sentencing recommendations to the judge, it is important to be cognizant of the fact that the court has the awesome responsibility of balancing between the needs of the community for protection and justice and those of the defendant for treatment and rehabilitation.

CRIMINAL RESPONSIBILITY AND INTOXICANTS

Although the connection between the use of intoxicants and crime has been universally recognized, the explosive increase in drug-related crime over the past two decades has had only minimal impact on substantive criminal law. The recognition (albeit equivocal) of substance use disorders as "diseases" and the growth of a professional field and industry around the field has had significant social and professional consequences and instructive (although surprisingly limited) effects on the legal rules.

Recent scientific research illuminating the distinction between mind and brain, mechanisms of cognition, the nature of rationality, the relationship between intention and action, mechanisms of emotional and behavioral control, and the distinctions between reaction, response, compulsion, and decision are of fundamental relevance to the criminal law. Yet, the law remains self-consciously nescient. Its reasoning remains grounded in long discarded models, disproved theories, and culturally dated assumptions about human rationality, intent (knowledge and volition), motivation, and the regulation of behavior (action). Moreover, although well-understood in the addictions field, the specific effects of all classes of intoxicants on these complex processes have been essentially ignored by the law. Legal reasoning about intoxication continues to be informed by eighteenth and nineteenth century understanding of the effects of alcohol on behavior (31).

Conceptual Problems

Definition, Description, and the Problem of DSM-IV-TR

Because the criminal law has a long history of difficulty defining the concepts of "mental disease" and "mental defect," it is perhaps not surprising that the American Psychiatric Association's *DSM-IV-TR* (32) has been adopted by the courts as a Rosetta Stone for recognizing a defendant's alleged "mental" problems as true diseases or defects. As clinicians, we know that *DSM-IV-TR* is not and was never intended to be a textbook of neuropsychiatry or addiction medicine. Despite the very explicit caveat about its limitations stated in the Introduction (32, pp. xxiii–xxiv) and the Cautionary Statement about its validity and application in forensic contexts (32, p. xxxii–xxxiii), expect to see a copy of *DSM-IV-TR* on counsel tables in every criminal case wherein a mental defense is anticipated. Also the addiction experts should expect to be examined and cross-examined about their findings and opinions in the constricting terminology of *DSM-IV-TR*. As one prosecutor remarked, "If it's listed in *DSM-IV-TR*, then it's a real mental illness; if it's not in *DSM-IV-TR*, then it isn't a real disease and should be given no credence." To challenge the unwarranted authority this publication has accrued so that the testimony is not bound by its serious limitations, simplifications, and omissions, it must make it clear that neither you (the expert), the psychiatric profession, nor the addiction medicine field recognizes *DSM-IV-TR* as the "authoritative" text. In preparing the testimony, it is vital that to anticipate and analyze all the ways that opposing counsel might use the language of *DSM-IV-TR* to try to make your testimony appear unreliable, inconsistent, or contradictory. Next, you must formulate strategy and tactics for thwarting this predictable assault on your credibility. Finally, you must make your attorney aware of all such potential problems so that the attorney will be prepared to help "rehabilitate" you on redirect examination. As the DSM-V is being revised; it appears that there will be changes to the current classification of substance use disorders diagnoses; however, these changes will not fundamentally alter current overall concepts expressed in *DSM-IV-TR*(33).

Disease, Disorder, Defect, and Dysfunction

Moving beyond the hurdle of *DSM-IV-TR*, the addiction specialist must be prepared to confront the distinctions between "disease," "disorder," and "dysfunction." The first two terms have long and tortuous histories in the law of every jurisdiction, whereas the concept of cerebral "dysfunction" has virtually none. And yet, it is precisely in terms of cognitive, emotional, and behavioral dysfunction that one can best explain (and even quantify) the effects of acute, subacute, and chronic intoxicant use. Most defendants seeking to avail themselves of an intoxicant-based defense will have grossly normal findings on objective neuropsychiatric diagnostic tests as the electroencephalogram, computed axial tomography scan, or magnetic resonance imaging scan. Even when administered using the latest enhanced techniques, these modalities are of limited value in demonstrating cerebral dysfunction (34–36). Although the newer brain imaging technologies, such as the quantitative electroencephalogram (34), single-photon emission computed tomography (35), and brain electrical activity mapping (36), promise considerable future utility, at present, valid norms for these modalities are still in the earliest stages of development. Because the legal tests applied by the courts for the admissibility of scientific evidence based on "newer" technologies are strict and narrow (21,22). Historically, the courts are slow to recognize the evidentiary validity of emerging scientific technologies, although facilitation of integrating scientific knowledge and evidence-based practice into forensic practices is an active topic of debate (37,38).

Use, Misuse, Abuse, Dependence, Addiction

Terminology in the field of addictive disease remains an unsettled area. Within *DSM-IV-TR*, for example, there is no formal definition or use of the word "addiction." That term as it is often used is referred to instead as "dependence," a word less likely to have pejorative connotations within the courtroom. One might argue that substance dependence is a medical disease whereas substance addiction is a social issue. It is crucial to be consistent with the use of terminology, making certain to define the usage of the term at the outset, recognizing that not all use qualifies as abuse. There is no reference to quantity of use within the definitions of abuse or dependence, but that has not stopped the lay public from assuming that any use of heroin constitutes abuse, whereas only high volumes of alcohol intake would amount to abuse. Use of a substance does not establish the presence of a disease, but it does establish the presence of potentially intoxicating effects. Again, be consistent with the use of terminology and the definition of the disease process so that the field remaining unsettled in this area will not cause significant difficulties. Finally, if appropriate, there may be need to educate participants regarding use of the "substance-induced" category as it applies to alteration of mood or perception, individuals with substance-induced disorders may often be mistakenly presumed to have substance use disorders. The substance-induced category should be used diagnostically, even if the substance to which it refers is not a drug of abuse. If, for example, an antihypertensive has caused depressive symptoms and secondary criminal action, one of the appropriate diagnoses would be a substance-induced mood disorder.

The Elements of the Offense

Definitions of both common law and statutory crimes require the voluntary commission of a bad act or harmful omission (*actus reus*) in conjunction with a bad state of mind (*mens rea*). However, these fundamental concepts have resisted enduring definition. Most older common law crimes have been redefined in modern criminal statutes. Criminal codifications often use adverbial qualifiers such as "knowingly," "willfully," or "intentionally" to designate as voluntary an act performed consciously as the result of effort or determination (39).

The Exculpatory Doctrine in Common Law

The early common law made no concession whatsoever because of impaired behavioral control. Justice Story, in an 1828 case involving alcohol intoxication, stressed the merit of "the law allowing not a man to avail himself of the excuse of his own gross vice and misconduct to shield himself from the legal consequences of such crime" (40).

Over time, scientific views of human behavior gradually supplanted moral ones. Concurrently, there was a substantial increase in the consumption of alcohol in all social and economic strata. In response to these societal changes, the common law evolved what came to be known as "the exculpatory doctrine." This doctrine permitted the presentation of evidence of specified mental conditions (including intoxication) in legal proceedings as a means of mitigating culpability, liability, or responsibility. Such evidence could be introduced in the form of an assertion of a defendant's insanity or lack of the "specific" intent required as an element of the offense charged. New and more difficult problems arose almost immediately.

The Enduring Problematic Concept of "Intent"

The early cases in which the exculpatory doctrine was applied involved alcohol intoxication. The courts gradually realized that "common sense" suggested that a distinction should be made between a crime committed by an intoxicated as opposed to a sober person. But traditional moral attitudes stigmatizing intoxication as a vice indicated the impropriety of complete exculpation. The criminal rules on "intent" provided an expedient, if inadequate, means of mediation.

These doctrines, which were the foundation for the exculpatory rule, imply that "specific intent" is distinguishable from "general intent." These also signify that certain crimes require only "general intent," whereas other offenses require certain "specific" intents. This dubious distinction persists at law, although neither the courts nor modern cognitive science has yet to formulate a reliable criterion or test for distinguishing "general" from "specific" intent. Today, "specific intent" most often refers to a "special" mental element that must be present in addition to the bad mental state required to accompany the bad act constituting the offense. For an analysis of the evolution and modern status of the legal premise of intent and its application to mental defenses (including intoxication), see Ref. 41 (§§3.5). When impulsive or compulsive behavior is involved, as in intoxicant use, this distinction is even more problematic.

The meaning of "intent" in the criminal law has always been obscure. Traditionally, intent was defined to include elements of both knowledge and volition. In the modern era, a statutory distinction generally is made between the mental states of knowledge and intent. Obviously, certain intoxicants, when used in certain ways by certain persons, affect certain cognitive, emotional, and behavioral functions in certain ways. Defining, distinguishing, and presenting these to the jury in nontechnical, readily intelligible language is the responsibility of the addiction expert. Successful communication of these clinical complexities to the jury by the expert is the cornerstone of a viable intoxicant-based defense.

Despite limited recognition by the courts and society that some degree of exculpation might be warranted in cases where an intoxicant-involved person commits a crime, neither the exculpatory doctrine of the common law nor modern statutory laws dealing with intoxication and related mental defenses has been even moderately satisfactory or equitable. One important reason for this is that both the exculpatory doctrine of the common law and our modern statutory laws were based on very early medical observations and common lay experience with the effects of alcohol. Despite the wealth of scientific knowledge about the specific cognitive, emotional, and behavioral effects of all the intoxicants, the substantive criminal law in this area has evolved very little and still reflects its alcohol-informed heritage.

The implicit public policy in the prevailing law reflects society's historical vacillation and expedient compromises between the punishment of intoxicant-influenced offenders in complete disregard of their condition (i.e., viewing them as ordinary criminals) and the total exculpation often suggested by the clinical evidence (i.e., viewing them as patients).

Intoxication as a Defense

Today, the effect of intoxication on criminal responsibility is well established but only precariously settled. At law, intoxication can be either (a) involuntary, where the intoxicant is ingested as the result of force or duress (42), deceit or trickery (43), medical advice (44), or lack of awareness of a susceptibility to a recognized atypical reaction to that substance (45), as in pathologic intoxication; or (b) voluntary, where the intoxicant is ingested for effect, as in recreational drug use. Many jurisdictions have recognized involuntary intoxication as a complete defense to criminal behavior in appropriate circumstances. Most jurisdictions, however, adhere to the view that voluntary intoxication does not excuse a criminal act unless the actor, because of his intoxication, could not form the intent required in the statutory definition of the crime. That is, voluntary intoxication may be raised to negative an element of an offense. Unfortunately, neither the distinctions between voluntary and involuntary intoxication nor those between general and specific intent are clear or consistent. See Ref. 41 for a review of intoxication-based defenses (§4.10).

In cases involving the ingestion of intoxicants, courts have consistently applied the same rules of analysis, mitigation, and exculpation derived from the common law and developed to deal with alcohol intoxication (46). One notable exception was expressed in the dissenting opinion in *State v. Hall* (47), which argued that drug and alcohol intoxication ought to be distinguished, and that "[o]ur intoxication rationale as applied to alcohol simply does not fit the use of modern hallucinatory drugs; and it was never meant to" (47, p. 213). Similarly, most legal commentators have not distinguished intoxication resulting from the ingestion of alcohol and from the other classes of intoxicants (48,49). In 1980, this problem was addressed in a remarkably comprehensive law review article (50). This scholarly commentary (a) examined in detail the specific effects of all of the intoxicants then in general use, (b) reviewed the traditional and prevailing legal reasoning on intoxication and intent, (c) discussed the resultant implications for intoxicant-based defenses against criminal responsibility, and (d) concluded with a recommendation that ". . . either the court or the legislatures must increase their expertise in these areas and respond to these potentially serious flaws in the criminal legal system" (50, p. 1145). Despite having been extensively cited in subsequent cases, its well-reasoned proposals have yet to be implemented. The criminal law continues to fail or refuse to recognize the fundamental differences between the effects of alcohol and those of other intoxicants (most importantly, cocaine) on human cognition, emotion, and behavior (51–53).

The law views alcohol as a neural depressant and disinhibitor that releases (cognitive and moral) inhibitions, thereby setting free ill-defined drives and putative "bad" impulses and traits, which are subsequently expressed in a criminal act. An analogy echoing through many judicial opinions regarding the mechanism of intoxication states: "drinking alcohol is like taking your foot off the brake [of a car]." Although this may not be an entirely ill-informed metaphor, it is surely an inadequate one, for it implicitly maintains that alcohol effects are stable, predictable, and consistent both across and within individuals. When applied to other intoxicants, this analogy is clearly out of touch with currently accepted principles of neuropsychopharmacology and the cognitive sciences. This disparity is most glaring for cocaine intoxication. After introducing the "removing the foot from the brake" analogy for alcohol intoxication for contrast, it is useful to explain to the jury that the effect of ingesting cocaine is better understood as being more like "stepping on the gas." The outcome may be the same: The metaphoric car moves forward, that is, the person commits a criminal act, but the mechanism is entirely different. It has been suggested that in a sense cocaine is that drug which supplies intent where otherwise there would have been none. Distinguishing the effects of cocaine (or other intoxicants) from those of alcohol is vital because it problematizes the legal concepts of intent and intoxication. This alone may lead the jury to find "reasonable doubt" about the defendant's having the required state of mind.

Consider, as an example, the conceptual problem posed for a jury in a case where a polydrug addict with a long history of robbing drugstores to get drugs (not money) now robs a drugstore while grossly intoxicated from high intravenous doses of phencyclidine (PCP), heroin, and cocaine. Eyewitness testimony states that although he looked and acted as if intoxicated, the defendant also appeared to have acted with purpose. His actions clearly demonstrated that he "knew" (at least) the following: (a) to rob a pharmacy (as opposed to, say, a grocery store) to get drugs; (b) which specific (desirably intoxicating) drugs to steal; and (c) how to commit a robbery and get to the controlled substances in the safe. In this scenario, it would be nonetheless possible that the extent and specific effects of the polydrug intoxication had rendered the defendant incapable of forming the specific intent required as an element of the offense of robbery in that jurisdiction. To succeed in negativing the elements of the offense of robbery, the defense would have to introduce expert testimony to attempt to explain at least the following: (a) that his "intent" was to get drugs, not specifically to commit the crime of robbery; (b) that his intoxication precluded him from forming the specific intent required for robbery, but (c) that the intoxication did not affect his previously well-learned ("overlearned") knowledge about intoxicating drugs and about how to rob drugstores. For such expert testimony to be accepted by the jury, it would need to tie together (a) the defendant's intoxicant history, (b) the specific effects of each intoxicant influencing the defendant at the time of the robbery, (c) his prior experience in robbing drug stores, and (d) the specific facts of the instant case.

Dependence as a Defense

Dependence on an intoxicant or active intoxication, absent more, does not provide a complete defense in any jurisdiction (54,55). The nature, course, and effects of dependence on specific substances on cognition, emotion, or behavior have not been recognized by the law.

Interestingly, opioid intoxication (but not dependence) may be of such extent as to negate the "knowingly" element of criminal intent. But neither opioid intoxication nor dependence has been held to negate the "willfully" element of criminal intent. Intoxication (but not dependence) induced by any substance may be sufficient to render a person incapable of the "deliberation" or "premeditation" required as an element of a specific degree of an offense, as in first-degree murder. In no jurisdiction has dependence on specific intoxicants been differentiated from that of alcohol, thereby warranting special consideration.

Until recently, attempts to use dependence as a defense to criminal responsibility were couched in terms of insanity, by characterizing dependence or addiction as a mental disorder that rendered the defendant insane and therefore not criminally responsible. For the most part, these attempts have been unsuccessful. In 1984, *United States v. Lyons* held that henceforth no defendant could base any defense of insanity on the claim that he lacked substantial capacity to conform his conduct to the requirements of law, supporting that opinion by citing "the present murky state of medical knowledge" about human volition (56).

A novel defense of "medical necessity" proposed in 1985 by Uelmen and Tennant sought to present addiction not as a mental disorder but, by reason of its involving a putative endorphin deficiency, as a physical condition requiring medical treatment (57). Analogizing the situation of the addict to that of the diabetic, the defense of "medical necessity" sought to conform to the contours of the well-established defenses of duress or necessity. Uelmen and Tennant suggested that "obviously, the legal profession is sleeping through the current revolution in Biochemistry" (57, p. 6). Although inconsistently successful in minor cases involving possession of small quantities of marijuana by persons using that substance to alleviate the symptoms of glaucoma (58), multiple sclerosis (59), or spasticity (60), the defense of "medical necessity" has otherwise been rejected by the courts. Many cases in which this novel defense was rejected relied upon the early case of *United States v. Moore*, which pointed to "the choice that each addict makes at the start as to whether or not he is going to take narcotics and run the risk of becoming addicted to them" (61).

Withdrawal as a Defense

Defenses based upon the argument that the criminal act at issue was the direct or indirect product of withdrawal from an intoxicant have not prevailed, except in the limited and infrequent circumstance where a defendant in withdrawal commits an act while semiconscious or unconscious. An action that, while purposive, is not spontaneous, and therefore is not voluntary, is defined at law as an "automatism" and does not incur criminal responsibility. See Ref. 41 for a discussion of the utilization of automatism in a criminal defense (§4.9).

Intoxicant-Induced Insanity as a Defense

An insanity defense asserts that at the time the accused committed the act for which he is charged, a mental illness precluded him from having the required bad state of mind to be convicted of the act. The insanity defense has been a part of English and American jurisprudence for several hundred years. It reflects a shared belief that only those individuals who have chosen to commit wrongful acts should be punished, and that those without the capacity to appreciate the wrongfulness of their conduct should be absolved. The roots of the insanity defense are ultimately embedded in the Judeo-Christian tradition of linking moral responsibility with punishment and absolution.

The elements of the legal definition of insanity that predominates today were shaped primarily by two famous cases: the 1843 English case of Daniel M'Naghten (62) and the 1982 acquittal of John Hinckley (63), who had shot President Reagan. In both instances, the public outcry over the successful employment of the insanity defense as it existed at those times resulted in a substantial conceptual redefinition and limitation of the availability of the defense. Most notably, the federal 1984 Insanity Defense Reform Act (18) and the Comprehensive Crime Control Act of 1984 (64), which followed in the wake of Hinckley's successful defense based on a legal test for insanity then in wide use, eliminated many types of mental illness as bases for a defense and reinstated the strict cognitive test of insanity set forth in M'Naghten (62). Temporary insanity caused by voluntary intoxication does not meet the requirements of the 1984 Act, nor does intoxicant dependence, absent more (65). However, where the insanity caused by the chronic use of intoxicants endures beyond any period(s) of intoxication, it may insulate a defendant, provided the resulting insanity otherwise conforms to the requirements of the 1984 Act (19, §§3:13;41, §§4.10(g)). Interestingly, neither intoxication nor dependence has been recognized as a uniquely aggravating factor to an antecedent or concurrent mental condition that by itself would not render a defendant insane as defined in the 1984 Act.

Insanity that arises from either acute or chronic intoxicant use has not been distinguished from insanity produced by other causes. Thus, whether temporary insanity caused by voluntary intoxication will be exculpatory largely depends on the legal test for insanity used in that jurisdiction. Several states have statutorily excluded this defense.

The Concept of Partial Responsibility

Partial responsibility, or diminished capacity, is a difficult and muddled concept in the law, with little coherence or consistency. Many courts appear to reject or not understand it.

Insanity of the legal type is considered a complete defense to criminal acts in most jurisdictions. A mental disorder that constitutes "something less than insanity" is not considered a complete defense to a crime, but is widely thought to lessen the degree of criminal responsibility, at least for crimes where there is a lesser degree of responsibility or severity available (as in murder, which might be reducible from first degree to second or a lesser degree). Today, mitigation, not exculpation, is the most common application of the concept of diminished capacity (19, §§3:16).

Argument asserting diminished capacity can also be made when a defendant claims that a mental illness precluded him or her from having the mental elements required for the crime. That is, because of a mental disorder, the severity of which did not render the defendant insane as provided by the test for insanity employed in that jurisdiction, the defendant nonetheless was unable to have committed the crime as charged because the defendant's mental disorder prevented the defendant from having the statutorily required elements of the offense charged (e.g., acting with "malice" or "premeditation"). That the effects of specific intoxicants can reach this threshold may be an undisputed clinical "fact"; nonetheless, courts continue to resist its acceptance (66).

Many states disallow any evidence of diminished capacity to be admitted during trial. By public referendum, the California Penal Code eliminated diminished capacity as a defense, but retained its availability as a mitigating factor (67). In *Bethea v. United States*, the court expressed the now widely held view that embracing the concept of diminished responsibility would lead to an unacceptable "sliding scale of sanity in criminal responsibility" (68). Moriarty provides an elegant analysis of the concept and a comparison of the positions taken by the American Bar Association, the federal courts, and the various state courts (19, §§3:19–21).

Intoxicant Use and Effects as Mitigating Factors

Although many states now require judges to adhere to legislatively prescribed sentencing guidelines, in some jurisdictions judges have retained limited discretion to consider a convicted defendant's complete drug history (including intoxication and dependence) as a mitigating factor. However, it is a general rule that the nature, extent, and effects of the intoxicant history must be introduced into evidence before being eligible for consideration at sentencing. There are marked differences between jurisdictions regarding the type of evidence (expert testimony, corroborating witnesses, etc.) required or admissible to establish the extent and effects of intoxication in support of mitigation.

Under the current Revised Federal Sentencing Guidelines, a federal judge may exercise a downward departure from the legislated guidelines for sentencing based on "diminished capacity" except where it is the result of voluntary intoxication with any substance (69). Nonetheless, in some federal jurisdictions, "addiction" has been accepted as evidence of diminished capacity and therefore as a basis for granting a downward departure at sentencing. This is the exception, however, not the rule.

THE ADDICTIVE PROCESSES

The concept of behaviors involving addictive processes, rather than intoxicating substances, as in "compulsive" or "pathologic" gambling, is of exceptional theoretical importance for the criminal law and the addictions field (70,71). The concept has required a reexamination of many fundamental legal postulates, precedents, and assumptions about criminal responsibility and intentionality. If viewed as addictive disorders (as in "compulsive gambling") in which no exogenous intoxicating substance is ingested, such processes raise profound questions about the paradigms that inform research, theory, and practice in the addictions field. If viewed as impulse control disorders (as in "pathologic gambling"), these processes raise difficult questions about the causal and temporal relationships between a person's impulses and the acts issuing therefrom (72). Unfortunately, in recent years, addiction terminology has been used to refer to everything from Internet usage ("Internet addiction") to dedication to one's career ("workaholic"), thus lessening its applicability and meaning with respect to physiologic addictive disease. To lessen the potential for difficulties, precise usage of terminology is called for.

Pathologic Gambling

Burglass has reviewed in depth the rationale, process, conceptual problems, and practical implications of introducing dysfunctional gambling behavior in defense or mitigation of criminal responsibility (72). One critical step toward the resolution of the conceptual problems would be for the field to formulate a classification of pathologic gamblers and the situations relevant to their behavior(s) that would be defensible empirically and relevant to the issue of criminal responsibility. For example, pathologic gamblers who commit crimes would be either normal or diseased, and their gambling behavior at the time of the commission of the crime charged would be pathologic in various degrees (72). Unfortunately, no such classification schema has been proposed.

What we find in the fact patterns of cases involving pathologic gambling is not a total or even substantial incapacity to carry out simple (or even complex) acts that can be reasonably attributed to the "disease." Nor do we find such a compromise of intellectual function as to entirely exclude purposeful conduct. Instead, we observe an apparent blunting of ethical sensitivity sufficient to destroy the understanding, appreciation, or regard for the moral quality of the criminal act, combined with a drastic, often protracted, lapse of inhibition. Rarely do we find a lapse of conscious awareness of the criminal act itself. Because pathologic gambling is a chronic disorder with a recognizable natural history (73,74), these mental elements typically can be identified before, during, and after the crime is committed. In this sense, the problem behavior seen in pathologic gambling is more like a process than like a state. In its effects, it more closely resembles "insanity" of both legally recognized varieties—the inability to distinguish right from wrong or the inability to resist an impulse—than it does any state of intoxication. Before being widely rejected, the "capacity to conform" test for an insanity defense highlighted the problem of defining a "mental disease or defect." The *Freeman* court held that "an abnormality manifested only by repeated criminal or otherwise anti-social conduct" was not a disease (65, p. 625).

Clinical and Forensic Distinctions

It is recognized clinically that at least some compulsive gamblers who commit crimes are impaired physically and psychologically, and thus may be only partially responsible for their misconduct. In this sense, at law they resemble the inebriate, whose reason has been temporarily compromised; and for them the rules governing intoxication often seem more applicable than do those for insanity. Although they are only very rarely psychotic, and only a few may even be neurotic (73), they are nonetheless considered abnormal by many clinicians (74,75), even though in ways of questionable relevance. Hence, for this subgroup of "impaired" compulsive gamblers, neither complete exculpation nor full responsibility seems appropriate. One might argue that as applied to pathologic gamblers who commit crimes, the legal rules should be applied not in terms of lack of intent, but in terms of lack of understanding of the ethical quality of the act and/or the ability to control behavior. But the legal rules have not adopted this view. As noted by Strassman, "[t]he link between compulsive gambling and a criminal offense is too tenuous to permit the court to find that the defendant lacks substantial capacity to conform his behavior to the requirements of the law as a result of his compulsive gambling disorder" (76, p. 201).

It must be conceded that many (possibly most) compulsive gamblers accused of crimes are simply persons who gamble to excess, not helpless victims of a "disease" of gambling that drives them to crime; and that such individuals should be accountable for their actions and the consequences thereof.

In practice, rather than raising an insanity defense, counsel for a pathologic gambler is more likely to attack the elements of the offense charged, arguing that the mental disorder of pathologic gambling rendered the defendant incapable of forming the specific intent requisite to the crime. *Wilson v. Commissioner* held that the defendant did not act "willfully" in filing an inaccurate tax return because his mental disorder prevented his forming a specific intent to violate the tax laws (77). For a comprehensive review of mental defenses in federal tax cases, see Ref. 78.

Most judges—unpersuaded by modern scientific knowledge—in exercising their broad discretion in evidentiary matters, hold many persons criminally liable even though they are clearly afflicted with recognized diseases. The general failure of pathologic gambling as a defense in most criminal prosecutions reflects precisely this point of view. Currently, governing case law in most, but not all, jurisdictions is based on *United States v. Shorter* (11).

The Implications of United States v. Shorter

In *Shorter*, Judge Greene clearly considered pathologic gambling to be an addictive disorder. He correctly identified the conceptual problem that arises when the state of mind caused by such disorders exists over a long period, during which time the disordered person commits one or more crimes but otherwise manages to behave in a controlled and rational manner (11). In such cases, the defense faces the daunting task of explaining how selected behaviors can be the substantially involuntary products of the intoxication or disorder, whereas other, relatively contemporaneous, behaviors need not be similarly affected. There is no satisfactory, unitary explanation for this. The elements of each offense must be analyzed in light of the facts of the case and the nature of the addictive process involved.

In *Shorter*, the judge also challenged the qualifications and legitimacy of clinicians specializing in compulsive gambling and refused to admit much of their testimony (11 [1985, p. 257]).

Sexual Addiction

In recent years, the diagnosis of "compulsive sexuality" or "sexual addiction" (79) has been offered as the basis for exculpation or mitigation in cases involving sexual, as well as less obviously related, offenses. Some few courts have admitted expert testimony about this controversial condition. In no jurisdiction has such a defense prevailed, absent more. A number of courts have admitted a defendant's alleged "sexual addiction" as a mitigating factor at sentencing. Limited treatment programs (most based on 12-step or other self-help principles) are available in the federal prison system and in that of most states.

Eating Disorders

There have been a few cases involving shoplifting and petty theft from groceries where an eating disorder (bulimia) was advanced as a defense. In none of these cases did the defense exculpate the accused. In two cases, after the defendants were convicted of the crimes charged, the sentencing judge recognized the eating disorder as a legitimate "mental disorder" that constituted a valid mitigating factor. Both defendants were sentenced to community supervision and service and to mandatory professional treatment instead of incarceration.

Compulsive Spending or Shopping

Recently, support groups based on 12-step principles and other self-help models have emerged for persons with the "diseases" of "compulsive spending" and "compulsive shopping." Advocates in these movements have adopted or endorsed addiction-derived explanations, language, and treatment approaches for these problems. The application of an addiction paradigm to these behaviors is of dubious validity, and neither problem has been widely recognized as an addictive disorder by professionals in the field (80,81).

Criminal defenses based on the "diseases" of compulsive spending or shopping have been rejected by the courts. In a few cases involving petty theft and shoplifting, expert clinical testimony about these excessive behaviors, although admitted, had little mitigatory impact at sentencing. A very thought-provoking feminist analysis of kleptomania and "compulsive shopping" as sexual disorders diagnosed only in women has been advanced by Camhi (82).

THE EFFECTS OF INTOXICANTS ON MEMORY

Expert Testimony About the Memory of Witnesses

Human memory is a complex phenomenon. One would expect the literature on the effects of intoxicants on human cognition, particularly memory, to be extensive—it is not. In cases where the defendant has been accused by persons who are or have been drug involved, an expert must assess the potential impact of their intoxicant use on their credibility as witnesses. The focus must be on the effect of the relevant intoxicant(s) on memory and its constituent cognitive processes (34–36,83–85). Although Federal Rule of Evidence 704(b) prohibits expert testimony on whether or not a defendant had the state of mind required for a particular crime (a decision reserved for the jury), it does not prohibit expert testimony about mental factors potentially affecting witnesses (20). To be an effective expert in this area, the addiction specialist requires a broad and deep understanding of human memory. Authoritative texts on research and theory about human memory written from both the clinical (86) and legal (19, Chapter 13) perspectives need to be studied closely.

Cocaine-Related Memory Dysfunction in Criminal Proceedings

Although any of the intoxicants can have potentially deleterious effects on selected memory functions, the effects of cocaine raise the most serious and frequent concerns (35,52,85,87,88). A significant number of today's large-scale cocaine trafficking cases are founded principally or solely on the testimony of alleged or self-styled coconspirators, who, more often than not, were themselves using large amounts of cocaine (and usually other intoxicants as well) during the period about which they will testify in great detail as to time, place, person, sequence, and events. In evaluating the credibility of such witnesses, it is critical to look for any possible effects of intoxicant use on their memory functions. It is always important and often productive to look for predicates and indicia of (cocaine-induced) confabulation that may taint their testimony. To establish the possibility that testimony may contain confabulated elements and therefore be subject to "reasonable doubt," it is necessary to assess the circumstances, frequency, extent, and detail of the witness's prior statements, depositions, narratives, or conferences with the authorities. Evidence of high-dose cocaine use, extensive "testimonial schooling" (19, §§13:18), and progressively detailed and inclusive recall provides a sufficient predicate for an addiction medicine expert to consider reasonably and responsibly the possibility that confabulation is present. See Ref. 19 for a discussion of the legal issues, problems, and concerns associated with witness confabulation arising from all causes (§§13:17–19).

The Phenomenon of Confabulation

Confabulation is a neuropsychiatric symptom that is characteristic of diffuse organic brain disease and/or dysfunction. It refers to the unconscious filling in of memory gaps by imagined experiences, fabricated stories, or grossly distorted accounts of recent or remote events. It is absolutely distinct from lying, which implies both motive and awareness of the distortion or untruth. Confabulatory recall is inconsistent; it may change from moment to moment; and it may be induced unwittingly by suggestion. Characteristically, isolated events and information from the past are retained in fragmented form but are at times related without regard for the intervals that separated these or for their proper temporal sequence. Sometimes, in confabulating, a person will telescope events, compressing time, thereby linking as cause and effect events that were widely separated in time and causally unrelated. These memory fragments may be cued, intentionally or unintentionally, during conversation (a) by suggestion, (b) by presentation of selected data about recent or remote events as if it were unequivocal fact, or (c) by provision of a cogent, internally consistent narrative explanation of some situation or event. The dysfunctional brain, in an attempt to maintain consistency with this apparent "reality," may fill in any memory gaps with associative, derivative, or suggested data.

Confabulation is never a consistent finding in any clinical condition. It is most frequently seen in cases of severe, nutrition-deficient alcoholism, head trauma, cerebral hypoxia, certain heavy metal poisonings, certain infections of the central nervous system (e.g., herpes or HIV encephalitis), or high-dose psychostimulant use.

Cocaine-Induced Confabulation

Confabulation may be seen in two phases of high-dose cocaine use. During the acute intoxication phase, the profound confusion, grandiosity, emotional lability, false sense of mastery, illusions, delusions, and hallucinations occasionally can induce certain users to confabulate "in real time." During the convalescent phase, after a period of abstinence from cocaine, the person gradually recalls fragments of past experience (many of which may have been originally misperceived) in a distorted way. In an attempt to preserve logical consistency, these may be linked with confabulated material. The more often such confabulated material is ratified by the social setting and in particular by authority figures (e.g., physicians, attorneys, or law enforcement officers), the more likely it is to become a fully integrated and unquestioned part of that person's self-history. It even may go on to become the basis for future thoughts, conclusions, and actions.

Although the U.S. Court of Appeals for the Sixth Circuit upheld the disallowance of such testimony in *United States v. Ramirez*, finding that such testimony went to the credibility, not the competence, of a witness (14), the exclusion of such testimony by a qualified addiction expert has been the rare exception, not the rule. A transcript of the direct and cross-examinations of the author about the effects of cocaine on the memory (confabulation) and credibility of a witness in a cocaine conspiracy case can be found in Ref. 19 (Appendix 3E).

REGULATORY AND ADMINISTRATIVE PROCEEDINGS

Members of licensed, regulated, or otherwise supervised professions (e.g., health care professionals, attorneys, airline pilots, interstate truckers) can find their licenses at risk for a number of reasons involving intoxicants. Two, however, are of exceptional importance and are discussed here: (a) allegations of "impairment" consequent to intoxicant use, and (b) for physicians, allegations of the "inappropriate" prescribing of opioids for the long-term management of chronic nonmalignant pain. In cases involving professional impairment, Burglass has identified two fundamental and very serious medical–legal issues: (a) the common presumption that "use equals abuse equals addiction equals impairment" and (b) that only a few regulatory agencies (e.g., the Federal Aviation Administration for pilots and the Department of

Transportation for interstate truck drivers) have normative data defining the cognitive, sensory, or motor skills required of a normal, that is, a "nonimpaired" practitioner (89,90). With the exception of the blood alcohol concentration, which, as a matter of public policy, has been adopted in every state as an objective, affirmative indicium of impairment for the operation of a motorized vehicle, there are no similarly established norms for any other intoxicants, nor for alcohol-mediated impairment in other contexts.

Characteristically, these investigations and prosecutions of professional impairment are undertaken in the name of public health and safety. However, the ill-specified nature of these causes, and the zeal and fervor with which intoxicant regulatory activities are pursued, have led some observers to characterize our present food and drug laws, all medical and scientific justifications aside, as ultimately religious in intent, purpose, and effect, that is, as being, in effect, the dietary and liturgical laws of the modern secular religion of science (2).

Professional Impairment

In the assessment of professional impairment, regulatory policies do not reflect the clinically significant, specific differences between intoxicants in terms of their effects, patterns of use, routes of administration, nature of the dependence and/or withdrawal syndromes (if applicable), or resultant substance-related disabilities. Although there are a few regulatory and legal cases where (limited) consideration was given to these crucial distinctions, such deliberations are clearly the exception, not the rule.

All too often the proverbial deck is stacked against the accused professional, who, upon being accused of even the mere use of an intoxicant, is presumed to be impaired consequent thereto. Contrary to the traditions of Anglo-American jurisprudence, the accused professional then has the effective burden of proving his or her "innocence" in the face of the presumption of guilt. These prosecutions are invariably legitimized and justified as necessary to protect patients or clients, institutions, or professions from the harmful actions of impaired practitioners. But in practice, the hearing panels are often biased, punitive, and easily influenced by professional or institutional interests and politics. Even the isolated or occasional use of an intoxicant is often conflated with impairment, and harsh sanctions are imposed. If the accused admits to any use of intoxicants, impairment is usually presumed. If the accused denies use of intoxicants, the conclusion that accused is in "denial" will likely be drawn and considered as evidence of "addiction" and, consequently, of "impairment."

Of course, some intoxicant-involved professionals are impaired and in need of treatment until they are able to resume practicing with the skill and safety required in their profession. In recent years, a virtual industry for the diagnosis and treatment of "impaired" professionals has emerged. One can detect therein a disturbing propensity to conceptualize and treat professional "impairment" as if it were itself a distinct disease entity; it is not (89,90). The determination of intoxicant-related impairment in professionals is a very complex assessment that requires extensive input from independent, unbiased addiction medicine specialists throughout the process. If injustices are to be avoided, specialists in addiction medicine must be willing to become involved in these unpopular and often unsavory cases. They need to offer expert testimony that (a) obligates the regulators (clinically, ethically, and legally) to recognize and consider all relevant intoxicant-specific distinctions and (b) requires the regulators to "prove" their case for impairment by specifying and quantifying the alleged deficiencies or disabilities of cognition, emotion, behavior, or professional skill that define the accused as impaired when measured against the standards of performance, skill, care, and safety required for professional practice in that jurisdiction or context.

As if this entire area was not already sufficiently troubling, Ackerman has identified an ominous trend toward requiring physicians who have been treated for chemical dependency to make informed consent disclosure to all patients (91).

Prescribing Opioids for Pain in Private Practice

Each year the prescribing profiles for controlled substances (class II opioids, in particular) of thousands of physicians are routinely (often automatically) monitored, sampled, or otherwise scanned, and evaluated by state regulatory bodies (92,93). Despite the dubious ethics and questionable purposes/efficacy of such monitoring programs, these practices are increasingly being "justified" by state regulatory bodies in the name of public health and safety, which are (presumptively) privileged over issues of individual privacy and confidentiality. The legal authority for these actions and the regulation of opioid prescribing for pain is provided by health (medical) practice acts legislated at the state level and by federal and state acts governing the use of controlled substances. Hundreds of physicians whose prescribing profiles are deemed "questionable" are then more thoroughly investigated. Such investigations and prosecutions may be initiated by even the brief treatment of a single patient! Of course, there are physicians whose prescribing of opioids is clinically inappropriate and/or unethical. Some in this group simply lack adequate current knowledge about the indications for opioid analgesia and/or the rational choice of appropriate opioid agents. Others are motivated by simple greed or sexual interest. Others are innocently duped, manipulated, or otherwise pressured by cunning and/or demanding patients. Regulatory agencies, in the main, have adequate procedures and appropriate sanctions to deal with these groups of physicians. Review of regulatory programs and new opioid technologies for chronic pain management is presented by Fishbain and colleagues (94). What the majority of the state regulatory agencies lack are provisions and procedures for dealing fairly with physicians whose prescribing of opioids is not inappropriate and/or unethical. Indeed, most of the standards of practice governing opioid use are based on myths, prejudice, and misinformation about opioids, and the unexamined belief that mere exposure to these drugs invariably results in addiction in all patients. The prevailing obsession of regulators with "police" activities intended to prevent diversion has blinded them to their coequal obligation to ensure adequate access to opioids for patients who require these drugs for legitimate medical purposes (93). Conscientious, compassionate physicians in the latter group face substantial forensic problems: (a) the investigatory process raises serious ethical questions of privacy and confidentiality for both the physician and the patient; and (b) the regulatory hearings not infrequently violate fundamental legal principles of due process. The language of most state medical practice acts is predominantly proscriptive in intent, overly broad and/or vague, and easily subject to misinterpretation (93). It is therefore not surprising that the majority of American physicians tend to be "opiophobic." As a consequence, many legitimate pain patients are undertreated, mistreated, or not treated at all (95,96).

Although the use of opioids for the treatment of chronic nonmalignant pain remains the subject of sociopolitical controversy, clinical debate, and research (96,97), the validity and utility of the modality have been recognized and conscientious clinical protocols have been developed and implemented (98–101). When such protocols are used by pain specialists based in prestigious academic medical centers or dedicated pain treatment programs, the legitimacy, knowledge, and competence of the prescribing physician(s) are presumed, and regulatory problems rarely arise. The situation in private practice, however, is markedly different. In the latter context, legitimacy, knowledge, and competence are not presumed. The physician in private practice who is charged with the "inappropriate" prescribing of opioids effectively bears the burden of establishing his or her "legitimacy" and proving that the questioned use of opioids was in fact clinically appropriate and/or otherwise in keeping with applicable standards of care and practice. Sadly, state regulators have little difficulty finding addiction medicine experts who do not hesitate to condemn the opioid prescribing practices of knowledgeable and ethical colleagues as "inappropriate" and/or "substandard."

Each year, dozens of well-informed, well-intentioned physicians are formally charged with violation(s) of a state medical practice act for having "inappropriately" prescribed opioid drugs to patients for chronic nonmalignant pain. They then must defend themselves (and their licenses) in a formal, adversarial hearing process, not unlike a criminal trial. Because such regulatory violations do not in themselves constitute acts of malpractice, medical malpractice insurance rarely provides counsel or funds the costs for the defense of such matters. The accused physician therefore must fund his or her own defense, the cost of which can easily exceed $100,000.

The two most frequent bases upon which regulators found allegations that a physician's use of long-term opioid therapy for chronic, nonmalignant pain is inappropriate are that such therapy "creates addicts" and that opioid therapy is contraindicated in any patient with a history of substance abuse. Both assertions are highly controversial, and the underlying assumptions, concerns, and issues of both have been comprehensively examined and challenged by specialists in pain management and addiction medicine (102,103). Although a 1992 review of the literature revealed reported prevalences of drug abuse, dependence, and addiction in chronic pain patients ranging from 3.2% to 18.9% (104), it has been suggested that the true prevalence of addictive disease in the chronic, nonmalignant pain population is unknown (105). In any event, every chronic pain patient being considered for long-term opioid therapy must undergo a comprehensive, multidimensional evaluation, which must include an analysis of their (a) pain (etiology, history, character), (b) prior experience with all modalities of pain management, including opioids, and (c) prior and current use of all classes of psychoactive drugs, prescribed or otherwise (105,106). The clinician in the pain clinic, private practice, or other settings must make a conscious effort to identify prior or current addictive disease, and must also attempt to identify those patients who are in active recovery (105).

For even the most-knowledgeable, best-intentioned, and best-prepared practitioner accused of opioid prescribing violations, exculpation is by no means assured, and ultimate vindication should never be assumed. However, documentation of the following material in the medical record often has proved to be the pivotal element in the successful defense of such cases:

1. A comprehensive evaluation and assessment of the etiology, history, and character of the patient's pain.
2. Clinical records or summaries from the specialists or subspecialists who have diagnosed and treated the primary medical or surgical conditions thought to be producing the patient's pain.
3. An appropriately executed (signed, witnessed, and notarized) document of the patient's "Informed Consent to Treatment with Opioid Drugs." Because the law on informed consent varies substantially from state to state and is subject to increasingly frequent review and revision (107), this critical document must be drafted in close consultation with an attorney who is experienced, and absolutely up-to-date in this area of the law. Moreover, the trend in the law of informed consent is in the direction of requiring increased specificity about alternatives and risks, broader comprehensiveness, and clearer evidence of the patient's practical understanding of both the proposed treatment and the meaning of the signed document of consent.
4. Frequent multidimensional assessment and documentation of the efficacy of opioid therapy, the absence of drug toxicity, and the absence of indicia of "addiction" (including periodic urine toxicology screening). Multidimensional assessment of the frequency and distress illuminates the impact of symptoms and the efficacy of treatment on a patient's quality of life (108).
5. Annual (or more frequent if indicated) "Letters of Indemnification" from an appropriate surgical or medical specialist stating that the specialist has reexamined the patient found that the underlying medical or surgical condition is still present and/or unchanged, that there have been no treatment innovations or technological breakthroughs from which the patient might be expected to benefit, and that therefore continued management of the patient's pain is clinically justifiable.

6. If the physician prescribing the opioids is not a credentialed expert or specialist in either pain management or addiction medicine, letters of consultation from a specialist in both of these areas are essential. Moreover, even if the prescribing physician is an expert in one of these two areas, a consultation letter from an expert in the other area is critical. These consultative reports should be updated at intervals appropriate to the patient's underlying diseases and/or reflective of the results of the regular multidimensional assessments described previously. Thus, patients who have exhibited behaviors that might be construed as "drug-seeking behavior" will need to be more frequently assessed by an addiction medicine specialist. Patients whose response to opioid therapy is untoward or inadequate (in terms of enhanced function and comfort) will require more frequent evaluation by a pain specialist.

Despite the application of scrupulous clinical "due diligence" and the maintenance of thorough, ongoing documentation, the use of long-term opioid therapy in patients with chronic nonmalignant pain is still fraught with potential pitfalls. Although articles in law reviews and clinical journals can provide insightful overviews of the policy and law governing the prescribing of opioids for pain (93,109,110), the interpretation and application of those laws by regulatory bodies change substantially from one case to the next. Therefore, for anyone who uses this treatment modality in private practice, knowledge of the current state of the law is absolutely essential!

To date, the attempt to define and control this complex area of medical practice by substituting regulations for clinical judgment has failed—resulting in grievous injustices for many practitioners and patients. The problem is neither "bad regulations" nor "incompetent regulators," and the solution is neither the drafting of more enlightened regulations nor the revision of biased regulatory procedures. The fundamental problem is that regulation is an inappropriate strategy for shaping policy and practice in this area. Clearly, a different approach is needed. The interests and concerns of all parties can be met by the promulgation of practice guidelines—specific, yet broad and flexible. Appropriate guidelines cannot possibly be formulated by bureaucrats, politicians, administrators, third-party payors, or any of the other marginally educated and/or nonclinically trained "watchdogs" of medicine and public health. The task demands comprehensive clinical knowledge and broad patient experience in pain management and addiction medicine. It needs to be an interdisciplinary, collaborative project initiated and directed by medical specialists in the fields of pain management and addictive disease. Fortunately, both fields are currently hard at work developing such guidelines. Input from practitioners (both specialists and generalists), as well as from patients, is being actively solicited and is an indispensable element of the process.

It is early yet to determine whether the availability of buprenorphine for the office-based practitioner will lead to significant legal difficulties. However, given the strict supervision being administered in terms of specialized Drug Enforcement Agency (DEA) certification, specialized training requirements, and limitations on patient quantity, it is certainly likely to be a closely examined process.

Administrative Proceedings

The effects of intoxicants of different classes have not been differentiated in administrative hearings or other proceedings involving employment eligibility, benefits, restriction, discrimination, supervision, discipline, or termination. In these venues, as in professional regulatory contexts, the prevailing presumption reflects the false and dangerous syllogism that "use equals abuse equals addiction equals impairment" (89). Moreover, routine screening for intoxicant use in the workplace is technically problematic (111) as well as legally and ethically questionable (112). Well-established principles of administrative law procedure are often violated and fundamental legal rights (e.g., due process) often ignored. Despite their being treated like criminal "defendants," the accused in these proceedings are neither guaranteed adequate legal representation nor provided with the funds and resources (e.g., expert witnesses) necessary to present an adequate defense. Data and conclusions from questionably valid screening protocols and dubious testing methods and procedures often go unchallenged. It is vital that an addiction medicine specialist (preferably one with added qualifications as a Medical Review Officer) (a) reviews all of the technical data, (b) examines the accused to assess the nature and extent of any intoxicant-related problems or disabilities that might be relevant to job performance, and (c) provides testimony to the administrative review body to explain the meaning, significance, and implications of the findings. There is no other way to assure fairness for all parties.

Given the cultural prejudices about intoxicant use and the pressures on employers to maintain a "drug-free workplace," an employee who is accused of intoxicant use cannot safely assume that he or she will get a fair hearing or receive an equitable disposition. Addiction medicine specialists must be aware of these prevailing inequities. The need and opportunities for professional involvement in intoxicant-related matters of administrative law are great.

CONCLUSION

Forensic issues involving addiction psychiatry encompass a wide range of problems within a complex clinical and biopsychosocial context. Substance-related problems with forensic implications may range from problems originating from an occasional problematic use to substance use disorders, such as abuse or dependence and a vast array of substances. Areas of forensic psychiatry may involve criminal, civil and administrative, professional and monitoring issues. The forensic arena presents a set of specific definitions, requirements, and criteria that the addiction specialist experts should become familiar with, including the role, expectations, and the court's consideration and view of the latitude of the expert testimony throughout the different phases of the trial. The role of the addiction expert in Forensics has become essential, given the expanding knowledge in the field of addiction psychiatry and substance use, the secular increase in the prevalence of substance abuse, and the periodic introduction of new trends of patterns and types of substance abuse. The multiplicity of conceptual problems in this field reflects the complexity of the historical and contextual social determinants that shaped these concepts over time. New discoveries in sciences and the interdisciplinary collaboration between the practitioners of law and the doctrines of jurisprudence and medical addiction sciences may ultimately help clarify these conceptual issues, although this may occur at what has been a slow pace. Practicing in the forensic arena presents a wide array of significant challenges for the addiction specialists; some of them, such as heightened adversarial role, are at odd with the predominant "helping" attitudes of the health profession. Other significant challenges include working within the constricting rules of criminal proceedings or facing ethical concerns, opinions, attitudes, and values. On the other hand, addiction experts, adhering to their role, may be instrumental in clarifying the many lingering stigmatizing misconceptions and help bring into focus modern concepts, based on knowledge and objective considerations, which would ultimately enhance the function of justice.

REFERENCES

1. Burglass ME, Shaffer H. The natural history of ideas in the addictions. In: Shaffer H, Burglass ME, eds. *Classic Contributions in the Addictions*. New York, NY: Brunner/Mazel; 1981:xvii–xlii.
2. Burglass ME, Shaffer H. Diagnosis in the addictions I: conceptual problems. *Adv Alcohol Subst Abuse*. 1984;3(1&2):19–34.
3. Shaffer H. Theories of addiction: in search of a paradigm. In: Shaffer H, ed. *Myths and Realities: A Book About Drug Users*. Boston, MA: Zucker; 1977:42–45.
4. *State v. Eldredge*, 773 P.2d 29 (Utah 1989).
5. *Commonwealth v. Baldwin*, 502 A.2d. 253 (Pa. Super. Ct. 1985).
6. *People v. Rogers*, 800 P.2d 1327 (Colo. Ct. App. 1990).
7. *State v. Peeler*, 614 P.2d 335 (Ariz. Ct. App. 1980).
8. *People v. Gallegos*, 644 P.2d 920 (Colo. 1982).
9. *United States v. Rea*, 958 F.2d 1206 (2d Cir. 1992).
10. *United States v. LeRoy*, 944 F.2d 787 (10th Cir. 1991); *aff'd. after remand*, 984 F.2d 1095 (10th Cir. 1993).
11. *United States v. Shorter*, 608 F. Supp. 871 (D. D.C. 1985); *aff'd.*, 18 F. Supp. 255 (D. D.C. 1987).
12. *United States v. Davis*, 772 F.2d 1339 (7th Cir. 1985).
13. *United States v. Berrios-Rodriguez*, 768 F. Supp. 939 (D. Puerto Rico 1991).
14. *United States v. Ramirez*, 871 F.2d 582 (6th Cir. 1989).
15. *Hall v. State*, 568 So. 2d 882 (Fla. 1990).
16. Simon R. *Clinical Psychiatry and the Law*. 2nd ed. Washington, DC: American Psychiatric Press; 1992.
17. Golding SL, et al. Specialty guidelines for forensic psychologists. *Law Hum Behav*. 1991;15:655–665.
18. Insanity Defense Reform Act of 1984, 18 U.S.C. sec. 17.
19. Moriarty JC. *Psychological and Scientific Evidence in Criminal Trials*. New York, NY: Clark Boardman Callaghan; 1996.
20. Federal Criminal Code and Rules, 18 U.S.C., 1996.
21. *Frye v. United States*, 293 F. 1013 (D.C. Cir. 1923).
22. *Daubert v. Merrell Dow Pharmaceuticals, Inc.*, 113 S. Ct. 2786 (1993).
23. *United States v. DiDomenico*, 985 F.2d 1159, 1163 (2d Cir. 1993).
24. *Arcoren v. United States*, 929 F.2d 1235 (8th Cir.), *cert. denied*, 112 S. Ct. 312 (1991).
25. *United States v. Rubio-Villareal*, 927 F.2d 1495, 1502 (9th Cir. 1991).
26. *United States v. Azure*, 801 F.2d 336, 340 (8th Cir. 1986).
27. *United States v. Schmidt*, 711 F.2d 595, 598 (5th Cir. 1983).
28. *United States v. Gilliss*, 645 F.2d 1269, 1278 (8th Cir. 1981).
29. *United States v. Zink*, 612 F.2d 511, 514–515 (10th Cir. 1980).
30. Burglass ME. The role of the medicalpsychiatric expert witness in drug-related cases. *Inside Drug Law*. 1985;2(3):1–6.
31. Nemerson SA. Alcoholism, intoxication, and the criminal law. *Cardozo L Rev*. 1988;10:423.
32. American Psychiatric Association. *Diagnostic and Statistical Manual of Mental Disorders*. 4th ed., text revision. Washington, DC: American Psychiatric Association; 2000.
33. Helzer JE, Bucholz KK, Gossop M. *A Dimensional Option for the Diagnosis of Substance Dependence in DSM-V. Int J Methods Psychiatr Res*. 2007;16(suppl 1):S24–S33.
34. Roemer RA, Cornwell A, Dewart D, et al. Quantitative electroencephalographic analyses in cocaine-preferring polysubstance abusers during abstinence. *Psychiatry Res*. 1995;58(3):247–257.
35. Strickland TL, Mena I, Villanueva-Meyer J, et al. Cerebral perfusion and neuropsychological consequences of chronic cocaine use. *J Neuropsychiatry Clin Neurosci*. 1993;5(4):419–427.
36. Herning RI, Glover BJ, Koeppl B, et al. Cocaine-induced increases in EEG alpha and beta activity: evidence for reduced cortical processing. *Neuropsychopharmacology*. 1994;11(1):1–9.
37. Silva JA. Forensic psychiatry, neuroscience, and the law. *J Am Acad Psychiatry Law*. 2009;37(4):489–502.
38. Glancy GD, Saini M. The confluence of evidence-based practice and Daubert within the fields of forensic psychiatry and the law. *J Am Acad Psychiatry Law*. 2009;37(4):438–441.
39. Cook J. Act, intention, and motive in the criminal law. *Yale Law J*. 1917;26:645–658.
40. *United States v. Drew*, 25 Fed. Cas. No. 14,993 (C. C. D. Mass. 1828).
41. LaFave WR, Scott AW. *Substantive criminal law*. St. Paul, MN: West; 1986 [suppl 1996].
42. *Burrows v. State*, 297 P. 1029 (Ariz. 1931).
43. *People v. Scott*, 146 Cal. App.3d 823, 194 Cal. Rptr. 633 (1983).
44. *City of Minneapolis v. Altimus*, 306 Minn. 462, 238 N.W.2d 851 (1976).
45. *Kane v. United States*, 399 F.2d 730 (9th Cir. 1968).
46. Burke SB. The defense of voluntary intoxication: now you see it, now you don't. *Ind L Rev*. 1986;19:147.
47. *State v. Hall*, 214 N.W.2d 205 (Iowa 1974).
48. Hall J. Intoxication and criminal responsibility. *Harv L Rev*. 1944;57:1056.
49. Schabas PB. Intoxication and culpability: towards an offence of criminal intoxication. *U T Fac L Rev*. 1984;42:147.
50. Benton EH, Bor A, Leech WH, et al. Special project. Drugs and criminal responsibility. *Vanderbilt L Rev*. 1980;33:1145–1218.
51. Verdejo-García AJ, López-Torrecillas F, Aguilar de Arcos F, et al. Differential effects of MDMA, cocaine, and cannabis use severity on distinctive components of the executive functions in polysubstance users: a multiple regression analysis. *Addict Behav*. 2005;30(1):89–101.
52. Foltin RW, Fischman MW, Pippen PA, et al. Behavioral effects of cocaine alone and in combination with ethanol or marijuana in humans. *Drug Alcohol Depend*. 1993;32(2):93–106.
53. Duffy JD. The neurology of alcoholic denial: implications for assessment and treatment. *Can J Psychiatry*. 1995;40(5):257–263.
54. *Evans v. State*, 645 P.2d 155 (Alaska 1982).

55. *Commonwealth v. Sheehan*, 376 Mass. 765, 383 N.E.2d 1115 (1978).
56. *United States v. Lyons*, 731 F.2d 243 (5th Cir. 1984) (*en banc*).
57. Uelmen GF, Tennant FS. Endorphins, addiction and the defense of medical necessity. *Champion*. 1985;9:6–11.
58. *United States v. Randall*, 104 Wash. Daily L. Rep. 2249 (1976).
59. *State v. Diania*, 604 P.2d 1312 (Wash. App. 1979).
60. *State v. Tate*, 477 A.2d 462 (N.J. Ct. App. 1984).
61. *United States v. Moore*, 486 F.2d 1139 (D.C. Cir. 1973) (*en banc*).
62. *M'Naghten's Case*, 8 Eng. Rep. 718 (1843).
63. *United States v. Hinckley* [No opinion issued], (D. D.C. 1982).
64. Comprehensive Crime Control Act of 1984 (18 U.S.C. sec 20).
65. *United States v. Freeman*, 804 F.2d 1574 (11th Cir. 1986).
66. *Commonwealth v. Mello*, 420 Mass. 375, 649 N.E.2d 1106 (Mass. 1995).
67. *West's Ann. Cal. Penal Code §§ 28.*
68. *Bethea v. United States*, 365 A.2d 64 (App. D.C. 1976).
69. United States Sentencing Commission. *Federal Sentencing Guidelines Manual, 1995–96 ed.* St. Paul, MN: West Publishing; 1996.
70. Sood ED, Pallanti S, Hollander E. Diagnosis and treatment of pathologic gambling. *Curr Psychiatry Rep*. 2003;5(1):9–15.
71. Potenza MN. Review. The neurobiology of pathological gambling and drug addiction: an overview and new findings. *Philos Trans R Soc Lond B Biol Sci*. 2008;363(1507):3181–3189.
72. Burglass ME. Pathological gambling: forensic update and commentary. In: Shaffer H, Cummins T, Gambino B, et al., eds. *Compulsive Gambling. Yesterday, Today, and Tomorrow*. Lexington, MA: Lexington Books/DC Heath; 1981:205–222.
73. Custer RL. Gambling and addiction. In: Craig RJ, Baker SL, eds. *Drug Dependent Patients*. Springfield, IL: Charles C Thomas; 1982:367–381.
74. Lesieur HR. *The Chase Career of the Compulsive Gambler*. New York, NY: Anchor Press/Doubleday; 1977.
75. Carlton PL, Manowitz P. Physiological factors as determinants of pathological gambling. *J Gambling Behav*. 1988;3:274–285.
76. Strassman HD. Forensic issues in pathological gambling. In: Balski T, ed. *The Handbook of Pathological Gambling*. Springfield, IL: Charles C Thomas; 1987:195–204.
77. *Wilson v. Commissioner*, 76 TC 623 (1981).
78. Ritholz J, Fink R. New developments and dangers in the psychiatric defense to tax fraud. *J Taxation*. 1970;32:322–330.
79. Carnes PJ. *Don't Call it Love*. New York, NY: Bantam Books; 1991.
80. Christenson GA, Raber RJ, deZwann M, et al. Compulsive buying: descriptive characteristics and psychiatric comorbidity. *J Clin Psychiatry*. 1994;55:5–11.
81. Bernik MA, Akerman D, Amaral JAMS, et al. Cue exposure in compulsive buying [letter]. *J Clin Psychiatry*. 1996;57:90.
82. Camhi L. Stealing femininity: department store kleptomania as sexual disorder. *Differences*. 1993;5(1):26–50.
83. Heffernan TM. The impact of excessive alcohol use on prospective memory: a brief review. *Curr Drug Abuse Rev*. 2008;1(1):36–41.
84. Yucel M, Lubman DI, Solowij N, et al. Understanding drug addiction: a neuropsychological perspective. *Aust N Z J Psychiatry*. 2007;41(12):957–968.
85. Bernal B, Ardila A, Bateman JR. Cognitive impairments in adolescent drug-abusers. *Int J Neurosci*. 1994;75:203–212.
86. Lezak MD. *Neuropsychological Assessment*. 3rd ed. New York, NY: Oxford University Press; 1995.
87. Withers NW, Pulvirenti L, Koob GF, et al. Cocaine abuse and dependence. *J Clin Psychopharmacol*. 1995;15(1):63–78.
88. Teoh SK, Mendelson JH, Woods BT, et al. Pituitary volume in men with concurrent heroin and cocaine dependence. *J Clin Endocrinol Metab*. 1993;76:1529–1532.
89. Burglass ME. Use equals abuse equals impairment: a false and dangerous syllogism [abstract]. *Alcohol Clin Exp Res*. 1988;12(1):190.
90. Burglass ME. Chemical dependence and impairment: conceptual problems [abstract]. *Alcohol Clin Exp Res*. 1989;13(1):147.
91. Ackerman TF. Chemically dependent physicians and informed consent disclosure. *J Addict Dis*. 1996;15(2):25–42.
92. Portenoy RK. Therapeutic use of opioids: prescribing and control issues. *NIDA Res Monogr*. 1993;131:35–50.
93. Hills S. Government regulatory influences on opioid prescribing and their impact on the treatment of pain of nonmalignant origin. *J Pain Symptom Manage*. 1996;11(5):287–298.
94. Fishbain D, Johnson S, Webster L, et al., Review of regulatory programs and new opioid technologies in chronic pain management: balancing the risk of medication abuse with medical need. *J Manag Care Pharm*. 2010;16(4):276–287.
95. Morgan J. American opiophobia: customary underutilization of opioid analgesics. *Adv Alcohol Subst Abuse*. 1985;5:163.
96. Portenoy RK. Chronic opioid therapy for persistent noncancer pain: can we get past the bias? *APS Bull*. 1991;1:4–5.
97. Reidenberg MM, Portenoy RK. The need for an open mind about the treatment of chronic non-malignant pain. *Clin Pharmacol Ther*. 1994;55(4):367–369.
98. Victor TW, Alvarez NA, Gould E. Opioid prescribing practices in chronic pain management: guidelines do not sufficiently influence clinical practice. *J Pain*. 2009;10(10):1051–1057.
99. Portenoy RK. Chronic opioid therapy in nonmalignant pain. *J Pain Symptom Manage*. 1990;5(1 suppl):S46–S62.
100. Savage SR. Opioid use in the management of chronic pain. *Med Clin North Am*. 1999;83(3):761–786.
101. Schofferman J. Long-term use of opioid analgesia for the treatment of chronic pain of non-malignant origin. *J Pain Symptom Manage*. 1993;8:279–288.
102. Wesson DR, Ling W, Smith DE. Prescription opioids for the treatment of pain in patients with addictive disease. *J Pain Symptom Manage*. 1993;8:289–296.
103. Savage SR. Management of acute and chronic pain and cancer pain in the addicted patient. In: Miller NS, ed. *Principles of Addiction Medicine*. Sec. VIII, Chap 1. Chevy Chase, MD: American Society of Addiction Medicine; 1995:1–16.
104. Fishbain DA, Rosomoff HL, Rosomoff RS. Drug abuse, dependence, and addiction in chronic pain patients. *Clin J Pain*. 1992;8: 77–85.
105. Savage SR. Addiction in the treatment of pain: significance, recognition, and management. *J Pain Symptom Manage*. 1993; 8(5):265–278.
106. Sees KL, Clark HW. Opioid use in the treatment of chronic pain: assessment of addiction. *J Pain Symptom Manage*. 1993; 8(5): 257–264.
107. Faden R, Beauchamp T. *A History and Theory of Informed Consent*. New York, NY: Oxford University Press; 1986.
108. Portenoy RK, Thaler HT, Kornblith AB, et al. The Memorial Symptom Assessment Scale: an instrument for the evaluation of symptom prevalence, characteristics and distress. *Eur J Cancer*. 1994;30A(9):1326–1336.
109. Tennant FS, Uelmen GF. Narcotic maintenance for chronic pain: medical and legal guidelines. *Postgrad Med*. 1983;73:81–94.
110. Clark HW, Sees KL. Opioids, chronic pain, and the law. *J Pain Symptom Manage*. 1993;8(5):297–305.
111. Osterloh J, Becker C. Chemical dependency and drug testing in the workplace. *West J Med*. 1990;152:506–513.
112. Burglass ME. Employee assistance and drug testing: striving for fairness [abstract]. *Alcohol Clin Exp Res*. 1988;12(1):190.

CHAPTER 80: Clinical and Societal Implications of Drug Legalization

Benjamin R. Nordstrom ■ Herbert D. Kleber

INTRODUCTION

The costs of America's struggle with the consequences of drug addiction have been enormous. In 2007, an estimated 19.9 million Americans aged 12 or older (approximately 8% of the population) were current users of illicit drugs. In addition, 6.9 million Americans over the age of 12 were classified as having either abuse of or dependence on illicit substances. This figure has been stable since 2002 (1). Other estimates have held that approximately 3% of the U.S. population will meet criteria for dependence on an illicit substance at some point in their lives (2).

Costs Caused by Addiction

Some of the costs are intrinsic to the physical, psychological, and social consequences of drug addiction. The Office of National Drug Control Policy estimates that the total cost of drug abuse on society in 2002 was $180.9 billion dollars including the costs of lost productivity, health care costs, and criminal justice costs (3). A study of children placed in foster care showed that 78% of the children came from homes where drug use was a primary reason for placement, and 94% of the mothers of infants in foster care had a history of drug use (4). Heavy and early use of marijuana in adolescence is associated with earlier onset of psychosis. Some drug-related crimes, namely those stemming from "behavioral toxicity" (i.e., disinhibition and poor judgment due to intoxication) are also a direct cost of addiction. Although it is impossible to get an accurate measure of exactly how much crime is caused by behavioral toxicity, it has been found that 27% of victims of violent crime state that their assailant was under the influence of drugs or alcohol at the time of the attack (5,6).

The intangible costs of addictions are well known to any clinician who treats these maladies. Addictions cause incalculable heartache, despair, and strain in the lives of those who have addictions, and in the lives of those who love them. Although it is impossible to monetize these harms, it is important to consider them in any discussion about the consequences of addictions.

Costs Caused by Drug Policy

Other costs are incurred as a consequence of the policies our society has put in place in response to perceived problems associated with drug use. Given that these costs must be accounted for in government budgets, these costs are much easier to directly measure compared to the sort of estimation of costs seen in the previous section. Nationwide in 2007, approximately 13% of the 14,209,365 total arrests were for drug violations. Only 17.5% of drug-related arrests were for the sale or manufacturing of drugs. The remaining 82.5% of drug-related arrests were for the possession of illicit substances only (7). It has been estimated that of the $38 billion spent on corrections in 1996, $30 billion was spent incarcerating drug users or drug offenders (8). As many as 400,000 people are in jails and prisons on drug-related charges (9). Currently 52.2% of the offenders in federal prisons are convicted of drug offenses (10).

One of the consequences of making drugs illegal is that the cost of drugs rises. This makes drug habits more expensive to maintain, which could potentially lead to more crime. Those crimes that are committed to generate revenue with which to acquire drugs are called "acquisitive crimes."

In 2004, 17% of state prisoners and 18% of federal inmates reported having committed their current offense in order to get money to purchase drugs (5,6). During 2002, 68% of offenders in local jails were found to be dependent on or abusing illicit drugs. The same survey revealed that approximately a quarter of convicted property and drug offenders serving time in local jails had committed their crimes to get money with which to purchase drugs. Only 5% of violent offenders in local jails had similarly committed their crimes in order to purchase drugs (11). Although violent drug-related crimes are less common than nonviolent drug-related crimes, they pose a greater cost to society due to the effects that such crimes impose on their victims (12).

Among state prisoners, 30% of property offenders, 26% of drug offenders, and 11% of violent offenders had committed their crimes to obtain money with which to buy drugs. In federal prisons, 25% of drug users (but only 11% of property offenders) reported they had committed their crimes to obtain drug money (13).

Another feature of an illegal market is the absence of any legal manner to adjudicate disputes. Thus, when one feels mistreated in a drug transaction, one can either resign oneself to the situation or retaliate, including using violence. Such crimes that occur from such disputes in drug selling are called "distributive crimes." According to the Uniform Crime Report, approximately 4% of the total 14,831 homicides that occurred in 2007 were coded as drug related (7). Distributive crime also includes dealers fighting other dealers in fights over turf.

There are intangible harms to our current drug policies as well. When a large number of people perform an act that is technically criminal, it reduces the legitimacy of the criminal code. Further, if arrest and incarceration are so common as to be routine features of life for certain families and communities, the stigma of violating social norms becomes reduced (14) and the bonds between a marginalized group and mainstream society are further weakened. A final intangible harm is the very large amount of suffering caused by long prison sentences, which disrupt families, relationships, and communities. Societal attitudes about drug use/abuse and the appropriate social response tend to go through cycles. Strong punitive responses calling for stiff penalties and prison instead of treatment are often followed by calls for relaxed enforcement, even legalization, and treatment instead of prison. We seem to be heading into that part of the pendulum swing. Occasionally the pendulum stops in the middle with a balanced approach of legal sanctions and treatment and prevention.

DEFINING TERMS

Discussions about drug control policy can be filled with similar-sounding jargon. To help facilitate this chapter, we are using the following definitions:

- *Legalization* means removing laws prohibiting the sale of drugs.
- *Decriminalization* means removing drug-related offenses from the criminal code, while maintaining the illegality of drug use. Speeding and parking violations are examples of behaviors that are illegal without being criminal.
- *Depenalization* means reducing the severity of penalties for drug-related offenses.
- *Harm reduction* means accepting that irrespective of policy remedies, drugs will cause a certain amount of harm to the individual and to society, and that sound public policy should be based on reducing the amount of that harm rather than reducing use.

However, some have argued that harm reduction should be parsed into two forms: micro-harm reduction and macro-harm reduction (15). Micro-harm reduction means reducing the harm per unit dose of drug, while macro-harm reduction means reducing aggregate harm caused by use of the drug. Thus, testing illicitly sold MDMA tablets (Ecstasy) at a dance club to ascertain the safety of their contents would be an example of micro-harm reduction. However, if this led to a greater sense of safety among potential tablet buyers, and more people were thus emboldened to participate in that drug market, this safety check could be inimical to macro-harm reduction. In other words, macro-harm reduction takes into the account the inherent danger in the drug and the prevalence of use. It has been noted that when people who favor legalization speak of harm reduction, they usually mean micro-harm reduction (16).

This chapter is not meant to be a thorough exposition on drug control policy as a whole. We will not take on the broader topic of comprehensive drug policy reform.

The relatively narrow focus of this chapter is on the clinical and societal implications of legalizing drugs.

PHILOSOPHICAL CONSIDERATIONS

It would be impossible to write about the consequences of legalizing drugs without mentioning the philosophical bases from which parties approach this issue. These philosophies basically break down into two broad categories: deontologic and consequentialist.

Deontologic arguments take their name from the Greek *deont*—"it is necessary." These arguments are based in abstract notions of right and wrong. For the purposes of a discussion about drug legalization, there are two main types of deontologic arguments. The first of these are the moralistic arguments that drug use is fundamentally wrong and should be opposed on this ground. The sociologist Howard Becker writes of how when marijuana use was increasing in the middle part of the 20th century, "moral entrepreneurs" stigmatized the behavior and made a moral case for making marijuana illegal (17). There are also deontologic arguments for legalizing drugs as well. An example of such thought can be seen in the platform of the Libertarian Party, which writes: "Only actions that infringe on the rights of others can be properly termed crimes. We favor the repeal of all laws creating 'crimes' without victims, such as the use of drugs for medicinal or recreational purposes." (18).

Consequentialist philosophies are more concerned with the consequences of, rather than the motives behind, a given policy. A form of consequentialist thought that is widely known is utilitarianism, which postulates that sound policy maximizes the best result for the largest number of people. Consequentialist thought forms the basis of much of our public health law. As this is a textbook for clinicians and not moral philosophers, we will limit our discussion of American drug control policy to consequentialist orientations. Although many people do oppose or support drug legalization for purely ideological reasons, we are not prepared to debate the strengths and weaknesses of these perspectives. Our discussion will only focus on how drug legalization would affect utility for the population as a whole.

THEORETICAL BASIS FOR LEGALIZATION

Consequentialist legalizers believe that, as harmful as addiction may be to individuals, the effect of policies attempting to control drug use lead to unintended consequences that are worse than what is likely to follow were drugs legalized. They note that because there will always be a demand for drugs, there will always be a supply of drugs. They speculate that efforts to reduce or control supply and demand are therefore illogic, create more harm than good, and are doomed to fail anyway. Moreover, a common feature of legalizer ideology is that once the drug trade is legalized it will be able to be taxed in such a way that sufficient revenue will be generated to offset the costs of the social ills that would follow from a hypothesized increase in the prevalence of addiction (19,20).

THEORETICAL BASIS FOR DRUG PROHIBITION

David Courtwright lists five reasons societies have historically objected to nonmedical drug use: (1) the drugs cause direct harm to the users and others, (2) the drugs cause unjustifiable social costs, (3) religious disapproval, (4) the drug is associated with a deviant or disliked group, and (5) widespread use of the drug endangers the future of the society (21). With respect to Courtwright's fourth point, the role outright racism played in various national moral panics that have been associated with drug control legislation has been noted by other authors as well (22,23). Insofar as racism was endemic to much of public thought in America at the time many of the first drug control laws were promulgated, it is not surprising that racism entered the discourse on drug policy.

Although Courtwright accurately describes the *historical* roots of drug prohibition, the *current* prohibitionist regime can be viewed as an attempt to limit or prevent drug addiction in the population. This can be viewed as a public health prevention effort in addition to a law enforcement endeavor. Empirically, we know that a certain small percentage of people who try any given drug will go on to develop an addiction to that drug. For example, 17% to 22% (snorting vs. smoked) of people who try cocaine will go on to develop a dependence syndrome to it. Similarly, about 23% of people who try heroin will become addicted. Conservatively, 9% to 10% of people who try cannabis will become addicted to it. Approximately 15% of people who try alcohol will become alcoholics, and 32% of people who try cigarettes will become nicotine dependent (24).

In order to limit the prevalence of drug addiction in the population, drug prohibition attempts to make the incidence of drug use as low as possible: the fewer people who try a drug even once, the fewer people who will become addicted. The logic behind this perspective is brought into relief when considering the societal implications of the legal status of alcohol. Even though the risk of getting addicted to alcohol is less than the risk of getting addicted to other drugs, the burden of suffering imposed by alcohol is much higher than that for cocaine, owing to the widespread prevalence of alcohol use and, therefore, dependence.

The decision to use drugs is influenced by a number of factors. First, the drug must be physically available. Second, the drug must be financially available, that is, it cannot be used if its price point is outside of the purchasing power of its intended market. Third, the person must have some curiosity or desire to use the drug. Fourth, there has to be a relative weakness in controls to *not* use the drug. These controls can be formal, such as police observation, or informal, such as an unacceptable social stigma for using the drug, for example, the Mormons' prohibition on alcohol and tobacco use.

As previously noted, legal prohibition attempts to disrupt the supply of drugs, causing the cost of the drug to increase. Also, legal prohibition assigns a criminal and social stigma to drug use. By increasing the cost of the drug in both economic and social terms, legal prohibition attempts to keep the demand for drugs lower than they would be in an unfettered marketplace. Attempting to prevent the initiation of any drug use is an example of primary prevention while the attempt to prevent occasional drug use from progressing into a dependence syndrome is an example of secondary prevention (25).

Legal prohibition also encompasses elements of tertiary prevention as well. Tertiary prevention is concerned with limiting the effects of a disease once it has already taken root (25). Prohibition allows for programs such as drug courts, Drug Treatment as an Alternative to Prison (DTAP), and Treatment Alternatives for Street Crime (TASC). These kinds of program use the authority of the criminal justice system to leverage addicts into drug treatment and, hopefully, abstinence. Also, legal prohibition helps keep informal social controls at maximum strength, which gives leverage to family members, employers, and friends who are attempting to get a substance abuser into treatment.

In short, consequentialist prohibitionists believe that the sum of the harms caused by prohibition are less than the sum of the harms that would be caused were the prevalence of addiction to rise when the controls on it are removed. Legalizers of the consequentialist variety believe the exact opposite. They hold that the current regime is causing so much harm that outright legalization of drugs would cause a net decrease in the burden of suffering in society. As drug legalization does not exist anywhere in contemporary America so its effects can be studied, neither side can assert its position with total certainty. Given the logistical and political constraints, it is unlikely that we will ever see a randomized controlled trial of drug legalization in this country. There are, however, important lessons that can be learned from studying economic models, our own country's past experience with drug policy as well as by paying attention to the experience of other countries.

ECONOMIC MODELS

Demand for a commodity is said to be "elastic" if it decreases as the price increases. Demand is said to be "inelastic" if it does not decrease as price increases (26). Therefore, the demand for novelty T-shirts is likely to be relatively elastic, while the demand for sewage removal is likely to be relatively inelastic. Drug prohibition is partially based on the rationale that increasing the price and risk associated with drug use will discourage consumption (27)—that is, that demand for drugs will be elastic.

There is evidence from laboratory studies of drug self-administration in nontreatment seeking drug users that implies that demand for drugs is relatively elastic. These studies offered subjects the choice between a dose of their drug of choice and money. As the magnitude of the alternative monetary reinforcer and/or the dose of drug decreases, the frequency of the choice to use drugs diminishes (28–33).

Working from data from the National Household Survey of Drug Abuse and the Drug Enforcement Agency's System to Retrieve Information from Drug Evidence (STRIDE)—which collects information on drug price and purity—economists Harry Saffer and Frank Chaloupka created models to investigate the relationship between drug use and price (34). They found that heroin and cocaine both showed elastic demand and that if they were legalized, heroin consumption would double and cocaine consumption would increase by 50%.

Another model was constructed using data from the Monitoring the Future survey of high-school drug use and the STRIDE data set (35). The researchers found that demand for cocaine among high-school students was very sensitive to price. Interestingly, they also found that decriminalizing marijuana did not affect marijuana use, perhaps because enforcement tends to be very lax.

In sum, the economic data show that, as with virtually any commodity, demand for illicit drugs is sensitive to price. While prolegalization advocates are certainly correct that there will always be *a* demand for illicit drugs, *how much* demand there will be is at least partially dependent on the supply of the drugs in question. Importantly, the economic models imply that this is especially true for youth. There are recent suggestions, for example, that as the price of heroin in New York market has become cheaper, some adolescent abusers of prescription opioids are switching from them to heroin.

HISTORICAL PRECEDENTS

Pre-Harrison Act

It is important to note that all manner of drugs used to be legal in this country. The Harrison Act, passed in 1914, was the first national law that outlawed the unfettered access to drugs such as cocaine, heroin, and morphine. The historian David T. Courtwright has described the pattern by which drugs (including distilled spirits, tobacco, opioids, cocaine, and amphetamine) are first used in medical practice for specific conditions, but once the drug is in the patients' hands, the medical use spreads into using the drug to treat an ever-increasing list of ailments, and soon social experimentation and later addiction follow. Once social use and addiction begin to manifest, agents of social control (e.g., law enforcement and legislators) take notice and begin to take steps to limit the availability of the drug (21). Two recent examples include the long-acting opioid Oxycontin and stimulants such as Ritalin.

At around the turn of the previous century the modal drug addict changed from the largely sympathetic image of a middle-class woman addicted to the opiate in a patent medicine to a frightening specter: cocaine and heroin using young, inner-city men, and racial or ethnic "others" (22,36,37). This shift in the demographics of drug users was partly made possible by advances in organic chemistry which allowed for the ready extraction of powerful alkaloids from the coca plant and the opium poppy, as well as by the invention of the hypodermic needle (21). Although record keeping from the era is less than adequate, there are data that the legalization regime produced a large number of addicts (22) and that these addicts frequently turned to crime to finance their legal habits (9,23,36). Although there were also economic and diplomatic reasons for the passage of the Harrison Act (22), and although racist and xenophobic hysteria certainly played a part in popularizing antidrug sentiment, it is important to note that it was the significant intrinsic harms associated with drug use that substantially led to prohibition rather than the other way around.

Alcohol Prohibition

In 1920, the 18th Amendment to the United States Constitution banned the "manufacture, sale, or transport of intoxicating liquors within, the importation thereof into, or the exportation thereof from the United States." The status of alcohol under Prohibition is not directly analogous to the status of drugs under the current regime because possession of alcohol for personal consumption was not illegal. However, people who support the legalization of drugs frequently point to the experience with Prohibition as evidence that supply-side efforts to control substance use are inherently ineffective (38).

While it is true that public support for Prohibition waned, and that the 18th Amendment was repealed by the passage of the 21st Amendment in 1934, whether Prohibition "failed" depends on what outcomes are considered in the analysis. Certainly, Prohibition was a massive political failure, but there are data that support the contention that Prohibition had a significant and salutatory impact on alcohol-related morbidity and mortality.

At the beginning of the 20th century Americans consumed an average of 2.6 gallons of alcohol per person. Over the next 20 years, the Temperance Movement gained in popularity, and 36 of the 48 states enacted some form of alcohol prohibition at the state level. By 1919, per capita alcohol consumption had dropped to 1.96 gallons per year. In 1934, per capita alcohol use stood at 0.97 gallons per year. From then on, consumption rose to roughly three times as high as that immediately after Prohibition (39).

Deaths from cirrhosis of the liver decreased from their peak in 1907 as the majority of states went dry (40). Cirrhosis deaths fell from 12 per 100,000 in 1916 to 5 per 100,000 in 1920, and then remained at that level throughout Prohibition, only to rise again after Repeal (41). Among men the cirrhosis rate declined even more sharply, from 29.5 per 100,000 to 10.7 per 100,000 in 1929 (42).

The decrease in consumption in alcohol was associated with other positive public health and social consequences as well. Admissions to psychiatric hospitals for alcohol-related psychosis dropped by 60% from 1919 to 1922. Arrests for drunkenness and disorderly conduct dropped 50% between 1916 and 1922, and public welfare agencies reported large declines in the number of alcohol-related family problems (42).

In the public imagination, these health benefits were offset by the increase in violence associated with the black market distribution and sales of alcohol during Prohibition. Movies such as *The Untouchables* and *Public Enemies* paint a vivid picture of gangster-driven "rum running." However, homicide rates increased faster before Prohibition than during Prohibition, and organized crime was established in cities well before the 18th Amendment was passed (42). It is worth noting again that even today only 4% of homicides are drug related (7).

This pattern of alcohol prohibition leading to significant public health benefits were repeated in 1994 when the residents of Barrow, Alaska voted to ban alcohol possession, sale, and importation. Immediately the town noticed a 70% reduction in crime. In the month before the ban went into effect there were 118 alcohol-related emergency room visits, while in the month after the ban went into effect there were 23 such visits. Despite these salutatory social benefits, the town voted to repeal the ban in 1995. Immediately after the ban was lifted, admissions to the detoxification center resumed and alcohol-related crime began to rise (43).

Neither national Prohibition nor the experience in Barrow was done experimentally, thereby weakening any attempt to ascertain a causal relationship between the public policy changes and public health benefits. That being said, tentative conclusions can be drawn. When societies increase formal and informal social controls around alcohol use, this is associated with less consumption of alcohol and less alcohol-related morbidity and mortality. Another conclusion is that once a substance becomes ingrained as part of a mainstream culture, the majority of substance users who do not use the substance problematically will not tolerate having their own behavior curtailed because of the expense and misery incurred by a minority of problem users.

EXPERIENCES OF OTHER COUNTRIES

Although it is inherently difficult to make comparisons across disparate cultures, there are some lessons that can be learned from observations of what transpires with respect to drug policy in other cultures.

Netherlands

Many people are under the impression that the Netherlands legalized or decriminalized cannabis. In fact, the Netherlands made no changes to any existing laws, but rather since 1976 has opted not to enforce the laws pertaining to cannabis, resulting in what some authors refer to as "*de facto legalization*" (9). Proponents of legalization state that this policy change did not result in increased drug use (19,44,45).

That the prevalence of marijuana use does not increase very much with decriminalization has also been demonstrated in economic models studying those states where marijuana possession has been decriminalized (35). Under the Dutch regime, unlike the American states that decriminalized marijuana possession, however, the coffee shops that sell marijuana could openly advertise their product. In fact, following this "commercialization" of marijuana, use of the drug did begin to significantly increase (46). Between 1984 and 1992, marijuana use by Dutch adolescents increased 200% (47) while over the same period marijuana use decreased by 66% in their American teenage counterparts. From 1991 to 1993 the Netherlands saw a 30% increase in the number of registered cannabis addicts (48). Between 1990 and 1995, the prevalence of Dutch cannabis users who had smoked cannabis for the previous 5 years increased from 2% to 5%, and that the number of adolescents who ever used cannabis increased from 7% to 17% (49).

In 1996, in response to domestic and international pressure, the Dutch Parliament passed restrictions to cut in half the number of cannabis-selling coffee houses and to reduce the amount of cannabis an individual could buy (50). Although the reduction in the amount of cannabis sold was enacted, the coffee shop proprietors fought the closings in the legal system, and only 10% of these establishments were shuttered (9).

One lesson that can be drawn from the Dutch experience is that advertising and commercialization of drugs, as with any commodity, can affect their consumption. A second lesson is that once a drug market becomes legitimated and can protect its own interests using the institutions and procedures available to all legitimate businesses, it is difficult to curtail or limit that market.

The widespread opening of so-called medical marijuana dispensaries in California and the ease of accessing them has been associated with hundreds of thousands of users, availability of very high-potency marijuana (over 15% THC), advertising by doctors offering the necessary card, and well-financed attempts by the dispensary owners both to legitimize them, and offers to pay taxes (which, again, makes them more legitimate and harder to close). Many flout the referendum that permitted them by making large sums of money while by law they are supposed to be not-for-profit (51). The Los Angeles city council has struggled to contain the number of marijuana dispensaries. Although several hundred are believed to exist, the city council wants to reduce the number of dispensaries to 70. As was seen in the Netherlands, those supporting dispensaries have availed themselves of the court system to protect their interests (52).

As noted above, once national policy and attitudes regarding cannabis changed in the Netherlands, adolescent cannabis consumption increased. It is interesting to note that as more and more U.S. states begin considering making "medical marijuana" available the attitudes and practices of U.S. adolescents seem to be changing in tandem. The 2009 Monitoring the Future study, an annual survey of adolescent drug use and drug-related beliefs, shows that after a decade of decline, the prevalence of adolescent cannabis use has increased over the past 2 years. At the same time, adolescents have begun to regard cannabis with less disapproval and perceive it as less risky than they did in the past (53). As our nation continues to conduct a large-scale, uncontrolled experiment with making cannabis legally available, attention to such trends will prove critical to the determination of whether the benefits of the policy change are justified by its costs.

United Kingdom

Some in the prolegalization camp speak approvingly of the ability of British doctors to maintain drug addicts on heroin. However, of the estimated 150,000 opioid addicts in Britain, only 17,000 are maintained on methadone and 400 are maintained on heroin (54). It is unclear why, even when available, physicians use heroin so infrequently if this treatment offers an advantage to methadone (55).

This question may be answered by one British study that sought to study the effects of heroin maintenance in an experimental fashion by randomizing subjects to maintenance on oral methadone or injectable heroin (56). Initially 44 participants were randomized to heroin and 52 to oral methadone, but due to attrition and death the analysis included data on only 42 participants receiving heroin and 46 receiving methadone. The study ran for 12 months and the average dose of both heroin and methadone was 60 mg. Those maintained on methadone were significantly more likely to reduce the frequency of injecting drugs illicitly and to cease use of other opioids than those maintained on heroin. There were no benefits to heroin maintenance in terms of crime or health outcomes. Disturbingly, 37% of those in the study admitted to diverting some of their heroin on the black market (55). Thus, in this study, heroin maintenance was, at best, slightly inferior to methadone maintenance. This may well account for part of the reason why British physicians are reluctant to resort to heroin maintenance.

Switzerland

In the third season of the HBO urban crime drama *The Wire*, a Baltimore police commander creates a zone within his district where drug dealing and drug using would be overlooked in an effort to siphon these problems away from residential areas and concentrate them in one small location. In this fictional account, public service agencies rush in to assist the addicted population, but the area, called Hamsterdam, becomes increasingly anarchic—albeit within circumscribed boundaries. Finally, the local news media publicizes what is going on, and Hamsterdam is closed with a massive police sweep, and the viewer is left to consider the mixed results of the social experiment.

In 1987, Zurich, Switzerland actually ran such an uncontrolled experiment. The year prior, heroin had moved into the previously cannabis endemic Platzspitz Park, which quickly earned the moniker "Needle Park." In response, the city council and police force made it unofficial policy not to enforce any laws regarding individual drug use or drug possession within the park, while vigorously enforcing such laws in the rest of the city and surrounding canton (9).

As in *The Wire*, multiple nonprofit agencies swept in and began offering needle exchange, medical help, resuscitation teams, and mobile kitchens. Users, the majority of whom came from outside Zurich, poured into the Platzspitz. The number of syringes distributed and the number of resuscitations performed each day increased out of proportion to the increased number of addicts, leading Swiss researchers to conclude that the addicts were injecting ever-larger amounts of heroin (57). Heroin-related deaths began to rise, and Switzerland attained the highest heroin-related mortality rate in Europe and North America (58).

Rather than leading to improved health and decreased crime among addicts, the Platzspitz appears to have caused generally the opposite effect. Although overdoses increased, the adjusted rate of HIV infection began to fall (9), thefts and robberies increased dramatically, and violence was endemic in the Platzspitz (57). Eventually, the citizens of Zurich could not tolerate the anarchic conditions in the midst of their city and the Platzspitz was closed in early 1992 (9). After the closure of the Platzspitz, the open-air heroin market reconstituted itself at an abandoned railway station called Letten. This site was also subsequently closed in 1995, thus ending Switzerland's experiment with tolerating an open-air drug market. Researchers have found that after closing the zones of tolerance, the number of opiate addicts seeking treatment in methadone maintenance clinics increased (59).

Whether the Platzspitz was a success or failure depends on what endpoints a person considers relevant. Politically, the experiment was a disaster. Crime rates and individual drug use increased and heroin-related deaths rose dramatically. On the other hand, HIV rates did start to fall with the extensive needle exchange program, and rates of drug use in the general population did not increase (9). Ultimately, concentrating a deviant population into one small area may lead to some public health benefits while producing other drawbacks.

After their experience with the Platzspitz the Swiss continued to struggle with finding the best response to heroin use. Initially the Swiss wanted to perform a randomized, controlled trial of heroin maintenance. Inclusion criteria were not stringent: users had to be at least 20 years old, have injected heroin for at least 2 years, and have failed treatment at least twice. The experiment called for assignment into one of three arms: injectable morphine, injectable heroin, and injectable methadone. Only at one site was assignment random. Discomfort associated with injectable morphine led to the abandonment of this arm, and patients did not accept injectable methadone. Thus, the vicissitudes of conducting research caused the study to become an essentially open trial of heroin maintenance. All heroin had to be used on site, thus preventing any leakage onto the black market. The participants could select their desired heroin dose, and average daily dose soared to between 500 and 600 mg a day—roughly 10 times the amount used by an average street user (55).

Without a true control group, the study was limited to a before-and-after study of the heroin recipients. There was no leakage of heroin to the black market and no heroin overdoses occurred. Treatment retention was impressive: 69% remained at 18 months, and half of the drop outs entered into some other form of drug treatment. Both self-reported criminal activity and rates of arrest decreased and unemployment fell from 44% to 20%, with employment described as permanent rising from 14% to 32%. Cocaine use did not diminish, but there were few new cases of HIV. In addition to being non-randomized and uncontrolled, the study was criticized for using primarily self-report outcomes (60). An analysis of the program showed that the heroin maintenance failed to demonstrate an ability to reduce criminal behavior (61). Because of these limitations, the Swiss data are hard to interpret with confidence.

Canada

Recently, researchers in Montreal, Quebec, and Vancouver, British Columbia performed a much more methodologically rigorous randomized controlled trial of heroin maintenance in opioid-dependent participants (62). In this trial, 111 participants were randomized to 12 months of treatment with oral methadone, 115 were randomized to injected heroin maintenance, and 25 were randomized to injected hydromorphone (Dilaudid). Methadone was dosed once daily (the average dose was 96 mg) and heroin was usually administered twice daily (the average daily dose was 392.3 mg). At 12-month follow-up significantly more participants in the heroin group were retained in treatment compared to the methadone group (87.8% vs. 54.1%, $P < 0.001$).

Other endpoints were measured by reduction in baseline scores of various subscales of the European Addiction Severity Index. The researchers found that more of the heroin maintained participants compared to the methadone maintained participants had at least a 20% reductions in illicit drug use or other illegal activities (67% vs. 48%, $P = 0.004$). This metric seems primarily accounted for by large reductions in days of illicit heroin use in the heroin maintenance group. **A major caveat to accepting this result is the fact that these reductions are based on self-report data only.** The heroin maintenance group also showed statistically significant reduction in subscale scores of psychiatric well-being, employment satisfaction, and social relations.

There were no statistically significant differences between the groups with respect to improvements in subscales for participation in illegal activities (decoupled from illicit drug use), days of cocaine use, medical status, economic status, family relations, or alcohol use. In addition, there were 18 serious adverse events in the methadone group (none were found to be the result of methadone use) while there were 51 adverse events in the heroin group (47% of which were caused by the study drug, including 11 opioid overdoses necessitating the administration of naloxone and hospital transfer, and seven seizures).

The study authors concluded that heroin maintenance is more effective than oral methadone. However, a more jaundiced take on these results would hold that the data showed that, based only on self-report data, when people are offered large amounts of free, legal heroin they will use less costly, illegal heroin. Lastly, the findings supporting improvements in other domains of functioning are offset by no improvement in other critical domains. Moreover, this is done at the cost of several life-threatening incidents and does not reduce other drug use (e.g., cocaine) or participation in other illicit activity.

The findings of this study raise the question of whether heroin maintenance can be considered a "treatment" at all. Methadone's once-daily dosing is supposed to allow for people to resume normal functioning, such as finding employment, and this schedule is already considered onerous by many patients (hence its moniker of "liquid handcuffs"). Heroin was given twice a day, at huge doses, and still did not prevent people from overdosing or allowing them to make convincing improvements in their overall psychosocial functioning. As drug policy experts MacCoun and Reuter point out, "Heroin maintenance has a contradiction at its heart. Having chosen to prohibit the drug, society then makes an exception for those who cause sufficient damage, to themselves and society..." If the barrier to getting into heroin maintenance is set too high, requiring individuals to incur severe damages before allowing them access to a supposedly useful solution it "is expensive... and inhumane. However, if it sets the barrier low, then access to heroin becomes too easy... This raises a fundamental ethical concern. [H]eroin maintenance itself is clearly social policy, not medicine... [S]ocial policy should not be dressed up as therapeutic activity." (9).

Sweden

From 1965 to 1967 Sweden also ran an uncontrolled experiment with maintaining addicts on their drug of choice. Starting around 1950, Sweden experienced an epidemic of amphetamine dependence. In response, the government provided legal, state-financed amphetamines. Between 1965, when the program started, and 1967, when the program ended, the prevalence of amphetamine dependence in Sweden doubled. There are data indicating that some of the spread of amphetamine use was due to young amphetamine-using men proselytizing about the benefits of amphetamines. In addition, there was substantial diversion of drugs from patients to friends and acquaintances. Interestingly, crime among legal users rose, rather than fell, when their drug of choice was made freely available to them (21,63).

Starting in 1972, Swedish policy remained lenient toward individual users, and focused on prosecuting "kingpins." The police allowed individual possession of up to a week's worth of drugs at a time, and arrests for drug possession fell. By 1980, legislative priorities changed, and possession of anything more than a single cannabis cigarette was punished. Drug arrests tripled in 3 years, and the government introduced mandatory drug treatment. Afterward, drug use—particularly among young people—fell. By 1998, the percentage of military conscripts using drugs fell by 75% and drug use by ninth graders fell 66%. In 1970, 37% of daily drug users had been under 25; by 1992 this number had fallen to 10% (63).

In Sweden, as in the United States, early policies of permissiveness toward drugs became incrementally more restrictive as the problems attendant to drug use became clearer, and as attitudes in the electorate changed over time.

China

Contrary to popular belief, the practice of smoking opium was not popular in China prior to the 18th century. It started as a practice of combining a weak opium gum with tobacco, and then smoking the resulting mixture, called *madak* (36). In 1773, in order to correct a trade imbalance, the British East India Company began to import pure opium into China. By the mid-1800s, the practice of opium smoking had progressed to the point that the Imperial government forbade the further import of the substance. When the British refused to comply, the Chinese destroyed 20,000 chests of opium the British had stored off shore.

This set off a series of battles from 1839 to 1842 known as the First Opium War. The British prevailed and forced the Chinese to open five ports to the opium trade and to pay restitution for the opium that had been destroyed. A Second Opium War was fought from 1856 to 1858 and another British victory resulted in the outright legalization of the opium trade in China. The result was that China imported 6 million pounds of opium in 1839, and 15 million pounds by 1879. Although estimates of the rates of opiate addiction vary wildly, China developed one of the highest rates of opiate addiction in the world throughout the 19th century (21,36,64).

Although the data from this period are very limited some broad conclusions can be reached. The Chinese experience with the Opium Wars lends support to the position that when drugs are commoditized in the marketplace they can be as effectively sold as any other good. Second, this historical period again shows the difficulty of making accurate predictions about how increasing the supply and availability of a drug will affect demand for the drug. Third, this is another example of how the financial interests of those dealing in addictive substances will override the interests of the public health. Fourth, as we will see, once a public develops a taste for drugs, getting widespread addiction under control is a difficult business.

By the early 1900s, the Chinese and British agreed to abolish the opium trade, and the Chinese government employed a vigorous poppy eradication campaign and instituted harsh consequences for violations (22). After World War II, the Chinese communists (who, along with their Nationalist rivals, had raised funds via the opium trade) attempted to suppress opium use in their population. This program included roundups, arrests, and executions of drug dealers as well as mass participation in antiopium rallies, and public confessions by ex-addicts (65). In all, relative increases in the 1980s not withstanding, China had one of the lowest crime rates in the world, and its rate of drug crime was particularly low (66). Although rates of drug use have been rising in China, it was recently found that in six provinces with "high prevalence" drug use, the lifetime prevalence of illicit drug use was only 1.6%, and the 1-year prevalence was 1.17% (67). China's main response to drug use has been to increase supply-reduction measures (68).

Afghanistan

After the Vietnam War, much of the world's poppy cultivation shifted to the Golden Crescent area of Iran, Pakistan, and Afghanistan. Poppy cultivation was particularly widespread in Afghanistan, and by the 1990s, Afghanistan was responsible for growing opium poppies that supplied 70% of the world's heroin. After the Soviet-client government collapsed, the Taliban took control in Afghanistan. Despite the high prices (relative to other crops) offered for poppy, the Taliban's harsh style of governance kept poppy cultivation to a minimum. By threatening punishment, punishing transgressors publicly, and close monitoring with tight local accountability, the Taliban reduced poppy cultivation by 99% in the areas they controlled. After the U.S.-led war that deposed the Taliban, poppy cultivation has returned to previous levels despite Western efforts to discourage the practice. Profits from the opium trade are used by the Taliban to fund their war against both the international forces (mainly the United States) and the Afghanistan government (69).

The experiences of China and Afghanistan hold important lessons for proponents of legalization and prohibition alike. In contradiction to the positions held by proponents of legalization, these examples lend evidence to the contention that supply-side interventions can be extremely successful in reducing drug use in a population. An equally important message exists for the advocates of prohibition: supply-side efforts alone can work, but potentially at the expense of civil liberties and a civil society. The amount of government intrusion, scrutiny, and coercion into the lives of citizens necessary to "win" a "war" on drugs may well be inimical to Western and democratic principles.

SUPPLY DISRUPTIONS

Another source of information about how drug supply can affect demand can be found in times when drug supply is temporarily severely reduced. Although these occurrences are not planned, some limited inferences can be made from studying their effects on a quasiexperimental basis (70).

World War II

During World War II, rates of heroin addiction fell dramatically throughout the United States. This was due, in part, to the large-scale disruption in heroin trafficking routes due to the war, and to the increased coastal defenses that prevented smuggling into the country. It is important to note that other factors such as the mobilization of young drug-using-age men into the military and the "aging out" of older addicts also contributed to this decline (21,22,36). Regardless, when considering the inevitability of drug use—pointed out by many who favor a legalization regime (e.g., Ref. 20)—it is important to also consider how the prevalence and magnitude of use can be sensitive to matters of both supply and demand.

New South Wales Heroin Drought

In January 2001, the heroin supply to the Australian state of New South Wales experienced an abrupt and unexpected disruption. This decrease was likely the result of record low prices of heroin combined with better interdiction. These factors led to low profits and high risk for drug traffickers (71). This "drought" peaked from January to April of 2001, and resulted in a dramatic increase in the difficulty of procuring heroin faced by addicts (72).

The shortage of heroin led to a significant reduction in the amount and frequency of heroin use, number of non-fatal heroin overdoses, heroin-related fatalities and heroin-related hospital visits. There was also a significant reduction in the amount and frequency of heroin use, number of nonfatal heroin overdoses, heroin-related fatalities, and heroin-related hospital visits (73–79). At the same time, there was a reduction in the number of people seeking treatment for opioid dependence (76–78). During the drought the price of heroin rose, while its purity fell. At the same time, there was a transient increase in the number of robberies in New South Wales early in the drought, but rates of theft fell overall (76–78). Although heroin use fell over the drought, the use of other drugs, such as cocaine and methamphetamine, increased (74,75). There was, however, no increase in the number of overdose deaths associated with these other drugs (76–78).

The conclusions that can be drawn from the Australian heroin drought are somewhat limited. The events that precipitated the supply reduction were unique, and the nature of the data gleaned prevents any firm causal inference from being made. However, a sudden, dramatic supply reduction appears to have been associated with reduced heroin use, purity and availability, and with increased price. At the same time, heroin-related injury and deaths fell and crime did not markedly increase. At minimum, were supply shortages to result in increased morbidity and mortality as hypothesized by some prolegalization advocates, such did not turn out to be the case in Australia.

TAXATION

As previously noted, one of the purposes of prohibition is to increase the price of illicit drugs in an attempt to discourage their use. Taxation is one approach that has been extensively used to increase the price of tobacco to decrease its consumption and to generate revenue to offset tobacco-related costs. Increasing the price of tobacco has been shown to decrease its consumption, particularly among lower-income groups and adolescents (80). It has been found that state tobacco taxes significantly decrease tobacco consumption, and that larger tax increases are associated with larger reductions in use (81). Tax increases on tobacco were a component of New York City's antismoking campaign that resulted in significant reductions in the prevalence of smoking in the city (82).

Interestingly, many proponents of drug legalization say a benefit of legalization would be that revenue could be generated to offset the harm caused by drug use (20). However, these same proponents also identify the black market nature of the drug trade as a source of significant drug-related harm. This puts them in the ideologically precarious position of saying that although meddling with the drug market causes the black market and, thus, harm—they will meddle in the market in such a way as to not produce a black market. History tells us this is probably a naive hope.

Drug markets historically tolerate very little interference before black markets emerge. Prior to the advent of any formal laws regulating cocaine sales, pharmacists attempted to limit dispensing the drug to those with legitimate medical concerns. The market of cocaine addicts did not tolerate even this mild disruption, and a black market emerged well before cocaine was even illegal (23). New York City officials noted that as their strict antitobacco policies went into effect, including the increased excise tax on cigarettes, the number of cigarettes bought outside the city limits to avoid that tax doubled (82). The black market for legal, but taxed, cigarettes in New York has created a violent, even deadly, traffic in bootleg tobacco (83). Canada had a similar experience in the early 1990s when its government raised tobacco taxes (21). Thus, any tax on a legal drug market would have to be set at just the right level: enough to generate sufficient revenue to offset the costs created by drug use, but not so much as to create a black market (9). As the historian, David Courtwright, notes:

> "The idea that the black market is the result of something called 'prohibition' is the central premise of the liberal view of drug history and the basis of the affiliated proposal called legalization. Licit, taxed sales of drugs…to adults could, theoretically, end the evils attendant to the black market while providing revenue for state-sponsored prevention and treatment programs. The catch, apart from increased addiction due to increased exposure is that retaining taxes (and restrictions like no sales to minors) means retaining, to some degree, the black market. Light taxes and few restrictions would make the black market a minor nuisance, but would increase the amount of compulsive use. Heavy taxes and many restrictions would mean fewer new addicts, but would create incentives for illicit manufacturing, smuggling, diversion and violence." (21).

Courtwright also identifies a second danger in taxation schemes of psychoactive drugs. He notes that whether governments taxed opium (as in the Dutch East Indies, Indochina, Brunei, Hong Kong, Singapore, or Java), alcohol (as in the United States, the Soviet Union, or post-colonial India), or tobacco, governments were forced to trade off the public health for pecuniary gain. Once the public developed an appetite for the drug in question, and the government developed an appetite for the relatively easy revenue stream, undoing unsound policy is, practically speaking, very difficult (21). A parallel experience can be seen with gambling: states, now well-hooked on lottery revenues, continue to promote their lotteries despite the regressive nature of the revenue they extract and the potential to stimulate problem gambling in the electorate (9).

SUMMARY

In closing, from a public health perspective, our national experience with the two drugs we have legalized, alcohol and nicotine, has been an unmitigated disaster. The interests of the corporations that produce and distribute these substances are defended by talented and well-funded lobbyists exercising the First Amendment right to petition the government for redress of grievances. The ineffectiveness of efforts to limit the marketing of these substances is attested to by noting the abundance of tobacco and alcohol advertising in any magazine, in any store, or at any sporting event.

Due to the widespread availability, low price, and persistent advertising of these products we experience 400,000 excess deaths a year due to tobacco and 100,000 excess deaths a year from alcohol (84). As much money as is spent on the so-called "War on Drugs," far greater sums are lost due to decreased productivity, increased health care consumption, excess deaths, and criminal justice costs associated with alcohol and tobacco use (85–87). And to what benefit have we incorporated these substances into the mainstream of our society? What quantifiable good have they wrought to offset the harms they have caused? Have they meaningfully and materially enriched and gladdened as many lives as they have destroyed? Ultimately, for alcohol and tobacco, these questions are moot. For good or for ill, these substances have been woven into our social fabric, probably permanently. Alcohol has been a part of the mainstream of our culture for thousands of years—tobacco, for hundreds. Those proverbial bells cannot be un-rung.

However, we do have an opportunity to prevent the ringing of other bells. We do have an opportunity to prevent the more widespread use of, and addiction to, illicit drugs were more people to be exposed to them. We do have an opportunity to prevent the rise of a legalized, legitimized, and organized, Big Cannabis, Big Cocaine, and Big Opium. The data from other places and other times tell us that the inherent good they would bring would not offset the misery that would follow in their wake. History also teaches us that bad policy, when linked to a politically palatable tax source, is hard to undo. Thankfully, the options before us are not limited to the false dichotomy of status quo or legalization. The point of this chapter has not been to dismiss the importance of comprehensive drug policy reform in America, or to imply that the status quo is efficient or even defensible. However, the implications of outright legalization are such that this option is best left off the table.

REFERENCES

1. Substance Abuse and Mental Health Services Administration. *Results from the 2007 National Survey on Drug Use and Health: National Findings. Office of Applied Statistics, Substance Abuse and Mental Health Services Administration.* Rockville, MD: Department of Health and Human Services; 2008.
2. Grant BF. Prevalence and correlates of drug use and DSM-IV drug dependence in the United States: results of the National Longitudinal Alcohol Epidemiologic Survey. *J Subst Abuse.* 1996;8:195–210.
3. Office of National Drug Control Policy. *The Economic Costs of Drug Abuse in the United States, 1992–2002.* Washington, DC: Office of National Drug Control Policy and Executive Office of the President; 2004.
4. Halfon N, Mendonca A, Berkowitz G, et al. Health status of children in foster care. The experience of the Center for the Vulnerable Child. *Arch Pediatr Adolesc Med.* 1995;149(4):386–392.
5. Bureau of Justice Statistics. *Criminal Victimization in the United States, 2005.* Statistical Tables. Washington, DC: Bureau of Justice Statistics, Office of Justice Programs and U.S. Department of Justice; 2006.
6. Bureau of Justice Statistics. *Drug Use and Dependence, State and Federal Prisoners, 2004.* Washington, DC: Bureau of Justice Statistics, Office of Justice Programs and U.S. Department of Justice; 2006.
7. Federal Bureau of Investigation. *Uniform Crime Report 2007.* Washington, DC: Federal Bureau of Investigation and U.S. Department of Justice; 2008.
8. National Center on Addiction and Substance Abuse. *Behind Bars: Substance Abuse and America's Prison Population.* New York: Columbia University; 1998:1.
9. MacCoun RJ, Reuter P. *Drug War Heresies: Learning From Other Vices, Times, and Places.* New York: Cambridge University Press; 2001.
10. Federal Bureau of Prisons. *Quick Facts about the Bureau of Prisons.* Washington, DC: Bureau of Prisons and U.S. Department of Justice; 2009.
11. Bureau of Justice Statistics. *Substance Dependence, Abuse, and Treatment of Jail Inmates, 2002.* Washington, DC: Bureau of Justice Statistics, Office of Justice Programs and U.S. Department of Justice; 2005.
12. Miller TR, Levy DT, Cohen MA, et al. Costs of alcohol and drug-involved crime. *Prev Sci.* 2006;7:333–342.
13. Bureau of Justice Statistics. *Substance Abuse and Treatment, State and Federal Prisoners, 1997.* Washington, DC: Bureau of Justice Statistics, Office of Justice Programs and U.S. Department of Justice; 1999.
14. Robinson PH. *Criminal Law: Case Studies and Controversies.* New York: Aspen Publishers; 2005.
15. MacCoun RJ. Biases in the interpretation and use of research results. *Annu Rev Psychol.* 1998;49:259–287.
16. Boyum D, Reuter P. *An Analytical Assessment of U.S. Drug Policy.* Washington, DC: AEI Press; 2005.
17. Becker HS. *Outsiders: Studies in the Sociology of Deviance.* Toronto, Ontario: Collier-Macmillan Canada, Ltd.; 1963.
18. Libertarian Party. *National Platform of the Libertarian Party.* Denver, CO; 2008.
19. Nadelmann E. The case for legalization. In: Inciardi, J. ed. *The Drug Legalization Debate.* Newbury Park, CA: Sage Publications; 1991:17–44.
20. Nadelmann E. Think again: drugs. *Foreign Policy.* 2007;162:24–30.
21. Courtwright DT. *Dark Paradise: A History of Opiate Addiction in America.* Cambridge, MA: Harvard University Press; 2001.
22. Musto DF. *The American Disease: Origins of Narcotic Control.* New York: Oxford University Press; 1999.
23. Spillane JF. *Cocaine: From Medical Marvel to Modern Menace.* Baltimore, MD: Johns Hopkins University Press; 2000.
24. Anthony JC, Warner LA, Kessler, RC, et al. Comparative epidemiology of dependence on tobacco, alcohol, controlled substances,

and inhalants: basic findings from the National Comorbidity Survey. *Exp Clin Psychopharmacol.* 1994;2(3):244–268.
25. Gordon RS. An operational classification of disease prevention. *Public Health Rep.* 1983;98(2):107–109.
26. Kleiman MAR. *Against Excess: Drug Policy For Results.* New York: Basic Books; 1992.
27. Pacula RL, Chaloupka FJ. The effects of macro-level interventions on addictive behavior. *Subst Use Misuse.* 2001;36(13):1901–1922.
28. Higgins ST, Bickel WK, Hughes JR. Influence of an alternative reinforcer on human cocaine self-administration. *Life Sci.* 1994;55(3):179–187.
29. Comer SD, Collins ED, Fischman MW. Choice between money and intranasal heroin in morphine-maintained humans. *Behav Pharmacol.* 1997;8(8):677–690.
30. Higgins ST. The influence of alternative reinforcers on cocaine use and abuse: a brief review. *Pharmacol Biochem Behav.* 1997;57(3):419–427.
31. Hart CL, Haney M, Foltin RW, et al. Alternative reinforcers differentially modify cocaine self-administration by humans. *Behav Pharmacol.* 2000;11(1):87–91.
32. Donny EC, Bigelow GE, Walsh SL. Choosing to take cocaine in the human laboratory: effects of cocaine dose, inter-choice interval, and magnitude of alternative reinforcement. *Drug Alcohol Depend.* 2003;69(3): 289–301.
33. Donny EC, Bigelow GE, Walsh SL. Assessing the initiation of cocaine self-administration in humans during abstinence: effects of dose, alternative reinforcement, and priming. *Psychopharmacology.* 2004;172(3):316–323.
34. Saffer H, Chaloupka FJ. The demand for illicit drugs. *NBER Working Paper Series.* Cambridge, MA: National Bureau of Economic Research; 1995.
35. Chaloupka FJ, Grossman M, Tauras JA. The demand for cocaine and marijuana by youth. *NBER Working Paper Series.* Cambridge, MA: National Bureau of Economic Research; 1998.
36. Jonnes J. *Hep-cats, Narcs, and Pipe Dreams: A History of America's Romance With Illegal Drugs.* New York: Scribner; 1996.
37. Courtwright DT. The road to H: the emergence of the American heroin complex, 1898–1956. In: Musto DF, ed. *One Hundred Years of Heroin.* Westport, CT: Auburn House; 2002.
38. Grinspoon L, Bakalar J. The war on drugs—a peace proposal. *N Engl J Med.* 1994;330:357–360.
39. Lender ME, Martin JK. *Drinking in America: A History.* New York: Macmillan; 1982.
40. Musto DF. *Drugs in America: A Documentary History.* New York: New York University Press; 2002.
41. Goldstein A. *Addiction: From Biology to Public Policy.* New York: W.H. Freeman; 1994.
42. Aaron P, Musto DF. *Alcohol and Public Policy: Beyond the Shadow of Prohibition.* In: Moore M, Gerstein D, eds. Washington DC: National Academy Press; 1981:127–181.
43. McCoy C. Booze flows back into Barrow, Alaska after a yearlong ban. *Wall Street J.* 1995.
44. Karel R. A model legalization proposal. In: Inciardi J, ed. *The Drug Legalization Debate.* Newbury Park, CA: Sage Publications; 1991:80–102.
45. McVay D. Marijuana legalization: the time is now. In: Inciardi J, ed. *The Drug Legalization Debate.* Newbury Park, CA: Sage Publications; 1991:147–160.
46. MacCoun RJ, Reuter P. Interpreting Dutch cannabis policy: reasoning by analogy in the legalization debate. *Science.* 1997;278:47–52.
47. de Zwart WM, Mensink C, Kuipers, SBM. *Key Data: Smoking, Drinking, Drug Use and Gambling among Pupils Aged 10 and Older.* Utrecht, Netherlands: Institute for Alcohol and Drugs; 1994.
48. Gunning KF. President, Dutch National Commission on Drug Prevention, Rotterdam, Holland; 1995.
49. Spanjer M. Dutch schoolchildren's drug-taking doubles. *Lancet.* 1996;347:534.
50. Kroon R. Interview with Dutch Prime Minister Kim Wok. *International Herald Tribune.* 1996.
51. Parloff R. How marijuana became legal. *Fortune.* 2009;160(6):140–142, 144, 146.
52. Emshwiller JR. Los Angeles set to close marijuana dispensaries. *Wall Street J.* 2010;A7.
53. Johnston LD, O'Malley PM, Bachman JG, et al. *Teen Marijuana Use Tilts Up, While Some Drugs Decline in Use.* Ann Arbor, MI: University of Michigan News Service; 2009.
54. Glaze J. *Letter to Michael Snell, Esq.* British Embassy in Washington, D.C.B.H. Office; 1992.
55. Reuter P, MacCoun RJ, eds. *Heroin Maintenance. One Hundred Years of Heroin.* Westport, CT: Auburn House; 2001.
56. Hartnoll RL, Mitcheson MC, Battersby A, et al. Evaluation of heroin maintenance in controlled trial. *Arch Gen Psychiatry.* 1980;37(8):877–884.
57. Huber C. Needle Park: what can we learn from the Zurich experience? *Addiction.* 1994;89:513–516.
58. Reuter P, Falco M, MacCoun RJ, et al. *Comparing Western European and North American Drug Policies: an International Conference Report.* Santa Monica, CA: RAND; 1993.
59. Falcato L, Stohler R, Duersteller-MacFarland KM, et al. Closure of an open drug scene—a case register-based analysis of the impact on the demand for methadone maintenance. *Addiction.* 2001;96:623–628.
60. Reuter P, MacCoun RJ, eds. *Heroin Maintenance. One Hundred Years of Heroin.* Westport, CT: Auburn House; 2002.
61. Kilias M, Uchtenhagen A. Does medical heroin prescription reduce delinquency among drug-addicts? On the evaluation of the Swiss heroin prescription projects and its methodology. *Studies Crime Crime Prev.* 1996;5(2):245–256.
62. Oviedo-Joekes E, Brissette S, Marsh DC, et al. Diacetylmorphine versus methadone for the treatment of opioid addiction. *N Engl J Med.* 2009;361:777–786.
63. Swedish National Institute of Public Health. *A Restrictive Drug Policy: The Swedish Experience.* Stockholm: Swedish National Institute of Public Health Health; 1993.
64. Courtwright DT. *Forces of Habit: Drugs and the Making of the Modern World.* Cambridge, MA: Harvard University Press; 2001.
65. Meyer K. From British India to the Taliban: lessons from the history of the heroin market. In: Musto DF, ed. *One Hundred Years of Heroin.* Westport, CT: Auburn House; 2002.
66. Bakken B. Crime, juvenile delinquency and deterrence policy in China. *Aus J Chin Aff.* 1993;30:29–58.
67. Hao W, Xiao S, Liu T, et al. The second National Epidemiological Survey on illicit drug use at six high-prevalence areas in China: prevalence rates and use patterns. *Addiction.* 2002;97:1305–1315.
68. Chen Z, Huang K. Drug problems in China. *Int J Offender Ther Comp Criminol.* 2007;51(1):98–109.
69. Farrell G, Thorne J. Where have all the flowers gone? Evaluation of the Taliban crackdown against opium poppy cultivation in Afghanistan. *Int J Drug Policy.* 2005;16:81–91.

70. Weatherburn D, Jones C, Freeman K, et al. Supply control and harm reduction: lessons from the Australian heroin "drought." *Addiction*. 2003;98:83–91.
71. Degenhardt L, Reuter P, Collins L, et al. Evaluating explanations of the Australian "heroin shortage." *Addiction*. 2005;100:459–469.
72. Day C, Topp L, Rouen D, et al. Decreased heroin availability in Sydney in early 2001. *Addiction*. 2003;98:93–95.
73. Degenhardt L, Day C, Dietze P, et al. Effects of a sustained heroin shortage in three Australian states. *Addiction*. 2005;100:908–920.
74. Longo MC, Henry-Edwards SM, Humeniuk RE, et al. Impact of the heroin "drought" on patterns of drug use and drug-related harms. *Drug Alcohol Rev*. 2004;23:143–150.
75. Roxburgh A, Degenhardt L, Breen C. Changes in patterns of drug use among injecting drug users following changes in the availability of heroin in New South Wales, Australia. *Drug Alcohol Rev*. 2004;23:287–294.
76. Degenhardt L, Conroy E, Gilmour S, et al. The impact of a reduction in drug supply on demand for and compliance with treatment for drug dependence. *Drug Alcohol Depend*. 2005;79:129–135.
77. Degenhardt L, Conroy E, Gilmour S. The effect of a reduction in heroin supply in Australia upon drug distribution and acquisitive crime. *Br J Criminol*. 2005;45:2–24.
78. Degenhardt L, Conroy E, Gilmour S, et al. The effect of a reduction in heroin supply on fatal and non-fatal drug overdoses in New South Wales, Australia. *Med J Aust*. 2005;182(1):20–23.
79. Degenhardt L, Day C, Dietze P, et al. Effects of a sustained heroin shortage in three Australian states. *Addiction*. 2005;100:908–920.
80. Townsend J. Price and consumption of tobacco. *Br Med J*. 1996;52(1):132–142.
81. Peterson DE, Zeger SL, Remington PL, et al. The effect of state cigarette tax increases on cigarette sales, 1955 to 1988. *Am J Public Health*. 1992;82:94–96.
82. Frieden TR, Mostashari F, Kerker BD, et al. Adult tobacco use levels after intensive tobacco control measures: New York City, 2002–2003. *Am J Public Health*. 2005;95(6):1016–1023.
83. Fleenor P. *Cigarette Taxes, Black Markets and Crime: Lessons from New York's 50-Year Losing Battle. Policy Analysis*. Washington, DC: Cato Institute; 2003.
84. McGinnis JM, Foege W. Actual causes of death in the United States. *J Am Med Assoc*. 1993;270(18):2207–2212.
85. Brenner TA. The legalization of drugs: why prolong the inevitable? In: Evans R, Berent I, eds. *Drug Legalization: For and Against*. La Salle, IL: Open Court Press; 1992:157–180.
86. Smith M. The drug problem: is there an answer? In: Evans R, Berent I, eds. *Drug Legalization: For and Against*. La Salle, IL: Open Court Press; 1992:215–220.
87. Wisotsky S. Statement before the Select Committee on Narcotics Abuse and Control. In: Evans R, Berent I, eds. *Drug Legalization: For and Against*. La Salle, IL: Open Court Press; 1992.

CHAPTER 81 Future Directions

Pedro Ruiz ■ Eric C. Strain

INTRODUCTION

Since the first edition of this textbook was published in 1981 (1), the field of addiction has grown tremendously. This growth has taken place in all areas of the field, that is, in all dimensions of the biopsychosocial aspects of these disorders. The field of substance abuse has changed a great deal since the early 1960s when a small group of scientists, physicians, and mental health professionals began to focus their interests on the medical and psychosocial consequences of substance abuse. The first edition of this textbook attempted to address all of those medical and societal problems related to the abuse of addictive substances from a clinical and scientific point of view. Specific substances were examined, as well as epidemiologic components, treatment approaches, and prevention models.

The second edition of the textbook was published in 1992 (2). This edition appeared after a decade of extraordinary challenges faced by the addiction field. During this decade, the understanding of substance abuse from a neurobiologic point of view became a necessity. New scientific knowledge evolved rather quickly in this area of the field. This new perspective in the understanding of addictive disorders opened a new window of opportunity for new treatment approaches and possibilities for the exploration of new etiologic factors related to the cause of addictive disorders. During the decade prior to the publishing of this second edition, new perspectives in the areas of prevention, treatment alternatives, and policy planning and implementation became viable. At the time of publication of the first edition of the book, there were only two medications approved for the treatment of substance use disorders in the United States: disulfiram and methadone. By the time the second edition was published, the number of approved medications had doubled, with the addition of oral naltrexone for the treatment of opioid dependence in 1984, and nicotine gum by prescription for the treatment of nicotine dependence also in 1984. These changes illustrate several forces in the field of addictions that would continue in subsequent years—including the entry of pharmaceutical companies into the field of addictions, the gradual shift of addictions treatment into general medical practice, and the tendency to focus upon licit drug use as an area of particular interest in the field of medicine. The idea of the second edition of this book was to provide a comprehensive and detailed description of the thinking and new development in both the basic sciences and clinical practice with respect to addictive conditions.

The third edition of the textbook was published just 5 years after the second edition—in 1997 (3). During the half of a decade that had passed since the publication of the second edition, new scientific advances had greatly impacted the understanding of addictive behaviors and its causes. New knowledge about the impact of substances of abuse on the brain and its behavioral outcomes had become a reality. Cloned receptors in the brain were identified as sites of action for many substances of abuse. Cellular mechanisms of action were also identified for drugs such as cocaine, marihuana, and opiates. Brain circuits were also found to have a role in behavioral manifestations like euphoria, as well as the process of addiction and drug withdrawal. The national emphasis on neurosciences research took place during this half of a decade, and its positive impact on new scientific discoveries vis-à-vis drug addiction was rewarding during this period. Concurrent with this growing awareness of the neuroscientific basis of addiction, the treatment field also was refining its methodologies and demonstrating the efficacy of different approaches—both pharmacologic and nonpharmacologic. Illustrating the growth in the field, six medications were approved in the United States for use in the treatment of substance use disorders during this period: the nicotine patch in 1992; LAAM in 1993; oral naltrexone for alcohol dependence in 1995; nicotine nasal spray in 1996; a nicotine inhaler in 1997; and bupropion for nicotine dependence; a seventh medication—sublingual buprenorphine—was first approved for the treatment of opioid dependence in France, in 1996. Given the limited availability of methadone treatment in that country, it quickly became a valuable treatment for patients who suffered from opioid dependence. In addition, it showed that a medication for an illicit drug use disorder could be a viable product for a pharmaceutical company. Also of note during this period was a major effort to identify cocaine pharmacotherapies (an effort that continues to the present), the growth of neuroimaging as a tool to better understand reward pathways and the differential effects of acute versus chronic drug use, and the efficacy of novel contingency management strategies such as voucher incentives to produce sustained periods of drug abstinence.

The fourth edition of this textbook was published in 2005 (4). This edition was published almost a decade later from the previous one; during this period, new challenges faced the field of addiction and they were fully addressed in this edition. These included issues pertaining to lack of parity between medical illnesses and addictive conditions, and cost containment via managed care, which has negatively impacted on the clinical care received by patients who suffer from addictive disorders. In addition, new medications such as buprenorphine was approved for use in the United States in 2002 and acamprosate was approved for use in the United States in 2004, but these were marketed in Europe for many years prior to its approval in the United States, offered new hopes in the addiction field; the role of neurosciences vis-à-vis addictive disorders clearly demonstrated its value and relevance in the field of addiction. However, despite the positive advances in the neurosciences, the psychosocial aspects of addictive disorders continued to be very relevant in the addiction field and were thoroughly addressed in that edition.

Obviously, since the first edition of this textbook almost three decades ago, the field of addiction has gained a great deal due to research advances along the lines of the biopsychosocial model, but particularly in the neurosciences area of the field. It is within this context that this fifth edition was produced and, hopefully, has appropriately and thoroughly addressed all major advances that have taken place in the field of addiction since the fourth edition was published almost a decade ago.

CURRENT PERSPECTIVES

A close view and analysis of what is relevant and current at the present time should permit us to elaborate on the most prominent aspects of the future of the addiction field. There are several points that can be highlighted about the current state of addictions, and while these may seem self-evident, it is useful to clearly state them as they have not always been fully acknowledged either in the health professions or by the broader culture.

The first of these is that addictive disorders are medical conditions. That is, the field of medicine is that discipline that addresses this area of science—it has a growing body of experience in the treatment of these disorders, their prevention, and research about these conditions. This is not meant to diminish in any way the expertise that other disciplines bring to our understanding of addictions. Clearly, sociology, economy, criminology, and other disciplines have made and will continue to make important contributions to our understanding of addictive disorders and their impact. However, we believe that medicine is that field of science where work in this area should primarily reside—and, while that may seem clear to the reader, it was not long ago when such a point would be debated. Furthermore, among the disorders in medicine, addictions seem to us to be the most intriguing—in part, because our understanding of them can range from studies of the neuroscience of brain function to cultural aspects of use that encompass broad numbers of populations. Addictions range from epigenetics to epidemiology and from circuits in the brain to cost–benefit analyses of treatments.

The second point regarding the current state of addictions is that addictive disorders are a pressing problem throughout the world, and it is unlikely that addictive disorders will be "cured" anytime soon. The problems of substance use are not a problem of the contemporary era; as noted in the Old Testament of the Bible:

> Who has woe? Who has sorrow? Who has strife? Who has complaints? Who has needless bruises? Who has bloodshot eyes? Those who linger over wine, who go to sample bowls of mixed wine. Do not gaze at wine when it is red, when it sparkles in the cup, when it goes down smoothly! In the end it bites like a snake and poisons like a viper. Your eyes will see strange sights and your mind imagine confusing things. You will be like one sleeping on the high seas, lying on top of the rigging. "They hit me," you will say, "but I'm not hurt! They beat me, but I don't feel it! When will I wake up so I can find another drink?" (Proverbs 23: 29–35)

No country is immune from addictions, and while rates of use may fluctuate over time (e.g., due to availability, changes in cultural norms, or economic conditions), substance use disorders persist and in many cases grow as new forms of drugs and delivery systems become available. For students contemplating an area to pursue in their career, understanding these disorders, and helping those who suffer from them holds the promise of intriguing work and satisfying patient care—despite these being conditions that have plagued humans for thousands of years.

We also are optimistic about this field. Advances in understanding all aspects of addictions continue to grow. These advances help in prevention and treatment; in addition, while research in addictions helps our understanding of these disorders, this work also provides insights into the broader topics of motivated behavior—that is, the neuroscientific basis of behavior, as well as the environmental circumstances and determinants of choice and consumption.

Regarding the area of neurosciences, this has been one aspect of the addictions field that has produced substantial and highly relevant scientific advances in the last decade. Mechanisms of memory, reward, and reinforcement have been clarified, and will continue to help drive the field and show the biology of addictions. However, this is not to say that the psychosocial aspects of addictive disorders are no longer important and necessary. On the contrary, nowadays, more than ever before we need to address all aspects of addiction from a psychosocial point of view. In this edition of the book, Section 1 (Foundations), Section 2 (Determinants of Abuse and Dependence), Section 6, Part 2 (Psychosocial and Other Treatments), Section 8 (Models of Prevention), Section 10 (Special Populations), Section 11 (Training and Education), and Section 12 (Policy Issues), all address very comprehensively and thoroughly the psychosocial aspects of the biopsychosocial model.

In addition to growth in our understanding of the neuroscience of addictive disorders, psychiatric genetics is an area full of opportunities for currently assessing the potential relationship between genetic factors and addictive disorders, although the processes underlying mental disorders from a genetic point of view is becoming a very complex one. The genes related to mental conditions appear to be very complex; however, "neural circuits" could be quite promising with respect to the understanding of mental disorders, including addiction.

Finally, current perspectives on addictions need to acknowledge the growth in our understanding of the treatment of these disorders. While it is now generally accepted, not long ago the statement that treatment for substance abuse is effective was not widely known—and the evidence for such a statement was not readily available. There is now a rich source of controlled clinical trials showing the efficacy of a variety of treatments, well-documented through reviews such as those provided by the Cochrane Database (5–10). These treatments take the form of both pharmacotherapies and nonpharmacologic treatments. As noted earlier in this chapter, there has been a marked increase in the number of approved medications for the treatment of substance use disorders, and this growth has helped health care professionals change their perspective on these conditions, and it has helped a tremendous number of patients. However, growth in treatment has not been limited to medications, and work has demonstrated the efficacy of psychosocial treatments for addictions (11) and that there is a substantial evidence base for particular forms of treatment (12). While there remain important questions about treatment, the field of addictions has provided well-controlled studies showing that interventions can work for these patients, helping in changing a cultural perception that substance abuse was best addressed through nonmedical means such as the criminal justice system.

FUTURE DIRECTIONS

With respect to future directions in the field of addiction, there are many aspects within the area of neurosciences that could be quite relevant to the etiologic understanding and appropriate treatment of addictive disorders.

For instance, preclinical studies indicate that neuroadaptations that take place among adolescents exposed to some substance of abuse like nicotine or cannabinoids are different than those observed during adulthood (13). Obviously, genetics play a major role in addictive conditions; it is estimated that 40% to 60% of the vulnerability to addictive behavior is related to genetic factors (14). For instance, genotypic vulnerability to addiction tends to reflect both variability in the metabolism of the substance of abuse and variability in the sensitivity to the reinforcing effects of the abused substance (15). However, addiction-driven and addiction-resistant phenotypes may also reflect sensitivity to various stressors and alternative reinforces in the individual's environment (16).

Excellent efforts have also been dedicated to study the nature of global versus regional hierarchical brain organization (17). This type of work has also led to the consideration of mental disorders being primarily perturbations in the optimal organization of the brain (18). Certainly, the use of simulation models of the brain from the perspectives of computational neurosciences can be a very promising approach to understand the relationship between brain structures, brain organization, and brain circuits vis-à-vis mental disorders, including addictive conditions. This approach can lead to the potential utilization of brain pacemakers or the optimization of neural plasticity to improve or cure mental/addictive disorders.

Future possibilities in the field of addiction can also include helping drug addicts to be less dependent or to be able to withdraw from their drug/drugs of dependence, as well as to have access to new medications that can assist them in avoiding relapses (19,20). There is also the possibility that if addiction could be perceived as a chronic, relapsing brain disorder, the moral view of addiction and its punitive social policy consequences can be changed in the near future and, thus, offering the potential for new and more humane policies with respect to the care of addicts. This approach will also eliminate the stigmatization and imprisonment of addicts (21). However, these new approaches can also lead to the justification of heroic treatments and intervention such as ultra-rapid opiate detoxification and/or neurosurgery for heroin dependence (22,23).

From a policy point of view, it is difficult to understand as to why alcohol and tobacco are considered legal drugs while others such as heroin, cocaine, and cannabis are not considered legal (24). Along the lines of policy, it appears that there will be no major changes in the future insofar as international policies toward addiction are concerned (25). Clearly, the neurobiologic research efforts in animals and humans during the last several decades have demonstrated that the most important psychoactive drugs of dependence act on key neurotransmitter systems of our brain and cause related behaviors (26). Twin and adoption studies have also depicted that genetics along with the environment contributes to our vulnerabilities to different types of addiction (26).

Obviously, the applications of neuroscience research on addiction are likely to bring benefits and possible harm as well in the future (26). While so far, neurobiologists have focused on the benefits, it is also important that we focus on the potential harm (26).

From a different point of view, recent research efforts have depicted potential beneficial effects; for instance, it looks that gamma-aminobutyric acid (GABA) transmission and GABA B receptors play a module role in the mechanism of action of different drugs of abuse (27). This discovery has very good future potentials. While there are many unknown aspects concerning the mode of action of abused drugs, a unifying theme for toxicity and addiction was advanced based on electron transfer (ET), reactive oxygen species (ROS), and oxidative stress (OS). This concept applies to nicotine, cocaine, alcohol, phencyclidine, ecstasy, amphetamines, morphine–heroin, tetrahydrocannabinol, and therapeutic drugs such as benzodiazepines, phenytoin, Phenobarbital, aspirin, and acetaminophen (28). This type of new knowledge will certainly help to better understand the neurobiologic mechanisms related to addictive behavior.

CONCLUSION

The field of substance use disorders has shown tremendous growth since the first edition of this textbook was published 30 years ago. Our understanding of the biologic determinants of drug use, and effective prevention and treatment interventions, has steadily improved over time. These accomplishments have helped change cultural attitudes about the nature of addictive disorders, and most importantly, they have brought these disorders into the field of medicine and created a dynamic interest by health care professionals dedicated to helping patients who suffer from these disorders. Despite these accomplishments, much work remains.

In the United States and in many other countries, there is a pressing need to expand services for those who need treatment. Hand-in-hand with such an expansion of treatment is the need to identify ways to encourage people to engage in treatment. There is also a need to identify and promulgate the most effective prevention programs to decrease the number of persons who develop substance abuse problems. For many classes of drugs, there are effective pharmacologic and nonpharmacologic treatments—it is the delivery systems for such treatments that need to be improved.

However, there remains a need to identify pharmacologic treatments for stimulant use disorders (i.e., cocaine and amphetamines). Despite decades of effort and testing, there is still no approved medication to treat these disorders.

There remain other areas that need to be addressed—the optimal treatment of women (including pregnant women), the growing body of older substance users, the seemingly intractable fifth of the population that continues to have nicotine dependence, and the optimal treatment of persons with co-occurring disorders, to name just a few. However, perhaps the most critical need in the future is to identify how the growing neuroscientific and genetic basis of addictions can be translated into clinical practice and improved treatment outcomes. Substance abuse is a clinical disorder. Bringing basic science findings into the clinical setting is an important step. How this will occur remains unclear at this time—it may be related to the study of memory and learning, of behavior and reinforcement, or of pharmacologic manipulation of reward circuits. Regardless of the next step forward, it will be important to remember that there is a patient who seeks our help through the understanding of the unique features of that person's life story.

REFERENCES

1. Lowinson JH, Ruiz P, eds. *Substance Abuse: Clinical Problems and Perspectives*. Baltimore, MD: Williams & Wilkins; 1981.
2. Lowinson JH, Ruiz P, Millman RD, et al., eds. *Substance Abuse: A Comprehensive Textbook*. 2nd ed. Baltimore, MD: Williams & Wilkins; 1992.
3. Lowinson JH, Ruiz P, Millman RD, et al., eds. *Substance Abuse: A Comprehensive Textbook*. 3rd ed. Baltimore, MD: Williams & Wilkins; 1997.
4. Lowinson JH, Ruiz P, Millman RD, et al., eds. *Substance Abuse: A Comprehensive Textbook*. 4th ed. Philadelphia, PA: Lippincott Williams & Wilkins; 1995.
5. Mattick RP, Breen C, Kimber J, et al. Methadone maintenance therapy versus no opioid replacement therapy for opioid dependence. *Cochrane Database Syst Rev*. 2009;(3):CD002209.
6. Gowing L, Ali R, White JM. Buprenorphine for the management of opioid withdrawal. *Cochrane Database Syst Rev*. 2009;(3):CD002025.
7. Stade BC, Bailey C, Dzendoletas D, et al. Psychological and/or educational interventions for reducing alcohol consumption in pregnant women and women planning pregnancy. *Cochrane Database Syst Rev*. 2009;(2):CD004228.
8. Amato L, Minozzi S, Davoli M, et al. Psychosocial and pharmacological treatments versus pharmacological treatments for opioid detoxification. *Cochrane Database Syst Rev*. 2008;(4):CD005031.
9. Hesse M, Vanderplasschen W, Rapp RC, et al. Case management for persons with substance use disorders. *Cochrane Database Syst Rev*. 2007;(4):CD006265.
10. Rigotti NA, Munafo MR, Stead LF. Interventions for smoking cessation in hospitalised patients. *Cochrane Database Syst Rev*. 2007;(3):CD001837.
11. McLellan AT, Arndt IO, Metzger DS, et al. The effects of psychosocial services in substance abuse treatment. *JAMA*. 1993;269(15):1953–1959.
12. Dutra L, Stathopoulou G, Basden SL, et al. A meta-analytic review of psychosocial interventions for substance use disorders. *Am J Psychiatry*. 2008;165(2):179–187.
13. Adriani W, Laviola G. Windows of vulnerability to psychopathology and therapeutic strategy in the adolescent rodent model. *Behav Pharmacol*. 2004;15(5–6):341–352.
14. Goldman D, Oroszi G, Ducci F. The genetics of addiction: uncovering the genes. *Nat Rev Genet*. 2005;6:521–532.
15. Crabbe JC. Genetic contributions to addiction. *Annu Rev Psychol*. 2002;53:435–462.
16. Ranaldi R, Banco P, McCormick S, et al. Equal sensitivity to cocaine reward in addiction-prone and addiction-resistant rat genotypes. *Behav Pharmacol*. 2001;12(6–7):527–534.
17. Mesulan M. From sensation to cognition. *Brain*. 1998;121:1013–1052.
18. Herz J, Krogh A, Richard GP. *Introduction to the Theory of Neural Computation*. Santa Fe, NM: Santa Fe Institute Addison Wesley Editorial; 1991.
19. Morris KA, Iverson LJ, Nutt DJ. *Foresight State of the Art Science Review: Pharmacology and Treatments*. London, England: Department of Trade and Industry; 2005.
20. Robbins TW, Cardinal RN, DiCiano P, et al-. *Foresight State of the Art Science Review: Neuroscience of Drugs and Addiction*. London, England: Department of Trade and Industry; 2005.
21. Dackis C, O'Brien C. Neurobiology of addiction: treatment and public policy ramifications. *Nat Neurosci*. 2005;8:1431–1436.
22. Hall W. UROD: an antipodean therapeutic enthusiasm. *Addiction*. 2000;95:1765–1766.
23. Hall WD. Stereotactic neurosurgical treatment of addiction: minimizing the chances of another "great and desperate cure". *Addiction*. 2006;101:1–3.
24. Capps B, Ashcroft R, Campbell AV. *Foresight State of the Art Science Review: Ethical Aspects of Development in Neuroscience and Drug Addiction*. London, England: Department of Trade and Industry; 2005.
25. Berridge V, Hickman T. *Foresight State of the Art Science Review: History and the Future of Psychoactive Substances*. London, England: Department of Trade and Industry; 2005.
26. Haw W. Avoiding potential misuses of addiction brain science. *Addiction*. 2006;101:1529–1532.
27. Filip M, Frankowska M. GABA(B) receptors in drug addiction. *Pharmacol Rep*. 2008;60(6):755–770.
28. Kovacic P. Unifying mechanism for addiction and toxicity of abused drugs with application to dopamine and glutamate mediators: electron transfer and reactive oxygen species. *Med Hypotheses*. 2005;65(1):90–96.

Index

Note: Page numbers followed *f* indicate figures; page numbers followed by *t* indicate tables.

AA. *See* African Americans (AA); Alcoholics Anonymous (AA)
α_{2A}-Adrenoreceptor, 247
α_{2A}-Antagonist atipamezole, 243
AADIS. *See* Adolescent Alcohol and Drug Involvement Scale (AADIS)
α-Adrenergic receptors, 243
β-Adrenergic receptors, 243
AAPM. *See* American Academy of Pain Medicine (AAPM)
A_{2A} receptor gene (ADORA2A)
 caffeine consumption and, 338, 339
AAS. *See* Anabolic-androgenic steroids (AAS)
Aberrant drug-related behaviors, 700–702, 701*t*
Abscess, 675
Absenteeism, group therapy, 581
Absorption, 143
Abstinence
 in individual psychotherapy
  co-occurring disorders and, 569
  establishment of, 568–569
  family interventions and, 569
  vs. harm reduction, 565–566
 in sexual addiction, 402–403
  couple therapy, 402
  sex therapy, 402–403
Abstinence-oriented religious group, 923
Abstinence-specific support, and SHG, 528–529
Abuse
 defined, 118
Abuse and harmful use
 comparison of, 119
Acamprosate, for alcohol dependence, 154–155, 480*t*, 483–485
 efficacy studies, 483–484
 FDA approval, 483
 impaired renal function and, 485
 mechanism of action, 483
 naltrexone and, 485
 optimal use of, 485
 safety issues, 484
ACC. *See* Addiction Counseling Competencies (ACC); Assertive continuing care (ACC)
Accreditation Council on Continuing Medical Education (ACCME), 943
Accreditation Council on Graduate Medical Education (ACGME), 939
Acculturation, 102
 defined, 102
 failure group, 924
Acculturation process and substance abuse, link between, 833–834
Acetaldehyde dehydrogenase (ALDH), 144, 477
Acetaminophen, 707
Acetone, 299–300
 abuse potential of, 300
ACOG. *See* American College of Obstetricians and Gynecologists (ACOG)
Acquired immune deficiency syndrome (AIDS), 307
Acquisitive crimes, 1034
ACRA. *See* Adolescent Community Reinforcement Approach (ACRA)

Active drug abusers, opioid therapy for, 718
Activities of daily living, 915
Acupuncture
 for alcohol addiction, 472
 as analgesia, 466–467
 animal experiment of, 468–469
 aversive side effects of, 472
 for cocaine addiction, 472–473
 and craving, 471
 defined, 466
 dependence liability of, 472
 electroacupuncture, 467–468
 history of, 466–467
 manual needling, 467
 for opiate withdrawal symptoms, 467
 for pain management, 467
 for relapse prevention, 471–472
 serendipitous clinical practice, 466
 for smoking, 472
 TEAS, 468
 use of, technical comments, 473–474
 for withdrawal syndromes, 469–471
Acute pain
 defined, 696–697
 overview, 695
 vs. chronic pain, 696–697
ADA. *See* Americans with Disabilities Act (ADA)
ADAMHA. *See* Alcohol, Drug Abuse, and Mental Health Administration (ADAMHA)
Addiction
 costs caused by, 1034
 counselor
  certification issue, 974–975
  history, 971–974, 972*t*–974*t*
  licensure issue, 974–975
  training and education, 971–977
 defined, 699–700
 gastrointestinal disease and, 669
 laboratory models of, 88–95
  validity of, 94–95
 nurses
  certification as, 981
  role of, 982
Addiction biology
 brain reward system, 998
 craving and relapse, 999
 immediate targets of drugs in the brain: receptors, 997–998
 policy lessons from modern brain biology, 999
  intervention, 1000
  prevention, 1000
  treatment, 1000–1001
 toxic effects of specific drugs, 999
 transition to the disease of addiction, 998–999
 withdrawal, 999
Addiction Counseling Competencies (ACC), 972, 974
Addiction disease and law enforcement, 5–6
Addiction-related impairment, 909
 secondary to substance use, 913–914
 under Social Security law, 915
Addiction Research Center (ARC), 161, 164
 psychiatry and clinical pharmacology at, 164

Addiction Research Center Inventory (ARCI), 249
Addiction Research Center Inventory-Morphine Benzedrine Group subscale (ARCG-MBG), 262
Addictions Committee, 965
Addiction severity index (ASI), 179
Addictions Nursing Certification Board (ANCB), 981
Addictions nursing specialty organizations, 958–959
Addiction specialists, 1019
 being qualified as an expert, 1019
 postconviction phase, 1021
 pretrial phase, 1020–1021
 rationale for the admission of expert testimony, 1019–1020
 role in addiction medicine, 1020–1021
 therapists, conflicts between, 564
 trial phase, 1021
Addiction Technology Transfer Centers (ATTC), 968, 972
Addiction treatment
 as harm reduction, 761–766
 settings, 960–961
Addictive disease, as disability, 908
Addictive disorders, 920
 among migrants and refugees, case examples, 919, 921–922
 life cycle, 910
 mainstream treatment modalities, 922
 religious conversion and recovery, 923
 self-help activities, 922–923
Addictive personality. *See also* Personality disorders
 concept of, 79
Addictive processes
 compulsive spending or shopping, 1027
 eating disorders, 1027
 pathologic gambling
  clinical and forensic distinctions, 1026–1027
  implications of United States v. shorter, 1027
 sexual addiction, 1027
Addressing Tobacco Through Organizational Change (ATTOC), 519, 520
Adenosine receptors, caffeine in, 339–340
ADH. *See* Alcohol dehydrogenase (ADH)
ADHD. *See* Attention-deficit hyperactivity disorder (ADHD)
Adherence, 664
Adkins Life Skills Program: Career Development Series, 780
Administrative law judge (ALJ), 916–917
Adolescence, and substance abuse risk, 744–745
Adolescent Alcohol and Drug Involvement Scale (AADIS), 791
Adolescent Community Reinforcement Approach (ACRA), 792
Adolescents
 buprenorphine for, 443–444
 Internet addiction in, 409
 motivational interviewing in, 627
 and SHG, 528

1051

Adolescent substance abuse, 786–796
　assessment of, 790–792
　comorbidity of, 788–790
　　attention-deficit hyperactivity disorder, 789
　　conduct disorder, 789
　　depressive disorders, 789–790
　　posttraumatic stress disorder, 790
　　psychotic and bipolar disorders, 790
　development and course of, 787–788
　Dutch, 1038
　epidemiology, 786–787
　peer influence and, 787
　prevalence of, 786–787
　protective factors, 787–788
　risk factors, 787
　screening, 790–792
　treatment of, 792–796, 977
　　aftercare, 794
　　outcome parameters, 793–794
　　pharmacotherapy, 794–796
　　psychosocial, 792–793
The Adonis Complex, 358–359
Adoption of a Federal Antimaintenance Policy, 5
Adoption studies
　alcoholism, 37
　tobacco dependence, 42–43
Adrenoleukodystrophy (ALD), 295
Advance Practice Nurses (APNs), 981
Afghanistan, 1041
African Americans (AA), 147, 813–817
　epidemiology, 814
　medical comorbidity, 815–817
　　HIV infection, 815
　　mental illness, 815–816
　overview, 813
　prevention, 814, 816
　risk factors, 814
　social consequences, 814–815
　sociocultural factors, 813
　treatment of, 816–817
2-AG. See 2-arachidonoylglycerol (2-AG)
Aggression, 82–83
Aging. See also Older adults
　with drug abuse, 804–805
　HIV and, 807–808
Agonist–antagonist drugs, 707. See also Opioid(s)
β–Agonists, for asthma, 367
Agoraphobia, 914
AI. See American Indians
AIDS. See Acquired immune deficiency syndrome (AIDS)
AIR dusters, 287
Air Force Alcohol Drug Abuse Prevention and Treatment (ADAPT) program, 933
Alanine aminotransferase (ALT), 126
Alaska Natives
　HIV/AIDS risk among, 843
　overuse of alcohol among, 837
　risk factors for smoking among, 844
　substance abuse problems among. See Substance abuse, among AI/ANs
　traumatic loss in, 843
Alcohol
　cancer and, 668
　cardiovascular disease and, 667
　consumption, determinants of, 143–148
　consumption, epidemiology of, 139–141
　　international drinking patterns, 139–140
　　prevalence of alcohol use problems, 140–141
　　in United States, 140
　current use, 19–20
　drug interactions between
　　benzodiazepines and, 737
　　bupropion and, 738
　　cocaine and, 738
　　methadone and, 738
　　methylphenidate and, 738

　effects on neurotransmission, 144–146
　　cholinergic system, 146
　　dopaminergic system, 145
　　GABAergic system, 145
　　glutamatergic system, 145
　　opioidergic system, 145–146
　　serotonergic system, 146
　history of, 138–139
　　American continent, 139
　　ancient eastern world, 138
　　era of distilled spirits, 139
　　Hellenic world, 138–139
　　prehistoric times, 138
　　Roman world, 138–139
　　temperance movement, 139
　HIV infections and, 682
　induced cognitive disorders, 157–158
　induced mood and anxiety disorders, 158
　induced sleep disorders, 158
　intoxication, 157
　low level of response to, 39
　nicotine and, 330
　overview, 138
　pharmacology of, 143–144
　　absorption of, 143
　　distribution of, 143
　　elimination of, 144
　　metabolism of, 144
　during pregnancy, information for clinicians, 651–652
　prenatal exposure on neonate, 651
　treatment demand for, 27
　in twins, 338
　usage among armed force personnel, 926
　use and development of alcohol dependence, 39
　use in older adults, 806
　withdrawal, 157
Alcohol, Drug Abuse, and Mental Health Administration (ADAMHA), 268
Alcohol, Smoking and Substance Involvement Screening Test (ASSIST), 809
Alcohol abuse, 126
　African Americans. See African Americans (AA)
　Hispanic Americans, 822
　motivational interviewing in, 625–626
　treatment of
　　social workers and, 965–966
Alcohol and Drug Education for Physician Training in primary care (ADEPT), 939
Alcohol and the Prohibition Movement, 1
Alcohol biomarkers, 126
Alcohol consumption
　comorbidity with
　　antisocial personality disorder (ASPD), 157
　　anxiety disorders, 157
　　mood disorders, 157
　　other psychiatric disorders, 156–157
　　other substance use disorders, 157
　complications of, 156–159
　in pregnancy screening for, 651–652
　psychiatric complications of, 157–158
Alcohol deglamorization campaigns, 933
Alcohol dehydrogenase (ADH), 40, 144, 832
Alcohol dependence
　acamprosate for, 483–485
　acupuncture for, 472
　baclofen for, 488
　caffeine and, 348
　disulfiram for, 477–478
　dopamine for, 489
　early onset of alcohol use and development of, 39
　FDA-approved pharmacotherapies for, 479t
　genetics of, 146–148
　　acetylcholine receptor genes, 148
　　ADH genes, 147
　　ALDH genes, 147
　　candidate gene studies, 147

　　GABAergic genes, 148
　　linkage studies, 147
　　opioidergic genes, 148
　　serotonergic genes, 148
　methadone and, 428
　naltrexone for
　　injectable, 482–483
　　oral, 478, 480–482, 480t
　non-FDA-approved pharmacotherapies for, 487t
　overview, 477
　serotonin reuptake inhibitors (SRI) for, 488–489
　topiramate for, 485–486, 488
　variables influencing of, 142
Alcohol disorders
　AA, 152–153
　acamprosate, 154–155
　alcohol breath test, 150–151
　baclofen, 155
　behavioral family therapy, 153
　blood alcohol level, 150–151
　CDT, 150
　cognitive-behavioral therapies, 152
　disulfiram, 155–156
　GGTP, 150
　laboratory tests, 150, 151
　liver function tests, 150
　MCV, 150
　miscellaneous laboratory tests, 151
　naltrexone, 153–154
　pharmacotherapy of anxious alcoholics, 156
　physical examination of, 149
　serotonergic medications of, 155
　topiramate, 154
　treatment, 151–152
　　of alcohol withdrawal, 152
　　settings in, 151
Alcoholic liver disease, 669–670
Alcoholic pancreatitis, 669
Alcoholic Rehabilitation Act, 971
Alcoholics Anonymous (AA), 152–153, 523, 922, 938, 945, 949
　group therapy management and, 581–582
　in network therapy, 554, 560
Alcoholics Anonymous recovery program, 778
Alcohol-induced mood disorder, 910
Alcoholism, 937
　ADH and ALDH, 40
　adoption studies, 37
　clinical and etiologic heterogeneity, 37–38
　comorbidity, 38
　deaths attributable to, 838
　dopaminergic system, 40–41
　electrophysiologic markers, 39
　family studies, 36
　GABA, 41
　GABAergic system, 41
　gender and epidemiology, 852
　gene, 41
　genetically mediated markers of, 37–38
　genetic contribution to development of, 832
　genetic influences in, 36–41
　intermediate phenotypes, 38
　issues among AI/ANs, 838
　molecular genetic studies, 40
　opioidergic system, 41
　pharmacotherapy of, 153–156
　psychosocial treatment of, 152–153
　serotonergic system, 41
　subjective and behavioral effects in women, 848
　subtypes, 38, 142–143
　telescoping effect, 852
　treatment for, 852
　triggers for, 852
　twin studies, 37
Alcoholism and Addiction (AAPAA), 939
Alcoholism (male-limited), 38
Alcohol Problems: A Report to the Nation, 938

Alcohol prohibition, 1037–1038
Alcohol-related birth defects (ARBD), 651
Alcohol-related neurodevelopmental disorder (ARND), 651
Alcohol use
  by AA/PIs, 829–830
  classification of, 141
  DSM-IV-TR criteria for, 142t
  morbidity and mortality associated with, 158–159
  phenomenologic presentation of, 141–142
  in pregnancy, 858
  prevalence in United States, 140–141
  psychiatric complications of, 157–158
Alcohol Use Disorder and Associated Disabilities Interview Schedule—Alcohol/Drug-Revised (AUDADIS-ADR), 102
Alcohol use disorders
  gender difference in prevalence of, 847
  naltrexone for, 448, 450–453
    clinical trials, 450–451
    doses and routes of administration, 452
    laboratory studies for, 451–452
    with other medications/ therapies, 452
Alcohol Use Disorders Identification Test (AUDIT), 149
Alcohol use relapse
  factors associated with, 838–839
ALD. See Adrenoleukodystrophy (ALD)
Aldehyde dehydrogenase (ALDH), 40, 144
Aldehyde dehydrogenase (ALDH2) deficiency and alcoholism, link between, 832
ALDH. See Acetaldehyde dehydrogenase (ALDH); Aldehyde dehydrogenase (ALDH)
Allodynia, 698
Allostasis, in ED
  genetic vulnerability for, 378
  model of, 377
Allostatic load, defined, 377
Allostatic state, defined, 377
Alpha-amino-3-hydroxy- 5-methylisoxazole-4-propionic acid (AMPA) receptors, 243
Alpha-methylfentanyl, 280
Alprazolam, 259, 260, 658, 659, 690, 727, 737, 993
ALT. See Alanine aminotransferase (ALT)
Alternative support groups, 523–524, 533–541
  considerations, 540–541
  contact information, 534b
  evidence of efficacy, 539, 540
  history, 533–534
  LifeRing, 538–539, 539b
  MM, 536–537, 537b
  SMART, 537, 538, 538b
  SOS, 535–536, 536b
  WFS, 534–535, 535b
Alzado, Lyle, 365–366
Amenorrhea, methadone side-effects, 427
American Academy of Addiction Psychiatry (AAAP), 939
The American Academy of Anti-Aging Medicine, 359
American Academy of Pain Medicine (AAPM), 700
American Association of Poison Control Centers, 287
American Board of Addiction Medicine (ABAM), 940
American Board of Psychiatry and Neurology (ABPN), 939, 943
American College of Obstetricians and Gynecologists (ACOG), 651
American College of Sports Medicine, 355
American Disabilities Act (ADA), 908
American Indians
  bicultural competence among, 840
  HIV/AIDS risk among, 843
  overuse of alcohol among, 837
  risk factors for smoking among, 844

substance abuse problems among. See Substance abuse, among AI/ANs
  traumatic loss in, 843
American Medical Association (AMA), AAS and, 356
American Medical Society on Alcoholism (AMSA), 938
American Nurses Association, 981
American Pain Society (APS), 699
American Psychiatric Association (APA), 307
American Psychological Association (APA), 979
American Society of Addiction Medicine (ASAM), 114, 202, 700, 939
American Society of Addiction Medicine Patient Placement Criteria (ASAM-PPC), 792
Americans with Disabilities Act (ADA), 784
Amino-3-hydroxy-5-methyl-4-isoxazole (AMPA), 259
AMPA. See Alpha-amino-3-hydroxy-5-methylisoxazole-4-propionic acid (AMPA) receptors; Amino-3-hydroxy-5-methyl-4-isoxazole (AMPA)
Amphetamine dependence
  preclinical investigations of potential treatments for, 242t
  randomized controlled clinical trials of, 248t
Amphetamines, 736
  acetylcholinergic receptor in, 244
  in adrenergic system, 243
  agonist pharmacotherapy, 247
  antidepressants for, 245–246
  antipsychotics, 246
  behavioral interventions for, 245
  calcium channel blockers, 246–247
  current use, 22
  defined, 238
  determinants of use, 241–245
    pharmacology of, 241
    physiology of, 244–245
    preclinical target systems, 241–244
  dopaminergic system, 241
  endocannabinoid system in, 244
  epidemiology of, 240–241
  evaluation and treatment approaches for, 245
  GABA enhancers in, 246
  in GABA receptors, 241, 243
  genetic mechanisms, in animal, 247
  in glutamatergic drugs, 243
  history of, 238–240
  human gene polymorphisms, 247, 249
  as medications, 245
  on military performance, 239
  nitric oxide in, 244
  in opioid, 244
  performance maintenance in, 239
  pharmacotherapy of, 245
  during pregnancy, information for clinicians, 656
  prenatal exposure on fetus and neonate, 655–656
  in psychosis, 240
  serotonergic system, 243
  stimulant-like medication, 247
  treatment demand for, 28
  used by athletes, 239
Amphetamines dependence
  methadone and, 428–429
Amphetamine-type stimulants (ATS), 238
Amphetamine use disorders (AUD), 240
Amphetamine users
  motivational interviewing in, 626
Anabolic-androgenic steroids (AAS) use, 354–370
  complications of, 362–365, 364f
  designer, 361–362
  epidemiology of, 356–357, 357f, 358t
  ethics of, 367–368
  by high school students, 356–357, 357f
  history of, 354–356, 355f
  indications for, 358–360

legal issues in, 368–369
metabolism, 360–361, 361f
psychiatric complications of, 365–366, 365f
related dietary supplements, 360
sex-specific effects of, 363–364, 364f
substances used concomitantly with, 366–367
testing for, 369
therapeutic use exemptions, 368
treatment of, 369–370
widely available, 358t
withdrawal, symptoms of, 365–366, 365f
Anabolic Steroids Control Act, 355
Analgesia, acupuncture as, 466–467
Analgesic pharmacodynamic tolerance, 698–699
ANCB. See Addictions Nursing Certification Board (ANCB)
AND. See Associate's degree in nursing (AND)
Androstenedione, 360
Anhalonium lewinii, 270
Animal experiment, of acupuncture
  physical dependence, 468–469
  psychic dependence, 469
Animal models, effect of DHEA on, 847–848
Anorexia in reverse, 358–359
Anorexia nervosa (AN), 373, 374t
  naltrexone in, 454
ANs. See Alaska Natives
Antabuse, 120, 155, 737, 923. See also Disulfiram
β-Antagonist timolol, 243
"Antiaging" clinics, 359
  Internet advertisement for, 359
Antiandrogenic agents, for criminal paraphiliacs, 404
Antibiotics
  interactions with methadone/buprenorphine, 734t, 735
Antibodies, vaccines and
  binding
    affinity, 458, 458f
    to antigen, 457
    to block uptake, 458
    mass action equilibrium, 457–458
    to small molecule, 457
  cocaine, 461–462
  heroin, 463–464
  methamphetamine, 462–463
  morphine, 463–464
  nicotine, 460–461
  and pharmacodynamics, 459
  and pharmacokinetics, 459
  phencyclidine, 462
Anti-craving medications, in co-occurring disorders, 727–728
Antidepressants, 245–246
  co-occurring disorders and, 726–728
  with mild stimulant, 246
  pharmacotherapies for amphetamine, 245–246
  in sex addiction, 400
Antidoping programs, defined, 367
Antihistamines, 427
Antiretroviral (ARV) medications
  interactions with opioids, 732–734, 732t
Antisocial behavior disorder with alcohol abuse, 38
Antisocial personality disorder (ASPD), 142
  with alcoholism, 38
Antivirals
  interactions with methadone/buprenorphine, 734, 734t
Anxiety, 909, 915–916
  caffeine and, 339, 341, 342, 346–347
  in HIV infection, 690–691
Anxiety disorders, 81
  gender differences in response to psychotherapeutic treatment for, 849–850
  prevalence among women, 849
  treatment of, 727
Anxious alcoholics, pharmacotherapy of, 156

APA. *See* American Psychiatric Association (APA); American Psychological Association (APA)
APNs. *See* Advance Practice Nurses (APNs)
Apollo, 38
APS. *See* American Pain Society (APS)
APS-AAPM Clinical Guidelines for the Use of Chronic Opioid Therapy, 914
2-Arachidonoylglycerol (2-AG), 219
2-Arachidonylglycerylether, 219
ARBD. *See* Alcohol-related birth defects (ARBD)
ARC. *See* Addiction Research Center (ARC)
ARCG-MBG. *See* Addiction Research Center Inventory-Morphine Benzedrine Group subscale (ARCG-MBG)
ARCI. *See* Addiction Research Center Inventory (ARCI)
Armed force
  alcohol abuse of, 926
  characteristics of substance users, 929–930
  comparison with civilians, 930–932
  comprehensive health behavior surveys among, 927–928
  cultural factors influencing substance use among, 934
  development of DoD policy on substance use and abuse, 927
  drug detection dogs, 933
  drug-testing program, 933
  environmental factors influencing substance use among, 934–935
  factors influencing substance use among, 934–935
  illicit drug use in, 926
  intervention and treatment of substance use, 933–934
  outpatient services, 933
  prevention of substance use, 933
  social factors influencing substance use among, 934
  sociodemographic characteristics, 928
  substance use and military readiness, 926
  tobacco use in, 926
  trends in substance use, 928–929
ARND. *See* Alcohol-related neurodevelopmental disorder (ARND)
ARV medications. *See* Antiretroviral (ARV) medications
"5 A's," for brief intervention, 328–329, 329t
ASAM. *See* American Society of Addiction Medicine (ASAM)
ASAM-PPC. *See* American Society of Addiction Medicine Patient Placement Criteria (ASAM-PPC)
ASI. *See* Addiction severity index (ASI)
Asian Americans
  ethnicity, 829
  population of, 829
  substance use issues among. *See* Substance abuse, among AA/PIs
Asian–Pacific Islanders, 918
ASPD. *See* Antisocial personality disorder (ASPD)
Assertive continuing care (ACC), 223
  in adolescents with SUD, 794
Assertiveness, 568
ASSIST. *See* Alcohol, Smoking and Substance Involvement Screening Test (ASSIST)
Associate's degree in nursing (AND), 981
Association for Medical Education and Research in Substance Abuse (AMERSA), 938, 939, 941
Association of American Medical Colleges (AAMC), 941
Association of Psychology Postdoctoral and Internship Centers (APPIC), 950
Atazanavir, 733–734
Athletes, AAS use by
  background of, 354–356, 355f

Ativan. *See* Lorazepam
ATS. *See* Amphetamine-type stimulants (ATS)
ATTC *See* Addiction Technology Transfer Centers (ATTC)
Attention-deficit hyperactivity disorder (ADHD), 82, 195, 238
  with adolescent SUD, 789
  and Internet usage, 415
  nicotine dependence in, 330
ATTOC. *See* Addressing Tobacco Through Organizational Change (ATTOC)
AUD. *See* Amphetamine use disorders (AUD)
AUDADIS-ADR. *See* Alcohol Use Disorder and Associated Disabilities Interview Schedule—Alcohol/Drug- Revised (AUDADIS-ADR)
AUDIT. *See* Alcohol Use Disorders Identification Test (AUDIT)
Automobile accidents
  cell phone use and, 413–414
AZT. *See* Zidovudine (AZT)

Bacchus, 38
Bachelor's degree in social work (BSW), 966
Bachelor's degree programs in nursing (BSN), 981
Baclofen, 145, 243, 246, 487, 709, 853
  for alcohol dependence, 488
  in alcohol disorders, 155
Bad trip, 272
BAER. *See* Brainstem auditory-evoked responses (BAER)
Bailey, Margaret, 965
BAL. *See* Blood Alcohol Level (BAL); British anti-Lewisite (BAL)
Baltimore Buprenorphine Initiative, 961
Barbiturates
  determinants of abuse, 263
  effects on $GABA_A$ receptors, 263
  overview, 262–263
  pharmacology of, 263
  toxicities of, 257
  for treatment of insomnia, 262
Barbituric acid, 262
Barriers to Employment Success Inventory, 779
BATF. *See* Bureau of Alcohol, Tobacco, and Firearms (BATF)
BCT. *See* Behavioral couple therapy (BCT)
BD. *See* Bipolar disorders (BD)
BDNF. *See* Brain- derived neurotrophic factor (BDNF)
Beard and Wolf's diagnostic criteria, for Internet addiction, 410t
BED. *See* Binge-eating disorder (BED)
Behavior, 88–97
Behavioral couple therapy (BCT), 588, 858
Behavioral family therapy, 792
  in alcohol disorders, 153
Behavioral model
  for family/couples therapy, 586
Behavioral patterns, sexual
  types of, 395–397, 396t
Behavioral pharmacology, 164–165
Behavioral Pharmacology Research Unit (BPRU), 165
Behavioral principles
  voucher-based contingency management, 603–604
Behavioral research, on human opioid use ARC, 164
  behavioral pharmacology, 164–165
  ethnography of, 165–166
  sociology of, 165–166
Behavioral Risk Factor Surveillance System (BRFSS), 17
Bell, Chris, 366
Belle de Jour, 397

Bennett Mechanical Comprehension Test, 779
Benoit, Chris, 365
Benzene, 306
Benzodiazepines (BZD), 255, 721, 914
  behavioral effects of, 259
  biotransformation in, 260
  determinants of abuse, 259–260
  drug interactions between
    alcohol and, 737
    opioids and, 735
  pharmacology of, 258–259
  during pregnancy, information for clinicians, 659
  prenatal exposure on fetus and neonate, 658–659
  toxicities of, 257
Benzodiazepines (BZD) dependence
  caffeine and, 348
  methadone and, 428
Benzodiazepines (BZD) discontinuation
  history of, 501
  minimal intervention programs for, 502
  overview, 501
  systematic discontinuation programs for, 502–505
    outcome determinants, 507
    pharmacotherapy for, 505–506, 505t
    psychotherapy for, 506
    treatment settings, 507–508
Benzoylecgonine, 130, 196, 459
Bereavement, 923
Beta-endorphin, 45
Betel nut chewing, 918
Binge-eating disorder (BED), 373, 374t
  naltrexone in, 454
  substance use and, 376
Bipolar disorders (BD)
  with adolescent SUD, 790
  in HIV infection, 683
Bipolar illness, 80
Birth defects
  in buprenorphine-treated women, 444
Bisexuality, 872–873
β–blockers, for hypertension, 367
Blood alcohol concentrations (BAC), 40
Blood alcohol level (BAL), 151
Blood pressure, caffeine-associated. *See* Hypertension
Body acupuncture, 466
  vs. ear acupuncture, 473
Body building products, AAS in, 360–361
Body fluids, choice of, 130–131
Boot camp programs, 885
Boston Medical Center model, 962
Boston Medical Center treatment model, 962
Boston Tea Party, 335
BPRU. *See* Behavioral Pharmacology Research Unit (BPRU)
Brain damage, 920
Brain- derived neurotrophic factor (BDNF), 249
Brainstem auditory-evoked responses (BAER), 301
Breadth
  clinical assessment, 111
Breakthrough pain, 697. *See also* Pain
Breast-feeding
  buprenorphine and, 654
  mother on, 444
  cocaine and, 655
BRFSS. *See* Behavioral Risk Factor Surveillance System (BRFSS)
Brief negotiation interview (BNI), 945
Brief strategic family therapy (BSFT), 222, 588, 792
British anti-Lewisite (BAL), 303
British Journal of Sexual Addiction, 393
Bromo-LSD, 271
Brown, Barry, 971
BSFT. *See* Brief strategic family therapy (BSFT)
BSN. *See* Bachelor's degree programs in nursing (BSN)

BSW. *See* Bachelor's degree in social work (BSW)
Bulimia nervosa (BN), 373, 374*t*
   naltrexone in, 454
Bupivacaine, 709
Buprenorphine, 1046, 1047
   drug interactions between
      antivirals/antibiotics and, 734–735, 734*t*
   interactions with
      HIV medications and, 732*t*, 733–734
   misuse, 32–33
   in network therapy, 558
   opioid-agonist therapy with, 718
   for opioid dependence, 731
      adolescents, 794–795
      during pregnancy, 654
Buprenorphine, for opioid-withdrawal syndrome
   clonidine *vs.*, 496
   lofexidine and, 495–496
Buprenorphine, in opioid dependence, 437–444
   for adolescents, 443–444
   birth defects and, 444
   doses, 439
   efficacy of, 439
   history of, 437–438
   legal issues, 440–442, 441*t*
      restrictions on, 442, 442*f*
   morphine *vs.*, 438–439
   NAS with, 444
   optimal use of, 439–440
      induction, 439–440
      stabilization, 440
      withdrawal, 440
   pharmacodynamics, 438–439
   pharmacokinetics, 438
   side effects from, 442–443
      cardiac arrhythmias, 443
      cognitive and psychomotor effects of, 442–443
      diversion of, 443
      hepatitis, 443
      respiratory depression, 442
   for special populations, 443–444
Buprenorphine maintenance, 181
Buprenorphine treatment, 961–962
Bupropion
   drug interactions between
      alcohol and, 738
   for smoking cessation, 323, 328
Bupropion SR, 323, 326, 328, 517
Bureau of Alcohol, Tobacco, and Firearms (BATF), 268
Bureau of Labor Statistics, 965
Bureau of Narcotics and Dangerous Drugs (BNDD), 9
Bureau of Substance Abuse Services in Massachusetts, 961
Butane gas, 299
   inhalation of, 287
Butorphanol, 707
BZD. *See* Benzodiazepines (BZD)

CADC certification. *See* Certified Alcohol and Drug Abuse Counselor (CADC) certification
Caffeine (1,3,7-trimethylxanthine)
   and alcohol dependence, 348
   annual per capita consumption, 338, 338*f*
   and anxiety, 346–347
   benzodiazepines dependence and, 348
   cocaine use and, 349
   dependence, 347–348, 347*t*
   epidemiology, 337–338
   genetic factors in, 338–339
   and health, 340–341
   history, 335
   intoxication, 345–346, 346*t*
   neuropharmacology, 339–340
      adenosine, 339–340
      dopamine, 340
   and nicotine and cigarette smoking, 348–349
   on performance, 342
   pharmacokinetics, 339
   physical dependence and withdrawal, 344–345, 344*t*
   physiological effects, 340
   reduction/elimination of, 349, 350*t*
   reinforcing effects of, 343
   and sleep, 342–343
   sources of, 335–337, 336*t*–337*t*
   subjective and discriminative stimulus effects, 341–342
   therapeutic uses, 340
   tolerance, 343–344
   withdrawal, 344–345, 344*t*, 349, 350*t*
Caffeine withdrawal syndrome, 344–345, 344*t*
   clinical implications, 349
   treatment, 349, 350*t*
CAGE-AID. *See* Cut Down, Annoyed, Guilty, Eye-Opener Tool, Adjusted to Include Drugs (CAGE-AID)
CAGE questionnaire, 944–945
Calcium balance, caffeine on, 341
Calcium channel blockers
   amphetamines, 246–247
California Society for the Treatment of Alcoholism and Other Drug Dependencies (CSTAODD), 939
Caminiti, Ken, 356
Campbell Collaboration, 968
Campral, 479. *See also* Acamprosate
Canada, 1040
   medical marijuana in, 769
Cancer
   alcohol and, 668
   tobacco and, 668
   viral causes of, 669
Candidate genes, 80
Candidate mediators, of PG, 387–388
Cannabinoid (CB) receptors, 46
Cannabinoid–dopamine interactions, 62–63
Cannabinoid receptor (CB-1), 207, 228
Cannabinoids, 46, 62–63
   and ethanol self-administration, 61–62
   genetic influences in, 46
   mechanisms of action, 62
   and nicotine self-administration, 65
   and opiate self-administration, 59–60
   self-administration, 63
Cannabis, 2. *See also* Marijuana
   abrupt cessation of, 218
   acute effects on psychomotor performance, 230
   administration of, 217–218
   cardiovascular disease and, 667
   chronic use of, 231
   cognitive functions of, 230
   comorbidity of, 225–228
   cultivation of, 217
   defined, 214
   determinants of use, 218–220
      environmental factors, 220
      genetics of, 219–220
      neurobiology of, 219
      pharmacological constituents of, 218–219
   epidemiology, 215–217
   evaluation of
      assessment tools for, 220–221
      screening tools for, 220–221
   functional significance of, 231–232
   history of, 214–215
   induced psychotic disorder, 790
   motivation of, 232–233
   nonpsychiatric health effects of, 228–233
      brain function and cognitive performance, 230–233
      in cancer, 229
      in cardiovascular system, 230
      in immune system, 229
      perinatal effects of, 229–230
      in reproductive system, 229–230
      in respiratory system, 228–229
   permanent or temporary deficits, 231
   pharmacotherapy for, 224–225
   phenomenology of, 217–218
   during pregnancy, 229
   psychosocial treatment approaches, 221–224
      interventions for adolescents, 222–224
      interventions for adults, 221–222
   secondary prevention of, 224
   treatment demand for, 27–28
   withdrawal: signs and symptoms, 218*t*
Cannabis abuse
   effective treatments for, 223
   motivational interviewing in, 626–627
Cannabis dependence
   methadone and, 429
Cannabis Expiation Notice system, 767
Cannabis sativa, 214
Cannabis use
   and course of psychiatric disorder, 228
   prevalence of, 215–216
Cannabis use disorders (CUD), 214
   comorbidity of, 225–228
      casuality effect of, 226–227
      drug use disorders, 225–226
      gateway effect of, 226–227
      psychiatric disorders of, 227–228
   increase in treatment admissions for, 216–217, 217*f*
   pharmacotherapy for, 224–225
      clinical trials of, 225
      laboratory analog studies, 224–225
   prevalence of, 216–217
      conditional dependence in, 216
      increase in, 216
      increase in treatment admissions for CUD, 216–217
Cannabis Youth Treatment (CYT) study, 226, 793
Canseco, Jose, 356
CAPS. *See* Career Ability Placement Survey (CAPS)
Carbamazepine, 727
Carbohydrate Deficient Transferring (CDT), 126, 150
Carboxyhemoglobin (COHb), 228
Cardiac arrests
   gambling problems and, 387
Cardiac arrhythmias, side-effects of AAS, 362
Cardiac death, side-effects of AAS, 362
Cardiotoxicity, 306
Cardiovascular disease
   alcohol and, 667
   cannabis and, 667
   cocaine, stimulants, MDMA and, 667
   opioid and, 667
   tobacco and, 666–667
Career Ability Placement Survey (CAPS), 779
Career Occupational Preference System (COPS), 779
Career Orientation Placement and Evaluation Survey (COPES), 779
Career Teacher Program in the Addictions, 938, 943–944
CareerZone, 779
CARN Examination Manual, 960
CARNs. *See* Certification for addictions Registered Nurses (CARNs)
CART. *See* Combination antiretroviral therapy (CART)
CASAC. *See* Credentialed Alcoholism and Substance Abuse Counselor certification (CASAC)
Casein kinase 1 epsilon gene (Csnk1e), 247

Case Presentation Method (CPM), 972
Casino gambling, plasma concentrations of cortisol in, 389
Catechol-*O*-methyl transferase (COMT) gene, 249
Catlin, Don, 361–362
CATOR. *See* Comprehensive Assessment and Treatment Outcome Research (CATOR)
"Causal" etiology hypotheses, for ED and SUD, 376
CB-1. *See* Cannabinoid receptor (CB-1)
CBI. *See* Combined behavioral intervention (CBI)
CB1 receptors, 46, 219
CB2 receptors, 46
CBT. *See* Cognitive-behavioral therapy (CBT)
CC. *See* Continuing care (CC)
C-CATODSW. *See* Certified Clinical Alcohol, Tobacco, and Other Drugs Social Worker (C-CATODSW)
CD. *See* Conduct disorder (CD)
CDC. *See* Centers for Disease Control and Prevention (CDC)
CDSA. *See* Controlled Drugs and Substances Act (CDSA)
CDT. *See* Carbohydrate Deficient Transferring (CDT)
Ceiling effect, 731
Cell phone
 use while driving, 413–414
Cellulitis, 675
Centaur, 397
Center for Addiction Research and Education (CARE), 939–940
Center for Substance Abuse Treatment (CSAT), 179, 562, 725, 972, 983
Centers for Disease Control and Prevention (CDC), 17, 177, 682
Central nervous system (CNS), 238
Central nervous system (CNS) infection
 HIV infections and, 684–691
  myopathy, 685
  neurological complications management, secondary, 685–686, 685t
  neuropsychiatric disorders, treatment of, 687–691
  peripheral nervous system pathology, 685
Cerebrospinal fluid (CSF) studies
 HIV-1 infection and, 686–687
Certificate of Proficiency, 953, 980
Certificate of Qualification in Social Work (CQSW), 983
Certification for addictions Registered Nurses (CARNs), 981
Certification in addictions nursing, 959–960
Certified Addictions Registered Nurse—Advanced Practice (CARN-AP), 959–960
Certified Addictions Registered Nurse (CARN), 959
Certified Alcohol and Drug Abuse Counselor (CADC) certification, 985
Certified Clinical Alcohol, Tobacco, and Other Drugs Social Worker (C-CATODSW), 969
CEU. *See* Continued Education Unit (CEU)
CEWG. *See* Community Epidemiology Work Group (CEWG)
CGMP. *See* Cyclic glucose monophosphate (cGMP)
Chantix. *See* Varenicline
Charity Organization Societies (COS), 965
Chewing gum, in NRT, 323
Child abuse, sex addiction and, 395
Childhood adversities, 83–84
Childhood trauma, sex addiction and, 395
Children
 AAS-related mood perturbations in, 365
 Internet addiction in, 409
China, 1041
 harm reduction in, 768b
China White, 280
Chlamydia trachomatis, 674

Chlordiazepoxide, 152, 255, 259, 260, 501, 658, 659
Chlorohydrocarbons, 300, 305
Chlorpromazine, 89, 273, 687, 738
 for AN, 379
Christopher, Jim, 535
Chronic inhalation abuse, 295
Chronic obstructive pulmonary disease (COPD), 228
Chronic pain
 acute pain *vs.*, 696–697
 defined, 697
 overview, 695
Chronic pain syndrome, 698
CIDI-SAM. *See* Composite International Diagnostic Interview–Substance Abuse Module (CIDI-SAM)
Cigarette smoking
 caffeine and, 348–349
 drug interactions of, 738–739
 in twins, 338
Cigarette use, defined, 928
Cipro. *See* Ciprofloxacin
Ciprofloxacin, 674, 676, 735
Cirrhosis of the liver, 1037
CIWA scale. *See* Clinical Institute Withdrawal Assessment (CIWA) scale
Classical conditioning
 addiction stimuli and, 593
 in cognitive behavioral therapy, 594
Clinical assessment
 characteristic of good
  cross-checks of self-report, 111
  patient involvement in identifying problems, 111
  treatment plan information, 110–111
 goals of, 107–110
  barriers to treatment, identification of, 109
  co-occurring problems, identification of, 108
  cover multiple domains, 108
  cultural sensitivity, 110
  evidence-based practice, 109
  involvement in other systems, identification of, 108–109
  monitoring change, 109
  sharable and usable, 108
  strength identification, 108
  validity and reliability, 109–110
 principles of, 107
 progressive approach to, 114–115
 report writing, 113–114
 for severity-based problem prioritization, 111–113
  recency, breadth, and prevalence assessment, 111
  treatment and problem history, 112–113, 113t
  use of scale scores, 111–112, 112f
 sources of
  clinical judgment, 107
  collateral reports, 107
  self-report, 107
Clinical drug testing, 132
Clinical Institute Withdrawal Assessment (CIWA) scale, 982
Clinical judgment, 107
Clinical Opioid Withdrawal Scale (COWS), 962
Clinical Practice Guideline on Treating Tobacco Use and Dependence, 322
Clinical psychologist, 979
Clinical training, 954
Clonazepam, 258, 260, 658
Clonidine, 180, 181, 224, 439, 449, 651–652, 709, 725, 832
 opioid-withdrawal syndrome, 494–495
 abuse, 495
 vs. buprenorphine, 496
 vs. lofexidine, 495

Cloninger's Tridimensional Personality Questionnaire (TPQ), 38
Clostridium tetani, 678
Club drugs
 current use, 21–22
CM. *See* Contingency management (CM)
CNR1 gene, 46
CNR2 gene, 46
CNS. *See* Central nervous system (CNS); Central nervous system (CNS) infection
Coca-Cola Company, 191, 991
Cocaethylene, 197, 208, 730–731
Cocaine, 130
 cardiovascular disease and, 667
 comorbidities and complications of, 207–211
  associated psychiatric disorders, 207–208
  cardiovascular system, 208–209
  in fetal development, 210–211
  impact on sexual function, 210
  medical complications, 208
  neuropathology, 209–210
  in pregnancy, 210–211
  pulmonary syndromes, 208–209
 current use, 21
 determinants of use, 196–200
  environmental features, 199–200
  neurobiology, 197–199, 198f
  pharmacologic considerations of, 196–197
  social features, 199–200
 drug interactions with, 736–737
  alcohol and, 738
 epidemiology of, 192–194
 evaluation and treatment approaches, 200–207
  agonist therapies, 205
  current treatment, 202–203
  future treatment, 202–203
  initial evaluation of, 200–202
  inpatient *vs.* outpatient care, 202
  management of, 200–202
  pharmacologic treatment, 203–205, 204t
  psychosocial treatments, 203
  reducing brain exposure to, 205
  relapse prevention, 205–207
 genetic factors, 45
 overview, 191
 phenomenology of, 194–195
 during pregnancy, information for clinicians, 655
 prenatal exposure on neonate, 654–655
 pulmonary complications of, 677
 reinforcement
  glutamate and, 57–58
  norepinephrine and, 57
  serotonin and, 57
 routes of administration, 196
 self-administration in DAT knockout mice, 57
 in smokable form, 197
 timeline of regular use in United States, 193f
 treatment demand for, 26–27, 28
 use
  in African Americans, 814
  in older adults, 804
Cocaine abuse
 comorbidities and complications of, 207–211
  associated psychiatric disorders, 207–208
  cardiovascular system, 208–209
  in fetal development, 210–211
  impact on sexual function, 210
  medical complications, 208
  neuropathology, 209–210
  in pregnancy, 210–211
  pulmonary syndromes, 208–209
 in United States, 192–193, 193f
Cocaine and drug intolerance, 10–11
Cocaine Anonymous (CA), 523
Cocaine—benzoylmethylecgonine, 196

Cocaine crash, 200
Cocaine dependence, 191, 197
  acupuncture for, 472–473
  caffeine and, 349
  clinical criteria for, 195t
  functional anatomy of, 198f
  methadone and, 428–429
  naltrexone in, 454
  pharmacologic treatment, 203–205, 204t
Cocaine hydrochloride, 10–11
Cocaine Selective Severity Assessment (CSSA), 201
Cocaine use
  in pregnancy, 859
Cocaine users
  motivational interviewing in, 626
Cocaine vaccines, 461–462
Coca leaves, 2, 191
  history of, 191–192
COCE. See Co-Occurring Center for Excellence (COCE)
Cochrane group, 206
COD. See Co-occurring disorders (COD)
Codeine, 2, 45, 707
  for opioid dependence, 496–497
Codependence, 586
COGA. See Collaborative Study on Genetics of Alcoholism (COGA)
Cognitive–behavioral interventions, 884–885
Cognitive–behavioral model of relapse, 638, 638f
  revised, 638–639, 639f
Cognitive-behavioral theory
  for Internet addiction, 412
Cognitive-behavioral therapy (CBT), 182, 380, 792, 923, 963, 975
  for alcohol disorders, 152–153
  for amphetamines, 245
  for cocaine treatment, 191
  for CUD, 221
  efficacy of, 596–597
  extrasession practice, 598–599
  features of, 594–596, 597
    common factors, 595
    durability, 594, 595f
    unique factors, 595
  history of, 593–594
  interventions of
    acceptable, 596
    essential and unique, 595
    prescribed, 596
    recommended, 595–596
  limitations of, 599–600
  network therapy technique, 552
  for paraphilias, 404
  for sex addiction, 400–401
  training and competence in, 599
  use, techniques and strategies of, 597–598
Cognitive distortions, with PG, 388
Cognitive impairment, 914
  HIV-1 infection and, 686
COHb. See Carboxyhemoglobin (COHb)
Collaborative Study on Genetics of Alcoholism (COGA), 147
Collateral reports, 107
College students
  substance abuse, 22
Combination antiretroviral therapy (CART), 683
  adherence to, 684
    HIV infections and, 684
Combined behavioral intervention (CBI)
  for alcohol use disorders, 451
Coming out, 873
Community education programs, 830
Community Epidemiology Work Group (CEWG), 17
Community method, 543. See also Therapeutic community

Community reinforcement, network therapy technique, 552
Community Reinforcement and Family Training (CRAFT), 552, 587
Community Reinforcement Approach (CRA), 587
Comorbidity
  conceptual issues and confounding factors in assessing, 375–376
  definition of, 375
  of ED and SUD, 375
    assessment of patients and, 378–379
    elements of treatment integration, 379
    hypotheses for, 376–378
    treatment delivery for, 379
  nicotine and psychiatric, 329–330
  substance abuse, 19
Competence
  enhancement of school-based programs, 747t, 750–751
Composite International Diagnostic Interview–Substance Abuse Module (CIDI-SAM), 349
Comprehensive Assessment and Treatment Outcome Research (CATOR), 634
Comprehensive Drug Abuse Prevention and Control Act of 1970, 9, 268
Comprehensive Textbook of Psychiatry, 192
"Compulsive gambling," 384
Compulsive Internet use. See Internet addiction
Computed tomography (CT)
  for inhalent toxicity, 293
COMT. See Catechol-O-methyl transferase (COMT) gene
Concerta. See Methylphenidate
Conditioned place preference (CPP), 297
Conduct disorder (CD)
  with adolescent SUD, 789
Consequentialist philosophies, 1035
Consortium of Behavioral Health Nurses Association, 959
Constipation, methadone side-effects, 426
Constituent-involving strategies, 104
Consultative exam (CE), 916
Contingency, reinforcement, 88
  parameters of, 90–91
Contingency management (CM)
  for amphetamines, 245
  for CUD, 221
  principles of, 603
  voucher-based, 603–619. See also Voucher-based contingency management
Continued Education Unit (CEU), 985
Continuing care (CC)
  in adolescents with SUD, 794
Continuing care groups, 579–580
Continuing medical education, 945–946
Controlled Drugs and Substances Act (CDSA), 769
Controlled Substances Act (CSA), 713, 714
  key elements of, 714
Controlled Substances Analogues Enforcement Act, 1986, 280
"Convergence hypothesis," 852
Co-Occurring Center for Excellence (COCE), 721
Co-occurring disorders (COD), 178, 721–728
  defined, 722
  epidemiology of, 523t, 722, 722t
  history of, 721–722
  patient evaluation with, 723–725, 724t
  tobacco use in, 728
  treatment of, 725–728
    antidepressants, 726–728
    cost of, 722, 722t
    depression, 726–728
    disulfiram and anti-craving medications, 727–728

    mood stabilizers, 726–728
    psychotropic medications use, 726, 726t
    quadrant model, 725, 726f
Co-occurring psychiatric disorders
  eating disorders, 850
  mood and anxiety disorders, 849–850
  personality disorders, 851–852
  posttraumatic stress disorder, 850–851
COPD. See Chronic obstructive pulmonary disease (COPD)
COPES. See Career Orientation Placement and Evaluation Survey (COPES)
Coping, 99–100, 637
Coping skills, and SHG, 529–530
COPS. See Career Occupational Preference System (COPS)
Corticotropin-releasing factor (CRF), 210, 219, 377
  cannabinoid interactions, 63
Cortisol, plasma concentrations of
  in casino gambling, 389
COS. See Charity Organization Societies (COS)
Costs
  caused by addiction, 1034
  caused by drug policy, 1034–1035
Council on Social Work Education (CSWE), 966
Counseling
  psychologist, 979
  vocational rehabilitation, 780–781
Counselors
  addiction
    certification issue, 974–975
    history, 971–974, 972t–974t
    licensure issue, 974–975
    training and education, 971–977
  competencies required for, 562
  defined, 984
  education and training, 985
  Evaluation of Competency and Ethical Conduct, 984
  licensed professional, 983
  OASAS-CASAC credentialing, 984
  role and scope of practice, 985
  specialty treatment program and, 562–563
  vs. therapists, 562
  work experience, 984–985
Couple therapy. See also Family/couples therapy
  in sex addiction, 402
CPM. See Case Presentation Method (CPM)
CPP. See Conditioned place preference (CPP)
CQSW. See Certificate of Qualification in Social Work (CQSW)
CRA. See Community Reinforcement Approach (CRA)
Crack
  babies, 210
  from coca leaves to, history of, 191–192
  current use, 21
  treatment demand for, 28
Crack lung syndrome, 209
CRAFFT, 791
CRAFT. See Community Reinforcement and Family Training (CRAFT)
C-rations, 926
Cravings, 637
  acupuncture for, 471
  management, 640–641, 642f
Credentialed Alcoholism and Substance Abuse Counselor certification (CASAC), 984
CREST. See National Institute of Drug Abuse's Cocaine Rapid Efficacy Screening Trial (CREST)
CRF. See Corticotropin-releasing factor (CRF)
Crime
  drug-related, 33–34
Criminal justice system
  drug users and drug-related offenders in, 18

Criminal responsibility and intoxicants, 1021–1022
  concept of partial responsibility, 1025–1026
  conceptual problems
    definition, description, and the problem of DSM-IV-TR, 1022
    disease, disorder, defect, and dysfunction, 1022
    use, misuse, abuse, dependence, addiction, 1022–1023
  dependence as a defense, 1024–1025
  elements of the offense
    enduring problematic concept of "intent," 1023
    exculpatory doctrine in common law, 1023
  intoxicant-induced insanity as a defense, 1025
  intoxicant use and effects as mitigating factors, 1026
  intoxication as a defense, 1023–1024
  withdrawal as a defense, 1025
Cross-training, 725
Cryptococcus neoformans
  HIV infections and, 686
CSA. *See* Controlled Substances Act (CSA)
CSAT. *See* Center for Substance Abuse Treatment (CSAT)
Csnk1e. *See* Casein kinase 1 epsilon gene (Csnk1e)
CSSA. *See* Cocaine Selective Severity Assessment (CSSA)
CT. *See* Computed tomography (CT)
Cuban Americans
  drinkings levels, 823t
  substance abuse
    research and treatment outcomes, 824–826
CUD. *See* Cannabis use disorders (CUD)
Cues
  management of, 640–641, 642f
Cultural competence
  substance abuse treatment and, 104
Cultural factors and substance abuse issues, link between, 833
Culturally specific interventions, substance abuse, 840–841
Culture, 99
  influence on drug use, 101–102, 103
Current prevalence
  clinical assessment, 111
Cut Down, Annoyed, Guilty, Eye-Opener Tool, Adjusted to Include Drugs (CAGE-AID), 715, 809
CyberPsychology and Behavior and *Computers in Human Behavior*, 407
Cyber-relationship addiction, 410
Cybersex addiction, 398, 410
Cyclic glucose monophosphate (cGMP), 300
CYP1A2 gene
  in caffeine metabolism, 338–339
  induction, by cigarette smoking, 738
CYP2A6 gene, in nicotine, 321
CYP 3A4 inhibitors
  classification of, 730, 731t
CYP enzymes. *See* Cytochrome P450 (CYP) enzymes
Cyproheptadine, for AN, 379
CYT. *See* Cannabis Youth Treatment (CYT) study
Cytochrome P-450, in caffeine metabolism, 339
Cytochrome P450 (CYP) enzymes, 730
Cytochrome P450 (CYP) system, 44
  and substance abuse, 832
CYT Study. *See* Cannabis Youth Treatment (CYT) Study

DA. *See* Dopamine (DA)
D-amphetamine, 56, 61, 243, 247, 249, 279, 342
  caffeine *vs.*, 342
DARE. *See* Drug Abuse Resistance Education (DARE)
DA receptor, 199
DAST. *See* Drug abuse screening test (DAST)
DAT. *See* DA transporter (DAT); Dopamine transporter (DAT) inhibitor
DATA. *See* Drug Addiction Treatment Act (DATA)
DAT gene, 249
DA transporter (DAT), 199
DAWN. *See* Drug Abuse Warning Network (DAWN)
DBD. *See* Disruptive behavior disorders (DBD)
DC. *See* Drug counseling (DC)
D2 dopamine receptor (DRD2), 40, 43, 45
DDR program, 933
DEA. *See* Drug Enforcement Administration (DEA); Drug Enforcement Agency (DEA)
Deaths
  drug-related, 34
"Deca-Dick," 364
Deca-Durabolin, 363–364. *See also* Nandrolonedecanoate
Decompensation, episodes of, 915
Decriminalization, defined, 1035
Degreaser's flush, 304
Dehydroepiandrosterone (DHEA), 360
Delayed grieving, 920
Delirium
  in HIV-1 infection, 687–688
    treatment of, 687–688
  tremens, 938
Delta receptors, 161
Delta-9-tetrahydrocannabinol (THC), 214
Dementia
  in HIV-1 infection, 688
Demerol. *See* Meperidine
Deontological philosophies, 1035
Depade. *See* Naltrexone
Department of Health and Human Services/Substance Abuse and Mental Health Services Administration (DHHS/SAMHSA), 124
Depenalization, defined, 1035
Depression
  in COD patient
    treatment of, 726–728
  in HIV infection, 683
  in methadone patients, 429–430
  naltrexone in, 453
  nicotine dependence in, 330
  withdrawal from AAS and, 365
Depressive disorders
  with adolescent SUD, 789–790
DEQ. *See* Drug effects questionnaire (DEQ)
Desensitization, 923
Designer drugs, 270
Designer steroids, 361–362
Desoxyn. *See* Methamphetamine
Detoxification method, 179–180, 961
  under anesthesia, 180
  coordination of care, 180
  goal of, 179
  traditional methods, 180
  comparison of, 180
Detrusor instability, with caffeine, 341
Dextromethorphan (DXM), 172, 181, 725, 736, 742
DHHS/SAMHSA. *See* Department of Health and Human Services/Substance Abuse and Mental Health Services Administration (DHHS/SAMHSA)
Diacetylmorphine. *See* Heroin
Diagnosis
  on clinical assessment report, 113
Diagnosis, Intractability, Risk, and Efficacy (DIRE) Score, 805–806
Diagnosis, Intractability, Risk and Efficacy Inventory (DIRE), 715
Diagnostic and Statistical Manual of Mental Disorders, Fourth Edition, Text Revision (DSM-IV-TR) criteria
  for AN, 373, 374t
  for anxiety disorder, 347
  for BN, 373, 374t
  for caffeine intoxication, 345–346, 346t
  caffeine withdrawal in, 345
  for EDNOS, 373, 374t
  for nicotine dependence, 320
  for pathological gambling, 384–385, 385t
  sleep disorder, 343
  for substance dependence, 347–348, 347t
Diagnostic and Statistical Manual of Mental Disorders, 4th Edition (DSM-IV), 117–121, 192, 238
  abuse and harmful use, 118–119, 119t
  course modifiers, 119–120
    on agonist therapy, 119–120
    in controlled environment, 120
    remission, 119
  dependence, 117–118, 118t
  substance-induced disorder, 120
  vs. ICD-10, 118t, 120
Diagnostic and Statistical Manual of Mental Disorders (DSM-V)
  changes under consideration for, 121
Diagnostic and Statistic Manual (DSM), 408
  for Internet addiction, 409, 416
Dianabol, 354. *See also* Methandrostenolone
Diazepam, 152, 259, 260, 484, 488, 501, 503–504, 507, 658–659, 914, 923
Dictionary of Occupational Titles (DOT), 779
Dietary Supplement Health and Education Act of 1994 (DSHEA), 356
Dietary supplements, AAS-related, 360–361
Differential Aptitude test, 779
Dihydrocodeine, 439, 707
  for opioid dependence, 496–497
Dimethoxymethylamphetamine (DOM), 267
Dimethyltryptamine (DMT), 267
DIRE. *See* Diagnosis, Intractability, Risk and Efficacy Inventory (DIRE)
DIRE Score. *See* Diagnosis, Intractability, Risk, and Efficacy (DIRE) Score
Disability, status of, 908
  and addiction, 909–910
    case example of, 913
  alcoholism, case example, 912–913
  cocaine use and mood disorder, case example, 911–912
  occupational limitations, 909
  risk of relapse of substance use, case example of, 913
  under Social Security law, 915
  thought disorder, case example, 910–911
Disability Determination Service (DDS), 916
Disability information, sources of, 909
Disease model beliefs, and SHG, 527
"Disordered gambling," 384
Disruptive behavior disorders (DBD), 788
Disruptive behaviors
  group therapy, 581
Dissociative anesthetics, 277
Distributive crimes, 1034–1035
Disulfiram, 206, 1046
  in alcohol disorders, 155–156
  in co-occurring disorders, 727–728
  drug interactions of, 737
  naltrexone and, 453–454
Disulfiram, for alcohol dependence, 477–478
  efficacy studies, 477
  FDA approval, 477
  mechanism of action, 477
  optimal use of, 478
  safety issues, 477–478
  side effects, 477–478
Divalproex, 485
  for mania, 727
Diversion risk reduction plan, methadone, 431–432
Divorce
  gambling problems and, 387

DMT. *See* Dimethyltryptamine (DMT)
Doctoral-level psychologists, 949
Doctor-patient relationship, 663–664
Dolophine. *See* Methadone
DOM. *See* Dimethoxymethylamphetamine (DOM)
Domestic violence
   gambling problems and, 387
Don Juanism, 397
Dopamine (DA), 241, 277
   for alcohol dependence, 489
   and cannabinoid self-administration, 63
   and ethanol self-administration, 60–61
   mesolimbic transmission
      ethanol and, 60
   neurotransmission, 197
   and nicotine self-administration, 64
   and opiate reinforcement, 58–59
   and opiate self-administration, 59
   in PG, 388–389
   and psychostimulant reinforcement, 55–56
Dopamine D3 (DRD3) receptor gene, 45
Dopamine D4 receptor (DRD4), 40
Dopamine receptors, 40, 43, 45, 145
   caffeine in, 340
   classification of, 56
   and psychostimulant reinforcement, 56
Dopaminergic neuronal function, in ED and SUD, 377–378
Dopaminergic system
   alcoholism, 40–41
   tobacco dependence, 43
Dopamine transporter (DAT) inhibitor, 241
Dose(es)
   opioid therapy, 709–713
      escalation, 711
      "fixed schedule" (around-the-clock) dosing, 709
      individualization, 710–712
      relative potencies and, 712
      side effects, 712–713
DOT. *See* Dictionary of Occupational Titles (DOT)
Double Trouble in Recovery (DTR), 523
DRD2. *See* D2 dopamine receptor (DRD2)
DRD3. *See* Dopamine D3 (DRD3) receptor gene
DRD4. *See* Dopamine D4 receptor (DRD4)
DRD2 Taq1A1, 412
Driving under the influence (DUI), of alcohol, 20
Driving while intoxicated (DWI), 126
Dronabinol, 225
Drug
   psychoactivity of, 131–132
   testing
      history of, 123
      rationale for, 123–124
Drug abuse
   club of, 125
   defined, 700, 926
   ethical considerations, 134–135
   panel groups of, 124*t*
   performance characteristics of different assays, 130*t*
   reference guide, 131*t*
   screening for, 123–136
   treatment of
      social workers and, 966
Drug Abuse Office and Treatment Act, 9
Drug Abuse Resistance Education (DARE), 749
Drug abuse screening test (DAST), 179, 723, 808
Drug Abuse Warning Network (DAWN), 17, 168, 192, 288
   mortality data by, 730
Drug addiction, 908
Drug Addiction Treatment Act (DATA), 441, 441*t*, 762, 961
Drug control agencies, 1015–1016
Drug counseling (DC), 222
Drug Demand Reduction (DDR), 927

Drug diversion
   defined, 700
Drug effects questionnaire (DEQ), 249
Drug Enforcement Administration (DEA), 278, 713, 714, 745, 754
Drug Enforcement Agency (DEA), 268
Drug interactions, 730–739
   adverse effects of, 735–736
   alcohol and other medications, 737–738
   cigarette smoke/nicotine and other medications, 738–739
   mechanisms for, 730–731
   opioid analgesics and other medications, 736
   opioids
      and antiretroviral medications, 732–734, 732*t*
      and antivirals/antibiotics, 734–735, 734*t*
      and benzodiazepines, 735
      used for opioid dependence and other medications, 731–732
   overview, 730
   stimulants and other medications, 736–737
Drug maintenance
   harm reduction models and, 761–762
   international developments in, 762–763
Drug misuse, 806
Drug overdose
   prevention of, 758
Drug policy
   context of, 991–994
   costs caused by, 1034–1035
   defined, 988
   and drug abuse, 988–989
   and drug czars, 989
   and drug epidemic, 989–990
      potential health impact of, 990
   goal of, 988
   history of, 990–991
   international perspective, 1001–1002
   web site, 990
Drug policy issues, central, 1006–1007
Drug policy reform
   as harm reduction, 766–769
Drug possession/dealing, 432
Drug prohibition
   theoretical basis for, 1036
Drug-related determinants
   for opioids
      nonpharmacological drug-related factors, 171–172
      pharmacokinetics, 171
      receptor activity, 170–171
Drug(s)
   addiction
      laboratory models of, 88–95
   intake, regulation of, 93
   reinforcement
      modulation by nondrug consequences, 93
   use. *See also* Substance abuse
      behavioral aspects of, 88–97
      HIV-1 infection and, 682–692
      maternal and neonatal complications of, 648–659
      medical complications of, 663–678. *See also* Medical complications
      operant modulation in clinical population, 95–96, 95*f*, 96*f*
      sociocultural factors of, 99–105
Drug seeking response, 92
Drug self-administration
   stimuli and, 91–92
Drug substitution
   harm reduction models and, 761–762, 763–764
Drug supply
   World War II, 1041–1042
Drug trafficking, 918
Drug Treatment as an Alternative to Prison (DTAP), 1036

Drug use
   and civil law, 860
   and criminal justice system, 860
Drug use and addiction
   magnitude of the public health problem, 994
      risk factors-developing brain in the adolescent, 996
      risk factors-environment, 995
      risk factors-individual, genetics, 995–996
      risk factors-the drug, 996–997
Drug use disorders
   gender difference in prevalence of, 847
Drunkenness, 937
DSHEA. *See* Dietary Supplement Health and Education Act of 1994 (DSHEA)
DSM-IV. *See Diagnostic and Statistical Manual of Mental Disorders, 4th Edition (DSM-IV)*
DSM-V. *See Diagnostic and Statistical Manual of Mental Disorders (DSM-V)*
DTR. *See* Double Trouble in Recovery (DTR)
"Dually diagnosed," 721
DUI. *See* Driving under the influence (DUI)
Dutch cannabis policy, 766–767
DWI. *See* Driving while intoxicated (DWI)
DXM. *See* Dextromethorphan (DXM)
Dynamic model of relapse, 638–639, 639*f*
Dynorphin, 61, 206, 207, 467, 468

EAPs. *See* Employee Assistance Programs (EAPs)
Ear acupuncture, 466, 472
   cocaine addiction and, 473
   vs. body acupuncture, 473
Early recovery groups, 579
Early remission
   categories, 119
Eating disorder not otherwise specified (EDNOS), 373, 374*t*
Eating disorders (ED), 373–381
   addiction, 378
   allostatic model of, 377
   classification of, 850
   comorbidity of
      conceptual issues, 375–376
      confounding factors in assessing, 375–376
      substance abuse and, 375, 376–379
   environmental and social factors for, 376–377
   evidence-based behavioral treatments for, 850
   genetic vulnerability for allostasis in, 378
   hypotheses for, 376–378
   individual factors, personality, and impulsivity, 377
   naltrexone in, 454
   neurobiologic dysregulation in, 377–378
   shared causation of, 376
   special considerations in, 378–379
   syndromes, 373
      anorexia nervosa, 373, 374*t*
      BED, 373, 374*t*
      bulimia nervosa, 373, 374*t*
      demographics of, 375
      EDNOS, 373, 374*t*
      general epidemiology of, 373, 375
   treatment approaches for, 379–381
      pharmacologic, 379–380
      psychological, 380–381
EBI. *See* Evidence-based intervention (EBI)
EBP. *See* Evidence-based practice (EBP)
Ecological momentary assessment (EMA), 174
Economic refugees, 918
Ecstasy. *See* 3,4-Methylenedioxymethamphetamine (MDMA)
ED. *See* Eating disorders; Emergency Department (ED)
Edema, methadone side-effects, 427
EDNOS. *See* Eating disorder not otherwise specified (EDNOS)

EDTA. *See* Ethylenediaminetetraacetic acid (EDTA)
Education
  addiction counselor, 971–977
    approaches to, 975–977
  affective
    school-based programs, 747, 747t
  counselors, 985
  nurses, 981
  physician assistant, 982
  psychologists, 980
  social workers, 966, 967, 983–984
EEG. *See* Electroencephalogram (EEG)
Efavirenz, 426, 664, 688, 689, 690, 733
Ego-dystonic homosexuality, 872
EIA. *See* Enzyme immunoassays (EIA)
Electroacupuncture, 467–468. *See also* Acupuncture
  vs. TEAS, 473–474
Electroencephalogram (EEG), 303
  alcoholism and, 39
Electrophysiologic markers
  alcoholism and, 39
Electrophysiology
  HIV-1 infection and, 687
ELISA. *See* Enzyme-linked immunoadsorbent assay (ELISA)
EMA. *See* Ecological momentary assessment (EMA)
EMCDDA. *See* European Monitoring Centre for Drugs and Drug Addiction (EMCDDA)
Emergency Department (ED), 192
Emotional distress, 920
Emotional states, 637
Employee Assistance Programs (EAPs), 104
Employment status, in substance use, 18–19
Endocarditis, infective, 676
Endogenous opioid peptides (EOP), 377
Enforcement of Underage Drinking Laws (EUDL), 933
Environmental availability, 101
Environmental determinants, for opioids, 173–174
  settings of, 173–174
  specific opioid-associated cues, 174
Enzyme immunoassays (EIA), 125, 127
  basic principles of, 127f
Enzyme-linked immunoadsorbent assay (ELISA), 125, 127
EOP. *See* Endogenous opioid peptides (EOP)
Epidemiological Catchment Area study
  COD studies of, 722
Epidemiology, European perspective
  pitfall due to abnormal treatment profiles, 32–33
Epidemiology, United States, 17–23. *See also* Substance abuse
  data, sources of, 17
  indicators, role, 23
Epitope, of vaccines, 459–460, 460f
Erectile dysfunction, methadone side-effects, 427
"Eroticized child," 395
ERP. *See* Event-related brain potentials (ERP)
Escitalopram, in Internet addiction, 414–415
Establishing operations, 92–93
Eszopiclone, 258, 261, 262
Ethanol, 60–62
  in alcohol abuse, 126
  mechanisms of action, 60
  mesolimbic dopamine transmission and, 60
  self-administration, 60–62
Ethnicity, 99, 101–102
Ethnic minority groups, and SHG, 528
Ethylenediaminetetraacetic acid (EDTA), 303
Ethyl glucuronide, 126–127
European Addiction Severity Index, 1040
European Monitoring Centre for Drugs and Drug Addiction (EMCDDA), 26
European perspective
  epidemiology of, 26–34
  infectious disease and drug use, 30

Evaluation of Competency and Ethical Conduct, 984
Event-related brain potentials (ERP)
  alcoholism and, 39
Evidence-based intervention (EBI), 968
  resources, 968
Evidence-based medical education, 943
Evidence-based practice (EBP), 967–968
  clinical assessment, 109
  defined, 968
  resources, 968
Evidence-based screening, 937
Evidence-based substance abuse treatments
  cultural considerations in, 841
  utilization and effectiveness of, 842–843
Evidential strategies, 104
Exercise, testosterone with, 359
Expert testimony
  law and, 1020
  rationale for the admission of, 1019–1020
Externalizing disorders, in adulthood, 920
Extrasession practice
  cognitive behavioral therapy and, 598–599

Fagerström test for nicotine dependence (FTND), 323
Family
  abstinence and, 569
  on children, 586
  definition of, 585
  forms of, 585
  preventive strategies and, 103
  problems
    substance abuse and, 585–586, 585f
  substance use and, 99–100
  and therapeutic community, 545–546
Family Association Programs, 546
Family/couples therapy, 584–591
  considerations in, 589–590
  couple-based approaches, 588
  efficacy of, 587–589
  family approaches, 587, 588–589
  foundational frameworks of
    behavioral model, 586–587
    family disease approach, 586
    family systems approach, 586
  future directions of, 590–591
  history of, 584–585
  implementation of, 589
  limitations of, 590
  mechanisms of action of, 590–591
  in stepped care approach, 591
Family disease approach
  to family/couples therapy, 586
Family factors and substance abuse issues, link between, 833
Family history, Internet use and, 412
Family history negative (FHN)
  alcoholism and, 39
Family history positive (FHP)
  alcoholism and, 39
Family Smoking Prevention and Tobacco Control Act, 331, 331t
Family studies
  alcoholism, 36
  tobacco dependence, 42
Family support network intervention, 222
Family systems approach
  to family/couples therapy, 586
Family therapy, 104. *See also* Family/couples therapy
Family violence, 83–84
FAS. *See* Fetal alcohol syndrome (FAS)
FASD. *See* Fetal alcohol spectrum disorder (FASD)
FBI. *See* Federal Bureau of Investigation (FBI)
FBT. *See* Fentanyl buccal tablet (FBT)
FDA. *See* Food and Drug Administration (FDA)

2007 FDA Amendments Act, 714–715
Fear of federal control on the part of health professions, 6
Federal Antimaintenance Policy, 5
Federal Bureau of Investigation (FBI), 745
The Federal Bureau of Narcotics (1930), 7
Federal demand departments and agencies, 1016–1017
Federal drug control bureaucracy, reorganization of, 9
Federal farms, 966
Federal narcotic farms, 7
Federal opioid treatment standards
  governing methadone treatment. *See* Opioid Treatment Program (OTP)
Federal policy agencies, 1013–1015
Federation of State Medical Boards, 715
Feedback
  group therapy, 580–581
Fentanyl, 162, 172, 280, 707, 913
Fentanyl buccal tablet (FBT), 709
FEP. *See* First-episode psychosis (FEP)
Fetal alcohol spectrum disorder (FASD), 651
Fetal alcohol syndrome (FAS)
  aspects of, 651
Fetal solvent syndrome, 307
Fetus
  amphetamine on, 655–656
  benzodiazepine on, 658–659
  cocaine on, 654–655
  marijuana on, 657
  nicotine/tobacco on, 658
  PCP on, 659
FHN. *See* Family history negative (FHN)
FHP. *See* Family history positive (FHP)
First-episode psychosis (FEP), 790
"Fixed schedule" (around-the-clock) dosing, 710
Flashbacks, 273–274
Fluconazole, with methadone, 423
Flumazenil, 261, 505
Fluorescent polarization immunoassay (FPIA), 125
Fluorocarbons, 287, 306
Fluoxetine, 61, 155, 156, 243, 246, 380, 400, 488, 689, 795
  for BN, 380
Fluvoxamine, 61, 155, 400
  with methadone, 423
Follicle-stimulating hormone (FSH)
  alterations, methadone and, 427
Food and Drug Administration (FDA), 713
Forensic drug testing, 123, 132–133
Four A's approach
  for opioid therapy, 713, 714t, 716
FPIA. *See* Fluorescent polarization immunoassay (FPIA)
"FRAMER" intervention, 893–894
Freebasing, 192
Free Inquiry, 535
Freons, 286
  use of, 287
Freud, Sigmund, 191
FTND. *See* Fagerström test for nicotine dependence (FTND)
Full agonist, 170
Functional family therapy, 222, 792
Functional magnetic resonance imaging (fMRI)
  neurobiological correlates of substance use disorders, 848–849
Furosemide, 427

GABA. *See* Gamma-aminobutyric acid (GABA); Gamma-aminobutyric acid (GABA) receptor
$GABA_A$ receptors, 258
GABA enhancers
  in amphetamines, 246

GABAergic system, 145
  alcoholism, 41
GAIN. *See* Global Appraisal of Individual Needs (GAIN)
GAIN-SS. *See* Global Appraisal of Individual Needs-Short Screener (GAIN-SS)
Gambling, defined, 384
Gamma-aminobutyric acid (GABA), 197, 241, 243
  dopaminergic activity in, 241
  and ethanol self-administration, 61–62
  and nicotine self-administration, 64
Gamma-aminobutyric acid (GABA) receptor, 255
  genes in alcoholism, 41
Gamma-glutamyltransferase (GGT), 126
Gamma-glutamyl-transpeptidase (GGTP), 150
Gamma-hydroxybutyrate (GHB), 22
Gamma-hydroxybutyrate (oxybate), 125, 255, 264–265
  determinants of abuse, 264–265
  pharmacology of, 264
Gamma vinyl-GABA (GVG), 246
Gas chromatography mass spectrometry (GC-MS), 123, 129–130
Gas chromatography tandem mass spectrometry (GC-MS-MS), 123
Gas-liquid chromatography (GLC), 125, 125*f*, 129–130
Gasoline, 303–304
  prenatal exposure on neonate, 657
Gastrointestinal complaints
  gambling problems and, 387
Gastrointestinal diseases
  addiction and, 669
Gateway theory, 21
Gay, lesbian, and bisexuals
  affectional and sexual needs, 875
  HIV-related infections and AIDS among, 876
  link between psychodynamic forces in developing, 875
  substance abuse among
    genetic predisposition, 874
    homophobia and, 875
    incidence of, 871
    pervasive internal and social pressures role in, 876
    psychodynamic forces role in developing, 875
    risk factors for, 871
    societal prohibitions and, 874–875
  treatment concerns for, 877–878
Gay people
  HIV-related infections and AIDS among, 876
  methamphetamine abuse, 876–877
  treatment concerns for, 877
Gay sexual orientation
  in adolescence, 875
  coming out, 873
  homophobia and heterosexism, 873–874
  lesbian issues, 874
  and substance abuse
    genetic link between, 874
    risk factors, 874
GC-MS. *See* Gas chromatography mass spectrometry (GC-MS)
GC-MS-MS. *See* Gas chromatographytandem mass spectrometry (GC-MS-MS)
GDR. *See* German Democratic Republic (GDR)
Gender differences
  substance abuse, 17–18, 28–29, 29*t*
  in tobacco dependence, 43
General Guidelines for Providers of Psychological Services, 979
Genetics
  alcoholism, 36–41
  cannabinoids, 46
  cocaine, 45
  nicotine dependence, 44–45
  opiates, 45

substance use disorders, 36–47
tobacco dependence, 42–45
Genital herpes, 674
German Democratic Republic (GDR), on AAS use, 354–355
GGT. *See* Gamma-glutamyltransferase (GGT)
GGTP. *See* Gamma-glutamyl-transpeptidase (GGTP)
GHB. *See* Gamma-hydroxybutyrate (GHB)
Glasser, William, 546
GLB. *See* Gay, lesbian, and bisexuals
GLC. *See* Gas-liquid chromatography (GLC)
Global Appraisal of Individual Needs (GAIN), 107, 111–112, 791
  clinical scales, structure of, 112, 112*f*
Global Appraisal of Individual Needs-Short Screener (GAIN-SS), 791
Global criteria
  defined, 972
  twelve core functions and, 972*t*–974*t*
Glucuronidation, 730
Glue sniffing, 284, 286
Glutamate
  and cocaine reinforcement, 57–58
  and nicotine self-administration, 64–65
  and opiate self-administration, 59–60
Glutamate system modulators, 206
Goldberg, Ivan, 408
Gonorrhea, 674
Goodman, Aviel, on sex addiction, 395
Graduate medical education, 944–945
Group identification, 100
Group leader, functions of, 580
Group therapy, 104, 825
  advantages of, 576
  defined, 575
  for different stages of recovery, 578–580
    early recovery groups, 579
    mixed-phase groups, 578–579
    phase-specific groups, 578
    relapse prevention and continuing care groups, 579–580
  efficacy of, 575–576
  limitations of, 576–577
  management
    leadership, 580
    peer confrontation, 580–581
    preparing new members, 580
    substance use by member, 582
  patient selection factors, 577–578
  for sexual addiction, 399–400
  vs. self-help group, 577
Growth hormone deficiency (GHD), AAS for, 358
Guides to the Evaluation of Permanent Impairment, 909
GVG. *See* Gamma vinyl-GABA (GVG)
Gynecomastia, side-effects of AAS, 363–364

HAART. *See* Highly active antiretroviral therapy (HAART)
Haemophilus influenzae, 458, 677
The Hague Treaty (1912), 3–4
Hair
  drug testing, 134*t*, 135*t*
Hallucinogens
  adverse reactions, 272–274
    acute reactions, 272–273
    drug interactions, 274
    long-term adverse effects, 273–274
    treatment of acute adverse reactions, 273
  chemical classification of, 269–270
  defined, 267
  effects of chronic use, 271
  epidemiology of, 268
  history of, 267–268
  mechanisms of action, 271–272
    with multiple neurotransmitter systems, 271

overview, 267
  phenomenology of, 268
  during pregnancy, information for clinicians, 659
  prenatal exposure on fetus and neonate, 659
  psychological effects of, 270–271
Handicap, 909
Hard-drug markets, 766
Harmful use, 118
Harmful use and abuse
  comparison of, 119
Harm reduction (HR), 754–769, 1035
  addiction treatment as, 761–766
  caveats, 755–756
  challenges, 754–755
  in China (case study), 768*b*
  drug consumer groups, 759–761
  drug policy reform as, 766–769
  drug substitution, 761–762, 763–764
  Dutch cannabis policy, 766–767
  heroin-assisted treatment, 764–765
  human rights, 755
  low-threshold maintenance, 763
  maintenance, 761–762
  marijuana policies, 766–769
  methadone
    in correctional settings, 763
  municipal zoning policies, 759–760
  nonopioid drugs, 765–766
  open drug scenes, 759–760
  overdose prevention, 758
  peer outreach and education, 758
  public health, 755
  reframing issue, 754–755
  safer drug use, 758–759
  safe spaces, 760–761
  syringe exchange programs (SEPs), 756–758
    outside U.S., 757–758
    in U.S., 757
  in U.S., 756
Harm reduction *vs.* abstinence
  individual psychotherapy, 565–566
The Harrison Act (1914), 4, 11
Harrison Narcotic Act of 1914, 192, 440
Hashish, 2
HAV. *See* Hepatitis A virus (HAV)
Hazardous drinking, 937
HBV. *See* Hepatitis B virus (HBV)
HCG. *See* Human chorionic gonadotropin (HCG)
HCSUS. *See* HIV Cost and Service Utilization Study (HCSUS)
HCV. *See* Hepatitis C virus (HCV)
2,5-HD. *See* 2,5-hexanedione (2,5-HD)
Health, caffeine on
  negative effects, 341
  positive effects, 341
Health and Human Services (HHS), 441
Health care professionals, substance use disorders among
  epidemiology of, 892
  ethical considerations for, 898
  evaluation of
    confidentiality, 894
    family history, 894
    "FRAMER" approach, 893–894
    laboratory testing, 895
    outcome of, 896
    physical examination, 894
  legal considerations for, 895, 897
  monitoring of, 895
  nurses, 892
  prevalence of, 892
  prevention of, 893
  risk factors for, 892
  signs and symptoms of, 893
  sociocultural considerations for, 895
  special considerations for, 898–899
  treatment for, 895

Health care settings, screening and brief interventions, 937
Health care use/costs, SHG and, 526
Health education, on addiction
  career teacher program, 943–944
  continuing medical education, 945–946
  in early- to mid-19th century, 937
  evidence-based practice, 943
  graduate medical education, 944–945
  history, 937–941
  in mid-20th century, 938
  requirements, 941–943
  substance use disorders (SUDs) education and training, 951–953
  undergraduate medical education, 944
Health promotion, 927
Hearing loss
  by different solvents, 302t
Heart disease, ischemic
  substance abuse and
    management of, 667–668
Hematologic toxicity, 306–307
Hepatitis, viral, 670–673
Hepatitis A virus (HAV), 177, 670
Hepatitis B Virus (HBV), 30, 177, 666, 669, 670–671, 673, 854
Hepatitis C virus (HCV), 177, 671–673
  medications
    interactions with opioids, 734, 734t
  substance abuse disorders and, 19
Hepatitis D, 673
Hepatocellular carcinoma, side-effects of AAS, 363
Heroin, 2, 714
  addiction
    epidemiologic black hole of, 32
  adverse consequences of, 854
  among AI/AN groups, 843
  current use, 21
  epidemiology of, 854
  gender difference in, 854
  maintenance, 181
  for opioid dependence treatment, 498
  restrictions on, 7
  treatment demand for, 26–27
  treatment of, 854
  triggers for, 854
  use by incarcerated individuals, 882
  vaccines, 463–464
Heroin-assisted treatment, 764–765
  studies related to, 764–765
Heroin use, 910
  incidence of, 167
  prevalence of, 167
Herpes simplex virus (HSV) encephalitis
  HIV-1 infection and, 686
Heterosexism, 873–874
Hexane, 301
2,5-hexanedione (2,5-HD), 302
HGH. See Human growth hormone (HGH)
HHS. See Health and Human Services (HHS)
High-density lipoprotein (HDL), AAS use and, 362–363
Highly active antiretroviral therapy (HAART), 682, 692, 732, 733, 808
Hispanic Americans, 819–827
  alcohol abuse, 822
  current trends, 822–823
  defined, 819–821, 820t, 821t, 822t
  ethnic and racial considerations, 825–826
  growth of, 819, 820t
  median family income, 821t
  overview, 819
  public policy, 826–827
  sociocultural factors, 823–825
Hispanics
  defined, 825
  female addicts, 825–826

HIV. See Human immunodeficiency virus (HIV)
HIV-1. See Human immunodeficiency virus type 1 (HIV-1) infection
HIV Cost and Service Utilization Study (HCSUS), 808
HIV infection. See Human immunodeficiency virus (HIV) infection
HIV medications
  interactions with methadone/buprenorphine, 732–733, 732t
Hmong, 920
Homelessness, 963
Homelessness, substance abuse problems among
  factors influencing, 903
  prevalence of, 901
  risk factors for, 901
  sociocultural considerations for, 902–903
  treatment of
    active, 905
    basic guidelines for, 904
    engagement step, 905
    housing modalities for, 904
    maintenance/relapse prevention, 905–906
    models of care in, 903–904
    Mueser's paradigm of integrated treatment, 904
    persuasion step, 905
Homophobia, 873
Homosexual behavior, 872
  substance abuse, HIV infections, and AIDS, 876
Homosexuality, 871
  nonprejudicial framework on, 872
Honesty, and therapeutic community, 547
Hoochinoo, 837
Hooton, Taylor, 365
Hormonal alterations, methadone side-effects, 427
Hostility
  group therapy, 581
House staff, 937
Housing modalities, 904
HPA. See Hypothalamic–pituitary–adrenal (HPA) axis
HPV. See Human papilloma virus (HPV) infections
HR. See Harm reduction (HR)
HSV. See Herpes simplex virus (HSV) encephalitis
5-HT. See Serotonin (5-HT)
5-HTT. See Serotonin transporter gene (5-HTT); Serotonin transporter (5-HTT)
5-HTTLPR. See Serotonin transporter–linked polymorphic region (5-HTTLPR)
Hughes Act, 965, 966
Human chorionic gonadotropin (HCG), 367
Human growth hormone (HGH), 359, 366
Human immunodeficiency virus/acquired immunodeficiency syndrome (HIV/AIDS)
  among gay, lesbian, and bisexuals, 878
  and homosexual behavior, 876
  risk among AI/ANs, 843
Human immunodeficiency virus (HIV), 177, 210
  muscle loss with, 358–359
  substance abuse disorders and, 19, 30
Human immunodeficiency virus (HIV) infection
  in African Americans, 815
  aging and, 807–808
Human immunodeficiency virus type 1 (HIV-1) infection
  alcohol use, 682
  central nervous system infection and, 684–692. See also Central nervous system (CNS) infection, HIV infections and
  intravenous drug use and, 682–683
  mechanisms of transmission, 682
  neurobehavioral evaluation in, 686–687
  prevalence of, 682
  psychiatric disorders in, 683. See also Psychiatric disorders, in HIV infection
  psychological issues in, 683–684. See also Psychological distress, HIV infections and

Human papilloma virus (HPV) infections, 675
Human rights
  harm reduction (HR) model, 755
Hydrocodone-combination products, 914
Hydrocodone (Vicodin), 21, 45, 707
Hydromorphone, 707, 709
11-Hydroxytetrahydrocannabinol (11-OH-THC), 219
5-Hydroxytryptamine (5-HT), 241
Hyperalgesia, 698
  opioid-induced, 711–712
Hyperhidrosis, methadone side-effects, 427
Hyperpathia, 698
Hypersexuality. See Sexual addiction
Hypertension, 927
  caffeine-associated, 339, 341
    tolerance to, 344
  gambling problems and, 387
Hypervigilance, 920
Hypocrisy, sex addicts families and, 395
Hypogonadism, AAS for, 358
Hypothalamic-pituitary-adrenal (HPA) axis, 197, 848

IAAF. See International Association of Athletics Foundations (IAAF)
ICD. See International Classification of Diseases (ICD)
ICD-10. See International Classification of Disease (ICD-10)
ICD-NEC. See Impulse Control Disorder Not Elsewhere Classified (ICD-NEC)
ICD-10 symptom checklist for mental disorders, 179
IC&RC. See International Certification and Reciprocity Consortium (IC&RC)
ICRC/AODA. See International Certification and Reciprocity Consortium/Alcohol Drug Abuse
I-Cup, 128, 128f
Idiopathic pain, 697. See also Pain
IDU. See Injection drug users (IDU)
IE. See Infective endocarditis (IE)
Ilicit substance, 648
Ill-advised policy for Ontario, 915
Illicit drugs, 256f, 257f
  Hispanic Americans, 822
  use in older adults
    interaction with medications, 804–805
    rates of, 802–803
Illicit drug use
  by AA/PIs, 829–830
  by AI/ANs, 838
  defined, 928
  and genetic transmission, 832
Immigrants, 918
  acculturation, impacts, 920–921
  continental origins, 918
  cultural diversity within groups, 921
  culturally competent evaluation, 919–920
  high-risk immigrant groups, 922
  obtaining patient's substance related problem, 919
  onset of substance abuse, 921–922
  prevention of drug abuse, 924
  and substance abuse, 918
  treatment and recovery, 922–924
  in United States, 918
  working with a translator, 918–919
Immigration
  and problem drug use, 29–30
Immunization, 666
Immunoassays
  on-site screen, 127–128
Impaired cognition, with PG, 388
Impaired Physician program, 913
Impairment, 908
  definition, 908
  IQ decline due to, 908

Impotence, side-effects of AAS, 363–364
Impulse Control Disorder Not Elsewhere
    Classified (ICD-NEC), 384
Impulsive–compulsive spectrum disorder, 387
Impulsivity, 81–82
    defined, 81
    with PG, 388
Incarcerated populations, substance use problem
        among
    epidemiology of, 881–882
    factors influencing, 888–889
    impact of, 881
    prevalence of, 881
    prevention strategies for, 882–883
    sociocultural considerations for, 887
    treatment interventions for
        boot camp programs, 885
        challenges associated with, 883
        cognitive–behavioral interventions, 884–885
        jail-based agonist, 885–886
        opioid agonist maintenance, 885
        prison-based agonist, 886–887
        therapeutic community modality, 883–884
INCB. *See* International Narcotics Control Board
    (INCB)
Individual psychotherapy. *See* Psychotherapy,
    individual
Indo-Europeans, 918
Indolealkylamines-hallucinogens
    structure of, 269f
Induction, 962
    buprenorphine, 439–440
Infectious disease
    and drug use
        European experience and Russian paradigm, 30
Infective endocarditis (IE), 676
Information dissemination
    school-based programs, 746–747, 747t
Information overload, 410
Inhalant abuse, 284
    diagnostic criteria for, 309
    drug screening for, 309
    DSM evaluations of, 307–308
        in adolescents, 308
        in adults, 308
    neuroimaging studies in animals, 310
    nonnervous system toxicity of, 304
    toxicology of, 293–294
    treatment of, 308–310
Inhalants, 284
    acetone, 299–300
    butane, 299
    cardiotoxicity, 306
    chemicals commonly found in, 285t
    chlorohydrocarbons, 300
    clinical neuropathology, 295–297
        myelopathy (nitrous oxide), 296–297
    clinical neurotoxicology
        encephalopathy, 294–295
    DSM evaluations of abuse, 307–308
    epidemiology of, 288–291
        abuse patterns, 289, 291
        modalities of, 291
        surveys of, 288–289
    hematologic toxicity, 306–307
    hepatotoxicity of, 305
    historical events of, 284–288
        deaths of, 286–287
        substances, 284, 286
        toxicities of, 286–287
        tracking of, 287–288
    laboratory studies of, 297–298
    lifetime use issue, 289, 290t, 291
    in neonatal syndrome, 307
    nitrous oxide, 300–301
    percentages of adolescents using, 290t
    peripheral neuropathies, 301–305

alcohol, 304
gasoline, 303–304
laboratory studies, 301–302
methyl butyl ketone, 302–303
methylene chloride (dichloromethane), 303
n-hexane, 302–303
nonnervous system toxicity of inhalant
    abuse, 304
ototoxicity, 301
renal toxicity, 304–305
1,1,1-trichloroethane, 303
during pregnancy, information for clinicians, 657
prenatal exposure on neonate, 656–657
    gasoline, 657
    toluene, 656
propane, 299
pulmonary toxicity, 305–306
recantation of, 289
in sample of 723 antisocial youth in residential
    care in Missouri, 292t
socialcultural issues for, 291–294
toluene, 298–299
treatment of, 308–310
Inhalant toxicity
criteria for, 293–294
Inhalant use disorders (IUD), 288
Inhaler, in NRT, 323
Injectable naltrexone, for alcohol dependence,
    482–483
    efficacy studies of, 482
    FDA approval, 482
    mechanism of action, 482
    optimal use of, 483
    safety issues, 483
    vs. oral formulation, 483
Injection drug users (IDU), 665, 756
Inpatient therapy, for sexual addiction, 399
InSite, 760, 760f
Insomnia
    caffeine-associated, 341, 342–343
    gambling problems and, 387
    in HIV infection, 689–690
Institute of Medicine (IOM), 940
    continuum of care model, 745, 746f
Insulin levels
    caffeine and, 340
Interferon
    interaction with opioids, 734, 734t
Interim maintenance, methadone, 434
Internalization, 402
International adoptees, 920
International Association of Athletics Foundations
    (IAAF), 367
International Certification and Reciprocity
    Consortium/Alcohol Drug Abuse
    (ICRC/AODA), 984
International Certification and Reciprocity
    Consortium (IC&RC), 974
International Classification of Disease (ICD-10), 117
    abuse and harmful use, 118–119, 119t
    course modifiers for, 120
    substance-induced disorder, 120
    vs. DSM-IV-TR, 118t, 120
International Classification of Diseases (ICD), 141
International Classification of Functioning,
    Disability, and Health (ICF), 908
International drinking patterns, 139–140
    alcohol use disorders around world, 140
    dry/wet culture dichotomy, 140
International Federation of Social Workers, 982
International Narcotics Control Board (INCB), 713
International Nurses Society on Addictions
    (IntNSA), 981
International Olympic Committee, 239
    AAS and, 355
Internet
    advertisement, for antiaging clinics, 359

Internet addiction, 407–416, 410
    Beard and Wolf's diagnostic criteria for,
        410t
    definition, 408
    environmental factors, 412–414
    epidemiology, 408–412
        children and adolescents, 409
        general population, 408–409
    etiology and predisposing factors, 412
        cognitive-behavioral theory, 412
        family history, 412
        social skills deficit theory, 412
    evaluation and treatment, 414–416
        ADHD and, 415
        recommendations for, 415–416
    evolution and development of diagnostic
        criteria for, 410–412, 410t, 411t
    history, 408
    neurobiology, 412
    phenomenology, 409
    pre-existing and concurrent psychiatric
        comorbidities, 413
    psychometric instruments for, 411t
    and sleep deprivation, 413
    special considerations, 416
    Young's diagnostic questionnaire for, 410t
Internet resources, on nicotine dependence, 520t
"Internet usage disorder," 414
Internet World Stats, 408
Interpersonal determinants, relapse, 637–638
Intimate partner violence (IPV), 83
IntNSA. *See* International Nurses Society on
    Addictions (IntNSA)
Intoxicants on memory, effects of
    cocaine-related memory dysfunction in
        criminal proceedings
        cocaine-induced confabulation, 1028
        confabulation, 1028
        expert testimony about the memory of
            witnesses, 1027–1028
Intrapersonal determinants, relapse, 637
Intravenous drug abuse
    adverse consequences of, 854
    among AI/AN groups, 843
    epidemiology of, 854
    gender difference in, 854
    treatment of, 854
    triggers for, 854
Intravenous drug use (IVDU), 682–683
Intravenous (IV) cocaine, 196–197
Intrusive thoughts, 920
IPV. *See* Intimate partner violence (IPV)
IQ, 908
IRMS. *See* Isotope ratio mass spectroscopy
    (IRMS) testing
Irritable bowel syndrome, 914
Isbell, Harris, 164
Ischemic heart disease, substance abuse and
    management of, 667–668
IScreen™, 128, 128f
Isobutyl nitrite, 307
Isotope ratio mass spectroscopy (IRMS)
    testing, 369
IUD. *See* Inhalant use disorders (IUD)
IV. *See* Intravenous (IV) cocaine
IVDA. *See* Intravenous drug abuse
IVDU. *See* Intravenous drug use (IVDU)

Jail-based agonist treatment, 885–886
Jails and prisons, difference between, 881
Jansen, Jon, 356
John Holland's trait–factor theory
    of occupational choice, 779
Johnson Institute Intervention, 587
Joint Commission on Accreditation of Health
    Care Organizations, 584

1064 Index

Journals
  on substance abuse, 968–969

Kaposi sarcoma (KS), 307
Kappaopioid system agonists, 207
Kappa receptors, 161–162
Kemstro. *See* Baclofen
Ketalar. *See* Ketamine
Ketamine, 21, 22, 125, 301
Kirkpatrick, Jean, 534
Kishline, Audrey, 536
Kleptomania
  naltrexone in, 454
Klonopin. *See* Clonazepam
Koinonia, 544, 545, 549
Kolb, Lawrence, 164
K-rations, 926
Kroc Foundation, 938
KS. *See* Kaposi sarcoma (KS)

LAAM. *See* Levo-alpha acetyl methadol (LAAM)
Lapse, 633
Large-group psychotherapy, 923
Lateness, group therapy, 581
Laughing gas, 284
Laws and regulations, of controlled prescription drugs use, 713–715
L.C.D.C. *See* Licensed chemical dependency counselor (L.C.D.C.)
L.C.S.W. *See* Licensed clinical social worker (L.C.S.W.)
Leadership, group therapy, 580
Learning, in cognitive behavioral therapy, 594
Legal issues, on buprenorphine, 440–442, 441t, 442f
Legalization
  defined, 1035
  theoretical basis for, 1035–1036
Legal refugees, 918
Lesbians, substance abuse issues among, 874
Levo-alpha acetyl methadol (LAAM), 419, 437, 494, 496, 731, 735
  maintenance, 180–181
Levorphanol, 707, 708
Liaison Committee on Medical Education (LCME), 941
Librium. *See* Chlordiazepoxide
Licensed chemical dependency counselor (L.C.D.C.), 984
Licensed clinical social worker (L.C.S.W.), 983
Licensed professional counselor (L.P.C.), 983
Licit substance, 648
LifeRing. *See* LifeRing Secular Recovery (LifeRing)
LifeRing Secular Recovery (LifeRing), 524
  contact information, 534b
  history, 538
  meeting format, 539, 539b
  program, 538–539
Life Skills Training (LST) program, 750–751
Life stress, 84
Linguistic strategies, 104
Lioresal. *See* Baclofen
Lipid profile abnormalities, side-effects of AAS, 362–363
Listeria monocytogenes, 460
Literature, voucher-based contingency management review, 605–606
  trends in, 607–615, 607t, 609t–612t, 614t–618t
Lithium, for mania, 727
Liver disease, alcoholic, 669–670
Liver function tests (LFT), AAS use and, 363
Lofexidine, for opioid-withdrawal syndrome
  naltrexone and, 495
  vs. buprenorphine, 495–496

  vs. clonidine, 495
  vs. methadone, 495
Loitering, 432
Long-acting opioids, 962
Long-term psychodynamic psychotherapy (LTPP), 572
Loop diuretics, 366
Lophophora williamsii, 270
Lorazepam, 152, 260, 503
  for delirium associated with HIV-1 infection, 687
Low-threshold maintenance, 763
Lozenges, in NRT, 323
L.P.C. *See* Licensed professional counselor (L.P.C.)
LSD. *See* Lysergic acid diethylamide (LSD)
LST. *See* Life Skills Training (LST) program
LTPP. *See* Long-term psychodynamic psychotherapy (LTPP)
Lubiprostone, 712
Lung cancer, tobacco and, 668
Lung disease, 677
Luteinizing hormone (LH)
  alterations, methadone and, 427
Luvox. *See* Fluvoxamine
Lysergic acid, chemical classification of, 269f, 270
Lysergic acid diethylamide (LSD), 8–9, 267, 273

MAC. *See* Master Addiction Counselor (MAC)
Macroenvironment, 100–102. *See also* Social structures, large
Magnetic resonance imaging (MRI)
  for inhalent toxicity, 294
  for toulene abuser, 296
Maintenance Clinics (1912 to 1925), 5
Major depression, 80–81, 914, 916
Major depressive disorder (MDD), 788, 789–790
Mallory–Weiss lacerations, 273
Mandatory Minimum Sentences (1951 to 1956), adoption of, 8
Mania
  in HIV infection, 683
  treatment of, 727
Manual needling, 466, 467
  needle staying *vs.*, 473
MAOI. *See* Monoamine oxidase inhibitors (MAOI)
Mariani, Angelo, 191
Mariel refugees, 922
Marihuana, 2
  current use, 20–21
Marihuana: The First Twelve Thousand Years, 214
The Marihuana Problem (1930 to 1937), 7–8
Marijuana, 130, 714. *See also* Cannabis
  harm reduction, 766–769
  medical, 767–769
    in Canada, 768–769
  during pregnancy, information for clinicians, 657–658
  prenatal exposure on fetus and neonate, 657
Marijuana-induced mood and anxiety disorders, 916
Marijuana transfer tax, 215
Marijuana use
  comorbidity, 855
  epidemiology of, 854
  gender difference in, 854
  and hormone, 855
  negative effects of, 855
  in pregnancy, 859
  treatment for, 855
Marital therapy. *See* Family/couples therapy
Markets, separation of, 766–767
Marriage
  definition of, 585
MAST. *See* Michigan Alcohol Screening Test (MAST)
Master Addiction Counselor (MAC), 985

Master of Science Degree in Nursing (MSN), 981
MAST-G. *See* Michigan Alcohol Screening Test-Geriatric Version (MAST-G)
Maternal complications, 648–660
MBK. *See* Methyl butyl ketone (MBK)
McGuire, Mark, 360
MCV. *See* Mean Corpuscular Volume (MCV)
MDA. *See* Methylenedioxyamphetamine (MDA)
MDE. *See* Methylenedioxyethylamphetamine (MDE)
MDFT. *See* Multidimensional family therapy (MDFT)
MDMA. *See* 3,4-Methylenedioxymethamphetamine (MDMA)
Mean Corpuscular Volume (MCV), 150
Mechanisms of action
  family/couples therapy, 590–591
Media, 102
Medical and Psychological Response to Addiction (1962 to 1970), 8–9
Medical complications, 663–678
  adherence, 664
  care of, 663–666
  doctor–patient relationship, 663–664
  immunization, 666
  injection drug use, 665
  overdose, 665–666
  overlapping symptoms and syndromes, 664
  prevention of complications, 664–665
  sexual risk behavior, 666
Medical disorders
  opioid dependence and, 430
Medically supervised injecting centre (MISC), 760
Medically supervised withdrawal, methadone, 427–428
Medical maintenance treatment, of methadone, 433–434
Medical management (MM) treatment
  for alcohol use disorder, 451
Medical marijuana, 767–769
  in Canada, 768–769
Medical model, 903
Medical records, 916
Medical Specialty Action Group (MSAG), 940
Medication-assisted treatment (MAT), 961–962
MEK. *See* Methyl ethyl ketone (MEK)
Memory impairment, 914
Menstrual cycle
  follicular phase link with responsivity to stimulants, 848
Mental health, drug use disorders and, 19
Mental health and substance abuse services, funding of, 903
Mental status, 919
Mentors, therapeutic community members as, 546–547
Men who have sex with men (MSM)
  sexual risk behavior, 666
Meperidine, 171, 448, 704, 707
  designer analog of, 280
Meprobamate, 255, 914
Mescaline
  chemical classification of, 270
Messenger RNA (mRNA), 259
MET. *See* Motivational enhancement therapy (MET)
Meta-analysis
  psychotherapy, 572
  voucher-based abstinence reinforcement, 95
Metaclopramid, 712
Methadone, 8, 419–434, 707, 708, 1046
  clinical use of, 422–428
  in correctional settings, 763
  diversion risk reduction plan, 431–432
  drug interactions, 423–426, 424t–425t
  drug interactions between

alcohol and, 738
antivirals/antibiotics, 734–735, 734t
HIV medications and, 732–733, 732t
epidemiology and history, 419
half-life, 708
induction, 422
interim maintenance, 434
medically supervised withdrawal and tapering, 427–428
medical maintenance treatment, 433–434
misuse, 32–33
for nonopioid substance use, 428–429
alcohol, 428
benzodiazepines, 428
cannabis, 429
cocaine and amphetamines, 428–429
tobacco, 429
for opioid dependence, 731
for opioid dependence during pregnancy, 653
pharmacodynamics, 421
pharmacokinetics, 421
pharmacology, 421
in pregnancy, 433
problematic behavior, managing, 432–433
serum levels, 423
side effects, managing, 426–427, 426t
stable dose of, determining, 423
take-home doses of, 431
treatment
efficacy, for opioid dependence, 420–421
federal opioid treatment standards governing. *See* Opioid Treatment Program (OTP)
urine testing for, 431
Methadone, for opioid dependence treatment, 494
and lofexidine, 495
vs. dihydrocodeine, 497
vs. heroin, 498
vs. LAAM, 496
vs. morphine, 497
Methadone maintenance, 9–10, 180
history of, 166–167
Methadone maintenance programs
opioid therapy in, 717
Methadone maintenance treatment (MMT), 692, 761–762, 854
Methadone treatment, 961
Methadose. *See* Methadone
Methamphetamine, 240, 462–463
abuse, 844, 852–853, 871
among gay men, 876–877
current use, 22
psychiatric disorders and, 683
prevalence of, 240
treatment demand for, 28
in United States, 240
Methandrostenolone, 354
Methanol neurotoxicity, 304
Methicillin-resistant *Staphylococcus aureus* (MRSA), 675
Methyl butyl ketone (MBK), 302–303
Methylene chloride (dichloromethane), 303
Methylenedioxyamphetamine (MDA), 124
3,4-Methylenedioxymethamphetamine (MDMA), 21, 124, 264, 736, 759
behavioral effects of, 279
epidemiology of, 279
history of, 278–279
miscellaneous designer drugs, 280
neurotoxicity of, 280
psychopharmacology of, 279
MDMA tablets (Ecstasy), 1035
toxicity of, 279–280
treatment demand for, 28
for treatment of PTSD, 279
Methyl ethyl ketone (MEK), 303

Methylnaltrexone, 712
in opioid-induced bowel dysfunction, 426
Methylphenidate (MPH)
current use, 22
formulations for ADHD, 238
interaction with alcohol, 738
1-Methyl-4- phenyl-1,2,3,6-tetrahydropyridine (MPTP), 280
Mexican Americans
drinking levels, 823t
substance abuse
research and treatment outcomes, 824–826
M-3-G. *See* Morphine 3-glucuronide (M-3-G)
M-6-G. *See* Morphine 6-glucuronide (M-6-G)
MI. *See* Motivational interviewing (MI)
Michigan Alcohol Screening Test-Geriatric Version (MAST-G), 808
Michigan Alcohol Screening Test (MAST), 723
MicroCog computerized battery
to assess cognitive performance, 203
Microenvironment, 99–100. *See also* Social groups
Midazolam, 260
Mildly intoxicated person, 909
Millar, Anthony, on AAS use, 366
Minimal interventions
defined, 501
in primary care settings, 502
for sedative-hypnotic drug usage, 502
Minnesota Model, 793
MISC. *See* Medically supervised injecting centre (MISC)
Misoprostol, 712
Missed grieving, 920
"Mississippi Mermaid," 395
Misuse
defined, 700
Mitchell, George, 359
Mixed agonist–antagonist, 162, 170
Mixed pain, 697
Mixed-phase groups, 578–579
MM. *See* Medical management (MM) treatment; Moderation Management (MM)
MMT. *See* Methadone maintenance treatment (MMT)
MMTP. *See* MMT program (MMTP)
MMT program (MMTP), 762
Modafinil, 247
Moderation management (MM)
contact information, 534b
history, 536
meeting format, 537
nine steps of, 537b
program, 536–537
Molecular fingerprinting, 129
Molecular genetic studies
alcoholism, 40
tobacco dependence, 43–45
Monitoring the Future (MTF)
survey, 279
University of Michigan, 17
Monoamine oxidase inhibitors (MAOI), 736
Mood disorders
gender differences in response to psychotherapeutic treatment for, 849–850
in HIV-1 infection, 688–689
prevalence among women, 849
Mood stabilizers
co-occurring disorders and, 726–728
MOR. *See* Mu-opioid receptor (MOR)
Morbidity, 914
Morphine, 2, 707, 709, 736
buprenorphine *vs.*, 438–439
vaccines, 463–464
Morphine 3-glucuronide (M-3-G), 707
Morphine 6-glucuronide (M-6-G), 707
Motivation, 637, 778–779

Motivational enhancement, 566–567
stages of, 566
interventions, 530
Motivational enhancement therapy (MET), 623, 793
for CUD, 221
Motivational interviewing (MI), 975
considerations in, 629–630
barriers to implementing, 630
evaluation challenges, 629–630
training, 629
efficacy in, 624–627
adolescents, 627
alcohol abuse, 625–626
amphetamine or stimulant users, 626
cannabis abuse, 626–627
cocaine users, 626
opiate abuse, 626
pregnant women, 627
psychiatric populations, 627
tobacco users, 626
history of, 622–623
optimal use of, 628–629
brief motivational interventions, 628
in pretreatment and addictions treatment, 629
in primary care, 628–629
for smoking cessation, 329
MPTP. *See* 1-methyl-4- phenyl-1,2,3,6-tetrahydropyridine (MPTP)
MRI. *See* Magnetic resonance imaging (MRI)
mRNA. *See* Messenger RNA (mRNA)
MRSA. *See* Methicillin-resistant *Staphylococcus aureus* (MRSA)
MS. *See* Multiple sclerosis (MS)
MSM. *See* Men who have sex with men (MSM)
MS-MS. *See* Tandem mass spectrometry (MS-MS)
MSN. *See* Master of Science Degree in Nursing (MSN)
MST. *See* Multisystemic family therapy (MST)
MTF. *See* Monitoring the Future (MTF); Monitoring the Future (MTF) survey
MTR MRI signal, 298
Mueser's paradigm of integrated treatment, 904–905
Multidimensional family therapy (MDFT), 222, 589, 792
Multiple sclerosis (MS), 293
Multisystemic family therapy (MST), 589
Multisystemic therapy, 222, 792
Mu-opioid receptor (MOR), 41
Mu receptor gene, 45
Mu receptors, 161
Murray, Thomas, on antidoping programs, 367
Muscle growth, by AAS, 354, 358–359
Muscle loss, associated with HIV, 358–359
Musculoskeletal injuries, side-effects of AAS, 363
Myelopathy (nitrous oxide), 296–297
Myocardial infarction, coffee-associated, 339, 341
Myopathy
in HIV-1 infection, 685
histologic findings, 685

NAACT. *See* National Association of Alcoholism Counselors and Trainers (NAACT)
NAADAC. *See* National Association for Alcoholism and Drug Abuse Counselors (NAADAC); National Association of Addiction Counselor (NAADAC)
NAc. *See* Nucleus accumbens (NAc)
N-acetyl cysteine, 206
NAChR. *See* Nicotinic acetylcholine receptors (nAChR)
NAD+. *See* Nicotinamide adenine dinucleotide (NAD+)
NADA. *See N*-arachydonyl-dopamine (NADA)

Index

NADAP. See National Association on Drug Abuse Problems (NADAP)
Naltrexone, 380, 447–455, 945
  for alcohol dependence
    injectable, 482–483
    oral, 478, 480–482, 480t
  in alcohol disorders, 153–154
  in anorexia nervosa, 454
  in binge eating disorder, 454
  for BN, 376
  in bulimia, 454
  disulfiram and, 453–454
  in eating disorders, 454
  efficacy of, 448–453
    for alcohol use disorders, 450–453
    for opioid dependence, 448–450
  in Internet addiction, 415
  in kleptomania, 454
  maintenance, 181
  for opioid dependence, 494
    with lofexidine, 495
  in other populations, 453–454
  other uses, 454
  pharmacology, 447–448, 448t
  in problem gambling, 454
  safety of, 453–454
    contraindications, 453
    side effect profile, 453
Nandrolone decanoate, 362–363
NAOMI. See North American Opiate Medication Initiative (NAOMI)
N-arachidonylethanolamide, 219
N-arachydonyl-dopamine (NADA), 219
Narcan. See Naltrexone
Narcotic Addict Treatment Act (NATA), 419, 441
Narcotic Drugs Import and Export Act (1922), 6
Narcotics, 1
Narcotics Anonymous (NA), 523
Narcotic Sentencing and Seizure Act, 10
NAS. See National Alcohol Survey (NAS); Neonatal abstinence syndrome (NAS)
Nasal spray, in NRT, 323
NASW. See National Association of Social Workers (NASW)
National Alcohol Survey (NAS), 17
National Ambulatory Medical Care Surveys, 806
National Association for Addiction Professionals, 975
National Association for Alcoholism and Drug Abuse Counselors (NAADAC), 975
National Association of Addiction Counselor (NAADAC), 985
National Association of Alcoholism Counselors and Trainers (NAACT), 975
National Association of Social Workers (NASW), 965, 969, 983
National Association on Drug Abuse Problems (NADAP), 781
National Board of Medical Examiners (NBME), 938
National Certified Addiction Counselor (NCAC), 985
National Clearinghouse for Alcohol and Drug Information, The, 969
National Commission on Certification of Physician Assistants, 982
National Comorbidity Survey Replication (NCS-R), 81, 788, 803
National Council on Alcoholism (NCA), 938
National Curriculum Committee, 972
National Drunk and Drugged Driving Awareness week, 933
National Epidemiological Survey on Alcohol and Related Conditions (NESARC), 17, 79, 80, 156, 157, 803
National Focal Points (NFP), 26
National Football League's retired Player's Association, AAS use and, 356
National Highway Traffic Safety Administration, 414
National Household Survey on Drug Abuse (NHSDA), 192
National Institute of Drug Abuse's Cocaine Rapid Efficacy Screening Trial (CREST), 203
National Institute of Mental Health (NIMH), 268
National Institute on Alcohol Abuse and Alcoholism (NIAAA), 17, 147, 268, 584, 965, 984
National Institute on Drug Abuse (NIDA), 17, 268, 965, 981
National Institutes of Health (NIH), 268
National Laboratory Certification Program (NLCP), 124
National Narcotics Leadership Act, 11
National Nurses Society on Addictions (NNSA), 981
National Occupational Information Network (O'Net), 779
National Poison Data System, 291
National Registry of Evidence-Based Programs and Practices (NREPP), 968
National Survey on Drug Use and Health (NSDUH), 17, 167, 194, 288, 965
2008 National Survey on Drug Use and Health (NSDUH), 802, 803
Native Americans, motivational interviewing for, 841–842
NCAC. See National Certified Addiction Counselor (NCAC)
NCS-R. See National Comorbidity Survey Replication (NCS-R)
"Near-misses," in gambling, 390
Needle-exchange programs (NEP), 182
Neighborhood, 101
Neisseria gonorrhoeae, 674
Neonatal abstinence syndrome (NAS)
  with buprenorphine, 444
Neonatal complications, 648–660
Neonatal syndrome, 307
Neonates
  alcohol on, 651
  amphetamine on, 655–656
  benzodiazepine on, 658–659
  cocaine on, 654–655
  gasoline on, 657
  marijuana on, 657
  nicotine/tobacco on, 658
  opioids on, 652–653
  PCP on, 659
  toluene on, 656
NEP. See Needle-exchange programs (NEP)
NESARC. See National Epidemiological Survey on Alcohol and Related Conditions (NESARC)
Net compulsions, 410
Netherlands, drug policy in, 1038–1039
Network therapy, 104, 945
  adapted therapy, 558–559
  agenda, 559–560
  defining membership, 553
  defining task, 553–554
  individual therapy, 555–556
  Internet, 558
  medication observation, 555
  meeting arrangements, 555
  pharmacotherapy, 554–555
  principles of, 559–560
  research on, 556–558
Network therapy technique
  cognitive-behavioral therapy, 552
  community reinforcement, 552
  description, 551
  key elements, 551–552
  social support, 552
Neuraxial analgesia, 709
Neuroactive gonadal steroid hormones
  effects on response to cocaine administration, 848
  excitatory and inhibitory effects, 847
  and responsivity to stimulants, 848
Neurobehavioral evaluation
  in HIV-1 infection, 686–687
Neuroimaging
  HIV-1 infection and, 687
Neurologic complications, secondary
  HIV-1 infections and, 685–686, 685t
Neurologic disease, 677–678
Neurologic syndromes
  by organic solvents, 294t
Neuropathic pain, 697. See also Pain
  defined, 698
Neuropsychiatric disorders
  HIV-1 infection and
    anxiety, 690–691
    delirium, 687–688
    dementia, 688
    mood disorders, 688–689
    pain, 691
    psychosis, 690
    sleep disorders, 689–690
Neuropsychological assessment
  HIV-1 infection and, 686
Nevirapine, 733
New York City Chapter, 965
New York City Medical Society on Alcoholism (NYCMSA), 938
New York State Office of Alcoholism and Substance Abuse (OASAS), 984
NFP. See National Focal Points (NFP)
N-hexane, 302–303
NHSDA. See National Household Survey on Drug Abuse (NHSDA)
NIAAA. See National Institute on Alcohol Abuse and Alcoholism (NIAAA)
Nicotiana tabacum, 319
Nicotinamide adenine dinucleotide (NAD+), 144
Nicotine, 63–65, 319–332. See also Tobacco
  and alcohol, 330
  dependence
    caffeine and, 348–349
    genetic influences on, 44–45, 320–321
    predictors of, 320, 321t
    tobacco addiction and, 320–321
  drug interactions of, 738–739
  environmental factors for, 322
  epidemiology, 319–320
  history, 319
  inhaler, 517
  lozenge, 516
  mechanisms of action, 63
  nasal spray, 516
  and other drug dependence, 330
  patches, 516
  pharmacokinetics and pharmacodynamics, 322
  pharmacology, 321–322
  during pregnancy, information for clinicians, 658
  prenatal exposure on fetus and neonate, 658
  prevalence, 319
  and psychiatric comorbidities, 329–330
  on public health, 319
  recent trends and patterns, 319
  regulation, 330–331
  screening and identification, 322–323
  self-administration, 64–65
  toxicity, 516
  treatment, 323–329, 324t–327t
    behavioral therapies, 328–329
    combination smoking treatment, 328
    non-nicotine medications, 323–328
    NRT, 323
  vaccines, 460–461
Nicotine dependence, management of
  ATTOC, 519, 520

history of, 510–511
Internet resources, 520*t*
overview, 510
pharmacotherapy
approaches, 512–513, 512*t*
efficacy of, 513–514
future directions, 514–515
nicotine-based, 513
non-nicotine-based, 513
optimal use, 515–517
safety concerns, 515–517
in smokers with psychiatric disorders, 514
special considerations in, 519
practice guidelines of, 511–512, 512*t*
psychosocial treatments, 517–519
Nicotine–dopamine interactions, 63–64
Nicotine gum, 515
side/adverse effects, 515–516
Nicotine replacement therapies (NRT), 323, 855, 858
Nicotine use
epidemiology of, 855
gender difference in, 855
prevalence of, 847
in pregnancy, 858–859
treatment for
behavioral treatments, 855–856
nicotine replacement therapy, 855
triggers for, 855
Nicotinic acetylcholine receptors (nAChR), 44–45, 320–321
NICU Network Neurobehavioral Scale (NNNS), 653
NIDA. *See* National Institute on Drug Abuse (NIDA)
NIDA-modified ASSIST, 179
NIH. *See* National Institutes of Health (NIH)
NIMH. *See* National Institute of Mental Health (NIMH)
Nitrous oxide, 300–301
clinical neuropathology, 296–297
history of, 284
use of, 287
NLCP. *See* National Laboratory Certification Program (NLCP)
NMDA. *See* N-methyl-D-aspartate (NMDA)
N-methyl-D-aspartate (NMDA), 243, 261, 277, 299
receptor, 708
NNNS. *See* NICU Network Neurobehavioral Scale (NNNS)
NNRTI. *See* Nonnucleoside reverse transcriptase inhibitors (NNRTI)
NNSA. *See* National Nurses Society on Addictions (NNSA)
Nociceptin, 162
Nociceptive pain. *See also* Pain
defined, 697
somatic, 697–698
visceral, 698
Nonadherence behaviors, 700
medical context, 700–702, 701*t*
opioid therapy and, 716–717
Nonbenzodiazepine sedative agents, 914
Non–Hodgkin lymphoma
HIV-1 infections and, 686
Nonnucleoside reverse transcriptase inhibitors (NNRTI)
for dementia in HIV patients, 688
Nonopioid drugs, 765–766
Nonrapid eye movement (NREM), 158
Non-substance-related disease, 910
NOP receptors, 162
Norbolethone, 361
11-nor- 9-carboxy-tetrahydrocannabinol (THC-COOH), 219
Norepinephrine
and cocaine reinforcement, 57
and nicotine self-administration, 65

and opiate self-administration, 59–60
in PG, 388
North American Opiate Medication Initiative (NAOMI), 765
Northern Plains tribes (NP), substance abuse issues among, 839
Nortriptyline, for smoking cessation, 328
NQO2. *See* Quinone oxidoreductase (NQO2) gene
NREM. *See* Nonrapid eye movement (NREM)
NREPP. *See* National Registry of Evidence-Based Programs and Practices (NREPP)
NRT. *See* Nicotine replacement therapies (NRT)
NRTI. *See* Nucleoside reverse transcriptase inhibitor (NRTI)
NSDUH. *See* National Survey on Drug Use and Health (NSDUH); 2008 National Survey on Drug Use and Health (NSDUH)
Nucleoside reverse transcriptase inhibitor (NRTI), 732, 733
Nucleus accumbens (NAc), 145, 197
Nurses
addiction
certification as, 981
role of, 982
defined, 980–981
education and training, 981
role and scope of practice, 981–982
substance use disorders among, 892
Nursing practice
in addiction, 958–961
addictions nursing specialty organizations, 958–959
and buprenorphine treatment, 961–962
CARN-AP credential certification, 959–960
and methadone treatment, 961
and nicotine addiction treatment, 963
nurse care manager model of care, 961
nursing education, 958
role in providing addiction treatment, 960
role of certified professional, 959–960
special populations and medical-assisted treatment, 962–963
and treatment settings, 960–961
Nymphomania, 393

O-arachinoyl-ethanolamine, 219
OASAS. *See* New York State Office of Alcoholism and Substance Abuse (OASAS)
Obsessive–compulsive disorder (OCD)
PG as addiction and, 387
Occam's razor, 910
Occupational Medicine Practice Guidelines, 909
Occupational Outlook Handbook (OOH), 779
OCD. *See* Obsessive–compulsive disorder (OCD)
ODD. *See* Oppositional defiant disorder (ODD)
Odorizers, 284
Office-based opioid treatment, 962
Office-based therapy
strengths and limitations of, 564–565
Office of Drug Abuse Law Enforcement (ODALE), 9
Office of National Drug Control Policy (ONDCP), 11, 268, 940
Office of National Narcotics Intelligence (ONNI), 9
Official Disability Guidelines, 909
11-OH-THC. *See* 11-hydroxytetrahydrocannabinol (11-OH-THC)
Olanzapine, for AN, 379
Older adults, 802–810
on AAS, 357
alcohol use in, 806
cocaine use in, 804
drug abuse
aging and, 804–805
health effects of, 804–805
HIV, aging and, 807–808
increased mortality risk, 805

neurodevelopmental abnormalities and, 804
warning signs for prescription drug abuse, 807*t*
epidemiology of, 802–804
illicit drug use
interaction with medications, 806–807
rates of, 802–803
pain medications use, 805–806
psychotropic medications use, 805
Treatment Episode Data Set (TEDS), 803–804, 803*f*
treatment of, 808–810
access to medical care, 809
older offenders, 809–810
outcomes, 810
prevention of illness, 809
screening and assessment, 808–809
Oligomenorrhea, methadone side-effects, 427
Ondansetron, for BN, 380
ONDCP. *See* Office of the National Drug Control Policy (ONDCP)
O'Net. *See* National Occupational Information Network (O'Net)
OOH. *See* Occupational Outlook Handbook (OOH)
Operant analyses, 89
Operant conditioning
in cognitive behavioral therapy, 594
elements of, 88
Operant modulation in clinical population, 95–96, 95*f*, 96*f*
Opiate(s), 58–60, 447
abuse, motivational interviewing in, 626
classification of, 58
current use, 21
defined, 161
and ethanol self-administration, 61–62
genetic factors, 45
mechanisms of action, 58
for pain in HIV patients, 691
reinforcement, dopamine and, 58–59
self-administration, 59–60
treatment demand for, 27
Opioid(s), 447, 448*t*
abuse, 168
past-year treatment for, 168
treatment admissions for, 168
addiction, 179
administration route of, 708–709
agonist maintenance treatment, 885
agonist therapies, 854
availability of, 168
cardiovascular disease and, 667
classification of, 161–163
cognitive factors for, 173
comorbid disorders, 174–178
complications of, 174–178
defined, 161
determinants of use, 170–174
drug interactions between
and antiretroviral medications, 732–734, 732*t*
and antivirals/antibiotics, 734–735, 734*t*
and benzodiazepines, 735
for opioid dependence and other medications, 731–732
drug-related determinants for
nonpharmacological drug-related factors, 171–172
pharmacokinetics, 171
receptor activity, 170–171
emergency department (ed) visits, 168
environmental determinants, 173–174
epidemiology of, 167–169
evaluation approaches, 178–179
genetics of, 172–173
history of, 163–164
human behavioral research on, 164
misuse with chronic pain patients, 805–806
and nicotine self-administration, 65
phenomenology of, 169–170

Opioid(s), (*Continued*)
   physical dependence, 699
   during pregnancy, information for clinicians, 653–654
   prenatal exposure on neonate, 652–653
   selection of, 707–708
   tolerance, 698–699
   treatment approaches, 179–183
     access to, 182
     behavioral therapies, 182
     contingency management, 182
     detoxification method, 179–180
     linkage of care, 182–183
     overview of, 179
     pharmacological approaches, 181
     reimbursement for, 183
     vaccines, 182
   use among youth, 167–168
"Opioid agreement," 716
Opioid analgesics
   characteristics of, 703*t*–706*t*
   drug interactions of, 736
Opioid antagonists, 448*t*
Opioid dependence
   buprenorphine in, 437–444
     efficacy in the treatment of, 439
   drug interactions of opioids for, 731–732
   longitudinal course of, 168–169
   and medical disorders, 430
   methadone treatment for, efficacy of, 420–421. *See also* Methadone
   and psychiatric disorders, 429–430
   psychosocial and ancillary services, 430–431
Opioid dependence, naltrexone for, 448–450
   doses, 449
   for maintenance therapy, 449
   routes of administration, 449–450
     implants, 449–450
     sustained- release injections, 450
   for withdrawal/detoxification, 449
Opioid dependence, treatment of, 494–498
   codeine for, 496–497
   dihydrocodeine, 496–497
   heroin for, 498
   LAAM for, 496
   morphine for, 497
   overview, 494
Opioid detoxification
   naltrexone for, 449
Opioid–dopamine interactions, 63
Opioidergic system
   alcoholism, 41
Opioid-induced hyperalgesia, 711–712
Opioid pain relievers, 913
Opioid prescribing patterns, 914
Opioid receptor knockout mice
   and opiate self-administration, 60
Opioid receptors
   heterodimerization of, 58
Opioid replacement therapy (ORT), 442
Opioid risk tool (ORT), 715
Opioid rotation, 162, 707
Opioid therapy
   for active drug abusers, 718
   with buprenorphine, 718
   dosing, 709–713
     escalation, 711
     "fixed schedule" (around-the-clock), 710
     individualization, 710–712
     relative potencies and, 712
     side effects, 712–713
   four A's approach for, 713, 714*t*, 716
   in methadone maintenance programs, 717
   nonadherence behaviors and, 716–717
   opioid selection for, 707–708
   outcomes of, 702–713
     monitoring, 713, 716–717
     overview, 698
   patients selection, 702
   principles of, 702–718
   with remote history of substance abuse, 717
   risk assessment and management, 713–717
   route of administration, 708–709
Opioid treatment program (OTP), 419. *See also* Methadone
   administration for, 420
   interim maintenance treatment, 420, 434
   medication administration, dispensing, and use in, 420
   patient admission criteria for, 420
   required services in, 420
Opioid use. *See* Prescription opioid use
Opioid use disorders
   COD, 178
   complications of, 174, 177
     injection drug use, 176*t*
   criteria for, 170
   history of, 174
   HIV risk factor assessment, 175*t*
   phenomenology of use, 169
   phenomenology of withdrawal, 169–170
   physical examination of, 174, 175*t*
   polysubstance use, 178
Opioid withdrawal
   naltrexone for, 449
Opioid-withdrawal syndrome, 494
   buprenorphine for, 495–496
   clonidine for, 494–495, 496
   lofexidine for, 495–496
   methadone for, 495
Opium, 1–2
   addiction, 937
Opium Poppy Control Act, 8
Opium smoking, 918
Oppositional defiant disorder (ODD), 789
OPPS. *See* Ottawa Prenatal Prospective Study (OPPS)
OPRM1 gene, 41
Oral fluid
   drug testing, 134*t*, 135*t*
   testing drugs in, 133
Oral naltrexone, for alcohol dependence, 480–482, 480*t*
   efficacy studies of, 480–481, 480*t*
   ethnic differences and, 481
   FDA approval, 478
   mechanism of action, 478, 480
   optimal use of, 481
   side effects, 481
Oral transmucosal fentanyl citrate (OTFC), 709
ORL1 receptors, 162
Orphanin FQ, 162
ORT. *See* Opioid replacement therapy (ORT); Opioid risk tool (ORT)
OTC medications. *See* Over-the-counter (OTC) medications
OTFC. *See* Oral transmucosal fentanyl citrate (OTFC)
Ototoxicity
   clinical nature of, 301
OTP. *See* Opioid Treatment Program (OTP)
Ottawa Prenatal Prospective Study (OPPS), 229
Outcome expectancies, 637
Outpatient treatment program (OTP), 961
Ovarian steroid hormones, 847
Overdose, 665–666
Over-the-counter (OTC) medications
   misuse of, 742
Oxazepam, 152, 260
Oxycodone (OxyContin), 21, 45, 448*t*, 707, 1037
OxyContin. *See* Oxycodone (OxyContin)

PA. *See* Physician assistant (PA)
Pacific Islanders
   population of, 829
   substance use issues among. *See* Substance abuse, among AA/PIs
PADT. *See* Pain Assessment and Documentation Tool (PADT)
Pain
   assessment of
     principles, 695–698, 696*t*
   etiology of, 697–698
   in HIV infection, 691
   opioid therapy for. *See* Opioid therapy
   pathophysiology of, 697–698
   sex differences in response to, 848
   and substance abuse, 698–702
     abuse and misuse, 700
     addiction, 699–700
     nonadherence behaviors, 700–702
     physical dependence, 699
     tolerance, 698–699
   syndromes, 698
Pain Assessment and Documentation Tool (PADT), 713
Pain management
   acupuncture for, 467
   overview, 695
Pain reliever
   nonmedical use of
     incidence of, 167
     prevalence of, 167
   use, in older adults, 805–806
Pancreatitis, alcoholic, 669
Panic attacks, 914
Paradoxical pain, 711
Parametric studies
   voucher-based contingency management and, 613
Paraphilias, 396, 403–404
Parenting, 99, 586
Parkinson disease
   pathology in, 280
   with PG, 388–389
Partial agonist, 170
Participation
   group therapy, 581
   self-help groups (SHG), 526
     adolescents in, 528
     ethnic minority groups, 528
     facilitating, 530
     obstacles to, 530
     in treatment, 525–526
     women in, 527–528
Partner-focused appraoches, 587
Partners as patients, 591
Passive smoking, impact of, 927
Paternal-history-positive (PHP), 146
Pathological gambling (PG), 384–391
   as addiction/impulsive–compulsive spectrum disorder, 387
   candidate mediators of, 387–388
   diagnosis of, 384–385
   epidemiology of, 385
   genetic studies, 389
   impaired cognition, impulsivity, and cognitive distortions, 388
   neuroanatomy, 389–390
   neurotransmitter systems, 388–389
   psychiatric disorders with, 386
   social and environmental factors, 385–386
   social and public health costs of, 387
   terms and definitions, 384
   treatment, 390–391
Pathophysiology, defined, 697
Patient Placement Criteria 2-R (PPC-2R), 202
Patients assessment, ED–SUD comorbidity and, 378–379
Patient selection
   group therapy, 577–578
   for opioid therapy, 702

Pavlovian, 164, 200
PCP. *See* Phenylcyclohexylpiperidine (PCP)
PCP-induced psychosis, 278
PCP/phencyclidine
    during pregnancy, information for clinicians, 659
    prenatal exposure on fetus and neonate, 659
PCR. *See* Polymerase chain reaction (PCR)
PCS. *See* Physical component summary (PCS)
PD. *See* Personality disorders
Peer confrontation
    group therapy, 580–581
Peers
    substance use and, 100, 787
    and therapeutic community, 546, 549
Pelioisis hepatitis, side-effects of AAS, 363
Pemberton, John, 191
Performance-enhancing drugs. *See* Anabolic-androgenic steroids (AAS)
Peripheral nervous system pathology
    in HIV-1 infection, 685
Peripheral strategies, 104
Persistent pain. *See* Chronic pain
Personal Experience Inventory, 790
Personal Experience Screening Questionnaire, 790
Personality, 79–80
Personality disorders, 80
    among individuals with substance use disorders, 851
    categories of, 851
    treatment for, 851–852
PET. *See* Positron emission tomography (PET)
Pethidine. *See* Meperidine
P-glycoprotein (P-gp), 730
    in absorption of methadone, 421
P-gp. *See* P-glycoprotein (P-gp)
Pharmaceutical stimulant
    current use, 22
Pharmacodynamics
    antibody effects on, 459
    of buprenorphine, 438–439
    of methadone, 421
    of nicotine, 322
Pharmacodynamic theory, 164
Pharmacokinetics
    antibody effects on, 459
    of buprenorphine, 438
    of caffeine, 339
    of methadone, 421
    of nicotine, 322
    of opioids, 171
Pharmacologic effects, of sedative-hypnotics, 914
Pharmacology, methadone, 421
Pharmacotherapy
    in adolescent substance abuse, 794–796
    agents, 832
    for sex addiction, 400
    voucher-based contingency management and, 613
Phase-specific groups, 578
Phencyclidine. *See* Phenylcyclohexylpiperidine (PCP)
Phenethylamine -hallucinogens
    structure of, 269f
Phenylcyclohexylpiperidine (PCP)
    current trends in use, 278
    epidemiology of, 278
    hepatic recirculation of, 277
    history of, 277
    intoxication, 278
    neurotoxicity of, 278
    vaccines, 462
Phenylisopropylamines hallucinogens
    chemical classification of, 270
PHP. *See* Paternal-historypositive (PHP)
Physical component summary (PCS), 178
Physical dependence. *See also* Addiction
    defined, 699
Physician assistant (PA)

defined, 982
    education and training, 982
    role and scope, 982
Physician Clinical Support System (PCSS), 940
Physician ownership, of prevention and treatment, 937
Physicians, substance use disorders among, 892
PIs. *See* Pacific Islanders
Pistorius, Oscar, 367
"Platform Zero," 759
PND. *See* Postnatal day (PND)
Pneumonia, 677
Polydrug abuse
    treatment demand for, 28
Polymerase chain reaction (PCR), 177
Polysubstance use
    with opioid use disorders, 178
POMS. *See* Profile of Mood States (POMS)
Pornography, in cybersex addiction, 398
Positron emission tomography (PET), 296
Postnatal day (PND), 297
Posttraumatic stress disorder (PTSD), 81, 279, 790, 919–920
    characterization of, 850
    prevalence of, 850
    treatments for, 851
Potency, defined, 712
PPC-2R. *See* Patient Placement Criteria 2-R (PPC-2R)
PPD. *See* Primary psychotic disorders (PPD); Purified protein derivative (PPD)
Practice Research Network (PRN) survey, 983
Prediabetes, 910
Prefrontal cortex (PFC), in PG, 389–390
Pregnancy
    alcohol and drug use in, 648–659, 858. *See also* Alcohol; specific drugs
        history of, 649–650
        prevalence of, 648–649, 649f
        social characteristics of, 650–651
    buprenorphine in, 444
    cocaine use in, 859
    marijuana use in, 859
    methadone in, 433
    motivational interviewing in, 627
    nicotine use in, 858–859
    opioid use in, 859
Pre-Harrison Act, 1037
Prehypertension, 910
Preincarceration behavior, 882
Prescription drug misuse, 928, 938
Prescription opioid use
    comorbidity, 853
    epidemiology of, 853
    gender difference in, 853
    in pregnancy, 859
    triggers for nonmedical, 853
Price, Gladys, 965
Primary psychotic disorders (PPD)
    with adolescent SUD, 790
Prison-based agonist treatment, 886–887
Prisoners, ORT for, 444
Prison settings, 104
PRN survey. *See* Practice Research Network (PRN) survey
Problematic behavior, managing, 432–433
Problematic Internet use. *See also* Internet addiction
    classification criteria for, 411t
Problem drug use, 26
    immigration and, 29–30
Problem gambling, 384
    naltrexone in, 454
Profile of Mood States (POMS), 249
Project COMBINE, 451
Project MATCH, 524
Propane, 299
Propoxyphene, 707

Prozac. *See* Fluoxetine
Pseudoaddiction, 700–701. *See also* Addiction
Psilocybe mexicana, 270
Psilocybin, psychotomimetic effects of, 273
Psychiatric comorbidities, nicotine and, 329–330
Psychiatric disorders, 838
    in HIV infection, 683
        bipolar disease, 683
        depression, 683
        mania, 683
        schizophrenia, 683
    methamphetamine and, 683
    opioid dependence and, 429–430
    with PG, 386
    sex addition with, 397
Psychiatric functions, assessment of, 909
Psychiatric in-patient facilities, 949
Psychiatric populations
    motivational interviewing in, 627
Psychoactive substances, use of, 910
Psychodynamic psychotherapy
    for sex addiction, 401
Psychological distress
    HIV infections and, 683–684
        adherence to CART, 684
        risk taking behavior, 683–684
        sexual abuse, 683
Psychological factors, 79–82
    anxiety disorders, 81
    attention deficit hyperactivity disorder, 82
    bipolar illness, 80
    impulsivity, 81–82
    major depression, 80–81
    personality, 79–80
    personality disorders, 80
    posttraumatic stress disorder, 81
    thought disorders, 81
Psychological inoculation
    school-based programs, 748
Psychological maladjustment, 834
Psychologists
    clinical, 979
    counseling, 979
    defined, 979–980
    education and training, 980
    role and scope of practice, 980
    school, 979–980
Psychomotor retardation, 914
Psychosis
    and antipsychotic medications, 727
    in HIV infection, 690
    treatment of, 690
Psychostimulants, 55–58
    cocaine reinforcement, 57–58
    cocaine self-administration in DAT knockout mice, 57
    for dementia associated with HIV-1 infection, 688
    dopamine and, 55–56
    dopamine receptors and, 56
    drug interactions of, 736–737
    mechanisms of action, 55
Psychotherapy, individual, 562–573
    controlled trials, 571–572
    engagement, 566–568
        connecting problems with substance abuse, 568
        goal setting, 568
        motivational enhancement, 566–567
        preparing patient for specialty treatment, 567
    features of, 565–566
    history of, 565
    principles and interventions, research-based, 571
    recovery issues, 571
    self-help programs, 569–571
    stabilization phase, 568–569. *See also* Abstinence, in individual psychotherapy

Psychotropic medications
  in co-occurring disorders, 726, 726t
  in older adults, 805
PTSD. See Posttraumatic stress disorder (PTSD)
Public health
  harm reduction (HR) model, 755
  strategies and legislations, 840
Public policy
  Hispanic Americans, 826–827
Puerto Ricans
  drinking levels, 823t
  substance abuse
    research and treatment outcomes, 824–826
Pulmonary complications, cocaine and, 677
Pulmonary toxicity, 305–306
Punishment, 93
  voucher-based contingency management, 604
Pure Food and Drug Act, 3
Purified protein derivative (PPD), 178
  skin test, 178

"Qahwa," 335
Qat chewing, 918
QTc prolongation
  buprenorphine and, 443
QT interval prolongation, methadone side-effects, 427
QTL. See Quantitative trait locus (QTL)
Quality of life outcomes, SHG and, 525
Quantitative trait locus (QTL), 247
"Quest" cigarettes, 331
Quetiapine
  for mania, 727
  for psychosis in HIV patients, 690
Quinone oxidoreductase (NQO2) gene, 249

Race/ethnicity, 99
  for substance abuse, 18
Radioimmunoassay (RIA), 125
Randomized controlled trials (RCT), 245
Rapid eye movement (REM), 158
Rapid plasma reagin (RPR), 177
"Raw Deal," 368–369
RCT. See Randomized controlled trials (RCT)
Readiness, 778
Recency
  clinical assessment, 111
Recovery
  defined, 633–634
  individual psychotherapy and, 571
  of sex addiction, 404–405
  value of work in, 777–778
Recovery-oriented religious group, 923
"Recreational gambling," 384, 385
  substance abuse and, 386
Red-flag behaviors, 700
Red Road to Wellbriety program, 842
Referral, vocational rehabilitation, 780–781
Refugee groups, 918
  health perspectives, 918
Regulatory and administrative proceedings, 1028
  administrative proceedings, 1031
  prescribing opioids for pain in private practice, 1029–1031
  professional impairment, 1029
Rehabilitation. See also Vocational rehabilitation
  defined, 778
Reinforcement, 88
  of alternative behaviors, 93–94
  contingency, parameters of, 90–91
  experimental demonstrations of, 89–90, 90f
  modulation by nondrug consequences, 93
  voucher-based contingency management, 604
Reinforcers, 88, 89–91
Reinstatement model, 92

Rejuvenation centers. See "Antiaging" clinics
Relapse, 633
  determinants, 636–638
    interpersonal, 637–638
    intrapersonal, 637
Relapse prevention (RP), 579–580
  acupuncture for, 471–472
  clinical interventions, 639–644
    adjunctive therapy, 643–644
    cognitive distortions, identification and coping, 643
    co-occurring psychiatric disorders, treatment of, 644
    cues and cravings, identification and management of, 640–641, 642f
    follow-up outpatient treatment, 644
    negative emotions, identification and management of, 642–643
    relapse management plan development, 643
    relapse process and event, understanding, 640, 640f
    risk identification and development of coping strategies, 640, 641f
    social network development, 641–642
    social pressures management to substance use, 641, 642f
  empirical studies of, 635–636
  models of, 638–639
    cognitive–behavioral model, 638, 638f
    cognitive–behavioral model, revised, 638–639, 639f
  outcome studies, 634–636
  relapse determinants and, 636–638
    interpersonal, 637–638
    intrapersonal, 637
Relapse risk, 913, 938
Relative potency, 712
Reliability, clinical assessment, 109–110
Religious/spiritual orientation, and SHG, 527
REM. See Rapid eye movement (REM)
Remission, 119
  early, 119
  sustained, 119
REMS. See Risk evaluation and mitigation strategies (REMS)
Remyelination, 296
Renal function, impaired
  acamprosate and, 485
  topiramate and, 486, 488
Renal impairment
  buprenorphine and, 438
Renal toxicity, 304–305
  during pregnancy, 305
Report, clinical assessment
  format, 113–114
Rescue dosing, 710
Rescue medication, 712
Residency Review Committees (RRC), 943
Resistance skills
  school-based programs, 747t, 748–750
Respiratory depression
  from buprenorphine, 442
Responsibility
  defined, 547
  therapeutic community and, 547–548
Revia. See Naltrexone
RIA. See Radioimmunoassay (RIA)
Ribavirin, 672
  interaction with opioids, 734, 734t
Richmond, Mary, 965
Rifadin. See Rifampin
Rifampin, 426, 664, 676, 731,
  interaction with opioids, 734, 734t
Risk evaluation and mitigation strategies (REMS), 709, 715
Risk taking behavior
  HIV infections and, 683–684

Risperdal Consta. See Risperidone
Risperidone, 61, 246, 273, 482
  for psychosis in HIV patients, 690
Ritalin, 22, 239t, 1037. See also Methylphenidate (MPH)
"Roid rage," 365
RP. See Relapse prevention (RP)
RPR. See Rapid plasma reagin (RPR)
Rush, Benjamin, 937
Russian paradigm
  infectious disease and drug use, 30

SAD. See Social anxiety disorders (SAD)
Safer injection facilities (SIF), 760
Safe spaces, 760–761
Saliva pH, buprenorphine absorption and, 438
SALOME. See Study to Assess Longer-term Opioid Medication Effectiveness (SALOME)
SAMHSA. See Substance Abuse and Mental Health Services Administration (SAMHSA)
Satyriasis, 393
Scale scores
  in clinical assessment, 111–112, 112f
Schedule II drugs, 192
Schizophrenia, 195
  in HIV infection, 683
  naltrexone in, 453
  nicotine dependence in, 329–330
School-based programs, 742–752
  affective education, 747
  alternatives, 747–748
  competence enhancement, 750–751
  current trends, 742
  information dissemination, 746–747
  major approaches, 747t
  prevalence, 742
  prevention, 743
    etiology and implications for, 743–745
    strategies for, 745–751
    types of, 745
  psychological inoculation, 748
  resistance skills training, 748–750
  risk factors, 743–744
    behavioral, 744
    cognitive and attitudinal, 743–744
    personality, 744
    pharmacologic, 744
    social, 743
  supply and demand reduction, 745
School psychologist, 979–980
Schools
  preventive strategies and, 103
  substance use and, 100
Scope of Practice
  counselors, 985
  nurses, 981–982
  physician assistant, 982
  psychologists, 980
  social workers, 984
Screener and Opioid Assessment for Patients with Pain (SOAPP), 715
Screener and Opioid Assessment of Pain Patients-Revised (SOAPP-R), 806
Screening, brief intervention, and referral to treatment (SBIRT), 940
Screening and brief intervention (SBI), 960
Screening Tool of Older Person's Prescriptions (STOPP), 806
SDS. See Severity of dependence scale (SDS)
Secular Organizations for Sobriety/Save Our Selves (SOS), 524
  contact information, 534b
  guidelines for, 536b
  history, 535
  meeting format, 536
  program, 535–536

Sedative-hypnotics, 914
  abuses, 258
  barbiturates, 262–263
  benzodiazepines, 258–260
  comorbidities of, 257–258
  complications of, 257–258
  epidemiology of, 255–257, 256f
  γ-hydroxybutyrate (oxybate), 264–265
  history of, 255
  overview, 255
  z-drugs, 260–262
Sedative-hypnotics discontinuation. *See also*
    Benzodiazepine (BZD) discontinuation
  history of, 501
  minimal intervention programs for, 502
  overview, 501
  systematic discontinuation programs for, 502–505
    additional therapies for, 505–506
    outcome determinants, 507
    pharmacotherapy for, 505–506, 505t
    psychotherapy for, 506
    treatment settings, 507–508
Sedative-induced mood disorder, 914–915
Selective serotonin reuptake inhibitors (SSRI), 243, 736
  in co-occurring disorders, 727
  in sex addiction, 400
Self-efficacy, 637
  and SHG, 529–530
Self-help activities, 922–923
Self-help groups (SHG)
  abstinence-specific support and, 528–529
  alternative self-help programs. *See* Alternative support groups
  brief interventions and, 530
  coping skills and, 529–530
  disease model beliefs and, 527
  general support and, 528–529
  goal direction in, 529
  and health care use and costs, 526
  ingredients of, 528
  network support treatment, 530
  participation, 526
    adolescents in, 528
    ethnic minority groups, 528
    facilitating, 530
    obstacles to, 530
    in treatment, 525–526
    women in, 527–528
  and quality of life outcomes, 525
  religious/spiritual orientation and, 527
  and rewarding activities, 529
  self-efficacy and, 529–530
  severity and impairment, 526–527
  12-step principles, 523, 530
  substance use outcomes, 524–525, 524f
  vs. group therapy, 577
Self-help programs, 569–571
Self-Management and Recovery Training (SMART), 524
  contact information, 534b
  history, 537
  meeting format, 538
  program, 538
  purposes and methods, 538b
Self-medication, 910
  hypothesis, 721
Self-report, 107
Semi-structured assessment, 110
Sensation seeking, 45
Seroquel. *See* Quetiapine
Serious and persistent mental illness (SPMI), 683
Serotonergic agents, for paraphilias, 404
Serotonergic medications
  for alcohol disorders, 155
Serotonergic neuronal systems, in ED and SUD, 378

Serotonergic system
  in alcoholism, 41
  tobacco dependence, 43–44
Serotonin (5-HT), 279
  and cocaine reinforcement, 57
  and ethanol self-administration, 61–62
  in PG, 389
Serotonin reuptake inhibitors (SRI), for alcohol dependence, 488–489
Serotonin transporter gene (5HTT), 41, 43–44, 249, 412
Serotonin transporter–linked polymorphic region (5-HTTLPR), 41, 43–44
Sertraline, 155, 156, 245, 246, 248, 380, 400, 487, 488, 689, 727, 795, 850
Serum glutamic oxaloacetic transaminase (SGOT), 150
Serum glutamic pyruvic transaminase (SGPT), 150
Seventh Generation Program, 840
Severity of dependence scale (SDS), 179
Sex addicts anonymous (SAA) program, 399–400
Sexaholics anonymous (SA) program, 399–400
Sex and love addicts anonymous (SLAA) program, 399–400
Sex differences, and drugs of abuse
  neuroactive gonadal steroid hormones, 847–848
  neuroimaging and neurobiologic correlates, 848–849
  in stress reactivity and relapse, 848
Sex therapy, in sex addiction, 402–403
"Sexting," 414
Sexual abuse, HIV infections and, 683
Sexual addiction, 393–405
  behavioral patterns, types of, 395–397, 396t
  comorbidity, 397–398
  criteria for, 394t
  cybersex addiction, 398
  diagnosis, 393–394, 394t
  etiology, 394–395
  paraphilias, 403–404
  recovery process, 404–405
  treatment, 398–403, 399t
    abstinence, 402–403
    CBI, 400–401
    group therapy, 399–400
    inpatient therapy, 399
    other therapy groups, 400
    pharmacotherapy, 400
    psychodynamic psychotherapy, 401
Sexual compulsives anonymous (SCA) program, 399–400
Sexual compulsivity. *See* Sexual addiction
Sexual crimes, 404
Sexual dysfunction, methadone side-effects, 427
Sexual impulsivity. *See* Sexual addiction
Sexually transmitted diseases (STD)
  substance use and
    chlamydia, 674
    genital herpes, 674
    gonorrhea, 674
    HPV infections, 675
    syphilis, 673–674
    trichomoniasis, 675
Sexually transmitted infections (STI), 177
Sexual-minority women
  definition of, 859
  substance use disorders among
    epidemiology of, 859–860
    risk factors for, 860
    treatment of, 860
Sexual orientation, definition of, 872
Sexual risk behavior, 666
SFCT. *See* Solution-focused couple therapy (SFCT)
SGOT. *See* Serum glutamic oxaloacetic transaminase (SGOT)
SGPT. *See* Serum glutamic pyruvic transaminase (SGPT)

The Shanghai Commission and the Smoking Opium Act (1909), 3
"Shared" etiology hypotheses, for ED and SUD, 376
SHG. *See* Self-help groups (SHG)
Short-acting opioids, 962
SIF. *See* Safer injection facilities (SIF)
SIGI³. *See* System of Interactive Guidance and Information Plus (SIGI³)
Signatures
  on clinical assessment report, 114
Silence, group therapy, 581
Single-photon emission computed tomography (SPECT), 273
Size and symbolism of the addiction problem, 4–5
Skin infections
  drug use and, 675–676
  prevention of, 675
Sleep, caffeine and, 342–343
Sleep deprivation, Internet addiction and, 413
Sleep disorders, in HIV infection, 689–690
"Sleeper effect"
  of cognitive behavioral therapy, 594, 595f
SMART. *See* Self-Management and Recovery Training (SMART)
SMART Recovery: News and View, 538
Smoking. *See also* Cigarette smoking
  acupuncture, 472
  cessation
    brief intervention for, 328–329, 329t
    bupropion for, 323, 328
    five A's for, 628
    naltrexone in, 454
    nortriptyline for, 328
    programs, 927
    varenicline for, 328
    voucher-based contingency management for, 604–605, 605f, 606f
  in depression, 330
  environmental factors for, 322
  nicotine dependence and. *See* Nicotine, dependence
  during pregnancy, 856
  prevalence, 319
  and psychiatric comorbidities, 329–330
  on public health, 319–320
  rates, 319
Smorgasbord approach, 924
Sniffers, 293
SOAPP. *See* Screener and Opioid Assessment for Patients with Pain (SOAPP)
SOAPP-R. *See* Screener and Opioid Assessment of Pain Patients-Revised (SOAPP-R)
Sobering Thoughts, 534
Sober living homes, 104
Social anxiety disorders (SAD), 790
Social attachment, 84
Social functioning, 915
Social groups
  family unit and parenting, 99–100
  group identification, 100
  peer group, 100
  schools, 100
  social networks and support, 100
  workplace, 100
Social model, 903
Social networks, 100
Social Security Administration, 916
Social Security Disability Insurance (SSDI), 914–915
Social Security law, 915
Social skills deficit theory, for Internet addiction, 412
Social structures, large
  acculturation, 102
  cultural influences, 101–102
  environmental availability, 101
  media, 102
  neighborhood disorganization, 101
  socioeconomic conditions, adverse, 101

Social support, 100
  network therapy technique, 552
Social treatment strategies, 104
Social workers
  alcohol abuse and, treatment of, 965–966
  defined, 982–983
  drug abuse and, treatment of, 966
  education, 966
    and training, 983–984
  evidence-based practice and, 967–968
  licensure and certification of, 966
  role and scope of practice, 984
  substance abuse and, treatment of, 965–969, 966f
    education and training in, 967
    services provided for, 967
  training, 966
Society, 99
Sociocultural strategies, 104
Sociocultural variations
  substance use disorders and, diagnosis of, 102–103
Sociodemographic factors, 17–19
Socioeconomic conditions, 101
Soft drinks
  caffeine in, 336t–337t, 337
    annual per capita consumption, 338, 338f
Soft-drug markets, 766
Soft-tissue infections
  drug use and, 675–676
  prevention of, 675
Solution-focused couple therapy (SFCT), 588
Somali refugees, 920
Somatic pain, 697–698
SOS. *See* Secular Organizations for Sobriety/Save Our Selves (SOS)
SOS International Newsletter, 535
Southwestern tribe (SW), substance abuse issues among, 839
Special Action Office for Drug Abuse Prevention (SAODAP), 9
Specialists, addiction. *See* Addiction specialists
Specialty treatment programs, psychotherapy
  selection considerations for, 563–564
  therapists and counselors in, 562–563
SPECT. *See* Single-photon emission computed tomography (SPECT)
The Spirituality of Imperfection, 548
SPMI. *See* Serious and persistent mental illness (SPMI)
Sports organizations, AAS by, 354
SSRI. *See* Selective serotonin reuptake inhibitors (SSRI)
Stabilization, of buprenorphine, 440
Stabilization phase, 568–569
Staphylococcus aureus, 675, 676
State Boards of Social Work, 966
Stavudine, 731
STD. *See* Sexually transmitted diseases (STD)
Stead, Eugene, Dr., 982
12-step programs, 104, 523, 569–570, 910, 913, 949. *See also* Self-help groups (SHG)
Steroids
  anabolic-androgenic. *See* Anabolic-androgenic steroids (AAS)
  designer, 361–362
STI. *See* Sexually transmitted infections (STI)
Stimulants. *See also* Psychostimulants
  agonist pharmacotherapy, 247
  cardiovascular disease and, 667
  common types of, 239t
  drug interactions of, 736–737
Stimulant use
  gender differences and epidemiology of, 852–853
  and hormones, 853
  treatment for, 853
Stimulant users
  motivational interviewing in, 626

Stimuli, discriminative
  drug seeking and, 91–92, 91f
STOPP. *See* Screening Tool of Older Person's Prescriptions (STOPP)
"Street methadone," 32–33
Stress-related disability, 909
Stress response, sex differences in, 848
Strychnine, 273
Students
  AAS use by, 356–357, 357f
  college, PG prevalence for, 385
Study to Assess Longer-term Opioid Medication Effectiveness (SALOME), 765
Sublingual tablets, in NRT, 323
Suboxone, 962. *See also* Buprenorphine
Substance abuse. *See also* Drug(s)
  European perspective
    drug-related crime, 33–34
    drug-related deaths, 34
    gender differences, 28–29, 29t
    immigration and, 29–30
    infectious disease and, 30
    methadone and buprenorphine misuse, 32–33
    treatment provision, 31
    treatment standards, inadequacy of, 32
    younger people, 29
  family problems and, 585–586
  HIV-1 infection and, 682–692
  resources on
    journals, 968–969
    websites, 969
  sociocultural factors of, 99–105
    management, 102–104
  training and education, 967
  treatment, 691–692
    clinical assessment of, 107–115
    cognitive behavioral therapy, 693–600
    family and couple-based approaches for, 584–591
    family/couples therapy, 584–591
    group therapy, 575–582
    individual psychotherapy, 562–572
    motivational interventions, 622–630
    relapse prevention, 633–644
    social workers and, 965–969, 966f
  in United states
    comorbidity, 19
    in criminal justice system, 18
    epidemiology of, 17–23
    gender differences, 17–18
    geographic factors, 19
    life cycle, 18–19
    race/ethnicity for, 18
    and treatment, 22–23
Substance abuse, among AA/PIs
  epidemiologic studies of
    illicit drug and alcohol use, 829–830
    national survey studies, 829–830
  factors influencing
    acculturation, 833–834
    family/cultural, 833
    genetic/biologic, 832–833
    psychological, 834
  prevention strategies against, 830–831
  treatment for
    cultural and practical barriers in, 831
    mental health assessment, 831–832
    prevention and maintenance, 832
    psychopharmacology, 832
    psychosocial, 832
Substance abuse, among AI/ANs
  childhood characteristics associated with, 839
  epidemiology of, 837
    alcohol use disorders, 838
    death rates, 838
    drug use relapse, 838–839
    traumatic exposure, 838

factors influencing, 843
marijuana use, 839, 840
prevention strategy for, 840
reasons for, 837
sociocultural considerations for, 839–840
special considerations for
  HIV/AIDS, 843–844
  methamphetamine and nicotine, 844
  urban areas, 844
tobacco use, 839
treatment strategies for
  culturally relevant, 840–841
  medications, 842–843
  motivational interviewing, 841–842
  Red Road to Wellbriety program, 842
  TPR model, 840
  traditional healing methods, 842
Substance Abuse and Mental Health Services Administration (SAMHSA), 17, 721–722, 829–830, 838, 966, 968, 969, 972
  TEDS, 21
Substance abuse policy development, 1011–1012, 1013
  implementation and execution, 1013
  problem definition, 1012
  solution deliberation, 1012–1013
Substance dependence, 347–348, 347t, 910
Substances
  alcohol, 19–20
  club drugs, 21–22
  cocaine, 21
  heroin and other opiates, 21
  history of, 284–286
  marihuana, 20–21
  methamphetamine, 22
  pharmaceutical stimulant, 22
  tobacco, 21
Substance treatment demand
  pattern of, 26–28
Substance use
  across life span, 79
  definitions, 928
Substance use disorders (SUD), 373–381, 730, 915. *See also* Eating disorders (ED); Substance abuse
  among health care professionals. *See* Health care professionals, substance use disorders among
  among homelessness. *See* Homelessness, substance abuse problems among
  among incarcerated populations. *See* Incarcerated populations, substance use problem among
  binge eating and, 376
  comorbidity of, 788–790
    attention-deficit hyperactivity disorder, 789
    conduct disorder, 788
    depressive disorders, 789–790
    posttraumatic stress disorder, 790
    psychotic and bipolar disorders, 790
  contingency management in, 603–619. *See also* Voucher-based contingency management
  determinants of, 36–47
  ED and
    comorbidity of, 375, 376–379
    patterns of, 376
  education and training, sample syllabus, 951–953
  environmental and social factors for, 376–377
  and gay identity formation, 874–876
  gender differences in, 847
  genetic factors in, 36–47
  individual factors, personality, and impulsivity, 377
  neurobiological correlates of, 848–849
  neurobiologic dysregulation in, 377–378

PG as addiction and, 387
pharmacotherapy for, 794–795
prevalence of, 786–787, 847
sex addition with, 397
shared causation of, 376
treatment approaches for, 379–381
pharmacologic, 379–380
psychological, 380–381
Substituted phenethylamines
chemical classification of, 269f, 270
Substituted tryptamines
chemical classification of, 269f, 270
Subutex, 437, 438, 773. See also Buprenorphine
"Such a Gorgeous Kid Like Me," 395
SUDs. See Substance use disorders (SUD)
SUD treatment, reality, 954
Suicide, AAS withdrawal and, 365
Summary recommendation
on clinical assessment report, 114
Sustained remission
categories, 119
Sweat
drug testing, 133, 134t, 135t
Sweden, 1040–1041
Swedish drug policy experience, 1002–1005
Switzerland, 1039–1040
Syphilis, 177, 673–674, 937
Syringe exchange programs (SEP), 756–758
outside U.S., 757–758
in U.S., 757
Systematic discontinuation programs, 502–505
additional therapies for, 505–506
defined, 501
pharmacotheapy for, 505–506, 505t
psychotherapy for, 506
purpose, 501
System of Interactive Guidance and Information Plus (SIGI³), 779
System to Retrieve Information from Drug Evidence (STRIDE), 1037

T-ACE
for alcohol consumption, detection, 651–652
Take-home doses
loss or misuse of, 432
of methadone, 431
Talbott, G. Douglas, 939
Tandem mass spectrometry (MS-MS), 129
TAP 21. See Technical Assistance Publication 21 (TAP 21)
Tapentadol, 707
Tapering, from methadone, 427–428
TaqA1 allele, in PG, 389
TAS certification. See Tobacco Addiction Specialist (TAS) certification
Taxation, 1042
TB. See Tuberculosis (TB)
TCA. See Tricyclic antidepressants (TCA)
TEAS. See Transcutaneous electrical acupoint stimulation (TEAS)
Technical Assistance Publication 21 (TAP 21), 974
TEDS. See Treatment Episode Data Set (TEDS); Treatment Episodes Data System
Teen Severity Addiction Index, 791
Telescoping, 387, 847, 852
Testicular atrophy, side-effects of AAS, 363
Testosterone. See also Anabolic-androgenic steroids (AAS)
anabolic effects of, 360
androgenic effects of, 360
biosynthesis and metabolism of, 360–361, 361f
Tetrahydrogestrinone (THG), 361–362
"That Guy" media campaign, 933
THC. See Delta-9-tetrahydrocannabinol (THC)
THC-COOH. See 11-nor- 9-carboxy-tetrahydrocannabinol (THC-COOH)

"The 400 Blows," 395
"The Mambo Kings Plays Songs of Love," 394
"The Man Who Loved Women," 395
Therapeutic alliance
psychotherapy, 572
Therapeutic community, 104, 562, 966
challenges to implementation and operation of, 883–884
in correctional setting, 883
defined, 543
in early Christian Church, 543–545
effectiveness of, 884
family and, 545–546
honesty, 547
mentors, members as, 546–547
multidimensional approach of, 545
overview, 543
peers and, 546, 549
religious roots of, 543–545
responsibility, 547–548
Therapeutic use exemptions (TUES), 368
Therapists
and addiction specialists, conflicts between, 564
in independent practice, 563–565
selection of, 563
specialty treatment program and, 562–563
vs. counselors, 562
"The Woman Next Door," 395
Thin-layer chromatography (TLC), 125
Thomas, Tammy, 361
Thought disorders, 81
TIAC. See Training Institute for Addiction Counselors (TIAC)
Tiagabine, 727
TIP. See Treatment improvement protocols (TIP)
TLC. See Thin-layer chromatography (TLC)
TMA. See Transcription-medicated amplification (TMA)
Tobacco. See also Nicotine
addiction, nicotine dependence and, 320
cancer and, 668
cardiovascular disease and, 667
current use, 21
genetic influences in, 42–44
during pregnancy, information for clinicians, 658
prenatal exposure on fetus and neonate, 658
use, in co-occurring disorders, 728
Tobacco Addiction Specialist (TAS) certification, 975
Tobacco dependence
adoption studies, 42–43
dopaminergic system, 43
family studies, 42
gender differences, 43
genetic influences in, 42–44
methadone and, 429
molecular genetic studies, 43–45
serotonergic system, 43–44
twin studies, 42
Tobacco public health policies, 840
Tobacco use, defined, 926
Tobacco users
motivational interviewing in, 626
Tolerance, defined, 698–699
Toluene, 286, 298–299
in brain glucose metabolism, FDG PET studies of, 298–299, 298f, 299f
inhalation, 294–295
by adults, 295
on CNS, 295
measure of radioactive binding in PET studies, 298, 298f
MRI studies for, 296
prenatal exposure on neonate, 656
in renal toxicity, 305
Toothache drops, 191

Topamax, 487. See also Topiramate
Topiramate, 727
for alcohol dependence treatment
efficacy studies, 486
impaired renal function and, 486, 488
mechanism of action, 485–486
optimal use of, 486
safety of, 486
side effects, 486
in alcohol disorders, 154
for BN, 380
Toxicology testing, 960
Toxoplasma gondii infection
HIV infection and, 685–686
TPH. See Tryptophan hydroxylase (TPH)
Traditional healing methods for substance abuse disorders, 842
Traditional radioligand competition assays, 297
Training
addiction counselor, 971–977
approaches to, 975–977
in cognitive behavioral therapy, 599
counselors, 985
motivational interviewing and, 629
nurses, 981
physician assistant, 982
psychologists, 980
social workers, 966, 967, 983–984
Training Institute for Addiction Counselors (TIAC), 985
Tramadol, 707
Transcription-medicated amplification (TMA), 177
Transcutaneous electrical acupoint stimulation (TEAS), 468
Transgo, 286
Trauma, 920
abstinence and, 569
Traumatic exposure, 838
AI/ANs, 843
Treatment Alternatives for Street Crime (TASC), 1036
Treatment demand
defined, 26
substance, pattern of, 26–28
for alcohol, 27
for amphetamine, 28
for cannabis, 27–28
for cocaine, 26–27, 28
for heroin, 26–27
for methamphetamin, 28
for opiates, 27
for polydrug abuse, 28
Treatment Episode Data Set (TEDS), 168, 803–804, 803f, 822
SAMHSA, 21
Treatment Episodes Data System, 856
Treatment improvement protocol (TIP), 977
number 42, 725
Treatment planning
clinical assessment report and, 114
Treponema pallidum, 673
Triazolam, 260
1,1,1-Trichloroethane, 303
Trichomonas vaginalis, 675
Trichomoniasis, 675
Tricyclic antidepressants (TCA), 243
in co-occurring disorders, 727
"Triggering," 401
Trimpey, Jack, 537
Trip, 270
Truffaut, Francois, 395
Tryptophan hydroxylase (TPH), 44
Tuberculosis (TB), 178, 676–677
medications
interaction with opioids, 734, 734t
TUES. See Therapeutic use exemptions (TUES)

Twins
    alcohol in, 338
    caffeine use in, 338
    cigarette smoking in, 338
Twin studies
    alcoholism, 37
    tobacco dependence, 42
Type A alcoholics, 38
Type 2 alcoholism (male-limited), 38
Type 1 alcoholism (milieu-limited), 38
Type B alcoholics, 38

UDP-glucuronosyltransferase (UGT) 2B7, 736
UFT. *See* Unilateral family therapy (UFT)
UGT 2B7. *See* UDP-glucuronosyltransferase (UGT) 2B7
Ultrarapid opioid withdrawal, naltrexone in, 449
UNDCP. *See* United Nations International Drug Control Program (UNDCP)
Undergraduate medical education, 944
Uniform State Narcotic Drug Act, 8
Unilateral family therapy (UFT), 587
United Kingdom, drug policy in, 1039
United Kingdom's Disability Discrimination Act (1995), 908
United Nations International Drug Control Program (UNDCP), 754
United Nations Office on Drugs and Crime (UNODC), 240
United States and international drug policy, future of, 1007–1008
United States Medical Licensing Examination (USMLE), 942
United States (U.S.)
    harm reduction in, 756
    syringe exchange programs in, 757
Universal precautions approach, 713
UNODC. *See* United Nations Office on Drugs and Crime (UNODC)
Urinalysis testing program, 927
Urinary incontinence, with caffeine, 341
Urinary urgency, with caffeine, 341
Urine drug screening, 716, 916
Urine drug testing, 134*t*, 135*t*
    in adolescent SUD, 791
Urine testing, for drugs, 431
U.S. Department of Education, 743
U.S. National Collegiate Athletic Association (NCAA), 355
Utilitarianism, 1035

Vaccines for substance abuse
    alternative design of, 459–460
    antibodies and. *See* Antibodies, vaccines and
    cocaine, 461–462
    epitope, 459–460, 460*f*
    heroin, 463
    methamphetamine, 462–463
    morphine, 463–464
    nicotine, 460–461
    overview, 457
    phencyclidine, 462
    self-adjuvanting vaccine, 459–460, 460*f*
Validity
    clinical assessment, 109–110
    laboratory model of drug addiction, 94–95
Valium. *See* Diazepam
Varenicline, 510, 517
    for smoking cessation, 328
The Variety of Religious Experience, 549
Vascular endothelial growth factor (VEGF), 307
VDRL. *See* Venereal Disease Research Laboratory (VDRL)

VEGF. *See* Vascular endothelial growth factor (VEGF)
Venereal Disease Research Laboratory (VDRL), 177
Venlafaxine, for anxiety in HIV infection, 691
Ventral tegmental area (VTA), 145, 197, 241
VESID. *See* Vocational and Educational Services for Individuals with Disabilities (VESID)
Veterans Administration Centers, 950
Vice disease, 937
Vicodin, 21. *see also* Hydrocodone (Vicodin)
Video game addiction, 409
Vietnam War, 927
Violence, 82–83. *See also* Intimate partner violence (IPV)
Violent video games, 413
Viral hepatitis, 670–673
    hepatitis A, 670
    hepatitis B, 670–671
    hepatitis C, 671–673
    hepatitis D, 673
Virus
    as cause of cancer, 669
Visceral pain, 698
Vivitrol, in alcohol use disorder, 451. *See also* Naltrexone
Vocational and Educational Services for Individuals with Disabilities (VESID), 782
Vocational rehabilitation, 778–783
    assessment, 778–780
    counseling and referral, 780–781
    illustrative cases, 782–783
    impediments to, 783–784
    improvement of, 784–785
    placement and follow-up, 781–782
    strategies, 778
Volatile solvent abuse, 286
Voucher-based abstinence reinforcement, 95–96, 95*f*, 96*f*
Voucher-based contingency management, 603–619
    behavioral principles in, 603–604
    elements of, 603–605
    features of, 604
    literature, trends in, 607–615, 607*t*, 609*t*–612*t*, 614*t*–618*t*
        combination with pharmacotherapies, 613, 614*t*
        conducting parametric studies, 613, 616*t*–617*t*
        extending to additional SUDs, 607–608, 607*t*
        extending use into community settings, 608, 611*t*–612*t*, 613
        longer-term outcomes, improvement in, 613, 615*t*
        as a research tool, 613, 615, 618*t*
        treatment of special populations, 608, 609*t*–610*t*
    literature review, 605–606
    results, 604*f*, 606–607
    for smoking cessation, 604–605, 605*f*, 606*f*
VTA. *See* Ventral tegmental area (VTA)

Washingtonian Center for Addictions, 965
Washington Physicians Health Program, 913
Web-based training programs, 945
Websites, on substance abuse, 969
Wechsler verbal scores, 293
Wellbutrin, 517. *See also* Bopropion SR
WFS. *See* Women for Sobriety (WFS)
White matter disorders, clinical disorder of, 295
WHO. *See* World Health Organization (WHO)
Wikler, Abraham, 164
Wild-type (WT) organisms, 247
Winick, Charles, 168
Withdrawal
    from AAS

depression and, 365
suicide and, 365
from buprenorphine, 440
caffeine, 344–345, 344*t*, 349, 350*t*
symptoms of, AAS use, 365–366, 365*f*
Withdrawal syndromes, acupuncture for, 469–471
Women, and SHG, 527–528
Women for Sobriety (WFS), 524
    contact information, 534*b*
    history, 534
    meeting format, 535
    program, 534–535, 535*b*
Women with substance use disorders
    alcoholism
        epidemiology of, 852
        subjective and behavioral effects of, 848
        treatment of, 852
    co-occurring psychiatric conditions
        eating disorders, 850
        mood and anxiety disorders, 849–850
        personality disorders, 851–852
        posttraumatic stress disorder, 850–851
    cultural issues associated with, 859
    legal issues and, 860
    risk factors for, 859
    treatment of, 859
        behavioral couples therapy, 858
        gender-specific, 857–858
        treatment seeking and utilization, 856–857
Woody, George, 571
Work
    defined, 777
    value in recovery process, 777–778
Working with translators, models
    black box, 919
    junior clinician, 919
    three partners, 919
Work Keys, 779
Workplace, 100
    testing, 132–133
World Anti-Doping Agency, 239
World Anti-Doping Association (WADA), 361, 369
World Drug Report 2009, 240
World Health Organization (WHO), 141, 240, 908
WT. *See* Wild-type (WT) organisms

Xanax. *See* Alprozolam

Yale Plan Clinics, 965
Yale Summer School of Alcohol Studies, 965
Young, Kimberly, 408
Young's diagnostic questionnaire, for Internet addiction, 410*t*
Youth Assistance Program (YAP), 545
Youth attitudes, opioid use, 167–168
Youth prevalence, opioid use, 167
Youth Risk Behavior Survey (YRBS), 17, 288
YRBS. *See* Youth Risk Behavior Survey (YRBS)

Zaleplon, 261
Z-drugs, 255, 914
    determinants of abuse, 262
    overview, 260–261
    pharmacology of, 261–262
Ziconotide, 709
Zidovudine (AZT), 730, 732–733
Zinberg's sample, for opioid, 173
Zoloft. *See* Sertraline
Zolpidem, 261, 914
Zopiclone, 261
Zyban, 323, 517. *See also* Bupropion SR